Georgiade
Plastic, Maxillofacial and Reconstructive Surgery

THIRD EDITION

Georgiade
Plastic, Maxillofacial and Reconstructive Surgery

THIRD EDITION

EDITORS

Gregory S. Georgiade, M.D., F.A.C.S.

Vice Chairman, Department of Surgery
Professor
General Surgery
Professor
Plastic, Maxillofacial, and Reconstructive Surgery
Duke University Medical Center
Durham, North Carolina

Ronald Riefkohl, M.D., F.A.C.S.

Clinical Associate Professor
Plastic, Maxillofacial, and Reconstructive Surgery
Duke University Medical Center
Durham, North Carolina

L. Scott Levin, M.D., F.A.C.S.

Chief
Division of Plastic, Maxillofacial and Reconstructive Surgery
Associate Professor
Plastic, Maxillofacial and Reconstructive Surgery
Associate Professor
Orthopedic Surgery
Duke University Medical Center
Durham, North Carolina

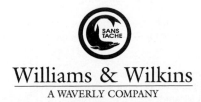

Williams & Wilkins
A WAVERLY COMPANY

BALTIMORE • PHILADELPHIA • LONDON • PARIS • BANGKOK
HONG KONG • MUNICH • SYDNEY • TOKYO • WROCLAW

Executive Senior Editor: Darlene Barela Cooke
Managing Editor: Sharon R. Zinner
Production Coordinator: Peter J. Carley
Book Project Editor: Jennifer D. Weir
Cover Designer: Cathy Cotter
Typesetter: The Clarinda Company
Printer: R. R. Donnelley & Sons
Digitized Illustrations: The Clarinda Company
Binder: R. R. Donnelley & Sons

ISBN 0-683-03455-3

90000>

9 780683 034554

Copyright © 1997 Williams & Wilkins
351 West Camden Street
Baltimore, Maryland 21201-2436 USA

Rose Tree Corporate Center
1400 North Providence Road
Building II, Suite 5025
Media, Pennsylvania 19063-2043 USA

Accurate indications, adverse reactions and dosage schedules for drugs are provided in this book, but it is possible that they may change. The reader is urged to review the pack-age information data of the manufacturers of the medications mentioned.

Printed in the United States of America

Third Edition,

Library of Congress Cataloging-in-Publication Data

Georgiade plastic, maxillofacial, and reconstructive surgery /
   consulting editor, Nicholas G. Georgiade : editors, Gregory S.
Georgiade, Ronald Riefkohl, L. Scott Levin.—3rd ed.
     p. cm.
   Rev. ed of: Textbook of plastic, maxillofacial and
reconstructive surgery / editors, Gregory S. Georgiade . . . [et al.].
2nd ed. c1992.
   Includes bibliographical references and index.
   ISBN 0-683-03455-3
   1. Surgery, Plastic. I. Georgiade, Nicholas G., 1918–   .
II. Georgiade, Gregory S. III. Riefkohl, Ronald. IV. Levin, L.
Scott. V. Textbook of plastic, maxillofacial, and reconstructive
surgery.
   [DNLM: 1. Surgery, Plastic—methods. 2. Surgery, Oral—methods.
WO 600 G352 1996]
RD118.E87 1996
617.9′5—dc20
DNLM DLC
for Library of Congress   96-14580
                          CIP

The publishers have made every effort to trace the copyright holders for borrowed mater-ial. If they have inadvertently overlooked any, they will be pleased to make the necessary arrangements at the first opportunity.

96 97 98 99
1 2 3 4 5 6 7 8 9 10

To purchase additional copies of this book, call our customer service department at **(800) 638-0672** or fax orders to **(800) 447-8438.** For other book services, including chapter reprints and large quantity sales, ask for the Special Sales department.

Canadian customers should call **(800) 268-4178,** or fax **(905) 470-6780.** For all other calls originating outside of the United States, please call **(410) 528-4223** or fax us at **(410) 528-8550.**

Visit Williams & Wilkins on the Internet: http://www.wwilkins.com or contact our customer service department at **custserv@wwilkins.com.** Williams & Wilkins cus-tomer service representatives are available from 8:30 am to 6:00 pm, EST, Monday through Friday, for telephone access.

To

Nicholas G. Georgiade, *D.D.S., M.D., Professor Emeritus*
Former Chief, Division of Plastic Surgery
Duke University School of Medicine

and

Ruth S. Georgiade
Former Research Associate, Department of Surgery

for their continued support and dedication
in the coordination and preparation of the
many manuscripts and bibliographies

Foreword

The mission of the Department of Surgery at Duke University Medical Center is to foster excellence and leadership in health care delivery, teaching, and research. In our quest to accomplish these goals, we recognize that our most important resources are people, and physicians Gregory and Nicholas Georgiade, Ronald Riefkohl, and Scott Levin are highly valued members of the Department of Surgery. Each is a skilled surgeon with broad and extensive experience in both the operating room and the clinic. In addition to these surgical skills, each is a productive scholar and gifted teacher who enjoys the respect and admiration of both colleagues and students.

If one defines creativity as the thinking of novel and appropriate ideas, then innovation is the successful implementation of those ideas within a discipline. *Textbook of Plastic, Maxillofacial and Reconstructive Surgery* has now reached its third edition. It has been highly successful and is widely recognized as a standard for the field, because it not only represents a synthesis of the most creative thinking in this rapidly evolving and important area of surgery but also provides the practical guidelines for translating this creative thought into innovative applications that benefit patients.

Through a careful process of editing and planning, the authors have selected contributors who patiently assessed the fundamental cognitive data in the field of plastic, maxillofacial, and reconstructive surgery and then formulated this data into a body of knowledge that is both current and useful to the student and practicing surgeon. This text has been refined by the hands-on experience not only of the authors but also the editors, and serves as a repository of state-of-the-art knowledge, which is the ultimate goal of all information transmission. Meticulous attention to detail in the preparation of the written text and illustrations is the hallmark of this text, which has been prepared with the same care that is required to perform the surgical procedures and evaluations described herein.

The synthesis of a comprehensive text covering such a wide variety of topics is indeed a labor of love. To each of the contributing authors and to the editors who have carefully planned and executed this work, I offer my sincerest congratulations and heartfelt thanks, on behalf of all who will benefit from this work and all the colleagues in the Department of Surgery who are privileged to work with them.

Robert W. Anderson, M.D.
The David C. Sabiston, Jr. Professor and Chairman
Department of Surgery
Duke University Medical Center

Preface

This third edition represents the continued dedication of the editors to supplying readers with the most up-to-date information available in a broad-based and expanding specialty area. The well-known authors of the various chapters have been selected because of their expertise in the field of plastic, maxillofacial, reconstructive, and aesthetic surgery. The 109 chapters have been prepared as comprehensively as is practical for the various subjects discussed. Suggested readings are included to provide the reader with necessary reference information. In spite of the extensive information available in this text, the material is presented in one readily manageable volume.

Acknowledgments

The third edition of this book would not have been possible without the generosity of the many contributing authors who willingly offered their expertise, time, and resources to provide the chapters for this textbook.

We want to thank our office staff—Judy Hall, Debbie Barber, Joyce Morris, and Alice Rainey—for their assistance in the production of this textbook.

Thanks also to Darlene Cooke, executive editor, Sharon Zinner, senior managing editor, Paula Mueller, associate managing editor, Pete Carley, production coordinator, and other members of the Williams & Wilkins staff, who have supported us in meeting deadlines and in the entire production of this textbook.

Contributors

Hussein S. Abul-Hassan, M.D.
Alexandria University, Cleopatra, Alexandria, Egypt

Christina Y. Ahn, M.D.
Los Angeles, California

Mary E. Albers, M.D.
Attending Physician, Head and Neck Cancer Clinic, Division of Hematology-Oncology, Duke University Medical Center, Durham Veterans Administration Medical Center, Durham, North Carolina

Mark A. Anton, M.D.
Newport Beach, California

Oleh Antonyshyn, M.D., F.R.C.S.(C.)
Assistant Professor, Department of Surgery, University of Toronto, and Head, Division of Plastic Surgery, Sunnybrook Hospital, Toronto, Canada

Louis C. Argenta, M.D., F.A.C.S.
Professor and Chairman, Department of Plastic and Reconstructive Surgery, Bowman Gray School of Medicine, and Director, North Carolina Center for Cleft and Craniofacial Deformities, Winston-Salem, North Carolina

Sherrell J. Aston, M.D., F.A.C.S.
Chairman, Department of Plastic Surgery, Manhattan Eye, Ear, and Throat Hospital, and Associate Professor, Plastic Surgery, New York University School of Medicine, New York, New York

Jane Lupton Bahor, A.S.
Facial and Digital Prosthetist, Dental Laboratory Technologist and Chief, Custom Restorations, Department of Surgery, Division of Plastic, Maxillofacial, and Oral Surgery, Division of Prosthetics and Orthotics, Duke University Medical Center, and Executive Board American Anaplastology Association, 1993–1995, Durham, North Carolina

Daniel C. Baker, M.D.
Associate Professor of Surgery (Plastic Surgery), New York University School of Medicine and Attending Surgeon, University Hospital, Bellevue Hospital Center, Manhattan Eye, Ear, & Throat Hospital and Manhattan Veterans Administration Hospital, New York, New York

Joseph C. Banis, Jr., M.D., F.A.C.S.
Associate Clinical Professor of Surgery, Division of Plastic Surgery, Department of Surgery, University of Louisville, Louisville, Kentucky

Munish K. Batra, M.D.
Department of General Surgery, St. Luke's Medical Center, Cleveland, Ohio

Bruce S. Bauer, M.D., F.A.C.S.
Associate Professor of Surgery, Northwestern University Medical School, Chicago, Illinois

A. J. Beard, F.R.A.C.S.
Consultant Hand and Upper Limb Surgeon, Sydney, Australia

Ellen Beatty, M.D.
Clinical Assistant Professor, Plastic Surgery, University of South Florida, Tampa, Florida

Patricia Bitter, M.D.
Minneapolis, Minnesota

Nan Boyer, O.T.R., C.H.T.
Bachelor of Science Degree in Occupational Therapy, Certified Hand Therapist and Coordinator, Occupational Therapy Department, Henry Ford Medical Center—Fairlane, Dearborn, Michigan

Michael J. Breiner, M.D.
Assistant Professor of Plastic Surgery, Baylor College of Medicine, and Director, St. Luke's Resident's Aesthetic Clinic, Houston, Texas

Jean Trimble Bried, P.A.
Department of Plastic Surgery, The Emory Clinic, Atlanta, Georgia

David M. Brizel, M.D.
Associate Professor, Department of Radiation Oncology, Duke University Medical Center, Durham, North Carolina

Louis P. Bucky, M.D.
Assistant Professor of Surgery, Division of Plastic Surgery, University of Pennsylvania Medical Center, Philadelphia, Pennsylvania

Gregory M. Buncke, M.D., F.A.C.S.
Assistant Clinical Professor in Surgery, University of California at San Francisco, San Francisco, California

Harry J. Buncke, Jr., M.D., F.A.C.S.
Clinical Professor of Surgery, University of California at San Francisco, Director, Replantation-Transplantation Service, Davies Medical Center, and Associate Clinical Professor, Stanford Medical School, San Francisco, California

A. Jay Burns, M.D., F.A.C.S.
Assistant Professor, University of Texas Southwestern Medical School and Director, Congenital Vascular Anomalies Clinic, Children's Medical Center, Dallas, Texas

H. Hollis Caffee, M.D., F.A.C.S.
Professor and Chairman, Division of Plastic Surgery, University of Florida, Gainesville, Florida

James H. Carraway, M.D., F.A.C.S.
Professor of Plastic Surgery, University of Eastern Virginia, Norfolk, Virginia

Culley C. Carson III, M.D., F.A.C.S.
Professor of Surgery, Chief, Division of Urology, University of North Carolina School of Medicine, Chapel Hill, North Carolina

Kristoffer Ning Chang, M.D., F.A.C.S.
Assistant Clinical Professor of Surgery, Univeristy of California at San Francisco, San Francisco, California

Hung-chi Chen, M.D., F.A.C.S.
Professor of Plastic Surgery, Chang Gung Medical College, Taipei, Taiwan, Republic of China

Norman L. Clark, M.D., D.M.D.
Director, Section of Plastic, Reconstructive, and Craniomaxillofacial Surgery, R. Adams Cowley Shock Trauma Center, Baltimore, Maryland

Patricia A. Clugston, M.D., F.R.C.S.(C.)
Clinical Instructor, Division of Plastic Surgery, Department of Surgery, University of British Columbia, Vancouver, British Columbia, Canada

Norman M. Cole, M.D., F.A.C.S.
Clinical Professor of Plastic Surgery, University of Louisville, Louisville, Kentucky, and Associate Clinical Professor of Plastic Surgery, University of Kentucky, Lexington, Kentucky

Larry B. Colen, M.D., F.A.C.S.
Associate Professor, Plastic and Reconstructive Surgery, Eastern Virginia Medical School, Norfolk, Virginia

Eugene H. Courtiss, M.D., F.A.C.S.
Associate Clinical Professor of Surgery, Harvard Medical School, and Consultant in Plastic Surgery, Massachusetts General Hospital, Boston, Massachusetts

Edwin B. Cox, M.D.
Consulting Assistant Professor, Department of Medicine, Duke University Medical Center, Durham, North Carolina

Court B. Cutting, M.D., F.A.C.S.
Associate Professor of Plastic Surgery, Institute of Reconstructive Plastic Surgery, New York University Medical Center, New York, New York

T. M. B. de Chalain, M.D., F.C.S.(SA)
Clinical Fellow in Plastic Surgery, Emory University, Atlanta, Georgia

Anthony J. DeFranzo, M.D., F.A.C.S.
Associate Professor of Plastic Surgery, Bowman Gray School of Medicine, Winston-Salem, North Carolina

A. Lee Dellon, M.D., F.A.C.S.
Professor of Plastic Surgery, and Professor of Neurosurgery, Johns Hopkins University School of Medicine, Baltimore, Maryland

John W. Derr, Jr., M.D., F.A.C.S.
Assistant Clinical Professor of Surgery, Division of Plastic Surgery, Department of Surgery, University of Louisville, Louisville, Kentucky

Donald M. Ditmars, Jr., M.D., F.A.C.S.
Division Head, Plastic and Reconstructive Surgery, Henry Ford Hospital, and Clinical Assistant Professor I, University of Michigan, Detroit, Michigan

Gregory A. Dumanian, M.D.
Chief Resident in Plastic Surgery, University of Pittsburgh Medical Center, Pittsburgh, Pennsylvania

Milton T. Edgerton, Jr., M.D., F.A.C.S.
Former Chairman and Currently Emeritus Professor, Department of Plastic and Maxillofacial Surgery, University of Virginia, and Former Director and Chief, The Gender Identity Clinics, Johns Hopkins Hospital, University of Virginia, Charlottesville, Virginia

Tarek Abdalla El-Gammal, M.D.
Clinical Fellow of Reconstructive Microsurgery, Department of Plastic and Reconstructive Surgery, Chang Gung Memorial Hospital and Medical College, Taipei, Taiwan, Republic of China

Richard Ellenbogen, M.D., F.A.C.S., F.I.C.S.
Clinical Instructor in Plastic Surgery, University of Southern California, Los Angeles, California

David L. Feldman, M.D.
Director, Division of Plastic and Reconstructive Surgery, Maimonides Medical Center, and Assistant Professor of Surgery, SUNY Health Science Center, Brooklyn, New York

Jack Fisher, M.D., F.A.C.S.
Assistant Clinical Professor, Department of Plastic and Reconstructive Surgery, Vanderbilt University, Nashville, Tennessee

Jack C. Fisher, M.D., F.A.C.S.
Professor of Surgery, University of California, San Diego, California

Peter B. Fodor, M.D., F.A.C.S.
Assistant Clinical Professor, Reconstructive and Plastic Surgery, UCLA Medical Center, Los Angeles, California

Gregory S. Georgiade, M.D., F.A.C.S.
Vice Chairman, Department of Surgery, and Professor, General Surgery and Plastic, Maxillofacial and Reconstructive Surgery, Duke University Medical Center, Durham, North Carolina

Nicholas G. Georgiade, D.D.S., M.D., F.A.C.S.
Professor Emeritus and Former Chief, Division of Plastic, Maxillofacial, and Oral Surgery, Duke University Medical Center, Durham, North Carolina

Mary K. Gingrass, M.D.
Institute for Aesthetic and Reconstructive Surgery, Baptist Hospital, Nashville, Tennessee

Jay A. Goldberg, M.D.
Attending Surgeon, Missouri Bone and Joint Clinic, St. Louis, Missouri

J. Leonard Goldner, M.D., D.Sc. (Hon.)
James B. Duke Professor Emeritus, Orthopaedic Surgery, Duke University Medical Center, Durham, North Carolina

Richard D. Goldner, M.D.
Associate Professor, Division of Orthopaedic Surgery, Duke University Medical Center, Durham, North Carolina

Mark S. Granick, M.D., F.A.C.S.
Professor and Chief, Division of Plastic Surgery, Medical College of Pennsylvania, Hahnemann University, Philadelphia, Pennsylvania

Richard O. Gregory, M.D., F.A.C.S.
Associate Clinical Professor of Plastic Surgery, University of South Florida, Orlando, Florida

James C. Grotting, M.D., F.A.C.S.
Clinical Professor of Plastic Surgery, University of Alabama at Birmingham, and McCollough, Grotting & Associates Plastic Surgery Clinic, P.C., Birmingham, Alabama

Dwight C. Hanna, M.D., F.A.C.S.
Clinical Professor Emeritus of Plastic Surgery, The University of Pittsburgh, and Western Pennsylvania Hospital, Pittsburgh, Pennsylvania

John M. Harrelson, M.D.
Professor of Orthopaedic Surgery, Associate Professor of Pathology, Chief, Musculoskeletal Oncology Section, and Chief, Diabetic Insensitive Foot Clinic, Duke University Medical Center, Durham, North Carolina

Richard H.C. Harries, B.M., B.S., B.Sc.
Plastic Surgical Registrar, Wound Healing and Injury Research Centre, The Queen Elizabeth Hospital, Adelaide, South Australia

Carl R. Hartrampf, Jr., M.D., F.A.C.S.
Clinical Professor, Department of Surgery, Division of Plastic Surgery, Emory University School of Medicine, Atlanta, Georgia

Tad Heinz, M.D.
Assistant Professor of Surgery and Associate Fellow, American College of Surgeons, Birmingham, Alabama

Gregory P. Hetter, M.D., F.A.C.S.
Assistant Clinical Professor of Surgery, Plastic, University of Nevada Medical School; and Private Practice, Las Vegas, Nevada

Philip E. Higgs, M.D., F.A.C.S.
Assistant Professor of Surgery, (Plastic and Reconstructive), Washington University School of Medicine, St. Louis, Missouri

David H. Hildreth, M.D.
Clinical Associate Professor of Orthopaedics, Department of Orthopaedics, UTHSC University of Texas Health Science Center; and Chief, Hand Section, Park Plaza Hospital, Houston, Texas

James G. Hoehn, M.D., F.A.C.S.
Clinical Professor of Surgery, Training Program Director, Division of Plastic Surgery, Albany Medical College, Albany, New York

Andrew T. Huang, M.D.
Professor of Medicine, Division of Hematology-Oncology, Duke University Medical Center, Durham, North Carolina

Thomas J. Hubbard, M.D.
Mladick Center for Cosmetic Plastic Surgery, Virginia Beach, Virginia

Steve Hughes, M.D.
Division of Plastic and Reconstructive Surgery, University of Missouri Medical Center, Columbia, Missouri

Norman E. Hugo, M.D., D, Sci (H.C.), F.A.C.S.
Professor, Division of Plastic Surgery, Columbia Presbyterian Medical Center, New York, New York

Dennis J. Hurwitz, M.D., F.A.C.S.
Attending Surgeon, University of Pittsburgh Medical Center and Children's Hospital of Pittsburgh, Pittsburgh, Pennsylvania

Jeffrey Scott Isenberg, M.D., M.P.H.
Assistant Professor of Plastic Surgery and Head, Microvascular Surgery, The University of Oklahoma Health Sciences Center, Oklahoma City, Oklahoma

Ian T. Jackson, M.D., D.Sc. (Hon.), F.R.C.S., F.A.C.S., F.R.A.C.S. (Hon.)
Southfield, Michigan

M.J. Jurkiewicz, D.D.S., M.D., F.A.C.S.
Professor Emeritus of Plastic Surgery, Emory University, Atlanta, Georgia

Morton L. Kasdan, M.D., F.A.C.S.
Clinical Professor of Surgery, University of Louisville and Clinical Professor of Preventive Medicine and Environmental Health, University of Kentucky, Louisville, Kentucky

Lowell R. King, M.D., F.A.C.S.
Head, Section on Pediatric Urology, Duke University Medical Center, Durham, North Carolina

Harold E. Kleinert, M.D., F.A.C.S.
Clinical Professor of Surgery, University of Louisville School of Medicine, Louisville, Kentucky, and Clinical Professor of Surgery, Indiana University–Purdue University School of Medicine, Indianapolis, Indiana

Phyllis J. Kornguth, M.D., Ph.D.
Chief, Breast Imaging Section, Associate Professor of Radiology, Duke University Medical Center, Durham, North Carolina

Thomas J. Krizek, M.D., F.A.C.S.
Professor and Vice Chairman, Department of Surgery and Director, Division of Plastic Surgery, University of South Florida, Tampa, Florida

Hamish Laing, M.B.B.S., F.R.C.S. (Plast)
Senior Registrar in Plastic Surgery, The Great Ormond Street Hospital for Children, London; and The Welsh Centre for Burns and Plastic Surgery, Morriston, Wales

Margaretha Willemina Langman, P.S., D.R.A.
Charlotte, Virginia

Don LaRossa, M.D., F.A.C.S., F.A.A.P.
Associate Professor, Division of Plastic Surgery, University of Pennsylvania, Philadelphia, Pennsylvania

Donald R. Laub, Sr., M.D., F.A.C.S.
Clinical Associate Professor of Surgery, Stanford University Medical School, Stanford, California

Donald R. Laub, Jr., M.D.
Chief Resident, Plastic and Reconstructive Surgery, Dartmouth–Hitchcock Medical Center, Lebanon, New Hampshire

David C. Leber, M.D., F.A.C.S.
Attending Surgeon, Harrisburg Hospital and Polyclinic Medical Center, Harrisburg, Pennsylvania, and Holy Spirit Hospital, Camp Hill, Pennsylvania, and Clinical Associate Professor of Plastic Surgery, Hershey Medical Center of The Pennsylvania State University, Harrisburg, Pennsylvania

Barry Lembersky, M.D.
Assistant Professor of Medicine, University of Pittsburgh Cancer Institute, University of Pittsburgh School of Medicine, Pittsburgh, Pennsylvania

L. Scott Levin, M.D., F.A.C.S.
Chief, Division of Plastic, Maxillofacial, and Reconstructive Surgery, and Associate Professor, Plastic, Maxillofacial, and Reconstructive Surgery, and Associate Professor, Orthopedic Surgery, Duke University Medical Center, Durham, North Carolina

Ted E. Lockwood, M.D., F.A.C.S.
Associate Clinical Professor of Plastic Surgery, University of Kansas Medical School and Assistant Clinical Professor of Plastic Surgery, University of Missouri–Kansas City Medical School, Overland Park, Kansas

Ralph T. Manktelow, M.D., F.R.C.S.(C.)
Professor and Chairman, Division of Plastic Surgery, Department of Surgery, The Toronto Hospital and The Hospital for Sick Children, Toronto, Canada

Paul N. Manson, M.D., F.A.C.S.
Professor and Chairman, Plastic Surgery, Johns Hopkins School of Medicine, and Professor of Plastic Surgery, The University of Maryland School of Medicine, and Attending Surgeon, The University of Maryland Shock Trauma Center, Baltimore, Maryland

Carl H. Manstein, M.D., F.A.C.S.
Chief, Plastic Surgery, Jeanes Hospital, and Chief, Plastic Surgery, The Hospital of the Philadelphia Geriatric Center, and Associate Clinical Professor in Plastic Surgery, Temple University, Philadelphia, Pennsylvania

Mark E. Manstein, M.D., F.A.C.S.
Chief, Plastic Surgery, and Attending in Plastic Surgery, Holy Redeemer Hospital, Meadowbrook, Pennsylvania, and Assistant Surgeon to Pennsylvania Hospital, and Clinical Associate, University of Pennsylvania Hospital, Philadelphia, Pennsylvania

Malcolm W. Marks, M.D., F.A.C.S.
Associate Professor, Plastic Surgery, Bowman Gray School of Medicine, Winston-Salem, North Carolina

Robert M. Mason, Ph.D., D.M.D.
Professor and Chief of Orthodontics, Duke University Medical Center, Durham, North Carolina

Alain Masquelet, M.D.
Professor of Orthopaedic Surgery, University of Paris, and Head of Department, Orthopaedic and Reconstructive Surgery, Hospital Avicenne, Bobigny, France

Stephen J. Mathes, M.D., F.A.C.S.
Professor of Surgery, Head, Division of Plastic and Reconstructive Surgery, University of California at San Francisco, San Francisco, California

G. Patrick Maxwell, M.D., F.A.C.S.
Assistant Clinical Professor, Department of Plastic Surgery, Vanderbilt University, and Director of the Institute for Aesthetic and Reconstructive Surgery, Baptist Hospital, Nashville, Tennessee

Joseph G. McCarthy, M.D., F.A.C.S.
Lawrence D. Bell Professor of Plastic Surgery, and Director, Institute of Reconstructive Plastic Surgery, New York University Medical Center, New York, New York

Kenneth S. McCarty, Jr., M.D., Ph.D.
Director of Endocrine Oncology, Professor of Pathology, and Professor of Medicine, University of Pittsburgh, Pittsburgh Cancer Institute, Pittsburgh, Pennsylvania

John B. McCraw, M.D., F.A.C.S.
Professor of Plastic Surgery, Eastern Virginia Medical School, Norfolk, Virginia

Robert M. McFarlane, M.D., M.Sc., F.R.C.S.(C.), F.A.C.S.
Professor Emeritus and Former Chair, Division of Plastic Surgery, The University of Western Ontario, London, Ontario, Canada

Mary H. McGrath, M.D., M.P.H., F.A.C.S.
Professor of Surgery and Chief, Division of Plastic and Reconstructive Surgery, The George Washington University Medical Center, and Attending in Plastic Surgery, Children's National Medical Center, Washington, D.C.

Thomas A. McGraw, D.M.D.
Assistant Professor, Oral and Maxillofacial Surgery, Duke University Medical Center, and Diplomate, American Board of Oral and Maxillofacial Surgery, Durham, North Carolina

Ann McMellin, M.D.
Virginia Beach, Virginia

Frederick J. Menick, M.D.
Associate Clinical Professor, and Chief, Division of Plastic Surgery, University of Arizona College of Medicine, Tucson, Arizona

Hano Millesi, M.D.
University Professor, Klinische Abteilung fur Wiederherstellende und Plastische Chirurgie, Vienna, Austria

Oktavijan Minanov, M.D.
Resident in Surgery, University of North Carolina Hospitals, University of North Carolina School of Medicine, Chapel Hill, North Carolina

Richard A. Mladick, M.D., F.A.C.S.
Director, Mladick Center for Cosmetic Plastic Surgery, Virginia Beach, Virginia

John B. Mulliken, M.D., F.A.C.S.
Associate Professor of Surgery, Harvard Medical School, and Director, Craniofacial Center, and Senior Associate Surgeon, Division of Plastic Surgery, Children's Hospital, Boston, Massachusetts

John C. Murray, M.D.
Associate Professor of Medicine, Division of Dermatology, Duke University Medical Center, Durham, North Carolina

David T. Netscher, M.D., F.A.C.S.
Associate Professor, Division of Plastic Surgery, Baylor College of Medicine, and Chief of Plastic Surgery Section, Department of Veteran Affairs, Medical Center, Houston, Texas

Suzanne M. Olbricht, M.D.
Director, Division of Dermatologic Surgery, Beth Israel Hospital, and Instructor, Harvard Medical School, Boston, Massachusetts

Fernando Ortiz-Monasterio, M.D.
Professor Emeritus, Universidad Nacional Autonoma De Mexico, and Professor of Plastic Surgery, Postgraduate Division, Universidad Nacional Autonoma De Mexico, Mexico City, Mexico

Bryan D. Oslin, M.D.
Southern Plastic Surgery, P.L.L.C., Nashville, Tennessee

Nicholas H. Papas, M.D.
Clinical Instructor in Plastic Surgery, Northeastern Ohio Universities College of Medicine, Akron, Ohio, and Former Fellow, Christine M. Kleinert Institute for Hand and Microsurgery, Louisville, Kentucky

Christoph Papp, M.D.
Prim. University Professor, and Head, Plastic and Reconstructive Surgery Unit, Hospital "Barmherzige Bruder", Salzburg, Austria

Pravin-Kumar K. Patel, M.D.
Assistant Professor of Surgery, Northwestern University School of Medicine, Division of Plastic Surgery, Children's Memorial Hospital, and Chief, Plastic, Reconstructive, and Maxillofacial Surgery Service, Shriners Hospital, Chicago, Illinois

George C. Peck, M.D., F.A.C.S.
Attending Plastic Surgeon, Department of Plastic and Reconstructive Surgery, St. Barnabas Hospital, Livingston, New Jersey; and Beth Israel Hospital, Passaic, New Jersey

George C. Peck, Jr., M.D.
Assistant Attending Plastic Surgeon, St. Barnabas Hospital, Livingston, New Jersey; and Attending Plastic Surgeon, Beth Israel Hospital, Passaic, New Jersey

William C. Pederson, M.D., F.A.C.S.
Clinical Associate Professor, Surgery and Orthopaedic Surgery, The University of Texas Health Science Center at San Antonio, and Attending Surgeon, The Hand Center of San Antonio, San Antonio, Texas

Joel E. Pessa, M.D.
Assistant Professor, Plastic and Reconstructive Surgery, Dartmouth–Hitchcock Medical Center, Lebanon, New Hampshire

H.D. Peterson, D.D.S., M.D., F.A.C.S.
Director, NC Jaycee Burn Center, and Professor of Surgery, University of North Carolina Hospitals, University of North Carolina School of Medicine, Chapel Hill, North Carolina

George J. Picha, M.D., Ph.D., F.A.C.S.
Research Associate, Biomedical Engineering, and Assistant Clinical Professor, Plastic and Reconstructive Surgery, Case Western Reserve University, Independence, Ohio

Joseph M. Pober, M.D., F.A.C.S.
St. Luke's–Roosevelt Hospital Center, Columbia University College of Physicians and Surgeons, and Clinical Instructor, Department of Surgery (Plastic), College of Medicine, SUNY Health Science Center, and Department of Surgery (Plastic), Cabrini Medical Center, The New York Medical College, New York, New York

Leonard R. Prosnitz, M.D.
Professor and Chairman, Department of Radiation Oncology, Duke University Medical Center, Durham, North Carolina

Thomas Pruzinsky, Ph.D.
Associate Professor of Psychology, Quinnipiac College, Hamden, Connecticut, and Adjunct Faculty, Institute for Reconstructive Plastic Surgery, New York University Medical Center, New York, New York

Charles L. Puckett, M.D., F.A.C.S.
Professor and Chairman Division of Plastic Surgery, and Vice Chairman, Department of Surgery, University of Missouri Medical Center, Columbia, Missouri

Peter Randall, M.D., F.A.C.S.
Emeritus Professor of Plastic Surgery, University of Pennsylvania School of Medicine, and Senior Surgeon, Children's Hospital of Philadelphia, Philadelphia, Pennsylvania

Robert Rehnke, M.D.
St. Petersburg, Florida

Ronald Riefkohl, M.D., F.A.C.S.
Clinical Associate Professor, Plastic, Maxillofacial, and Reconstructive Surgery, Duke University Medical Center, Durham, North Carolina

John E. Riski, Ph.D., F.A.S.H.A., A.S.H.A.
Director, Speech Pathology Laboratory, Scottish Rite Children's Medical Center, and Adjunct Associate Professor, University of Georgia, Atlanta, Georgia

Edmond F. Ritter, M.D.
Assistant Professor of Plastic, Reconstructive, Oral, and Maxillofacial Surgery, Duke University Medical Center, Durham, North Carolina

Cary N. Robertson, M.D., F.A.C.S.
Associate Professor of Urology, Division of Urology, Duke University Medical Center, Durham, North Carolina

Martin C. Robson, M.D., F.A.C.S., F.R.A.C.S.(Hon.)
Professor of Surgery, University of South Florida, and Chief of Surgery, Veterans Administration Medical Center, Bay Pines, Florida

M. Claudia Romana, M.D.
Chirurgien des Hopitaux, Service de Chirurgie Orthopedique et Reparatrice de L'Enfant, Hopital Trousseau, Paris, France

Craig Rubinstein, M.B., M.S., F.R.A.C.S.
Plastic Surgeon, Western Hospital, Footscray-Melbourne, Australia, and Plastic Surgeon, Austin Hospital, Heidelberg-Melbourne, Australia

Ross Rudolph, M.D., F.A.C.S.
Associate Clinical Professor of Plastic Surgery, University of California at San Diego, and Head, Division of Plastic Surgery, Scripps Clinic and Research Foundation, San Diego, California

Cameron S. Schaeffer, M.D.
Fellow in Pediatric Urology, Duke University Medical Center, Durham, North Carolina

Luis R. Scheker, M.D.
Assistant Clinical Professor of Surgery (Plastic and Reconstructive), Department of Plastic Surgery, University of Louisville School of Medicine, Louisville, Kentucky

Gerald Schneider, M.D., F.A.C.S.
Division of Plastic Surgery, Scripps Clinic and Research Foundation, LaJolla, California

Mark A. Schusterman, M.D., F.A.C.S.
Associate Professor and Chairman, Department of Plastic Surgery, M. D. Anderson Cancer Center, Houston, Texas

Hilliard F. Seigler, M.D., F.A.C.S.
Professor of Surgery and Professor of Immunology, Duke University School of Medicine, Durham, North Carolina

John M. Shamoun, M.D., F.A.C.S.
Newport Institute of Plastic and Reconstructive Surgery, Newport Beach, California

William W. Shaw, M.D., F.A.C.S.
Professor and Chief, Division of Plastic and Reconstructive Surgery, University of California at Los Angeles, Los Angeles, California

Randolph Sherman, M.D., F.A.C.S.
Associate Professor of Plastic, Orthopedic, and Neurological Surgery, University of Southern California, Los Angeles, California

Paul J. Smith, F.R.C.S.
Consultant Plastic and Hand Surgeon, The Hospital for Sick Children, Mount Vernon Hospital, and Senior Lecturer, Child Health, Institute of Child Health, London, England

Mark Vincent Sofonio, M.D.
Desert Hospital and Eisenhower Hospital, Indian Wells, California

Mark P. Solomon, M.D., F.A.C.S.
Associate Professor of Surgery and Co-Chief, Division of Plastic Surgery, Medical College of Pennsylvania, Hahnemann University, Philadelphia, Pennsylvania

Mary Scott Soo, M.D.
Assistant Professor of Radiology, Department of Radiology, Duke University Medical Center, Durham, North Carolina

Melvin Spira, M.D., D.D.S., F.A.C.S.
Professor, Division of Plastic Surgery, Cora and Webb Mading Department of Surgery, Baylor College of Medicine, and Chief of Plastic Surgery, St. Luke's Episcopal Hospital, Houston, Texas

Samuel Stal, M.D., F.A.C.S.
Chief of Plastic Surgery, Texas Children's Hospital, and Division of Plastic Surgery, Baylor University Medical School, Houston, Texas

John K. Stanley, M.Ch. Orth., F.R.C.S.E., F.R.C.S.
Director, Centre for Hand and Upper Limb Surgery, Wrightington Hospital, Wigan, United Kingdom, and Honorary Lecturer, University of Manchester, Department of Orthopaedics, Lancashire, United Kingdom

Alexander C. Stratoudakis, M.D., F.A.C.S.
Athens, Greece

Mark R. Sultan, M.D., F.A.C.S.
Assistant Professor of Plastic and Reconstructive Surgery, Columbia Presbyterian Medical Center, New York, New York

Michael J. Sundine, M.D.
Assistant Professor, Division of Plastic and Reconstructive Surgery, University of Louisville, Louisville, Kentucky

John Taras, M.D.
Assistant Clinical Professor of Orthopaedic Surgery, Thomas Jefferson University, Jefferson Medical College, Philadelphia, Pennsylvania

Edward O. Terino, M.D., F.A.C.S., L.L.D.
Medical Director of Plastic Surgery, Institute of Southern California, Agoura, California

Allen L. Van Beek, M.D., F.A.C.S.
Clinical Associate Professor, Department of Surgery, Division of Plastic Surgery, University of Minnesota, Minneapolis, Minnesota

Nancy Van Laeken, M.D., F.R.C.S.(C.)
Clinical Associate Professor, Division of Plastic Surgery, Department of Surgery, University of British Columbia, Vancouver, British Columbia, Canada

Michael P. Vincent, M.D., F.A.C.S.
Associate Professor of Surgery, Uniformed Services University of the Health Sciences, Bethesda, Maryland, and Chief, Plastic Surgery, Shady Grove Adventist Hospital, Rockville, Maryland

Robin T. Vollmer, M.D.
Clinical Assistant Professor, Duke University Medical Center, Durham, North Carolina

Ruth Walsh, M.D.
Associate, Department of Radiology, Duke University Medical Center, Durham, North Carolina

James Watson, M.D.
Assistant Professor of Surgery, Division of Plastic and Reconstructive Surgery, UCLA School of Medicine, Los Angeles, California

Paul M. Weeks, M.D., F.A.C.S.
Professor of Surgery (Plastic and Reconstructive) and Chief, Division of Plastic Surgery, Washington University School of Medicine, St. Louis, Missouri

Fu-Chan Wei, M.D., F.A.C.S.
Professor and Chairman, Department of Plastic and Reconstructive Surgery, Chang Gung Memorial Hospital, Taipei, Taiwan, Republic of China

Paul M.N. Werker, M.D., Ph.D.
Attending Staff Plastic Surgeon, Department of Plastic, Reconstructive, and Hand Surgery, University Hospital, Utrecht, Utrecht, The Netherlands

Tolbert S. Wilkinson, M.D., F.A.C.S.
Director, Institute for Aesthetic Plastic Surgery, and Editor, *Technical Forum*, San Antonio, Texas

Margaret E. Williford, M.D.
Assistant Clinical Professor, Department of Radiology, Duke University Medical Center, Durham, North Carolina

S. Anthony Wolfe, M.D., F.A.C.S.
Clinical Professor, Plastic and Reconstructive Surgery, University of Miami School of Medicine, and Chief, Division of Plastic Surgery, Cedars Medical Center, Miami Children's Hospital, Miami, Florida

Kevin Yakuboff, M.D.
Associate Professor, Division of Plastic and Reconstruction Surgery, Head, Hand Surgery Section, Division of Plastic Surgery, University of Cincinnati, Cincinnati, Ohio

Lawrence S. Zachary, M.D., F.A.C.S.
Assistant Professor of Surgery, University of Chicago, Chicago, Illinois

George Zavitsanos, M.D.
Resident in Plastic Surgery, Duke University Medical Center, Durham, North Carolina

Contents

FOUR: Aesthetic Surgery

FIVE: Breast and Chest

SIX: Genitalia

SEVEN: Microsurgery

EIGHT: Hand

NINE: Trunk & Lower Extremity

TEN: Practical Concepts for the Plastic Surgery Practice

ONE

Basic Principles

1

Biology of Tissue Injury and Repair

Thomas J. Krizek, M.D., F.A.C.S., Richard H.C. Harries, B.M., B.S., B.Sc., and Martin C. Robson, M.D., F.A.C.S., F.R.A.C.S. (Hon.)

Definitions

The complexity of the healing wound is only just starting to be unravelled. For over 3500 years physicians have been writing about wounds, but progress has been slow. However, with advances in the fields of molecular biology and immunocytochemistry, medical science will soon be able to understand the metabolic, humoral, and cellular cascades that promulgate wound healing and tissue repair.

Unlike many lower life forms, few mammals and primates enjoy the luxury of being able to regenerate injured tissues. In order to survive in a hostile environment, the more rapid process of wound repair is utilized. While the terms *regeneration* and *repair* are frequently used in medical vocabulary, their specific meanings are often interpreted differently by different physicians. As a result, Lazarus and colleagues (1) proposed some basic definitions and guidelines for researchers and clinicians who have an interest in the wound healing field. A *wound* can be defined as a disruption of normal anatomic structure and function. Wounds are frequently classified into those that are acute and those that are chronic. Rather than define these two terms with an arbitrary and sometimes inappropriate temporal separation, Lazarus and colleagues (1) expanded on the concept of time and introduced the idea of orderliness. An *acute wound* can now be defined as any wound that proceeds through an orderly and timely reparative process that results in a sustained restoration of anatomic and functional integrity. *Chronic wounds* are therefore defined as wounds that do *not* proceed through an orderly and timely reparative process to produce sustained restoration of anatomic and functional integrity, or proceed through the repair process without establishing a sustained anatomic and functional result. To differentiate more fully between acute and chronic wounds, we must look at both orderliness and timeliness. *Orderliness* refers to a sequence of biologic events, including the following: control of infection, resolution of inflammation, angiogenesis, restoration of a functional connective-tissue matrix, contraction, resurfacing, differentiation, and remodeling. *Timeliness* remains relative and is determined by the nature and degree of the pathologic process that caused the wound, and the medical condition of the patient (including their prescribed drug history and any relevant environmental factors, e.g., need and access to community supports and socioeconomic status). All of the above factors must be taken into account when gauging the time it should take any given wound to heal. In brief, acute wounds are those that heal in an orderly and appropriately timed manner, while chronic wounds are those that are neither orderly nor timely.

Just as the definition of a wound necessarily covers a spectrum of situations, so must the definition of a *healed* wound. Healing is a complex process that results in the restoration of anatomic continuity and function in an orderly and timely manner. Lazarus and colleagues (1) suggest this process can lead to one of three outcomes. First, an *ideally* healed wound is one that has returned to normal anatomic structure, function, and appearance, i.e., there is no evidence of scar tissue. Restoration of the parenchymal tissue of the liver would be an example of ideal healing. Second, a wound may be *acceptably* healed; i.e., where scar is present but sustained anatomic continuity and function is achieved. Finally, a *minimally* healed wound is characterized by the restoration of anatomic continuity, but without a sustained functional result. Such wounds frequently recur. The recurrent breakdown of burn wounds covered with cultured keratinocytes would be an example of a minimally healed wound.

As our understanding of the wound healing process evolves so should the terms used to define the process. The definitions given above can be thought of as nomenclature guidelines that will necessarily change as research into the field of wound healing progresses.

Basic Anatomic Concepts

A detailed review of the anatomic features of various tissues is beyond the scope of this review, yet wound management cannot be approached thoughtfully or accomplished meaningfully in the absence of the following considerations.

SKIN

The skin has two layers that constitute its basic anatomy, each playing a significant role in wound management.

Epidermis

The outer epidermis is our protective, waterproofing layer and the part of us that the world sees. Its color, texture, and particularly any deformity or scar, are manifest here. The germinal or basal layer is constantly replenishing itself, pushing dying cells and keratin to the surface. Any superficial injury, such as an abrasion or burn, may destroy this outermost waterproofing layer and allow both weeping of tissue fluids from within and the absorption of medications or the invasion of bacteria from without. Because the germinal layer is intact in superficial wounds, such as scrapes and superficial burns, healing usually occurs without scarring. Because the melanocytes are also in the germinal layer, discoloration may occur (lighter after some superficial burns, darker as in tanning after sunburns). Because the naked nerve fibers end in the germinal layer, superficial injuries are irritating to large numbers of nerve endings and are particularly painful. The epidermis has no collagen fibers and therefore has little inherent tensile strength. When a wound is carefully coapted, epithelial cells migrate quickly and will often seal a wound within a few hours (and thus waterproof it).

Dermis

Collagen in the dermis is a fibrous protein deposited by fibroblasts that, through its intrinsic fiber strength and its complex cross-linkages (weave), holds us together. The epidermis rests on the collagenous dermis in an irregular surface interface (papillary ridges) that makes them mechanically difficult to separate. In a coapted wound, the epidermis rapidly seals the wound, but it is the collagen in the dermis that must be laid down across the wound to give it strength. The dermis contains the epithelial-lined skin appendages that include the eccrine or sweat glands and the sebaceous oil glands. Each empties into a hair follicle. The major blood supply to the skin is through vessels in the dermis; there are none in the epidermis.

Wound Healing

Traditionally, wound healing has been said to proceed through several stages. Commonly, these are referred to as hemostasis, inflammation proliferation, and maturation. Hemostasis is the initial stage, preventing excessive blood loss and generating a fibrinous network that traps platelets and triggers events that lead into the inflammatory phase of wound healing. Following a cascade of humoral events a cellular response occurs, leading to an influx of different populations of cells and the laying down of a new extracellular matrix and blood vessels. It is during this phase that epithelialization, contraction, and collagen production occur. The final phase of wound healing involves maturation, or remodeling, whereby collagen is organized and consolidated and angiogenesis subsides as the resting metabolic needs of the maturing scar diminish. This process is a dynamic one and can proceed for as long as two layers post wounding. It is this sequence of events that the definitions provided above tried to encapsulate.

HEMOSTASIS

Following disruption of the normal anatomic structure of tissue, blood vessels are divided and, at the cellular level, cells are either lethally disrupted or damaged but survive. Basement membranes are similarly damaged, exposing underlying extracellular matrix molecules. This cataclysmic series of events initiates the clotting cascade, as well as the complement cascade. Damage to all membranes initiates the arachidonic acid pathway. The clotting cascade terminates as a fibrin plug, preventing excessive blood loss, and this matrix traps platelets. The platelets are then stimulated to release a wide range of humoral factors, called *growth factors,* including: platelet-derived growth factor (PDGF); transforming growth factor β (TGF$_\beta$); and fibroblast growth factor (FGF) (2). The complement cascade helps initiate the migration of cells into the wounded area and plays a role in eliminating foreign material (e.g., bacteria or membrane-coated viruses) from the wound. The end products of the arachidonic acid pathway are a whole series of leukotrienes and prostagrandins, which are vasoactive and mitogenic (3).

INFLAMMATORY PHASE

These largely humoral events provide the foundation for the inflammatory phase of healing. This phase is classically represented by the signs and symptoms of rubor (redness), tumor (swelling), calor (heat), and dolor (pain). Rubor, or redness, is caused by vasodilation. The most potent prostanoid vasodilator is prostacyclin (PGI$_2$). Others include prostaglandins A, D, and E (PGA, PGD, and PGE). While prostaglandins G$_2$ and H$_2$ (PGG$_2$ and PGH$_2$) initially evoke a vasoconstrictive activity, they are responsible for a secondary vasodilatory response (3).

Tumor, or swelling, is primarily caused by the leakage of plasma proteins through gaps in the vascular spaces of the tissue endothelium. While most prostanoids do not evoke this edematous process, they do have an enhancing effect. The prostanoids most frequently implicated in potentiating edema are PGE$_2$ and PGF$_{2a}$, PGI$_2$, and PGE$_2$ have little direct effect on vascular permeability, but they markedly enhance edema formation and leukocyte infiltration by promoting blood flow into the area of injured tissue (3). While arachidonic and prostaglandins E and E$_2$ can produce fever, calor around a wound refers to the increased local tissue temperature secondary to both increased blood flow and elevated metabolic rates.

Dolor, or pain, is provoked by arachidonic in the experimental situation. The eicosonoid derivatives initiate or provoke varying degrees of hyperalgesia, especially PGI$_2$, PGE, and PGE$_2$. The homeostatic mechanisms that guide these cascades toward constructive wound repair, rather than prolonged and injurious inflammation, are yet to be fully understood. A steady-state relationship between PGE$_2$ and PGF$_{2a}$ apparently maintains the flow and balance of intracellular and extracellular nutrients and waste fluids for cell and tissue viability and integrity (3). Through control of the vasoactive and vasoconstrictive activities of these two prostanoids, cell viability and permeability and microvasculature patency are maintained. This mechanism points out the vital role of the inflammatory mediators in the early wound-healing process.

Within hours of wounding, the cellular aspect of the inflammatory response occurs. Polymorphonuclear leukocytes (PMNs) appear and remain the predominant cell for approximately forty-eight hours. The activated PMN is the origin of many inflammatory mediators and bactericidal oxygen-derived free radicals (3). Since the absence of neutrophils does not prevent wound healing, they do not appear to be essential cells. However, the macrophages are essential. Monocytes enter the wound after the PMNs and reach maximum numbers approximately 24 hours later. They quickly evolve into macrophages, the main cells involved in wound débridement. Macrophages persist for several weeks in wounds healing by primary intention and are numerous in chronic open wounds (3). Macrophages secrete substances, e.g., basic fibroblast growth factor (bFGF), that are chemotactic and mitogenic for fibroblasts and endothelial cells and increase angiogenesis (3).

The fibroblast is the workhorse of the wound-repair process. It is the cell responsible for the formation of all the connective-tissue components in the healing wound, including collagen, glycosaminoglycans, and elastin fibers.

Epithelialization is a prominent process in wound healing. The basal epithelial cell at the wound margin flattens and migrates into the open wound area. As the basal cells at the wound margin multiply in a horizontal direction, the basal cells behind this margin assume a vertical growth column characteristic of a normal epithelial barrier (3). Although this process is accomplished with relative ease in wound healing by primary intention, in those healing by secondary intention or in partial-thickness burns the epithelium must often migrate over great distances, which requires much more time. Migration of epithelial cells occurs only over viable tissue and only if the wound is not infected. An open wound remains in the inflammatory phase of healing with no effective collagen production until it has been covered with an epithelial element (3).

It is of particular importance to realize that inflammation continues until wound closure occurs. Only after successful wound closure can the wound progress into the next stages of healing. The longer a wound remains in the inflammatory phase, the more extensive the eventual scar tissue. This is readily understood when one realizes that the inflammatory phase stimulates the release of most of the humoral factors of repair. Prolonging this step can lead to more extensive repair, or scar.

Much work is yet to be done before all the humoral messengers of repair are understood. These messengers include a range of peptide growth factors that effect cellular responses, including cell migration and proliferation.

In the past, growth factors were thought to start acting following coagulation and the formation of a platelet plug, but it now appears they play a much earlier role. PDGF and bFGF are produced by the injured cell at the time of wounding. Indeed, because bFGF is detectible so early within the wound milieu, it is now thought that bFGF is also stored in the extracellular matrix, bound to heparin, and hence is readily available at the time of wounding (4). Once the platelet plug is in place, several growth factors are released that are chemotactic to and mitogenic for inflammatory cells. TGF$_\beta$ and PDGF are released from the platelet and mediate chemotaxis of neutrophils, macrophages, and fibroblasts into the wound (2). PGDF is the more important peptide during the period of inflammation and is responsible for the directed and sequential migration of neutrophils, macrophages, and fibroblasts into the wound over the first several days following wounding.

PROLIFERATIVE PHASE (EPITHELIAL REGENERATION, CONTRACTION, AND FIBROPLASIA)

The second phase of wound repair takes place from day 5 through the 3rd week after wounding. During this period, epithelial and connective tissue proliferate. Epithelial regeneration plays an essential part in the restoration of the tissue by providing an efficient barrier against invasive bacteria. The process includes mobilization, or loosening of the basal cells from their dermal attachments, and migration to the place of defect with proliferation and replacement by mitosis of pre-existing cells. Finally, by differentiation, cell function is re-

stored. The epithelial cell movement across a denuded area is predictable and relentless. It continues as long as the wound is denuded of epithelial cells. The fundamental process that initiates division and migration has not been elucidated, but the process continues until the epithelial cell comes into contact with another epithelial cell. In the past, it was thought that dedifferentiation and migration of cells played the major role, but it is now believed that mitosis involving basal cell layers is also important.

In wounds closed by first intention in which margins are coapted, the process of epithelialization may be complete in 24 to 48 hours. Wounds that close by secondary intention exhibit a more involved process. Little early mitotic activity exists at the donor site for a split-thickness skin graft. By 36 to 48 hours, however, there is increased mitotic activity with thickening of the epithelial layers. The proliferation arises from the margins, as well as from epidermal appendages in the dermis (the rete or papillary ridges). In the full-thickness wound, there is little migratory effort for 3 to 5 days, until an adequate granulation bed exists. The migration of epithelial cells follows in close relation to the granulation bed. Proliferation starts on either side and follows along the cut edge of the dermis across the granulation bed until the edges meet. The deep epithelial surface gradually thickens, with ultimate junction in the line of repair. Thickness may increase in some as much as 1 mm/day (5).

The second major event in the proliferative phase is wound contraction or "intussusceptive growth," by which large wounds close without scarring. This phenomenon is a form of tissue remodeling and may represent the vestige of a function now lost. Because a wound must be closed before it can begin the remainder of the healing phase, the body attempts to accomplish this by epithelialization and contraction. Epithelial cells, by multiplying and migrating across the surface of an open wound, will help to cover the open wound. Wound shrinking at the edges also serves the attempt at closure. All wounds contract from end to end, not from side to side. If an excised wound is 2 cm long when it is closed, it may be 1.8 cm long when it has finished healing. If the wound is a curve or a circle, the tissue within the curve may be bunched up as contraction occurs (the "trapdoor"). If the wound is allowed to remain open for a long time and inflammation is severe, the contraction processes may become far advanced. Contraction is aggravated by stress on the wound. An inflamed chronic wound running across a joint may be so shortened when healed as to limit motion; this is called a *contracture*. Contraction is normal; contracture is the joint-limiting, pathologic end result of excess contraction.

At the cellular level, the proliferative phase of wound healing is represented primarily by macrophages, fibroblasts, myofibroblasts, and endothelial cells. These cells proliferate, bringing about the synthesis and assembly of extracellular matrix and new blood vessels. These processes, each unique, when coordinated bring about the macroscopic events of wound contraction, epithelialization, and scar contraction or contracture. How all these entities are initiated and coordinated remains incompletely understood. Certainly, peptide growth factors are important. PDGF is produced by platelets, macrophages, fibroblasts, and endothelial cells, all of which are now present within the wound. PDGF stimulates the synthesis of extracellular matrix and is mitogenic for fibroblasts

(6,7). bFGF is produced by fibroblasts and endothelial and other mesenchymal cells, and is chemotactic and mitogenic for fibroblasts and endothelial cells (5). Therefore, bFGF is involved intimately with angiogenesis and the synthesis of collagen matrix. TGFβ synthesized by a wide range cells (fibroblasts, macrophages, lymphocytes, platelets, and keratinocytes) is only weakly mitogenic for fibroblasts and, indeed, can inhibit the replication of many cell types (8). TGFβ is, however, a potent activator of extracellular matrix protein synthesis, especially collagen; in addition it is a strong chemotactic agent. These two actions reflect the fact that TGFβ is an important regulator of wound healing in vivo. Of the peptide growth factors, as they pertain to wound healing, PDGF-BB, bFGF and TGFβ are by far the most extensively studied. There is a wide range of other growth factors, such as insulin-like growth factor (IGF), epidermal growth factor (EGF), vascular endothelial growth factor (VEGF), keratinocyte growth factor (KGF), and other transforming growth factors (TGF), discovered and yet to be discovered, that may have similarly important roles to play in the proliferative stage of wound healing. Keratinocyte replication and migration are thought to be coordinated by TGF, EGF and PDGF (9,10).

The fibroblast plays an important role in the proliferative phase, not only producing peptide growth factors but also providing collagen and other extracellular matrix molecules in response to these growth factors. It follows that bFGF and PDGF should stimulate wound contraction. This has been shown in clinical trials involving pressure sores, where contraction is the primary mechanism of wound closure (11,12). The specific cellular mechanisms are still not fully elucidated.

One of the more recent significant findings in wound healing has been the discovery of a cell that has both fibroblast and smooth-muscle characteristics. In 1971, Gabbiani and colleagues (13) first postulated the presence of myofibroblast cells in a contracting wound. Further studies by Rudolph and coworkers (14) demonstrated that the rate of wound contraction partly depended on the number of myofibroblasts within the wound. Additional work (15) indicated that the myofibroblasts are distributed throughout the wound, not just at the margins. Thus, the entire granulation surface serves as a contractile organ wherein the myofibroblasts shorten the wound and then collagen deposition and cross-linking maintain the degree of contraction. Through such a lock-step mechanism, the bed of the contracting wound shortens in progressive fashion. Note, however, that collagen formation is not essential for wound contraction. Even with vitamin C deficiency, wound contraction proceeds normally.

The 3rd major development in the proliferative phase is the production of substances of connective-tissue repair. Early histologists were impressed by the increase in fibroblasts and collagen during healing and suggested that a correlation might exist between the number of fibroblasts, the quantity of collagen, and the tensile strength of the scar (16). Indeed, scar tissue would seem to develop from the production of collagen molecules by fibroblasts. These molecules aggregate to form fibers, followed by a weaving of the fibers and fibrils into a purposefully ordered pattern. The molecule in the appropriate environment of the ground substance is formed into a larger, more stable collagen by intra- and inter-

molecular bonds. The protein from fibroblasts (procollagen) has a high proline content. Collagen that forms the fibers and fibrils is an extracellular substance. To become extracellular requires a special hydroxylation step from the peptide proline to the unique collagen amino acid hydroxyproline. With the hydroxylation of proline and lysine, final assembly can take place.

The solubility of collagen and the nature of its polymerization have been extensively studied. Tropocollagen is composed of three chains, each with a molecular weight of about 94,000. In native proteins, the individual chains are arranged as a left-handed helix, producing a ropelike structural molecule. Intramolecular and intermolecular cross-linking by aldehyde groups develops early during fibroplasia. Secondary gain in tensile strength during the period of remodeling is related to the intermolecular bonds.

Fibroblasts also produce glycosaminoglycans (mucopolysaccharides) once they have migrated into the wound. The precise role of the mucopolysaccharides in wound healing is not fully understood. Most of the glycoprotein in the wound during the first few days appears to be derived from serum glycoproteins. The production of new polysaccharides in the wound is closely related to the period of collagen formation and fibroplasia. Bentley (17) demonstrated that chondroitin sulfate, with its concentration of hyaluronic acid, appears early in the wound at about days 4 to 6, and rises again at the end of fibroplasia.

The glycosaminoglycans are repeating disaccharide units attached to the protein core. As they are secreted by fibroblasts, these substances are hydrated to contribute to the "ground substance, an amorphous gel that may play a role in subsequent aggregation of collagen fibers" (18).

At the end of the inflammatory stage (5 to 7 days in clean, primarily closed wounds) the wound has about 10% of its ultimate tensile strength. After 15 to 20 days, the wound can resist normal stress. Much more collagen is formed than is ultimately needed and wound tensile strength continues to increase for several weeks. By 3 weeks, the synthesis of wound collagen remains high, but the net collagen accumulated is matched by collagen degradation. At 6 weeks, the wound has reached about 60% of strength. It will reach its maximum in 3 to 6 months. However, healed wounds rarely regain more than 70 to 80% of intact skin strength.

MATURATION OR REMODELING PHASE

Although a wound probably never becomes as strong as intact skin, the scar matures over time and the collagen fibers, laid down in disarray in the fibroplasia phase (they are like steel wool, potentially strong but poorly organized), begin to be rewoven in response to stress. The fibers are lined up (like weaving steel wool into a cable) along stress lines, and the more stretch on the wound, the more cablelike the scar will be. Big scars may seem to be stronger, but in actuality, because strength is dependent on weave rather than amount of collagen, a fine hairline scar may be stronger than a thick scar.

During this maturation phase, which may last a year or longer, the scar will flatten, the redness will fade, and the pruritus will disappear. When this happens, one can accept that the wound has reached its maximum healing and time will contribute no more. The fibroblasts appear to be responsible for reabsorption and production of new collagen. The zone of activity in which this chemical process takes place is localized in an area approximately 0.75 mm on either side of the wound edge (19). If tension is placed on the wound, it is noted that the random collagen fibers appear to line up parallel to the forces of tension. Within 3 months, the scar becomes flatter, softer, and lighter in color. The collagen becomes thicker and denser, and the blood vessels constrict and disappear. The number of fibroblasts is gradually reduced and the scar tissue becomes almost acellular.

Obviously, a fresh wound that is ill-placed or poorly aligned can be no more than an ill-placed or poorly aligned mature scar a year later. Although vitamins and a nutritious diet may be prudent for healthy living, there is no evidence that the supplementation of vitamins (e.g., C, E) or additional nutritious food will make a difference in the healing of the usual wound in an otherwise healthy person.

Once again, emphasis must be placed upon the ideal milieu and stimuli for wound healing to progress in an orderly fashion with minimal connective-tissue formation.

Factors Affecting the Wound Healing Process

Although the phenomenon of wound healing is relatively fixed in an orderly progression of events, the rate of wound healing in any of the phases can be regulated by many factors. A healing wound does not develop separately from the organism or its environment.

For years, mankind has hoped to accelerate wound healing, but we have learned that very little can be done therapeutically to hasten repair beyond the normal. A variety of substances have been purported to hasten tissue repair, including scarlet red, gentian violet, balsam of Peru, powdered cartilage and bone, zinc oxide, and oxygen. Most of these agents probably restore healing to a more optimal level rather than accelerate the process.

NUTRITION

All else being equal, wounds in the young heal more rapidly than those in the elderly, whether this be by increased fibroplasia, decreased susceptibility to infection, increased general cell proliferation, or just better nutrition. Protein deficiency is believed to retard vascularization and lymphatic formation, to lower resistance to infection and to inhibit several phases of wound healing. In such an environment, there is a delay in both fibroplasia and the development of tensile strength. In 1949, Localio and associates (20) reported that the feeding of d1-methionine to protein-depleted animals restored the substrate period to is normal length and increased the rate of fibroplasia. This suggests that this single amino acid is necessary for synthesis by fibroblasts of both mucopolysaccharides and collagen. Although administration of methionine does appear to restore the healing process to a normal rate, the reversal of protein starvation requires time. Protein deficiency states should be corrected before the operation.

Trauma abruptly alters the metabolic status quo. The post injury state is marked by increased heat production gluconeogenesis; negative nitrogen, potassium, sulfur, and phosphorus balance; early hyperglycemia, and modification in carbohydrate utilization. Also occurring are elevated serum concentrations of free fatty acids with ketosis; sodium, chloride and water retention; potential depletion of ascorbic acid, thiamine, riboflavin, nicotinamide and vitamin A; and possible deficiencies of trace metals such as zinc, copper, and iron. Coupled with these events are potentially great caloric requirements associated with multiple injuries, burns, and sepsis. When postoperative nutritional problems (e.g., malignancy, increased age, diabetes, or gastrointestinal disorders such as Crohn disease or cirrhosis), the potential for nutritional disaster exists. If malnutrition does occur, patients exhibit a potential for weakness, greater susceptibility to anesthetics and shock, impaired liver and GI tract function, retarded wound healing, serious infections, prolonged hospitalization, and death. It should also be noted that a given wound will heal more slowly in an individual who has another significant injury (e.g., a burn with a concomitant long-bone fracture).

Vitamin C

The importance of vitamin C as a cofactor necessary for collagen synthesis has been recognized since it was used for the prevention of scurvy in sailors centuries ago. Humans cannot synthesize vitamin C, and normally store it for only 4 or 5 months. Ascorbic acid is an active reducing agent involved in the production of superoxide radicals, and an important intermediary in respiration and in the synthesis of an antibacterial substance from leukocytes. In addition, vitamin C (or rather its ester equivalent, ascorbate) is required for the hydroxylation of proline and lysine. In the scorbutic individual, collagen lysis outstrips synthesis, causing a weakening of collagen, increased capillary permeability, fragility, and rupture and hemorrhage of vessels. It has not been established whether the increased requirement for vitamin C reflects an accumulation of ascorbic acid at the wound site or an increased rate of vitamin C metabolism. Excessive doses of vitamin C do not further accelerate wound healing.

Vitamin A

Vitamin A is important in vision, reproduction, epithelium maintenance and multiplication, synthesis of proteoglycans, stabilization of lysosomal membranes, and the enhancement of cellular immunity. Experiments have shown vitamin A accelerates healing of skin lesions, whereas deficiencies retard epithelialization, wound closure, collagen synthesis rates, and cross-linking of new collagen. In addition, vitamin A deficiency causes depletion of vitamin C reserves. It now appears that vitamin E enhances absorption, storage, and utilization of vitamin A. Importantly, vitamin A offsets the inhibitory effects of adrenal steroids on wound repair, even when applied locally. Large stores are maintained in the liver and supplementation is not required with routine surgical procedures. In the malnourished patient, 25,000 IU/day is adequate for normal wound repair.

Vitamin E

The role of vitamin E in wound healing is unknown. Ehrlich and others (21) observed that vitamin E inhibited wound healing by decreasing tensile strength and hampering accumulation of collagen. It had no effect on glucocorticoid inhibition of wound healing, and its actions were reversed by vitamin A. It is believed that vitamin E may act through its membrane-stabilizing effects.

Oxygen

Oxygen is considered an essential substrate for effective wound healing. During healing, the wound consumes a greater amount of oxygen than normal tissues (22,23). The partial pressure of oxygen (pO_2) within tissue is dependent upon several physical properties, including distance from the nearest capillary, intercapillary distance, rate of oxygen consumption, and a diffusion coefficient specific for that issue. When a wound occurs, local capillaries are injured, reducing the availability of oxygen. Thus, the oxygen requirement for repair is greatest when the local circulation is least able to satisfy the need. Although the tissue pO_2 in the healed wound is measured at 30 to 50 mm Hg, the minimal pO_2 necessary for healing is not known. Hunt and Pai (24) clearly observed that fibroblast replication was potentiated at partial pressures of 30 to 40 mm Hg. However, collagen synthesis required higher oxygen partial pressures.

Recent studies (25) indicate that the rate of epithelial cell proliferation in wounds is directly proportional to the arterial oxygen tension at the wound site. Oxygen increases the efficiency of collagen formation. Collagen cannot escape from the fibroblast unless a specific portion of the proline and lysine has been hydroxylated. Other studies (26) indicate that reduced oxygen may result in the formation of underhydroxylated collagen, causing a weakening of the tensile strength in wounds.

MICROENVIRONMENT, HOST RESISTANCE AND INFECTION (27–29)

The humoral and cellular defense mechanisms of the body are usually sufficient to control infection and promote wound healing. However, they cannot function efficiently in an environment of debris, necrotic tissue, hematoma, and virulent and numerous bacteria. In all these instances, bacteria may compete effectively with phagocytes, fibroblasts, endothelial cells, and epithelium, leading to infection and delayed wound healing.

Although leukocytes are necessary for efficient killing of most microbes, certain gram-negative organisms are lysed directly by an antibody and complement complex in serum (3). Another humoral mechanism is responsible for direct kill of gram-positive and gram-negative species. Wound fluid is not a medium for bacterial growth as hematoma is, and in fact it is actually independently bactericidal to a number of organisms (3).

The amount of bacterial inoculum introduced into a wound is critical for appropriate management of the wound. A dynamic equilibrium exists between the bacteria in the wound and the host. This relationship is best described as a balance (29). With adequate wound host defenses and without interference by such factors as hematomas or foreign bodies, a wound can withstand a level of up to 100,000 (10^5) organisms per gram of tissue and still heal or be repaired successfully (3). If greater than 10^5 bacteria per gram are present, wound closure is likely to lead to clinical wound infection. The only exception to this occurs in the case of β-hemolytic streptococci, which can produce clinical wound infection if present in any number. Although bacterial balance in a wound can be surmised by a careful history and physical evaluation, it can only be confirmed by quantitative and qualitative bacteriology performed on a tissue-biopsy specimen from the wound (3).

Conclusion

Wound healing has been studied for thousands of years. Despite this, clinicians still have only a rudimentary understanding of how a wound heals or, conversely, why a wound fails to heal. Recent advances in molecular biology, especially the availability of peptide growth factors in commercial quantities, has accelerated research into wounds. Now that wounds and wound healing have been defined in a universal manner, efforts can be concentrated on understanding underlying mechanisms. The scheme that has been discussed represents a foundation to which elements will be added and removed as the complex cascade of events that contribute to wound healing are unraveled. The observation that wound healing is inevitable should not encourage complacency among clinicians. Indeed, the possibility of clinical intervention leading to accelerated, scar-free wound healing now exists. Clinicians should now review wounds and wound healing as an area of clinical practice where they can positively change outcomes.

References

1. Lazarus GS, Cooper DM, Knighton DR, et al. Definitions and guidelines for assessment of wounds and evaluation of healing. *Arch Dermatol* 1994; 130:489.
2. McGrath MH. Peptide growth factors and wound healing. *Clin Plast Surg* 1990; 17:421.
3. Robson MC, Burns BF, Phillips LG. Wound repair: principles and applications. In: Ruberg RL, Smith DJ Jr, eds. *Plastic surgery: a core curriculum.* 1993; 3–30.
4. Bennett NT, Schultz GS. Growth factors and wound healing: biochemical properties of growth factors and their receptors. *Am J Surg* 1993; 165:728.
5. Dingman RO. Factors of clinical significance affecting wound healing. *Laryngoscope* 1973; 83:1540.
6. Greenhalgh DG, Sprugel KH, Murrary MJ, et al. PDGF and FGF stimulate wound healing in the genetically diabetic mouse. *Am J Pathol* 1990; 136:1235.
7. Robson MC, Phillips LG, Thomason A, et al. Platelet-derived growth factor BB for the treatment of chronic pressure ulcers. *Lancet* 1992; 339:23
8. Olashaw NR, O'Keefe EJ, Pledger NJ. Platelet-derived growth factor modulates epidermal growth factor receptors by a mechanism distinct from that of phorbol esters. *PNAS* 1986; 83:3834.
9. Burgess AW. Epidermal growth factor and transforming growth factor. *Br Med Bull* 1989; 45:401.
10. Schultz GS, White M, Mitchell R, et al. Epithelial wound healing enhanced by transforming growth factor and vaccinia growth factor. *Science* 1987; 235:350.
11. Robson MC, Phillips LG, Thomason A, et al. Recombinant human platelet-derived growth factor—BB for the treatment of chronic pressure ulcers. *Ann Plast Surg* 1992; 29:193.
12. Robson MC, Phillips LG, Lawrence T, et al. The safety and effect of topically applied recombinant basic fibroblast growth factor on the healing of chronic pressure sores. *Ann Surg* 1992; 216:401.
13. Gabbiani G, Hirschel BJ, Ryan GB, et al. Granulation tissue as a contractile organ: a study of structure and function. *J Exp Med* 1972; 135:719.
14. Rudolph R, Guber S, Suzuki M, et al. The life-cycle of the myofibroblast. *Surg Gynecol Obstet* 1977; 145:389.
15. Rudolph R. Location of the force of wound contraction. *Surg Gynecol Obstet* 1979; 148:547.
16. Madden JW, Peacock EE. Studies on the biology of collagen during wound healing. I. Rate of collagen synthesis and deposition in cutaneous wounds of the rate. *Surgery* 1968; 64:288.
17. Bentley JP. Rate of chondroitin sulfate formation in wound healing. *Ann Surg* 1967; 165:186.

18. Bryant WM. Wound healing. *Diba Found Symp* 1977; 29:2.
19. Adamsons RJ, Musco F, Enquist IF. The chemical dimensions of wound healing: effect of d1-methionine on healing surface wounds. *Surg Gynecol Obstet* 1966; 123:515.
20. Localio SA, Gillette L, Hinton JW. Biological chemistry of wound healing: effect of d1-methionine on healing surface wounds. *Surg Gynecol Obstet* 1949; 89:69.
21. Ehrlich P, Tarver H, Hunt TK. Inhibitory effects of vitamin E on collagen synthesis and wound repair. *Ann Surg* 1972; 175–235.
22. Hunt TK, Zederfeldt B, Goldstick TK. Oxygen and healing. *Am J Surg* 1969; 118:521.
23. Hunt TK, Twomey P, Zederfeldt B, et al. Respiratory gas tensions and pH in healing wounds. *Am J Surg* 1967; 114:302.
24. Hunt TK, Pai MP. The effect of varying ambient oxygen tensions on wound metabolism and collagen synthesis. *Surg Gynecol Obstet* 1972; 135:561.
25. Silver IA. Oxygen tension and epithelialization. In: Maibach HI, Rovee, DT, eds. *Epidermal Wound Healing.* Chicago: Year Book, 1972; 291–305.
26. Uitto J, Prockop DJ. Synthesis and secretion of under-hydroxylated procollagen at various temperatures by cells subject to temporary anoxia. *Biochem Biophys Res Commun* 1974; 60:414.
27. Bierens de Haan B, Ellis H, Wilks M. The role of infection on wound healing. *Surg Gynecol Obstet* 1974; 138:693.
28. Burke JF, Morris PJ, Bondoc CC. The effect of bacterial inflammation on wound healing. In: Dunphy JE, VanWinkle W, eds. *Repair and regeneration.* New York: McGraw-Hill, 1969; 19–30.
29. Krizek TJ, Robson MC. Evolution of quantitative bacteriology in wound management. *Am J Surg* 1975; 130:579.

2

Basic Principles of Surgical Techniques

Malcolm W. Marks, M.D.

The success of a surgical procedure is determined by the surgeon's understanding of orderly wound healing and the principles of precise surgical technique. Wound healing begins at the moment of injury or surgical incision and follows an orderly sequence of vascular, cellular, humeral, and biochemical processes. Factors that interfere in the natural progression and speed of healing will compromise the ultimate result. Foreign bodies and bacterial organisms change the inflammatory process while motion and wound tension interfere with vascularity.

In the 1500s Paré stressed the importance of good surgical technique (1). In the late 1700s John Hunter was instrumental in introducing modern pathology and experimental surgery. He was also the first to notice the importance of inflammation in healing (2). In the early 1800s surgery still remained unusual, however, because of the inability to control pain, hemorrhage, and infection. The modern era of surgery began in 1846 with the advent of general anesthesia, when a patient was first anesthetized with ether at the Massachusetts General Hospital (3). In the mid-1800's Louis Pasteur recognized the germ theory of disease (4). Joseph Lister, aware of Pasteur's work, introduced the modern concept of surgical asepsis (5,6). In the early 20th century. William Halsted introduced the basic principles of surgical techniques, stressing (a) asepsis, (b) hemostasis, (c) obliteration of dead space, (d) preservation of blood supply, (e) gentleness, and (f) avoidance of tissue tension at the suture line (7). The Halstedian principles, combined with today's understanding of preoperative planning, wound preparation, scar placement, suture technique, and postoperative management, enable modern aesthetic and reconstructive procedures. These procedures require an understanding of three-dimensional contour, symmetry, and skin color and texture, and mandate attention to meticulous surgical technique.

Preoperative Planning

The objective of a surgical procedure is to treat an underlying problem in a manner that maximizes a correction while minimizing scarring and limitation of function. A detailed understanding is required of the region's vascular supply, soft-tissue cover, skeletal stability, innervation, and mobility. The surgeon assesses the physiology and function of the area so that a procedure may be devised for its restoration or preservation.

Reconstructive procedures are directed not only at correcting an anatomic deformity but also at restoring a patient's sense of physical and psychologic well being. The operative plan, the timing and sequence of procedures, must

be worked out with this in mind and a dialog established with the patient and family. Complex reconstructions may need a team approach and consultation with other specialists. Optimal timing of repair must be determined. Certain congenital deformities such as craniosynostosis are best repaired in the early months of life (to advantage of rapid brain development), while congenital ear deformities are delayed until 4 or 5 years of age when rapid growth of the ear has plateaued. A secondary correction of scars is postponed until sufficient scar maturation has taken place, 6 to 12 months after original wounding or surgery. During this period scars soften and tissues become better vascularized. However, an unstable wound that is painful or results in exposure of vital structures may need immediate revision regardless of the stage of healing.

Placement of incisions is planned to provide optimal exposure as well as an ideal postoperative scar that does not limit mobility or function. It is also important that the incision and subsequent scar not compromise future procedures. X rays, scans, dental models, laboratory studies, and preoperative photographs are reviewed.

Appropriate surgical instruments, including loupes and a microscope if necessary, must be available and adequate lighting ensured. The patient is positioned in a safe and comfortable fashion that allows the surgeon access to the surgical site. The type of anesthesia—local, regional, or general—is chosen. Head and neck procedures require careful positioning and securing of the endotracheal tube to ensure both safe anesthesia and access to the operative site. If a local procedure with intravenous sedation is planned, an oxygen-delivery system should be secured.

Preparation of the Wound

An open wound is evaluated for bacterial and foreign-body contamination, amount of contusion or tissue necrosis, vascularity, and condition of surrounding and underlying tissue. Foreign material must be removed and necrotic material débrided. Irrigation with sterile saline will help in removal of debris. Irrigation of a wound requires large volumes of solution and is best delivered by a pulsatile jet lavage. If that is not available, irrigation through a syringe provides an effective means of removing debris from a small wound. The amount of débridement is determined by degree of tissue injury and location. If the wound is in an area with abundant soft tissue and soft-tissue laxity, an aggressive débridement may be carried out. If the wound is in an anatomically sensitive area where excessive removal of tissue may result in subsequent functional compromise (e.g., over a joint) or aesthetic compromise (e.g., on the face), a more conservative débridement is warranted.

The surgeon determines both how best to close a wound and the best timing of closure. The wound may be closed primarily and immediately, or closure may be delayed, with the wound left to heal. In a delayed closure, the wound is treated by serial dressing changes, at which time further débridements are carried out. The wound is finally closed when it is determined that all necrotic tissue has been removed and bacterial contamination has been minimized. If the wound is left to heal by secondary intention, dressing changes are continued until the wound has closed through contraction and epithelialization.

Asepsis

An operative site is prepared by the application of antiseptics and antimicrobial agents. These agents provide a mechanical cleansing of the area as well as bacteriocidal activity; they are toxic to cells and should not be introduced directly into open wounds. When dealing with open wounds, cleansing is provided by irrigation with a balanced saline solution.

Hair need be trimmed only to provide expeditious operative exposure. If hair is to be shaved, it is best done immediately prior to surgery (shaving the night before may increase the risk of wound infection). It is not necessary to remove hair from cosmetically sensitive areas such as the beard, the eyebrows, or the scalp. It is not possible to sterilize the operative area when entering the oral or nasal cavity, sinuses, or pharynx. Good surgical technique preserving the abundant blood supply to these areas combined with perioperative antibiotics reduces the risk of postoperative infection.

Hemostasis

Excessive bleeding will compromise wound healing by causing ischemia or hematoma that can become a focus for infection. A dry surgical field may be obtained by the injection of epinephrine, which is a potent vasoconstrictor. Although epinephrine solutions are commercially available in strengths of 1:100,000 and 1:200,000, dilute solutions of 1:400,000 are effective. Epinephrine may be directly infiltrated into a wound or applied topically to an open wound on a soaked sponge.

Bleeding from small vessels is controlled through electrocautery. These units provide a pinpoint electrical current of high frequency and amperage combined with low voltage, producing thermocoagulation. Electrocautery units may be unipolar or bipolar. Bipolar coagulation is directed only at the tissue between the teeth of the forceps, is not conducted to surrounding tissues, and is to be used if a conduction of electrocautery will damage adjacent nerves, vessels, or tissues. Larger vessels are clamped and tied with sutures. Hemostatic agents such as thrombin or gel foams are helpful in providing hemostasis to large, oozing areas. If there is any doubt as to hemostasis, drains are placed to minimize accumulation of serum and blood. Hematomas must be evacuated upon recognition to avoid secondary sequelae including infection, compromise of overlying flaps, and subcutaneous scarring.

Placement of Incisions

Elective incisions are ideally placed in lines of minimal tension or resting skin-tension lines. These lines run perpendicular to the pull of the underlying musculature. Placement of scars in or parallel to these lines will minimize the propensity to form hypertrophic scars. The lines of expression in the face also lie perpendicular to the long axis of the underlying muscles, and both incisions and excisions should be designed so that the scar falls within or parallel to these lines of expression (8). Incisions may also be well hidden at the junction of aesthetic units.

Scars should be placed where they will not be visible or will be as inconspicuous as possible. The forehead is ideally approached through a transcoronal incision, the breast through an inframammary incision, the nose through a transcolumella incision. The skin is incised perpendicular to the surface of the skin except in hair-bearing tissue; here the incision is beveled away from the hair follicle to avoid injury and subsequent hair loss. The incision is long enough so that the surgical procedure may be carried out with ease, without unnecessary traction on wound edges, but should be no longer than needed.

Handling of Tissue

Tissues must be handled gently to preserve cellular integrity. Excessive pressure with pickups will crush the tissue, causing ischemia, necrotic debris, and compromise of wound healing. Ideally, the skin is retracted with hooks, and when forceps are used they should be fine-toothed forceps that are closed with minimal tension. Once the skin and subcutaneous tissues have been incised, dissection should be carried out along anatomic planes. This provides a relatively bloodless field and avoids unnecessary trauma to tissues above and below these planes. Tissues are kept moist by irrigation or application of wet packs, avoiding tissue desiccation. Fascial integrity is preserved if possible, minimizing herniation of fat and soft tissues into the operative field. Vascularity to the tissues is carefully preserved. Vessels that do not have to be ligated are spared. Traction on nerves is avoided to prevent neuropraxic injury. Muscles are elevated in a subperiosteal plane if possible, avoiding unnecessary transection with subsequent fibrosis and shortening.

Careful preoperative planning will prevent unnecessary incision and dissection and avoid compromise of blood supply. Old scars and incisions must be recognized and their effect on subsequent operative procedures determined. A Doppler probe may be helpful in identifying arteries when dissecting the blood supply to a flap or a recipient vessel for free tissue transfer. Mapping of the vessels with the Doppler probe, dissection with loupe magnification, and use of bipolar coagulation are all important techniques in the preservation of small vessels that might be critical to the successful outcome of a tissue transfer.

Handling of bone, as with soft tissue, is directed at the preservation of its structural and cellular integrity and its vascularity. Meticulous technique will accomplish this goal, expediting healing and minimizing infection. Rigid fixation is the most important technique that promotes fracture union and incorporation of a bone graft. Although wire fixation may suffice, rigid fixation generally is accomplished by plate-and-screw or lag-screw fixation. Rigid fixation ensures anatomic reduction and immobilization, and thus prevents displacement. It also enables early mobilization while protecting surrounding soft tissues.

Implants and grafts are selected to restore contour and symmetry. These may include synthetic materials such as proplast or silicone, autograft or allograft. Donor source, bed vascularity, and risk of infection must be evaluated in order to select which type of implant or graft is best.

Technique of Closure

Wounds are closed in layers to obliterate or minimize dead space. Failure to eliminate dead space results in the formation of hematoma or seroma. When dead space is unavoidable, drains for postoperative evacuation are mandatory. Layered closure requires approximation of fascia. Fascia has sufficient strength to hold the stitch and is less sensitive to ischemia caused by a knot. Sutures in fat tend to cause fat necrosis, while sutures in muscle tend to tear, allowing separation with secondary dead space. Skin is approximated with buried dermal sutures. These sutures should be absorbable, dissolving within 3 to 4 weeks. When nonabsorbable sutures are used in the dermis, they act as foreign bodies and are more likely to become nidi of infection. The knot of the buried dermal suture should be inverted to minimize risk of surface erosion. The skin is closed with monofilament suture with eversion of wound edges. Sutures are tied loosely to avoid skin necrosis, and subsequent scar should be removed early. If a skin suture is expected to remain in place for longer than would be ideal, a subcuticular stitch that leaves no marks is used. Skin sutures are placed at identical levels on each side and small bites are taken to minimize the amount of tissue constricted by the suture. Tension on tissues and suture lines is to be avoided, because it compromises blood flow and increases the fibroplastic response. Tension on a flap may obstruct arterial inflow or venous egress, with tissue necrosis. In a similar fashion, tension on a vascular anastomosis will induce vessel spasm, disrupt flow, and lead to thrombogenesis. Tension on a nerve repair will inhibit axonal regeneration at the site of repair, while distracting forces on a fracture site will delay bony union. Tension is avoided by adequate dissection of tissues to be mobilized and bone, vessel, or nerve grafts. If closure of the skin requires excessive tension, an alternate method of closure must be considered. If primary closure is not possible because of lack of adequate tissue, repair with split-thickness or full-thickness skin graft may be necessary. If an adequate vascular bed is not available, the wound is closed with a flap. A skin flap may be advanced, transposed, or rotated into the defect. Alternately, muscle, musculocutaneous flaps, or fasciocutaneous flaps may be transferred. The Z-plasty is an effective means of gaining length along the direction of a scar and geometrically reorienting scar (9). Although best avoided in the primary closure of a wound, the technique has numerous applications and is one of the most widely used procedures in plastic surgery. A Z-plasty may be used as a single Z or as multiples. Most cleft lip repairs are modifications of the Z-plasty principle. The angles of the Z should be about 60° so that two equal triangles may be elevated and transposed as interdigitating flaps.

Postoperative Management

Postoperative care is directed at minimizing pain and promoting healing. Open wounds should be kept clean and moist with changes of balanced saline dressing. Skin wounds closed with subcuticular sutures are steristripped to maintain coaptation of the skin. Wounds with interrupted sutures may be cleansed with gauze and hydrogen peroxide followed by application of a topical antibiotic ointment. Dressings are changed to maintain a clean wound and maximize patient comfort. Nature and quantity of drain output is recorded and drains are removed once drainage is acceptable. Skin grafts to ideal beds are stented with a bolster, or circumferential dressings, minimizing serous buildup beneath the graft. A questionable graft site may be treated by a fine-mesh gauze layer over which dressing changes are continued. Flaps are carefully monitored for vascular viability. A compromised flow may require removal of sutures, adjustment of dressing or patient position, or reexploration in the case of free-tissue transfer. Free flaps are monitored by temperature probes or laser Doppler. Extremities are immobilized or splinted, and motion reinstituted when appropriate. Antibiotics are used both to treat infections and prophylactically if operating in a contaminated area. There is reason for antimicrobial prophylaxis when foreign materials or nonvascularized grafts are implanted. The use of prophylactic antibiotics in routine procedures remains controversial.

Attention to the details of preoperative planning, intraoperative technique, and postoperative management will determine the surgical result. Surgeons who have mastered these techniques will avoid intraoperative adventures and postoperative complications. They will routinely obtain good results, provide the best care for their patients, and advance the art of their surgical specialty.

Acknowledgement

The author acknowledges the work of Robert M. Pearl and Robert A. Chase, who wrote the chapter "Basic Principles of Surgical Technique" in the second edition of this text.

Bibliography

1. Paré A. *The workes of that famous chirurgion Ambrose Paréy,* trans. Thomas Johnson. London, 1634; 324, 429, 457–464. Johnson's translation was from the 1582 Latin edition of Parés' 1579 collected works, the second French edition.
2. Garrison FH. *History of medicine.* 4th ed. Philadelphia: WB Saunders, 1929.
3. Keys TE. *The history of surgical anesthesia.* New York: Dover, 1963.
4. Pasteur L, Joubert JF, Chamberland CE. La theorie des germes et ses applications á la médecine et à la chirurgie. *CR Acad Sci* 1878; 86:1037.
5. Lister J. On a case illustrating the present aspect of the antiseptic system of treatment in surgery. *Br Med J* 1871; 1:31.
6. Lister J. On a new method of treating compound fracture, abscess, etc. *Lancet* 1867; 1:326–329, 357–359, 387–389, 507–509; 2:95–96.
7. Halsted WS. *Surgical papers.* In: Burket WC, ed. Baltimore: The Johns Hopkins Press, 1924; 311–586.
8. Burgess AF. *Elective incisions and scar revision.* Boston: Little, Brown, 1973.
9. McGregor IA. *Fundamental techniques of plastic surgery.* 2nd ed. Edinburgh: Livingstone, 1962.

3

Skin Grafting

Jack C. Fisher, M.D., F.A.C.S.

When the history of 20th-century plastic surgery is written, ample reference will be made to microsurgery, myocutaneous flaps, tissue expansion, and perhaps even to the pharmacologic control of graft rejection. Nevertheless, skin grafting will continue to stand as this century's most significant technical advance in plastic surgery.

Credit is usually given to Reverdin (1) for the first biologic transfer of skin, which was reported in 1870. Pollock (2) applied the first successful autograft to a burn wound. However, the common clinical use of grafted skin awaited 20th-century refinements. Before World War I, only very thin (Thiersch) or full-thickness (Wolff) grafts were used. Halsted applied large, full-thickness grafts to his mastectomy wounds. Blair and Brown first reported their clinical use of split skin grafting in 1929 (3). Widespread acceptance of split-skin grafting was later assured by invention of the dermatome by Earl Padgett and George Hood (4). Blair, however, continued to prefer a scalpel for graft harvest.

Surgeons can intervene with skin grafts or skin flaps rather than depend on natural healing processes. There is good reason to graft well in advance of active contraction in order to limit deformity and disability. Partial-thickness (split) skin grafts will slow the rate of contraction in a wound but not eliminate it altogether. Full-thickness grafts and skin flaps can stop contraction if applied early to surface defects (Fig. 3–1).

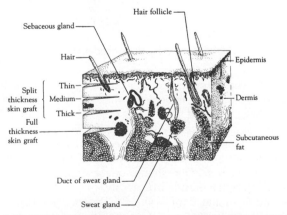

FIG. 3–1. Schematic demonstration of the histology of normal skin, emphasizing the skin appendages (hair follicles and sweat glands) that yield new epithelium following split-graft harvest. On the left are skin grafts of varying thicknesses. (From *Skin Grafting,* R Rudolph, JC Fisher, JL Ninnemann. Boston: Little, Brown, 1980).

Preparing Wounds for a Skin Graft

Skin grafts require a living regenerative surface for successful neovascularization. Grafting means tissue transfer without preservation of blood supply; therefore vascular union must develop promptly in order for the graft to survive.

Cortical bone denuded of its periosteum cannot accept a skin graft; neither are tendons, nerves, or cartilage suitable surfaces for grafting. Most other tissues (e.g., muscle, fat, fascia—even dura and periosteum) can readily accept skin grafts if certain criteria are met:

1. *Viability.* The wound surface must be viable. It must have a blood supply and it must be débrided of all nonliving tissue. Following débridement, chronic wound surfaces must be protected by a dressing or biologic membrane to prevent further necrosis.
2. *Hemostasis.* Following débridement, all bleeding must be controlled or a graft cannot be expected to survive. More skin grafts fail because of a hematoma than many surgeons recognize or are willing to admit.
3. *Bacterial equilibrium.* All granulating surfaces are contaminated with bacteria. However, quantitative microbiologic studies show that wounds with bacterial densities less than 10 (55) organisms/gram will accept grafts more readily than wounds with higher levels of contamination (5). Quantitative (biopsy) culture of the wound surface can be a useful diagnostic aid prior to skin grafting. The traditional swab culture is unreliable and does not tell the surgeon anything about bacterial density within the wound.
4. *Systemic equilibrium.* Patients with certain illnesses are not suitable candidates for grafting. For example, those who receive steroid medication do not vascularize grafts well. Venous stasis can be as disabling to graft viability as is arterial insufficiency. Diabetes and prior radiation provide their own handicaps to graft acceptance. Some of these preconditions can be treated and stabilized before grafting; others cannot.

Inexperienced skin grafters often ask what can be applied on the wound surface to make it ready for a graft. The answer is that no applied substance can substitute for blood supply or meticulous débridement. Preparatory solutions like the organic iodines (e.g., Povidone) are probably without biologic advantage, or contain inflammatory ingredients like detergents, or are so deeply pigmented that they obscure the surgeon's ability to examine the wound surface. Topical antibacterial creams commonly used for burn treatment may inhibit graft healing.

A physiologic saline solution is adequate. However, we prefer to use a very dilute solution of sodium hypochorite (l0% in saline). Known as Dakin's solution when introduced during World War I, it can be prepared easily by diluting laundry bleach 1:10. Dakin's solution releases free chlorine and oxygen and dissolves thin residual layers of fibrin; it can neutralize the foul odor that accompanies a chronic wound. Dressings for a wound surface should be moistened at the time of application and again at the time of removal. The time-honored wet-to-dry dressing deserves no recognition or use; it is unnecessarily painful as well as damaging to migrating epithelium.

Selecting the Appropriate Donor Site(s)

Selection of a suitable donor site must take into account whether the graft will be of split- or full-thickness skin, as well as the size of the area to be grafted.

SPLIT-THICKNESS SKIN

For the smallest requirements (e.g., a finger tip), a postage stamp–sized split graft from the upper inner arm is ideal. For larger defects, it is best to begin with the lateral buttock, which will be less painful when the patient is supine and can easily be hidden by swimwear or sportswear. When a greater need must be met, extend into the posterior buttock, then onto the more-visible thigh. For very extensive burns, the additional choices in order of preference include abdomen, back, scalp, anterior chest wall, arms, and last, the lower leg. (Lower-extremity donor sites heal less well than do other locations.)

Visible areas should be avoided for small grafting needs because all patients tend to feel embarrassment when evidence of skin grafting is emblazoned on thighs or other visible zones.

Buttock and thigh are appropriate when thick split skin is needed for durability. Avoid the groin and antecubital regions, where grafts cannot be harvested without risking exposure of subcutaneous fat, and subsequent contracture.

Facial grafting requires special attention to color matching (Fig. 3–2). Hip and leg skin will assume a tawny hue when grafted to the face. This principle applies equally to patients of all ethnic origins. The scalp is an excellent site for facial grafting; no hair follicles need be transferred. We have replaced deeply pigmented facial grafts with shoulder skin and achieved an acceptable color match. Unfortunately, scalp skin can be too red for pale-skinned individuals, leaving no ideal choice.

FULL-THICKNESS SKIN

Only limited grafting needs can be served by a full-thickness skin graft. The resulting defect must always be repaired. The thinnest skin is the eyelid, followed by postauricular (Figs. 3–3 and 3–4), preauricular, supraclavicular, antecubital, and groin skin.

Skin Harvest

Plastic surgeons have adopted the agricultural term *harvest* when they refer to cutting skin grafts. A variety of instruments are used, depending on quantity and thickness of the graft(s) required.

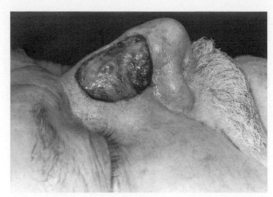

FIG. 3–2. Nasal skin defect following excision of basal cell carcinoma.

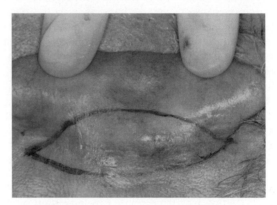

FIG. 3–3.   Postauricular graft donor site.

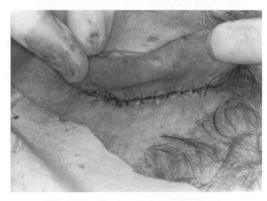

FIG. 3–4.   Donor site closed primarily.

Full-thickness grafts may be excised by dissection. Experienced surgeons should separate the skin from the underlying fat. Whenever fat is excised in continuity with skin, it must be carefully removed (defatted) prior to application. (Fig. 3–5). Donor defects are closed in two layers, using an absorbable suture for deeper closure and a running pull-out suture for the skin. One should never scrape away the fat; this can injure the dermis irreparably.

Invention of the dermatome by Padgett and Hood contributed to the popularity of split-skin grafting during and after World War II. Skin grafting technique is often learned today using the Brown electric or air-powered dermatome (6) (Fig. 3–6). We prefer the air-drive model because of its faster blade. Split grafts are cut between 12/1000 and

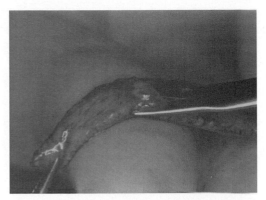

FIG. 3–5. Full-thickness graft defatted with fine scissors.

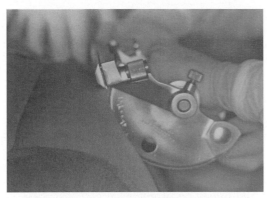

FIG. 3–7. Reese drum dermatome: split graft taken across buttock.

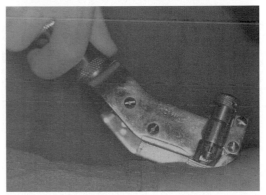

FIG. 3–6. Brown dermatome (air-driven): correct angle for taking split grafts.

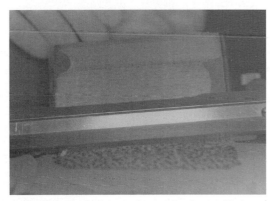

FIG. 3–8. Split graft adherent to drum adhesive as blade cuts at selected skin thickness.

l8/1000 inch in thickness. Application of very thin grafts may close the wound but will not halt contraction. Thicker grafts are more durable and contract less, but must be taken from sites where the skin is of sufficient thickness (e.g., buttock, thigh, back).

Power dermatomes are best used on surfaces with underlying muscle padding. Skin is more effectively removed from the abdomen or chest wall using a drum dermatome (Fig. 3–7). Drum dermatomes rely on the principle that adhesive surfaces will bind to the skin sufficiently for a manually operated blade to cut a satisfactory split graft (Fig. 3–8). Errors in use of a drum dermatome are usually related to inadequate preparation. Always use a fat-dissolving solvent (e.g., ether, acetone, or alcohol) before applying the dermatome. Drum dermatomes should not be used on the scalp; hair shafts are too dense for the adhesive to stick. The donor scalp should be infiltrated with saline so that the power dermatome can function against a padded surface. Drum dermatomes are favored for the most precise harvest of skin grafts of predictable thickness. The popular Rees and Padgett models operate on the same principle.

Not to be forgotten is the fine art of free-cutting skin grafts. Many of our British colleagues maintain facile skills with the Humby, Ferris Smith, or similar grafting knives. Whether or not you choose to develop skill with a long-bladed knife, you must achieve skill with small knives like the Goulian (made by Weck), an instrument useful for taking small split grafts of consistent thickness.

The trick with free cutting skin is (a) concentration to maintain blade angle and graft thickness, and (b) remembering to *slice*—like roast beef—rather than to push.

Pinch grafting, an old technique, should be discarded completely. Surgeons used to pierce the skin with a needle, draw the skin to a point, and slice off a piece with a scalpel blade. The resulting graft was unsatisfactory, producing full-thickness skin in the middle but only partial thickness at the borders. Pinch grafts don't take well, and the donor sites often heal with hypertrophic scars.

Skin Graft Storage

Both skin autografts and allografts can be stored at 4° C for a limited period of time. This technique is useful when the graft is to be used within a few days of harvesting. The graft should be spread on moist cotton gauze. The addition of tissue-culture medium may enhance viability. Antibiotics can help to prevent microbial growth.

Storage for up to 2 weeks is an acceptable clinical practice. For longer periods of time, skin banking conditions must be developed, with grafts being stored in a frozen or lyophilized state.

Delayed Graft Application

After lesion excision and skin graft harvesting, hemostasis can occasionally be a problem. When this occurs, the harvested graft may be stored, either on the donor site or at 4° C for several days, then applied as a delayed graft, perhaps at bedside. It is our usual practice to delay skin grafting of free muscle-flap surfaces for 2 to 3 days and to cover them once it becomes apparent that there are no problems with flap circulation (6).

Donor Site Care

Split-graft donor sites can be expected to heal like any partial abrasion. Following bleeding and hemostasis, an inflammatory reaction develops and a protective fibrin shield forms over the wound surface. After 2 or 3 days, active epithelial proliferation can be observed. Epidermis regenerates by growth and migration of epithelial cells from the hair follicles and skin appendages. The dermis should be covered by new epithelium in 5 to 10 days, depending on the thickness of graft taken.

As soon as the graft is harvested, apply to the donor site a wrung-out sheet of lubricated gauze followed by a lap pad. Do not remove the gauze layer, as removal may cause new bleeding. After securing the skin graft, return to the donor site, remove the lap pad, express any accumulated clot from beneath the gauze, apply a layer of Telfa or Xeroform, and then wrap with gauze. On the following day remove all but the first layer, leaving the lubricated gauze to come off spontaneously, just as a scab does. Exposing a donor site decreases surface temperature from 98° F to 91° F, thereby decreasing the potential for accelerated bacterial growth.

Conversion of a donor site to a full-thickness wound requiring its own graft is a complication of grafting, caused either by cutting to an excessive depth or by inattention to postoperative wound care. If during the harvest of a graft subcutaneous fat is observed, sew that graft back in place and choose another site. These inadvertent avulsions will usually revascularize quickly, albeit with a scar that must later be explained to the patient.

The differences between lubricated gauzes are subtle; select your favorite. Available synthetic skin substitutes offer any advantage over time-honored methods for donor site care. Some will even stick to the donor site. Biobrane, an extremely effective temporary wound coverage, is expensive and inhibits both wound contraction and epithelial migration, which is undesirable in a donor site.

Graft Immobilization

If a graft is not held immobile long enough to receive its new blood supply, then it cannot live. The failed graft that becomes infected may be the graft that was inadequately secured.

Grafts may be sutured, stapled, or taped to the wound margin or to each other (Fig. 3–9). Grafts are fragile, and sheering forces will tear them if they are affixed under tension. For prevention of troublesome sheering forces, we prefer either no dressing at all or a tie-over dressing.

Leaving a graft open to view sounds more daring than it is. It does require a cooperative patient and a nursing staff willing to observe and take action when serum or clot accumulation occurs or subtle graft movement is seen. This is obviously not a suitable technique for a child, for an uncooperative adult, for certain body regions, or for an inat-

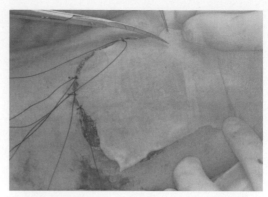

FIG. 3–9. Split graft applied to wound surface.

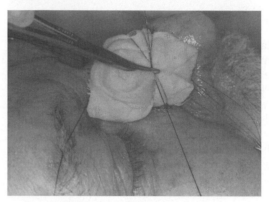

FIG. 3–10. Tie-over dressing.

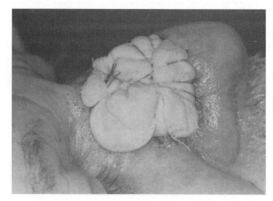

FIG. 3–11. Tie-over dressing completed.

tentive nursing staff. A tie-over dressing, sometimes called a *stent,* can be the best insurance for graft fixation (Fig. 3–10). Conventional dressings seem to loosen with time no matter how expertly applied.

Some surgeons assert that a tie-over dressing takes too long, but they may spend more time on a second graft after the initial attempt fails. A tie-over dressing ought to be done quickly, without fuss over tiny sutures. Use 4-0 silk (faster handling), big needles (also faster), quickly tie ends long, and go on to the next stitch (Figs. 3–11 and 3–12). If the scrub nurse can stay ahead of you, then you are probably not suturing fast enough.

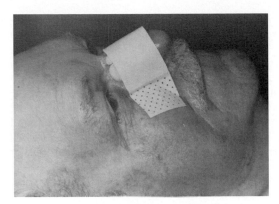

FIG. 3–12. Simple dressing.

Other bad habits to avoid include:

1. Placing the wrong side down (inverted grafts won't grow).
2. Leaving clots beneath the graft before applying a dressing.
3. "Pie-crusting" (i.e., making multiple small holes in the graft, presumably for drainage). It is much preferable to allow more time for hemostasis.

How Grafts Heal

If a graft is successfully held immobile on its wound bed, it will gradually regain the pink color it lost at the time of harvest. This return of color begins within a few hours as passive absorption of red cells takes place from the wound into the preexistent but vacated vascular channels of the graft.

The graft in this tentative status is also nourished by an exchange of nutrients. Fluid is passively absorbed by the graft, leading to edema within 2 to 3 days. Finally, the proliferating capillary tufts of the granulating bed unite with the vascular spaces of the graft; with resulting revascularization.

Grafts slowly gain durability and eventually lose their edema. They then enter the maturing phase of healing characterized by changes in dimension, pigmentation, and sensibility. We speak in error of a graft's "contracting." Contraction is a characteristic of the wound surface, not of the graft. Nevertheless, skin grafts will themselves "shrink" if they have been drawn too tightly across a defect. Grafts should therefore cover a defect abundantly and without tension. A wound will always contract to some degree following grafting (only a trace following a full-thickness graft, but as much as 30 to 35% after a split-thickness graft application).

Pigment cells of the skin are highly sensitive to injuries like skin transfer. Therefore, most grafts undergo an initial loss of pigmentation, followed by hyperpigmentation and then gradual return to normal color. Donor sites will pass through a similar pigment transition.

Reinnervation is incomplete for most grafts, although better in split grafts than in full-thickness grafts or flaps. Pontén (7) has determined by two-point discrimination testing that skin grafts will assume sensibility characteristics of the recipient wound, not of the original donor site.

Even under ideal vascularization and maturation conditions, certain unwanted sequelae may result (e.g., scaling because the graft cannot yet self-lubricate, or milia due to obstructed of buried sweat glands). Scaly skin can be lubricated daily with a lanolin-containing moisturizing lotion. Milia should be excised.

Special Techniques

MESH GRAFTING

A mechanical device can multiply pierce a graft, allowing it to be expanded into a mesh of varying size (the longer the slits, the greater the expansion ratio). Certain wounds lend themselves to meshing (e.g., an irregular concave surface in which exudate puddles or an enormous burn wound with donor-site scarity).

Readers aware of wound contraction and epithelization will immediately recognize the disadvantage of meshing: It leaves an incompletely covered surface that must contract further to achieve closure.

Those who make a habit of meshing every graft do not yet understand the principles of wound coverage. The quality of a healed surface is dependent on the thickness and integrity of the graft applied. Always avoid applying meshed grafts to a face, a hand, or any flexor surface (e.g., neck, knee).

DERMAL-FAT GRAFTING

For padding, composite grafts of dermis and fat have been successfully used. Their limitation is that much of the fat will resorb. Surgeons who use this old technique tend to rely on the grafted dermis, not the fat.

MUCOSAL GRAFTING

Skin does not do well inside the mouth. Like all grafts, skin retains its original characteristics. Whenever a secretory surface is required (e.g., conjunctiva, nasal lining, buccal mucosa), a mucosal graft is ideal.

Grafts of mucosal membrane may be transferred as a full-thickness or split-thickness graft. A special dermatome (Castroviejo) is available for harvesting small split-mucosal grafts. Full-thickness mucosa contracts after harvest, so it is best to take more than you expect to need.

The best sources for mucosal grafts are the buccal surface, nasal septum, and conjunctiva. The conjunctiva is thinnest; the septum is thickest.

COMPOSITE GRAFTING

A composite graft includes more than one kind of tissue. For example, a wedge of ear, including skin and cartilage, is ideal for reconstructing alar defects. A graft of nasal septum and overlying mucosa can be used for eyelid reconstruction.

Composite grafts are necessarily limited in dimension because they must derive blood supply from the recipient wound. Furthermore, the donor site must be closed primarily. Recipient wound preparation, suture immobilization, and graft handling must be flawless or else vascularization will not take place.

HAIR TRANSPLANTS

For hair transplants, see Chapter 56.

CULTURED SKIN GRAFTS

As techniques for tissue culture improved during the 1970s, attempts were made to create cultured skin substitutes that might help large defects to heal permanently. Whenever autologous skin is in short supply for extensive 3rd-degree burns or giant hairy nevi treatment, cultured skin-grafting techniques may be another alternative for coverage of such large deficiencies. In vitro cultivation and serial culturing of keratinocytes make production of viable epithelial sheets possible. Cultured epithelium alone, however, does not provide mechanically and aesthetically satisfactory long-term coverage.

Why Skin Grafts Fail

As surgeons, we always want a perfect graft take, but sometimes perfect results elude us and only part—or none—of the graft remains viable. On those occasions, the surgeon must take full responsibility for imperfect results. Clinical success requires that the entire graft become revascularized. To achieve success routinely, establish a high standard and consider anything less than 100% revascularization to be a failure for which you must find an explanation in your own management. By the time a graft has clearly failed, decomposing skin will have led to formation of pus. Infection must not be used as an excuse to imply that graft loss was beyond the surgeon's control.

The most common reason for graft loss is hematoma, followed closely by inadequate graft fixation. Each of these factors is within the surgeon's control. Extra moments taken to achieve complete hemostasis will save many hours of a surgeon's time and days of patient hospitalization that would be required for regrafting. The difference between a firmly held graft and a dressing that allows graft movement is the life of that graft.

Misjudgement of the wound, its vascularity, and its inherent bacterial density may also lead to failure. Less common errors include application of the graft epidermal-side down; always place the dermal (shiny) surface down. Vascularization requires union between a granulating surface and the graft dermis.

Grafted skin cannot maintain its neovasculature if held in a dependent position. Lower-extremity wounds must be elevated for 2 weeks after graft application; for several more weeks external elastic compression is needed whenever the leg is in dependent position. Small blisters on a newly grafted surface indicate excessive hydrostatic pressure.

Summary

Develop your biologic understanding of the grafting process. Perfect your skin grafting skills. Free transfers of tissue are likely to remain this century's most significant gift to reconstructive surgery. For a more detailed understanding of skin grafting principles and methods, consult a comprehensive monograph on the subject. (8)

Bibliography

1. Klasen HJ. *History of free skin grafting.* Heidelberg: Springer-Verlag, 1981.
2. Freshwater FM, Krizek TJ. Skin grafting of burns: a centennial. *J Trauma* 1971; 11: 862.
3. Blair VP, Brown JB. Uses of large split skin grafts of intermediate thickness. *Surg Gynecol Obst* 1929; 49: 82.
4. Padgett EC. Skin grafting in severe burns. *Am J Surg* 1939; 43: 626.
5. Robson MC, Krizek TJ. Predicting skin graft survival. *J Trauma* 1973; 13: 213.
6. James MI, McGrouther DA. Delayed exposed skin grafting: a 10-year experience of the technique. *Brit J Plast Surg* 1985; 38: 124.
7. Pontén B. Grafted skin—observations on innervation and other qualities. *Acta Chir Scand* (Suppl) 1960; 257: 1.
8. Rudolph R, Fisher J-C, Ninnemann JL. *Skin grafting.* Boston: Little, Brown, 1979.

4

Basic Principles of Skin Flaps

Jack Fisher, M.D., F.A.C.S., and Mary K. Gingrass, M.D.

In the past, a discussion on skin flaps in reconstructive plastic surgery would have devoted considerable space to the random pattern flap, the tubed pedicle flap, waltzing of tissue to distance sites, and the delay phenomenon. However, with our present understanding of blood supply to skin and the clinical development of new types of flaps, there is less need for use of random tissue and less dependence on the delay phenomenon. Free-tissue transfer has further decreased the need for waltzing tissue over multiple stages to distant sites. Nevertheless, knowledge of the anatomy and physiology of skin and skin flaps is essential.

The design and execution of well-planned skin flap procedures, often randomly based in such areas as the head and neck, remain important. Now, however, many new flaps with defined vascular anatomy have been described in other areas of the body. This has been especially true with the advent of free-tissue transfer, because there is increasing interest in identifying specific sites from which skin can be raised with a known dominant vascular pedicle.

This chapter will present topics important to a basic understanding of skin flaps, including the vascular anatomy of skin. Our present understanding of the blood supply to the skin, in association with the underlying muscle and fascia, has produced a fundamental change in the practice of plastic and reconstructive surgery. Advances in knowledge have led to the development of musculocutaneous, osteocutaneous, and fasciocutaneous flaps, and provided the foundation for the field of microvascular free-tissue transfer (1).

Although newer techniques have superseded many of the skin flap procedures, pathogenesis of skin-flap necrosis, the delay phenomenon, and revascularization of skin remain important topics. Much research has been devoted to the pharmacologic manipulation of skin flaps in order to improve survival. Methods of monitoring skin-flap viability remain of great interest to both researchers and clinicians.

Skin Flap Classification by Vascular Anatomy

Understanding the vascular anatomy of skin flaps requires a basic knowledge of the blood supply throughout the body. The subdermal vascular plexus and its relationship to skin perfusion must be considered in the context of the blood supply to the underlying muscle and fascia and of the body as a whole (Fig. 4–1). Accurate knowledge of vascular anatomy is an important prerequisite to successful skin-flap transfer. Numerous methods have been described for di-

rectly or indirectly manipulating and augmenting the blood flow to an area of skin. However, these manipulations can do little to salvage a flap poorly designed with respect to vascular anatomy.

A simplified scheme of the blood supply to skin has been described as consisting of three major components. First is the segmental vasculature, which consists of branches of the aorta (e.g., the femoral and intercostal vessels). Second is the perforating vessels, which are supplied by the segmental vessels and connect to the third group, the cutaneous vasculature. There are two major subgroups within the cutaneous vasculature: the musculocutaneous perforators, which supply blood to most of the body's skin, and the direct cutaneous vessels, which supply a limited number of anatomic sites. The direct cutaneous vessels form the axial pattern or arterial flaps, which will be discussed below.

The main blood supply to the skin comes from the musculocutaneous perforators, a fact that has gained great clinical importance in the last decade. These musculocutaneous vessels are arranged perpendicularly and supply a limited territory of overlying skin. This is in contrast to the direct cutaneous vessels that run parallel to the skin at a limited number of anatomic sites. Thus, one method of classification of skin flaps is based on their vascular anatomy.

Ian Taylor and colleagues have made a major contribution in defining the vascular anatomy of the skin. Their many elegant studies over the years led to the concept of *angiosomes,* which are defined as composite blocks of tissue supplied by a named source artery. The work of Taylor and associates evolved from mapping of localized vascular territories in pursuit of new free-flap donor sites to defining the arterial network for the entire human body. This has contributed greatly to the evolution of clinical skin flap design.

RANDOM PATTERN (CUTANEOUS) FLAP

The random pattern flap has no specific arterial–venous system (2). This flap has significant limitations that formerly were determined by length/width ratios. However, experimental work has shown that it is the blood supply of the flap, and not the width of it, that determines the allowable length of the surviving piece (1,3). The concept of the musculocutaneous perforater not only allowed for development of the musculocutaneous flap but also provided an understanding of the blood supply to the skin of the random pattern flap. Perfusion by musculocutaneous perforators in the base of the flap provides perfusion of the dermal–subdermal plexus of the flap (Fig. 4–2).

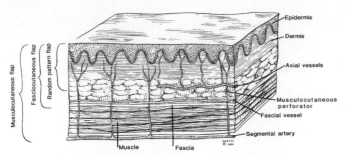

FIG. 4–1. A simplified representation of skin blood supply with both random and axial pattern distributions.

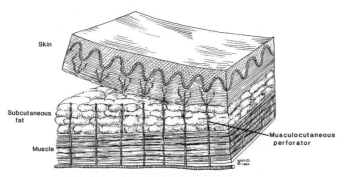

FIG. 4–2. A random pattern (cutaneous) flap. The intact musculocutaneous perforators in the base of the flap perfuse the dermal–subdermal plexus of the elevated portion of the flap.

AXIAL PATTERN (ARTERIAL) FLAP

The axial pattern flap is a skin flap with a defined anatomic arterial–venous system (2). It includes a specific direct cutaneous artery in its longitudinal axis *a* (Fig. 4–3). This vessel runs superficial to the muscle within the subcutaneous tissue. The axial pattern flap may be raised at least to the length of the arterial-venous system that runs within it and can be even longer (2). This is because a portion of the flap distal to the vessels survives as random skin. The axial pattern flap includes the underlying subcutaneous tissue that contains the direct cutaneous vessel and there is significant variation of flap thickness depending upon the amount of surface fat. An axial pattern flap in which the skin-bridge base has been divided and is only attached by its vascular pedicle is referred to as an "island flap" (Fig. 4–4). The axial pattern island flap has evolved into the model for potential free-tissue transfer by microvascular techniques (4).

Two of the early axial pattern flaps used clinically were the deltopectoral flap popularized by Bakamjian and the groin flap described by McGregor and Jackson (5). However, many axial pattern flaps have been described and used clinically (Table 4–1).

Skin Flap Classification by Mobilization

A simple classification of skin flaps into local or distant has been developed and is well known (6).

LOCAL FLAPS

Local flaps can be divided into two groups: those that rotate about a point to reach the defect, and those that advance into the defect.

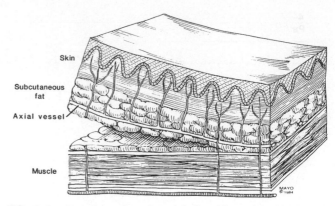

FIG. 4–3. An axial pattern (arterial) flap. The axial vessel is elevated with the flap; as depicted, there may be an overlap between territories of direct cutaneous vessels and musculocutaneous perforators.

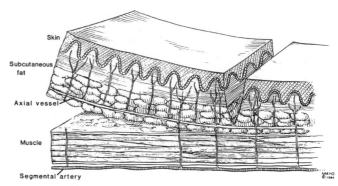

FIG. 4–4. An island flap. The axial vessel is elevated with the flap, and the skin bridge at the base is divided, isolating the flap on its vascular pedicle.

Flaps That Move Around a Fixed Point

Rotation Flaps

The movement of a rotation flap is in an arc around a fixed point and primarily in one plane. This is a semicircular flap (Fig. 4–5).

Transposition Flaps

These rectangular flaps rotate on a pivotal point. The more it is rotated, the shorter the flap effectively becomes (Fig. 4–6). The rhomboid (Limberg) flap is an example of the transposition flap (Fig. 4–7).

Interpolated Flaps

With the interpolated flap, the donor site is separated from the recipient site, and the pedicle of the flap must pass over or under the tissue to reach the recipient area (Fig. 4–8). An example is a nasolabial flap for reconstruction of the nose.

Advancement Flaps

The primary motion of an advancement flap is in a straight line from donor site to recipient site without rotation or lateral movement. Advancement flaps include the following.

Table 4–1
Axial Pattern Flaps

Flap	Blood Supply
Median forehead	Supratrochlear vessels
Nasolabial	External nasal angular vessels
Deltopectoral	Internal mammary perforators
Groin	Superficial circumflex iliac artery
Dorsalis pedis	Dorsalis pedis artery

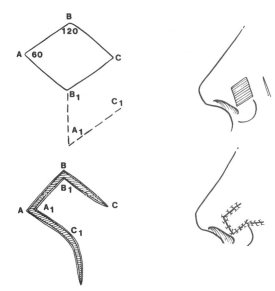

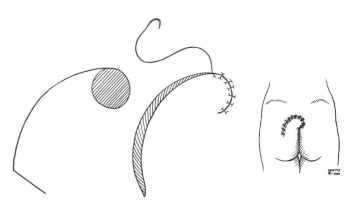

FIG. 4–5. A rotation flap. Movement is in an arc around a fixed point.

FIG. 4–7. A Limberg's flap (rhomboid flap). It is used for closure of rhomboid defects with angles at 60° and 120° and sides of equal length. The short diagonal of the rhomboid is extended equal to its own length (B₁ to A₁) and then back-cut at 60° (A₁ to C₁). The base of the flap is parallel to the lines of maximal extensibility, and the secondary effect is closed by a shift of tissue.

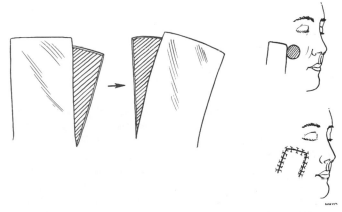

FIG. 4–6. A transposition flap. The rectangular flap is rotated on a pivot point.

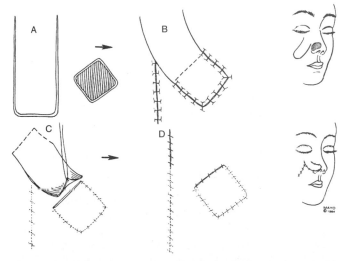

FIG. 4–8. An interpolated flap is shown. **A,** the flap is outlined and elevated. **B,** the donor site is closed, and flap is inset into the defect. **C,** once the flap is revascularized, its pedicle is divided. **D,** insetting is completed.

Single-Pedicle

With these flaps, a rectangle of skin is moved forward by virtue of its elastic properties (Fig. 4–9).

Bipedicle

Here an incision is made parallel to the defect and the flap is undermined and advanced. Often, this type of advancement requires skin grafting to close the donor site (Fig. 4–10).

V–Y

With these flaps, a V-shaped incision in the skin is closed by advancing the sides of the "V" and closing it in the shape of a "Y" (Fig. 4–11). This technique is commonly used to repair defects resulting from fingertip injuries.

DISTANT

As with local flaps, distant flaps can be based on blood supply of either a random or an axial pattern. Distant flaps are those that are separated from the defect. They can be based on a pedicle and transferred directly to the defect, as in the use of a groin flap to cover a defect of the hand (Fig. 4–12) or the deltopectoral flap for head and neck reconstruction. Today microvascular free-tissue transfer has virtually replaced the indirect flap.

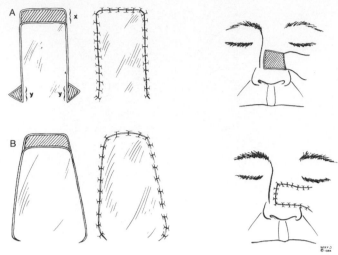

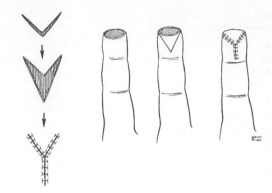

FIG. 4–11. A V–Y advancement flap.

FIG. 4–9. An advancement flap is shown. **A,** in the advancement flap, triangles *y* (Burrow's triangle) of skin have been removed lateral to the base equal to the distance of the advancement (*x* = *y*). **B,** incisions are made into base of flap to assist in advancement.

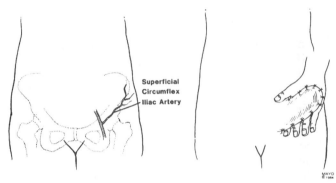

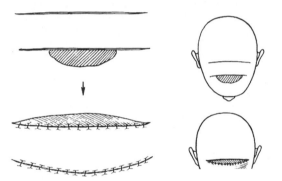

FIG. 4–12. A groin flap can be used as a distant pedicle flap to cover the defects of the hand. The pedicle is divided after adequate revascularization by the recipient bed of the hand.

FIG. 4–10. A bipedicle advancement flap with incisions parallel to the defect.

Delay Phenomenon

Delay is defined as a method of augmenting the surviving length of a flap (7). With the development of axial pattern, musculocutaneous, fasciocutaneous, and microvascular free flaps in recent years, the importance of the delay phenomenon has been dramatically reduced. Although there is less clinical dependence on the delay phenomenon now, it remains important to the mechanisms of tissue perfusion and viability.

MECHANISMS

Surgeons have long known that raising a skin flap in several stages allows a greater length to survive than transferring the flap in a single stage. It has been thought that partial interruption of the blood supply to a skin flap before its complete elevation and transfer either enhances its blood supply or increases its tolerance to ischemia. Clinical success not withstanding, confusion remains as to the exact mechanism of the delay phenomenon.

Because of its importance in reconstructive surgery, the delay phenomenon has attracted a great deal of research. Findings have been contradictory or nonreproducible. Early

work in this field attributed the benefits seen in delay to increased vessel size, reorientation of vessels along the axis of the flap, increased numbers of vessels, and improved blood flow (8, 9). Other research has shown only a temporary increase in the number of vessels during delay (10). It has also been stated that delay conditions the flap to survive in a state of relative hypoxia (10). This is in contrast to the concept that delay works by improving vascularity in the flap (11).

Ischemia appears to be an important factor in the delay phenomenon (12). It has been shown that increased P_{CO_2} reflects greater ischemia. Ischemia also appears to be an important factor in skin flap revascularization.

Another important concept with conflicting experimental results is that of arteriovenous shunting. In one series of experiments, blood flow was demonstrated in areas of skin flaps destined to become necrotic (13). In this work, angiography showed filling of blood vessels in areas that did not fluoresce after injection of fluorescein dye into the vascular system. The assumption made was that, because of open arteriovenous shunts, nutrient blood flow did not reach the distal skin even though the area was perfused. On the basis of this model, the delay phenomenon was attributed to fewer patent arteriovenous shunts after delay, compared to acutely elevated flaps.

Further research in the area of arteriovenous shunting and the delay phenomenon has produced varying results. (14) Although further investigations questioned the validity of the arteriovenous shunt concept as a major factor in the delay phenomenon and in the pathogenesis of skin flap failure, there is some evidence that arteriovenous shunting does occur at least in the proximal portion of the flap. (15) Whether the delay phenomenon is due to a decrease in arteriovenous shunting, the stimulus of hypoxia, or reorientation of blood supply, delay does increase blood flow to skin flaps. (16)

It is known that arteriovenous shunts are under sympathetic control, and there is the possibility of closing these shunts to enhance nutrient blood flow to the distal flap by appropriate pharmacologic agents. (13) Whatever the mechanism of the delay phenomenon, if it could be mimicked pharmacologically, multiple surgical steps might be avoided. Arteriovenous shunting is discussed further in the sections on Pathogenesis of Skin Flap Failure and Improving Skin Flap Survival.

TIMING OF DELAY

Data concerning the timing of delay procedures are inconsistent. Recommendations vary from 10 days to 3–4 weeks (17,18). Experimental data indicate that the increase in blood flow reaches a maximum as early as 1 week after the delay procedure (19).

SURGICAL TECHNIQUE

The method of generating a surgical delay varies with the blood supply of the skin to be elevated. In those areas with significant musculocutaneous perforators, cutting the skin on each side of a potential flap will accomplish little. In such an area it is necessary to undermine the flap in order to decrease blood flow significantly and initiate the delay phenomenon (Fig. 4–13). Where there are direct cutaneous vessels or few deep perforators, undermining may not be critical because blood flow is primarily in an axial pattern and dividing the skin parallel to the blood supply may be adequate (Fig. 4–14). Thus, the type of flap and its relationship to perforating or axial vessels must be considered when performing a delay procedure.

Pathogenesis of Skin Flap Failure

In spite of improved understanding of skin blood supply and advances in reconstructive techniques, skin-flap failure is still a significant problem. Potential factors contributing to unsuccessful outcomes are both intrinsic and extrinsic (15). Extrinsic factors, more obvious and potentially controllable, include wound infection, systemic hypotension, and compression or tension of the flap. With appropriate intervention these factors may be altered, thereby decreasing flap necrosis. However, the major cause of skin flap failure is inadequate blood supply (15,20), an intrinsic factor. The most likely cause of inadequate blood supply is poor planning by the surgeon.

Initially, flap necrosis was attributed primarily to poor venous drainage, and the length/width ratio was considered the critical factor in flap survival. This clinical rule prevailed until research proved otherwise (in animal models, similar flaps of differing widths survived to the same lengths (1). If a large artery and a large vein run through a flap, the surviving length of the flap is limited only by the length of the axial blood supply (3). Thus current evidence points to insufficient arterial inflow as the primary cause of skin flap failure (15).

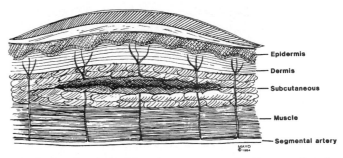

FIG. 4–13. Surgical delay in an area of skin supplied by musculocutaneous perforators requires undermining as well as division of the flap sides.

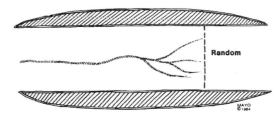

FIG. 4–14. Surgical delay of an axial pattern flap requires division of the skin parallel to and beyond the direct cutaneous vasculature. Undermining may be less important here.

Because it is believed that flap necrosis is secondary to arterial insufficiency, any arteriovenous shunting that occurs within a flap is likely to impede perfusion and contribute to necrosis (21). A marked increase in erythrocyte volume in the distal region of pedicle flaps has been found and suggests that, owing to open vascular shunts, the blood has bypassed the nutrient vessels of the skin (22). Other work showing increased hematocrit values in the poorly supplied distal areas of skin flaps has been interpreted as demonstrating a stasis phenomenon in ischemic tissue, not arteriovenous shunting (23). It is safe to say that arteriovenous shunting plays some role in skin flap necrosis but arterial insufficiency is the primary intrinsic cause.

One of the extrinsic factors associated with skin flap necrosis is hematoma. The pressure of an underlying hematoma has been thought to compromise the dermal–subdermal circulation and thus lead to necrosis. Although pressure from an extensive hematoma may be a factor, it appears that a direct toxic effect within the blood contributes to skin flap necrosis (24). This toxic effect is not related to bacterial contamination, and if the hematoma is removed within 24 hours, the flap can be salvaged (also, a delay procedure protected these experimental flaps from hematoma-associated necrosis.) Further studies have demonstrated a substance in whole blood that acts on vascular smooth muscle to influence blood flow to skin (25). The hematoma itself is not toxic to cells of the skin, but some substance in it causes vasoconstriction of the microcirculation (25). Tension has also been implicated in skin flap necrosis; however, skin with a good blood supply can withstand high tension without necrosis (20).

Another potentially significant external factor in the pathogenesis of skin flap necrosis is cigarette smoking, because it may act on blood supply. Tobacco smoke has numerous constituents, including nicotine, particulate matter, and gaseous components (e.g., carbon monoxide, carbon dioxide, and nitrous oxide) (26). Research over many years shows that cigarette smoking causes diminished blood flow (27), and this effect on the circulation is attributed primarily to nicotine acting directly on the vasculature (28,29). It may also be due to stimulation of the sympathetic ganglia and the adrenal medulla (30) by nicotine as it causes increased levels of circulating epinephrine and norepinephrine (31).

The carbon monoxide in cigarette smoke (3 to 6% of the smoke) is bound by hemoglobin to produce carboxyhemoglobin, which can limit the oxygen-carrying capacity of blood (32). Increased carboxyhemoglobin concentration and smoking are also associated with endothelial changes in the vasculature (33) and increased platelet adhesiveness (34,35).

Investigators have looked into the acute effects of smoking on the cutaneous microcirculation in elevated skin flaps (26). Studies showed decreased blood-vessel diameter and erythrocyte velocity during smoking. These effects disappeared within 10 minutes after cessation of smoking. Although there is evidence that smoking decreases blood flow, the important question is whether it also decreases skin flap survival. Experiments using nicotine revealed no effect on skin flap survival (36), but others using cigarette smoke have shown a significant decrease in survival of skin flaps (32,37). Clinical studies have confirmed experimental evidence of the detrimental effect of cigarette smoking. Rees (38) retrospectively reviewed 1186 facelift patients and concluded that smoking adversely effected skin flap survival. Results showed that 74% of skin sloughs were due to smoking, and that smokers have a 7.5% chance of developing skin slough compared to a 2.7% chance for nonsmokers (38). Riefkohl (39) prospectively studied 83 rhytidectomy patients and found that there was a significantly greater incidence of skin slough in smokers as compared to ex-smokers and nonsmokers. Based on the available data, it is not unreasonable to implicate cigarette smoking in skin flap failure.

Revascularization of Skin Flaps

There are three important questions concerning the revascularization of flaps: (a) When is the flap adequately vascularized from its recipient bed to tolerate division of its base or pedicle? (b) Where in the recipient bed does the revascularization originate? (c) What is the stimulus that initiates this revascularization? Each of these factors is important in planning the division of a pedicle skin flap.

RATE OF REVASCULARIZATION

What is the rate at which revascularization occurs and becomes adequate to sustain a flap independent of its original blood supply? Experimental data do not always correlate with clinical experience. Surgeons traditionally wait 2 to 3 weeks before dividing the pedicle, but much of the experimental data indicates that adequate revascularization occurs sooner. Considerable variation exists among the experimental results, with revascularization to sustain skin flaps in various animal models varying from 5 to 10 days (22,40,41).

Data from experimental work on free flaps give useful information relating to pedicle skin flaps. In these models,

revascularization adequate to sustain the tissue occurred in 5 to 6 days (42,43). This research in animals (pigs, rats, rabbits) may not correlate with the human clinical situation because, especially in smaller animals, revascularization occurs in just a few days.

Recent clinical experience with free-tissue transfers has given further insight into the rate of revascularization. Several clinical cases have been reported in which microvascular free skin flaps lost their vascular pedicle within days of transfer, with varying degrees of survival. In one case, a free deltopectoral flap lost its vascular pedicle at 14 days and 75% of the flap survived (44). In another report, loss of the pedicle at 10 days resulted in 30% survival of the flap (42). Based on clinical judgment, most surgeons wait at least 2 to 3 weeks before dividing the pedicle of a skin flap.

Animal research has evaluated the relative contributions of the wound edges and the wound bed in the revascularization process (40). It appears that both are important. Because of the source of the blood supply, an axial pattern flap may have a different route of revascularization than a random pattern flap. The quality of the recipient bed is also important in flap revascularization. Irradiated or scarred recipient areas are likely to contribute less than a healthy bed to revascularization. Studies also show that denervation of skin flaps results in a delay of revascularization. Sympathetic denervation has been found to increase oxygen free-radical production, which seems to contribute to delayed revascularization (41).

STIMULUS OF REVASCULARIZATION

It appears that ischemia is the critical factor in initiating this process (45). Experiments show that revascularization of skin flaps occurs first in the region of slowest isotope clearance, suggesting that the stimulus for revascularization is greater in the more-hypoxic distal area of the flap (22). Studies have demonstrated an initial increase (lasting 7 to 10 days) in uptake of intravenously injected dye in the relatively ischemic distal portion of the pedicle flap; then the entire flap stains with dye. Revascularization between the flap and its recipient bed begins 3 or 4 days after the operation at the most-hypoxic distal portion of the flap. Other research has shown that ischemia results in an increase in both size and density of the vessels associated with skin flap revascularization (46).

Benefits of Staged Division of Pedicle Flap

There is microangiographical evidence that, when the flap pedicle is divided in stages, there is an increase in the number and size of vessels compared to cases in which flaps are divided acutely (46). Once the pedicle of a flap is divided, the flap is completely dependent on the recipient bed for its blood supply; thus the purpose of staged division of the pedicle is increased flap survival, which has been confirmed both clinically and experimentally. In addition to making the division safer, staged division of the pedicle may be done earlier because it results in relative ischemia and stimulates the revascularization process. However, it is possible that the well-vascularized flap in an ischemic bed may undergo less revascularization because of the lack of stimulation for vessel growth (47).

Improving Skin Flap Survival

The volume of research on improving skin flap survival is impressive, but many of the results have been inconsistent, nonreproducible, or poorly documented. A study looking at the McFarlane dorsal-flap rat model may explain the contradictory results of many flap physiology studies (47). It appears that a significant portion of the McFarlane dorsal rat flap survives independent of nutrient blood flow and behaves as a full-thickness skin graft (48). Numerous pharmacologic agents have been proposed to improve skin flap survival. Despite improved animal models and further understanding of the mechanisms of skin flap failure, surgeons are still hesitant to use the drugs clinically, and there is little direct evidence that any of the agents has actually improved survival of a flap in which there was compromised circulation (49). For these agents to be used in humans, they should reproducibly increase flap survival in several different species under controlled conditions. Also, there must be a clear understanding of their mechanism of action, they must be safe to administer to humans, and they must have reasonably low complication rates. Despite improved understanding of skin-flap blood supply and better flap design, failure of flaps remains a clinical problem.

Work in this field has taken two directions: attempts to improve the blood flow to the flap and attempts to improve the flap's ability to tolerate an ischemic insult (50). In addition, noxious substances that have a negative influence on skin flap survival need to be identified.

IMPROVING BLOOD FLOW PHARMACOLOGICALLY

Agents used to improve skin-flap blood flow generally have a complex mode of action, and it is difficult to isolate their effects. Results have been inconsistent from one species to another with the same drug, and extrapolating pharmacologic effects from animal to humans is even more difficult. Further, some of the theories on which drug use are based may be flawed or incorrect.

A popular theory on improving blood flow involves manipulation of the autonomic nervous system. Studies using sympatholytic agents (reserpine, guanethidine) have produced widely varying results, reviewed elsewhere (50). These agents generally must be administered preoperatively in order to be effective. Since sympatholytic agents are not without adverse effects, it is difficult to justify their use prophylactically.

Sympathetic receptor blockers have also been used to improve blood flow. There are two main categories of sympathetic receptors: α- and β-receptors. Skin blood flow is primarily regulated by α-receptors, and cardiac muscle by β-receptors. Skeletal muscle may be regulated by either α- or β-receptors and is therefore somewhat more difficult to manipulate. In general, α-receptor stimulation causes peripheral vasoconstriction and beta-2 receptor stimulation causes peripheral vasodilation.

Most pharmacologic intervention regarding flap blood flow has centered around α-receptor blockage, which theoretically dilates skin blood vessels (51). Alpha blockers proposed for this purpose include phenoxybenzamine (52), chlorpromazine (53), and phentolamine (54). Isoxsuprine has received particular attention; some reports showed increased skin flap survival and others did not (25,50-58). One of the problems with animal research is that most laboratory animals have a panniculus carnosus. In the rat, the panniculus is an integral part of the skin's blood supply, and what is thought to be a skin flap may be a musculocutaneous flap. In the pig, the skin is not as dependent on the blood supply of the panniculus (1). Pigs pretreated with isoxsuprine had better muscle flap survival but no improvement in skin flap survival. The most likely explanation for this finding is that isoxsuprine has a greater effect on skeletal muscle blood supply than on the blood supply of the skin (56). Other work has shown increased skin flap survival in the rat, with hematoma-induced necrosis when treated with isoxsuprine (25); however, the flap was probably musculocutaneous, and the isoxsuprine may have been working primarily on the underlying muscle and indirectly affecting the overlying skin.

There are also vasodilators that act by direct relaxation of smooth muscle. The main drugs in this class, which are postulated to enhance skin flap survival, are nitroglycerin, hydralazine, and various prostaglandin-related compounds. Studies suggest nitroglycerin for both topical and systemic administration in multiple animal models (59-63); however, its efficacy in increasing skin flap survival in clinical studies has not been adequately tested. Hydralazine is a potent vasodilator with strong systemic effects on human blood pressure, and studies suggest its use for enhancing skin flap survival (64). Several prostaglandin-related compounds have been shown to have vasoreactive properties. PGE_1 and PGE_2 (prostacyclin) have been shown to have both vasodilatory and antithrombotic effects, whereas thromboxane A_2 is a potent vasoconstrictor and promotes platelet aggregation. Experimental studies (65-67) and clinical reports (66-68) have shown positive effects of PGE_1 on skin flap survival. Iloprost, a prostacyclin analog, has been shown to improve survival of ischemic skin flaps in rats (69), and is currently being investigated in clinical trials for vascular disease and myocardial infarction. Encouraging experimental work has also been done on thromboxane inhibitors (70). Agents that interfere with arachidonic acid metabolism, including ibuprofen and indomethacin, have also been found to enhance skin flap survival (61,71).

Changing the Rheological Properties of Blood

Another approach to improving skin-flap blood flow is based on the flow mechanics of liquids; studies have attempted to alter characteristics of blood components or solution viscosity. Experimenters have added chemical agents to the blood, or decreased the concentration of one or more components. Drugs used both experimentally and clinically include pentoxifylline, heparin, and dextran. Pentoxifylline has several modes of action, including altering deformability of erythrocytes, decreasing platelet aggregation, and lowering blood viscosity (72). It is believed that its main value in increasing flap survival is pentoxifylline's ability to increase erythrocyte deformability and flexibility (70). Although it was shown experimentally to increase flap survival, the success of pentoxifylline in clinical application is less certain. Heparin has been shown to increase flap survival experimentally (73,74).

Results with low-molecular-weight dextran have been less favorable (65,75).

Changing the viscosity of blood involves depleting protein, lowering hematocrit levels, and perfusion with solutions of varying viscosities. Although anemia potentially decreases the amount of oxygen carried to the tissues, experimental evidence shows that the associated decreased viscosity improves skin flap survival (76). Similarly, protein depletion lowers serum viscosity and enhances experimental skin flap survival (77). As with other approaches to increased flap survival, results are variable, and it is unlikely that making patients anemic or hypoproteinemic will have clinical acceptance.

ENHANCING TOLERANCE TO ISCHEMIA

Methods to improve the flap's ability to tolerate ischemic insult have included hyperbaric oxygen, hypothermia, moist environment, and systemic corticosteroid therapy. Another approach is to use drugs that alter cellular metabolism and protect against ischemia (78); this originates from research in organ storage and preservation and may be promising. Hyperbaric oxygen (79-83), hyperthermia (83), and moist dressings (84-86) have all produced improved survival of experimental skin flaps. Systemic administration of steroids are known to stabilize cell membranes, cause vasodilation with presumed improved oxygen consumption, and produce complex action of enzyme biosynthesis. The specific mode of action of steroids on the microcirculation is unknown. The no-reflow phenomenon states that prolonged ischemia leads to irreversible cell damage (87) It is now well known that ischemic tissue generates oxygen free-radicals and that these free radicals have toxic effects on vascular endothelium. Studies have shown in numerous skin flap models that cells can be protected by certain free-radical scavengers including superoxide dismutase (88-90), allopurinol (89,90), chlorpromazine (53), and defuroxime (91). Russell and colleagues (92) and Angel and coworkers (93) have published review articles on reperfusion injury and oxygen free-radicals.

Monitoring Skin Flap Viability

Skin flap failure is a significant clinical problem, and objective methods of assessing flap viability would be useful. Pedicle skin flaps traditionally have problems in their distal portion. To salvage this portion of the flap, the surgeon must either move rapidly to change external factors like kinking or hematoma, or institute early pharmacologic treatment. With greater accuracy in predicting the survival length of flaps, complications could be reduced. Subjective methods, like assessment of flap viability by color, capillary refill, and dermal bleeding, require significant clinical experience. Variables such as oxygen content of blood, dilation of the capillaries, blood flow, and skin pigmentation can affect these subjective evaluations (23)

In addition to clinical assessment, fluorescein dye is commonly used to determine viability. Traditionally, this method gives only intermittent data over time and is dependent on the impressions of the observer.

The ideal test of skin flap viability should be safe for both the patient and the flap. It should be an accurate, reliable method that provides results rapidly and can be repeated (94). Methods for assessing blood flow and viability in skin flaps can be divided into four categories: clinical tests, chemical tests, radioisotope methods, and instrument-based methods (95).

Of the chemical tests, intravenous injection of the vital dye fluorescein is the most commonly used. Fluorescein diffuses out of the capillaries and into the interstitial fluid, producing a yellow-green color in skin exposed to ultraviolet light (96). It is important to remember that fluorescein is considered a safe substance, and complications have been infrequent considering its widespread use. Vomiting and nausea are the most-reported side effects, although pruritus and urticaria have occurred (97). Close monitoring of patients during bolus administrations of fluorescein has shown a significant incidence of hypotension (98). Whether this is a vasovagal reaction, a direct vasospastic effect of the dye, or an anaphylactoid reaction is unknown. Although there is a component of subjectivity in the traditional use of fluorescein, it is a relatively reliable reflection of the limits of the functional microcirculation (96).

An attempt has been made to reduce the subjective component of the fluorescein method by using fiberoptic dermofluorometry (99). This technique allows for more frequent examinations with smaller volumes of fluorescein, and it may provide objective data by which tissue fluorescence can be quantified.

Radioisotopes can give a measurement of blood flow limited to a particular point in time. Although this technique is useful experimentally, it does not meet the need for continuous, efficient monitoring in a clinical case.

The possibilities of monitoring skin flap viability with sophisticated instrumentation have been based on temperature, transcutaneous gas (PO_2 or PCO_2), tissue pH, photoplethysmography, Doppler-shift flow metering, electromagnetic flow metering, and interstitial fluid-pressure measurements (23,95,99-101). Results with these techniques have been variable. At present, clinical assessment and intravenous fluorescein dye are the most commonly used methods of assessing skin flap viability.

Bibliography

1. Daniel RK, Williams HB. The free transfer of skin flaps by microvascular anastomoses: an experimental study and reappraisal. *Plast Reconstr Surg* 1973; 52:16.
2. McGregor IA, Morgan G. Axial and random pattern flaps. *Br J Plast Surg* 1973; 26:202.
3. Milton SH. Pedicled skin-flaps: the fallacy of the length:width ratio. *Br J Surg* 1970; 57:502.
4. Daniel RK, Taylor GI. Distant transfer of an island flap by microvascular anastomoses. *Plast Reconstr Surg* 1973; 52:111.
5. Jackson IT. Flaps design and management. In: Calnan J, ed. *Recent advances in plastic surgery*. New York: Churchill-Livingstone, 1976; 153–172.
6. Grabb WC. Classification of skin flaps. In: Myers MB, Grabb WC, eds. *Skin flaps*. Boston: Little, Brown, 1975; 145–154.
7. Blair VP. *Surgery and diseases of the mouth and jaws: a practical treatise on the surgery and diseases of the mouth and allied structures*. St. Louis: CV Mosby, 1912.
8. German W, Finesilver EM, Davis JS. Establishment of circulation in tubed skin flaps: an experimental study. *Arch Surg* 1933; 26:27.
9. Bardach J, Kurnatowski A. Blood supply of a Filatov's skin flap. *Acta Chir Plast* 1961; 3:290.
10. McFarlane RM, Heagy FC, Radin S, et al. A study of the delay phenomenon in experimental pedicle flaps. *Plast Reconstr Surg* 1965; 35:245.
11. Myers MB. Attempts to augment survival in skin flaps—mechanism of the delay phenomenon. In: Grubb WC, Myers MB, eds. *Skin flaps* Boston: Little, Brown, 1975; 65–79.

12. Myers MB, Cherry G, Milton S. Tissue gas levels as an index of the adequacy of circulation: the relation between ischemia and the development of collateral circulation (delay phenomenon). *Surgery* 1975; 71:15.

13. Reinisch JF. The pathophysiology of skin flap circulation (the delay phenomenon). *Plast Reconstr Surg* 1974; 54:585.

14. Prather A, Blackburn JP, Williams TR, et al. Evaluation of tests for predicting the viability of axial pattern skin flaps in the pig. *Plast Reconstr Surg* 1979; 63:250.

15. Kerrigan CL. Skin flap failure: pathophysiology. *Plast Reconstr Surg* 1983; 72:766.

16. Guba AM. Study of the delay phenomenon in axial pattern flaps in pigs. *Plast Reconstr Surg* 1979; 63:550.

17. Gillies HD, Millard DR. *The principles and art of plastic surgery.* Boston: Little, Brown, 1957.

18. Myers MB, Cherry G. Differences in the delay phenomenon in the rabbit, rat and pig. *Plast Reconstr Surg* 1971; 47:73.

19. Guba AM, Callahan J. Nutrient blood flow in delayed axial pattern skin flaps in the pig. *Plast Reconstr Surg* 1979; 64:372.

20. Myers MB. Investigations of skin flap necrosis. In: Grabb WC, Myers MB, eds. *Skin flaps.* Boston: Little, Brown, 1975; 3–10.

21. Reinisch JF. Discussion. *Plast Reconstr Surg* 1983; 72:775.

22. Young CMA. The revascularization of pedicle skin flaps in pigs. A functional and morphologic study. *Plast Reconstr Surg* 1982; 70:445.

23. Kerrigan CL, Daniel RK. Monitoring acute skin-flap failure. *Plast Reconstr Surg* 1983; 72:775.

24. Mulliken JB, Healey NA. Pathogenesis of skin flap necrosis from an underlying hematoma. *Plast Reconstr Surg* 1979; 63:540.

25. Hillelson RL, Glowacki J, Healey NA, et al. A microangiographic study of hematoma-associated flap necrosis and salvage with isoxsuprine. *Plast Reconstr Surg* 1980; 66:528.

26. Reus WF, Robson MC, Zachary L, et al. Acute effects of tobacco smoking on blood flow in the cutaneous micro-circulation. *Br J Plast Surg* 1984; 37:213.

27. Franke FE, Hertzman AB. Effects of cigarette smoking on the skin circulation (abstract). *Am J Physiol* 1940; 129:357.

28. Sarin CL, Austin JC, Nickel WO. Effects of smoking on digital blood-flow velocity. *JAMA* 1974; 229:1327.

29. Roth GM, McDonald JB, Sheard C. The effect of smoking cigarettes and of intravenous administration of nicotine on the electrocardiogram, basal metabolic rate, cutaneous temperature, blood pressure and pulse rate of normal persons. *JAMA* 1944; 125:761.

30. Gebber GL. Neurogenic basis for the rise of blood pressure evoked by nicotine in the cat. *J Pharmacol Exp Ther* 1969; 166:225.

31. Cryer P, Haymond MW, Santiago JV, et al. Norepinephrine and epinephrine release and adrenergic mediation of smoking-associated hemodynamic and metabolic events. *N Engl J Med* 1976; 295:573.

32. Lawrence WT, Murphy RC, Robson MC, et al. The detrimental effect of cigarette smoking on flap survival: an experimental study in the rat. *Br J Plast Surg* 1984; 37:216.

33. Astrup P, Kjeldsen K. Carbon monoxide, smoking, and atherosclerosis. *Med Clin North Am* 1974; 58:323.

34. Birnstingl MA, Brinson K, Chakrabarti BK. The effect of short-term exposure of carbon monoxide on platelet stickiness. *Br J Surg* 1971; 58:837.

35. Davis JW, Davis RF. Acute effect of tobacco cigarette smoking on the platelet aggregate ratio. *Am J Med Sci* 1979; 278:139.

36. Falcone RE, Ruberg RL. Pharmacologic manipulation of skin flaps: lack of effect of barbiturates or nicotine. *Plast Reconstr Surg* 1980; 66:102.

37. Schultz RC, Nolan JT, Jenkins R, et al. Acute effects of cigarette smoke exposure on experimental skin flaps. Presented at the meeting of the American Association of Plastic Surgeons, Chicago, May 6–9, 1984.

38. Rees TD, Liverett DM, Guy CL. The effect of cigarette smoking on skin flap survival in the facelift patient. *Plast Reconstr Surg* 1984; 73:911.

39. Riefkohl R, Wolfe JA, Cox EB, et al. Association between cutaneous occlusive vascular disease, cigarette smoking and skin slough after rhytidectomy. *Plast Reconstr Surg* 1986; 92:592.

40. Tsur H, Daniller A., Strauch B. Neovascularization of skin flaps: route and timing. *Plast Reconstr Surg* 1980; 66:85.

41. Im MJ, Biel RJ, Wong L, et al. Effects of sympathetic denervation and oxygen free radicals on neovascularization in skin flaps. *Plast Reconstr Surg* 1993; 92:736.

42. Serafin D, Shearin JC, Georgiade NG. The vascularization of free flaps: a clinical and experimental correlation. *Plast Reconstr Surg* 1977; 60:233.

43. Strauch B, Sharzer L, Glaser B, et al. Neovascularization: what is the relationship between contact surface area and volume of tissue? *Plast Reconstr Surg* 1979; 2:225.

44. Gilbert A, Beres J. Une complication inhabituelle d'un lambeau libre. *Ann Chir Plast Esthet* 1976; 21:151.

45. Myers MB, Cherry G. Blood supply of healing wounds: functional and angiographic. *Arch Surg* 1971; 102:49.

46. Cohen BE. Beneficial effect of staged division of pedicle in experimental axial-pattern flaps. *Plast Reconstr Surg* 1979; 64:366.

47. Fisher J, Wood MB. Late necrosis of a latissimus dorsi free flap. *Plast Reconstr Surg* 1984; 74:274.

48. Hammond DC, Brooksher RD. An isolated dorsal skin flap model in the rat. Unpublished paper, Department of General Surgery, Blodgett/St. Mary's Hospitals, Grand Rapids, Michigan.

49. Cherry GW. Discussion. *Plast Reconstr Surg* 1982; 70:549.

50. Kerrigan CL, Daniel RK. Pharmacologic treatment of the failing skin flap. *Plast Reconstr Surg* 1982; 70:541.

51. Finseth F, Adelberg MG. Prevention of skin flap necrosis by a course of treatment with vasodilator drugs. *Plast Reconstr Surg* 1978; 61:738.

52. Myers MB, Cherry G. Enhancement of survival in devascularized pedicles by the use of phenoxybenzamine. *Plast Reconstr Surg* 1968; 41:254.

53. Bibi R, Ferder M, Strauch B. Prevention of flap necrosis by chlorpromazine. *Plast Reconstr Surg* 1986; 77:954.

54. Jonsson CE, Jurell G, Nylen B, et al. Effects of phentolamine and propranolol on the survival of experimental skin flaps. *Scand J Plast Surg* 1975; 9:98.

55. Finseth F, Adelberg MG. Experimental work with isoxsuprine for prevention of skin necrosis and for the treatment of failing flap. *Plast Reconstr Surg* 1979; 63:94.

56. Finseth F. Clinical salvage of three failing skin flaps by treatment with a vasodilator drug. *Plast Reconstr Surg* 1979; 63:304.

57. Cherry GW. The differing effects of isoxsuprine on muscle flap and skin flap survival in the pig. *Plast Reconstr Surg* 1979; 64:670.

58. Sasaki A, Harii K. Lack of effect of isoxsuprine on experimental random flaps in the rat. *Plast Reconstr Surg* 1980; 66:105.

59. Rohrich RJ, Cherry GW, et al. Enhancement of skin flap survival using nitroglycerin ointment. *Plast Reconstr Surg* 1984; 73:943.

60. Blomain EW, Manders EK, Saggers G, et al. Topical nitroglycerin ointment enhances the survival of skin flaps. *Surg Forum* 1982; 33:594.

61. Nicter LS, Sobieski MW, Edgerton MT. Efficacy of topical nitroglycerin for random pattern skin flap salvage. *Plast Reconstr Surg* 1985; 75:847.

62. Waters LM, Pearl RM, Macauley RM. A comparative analysis of the ability of five classes of pharmacologic agents to augment skin flap survival in various models and species: an attempt to standardize skin flap research. *Ann Plast Surg* 1989; 23:117.

63. Price MS, Pearl RA. Multiagent pharmacotherapy to enhance skin flap survival: lack of additive effect of nitroglycerin and allopurinol. *Ann Plast Surg* 1994; 33:52.

64. Hendel PM, Lilien DL, Buncke HJ. A study of pharmacologic control of blood flow to delayed skin flaps using xenon washout. Parts I and II. *Plast Reconstr Surg* 1983; 71:387–410.

65. Ogowa Y, Suzuki S, Kusumoto K. The effect of isoxsuprine, pentoxifylline, low-molecular-weight dextran, insulin and PGE_2 on flap survival in rats. *Jap J Plast Reconstr Surg* 1982; 2:318.

66. Suzuki S, Isshiki N, Ogowa Y, et al. Effect of intravenous prostaglandin E_1 on experimental skin flaps. *Ann Plast Surg* 1987; 19:49.

67. Okamoto Y, Nakajima T, Yoneda K. Augmentation of skin flap survival by selective intraarterial infusion of prostaglandin E_1: experimental and clinical studies. *Ann Plast Surg* 1993; 30:154.

68. Suzuki S, Isshiki N, Ogawa Y, et al. The effect of intravenous PE_1 on clinically critical flaps. *Jap J Plast Reconstr Surg* 1986; 6:933.

69. Seneroff DM, Isreali D, Zhang WX, et al. Iloprost improves survival of ischemic experimental skin flaps. *Ann Plast Surg* 1994; 32:490.

70. Zachary LS, Heggers JP, Robson MC, et al. Combined prostacyclin and thromboxane synthetase inhibitor UK38485 in skin flap survival. *Ann Plast Surg* 1986; 17:112.

71. Knight KR, Crabb DJ, Niall M, et al. Pharmacologic modification of blood flow in the rabbit micromusculature with prostacyclin and related drugs. *Plast Reconstr Surg* 1985; 75:672.

72. Takayanagi S, Ogawa Y. Effects of pentoxifylline on flap survival. *Plast Reconstr Surg* 1980; 65:763.

73. Sawhney CP. The role of heparin in restoring the blood supply in ischemic skin flaps: an experimental study in rabbits. *Brit J Plast Surg* 1980; 33:430.

74. Wong L, Im MJ, Hoopes JE. Increased survival of island skin flaps by systemic heparin in rats. *Ann Plast Surg* 1991; 26:221.

75. Myers MB, Cherry G. Design of skin flaps to study vascular insufficiency: failure of Dextran 40 to improve tissue survival in devascularized skin. *J Plast Res* 1967; 7:399.

76. Earle AS, Fratianne RB, Nunez FD. The relationship of hematocrit levels of skin flap survival in the dog. *Plast Reconstr Surg* 1974; 54:341.

77. Ruberg RL, Falcone RE. Effect of protein depletion on the surviving length in experimental skin flaps. *Plast Reconstr Surg* 1978; 61:581.

78. Mes LB. Improving flap survival by sustaining cell metabolism within ischemic cells: a study using rabbits. *Plast Reconstr Surg* 1980; 65:56.

79. Arturson G, Khanna NN. The effects of hyperbaric oxygen dimethyl sulfoxide and complamin on survival of experimental skin flaps. *Scand J Plast Reconstr Surg* 1970; 4:8.

80. Nemiroff PM, Lungu AL. The influence of hyperbaric oxygen and irradiation on vascularity in skin flaps: a controlled study. *Surg Forum* 1987; 38:565.

81. Nemiroff PM. HBO and irradiation on experimental skin flaps in rats. *Surg Forum* 1984; 35:549.

82. Zamboni WA, Roth AC, Russell RC, Nemiroff PM, et al. The effect of acute hyperbaric oxygen on axial pattern skin flap survival when administered during and after ischemia. *J Reconstr Microsurg* 1978; 61:256.

83. Kiehn CL, DesPrez JD. Effects of local hypothermia on pedicle flap tissue. I: Enhancement of survival of experimental pedicles. *Plast Reconstr Surg* 1960; 25:349.

84. Sasaki A, Fukuda O, Soeda S. Attempts to increase the surviving length in skin flaps by moist environment. *Plast Reconstr Surg* 1979; 64:526.

85. McGrath MH. How topical dressings salvage "questionable" flaps: experimental study. *Plast Reconstr Surg* 1981; 67:653.

86. Mendelson BC, Woods JE. Effect of corticosteroids on the surviving length of skin flaps in pigs. *Br J Plast Surg* 1978; 31:293.

87. May JW, Chait LA, O'Brien BM, et al. The no-reflow phenomenon in experimental free flaps. *Plast Reconstr Surg* 1978; 61:256.

88. Sagi A, Ferder BS, Levens D, et al. Improved survival of island flaps after prolonged ischemia by perfusion with superoxide dismutase. *Plast Reconstr Surg* 1986; 77:639.

89. Manson PN, Anthenelli RM, Im MJ, et al. The role of oxygen free radicals in ischemic tissue injury in skin island flaps. *Ann Surg* 1983; 198:87.

90. Im Mj, Manson PN, Buckley GB, et al. Effects of superoxide dismutase and allopurinol on the survival of acute island skin flaps. *Ann Surg* 1985; 201:357.

91. Angel MF, Narayanan K, Swartz WM, et al. Defuroxime increases skin flap survival: additional evidence of free radical involvement in ischemic flap surgery. *Br J Plast Surg* 1986; 39:469.

92. Russell RC, Roth AC, Kucan JO, et al. Reperfusion injury and oxygen free radicals: a review. *J Reconstr Microsurg* 1989; 5:79.

93. Angel MR, Ramasastry SS, Swartz WM, et al. Free radicals: basic concepts concerning their chemistry, pathophysiology, and relevance to plastic surgery. *Plast Reconstr Surg* 1987; 79:991.

94. Creech BJ, Miller SH. Evaluation of circulation in skin flaps. In: Grabb WC, Myers MB, eds. *Skin flaps*. Boston: Little, Brown, 1975; 21–38.

95. Jones BM. Monitors for the cutaneous microcirculation. *Plast Reconstr Surg* 1984; 73:843.

96. McGraw JB, Myers B, Shanklin KD. The value of fluorescein in predicting the viability of arterialized flaps. *Plast Reconstr Surg* 1977; 60:710.

97. Stein MR, Parker CW. Reactions following intravenous fluorescein. *Am J Ophthalmol* 1971; 72:861.

98. Buchanan RT, Levine NS. Blood pressure drop as a result of fluorescein injection. *Plast Reconstr Surg* 1982; 70:363.

99. Silverman DG, LaRossa DD, Barlow CH, et al. Quantification of tissue fluorescein delivery and prediction of flap viability with the fiberoptic dermofluorometer. *Plast Reconstr Surg* 1980; 66:545.

100. Serafin D, Lesesne DB, Mullen RY, et al. Transcutaneous PO_2 monitoring for assessing viability and predicting survival of skin flaps: experimental and clinical correlations. *J Microsurg* 1981; 2:165.

101. Fischer JC, Parker PM, Shaw WW. Laser Doppler flowmeter measurements of skin perfusion changes associated with arterial and venous compromise in cutaneous island flaps. *Microsurg* 1985; 6:238.

5

Muscle and Musculocutaneous Flaps

Kristoffer Ning Chang, M.D., F.A.C.S., and Stephen J. Mathes, M.D., F.A.C.S.

Muscle and musculocutaneous flaps are now well-established tools for the reconstruction of many complex wounds. These wounds may be difficult to manage because of (a) exposed vital structures such as bones, tendons, vessels, mediastinal structures, or meninges; (b) compromised ability to heal, owing to such factors as prior irradiation; (c) extensive loss of skin, subcutaneous tissue, and mucosal lining; or (d) exposed prosthetic materials and grafts. Examples of these types of wounds include median sternotomy wounds, lower-extremity trauma, head and neck cancer defects, chronic osteomyelitis, and osteoradionecrosis. Muscle and musculotaneous flaps have found diverse applications in multiple surgical specialties, including general surgery, orthopedic surgery, cardiothoracic surgery, gynecologic surgery, neurosurgery, urology, and peripheral vascular surgery (1-14).

Muscle and musculocutaneous flaps offer several important advantages. The flaps can provide large amounts of skin and bulk. They have constant vascular anatomy that allows safe elevation and predictable arc of rotation. These flaps are less susceptible to infection and more likely to achieve wound healing compared to commonly used skin flaps. A large muscle flap can often be transposed while leaving minimal external contour defect. The efficacy of muscle and musculocutaneous flaps is enhanced by the use of microsurgery, with a high degree of success (15,16).

Vascular Anatomy of Muscles (17-20)

Muscle blood supply is based on one or more vascular pedicles that enter the muscle belly between origin and insertion. The dominant pedicle is defined by (a) anatomic study using angiographic technique, and (b) clinical observation of circulation in the muscle after its surgical manipulation for use as a flap. Division of the dominant vascular pedicle of the muscle generally results in avascular necrosis. When divided, the muscle circulation is sustained by the larger dominant vascular pedicle, while the minor pedicle contributes a smaller vascular supply.

The muscles of the human body vary greatly in size, shape, and function. Five patterns of vascular anatomy are recognized in muscles (Fig. 5–1).

Muscles of Type I pattern contain a single vascular pedicle. An example is the tensor fascia lata, which is supplied by the transverse branch of the lateral circumflex femoral artery.

Type II–pattern muscles contain both dominant and minor vascular pedicles. The larger dominant vascular pedicle will sustain circulation in the muscle after division of the minor pedicles. This is the most common pattern of circulation observed in human muscle. An example is the gracilis, which is supplied by the medial circumflex femoral artery (the dominant pedicle) and branches from superficial femoral arteries (the minor pedicles).

Type III–pattern muscles have two major pedicles. These pedicles either have separate regional sources of circulation or are located on opposite sides of the muscle. An example is the gluteus maximus, which is supplied by inferior and superior gluteal arteries.

Type IV–pattern muscles are supplied by multiple vascular pedicles. The sartorius, for example, receives multiple branches from the superficial femoral artery. Each pedicle provides circulation to a portion of the muscle. Division of more than two or three of these pedicles during elevation results in distal muscle necrosis.

Type V pattern consists of one major vascular pedicle and several secondary segmental vascular pedicles. Both types of pedicles provide significant sources of circulation to the muscles. A selected list of the vascular anatomy of muscles, including some of the more commonly used ones, is provided in Table 5–1.

Arc of Rotation

The extent of elevation of the muscle from its normal anatomic position without devascularization and its subsequent ability to reach an adjacent defect determine the arc of rotation. The point of rotation is determined by the site of entrance of the dominant pedicle into the muscle. Muscle distal to the point of rotation is useful as a transposition flap. The points of rotation for muscles of Types I, II, III, and V are located at one end, or the proximal one-third, of the muscle. Muscles of Type IV, with segmented vascular pattern, have a very limited arc of rotation. Type V muscles have two arcs of rotation: The latissimus dorsi can be elevated on the thoracodorsal artery to cover a large defect in the anterior chest; posteriorly, it can be elevated and rotated based on paramedian vessels to cover a midline defect (Fig. 5–2).

In addition to rotational movement, muscles can be used as turnover flaps. An example is the reconstruction of a median sternotomy wound using pectoralis major muscle based on perforators from internal thoracic artery. Musculocutaneous flaps can also be used as advancement flaps. Examples are V–Y advancement of gluteus maximus musculocutaneous flap for reconstruction of sacral defect and V–Y advancement of hamstring musculocutaneous flap for an ischial defect (21,22). Using transverse rectus abdominis flap in breast reconstruction

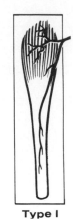
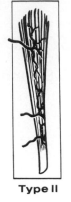
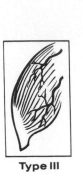
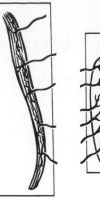
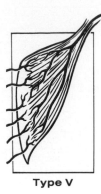

Type I **Type II** **Type III** **Type V**

FIG. 5–1. Patterns of vascular anatomy of muscle; see text for description. (Reproduced with permission from SJ Mathes, F Nahai. Classification of the vascular anatomy of muscles: experimental and clinical correlation. *Plast Reconstr Surg,* 1981; 67:177).

Table 5–1
Classification of Vascular Anatomy of Muscles

Type I pattern	Gastrocnemius (medial head)
	Gastrocnemius (lateral head)
	Rectus femoris
	Tensor fascia lata
Type II pattern	Biceps femoris
	Gracilis
	Peroneus brevis
	Peroneus longus
	Platysma
	Semimembranosus
	Semitendinosus
	Soleus
	Sternocleidomastoid
	Trapezius
	Vastus lateralis
	Vastus medialis
Type III pattern	Gluteus maximus
	Rectus Abdominis
	Temporalis
Type IV pattern	Extensor digitorum longus
	Extensor hallucis longus
	Flexor digitorum longus
	Flexor hallucis longus
	Sartorius
	Tibialis anterior
Type V pattern	Latissimus dorsi
	Pectoralis major

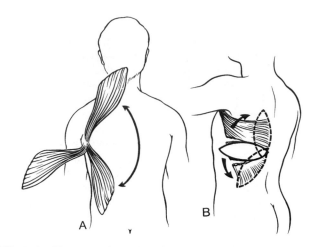

FIG. 5–2. Two arcs of rotation of the latissimus dorsi based on **A,** the thoracodorsal artery, and **B,** the posterior intercostal perforators. (Reproduced with permission from SJ Mathes, F Nahai. Classification of the vascular anatomy of muscles: experimental and clinical correlation. *Plast Reconstr Surg* 1981; 67:177.)

requires execution of complicated three-dimensional rotation, with twisting and folding of the muscle (23). In extensive craniofacial defect, three-dimensional folding with multiple skin islands is used to fulfill the reconstructive requirement (24). Muscle flaps can also be split to increase area of coverage.

Musculocutaneous Perforators and Flaps (20,25)

The vascular supply of the skin comes from direct cutaneous arteries and musculocutaneous arteries. Direct cutaneous arteries include those vessels that travel through intermuscular septums and deep fascia to reach the skin. Direct cutaneous vessels predominate in the head region send and around the limb girdles, joints, digits, and genitalia. In the trunk area, muscu-

locutaneous perforators from the flat and broad muscles predominate. In thighs and legs, both types of vessels contribute to cutaneous circulation.

Arteries enter the muscle, ramify, and give off musculocutaneous perforators to the skin. The musculocutaneous perforators arborize in the dermal plexus and supply the cutaneous territory overlying the muscle (Fig. 5–3). The location and size of the musculocutaneous perforators have been studied both clinically and through dye injection in cadavers. Figure 5–4 illustrates the location of the musculocutaneous perforators in the anterior truncal region, which reach the skin from pectoralis major and rectus abdominis muscles.

The pattern of the blood supply to the underlying muscle must be taken into account when designing the overlying skin island. In general, the Type I blood supply will support all the overlying skin of the muscle unit. With Type II blood supply, the proximal area of skin, or that over the dominant pedicle, is far more reliable than the skin over the distal pedicle. With Type III blood supply, each half of the muscle can be elevated separately with overlying skin. Muscles with Type IV blood supply are not suitable for musculocutaneous flaps. The Type V blood supply is quite useful because skin islands can be based either on the major proximal blood sup-

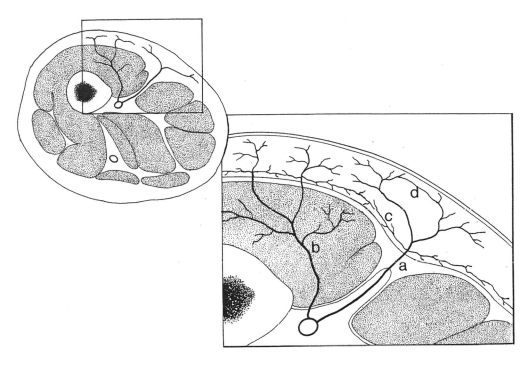

FIG. 5–3. Cross-section of the thigh showing skin blood supply from **A,** direct cutaneous artery, and **B,** musculocutaneous arteries. Both types of vessels ramify to form **C,** fascial plexus, which connects with **D,** dermal–subdermal plexus.

ply or the secondary segmental blood supply to the muscle. Figure 5–5 illustrates the use of rectus abdominis as a muscle transposition flap for (a) a median sternotomy wound, and (b) breast reconstruction.

The area of skin island that can be safely elevated beyond the muscle is variable. In addition to the primary consideration regarding the vascular supply of the underlying muscle, other determining factors include: (a) the size of the musculocutaneous perforators; (b) the distance they reach beyond the border of the muscle; and (c) the axial orientation of the vessels. In general, the broad, flat truncal muscles with large perforators are able to carry some skin beyond the muscle. In breast reconstruction, large amounts of lower-abdominal skin are carried by the rectus abdominis muscle. In contrast, skin over the distal aspect of muscles such as the gracilis is unreliable. Many narrow and long muscles have no suitable skin for carrying. Survival of skin over muscle flap is related to the concept of angiosomes: The body consists of networks of linked vascular territories (angiosomes), each having a source vessel; while skin from the adjacent angiosome may be carried by a muscle flap via interconnecting vessels, skin from the next territory will not survive (26).

Functional Preservation in Flaps

If the muscle origin or insertion or the motor nerve is divided during the flap elevation, the muscle will no longer serve its original function. This may result in functional disability or alteration of form and function. Several techniques can be used to minimize the detrimental effects by (a) choosing a muscle from a group of synergistic muscles, and (b) using only a portion of the muscle as needed. Gracilis, for example, is expendable because the remaining and more powerful adductor muscles will preserve function. In flat, broad muscles of the trunk (e.g., latissimus dorsi, pectoralis major, trapezius), only part of the muscle may have to be transposed, leaving the motor nerve and a major portion of the origin and insertion intact (27). In sternal wound reconstruction, the lateral

portion of the pectoralis muscle can be left intact in order to preserve the anterior axillary fold. In breast reconstruction using transverse rectus abdominis flap, leaving intact medial and lateral portions of the rectus muscle facilitates closure of the donor defect and reduces the use of synthetic mesh. In microsurgical transfer of serratus anterior, harvesting only the lower slips preserves its function in stabilizing the scapula. Muscles of the extremities, such as tibialis anterior, flexor digitorum longus, or extensor digitorum longus, have long tendons. For coverage of a small defect, careful dissection of part of the muscle from the tendon allows transposition without disruption of the muscle–tendon unit.

Motor Innervation

The motor nerve generally enters the proximal muscle near the origin; it is often closely associated with the dominant vascular pedicle to the muscle. Muscle denervation noted on preoperative evaluation may indicate an associated injury to the vascular pedicle. Location and preservation of the motor nerve are essential in free functional muscle transplantation. Specific effort to divide the motor nerve will not always significantly reduce muscle bulk in the denervated muscle. Required proximal dissection subjects the vascular pedicle to risk of injury.

Muscle with Skin Graft or Musculocutaneous Flap

Superficial muscle may be elevated as a muscle flap and skin grafted, or elevated with overlying skin as a musculocutaneous flap. This depends on both the reconstructive need of a particular defect and the aesthetic and functional considerations of each method. In general, the use of muscle flap alone, without the overlying skin island, is less likely to cause external contour deformity. The inclusion of skin island in the muscle flap may result in unacceptable donor-site deformity in certain parts of the body, where muscle flap alone is to be pre-

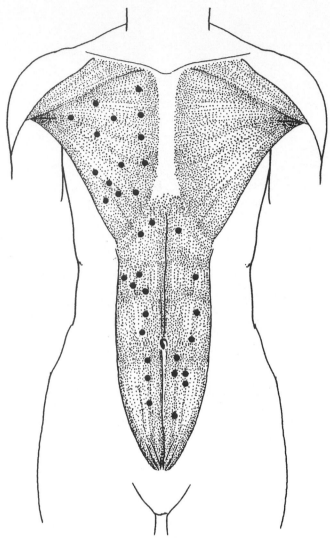

FIG. 5–4. Musculocutaneous perforators through pectoralis major and rectus abdominis into skin of anterior trunk. Dots indicate location of large and small perforators. (Modified from Mathes and Nahai,[20] p 100.)

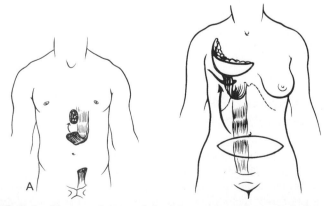

FIG. 5–5. The use of rectus abdominis muscle as **A,** a muscle flap, and **B,** extended skin island musculocutaneous flap. (Modified from Mathes and Nahai,[20] p 230.)

ferred. Certain complex wounds can be filled better by using muscle alone (e.g., osteomyelitis cavities). Muscle flaps make excellent recipient sites for skin grafts. Skin-grafted muscle can offer durable surfaces (e.g., in microsurgical reconstruction of plantar surface of the foot when the muscle flap is skin grafted) (28). In some situations, the inclusion of overlying skin is either required or preferable. Examples include postmastectomy chest-wall deformity, pressure sores, and extirpative defect around the head and neck region in which skin or mucosal surface is missing.

Specialized Application of Muscle Flap

Muscle flaps can restore specialized body function. For example, motor function can be restored when the muscular motor nerve is coapted to a suitable donor motor nerve at the recipient site during microsurgical transplantation of a muscle flap (29). Serratus anterior, pectoralis minor, and other muscles are used for reanimation of the paralyzed face (30, 31). Gracilis muscles are transplanted to the forearm to achieve finger flexion in Volkmann's ischemic contracture (32). A neurosensory flap can be designed by incorporating a cutaneous sensory nerve into a musculocutaneous flap. Such a flap has been used successfully for replacement of extensive plantar foot and heel defects (33). Muscle flaps can also be transferred in conjunction with other specialized tissue (e.g., bone) for complex reconstruction.

Healing and Infection in Flaps

Heavy contamination, the presence of infection, and decreased vascularity are often encountered in a wound to be reconstructed. Successful outcomes depend on the ability of the flap to bring in well-vascularized tissue. Musculocutaneous flaps and muscle flaps have been demonstrated to be effective in the management of difficult wounds such as those occurring in chronic osteomyelitis, osteoradionecrosis, and massive lower-extremity injuries. Such clinical observation has been confirmed by animal experiments in which musculocutaneous, random-pattern, and fasciocutaneous flaps were subjected to bacterial inoculation in both the dermal portion and the wound space under the flaps. Intradermal injection of staphylococci resulted in the most extensive skin necrosis in random-pattern flaps. The cutaneous portion of the musculocutaneous flap was the least affected. The musculocutaneous flap was most effective in containing bacterial proliferation in the wound space after bacterial inoculation; next most effective was the fasciocutaneous flap. Introduction of bacteria into the wound space underneath the random-pattern flap led to high bacterial concentration in the wound space and frequent flap necrosis. The greatest amount of collagen was deposited in the wound space within musculocutaneous flaps (34-37). Several factors have been demonstrated to account for the difference observed in the various types of flaps, including dermal blood flow, tissue oxygen tension, blood flow in the muscles, effective mobilization of leukocyte, and effective bacterial killing by the leukocytes. Tissue hypoxia has been shown significantly to impair the bacteriocidal capability of leukocytes; it also leads to impaired collagen deposition. Successful management of a difficult wound with a flap depends on the proper selection of the flap as well as optimization of tissue perfusion and tissue oxygenation of the body (38).

Considerations in Optional Flap Surgery

Muscle and musculocutaneous flaps have proven to be useful and versatile reconstructive tools. However, successful outcome requires attention to certain basics: (a) thorough excisional preparation of the recipient bed; (b) accurate knowledge of anatomy of the muscle(s) and the vascular pedicle(s); (c) accurate assessment of arc of rotation of the flaps; (d) accurate assessment of the amount of skin and muscle required; (e) avoidance of harmful twisting and compression of the pedicle and the muscle; (f) maximization of blood supplied to the skin portion of the flap. In making the incision through the skin and subcutaneous tissue, the skin incision can be beveled away from the skin unit to capture a maximal number of musculocutaneous perforators. During elevation of the musculocutaneous flap, the skin may be anchored to the underlying muscle with temporary stitches to protect the musculocutaneous perforators; (g) sufficient anchoring of the muscle underlying the skin island so that it does not pull away from the overlying skin portions. In wound closure, both the muscle and cutaneous portions should be closed without tension; (h) avoidance of raising muscle or musculocutaneous flap from an irradiated area, because there is higher incidence both of failure to heal and of flap necrosis (39).

Bibliography

1. Mathes SJ, Feng L-J, Hunt TK. Coverage of the infected wound. *Ann Surg* 1983; 198:420–429.
2. Nahai F, Rand R, Hester TR, et al. Primary treatment of the infected sternotomy with muscle flaps: a review of 211 consecutive cases. *Plast Reconstr Surg* 1989; 84:434–441.
3. Ariyan S. The pectoralis major sternomastoid and other musculocutaneous flaps for head and neck reconstruction. *Clin Plast Surg* 1980; 7:89–109.
4. Mathes SJ, Alpert B, Chang N. Use of the muscle flap in chronic osteomyelitis: experimental and clinical correlation. *Plast Reconstr Surg* 1982; 69:815–829.
5. Godina M. Early microsurgical reconstruction of complex trauma of the extremity. *Plast Reconstr Surg* 1986; 78:285–292.
6. Khouri RK, Shaw W. Reconstruction of the lower extremities with microvascular full flap. A ten year experiment. *J Trauma* 1985; 29: 1086–1094.
7. Arnold PG, Pairolero PC. Introthoracic muscle flaps: 10-year experience in management of life threatening infection. *Plast Reconstr Surg* 1989; 84:92–98.
8. Lesavoy MA, Dubrow TJ, Wackym PA, et al. Muscle flap coverage of exposed endoprosthesis. *Plast Reconstr Surg* 1989; 83:90–96.
9. McCraw JB, Massey FM, Shanklin KD, Horton CG. Vaginal reconstruction with gracilis myocutaneous flaps. *Plast Reconstr Surg* 1976; 58:176–183.
10. Tobin GR, Day TG. Vaginal and pelvic reconstruction with distally based rectus abdominis myocutaneous flap. *Plast Reconstr Surg* 1988; 81:62–70.
11. Ryan JA Jr, Gibbons RP, Correa RJ Jr. Urologic use of gracilis muscle flap for non-healing perineal wounds and fistulae. *Urology* 1985; 26:456–459.
12. Ramirez OM, RamAsastry SS, Granick MS. A new surgical approach to closure of larger lumbosacral meningomyelocell defects. *Plast Reconstr Surg* 1987; 88:799–807.
13. Evan GR, Francel TJ, Manson PL. Vascular prosthetic complications: success of salvage with muscle flap reconstruction. *Plast Reconstr Surg* 1993; 911294–1302.
14. Seartes JM Jr, Colen LB. Foot reconstruction in diabetes mellitus and peripheral vascular insufficiency. *Clin Plast Surg* 1991; 18:467–483.
15. Khouri RK. Free flap surgery—the second decade. *Clin Plast Surg* 199;2; 19:757–761.
16. Chang KN, Kenefick TP, Toth BA. Use of long interposition vein grafts in microsurgical reconstruction of lumbosacral defects. *Perspectives in Plastic Surgery* 1992; 6:118–122.
17. McCraw JB, Dibbell DG, Carraway JH. Clinical definition of independent myocutaneous vascular territories. *Plast Reconstr Surg* 1971; 60:341–352.
18. Mathes SJ, Nahai F. *Clinical atlas of muscle and musculocutaneous flaps*. St. Louis: CV Mosby, 1979.
19. Mathes SJ, Nahai F. Classification of the vascular anatomy of muscles: experimental and clinical correlations. *Plast Reconstr Surg* 1981; 67:177–187.
20. Mathes SJ, Nahai F. *Clinical applications for muscle and musculocutaneous flaps*. St. Louis: CV Mosby, 1982.
21. Hurteau JE, Bostwick J, Nahai F, et al. V–Y advancement of hamstring musculocutaneous flap for coverage of ischial pressure sore. *Plast Reconstr Surg* 1981; 68:539–542.
22. Fisher J, Arnold PG, Waldorf J, et al. Gluteus maximus musculocutaneous V–Y advancement flap for large sacral defect. *Ann Plast Surg* 1983; 11:517–522.
23. Hartrampf CR, Michelow BJ, Casas LA. Concepts in TRAM flap design and execution. In: Hartrampf CR, ed. *Hartrampf's breast reconstruction with living tissue*. New York: Raven, 1991; 47–70.
24. Pribaz JS, Morris DJ, Mulliken JE. Three-dimensional folded free flap reconstruction of complex facial defects using intraoperative modeling. *Plast Reconstr Surg* 1994; 93:285–293.
25. Cormack GC, Lamberty BG. *The arterial anatomy of the skin flap*. 2nd ed. New York: Churchill Livingstone, 1994.
26. Tayle GI, Palmer JH. The vascular territories (angiosomes) of the body. In: McCarthy JG, ed. *Experimental study and clinical applications—plastic surgery*. Philadelphia: WB Saunders, 1990; 329–337.
27. Tobin GR, Schusterman ML. Anatomy of the intramuscular latissimus dorsi muscle. The basis for splitting the flap. *Plast Reconstr Surg* 1981; 67:637–641.
28. May JW, Halls MJ, Simon SR. Free microvascular muscle flaps with skin graft reconstruction of extensive defects of the foot. *Plast Reconstr Surg* 1985; 75:627–639.
29. Zhu SX, Zhang BX, Yao JX, et al. Free musculocutaneous flap transfer of extensor digitorum brevis muscle by microvascular anastomosis for restoration of function of thenar and adductor pollicis muscles. *Ann Plast Surg* 1985; 15:481–488.
30. Buncke HJ, Buncke GM, Oliva A, et al. Secondary procedures in facial reanimation. In: Grotting JC, ed. *Reoperative aesthetic and reconstructive surgery*. St. Louis: Quality Medical Publishing, 1995; 629–655.
31. Terzis JK. Pectoralis minor: a unique muscle for correction of facial palsy. *Plast Reconstr Surg* 1989; 83:767–776.
32. Zuker R. Volkmann's ischemic contracture. *Clin Plast Surg* 1989; 16:537–545.
33. Chang KN, DeArmond SJ, Buncke HJ. Sensory reinnervation in microsurgical reconstruction of the heel. *Plast Reconstr Surg* 1986; 78:652–663.
34. Chang KN, Mathes SJ. Comparison of the effect of bacterial inoculation in musculocutaneous and random pattern flaps. *Plast Reconstr Surg* 1982; 70:1–9.
35. Calderon W, Chang KN, Mathes SJ. Comparison of the effect of bacterial inoculation in musculocutaneous and fasciocutaneous flaps. *Plast Reconstr Surg* 1986; 77:785–792.
36. Gosain A, Chang KN, Mathes SJ, et al. A study of the relationship between blood flow and bacterial inoculation in musculocutaneous and fasciocutaneous flap. *Plast Reconstr Surg* 1990; 86:1152–1161.
37. Eshima I, Mathes SJ, Paty P. Comparison of the intracellular bacterial killing activities of leukocytes in musculocutaneous flap and random pattern flaps. *Plast Recounts Surg* 1990; 86:541–547.
38. Hunt TK, Halliday B, Kingston DR, et al. Impairment of microbicidal function in wound: correction with oxygenation. In: Hunt TK, Hepenstal RB, Pin E, Rovee D, eds. *Soft and hard tissue repair—biological and clinical aspects*. New York: Praeger 1984; 455–468.
39. Arnold PG, Lovich SF, Pairolero PC. Muscle flaps in irradiated wounds: an account of 100 consecutive cases. *Plast Reconstr Surg* 1994; 93:324–327.

6

Composite Grafts

Daniel C. Baker, M.D.

A composite graft can be defined as a free graft composed of two or more tissue components. In this context, several types of grafts may be considered as composite grafts (Table 6–1). These include skin and cartilage, skin and fat, full-thickness of lip (1), full-thickness of eyelid, digital composites (2), free nipple grafts, and the combined hairbearing and whole-thickness graft for eyebrow reconstruction (3).

The term *composite graft* has become almost synonymous with a free graft from the external ear and involves the transfer of a section composed of auricular cartilage, fat, and connective tissue covered by skin on one or both sides of the graft. It therefore involves the transplantation in one stage of tissues containing more than one germinal layer (Fig. 6–1).

The use of composite grafts for the repair of alar defects was first described by König (4) in 1902 and again (5) in 1914. Joseph (6) used this method and quoted König in his book *Nasenplastik and sonstige Gesichtsplastik* in 1931.

Despite early enthusiasm, composite grafts did not gain widespread clinical acceptance, and were abandoned as a practical technique in many clinics because of a high incidence of partial or total failure. A complete take is necessary to achieve the desired cosmetic result. This is particularly true in the nasal tip and alar region. Other reasons for disappointment were the limitations of graft size, excess shrinking, and contour distortion from warping and curling. Necrosis in composite grafts is almost always the result of congestion, stasis, and "wet gangrene," because of insufficient venus and lymphatic drainage—rarely arterial insufficiency.

During World War II, the method was revived and popularized by Brown and Cannon in 1946 (7) with great success. Since then the results have been uniformly good in properly selected cases, as reported by Converse (8), Dufourmentel (9, 10), McLaughlin (11), Conley and Von Fraenkel (12), Robinson (13), and Davenport and Bernard (14).

Success depends on the early establishment of blood flow in the graft to maintain homeostasis. A number of factors are important to insure functional hemodynamics. The graft itself must not be traumatized in any way. Atraumatic technique and careful handling without crushing instruments is mandatory. The recipient wound should have a vascularized bed devoid of scar tissue. The margins of the wound should be cut well back to include all scar and radiation damage whenever possible.

The exact mechanism by which active circulation is established in a composite graft has not been demonstrated.

The nutritional status of a composite graft is tenuous from the time the graft is separated from the donor tissue until it is revascularized. Nourishment of the graft is thought to occur by three mechanisms: (a) plasmatic circulation; (b) inosculation (mouth to mouth anastomosis of blood vessels), and (c) penetration of the graft by vessels from the recipient site.

Considerable experimental work has been performed to determine the precise healing phases of composite grafts.

McLaughlin (11) described the clinical appearance of a composite graft during its first days of revascularization. The initial dead white color is replaced some 6 to 24 hours later by the pale pink tinge representing erythrocyte invasion. At approximately 24 hours the graft becomes cyanotic from venous congestion but, if the graft is destined to survive, the cyanosis gradually turns into a healthy pink color in 3 to 7 days.

Evidence of inosculation was shown by Ballantyne and Converse (15) in 1958, when they transplanted auricular composite grafts onto the chorioallantoic membrane of the chicken embryo. It is now assumed that the cartilagenous portion of the composite graft maintains the patency of the graft vessels during the critical first postoperative days until there is ingrowth of capillaries from the host. Many other studies have been performed and recommendations made to increase the likelihood of graft survival.

Medawar (16) hypothesized that reducing the temperature of a graft would lower its metabolic activity and catabolism during the period of revascularization. Conley and Von Fraenkel recommended cooling of the composite grafts immediately after placement in order to decrease tissue metabolism. It is also well established that a well-nourished recipient bed is critical for composite graft survival.

It is common to see cyanosis of the graft during the 1st week owing to a venous stasis. The auricle, nose, and eyelids have a large capillary network, which makes them ideal donor and recipient sites for composite grafts.

The size of the graft is also important. In larger grafts, survival of the graft is determined by the rate of revascularization versus the rate of the tissue's destructive processes.

Therefore, it is important to increase raw surface available for revascularization. This is accomplished by harvesting a composite graft with an excess of skin over cartilage. Doing this produces overlapping with multiple vascular anastomoses in the dermis, which helps in transmitting blood flow. Usual recommendations are that the center of the composite graft should be no greater that 1 cm from the source of its blood supply. Therefore, the total graft should be 2 cm or less in its greatest dimension for survival. The contact area may also be increased by making a hinged flap from the skin at the margin of the defect, as well as from the inside of the nose. A more recent technique utilizes a large extension of

Table 6–1
Common Uses of Composite Grafts

Defect	Donor Site	Comments
Nose		
Alar rim	Helical rim	Most popular for alar repair
	Ear lobe	For soft-tissue defect only
	Opposite ala	Useful for small defect when reduction of opposite nostril would give symmetrical appearance to the nose
Columella	Helical rim or crus	
Lateral nasal wall	Concha of ear	Concha grafted to forehead flap to provide lining and support for nasal wall
	Nasal septum	Mucosa of one side of septum with underlying cartilage grafted to forehead flap
Short nose with full-thickness tissue defect	Concha of ear	Conchal graft to forehead flap to provide lining and support for graft to nasal dorsum
Nasal lining and cartilagenous support	Concha or scapha of ear	Utilized to repair nostril stenosis, alar collapse, short nose
Skin and soft tissue of tip or dorsum	Ear lobe	
	Postauricular skin and cartilage	
Septal perforation	Lower lateral cartilage	Utilize graft on each side of septum or place buccal mucosa graft on one side
	Concha	
Ear		
Helical rim	Wedge from opposite auricle	Provides anterior skin and cartilagenous framework for helical rim
	Concha from opposite ear	
Concha	Concha from opposite ear	
Tragus	Antitragus from opposite ear	
Eyebrow	Scalp	Taken as a strip graft
Nipple	Opposite nipple sharing	
	Ear lobe	

(Adapted from Smith RO, Dickinson JR, Cipcic JA. Composite grafts in facial reconstructive surgery. *Arch Otolaryngol* 1972; 95:252.)

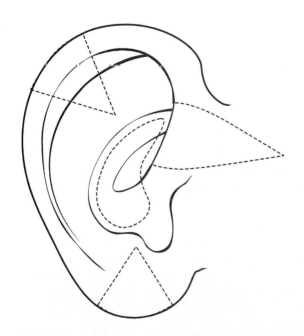

Donor Areas of the Ear

FIG. 6–1. Common donor sites for composite auricular grafts.

periauricular skin in addition to the composite graft, in an effort to increase the potential size of the available composite graft. The logic behind this design is that the large full-thickness skin graft physiologically supports the composite graft during healing and lessens the dependence of the graft on vascular ingrowth from the periphery alone.

Support for the success of composite grafts was provided by the publication of large series of cases in which an acceptable percentage of the grafts survived. Symonds and Crikelair (17) reported 36 cases with 89% graft survival; in 1959, Meade (18) reviewed 50 cases with survival of 92% of the grafts; and Douformentel and Pesteur (19) reported 43 cases in 1973 with a 90% survival.

Preparing the Recipient Site

Preparation of the recipient site should be complete before harvesting the composite graft. This includes removal of local disease and of any scar tissue to provide as healthy a recipient site as possible for the composite graft.

Techniques to increase surface contact include: (a) "tongue-in-groove" apposition of tissues, and (b) development of a hinge flap in the recipient area.

The tongue-in-groove technique, described by Davenport and Bernard in 1959, is accomplished by converting the recipient site tissues into a wedge that fits into a groove created in

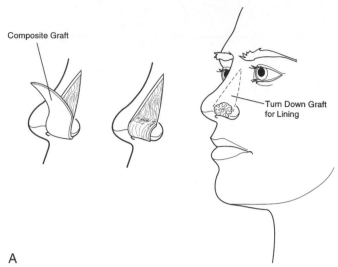

Composite Graft

Turn Down Graft for Lining

A

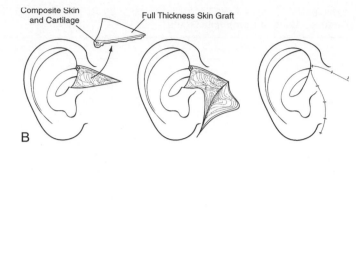

Composite Skin and Cartilage

Full Thickness Skin Graft

B

FIG. 6–2. A, B, Baker composite grafts. Composite graft from base of helix to reconstruct alar defect. Surface area is increased by a vas- cularized turn-down flap. The composite portion reconstructs the ala, and full-thickness skin covers the upper nasal defect.

the apposing composite graft, thereby increasing the contact area about 50%.

Preparation of a hinge flap at the recipient site is achieved by turning down a portion of the rim of the defect. In electing to utilize this technique, the surgeon should be certain that the flap provides a healthy vascular bed for the graft (Fig. 6–2). Meticulous hemostasis is essential, as hematoma is a common cause of graft failure.

Harvesting the Graft

A template of the defect is taken and transferred to the donor site. The graft is usually excised as a wedge-shaped portion by a "V" excision that extends through the helix and includes the outlined graft. The graft is then trimmed to fit the contour of the nasal wound. The surgeon must take care not to traumatize the graft with rough handling of sharp instruments, and it should be kept moist at all times. Intranasal closure of the mucus membrane is performed first with 4-0 or 5-0 chromic suture. The skin surface is then closed with 5-0 or 6-0 nylon suture.

Grafting Specific Areas

NASAL DEFECTS

Alar Rim

Reconstruction of the alar rim is the most common use for composite grafts. Grafts from the helix have been used most frequently. The auricular graft provides tissue with a contour similar to that of the ala, and the cartilage gives stability to the reconstructed rim (Fig. 6–3). An excellent survival (approximately 90%) has been reported for this graft, particularly when it measures 2 cm or less in width.

Base of Ala and Adjacent Nasolabial Area

This technique is employed to reconstruct the nasolabial area after excision of carcinoma and for defects resulting from injury (Fig. 6–4). The graft has a wider surface of contact with the edges of the defect than by simple edge-to-edge approximation, and revascularization is facilitated. A

template of the defect is made with the location of the nasolabial lane outlined on the pattern. The composite graft is designed so that the postauricular skin crease recreates the nasolabial line and the conchal cartilage and anterior skin line and supports the nasal wall. Repair of the donor site is accomplished by direct approximation of the postauricular skin, followed by application of a full-thickness skin graft to the anterior defect.

The composite graft, after fat is trimmed from the base of the dermis, is sutured to the edge of the defect; the edges of the conchal skin are sutured to the edges of the vestibular skin, and the edges of the graft are sutured to the edge of the defect. The conchal skin is sutured to the postauricular skin along the anterior border of the nostril. The color match is usually good, and restoration of the full-thickness of the ala and nasolabial area is achieved. Converse (1950) reported the successful use of this method in four cases.

Alar Base

Another type of composite graft is removed from the base of the ala on the unaffected side, turned upside-down, and employed as a wedge in the base of the deformed ala on the opposite side to provide increased length (Fig. 6–5).

The opposite nasal ala provides ideal tissue for repair of an alar defect, particularly if the uninvolved ala is long and can be improved by reduction; however, the usefulness of such a graft is limited by the small amount of tissue that can be obtained without creating a new deformity.

Nasal Tip

Grafts of skin and fat removed from the lobe of the ear are employed for the repair of small defects of the nasal tip, the medial portion of the ala, and the columella when cartilaginous support is not needed. Dupertuis (20) reported graft survival in 15 of 15 composite ear lobe grafts.

Columella

In 1959, Meade (18) described utilization of a helical-rim composite graft to repair the short columella associated with unilateral or bilateral cleft lip (Fig. 6–6). The columella is

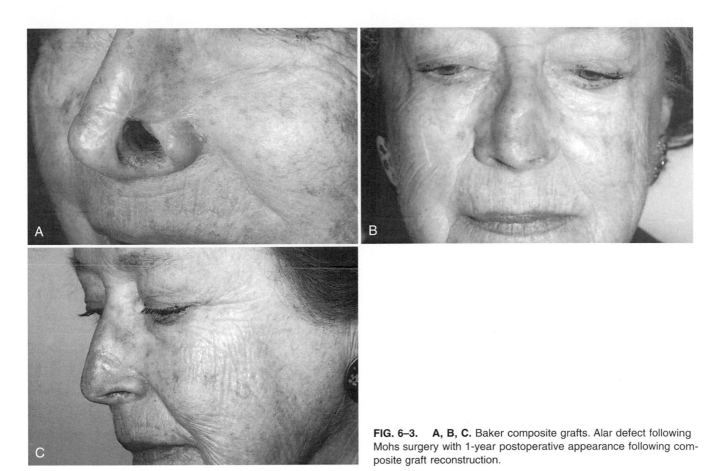

FIG. 6–3. **A, B, C.** Baker composite grafts. Alar defect following Mohs surgery with 1-year postoperative appearance following composite graft reconstruction.

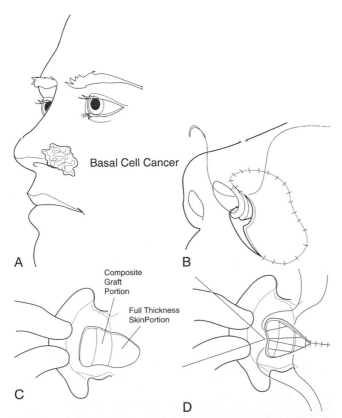

FIG. 6–4. **A,** retroauricular composite graft to reconstruct alar base and nasolabial defect following excision of basal cell cancer. **B, C, D.** Baker composite grafts.

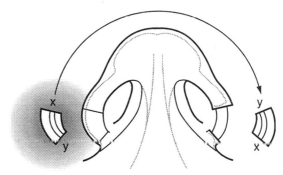

FIG. 6–5. Alar base reduction to reconstruct stenosed contralateral nostril.

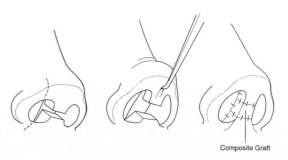

FIG. 6–6. Composite auricular graft to reconstruct short columella.

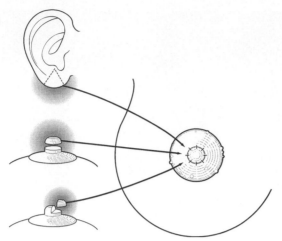

FIG. 6–7. Various donor sites for reconstructing nipple.

freed by dividing its base and extending the incision superiorly through the membranous columella. The columella is then advanced outward and fixed in its new position by sutures to the septum. Meade found this advancement produced a defect in the lower columella. A wedge-shaped auricular graft was utilized for the columellar reconstruction. The graft was designed so that the length of helical rim removed equalled the height of the columellar defect. Meade reported employment of this technique in nine cases; two patients had superficial tissue loss, which did not prevent an acceptable result, and the remainder had total survival of grafts.

Ear

Composite grafts also have application in auricular reconstruction. Grafts from the helical rim are used in cases of partial reconstruction of the auricle. The auricle can be used as a donor site for a composite graft at 7 years of age. Grafts from the concha or inner helix are much superior to free strips of cartilage, since they better resemble the normal appearance of the helix.

In microtic ears, Brent (21,22) and Tanzer (23) have used segments of the opposite ear, including cartilage and skin, either to add a tragus or to reconstruct a semblance of conchal cupping.

Eyebrow

Byars (24) and Rees (3) have reported successful use of composite grafts consisting of hair-bearing skin and its underlying fat for reconstruction of the eyebrows. The graft should be designed so that, when transferred to the supraorbital area, the hairs are oriented to grow upward and outward, as in a normal eyebrow. This procedure is simpler than reconstruction of an eyebrow with a flap, and is highly successful. If the graft should fail, then the surgeon can resort to the use of more complicated hair-bearing grafts.

Nipple

The best tissue for nipple reconstructions is a composite graft from the opposite nipple. This offers the most realistic aesthetic result with only minimal donor site scarring (Fig. 6–7). Auricular composite grafts have also been described (25).

Adequate nipple projection of the opposite, normal breast is the major factor influencing donor-site selection. If there is

adequate projection, the opposite nipple offers a tissue graft of similar texture, size, and color. Approximately half of the normal nipple can be excised and transferred as a composite graft, using either the upper or lower half. A graft up to 7 mm will survive, and the donor site is allowed to reepithelialize (26).

In conclusion, it is important to realize that composite grafts are an extremely valuable alternative to flaps in selective cases of small defects. Their advantages are one-stage reconstruction, high success rate, and minimal donor-site deformity. Certain basic principles must be followed to assure the highest graft survival: increase surface area for revascularization, atraumatic tissue handling, minimal electrocautery, and cooling the graft for 48 to 72 hours postoperatively.

References

1. Flanagin WS. Free composite grafts from lower to upper lip. *Plast Reconstr Surg* 1956; 17:376.
2. Douglas B. Successful replacement of completely avulsed portions of fingers as composite grafts. *Plast Reconstr Surg* 1959; 23:213.
3. Rees TD. Transfer of free composite grafts of skin and fat. *Plast Reconstr Surg* 1960; 25:556.
4. König F. I. Zur deckung von defecten der nasenflugel. *Berl Klin Wehnschr* 1902; 7:137–138.
5. König F. Ueber nasenplastik. *Beitr Klinisch Chir* 1914; 94:515.
6. Joseph J. *Nasenplastik und sonstige gesichtsplastik.* Leipzig: C. Kabitzch, 1931; 383.
7. Brown JB, Cannon B. Composite free grafts of two surfaces of skin and cartilage from the ear. *Ann Surg* 1946; 124:1101.
8. Converse JM. Reconstruction of the nasolabial area by composite graft from the concha. *Plast Reconstr Surg* 1950; 5:247–251.
9. Dufourmentel C. Reparation de l'aile du nez par greffe libre de pavillon de l'oreille. *J Chir* 1951; 67:485–490.
10. Doufourmentel C. Les greffes composees de pavillon de l'oreille dans le graitement des pertes de substance de l'aile et de la pointe du nez. *Ann Chir Plast* 1957; 1:59–66.
11. McLaughlin CR. Composite ear grafts and their blood supply. *Br J Plast Surg* 1954; 7:274.
12. Conley JJ, Vonfraenkel PH. The principal of cooling as applied to the composite graft in the nose. *Plast Reconstr Surg* 1956; 17:444.
13. Robinson F. A large composite auricular graft. *Brit J Plast Surg* 1956; 8:330–332.
14. Davenport G, Bernard FD. Improving the take of composite grafts. *Plast Reconstr Surg* 1959; 24:175.
15. Ballantyne DL, Converse JM. Vascularization of composite auricular grafts transplanted to the chorio-allantois of the chick embryo. *Plast Reconstr Surg* 1958; 22:373–377.
16. Medawar PD. Notes on the problems of skin homographs. *Bull War Med* 1942; 4:1.
17. Symonds FD, Crikelair GF. Auricular composite grafts in nasal reconstruction. *Plast Reconstr Surg* 1966; 37:433.
18. Meade RJ. Composite ear grafts for construction of columella. *Plast Reconstr Surg* 1959; 23:134.
19. Dufourmentel C, Pesteur J. Les greffes auriculaires composees dans la reconstruction de l'etage inferieur de la pyramide nasale. *Ann Chir Plast* 1973; 18:199–212.
20. Smith RO, Dickinson JR, Cipcic JA. Composite grafts in facial reconstructive surgery. *Arch Otolaryngol* 1972; 95:252.
21. Dupertuis SM. Free earlobe grafts of skin and fat: their value in reconstruction about the nostrils. *Plast Reconstr Surg* 1946; 1:135.
22. Brent B. The correction of microtia with autogenous cartilage grafts. I. The classic deformity. *Plast Reconstr Surg* 1980; 66:1.
23. Brent B. The correction of microtia with autogenous cartilage grafts. II. Atypical and complex deformities. *Plast Reconstr Surg* 1980; 66:13.
24. Tanzer RC. Microtia—a long-term follow-up of 44 reconstructed auricles. *Plast Reconstr Surg* 1978; 61:161.
25. Byars LT. Free full thickness skin grafts. *Surg Gynecol Obstet* 1942; 75:8–20.
26. Brent B, Bostwick J. Nipple-areola reconstruction with auricular tissues. *Plast Reconstr Surg* 1977; 60:353.
27. Musgrave RH, Lehman JA. Composite grafts. In: Georgiade GS, Georgiade NG, Riefkohl R, Borwick WJ, eds. *Textbook of Maxillofacial and Reconstructive Surgery.* Baltimore: Williams & Wilkins, p. 7.

7

Principles of Bone Transplantation

Alexander C. Stratoudakis, M.D., F.A.C.S.

The earliest attempt to transplant bone was published by Van Meek'ren in 1682 (1). Credit is generally given to Duhamel (1742) for the earliest scientific approach to osteogenesis. He placed silver wires subperiosteally and found, weeks later, that they were covered with bone. Duhamel believed this to be the result of the osteogenic properties of periosteum. Von Haller (1763) regarded the periosteum chiefly as the support of blood vessels, which were agents for osteogenesis in the healing of fractures. He believed that osteogenesis was due to an exudation from arteries. Two sharply divided schools of thought arose, based on the views of these two men. Although Heine totally resected ribs subperiosteally and found that they grew back, the controversy was not settled until Flourens (1842) conclusively showed that periosteum is osteogenic and is the chief agent responsible for the healing of bone defects.

In 1867, Ollier reviewed the earlier literature and reported on his own experiment, concluding that the transplanted periosteum and bone remained alive and could, under proper circumstances, become osteogenic. He believed that viable bone with attached periosteum was the best form of graft to use; however, he also believed that the contents of the Haversian canals and the endosteum were important in bone regeneration.

Barth (1893–1898), a student of Marchand, claimed that all transplanted bone marrow and periosteum die and are replaced by surrounding tissue. He and Marchand were the first to use the term "creeping substitution" (*schleichender ersatz*) to describe the invasion of old bone by budlike masses of new bone, without previous resorption of the old bone. They did not consider this to be the only method of replacement, admitting the occurrence of the usual method of resorption and apposition, but they felt that it was by far the most important process. The term *creeping substitution* has been frequently used, erroneously, to describe a process that is really resorption and apposition.

Axhausen (1907, 1909) made a major contribution to the problem of osteogenesis and bone transplantation from his experiments, upon which he formulated his principles that periosteum has a high degree of survival and osteogenic activity in autografts, markedly less in homografts, and practically none in heterografts. He believed that all transplanted bone died, although most of the periosteum survived, to become a source of osteogenesis.

Later investigators concerned themselves with the problem of the contribution of the host bed to the regeneration of a graft, a subject that was complicated by the controversy between those who believed that bone can arise by metaplasia from surrounding connective tissue and those who believed it arises only from soft tissues associated with bone (2,3).

Biology of Bone Transplantation

TERMINOLOGY

Autologous bone is the bone transplanted from one anatomic area to another.

Isograft is a graft transplanted from one individual to another of the same inbred strain. The only clinical situation in which this could arise is in identical twins.

Homograft is a graft transplanted from one individual to another of the same species. This type of graft is also referred to as *allogeneic or allograft*.

Heterograft is a graft transplanted from an organism of one species to another. This type of graft is also referred to as a *xenograft*. The use of heterologous bone has by and large been discontinued. The fate of xenoimplants is sequestration or envelopment in a fibrous capsule. This has been shown both experimentally (4) and clinically (5).

Nonviable bone processed by various methods and used for clinical or experimental applications, as well as synthetic or nonbiologic materials used for the same purposes, are referred to as *implants,* while the combination of autologous marrow with frozen or lyophylized banked bone is termed a *composite bone graft* (6).

CELL SURVIVAL

In the case of an autograft, there is little question that both the transplanted bone and the recipient tissues participate in the formation of new bone. The fact that osteogenic cells survive the transplantation of autogenous bone has been convincingly demonstrated (7,8). In fact, it has been shown that bone regeneration occurs from osteoprogenitor cells and not from mature osteocytes, which degenerate by autolysis following transplantation, leaving empty lacunae. Preosteoclasts may also survive and initiate resorption of donor bone (9).

Stutzmann and Petrovic (10–14) believe that periosteum contains two cell types able to divide, the so-called skeletoblast and the preosteoblast. The skeletoblast, histologically a fibroblastlike cell, may divide up to 50 times, but its intermitotic interval is relatively long. The skeletoblast is the precursor of the preosteoblast, the secondary-type prechondroblast, and the preosteoclast. These three cell varieties divide relatively frequently but never more than 10 times. When the preosteoblast matures into an osteoblast, it stops dividing. The so-called secondary-type prechondroblast is a cell present in the condylar cartilage of the mandible and also in the post-fracture cartilaginous callus, as well as in some varieties of bone sarcomas. When transformed into the secondary-type prechondroblast, the cell stops dividing. Bone regeneration therefore occurs primarily from skeletoblast-derived cells. According to these authors, an osteoprogenitor cell, strictly speaking, does not exist. The only stem cell is the skeletoblast. Finally, several authors (12-13) demonstrated that bone-resorbing cells are of extrinsic origin, originating from bone marrow and delivered through the blood as monocyte-type cells. In fact, what Trueta has described as cells originating from vessel walls are "blood monocyte–type" cells, which leave the bloodstream and enter the tissues.

OSTEOCONDUCTION

The process of growth of sprouting capillaries, perivascular tissue, and osteoprogenitor cells from the recipient bed into the three-dimensional structure of a bone graft or an implant is called *osteoconduction*. Osteoconduction may occur in a framework of nonbiologic materials such as glass, ceramics, or plastics, as well as within nonviable biologic materials such as autoclaved bone, demineralized bone, and frozen or freeze-dried allogeneic bone (9).

OSTEOINDUCTION

The process of differentiation of stem cells into osteoprogenitor cells on calcified tissue matrices that are either demineralized in the course of resorption or predemineralized in vitro is called *osteoinduction*. The concept of osteogenic induction was first formulated by Levander in 1938 (15) and has been studied very extensively by Urist (9), who determined the critical components to be an insoluble noncollagenous bone morphogenetic protein (BMP), a proteolytic enzyme (BMPase), and a bone hydrophobic glycopeptide (HGP). To date, BMP remains the only known molecule capable of promoting osteoinduction.

So far, eight BMPs (BMP-1 through BMP-8) have been cloned with recombinant DNA technology, and additional growth factors have been identified as being important for bone repair and maintenance, including platelet-derived growth factor (PDGF), transformation growth factor (TGF), insulin-like growth factors, basic fibroblastic growth factor, and epidermal growth factor (16).

The osteoinductive properties of bone are destroyed by autoclaving and by irradiation sterilization, and are affected to various degrees by other manipulations in the processing of bone. Freeze drying, for example, preserves enzymes that degrade constituents of bone matrix essential for the bone morphogenetic response. Sterilization with other chemical methods used in bone banks (e.g., 8-propiolactone and hydrogen peroxide), destroy the BMP, whereas thimerosal, which incidentally was used almost 25 years ago by Reynolds, inhibits BMPase without denaturation of BMP (9). Irradiation also reduces the breaking strength of bone in doses above 3 megarads; lower doses do not appear to have a significant effect on the mechanical properties of bone (17).

BONE HEALING AND REGENERATION

The healing and regeneration of bone are cell-mediated events (in contradistinction to dystrophic calcification, which is a process of nucleation of calcium and phosphate ions around tissue macromolecules). Competence factors (such as PDGF and fibroblast-like growth factor) regulate cell cycles (i.e., cell proliferation, maturation, and differentiation), while BMPs function as maturation factors, inducing the differentiation of pluripotential cells to osteoblast phenotypes (16). Other substances (e.g., prostaglandins) play a significant role in bone formation and bone resorption (18). In bone embryogenesis and regeneration the cells and biochemical mediators act in a strict time sequence. Furthermore, the same mediators may have different effects depending on their concentration.

VASCULARIZATION OF BONE GRAFTS

Whether the initial revascularization of a bone autograft occurs by formation of anastomoses between vessels of the graft and those of the recipient bed, as occurs in split-thickness skin grafts, or by invasion of the graft by newly formed vessels, is a matter of debate. Deleu and Trueta (19), having studied the phenomenon of bone revascularization in the anterior chamber of the eyes of the guinea pig and the rat, concluded that such anastomoses do indeed occur. However, Albrektsson and Albrektsson (20), using an ingenious transparent chamber for direct, in vivo observation of autograft revascularization in the rabbit, failed to observe any reutilization of preexisting graft vessels. Vascularization then must proceed by gradual penetration of the graft by host vessels while osteoclastic activity and apposition of new bone are taking place. The rate of vascularization depends on the species, on the size of the bone graft, and on the type of bone implant used (2). Cancellous grafts revascularize faster than cortical (19), and membranous bone revascularizes faster than mixed corticocancellous endochondral grafts (21).

INCORPORATION OF THE BONE GRAFT

The process of envelopment and interdigitation of the donor bone tissue with new bone deposited by the individual is termed *incorporation* (22). The quantity of donor bone resorbed is greater in cancellous than in cortical bone autografts and greater in autografts than in alloimplants. In all instances, the endpoint of incorporation generally falls short of complete replacement with living bone. When cortical bone is grafted in an adult, as much as 90% of the volume of the graft may be of donor origin. The donor tissue may remain unresorbed for as long as 13 years after the operation. In growing bones in children, tissue remodeling is so much more rapid than in adults that only microscopic quantities of the structure of the donor may be recognizable by the second year after transplantation (9). In dog experiments, Enneking (23) arrived at the following conclusions: (a) resorption of the necrotic bone transplant is independent of physiologic skeletal metabolism; (b) appositional bone formation is influenced by the skeletal renewal rate; (c) torsional stress failure is correlated more with porosity than with microanatomical features; and (d) in autografts, at 48 weeks of healing, when physical resistance to torsional stress is nearly normal, only 60% of the transplant is resorbed and replaced by new bone. The same group of investigators studying cortical bone allografts in dogs concluded that the incidence of nonunion, fatigue fracture, increased porosity, increased cumulative new-bone formation, decreased cross-sectional area, and decreased mechanical strength were significantly different when either fresh or freeze-dried allografts were compared to fresh autografts (24).

ANTIGENICITY OF BONE

Bone allografts elicit both humoral- and cell-mediated antigenicity (25,26) proportional to the genetic disparity between host and donor. Bone allotransplantation is followed by a sequence of events that leads, either to vascularization and eventual incorporation of the allograft or alloimplant, or to sequestration. The intensity of this reaction seems to depend on the genetic transplantation differences between donor and recipient, although in Muscolo's study (27), no clear relation could be established between the histocompatibility and the incorporation of the graft.

The events leading to incorporation of allografts proceed at a much slower rate than those of autografts (27), and they appear to be much more prone to infection, fracture, and nonunion (28). Antigenicity is reduced by various methods used to process and preserve the allograft, such as freezing or freeze drying (29). Unfortunately, the above methods also have an adverse effect, reducing the mechanical (torque) strength of bone (30). In the clinical use of processed allografts, antigenicity exerts only a limited effect on the outcome, and tissue typing has not been practiced in the reported clinical series. However, Mankin and coworkers (28) acknowledge that further studies are needed. Stevenson (25), in her experimental work, has detected antibodies in synovial fluid when no systemic antibodies could be detected, implying that matching for tissue antigens may reduce sensitization of the host. This would improve incorporation and reduce degenerative changes in the joint after implantation of an allograft.

Rejection becomes a much more serious problem in vascularized bone transfers, in which the musculoosseous grafts are rejected similarly to visceral organ grafts (31). The chronic immunosuppression that allows visceral organ transplantation carries an obligate morbidity. This morbidity is acceptable in the patient threatened by hepatic or renal failure, but it is unjustifiable in the patient requiring skeletal reconstruction of a nonvital body part (32). Efforts are continuing in the laboratory to elucidate the antigenic stimulus and to investigate methods of inducing tolerance through treatment of the graft rather than through the patient as a whole. Transplantation immunity is inhibited by the development of serum-blocking factors (enhancement), and eventually a stable state is reached between donor and recipient. The immune response to allografts or frozen bone alloimplants destroys the osteoinductive property (9).

Autograft Substitutes

In the reconstruction of skeletal defects, autografts should be used whenever possible. Although allografting may be a less than optimal solution, it has become an important method in dealing with major skeletal loss when factors such as the size of the defect, donor-site morbidity in patients already severely impaired by their disease and/or surgery, or the need to reconstruct an articular surface preclude the use of autografts (28). There are several reports of their use with high success rates. (28,33,34)

XENOGENEIC BONE

The use of xenogeneic transplants has been abandoned. The genetic transplantation differences between human tissue and that of other species (e.g., bovine) are such that the fate of such grafts is their eventual sequestration without any new bone formation.

FROZEN BONE

Bone harvested under sterile conditions and kept frozen at −80° C does not undergo enzymatic destruction (35) and may be stored for long periods of time with seemingly little adverse effect on its function (36).

FREEZE-DRIED (LYOPHYLIZED) BONE

Lyophylized bone is used mainly as a composite graft (i.e., in combination with marrow from the recipient). In orthopedic surgery, it is used to fill defects resulting from the extirpation of bone tumors or cysts or as an adjunct in spinal fusions. It has also been used extensively by periodontists to fill alveolar defects and by oral surgeons for reconstruction in the maxillofacial region. However, lyophylized bone has been shown to retain its antigenicity, and in applications where larger segments of bone are required to have the ability to withstand stress, the results have been very unfavorable, showing incomplete incorporation and decreased ability to withstand torsional stress (23). The bending strength was shown to be lowered to 55–90% of controls (37). Longitudinal cracks have also been observed when freeze-dried bone is rehydrated (38). It is suggested that freeze-dried bone be supplemented with generous amounts of autogenous iliac bone (9).

DEPROTEINIZED BONE

Such bone preparations lack osteoinductivity. Despite one report in which good results are claimed (39), experimental results indicate the failure to incorporate deproteinized bone into the host skeleton (15).

DEMINERALIZED BONE

In contrast to deproteinized bone, demineralized bone retains its osteoinductive properties and has been used by Mulliken and colleagues for reconstruction in the craniofacial region (40-42) and by Upton for hand reconstruction (43). It is acknowledged, however, that the use of radiation for sterilization diminishes osteoinductivity, and other ways to sterilize the implant are being investigated.

CHEMOSTERILIZED AUTOLYSED, ANTIGEN-EXTRACTED, ALLOGENEIC (AAA) BONE

This AAA alloimplant has been described and is being used by Urist and Dawson (44). Cadaver bone is harvested as soon as possible after death and processed so that the BMP is preserved while nearly all the stainable intralacunar material is enzymatically digested. It is then freeze dried. The breaking strength is claimed to be about one-half that of whole, undemineralized wet bone. The highest success rates come from operations on young children with a high proliferative bone-growing capacity. Urist advises rigid immobilization of the recipient bone and onlaying rather than inlaying the graft in order to assure maximal contact with the host vascular bed. A series has been published on spinal fusions utilizing this alloimplant. The incidence of pseudarthrosis was slightly higher than that of a control series in which autogenous iliac bone was used, but the number of operations was too small to draw any conclusions (9,44).

INORGANIC, NONBIOLOGIC IMPLANTS

Research in inorganic implants began in the mid-1970s, mainly based on the proposition that bone mineral was hydroxyapatite (HA), and therefore synthetic implants of the same material would be biocompatible with osseous tissue. Significant structural and chemical differences exist between bone mineral that is calcium-deficient carbonate apatite, and HA, and several new bioceramics are being developed and investigated for use as bone graft substitutes. It has still not been possible to produce a substance that has the same composition and structure as bone mineral (45). Such implants are intended to function as matrices allowing the ingrowth of bone, and they are generally used as vehicles for deployment of bioactive molecules or cells, which greatly enhance bone formation.

Their clinical performance depends on their biological and mechanical properties. Ideally they should allow bonding of the adjacent bone to their surface with eventual incorporation and replacement by bone. They should possess a modulus of elasticity appropriate for effective remodeling of the surrounding bone. Their resorbability is an advantage but should not occur so rapidly as to prevent incorporation.

Disadvantages so far include brittleness, low fatigue strength, high modulus of elasticity and difficulty in fabrication (45).

BIODEGRADABLE SYNTHETIC IMPLANTS

Polymers of the lactic and glycolic acids are currently being used for fabrication of absorbable rigid-fixation devices. (16,46,47) They are also being investigated as vehicles for deployment of bioactive molecules or cells. Implantation of bulk volumes of these materials may present problems, however, including the development of aseptic draining sinuses, which are not seen when sutures made from the same materials (Vicryl) are used. It is evident that the quantity of implant introduced should be minimized. Since such materials biodegrade into carbon dioxide and water when they react with interstitial fluid, it follows that an extremely porous (to increase the contact surface) polymer construct can be fabricated as an implant to be used as a delivery vehicle for cells or bioactive factors in non-weight-bearing applications or for prefabrication of tissues of customized shape (16).

Bone Autografts

In 1972 an estimated 100,000 bone grafting operations were being performed in the United States annually (48). Since then, their increased application in all related surgical specialties has greatly increased this number, and Burchardt (22), in a more recent publication, brings it up to 200,000. Autogenous bone is used in the vast majority or these cases. Fusion of joints, replacement of missing segments of bone, induction of healing in nonunited fractures, stabilization and retention of the facial skeleton in a displaced position (49), augmentation and normalization of facial contour, and creation of congenitally missing parts of the skeleton are clinical problems to which bone grafting provides the solution. The requirements of the bone graft vary greatly depending on the situation. Whereas one graft must be able to withstand torsional stress, a different graft will be chosen when early revascularization is the prime consideration. In a joint fusion, the contour of the graft may not be important, but in a craniofacial reconstruction, the shape is of particular relevance.

DONOR SITES AND THEIR MORBIDITY

A thorough working knowledge of each donor site with regard to the nature and properties of the bone it provides, as well as of the different possibilities in relation to the patient's age, is required if the surgeon is to utilize the transference of bone optimally and with the fewest possible sequelae. A description of the different donor sites follows.

The Cranium

Originally limited to a source of bone grafts for the cranial region during neurosurgical procedures, use of calvarial bone grafts was extended to the reconstruction of the facial region by Tessier with excellent results (49). Calvarial bone is now being used with increasing frequency for congenital, traumatic, or surgically created deficits of the facial skeleton. Smith and Abramson (50) demonstrated in the rabbit that membranous bone underwent less resorption than endochondral bone. The experimental work of Zins and Whitaker (51) has confirmed their findings and the clinical impression regarding the superiority of cranial bone for craniofacial reconstruction. Tessier (49) described in detail the technique of obtaining a cranial bone graft.

In children, because of the tremendous capacity of the dura and, to a lesser extent, of the pericranium to generate bone, cranial bone grafts are used almost exclusively for reconstruction of the cranium and face. In infants and young children, defects created by the harvesting of cranial bone are reconstituted, either totally or in part. In older children, when the calvaria is still too thin to split into inner and outer table, the donor defect should be covered either with autogenous graft from a different source or with an allogeneic implant. In adults, the cranial bone can easily be split into inner and outer tables. Generally, the outer table is used as the graft, and the inner table is returned to cover the donor site (49).

The location of the donor site is determined by the desired curvature. Generally, the parietal areas constitute the most appropriate donor sites. Small grafts may be obtained by burring the circumference of the outer table around the desired graft and carefully separating the outer from the inner table with a chisel at the level of the diploe. The harvesting of larger grafts requires a formal craniotomy.

Advantages of cranial bone grafts are: (a) the large quantity of bone available in children, in whom availability from other sources is limited; (b) less resorption as compared to endochondral bone grafts; (c) superior aesthetic results with proper selection of the curvature; (d) lack of significant postoperative pain; and (e) easy accessibility of the donor site, which either is part of the operative field, in cranial or craniofacial procedures, or can be draped out with the face when small grafts are needed during smaller procedures, such as the repair of an orbital floor defect. The disadvantages are few. Due to their rigidity, cranial bones do not conform to fill dead spaces and therefore may have to be combined with grafts from other sources such as the iliac crest or tibia. (49) The possibility of a dural tear or an epidural hematoma exists, although in a recent review the morbidity of cranial bone-graft harvesting was found to be very low when carried out by surgeons with proper training (52).

The Thorax

The first rib graft was apparently performed as early as 1912 (53) in the reconstruction of a mandible using autogenous rib strips. The use of split-rib grafts was popularized by Longacre, in a large number of reconstructions of defects of the cranial and facial skeleton. He noted that, in children, those crania reconstructed with split ribs developed at a normal rate, and that at 2 years new bone had formed large bony plates, with only vestiges of the original ribs. He also commented on the rapid regeneration of ribs and on the fact that he had used the same regenerated rib on occasion within 6 months to 1 year (54).

While split ribs are still used occasionally in craniofacial reconstruction, they have by and large been replaced by cranial bone. The regenerated rib in particular consists of dense cortical bone that Tessier (49) considers unsuitable for grafting.

In harvesting autogenous ribs, an incision is made over the seventh rib; a submammary incision is used in the female patient. The dissection then proceeds under the latissimus dorsi muscle, splitting the fibers of the serratus as needed anteriorly. The ribs are harvested subperiosteally, with care to preserve the integrity of the pleura. Only alternate ribs are harvested. Following their removal, each rib bed is closed with a continuous absorbable suture. For small pleural tears, closure of the pleura under positive pressure is usually adequate. If a larger tear has occurred, temporary insertion of a thoracostomy tube should be carried out. Rib grafts should be avoided in children (49).

The Iliac

The iliac bone is an excellent source of large quantities of cancellous and corticocancellous bone. The technique described by Tessier and published by Wolfe and Kawamoto (55) has yielded consistently good results with very little postoperative discomfort and minimal complications. With the hip elevated on a folded towel, the skin is retracted medially by an assistant. An incision is then carried out through skin and periosteum over the iliac crest, behind the anterior superior iliac spine. The iliac spine and the bone adjacent to it are left intact while the iliac crest is split sagittally, leaving the muscle attachments intact.

If a full-thickness bone graft is required, both medial and lateral halves of the iliac crest are reflected and retracted in continuity with the periosteum and muscle attachments. The graft is then taken in the desired shape and size. If only partial-thickness corticocancellous bone is needed, the medial portion of the crest is reflected, and the bone harvested. Additional quantities of cancellous bone can be harvested easily with a curette. The iliac crest is then reconstructed by direct wiring. A drain is generally not used. When properly carried out, this method allows the harvesting of a large quantity of bone without any aesthetic deficit. Young patients are usually able to ambulate on the day following the procedure with only a moderate amount of discomfort. This technique is not suitable for patients younger than 9 or 10 years of age because of incomplete ossification. Bone can be reharvested from the same area in 18–24 months (49).

In the younger child, the technique described by Crockford and Converse (56) may be used in the rare instance that an iliac bone graft will become necessary. The crest is left undisturbed, while the fascia lata and muscles are incised on the lateral surface down to bone and reflected. Bone is then harvested from the lateral surface, beneath the growth centers.

Published complications of iliac bone-graft harvesting include:

1. Herniation of abdominal contents through the scar (57, 58) is probably the result of disruption of the attachment of muscles on the iliac crest and harvesting of large full-thickness grafts. With preservation of the iliac crest and the periosteum, herniations should be totally preventable.
2. "Gluteus gait" is a persistent type of dragging limp caused by extensive stripping of the lateral surface of the ilium, with weakening of the attachments of the gluteal musculature and fascia lata. A clicking sound when the patient walks may be produced if the fascia lata slips suddenly over the greater trochanter instead of sliding smoothly over it. A strong repair of the fascia lata and accurate apposition of the edges of the periosteum should prevent any gait problems (53).
3. Meralgia paresthetica (neuropathy of the lateral femoral cutaneous nerve of the thigh) is a complication that can be prevented by avoiding injury to the iliac spine and to the periosteum (59). The lateral femoral cutaneous nerve lies on the deep surface of the iliacus muscle. It leaves the pelvis just deep to the attachment of the inguinal ligament to the anterior superior iliac spine, but sometimes through the ligament or through the spine itself (60).
4. Fracture of the iliac crest occasionally occurs (61).
5. Hematoma formation is considered the most frequent complication, and most authors recommend leaving a drain in the wound. Tessier, however, feels that this is not necessary and closes the incisions without leaving a drain, claiming a very low incidence of hematoma formation (P. Tessier, personal communication).

The Tibia

The importance of the tibia as a source of autologous bone has declined because primary bone grafts of clefts have generally been abandoned and osteoperiosteal grafts are no longer in vogue. The tibia is still useful, however, in providing a strip of cortical and some highly osteogenic cancellous bone. The technique of harvesting bone from the tibia was originally published by Breine and Johanson (62) and will be described here as currently performed by Tessier.

An Esmarch bandage is applied to provide a bloodless field. Through a long, curved incision the skin and subcutaneous tissues are dissected from the anteromedial surface of the tibia, and the periosteum is incised medially, laterally, and distally, remaining attached only proximally from the level of the epiphysis to the midshaft of the tibia. With a very sharp osteotome, the periosteum with a thin layer of attached cortical bone is elevated in a distal-to-proximal direction, remaining attached as a proximally based osteoperiosteal flap. The underlying cortical bone of the medial surface of the tibia is then removed with the help of the osteotome, and the medullary cavity entered. Cancellous bone is curetted from the area of the proximal epiphysis, and the osteoperiosteal flap is sutured back in place. The skin is closed, and a snug dressing is applied. The harvested bone is generally used to supplement cranial grafts and to fill dead spaces, sparing the ilium for future use where multiple stages are planned. There is no deformity other than the surgical scar, and the patient experiences only temporary difficulty in walking.

Other Autogenous Donor Sites

For procedures involving the upper extremity, it is obviously advantageous to obtain the grafts from bones in the same surgical field. The distal radius and the proximal ulna have been used as a source of both cortical and cancellous bone with good results by McGrath and Watson (63). An oval-to-elliptical segment of cortical bone is removed by outlining the segment with multiple drill holes. Cancellous bone can then be curetted. When the ulna is used, the graft should be taken at least 2 inches below the olecranon to avoid weakness over the elbow joint. The radius is exposed between the 1st and 2nd dorsal extensor compartments, and periosteum is reflected off its lateral aspect.

The fibula is the most suitable bone graft to bridge defects in the long bones that result either from traumatic losses or from the resection of tumors. Harvesting the fibula as a bone graft does not cause major functional deficits, provided the fibular head as well as the distal quarter of the fibula are not disturbed (in order to maintain knee and ankle stability). Enneking (64) analyzed the results obtained in 40 patients who underwent such grafting operative procedures. Thirty-three patients had dual grafts, while seven had a single fibular graft. Dual grafts were used for major bones (humerus, femur, and tibia without fibula), while single grafts were used for the radius and for the tibia when the ipsilateral fibula was intact. In 25 patients, union was achieved in 12 months and in 2 in 20 months, while 12 patients required a supplementary cancellous graft at the site of nonunion to obtain stability. One patient required removal of an infected graft. Stress fractures of the grafts occurred in 18 of the 40 patients after union had occurred. The stress fractures healed in 15 of these patients; in 7 with no treatment, in 7 with external immobilization, and in 2 after bone grafting of the ununited fracture. There were three persistent nonunions of stress fractures despite bone grafting, internal fixation, and electrical stimulation. The length of the graft did not affect the incidence of nonunion, but it did affect the number of fatigue fractures. The shorter grafts (7.5–12 cm) were associated with a 33% incidence of nonunion, while the longer grafts (12–25 cm) had a 32% rate of nonunion. The incidence of fatigue fractures in the longer grafts (58%) was much greater than in the shorter grafts (17%). The grafts decreased in density during the first 6 months but gradually regained their mass and were generally comparable to normal cortical bone at 2 years. As the patients became functional, most (55%) of the grafts became more dense than normal. Some (34%) remained the same size, and a few (9%) atrophied (64).

Free Vascularized Bone Grafts

The first clinically successful free bone graft was reported by Taylor in 1975 (65). In selected patients, free vascularized bone grafts may offer considerable advantages over conventional bone grafting because large segments of bone transferred with their blood supply should heal to the recipient bone without the usual replacement by creeping substitution. The endosteal (nutrient) blood supply, however, must be preserved if predictable bone survival is to be achieved (66,67).

It has been shown that epiphyseal growth is preserved following transfer of a vascularized bone segment (68,69). When compound anterior rib segments were transferred with only their periosteal blood supply preserved, they showed no improved osteocyte survival or bone union as compared with conventional free grafts of the rib (70). More recently, Berggren and colleagues (71) used bone grafts in dog mandibles and compared free vascularized bone grafts that had intact medullary and periosteal blood supply with grafts with only periosteal supply intact. They concluded that, in grafts with only periosteal blood supply, survival of the osteocytes and marrow is not as complete as in grafts with both medullary and periosteal blood supply. No difference in the ability to participate in healing to a recipient bone defect could be demonstrated (71). Moore and others (72) compared vascularized and conventional rib grafts by biomechanical torsional testing and concluded that vascularized grafts were significantly stronger after 3 months of healing in the dog ulna model. These findings were confirmed by Goldberg. In the clinical setting, however, the same complications reported by Enneking in his retrospective study of conventional bone grafts have also followed free vascularized bone grafts. Fatigue fracture, nonunion, and infection have been reported (73-75).

Pedicled Vascularized Bone Grafts

In the craniofacial region, vascularized calvarial bone may be transferred, retaining a vascular pedicle based on the temporalis muscle, either including the galea as recommended by McCarthy and Zide (76), or simply retaining periosteal continuity, which also preserves the blood supply as shown by Antonyshyn and others (77). Such vascularized bone grafts (or, more appropriately, flaps) have been shown to resorb less than free grafts (78) and to retain significant growth potential (79). If a suture is included in the flap, it also continues to grow, in contrast to a nonvascularized bone graft (80). However, if the blood supply to the transposed bone segment is interrupted, it resorbs to a greater degree than a nonvascularized bone graft, presumably because of the avascular sleeve of tissue that surrounds it (81). This method should probably be reserved for bone grafting in clinically unfavorable recipient sites (69).

Handling and Machining of Bone Grafts

The least possible time should be allowed to lapse between the harvesting and the placement of the bone graft. During that time the graft should not be allowed to dry out, but should be kept in a liquid medium to ensure viability of the maximum number of cells. In a comparative study of the various media for temporary storage of autografts, Marx and colleagues (82) have determined that the best storage medium is either D_5W or normal saline. The ability of the patient's serum to sustain cellular viability was extremely poor, and more elaborate tissue-culture media offered no advantage over D_5W or normal saline (82).

Cortical and corticocancellous bone grafts are cut to the desired shape with a combination of bone-cutting forceps and electrical or air-powered saws and drills. It has been shown that the proper configuration of drill points and selection of appropriate drilling speeds are important in reducing the amount of mechanical and thermal damage to bone.

Jacob and others (83) made the following recommendations: (a) bone drills must have an appreciable rake angle (cutting-edge angle); (b) a point angle on the drill is desirable to prevent the drill from "walking" on the surface; (c) drilling should be done in the 750–1250 rpm range; (d) coolant in the form of saline should flood the entire drilling field (cold saline would possibly allow drilling at higher speeds); (e) the periosteum should be reflected away from the point where the drill will enter the bone to prevent the chips that are being ejected from the hole from being forced under the tissue and clogging the flutes of the drill; and (f) drill flutes should, for compact bone, be steep enough to remove chips at an even rate (83). Thompson (84) considers the optimal drilling speed to be about 500 rpm. He found that drilling at lower speeds causes fragmentation of the edges of the hole, while drilling at higher speeds increases the thermal changes in the bone. At 500 rpm, Thompson found the temperature was about 43° C at 2.5 mm from the extraoral skeletal pin used for drilling, while at 1000 rpm, the temperature was above 65.5° C (84). While the optimal drilling speed has not been universally agreed upon, the available studies indicate that it is in the vicinity of 500–1000 rpm and that the use of high-speed air-powered drills should be avoided.

Bibliography

1. Jobi a Meek'ren. *Observationes medico chirurgicae.* Ex officina Henrici et Theodore Boom, Amstelodami, 1682.
2. Chase SW, Herndon CH. The fate of autogenous and homogenous bone grafts. A historical review. *J Bone Joint Surg [Am]* 1955; 37:809.
3. Burchardt H, Enneking WF. Transplantation of bone. *Surg Clin North Am* 1978; 58:403.
4. Anderson KJ, Dingwal JA, Schmidt J, et al. The effect of particle size of the heterogenous bone transplant on the host tissue. *J Bone Joint Surg [Am]* 1961; 43:996.
5. Ramani PS, Kalbag RM, Gengupta RP. Cervical spinal interbody fusion with Kiel bone. *Br J Surg* 1975; 62:147.
6. Simmons DJ, Elisasser JC, Cummins H, et al. The bone inductive potential of a composite bone allograft-marrow autograft in rabbits. *Clin Orthop* 1973; 97:23.
7. Ray RD. Vascularization of bone grafts and implants. *Clin Orthop Rel Res* 1972; 87:43.
8. Amsel S, Dell ES. Bone marrow repopulation of subcutaneously grafted mouse femurs. *Proc Soc Exp Biol Med* 1971; 138:550.
9. Urist M. Practical applications of basic research in bone graft physiology. *Instruc Course Lect* 1976; 25:1.
10. Stutzmann J, Petrovic A. Bone cell histogenesis: the skeletoblast as a stem cell for preosteoblasts and for secondary type prechondroblasts. *Progr Clin Biol Res* 1982; 101:29.
11. Petrovic A, Stutzmann J, Oudet C. Craniofacial growth research. In: *Cybernetics, theory of catastrophy.* Symposium on Skull Growth, Academic Medical Center of Amsterdam, 1985.
12. Lemoine C, Petrovic, A, Stutzmann J. Inflammatory process of the rat maxilla after molar autotransplantation. *J Dent Res* 1970; 49:1175.
13. Petrovic A. Cellules sanguines, plasma et coagulation. In: Kayser C, et al, eds. *Traite de physiologie.* Paris: Flammarion, 1970; 138–208.
14. Stutzmann J, Petrovic A, Shaye R. Analyse en culture organotypique de la vitesse de formation-résorption de l'os alveolaire humain prélève avant et pendant un traitement comprenant le déplacement des dents: nouvelle voie d'approche en recherche orthodontique. *L'Orthodontie Française* 1979; 50:399.
15. Levander G. A study of bone regeneration. *Surg Gynecol Obstet* 1938; 67:705.
16. Hollinger JO, and Seyfer AE. Bioactive factors and biosynthetic materials in bone grafting. *Clin Plast Surg* 1994; 21:415.
17. Pelker RR, Friedlaender GE. Biomechanical aspects of bone autografts and allografts. *Orthop Clin North Am* 1987; 18:235.
18. Miller SC, and Marks SC Jr. Effects of prostaglandins on the skeleton. *Clin Plast Surg* 1994; 21:393.
19. Deleu J, Trueta J. Vascularization of bone grafts in the anterior chamber of the eye. *J Bone Joint Surg [Br]* 1965; 47:319.
20. Albrektsson T, Albrektsson B. Microcirculation in grafted bone: a chamber technique for vital microscopy of rabbit bone transplants. *Acta Orthop Scand* 1978; 49:1.
21. Kusiak JK, Zins JE, Ring E, et al. Early revascularization of membranous bone grafts. *Surg Forum* 1981; 32:567.
22. Burchardt H. Biology of bone transplantation. *Orthop Clin North Am* 1987; 18:187.
23. Enneking WF, Burchardt H, Puhl JJ, et al. Physical and biological aspects of repair in dog cortical bone transplants. *J Bone Joint Surg [Am]* 1975; 57:237.
24. Burchardt H, Jones H, Glowczewskie F, et al. Freeze-dried allogeneic segmental cortical bone grafts in dogs. *J Bone Joint Surg [Am]* 1978; 60:1082.
25. Stevenson S. The immune response to osteochondral allografts in dogs. *J Bone Joint Surg [Am]* 1987; 69:573.
26. Friedlander GE. Immune responses to osteochondral allografts. Current knowledge and future directions. *Clin Orthop* 1983; 174:58.
27. Muscolo DL, Caletti E, Schajowich F, et al. Tissue-typing in human massive allografts of frozen bone. *J Bone Joint Surg [Am]* 1987; 69:583.
28. Mankin HJ, Gebhardt MC, Tomford WW. The use of frozen cadaveric allografts in the management of patients with bone tumors of the extremities. *Orthop Clin North Am* 1987; 18:275.
29. Friedlander GE, Strong DM, Sell KW. Studies on the antigenicity of bone. 1. Freeze-dried and deep frozen allografts in rabbits. *J Bone Joint Surg [Am]* 1976; 58:854.
30. Pelker RR, Friedlander GE, Markham TC. Biomechanical properties of bone allografts. *Clin Orthop* 1983; 174:54.
31. Yaremchuk MJ, Nettlebad H, Randolph MA, et al. Vascularized bone allograft transplantation in a genetically defined rat model. *Plast Reconstr Surg* 1985; 75:355.
32. Paskert JP, Yaremchuk MJ, Randolph MA, et al. Prolonging survival in vascularized bone allograft transplantation. Developing specific immune unresponsiveness. *J Reconstr Microsurg* 1987; 3:253.
33. Jasty M, Harris WH. Total hip reconstruction using frozen femoral head allografts in patients with acetabular bone loss. *Orthop Clin North Am* 1987; 18:291.
34. Urbaniak JR, Aitken M. Clinical use of bone allografts in the elbow. *Orthop Clin North Am* 1987; 18:311.
35. Ehrlich MG, Lorenz J, Tomford WW, et al. Collagenase activity in banked bone. *Trans Orthop Res Soc* 1983; 8:166.
36. Mankin HJ, Doppelt SH, Sullivan TR, et al. Osteoarticular and intercalary allograft transplantation in the management of malignant tumors of bone. *Cancer* 1982; 50:613.
37. Triantafyllou N, Sotiropoulos E, Triantafyllou J. The mechanical properties of lyophylized and irradiated bone grafts. *Acta Orthop Belg* 1975; 41:35.
38. Pelker RR, Friedlaender GE, Markham TC, et al. Effects of freezing and freeze-drying on the biomechanical properties of rat bone. *J Orthop Res Soc* 1986; 11:272.
39. Hurley LA, Zeier FG, Stinchfield FE. Anorganic bone grafting; clinical experiences with heterografts processed by Ethylenediamine extraction. *Am J Surg* 1960; 100:12.
40. Mulliken JB, Glowacki J. Induced osteogenesis for repair and construction in the craniofacial region. *Plast Reconstr Surg* 1980; 65:553.
41. Mulliken JB, Glowacki J, Kaban LB, et al. Use of demineralized allogeneic bone implants for the correction of maxillocranial deformities. *Ann Surg* 1981; 194:366.
42. Mulliken JB. The use of demineralized bone for reconstruction of a large cranial defect. *Surg Rounds* 1982; 5:16.
43. Upton J, Glowacki J. Hand reconstruction with allograft demineralized bone: twenty-six implants in twelve patients. *J Hand Surg Am* 1992; 17:704.
44. Urist MR, Dawson E. Intertransverse process fusion with the aid of chemosterilized autolyzed antigen-extracted allogeneic (AAA) bone. *Clin Orthop Rel Res* 1981; 154:97.
45. Spector M. Anorganic bovine bone and ceramic analogs of bone mineral as implants to facilitate bone regeneration. *Clin Plast Surg* 1994; 21:437.
46. Makela P, Waris T, Serlo W, et al. The new poly-L-lactide (PLLA)–wire in craniectomy closures. An experimental study in rabbits and pigs. Paper presented at the 5th International Congress of the International Society of Craniofacial Surgeons, Oaxaca, Mexico, October 1993.
47. Losken HW, Tschakaloff A, Mooney M, et al. Experimental studies on biodegradable plates and screws: memory relapse and degradation kinetics. Paper presented at the 5th International Congress of the International Society of Craniofacial Surgeons, Oaxaca, Mexico, October 1993.

48. Ray RD. Bone grafts and bone implants. *Otolaryngol Clin North Am* 1972; 5:389.

49. Tessier P. Autogenous bone grafts taken from the calvarium for facial and cranial applications. *Clin Plastic Surg* 1982; 9:531.

50. Smith JD, Abramson M. Membranous versus endochondral bone autografts. *Arch Otolaryngol* 1974; 99:203.

51. Zins JE, Whitaker LA. Membranous versus endochondral bone: implications for craniofacial reconstruction. *Plast Reconstr Surg* 1983; 72:778.

52. Kline RM, and Wolfe SA. Complications associated with the harvesting of cranial bone grafts. *Plast Reconstr Surg* 1995; 95:5.

53. Longacre JJ, Converse JM, Knize DM. Transplantation of bone. In: Converse JM, ed. *Reconstructive Plastic Surgery*. 2nd ed. Philadelphia: WB Saunders, 1977; 1:334.

54. Longacre JJ, DeStefano GA. Further observations of the behavior of autogenous split-rib grafts in reconstruction of extensive defects of the cranium and face. *Plast Reconstr Surg* 1957; 20:281.

55. Wolfe SA, Kawamoto HK. Taking the iliac bone graft. *J Bone Joint Surg* [*Am*] 1968; 60:411.

56. Crockford DA, Converse JM. The ilium as a source of bone grafts in children. *Plast Reconstr Surg* 1972; 50:270.

57. Reid RL. Hernia through an iliac bone graft donor site. *J Bone Joint Surg* [*Am*] 1968; 50:757.

58. Lotem M, Maor P, Haimoff H, et al. Lumbar hernia at an iliac bone graft donor site. *Clin Orthop* 1971; 80:130.

59. Massey EW. Meralgia paresthetica secondary to trauma of bone graft. *J Trauma* 1980; 20:342.

60. Ghent WR. Further studies on meralgia paresthetica. *Can Med Assoc J* 1961; 85:871.

61. Reale F, Gambacorta D, Mencattini G. Iliac crest fracture after removal of two bone plugs for anterior cervical fusion. *J Neurosurg* 1979; 51:560.

62. Breine U, Johanson B. Tibia as donor area of bone grafts in infants. *Acta Chir Scand* 1966; 131:230.

63. McGrath MH, Watson HK. Late results with local bone graft donor sites in hand surgery. *J Hand Surg* 1981; 6:234.

64. Enneking WF, Eady JL, Burchardt H. Autogenous cortical bone grafts in the reconstruction of segmental skeletal defects. *J Bone Joint Surg* [*Am*] 1980; 62:1039.

65. Taylor GL, Miller GDH, Ham FJ. The free vascularized bone graft. A clinical extension of microsurgical technique. *Plast Reconstr Surg* 1975; 55:533.

66. Ostrup LT, Fredrickson JM. Distant transfer of a free living bone graft by microvascular anastomoses. *Plast Reconstr Surg* 1974; 54:274.

67. Goldberg VM, Shaffer JW, Field G, et al. Biology of vascularized bone grafts. *Orthop Clin North Am* 1987; 18:19.

68. Brown K, Marie P, Lyszakowski J, et al. Epiphyseal growth after free fibular transfer with and without microvascular anastomosis. *J Bone Joint Surg* [*Br*] 1983; 65:4.

69. Zaleske DJ, Ehrlich MG, Pilliero C, et al. Growth plate behavior in whole joint replantation in the rabbit. *J Bone Joint Surg* [*Am*] 1982; 65:2.

70. Adelaar RS, Soucacos P, Urbaniak JR. A study of autologous cortical bone grafts with microsurgical anastomosis of periosteal vessel. Paper presented at the Surgical Forum, American College of Surgeons Meeting, Miami, Florida, 1974. Quoted in: Taylor GL: Microvascular free bone graft transfer, a clinical technique. *Orthop Clin North Am* 1977; 8:425.

71. Berggren A, Weiland AJ, Dorfman H. Free vascularized bone grafts: factors affecting their survival and ability to heal to recipient bone defects. *Plast Reconstr Surg* 1982; 69:19.

72. Moore JB, Mazur JM, Zehr D. A biomechanical comparison of vascularized and conventional autogenous bone grafts. *Plast Reconstr Surg* 1984; 73:382.

73. Taylor GL. Microvascular free bone transfer: a clinical technique. *Orthop Clin North Am* 1977; 8:425.

74. Weiland AJ, Daniel RK. Microvascular anastomoses for bone grafts in the treatment of massive defects in bone. *J Bone Joint Surg* [*Am*] 1979; 61:98.

75. Weiland AJ, Kleinert HE, Kutz JE, et al. Free vascularized bone grafts in surgery of the upper extremity. *J Hand Surg* 1979; 4:129.

76. McCarthy JG, Zide BM. The spectrum of calvarial bone grafting: introduction of the vascularized calvarial bone flap. *Plast Reconstr Surg* 1984; 74:10.

77. Antonyshyn O, Colcleugh RG, Hurst LN, et al. The temporalis myoosseous flap: an experimental study. *Plast Reconstr Surg* 1986; 77:406.

78. Cutting CB, McCarthy JG. Comparison of residual osseous mass between vascularized and nonvascularized onlay bone transfers. *Plast Reconstr Surg* 1983; 72:672.

79. LaTrenta GS, McCarthy JG, Cutting CB. The growth of vascularized onlay bone transfers. *Ann Plast Surg* 1987; 18:511.

80. Antonyshyn O, Colcleugh RG, Anderson C. Growth potential in suture bone inlay grafts: a comparison of vascularized and free calvarial bone grafts. *Plast Reconstr Surg* 1987; 79:1.

81. Bos KE. Bone scintigraphy of experimental composite bone grafts revascularized by microvascular anastomoses. *Plast Reconstr Surg* 1979; 64:353.

82. Marx RE, Snyder RM, Kline SN. Cellular survival of human marrow during placement of marrow-cancellous bone grafts. *J Oral Surg* 1979; 37:712.

83. Jacob CH, Berry JT, Pope MH, et al. A study of the bone machining process-drilling. *J Biomechanics* 1976; 9:343.

84. Thompson HC. Effect of drilling into bone. *J Oral Surg* 1958; 16:22.

8

Basic Principles of Tendon Grafting

Philip E. Higgs, M.D., F.A.C.S., and Paul M. Weeks, M.D., F.A.C.S.

Historically, repair of lacerations within the flexor tendon sheath produced poor outcomes. This led to the common practice of using tendon grafts to bridge the flexor tendon sheath, producing improved results. Today tendon function is best restored by direct repair of the severed tendon, followed by induction of early motion under the supervision of a physical therapist. Flexor tendon grafts play a part in the management of flexor tendon injuries when primary repair is precluded by wound or tendon/tendon sheath conditions. The factors precluding primary repair include: (a) infection; (b) loss of the A2 or A4 pulleys; (c) loss of more than one centimeter of tendon length; (d) inadequate soft tissue coverage; (e) swelling of the proximal end of the tendon, preventing passage through the A2 and A4 pulleys; (f) collapse and obliteration of the tendon sheath by scar; and (g) the presence of stiff joints. Delayed primary repair may be accomplished up to 5–6 weeks after injury if there is no significant scarring or loss of tendon substance. At later stages it is usually precluded by thickening of the proximal tendon end (preventing passage through the digital sheath) and shortening of tendon length; however, delayed primary repair at 48 years after injury has been reported (1). We will discuss indications, contraindications, procedures, and results for primary, secondary, and staged flexor tendon grafts.

Indications for Staged Flexor Tendon Grafts

The surgeon considers flexor tendon grafting only if primary, or delayed primary, repair is not feasible. If only profundus function has been lost, other methods of management are available, including: (a) fusion of the distal interphalangeal (DIP) joint, or (b) tenodesis of the profundus distal stump across the DIP joint. Patient selection depends upon age, occupation, and finger involved, as well as patient acceptance of the time commitment and realistic expectations of the outcome. The primary consideration is expectation of improved function after a successful graft. Those with joint problems (e.g., arthritis or stiffness that cannot be improved with corrective procedures) or the very elderly may be better served with alternative procedures.

The two most common indications for tendon grafting are (a) loss of more than one centimeter of tendon substance, or (b) collapse and scarring of the flexor tendon sheath. In the acute situation, when only tendon substance is lost, flexor tendon grafting can be performed immediately. More often loss of tendon substance is accompanied

by loss of the A2 or A4, which is an indication for a staged graft. This circumstance requires reconstruction of the pulleys over a silastic rod prior to grafting. Collapsed and scarred flexor tendon sheath will preclude delayed primary repair or tendon graft and is an indication for staged tendon graft. Immediate flexor tendon grafting is precluded by a scarred tendon bed, stiff joints, or loss of the A2 or A4 pulleys.

Contraindications for Staged Flexor Tendon Grafts

Contraindications to flexor tendon grafting include stiff joints, adherent extensor tendons, loss of A2 or A4 pulleys, and inadequate soft-tissue coverage. If flexor tendon grafting is indicated but cannot be accomplished acutely, then grafting should be delayed until the tissues have softened and the joints are supple. This usually requires 6 to 8 weeks but can be longer, depending upon the injury. Occasionally joint stiffness is due to extrinsic factors (e.g., tendon adhesions or skin loss) that prevent obtaining supple joints preoperatively. The postoperative function of a tendon graft will depend first on passive range of motion (ROM) of the effected joints. Joints that do not have adequate preoperative passive ROM cannot be expected to function better after tendon graft. Adequate passive ROM must be obtained before grafting; satisfactory rehabilitation efforts depend upon its completion and maturation before the tendon graft (2). If joint stiffness is due to intrinsic factors (e.g., collateral ligament shortening, volar plate adherence, or dorsal pouch fibrosis), a capsulotomy is performed. Range of motion obtained at surgery must be maintained with aggressive therapy. Tendon grafting is delayed until the joints are supple.

In addition to obtaining supple joints before grafting, it is necessary to have adequate soft tissue coverage. Attempts to place tendon grafts directly beneath skin grafts or through dense scar will lead to poor results. Adequate coverage with distant or local flaps should be accomplished before graft placement. Coverage procedures may be effectively combined with placement of silastic rods or with pulley reconstruction. Joint contracture due to adhesions about injured flexor tendons can be released by tenolysis or excision of the scarred tendon and either tendon graft or rod insertion. These are removed while preparing the bed for tendon grafting, and allow a single-stage final tendon reconstruction. Salient operative features in flexor tendon grafting are summarized in Table 8–1.

Table 8–1
Flexor Tendon Grafting

Timing
    Edema has subsided
    Scar soft
    Joint supple

Incision
    Bruner incorporating laceration site

Digital Sheath
    Preserve normal sheath
    Preserve all pulleys

Superficialis Tendon
    Minimal gap
        Distal repair of tendon
        Nerve repair
        Proximal repair of tendon
    Large gap
        Distal repair of tendon
        Nerve graft
        Proximal repair of tendon

Tendon Graft
    Palmaris
    Plantaris

Repair
    Distal
        Equal-size tendons (end-to-end)
        Unequal-size tendons
            Drill hole
            Bunnell suture
            Pullout wire
    Proximal
        Equal-size tendons (end-to-end)
        Unequal-size tendons (Brand repair)

Operative Procedures for Flexor Tendon Grafts

GRAFTS TRAVERSING THE DIGITAL SHEATH

Skin Incisions

All previous incisions and lacerations are marked before planning the incision required for tendon grafting. The surgeon plans to utilize, if possible, part or all of the previous laceration sites and to avoid basing flaps on previous lacerations or incisions. We have abandoned the mid-lateral approach for the volar zig-zag incision. The latter provides excellent exposure and, if a tenolysis is required, the same volar zig-zag incision provides rapid, safe, clear visualization under local anesthesia. A dart is used to prevent formation of an annoying scar contracture across the flexion crease at the web space (see Fig. 8–1). A semilunar incision is continued into the palm to the level of the superficial vascular arch.

RETRIEVING THE TENDON ENDS

Tendon ends within the tendon sheath are at the level of the distal interphalangeal (DIP) joint and the palm. The surgeon reflects the skin flaps to expose the digital sheath throughout the finger; when tendon ends are lying in the proximal interphalangeal (PIP) joint area, a flap of sheath, which includes

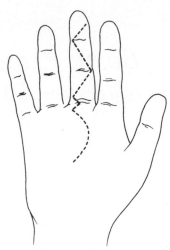

FIG. 8–1. A dart is incorporated in the volar zig-zag incision to preclude scar contracture across the crease.

the C1 and A3 pulleys, is reflected between the A2 and A4 pulleys. The surgeon must be careful to enter the sheath palmar to its reflection from the volar plate rather than cutting into the volar plate or entering the joint space by cutting through the accessory collateral ligaments. The plane of dissection is not clear when there is extensive scarring in this area. If the tendons are adherent beneath the A1 or A2 pulley, the interval between the A1 and A2 pulleys is opened. Proximally, the surgeon excises a window of palmar fascia over the flexor tendons of the involved finger. Frequently there is exuberant synovium within the palm, particularly when the proximal end of the tendon has withdrawn into the palm. This synovium is resected and the proximal end of the tendon is drawn into the palm. It is necessary to determine the excursion of the muscle.

The surgeon similarly retrieves the distal tendon end. If the distal tendon is beneath the A4 pulley, the sheath is opened over the DIP joint and the tendon drawn distally from beneath the A4 pulley. If the profundus tendon is adherent beneath the A4 pulley, the adhesions are divided, with a Freer elevator and the tendon advanced distally under gentle traction. A2 and A4 pulley are always preserved.

SOURCE OF TENDON GRAFTS

The sources of tendon grafts, in descending frequency of preference, are the palmaris longus, the plantaris, the long extensors of the middle three toes, and all others (3). Thick tendons are undesirable because they undergo greater central necrosis and form denser nonyielding adhesions. The palmaris longus is preferred because (a) it is thin; (b) its internal structure permits its fibers to be spread laterally to aid in repair; and (c) it is readily accessible in the field of surgery. Its presence is determined by active opposition of the thumb to the little finger and flexion of the wrist. Harvey and colleagues (4) examined 658 cadavers for presence of the palmaris and/or plantaris tendons. In 20.3% of the cadavers the palmaris was absent in one or both forearms; 12.5% had no palmaris in either forearm; the palmaris was absent in 20.9% of all forearms. One should always remember that the median nerve has been harvested, inadvertently, thinking it was the palmaris longus tendon (5). The tendon may be thin, or the muscle belly long, reducing its usefulness as a graft. The muscle arises from the medial epicondyle of the humerus and inserts into the palmar aponeurosis and the transverse carpal ligament. Its insertion is exposed through a transverse incision in the distal wrist crease. The surgeon must identify all fibers of the palmaris before attempting removal with a stripper. After removal, a clamp is placed on each end of the specimen and the muscle trimmed from the graft. Usually, it is of sufficient length for one palmar or distal wrist-to-fingertip graft.

The plantaris tendon is used when a longer graft or several grafts are needed. In Harvey's study, the plantaris tendon was absent either bilaterally or unilaterally in 22% of the cadavers (bilaterally in 12.8%). If the plantaris tendon was absent on one side, the chance of finding it on the other side was found to be 1 in 3, with no difference between males and females. No statistical correlation occurred between the presence of palmaris and plantaris tendons, and one cannot predict or determine the presence of the plantaris preoperatively. The plantaris may not be suitable for a graft because of variability in diameter or muscular attachments that make intact retrieval difficult. It usually provides sufficient length for two or three palm-to-fingertip grafts or one forearm-to-fingertip graft. Its tendon (frequently three to four times the length of the muscle belly) traverses the leg, passing medially between the gastrocnemius and soleus muscles. Distally the tendon emerges from beneath the deep fascia on the medial aspect of the Achilles tendon before inserting into the calcaneus. The surgeon exposes the tendon through a transverse incision posterior to the medial malleolus. The deep fascia should be split proximally as far as possible before using the tendon stripper.

The extensor digitorum longus arises as a common muscle from the anterior crest of the fibula, the interosseus membrane, and the crural fascia, and inserts into the dorsal aponeurosis of the second through fourth toes. The common tendon splits into individual tendons after passing under the cruciform ligament. The middle three toes have both long and short extensors, permitting removal of the long extensors for grafting. These tendons are always present and are of good quality and diameter as grafts. Occasionally the tendons fuse proximally, making harvesting difficult. The long toe extensors will provide three, and possibly four, tendon grafts. Removal of the long extensor of the little toe is usually avoided because there is no short extensor. There is little functional loss from using the toe extensors, although some flexion deformity and lateral deviation occurs when shoes are not worn.

Aulicino and colleagues (6) reported an independent long extensor of the fifth toe in 39 (50%) of 78 extremities. The length of usable tendon (range, of 16–29 cm; mean, 23 cm) was greater than that obtainable from the commonly fused long toe extensors. As a last resort, Aulicino and others suggested harvesting this tendon and preserving fifth toe extension by transfer of the fourth toe long extensor.

We avoid use of the superficialis tendons as grafts. The little-finger superficialis tendon can be used but is not sacrificed if intact. The remaining superficialis tendons are not suitable for use as free grafts because of size. The extensor indicis proprius and the extensor digiti minimi provide flat but short tendons that can be used as free grafts. There is no reason to sacrifice function when other tendons are available.

GRAFTS FOR ISOLATED PROFUNDUS INJURY

Many hand surgeons have decried the use of tendon grafts for isolated profundus injury (7). Other authors (8) have recommended a two-stage approach, as originally discussed by Gaisford and colleagues (9). For individuals that require or desire flexion of the DIP joint, tendon graft through a suitable bed, or staged graft when the bed is in question, can provide satisfactory results.

The surgeon proceeds by exposing and isolating the tendon ends, as described earlier. To facilitate passage of the proximal tendon, a 3-mm silastic rod or rubber catheter is inserted into the digital sheath from the palm to the distal phalanx. If the decussation of the superficialis tendon is obliterated, the rod is placed along the superficialis tendon; if the decussation of the superficialis tendon is open, the surgeon may elect to pass the rod through it. The tendon graft is sutured to the proximal end of the silastic rod or catheter. Then the rod is advanced distally, pulling the tendon graft through the sheath.

From this point, the surgeon may first repair either the proximal or distal attachment. The distal attachment is described below and will be the same whether done first or last. The proximal repair is typically a Pulvertaft weave type of repair.[10] We will describe the proximal-first procedure; the distal-first procedure is the same.

The distal end of the graft is temporarily sutured to the pulp skin for support while the proximal repair is being performed. The method of proximal suture depends upon the size discrepancy between the graft and the profundus tendon. If there is no discrepancy, an end-to-end repair with a modified Bunnell suture is preferred. If the graft is significantly smaller than the profundus, the suture technique of Pulvertaft (10) is useful. This weaving technique is easy to perform, provides a smooth transition from profundus tendon to graft, and has excellent holding power. The palmar and digital skin wounds are closed to the level of the PIP joint, leaving the distal incision open over the middle and distal phalanges before tension is adjusted in the graft.

ADJUSTING TENSION IN A TENDON GRAFT

There are several methods for determining proper graft tension. The following two have proven reliable in our experience. In the first, the finger is fully extended, a clamp is placed on the distal end of the tendon graft, and tension is applied to fully extend the muscle. The repair site is marked on the graft. A modified Bunnell suture is inserted so that the mark is between the criss-crosses. This compensates for the accordion effect that occurs when the suture is tied. The digital cascade of the injured hand serves as a guide to appropriate resting tension. A tendon graft should never be left too long. It is acceptable (and some even consider it desirable) to leave slight tension because the repair site can elongate several millimeters.

In the second method, the surgeon places a clamp on the distal end of the tendon graft and marks the excursion of the tendon under maximal and minimal tension at the level of the proximal end of the distal phalanx with the fingers in repose. The graft is attached distally at the midpoint. The wrist and metacarpal phalangeal (MP) joints are flexed, allowing the tendon graft to be advanced distally for easy suture. Methods

FIG. 8–2. A, a drill hole is made in the distal phalanx from the site of profundus attachment angling dorsally and exiting distal to the lunula. **B,** the profundus stump is split, a hole drilled in the distal phalanx, and the tendon advanced into the hole. The profundus slips can be sutured to the graft for added fixation, **C,** the site of tendon repair must not impinge on the A4 pulley when the DIP joint is fully flexed.

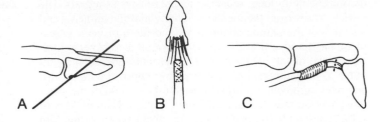

for distal attachment of a tendon graft are described below. Remember that, if the tension is too loose (i.e., graft is too long) the result will be poor. If the finger is extended relative to its appropriate stance, the distal suture can be removed and the tension readjusted.

When adjusting tension with the distal tendon attached first, the surgeon inserts the first interdigitation of the Pulvertaft weave. The wrist is placed in a neutral position and tension applied to the graft so as to flex the finger slightly more than the normal cascade. The surgeon then inserts a tacking suture in the tendons and verifies the positioning of the finger from extended to flexed position with wrist flexion and extension. If the finger remains markedly flexed with wrist flexion, the graft is too tight. If the finger does not flex into a normal cascade and remains extended when the wrist is extended, it is too loose.

DISTAL ATTACHMENT OF THE TENDON GRAFT

The method of distal attachment is determined by the length of profundus stump remaining attached to the distal phalanx.

No Profundus Stump Available

A drill hole is placed through the base of the distal phalanx at the site of profundus insertion. This hole is angled distally so that the germinal matrix of the nailbed will not be injured (Fig. 8–2A). The suture is attached to the tendon, threaded through the drill hole with a Keith needle, and tied over a padded button.

Less than 1 cm of Profundus Stump

The stump is split longitudinally to the bone. The bone is roughened and slightly grooved with a chisel. A drill hole is made between the split tendon ends that exits dorsally distal to the germinal matrix (Fig. 8–2B). A suture is secured to the tendon graft, passed through the drill hole, and tied over a padded button. The split ends of the profundus are sutured to the tendon graft while being careful to avoid cutting the tendon suture with the needle.

At Least 1 cm of Profundus Stump

After the suture has been attached to the tendon graft, it is criss-crossed through the tendon stump using only the distal 5 mm for suture attachment. Thus, the normal tendon insertion is preserved. The repair site must not impinge on the A4 pulley when the DIP joint is fully flexed (Fig. 8–2C).

If the proximal repair has been accomplished prior to this step, a single throw is placed in the tendon suture and held taut while the wrist is flexed and extended. The graft is not trimmed. The fingers should flex and extend in concert. If the operated finger is extended relative to its normal position in

the digital cascade, the surgeon takes down the distal tendon attachment because the tendon graft is too long and the distal suture must be placed more proximally on the graft. The maneuvers outlined above are repeated until proper tension has been obtained. If the tendon graft is too short (a slight discrepancy is tolerated, and even preferred by some), the suture is removed, tension determined, and the suture reinserted. If the distal tendon had been cut off initially (there would not be enough tendon to make the necessary adjustments), a second graft would have to be harvested. If the DIP joint assumes a 30–40° of flexion attitude after the tendon graft has been attached distally, the DIP joint is transfixed in extension with a K-wire, or splinted in extension. The joint is left extended for 6 to 10 weeks. DIP joint flexion deformity occurring at the operating table only becomes more pronounced over time.

Once the tendon is marked under the desired tension, the suture must be placed to ensure that tension is preserved. The surgeon starts a modified Bunnell suture 8 mm proximal to the mark and exits 3 mm distal to the mark. As the suture is tied, the tendon is compressed, maintaining proper tension. The wrist and MP joints are flexed and the forearm held midway between pronation and supination to allow excellent exposure for closure of the skin wound over the middle and distal phalanges without placing tension on the graft.

RESULTS AFTER GRAFTING FOR ISOLATED PROFUNDUS INJURY

Stark and others (11), utilizing the palmaris tendon preferentially, passed the graft through the superficialis in 22 fingers and alongside in three. If the superficialis bifurcation was scarred, the graft would be placed alongside. The distal end of the graft was attached to the terminal phalanx with a pull-out suture. Postoperatively, the wrist was immobilized in 30° of palmar flexion with digital extension blocked. The splint was maintained for 4 weeks, the pullout wire removed after 3 weeks. Flexion against resistance was not allowed until 8 weeks postoperatively. Two fingers obtained flexion to the midpalmar crease, eleven to 1.25 cm, nine to 2.5 cm, and one to 3.2 cm. Two fingers had less flexion after operation. In 22 of the 25 patients, useful active flexion of the DIP joint was present and active independent flexion of the DIP joint was possible. Stark and colleagues felt that 20 of 25 patients (80%) had a satisfactory result.

McClinton and colleagues (12) reported 100 tendon grafts for isolated flexor digitorum profundus injuries in 96 patients, 86% of whom were 40 years of age or younger. Preoperatively, all fingers had full passive ROM. The palmaris longus tendon was used in 80 cases, and the extensor digitorum communis in 10. The tendon graft was passed around the superficialis decussation in 93 cases and through it in seven cases. They used a Bunnell pullout wire at the distal juncture and either a Pulvertaft tendon weave or Bunnell tendon suture proximally. Tension was set to maintain normal digital cascade with the hand in repose. They preferred 30 mm of passive excursion of the muscle tendon unit as a prerequisite to grafting so as to minimize PIP joint flexion contracture. They immobilized the hand for 1 week postoperatively, after which they began full passive motion of the PIP joint with the MP joint flexed. Rehabilitation was advanced with full flexion and extension at 4 weeks and resisted flexion at 8 weeks. Forty-five patients were able to flex to the distal palmar crease; an additional 24 could flex to within 1.3 cm. More than 90% of the fingers obtained greater than 20° of flexion at the DIP joint. Fifty-five patients lost less than 10% of PIP joint extension, three lost 11 to 20%, and six lost 21 to 30%. According to Stark's criteria, more than 90% of patients had a satisfactory result.

Bora (13) reported flexor tendon grafting in twenty fingers of children ranging from 4 months to 13 years of age. Full passive ROM was present before surgery. The plantaris was used in 19 patients, the profundus in one. The graft was placed through the bifurcation, after which Bora immobilized the hand with an axilla-to-fingertip cast for 3 weeks. He obtained 17 satisfactory and three unsatisfactory results.

Pulvertaft (14) reported 68 cases, using the plantaris in 46 and the long toe extensor tendon in the remainder. Pulvertaft attempted to place the graft through the superficialis decussation; however, if it was too tight, one slip of the superficialis was excised. Tension was set to slightly increase flexion in repose. The hand was immobilized for 3 weeks with the digit in repose. Sixty-eight percent (33 grafts) were good or excellent, and 83% (57 grafts) were worthwhile. There were 11 poor results and the digital function was worse in 2 patients. Results were not as good in patients past 31 years of age.

Single-stage profundus grafting in the presence of an intact superficialis provides a reasonable opportunity to improve function. The digit must be supple and the patient should exhibit the need and possess the commitment to obtain a satisfactory result. Aggressive postoperative therapy is a necessity.

GRAFT WHEN PROFUNDUS AND SUPERFICIALIS TENDONS ARE INJURED

Exposure is gained through a volar zig-zag incision. A rectangular flap of digital sheath is reflected between the A2 and A4 pulleys. The surgeon takes care to preserve the distal stump(s) of the superficialis tendon. The volar plate is exposed. The surgeon determines the level of tendon laceration by inspection of the sheath and knowledge of the digital position at the time of injury. The distal end of the profundus tendon is usually between the A2 and A4 pulley, or it may have retracted distally beneath the A4 pulley. The surgeon opens the synovial lining of the sheath distal to the A4 pulley and identifies the distal end of the tendon.

The superficialis and profundus tendons and the opening of the A1 pulley are exposed by excising a window of palmar fascia. Scar about the tendons is excised and the proximal end of the tendons may be retrieved into the palm. If this cannot be easily done, either the vinculum longus or scar is responsible. Adhesions beneath the A1 or A2 pulleys are released with a Freer elevator or tenotomy scissors. If the su-

perficialis tendon has been cut distal to its decussation, excellent flexion at the PIP joint can be obtained by repairing the superficialis. If the vinculum is intact, the surgeon can repair the superficialis directly and graft the profundus, if needed, as described in the section titled "Grafts for Isolated Profundus Injury." If the superficialis cannot be repaired, the surgeon sutures the proximal ends of the distal segment to the distal edge of the A2 pulley with the PIP joint in 10° flexion to prevent hyperextension deformity of the PIP joint. If the distal stump of the superficialis is too short, the surgeon resects and sutures a slip of superficialis across the PIP joint to prevent hyperextension. Tendon grafting to the profundus is described in the section for intact superficialis.

GRAFTS NOT TRAVERSING THE DIGITAL SHEATH (BRIDGE GRAFTS)

Infrequently, there is loss of flexor tendon length proximal to the A1 pulley and the distal tendons are free of adhesions within the digital sheath. Then the surgeon exposes only the proximal portion of the digital sheath through a semilunar palmar incision. The skin flaps are reflected from the palmar fascia and the palmar fascia resected over the involved tendons. The proximal and distal ends of the tendons are identified. The surgeon cuts the distal stump of the superficialis to allow its retraction into the sheath. If the superficialis is already within the sheath and joint extension is not restricted, the tendon is left undisturbed. If the profundus has been cut distal to the lumbrical (and the lumbrical has not been severed), the proximal end of the tendon can be retrieved through the palmar incision. If the tendon has been cut proximal to the lumbrical, or the latter severed, the proximal end usually retracts into the carpal canal or forearm. Under these circumstances, two incisions (palmar and distal forearm) are preferred to opening the carpal canal. The surgeon identifies the profundus tendon in the forearm and passes a Hager dilator in the proper plane through the carpal canal into the palm and directed toward the involved finger. The tendon graft is sutured to the profundus tendon and its distal end sutured to the proximal end of the dilator and guided through the carpal canal into the palm. Tension is determined as follows: (a) gentle traction is placed on the distal segment of profundus tendon but the finger is held in full extension; (b) traction is placed on the tendon graft to provide maximal extension of the muscle belly; (c) the tendons are marked where they overlap proximal to the edge of the A1 pulley; and (d) the tendon ends are repaired with a modified Bunnell suture.

If the tendons are not gliding freely within the digital sheath, the tendon graft should be extended to the distal phalanx. The digital sheath is exposed throughout the finger by a volar zig-zag incision. The surgeon reflects a rectangular flap of sheath over the PIP joint and opens it over the DIP joint. A tenolysis is performed and the profundus extracted distally, maintaining its insertion. The superficialis insertion is left intact. The decussations are sutured to the distal edge of the A2 pulley to prevent PIP joint hyperextension. Tendon grafting is performed as described in the section on profundus tendon injury.

GRAFTS IN CHILDREN

Some surgeons defer tendon grafting until a child is 3 to 4 years of age or older, when control is possible (15,16). Our experience has been that the younger child uniformly develops an excellent result if prevented from breaking the tendon repair. Indications and operative procedure for tendon repair or grafting are the same for children and adults.

Postoperative Care

DRESSINGS

In Cooperative Adults

Hold the wrist in 30° flexion with the MP joints at 70 to 90° of flexion and the PIP and DIP joints in full extension. Place opened 4 × 4 sponges between the fingers. The PIP joint(s) of the operated finger(s) is maintained in slight (15 to 20°) flexion. Cut an ABD pad with a thumb hole and wrap it around the wrist. A second pad is required around the wrist and forearm. Place cotton or Dacron batting in the palm and put more opened 4 × 4's between the fingers and over the batting. Wrap a Kling gauze snugly to cover the entire dressing. Coban is applied to provide gentle even pressure.

In Children

Immobilization is accomplished with a small, snug, bulky dressing incorporating an aluminum splint. After the tendon graft has been performed, tape the remaining fingers in extension to a padded aluminum splint without intervening dressings. Flex the operated finger to 70° at the MP joint. Pad the palm and apply a strip of tape dorsally, extending it over the fingertip into the palm and up the volar forearm. This holds the grafted finger in flexion (45° at the PIP and 30° at the DIP joint); this is certainly a position to be avoided in adults, but of no deleterious effect in young children. The dressing is reinforced weekly as needed. At 4 weeks, the dressings are discarded and the parents or caregivers instructed in gentle extension exercises and told to encourage the child to grasp objects. No formal therapy is given and the child is allowed normal use of the hand. We have not had rupture of a tendon graft with this treatment.

MANAGEMENT AFTER GRAFTING (ADULTS)

Postoperative management is determined by the status of the superficialis tendon. If it is intact, the dressing is discarded after 3–5 days and a splint fabricated to hold the wrist in 20° to 30° of flexion and all fingers in the protective (intrinsic plus) position with the PIP joint of the operated finger held in slight (10° to 15°) flexion. Active isolated flexion of the grafted finger superficialis tendon is begun. The hand therapist begins passive ROM of the DIP under supervision the first week, removing the splint frequently to exercise the nonoperated fingers. At 2 weeks, active extension/passive flexion is initiated with a dynamic splint.

If the superficialis is not intact, a gentle dressing extending from the fingertips to the antecubital fossa is applied. The wrist is in a 20–30° flexed position and the digits are maintained in repose. Supervised passive motion is permitted. After 2 weeks, active extension/passive flexion is started; it is carried out for 2 more weeks, along with continued passive exercise.

Splints are fabricated as soon as the dressing is removed. A static dorsal protective splint maintains the operated finger in flexion and prevents extension. With the splint in place, the patient can continue to work on active flexion and move the other fingers freely.

During the second week of rehabilitation, gentle passive extension of the PIP joint is obtained with the MP and DIP joints flexed. Similarly, the DIP joint is extended with the MP and PIP joints flexed. Active flexion of the PIP and DIP joints with the MP joint stabilized in flexion is initiated. During the 3rd week, gentle passive extension of both the PIP and DIP joints is encouraged, with the MP joint first in flexion, then in increasing amounts of extension.

During the 4th week, the following exercises are begun: (a) passive flexion of the MP, PIP, and DIP joints; (b) gentle active PIP joint flexion with the MP joint stabilized in flexion; (c) gentle active DIP joint flexion with the MP and PIP joints stabilized in flexion; (d) massage of the fingers and hand without forcing the fingers into extension; and (e) massage of the palmar or wrist scar in a proximal-to-distal direction during active finger flexion.

The 5th week, the splint is brought to neutral at the wrist. In the 6th week, resistance is applied to these flexion exercises. During this time, massage is applied with increasing force. These basic exercises are continued until the patient has reached full recovery.

Within 4 weeks after removal of the dressing, individual patient problems begin to appear. Often passive extension of the PIP and DIP joints is not possible. Dynamic splinting of these joints is begun when indicated during the 6th week after surgery. Dynamic force is applied through the use of a rubber band in an outrigger hand splint or with piano wire in a spring-type finger extension splint. Dynamic splinting does not exceed 7 to 8 ounces of pull with a rubber band splint, or 9 to 10 ounces with a piano wire splint. Patients are encouraged to use their hands gradually for functional activities and to perform daily activities as soon as they can tolerate them.

Results

RATE OF TENDON GLIDING RECOVERY

Rate of recovery has been documented only when the superficialis and profundus are severed and the profundus grafted (17). In a series of 24 tendon grafts, within 6 weeks the average patient regained 50% of preoperative gross grip strength and 115° total active motion, which was 50% of the motion obtained at 1 year. By 12 weeks after grafting, the average patient had regained 66% of preoperative gross grip strength and 176° of total active motion (77% of the motion attained at 1 year). The rate of recovery was greatest during the first 4 months. As expected, motion at the MP joint approached normal within 6 to 8 weeks after surgery. DIP joint motion recovered more slowly than PIP joint motion.

AFTER FLEXOR TENDON GRAFT

Boyes and Stark analyzed the results of graft flexor reconstruction in 607 fingers (18). They found that the most important factor was the preoperative condition (scarring, joint contracture, multiple injuries) of the finger. Patients age 40 years and older had poorer results. A similar analysis by Kunzle and colleagues (19) confirms these findings.

AFTER BRIDGE GRAFT

Stark and others reported 41 flexor tendon grafts in 31 patients aged 3 to 69 years (20). There was loss of tendon substance between the musculotendinous junction and the distal palmar crease outside the digital sheath. They modified assessment criteria so that satisfactory results included finger flexion to within 5 cm or less of the midpalmar crease. Seven of the thirty-five were unsatisfactory due to limited extension, though 5 of the 7 patients felt that the operation had improved use of their hand. Satisfactory function was obtained in 8 of 10 thumbs.

Management of Unsatisfactory Results After Flexor Tendon Graft

To determine progress properly, active and passive ROM should be recorded at least every 4 weeks. A plateau in the rate of recovery should be verified over 1 to 2 months. If the patient is displeased with the functional result, we recommend use of an algorithm to provide an orderly approach to the problems (Fig. 8–3).

INDICATIONS FOR TENOLYSIS AND/OR CAPSULOTOMY

The surgeon must determine whether lack of function is due to adhesions limiting tendon gliding, rupture of the tendon graft, or stiff joints. This decision is based on the total ROM and the relationship between passive and active joint motion. Individual motivation is a consideration in adults, who must work diligently to maintain the gains accomplished at surgery. Children usually form soft adhesions following tenolysis and capsulotomy and these procedures are routinely used when indicated without consideration of cooperativeness. If passive joint flexion is limited but exceeds active motion, adhesions are restricting flexor tendon gliding. The surgeon must determine the cause of limited passive joint flexion. It may be due to adhesions around the extensor tendon, or scarring of the dorsal joint capsule and/or the dorsal one-third of the collateral ligaments. The extent of involvement can only be determined at the time of surgery.

If passive joint flexion is normal and exceeds active joint flexion, a flexor tenolysis is required. If passive and active joint motion are equal but inadequate, a tenolysis and capsulotomy are required. Both flexor and extensor systems may require tenolysis. If passive PIP joint extension is normal and exceeds active PIP joint extension, an extensor tenolysis is required. Thus, the operative procedure required may be: (a) capsulotomy; (b) capsulotomy and extensor tenolysis; (c) capsulotomy and flexor tenolysis; (d) capsulotomy with flexor and extensor tenolysis; (e) extensor tenolysis; (f) extensor and flexor tenolysis; or (g) flexor tenolysis.

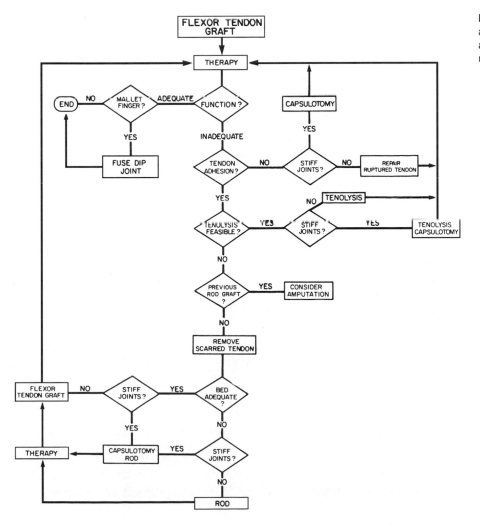

FIG. 8–3. An algorithm for management after flexor tendon graft. The authors use this approach as an aid to orderly evaluation and restoration of function.

CAPSULOTOMY THERAPY AFTER LOCAL TENOLYSIS

This operative procedure is routinely performed under local anesthesia on an outpatient basis. Digital or wrist-block anesthesia is established utilizing 1% Xylocaine (without epinephrine). If wrist-block anesthesia is used, the intrinsic contribution to digital function will not be present. After blood has been expressed from the upper extremity, an arm tourniquet is inflated to 75–100 mm Hg above the patient's systolic pressure. A dorsal serpentine incision over the PIP joint is used if the joint is stiff in extension. A volar zig-zag incision over the proximal and middle phalanges is used if the PIP joint is stiff in flexion. The surgeon marks to the level of the distal palmar crease but initially makes only the distal portion of the incision. If the joint is stiff in flexion and extension, only a volar approach is used.

The procedure usually takes 20 to 30 minutes and the patient is able to extend and flex the fingers actively. If the tourniquet becomes uncomfortable, it is released and reinflated in 10 minutes, or alternately a sterile forearm tourniquet may be used and inflated just before arm tourniquet release (21). At the end of the procedure, bleeding is controlled by coagulation of vessels and elevation and compression of the hand for 15 minutes. The surgical drapes are lowered and the ROM under anesthesia is demonstrated to the patient as a realistic goal. The wounds are closed and a light dressing applied. A plaster splint may be used to maintain digital positioning until a plastic splint is fabricated at the first rehabilitation session—usually later that day.

PROCEDURE IF JOINT IS STIFF IN EXTENSION

A dorsal serpentine incision is made over the proximal interphalangeal joint. The skin flaps are reflected and the free edges of the extensor hood identified. An incision is made along the free edge of the lateral bands from the midproximal phalanx to the midmiddle phalanx. The surgeon frees the lateral bands and identifies and preserves the insertion of the central slip. The extensor tendon is inspected proximally and a tenolysis performed if necessary (Fig. 8–4A) An incision is made into the dorsal capsule of the joint. (Fig. 8–4B). After each structure is freed of adhesions, the surgeon evaluates the patient's ability to flex the finger actively. If flexion is inadequate, the dorsal one-third of the collateral ligaments are incised (Fig. 8–4C). At this point, full passive flexion is possible. If the patient cannot fully flex the finger actively, a flexor tenolysis is performed as described later (Fig. 8–4D). When 90° of active PIP joint

flexion has been obtained, it is demonstrated to the patient. The wounds are sutured and a light dressing applied. Therapy begins later that day.

PROCEDURE IF JOINT IS STIFF IN FLEXION

The surgeon makes a volar zig-zag incision, extending from the midproximal phalanx to the midmiddle phalanx. The flexor tendon sheath is identified and the collateral ligaments of the PIP joint exposed by transecting Cleland's ligaments. The digital sheath over the PIP joint is opened and tension placed on the flexor tendons to see if they are adherent (Fig. 8–5). If the tendons are adherent, a flexor tenolysis is performed. If full extension is not possible after flexor tenolysis is complete, the accessory collateral ligaments are divided, including the volar one-third of the collateral ligaments. The surgeon tests the passive extension again and, if it is inadequate, inspects the volar plate. If it is taut with the joint extended, the periosteum of the proximal phalanx is freed maintaining attachment of the volar plate to the periosteum proximally. Care is taken to prevent hyperextension instability of the PIP joint, which is caused by resecting too much collateral ligament and overreleasing the volar plate. If hyperextension occurs, it is corrected by suturing a distally attached slip of the superficialis to the A2 pulley or the periosteum of the proximal phalanx, or by maintaining the PIP joint in slight flexion by dorsal splinting with advancement to full extension over 2 to 3 weeks (as in treatment of a complete PIP dislocation). If active extension is inadequate after full passive extension has been obtained, the surgeon inspects the extensor tendon and performs tenolysis through the volar incision.

CAPSULOTOMY THERAPY AFTER LOCAL TENOLYSIS

Active digital motion is begun during the first 24 hours with a light dressing in place. All patients are instructed in the therapy plan at this time. If visiting a therapy unit 2 to 3 times per week is not feasible, a home therapy program must be developed. Such patients are seen as often as possible. Gentle, active flexion and extension exercises are outlined for hourly performance. Exercise equipment (e.g., a black roll, dowel stick, exercise board) is used. Dynamic and/or static splints are fabricated within the first postoperative day to maintain the gains obtained at surgery. The patient is encouraged to use the hand for light everyday activities. Precautions against sports and heavy lifting must be stressed.

FINGER STIFF IN EXTENSION

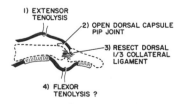

FIG. 8–4. The order of procedure for releasing the PIP joint stiff in extension is noted.

FINGER STIFF IN FLEXION

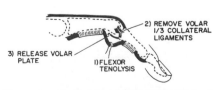

FIG. 8–5. The order of release of PIP joint stiff in flexion is presented.

During the 2nd week, edema is controlled by a compression stockinette, COBAN wrapping, and massage. Hourly active exercise sessions continue, with light resistance added. Additional splints are fabricated if necessary. The patient continues using the hand for light activities. During the 3rd week, scar massage becomes more vigorous. The patient continues hourly active exercises and more resistance is added. Splinting is advanced as needed and the patient is encouraged to use the hand for most everyday activities. During the 4th to 6th weeks, scar massage is vigorous. Distal-to-proximal massage is begun. Resistive exercise continues. Appropriate splinting continues, and the patient is encouraged to return to work using the hand without restrictions. In our series of 185 fingers (146 patients) change in active ROM varied from a loss of 42° to a gain of 100° (22). The average gain in active motion, respectively, was 23°, 39°, and 12° for the MP, PIP, and DIP joints (capsulotomy was limited to the PIP joints). The average gain in passive motion, respectively, was 20°, 33°, and 13° for the MP, PIP, and DIP joints.

EXTENSIVE TENOLYSIS AFTER FLEXOR TENDON GRAFT

The indications for tenolysis after flexor tendon graft are: (a) passive joint ROM exceeds the active joint ROM, and (b) the active joint ROM is insufficient to meet the patient's requirement. Satisfactory skin coverage, skeletal stability, adequate joint function, and at least protective sensation, are prerequisite.

It is important to determine as accurately as possible the level of the most significant adhesions that are preventing gliding. The adhesions are almost always more extensive than preoperative examination implies, and the surgeon must be prepared to explore the entire length of the tendon at the time of surgery.

The ideal interval between tendon grafting and tenolysis is unknown. Verdan (23) states that if a satisfactory ROM is not obtained, tenolysis should be performed 3 months after repair (17,24,25). Others have recommended waiting 6 months before performing a tenolysis. The reasons for the delay are twofold: (a) tendon function may improve spontaneously up to 6 months after tendon graft, and (b) tendon graft rupture may be a greater risk when tenolysis is done only 3 to 4 months postoperatively. Tenolysis in a chicken-tendon graft model weakened the tendon at 6 weeks; at 12 weeks tenolysis did not weaken the tendon and resulted in increased blood supply (26). In our experience, tendon graft rupture does not occur if the tenolysis is delayed for 6 months.

If the joints are supple, evaluation of tendon gliding is made easier. If the joints are stiff, tendon gliding can only be evaluated after the joints have been mobilized. Capsulotomy is performed under local anesthesia. This permits evaluation of active tendon gliding at the operating table. If there are restricting tendon adhesions, a volar zig-zag incision is made from the DIP joint crease to midpalmar area. The digital sheath is exposed along the length of the skin incision. A flap of sheath is raised at the PIP joint. Flexor tendons are freed from local adhesions. The surgeon identifies the interval between the A1 and A2 pulleys, visualizes the tendons, and applies traction to the tendons at the PIP level to determine the site of adhesions (Fig. 8–6). Most often, the tendons are ad-

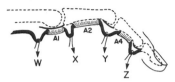

FIG. 8–6. Tendon gliding is tested at W, X, Y, and Z to determine the level of tendon adhesions.

Table 8–2
Flexor Tendon Tenolysis

1. Local anesthesia
2. Open digital sheath at W, X, Y, and Z (see Fig. 8–6)
3. Traction at W, X, Y, and Z (see Fig. 8–6)
4. Evaluate tendon gliding proximal and distal to traction point
5. Release adhesions
6. Test passive range of joint motion
7. Extensor tenolysis?
8. Capsulotomy?
9. Have patient actively flex and extend finger(s)
10. Show patient result of surgery

herent under the A2 pulley. If tension on the tendons over the PIP joint fails to produce full DIP joint flexion, the sheath over the DIP joint is opened and the tendon elevated with tension applied to it. Frequently the site of adhesions between the tendon and the middle phalanx becomes obvious and can be divided. A Freer elevator or Lorenz gauze packer is helpful in dividing adhesions beneath the A2 and A4 pulleys. Care is essential, because it is easy to damage or divide the tendon inadvertently beneath the pulleys. Full active tendon gliding must be obtained. The active ROM is demonstrated to the patient at the operating table to provide added motivation postoperatively. Care must be taken to preserve a pulley mechanism. Tenolysis should be continued until the active ROM is equal to the passive ROM. Tendon strippers are not helpful and may actually damage the tendon or surrounding structures. Mobilization, rather than devascularization of the tendon, is the goal. The operative procedure is summarized in Table 8–2.

POSTOPERATIVE THERAPY

Active ROM exercises are begun immediately after surgery. Early active exercises are important in obtaining a satisfactory result. Dynamic splints may aid in the restoration of extension. Active MP, PIP, and DIP joint flexion and extension exercises are performed frequently to prevent recurrent adhesions from restricting motion. Patient education is essential as to the importance of continuing to exercise throughout the day. The hand is kept elevated over the first 48 to 72 hours to reduce edema. An elastic finger stocking made from an Ace wrap is used at night or when the patient is not exercising. An inflatable finger cuff or Coban wrapping can be used to reduce edema. Cold packs may be applied intermittently to reduce the inflammatory response to exercise. Passive exercises are used to prevent joint stiffness. Dynamic splinting is initiated if the patient displays limited motion in flexion or extension of any joint. Scar massage is begun when the incision is healed. As the patient progresses and tolerance improves, more vigorous and resistive exercises are used to increase hand strength. The goal of therapy is to maintain tendon gliding and joint motion and to promote maximum functional use of the hand.

RESULTS OF TENOLYSIS AFTER TENDON GRAFTING

Kelly (27) reported on the indications for and effectiveness of tenolysis after tendon grafting. In 71 patients requiring flexor tendon grafts, there were 10 secondary tenolyses. Four had improvement of function following tenolysis, but the degree of improvement was not noted. McCash (28) reported 9 tenolyses out of a total of 33 secondary tendon repairs and tendon grafts. Fetrow (29) published the most extensive paper on tenolysis. He reported 220 flexor and extensor tenolyses in 134 patients; 24 patients had tenolysis performed more than once on a given tendon, and 31 patients had simultaneous tenolysis of two or more tendons. Tenolyses were required in 91 of 374 flexor tendon grafts (24%). Almost all tendon grafts were performed after repair of tendon lacerations in flexor zone II. Follow-up was obtained on 68 of the 91 tenolyses. A good or excellent result was classified as one in which the fingertip flexed to within ½ inch (about 13 mm) of the palm; a fair result was classified as one in which the fingertip flexed to between ½ and 1½ inches (about 38 mm) of the palm, and the remainder were classified as poor results. Of the 68 tenolyses, 26% of the patients were improved; 44% were greatly improved; and 30% were unchanged or made worse.

DETERMINING TENDON RUPTURE

Patients usually know when they have ruptured the tendon graft. Though a specific event may initially be denied, if pressed the patient frequently recalls one. When the graft has ruptured, the finger assumes a pronounced extension deformity. DIP joint motion is minimal or nil. There may be discoloration in the subcutaneous tissues due to hemorrhage. Tenderness at the site of disruption often persists for several days.

Occasionally a patient gives a history of loss of motion after exercising, accompanied by mild discomfort in the digit. We have waited and reexamined patients in 2 days, at which time they again were able to flex the finger actively; thus, this appears to be a fatigue phenomenon with recovery within 2 days. Exploration is recommended if recovery has not occurred by this time. Surgery is recommended immediately when there is obvious rupture. At surgery, the wound over the volar surface of the distal phalanx is opened. If the distal end is not disrupted, the surgeon makes an incision over the site of proximal repair. Distal disruptions can be resutured, but only if advancement of the tendon graft is minimal and does not significantly alter the balance among the fingers. Proximal disruptions usually require either a tendon graft or a rod graft.

Indications for a Two-Stage Reconstruction of the Flexor Tendon Mechanism

Flexor system grafting in the presence of extensive scarring of the flexor sheath, stiff joints, or an adherent extensor system, will not provide an optimal result. Reconstruction of an

Table 8–3
Stage 1: Flexor Tendon Reconstruction—Rod-Graft

Pulleys
   Preserve—all
   Reconstruct—A2 and A4
      Tendon weave through sheath remnants

PIP Joint
   Capsulotomy as required

Tendon Management
   Superficialis
      Intact without adhesions
      Intact with adhesions—tenolysis
      Disrupted—suture distal slips to prevent joint hypertension
   Profundus
      Respect proximal to lumbricate
      Leave 1.5 cm distal stump

Prosthesis
   Attachment
      Distal—suture beneath profundus stump
      Proximal—none
   Material
      Silastic tube (3 mm)
      Woven Dacron—silicon (5 mm)

Nerve Management
   Direct repair
   Surval nerve graft

extensively damaged pulley system is best accomplished over a silastic rod. Hunter has popularized the staged flexor tendon reconstruction (30). He suggests that its main use is in the area of failed flexor tendon surgery or in crushing injuries where the flexor system has been destroyed. A silicone rubber implant is inserted during the first stage, to be replaced by a tendon graft at a second stage.

A smooth-walled, mesothelium-lined sheath forms about the silastic rod (31). The fluid produced by this synovial pseudo-sheath supplies metabolic substrate to the graft while a blood supply develops. Adhesions are vastly reduced. The salient features of the first stage are outlined in Table 8–3.

FIRST-STAGE FLEXOR RECONSTRUCTION

A volar zig-zag skin incision is utilized to expose the tendon sheath. All remaining pulley mechanism is preserved. If the superficialis tendon is intact, it is preserved; if it is adherent, a tenolysis is performed. If disrupted, a distal slip is sutured to the periosteum of the proximal phalanx or to the digital sheath to prevent PIP joint hyperextension. The level of proximal profundus tendon resection is controversial. We resect the profundus proximal to the lumbrical origin because we prefer to do our proximal tendon graft repair in the distal forearm. It is imperative that a distal stump be preserved so that the rod can be sutured between the tendon and distal phalanx to prevent migration of the rod and erosion through the pulp. If the A2 or A4 pulleys are absent, they must be reconstructed. Synthetic materials have proven to be inadequate. Reconstruction with a tendon graft or extensor retinaculum are current favorites (32,33). We prefer the former method, using a 2-mm thick slip of the resected profundus tendon. The rod is placed through the carpal tunnel with sev-

Table 8–4
Stage II: Flexor Tendon Reconstruction—Rod-Graft

Incisions
    Distal—over profundus insertion
    Proximal—distal forearm

Tendon Graft (according to level of repair)
    Palm—palmaris
    Forearm—plantaris, toe extensor

Tendon Attachment
    Distal—Drill hole (Bunnell button—pull-out suture)
    Proximal
        Tendon ends equal, end-to-end repair
        Tendon ends unequal, brand repair

---

eral centimeters left free in the forearm to make later identification easier. If the digital nerves are injured, direct repair is preferred but grafts are usually required. Dressings are discarded 2 days post rod placement and active and passive motion begun.

Duration of Rod Implant

In our series of 29 rod implants followed by tendon grafting, the rod was left in place from 70 to 168 days (median, 110 days). When the percent recovery in ROM was plotted against the duration of rod implant, there was no significant difference in the final functional result if the rod had been in place any time between 70 and 168 days (18).

SECOND STAGE OF FLEXOR MECHANISM RECONSTRUCTION

If the rod cannot be palpated at the distal phalanx preoperatively, a lateral x ray can be helpful in locating the distal end of the rod. If it has retracted into the palm, the operative procedure will be replacement of the rod. If the rod is in proper position, the operative procedure is outlined in Table 8–4. The surgeon reenters the skin incision over the DIP joint and identifies the distal end of the rod. An L-shaped incision is made over the distal forearm. The forearm fascia is opened, the median nerve and superficialis tendons retracted, and the appropriate profundus tendon identified. The proximal rod end is identified. The proximal end of the tendon is drawn into the wrist. The end may be trimmed, but is left as long as possible. If the proximal end of the profundus tendon has been left long, the palmaris will reach the distal phalanx. If the profundus tendon has been resected in the distal forearm, the plantaris or a toe extensor is required to provide adequate length. After the proximal repair has been accomplished, the graft is sutured to the proximal end of the rod and advanced to the distal phalanx. Tension is determined and attachment of the graft distally is accomplished as described earlier. Postoperative management is as described under tendon grafting.

RESULTS OF TWO-STAGE FLEXOR TENDON RECONSTRUCTION

Hunter and Salisbury (34) reported results significantly better than the average results following primary repair in zone II injuries. Grafts were placed in 69 fingers (of 63 patients)

with varying severity of injury, though all required two-stage grafting. After recovery, 59 (85.5%) were able to flex to within 3.2 cm of the distal palmar crease, 35 (50%) to 1.9 cm or less.

Wehbe and others (35) performed two-stage reconstructions in 150 fingers of 136 patients. Of these, 45% were of the most severe level, presenting initially with additional nerve or vascular injury and/or contraction greater than 10° at any joint. The plantaris tendon was used preferentially (49.3%), with toe extensors a second choice (38.7%). The graft was attached to the distal phalanx by a pullout wire tied over a button in 91.8%, and a Pulvertaft weave was used for the proximal anastomosis in 93.3%. Preoperatively, the mean palm to pulp active distance was 41 mm. At final follow-up, this had improved to 15 mm. The mean grip strength increased from 21 to 70% of normal. Patients less than 21 years of age obtained better results. Results were worse in more severely damaged fingers and in patients with multiple injured rays. The complication rates were 28.7% and 43.0% for stages I and II respectively. The most common complication after stage I was synovitis (27% of fingers); after stage II it was bowstringing at the PIP joint (21.5%) followed by tendon rupture and adhesions requiring tenolysis (14.1% and 12.4%).

In our series (18) of 29 two-stage reconstructions, 62% obtained fair to excellent results and 38% poor results. All patients were followed for at least 52 weeks. One patient was considered a graft failure because of extensive scar. He regained only 99° of total active ROM. One patient sustained a disruption of the insertion of the tendon graft into the distal phalanx on the 25th day after surgery; this was reattached 2 days later. At 52 weeks he had regained 240° of total active ROM in the finger. One rod became exposed and required removal. The rod was reinserted after the skin wound had been healed for 3 months, and the patient gained 188° of total active ROM at 52 weeks.

TWO-STAGE TENDON GRAFTING FOR ISOLATED PROFUNDUS INJURY

Gaisford and colleagues (9) first suggested two-stage reconstruction after isolated profundus injury. Versaci (36) reported a series of five patients in which three obtained a near normal DIP active ROM, a 4th patient had nearly as good a result (though a pulley reconstruction was required), and a 5th patient obtained approximately twenty percent of active DIP flexion. It was noted that the patients obtaining the best results had the least damaged fingers preoperatively. Wilson and others (8) performed 12 profundus grafts in 11 patients. The mean total active ROM after operation was 166°; post–second stage grafting, this had increased to 240°. Digital pad-to-palm distance with active flexion was not reported. Eight patients presented with weakened grip compared to the normal hand; postoperatively, all were improved. One patient experienced a tendon graft rupture. All patients were young and highly motivated.

The three patients obtaining the best results in Versaci's series had the best preoperative digital condition. The patients in Wilson's series all had profundus avulsions or lacerations. In Sullivan's series (37), 4 sustained profundus avulsions and 12 sustained zone I lacerations. These injuries are limited to the injured tendon (38). The best results were obtained in the younger patients. These results are not clearly better than those obtained in a similar patient population utilizing single-stage grafting. The cost of this option is a longer treatment period, a second operation, and the possibility of additional complications associated with the second stage of the procedure.

INADEQUATE FUNCTION AFTER TWO-STAGE REPAIR

The primary causes of inadequate function after rod-graft repair are mallet deformity (here resulting not from extensor disruption but from mechanical factors contributing to increased flexion moment at the DIP joint), stiff joint, and tendon adhesions. The only treatment we have found adequate for the mallet deformity is fusion of the DIP joint. Before fusion, the patient makes a decision regarding the amount of flexion needed to provide the best function.

TENDON ADHESIONS OR STIFF JOINTS

Tendon adhesions and/or stiff joints may develop after a two-stage reconstruction. Hunter and Salisbury (34) report a 6.7% tenolysis rate; Chamay (39) performed tenolysis in 21% of patients undergoing two-stage reconstruction. Neither study reported results of this procedure. As noted earlier, LaSalle and Strickland's (40) series reported a 46.5% tenolysis rate with one rupture and significant improvement in 60% of these fingers.

We recommend capsulotomy or tenolysis, with the recognition that this is the last alternative. If unsuccessful, amputation should be discussed; but the decision is delayed until the patient requests amputation, often only reaching acceptance after a return to work. Unfortunately, some patients enter a repetitive cycle of operation and reoperation, undergoing many procedures that do little toward improving function. Use of a second rod, then graft, requires much discussion with the patient because of the time, expense, and generally disappointing ultimate outcome. At this point in management, judgment has its greatest impact—judgment gained by experience, both good and bad. Knowing the appropriate time to call a halt to operative intervention can only be gained through experience and concern for the patient.

Extensor Tendon Grafting

Extensor tendon grafting is a less frequently utilized procedure than that for flexor tendon defects. The very delicate nature of the balance of forces in the extensor hood mechanism makes the use of extensor tendon grafts in this area much more difficult. While free tendon material has been used in the reconstruction of boutonniere deformities and to reconstruct the extensor hood mechanism, these are infrequently applied procedures and do not constitute true intercalated tendon grafts. More commonly, extensor tendon grafts have been used in the extensor zones VI and VII for the reconstruction or repair of ruptured extensor tendons. The most common application of tendon grafting is for the extensor pollicis longus following rupture within the third dorsal compartment. While we find the extensor indicis proprius transfer remains a favorite procedure for this problem, other authors (41) have successfully applied free tendon grafts in dealing with the ruptured extensor pollicis longus. Common extensor tendon ruptures in patients with rheumatoid arthritis have also been effectively treated with free tendon grafts in the extensor zones VI and VII.

Traumatic injuries in zones V and VI have been successfully treated with free tendon grafts placed beneath soft tissue flaps attached to the dorsum of the hand (42,43). The use of Silastic rods for the development of a pseudo tendon sheath has also proven useful in selected cases. This technique has also been employed in injuries to zones I through V with inconsistent results.

An additional use of free tendon grafts has been to lengthen tendons in tendon transfer procedures where the length of the donor tendon is insufficient to reach the recipient.

EXTENSOR POLLICIS LONGUS RECONSTRUCTION

Surgical Technique

The most common rupture site of the extensor pollicis longus is at or in the third dorsal compartment. These injuries are seen in individuals with rheumatoid arthritis or following trauma, in particular as a late complication of a Colles' fracture. An incision is usually made just distal to Lister's tubercle, which allows access to an area where the surgeon is most likely to find the distal extensor tendon end. An incision may be carried proximally to the proximal edge of the extensor retinaculum where the proximal end of the extensor pollicis longus tendon may be located. In general, we recommend that the tendon graft be placed in a subcutaneous plane rather than through the third dorsal compartment; this will help avoid any problem of recurrence due to anatomical abnormalities within the third dorsal compartment. Once the proximal and distal ends of the extensor tendon have been isolated, a free graft is harvested.

Postoperative Management

Our initial operative dressing includes one that places the wrist in 20° to 30° of extension and holds the thumb in full extension. In the early postoperative period the surgeon refers the patient to the hand rehabilitation specialist, and a thermoplastic splint is fabricated that maintains the thumb in the position established at the time of the operation (Fig. 8–7). Our protocol requires that the thumb be maintained in extension for 3 weeks, at which point we begin mobilization. Between weeks 3 and 4, the patient's splint is brought down to neutral and active flexion is begun with the thumb. Protective splinting is continued between exercise sessions. Between weeks 4 and 5, passive motion is initiated, if necessary, to achieve full mobilization of the thumb. The splint is discontinued at the start of the 6th week. Active and passive ROM exercises and, if necessary, dynamic splinting are continued until week 7 or 8, as necessary to achieve full mobilization of the thumb.

An alternative rehabilitation protocol that we have used on occasion includes an active flexion–passive extension dynamic splinting in the early postoperative period (44,45). The use of static splinting for 3 weeks has provided good results, even though initially the patients are quite stiff in extension. The dynamic splinting was initiated in an attempt to accelerate the return to normal ROM and has been used, infrequently, at our institution. Both methods have provided good long-term results.

EXTENSOR TENDON GRAFTS IN MULTIPLE EXTENSOR TENDON RUPTURES

The next most common problem where tendon grafts may be useful is rupture of multiple extensor tendons. This is usually seen in the patient with rheumatoid arthritis, the ruptures of

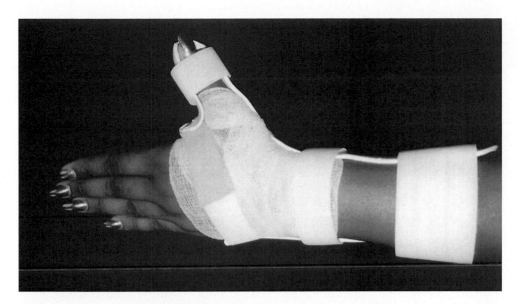

FIG. 8–7. We have found the thermoplastic splint to be the most comfortable method of maintaining extension and immobilization of the thumb.

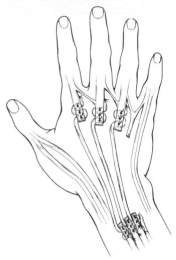

FIG. 8–8. Extensor tendon grafts sutured individually are useful for more distal traumatic loss.

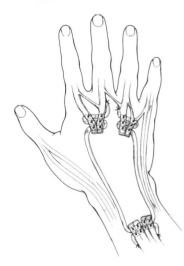

FIG. 8–9. Suturing in pairs minimizes the amount of donor graft needed and provides satisfactory results.

the extensor tendons often beginning at the little finger and then progressing radially across the hand to involve the ring, the long, and sometimes the index, finger. With a single extensor tendon rupture, reconstruction can be handled either by a free tendon graft or a side-to-side transfer. With patients who have rupture of multiple extensor tendons involving two or more fingers, the use of side-to-side transfers is often inadequate. In this case, reconstruction can proceed with multiple tendon transfers or with one or more extensor tendon grafts to the common extensors of the fingers. As in other tendon grafting procedures, the first choice for a tendon graft donor will be the palmaris longus. When looping or multiple tendon grafts are required, the plantaris tendon may prove to be more useful because of its extended length.

Surgical Technique

The tendon graft may be sutured individually, intercalated between each of the common ruptured tendons (Fig. 8–8). More commonly, if all four fingers are involved we will apply a single tendon graft to pairs of tendon slips, weaving each attach-

ment (Fig. 8–9). A common looped procedure has been described by Bora (46) that incorporates all the common ruptured tendons as a single conjoined tendon, interdigitating through the proximal and distal tendon stumps and itself.

Tension on the tendon graft incorporating multiple extensor tendons needs to be adjusted carefully. One must be certain that all fingers are under roughly comparable tension so that one digit does not lag behind the others when extending the fingers.

Postoperative Management

As in the flexor tendon grafting and the previously mentioned extensor tendon grafting for the thumb, one of the most critical areas of concern is the postoperative management of these tendons. Our typical protocol is to maintain the tendons in a static extension splinting for 3 weeks. During the 4th week, dynamic active motion is begun that includes an active flexion and passive extension (Fig. 8–10). The patient is maintained with the dynamic splinting for 2 to 3 weeks, and then the splinting is weaned and motion is in-

FIG. 8–10. We have successfully used the active flexion–passive extension protocol with the illustrated splint for earlier mobilization.

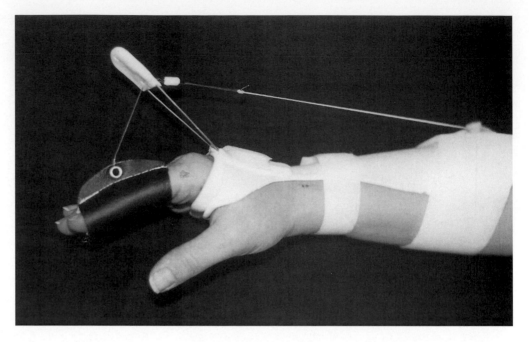

creased. Full active flexion with the wrist in neutral is allowed at 5 weeks. Rehabilitation therapy continues for 7 to 8 weeks until function is maximized.

EXTENSOR TENDON GRAFTS BENEATH FLAPS

In patients who have avulsion injuries to the dorsum of the hand with missing skin, soft tissue, and extensor tendons, extensor tendon reconstruction is generally preceded by soft-tissue coverage. For those with bony involvement, skeletal stabilization is achieved first and followed by soft-tissue reconstruction. If complete loss of soft tissue is present, the most appropriate coverage will be that of a pedicled or free flap. Pedicle flaps (e.g., a reversed radial-artery forearm flap) are convenient and reliable. Free flaps provide a wide variety of reconstructive choices that include adequate tissue coverage for future extensor tendon reconstruction. Studies show mixed results on immediate reconstruction with tendons grafts placed through free flaps at the time of flap coverage (42). Our practice has been to establish the soft-tissue coverage before tendon grafting and to perform the tendon grafting at a separate procedure. Grafting may be achieved using multiple tendon strips, especially when extensor tendon loss extends to the level of the extensor hoods. For more proximal losses, the reconstruction can be done in a conjoined or looped fashion, as described above, for those patients who have rheumatoid arthritis. In cases where significant scarring is anticipated on the dorsum of the hand after soft tissue coverage, placement of Silastic rods may be useful to form tunnels into which the planned grafts may be routed.

Extensor tendon graft after soft tissue closure is postponed until the flap or soft-tissue reconstruction has softened and matured. If Silastic rods were used, we like to wait a minimum of 8 to 12 weeks before grafting. Tension is established using the previously mentioned techniques to allow for full extension of the fingers when the wrist is flexed and nearly full flexion of the MP joints when the wrist is fully extended. Postoperative management of these patients generally calls for a static splint for 3 weeks and then initiation of protected

active motion. Sometimes enough scar forms that rods may be removed with adequate function assured and no need for second-stage tendon graft.

OTHER EXTENSOR TENDON GRAFTS

There are other potential uses for extensor tendons grafts that are more fully explained in the appropriate sections. These include extensor tendon grafts used to elongate tendons for extensor tendon transfers. The harvest and tension-adjustment procedures are similar to those described above. The particulars of the operative procedure would depend on the exact tendon transfers being used.

Additionally, free tendon grafts may be used to reconstruct extensor tendon hoods, such as cases of chronic boutonniere deformities or rupture of the extensor hood at the MP joints. In these cases the tendons are being used more as a suture or fascial retaining material than as free tendon grafts.

There have been anecdotal reports of the use of Silastic rods extending to the distal interphalangeal joints followed by free tendon grafts placed into the pseudo-sheath; results are mixed. Microvascular grafts have been described for complex injuries (47).

Results

Results of extensor tendon grafting for reconstruction of a ruptured extensor pollicis longus have, in general, been excellent. We have found little difference long-term in the outcome of those individuals who have undergone extensor tendon postoperative management in either a static or a dynamic protocol. Recent reports in the *Journal of Hand Therapy* found no significant differences between these two protocols for extensor tendon management in zone III and IV injuries (48). A series of 21 patients treated with flexor tendon grafts for reconstruction of the extensor pollicis longus was reported by Magnell and colleagues in the *Journal of Hand Surgery* in 1988 (41). They compared the final ROM of the involved hand with that of the opposite side and reported excellent results almost uniformly. Their outcomes were reported in terms of loss of motion. They reported losses of 6° at the interphalangeal joint, 3° at the MP joint, and 10° with composite flexion–extension. In addition, they found only a 7% decrease in pinch strength compared to the opposite side. All were considered to be excellent results. The obvious advantage of the tendon graft for this disorder is that it precludes the need to sacrifice the extensor indicis proprius. The results for tendon grafts to multiple digits have not been quite as satisfactory, with long-term results quite varied. This may reflect the fact that the patient is typically one with advanced rheumatoid arthritis. Bora and others reported an average of 65° total motion at the MP joints in twenty patients (46). This was achieved with an average extensor lag of 30° and average flexion of 95°.

Summary

Flexor and extensor tendon grafting is a useful technique for restoring function to damaged fingers. The surgical techniques are not overly complicated but do require attention to detail in handling tissue, establishing the proper tension, and obtaining a satisfactory environment for the graft before surgery. Adequate hand therapy is necessary to obtain best results. We point out that improved results can be obtained in patients with unsatisfactory outcomes in selected cases with tenolysis, capsulotomy, and (as always) aggressive and expert hand therapy. All of these factors combined often produce rewarding results.

Bibliography

1. Jones MW, Matthews JP. Flexor tendon grafting 48 years after injury. *J Hand Surg [Br]* 1988; 13:284.
2. Young VL, Wrap C, Weeks PM. The surgical management of stiff joints in the hand. *Plast Reconstr Surg* 1978; 62:835.
3. White WL. Tendon grafts: a consideration of their source, procurement and suitability. *Surg Clin North Am* 1960; 40:403.
4. Harvey FJ, Chu G, Harvey PM. Surgical availability of the plantaris tendon. *J Hand Surg* 1983; 8:243.
5. Vastamaki M. Median nerve as free tendon graft. *J Hand Surg [Br]* 1987; 12:187.
6. Aulicino PL, Ainsworth SR, Parker M. The independent long extensor tendon of the fifth toe as a source of tendon grafts for the hand. *J Hand Surg [Br]* 1989; 14:236.
7. Holm CL, Embrick RR. Anatomical consideration in the primary treatment of tendon injuries of the hand. *J Bone Joint Surg [Am]* 1959; 41: 599.
8. Wilson RL, Carter MS, Holdeman VA, et al. Flexor profundus injuries treated with delayed two-staged tendon grafting. *J Hand Surg* 1980; 5:74.
9. Gaisford JC, Hanna DC, Richardson GS. Tendon grafting: a suggested technique. *Plast Reconstr Surg* 1966; 38:302.
10. Pulvertaft RG. Suture materials and tendon junctures. *Am J Surg* 1965; 109:346.
11. Stark HH, Zemel NP, Boyes JH, et al. Flexor tendon graft through intact superficialis tendons. *J Hand Surg* 1977; 2:456.
12. McClinton MA, Curtis RM, Wilgis EF. One hundred tendon grafts for isolated flexor digitorum profundus injuries. *J Hand Surg* 1982; 7:224.
13. Bora FW. Profundus tendon grafting with unimpaired sublimus function in children. *Clin Orthop Rel Res* 1970; 71:118.
14. Pulvertaft GR. Tendon grafting for the isolated injury of flexor digitorum profundus. *Bull Hosp Jt Dis Orthop Inst* 1984; 44:424.
15. Entin MA. Flexor tendon repair and grafting in children. *Am J Surg* 1965; 109:387.
16. Wakefield AR. The treatment of tendon injuries in children. Presented at the annual meeting of the American Society for Surgery of the Hand, Chicago, January 17, 1964.
17. Weeks PM, Wray RC. Rate and extent of functional recovery after flexor tendon grafting with and without silicone rod preparation. *J Hand Surg* 1976; 1:174.
18. Boyes JH, Stark HH. Flexor-tendon grafts in the fingers and thumb. *J Bone Joint Surg [Am]* 1971; 53:1332.
19. Kunzle AL, Brunelli G, Orsi R. Flexor tendon grafts in the fingers. *J Hand Surg [Br]* 1984; 9:126.
20. Stark HH, Anderson DR, Zemel NP, et al. Bridge flexor tendon grafts. *Clin Orthop Rel Res* 1989; 242:51.
21. Strickland JW. Flexor tenolysis. *Hand Clinics* 1985; 1:121.
22. Young VL, Clement R, Weeks PM, et al. Effectiveness of the proximal interphalangeal joint capsulotomy. Proceedings of the American Society for Surgery of the Hand. *J Hand Surg* 1984; 9:671.
23. Verdan CE. Primary and secondary repair of flexor and extensor tendon injuries. In: Flynn JE, ed. *Hand surgery.* Baltimore: Williams & Wilkins, 1966; 220–274.
24. Kleinert HE, Kutz JE, Ashbell TS, et al. Primary repair of lacerated flexor tendons in "no-man's land." *J Bone Joint Surg [Am]* 1967; 49:577.
25. Pulvertaft RG. Tendon grafts for flexor tendon injuries in the fingers and thumb. *J Bone Joint Surg [Br]* 1956; 38:175.
26. Wray RC, Moucharafafieh B, Braitberg R, et al. The optimal time for tenolysis. *Plast Reconstr Surg* 1978; 61:184.
27. Kelly AP Jr. Primary tendon repairs. *J Bone Joint Surg [Am]* 1959; 41:581.
28. McCash CR. The immediate repair of flexor tendons. *Br J Plast Surg* 1961; 14:53.
29. Fetrow KO. Tenolysis in the hand and wrist. *J Bone Joint Surg [Am]* 1967; 49:667.
30. Hunter JM. Staged flexor tendon reconstruction. *J Hand Surg* 1983; 8:789.
31. Rayner CR. The origin and nature of pseudo-synovium appearing around implanted silastic rods: An experimental study. *The Hand* 1976; 8:101.
32. Kleinert HE, Bennett JB. Digital pulley reconstruction employing the always present rim of the previous pulley. *J Hand Surg* 1978; 3:297.
33. Lister GD. Reconstruction of pulleys employing extensor retinaculum. *J Hand Surg* 1979; 4:461.
34. Hunter JM, Salisbury RE. Flexor-tendon reconstruction in severely damaged hands: a two-staged procedure using a silicone–Dacron reinforced gliding prosthesis prior to tendon grafting. *J Bone Joint Surg* 1971; 53:829.
35. Wehbe MA, Hunter JM, Schneider LH, et al. Two-stage flexor-tendon reconstruction. *J Bone Joint Surg [Am]* 1986; 68:752.
36. Versaci AD. Secondary tendon grafting for isolated flexor digitorum profundus injury. *Plast Reconstr Surg* 1970; 46:57.
37. Sullivan DJ. Disappointing outcomes in staged flexor tendon grafting for isolated profundus loss. *J Hand Surg [Br]* 1986; 11:231.
38. Chang WH, Thoms OJ, White WL. Avulsion injury of the long flexor tendons. *Plast Reconstr Surg* 1972; 50:260.
39. Chamay A, Verdan C, Simonette C. The two-stage graft: a salvage operation for the flexor apparatus (a clinical study of 28 cases). In: Verdan C, ed. *Tendon surgery of the hand.* London: Churchill Livingstone, 1979; 109–112.
40. LaSalle WB, Strickland JW. An evaluation of the two-staged flexor tendon reconstruction technique. *J Hand Surg* 1983; 8:263.
41. Magnell TD, Pochron MD, Condit DP. The intercalated tendon graft for treatment of extensor pollicis longus tendon ruptures. *J Hand Surg [Am]* 1988; 13:105–109.
42. Scheker LR, Langley, SJ, Martin DL, et al. Primary extensor tendon reconstruction in dorsal hand defects requiring free flaps. *J Hand Surg [Br]* 1993; 18:568–575.
43. Reid DAC. Hand injuries requiring skin replacement and restoration of tendon functions. *Brit J Plastic Surgery* 1984; 27:5–18.
44. Hung LK, Chan A, Chang J, et al. Early controlled active mobilization with dynamic splintage for treatment of extensor tendon injuries. *J Hand Surg [Am]* 1990; 15:251–257.
45. Browne EZ, Ribik CA. Early dynamic splinting for extensor tendon injuries. *J Hand Surg [Am]* 1989; 14:72–76.
46. Bora FW, Osterman AL, Thomas VJ, et al. The treatment of ruptures of multiple extensor tendons at wrist level by a free tendon graft in the rheumatoid patient. *J Hand Surg [Am]* 1987; 12:1038–1040.
47. Desai SS, Chuang DC, Levin LS. Microsurgical reconstruction of the extensor system. *Hand Clin* 1995; 11:471.
48. Walsh MT, Rinehimer PT, Muntzer E, et. al. Early controlled motion with dynamic splinting versus static splinting for zones III and IV extensor tendon lacerations: a preliminary report. *J Hand Therapy* 1994; 7:232–236.

9

Principles of Cartilage Grafting

Joel E. Pessa, M.D., F.A.C.S., and Ronald Riefkohl, M.D., F.A.C.S.

Autogenous Cartilage

Autogenous cartilage is a versatile, dependable tissue that is readily available from a number of donor sites. Cartilage, like other autogenous tissues, has an extremely low infection rate, even when transplanted into a relatively avascular area. It is malleable and can be shaped and contoured by current techniques to match almost any existing structure. These qualities make cartilage grafting an indispensible technique for the reconstructive plastic surgeon.

TYPES OF CARTILAGE

Cartilage is categorized into three types according to the characteristics of its intercellular matrix: hyaline, elastic, and fibrocartilage. Although the different types of cartilage behave similarly when transplanted, in that volume is maintained without stress or vascular ingrowth, each has intrinsic properties that help meet specific goals. For example, hyaline cartilage, of which septum is the best example, is relatively rigid and lends itself best to structural support. Lower lateral cartilage, a type of elastic cartilage, is more malleable and is excellent for restoring form and shape on the nasal tip.

In general, autogenous cartilage grafts can be used by the plastic surgeon to achieve 3 different goals: (a) simple volume replacement, (b) structural support, and (c) as architectural support to create new form. Various techniques are available to adapt cartilage to fulfill these goals.

HISTORICAL REVIEW

Although it is presently taken for granted that autogenous cartilage readily survives transplantation, this is a relatively recent development. Bert (1) is credited with being the first, in 1865, to transplant cartilage in animals, and Koenig (2) was the first, in 1896, to use autogenous cartilage in humans to repair damaged tracheal cartilage. However, the modern era of cartilage transplantation was ushered in by Peer in 1941 (3). The results of several studies were later published in his classic treatise *Transplantation of Tissues* (4). Before that, neither otolaryngologists nor plastic surgeons believed that transplanted cartilage would survive. The reliability and survival of transplanted cartilage has since been confirmed in long-term studies (5,6).

SOURCES OF CARTILAGE

The most common uses of autogenous cartilage encountered by the plastic surgeon include ear reconstruction, eyelid reconstruction, and aesthetic and reconstructive rhinoplasty.

The donor site is determined primarily by the intended use of the cartilage graft.

Ear reconstruction relies heavily on autogenous costal cartilage taken from the 7th, 8th, and 9th ribs (7–13) (Fig. 9–1). Costal cartilage can be harvested subperichondrially to allow for regeneration in the young patient (14). This cartilage can also be used for nasal alar and dorsum reconstruction (15–17), provided the patient's skin is relatively thick so that a step-off deformity is not created. A disadvantage of costal cartilage is its tendency to warp with time unless trimmed to balance the intrinsic tension forces (18).

Elastic ear cartilage has found widespread use for lower eyelid support (19–21), and can be taken as a simple graft or as a composite chondromucosal graft. Other uses of ear cartilage include nipple areola reconstruction (22), reconstruction of the orbital floor (23,24), and temporomandibular joint (TMJ) repair (25). Conchal cartilage can be harvested by either an anterior or posterior approach (Fig. 9–2), although the authors favor the posterior approach due to the inconspicuous scar. When harvesting conchal cartilage, the use of a postoperative drain can be obviated by using a firm dressing (26). One must also be careful in harvesting the conchal cartilage graft to avoid a visible step-off deformity (27).

Nasal septal cartilage, an example of hyaline cartilage, is

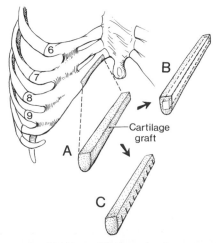

FIG. 9–1. A, appropriate chondral area showing an excellent source of varied sizes of cartilage. To minimize distortion of cartilage, the center of the cartilage graft is used **(B),** or scoring of the opposite side of the expected distortion is carried out **(C).**

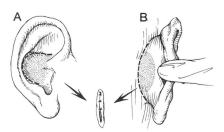

FIG. 9–2. **A,** anterior approach to the chondral cartilage. The curvature of the cartilage in this area is suitable for replacing an orbital defect. **B,** posterior auricular approach to the ear cartilage. Note the possibility of contouring cartilage for a nasal dorsal graft.

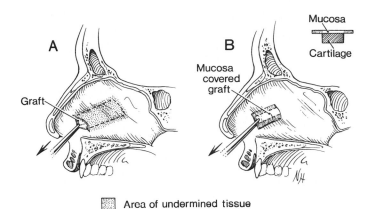

Area of undermined tissue

FIG. 9–3. **A,** septal cartilage graft being harvested. Care is taken to use a suitable graft from the lower septum to minimize the possibility of collapse of overlying cartilage. **B,** chondromucosal graft is satisfactorily obtained from the septum as the donor area.

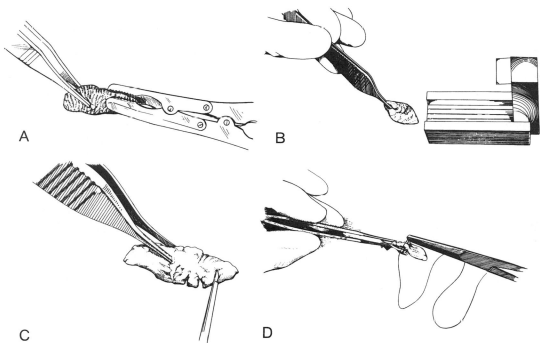

FIG. 9–4. **A,** technique of morselizing and softening the cartilage graft. **B,** use of the linear morselizer. **C,** technique of cross-cutting the cartilage. **D,** morselized cartilage can be shaped and tied with 5.0 nylon sutures.

most readily adapted to nasal reconstruction (28,29). Septal cartilage is harvested by a submucosal dissection; care must be taken to leave a 1-cm strut anteriorly and caudally to avoid a postoperative saddle-nose deformity or retrusive columella (Fig. 9–3).

TECHNIQUES

A number of techniques exist to modify the shape of the cartilage graft (30,31) (Fig. 9–4A, B). Perichondrium can be scored and, when performed on the concave surface, allows the graft to straighten (Fig. 9–4B). Alternately, cartilage can be abraded with similar effect. A more pronounced effect can be obtained by cross-cutting the edges of the cartilage (Fig. 9–4C). Cartilage can also be diced to be used as a volume

filler (32) or to reconstruct Montgomery tubercles (22). Cartilage can be used as single or multitiered grafts (Fig. 9–4D), further extending its role in volume augmentation. Cartilage can also be modified by combining it with other tissues as a composite graft (33,34), or by wrapping it with temporalis fascia to soften the result (35,36).

Many techniques hold promise for the future of cartilage transplantation, including banked cartilage, homologous and treated xenograft cartilage (37,38), and the perichondrocutaneous graft (39). Bioengineered and prefabricated cartilage seem likely to become a clinical tool in the near future (40,41). All these techniques stem from our basic understanding that cartilage reliably survives transplantation, and is readily adapted by the surgeon to fulfill a myriad of reconstructive procedures.

References

1. Bert P. Sur la greffe animale. *CR Acad Sci* 1865; 51:587.
2. Koenig F. Uber reaktive vorgange am knorpel nach verschieden schadigungen. *Arch Klin Chir* 1923; 124:1.
3. Peer LA. Fate of autogenous septal cartilage after transplantation in human tissues. *Arch Otolaryng* 1941; 34:696.
4. Peer LA. *Transplantation of tissues.* Baltimore: William & Wilkins, 1955.
5. Peer LA. Cartilage grafting. *Surg Clin North Am* 1944; 24:404.
6. Sheen JH. Tip graft: a 20-year retrospective. *Plast Reconstr Surg* 1993; 91:48.
7. Tanzer RC. Total reconstruction of the external ear. *Plast Reconstr Surg* 1959; 23:1.
8. Brent B. The correction of microtia with autogenous cartilage grafts: the classic deformity. *Plast Reconstr Surg* 1980; 66:1.
9. Brent B. The correction of microtia with autogenous cartilage grafts: atypical and complex deformities. *Plast Reconstr Surg* 1980; 66:13.
10. Fukuda O, Yamada A. Reconstruction of the microtic ear with autogenous cartilage. *Clin Plast Surg* 1978; 5:351.
11. Nagata S. Grafting the three-dimensional costal cartilage framework for lobule type microtia. *Plast Reconstr Surg* 1994; 93:221.
12. Nagata S. Grafting the three-dimensional costal cartilage framework for concha type microtia. *Plast Reconstr Surg* 1994; 93:231.
13. Nagata S. Grafting the three-dimensional costal cartilage framework for small concha-type microtia. *Plast Reconstr Surg* 1994; 93:243.
14. Lester CW. Tissue replacement after subperichondrial resection of costal cartilage: two case reports. *Plast Reconstr Surg* 1959; 23:49.
15. Chait LA, Fayman MS. Treatment of postreconstructive collapsed nasal ala with a costal cartilage graft. *Plast Reconstr Surg* 1988; 82:527.
16. Furlan S. Correction of saddle nose deformities by costal cartilage grafts: a technique. *Ann Plast Surg* 1982; 9:32.
17. Gunter JP, Rohrich RJ. Augmentation rhinoplasty: dorsal onlay grafting using shaped autogenous septal cartilage. *Plast Reconstr Surg* 1990; 86:39.
18. Gibson T, Davies WB. The distortion of autogenous cartilage grafts: its cause and prevention. *Br J Plast Surg* 1958; 10:257.
19. Jackson IT, Dubin B, Harris J. Use of contoured and stabilized conchal cartilage grafts for lower eyelid support: a preliminary report. *Plast Reconstr Surg* 1989; 83:636.
20. Matsuo K, Hirose F, Takahashi N. Lower eyelid reconstruction with a conchal cartilage graft. *Plast Reconstr Surg* 1987; 80:547.
21. Marks MW, Argenta LC, Fiedman RJ. Conchal cartilage and composite grafts for correction of lower eyelid retraction. *Plast Reconstr Surg* 1989; 83:629.
22. Brent N, Bostwick J. Nipple-areola reconstruction with auricular tissues. *Plast Reconstr Surg* 1977; 60:353.
23. Stark RB, Frileck SP. Conchal cartilage grafts in augmentation rhinoplasty and orbital floor fracture. *Plast Reconstr Surg* 1969; 43:591.
24. Constantian MB. Use of auricular cartilage in orbital floor reconstruction. *Plast Reconstr Surg* 1982; 69:951.
25. Tucker MR, Ingeborg MW. Autogenous auricular cartilage graft for temporomandibular joint repair. *J Cranio Max Fac Surg* 1991; 19:108.
26. Peck GC. *Techniques in aesthetic rhinoplasty.* New York: Thieme-Stratton, Gower Medical Publishing, 1984.
27. Guyuron B. Simplified harvesting of the ear cartilage graft. *Aesthetic Plast Surg* 1986; 10:37.
28. Teichgraeber MD, Wainwright MD. The treatment of nasal valve obstruction. *Plast Reconstr Surg* 1974; 93:1174.
29. Sheen JC. *Aesthetic rhinoplasty.* St. Louis: CV Mosby, 1981.
30. Aiach G. Simple and useful instruments in cartilage grafting. *Plast Reconstr Surg* 1995; 95:572.
31. Hoffman S. A silicone template to facilitate cartilage grafting in the nose. *Plast Reconstr Surg* 1989; 83:168.
32. Peer LA. Diced cartilage grafts. *Arch Otolaryng* 1943; 38:156.
33. Lehman JA, Garrett WS, Musgrave RH. Earlobe composite grafts for the correction of nasal defects. *Plast Reconstr Surg* 1971; 47:12.
34. Cosman B. Piggyback composite ear grafts in nasal ala reconstruction. *Ann Plast Surg* 1980; 5:293.
35. Siemian WR, Samiian MR. Malar augmentation using autogenous composite conchal cartilage and temporalis fascia. *Plast Reconstr Surg* 1988; 82:395.
36. Guerrerosantos J. Recontouring the middle third of the face with onlay cartilage plus free fascia graft. *Ann Plast Surg* 1987; 18:409.
37. Sailer HF. Experiences with the use of lyophilized banked cartilage for facial contour correction. *J Max Fac Surg* 1976; 4:149.
38. Ersek RA, Delerm AG. Processed irradiated bovine cartilage for nasal reconstruction. *Ann Plast Surg* 1988; 20:540.
39. Brent B. The versatile cartilage autograft: Current trends in clinical transplantation. *Clin Plast Surg* 1979; 6:163.
40. Bujia J, et al. Engineering of cartilage tissue using bioresorbable polymerfleeces and perfusion culture. *Acta Otolaryngol Stockh* 1995; 115:307.
41. Kim WS, et al. Cartilage engineered in predetermined shapes employing cell transplantation on synthetic biodegradable polymers. *Plast Reconstr Surg* 1994; 94, 223.

10

Basic Principles of Nerve Grafting

Hano Millesi, M.D.

To achieve function, axons must enter the graft at the proximal site of coaptation, proceed along the graft, cross over to the distal stump, and proceed to the end organ. The nerve graft is not a substitute for the lost segment of a nerve; rather, it provides an environment in which axons of the proximal stump can cross the defect. Thus, nerve grafts are akin to a guiding rail. Even though this conceptualization is basically correct, it has been the source of a number of mistakes. Materials other than living nerve tissue might be just as suitable and more efficient if nerve grafts functioned only as a bridging mechanism. Based on this theory, nonvital nerve grafts and alloplastic materials have been used, with consistently poor results to date.

Although the nerve graft *is* a guiding rail, this statement must be augmented by specifying those tissues for which it provides a passageway. Axons and axon branches need an environment provided by Schwann cells. A necessary additional function of these cells is the production of myelinated nerve fibers. Only if the Schwann cells have survived the grafting procedure can a graft serve as a railway for axons and thereby contain all of the necessary elements identical to the distal nerve stump.

In contrast, a nonviable (preserved) nerve graft provides a rail for a neuroma, with new growth occurring along the preserved graft. This method of nerve regeneration was studied by Schröder and Seiffert (1), who referred to it as "neuromatous neurotization." For return of function, there is little doubt that this approach offers a less optimal chance of success.

Return of function can only be expected after the axons have crossed both sites of coaptation—the proximal and distal ends of the graft. Because of this requirement, nerve grafting did not become widely accepted for some time. The basic argument was that if there was difficulty in axons crossing from one stump to another in an end-to-end nerve repair, it would only be compounded by the need to cross two coaptation sites.

This chapter covers some basic principles of nerve grafting, including the anatomy of peripheral nerves, principles of nerve regeneration, and essentials of nerve repair. A basic understanding of concepts is required because a generally accepted lexicon has not yet evolved and different authors use the same term without a common meaning.

Anatomical Structure of Peripheral Nerves

A *nerve trunk* consists of from one to many *fascicles* embedded in loose connective tissue (interfascicular epineurium) and surrounded by connective tissue (epifascicular epineurium). The *perineurium* consists of layers of mesothelial-like cells and collagen connective tissue. It envelopes the endoneurium and represents the demarcation between nonfascicular and fascicular tissues. It is responsible for the difference between the intrafascicular and extrafascicular environment of the nerve (the barrier function).

The endoneurial tissue within the fascicle contains *nerve fibers* with their endoneurial sheath. The central feature is the *axon,* surrounded by axolemma. In addition, the nerve fiber consists of Schwann cells with myelin sheath in myelinated nerve fibers, a basal lamina, and a loose collagen framework.

The individual fascicles must be able to move against each other in order to adapt to the deformations during movements of the limb. This possibility is provided by the loose connective tissue of the interfascicular epineurium.

To avoid mechanical irritations, the nerve trunk has to be able to move against the surrounding tissue during joint motions. This possibility is provided by layers of a loose connective tissue called the paraneurium or adventitia that surrounds the whole nerve trunk and links the nerve to the surrounding structures. This tissue is regarded as a part of the epifascicular epineurium by some authors, but it can be easily differentiated by its different structure.

The relationship between fascicular and nonfascicular tissue in cross-section is of practical importance. The fascicular pattern changes along the course of a nerve and has great individual variation. Five basic types of fascicular patterns can be distinguished:

1. *Monofascicular pattern.* The nerve consists of one large fascicle (Fig. 10–1A).
2. *Oligofascicular pattern with few large fascicles (up to five).* There is only minimal epineurial tissue between the fascicles. The individual fascicles can be handled easily from outside, and exact fascicular coaptation is provided by careful trunk-to-trunk coaptation.
3. *Oligofascicular pattern with more than five fascicles.* If the nerve segment consists of more than five large manageable fascicles, an exact fascicular coaptation is not guaranteed by trunk-to-trunk coaptation. The central fascicles cannot be controlled from the margin. A large quantity of interfascicular epineurium separates the individual fascicles. There is the danger that fascicular tissue may contact nonfascicular tissue. In a nerve trunk the fascicles are large enough to be separated and prepared individually for fascicular coaptation. A digital nerve with more than five fascicles does not meet this criterion; rather, it corresponds to a fascicle group (Fig. 10–1B, C).

4. *Polyfascicular pattern with group arrangement.* The nerve consists of many fascicles of different sizes, arranged in groups with wider spaces of epineural tissue between the groups (Fig. 10–1D).
5. *Polyfascicular pattern without group arrangement.* This pattern is one in which there are many fascicles of different sizes, diffusely arranged over the cross-section without group formation (Fig. 10–1E).

For surgical repair, the actual fascicular pattern must be known, and the distribution of motor and sensory fibers over the cross-section of the peripheral nerve is particularly important. Some investigators (2–4) have used electrical stimulation for sensory and motor fiber differentiation. This technique can only be applied during primary repair of the distal stump or with repair of the proximal stump in a conscious patient.

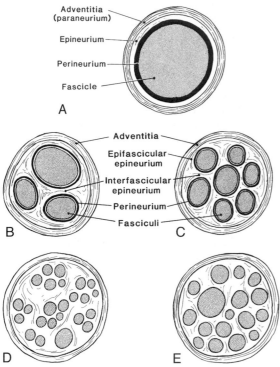

FIG. 10–1. Basic types of fascicular patterns are shown. **A,** the nerve segment consists of only one large fascicle. There is only marginal epineurial tissue (monofascicular structure). **B,** the nerve segment consists of a few large fascicles. There is only minimal epineurial tissue between the fascicles. Each fascicle can be handled easily from the margin (oligofascicular structure with 2–5 fascicles). **C,** The nerve segment consists of a certain number of fascicles (6 or more). The number is limited and the size of the fascicles is such that handling is easy. The central fascicle cannot be controlled from the margin. A large quantity of interfascicular epineurium separates the individual fascicles (oligofascicular pattern with 6 or more fascicles). **D,** the nerve segment consists of many larger and smaller fascicles. Size and number make handling difficult. There is a good quantity of interfascicular epineurium between the fascicles. The fascicles are arranged in groups (polyfascicular) pattern with group arrangement. **E,** there are many fascicles, varying in size, distributed diffusely over the cross-section, which makes surgical manipulation difficult (polyfascicular pattern without group arrangement).

Several investigators (5–7) have used staining techniques in differentiating motor and sensory fibers; a higher content of acetylcholinesterase is indicative of motor fibers. In many cases, a satisfactory image of the fascicular pattern can be obtained by retrograde tracing of the fascicles from the next branching back to the site of transection (8).

Principles of Nerve Regeneration

During nerve regeneration, there are two separate processes that develop simultaneously: (a) both stumps must heal to reestablish continuity, and (b) axon sprouts must cross from proximal to distal stump to reach the end organs. The gap between the two stumps is filled by fibrin, migrating fibroblasts, and outgrowing capillaries. After a period of 3 to 4 days, collagen fibers are produced. Fibroblasts originate from epifascicular and interfascicular epineurial tissue, the perineurium, and endoneurial tissue.

There are good reasons to believe that endoneurial and perineurial fibroblasts are more specialized for nerve tissue than epineurial fibroblasts. Schwann cells also migrate into the gap. In the normal environment of the axon (the endoneurium), there is a 9:1 ratio of Schwann cells to fibroblasts (9). If it can be assumed that this is an optimal relation, then the conclusion may be drawn that it is more favorable to axon sprouts when the tissue between the two nerve stumps contains a considerably higher quantity of Schwann cells than fibroblasts. Among the latter, endoneurial or perineurial fibroblasts are probably more desirable than epineurial fibroblasts. Based on the above analysis, it has been suggested that a strip of epineurial tissue be removed when repairing nerve segments of oligofascicular or grouped polyfascicular patterns (10–14).

Optimal conditions exist for nerve regeneration when axon sprouts can cross the gap between the nerve stumps in the early days after surgery (15). This can only occur when the axon sprouts originate close to the gap. Therefore, all damaged tissue of the proximal stump should be resected; otherwise it becomes fibrotic. Depending on the amount of retrograde degeneration, axon sprouts will then originate far more proximally and must grow along the fibrotic tissue of the stump before a delayed arrival at the gap. In the interim, the gap may be filled with collagen tissue, and the best opportunity for crossing has been lost.

If the axon sprouts do not meet a distal stump, they will form minifascicles with accompanying Schwann cells, fibroblasts, and capillaries, which have the potential to grow over some distance. A regeneration neuroma will be the result. Should the minifascicles meet the distal stump by random chance, there is some possibility of spontaneous healing of a transected nerve. Outgrowth of the minifascicles may be directed toward the distal stump by implanting a segment of an artery, an alloplastic tube, a mesothelial chamber (16), an empty perineurial tube (17), a vein (18), or a freeze-thawed muscle (19). It is an open question whether neurotization along a preformed structure, or within an empty space, corresponds in some way to the neuromatous nerve regeneration (1; Schröder and Seiffert) or whether it is a new way of nerve regeneration. When minifascicles meet a preserved nerve graft, the possibility of bridging a short defect occurs. Schröder and Seiffert refer to the latter event as "neuromatous nerve regeneration" (1).

Basic Principles of Nerve Repair

In the early days of peripheral nerve surgery, repair was by direct coaptation (cum carne). At that time, surgeons were unwilling to manipulate nerve stumps primarily. Coaptation was achieved by carefully adjusting the edges of other structures to each other. Hueter (20) sutured the tissue around the nerve. It is not clear whether the paraneurium or the epineurium was used for anchoring stitches.

A number of techniques have been developed for end-to-end repair of a transected nerve (neurorrhaphy), including:

1. Epineurial suture
2. Perineurial suture
3. Epiperineurial suture
4. Intrafascicular suture
5. Interfascicular guide suture

It becomes evident that the emphasis in labeling these techniques of neurorrhaphy was based on the type of tissue in which the anchoring stitches were placed. Actually, this is of little significance because sutureless techniques have been developed and compare favorably with a suturing approach. Further, to focus on the site of suture anchoring is an oversimplification. The main point is how well the fascicles of the cross-section coapt, and not so much where sutures are placed or whether sutures or glue are used to secure the coaptation.

Basically, a neurorrhaphy is performed in four steps: (a) preparation of the stumps, (b) approximation, (c) coaptation, and (d) maintaining the coaptation.

PREPARATION OF STUMPS

There are essentially two ways in which nerve stumps can be prepared: by resection or by interfascicular dissection.

Resection

Partial excision of the damaged sections of both stumps may be the approach selected in preparing the severed nerve for the next step of the procedure (Fig. 10–2). In secondary nerve repair, in which the damage of the stumps has become apparent by fibrosis, it is important to know whether the initial resection was performed until completely normal tissue was reached or until tissue showing fibrosis but preserved fascicular pattern was apparent in the cross-section (resection

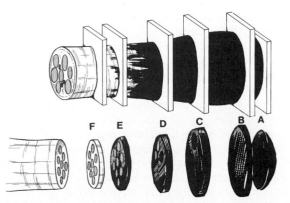

FIG. 10–2. Nerve stump with 8 fascicles and oblique damage. Preparation of the stump is done by resection.

into an area of 3rd-degree damage). In some cases, a very limited resection might reach tissue that does not show a fascicular pattern (damage of 4th degree).

Interfascicular Dissection

In contrast to resection, the two stumps can be prepared by interfascicular dissection, resecting the epifascicular epineurium and separating individual large fascicules in an oligofascicular nerve segment, or fascicle groups in a polyfascicular nerve segment, with group arrangement.

APPROXIMATION

At this stage of the procedure, the edges of the two stumps are fitted together such that the surfaces of the segments correspond optimally (keeping in mind the topography or fascicular pattern of the severed nerve). Tension at the suture anchoring site(s) is an important consideration when sutures are used. Every effort should be made to keep the tension to a minimum.

COAPTATION

In the nerve repair, coaptation can refer to apposition of various anatomic components. For example, the cross-section of two nerve stumps can be coapted; the cross-section of individual fascicles can be coapted; and the cross-section of groups of fascicles can be coapted. The goal of nerve repair is that of coapting the fascicular tissue of one stump as completely as possible with the fascicular tissue of the opposite stump to attain an optimal result. The ideal situation would be that of coapting fascicle to fascicle.

In dealing with a transected monofascicular nerve segment, stump-to-stump coaptation is synonymous with fascicle-to-fascicle coaptation. With oligofascicular nerve segments of up to five fascicles, stump-to-stump coaptation usually leads to a nearly ideal coaptation of the fascicles. However, in oligofascicular nerve segments with six to ten fascicles, the trunk-to-trunk approach does not attain ideal coaptation of the center fascicles of the cross-section. In this situation, interfascicular dissection is executed to separate the fascicles, with subsequent coaptation of the larger ones.

We believe that group-to-group coaptation is the most suitable approach for nerve segments with a polyfascicular grouped pattern. In the event of a defect, the ideal coaptation of fascicles within groups would not be feasible because the groups in each stump may be comprised of different numbers of fascicles as a result of a change in pattern over the length of the defect. However, clinical experience has proven that the lack of ideal fascicular coaptation does not influence results (21).

If individual fascicles were isolated and fascicle-to-fascicle coaptation attempted, the surgical trauma would be prohibitive and result in fibrosis and proliferation of connective tissue. Further, it would be very difficult to identify corresponding fascicles.

In a nerve segment with a nongrouping polyfascicular pattern, separation of individual fascicles would, again, result in too much surgical trauma. Similarly, identification of individual fascicles would present great difficulty, and with a segmental defect, the number of fascicles is not congruent. Group-to-group coaptation is obviously not realistic in the absence of group formation with this fascicular pattern. Two options remain. A stump-to-stump coaptation may be performed with eventual use of guide stitches. Alternately, the nerve stumps may be arbitrarily divided into sections, and each coapted with a corresponding section of the opposite stump.

MAINTAINING COAPTATION

Sutures are used to maintain coaptation wherever they are anchored; in the interfascicular epineurium, in the perineurium, or in both the perineurium and the epineurium.

Tissue glues have been used as an alternative to sutures in maintaining coaptation. Concentrated solutions of fibrinogen have been applied to coaptation sites with some success (22,23). A problem with this technique is fibrinolytic activity, which compromises the intended result. In addition, this technique does not allow for tension; therefore, it has been used most recently only in conjunction with anchoring sutures (24).

Coaptation can also be maintained by placing the two nerve stumps at the ends of a tube (e.g., a vein) some distance from the coaptation site. The tube may be split in a longitudinal direction or remain closed. Application of a tube to the suture site has likewise been suggested as a protective mechanism in preventing adhesions to surrounding tissue. However, no demonstrable advantage has yet been clinically proven.

THE GAP BETWEEN NERVE SEGMENTS (STUMPS)

As applied to nerve repair, *gap* may be defined as the distance between two stumps before restoration of continuity is attempted. When there is a clean transection at the time of primary repair, the distance may simply be a function of elastic retraction. Only the elasticity of the nerve must be overcome to achieve approximation in this case. When there is damaged nerve tissue, fibrotic retraction may result from tissue fibrosis and loss of elasticity. Where there is a nerve defect, a segment of nerve tissue has been lost, and the gap will be greater and more difficult to remedy.

Although the terms are often used synonymously, it should be clear that *gap and nerve defect are not the same.* When a segment of fibrotic nerve tissue must be resected during the preparation of two stumps, an additional defect is created. This, too, increases the gap. A retrospective analysis of factors that have contributed to a final gap may be indeed complex when a secondary repair is being undertaken.

Some methods for remedying gaps between two nerve stumps are:

1. Expand the nerve to its original length to compensate for elastic retraction.
2. Extend nerve tissue beyond its original length to remedy a nerve defect.
3. Mobilize the two stumps to distribute the extension of nerve tissue over a greater distance.
4. Transport the nerve to provide a shorter route.
5. Change the joint position to approximate two nerve stumps on the flexion side of the joint combined with transposition.
6. Shorten the adjacent bones.
7. Graft the nerve.
8. Interpose a nonvital graft or some type of tube to accomplish neuromatous neurotization.

Basic Concepts of Nerve Grafting

There are a number of aspects of, and many ways to perform, a nerve grafting procedure. The different conceptual aspects may be classified according to the following criteria: (a) mechanical aspects; (b) source of nerve grafts; (c) blood supply; and (d) donor nerves.

MECHANICAL ASPECTS

The distance between two nerve stumps can be bridged in two different ways:

1. The length of the graft is selected according to the minimal defect after the two stumps have been approximated to the extent possible by exhausting all other methods (mentioned above) for overcoming a gap. The remaining distance is then bridged by nerve grafts. Shorter grafts can be used, but the sites of coaptation offer the same unfavorable conditions for nerve regeneration and end-to-end repairs under tension.
2. The length of the graft is selected according to the maximal gap between the two stumps when the involved limb is in a functional position. Although longer grafts are necessary, optimal conditions are provided at the sites of coaptation. In addition, when mobilization of the limb is resumed, the graft is not exposed to tension, and reengagement of longitudinal movements is not necessary.
3. The trend to apply grafts as short as possible derives from the incorrect idea that the results are significantly better with shorter nerve grafts. At first glance this seems logical. There are reports showing a significant relationship between the length of the graft and the result, with the results becoming worse with increasing length of the graft. However, the surgeon has to consider that long grafts are needed when there are long defects, and the poorer results may be linked not so much to the long graft but to the long defect, making a long nerve graft necessary. In our clinical experience, we have good evidence to believe that with an equal length of defect within certain limits the length of the graft is not important. In a recent paper (25) it was demonstrated that the length of the graft as such is not a limiting factor. In this connection, it is even better to use a longer graft with two optimal sites of coaptation than a shorter graft.

SOURCE OF NERVE GRAFTS

Autogenous nerve grafts do not present the immunological problems of the allogenous or xenogenous grafts. The latter types are still in the experimental stage for peripheral nerves. In preserving nerve grafts, the following processes have been used: freezing, irradiation, lyophilization, and cialite solution (1). Allografts are less immunogeneic when preserved by one of the methods listed. Even though they are not vital, they are invaded by nerve fibers (neuromatous neurotization). During the 1960s and early 1970s, experimentation with preserved allografts did not meet with success. Under immunosuppressive therapy with cyclosporine A, allografts survive (26–29). Because even successful surviving allografts are not completely neurotisized, the results will always be inferior to an autograft transplanted under favorable conditions.

BLOOD SUPPLY

Restored Circulation by Spontaneous Vascularization

After free grafting, a nerve segment is initially without blood supply. As with a free skin graft, spontaneous anastomoses take place between vessels on the surfaces of both the graft and the recipient site. Vessels from the recipient site grow into the graft. When the avascular period is short, the graft survives well. During this period, no wallerian degeneration occurs within the graft, and there is no connective-tissue proliferation. After circulation has been reestablished, the graft behaves like a distal stump.

When there is a delay in spontaneous revascularization, the fibroblasts survive, but the Schwann cells and other special structures are lost. Such a graft segment becomes fibrotic and can be innervated only by neuromatous neurotization. If spontaneous revascularization fails to occur, the graft becomes necrotic. After free grafting, survival is a function of tissue mass (diameter), surface contact between graft and recipient site, and recipient site vascularity. When the relation is favorable, as with cutaneous nerve grafts, survival is enhanced. If the relation between diameter and surface area is not favorable (e.g., with a thick trunk graft), fibrosis of the graft occurs. Smaller elements of a trunk graft provided by isolating individual fascicle groups of the longitudinal microsurgical dissection (split nerve grafts) survive free grafting very well (30,31).

Preservation of Circulation

Continuity of a nerve can be restored by the two-stage transfer of a pedicled graft from a parallel nerve, as in a flap procedure. Circulation within the grafts is preserved during the transfer, and favorable results have been reported to the extent of protective discrimination (32–34).

A nerve segment on its vascular pedicle can be transferred as an island flap without interruption of blood supply if the recipient nerve is within range of the pedicle. Many cases discussed as vascularized nerve grafts are, in reality, island flap transfers of peripheral nerves (35,36).

Restored Circulation by Microvascular Anastomosis (Vascularized Nerve Graft)

The free vascularized nerve graft was introduced by Taylor and Ham (37). If vessels remain patent, the graft behaves like a distal stump at the onset. Important dimensions of the process seem to be that of survival of the paraneurium and the absence of adhesion formation in achieving spontaneous vascularization. The vascularized nerve is independent of vascularity in the recipient site.

Vascularized nerve trunk grafts have been used to bridge large defects. With the reestablishment of circulation, the danger of fibrosis does not occur as it does when using trunk grafts as free grafts. The disadvantage of a trunk graft is that the changing fascicular pattern makes it impossible to predict where the nerve fibers at a certain point in the proximal end will leave the graft at the distal end. The superficial branch of the radial nerve has been used successfully alone (37) and in conjunction with free grafts. Microvascular techniques have been developed for use with the sural nerve as a vascularized graft (38,39). The expectation that vascularized nerve grafts would significantly improve the quality of nerve regeneration over considerable distances has not yet been borne out (Gilbert, personal communications, 1981, 1982; 40). The majority of authors report a somewhat faster regeneration but an equal final result whether free nerve grafts or vascularized nerve grafts have been used (41–44). Only Terzis and colleagues (45) reported superior final results. In my experience, there was no significant difference. I could demonstrate this in a series of brachial plexus cases in which the biceps brachii was neurotised using vascularized nerve grafts and the triceps muscle neurotised by free nerve grafts. Thus, each patient was a self control. There was no significant difference between the two groups. Careful animal experiments with large animals (46,47) could demonstrate that, in spite of a better appearance of the vascularized nerve grafts compared to the free nerve grafts, the regeneration of the muscle and the axon count in the distal stump did not differ between the two groups. Undoubtedly, the major advantage of vascularized nerve grafts is the fact that the paraneurium, and consequently the gliding capacity of the nerve graft, is preserved. In contrast, a free graft has to survive by developing adhesions with the surrounding tissue. Also, nerve regeneration is unquestionably better if, along with the nerve graft, the overall circulation (e.g., in an injured finger) is improved by performing a vascularized graft (48).

DONOR NERVES

Nerve Trunk Grafts

The use of nerve trunks as grafts is limited. A major consideration is the functional loss the nerve undergoes when employed as a graft. If two parallel nerves are injured, one may be restored at the expense of the other (as with a pedicled nerve graft). Where there is extensive functional loss in selected nerve repairs (e.g., brachial plexus lesions), nerve trunk grafts may be used to advantage.

Nerve trunks cannot be used as free grafts, as noted above, because circulation must be maintained or immediately reestablished. An important disadvantage is the changing fascicular pattern over the length of the graft such that the course of regenerated fibers cannot be predicted from the proximal to the distal end.

The concept of the plexiform arrangement of peripheral nerve trunks (49,50) was a strong argument against the possibility of splitting a nerve trunk into fascicle groups and using them as free nerve grafts. We have done this in brachial plexus cases since 1980 if the ulnar nerve was available as a graft donor due to avulsion of C8 and T1 and for various reasons the ulnar nerve was not to be used as a vascularized nerve graft. We have learned that it is easy to resect rather long segments of fascicle groups without many intergroup connections. A follow-up study (52) demonstrated that the result of 25 cases (38 nerves) were equally good as the results using other types of nerve graft.

Cutaneous Nerve Grafts

Cutaneous nerve grafts have an ideal diameter-to-surface ratio for free grafting and may be regarded as a fascicular group. The ideal donor nerve should have only a few branches. A salient aspect of using cutaneous nerves as donor grafts is the difference in thickness contrasted with that of the nerve trunk to be repaired. Two possible solutions exist:

1. A composite nerve graft may be formed by suturing or gluing together several segments of cutaneous nerve. A cable is designed by uniting several segments of a cutaneous nerve to reach the same size as the nerve to be repaired (53). However, grafts so devised experience a loss in surface dimension available for contact with the recipient site. Further, in the event of a defect, the cross-sections of the two nerve stumps do not correspond, and only a random guiding of axons along the cable graft can occur.
2. Individual grafts of cutaneous nerve segments can be used to unite specific sites of the two stumps (10,54,55). The entire circumference of the individually placed grafts has good contact with surrounding tissue, and thereby an optimal chance of survival exists. If the topography is known, specific points of the two cross-sections can be connected with individual grafts.
3. Narkas (56) suggested a compromise between these two possibilities. The very ends of the nerve grafts were glued together to minimize the cross-sectional area and to allow bringing as much fascicular tissue as possible in contact with the stumps. The greater part of the length of the nerve graft remained isolated and optimal survival was possible.

The following nerves have been used as free cutaneous nerve grafts: (a) sural, (b) saphenous, (c) lateral femoral cutaneous, (d) medial antebrachial cutaneous, (e) medial brachial cutaneous, (f) lateral antebrachial cutaneous, (g) dorsal antebrachial cutaneous, (h) superficial radial, (i) cutaneous nerve of the cervical plexus, and (j) intercostal nerve.

Techniques of Interfascicular Nerve Grafting

Interfascicular nerve grafting differs significantly from other techniques as follows:

1. The length of the graft is selected to bridge the maximal defect in extending position. (See the earlier section on mechanical aspects). No attempt is made to diminish the distance by other methods.
2. If necessary, the nerve stumps are prepared by interfascicular dissection to reduce the amount of nonfascicular tissue.
3. The individual grafts are placed between corresponding fascicles or fascicular groups if the fascicular pattern of the stumps permits.
4. The nerve grafts are individually placed along the entire course to enhance the chance of survival. Since the early days of fascicular nerve grafting, this has been regarded as one of the most important factors for a successful outcome.

Individual steps of the technique are essentially the same as those described for neurorrhaphy (i.e., stump preparation, approximation, coaptation, and securing coaptation).

Cutaneous nerve grafts are provided by excision of one or several of the donor nerves. The two sural nerves are the first choice. Regardless of the anticipated lengths of nerve grafts, the sural nerve is always excised in its total length and transected just below the popliteal area. This locates the transsection site nearest the point of nerve attachment underneath the fascia. Thus, protection is provided for the neuroma that always forms at any site of nerve transsection and exposure

to irritation is prevented. The donor nerve is segmented according to the distance between the two stumps. The cut ends of the grafts should not be covered with epineurial or perineurial tissue; therefore, they are removed from the cross-sections. Resection of the ends is not necessary because these are free grafts, and connective-tissue proliferation is delayed. Hence, there is no interference with the coaptation site.

The donor nerve can usually be extended above 10% in length. However, each segmental length is selected in the relaxed state, which allows for additional extension of about 10%.

PREPARATION OF STUMPS

The nerve stumps are prepared in the usual way. Monofascicular and polyfascicular stumps without group arrangements are prepared by resection.

Nerve stumps with an oligofascicular pattern and a few large fascicles that are approximately the same size as the nerve grafts are prepared by resection of the epifascicular epineurium and interfascicular dissection, thus isolating the individual fascicles (Fig. 10–3).

Nerve stumps with a grouped polyfascicular pattern are prepared by resection of the epineurium and separation of the individual fascicle groups by interfascicular dissection. The technique of interfascicular dissection makes it possible to transect the fascicles or groups of fascicles exactly at the point of transition from normal to damaged tissue. Donor nerves, such as the sural nerve, have a changing fascicular pattern along their course. It is therefore possible to select segments that closely correspond to the individual fascicle groups of the recipient nerve and thus achieve an optimal match.

APPROXIMATION

The ends of each graft are approximated to corresponding cross-section sites of the two stumps. Site congruency is attained by exploiting all the possibilities previously outlined for defining intraneural topography.

COAPTATION

After approximation has been achieved, maximum care is taken to coapt the fascicular cross-sections as effectively as possible without displacement in either the longitudinal or lateral direction. If the approximation suture is placed ideally and if there is no tension, an optimal contact can be achieved without any deviation in a lateral direction. In this event, approximation and coaptation are performed in a single step. If the graft has a tendency to rotate or deviate laterally and if optimal coverage of the cross-sections cannot be achieved, two or three additional sutures may be necessary to attain and maintain optimal coaptation. The procedure of coaptation between oligofascicular or polyfascicular nerve segments with group arrangement is facilitated if individual fascicles or groups of fascicles have been transected at different levels. In this case, interdigitation between fascicles (or fascicle groups) and grafts occurs and provides side-by-side contact with neighboring fascicles, fascicle groups, and grafts. This is beneficial in preventing dislocation or disruption. Under such ideal conditions, the number of sutures can be reduced to a minimum (Fig. 10–4).

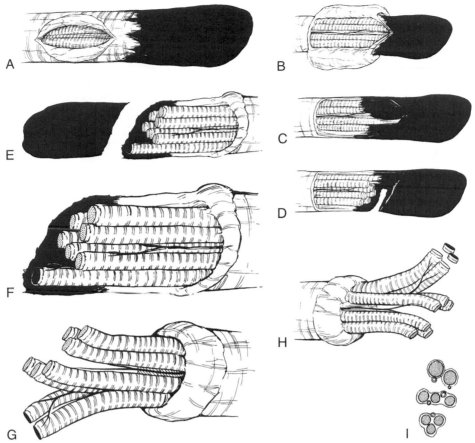

FIG. 10–3. Nerve stump with 8 fascicles and oblique damage. Preparation of the stump is by interfascicular dissection. **A,** longitudinal incision of the epifascicular epineurium proximal to the neuroma. **B,** the epifascicular epineurium is elevated. A space between the fascicles is seen indicating the border between groups. **C,** dissection is extended toward the neuroma. **D,** fascicles are transected at the point of transition from normal to abnormal appearance. **E,** neuroma is resected. **F,** exact inspection reveals the presence of fibrotic tissue around some fascicles and fibrosis of 2 fascicles. **G,** epifascicular and interfascicular resection at the back of the stump. The group arrangement becomes clearly apparent. The interfascicular tissue between the fascicles of each group is saved in each vessel. **H,** 2 fibrotic fascicles are resected. Finally, a stump is prepared with 3 fascicular groups. **I,** only minimal epineurial tissue remains.

MAINTAINING COAPTATION

If optimal coaptation has been achieved and tension eliminated, it is not necessary to use additional sutures or glue to maintain the coaptation. Extreme care must be taken to avoid shearing forces during wound closure and to prevent longitudinal traction. The involved limb is immobilized in the exact position it assumed during the operation.

Using a tissue glue, the tensile strength of a coaptation can be enhanced. As mentioned above, the tension between the two ends of a proximal stump and the graft should be zero. If this is really observed, there is no good reason to increase tensile strength, so I do not believe glue is really needed to help maintain coaptation. A long list of clinical and experimental work has demonstrated that gluing does no harm; even if glue enters between the cross sections, it does not prevent regeneration.

ALTERNATIVES TO NERVE GRAFTS

As alternatives to nerve grafts, alloplastic nerve conduits (57), venous grafts (Brunelli, personal communication, 1986; 58–62), and degenerated muscle tissue (19) have been used to provide pathways for neuromatous neurotization. In my experience, the results remain below the level of an autogenous free nerve graft performed under favorable conditions.

Postoperative Care and Follow-Up

Immobilization of the affected limb is maintained for 8 days. After this, careful mobilization is initiated without concern for rupture or dislocation. Electrotherapy can be used with exponential current if indicated. Follow-up is extremely important. After 2 to 3 weeks, advancement of the Tinel and Hoffmann signs along the graft can be observed. It may pause temporarily at the distal end of the graft and then proceed along the distal stump. This is an indication that at least some axon sprouts have crossed the site of coaptation and reached the distal stump. In some instances, a block develops at the distal suture site, and the axon sprouts cannot proceed. The Tinel and Hoffman signs then remain, with the maximal point at the distal end of the graft. In some cases, after proceeding along the distal stump, the Tinel and Hoffmann signs stop and subsequently retreat to the distal site of coaptation. This phenomenon means that changes within the scar tissue at the distal site of coaptation or along the graft itself have damaged the axon and caused a new axolysis.

60. Rigoni G, Smahel J, Chiu DTW, et al. Veneninterponat als leitbahn für die regeneration peripherer nerven. *Handchirurgie* 1983; 15:227.
61. Strauch B, Rosenberg B, Brunelli F, et al. Autogenous vein graft substitute in long segment nerve defects. Presented at the Inaugural Meeting of the American Society for Reconstructive Microsurgery, Las Vegas, Nevada, January 1985.
62. Sparmann M. Die bedeutung des sogenannten leitschienendefektes für die regeneraetion peripherer nerven über defektstrecken. Eine tierexperimentelle untersuchung am N. peronaeus des kaninchens. Habilitationsschrift aus dem Fachbereich 3—Klinikum Charlottenburg—der Freien Universität Berlin, 1987.
63. Bsteh FX, Millesi H. Zur kenntnis de zweizeitigen nerveninterplantation bei ausgedehntem peripherem nervendefekt. *Klin Med* 1960; 5:571.
64. Bosse JP. Discussional remark. In: Gorio A, Millesi H, Mingrino S, eds. *Posttraumatic peripheral nerve regeneration. Experimental basis and clinical implication.* New York: Raven, 1981; 347.
65. Smith JW. A new technique of facial animation. In: Hueston JT, ed. *Transactions of the 5th International Congress of Plastic and Reconstructive Surgery* (Melbourne, Australia). London: Butterworth, 1971; 83.
66. Scaramella L. L'anastomosi tra i due nervi faciali. *Arch Neurol* 1972; 82:209.
67. Anderl H. Reconstruction of the face through cross face nerve transplantation in facial paralysis. *Chir Plast* 1973; 2:117.

11

Biomaterials in Plastic Surgery

George J. Picha, M.D., Ph.D., F.A.C.S., Munish K. Batra, M.D., and
Mary H. McGrath, M.D., M.P.H., F.A.C.S.

The field of biomaterials and biocompatibility interfaces with all subspecialties. From Fallopius' repair of a calvarial defect using a gold plate in 1600 (1) to modern-day application of synthetic implantables, the field of biomaterials has undergone dramatic expansion. Advantages of alloplasts include absence of donor-site morbidity or donor-site scarring; however, substitutes for autologous tissue (2,3) have been challenged by issues such as toxicities (4-6), immunogenicity (7,8), degradation (9,10), and theoretical concerns of carcinogenicity (11,12). Researchers continue the search for biomaterials that provide mechanical durability, biocompatibility, and ease of processing and manufacturing. Advances in our understanding of the complex interaction between the body and a foreign material combined with society's changing needs (i.e., the expanding proportion of the geriatric population), will increase the demand for alloplast materials for prosthetic devices.

Biocompatibility

The surgical trauma associated with the implantation of a device initiates a wound healing response that is dependent on the clinician's expertise, the technique, the site of implantation, and the material's composition (14-16). The acute response is characterized by the influx of proteins, polymorphonucleocytes, and phagocytic cells, and is soon followed by release of various mediators of inflammation with the subsequent potential influx of immune cells (16). Recent studies show involvement of the complement pathway, the cytokine cascade, eicosanoids, reactive oxygen intermediates, and electrochemically mediated reactions to the implant (7,17,18). In addition to the above, chemical and physical properties of the implant, immunogenicity, the site of implantation, interfacial behavior, and genetic determinants comprise the body's response to the biomaterial (19,20,21). The result may vary from a stable synergism to a chronic inflammatory response, degradation, or rejection of the implant. Specifically, the surgeon must assess certain fundamental properties of the implant before its clinical application. These include: toxicologic evaluation (i.e., tissue culture); biochemical analysis; in vivo testing (i.e., cell growth); mutagenicity; and teratogenicity. Other tests would include durability testing, tensile strength, elastic modulus, conductivity, hydrolytic resistance, fatigue testing, and electrical stability, as well as oxidative degradation (6,13,22,23).

Synthetic Polymers (Plastics and Elastomers)

As a representative group, elastomers are widely used for medical implants that include silicone and polyurethane. Another group, thermoplastic polymers (plastics), includes polyamides, polyesters, polyethylenes, polyfluoroethylenes (PTFEs), epoxies, and polypropylene, to name a few. Many of the polymer's properties depend on the chemistry of the polymer chain backbone, the average number of repeating units in the chain, cross link density, and its molecular weight. These materials have a moderate cost of fabrication and methods of synthesis are well established (22,24). Most can be designed to be relatively biostable; however, all stimulate fibrous encapsulation. Others, such as nylon, polyesters, and some polyester polyurethanes, may undergo substantial degradation (25,26). Materials like PTFE and silicone have been configured both as injectables and in solid form for soft-tissue applications. Clinical sites of application include the ear, nose, chin, trachea, breast, and chest; they are also used as artificial skin and in tendon prostheses (ligaments), wound dressings, vascular prostheses, and structural support devices including mesh, sutures, and tissue glue (22,27-31).

The tissue reaction to an implant is influenced by its chemical composition, molecular weight, physical structure, and interfacial biocompatibility. A phenomenon noted in the 1940s, and explored further in the 1950s by Oppenheimer, was the development of sarcomas in mice implanted with plastic disks (11). The development of foreign-body sarcomas in mice may be influenced by the degree and chronicity of fibrosis, the size and shape of the implant, the surface charge, the chemical properties of the implant, its porosity, and the genetic makeup of the host (13,32-34). The "Oppenheimer Effect" was noted to occur frequently in murine species but rarely in humans. By example, no tumors were noted among nearly 11,000 women who underwent augmentation mammoplasty with varying techniques and materials (35). Other studies by Rubin and colleagues, and more recently by Deapen, showed similar results (36,37).

Silicone $\left[\begin{array}{c} CH_3 \\ | \\ -Si-O- \\ | \\ CH_3 \end{array}\right]$

erythema, pruritus, swelling, and pain at the site of injection (58). While no adequate studies have been done to assess the immunogenicity of this implant, it appears to be less immunogenic than bovine collagen (138).

Hard Tissue Replacements

CERAMICS

Formed from a combination of metallic and nonmetallic elements, the ceramics are the most clinically and biologically inert of all biomaterials (139). Their nonreactivity derives from the very strong bonds that form between the crystals as they are processed at 10,000 PSI and subsequently "sintered" at 800 to 1300° C to join the particles and eliminate pores (139,140). The result is a hard and strong compound that is resistant to compression forces and chemical alteration and has poor electrical and thermal conduction (2). Bioceramics have a high elastic modulus compared to bone, which may lead to fracture of bone or early loosening of the implant (141). In addition, bioceramics tend to have low resilience, are weak under tension and shear stresses, and are generally brittle. Anticipation of brittle fracture is the reason that ceramics have not been incorporated more avidly into clinical practice (139).

From the body's perspective, a single material design may be inadequate to fulfill all mechanical requirements, as the majority of autogenous tissues behave in a viscoelastic fashion. Thus composite materials with varying viscoelastic properties have been designed to meet a variety of compressive or tensile forces. Finally, regeneration of the biologic composite is provided by cells, and these cells will ultimately determine the interface between implant and body. Alloplastic material does not possess this regenerative capability because of an absence of viable cells, which often accounts for the interfacial failures.

The ceramics used as medical implants are generally divided into an inert group, the bioactive or surface-active ceramics, the resorbable ceramics, and the carbon-based compounds. Ceramics are now used mainly in the fields of dentistry, maxillofacial surgery, and orthopedics, but continued investigation is underway to broaden their applications.

INERT (UNREACTIVE) CERAMICS

Alumina (Al_2O_3) is the prototype of this group, which also includes titanium and zirconium oxides. Alumina is relatively inexpensive and easy to fabricate, and is among the most wear-resistant of all materials (142). Thus it has been used for structural forms in which biostability and resistance to mechanical compressive stress is important (143). It does not appear to elicit a biochemical reaction and its oncogenic potential is equal to or less than other implant materials (144). The nonporous inert ceramics undergo fibrous capsule formation after implantation, which helps achieve implant fixation to tissue. Porous implants were introduced to allow "osteointegration" at the implant–tissue interface in an attempt to achieve better fixation. It is believed that these implants are quickly infiltrated by osteoblast precursors at the tissue interface, and therefore prevent the infiltration of macrophages and multinucleated giant cells, as seen with nonporous implants (145). Therefore, the surface topography appears to influence the cellular response to these foreign bodies. Clinically, Alumina

has been applied in orthopedic hip implants since 1972 (146). These implants have undergone many modifications in attempts to improve wear mechanisms and tensile strength and are currently used as composites for orthopedic hip implants and tooth-root replacements in dentistry. Zirconium-oxide ceramics are also being investigated as femoral head replacements to decrease articulation wear.

BIOREACTIVE CERAMICS

Bioactive ceramics were conceived with the idea that an implant should induce and direct chemical bonding between itself and the surrounding tissue (147,148). This phenomenon appears to be a result of ion exchanges between the implanted material and the surrounding fluids. Researchers hypothesize that bioactive ceramics undergo surface dissolution with subsequent precipitation of bone mineral to create a contiguous interface between implant and tissue. In addition, the interfacial bonding appears to enhance new bone formation, possibly through stem-cell differentiation to osteoblasts (149).

The body's typical response to these ceramics includes and functional integration with bone without alteration of the natural mineralization process and absence of systemic toxicity. The bond between the ceramic and bone is strong.[144] In soft tissue, collagenous bonding occurs between implant and both muscular and subcutaneous tissue. These interfacial reactions occur only under optimal conditions, and any adverse biomechanical forces (e.g., movement) will shift the tissue response irreversibly from bonding to capsule formation (2). Solid and porous particulates of these bioactive ceramics have been used as bone substitutes, space fillers for crypts in alveolar sites of the mandible, adjacent to prostheses, orbital rehabilitation following enucleation, and carriers for medications (antibiotics) (143). Their brittle nature disallows use as structural support where significant compressive forces occur. An active area of investigation is their use as bioactive coatings to enhance prosthetic binding to bony matrix and improve mechanical force transfer at the interfacial level.

BIOACTIVE COATINGS

This is a rapidly expanding field in ceramic application. Hydroxyapatite (HA) has been used to coat metal orthopedic prostheses with the aim of providing a chemical bond between the bone and prosthesis (150). HA was chosen because it is considered the primary mineral constituent of bone (19). The mechanism of bone bonding appears to be due to precipitation of biologic apatite from body fluid onto the surface of the bioactive HA implant (51,152). It is believed that proteins adsorb to this biologic mineral layer and provide a scaffold for osteoblast attachment with subsequent production of osteoid directly onto the implant. HA-coated titanium and chromium cobalt subperiosteal and endosteal implants have been used clinically by dentists and oral surgeons for some time, while plasma spraying of orthopedic prostheses with an HA coating is still under investigation (153).

Histologically, these HA-coated implants demonstrate direct bone mineralization on the coating surface, unlike the noncoated implants, which show a fibrous tissue interface. In fact, the HA coating allows bony ingrowth even with a gap of 2 mm between implant and bone, while a noncoated prosthesis shows fibrous capsule formation with any gap greater than 300μ (150-154). Histological specimens from animals and humans show a new bone layer about 100 μ thick covering the hydroxyapatite surface within weeks of implantation (154,155).

Clinically, this would suggest more rapid and improved osteointegration with increased interfacial stability that may be further optimized with surface texturing. Testing of hydroxyapatite coating applied to metals has demonstrated that mechanical properties of the coating are greatly improved in tension, shear strength, and maximal fixation strength. The outcome is an implant that heals more rapidly, is less susceptible to fixation failure, and has a potentially longer life span because it permits more physiologic stress transfer (150,156).

RESORBABLE CERAMICS

These ceramics are calcium based and have found their applicability as osteophillic scaffolding on which bone can proliferate and bond chemically (157,164). Bioresorbtion occurs through combination of physiochemical dissolution and fragmentation, and is influenced by the degree of porosity (139,149). The major constituents of this group in current use are tricalcium phosphate (TCP) $[Ca_3(PO_4)_2]$, resorbable HA cement, calcium aluminate $[CaO \, Al_2O_3]$, Whitlockite $(3CaO \, P_2O_5)$, and plaster of paris $(CaSO_4)$.

The resorbable ceramics have found their mainstay in dentistry, where particulate HA has been used to restore the alveolar ridge in edentulous patients and TCP has been used to repair periodontal bony defects. HA cement is composed of tetracalcium phosphate and dicalcium phosphate and has been shown to be appropriate for a number of applications in the craniofacial skeleton. It is slowly replaced by bone without loss in volume or change in shape. It is currently undergoing clinical trials as a replacement for orbital floor defects, calvarial defects and frontal sinus obliteration; approval by the FDA is expected soon (92).

The advantage of these biosorbable ceramics is absence of long-term instability or compatibility problems, yet the unknown consequences of the release of their constituent elements warrants further investigation (2).

CARBON/CARBON COMPOSITES

This element is often included in the family of ceramics because of its ceramiclike properties and relative inertness in vivo (139). The strong carbon bonds confer great strength, while weaker bonding between atomic layers confers an elastic modulus close to bone (159). Pyrolysis, a method of producing pure carbon fibers by slow heating of polymeric fibers with rayon and polyacrylanitrile, results in a material with good strength and handling properties that is used in dental implants, thromboresistant cardiac valves, and composites for orthopedics (2,139).

Composites are formed to achieve performance greater than that of either material individually; the combination also allows materials to be customized to meet specific needs and applications (150). Carbon composites are formed by combining carbon fibers with a polymer matrix (160) (i.e., polysulfone, polyethylene, polyetheretherketone). These composites show excellent biocompatibility, good strength, and elastic modulus that approximates bone (150,156). Animal studies have substantiated the biocompatibility and biomechanical stability of these composites in orthopedic application (161,162).

Metals

Metallic implants have found their mainstay in orthopedics, but are being used more frequently in plastic surgery, ENT, and dental applications. They can exist as "pure" metal implants or alloys based on stainless steel, titanium, cobalt–chromium, tantalum, and nickel. Alloys generally have greater mechanical properties and higher biocompatibility.

Their applications include fixation (e.g., bone plates, rods, trays), support (e.g., suture, stainless-steel meshes), and electrical conductance (e.g., pacemaker wires, nerve stimulators) (2). Requirements of the metallic implants include mechanical strength, resistance to flexion fatigue, resistance to corrosion, and a density and weight comparable to surrounding tissue. In addition, interfacial behavior greatly influences the biointegration and longevity of these implants (16,25). This is evidenced by the recent interest and influx of textured implants, which "osteointegrate" with the surrounding tissue. Osteointegration allows the implant to bond mechanically to bone, thereby improving the rate and strength of fixation, decreasing the incidence of infection, and preventing a fibrous tissue interface that can lead to implant loosening (16,19,150,163). Osteointegrative metals are primarily limited to titanium and chromium–cobalt alloys.

Most metallic implants incite only limited antigenic or inflammatory response (2). Wear, from metal on metal or metal on polymer, results in particulate debris with chronic granulomatous formation and fibrosis that has the potential for bone destruction and implant failure (19,164); however, the two main factors contributing to implant failure are corrosion and implant fracture (2). Factors contributing to corrosion include tissue pH, various organic molecules, implant motion, and electrochemical dissolution with resultant metal ions (2,19,165). The in-vivo release of metal ions secondary to corrosion has been documented since the early 1960s. (166) These ions can be found in the serum of patients with metallic implants (167,168), yet the majority appear to be excreted in the urine (169). In-vivo metal ion release may lead to macrophage activation and stimulation of metalloproteinases and collagenases. Ultimately, a fibrous interface may develop, with inflammatory cellular elements that can lead to bone absorption and implant loosening and its associated pain and inflammation (170). Other concerns with release of metal ions include systemic allergic reactions seen with nickel (171,172), and theoretical risks of carcinogenicity associated with chromium, nickel, and possibly cobalt (173,174). Corrosion can be limited by coating the metal with an oxide film (passivation) that protects the metal and aids in biointegration (9).

Implant fracture may result from:

1. Improper implant design.
2. Manufacturing defects such as inclusions, insufficient electropolishing, or mixed metal devices that favor galvanic corrosion.
3. Improper stress distribution in the bone, causing atrophy and resorption of cortical bone.
4. Surgical handling that bends (works) the material until brittle spots develop.

170. Sunderman FW Jr. Carcinogenicity of Ni, Co and Cr. In: Hildebrand HF, Champy M, eds. *Biocompatibility of Co-Cr-Ni alloys.* New York: Plenum Press, 1988.

171. Elves MW, Wilson JM, Scales JT, et al. Incidence of metal sensitivity in patients with total joint replacements. *Br Med J* 1975; 4: 376–378.

172. Evans EM. Metal sensitivity as a cause of bone necrosis and loosening of the prostheses in total joint replacement. *J Bone Joint Surg [Br]* 1974; 56B:626–642.

173. Sunderman FW Jr. Carcinogenicity of Ni, Co and Cr. In: Hildebrand HF, Champy M, eds. *Biocompatibility of Co-Cr-Ni alloys.* New York: Plenum Press, 1988.

174. Gillespie WJ, Frampton CM, Henderson RJ, et al. The incidence of cancer following total hip replacement. *J Bone Joint Surg [Br]* 1988; 70:539–542.

175. Destefani FD. Ion implantation update. *Adv Mater Proc* 1988; 134:39–43.

176. Wagner WC. A brief introduction to advanced surface modification technologies. *J Oral Implantology* 1992; 18:231–235.

177. Brown SA, Devine SD, Merritt K. Metal allergy, metal implants and fracture healing. *Biomater Med Devices Artif Organs* 1983; 11:73–81.

178. Visuri T, Koskenvuo M. Cancer risk after McKee-Farrar total hip replacement. *Acta Ortho Scand* 1989; 60 [Suppl 231]:25.

179. Ward JJ, Thornbury DD, Lemons JE, et al. Metal-induced sarcoma. A case report and literature review. *Clin Orthop* 1990; 252:299–306.

180. Bagambisa FB, Kappert HF, Schilli W. Cellular and molecular biological events at the implant interface. *J Craniomaxillofac Surg* 1994; 22:12–17.

181. Matter P, Burch HB. Clinical experience with titanium implants, especially with the limited-contact dynamic compression plate system. *Arch Orthop Trauma Surg* 1990; 109:311–313.

182. Hille GH. Titanium for surgical implants. *J Mater* 1966; 1:373.

183. Ellerbe DM, Frodel JL. Comparison of implant materials used in maxillofacial rigid internal fixation. *Otolaryngol Clin North Am* 1995; 28:365–372.

184. Schliephake H, Lehmann H, Kunz U, et al. Ultrastructural findings in soft tissues adjacent to titanium plates used in jaw fracture treatment. *Int J Oral Maxillofac Surg* 1993; 22:20–25.

12

Tissue Expansion

Louis C. Argenta, M.D., F.A.C.S.

Reconstructive surgical procedures are frequently limited by the availability of adequate soft tissue. Over the past 15 years, mechanical tissue expansion has become a versatile and dependable technique for overcoming soft-tissue limitations.

Living tissues respond to the application of distracting mechanical force with an increase in the rate of mitosis of the overlying tissue migration of adjacent tissue and a realignment of collagen. In the process of tissue expansion, a silicone prosthesis is placed beneath the skin and gradually inflated, thus allowing for the development of new tissue that can be used for reconstructive surgery.

Tissue expansion possesses the unique ability to generate skin with an almost perfect match of color, texture, sensation, and special adnexal characteristics needed for reconstruction within a specific area. When adequately planned, the procedure results in minimal scarring and no donor defect. In addition to expansion of standard rotation or advancement flaps, tissue expansion can be used as an adjunct to myocutaneous and fasciocutaneous flaps, free flaps, and skin grafts. Tissue expansion has also been applied to other tissues of the body including bladder, intestine, ureter, blood vessels, and nerves (1). The ability of the body to generate new tissue in response to mechanical force appears universal and is an area for considerable future investigation.

The first published clinical case of tissue expansion was by Neumann in 1957 (2). Neumann placed an inflated balloon subcutaneously to facilitate an ear reconstruction. No further development occurred until 1976, when Radovan (3) reported using a sophisticated silicone implant with a self-sealing valve that could be placed entirely inside the body without external ports. Following Radovan's presentation, numerous clinical series (2-9) and experimental studies (10-12) were published, leading to the wide acceptance and use of the technique.

Tissue Response to Mechanical Expansion

The response of living tissue to mechanical expansion has been extensively studied in both animals and humans (13,14). Considerable variation occurs in tissue, depending on the rate, volume, and duration of the expansion. In general, gradual low-pressure and low increment expansion over many weeks results in fewer conspicuous changes than rapid high-pressure, large-volume expansions. These changes seem to relate directly to the body's ability to react to and compensate for the mechanical effects of the expansion. Overaggressive expansion may result in irreversible damage to the overlying tissue, including disruption of skin, fat necrosis, muscle atrophy, collagen and elastic fiber rupture, and neurapraxia.

After the expander has been removed and the reconstructive procedure accomplished, tissue that has been expanded normalizes with progressive dissolution of the capsule and a return of relative thickness and structure of the adjacent tissue.

EPIDERMIS

The epidermis becomes slightly thickened with cellular hyperplasia during expansion (11). Occasionally, hyperkeratosis and parakeratosis occurs. Electron microscopy reveals a narrowing of intercellular spaces and an increase in basal lamina undulation that is suggestive of increased mitosis (12). Animal studies using tritiated thymidine have demonstrated a 500% increase in mitotic activity of the basal layer during the process of expansion (15). Basal cellular phenotype is altered, as occurs in many other conditions with increased proliferative activity (16).

DERMIS

Tissue expansion dramatically changes the dermis over the implant. Increased fibroplasia with increased deposition and realignment of collagen fibers is evident. The overall thickness of the dermis is decreased 30 to 50%, resulting in increased compactness of collagen in both papillary and reticular dermis. Elastic fibers are fragmented, particularly in rapid expansion, and myofibroblasts increase significantly.

DERMAL APPENDAGES

No significant morphologic changes have been observed in nerve end receptors, sebaceous glands, hair follicles, or sweat glands. These structures are distracted from one another, but remain viable and active. Necrosis of adnexal structures with permanent dysfunction may occur in excessively rapid tissue expansion.

MUSCLE

Skeletal muscle is thinned and compacted with tissue expansion. Sarcomeres become abnormal and are increased during expansion, although the myofibrils become irregular. Mitochondria increase in number and size within the muscle, probably as an attempt to compensate for the relative anoxia during expansion. Functional activity of overlying muscle is generally unchanged.

ADIPOSE TISSUE

Pressure resulting from tissue expansion results in a significant atrophy of overlying fat cells that may be permanent.

With aggressive expansion, fat necrosis and fibrosis may occur. After expansion, ingrowth of adjacent fat cells may compensate for some contour defects, but most fat cells injured with expansion do not appear to recover significantly.

VASCULAR RESPONSE

Dramatic changes occur in the involved vasculature during expansion. There is an increase in number as well as in caliber of capillaries in the expanded tissue, with the greatest increase occurring in the dermal papillae. A significant increase in vascularity occurs at the junction of the capsule formed around the prosthesis and the adjacent dermal tissue (Fig. 12–1). Removal or injury to the capsule can significantly decrease the blood flow in expanded flaps.

The increase in vascularity has functional significance, in that random flaps that have been expanded show better survival than nonexpanded flaps (17). Clinically, expanded flaps can be rotated much more aggressively than nonexpanded tissue and are more resistant to infection (18).

The mechanism of increase of vascularity is poorly understood. Simple mechanical stretch results in new vessel growth proportional to the mechanical force applied to the membrane (19). Ischemia and hypoxia resulting from the ex-

pander are also stimuli for the increase in blood vessels, either by the opening of new vessels or by angiogenesis.

Tissue Expanders and Technique

Tissue expanders are basically silicone envelopes with a self-sealing reservoir through which percutaneous injections of saline are made (Fig. 12–2). The reservoir may be integrated into the envelope itself or may be connected to the envelope with a tube to allow remote positioning. Textured surfaces on implants have resulted in less migration of the device during inflation. Less capsule seems to form around textured implants, which allows for the more rapid generation of tissue with lower pressures. Directional and self-expanding prostheses have been developed.

Most manufacturers have a large variety of stock expanders in round, rectangular, and crescent shapes, with varying volumes. Custom-shaped implants of any size can also be fabricated. Almost all implants will tolerate 2 to 3 times their recommended volumes without rupture.

Tissue expansion is an adjunct for standard procedures in plastic surgery. The object of tissue expansion is to generate a specific quantity of a particular quality of tissue. Planning is critical, so that the proposed area of expansion can be ro-

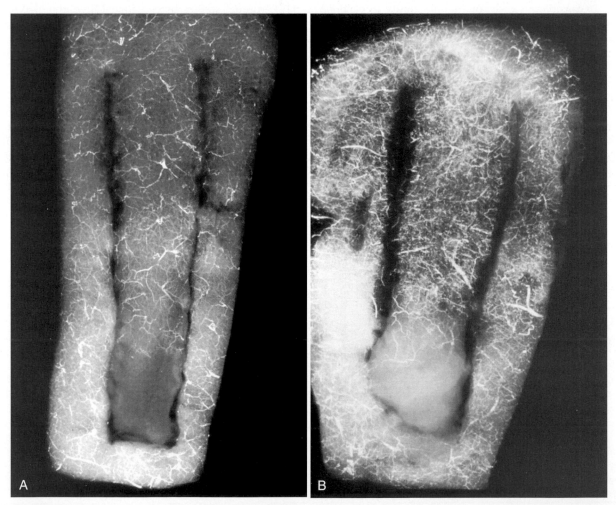

FIG. 12–1. Barium injections of flaps that have been elevated acutely. **A,** versus flaps that have been expanded. **B,** note the dramatic increase in vascularity throughout the expanded flap as well as the adjacent tissue.

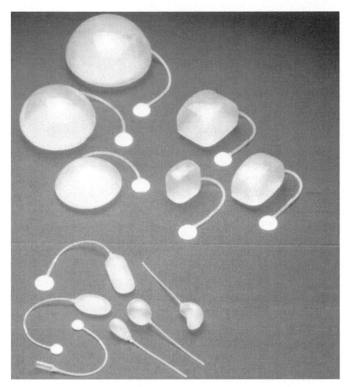

FIG. 12–2. Tissue expanders are available in many sizes and shapes. Custom implants can be specifically fabricated.

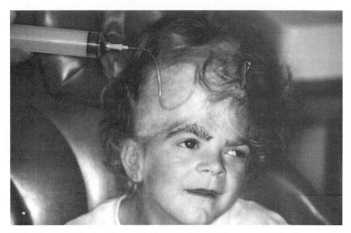

FIG. 12–3. Inflation is carried out with a 23-gauge butterfly needle under sterile conditions. Enough saline is inserted to develop tension of the skin overlying the prosthesis.

tated, advanced, or transposed to the recipient site with minimal risk and deformity. Planning results both in minimizing scars and situating scars in the least noticeable position. An excess of normal adjacent tissue should be expanded so that adnexal structures are evenly distributed and the flap moved with minimal tension and distortion. Implant selection depends more on the surface area to be expanded than on the actual volume of the device. The use of multiple expanders around the recipient site frequently facilitates the speed and safety of the reconstruction.

Expanders are placed under normal adjacent tissue through any incision that will not interfere with the subsequent reconstructive procedure; existing scars, or incisions in nonobvious areas, are preferred. Dissections should be carried on in the subcutaneous space as homogeneously as possible to minimize erosion and extrusion. Dissection should be wide so as to comfortably situate the prosthesis. Folds in the prosthesis, and abutment of the prosthesis to the wound edges, are meticulously avoided because they result in extrusion. As many adjacent nerves and vessels as possible are preserved during the dissection. After meticulous hemostasis is obtained, the wound is closed with or without drains in multiple layers.

If remote valves are used, they are placed subcutaneously at distant sites, avoiding underlying prominences. External reservoirs with long connecting silicone tubes may be helpful in infants or when inflation is to be carried on by the patient at home (20). Enough fluid is placed in the implant at the time of wound closure to avoid dead space around the implant without undue tension to the adjacent tissue.

After 7 to 10 days of wound healing, inflation is begun. A 23-gauge or smaller needle is inserted into the reservoir and

isotonic saline injected to produce tension of the overlying tissue (Fig. 12–3). Overaggressive inflation may result in extrusion of the prosthesis or loss of the overlying tissue, while insufficient inflation may result in protracted expansion. Some hyperemia is visible during the process of expansion; this generally indicates an increase in vascularity rather than infection. Blanching and excess pain should be avoided. Approximately twelve to twenty-four hours after inflation the tension of the overlying tissue will progressively decrease.

Frequent and small inflations separated by 2 to 3 days result in a more rapid tissue expansion than infrequent large-volume inflation. When tissue is needed in a limited period of time, continuous infusion at low volumes and low pressures can be performed. The surgeon should set no precise timetable for inflation, as this process depends on tolerance of the local tissues. Compromised tissue or tissue of debilitated patients may take longer to expand than others. With proper education, selected patients may be able to inflate their prostheses alone or with help from their families. An excess of tissue should be generated so that an adequate amount is available at the time of the reconstruction procedure.

Reconstruction

BREAST

Multiple procedures are available for reconstruction of the breast. The surgeon should tailor the reconstructive procedure to the needs of the patient, taking into account the quality and quantity of chest-wall tissue available, previous radiation, systemic factors, potential problems the patient may encounter later, and patient wishes. With this information, a logical decision can be made—to not reconstruct the patient, to reconstruct with an implant, or autologous tissue, or a combination of both.

Between 70 and 80% of post-mastectomy breast reconstructions in 1995 were performed using tissue expansion procedures. Excellent results, reliability, simplicity, minimizing of complications, and patient acceptance, have made tissue expansion breast reconstruction the choice of most patients and plastic surgeons (21-25). The advent of the Becker permanent expander has minimized the need for secondary implant exchanges, with high percentages of acceptable results and patient satisfaction (26). The use of a textured expander has improved the inframammary fold and projection of the nipple areolar complex, while expediting the rate at which expansion can be accomplished. Directional expanders have also proven useful to increase projection of the breast mound (27).

Immediate Breast Reconstruction

Select patients undergoing mastectomy for carcinoma with small tumors for whom the risk of metastatic disease is minimal are good candidates for immediate breast reconstruction (28,29). Textured expanders are preferred, in that they migrate less and seem to expand with less pressure. The surgeon places the expander under the pectoralis and serratus muscles, taking care to isolate totally the implant from the mastectomy dissection plane; seroma in the mastectomy plane encourages migration of the implant and increases the rate of infection when a separate, totally subpectoral position is not achieved. Patients should be maintained on antibiotics and the mastectomy site drained during the perioperative period until all seroma accumulation has ceased. Inflation begins 7 to 10 days following surgery and is carried on in a process similar to delayed breast reconstruction.

Patients with expanders may require adjunctive radiation therapy or systemic chemotherapy. In these cases, tissue expansion is carried on during the course of chemotherapy or radiation therapy using a small-volume frequent-fill regimen. Expansion during radiation therapy carries a higher risk of capsular contracture and wound complication (30). Patients who have failed radiotherapy as a primary therapy for breast carcinoma are in general poor candidates for reconstruction with expansion. Although some series report success, the incidence of undesirable contracture and wound complication is significant.

Delayed Breast Reconstruction

Reconstruction of the breast may be performed any time after healing of the mastectomy flaps and cessation of seroma collection. Optimally, reconstruction is done 6 weeks or later following ablative surgery (22,23,31). In secondary reconstruction, a permanent Becker, a high-profile directional expander, or a textured teardrop-shaped expander can be used. The prosthesis is placed in the subpectoral plane, covering as much of the implant as possible with muscle (Fig. 12–4). In patients with thin subcutaneous tissue, it is best to place the prosthesis entirely under muscle, mobilizing the serratus laterally; breast expanders placed above the muscle have a higher incidence of capsular contracture. Textured implants may alter this rate of contracture.

The prosthesis is usually placed through an incision in the previous scar, thus avoiding a second scar. Dissection is carried down to the pectoralis muscle, which is split laterally in the direction of its fibers so that the muscle incision does not lie over the apex of the implant. Dissection is then carried subpectorally and with sharp dissection extended under the serratus laterally and inferiorly. When the lateral portion of the pectoralis has atrophied, secondary to nerve damage during the mastectomy, as much of the prosthesis as possible is placed under the remaining pectoralis muscle, leaving the lateral inferior one-third of the implant subcutaneous. The in-

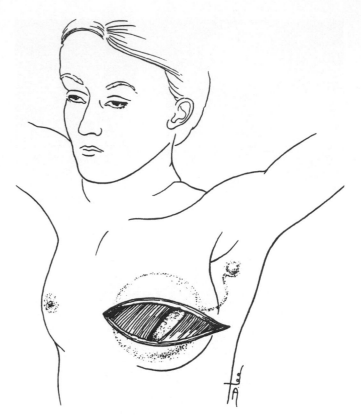

FIG. 12–4. Reconstruction after mastectomy using tissue expander. The prosthesis is placed submuscularly through the original mastectomy wound. The reservoir is placed in the axilla in the subcutaneous tissue. From Argenta LC. Reconstruction of the breast by tissue expansion. *Clin Plast Surg* 1984; 11:257.

flation reservoir is positioned in the axilla or, less optimally, on the anterior chest wall below the brassiere line.

Inflation is usually started at the time of implant placement, thus closing dead space. Frequent serial inflations are then begun 1 week following surgery and carried on at regular intervals so as to overexpand the breast to approximately twenty percent larger than the opposite side (22,23). More breast ptosis can be obtained if the implant is overexpanded, and the incidence of capsular contracture appears to be less after an overexpansion. The overexpanded breast is allowed to mature for 3 to 4 months. The implant is then deflated until symmetry is reached with the opposite side. Excellent stable aesthetic results can be obtained with this technique (24).

If a permanent expander becomes malpositioned during the process of expansion, if a permanent prosthesis is to be placed, or if the inframammary fold is not adequately defined, a secondary procedure is necessary. A better-defined inframammary fold can be achieved with an abdominal advancement procedure, as described in Figure 12–5 (23). The expander is replaced at the secondary procedure with a permanent smaller prosthesis and regular massage begun as soon as possible after surgery. Reconstruction of the nipple can be performed at the same procedure.

CONGENITAL ABNORMALITIES

Tissue expansion has revolutionized the reconstruction of congenital deformities (32). Asymmetries are not uncommon in pubescent females and minor asymmetries are

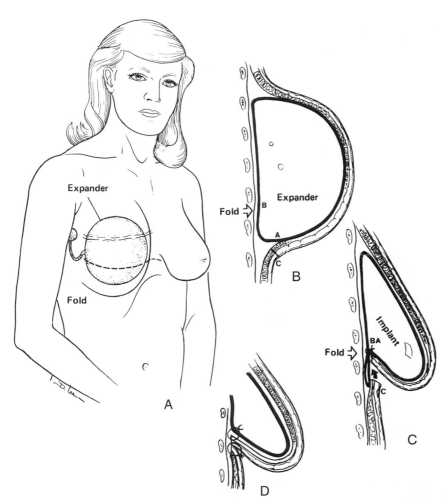

FIG. 12–5. The procedure for defining the infra-mammary fold after expansion. **A,** the prosthesis is overinflated and left in place for 3 to 4 months. **B,** an incision is made at point **C** and the expander replaced with a permanent prosthesis whose volume matches the opposite breast. Point A is moved to an appropriate position along the anterior chest wall (B) to create an appropriate ptotic breast. **D,** the abdominal skin is advanced in a cephalad direction to close the defect. (Reproduced with permission from Argenta LC. Reconstruction of the breast by tissue expansion. Clin Plast Surg 1984, 11:257. *Clinics in Plastic Surgery*)

best not treated. Significant asymmetries following burns, trauma, Poland syndrome, or any other condition, may be treated as soon as the asymmetry becomes a problem for the patient. Through a transaxillary incision, to avoid scars on the breast itself, a round tissue expander is placed beneath the pectoralis muscle and hypoplastic breast (Fig. 12–6). If the pectoralis is absent, as frequently occurs in Poland syndrome, the prosthesis is placed in the subglandular space under the hypoplastic breast. The prosthesis is then inflated at appropriate intervals to maintain symmetry until development of the opposite breast stabilizes. Most breasts continue to grow until the patient reaches 18 or 19 years of age, at which time the expander can be replaced with a permanent implant or an autologous soft-tissue transfer. When extensive reconstruction is necessary, as in Poland syndrome, the latissimus dorsi muscle can be transposed to correct the infraclavicular hollow at the time of the permanent implant procedure. This technique has been extremely successful in minimizing psychologic trauma in adolescent females. It carries the advantage of recapitulating normal growth of the breast as it results in enlargement and displacement of the nipple areolar complex to a more normal mature position. Tuberous breast deformities in which there is abnormal shape of the breast and nipple areolar complex can also be very successfully reconstructed by this technique (33).

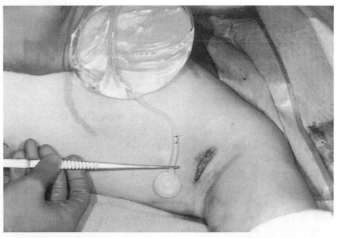

FIG. 12–6. Placement of an expander prosthesis through an axillary incision for reconstruction of congenital asymmetry of the breast. Redundancy is left in the connection tubing to avoid tearing the prosthesis during exercise.

Women who present after they have achieved complete breast development and have severe unilateral hypoplasia are also excellent candidates for reconstruction with tissue expansion. A Becker or textured expander is placed through an inframammary or transaxillary incision in the subpectoral space. The expander is then gradually inflated until symmetry is achieved. In women who have significant ptosis on the opposite side, a mastopexy may need to be performed.

HEAD AND NECK RECONSTRUCTION

Scalp

The scalp, among all the tissues of the human body, has unique hair-bearing qualities. All reconstructions of the scalp require rearrangement of a finite amount of hair-bearing tissue over a finite area. Tissue expansion has radically facilitated reconstruction of large scalp defects associated with congenital abnormalities, tumor, trauma, or male baldness (Fig. 12–7) (34,35).

The use of tissue expanders allows an increase in the available surface area of hair-bearing scalp tissue, thus permitting reconstruction in previously impossible situations. The process of expansion results in distraction of individual follicles from one another, rather than creation of new follicles. Distraction of hair follicles by a factor of 2 usually produces no discernable thinness of hair, but a significant increase in the possible alternatives for reconstruction. Planning is critical in scalp expansion. The implant should be placed so as to expand homogeneously as much as the normal hair-bearing scalp as possible. Multiple expanders, particularly in cases of burn alopecia, are particularly helpful

(179). Expanders are placed beneath the galea through what will be the advancing edge of a particular flap. Distant incisions may occasionally be useful, but require more preoperative planning so as not to compromise alternatives. Judicious scoring of the galea at the time of implant placements facilitates the rate of expansion and decreases pain. Expansion of the scalp may initially be uncomfortable and require multiple frequent small-volume injections. Pain and tension usually subside within a few hours.

Once adequate expansion has been achieved, the expanders are removed and the appropriate rotation, advancement, or specialized flap is created. Preservation of the major axial vessels to the scalp is vital to ensure viability and minimize ischemic hair loss (37). Direction of hair growth, particularly when the anterior hairline is reconstructed, requires attention. Selective incisions in the expanded capsule may be necessary in large defects, but should usually be avoided because significant compromise of blood supply may occur. Beveling the skin incision and moderating use of cautery will also minimizes injury to follicles. The abnormal scalp tissue to be replaced should be removed *after* mobilization of flaps in the event that insufficient tissue has been generated. The surgeon should make every attempt to preserve the pericranium. If defects cannot be completely closed, the expander may be left in place for a secondary expansion. This may be necessary in young infants where large nevi or complicated wounds are encountered. Serial expansions are very well tolerated in both children and adults. Fear of cranial deformity

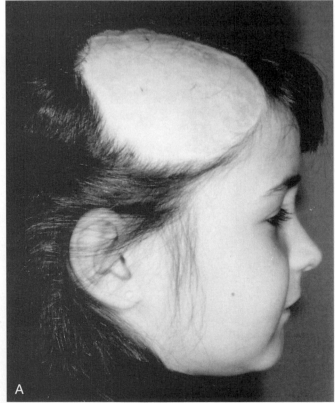
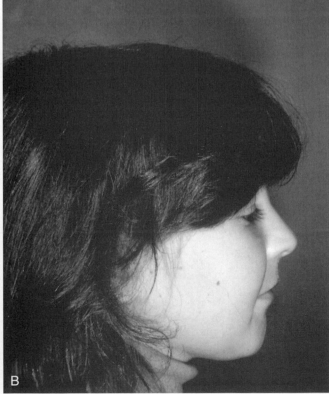

FIG. 12–7. Correction of traumatic alopecia using tissue expansion. **A,** a 6 × 8 cm defect in the scalp is covered with a split-thickness skin graft. **B,** the postoperative result after expansion to 600 cc with a single prosthesis and advancement of a hair-bearing flap.

in children can be avoided if the expansion procedure can be delayed until the child is 6 to 8 months of age. With gradual small-volume inflation, the amount of cranial distortion is minimal.

Male Pattern Baldness

Multiple procedures are available for reconstruction of male pattern baldness. Individuals with extensive baldness may benefit from tissue expansion to distribute the remaining follicles more homogeneously. The deformity that occurs during expansion, however, can be significant, and a highly motivated patient is required.

Scalp reduction to correct vertex male-pattern baldness can be significantly expedited with expansion. Prostheses are placed beneath the galea in the temporal or posterior occipital areas. Implants are placed through an incision in what will be the advancing edge of the lateral flap that is to be moved to the vertex. Once expansion has been achieved, the prostheses are removed and the hair-bearing scalp advanced to the vertex. The recipient bald areas are excised after the flaps have been mobilized appropriately so that excessive tissue is not removed. Tension is minimized to avoid scar alopecia.

Frontal hairline reconstruction calls for the use of expanded Juri flaps or the Bilateral Advancement Transposition (BAT) flap (Fig. 12–8) (39). Wide, anteriorly or posteriorly based, expanded flaps are created and transposed to reconstruct the anterior hairline. The expanded temporal scalp is then advanced to close the donor defect.

"Dog-ears" often occur after flap transposition in the scalp. They should not be excised at the time of reconstruction be-

cause excision may result in compromise of blood flow to the flaps. Most dog-ears resolve over several months, although some may require later correction. Relative alopecia occurs frequently after transposition and advancement flaps. As long as the follicle has not been injured, recovering of this alopecia will occur in 4 to 6 months.

Forehead

The forehead interfaces the soft tissues of the face and scalp and is anatomically similar to the scalp. Defects of the forehead area are best reconstructed by expanding the remaining forehead on either side of the recipient site. Prostheses are placed through an incision in the scalp under the frontalis muscle. The frontal branch of the facial nerve is avoided, particularly at the rotation stage, so that forehead animation is preserved. Defects can usually be removed, leaving a single vertical or transverse scar in the forehead. Expansion and cephalad advancement of the lateral face can facilitate correction of lateral forehead defects. Complex expansions and translocations of the forehead have been described, but they result in significant scar (40). It is important to remember that considerable hair-bearing scalp can be moved in forehead reconstruction with minimal deformity in large defects. Symmetrical positioning of the brow is critical in all reconstructions.

Expansion of the Face and Neck

Optimal reconstruction of large defects of the face requires the availability of adequate local tissue (8,9,35). Color, hair-bearing quality, and texture of facial skin make optimal the use of local tissues in reconstruction of difficult facial defects. Tissue expansion has become an important modality in the management of these defects. Consideration must be given to hair-bearing quality of skin and the potential for hair bearing in children. Flaps should be carefully thought out prior to placement of the tissue expanders so that the suture lines will ultimately come to rest in areas where they will be minimally visible. All reconstruction should be carried out, as possible, in anatomic units to minimize patchwork final results.

Expansion is achieved by placing prostheses in the subcutaneous tissue over the superficial fascia of the face and neck. A standard facelift plane is used, keeping the surgical plane as homogenous as possible to minimize the risk of nerve damage and compromise of the overlying skin. Standard or custom expanders with large surface areas are optimal for use in the face. Low-volume, frequent-interval expansion, particularly in children, results in homogenous and safe expansion of facial and neck tissues.

The neck is an extremely important source of tissue for reconstruction of the lower face. Neck skin is identical to most skin in the lateral and central face. Implants are best placed above the platysma to avoid damage to the branches of the facial nerve. Expanded neck flaps may be moved in a cephalad direction as far as the infraorbital rim. The neck and face can be expanded to extraordinary proportions using multiple large-surface expanders without compromise of the underlying vital structures (Fig. 12–9). When advanced or rotating expanded flaps are used, they should be secured to the underlying fascia or periosteum to minimize subsequent retraction, particularly around the mouth and eyes. The surgeon

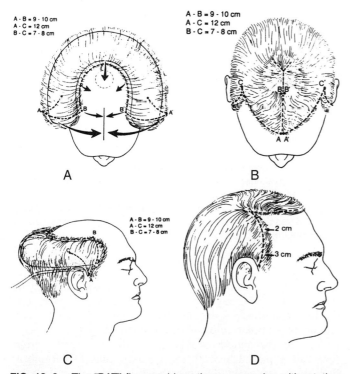

FIG. 12–8. The "BAT" flap combines tissue expansion with rotation advancement of tempoparietal flaps for the reconstruction of male pattern baldness. (Reproduced with permission from Anderson R, *Annals of Plastic Surgery,* 1993, 31:388.)

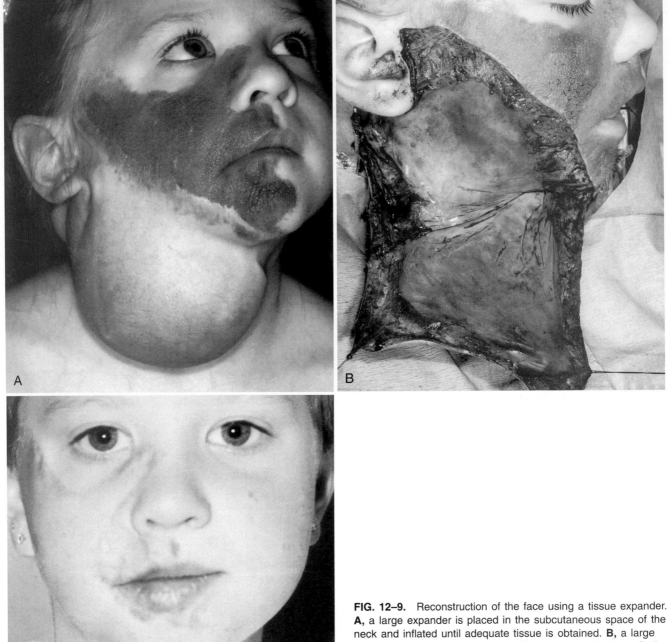

FIG. 12–9. Reconstruction of the face using a tissue expander. **A,** a large expander is placed in the subcutaneous space of the neck and inflated until adequate tissue is obtained. **B,** a large neck/face flap is generated that will cover the entire face. **C,** the patient 3 years after surgery. A full-thickness skin graft was used to reconstruct the upper lip.

plans reconstruction so that the final suture lines lie at the margin of aesthetic units.

Tissue expansion has been used successfully to expand both the skin and musculature in rare facial clefts (41), as well as to achieve closure of difficult cleft lips (42). Long-term results have been excellent with this technique, allowing normal animation and closure of the cleft.

NOSE

Total nose reconstruction is limited by sufficient soft tissue and skin to create internal and external lining. The problem is particularly complicated in burns, extensive neoplasms, and children with congenital nasal deformities. Expansion of the forehead greatly increases the amount of tissue available and enables primary closure of the donor defect.

A large rectangular prosthesis encompassing the entire forehead is placed beneath the frontalis muscle through an incision in the scalp. The prosthesis is inflated until an excess of tissue has been generated, usually over a period of 6 weeks. Expansion results in a significant thinning of the forehead flap that allows reconstruction of a more refined nose. The reconstruction of appropriate supporting struc-

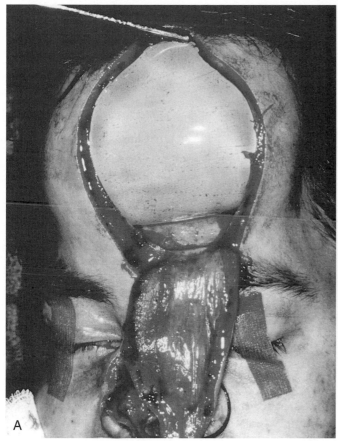

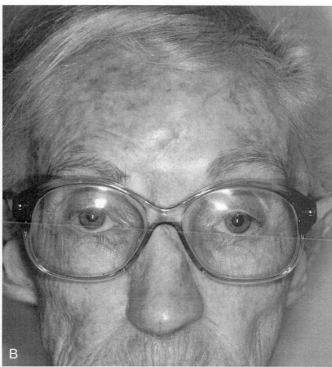

FIG. 12–10. **A,** total nose reconstruction can be achieved by expanding the forehead to develop a large forehead flap. The flap is doubled upon itself over a cantilever graft. **B,** functional aesthetic results in this patient have been stable over 8 years.

tures is vital or retraction of the expanded flap will occur. A cantilever cranial bone graft is secured to the nasofrontal area and used to support the forehead flap. Conchal cartilage grafts give refinement and support to the tip. The distal expanded forehead flap that is to line the nose is then thinned down to the dermis removing of the capsule. The flap is rotated down over the supporting bone and cartilage grafts, folded upon itself in the manner of Converse, and sutured to the remaining mucosal defects to reconstruct the nasal lining. The forehead flap is secured in place without undue tension. The flap is divided and inset 2 to 3 weeks following the initial procedure. Stable long-term functional nose reconstructions can be achieved with this technique (Fig. 12–10).

EAR

Tissue expansion can be used in a large variety of complicated ear reconstruction to minimize the need for a temporoparietal flap and skin grafts. Custom prostheses may be necessary if there are ear remnants to be preserved. If the ear is completely absent, a 100-cc crescent prosthesis is usually adequate. The prosthesis is inserted through an incision in the scalp, avoiding damage to the temporoparietal flap, which may be needed later. Inflation is carried out gradually in small increments because of the thinness of the overlying tissue. It is best to let this tissue mature for approximately three to four weeks after adequate expansion has been achieved, since the capsule is usually removed at the second procedure.

Removal of the capsule allows a better definition of the cartilage framework. Any of the standard cartilage frame work techniques can be used. Adhesion of the expanded tissue to the cartilage is achieved with suction drains rather than overlying pressure (43-45).

EXPANSION OF EXTREMITIES

Tissue expansion is well tolerated in both upper and lower extremities, provided certain guidelines are followed. Expansion facilitates excision of nevi, tattoos, scars, skin grafts, and damaged skin. The skin over the dorsum of the hand and foot expands readily; however, the palm and plantar surface of the foot expand very poorly and with great pain. The dorsum of the hand and fingers can be expanded with custom implants for the correction of syndactyly, thus avoiding all skin grafts (46,47).

Multiple prostheses are best placed radially to the defect, with tissue brought together so as to leave a longitudinal scar. The contour deformity that occurs with closure of radially placed prostheses corrects spontaneously and rapidly. Considerably more expansion is necessary if the surgeon desires to close flaps from the long access of the extremity.

The complication rate of prostheses placed below the knee is significant (48). Patients who have had extensive degloving or crush injuries below the knee are particularly poor candidates for expansion, probably owing to compromise of lymphatic drainage. Patients who have suffered clean, isolated defects of the lower extremity below the knee can be successfully reconstructed. We recommend the use of multi-

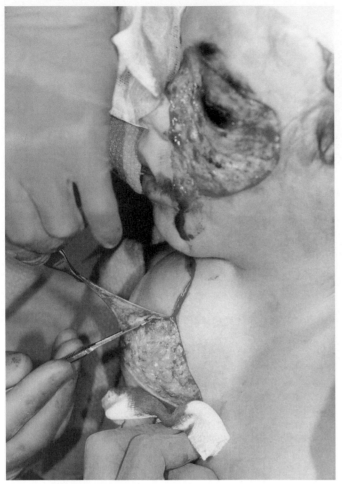

FIG. 12–11. Full-thickness skin grafts can be expanded and harvested for difficult reconstructive problems such as the periocular area. These grafts are stable over time and retain growth potential with excellent cosmetic results.

ple expanders around the defect to minimize excessive distortion and problems wearing clothing. Expanders have been very helpful in expanding overlying soft tissue for the placement of implants in the extremity (49). Reconstruction of polio victims and individuals who have lost extensive soft tissue is expedited by this technique.

TRUNK

The back and abdomen have very large surface areas that can be very rapidly expanded with a low risk of complication. Standard myocutaneous flaps on the trunk and extremities can be expanded before rotation (50), or before their harvesting as free flaps (51). Tissue expansion increases the adjacent random area of such flaps, so that extremely large tissue transfers can be accomplished safely. The latissimus dorsi muscles can be expanded bilaterally and mobilized medially and inferiorly for closure of large midline defects. The latissimus can also be expanded in its anatomic position and transposed anteriorly to cover the entire chest wall.

Tissue expansion of the skin alone can be achieved by placing multiple prostheses around the defect in the subcutaneous plane above the underlying fascia. Large expanders

(up to 500 cc) can be used with minimal risk. Studies describe the use of expanders to cover pressure sores (52). However, the rate of infection of prostheses adjacent to the such chronic infected wounds is significant.

Muscle and overlying skin can be successfully expanded for closure of a large abdominal-wall defect by placing the prosthesis beneath the muscle and fascia (53). Gradual expansion is useful to minimize pressure on underlying visceral organs.

Tissue expansion can be used to expand fasciocutaneous flaps for reconstruction of large defects of the back, particularly in myelomeningoceles. Expansion of skin and subcutaneous tissue is particularly useful in the division of conjoined twins, as it allows coverage of the conjoined area (54).

EXPANDED FULL-THICKNESS GRAFTS

Preexpansion of a donor site for full-thickness graft harvest, will dramatically increase the potential size of tissue available for such grafts (55,56). The survival of expanded full-thickness grafts is equal to that of nonexpanded grafts. A prosthesis is placed beneath the prospective donor site and inflated over a period of 4 to 6 weeks.

Reconstruction of the perioral and periorbital area with expanded full-thickness grafts is extremely useful, particularly in children. The supraclavicular area is especially well suited for this purpose and provides ideal color and texture match with minimal donor-site morbidity. The abdomen between the symphysis and the umbilicus can easily be expanded, even in young children, to provide a large surface area for harvest of extensive grafts. Reconstruction of the plantar foot and palmar hand can be accomplished with expanded full-thickness grafts harvested from the lower abdomen. At harvest, the prosthesis is left in place to facilitate removal of the full-thickness graft (Fig. 12–11). After the full-thickness graft has been transferred, the prosthesis is removed and the donor site closed primarily. Expanded full-thickness skin grafts covering much of the face have been successfully accomplished (56).

Special Uses of Tissue Expansion

NERVE EXPANSION

Sensory nerves are routinely lengthened with little risk during normal tissue expansion. The Ilizarov technique of bone lengthening demonstrated that major sensory and motor nerves can be successfully elongated. Both laboratory and clinical work in humans have shown that expansion of the proximal or distal segments can create sufficient nerve to bridge defects (57). Extensive work is still necessary in nerve expansion to enable comparison of its effectiveness with standard procedures.

SUSTAINED INTRAOPERATIVE EXPANSION

Expanders have been tried intraoperatively to harvest the vasoelastic properties of skin (58,59). Sequential load cycling of skin by expanding prostheses for several 10-minute intervals may be useful in closing of small tissue defects per primam. Several conflicting studies as to the long-term success of the procedure have been published (60-62). Also available are studies on the use of this technique to maximize results in facial cosmetic surgery (63).

Complications of Tissue Expansion

A high rate of complications can be expected by surgeons early in the learning process. With development of expertise, and appropriate selection of patients, complication rates can be minimized. Of significance, is the fact that even with complications, the vast majority of patients ultimately will achieve successful reconstruction using tissue expansion.

PAIN

Inflation of the expansion implant results in transient pain. Minimal analgesics administered for several hours after inflation are usually sufficient. The forehead, palm, sole of the foot, and genital areas are particularly uncomfortable during expansion. The use of small-volume injections at frequent intervals is recommended to minimize significant pain. Excessive pain may be an indication of tissue ischemia. The use of intraluminal analgesics that diffuse through the prosthesis over time is not recommended (64).

SEROMA

Seromas occur most often during expansion in the lower extremity and with immediate breast reconstruction. Partial inflation of the implant to fill dead space will minimize fluid collection. Seromas are likely to be a problem in immediate breast reconstruction if a completely separate submuscular plane has not been achieved for the prosthesis; suction drains and antibiotics until seromas have subsided are recommended. Placing a reservoir externally allows seromas to drain through the skin, but it also significantly increases risk of bacterial colonization.

HEMATOMA

Hematomas are major complications, potentially resulting in necrosis of the overlying tissue. They are usually the result of inadequate hemostasis when the prosthesis was placed, although some have described erosion of vessels during the process of expansion. Meticulous hemostasis will minimize this complication. Drains should not be depended upon to prevent hematomas.

INFECTION

Prosthesis within the body are predisposed to infection. Prostheses infected early in the course of expansion should be removed and adequately drained. They may be replaced 4 to 6 months later and the expansion repeated. If infection occurs as a result of extrusion late in the course of expansion, one may continue filling the prosthesis with low-volume frequent inflations until the expansion is completed. When the expanders are removed, the wound is copiously irrigated and the flaps are rotated. Expanded tissues have remarkable propensity to resist infection and excellent reconstructive results have been achieved despite infection of the prosthesis.

EXPOSURE

Implants that become exposed early in the course of expansion do so usually through a suture line or a preexisting scar. When early exposure occurs, it is best to abort the procedure, remove the expander, and repeat the procedure later. When exposure occurs late in the course of expansion, the prosthesis is sequentially filled until adequate tissue can be generated for reconstruction.

Bibliography

1. Manders EK, et al. Elongation of peripheral nerve and viscera containing smooth muscle. *Clin Plast Surg* 1987; 14:551.
2. Neumann CG. The expansion of an area of skin by progressive distention of a subcutaneous balloon. *Plast Reconstr Surg* 1957; 19:124.
3. Radovan C. Adjacent flap development using expandable silastic implants. Presented at the annual meeting of the American Society of Plastic and Reconstructive Surgeons, Boston, September 1976.
4. Radovan C. Breast reconstruction after mastectomy using the temporary expander. *Plast Reconstr Surg* 1982; 69:195.
5. Radovan C. Tissue expansion in soft-tissue reconstruction, *Plast Reconstr Surg* 1984; 74:482.
6. Argenta LC, Marks MW, Grabb WC. Selective use of serial expansion in breast reconstruction, *Ann Plast Surg* 1983; 11:188.
7. Argenta LC, Watanabe MJ, Grabb WC. The use of tissue expansion in head and neck reconstruction. *Ann Plast Surg* 1983; 11:31.
8. Argenta LC, Marks MW, Pasyk KA. Advances in tissue expansion. *Clin Plast Surg* 1985; 12:159.
9. Manders, EK, et al. Soft-tissue expansion: concepts and complications. *Plast Reconstr Surg* 1984; 74:493.
10. Austad E, Rose GL. A self-inflating tissue expander. *Plast Reconstr Surg* 1982; 70:107.
11. Austad E, et al. Histomorphologic evaluation of guinea pig skin and soft tissue after controlled tissue expansion, *Plast Reconstr Surg* 1982; 70:704.
12. Pasyk KA, et al. Electron microscopic evaluation of guinea pig skin and soft tissues "expanded" with a self-inflating silicone implant. *Plast Reconstr Surg* 1982; 70:37.
13. Pasyk KA, Argenta LC, Hassett, C. Quantitative analysis of the thickness of human skin and subcutaneous tissue following controlled expansion with a silicone implant. *Plast Reconstr Surg* 1988; 81:516.
14. Pasyk KA, Argenta LC, Austad E. Histopathology of human expanded skin. *Clin Plast Surg* 1987; 14:435.
15. Austad ED, Thomas SB, Pasyk K. Tissue expansion: dividend or loan. *Plast Reconstr Surg* 1986; 78:63.
16. Wollina U, Berger U, Stolle H, et al. Tissue expansion in pig skin—a histochemical approach. *Anat Hist Embr* 1992; 21:101.
17. Cherry GW, Austad E, Pasyk K, et al. Increased survival and vascularity of random-pattern skin flaps elevated in controlled, expanded skin. *Plast Reconstr Surg* 1983; 72:680.
18. Baker D, Dedrick D, Burney R, et al. Resistance of rapidly expanded random skin flaps to bacterial invasion *J Trauma* 1987; 27:1061.
19. Ryan T, Barnhill R. Physical factors and angiogenesis. In: Nigent P, ed. *Development of the vascular system*. CIBA Foundation Symposium 100, Pitman, 1983.
20. Dickenson W, Sharp D, Jackson I. Experience with an external valve in small-volume tissue expanders. *Brit J Plast Surg* 1988; 41:373.
21. Argenta L. Reconstruction of the breast by tissue expansion. *Clin Plast Surg* 1984; 11:257.
22. Versaci AD. Reconstruction of a pendulous breast utilizing a tissue expander. *Clin Plast Surg* 1987; 14:499.
23. Versaci AD. A method of reconstructing a pendulous breast utilizing the tissue expander. *Plast Reconstr Surg* 1987; 80:387.
24. Woods JE, Mangan MA. Breast reconstruction with tissue expanders: obtaining an optimal result. *Ann Plast Surg* 1992; 28(4):390.
25. Maxwell GP, Falcone PA. Eighty-four consecutive breast reconstructions using a textured silicone tissue expander. *Plast Reconstr Surg* 1992; 89(6):1022.
26. Becker H. The permanent tissue expander. *Clin Plast Surg* 1987; 14:519.
27. Hammmond D, Perry L, Maxwell G, et al. Morphologic analysis of tissue expansion shape using a biomechanical model. *Plast Reconstr Surg* 1993; 92:255.
28. Ward J, Cohen I, Knayoi F, et al. Immediate breast reconstruction with tissue expansion. *Plast Reconstr Surg* 1987; 80:559.
29. Artz J, Dinner M, Foglietti D, et al. Breast reconstruction using subcutaneous tissue expansion followed by polyurethane-covered silicone implants. *Plast Reconstr Surg* 1991; 88:635.
30. Paulhe P, Aubert JP, Magalon G. Forum on tissue expansion. Are tissue expansion and radiotherapy compatible? Apropos of a series of 50 consecutive breast reconstructions. *Ann de Chir Plast Esthe* 1993; 38(1):54.

31. Gibney J. Use of a permanent tissue expander for breast reconstruction. *Plast Reconstr Surg* 1989; 84:607.
32. Argenta L, VanderKolk K. Refinements in reconstruction of congenital breast deformities. *Plast Reconstr Surg* 1985; 76:73.
33. Versaci AD, Rozzelle AA. Treatment of tuberous breasts utilizing tissue expansion. *Aesth Plast Surg* 1991; 15:307.
34. Manders EK, et al. Skin expansion to eliminate large scalp defects *Ann Plast Surg* 1984; 12:305.
35. Argenta LC, Marks MW. Systematic approach to reconstruction of the head and neck by tissue expansion: In: Vistnes LM, ed. How They Do It. Boston: Little, Brown, 1990.
36. Wang SC, Chen FL, Li JY. Soft tissue expansion in the treatment of scar alopecia in preschool children. *Chinese Med J* 1991; 104(2) 164.
37. Dingman R, Argenta L. The surgical repair of traumatic defects of the scalp. *Clin Plast Surg* 1982; 9:131.
38. Adson M, Anderson R, Argenta L. Scalp expansion in the treatment of male pattern baldness. *Plast Reconstr Surg* 1987; 79:906.
39. Anderson R. The expanded "BAT" flap for treatment of male pattern baldness. *Ann Plast Surg* 1993; 31:385.
40. Iwahiri Y, Maruyama Y. Expanded unilateral full forehead flap for coverage of the opposite forehead defect. *Plast Reconstr Surg* 1993; 92:1052.
41. Moore MH, Trott JA, David DJ. Soft tissue expansion in the management of the rare craniofacial clefts. *Brit J Plast Surg* 1992; 45:155.
42. Sagehashi N. Cleft lip repair by soft tissue-tissue expansion. *Ann Plast Surg* 1992; 29:164.
43. O'Neal R, Rohrick R, Izenberg P. Skin expansion as an adjunct to reconstruction of the external ear. *Brit J Plast Surg* 1984; 37:517.
44. Kaneko T. A system for three-dimensional shape measurement and its application in microtia ear reconstruction. *Kei J Med* 1993; 42(1):22.
45. Hata Y, Hosokawa K, Yano K, Matsuka K. Correction of congenital microtia using the tissue expander. *Plast Reconstr Surg* 1989; 84:741.
46. Morgan R, Edgerton M. Tissue expansion in reconstructive hand surgery. Case report. *J Hand Surg* 1985; 10(A):754.
47. Van Beek A, and Adson M. Tissue expansion in the upper extremity. *Clin Plast Surg* 1987; 14:535.
48. Borges Filho PT, Neves RI, et al. Soft-tissue expansion in lower extremity reconstruction. *Clin Plast Surg* 1991; 18(3):593.
49. Serra J, Mesa F, Paloma V, et al. Use of calf prosthesis and tissue expansion in aesthetic reconstruction of the leg. *Plast Surg* 1992; 89:684.
50. Thornton J, Marks M, Izenberg P, et al. Expanded myocutaneous flaps: their clinical use. *Clin Plast Surg* 1987; 14:529.
51. Leighton W, Russell R, Feller AM, et al. Experimental pretransfer expansion of free flap donor sites: II. Physiology, histology, and clinical correlation. *Plast Reconstr Surg* 1988; 82:76.
52. Esposito G, di Caprio G, Ziccardi P, et al. Tissue expansion in the treatment of pressure ulcers. *Plast Reconstr Surg* 1991; 87:501.
53. Byrd HS, Hobar PC. Abdominal wall expansion in congenital defects. *Plast Reconstr Surg* 1989; 84:374.
54. Zubowicz B, Ricketts R. Use of tissue expansion in separation of conjoined twins. *Ann Plast Surg* 1988; 20:272.
55. Argenta LC, Marks MW, Iacobucci JJ, et al. Expanded full thickness skin grafts. *Plast Surg Forum* 1988; 11:136.
56. Bauer BS, Vicari FA, Richard ME, et al. Expanded full thickness skin grafts in children: case selection, planning, and management. *Plast Reconstr Surg* 1993; 92:59.
57. Wintner MS. Surgically assisted palatal expansion: an important consideration in adult treatment. *Amer J Orthod Dento Orthop* 1991; 99:85.
58. Sasaki GH. Intraoperative sustained limited expansion (ISLE) as an immediate reconstructive technique. *Clin Plast Surg* 1987; 14:563.
59. Wee SS, Logan SE, Mustoe TA. Continuous versus intraoperative expansion in the pig model. *Plast Reconstr Surg* 1992; 90:808.
60. Mackaz D, Saggers G, Kotwal N, et al. Stretching skin; undermining is more important than intraoperative expansion. *Plast Reconstr Surg* 1990; 86:722.
61. Hochman M, Branham G, Thomas J. Relative effects of intraoperative tissue expansion and undermining on wound closing tension. *Arch Otolarg* 1992; 118:1185.
62. Machida B, Liu M, Sasaki G, et al. Immediate vs. chronic tissue expansion. *Ann Plast Surg* 1991; 26:227.
63. Man D. Stretching and tissue expansion for rhytidectomy: an improved approach. *Plast Reconstr Surg* 1989; 84:561.
64. Derby L, Sinow J, Bowers L, et al. Quantitative analysis of lidocaine hydrochloride delivery by diffusion across tissue expander membranes. *Plast Reconstr Surg* 1992; 89:900.

13

Lasers in Plastic Surgery

Richard Gregory, M.D., F.A.C.S.

Einstein outlined the theory of laser operation in 1917, but only after Maiman made the first laser in 1959 did the application of lasers to medicine begin to be appreciated. Lasers continue to gain value in the fields of plastic and reconstructive surgery; the past 5 years have seen a huge increase in the use of lasers in a variety of cosmetic and reconstructive roles. This will not be a comprehensive review of the subject—simply a broad summary of the most salient points. Surgeons are encouraged to read a comprehensive text on the subject, attend training symposia/courses, and participate in the meetings of the American Society for Laser Medicine and Surgery.

Currently, the most popular subject in laser plastic surgery is the rejuvenation of weathered and aged skin with the high-powered, extremely short-pulsed carbon dioxide (CO_2) laser. This technique will largely replace some peels, as well as dermabrasion. New techniques have also been added to the repertoire of some earlier lasers and their indications have been refined.

The laser is not a panacea or a miracle machine, simply another tool in the armamentarium of the surgeon, as was recognized by the American College of Surgeons in a recently published *Guidelines for Laser Usage*. Likewise, it is neither an expensive electrocautery nor a marketing gimmick; the motivation for using the laser should be improved service to patients.

Laser Physics and Physiology

Lasers have several unique properties that are widely recognized as being collimated, coherent, and monochromatic. Lasers are characterized by wavelength, or the color of light emitted. Many lasers fall within the visible spectrum, from 400 nm in the blue range to 700 nm in the red range. A number of lasers also fall in the infrared and ultraviolet portions of the visible spectrum.

Laser light has energy when it strikes an object where it can be absorbed, transmitted, or refracted. However, the only energy capable of doing light work is that which is absorbed. But transmission through the tissue to the target must be adequate, so penetration of laser light also becomes a factor. When light photons strike an object, they are either absorbed or refracted. Different molecules absorb laser light differently. Absorption curves for a variety of absorbers (chromophores) can be plotted, depicting the percentage of absorption vs. the wavelength of the light. It should be noted that absorption is not linear and, in fact, hemoglobin has at least three major absorption peaks where the absorption is

greatest. Curves of hemoglobin, melanin, xanthophyll, and water absorption can be plotted along an axis of wavelength. Since tissue is not homogenous, there is competition by the various chromophores for absorbing the laser light. To minimize complications, such as pigmentation changes and scarring, the goal of any procedure should therefore be to maximize absorption in the target tissue and minimize it in the competing chromophores.

Light striking tissue can cause thermal, photoacoustic, or photobiochemical effects. By far the vast majority of tissue response to laser light is thermal, although photoacoustic and photobiochemical responses are assuming increasing importance in medicine.

Thermal energy created when laser light strikes a tissue will begin raising the temperature of the tissue at a rate dependent upon the amount of energy and the rate of energy delivery. Tissue effects are at first reversible, but protein denatures at approximately 60° C, causing irreversible effects in the tissue. At 100° C, vacuolizations (i.e., steam bubbles) form, followed by char, and eventually a plume is created as the tissue is evaporated. These effects are, of course, time dependent, and a given amount of energy will have significantly different effects when delivered in an extremely short period of time as contrasted to a long duration of energy delivery.

One of the more important concepts of laser usage advanced in recent years has been that of selective photothermolysis. This concept proposes that, after the appropriate wavelength or color of laser light has been chosen, the prime factor in optimizing results is the *pulse duration* (time/rate of delivery of the energy). Nearly every substance will have a brief period of time during which the thermal effects are confined to the target tissue, and there is very little heat conduction in the surrounding tissue substance. This time is termed the *thermal relaxation time,* and for water is about 200 microseconds. For melanosomes, the thermal relaxation time may vary from 250 to 1000 nanoseconds, depending on the size of the structure. The thermal relaxation time of hemoglobin, and in particular the hemoglobin-containing vessels of the port-wine stain, probably is in the range of 1 millisecond but may be higher for larger vessels. It is evident that the thermal relaxation time varies not only on the nature of the absorber but also in the size of the absorbing structures. Finally, enough energy must be delivered to the target in a period of time less than the thermal relaxation time in order to heat the absorber to a critical temperature. This is termed the *vaporization threshold.*

Using the concept of selective photothermolysis, many lasers have been designed that greatly facilitate the treatment of port-wine stains, pigmented structures (e.g., benign lentigo), other vascular structures and—in the most recently introduced laser—resurfacing with the CO_2 laser.

Indications

Benefits sufficient to justify using the laser must counterbalance the associated inconvenience, expense, and training. Among the advantages attributed to lasers are (a) decreased blood loss because the lasers readily seal vessels of a small caliber, (b) reduced pain resulting from sealing of the nerve endings, (c) reduced edema secondary to sealing of lymphatics; and, in appropriate circumstances, (d) reduced scarring owing to decreased damage to surrounding tissue. Disadvantages include expense of the laser and accessories, and a learning curve that may in some cases be lengthy. Inconvenience has often been associated with laser usage, but is a rapidly diminishing factor since design of the instruments has been improved.

Finally, the safety factors involved in laser usage are similar to those of other instruments and require protection from fire, plume or smoke generation, and eye hazards.

Indications for laser usage include the applications summarized below.

Definitions

It is important to understand both terminology and laser physics. Power from the laser is measured in terms of watts or milliwatts. The power per unit area, which determines the concentration of the laser energy striking the tissue, is termed *power density* or *irradiance* and is measured in terms of watts per cm^2. It should be noted that the power density is inversely proportional to the square of the diameter, and thus great changes in this value are created by changing the spot size only a small amount. Energy delivered to the tissue is time dependent and is defined as power × time. The energy is measured in joules and is equal to the watts × seconds. For instance, 1 joule equals 1 watt-second. The *fluence* is the irradiance × time, or measured in watt-seconds per cm^2. It is important to understand these terms because tissue effect is proportional to both power and time of delivery (Table 13–1).

Table 13–1
Laser Parameters

Target	Laser	Wavelength
Hemoglobin	Dye	577 and 585
	Copper vapor	578
	Krypton	568
Hemoglobin melanin	Krypton	521 and 530
	Copper vapor	511
	Argon	488 and 514
Melanin	Dye (TLDL)	510
Melanin and tattoos	Ruby	694
	Frequency-Doubled YAG	532
	Alexandrite	755
Protein and tattoos	Neodymium YAG	1064
H_2O	CO_2	10,600

Applications

COSMETIC

Cosmetic applications are the fastest growing area in laser use for plastic and reconstructive surgery. The high-power, rapidly pulsed laser has made resurfacing of badly weathered and aged skin both precise and predictable.

According to the theory of selective photothermolysis, the target of the CO_2 laser is primarily water. By pulsing it very rapidly below the thermal relaxation time of skin (less than 1 millisecond), precise layers of skin can be treated with minimal risk of scarring. Also, according to the concept of selective photothermolysis, enough laser energy has to be loaded into the tissue in a short enough period of time in order to achieve the desired goal. This has been found to be 4 to 5 joules per cm^2. To give a smooth and uniform effect, a 3-mm collimated (nondivergent) handpiece is frequently used to apply this laser energy. Recently approved by the FDA, a robotized handpiece known as a *computerized pattern generator* will allow rapid, precise application of the CO_2 laser. Another application involves an oscillating mirror directing a continuous wave CO_2 laser. Preliminary studies seem to indicate that this is capable of producing a similar clinical result—but with somewhat deeper thermal damage and perhaps more risk.

The energy per pulse (joules/cm^2) is determined by the laser and dictated by the area of the skin being treated. Generally speaking, more thickly keratinized and wrinkled skin requires a higher energy per pulse, whereas lower eyelid skin requires less. Because of the need to achieve a certain vaporization threshold, it is necessary to keep the energy per pulse above 200 millijoules per cm^2. Otherwise, sufficient energy is not delivered to vaporize the tissue; instead, it simply heats the tissue, thereby increasing the risk of scarring. Therefore, the range from 200 to 500 millijoules per pulse (500 is maximum power output for the laser) is used on various areas of the face. For a heavily weathered patient, 400 to 500 millijoules per pulse would be used around the mouth, where for a lightly affected patient perhaps 250 millijoules on the lower eyelids would be sufficient.

Another factor in laser resurfacing is the number of passes to be made. The first pass with the laser over the designated area generally removes most if not all of the epithelium. The epithelial debris is then brushed away, and a 2nd, 3rd, or 4th pass is achieved. Because of the exposure of the upper dermis, and thermal coagulation of the dermal collagen, there is less debris removed with subsequent passes. In fact, the surgeon can readily observe the tightening of the collagen bundles as the laser impacts the skin. It is essential to remove any debris between each pass to facilitate the laser light absorption. In most instances, three to four passes is the maximum possible without increasing the risk of scarring. Treated areas should be feathered into the surrounding untreated areas by lessening the energy per pulse or decreasing the number of passes and the spacing of laser spots. The laser impact spots should be overlapping by about 10% in the treated areas.

It is recommended that the laser treatment be concentrated into the area of the heaviest wrinkling by treatment of the isolated wrinkles during one of the passes.

The histology of the treated areas shows that the first pass with the laser generally coagulates the epithelium with little damage to the other underlying dermis. This then is wiped away and the second pass is made. Perhaps 20 to 50 microns of thermal coagulation is seen on the second pass, which may extend up to 100 to 150 microns, depending on the number of passes. Although long-term histologic follow-up of these patients is scant at present, it would seem that the residual thermal coagulated protein is incorporated into the new matrix of tissue created by the laser treatment and contributes to the resolution of the wrinkles and aged skin.

A full description of this process can be found in *Clinics in Plastic Surgery*.

VASCULAR LESIONS

A variety of vascular lesions can be treated with the laser (Table 13–2). Nearly any vessels small enough and superficial enough can be collapsed to allow permanent closure with a vascular lesion laser. Factors other than depth and size of the vessel must be considered, including the flow rate as well as the location on the body and a variety of laser parameters. Energy fluence and pulse duration influence the effectiveness of the laser. In many lasers, parameters have already been preset and cannot be changed by the therapist. The preset laser parameters are both a blessing and a curse.

Lasers can be of two varieties, one emphasizing simplicity of use and the other diversity of adjustable parameters. Many of the new, rapidly pulsed lasers (e.g., the pulsed dye laser, the Q-switched laser) can be adjusted only as to fluence and spot size, and both of these variables have distinct limitations. This simplicity of use translates into an element of safety: The fewer the adjustments, the less experience and judgment are required of surgeons to provide a safe treatment. But this simplicity limits the effectiveness of the laser therapy. Thus, the Argon and copper vapor lasers, for example, can effectively treat a more diverse group of lesions but require more of the surgeon. In either case, nothing substitutes for experience and good judgment.

Vascular lesions would include port-wine stains, also called capillary malformations, as well as telangiectasias and a variety of other arteriovenous malformations. Hemangiomas, which are grouped separately according to the Mulliken classification, have different considerations of treatment simply because of their inherent tendency to regress on their own and because of their complex nature.

Table 13–2
Depth of Pigment in Cutaneous Lesions

Epidermal	Combined dermal/epidermal	Dermal
Lentigines	Posttraumatic	Nevus of Ota
Café au lait macules	Becker nevus	Nevus of Ito
Ephelides	Compound nevus	Blue nevus
Nevocellular nevi		Postsclerotherapy
Nevus spilus		Hyperpigmentation
Seborrheic keratosis		
Pigmented actinic keratosis		

PORT-WINE STAINS

Port-wine stains are found in 0.3 to 0.5% of the population. Most are found on the face in the 1st and 2nd trigeminal nerve distribution and are quite shallow. Childhood port-wine stains have an average vessel diameter of 10 to 50 microns, while in the adult these can dilate up to 300 microns in diameter, which dictates different treatment and response.

The port-wine stain is associated with a variety of other disorders including Sturge-Weber syndrome, which can be expressed in seizures, glaucoma, and sometimes mental retardation. The Klippel-Trenaunay syndrome consists of port-wine stain and hypertrophy of a portion of the anatomy and is thought to be caused by increased metabolism secondary to increased blood flow. As mentioned above, the vessels in the port-wine stain enlarge as the patient ages. Two-thirds of the patients will have a nodularity or bleb formation by 46 years of age; this is thought to be the result of arteriovenous shunts.

Port-wine stain birthmarks can be treated by a number of laser types including the pulsed dye laser, the Argon laser, the copper vapor and copper bromide lasers, the Argon-pumped dye laser, and others. Hobby found that, with proper patient selection, he was able to treat some port-wine stains with good resolution and relatively few complications using an Argon laser. In other reports, the Argon laser treatment of port-wine stains had a high rate of complications secondary to improper patient selection and poor laser parameter selection. Because of this high complication rate, there was a strong determination to develop new lasers for treating young patients with port-wine stains. The theory of selective photothermolysis was born out of an attempt to reduce complications in port-wine stain treatment in infants and children. This theory, as previously noted, led to the development of the pulsed dye laser, which had a preset pulse duration (450 microseconds) and a preselected wavelength (initially 577 nm, later changed to 585 nm). Additionally, the fluence was limited to a relatively safe range. The complication rate and the treatment of pediatric port-wine stains was drastically reduced coincidental with limiting the diversity of lesions that can be effectively treated with this laser. The bottom line is that there is no one laser that is ideal for treating all port-wine stain birthmarks or other vascular lesions.

It was found that starting earlier in the treatment of these port-wine stains led to an improved clearance rate. In fact, if treated before 18 months of age, approximately eight treatments were needed for complete clearance in 25% of the patients and marked lightening in others, whereas waiting until the patient was much older reduced this clearance rate dramatically.

Port-wine stains on the extremities seem to respond less well, with good to excellent response in 84%. Generally speaking, the darker and more granular the lesion, the better would be the response to laser treatment.

In addition to the development of the pulsed dye laser, other attempts to reduce the complication rate led to the introduction of scanning devices that could be attached to the Argon laser and others so that the thermal effect on the tissue would be more readily controlled. This also reduced the incidence of complications.

The choice of lasers to treat an individual vascular lesion should be guided by the age of the patient, the location on the body, and the darkness of the lesion, which relates to the size of the vessels and other factors. A general guideline relating to laser selection should be as follows. In infants, the choice is almost always the pulsed dye laser for homogeneous pink port-wine stains. As the patient approaches adulthood, the vessels tend to enlarge and get darker as the result of stagnation of blood inside the vessels. In this population of patients, although the pulsed dye laser can be used initially, other lasers such as the copper vapor laser, the Argon-pumped dye laser, and those fitted with a scanning device may be more effective on the larger, deeper vessels. When this choice of lasers is not available, the surgeon must judge whether to treat or refer the patient.

Even more recent advances in the treatment of vascular lesions have led to lengthening of the pulse duration (1 to 10 msec seems to be acceptable) in order to effectively treat larger and deeper vessels. In addition, the spot size has been increased to 10 mm, which means not only that a larger area can be covered more quickly but also, because of a refraction of the energy, more effective ablation of vessels may be possible.

TELANGIECTASIAS

Telangiectasias, although most commonly treated on the face, can be seen anywhere on the body. A variety of influences can contribute to telangiectasias (e.g., acne rosacea, spider angioma, poikiloderma of Civatte). Many of these telangiectatic disorders have very high pressure of vessels of varying depths and require considerable laser fluence. As individual vessels are identified under magnification, a vessel-tracing technique can be used with an extremely small spot size. More diffuse, smaller vessel disease (e.g., poikiloderma) can be treated over an area (large spot size overlapping or a robotic scanner) with good resolution. Resolution of telangiectasias frequently requires more than one treatment.

OTHER VASCULAR LESIONS

Generally speaking, most superficial vascular lesions on the lower extremities respond poorly, often because of increased intravascular pressure. The laser can sometimes be used in combination with sclerotherapy for an improved response rate.

Vascular lesions are said to be the most common birth disorder, and many of these will be hemangiomas. Hemangioma is a lesion of infancy that has a high incidence of spontaneous resolution. This is thought to be due to the embryonal lining cells of the vessels, which are generally steroid responsive.

While many of these may not be present at birth, up to 90% are apparent by 1 month of age. Sixty percent of hemangiomas are on the head and neck, with many of those remaining appearing on the perineum. There is a 3:1 female:male incidence. Hemangiomas vary widely with regard to the depth and size of the vessel. Varying from a bright red cutaneous vessel to a deep dark-blue or purple larger-vessel disorder, many of them will undergo spontaneous regression. This is usually evidenced by a grey filmy discoloration in the surface. Although it has been said that 50% will have complete resolution by 5 years of age and 70% by 7 years of age, nevertheless many times there are residual disorders such as pigmentary changes, scars, and

minor vascular lesions left. Somewhere between 15 and 15% do not completely involute.

Hemangiomas are fraught with complications, including ulceration, bleeding, infection, deformity, airway obstruction, and visual deterioration secondary to suppression amblyopia. The Kasabach-Meritt syndrome is associated with a coagulopathy secondary to platelet trapping in the hemagioma and requires aggressive therapy.

Forty to sixty percent of hemagiomas are noted to be steroid responsive and can be treated orally or parenterally. Many times the shallow lesions will respond to a laser treatment, which probably should be done with the pulsed dye laser. This, however, will require several treatments spaced at 2- to 4-week intervals. Intralesional or percutaneous treatment with the neodymium YAG laser has been successful in shrinking some hemangiomas.

Other disorders that have a minimal vascular component will also respond to lasers. Verruca vulgaris (warts) and a variety of other lesions can be treated by lasers with minimal scarring. It is thought that coagulation of the blood vessels produced by lasers contributes to the resolution of the lesions.

Tattoo Treatment

The popularity of tattoos rises and falls with fashion. It is estimated that about 10% of adult men in the United States have tattoos, and between 50,000 and 100,000 women are being tattooed annually.

Tattoo dye is comprised largely of heavy-metal chemicals that we would consider too toxic for our landfills, and yet some people readily accept them for implantation into the body. Mercury, cadmium, cobalt, and chromium are among the dye substances used for decorative tattooing.

The tattoo particles vary from 2 to 400 microns in diameter. The depth initially is in the deep epidermis/shallow dermis, where the tattoo particles are implanted by repeated punctures with the needle. The healing of the wound at about 1 month seems to seal the tattoo pigment particles intracellularly by phagocytosis, and healing of the basement membrane prevents leaching of the tattoo dye. With the passing of years the dye appears to penetrate more deeply and indeed has been found in draining lymph nodes.

There is a great deal of variation in depth and size of the particle and density of the tattoo pigment, both in amateur and professional tattoos. Although superficial surveys indicate an acceptance, and indeed enthusiasm, for tattooing, fully 38% of tattooed people in one survey reported difficulties, primarily social in nature, and many wanted the tattoos removed.

Tattoo removal has been done nearly as long as tattooing itself. Mechanical abrasion of the tattoo particles has in the past been the primary mode of removal. This might have included salabrasion with common salt, but dermabrasion was also attempted. These mechanical removal techniques might have been combined with chemical destruction (e.g., urea or tannic acid), which improved the leaching. Additionally, thermal destruction with coagulators as well as liquid nitrogen were tried with limited success. The almost universal result of these techniques was scarring of the tattoo site. In many instances, the scarring was hypertrophic and almost as objectionable as the tattoos themselves.

The laser treatment of tattoos began in 1965, shortly after the laser became available. Many lasers have been used for the destruction of tattoo dye, but most of the early lasers—including argon, conventional carbon dioxide, and continuous-wave ruby lasers—also resulted in considerable scarring when the procedure was deep enough to remove the deep dermal pigment by thermal necrosis. Once again, urea paste was used in combination to improve the results.

Laser treatment of tattoos improved markedly when the rapidly pulsed lasers became available. The tattoo dye absorbs the laser light, which is pulsed extremely rapidly, causing a rapid buildup of heat and subsequent fracturing of the tattoo pigment particles. Much of the pigment removal is by macrophages, although it has been hypothezied that a chemical reaction leading to an optical change in the pigment causes the tattoo to lighten.

The Q-switched ruby, Q-switched alexandrite, Q-switched neodymium YAG, and pulsed dye lasers have all been used for tattoo removal with varying success. As one would expect, the differing color of the light available from the various lasers is absorbed differently by the colors of tattoo pigment. This causes a differential resolution of the various colors with each of the lasers. Many studies have been done using various lasers at differing pulse durations as well as differing fluences, sometimes doing side-by-side comparisons on the same tattoo. Generally speaking, shorter pulses (< 40 μsec) and higher fluences (> 6–10 joules/cm^2) gave better clearing of tattoo pigment but were also more disruptive of tissue. Fortunately, the incidence of permanent scarring has been small, being only rarely reported with the Q-switched ruby laser and not at all with the others. Hypopigmentation, usually transient, was very common, however, and hyperpigmentation was occasionally encountered. It should be noted that most of these lasers also react with other skin pigments such as melanin, as will be noted below in the discussion of laser treatment of pigmented lesions.

The differential clearing with regard to the laser light was quite noticeable. For instance, nearly all lasers treated black tattoo ink very well. The ruby was ineffective on red pigment. The neodymium YAG tended to treat green and red pigments poorly at 1064 nm; fortunately, this laser has a frequency-doubling crystal allowing the production of 532 nm (green) light, which was found to be effective on red ink. Blue, green, and yellow, however, continued to be resistant to the neodymium YAG laser. The alexandrite laser, at 755 nm, was found to be extremely useful in treating green tattoo dye as well as black and blue, but was uniformly ineffective in treating red tattoo dye.

Nearly all tattoos will require multiple treatments (from 4 to 10), and even then may leave behind some particularly resistant dye.

Most authors feel it is wise to wait 4 to 8 weeks between treatments, and an occasional rest period of 2 to 3 months between treatments is advisable. Fewer treatments seem to be necessary on the amateur tattoos. Although ideally the surgeon would have three or four different lasers to treat various tattoos, this is not generally practical. I have found that the Q-switched neodymium YAG laser with the frequency-doubling feature (i.e., both 1064 nm and 532 nm) was the best individual laser for my practice, but even it has its limitations.

Two special categories of tattoos should be mentioned. Traumatic tattoos with imbedding of foreign-body particles have been treated with the laser. The Q-switched laser gives an excellent result with many of these traumatic tattoos and with nearly 100% clearing in three or fewer treatments.

Finally, tattoos applied for eye liner, lip liner, and so on, should be discussed. Misapplication of the tattoo dye or dispersion due to migration occurs in 4 to 5% of these patients. Many patients have successful removal of their tattoo dye through a variety of lasers. Unfortunately, many flesh tones, as well as some red and white ones, contain dyes that will convert from their baseline color to a very dark tattoo color when treated with the laser. This is thought to result from reduction of the ferric oxide pigment, which is then extremely difficult to remove. Test areas are recommended.

The ultrapulsed carbon dioxide laser has been found to remove pigment granules in all forms of tattoos, but especially in the decorative facial tattoos. This laser evaporates tissue, thereby removing the pigment. It has been found to have excellent results with minimal scarring, very acceptable when used on tattoos. As always, the surgeon is encouraged to try a small, obscure test area before generalized treatment if there is any question about the response.

Pigmented Cutaneous Lesions (Table 13–2)

Pigmented lesions have been treated in a variety of ways, including cryosurgery, chemical peels, and bleaching with hydroquinone, a compound known to block tyrosine conversion to melanin. Unfortunately, mechanical and chemical methods of treatment will result in hyper and hypo pigmentation as well as recurrence in many instances.

For the above reason, the laser has been used to treat a variety of benign pigmented nevi. In this group, however, one of the largest concerns is that many of these lesions—including the nevocellular nevi, both congenital and acquired—have a potential for malignancy. Because of the possibility of malignant pigmented lesions masquerading as benign, it is generally wise to perform a biopsy on any suspicious lesion before treatment with the laser. We do not know what the long-term effects of laser treatment would be on the potential malignancy of these transitional, pigmented lesions.

Melanin absorption demonstrates a downward sloping curve from the ultraviolet to the infrared portion of the electromagnetic spectrum. Generally the lower wavelengths are more effectively absorbed by the melanin, and thus less energy is usually required to disrupt the melanin particles in the skin at the lower wavelengths. A variety of lasers have been used to treat these pigmented lesions, including the argon and a number of Q-switched lasers. Unfortunately, as the pulse duration increases the selectivity for the absorption in the melanin-containing structures is lost. At higher pulse durations (greater than 1 msec), generalized disruption of the tissue from thermal effects is commonly seen. For that reason, most recent clinical studies treating pigmented lesions have been with the Q-switched, pulsed lasers (e.g., the ruby, neodymium YAG, alexandrite, and pulsed dye lasers). Since the ruby wavelength, at 694 nm, is known to penetrate quite deeply, it is considered the laser of choice for the deeper pigmented lesions. In many instances, however, other lasers have been found to be equally effective.

Another quandary arises from these treatments. Since the melanocyte represents the manufacturing cell of the melanin and the keratinocyte is found to be the storage cell for the malanin, the question naturally arises, What is the target? Indeed, it has been found in treating some pigmented lesions where the melanin is largely found in the keratinocyte, selective destruction of the melanin-containing cells fails to prevent recurrence because of the lack of melanin in the melanocytes, which are therefore spared the laser effect. It has been found that subthreshold exposures of laser light (less than 1.5 to 2.5 joules/cm^2) may even stimulate melanogenesis, although the reason is not known. Melasma lentigines and café au lait macules are particularly inclined to experience this melanogenesis.

Among the superficial pigmented lesions, the café au lait macules are the most difficult to treat because of the marked recurrence rate. These broad, flat, tan-to-brown lesions frequently are present at birth and may be associated with neurofibromatosis. Although nearly all of the lasers are effective in removing the pigmentation from a café au lait macule in three or fewer treatments, recurrences may occur. Other superficial lesions (e.g., the lentigo simplex, solar lentigo, and labial melanotic macule) will respond to the laser treatment. The melanotic macule must be differentiated from malignant lesions before treatment.

Nevocellular nevi, either congenital or acquired, represent an increasingly important category of lesions with potential for laser treatment. Congenital nevocellular nevi may have a 1 to 5% (or more) likelihood of malignant transformation. Pretreatment biopsy is imperative, as is frequent follow-up of these lesions. In fact, it may not be possible adequately to follow these patients after laser treatment because some of the clinical indicators of malignant potential may have been lost.

Acquired nevocellular nevi respond somewhat better than the congenital variety, simply because the pigment tends to be more shallow. A variety of pulsed lasers have been used successfully in removing these lesions. One to three treatments were necessary and since many of these lesions, especially the congenital variety, are quite deep, the laser frequently will not reach the deepest portion of the lesion.

Nevus spilus, a café au lait–like macule with darker speckles, are unlikely to be premalignant. Unfortunately, many of these also exhibit a poor response to the pulsed lasers.

Seborrheic keratoses can be removed in a variety of ways. Depending on depth, a number of laser treatments may be necessary, and the surgeon might consider using the ultrapulsed carbon-dioxide laser for the thicker lesions. Pigmented actinic keratoses likewise respond to lasers, probably decreasing the malignant potential of this dysplastic lesion.

Nevus of Ota and nevus of Ito are very similar in appearance, both occurring more commonly in Asians. The primary difference between them is that the nevus of Ota usually occurs in the 1st and 2nd trigeminal nerve divisions of the face, whereas the nevus of Ito is generally on the shoulder or arm. Melanin pigmentation in these lesions is deep, but the lesions do respond well to both the Q-switched ruby and the Q-switched neodymium YAG lasers. Usually several treatments are necessary and recurrence is sometimes seen.

Becker nevi, commonly seen in children or young adults, with variable pigmentation and, frequently, dark coarse hair,

are usually very thick pigmented lesions. Although there are several encouraging reports on treatment of these lesions with the laser, there appears to be some variability in responsiveness.

Postsclerotherapy hyperpigmentation is most commonly seen with hypertonic saline and sodium tetradecyl sulfate injection, although it can be seen with polidocanol. This hemosiderin may result from leakage of hemoglobin into the tissue. Although the mechanism of action is not known, most of the above lasers, as well as the copper vapor laser, are effective in treating this condition.

Among the most resistant of all pigmented lesions to treat is melasma. This variable pigmentation, occuring in response to pregnancy or other hormonal stimulations such as oral contraceptives, is very common. Unfortunately, it tends to be persistent in many patients even beyond the cessation of hormonal stimulation. In fact, there seem to be two types, one showing a superficial epidermal pigmentation and the other being dermal in nature. Ultraviolet light examination shows enhancement of pigmentation in the superficial melasma. It has been found that most of these lasers improve the melasma, but for unknown reasons, perhaps the melanogenic stimulation, recurrence is extremely common. Therapy should include treatment with pigment-blocking drugs such as hydroquinone.

Posttraumatic hyperpigmentation, melanin deposited in postoperative scars and other traumatized areas, respond positively to a variety of laser treatment options.

Other Uses for the Laser in Plastic Surgery

Although the applications of the laser already mentioned are the most common, other uses for the laser in plastic surgery seem to have an important future.

There are incisional procedures in which the attributes of the laser are helpful. In these instances, the contact use of the neodymium YAG laser offers the benefits of superior coagulation without the electrical damage of electrocautery. Excision of tumors, as in breast surgery, may decrease the possibility of tumor emboli. Raising flaps, as in TRAM flap reconstruction of the mastectomy, has proven useful for the above reasons as well as the fact that there is little muscle stimulation during incision with the laser.

The CO_2 laser in the ultrapulsed mode is capable of incising the skin with a scar comparable to a scalpel but with less blood loss. This advantage would be important in precisonal surgery such as blepharoplasty and other periorbital procedures. Many surgeons are now combining a transconjunctival blepharoplasty with lower eyelid resurfacing, with excellent results.

New and Future Uses of the Laser

Photodynamic therapy of cancer, although in development for many years, soon will be released in this country. It is already in use in Canada and elsewhere for a variety of GI, GU, and pulmonary tumors. It has broad applicability, however, and can be used to treat a variety of skin and metastatic malignancies.

Ironically, the laser is being used to both transplant hair and remove unwanted hair. In hair transplantation, the recipient sites have been made with the laser for some time. The rapidly pulsed CO_2 laser decreases the bleeding and the tissue damage in the scalp, promoting good graft take. A new device to create the slit patterns for receiving the micrografts should greatly facilitate this process.

Hair removal with the laser is still in the early development stages. Several different techniques are being studied. One uses a dye that couples laser energy to the hair follicles, destroying them. Other laser wavelengths, still under investigation, directly target the follicles.

Telangiectatic veins of the legs are difficult to treat. Sclerotherapy on the midsized veins is effective, and ligation or stripping of the larger is preferred. The small "starburst" or matted telangtasias have not been readily treated in the past. New lasers are addressing this ubiquitous problem with excellent results.

Finally, investigations are underway to determine if the laser may be used to stimulate the healing of tissue. This biostimulation probably does occur, and may be useful clinically, but the procedure lacks a solid scientific foundation at present. Along this line, certain lasers are being used to treat striae (stretch marks), but it is too early to determine the effectiveness of this procedure.

Certainly the dawn of widespread laser use has come. It is long overdue, and there is much work to be done in developing this instrument for our profession.

Suggested Readings

Anderson RR. Laser-tissue interactions. In: Goldman MP, Fitzpatrick RE, eds. *Cutaneous laser surgery, the art and science of selective photothermolysis.* St. Louis: CV Mosby, 1994.

Anderson RR, Parrish JA. Microvasculature can be selectively damaged using dye lasers: a basic theory and experimental evidence in human skin. *Lasers Surg Med* 1981; 1:263.

Apfelberg DB. *Evaluation and installation of surgical laser systems.* New York: Springer-Verlag, 1987.

Fitzpatrick RE, Goldman MP, Ruiz-Esparza J. Laser treatment of benign pigmented epidermal lesions using a 300 nsec pulse and 510 nm wavelength. *J Dermatol Surg Oncol* 1993; 18:341.

Goldman MP, Fitzpatrick RE. *Cutaneous laser surgery: the art and science of selective photothermolysis.* St. Louis, CV Mosby, 1994.

Gregory RO, Baker SS. Laser blepharoplasty. *Aesthetic Surgery Quarterly* 1995; 15:2, 22.

Rosenberg GJ, Gregory RO. Lasers in aesthetic surgery. In: Habal MB, ed. *Clinics in Plastic Surgery* 23:1. Philadelphia: WB Saunders, 1966.

van Gemert MJC, Huldsbergen-Henning JP. A model approach to laser coagulation of dermal vascular lesions. *Arch Dermatol Res* 1981; 270:429.

Tan OT, Sherwood K, Gilchrest BA. Treatment of children with port-wine stains using the flashlamp pulsed tunable dye laser 3. *N Engl J Med* 1982; 20:416.

TWO

Skin and Soft Tissues

14

Repair of Traumatic Cutaneous Injuries Involving Skin and Soft Tissue

Martin C. Robson, M.D., F.A.C.S., Lawrence S. Zachary, M.D., F.A.C.S., and Richard H.C. Harries, B.M., B.S., B.Sc.

A wound can be defined as a disruption of normal anatomic structure and function; specifically, it involves a breach in the epithelial lining of whatever tissue is involved. Wounds may arise from surgical incisions, accidental trauma, or even prolonged bed rest. An *acute wound* is any wound that proceeds through the healing processes in a timely and orderly way, such that sustained anatomic function and integrity are restored (e.g., a laceration of the face that is repaired and heals without complication within 7 to 10 days is an example of an acute wound). A *chronic wound* is a wound that does not proceed to healing in a timely or orderly manner and/or fails to produce a sustained restoration of anatomic function and structure (e.g., a deep, partial-thickness wound that heals with dressings in 2 to 3 weeks is an acute wound; but if the same wound, for whatever reason, failed to heal after a period longer than expected or kept forming ulcers over previously healed sites, it could be regarded as chronic).

Because the human biologic state is not germ-free, there exists a delicate balance that allows survival in the presence of myriad species of bacteria, all with the potential of causing infection. There is an equilibrium between the factors of host resistance and the bacteria when no infection is present. Once the equilibrium is breached, either by an impairment in host resistance or an increase in the bacterial inoculum, clinical infection results. In any wound, the normal equilibrium between bacteria and host is endangered. Local defense mechanisms are challenged by disruption of the cutaneous barrier, which ordinarily provides protection. Impediments to local defense mechanisms (e.g., debris, blood clots, or necrotic tissue) often accompany a large bacterial inoculum in traumatic wounds.

The major advance in the prevention and management of infection in soft tissue has been the understanding that the mere presence of microorganisms in a wound is less important than the level of bacterial growth. A wealth of clinical and experimental data show that a level of bacterial growth of greater than 100,000 organisms per gram of tissue is necessary to cause a wound infection and the potential for invasive sepsis for most species of bacteria (1). Only the β-hemolytic streptococcus appears capable of routinely causing infection at levels of less than 100,000 organisms per gram of tissue (2).

The role of the surgeon in managing any soft-tissue wound is, first, to evaluate whether or not the patient's balance is in equilibrium. If it is, all efforts must be expended to maintain this status and prevent an ensuing infection; if it is not, in-fection is present and the management is directed at reestablishing the equilibrium.

Infection can be prevented by maintaining the patient's (host's) defenses at peak levels. The effect of the interaction between the bacteria and the host, although under systemic influence, is ultimately determined by local factors in the wound. Among these are necrotic tissue, decreased local wound perfusion, foreign bodies, hematoma, and dead space. Generally the patient presenting with a traumatic wound will not have immune defect due to systemic factors—and the surgeon could do little to influence this defect if it were present. However, the surgeon does play a significant role in eliminating local deterrents to effective host defense in the wound (3). If local wound factors are not controlled, there is potential for a subinfectious inoculum of bacteria to grow to sufficiently to produce infection.

All traumatic wounds are contaminated, at least to the extent that bacteria can always be identified by cultures performed on tissue biopsies of specimens (4). Because bacteria reside both on the surface of the skin and deep in the hair follicles and sweat glands, the bacterial count of skin is generally high; the numbers of bacteria normally present in the recesses is 1000 organisms per gram of tissue (1).

In 1941 Pulaski and colleagues (5) found, on culturing 200 fresh traumatic wounds aerobically and anaerobically, that all contained organisms, the dirty wounds more than the clean. Even clean-appearing wounds harbor organisms with sufficient frequency to suspect their presence in every case. No one can tell which of these wounds is going to develop infection. In a seris of 80 wounds, 20% yielded at least 10^5 organisms per gram of tissue (6). However, the mere presence of bacteria is less important than their potential for causing wound sepsis. Mechanical contamination in the form of debris, necrotic tissue, or sutures can provide the nidus for multiplication of initially small numbers of bacteria to significant levels of growth. Elek (7) has shown that the presence of a single silk will reduce by 10,000 times the number of staphylococci necessary to cause a wound infection. Conversely, the initial inoculum into a wound may be so massive that the local defense mechanisms are overwhelmed from the outset.

It is apparent that a working definition of a "contaminated" wound is necessary when dealing with traumatic injuries. A *contaminated wound* may be defined and identified both by its bacterial flora and by local wound factors. The bacterial level in the tissue is a reflection of the balance between the bacterial invaders and the host defense mechanisms. Contamination leads to wound infection and the potential for invasive sepsis when the level of bacterial growth exceeds 100,000 organisms per gram of tissue.

Evaluating the Patient and the Wound

Overall care of the individual with a soft-tissue injury must begin with a complete evaluation of the patient and a history of the accident. The history provides the treating physician a framework for assessing the severity of the injury. Obviously, a patient involved in a high-speed motor vehicle accident with multiple fractures will be at greater risk of associated injuries to other organ systems than will the patient who sustains a laceration from a piece of glass. From a thorough physical examination, the physician formulates a clear picture as to the level of the injury (i.e., a superficial laceration with no underlying injury versus a deep laceration with disruption of skin, soft tissue, muscle, and related adnexal structures). Once these parameters have been thoroughly investigated, a plan of management can be initiated.

Radiographic studies, including x-rays, tomography, xeroradiography, and computed tomography (CT) scanning, should be used when appropriate to aid in diagnosis. A patient with a foreign body of wood will benefit from xeroradiography for localization of the fragment, which may be missed on routine x-rays.

The diagnosis of the degree of contamination in a traumatic wound is made on the basis of history and clinical observation and may be confirmed by quantitative bacterial studies. The circumstances of the wounding and character of the wounding agent provide important clues. It is well known that a clean, dry windshield will support little bacterial growth, and such a laceration will have a small inoculation. Similarly, a sharp laceration from a clean butcher knife will be unlikely to lead to infection. A crush injury from a machine part that has been well greased presents a different problem, as does a puncture wound from a stake contaminated with soil. The bacterial inoculum from a non-meat-eating dog bite may be low and allow primary closure, whereas the inoculum from a human bite would be large because human saliva contains as many as 10^8 bacteria per millileter.

The location of the wound will reflect the potential of local defense mechanisms to withstand contamination. The excellent blood supply to the face and scalp provides more inherent resistance than is present in the lower extremities. This is why a facial wound with excellent blood supply would be expected to handle an inoculum for a longer period of time than the area at the juncture of the middle and lower thirds of the leg overlying the tibia, where poor blood supply might allow rapid bacterial multiplication.

Elapsed time since injury is an important factor in diagnosing the potentially contaminated wound. In a report on a series of wounds, the mean time since injury was 2.2 hours for patients with less than 10^2 bacteria per gram of tissue in their wounds; the mean time was 3 hours for a group with 10^2–10^5 organisms per gram of tissue; and, in those with greater than 10^5 organisms per gram of tissue before being seen, the mean time was 5.17 hours (6). More important, only those in the last group developed infection that prevented primary healing. The "period of grace" or "golden period" of which Pulaski (10) speaks is the amount of time required before an inoculum into a wound reaches the critical level of 10^5 bacteria per gram of tissue.

Bacterial Evaluation of the Wound

Because bacteria are present in all traumatic wounds and there appears to be a critical number that results in clinical infection, quantitative as well as qualitative surveillance of the wound is indicated. This is especially true for those wounds suspected of having a heavy initial inoculum, those occurrinng in patients with impaired host defenses, or those presenting more than 5 to 6 hours after injury. Surface swabs and cultures of purulent exudates have proven to be unreliable. Surface swabs yield many organisms that have not gained entrance into the tissues. If surface organisms are removed, only a single species appears to reach significant tissue levels. Heggers and others,[9] in studying 100 war wounds of the extremities, found 92% yielded single-species isolates. The bacteria of concern are those reaching significant tissue levels.

A tissue culture may be obtained by cleansing the wound surface, removing a specimen and, after diluting it tenfold, weighing, flaming, and homogenizing it. Serial tube dilutions and pour plates or back plating can then yield an accurate colony count related to a gram of tissue (3). Such detailed analyses are of little value in the emergency department because they would require 24 to 36 hours for completion. However, the immediately important information derived from such a technique can be obtained in 15 minutes with a rapid slide method (3). A specimen is removed from a wound, weighed, diluted, and homogenized. An aliquot of the suspension is then placed on a glass slide, Gram-stained, and examined under a microscope. If a single organism is seen on the slide, the bacterial count is greater than 10^5 organisms per gram of tissue in the original biopsy. If no organisms are seen on the slide, the bacterial count is 10^5 or fewer per gram.

Qualitative bacterial cultures are also important. At the time the tissue is homogenized, the homogenate is smeared, Gram-stained, and cultured aerobically and anaerobically. The Gram-stained smear helps to identify streptococci or clostridia, and the culture allows identification of the organisms and performance of antibiotic sensitivities. It is important to identify streptococci and the various clostridia species early. It has been demonstrated that β-hemolytic streptococci prevent satisfactory wound closure primarily, secondarily, or by a graft or flap, when they are present in a wound at any level. Clostridium tetani or perfringens must be identified as early as possible to allow for radical débridement and to prevent premature wound closure.

TETANUS IMMUNOPROPHYLAXIS

Guidelines for tetanus immunoprophylaxis have been established by the American College of Surgeons, Committee on Trauma, and are summarized below. Patients fully immunized who have received a booster injection within the last 10 years need no booster unless the wound is tetanus prone. Immunized patients with tetanus-prone wounds should receive a 0.5-cc tetanus toxoid booster if their last booster injection was given more than 5 years before injury. Immunized patients who have received no booster injection within the last 10 years need to receive a booster injection for any wound.

Individuals not previously immunized should receive a tetanus booster injection, followed by a full course of immunization, for even the most minor wounds. Patients with tetanus-prone wounds should receive a 0.5-cc booster injection of tetanus toxoid, plus 250 units of tetanus immune globulin, followed by a full course of immunization.

Preparing the Wound for Closure

The sine qua non of any wound is closure and in all instances the surgeon must determine if the wound is ready for closure. One criterion is the bacterial level in the wound. Another is the presence of nonviable or potentially nonviable tissue in the wound as well as any detrimental clot or foreign debris. Sharp débridement remains the most efficient way to prepare a traumatic wound for closure. Débridement removes a large proportion of contaminating bacteria as well as many local deterrents to normal host resistance. If the viability of the tissue remains in question after débridement, intravenous fluorescein can be given and the wound tissue inspected under ultraviolet light. Tissue fluorescence suggests viability.

Irrigation may be an important adjunct to sharp débridement. Wound irrigation, as normally delivered, even with voluminous amounts of solutions removes little but surface contamination; a pulsating jet lavage is better. In experimental animals, when compared to more standard types of irrigation the pulsating lavage removed significantly more bacteria and resulted in significantly fewer wound infections (10). If a pulsating jet lavage is not available, studies have shown that injection through a high-pressure system with a small-gauge needle approximates the results obtained with the lavage and is far superior to standard wound irrigation. Irrigation is probably best performed with a balanced saline solution. In 1919, Fleming (11) observed that disinfectants that kill bacteria also kill tissue and, therefore, the solution used to prepare the wound edges should not be used in the wound itself.

Systemic antibiotics have practical and potential value only if a therapeutic blood or, more important, tissue level is achieved within the first 4 hours after wounding. Burke (12) has shown that bacterial lodgment is not influenced after that time frame. When antibiotics are begun after the time required for bacterial lodgment, infection rates are higher. Surgical débridement and freshening the wound would render this restriction less rigid and make antibiotics more effective. However, in traumatic wounds, tissue levels of antibiotics are difficult to achieve rapidly. Adequate tissue levels are further hindered by conditions within the wound such as ischemia or necrotic tissue. Therefore, systemic antibiotics may not be of much use.

Closure of Acute Traumatic Wounds

Wound closures can be classified as primary, spontaneous, or tertiary. Primary repair means immediate reapproximation of the wound layers, which can be accomplished by a variety of techniques. After evaluation of the wound, the edges are sharply trimmed to allow for accurate coaptation. The deeper layers (e.g., the fascia) are closed with absorbable sutures. No sutures are placed in the subcutaneous tissue, because they promote fat necrosis, act as foreign bodies, and may facilitate wound infections. The dermal layer can be closed with simple inverted-interrupted sutures, and a very fine epidermal stitch is used to align the surface. Alternately, a continuous pull-out suture can be placed, or the edges can be approximated with micropore tape. When the edges of the wound cannot be reapproximated directly without tension, a local flap may be used to close the defect. In certain locations, primary closure can also be obtained by widely undermining the adjacent soft tissue. When this is done, traction on adjacent structures should not result in a subsequent deformity (e.g., an ectropion).

After adequate débridement, wounds that cannot be closed primarily, owing to contamination or tissue loss, can undergo delayed closure or be allowed to close spontaneously. Early reports of delayed closure stressed the necessity of not disturbing the dressing placed on a wound between the time of débridement and the time of delayed closure. Experimentally, the optimal time for a closure has been shown by Edlich and others (13) to be on or after the 4th postwounding day. We found that, if the bacterial level in the wound is 10^5 or fewer organisms per gram of tissue, successful wound closure can be expected (14). Treatment of the soft tissue should be initiated during the period of delay to hasten the decrease in bacterial levels. Occasionally, a wound will be allowed to close spontaneously. This may be preferable in wounds with heavy inocula of streptococci or clostridia. Wound contraction and epithelization will close most defects. Once closure has been accomplished, the need for secondary scar revision can be assessed.

Chronic Wounds

Chronically contaminated wounds (as opposed to the acute, potentially contaminated, wound) all contain bacterial flora in the tissue. Examples are thermal burns and traumatic wounds that were not closed acutely. The characteristic of such wounds is granulation tissue. Granulation tissue does not occur in the absence of bacteria. It is not found beneath the surface of a successfully closed wound. It has been likened to a pyogenic granuloma, and successful closure is predicated on the surgeon's ability to control the level of bacterial flora.

Biopsy cultures have revealed the clinical difficulty in identifying bacteriologically healthy granulation tissue (tissue that contains 10^5 or fewer bacteria per gram). Experimentally and clinically, successful closure of a contaminated wound (by spontaneous epithelialization, wound-edge approximation, application of skin grafts, or pedicle flaps) is directly and consistently related to the surgeon's ability to decrease the bacterial flora in the tissue to 10^5 or fewer bacteria per gram (1,3). In a series of 50 skin grafts applied to chronically contaminated wounds (regardless of the technique used to prepare the granulations for grafting), a bacterial count of 105 or fewer bacteria on the day of grafting resulted in a 94% graft take, as opposed to 19% when the bacterial counts were above 105 per gram of tissue on the day of grafting (15).

Reduction of the bacterial flora is best accomplished by meticulous attention to surgical detail. Frequent débridement and surgical cleansing are critical. Enzymatic débridement may be of some value, but it tends to allow rapid bacterial proliferation simultaneously (16). This is of potential danger, particularly when large areas are involved (e.g., in thermal burns). Systemic antibiotics do not reach adequate tissue levels in chronic granulation tissue and have been shown experimentally to have no effect on the bacterial level in granulating wounds (17). Conversely, water-based topical antibacterial creams do penetrate the depths of such wounds and have a direct effect on bacterial growth.

Because true bacterial control is only achieved by wound closure, the use of temporary biologic dressings for cleansing and temporary closure has been shown to be of value. In a randomized study of 100 delayed wound closures, we compared several methods for decreasing the bacteria to below critical level. Temporary biologic dressings proved to be the most effective. It appears that the biologic dressings adhered to the wound surface and effected a "biologic closure" that allowed the inflammatory tissue to function at peak efficiency and phagocytosis to proceed effectively. Porcine xenografts failed to establish biologic union with the underlying tissue and therefore were less effective than allografts or amniotic membranes (18). However, the true control of infection in a granulating wound is closure of the wound with autograft tissue.

Techniques of closure in chronically contaminated wounds vary widely, depending on the circumstances. In some wounds, approximation of the wound edges may be accomplished. In others, cutaneous defects may require coverage with skin grafts. Local wound factors other than bacteria (e.g., exposed bone, marginal blood supply in the recipient site, or previous radiation) may require the use of pedicled flap tissue or free flap coverage.

Finally, it seems likely that in the future operative wound closure may not be the only, or even the preferred, answer for the management of chronic wounds. A recent report[19] has shown flap closure of pressure ulcers is less than satisfactory. These authors reported greater than 75% ulcer recurrence in paraplegics within 2 years of surgery.

With the availability of recombinant human growth factors in commercial quantities, the management of chronic wounds may change dramatically. There are a growing number of clinical trials examining the efficacy of topically applied recombinant human growth factors on the closure of chronic wounds (20-28). The results of these trials, involving pressure sores, diabetic foot ulcers, and venous ulcers, have been promising. As more work is done in this area, the closure of chronic wounds—once bacterial balance has been achieved—may involve topical pharmacotherapy rather than operative intervention.

Dressings

After wound closure, an adequate dressing is applied to the wound. Understanding the function of dressings will help dictate their design and selection. Functions of dressings include: (a) protection, (b) absorption, (c) compression, (d) immobilization, and (e) provision of an aesthetic wound covering. It is necessary to protect the wound from mechanical injury of the wound edges and from desiccation. Also, during the first few hours, until the wound is sealed by fibrin, protection from exogenous bacterial contamination is essential. Because all wounds weep during the inflammatory stage of wound healing, absorption of this inflammatory exudate is useful. Likewise, any bleeding from the wound margins needs to be absorbed to prevent maceration. Edema is also part of the inflammatory process; compression, but not excessive pressure, is helpful. Attempts to prevent this obliga-

tory edema completely by a pressure dressing or cast should be avoided. Preventing excess motion of the approximated skin edges or of an applied flap or skin graft is a therapeutic imperative. A properly constructed dressing gives the optimal degree of immobilization. This will also decrease the pain associated with the wound. Finally, the dressings should be aesthetically acceptable; this is the portion of wound management that a surgeon first presents to the patient and others and is the surgeons' signature.

To accomplish the functions addressed above, dressings should be carefully constructed, from a variety of materials, and thoughtfully applied. The inner layer, in contact with the wound, should be fine-meshed gauze, either plain or impregnated. The purpose of impregnating gauze is not to prevent sticking to the wound, because macerating amounts of impregnate are necessary to accomplish this; rather, it provides a coating to the fibers and promotes drainage to the absorptive layers of the dressing. Plain gauze tends to entrap the drainage and form a coagulum at the innermost layer. Commercially impregnated gauze must be "wrung out" because its heavy impregnation tends to prevent drainage and to macerate tissue. The remainder of the dressing consists of bulky absorptive materials; however, cotton-containing gauze should not be applied next to a weeping wound because later removal is difficult. The dressing can then be completed by the application of firm, even compression using a roller bandage. The use of an Ace or elastic bandage is mentioned only to be condemned. An even, controllable amount of compression is not possible with such a bandage, and dangerously constrictive dressings may result as the wound proceeds through the obligatory edema phase. The dressing is completed by proper positioning and immobilizing in the appropriate position. This may require the use of plaster splints.

Summary

Basic principles of repair of traumatic cutaneous injuries involving the skin and soft tissue are similar to the principles of an operative incision. The differences are that all traumatic wounds are contaminated and all contain some deterrents to normal wound healing. Therefore, principles must be expanded to include ascertainment of level of contamination, identification and removal of deterrents to wound healing, and prevention of invasive infections. Once a proper assessment of the level of contamination is made, the bacterial balance of a given wound can be determined. If a wound is in bacterial balance, débridement and irrigation remove necrotic tissue, clots, and debris, and wound closure can proceed. Wound closure can be achieved surgically by wound approximation or by application of a flap or skin graft. In the case of chronic wounds, secondary healing might be stimulated pharmacologically with the use of cytokines. If a wound is not in bacterial balance, it must be attained while other deterrents to wound healing are being removed. Only then can successful closure of the traumatic soft-tissue wound be accomplished and healing proceed.

Bibliography

1. Robson MC, Krizek TJ, Heggers JP. Biology of surgical infection. In: *Current Problems in Surgery,* Chicago, Year Book Medical Publishers, 1973.
2. Robson MC, Heggers JP. Surgical infection. II. The β-hemolytic streptococcus. *J Surg Res* 1969; 9:289.

3. Robson MC. Infection in the surgical patient: An imbalance in the normal equilibrium. *Clin Plast Surg* 1979; 6:493.
4. Altemeier WA, Gibbs EW. Bacterial flora of fresh accidental wounds. *Surg Gynecol Obstet* 1944; 78:164.
5. Pulaski EJ, Meleney FL, Spaeth WLC. Bacterial flora of acute traumatic wounds. *Surg Gynecol Obstet* 1941; 72:982.
6. Robson MC, Duke WF, Krizek TJ. Rapid bacterial screening in the treatment of civilian wounds. *J Surg Res* 1973; 14:426.
7. Elek SD. Experimental staphylococcal infections in the skin of man. *Ann NY Acad Sci* 1956; 65:85.
8. Pulaski EJ. *Surgical Infections.* Springfield, IL. Charles C. Thomas, 1954.
9. Heggers JP, Barnes ST, Robson MC, et al. Microbial flora of orthopedic war wounds. *Milit Med* 1969; 134–602.
10. Hamer ML, Robson MC, Krizek TJ, et al. Quantitative bacterial analysis of comparative wound irrigations. *Ann Surg* 1975; 181–819.
11. Fleming A. The action of chemical and physiological antiseptics in a septic wound. *Br J Surg* 1919; 7:99.
12. Burke JF. The effective period of preventive antibiotic action in experimental incisions and dermal lesions. *Surgery* 1961; 60:161.
13. Edlich RF, Rogers W, Kasper G, et al. Studies in the management of the contaminated wound. I. Optimal time for closure of contaminated open wounds. II. Comparison of resistance to infection of open and closed wounds during healing. *Am J Surg* 1969; 117:323.
14. Robson MC, Heggers JP. Delayed wound closures based on bacterial counts. *J Surg Oncol* 1980; 2:379.
15. Krizek TJ, Robson MC, Kho E. Bacterial growth and skin graft survival. *Surg Forum* 1967; 18:518.
16. Krizek TJ, Robson MC, Groskin MG. Experimental burn wound sepsis-evaluation of enzymatic débridement. *J Surg Res* 1974; 17:219.
17. Robson MC, Edstrom LE, Krizek TJ, et al. The efficacy of systemic antibiotics in the treatment of granulating wounds. *J Surg Res* 1974; 16:299.
18. Robson MC, Samburg JL, Krizek TJ. Quantitative comparison of biological dressings. *J Surg Res* 1973; 14:431.
19. Disa JJ, Carlton JM, Goldbert NH. Efficacy of operative cure in pressure sore patients. *Plast Reconstr Surg* 1992; 89:272.
20. Brown GL, Curtzinger L, Jurkiewica JR, et al. Stimulation of healing of chronic wounds by epidermal growth factor. *Plast Reconstr Surg* 1991; 88:189.
21. Falanga V, Eaglstein WH, Bucalo B, et al. Topical use of recombinant epidermal growth factor (h-EGF) in venous ulcers. *J Dermatol Surg Oncol* 1992; 18:604.
22. Robson MC, Phillips LG, Thomason A, et al. Recombinant human platelet-derived growth factor-BB for the treatment of chronic pressure ulcers. *Ann Plast Surg* 1992; 29:193.
23. Mustoe TA, Cutler NR, Allman RM, et al. Phase II study to evaluate recombinant PDGF-BB in the treatment of pressure sores. *Arch Surg* 1994; 129:213.
24. Steed DL. Clinical evaluation of recombinant human platelet-derived growth factor for the treatment of lower extremity diabetic ulcers. Diabetic Ulcer Study Group. *J Vasc Surg* 1995; 21:71.
25. Robson MC, Phillips LG, Lawrence WT, et al. The safety and effect of topically applied recombinant basic fibroblast growth factor on healing of chronic pressure sores. *Ann Surg* 1992; 216:401.
26. Robson MC, Phillips LG, Cooper DM, et al. The safety and effect of transforming growth factor-b_2 for the treatment of venous stasis ulcers. *Wound Repair and Regeneration* (in press).
27. Rasmussen LH, Karlsmark T, Avnstrorp C, et al. Topical human growth hormone treatment of chronic leg ulcers. *Phlebology* 1991; 6:23.
28. Robson MC, Abdullah A, Burns BF, et al. Safety and effect of topical recombinant human interleukin-1b in the management of pressure sores. *Wound Repair and Regeneration* 1994; 2:177.

15

Scar Revision

Ross Rudolph, M.D., F.A.C.S., and Gerald Schneider, M.D., F.A.C.S.

The most frequent cause of failure in scar revision lies in unrealistic expectations on the part of the patient. Thus, each attempt at scar improvement must begin with an assessment of the patient's understanding and expectations of the likely results. An honest recounting of the benefits and limitations of scar revision as it applies to the scar in question must be carried out with the patient and concerned family before undertaking surgical modification.

The objectives of scar revision are to apply techniques that provide restoration of a smooth skin surface resembling the surrounding skin in all respects. A good scar should be (a) a fine line (or series of lines) that falls within or is parallel to a naturally occurring line such as a wrinkle, contour junction, or relaxed skin tension line (RSTL); (b) free of contour irregularity; (c) without abnormal pigmentation; and (d) void of contractures or distortion of adjacent structures.

These objectives may be accomplished by improving the scar's direction if it is not parallel to a RSTL, decreasing the scar's width, dividing the scar into smaller segments, correcting malalignment or distortion of adjacent anatomic units, improving surface irregularities, and improving pigment discrepancies.

Each scar is evaluated in the context of time, place, person, and nature of injury. Since not every scar is appropriate for revision, precise analysis of history and physical findings is essential to determine which scars are likely to be improved. Following this review, the surgeon must develop a plan and frankly communicate a reasonable estimate of the most likely outcome. There are several factors to be considered before proceeding, not the least of which is an assessment of the patient's acceptance of the limitations of any proposed correction.

1. *Time Since Injury.* Time is both enemy and friend to the patient with an unwanted scar. Time will improve most scars, and sufficient time should elapse for the 3rd phase of wound healing (maturation) to run its full course before a scar is considered for revision. In contrast, some scars will not materially improve with time, and waiting to revise them offers no advantage. For example, no amount of time will realign an eyebrow reapproximated without care or a lip vermilion with a stepoff, and an embedded foreign body may cause continuing inflammation that prevents maturation.

   Generally, wounds in adults require a minimum of 6 and as many as 24 months to show characteristics of maturation: pliability and fading of redness. Such characteristics may appear earlier in scars of the elderly due to a lack of biologic vigor, and at 6 to 12 weeks are unlikely to exhibit the raised and red appearance associated with wounds in young people. In contrast, scars in children may require 24, 36, or even 48 months to soften and fade. Time allows nodules to soften, and ridges and wrinkles to flatten. Waiting may minimize the need for revision or even render it unnecessary. The surgeon must be confident in this knowledge in order to resist the inevitable pressure brought by the patient or family to intervene earlier than is prudent. While some may dissent (1), the case for patience cannot be overemphasized.

   Waiting need not be passive. The process of maturation may be speeded by *judicious* injection of a low-solubility depot glucocorticoid, usually triamcinolone acetonide (Kenalog. Low concentrations (e.g., 2.5–3.3 mg/mL), should be used to avoid overcorrecting, that is, atrophy of a scar as it continues to mature. Care should be taken to keep the injection within the scar in order to avoid atrophy or hypopigmentation of the surrounding skin. The use of silicone gel sheeting (2) has minimal risk and may be considered an additional method to promote softening and smoothing of a maturing scar. Poor compliance and, rarely, scar ulceration and dermatitis, represent the only disadvantages to its use.

2. *Nature of the Injuring Agent and Wound Management.* Knowledge of the original injury is helpful in determining whether a reasonable chance exists to improve a scar. In a given area, a better outcome would be expected in a surgical scar made by an experienced surgeon vis à vis one following a tearing injury inflicted by a protruding nail, closed hours after injury without débridement, and complicated by subsequent infection. Variation in mode of injury and subsequent management can produce different outcomes, the former unlikely to benefit from revision and the latter suited for an attempt.

3. *Location.* Certain areas of the body are especially prone to scar thickening and spreading after revision (Fig. 15–1). The triangular area of the shoulders, upper chest, and lower midsternum reacts poorly to scar revision. Techniques of scar revision are applied most successfully in the head and neck, while less satisfactory results are obtained with the same techniques when applied below the level of the clavicles. Scar revision on the extremities and trunk is aided by relieving tension when possible, as with a Z-plasty that changes scar direction. Scars placed perpendicular to the line of muscular pull (and thus parallel to RSTL) are predictably less obvious.

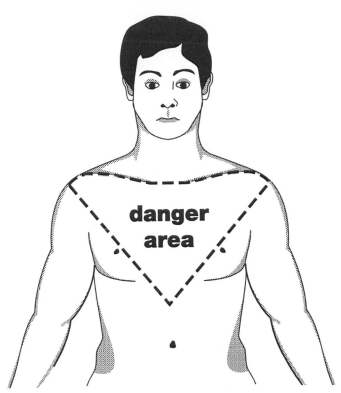

FIG. 15–1. The thick skin and underlying muscular pull in this area and similar but smaller area on the back are at high risk for hypertrophic scars.

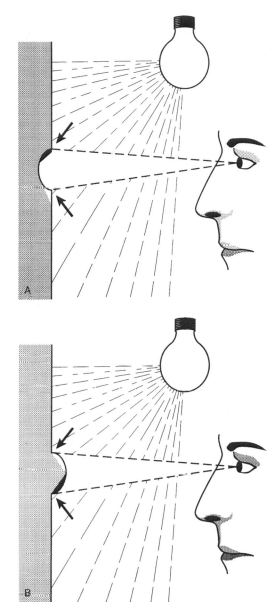

FIG. 15–2. A, concave surface causes light reflex at lower margin and shadow within overhanging margin. **B,** convex surface causes high light at point of light reflex and shadow beneath.

4. *Age of the Patient.* The vigor of healing appears to be inverse to chronologic age, all other variables being constant. For any given technique, an older individual will likely have a better result than a younger individual.

5. *Ethnic Background.* Science has yet to identify the precise factors that govern the quality of scars, yet this much is known: generally, the greater an individual's pigment, the more obvious the scar. However, the variation is so great that this observation must not be applied in any single case without further inquiry as to the history of scars in the individual in question. While light-skinned, blue-eyed individuals with fair hair will often exhibit nearly invisible scars from even the most noxious stimulus, darkly pigmented persons with dark hair often make scars that are both hyperpigmented and hypertrophic. We have only to consult articles from Japan or China to note elegant and precisely executed procedures resulting in extremely obvious scars. The majority of true keloids occur in blacks, and scar revision alone will not alter them. However, in darkskinned patients, a mediocre result is more often the result of scar hypertrophy than a true keloid.

6. *Skin Tone and Light Effect.* Scars are visible either because they are of a different color than the surrounding skin or because light is reflected differently from the scar's surface. Most light sources, whether artificial or sunlight, produce full-spectrum white light. When reflected from a nonwhite surface, this white light causes a white spot or reflex that is seen in contrast to the surrounding, darker surface. Moreover, the majority of light that strikes the skin at an angle to our view causes both highlight and shadow (Fig. 15–2). This is the mechanism by which scars in darkly pigmented individuals may be perceived as more obvious than scars of similar *surgical quality* in fair-skinned individuals. Thus, it is more difficult to obtain a cosmetically acceptable scar in pigmented patients because reflected white light from even minor surface irregularities is seen against the dark surrounding background of the uninjured skin.

7. *Healing of Previous Scars.* If the patient planning scar revision has other scars, the way they healed may help guide the surgeon.

8. *Nature of the Scar.* Patients wishing scar revision often complain of "keloids"; however, they may in fact have other types of scars, such as spread wide or hypertrophic scars (3). Spread wide scars are very amenable to the surgical scar revision techniques described below. Hy-

pertrophic scars may be managed with surgery when properly chosen. True keloids must be approached very gingerly with surgery. Large keloids and certain hypertrophic scars may be better managed with pressure, Kenalog injections, or upcoming biochemical approaches rather than with surgery (3).

9. *Whether Any Skin Was Lost.* The surgeon performing scar revision may first recognize deficiency in the amount of tissue when a large wound gap appears unexpectedly following scar excision. A thorough review of the history of injury should alert the surgeon to the possibility of missing tissue and the avoidance of intraoperative epiphany.

10. *Perceptions and Expectations of the Patient and Family.* As with all surgery, understanding what the patient foresees as a result of surgery is vital. A superb technical result may produce misery if the patient expects miraculous obliteration of scarring. In some ethnic groups, any facial scarring may be viewed as a mark of marital infidelity, leading to unrealistic expectations about surgical outcome (4). It is usually fairly easy to learn what the patient expects through gentle and sympathetic questioning, yet occasionally mutual misunderstanding and, rarely, outright lying can occur, leading to much unhappiness after surgery.

Surgical Techniques of Scar Revision

When surgical treatment is selected, scars are most often excised, and the wound sutured or revised with Z-plasty or W-plasty. Rarely is a large scar excised and the wound resurfaced with a skin graft or a skin flap, unless function is less important than appearance. Finally, dermabrasion has a role in the management of specific types of scars.

FUSIFORM SCAR REVISION

Assuming that criteria have been met for scar revision, a number of technical aspects must be considered. The scar revision should be planned, if possible, so that the final scar will lie in a natural wrinkle, crease, or boundary. Even if wrinkles are not yet present, scars do best when at right angles to muscle pull (which is where wrinkles form) (Fig. 15–3).

Natural creases, such as the nasolabial fold, should be paralleled rather than crossed at right angles, while natural boundaries such as the jaw line disguise parallel scars. The semicircular "trapdoor" scar may be best handled by complete excision if the final scar can be placed in a skin crease. Linear scar excision will be of little help to a poorly oriented scar, such as a vertical forehead scar that crosses multiple deep skin wrinkles. In this case, a Z-plasty or W-plasty may be done to change the direction of the scar (5).

In hair-bearing areas, placing incisions parallel to the angle of the hair follicles can preserve hair and disguise the final scar. Given a choice, scars should be placed within the hair rather than in visible skin. Avoid shaving hair, if possible, to preserve landmarks. Eyebrows and eyelashes in particular should not be shaved.

Planning should also serve to avoid tension. While it is not always possible, reducing tension to a minimum promotes a fine thin scar (6).

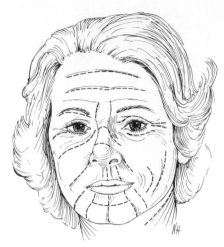

FIG. 15–3. Locations of the constant facial crease line. These are important in planning scar revision procedures.

ANESTHESIA

Ideally, the patient undergoing facial scar revision should be awake to cooperate in animating the face and demonstrating skin folds. Certain details of local anesthesia assist in obtaining a relaxed and cooperative patient. We prefer to use lidocaine with epinephrine, buffered with sufficient sodium bicarbonate to return the pH of the injected solution to neutral (i.e., 8 mL of commercial 1% lidocaine 1:100,000 epinephrine with 2 mL of 8.4% sodium bicarbonate). This minimizes the pain of injection when a small (27 or 30) gauge needle is used. Bupivacaine 0.25% with epinephrine, mixed with the above solution, can be used to provide longlasting pain relief.

Avoid the use of epinephrine in the fingers because it may cause ischemia. Skin markings, particularly those of the lip vermilion's white roll, should be carefully marked before injection as blanching and swelling after the injection may distort or obliterate important landmarks.

Planning the Revision

No absolute rules can be made, and the surgeon's experience and creativity are vital. In a linear scar revision, the goal should be to remove the old scar with a minimum of normal tissue yet orient the final scar in an ideal direction.

A valuable basic principle is that obvious landmarks should be preserved (or restored). These include lip vermilion border, hairlines (e.g., eyebrows, eyelashes, scalp), skin creases, and tissue borders (e.g., nasal alar rim, ear helix).

EXCISION AND UNDERMINING

The scar is excised with a scalpel. The choice of blade is by personal preference but it should ensure the ability to perform a smooth, perpendicular cut (Fig. 15–4A,B). Generally, the larger the scar the larger the blade should be. A more accurate cut of the corners may be facilitated by the use of an 11 blade. The entire depth of the scar need not be removed in all cases and, in fact, leaving some behind to act as filler in the case of subcutaneous tissue loss may raise the scar flush to the surrounding skin (Fig. 15–5A-D).

Top View   End View

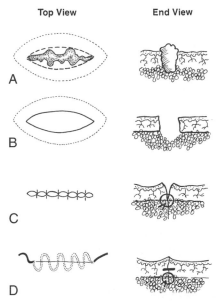

FIG. 15–4. Linear scar revision. **A,** elliptical (actually lens-shaped) excision outlined around jagged hypertrophic scar is designed to remove all the scar and lie in a natural skin fold. The outer dotted line marks the extent of undermining. **B,** lesion is excised, and undermining is completed. **C,** deep layer is closed with absorbable suture, knot is buried, and dermis is opposed (left). The end view (right) shows that the wound should be almost fully closed. **D,** final closure with a buried running subcuticular Prolene suture, superficial in the dermis (left). The top view left shows suture weaving back and forth across wound in dermis, piercing the epidermis only at each end. The thickness of the suture is exaggerated for clarity.

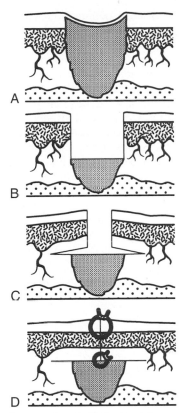

FIG. 15–5. **A,** depressed scar. **B,** incomplete removal of the scar base allows both **C,** filling of a depressed scar and **D,** anchoring to discourage spreading.

In the face and neck, undermining is in the fat close to the skin, whereas on the trunk and extremities more fat is left on the flaps. In either case, the subdermal vascular plexus should be preserved (see Fig. 15–4C). As a rough guideline, the combined width of the undermining (i.e., on both sides of the wound) should equal the open wound width. Undermining frees the normal skin from deep tissues and from remaining scar to allow free movement without tension.

Hemostasis should be obtained with conservative measures. With proper use of epinephrine, allowing 7 to 15 minutes to elapse from injection to incision, bleeding is minimal. The small amount of bleeding that occurs can often be controlled by pressure. If not, selective electrocautery can help. Random heavy electrocautery is avoided because it will compromise healing. Rarely, ligation of bleeding vessels may be used, especially if the vessel has retracted into fat or muscle. Hemostasis substances like oxidized cellulose should be avoided.

For precision, the wound closure should be with layers of sutures (see Fig. 15–4D). Staples may cause misalignment and surface scars. Paper strips may be used in place of skin sutures if perfect subcuticular alignment is achieved (which is rarely the case).

The subject of which sutures to use is fraught with legend and strongly held personal opinions. We prefer to close the deep layers with absorbable sutures, usually 4-0 Vicryl (Ethicon Corp., Somerville, NJ) or Dexon (Davis and Geck, Inc., Danbury, CT). Chromic catgut (but not plain) may be

used for the rare patient who is allergic to the synthetic sutures. The most superficial layer of deep sutures (see Fig. 15–4D) should be placed into the dermis, with the knot buried, and as close to the dermal–epidermal junction as possible. This will close the wound almost fully so that skin sutures have little or no tension. Drains are rarely used, but should be if fluid collection is feared.

Skin sutures ideally should be running subcuticular to avoid suture marks yet allow prolonged wound support (see Fig. 15–4D). Usually we use 4-0 Prolene (Ethicon Corp., Somerville, NJ). This suture is usually nonreactive. The subcuticular suture can be left for 2 to 3 weeks, and sometimes even longer if not irritated, because this prolonged support may reduce scar spreading. Suture tract epithelial ingrowth can occur where the sutures enter and exit the skin; in practice, this is usually not a major problem except around the eyelids, where sutures should be removed early. Clear Prolene makes the suture less obvious. The ends of the suture can be tied or anchored with sterile paper-tape strips, which further support the wound (7). If the incision is long and removal of subcuticular Prolene would be painful, subcuticular running Vicryl may be used instead.

When the wound is curved, gapped, or the sides are unequal lengths, it is best to use fine interrupted sutures with a careful everting technique of either simple or vertical mattress sutures. Interrupted sutures are also required in areas where movement may loosen a running subcuticular stitch (e.g., around the mouth, lips, eyelids, and possibly forehead) and may also be used in conjunction with the subcuticular suture to obtain better epidermal approximation. If used, they should be removed earlier than others, usually at 2 or 3 days. Since suture marks are dependent upon tension and the time sutures are in place, gentle tissue approximation and early suture removal are important to obtain the best result. To ensure wound integrity against the unexpected, wound tapes such as Steri-Strips (Minnesota Mining & Mfg., St. Paul, MN) or Suture Strips (Genetic Laboratories Wound Care, Inc., St. Paul, MN) should be applied when possible. Facial sutures may be removed in 4 to 5 days, while at least 7 days are required for extremity sutures, and longer (up to 3 weeks) for sutures on the palms and soles.

At the time of closure, a long-acting steroid like Kenalog (5–10 mg/mL) can be instilled; or, a trial of silicone gel sheeting can be employed if the patient is at risk because of history or ethnic grouping to form (or re-form) keloids or hypertrophic scars. If Kenalog is used, wound support with subcuticular sutures and/or external tapes is needed to reduce the risk of dehiscence.

"DOG-EAR" EXCISION

The bunching of tissue at the ends of elliptical wound closure describes geometrical *standing cones*. While very small dog-ears may eventually remodel and lie flat, larger ones will not and must be modified as the wound is closed. Angular excision, M-plasty, and other techniques have been described to deal with these deformities, but simple excision by equalling the length of the two sides works best, being sure to respect the line of closure or major skin creases (Fig. 15–6).

BURIED DERMAL FLAP FOR SUPPORT

Ideally, scar revision should be tension-free, yet this is not always possible, especially in the case of a wide scar. As shown in Figure 15–7, a dermal flap can be constructed of the deepithelialized scar, which can then be used to anchor and reinforce the scar revision against tension (3). The flap, actually made of scar, has sufficient strength to help prevent scar spread. This technique is especially useful in scars of the trunk and extremities. If the scar is depressed, the entire deepithelialized scar can be left in place and surrounding normal skin advanced over it, to provide more bulk (see Fig. 15–5A-D) and act as an anchor against spreading.

THE Z-PLASTY

The double flap rotation known as Z-plasty because of the shape of the design and final scar is an essential component of scar revision (8) It is used primarily to achieve two goals: (a) to change the direction of a scar by 90% and, simultaneously, (b) to gain length in a scar.

Scars at right angles to skin folds or creases become shortened and thick, and Z-plasty both relieves these deformities and makes recurrence after revision less likely. Innumerable variations have been described, but the most useful is the design in which the limbs of the Z-plasty are equal to the length of the scar (Fig. 15–8) and the limbs make an angle of 60° to the original scar.

When designing the Z-plasty, care must be taken to avoid basing it on avascular scar. After the flaps are cut, undermining around the bases helps mobility. The flaps are rotated 90° and sutured (see Fig. 15–8).

A major consideration of Z-plasty is that the total amount of scar is lengthened. Obviously, the anticipated improvement must be worth the lengthening of scar. In a child, where any scar may hypertrophy and be highly visible, the prominent Z scar may be unacceptable. A hypertrophic scar (or worse, a keloid) may not be suitable for Z-plasty because of

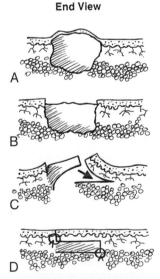

End View

FIG. 15–7. Buried dermal flap technique. **A,** a wide hypertrophic scar extends below the skin surface. **B,** scar is deepithelialized, with removal of epidermis and a small amount of contiguous scar. **C,** flap of scar "dermis" is elevated; opposing skin flap is elevated to accept the dermal flap. Deeper scar may be left, should be excised if too bulky. **D,** flap of dermis (actually scar) is advanced under the skin. It is anchored at both sides with absorbable sutures. A running subcuticular suture can be used for the final skin layer.

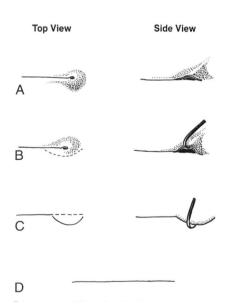

Top View   Side View

FIG. 15–6. Dog-ear excision. **A,** dog-ear is shown at end of linear scar revision. **B,** dog-ear is elevated with a hook, and one edge is marked for excision. **C,** one edge is incised, and excess tissue is gently drawn across wound. **D,** excess tissue is excised, and the wound is closed, extending the scar in the same direction.

Top View

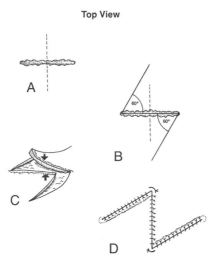

FIG. 15–8. The classic Z-plasty. **A,** a thick, contracted scar crosses a skin fold. Design is begun by drawing a perpendicular line at the midpoint of the scar; this line helps establish flap incisions, but it is not itself incised. **B,** completing the design, the limbs of flaps are equal to each other and to the length of the scar. Angles of the flaps are 60°. **C,** flaps are elevated, preserving the subdermal plexus. Undermining is accomplished around flap bases. The scar is excised unless it is too wide; here a portion of scar is left for clarity in showing flap transposition. **D,** flaps are transposed and sutured. A 3-corner suture (half-buried horizontal mattress) is used to anchor narrow tips, avoiding necrosis that could result from simple sutures near tips.

the risk of the new scar's becoming as prominent as the smaller, old scar. Especially on the face, multiple small Z-plasties may be superior to one large one.

THE W-PLASTY

Much the same may be true of the W-plasty, which has been overused. This technique substitutes a zig-zag scar for a linear one, and has the potential advantages of disguising a straight scar and of removing wide suture scars (5). Besides discarding normal tissue, multiple W-plasties can be highly visible on a young face, making the scar revision worse than the original deformity. In the facial area, the W-plasty is most useful in the older patient, who may be expected to heal scars well, and appears to have its major value in revision of long, depressed forehead scars. The limbs should be about 5 mm and the angles should be between 60° and 90°, depending on the relationship of the scar to the RSTL (Fig. 15–9). The W-plasty is less likely to produce alternative small ridges and depressions in some areas than multiple Z-plasties.

OTHER TECHNIQUES

Practically all techniques of plastic surgery may be called into use in scar revision, especially revision of complex scars. Some of the most useful are local flaps, full-thickness skin grafts, and dermabrasion; tissue expansion, tissue recruitment, and laser have lesser roles.

LOCAL FLAPS

When considering the treatment of a wide area of scar or a gap from missing tissue, it may be wiser to replace an entire aesthetic unit or subunit with a flap than to deal with indi-

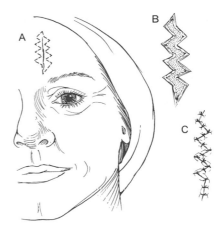

FIG. 15–9. The W-plasty. **A,** dotted lines show the design for the excision of the scar. **B,** flaps have now been developed and are ready for interdigitation. The W-flaps are in position.

vidual scars within the field or close the wound under unacceptable tension. For example, the residual scarring left from an incompletely laser-treated port wine stain of the second division of the trigeminal nerve may be more amenable to a cheek rotation flap (with or without tissue expansion) than to an attempt at excision of the many scars and residual hemangioma. A field of scar after a mixed-partial and full-thickness abrasion of the upper lip may be far more noticeable than an appropriately designed island advancement, cross-lip, or rotation flap. Since flaps are more suitable for older than younger patients, local tissue characteristics must be more carefully assessed before embarking upon flap reconstruction. Still, once flap reconstruction is selected all manner of flaps may be considered. In the case of missing tissue or large areas of scar, only the surgeon's ingenuity and skill limit the application of flap reconstruction.

FULL-THICKNESS SKIN GRAFTS

Full-thickness grafts are an alternative and often satisfactory way to close a gaping wound if local flaps are unavailable, and should always be considered when performing scar revision of the eyelids and adjacent areas. Full-thickness skin is preferable to split-thickness skin because it retains the natural feel, texture, and color of its native area (8). It is harvested from a hairless area and sutured with a bolus tie-over dressing.

For the face (the usual location), skin can be successfully obtained from behind the ear in all age groups and alternately in front of the ear in older patients. Of course, no other skin can replace eyelid skin; unfortunately, there is limited availability of this unique, thin tissue. For larger amounts of graft to be transferred to the face, the supraclavicular fossa offers skin of similar quality without much risk of an unacceptable donor-site scar. Full-thickness grafts from the upper inner arm may on occasion mimic facial and even eyelid skin, since it is usually very thin. Except in the most extreme circumstances, groin and abdominal full-thickness grafts are not acceptable for facial reconstruction.

TISSUE EXPANSION AND RECRUITMENT

When a shortage of tissue can be determined during preoperative assessment, a field of scar may best be replaced with expanded or recruited tissue from the local area. A two-staged operation must be acceptable to the patient and surgeon if tissue expansion is selected. Surgical planning includes consideration of the expander's placement to minimize new scars and anticipate the final location of scars, if secondary linear scar contractures are to be avoided. Recent developments in perioperative tissue recruitment allow the planned stretching of soft tissue to avoid the use of flaps or grafts (9). Since these techniques have a high scar burden themselves, they are best reserved for functional rather than aesthetic scar revision (e.g., replacement of a split-thickness skin graft used as a temporary dressing).

DERMABRASION

Dermabrasion is a useful adjunct to scar revision and differs from laser only in the method of destroying surface tissue and the associated heat byproduct. Recalling the discussion of light's influence on the visibility of scars will assist in understanding dermabrasion's potential to improve a scar's surface appearance. Since surface irregularities are more easily managed by abrasion than excision, this important technique should be considered when shadow or highlight are the cause of a scar's visibility.

While scar dermabrasion can be performed at any time after surgical modification, evidence points to greater efficacy when done early. One study indicates dermabrasion may give better results when performed at 4 rather than 8 weeks (10) and some surgeons even perform abrasion of the incision margin at the time of scar revision. Caution should be exercised when dermabrasion is performed in areas spare or void of accessory skin appendages that are the source of regenerative epithelium. Furthermore, patients who have recently been treated with iso-tretinoin (Accutane) have a greatly increased risk of hypertrophic scarring after either dermabrasion or laser treatment (11). They should not be considered candidates for either procedure for at least 1 year after cessation of treatment.

We prefer the use of the diamond fraise or fine-wire brush powered by a high-torque motor to hand sanding in dermabrasion after scar revision. Deep dermabrasion should be avoided to prevent extending the zone of injury to the deeper levels of the dermis where scarring is more likely.

LASER

The unique properties of photothermolysis produced by coherent laser energy offers advantages in the treatment of red, hyperpigmented, and hypertrophic scars, as well as keloids. The potential for scar improvement by laser energy relates to the selectivity of specific wavelength absorption by different tissues. When impacting the oxyhemoglobin-rich environment of the red hypertrophic scar, the light of a blue-green argon laser causes photocoagulation of capillaries, an increase in wound collagenase, and a possible alteration in the balance of collagen lysis and synthesis. The flashlamp-pumped pulsed dye laser (Candela) may also have clinically significant, observable benefits in treatment of objectionable scars (12).

The ability of the digitally controlled pulsed and scanning carbon-dioxide laser to vaporize thin skin-surface layers precisely may have a role in the heretofore disappointing area of acne scar treatment. Traditionally, this has been the realm of dermabrasion, and more recently dermabrasion coupled with punch skin grafting (13), but by selectively vaporizing the skin margin of a pitted scar and feathering the treatment into the surrounding area it is possible to decrease the contrast of darkly shadowed scars with this device. Expect further development of so-called laserabrasion technique for this and other skin-surface problems.

As with any resurfacing technique, including dermabrasion and chemical peel, the possibility of herpes simplex reactivation exists with laserbrasion. For this reason we consider prescribing oral acyclovir (Zovirax) for every patient undergoing such a procedure, immediately for any patient suspecting an imminent breakout of a cold sore or fever blister, and for any patient reporting an unexplainable increase in postprocedure pain.

Nonsurgical Modalities

Until recently, nonsurgical treatments of aesthetically unacceptable scar has been limited to (a) ionizing radiation, (b) injected glucocorticoids, (c) pressure, and (d) time. Now, silicone gel sheeting can be added to the list. Radiation has been reserved for scars of intractable and otherwise untreatable character in the organizational phase of scar production. Because of potential long-term injurious effects, its use must be questioned in the treatment of a nonlethal condition such as hypertrophic scar. Administering depot glucocorticoids requires both judgement and skill and they have potential disadvantages of subcutaneous atrophy, hypopigmentation, scar spreading, and visible precipitates; moreover, patients having suffered through one injection are sometimes reluctant to be injected again. This is particularly true of younger patients.

PRESSURE AND SPLINTS

Constant and unrelenting pressure, as well as mechanical splints, are essential adjuncts to burn scar treatment. Custom-tailored elastic garments worn without interruption diminish both burn scar contracture and subjective symptoms. Molded splints placed between the scar surface and the pressure garment increase the garment's efficacy. Because social stigma raises compliance issues, these garments are more often effective when a scar's nuisance quotient and discomfort exceed that of wearing the garment. Practically speaking, this limits the pressure garment's role to the treatment of large and debilitating scars caused by burns. Daily intermittent massage with lubricants has been recommended by experienced surgeons for many years, perhaps recalling Osler's admonition that "the purpose of the physician is to amuse the patient while nature effects the cure." Certainly, intermittent massage does no harm and can be applied to any surface scar.

SILICONE GEL SHEETING

Silicone gel sheeting appears to work by a mechanism other than pressure and is easier to use than pressure garments. Furthermore, its use is not associated with the pain of injection or need for expensive equipment. This therapy has no known significant risk but may lead to dermatitis, scar ulceration, or folliculitis if the sheeting is worn for prolonged periods without change or cleansing. Patients may find its use inconvenient if worn on highly convex or hairy surfaces and it may be considered unattractive on a visible area. Daily care is required for up to 18 months, making compliance difficult in some patients. Treatment with silicone gel sheeting may be started early after surgery when scar proliferation and remodeling are dominant, to prevent hypertrophy in susceptible wounds.

Undesirable Results From Scar Revision

The most common problem after scar revision is a recurrence of either hypertrophy or increasing scar width. If patient selection is not ideal, this is not a complication, but it is to be expected. As an extreme example, scar revision of a 3-week-old scar located on the deltoid area in a dark-skinned, 6-year-old patient is doomed to turn out poorly. Yet even with the best of selection and technique, scars may not become thin and inconspicuous. Patients should never be guaranteed results.

HEMATOMA

Hematoma may result if a dead space is not closed by sutures or dressing compression. Small Penrose drains, rubber-band drains, or small suction drains (made from butterfly scalp-vein needles or blood-drawing vacuum tubes) may be used to avert this problem.

INFECTION

Infection is rarely a problem in scar revision of the face, but can be on the trunk or extremities. Antibiotic coverage is rarely used, unless the revision is quite large; even then the value of antibiotics is questionable. Some wounds with retained foreign bodies appear to be prone to infection; at scar revision, all such foreign bodies should be removed if possible.

HYPERPIGMENTATION

Hyperpigmentation of the involved area may be transient after scar revision, dermabrasion, laser treatment, or other trauma. It may be inevitable based upon the individual patient's scarring history and hormonal status. While prevention by strict sun avoidance is counseled, even small amounts of reflected light may trigger the dispersion of pigment within and around a treated area. For this reason, we favor the use of sun block (SPF-15) after scar revision. At this time we believe those containing titanium dioxide to be best. When hyperpigmentation occurs, it may be treated by topicals containing both tretinoin and hydroquinone (11).

MILIA

Milia ("white-heads") are small sebaceous or inclusion cysts. They commonly occur on the face when epithelium grows down suture tracts. Eyelids are especially prone to milia formation; for prevention, sutures are removed as early as 4 days postoperatively. After abrasions, milia can form as regenerative epithelium grows over sebaceous duct openings. Treatment consists of unroofing the milia by having the patient scrub the area daily with a rough washcloth. Persistent milia can be unroofed with an 18-gauge needle tip or an 11 blade. After the milia are unroofed and their small sebaceous pellets expressed, they rarely recur.

Dehiscence

Dehiscence, or wound separation, rarely occurs when sutures are in place unless there is excess tension on the wound edges. More commonly, separation is due to direct trauma after sutures are removed. When sutures are removed early, patients (or caregivers of young children) should be informed that the wound is not fully healed and should be protected for another 5 to 7 days. Often reinforcing skin tapes are placed on the wound to protect it once sutures have been removed.

Bibliography

1. Borges AF. Timing of scar revision techniques. *Clin Plast Surg* 1990; 17:71–76.
2. Ahn ST, Monfans WW, Mustoe TAM. Topical silicone gel for the prevention and treatment of hypertrophic scar. *Arch Surg* 1991; 126: 499–504.
3. Rudolph R. Wide spread scars, hypertrophic scars, and keloids. *Clin Plast Surg* 1987; 14:253–253.
4. Crikelair GF, Cosman B. Facial scars in Puerto Rican females. *Plast Reconstr Surg* 1964; 33:556–557.
5. Borges AF. Revision of linear scars. In: Goldwyn RM, ed. *The unfavorable result in plastic surgery.* Boston: Little, Brown, 1972; 97–114.
6. Wray RC. Force required for wound closure and scar appearance. *Plast Reconstr Surg* 1983; 72:380–382.
7. Taube M, Porter RJ, Lord PH. A combination of subcuticular suture and sterile micropore tape compared with conventional interrupted sutures for skin closure. *Ann R Coll Surg Engl* 1983; 65:165–167.
8. McGregor IA. *Fundamental techniques of plastic surgery.* 3rd ed. London: Churchill Livingstone, 1965: 3.
9. Hirshowitz B, Lindenbaum E, Har-Shai Y. A skin stretching device for the harnessing of the viscoelastic properties of the skin. *Plast Reconstr Surg* 1993; 92:260–270.
10. Katz BE, Oca MAGS. A controlled study of the effectiveness of spot dermabrasion ("scarabrasion") on the appearance of surgical scars. *J Am Acad Dermatol* 1991; 24:462–466.
11. Dzabow CM, Miller WH Jr. The effect of 13*cis*-retinoic acid on wound healing in dogs. *J Dermatol Surg Oncol* 1987; 13:265–268.
12. Goldman MP, Fitzpatrick RE. *Cutaneous laser surgery.* Mosby–Year Book, 1994; 80–82.
13. Johnson WC. Treatment of pitted scars: punch transplant techniques. *J Dermatol Surg Oncol* 1986; 12:260.

16

Cutaneous Carcinomas

Suzanne M. Olbricht, M.D.

Basal Cell Carcinoma

More than 900,000 new cases of nonmelanoma skin cancer and 2300 nonmelanoma skin cancer deaths are identified in the United States per year (1), an increase of 15 to 20% each decade for the past several decades. Basal cell carcinomas (BCC) constitute 65 to 80% of new cases and as many as 20% of the deaths (2). Local skin cancer detection programs identify presumptive BCC in as many as 28% of participants (3).

The BCC is thought to arise from a pluripotential cell residing in the basal layer of the epidermis or appendigeal epithelium. Although it has been reported from any cutaneous surface, 85% are found on the head or neck areas. Usually a BCC is a stable, slow-growing lesion that is present for years. Rapid and destructive growth ("aggressive" tumors) may occur infrequently, massive silent penetration along deep tissue planes or along nerves is rarely reported (4), and metastasis is quite rare (0.025%) (5).

Factors that induce growth and dictate the behavior of BCC are being elucidated. Sunlight has a major role, although the exact mechanism remains undefined. Lymphocytes of patients who have BCC show reduced capacity for repair of UV light-induced DNA damage (6). Chronic cumulative sun exposure, as estimated by the age of the patient, vocational and recreational exposure history, and complexion (fair, poor tanning ability, red hair) (7,8), as well as childhood sunburns (9), are prominent risk factors. Markers for sun-damaged skin, including actinic keratoses, elastosis, localized pigmentary disorders, senile lentigines, freckles, spider nevi, telangiectasia, dry skin, wrinkled skin, and arcus senilis, define a population at greater risk for BCC than those without evidence of sun damage (11.3% vs. 1.0% in men 65 to 74 years old) (10). Therapeutic, diagnostic, or accidental exposure to radiation has led to development of BCC with latent periods reported as short as 7 years (11), but with an average of 20 to 25 years (12,13). Long-term psoralens and UVA (PUVA) radiation therapy, used in the treatment of chronic skin diseases such as psoriasis, increases the risk of BCC in a dose-dependent fashion (14), as does chronic arsenical intoxication from medicaments (15) or well water (16). Immunosuppressed patients (17,18), including those with AIDS (19), have both increased incidence and metastatic rate of cutaneous tumors. Miscellaneous predisposing lesions include old burn scars, tattoos, vaccination scars, chronic ulcers and sinuses, dermatofibromas, epidermal nevi, nevus sebaceous of Jadassohn, and areas of trauma. For unknown reasons, BCC may be diagnosed in unexpected patients, those less than 29 years old

(20), or black (21). The risk of a second cutaneous carcinoma, either BCC or squamous cell carcinoma (SCC), is reported to be 20% within 18 months in one study (22), as high as 30% within 2 years in an Anglo-Saxon ethnic group in New York state (23), and 36 to 50% within 5 years in other studies (24,25).

Physical examination readily identifies BCC in most patients (26). The most common BCC on the face is a slightly translucent, waxy, or pearly papule or nodule with surrounding and overlying telangiectasia and an easily defined border (Fig. 16–1). The superficial (often misnamed "multicentric") BCC, typically present on the back, is an erythematous, telangiectatic, well-demarcated macule with a fine scale (Fig. 16–2). A primary sclerosing BCC (also called a morpheaform or an infiltrating BCC) is relatively rare, and appears as an ill-defined flat, hypopigmented or yellowish indurated plaque, sometimes with overlying telangiectasia (Fig. 16–3). On occasion, a BCC may be fibromalike (fibroepithelioma of Pinkus), presenting as a moderately firm, often slightly pedunculated soft nodule with a smooth, pink surface. Secondary changes may include ulceration, crusting, scaling, pigmentation (Fig. 16–4), erythema, cystic collection, and scarring. A rodent ulcer is a BCC with prominent ulceration and inapparent tumor mass, commonly present around fusion planes of the nose and cheek. Cystic BCC may yield extrusion of mucinous material on puncture. A pigmented BCC mimics a malignant melanoma. A field-fire BCC is a lesion in which the center resolves with scarring and loss of appendages, while tumor is found at the edge.

The differential diagnosis of a BCC includes a host of benign tumors (usually nevocellular or appendigeal in origin), actinic keratoses, squamous cell carcinomas, malignant melanoma (especially amelanotic tumors), and inflammatory conditions (e.g., acneiform papule or granuloma fissuration from constant pressure of eyeglasses), or traumatic events, (e.g., excoriation, shaving cut).

The presence of a BCC is documented by pathologic examination of a tissue specimen obtained by curettage, shave biopsy, punch biopsy (a 2-mm disposable Keyes punch is sufficient), an incisional biopsy, or excision in toto. Curettage yields fragments of disoriented tissue that are adequate only for documenting a BCC and not for excluding other tumors or disease processes. Shave biopsy is easy to perform and the site heals well. In addition, the specimen generally contains enough material to enable the pathologist to diagnose an alternative process. If melanoma is being considered in the differential diagnosis, only a punch biopsy of at least 4 mm in

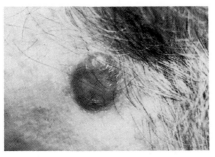

FIG. 16–1. Nodular basal cell carcinoma.

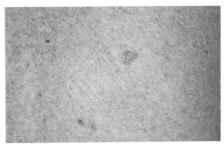

FIG. 16–2. Superficial basal cell carcinoma.

FIG. 16–3. Morpheaform basal cell carcinoma.

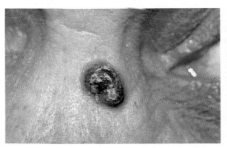

FIG. 16–4. Pigmented basal cell carcinoma.

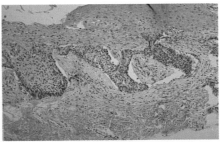

FIG. 16–5. Basal cell carcinoma, histology, tumor mass.

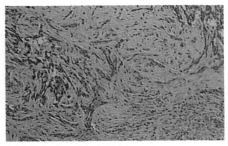

FIG. 16–6. Basal cell carcinoma, histology, fibrosis.

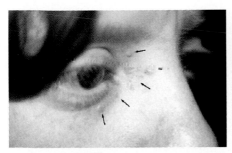

FIG. 16–7. Basal cell nevus syndrome.

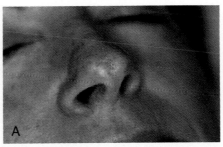

FIG. 16–8. Mohs micrographic surgical procedure. **A,** BCC, tip of nose, preoperative photograph.

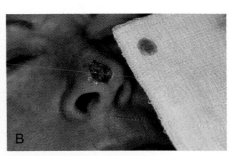

FIG. 16–8. B, stage I, Mohs micrographic surgery, thin layer of tissue removed around curettage site.

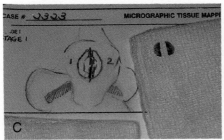

FIG. 16–8. C, stage I, micrographic mapping.

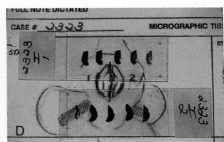

FIG. 16–8. D, stage I, frozen sections overlying map marked for presence of tumor.

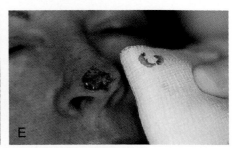

FIG. 16–8. E, stage II, excision of tumor-laden margins.

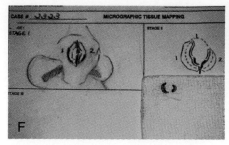

FIG. 16–8.   **F,** stage II, micrographic mapping.

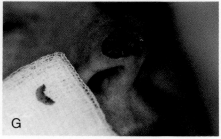

FIG. 16–8.   **G,** stage III, excision of tumor-laden margin. There was no tumor found at the margin of this specimen. The defect is ready for closure.

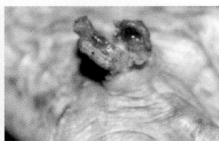

FIG. 16–10.   Cutaneous horn.

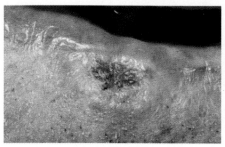

FIG. 16–11.   Squamous cell carcinoma of lower lip.

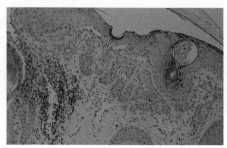

FIG. 16–13.   Actinic keratosis, histology.

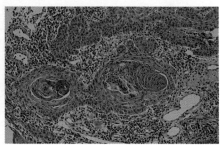

FIG. 16–14.   Squamous cell carcinoma, histology

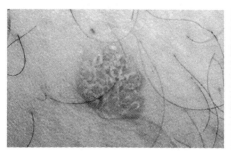

FIG. 16–15.   Bowen disease.

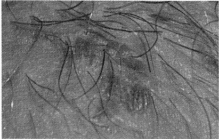

FIG. 16–16.   Bowenoid papulosis.

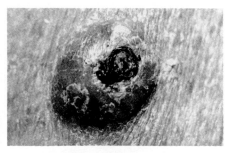

FIG. 16–17.   Keratoacanthoma.

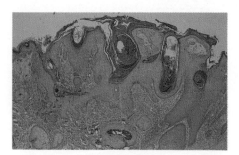

FIG. 16–18.   Keratoacanthoma, histology.

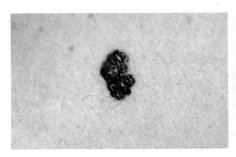

FIG. 16–19. Superficial spreading melanoma.

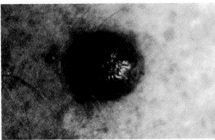

FIG. 16–20. Nodular melanoma.

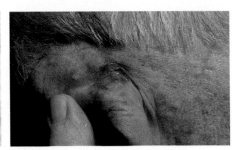

FIG. 16–21. Lentigo maligna melanoma.

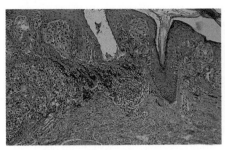

FIG. 16–22. Superficial spreading melanoma, histology.

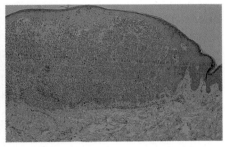

FIG. 16–23. Nodular melanoma, histology.

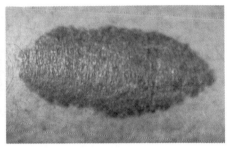

FIG. 16–24. Small congenital nevus.

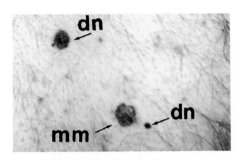

FIG. 16–25. Dysplastic nevus.

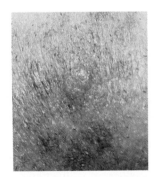

FIG. 16–26. Lentigo maligna.

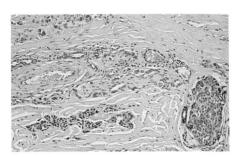

FIG. 16–27. Microscopic satellites.

diameter or an incisional or excisional biopsy will obtain a specimen appropriate for evaluation.

Microscopic evidence of BCC includes cytologically atypical cells with darkly staining, large, oval, elongated nuclei and little cytoplasm, collected in masses of various sizes with palisading of the cells at the periphery of the masses and retraction artefact about the masses (Fig. 16–5). Stromal changes include mucin deposition and fibrosis (Fig. 16–6). A cystic BCC will contain large masses of mucin, while fibrosis may be so striking in a morpheaform BCC that the tumor cells are difficult to detect. The tumor may differentiate toward hair structures, sebaceous glands, apocrine glands, or eccrine glands. Trichoepithelioma, both typical and desmoplastic, may be difficult to differentiate pathologically.

Three hereditary syndromes of multiple BCC are currently recognized. The basal cell nevus syndrome (27), whose genetic defect has been mapped (28), is inherited in an autosomal dominant fashion, and is characterized by multiple BCC (Fig. 16–7), palmar pits, and extreme sensitivity to radiation, with a short latency period of 4 to 5 years to the onset of numerous tumors (29). Hundreds of BCC, with disastrous consequences, can be seen in these patients (30). Other manifestations include jaw cysts, hypertelorism, calcification of the falx cerebri, spina bifida, bifid ribs, ovarian fibromas with rare malignant degeneration, cardiac fibromas, milia, epidermal cysts, mesenteric cysts, and gastric polyps, as well as tumors such as medulloblastomas, meningiomas, and fatal rhabdomyomas. The Basex syndrome (31), whose gene defect is also known (32), may be inherited as an X-linked dominant trait, and is comprised of a triad of cutaneous findings: multiple BCC developing between the ages of 15 and 25 years, follicular atrophoderma on the dorsum of the hands and elbows, and localized areas of anhidrosis. Xeroderma pigmentosum (33), a disorder of excision repair of ultraviolet (UV) light-induced pyrimidine dimers in DNA or in synthesis of DNA after UV irradiation, has six known genetic forms. Clinically, the patients manifest acute photosensitivity, photophobia, conjunctivitis, and multiple cutaneous neoplasms (usually before 10 years of age), often with horrifying results. Some forms also involve microcephaly, progressive mental deterioration, and sensorineural deficits.

Treatment of BCC is primarily surgical and destructive—and, in most cases, curative (i.e., with no recurrence). Optimal therapy for a primary lesion may depend on multiple factors, including size and location of the tumor, possibility of invasion of vital structures, age and general health of the patient, and the patient's cosmetic concerns. Possible modalities include excision, excision by Mohs micrographic technique, cryosurgery, electrodesiccation and curettage, radiation, laser surgery, and topical application of 5-fluorouracil (5FU).

Of special note in planning therapy is the consideration of adequate margins. In one study of 101 consecutive tumors less than 2 cm in diameter (34), gross margins (marked by electrodesiccation before excision) when compared with the histologic margins showed concordance within 1 mm in 94% of tumors and within 2 mm in 95%. A later study of 117 cases of untreated, well-demarcated BCC less than 2 cm in diameter determined that a minimum margin of 4 mm was necessary to eradicate the tumor totally in more than 95% of cases (35). Sclerosing BCC present a special problem, with a much greater discrepancy between clinically appreciable margins and tumor-free margins documented histologically (as noted in the first study), and corroborated by a report (36) in which a staged progressive surgical procedure documented subclinical extension of 7.2 ± 3% mm in 51 biopsy-proven primary morpheaform BCC.

Surgical excision is often the treatment of choice. The recurrence rate after primary excision is 5 to 6% (37). BCC is most likely to recur if the lesion is greater than 2 cm in diameter, morpheaform (sclerosing), or located in areas of embryonal fusion planes (nasolabial folds, nose-cheek angle, posterior ear sulcus, canal of the ear, periorbital area, and scalp) (38). Thirty-five percent of BCC recur that were histologically present at the margin of the surgical specimen (39), and recurrence is more common when both lateral and deep margins are involved (40). Reexcision of a pathologically diagnosed inadequate excision is preferable in most cases, especially if the tumor is located in a cosmetically or functionally significant area where a recurrence would be problematic.

Standard surgical excision and repair technique applies to the excision of a BCC. The tumor is outlined with a marking pen before the instillation of local anesthesia, because resulting vasoconstriction and edema may obscure the edge of the tumor. Finding the tumor edge may also be facilitated by curettage, because the mucinous stroma surrounding a BCC allows for easy separation of the diseased tissue from normal skin. A margin appropriate to the type of tumor and anatomic location is then marked surrounding the tumor, and an elliptical excision encompassing the tumor and margin is planned so that the repaired linear wound follows relaxed skin tension lines or hides in a normal wrinkle or anatomic structure. With tension applied to the surgical site, a scalpel is used to incise the planned ellipse perpendicular to the skin surface, deep to upper subcutaneous fat. The ellipse is removed with the aid of a curved scissors. Undermining in the upper subcutaneous fat beneath the subepidermal vascular plexus facilitates closure of the wound by sutures or staples. The specimen is sent to pathology. Placing a stitch in the most superior position (i.e., 12 o'clock) with a notation on the pathology requisition as well as on the operative report, facilitates correlation with the resulting scar should one of the margins be reported as positive. The treatment of difficult or high-risk BCC should be dealt with in two stages: first, removal of the entire tumor with adequate surgical margins, and second, construction of a plan for wound reconstruction (41,42). Minor modifications in surgical procedures for cosmetic considerations may have devastating consequences for recurrence, requiring secondary procedures or even limiting patient survival.

Dealing with the problem of difficult, large, high-risk, and recurrent BCC, Frederick Mohs in 1936 developed a staged procedure (43) in which he removed small amounts of accurately mapped tissue under local anesthesia after fixing the skin in vivo with zinc chloride. He then microscopically examined the inferior margin by horizontal section of tumor, and reexcised as necessary. He allowed these wounds to heal by secondary intention.

As practiced today, Mohs micrographic surgery (Fig. 16–8) is a fresh-tissue technique. It is generally performed in Mohs surgical units by physicians who have trained in dedicated one- to two-year fellowships after completing dermatologic or surgical residencies. Special staffing requirements include a laboratory technician who can map and process the specimen in oblique sections, and surgical assistants who can deal both with large, open wounds and with anxious patients who have to endure some waiting time between stages. Under local anesthesia, the tumor is assessed and debulked by curettage. The defect is then excised by saucerization of 1 to 2 mm of tissue. The lateral edge of the excision must have a 45° angle to facilitate histologic processing. Hemostasis is accomplished by electrodesiccation. Saucerized tissue is mapped and frozen and cut in oblique sections. The entire undersurface of the lateral and inferior margin is systematically reviewed for presence of tumor. This microscopic review differs from the usual vertical frozen sections of the pathologist and allows for evaluation of all the margins rather than a sampling (44). Repeat saucerizations are performed the same day until the margins are clear, requiring 30 to 60 minutes per stage. When the margins are tumor free, a decision about closure can be made depending on the site, size, and depth of the defect. For some wounds, the best cosmetic result is achieved with healing by secondary intention. Wounds can also be repaired by side-to-side closure, random-based cutaneous flaps, or grafts. Large defects may require major soft-tissue reconstruction. The advantages of the Mohs surgical procedure include maximal preservation of normal tissue and precise delineation of the track of the tumor. Cure rate is enhanced (45–48); for previously untreated tumors, the recurrent rate is 1 to 2%, and for recurrent tumors 4 to 9% (recurrence rate for use of other modalities to treat recurrent tumors is 20 to 50%). Indications for the procedure, therefore, are: (a) recurrent tumors; (b) primary tumors known to have high recurrence rates (greater than 2 cm in diameter, poorly demarcated margins, sclerosing or micronodular histology, and sites where deep penetration along fusion planes are common); and (c) primary lesions where maximal preservation of tissue is necessary such as the eyelid, nose, finger, genitalia, and areas around major facial nerves. Mohs surgical excision should also be considered when the excision of the primary lesion will require a flap or graft for closure, since recurrence under the plane of reconstruction can be difficult to diagnose.

Alternatives to excision include therapies that deliver a lethal physical insult to tissue within the area to be treated (field destructive techniques). Because these modalities destroy the tumor, biopsy confirmation before treatment is essential. In addition, no specimen will be obtained for histologic examination of the surgical margins. Some physicians frequently employ cryosurgery, in which liquid nitrogen (−196° C) is delivered to the anesthetized site via spray from a commercially available handheld instrument. The field (tumor and margins) is sprayed to complete freezing (−40° C to −60° C) of the tissue several millimeters deep, as measured either by thermocouple-tipped needles placed in the tumor (49) or by standardized timing of the freeze-and-thaw cycle (50). The result of cryotherapy is a local frostbite reaction: swelling, pain, and bulla formation for 1 to 2 days, then an ulcer covered by a crust that separates in 2 to 6 weeks. Erythema at the site may persist for months. The mature scar, cosmetically acceptable to selected patients in some locations, is hypopigmented, flat or somewhat depressed, and sclerotic. It softens and elevates with time but does not regain normal aging lines. Complications are few; there may be temporary massive local edema, permanent alopecia, or rare temporary paralysis of the facial nerve if it underlies the treated site (51). The recurrence rate is 2 to 6% in skilled hands (50,52,53).

Curettage and electrodesiccation (54) may also be used for field destruction. Under local anesthesia, a curette is used to remove the tumor mass, a procedure facilitated by the mucinous stroma of BCC, which easily separates from normal tissue. Heat via electrodesiccation is used to destroy a 1- to 2-mm rim of tissue in and about the defect. Generally, the eschar is then curetted and a second 1- to 2-mm rim of tissue electrodessicated. Healing is by secondary intention over a 2–6 week period and results in a flat, hypopigmented scar, sometimes with a hypertrophic center. The recurrence rate is 6 to 10% (55). In a study of BCC treated first by curettage and electrodesiccation, repeated three times in rapid succession and the wound then excised by shave, residual tumor was found in 8.3% of lesions treated on the trunk and extremities and 46.6% of lesions of the face (56). It may therefore be best to reserve this treatment for tumors of the trunk and extremities.

When curative superficial radiotherapy is used, the result is a hypopigmented, atrophic, telangiectatic scar that tends to worsen cosmetically with time. Because of the high risk of radiation-induced secondary cutaneous carcinoma (average lag time of 15 years) and worsening appearance of the scar, this method of treatment is inadvisable for patients less than 60 years old. Some authors feel that it is an excellent therapy for eyelid lesions (57) or nose (58). In general, the reported recurrence rate is 5 to 11% (59).

Laser light (argon, dye, or heavy-metal lasers) has been used to treat lesions made photosensitive by hematoporphyrin derivative (HPD) or 5-aminolaevulinic acid administered systematically, by local injection, or by topical application. This technique, called photodynamic therapy (PDT), has been used only for a small number of patients and does not have the cure rate of Mohs micrographic surgery (60,61), but may be useful for treatment of multiple, difficult, metastatic, or end-stage invasive lesions.

One useful chemotherapeutic agent is available for the treatment of BCC: 5-fluorouracil (5-FU) in a 5% cream is applied twice a day to a superficial BCC for 3 to 6 weeks. The lesion will be red, sore, and swollen, and may ulcerate toward the end of the treatment course. Healing time is generally 3 to 6 weeks and results in a slightly hypopigmented, soft, flat macule. The recurrence rate is estimated to be 20 to 50% and is highest for lesions with nodularity or deep foci (62,63). Better results were obtained in patients in whom curettage of the lesion was performed immediately before chemotherapy was instituted (64). Chemotherapy with 5-FU is primarily indicated for the patient with multiple superficial lesions, such as superficial spreading BCC of the back. In addition to 5-FU, it is possible that in the future retinoids may prove useful as primary or as adjunctive therapy. Systemic isotretinoin and etretinate, and topical tretinoin have been used to treat BCC but have a response rate of 30 to 40% and a significant incidence of troublesome adverse effects (65–67).

Persistent long-term follow-up care (68) of patients who have had a BCC is important. Visible recurrence at the site of a treated lesion may be delayed; 33% of recurrences are noted at 1 year, 50% at 2 years, and yet only 66% at 3 years (69). Patients are, however, much more likely to develop a second primary than a recurrence of the originally treated lesion, and their entire cutaneous surface should be examined every 6 to 12 months, with particular attention paid to sun-exposed surfaces, sites previously treated with radiotherapy, and areas difficult for the patient to examine. Patients with special risks, such as immunosuppression or hereditary disease, may need reexamination even more frequently. Most important, patients need instruction concerning risky behavior in the sun, since cumulative sun exposure is the most common—and only preventable—inciting factor. Patients are advised to minimize sun exposure from 10 AM to 2 PM (11 AM to 3 PM daylight savings time), to wear a wide-brimmed hat, long-sleeved shirt, and long pants when outside, and to apply a sunscreen with a sun protection factor (SPF) of 15 or more before any exposure to the sun and at least every 2 hours as long as the outdoor activity is continued. Water-repellant or water-resistant sunscreens are especially helpful during sweaty or wet outdoor activities. Significant sun exposure occurs even with brief exposures on overcast days (such as a 30-minute outdoor lunch at work). In addition, exposure to artificial sources of UV radiation, including tanning parlors, should be strictly avoided.

All children, outdoor workers, or fair-skinned individuals who have a tendency to burn should follow these guidelines. It has been calculated that the regular use of a sunscreen with an SPF of 15 for the first 18 years of life would reduce the lifetime incidence of BCC and squamous cell carcinoma by 78% (70). It is generally thought that decreasing sun exposure, even after the first skin cancer has been noted, will decrease the number of new primary cancers diagnosed. Certainly the use of sunscreen prevents tumor production in animal models (71). Preventive actions will eventually become universally mandatory, since the trend toward ozone depletion will give rise to greater intensity of UV radiation at the earth's surface (72). No adequate or generally useful chemopreventative agent has yet been developed. Oral isotretinoin may prevent carcinomas in some patients with overwhelming risk factors such as arsenic exposure, xeroderma pigmentosum, or the basal cell nevus syndrome, but it has numerous adverse effects (66,73). Sparse data exist for etretinate, another oral retinoid (67), and there are no in vivo data in humans substantiating the theoretical chemopreventative properties of tretinoin, a topical retinoid. On the contrary, in one study (74), mice treated with tretinoin and receiving UV radiation developed more tumors than mice treated with UV radiation alone. This result is controversial; however, patients using tretinoin to treat photoaging need to be warned so they can exercise appropriate care in avoiding sun exposure and in making follow-up appointments for examination.

Squamous Cell Carcinoma

Squamous cell carcinoma (SCC) is the second most common type of skin cancer; about 200,000 new cases are diagnosed in the United States each year. Sixty percent of the estimated 2300 nonmelanoma skin cancer deaths per year are owed to SCC arising from cutaneous sites (2). SCC may occur any-where on the skin or mucous membranes, where it arises from atypical epidermal keratinocytes. Rarely occurring in normal skin, it usually appears on sun-damaged skin or in actinic keratoses as a rapidly growing lesion. Up to 14% of older or quickly growing lesions may invade deeply, even extending along nerves (75,76). The rate of metastasis is debated. Lund (77,78) estimates that less than 0.1% of SCC arising in sun-damaged skin metastasize, while two other studies (79,80) suggest a metastatic rate of 2 to 3%. Large lesions of the ear, forehead, temple, and dorsa of the hands have a much greater metastatic rate, calculated to be 10 to 36% in a group of patients referred for Mohs micrographic surgery (81). Lip lesions may metastasize at a rate of 11 to 20% (81,82).

Conditions predisposing to BCC also predispose to the development of SCC. In particular, the direct relationship to sun exposure and actinically damaged skin is even more striking. Individuals over 50 years of age have a higher SCC:BCC ratio than younger individuals, probably due to greater cumulative sun exposure (83). Using mannequin heads and a chemical system of dosimetry for UV light measurement (84), it has been established that the areas of the greatest sun exposure had the highest incidence of SCC. UV-B light has been more strongly implicated, but UV-A probably also plays a role (85). Certainly patients receiving PUVA therapy develop SCC in a dose-dependent relationship (14) within 5 years. The risk of SCC in immunosuppressed patients is 18 times the general population (for BCC, 3 times) (86), and also correlates with sun exposure and evidence of photodamage (87). Actinic keratoses may be premalignant lesions (88); 20 to 25% of patients with actinic keratoses will develop at least one SCC.

Multiple mechanisms of tumorigenesis have been proposed, including faulty DNA repair after UV light exposure (89), induction of carcinogens from sterols in the skin (90), hyperplasia-inducing factors (91), and immunological alterations (92). Viral infection, particularly with specific subtypes of human papillomavirus, has been incriminated (93). Occupational exposure to tars and polycyclic aromatic hydrocarbons (94) and smoking (95) also predispose to the development of SCC. Chronic scarring processes produce SCC, which may act more aggressively with a metastatic rate of 20 to 30% (96–98). Such chronic scarring processes include burn scars, draining sinuses, pilonidal sinuses, lichen sclerosus et atrophicus, discoid lupus erythematosus, porokeratosis of Mibelli, dystrophic epidermolysis bullosa, and repeated abrasion. Theoretically, they give rise to SCC by inducing a constantly proliferating epidermal unit.

The primary clinical appearance of SCC is a poorly defined firm nodule, flesh-colored to red, with a hyperkeratotic crust (Fig. 16–9). The lesion may ulcerate as it grows. Production of large amounts of compacted parakeratosis may mimic a wart, or a so-called cutaneous "horn" (Fig. 16–10). Lesions of the lower lip can be difficult to diagnose, both clinically and histologically, appearing as a nonhealing sore, a white plaque (Fig. 16–11), or a rapidly growing inflammatory nodule. The differential diagnosis of SCC includes actinic keratosis, especially the hypertrophic variety commonly on the dorsum of the hand (Fig. 16–12), keratoacanthoma, an irritated seborrheic keratosis, and wart. Pathologic examination is again essential for documentation of the exact tumor

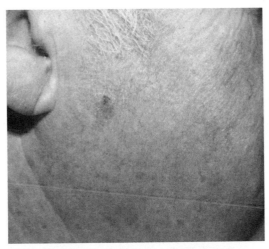

FIG. 16–9. Squamous cell carcinoma.

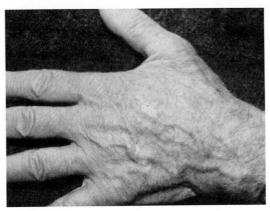

FIG. 16–12. Hypertrophic actinic keratosis.

type. Both clinical and histologic differences between SCC and actinic keratosis are in degree, rather than type, of change. In an actinic keratosis, atypical keratinocytes proliferate in the lower epidermis in buds that usually grow downward (Fig. 16–13). The upper epidermal cells may be normal, however, indicating the retained ability of the cells to mature. Invasive SCC occurs when the atypical cells invade the dermis in tumor masses that may contain keratin pearls (Fig. 16–14). It is generally accepted that the changes are progressive with time (99).

Several variants of SCC are recognized. SCC in situ, arising in an actinic keratosis is a histologic variant, clinically appears as a poorly demarcated inflammatory scaling papule or plaque in the midst of marked actinic damage. Bowen disease (Fig. 16–15), a single lesion of intraepidermal SCC that may occasionally develop invasive foci, is clinically manifested as a well-demarcated macule or slightly indurated plaque with a sharp but irregular outline, often with gray-brown hyperpigmentation erythema and fine superficial scaling. By definition, it does not arise from an obvious preexisting lesion or from skin with actinic damage. It is unclear whether Bowen disease is associated with a higher incidence of internal malignancy, as suggested in older literature (100). Bowenoid papulosis is the name used for single or multiple genital and verrucous papules (Fig. 16–16) that are resistant to therapy, have atypia reminiscent of Bowen disease on histologic examination, and are probably viral-induced with significant malignant potential (101–103). Specific subtypes of human papillomavirus (the "wart" virus), usually type 16, are isolated from both invasive cervical cancer and Bowenoid papulosis (104). Erythroplasia of Queryat (105) signifies an asymptomatic, sharply demarcated, bright red, shiny, slightly indurated plaque on the glans penis with the histologic picture of SCC in situ. It develops almost exclusively in uncircumcised men. Progression into invasive SCC has been observed in up to 30% of patients (105) with metastases in up to 20% (106). Carcinoma cuniculatum (107), or verrucous carcinoma, is a warty, slow-growing plaque, most commonly found on the feet. It has no cytologic atypia on histologic section and may be difficult to diagnose without a deep biopsy to identify the

characteristic broad invading tumor masses at the base of the lesion. Metastases have been reported (108).

The nosology of keratoacanthoma, sometimes called self-healing SCC, remains controversial. Clinically, it is a well-demarcated nodule with rolled firm borders and a central cup filled with keratinaceous debris (Fig. 16–17). An excision in toto, or central wedge incisional biopsy, may reveal the hallmarks of the histologic diagnosis (Fig. 16–18), which include cup-shaped acanthosis, glassy and mildly atypical keratinocytes pushing into the dermis in strands that may even invade perineural space, a pronounced inflammatory infiltrate, horn pearls, intraepithelial abscesses, and elimination of elastic tissue in the epithelial tongues. Clinically and histologically, it is difficult to differentiate between a keratoacanthoma and SCC (109), though immunoperoxidase markers may prove useful (110). Some authors advise full excision in each case (111,112), while others (113,114) will consider careful observation and conservative therapy for selected classic lesions. Data suggest that daily application of 5-FU topically (115) or weekly intralesional injection of 5-FU (116) may be effective over a 3-week period and thus avert a surgical or destructive procedure. Multiple keratocanthomas have been related to internal malignancies (117), photochemotherapy for psoriasis (118), and chronic sun exposure (119).

Hereditary syndromes associated with an increased incidence of SCC are rare. Xeroderma pigmentosum (see above) may develop widely destructive SCC. Epidermodysplasia verruciformis (120) is a rare autosomal recessive disorder with defects in cell mediated immunity (121,122) in which several subtypes of human papillomavirus induce widespread, polymorphic, and verrucous lesions beginning in childhood. The warts may develop carcinomatous changes within 2 years of onset. Metastasis from SCC and death have been reported. Muir-Torre syndrome (123,124) is an autosomal dominant disorder, manifested by multiple internal malignancies, cutaneous sebaceous proliferation (adenomas and carcinomas), and keratoacanthomas.

Treatment of SCC follows the same guidelines as discussed for BCC. Most data regarding success of therapy for BCC (as detailed above) include small numbers of SCC with similar results, excluding mucous membrane lesions and lesions already metastatic. Factors predisposing to recurrence

(125) include size greater than 1 cm in diameter, poorly differentiated cytological features, and histologic invasion into deep dermis or fat. Of note is the success of Mohs surgery in difficult cases with a recurrence rate of 3.3% on the head and neck and 12.5% on the lower extremity in 414 patients (126). Advanced and multiple SCC have been treated in small numbers with oral isotretinoin, which was helpful in 11 of 15 reported cases (127,128).

As with patients who have BCC, much morbidity from actinic damage may be preventable. Individual actinic keratoses can be treated with light cryotherapy (liquid nitrogen applied with a cotton swab for a total freeze-and-thaw time of 15 to 30 seconds), for cosmetic control of the lesions. Topically applied 5-FU over large areas of exposed skin, dermabrasion, laser resurfacing, or chemical peeling may eradicate premalignant lesions and delay the development of new lesions. Daily use of sunscreens (129) and a low-fat diet (130) may also reduce new development of actinic keratoses. Repeated follow-up examinations of the patient's entire cutaneous surface are also warranted on a long-term basis.

Malignant Melanoma

Malignant melanoma, a neoplasm of neural crest–derived cells that have differentiated toward melanocytes, is a common and sometimes lethal cutaneous tumor. In 1994 an estimated 32,000 melanomas were diagnosed in the United States, resulting in 6900 deaths (131). It was the second greatest killer among cancers of males 15 to 34 years of age, and accounted for 1% of all deaths from cancer. In countries populated by fair-skinned whites, its incidence and mortality rate have risen rapidly, 4 to 15% per year, more than doubling over the past decade (132–135) and the fastest of any cancer (136). Current age-adjusted annual incidence rates per 100,000 whites in the United States is 12.0 (14.3 for men and 10.4 for women) (137). By the year 2000, it is estimated that the cumulative lifetime risk for melanoma will be 1 in 75 Americans (138). In spite of this grim forecast, the 5-year survival rate has improved from 60% in 1960–1963 to 80% in 1979–1984 (139), probably because of earlier detection and improved diagnostic accuracy. A public-education campaign in Scotland was documented to produce a statistically significant rise in the diagnosis of thin melanomas, with a good prognosis and a concomitant fall in the proportion of thick lesions (140). Physicians are also alerted to the need for a complete skin examination, which may detect 6.4 times more melanomas than partial examinations (141).

Like other skin cancers, melanomas have been reported in the setting of immunosuppression (142–144), xeroderma pigmentosum (145), and radiation therapy (146). Likewise, exposure to solar radiation is related to the development of melanomas (147). A large Canadian study (134) comparing patients with melanoma and age-, sex-, and province-matched controls, identified blond hair, light color, sun-damaged skin, and severe freckling to be significant risk factors for melanoma. Significantly increased risk has been associated with severe sunburns before age 15, sunbathing, boating, and vacations spent in the sun (148). The incidence of melanoma is higher in patients who were children in sunny climates than in those who moved there as adults (149). In New York, a large case control study found a seventeen times increase in risk of melanoma of all types in patients who have had basal cell carcinomas and squamous cell carcinomas but no personal or family history of melanoma (150). The incidence of intraocular melanoma has also been correlated with sunlight exposure (151). It is likely that a combination of intermittent and total accumulated exposure to sunlight contributes to risk (152).

Two major types of melanoma are recognized clinically: superficial spreading melanoma (Fig. 16–19) and nodular melanoma (Fig. 16–20); the former grows radially, with or without a vertical growth phase, and the latter primarily grows vertically. Characteristics (153–155) that differentiate early melanomas from benign pigmented lesions include variegated color (red, white, and blue) or disarray of pigment (reticulated, clumped, and absent all in one lesion), irregular borders (angular indentation or notching), an irregular surface (verrucous or mixed verrucous and smooth), and a history of recent change in size or color. Elevation, bleeding, ulceration, tenderness, and itching are symptoms noted with deeply invasive lesions (156). Loss of skin markings through the lesion also constitutes a late sign associated with deep invasion (157). Melanoma may present without pigmentation (amelanotic melanoma), resulting in great diagnostic difficulty.

Other clinical types of melanoma are relatively less common. Lentigo maligna melanoma (Fig. 16–21) occurs in elderly patients and usually develops on the head and neck in actinically damaged skin. Clinically, it is manifested by induration or blue-black nodules within a previously slow-growing lentigo maligna. Acral-lentiginous melanoma (158, 159), the most common melanoma in blacks and other pigmented peoples, arises principally on the palm and soles. It may be difficult to differentiate from lentiginous nevi, but the same criteria of change in size, shape, color, and surface, and irregular borders, apply. Desmoplastic melanoma (160,161), or its variant neurotropic melanoma, is difficult to diagnose both clinically and histologically. The lesion tends to be located on a sun-exposed site, presenting as a poorly defined sclerotic mass only occasionally associated with abnormal pigmentation. Melanomas present on genital skin are also found in nonwhites as well as whites, and diagnosis is often delayed (162,163).

The differential diagnosis of melanoma includes a dysplastic nevus, Spitz nevus (benign juvenile melanoma), pigmented BCC, seborrheic keratosis, blue nevus, dermatofibroma, pyogenic granuloma, venous lake, and Kaposi sarcoma. Biopsy of any suspicious lesion is recommended, because accuracy of clinical diagnosis by specialized clinicians is only 60% (164), improved to 70% by the use of epiluminescence microscopy by formally trained users (165,166). Incisional biopsy and/or use of local anesthesia has not been shown to disseminate tumor or worsen the patient's prognosis (167). However, excision with narrow margins enables the pathologist to study the tumor in a step-wise fashion and improves diagnostic and prognostic accuracy, enabling the surgeon to plan definitive therapy more precisely. Shave biopsy and curettage are not advised, because they may not yield adequate material for diagnosis and will not allow measurement of the depth of penetration of the tumor.

Histologically, malignant melanoma is composed of dyshesive, polymorphous, and atypical melanocytes of principally epithelioid and spindle-cell type that proliferate along the dermoepidermal junction and spread as small nests or single cells (Pagetoid array) into the upper epidermis (Fig. 16–22). By definition, nodular melanoma pushes into the dermis as a single-tumor mass (Fig. 16–23) with lateral extension in the epidermis less than three rete pegs from the nodule, while in superficial spreading melanoma the lateral spread is more extensive. Frequent mitoses may be present, with or without lymphocytic infiltrate and fibrovascular response. Malignant melanoma in situ (i.e., lesions in which all atypical cells are confined to the epidermis) is thought to be biologically benign, and some pathologists prefer to use the term "severely atypical melanocytic hyperplasia" or "dysplastic nevus with severe atypia of the intraepithelial component". Borderline melanoma and minimal deviation melanoma are rare pathologic diagnoses and their biologic behaviors have not been defined. The Spitz nevus may be difficult to distinguish from malignant melanoma histologically because it contains large typical spindle and epithelioid melanocytes and mitotic figures. Spindle cell and desmoplastic melanomas may be difficult to differentiate from spindle cell SCC because of the relative lack of pigment within the lesion and the abundance of fibroblastic response.

Primary cutaneous melanomas are reported to occur at the site of preexisting pigmented lesions in 18 to 85% of cases clinically and 18 to 72% of cases histologically (168). Because 65% of white adults have at least one nevus, averaging 15 per person (169), much attention has been focused on the morphologic characteristics of precursor lesions. The number of benign nevi over 2 mm in diameter is directly proportional to risk of melanoma, although no direct site specificity has been seen (170,171). Large numbers of nevi (100 or more) indicate a patient in a high-risk group for melanoma, although that melanoma may not arise directly from any of the nevi (172). In contrast, at least 6% of giant congenital nevi (nevocellular pigmented plaques greater than 10 cm in diameter) degenerate over a lifetime (173). They account for one-third of prepubertal melanomas (174), and 50% of the resulting malignancies develop before 3 years of age (175). These melanomas may be difficult to diagnose early, because even benign areas of congenital nevi tend to have surface lobulation, dark coloration, and hamartomatous nodules. Small congenital nevi (Fig. 16–24) are defined as easily excisable lesions, noted by the parents within the first 2 weeks of life; they occur in 1% of newborns (176). Their rate of degeneration is hotly debated, but it is generally agreed to have increased, perhaps by as much as 5% (177).

A significant precursor of melanoma is the dysplastic nevus, which is generally acquired in adolescence and appears as a pigmented lesion, often greater than 5 mm in diameter, with irregular or poorly demarcated borders, irregular or very dark coloration (shades of brown and red), and an irregular surface (Fig. 16–25) (178), often occurring on sun-exposed sites in sun-sensitive individuals (179). The significance of these disorderly appearing nevi was first appreciated in the B-K mole syndrome (180), now called the familial dysplastic nevus syndrome, probably an autosomal dominant disorder in which individuals with dysplastic nevi and a family history of melanoma have a relative risk for cutaneous melanoma 148 times that of the general population (approaching 100%), while the risk in the same family of members without dys-

plastic nevi is not increased (181). Families with melanoma and dysplastic nevus syndrome have deletions in the chromosome region 9p21, which may be a specific melanoma susceptibility locus (182). Sporadic cases of melanoma are also related to dysplastic nevi (183,184), accounting for as many as 32% of all nonfamilial melanomas (185). The incidence of individuals with a single dysplastic nevus is about 4% and its significance remains unclear, but patients with multiple dysplastic nevi may have as much as a 7.7 times relative risk for melanoma (185) and need to be followed carefully, probably by sequential photographs that can document early invasive melanoma by facilitating recognition of subtle morphologic changes within a dysplastic nevus (186). Vigilance of high-risk patients cannot be relaxed: 10% of all melanoma patients develop second primary malignant melanomas (187). Multiple dysplastic nevi and melanomas may also be associated with personal or family history of germ cell tumors (188) and pancreatic cancer (189).

Melanomas are not known to develop in other congenital and acquired pigmented lesions such as café au lait macules, mongolian spots, Becker nevus, lentigines, and epidermal nevi. However, lentigo maligna (Hutchinson freckle), is considered premalignant. It is an irregularly pigmented and growing macule, occurring on sun-exposed skin of elderly patients (Fig. 16–26). Thought to give rise to frank invasive melanoma (lentigo maligna melanoma) in at least one-third of cases (190), progression is very slow, perhaps over 5 to 10 years.

The biologic behavior of melanoma, in relation to the risk of recurrence and death, is predictable (191,192). Superficial spreading melanoma has a long period (months to years) of lateral spread (radial growth). Lentigo maligna melanoma may have a decade of radial growth. Acral-lentiginous melanoma is thought to have a shorter period of radial growth before vertical growth. The malignancy at first remains localized to the skin, then spreads to regional lymph nodes, and/or metastasizes to distant sites, usually skin, brain, lungs, and liver. At the time of diagnosis of the initial primary cutaneous melanoma, staging can be adequately accomplished by a complete physical examination and a baseline chest x ray; without symptoms or signs of advanced disease, liver function tests, radionucleide liver-spleen and bone scans, whole-lung tomograms, CT chest scans, and CT brain scans do not furnish additional information (193). Nearly all patients with distant metastases die within 3 years (median survival 7.5-months) (194). Five-year survival in patients with lymph-node metastases is 30%, but 10-year survival is rare.

A combination of histologic factors studied by multivariate analysis predicts survival reproducibly. Of these factors, and regardless of tumor type or the presence of microscopic lymph-node metastases (195), depth as measured histologically in millimeters from epidermal surface (epidermal granular layer) to deepest tumor margin (Breslow measurement) is by far the most important. The second-most important variable is location. Ear and scalp melanomas (196,197), acral-lentiginous melanomas (191), and melanomas on genital or anorectal mucosa (198,199) have an extremely grave prognosis unexplained by any microstage factors. Lesions on the upper thorax, posterolateral arms, posterolateral neck, and posterior scalp (TANS locations) also have a relatively poorer prognosis (200). Other factors associated with unfavorable prognosis include ulceration; deeper level of invasion (Clark levels: II, focal papillary dermis; III, papillary dermis replacement; IV, reticular dermis; and V, subcutaneous fat); high mitotic rate; poor lymphocyte response; presence of microscopic satellites (201); and presence of greater than 20% of removed lymph nodes involved with microscopic metastases. The prognostic information yielded by the Clark levels of invasion is minimal if the depth of invasion has already been measured. The presence of microscopic satellites (nests of tumor cells below the principal invasive mass of primary tumor) (Fig. 16–27) is the best predictor of clinically occult metastases in lymph nodes (202). The role of regression as a prognostic factor is debated (203,204). In summary, the two most important and powerful factors in predicting the outcome in malignant melanoma are the measured depth of invasion of the primary tumor and the location of the primary tumor (Table 16–1).

Surgical excision is the treatment of choice for melanoma; there is no role at present for treating the primary lesion with chemotherapy, radiation, or other destructive techniques. The issue of resection margins has been addressed in several studies. Several reports (198,199,205–209) have shown that the magnitude of surgical resection margins has no effect on survival, even for high-risk melanomas, although a higher incidence of local recurrences was noted when thicker lesions were excised with less than 3 cm margins. Previous standard surgical practice had dictated excision of most melanomas with a border of normal skin at least 3 cm to 5 cm from the edge of the melanoma, but the historical basis for this recommendation is unclear. Some authors (210–212) suggest much narrower margins based on retrospective data: a 1.5 cm margin for all lesions less than 0.85 mm thick and lesions in the non-TANS locations 0.85 mm to 1.69 mm thick, with all other melanomas excised with a 3.0-cm radius. The National Institute of Health in Milan, Italy, in conjunction with five other countries, recently accomplished a randomized prospective study (213) of 612 patients with melanomas no thicker than 2.0 mm, divided into two treatment groups: excision with 1 cm margins and excision with margins of 3 cm or more. With a mean follow-up period of 55 months, there was no difference in disease-free survival rates, overall survival rates, and subsequent development of metastatic disease. Duration of follow-up time may, however, have been too brief to be an absolutely definitive study, as three patients, all with narrow excisions and a primary melanoma thicker than 1.0 mm, developed local recurrence. A 1.0-cm margin is therefore probably sufficient for all lesions less than 1.0 mm thick, and possibly sufficient for lesions less than 2.0 mm thick in the non-TANS locations. All other melanomas should be excised with a 3.0-cm radius. This recommendation should be weighted against cosmetic and functional considerations when dealing with melanomas on the face near vital structures such as the eye, eyelid, nose, ear, or facial nerve, which should not be sacrificed unless they are directly invaded. There are no data that show any advantage to removing the deep fascia. Hence, the usual extent of surgery for the primary tumor is the epidermis, dermis, and all the fat down to but not including the fascia. Likewise, there are no data showing an advantage to skewing an elliptical excision in the direction of the lymphatic drainage from the site; the orientation of the ellipse, therefore, may be placed for best cosmetic and functional advantage, including lymphatic drainage, where feasible.

Surgical excision of the primary tumor is the mainstay of treatment. Lymph-node dissection is performed if palpable metastases have developed in regional nodes. Surgical removal of recurrent tumor or easily excisable metastases to lymph nodes or viscera decreases morbidity and prolongs survival (214,215). Nodal disease may also respond to radiation therapy in 70 to 85% of cases (216). In the absence of easily detectable lymph node or distant metastases, there is no consensus about the value of additional surgical or medical therapies such as elective regional lymph node dissection (ERND), isolated regional perfusion, and adjuvant immunotherapy or chemotherapy. No large, definitive, long-term prospective studies have been done to delineate the effectiveness of ERND. General agreement exists that ERND does not benefit patients with either thin (less than 1.5 mm) lesions or thick (greater than 4.0 mm) lesions (217). Three studies (218–220) with fewer than 200 patients and one study of 1300 patients (221) with lesions of intermediate thickness did not detect a beneficial effect of ERND, while two other studies (222,223) appreciated a marked increase in death from melanoma after 5 years for patients with intermediate-thickness lesions treated with wide local excision only as compared to those who also underwent ERND. A report (224) of a prospective randomized study of 171 patients with lesions of all thicknesses treated with local excision with or without ERND revealed no statistical improvement in mortality with ERND in any subset of patients, but it included only 28 patients with lesions of intermediate thickness. These studies, the rationale for ERND, and a description of ongoing studies, have been reviewed recently (225). If ERND is to be performed, sentinel node examination (226), lymphoscintigraphy (227), or a combination of both (228) is useful in planning the surgical procedure.

Because unresectable melanomas of the limbs have been treated by isolated regional perfusion with melphalan (229) or cisplatin (230), yielding long-term responses of greater than 40%, it has also been used as an adjuvant therapy for primary melanomas of the extremity that are thicker than 1.5 mm. The technique (231) requires a surgically created perfusion circuit, anticoagulation, induction of regional hyperthermia, and often a fasciotomy to prevent development of a compartment syndrome. Prior ERND is advisable, particularly in the axillae, where postperfusion scarring may preclude adequate evalua-

Table 16–1
Prognostic Features of Primary Melanoma: Estimated 7½-Year Survival*

Thickness (mm)	Non-TANS**				TANS**
	Extremities	Head and Neck	Trunk	Hands and Feet	
<0.85	99+	99+	99+	99+	98
0.85–1.69	99+	99+	97	99+	78
1.70–3.64	86	64	77	60	58
3.63	83	65	22	0	33

*Adapted from Day, et al. (191).
**TANS—upper thorax, posteriolateral arms, posteriolateral neck, posterior scalp.

tion of lymph nodes by physical examination. A large retrospective study with well-matched controls (232) found no significant difference in patients of any subgroup treated with adjuvant isolated regional perfusion, however, a small prospective study (231) of 37 patients found recurrences to be markedly diminished in the perfused group. Since the data do not uniformly document a survival benefit for perfusion as an adjuvant therapy, the procedure is generally reserved for palliative treatment of selected patients with localized advanced disease.

Adjuvant immunotherapy and chemotherapy have been studied in many centers, but usefulness has never been documented (233). At best, nonspecific agents are palliative in the setting of metastatic disease (234). Vaccine therapy may be effective in slowing the progression of melanoma in some patients (235). It is possible that specific immunostimulatory agents derived by techniques utilizing the patient's own tumor cells will prove useful in the future (236).

The management of any patient who has had a melanoma includes rigorous repeated examination of the surgical site as well as the entire skin surface including the scalp and genitalia. As noted above, the patient with a thin melanoma has a greater lifetime risk of developing a second melanoma than metastases from his first melanoma. Examinations of the skin should be performed every 6 months for several years, then annually. If the patient has numerous severely atypical nevi and a family history of melanoma, the nevi should be self-examined monthly, and examined and carefully charted or photographed by the physician every 3 months for a lifetime (237). Computerized image analysis may also be useful in following high-risk patients (238). In addition, family members should be examined for precursor lesions and melanomas. The patient and family need to refrain from excessive sun exposure, which may entail a change in lifestyle as well as daily attention to the use of sun-protective topical preparations and clothing. A complete physical examination and annual chest x ray are sufficient information to exclude metastatic disease in a patient who is otherwise well. Specific complaints can be evaluated as indicated by their nature.

Surgical treatment is recommended frequently for precursor lesions. Congenital nevi are difficult to follow (especially the large lesions) and have a known high rate of malignant degeneration. Excision in toto with less than 1.0-cm margin is frequently performed; the surgeon must balance the costs and risks of surgery, general anesthesia, and functional or cosmetical disability against the risk of development of melanoma. Of note, in these lesions nevus cells are present in the dermis and subcutaneous fat and have been documented to give rise to deep melanomas (239); dermabrasion or superficial laser destruction would not be expected to sufficiently ameliorate the risk of malignancy. Biologically malignant lesions also arise in dysplastic nevi, melanoma in situ, and lentigo maligna, so that the treatment of choice of these lesions is excision in toto. Just as dysplastic nevi vary clinically from slightly atypical to severely atypical, a range of atypicality is also appreciated histologically in the characteristics of the nevus cells (cytological atypia) as well as their arrangement (architectural atypia). It is preferable to remove moderately to severely atypical nevi completely, because progression may occur. A 4- to 5-mm margin into midsubcutaneous fat is generally sufficient.

References

1. Miller DL, Weinstock MA. Nonmelanoma skin cancer in the United States: incidence. *J Am Acad Dermatol* 1994; 30:774–778.
2. Weinstock MA. Epidemiologic investigation of nonmelanoma skin cancer mortality: the Rhode Island follow-back study. *J Invest Dermatol* 1994; 102:6S–9S.
3. Olsen TG, Feeser TA, Conte ET, et al. Skin cancer screening—a local experience. *J Am Acad Dermatol* 1987; 16:637.
4. Hanke CW, Wolf RL, Hochman SA, et al. Perineural spread of basal cell carcinoma. *J Dermatol Surg Oncol* 1983; 9:742.
5. Paver K, Doyzen K, Burry N. The incidence of basal cell carcinomas and their metastases in Australia and New Zealand. *Aust J Dermatol* 1973; 14:53.
6. Wei Q, Matanoski GM, Farmer ER, et al. DNA repair capacity for UV light-induced damage is reduced in peripheral lymphocytes from patients with basal cell carcinoma. *J Invest Dermatol* 1995; 104:933–936.
7. Vitaliano PP, Urbach F. The relative importance of risk factors in nonmelanoma carcinoma. *Arch Dermatol* 1980; 116:454.
8. Giles CG, Marks R, Foley P. Incidence of non-melanocytic skin cancer treated in Australia. *Br J Med [Clin Res]* 1988; 296:13.
9. Gallagher RP, Hill GB, Bajdik CD, et al. Sunlight exposure, pigmentary factors, and risk of nonmelanocytic skin cancer. *Arch Dermatol* 1995; 131:157–163.
10. Engel A, Johnson ML, Haynes SG. Health effects of sunlight exposure in the United States. Results from the first National Health and Nutrition Examination Survey, 1971–1974. *Arch Dermatol* 1988; 124:72.
11. Ridley CM. Basal cell carcinoma following x-ray epilation of the head and neck. *Br J Dermatol* 1962; 74:222.
12. Martin H, Strong E, Spiro RH. Radiation-induced skin cancer of the head and neck. *Cancer* 1970; 25:61.
13. Conway H, Huygo NE. Radiation dermatitis and malignancy. *Plast Reconstr Surg* 1966; 38:255.
14. Stern RS, Laird N. The carcinogenic risk of treatments for severe psoriasis. Photochemotherapy follow-up study. *Cancer* 1994; 73:2759–2764.
15. Montgomery H, Waisman M. Epithelioma attributable to arsenic. *J Invest Dermatol* 1941; 4:365.
16. Wagner SL, Maliner JS, Morton WE, et al. Skin cancer and arsenical intoxication from well water. *Arch Dermatol* 1979; 115:1205.
17. Glover MT, Niranjan N, Kwan JT. Nonmelanoma skin cancer in renal transplant recipients: the extent of the problem and a strategy for management. *Br J Plast Surg* 1994; 47:86–89.
18. Parnes R, Safai B, Myskowski PL. Basal cell carcinomas and lymphoma: biologic behavior and associated factors in 63 patients. *J Am Acad Dermatol* 1988; 19:1017.
19. Lobo DV, Chu P, Grekin RC, et al. Nonmelanoma skin cancers and infection with the human immunodeficiency virus. *Arch Dermatol* 1992; 128:623–627.
20. Rabbari H, Mehregan AH. Basal cell epithelioma in children and teenagers. *Cancer* 1982; 49:350.
21. Chorum L, Norris JEC, Gupta M. Basal cell carcinoma in blacks: a report of 15 cases. *Ann Plast Surg* 1994; 33:90–95.
22. Bergstrasser PR, Halprin KM. Multiple sequential skin cancers: the risk of skin cancers in patients with a previous skin cancer. *Arch Dermatol* 1975; 111:995.
23. Biro L, Price E, MacWilliams P. Basal cell carcinoma in office practice. *NY State J Med* 1975; 75:1427.
24. Robinson JK. Risk of developing another basal cell carcinoma. A 5-year prospective study. *Cancer* 1987; 60:118.
25. Karagas MR. Occurrence of cutaneous basal cell and squamous cell malignancies among those with a prior history of skin cancer. *J Invest Dermatol* 1994; 102:10S–13S.
26. Koff AW, Bart RS, Andrade R. *Atlas of tumors of the skin.* Philadelphia: WB Saunders, 1978.
27. Gorlin RJ. Nevoid basal-cell carcinoma syndrome. *Medicine* 1987; 66:98.
28. Goldstein AM, Stewart C, Bale AE, et al. Localization of the gene for the nevoid basal cell carcinoma syndrome. *Am J Hum Genet* 1994; 54:765–773.
29. Golitz LE, Norris DA, Leukens CA, et al. Nevoid basal cell carcinoma syndrome: multiple basal cell carcinomas of the palms after radiation therapy. *Arch Dermatol* 1980; 116:1159.
30. Southwick GJ, Schwartz RA. The basal cell nevus syndrome: disasters occurring among a series of 36 patients. *Cancer* 1979; 44:2294.

31. Goeteyn M, Geerts ML, Kint A, et al. The Basex-Dupré-Christol syndrome. *Arch Dermatol* 1994; 130:337–342.

32. Vabres P, Lacombe D, Rabinowitz LG, et al. The gene for Basex-Dupré-Christol syndrome maps to chromosome Xq. *J Invest Dermatol* 1995; 105:87–91.

33. Kraemer KH, Lee MM, Scotto J. Xeroderma pigmentosum: cutaneous, ocular, and neurologic abnormalities in 830 published cases. *Arch Dermatol* 1987; 123:241–250.

34. Epstein E. How accurate is the visual assessment of basal cell carcinoma margins? *Br J Dermatol* 1973; 89:37.

35. Wolf DJ, Zitelli JA. Surgical margins for basal cell carinoma. *Arch Dermatol* 1987; 123:340.

36. Salasche SJ, Amonette RA. Morpheaform basal cell epitheliomas: a study of subclinical extension in a series of 51 cases. *J Dermatol Surg Oncol* 1981; 7:387.

37. Bart R, Schrager D, Kopf AW, et al. Scalpel excision of basal cell carcinomas. *Arch Dermatol* 1978; 114:739.

38. Panje WR, Ceilley RI. The influence of embryology of the midface on the spread of epithelial malignancies. *Laryngoscope* 1979; 89:1914.

39. Pascal R, Hobby L, Lattes R, et al. Prognosis of "incompletely excised" versus "completely excised" basal cell carcinoma. *Plast Reconstr Surg* 1968; 41:328.

40. Richmond JD, Davie RM. The significance of incomplete excision in patients with basal cell carcinoma. *Br J Plast Surg* 1987; 40:63.

41. Stanley RB Jr, Burres SA, Jacobs JR, et al. Hazards encountered in management of basal cell carcinomas of the midface. *Laryngoscope* 1984; 94:378.

42. Riefkohl R, Pollack S, Georgiade GS. A rationale for the treatment of difficult basal cell and squamous cell carcinomas of the skin. *Ann Plast Surg* 1985; 15:19.

43. Mohs FE: Chemosurgery. *Microscopically controlled surgery for skin cancer.* Springfield, IL: Charles C Thomas, 1978.

44. Rapini R. Comparison of methods of checking surgical margins. *J Am Acad Dermatol* 1990; 23:288–294.

45. Cottel WJ, Proper S. Mohs' surgery, fresh tissue technique. *J Dermatol Surg Oncol* 1982; 8:576.

46. Roenigk RK. Mohs micrographic surgery. *Mayo Clin Proc* 1988; 63:175.

47. Greenway HT, Dobes WL, Goodman MM, et al. Guidelines of care for Mohs micrographic surgery. *J Am Acad Dermatol* 1995; 33:271–278.

48. Rigel DS, Robins P, Friedman RJ. Predicting recurrence of basal cell carcinomas treated by microscopically controlled excision. *J Dermatol Surg Oncol* 1981; 7:807.

49. Torre D. Cryosurgery of basal cell carcinoma. *J Am Acad Dermatol* 1986; 15:917.

50. McLean DI, Haynes HA, McCarthy PL, et al. Cryotherapy of basal cell carcinoma by a simple method of standardized freeze-thaw cycles. *J Dermatol Surg Oncol* 1978; 4:175.

51. Elton RF. The course of events following cryosurgery. *J Dermatol Surg Oncol* 1977; 3:448.

52. Graham FG. Statistical data on malignant tumors in cryosurgery 1982. *J Dermatol Oncol Surg* 1983; 9:238.

53. Holt PJ. Cryotherapy for skin cancer: results over a 5-year period using liquid nitrogen spray cryosurgery. *Br J Dermatol* 1988; 119:231.

54. Knox JM, Lyles TW, Shapiro EM, et al. Curettage and electrodesiccation in the treatment of skin cancer. *Arch Dermatol* 1960; 82:197.

55. Kopf AW, Bart RS, Shrager D. Curettage-electrodesiccation in the treatment of basal cell carcinoma. *Arch Dermatol* 1960; 82:197.

56. Suhge-d'Aubermont PC, Bennett RG. Failure of curettage and electrodessication for removal of basal cell carcinoma. *Arch Dermatol* 1984; 120:1456.

57. Goldschmidt H, Breneman JC, Breneman DL. Ionizing radiation therapy in dermatology. *J Am Acad Dermatol* 1994; 30:157–182.

58. Childers BJ, Goldwyn RM, Ramos D, et al. Long-term results of irradiation for basal cell carcinoma of the skin of the nose. *Plast Reconstr Surg* 1994; 93:1169–1173.

59. Bart RS, Kopf AW, Petratos MA. X-ray therapy of skin cancer, evaluation of a "standardized" method for treating basal cell carcinoma. Sixth National Cancer Conference. Philadelphia: JB Lippincott, 1970; 559–570.

60. Wilson BD, Mang T. Photodynamic therapy for cutaneous malignancies. *Clin Dermatol* 1995; 13:91–96.

61. Cairnduff F, Stringer MR, Hudson EJ, et al. Superficial photodynamic therapy with topical 5-aminolaevulinic acid for superficial primary or secondary skin cancer. *Br J Cancer* 1994; 69:605–608.

62. Reymann F. Treatment of basal cell carcinoma of the skin with 5-Fluorouracil ointment: a ten year followup study. *Dermatologica* 1979; 158:368.

63. Mohs FE, Jones DL, Bloom RF. Tendency of fluorouracil to conceal deep foci of invasive basal cell carcinoma. *Arch Dermatol* 1978; 114:1021.

64. Epstein E. Flouroucil paste treatment of thin basal cell carcinomas. *Arch Dermatol* 1987; 121:207.

65. Lippman SM, Shimm DS, Meyskens FL. Nonsurgical treatments for skin cancer: retinoids and alpha-interferon. *J Dermatol Surg Oncol* 1988; 14:862.

66. Peck GL, DiGiovanni JJ, Sarnoff DS, et al. Treatment and prevention of basal cell carcinoma with isotretinoin. *J Am Acad Dermatol* 1988; 19:176.

67. Hughes BR, Marks R, Pearse AD, et al. Clinical response and tissue effects of etretinate treatment of patients with solar keratoses and basal cell carcinoma. *J Am Acad Dermatol* 1988; 18:522.

68. Robinson JK. What are adequate treatment and follow-up care for nonmelanoma cutaneous cancer? *Arch Dermatol* 1987; 123:331.

69. Rowe DE, Carroll RJ, Day CL. Longterm recurrence rates previously untreated (primary) basal cell carcinoma: implications for patient follow-up. *J Dermatol Surg Oncol* 1989; 15:315.

70. Stern RS, Weinstein MC, Baker SG. Risk reduction for nonmelanoma skin cancer with childhood sunscreen use. *Arch Dermatol* 1986; 122:537.

71. Kligman LH, Akin FJ, Kligman AM. Sunscreens prevent ultraviolet photocarcinogenesis. *J Am Acad Dermatol* 1980; 3:30.

72. Jones RR. Ozone depletion and cancer risk. *Lancet* 1987; II:443.

73. Kraemer KH, DiGiovanni JJ, Moshell AN, et al. Prevention of skin cancer in xeroderma pigmentosum with the use of oral isotretinoin. *N Engl J Med* 1988; 318:1633.

74. Forbes PD, Urbach F, Davies RE. Enhancement of experimental photocarcinogenesis by topical retinoic acid. *Cancer Lett* 1979; 7:85.

75. Bourne RG. The spread of squamous cell carcinoma of the skin via the cranial nerves. *Austral Radiol* 1980; 24:106.

76. Goepfert H, Dichtel WJ, Medina JE, et al. Perineural invasion in squamous cell carcinoma of the head and neck. *Am J Surg* 1984; 148:542.

77. Lund HZ. How often does squamous cell carcinoma of the skin metastasize? *Arch Dermatol* 1965; 92:635.

78. Lund HZ. Metastasis from sun-induced squamous cell carcinoma of the skin: an uncommon event. *J Dermatol Oncol Surg* 1984; 10:169.

79. Moller R, Reymann F, Hou-Jensen K. Metastases in dermatologic patients with squamous cell carcinoma. *Arch Dermatol* 1979; 115:703.

80. Katz AD, Urbach F, Lilienfield AM. The frequency and risk of metastasis in squamous cell carcinoma of the skin. *Cancer* 1957; 10:1162.

81. Dinehart SM, Pollack SV. Metastases from squamous cell carcinoma of the skin and lip. *J Am Acad Dermatol* 1989; 21:241.

82. Mora RG, Perniciaro C. Cancer of the skin in blacks. A review of 36 black patients with squamous cell carcinoma of the lip. *J Am Acad Dermatol* 1982; 6:1005.

83. Yiannias JA, Goldberg LH, Carter-Campbell S, et al. The ratio of basal cell carcinoma to squamous cell carcinoma in Houston, Texas. *J Dermatol Surg Oncol* 1988; 14:886.

84. Urbach F. Ultraviolet radiation and skin cancer. In: Montagna W, Dobson RL, eds. *Advances in biology of the skin.* Vol. VII. New York: Pergamon, 1966; 195–214.

85. Epstein JH. Photocarcinogenesis, skin cancer and aging. *J Am Acad Dermatol* 1983; 9:487.

86. Gupta AK, Cardella CJ, Haberman HF. Cutaneous malignant neoplasms in patients with renal transplants. *Arch Dermatol* 1986; 122:1288.

87. Boyle J, Mackie RM, Briggs JD, et al. Cancer, warts, and sunshine in renal transplant patients. A case control study. *Lancet* 1984; I:702.

88. Marks R, Rennie G, Selwood TS. Malignant transformation of solar keratoses to squamous cell carcinoma. *Lancet* 1988; I:795.

89. Epstein WL, Fukuyana K, Epstein JH. Ultraviolet, DNA repair and skin carcinogenesis in man. *Fed Proc* 1971; 30:1766.

90. Black HS, Douglas DR. Formation of a carcinogen of natural origin in the etiology of ultraviolet light-induced carcinogenesis. *Cancer Res* 1973; 33:2094.

91. Blum HF, McVaugh J, Ward M, et al. Epidermal hyperplasia induced by ultraviolet radiation. *Photochem Photobiol* 1975; 21:255.

92. Kripke ML, Fisher MS. Immunologic parameters of UV carcinogenesis. *J Natl Cancer Inst* 1976; 57:211.

93. Drolet BA, Neuberg M, Sauger J. Role of human papillomavirus in cutaneous oncogenesis. *Ann Plast Surg* 1994; 33:339–347.

94. Everall JD, Dowd PM. Influence of environmental factors excluding ultraviolet radiation on the incidence of skin cancer. *Bull Cancer (Paris)* 1978; 65:241.

95. Grodstein F, Speizer FE, Hunter DJ. A prospective study of incident squamous cell carcinoma of the skin in the nurses' health study. *J Natl Cancer Inst* 1995; 87:1061–1066.

96. Arons MS, Lynch JB, Lewis SR, et al. Scar tissue carcinoma. I. A clinical study with special reference to burn scar carcinoma. *Ann Surg* 1965; 161:170.

97. Sedlin ED, Flemming JL. Epidermal carcinoma arising in chronic ostemyelitic foci. *J Bone Joint Surg* 1963; 45:827.

98. Johnston WH, Miller TA, Frileck SP. Atypical pseudoepitheliomatous hyperplasia and squamous cell carcinoma in chronic cutaneous sinuses and fistulas. *Plast Reconstr Surg* 1980; 66:395.

99. Pearse AD, Marks R. Actinic keratoses and the epidermis on which they arise. *Br J Dermatol* 1977; 96:45.

100. Arbesman H, Ransohoff DF. Is Bowen's disease a predictor for the development of internal malignancy? *JAMA* 1987; 257:516.

101. Wade TR, Kopf AW, Ackerman AB. Bowenoid papulosis of the genitalia. *Arch Dermatol* 1979; 115:306.

102. Kimura S. Bowenoid papulosis of the genitalia. *Int J Dermatol* 1982; 21:432.

103. Carpenter-Kling JT, Jacyk WK. Anogenital flat papules. Bowenoid papulosis of the genitalia. *Arch Dermatol* 1994; 130:1311,1314.

104. Kato T, Saijyo S, Hatchome N, et al. Detection of human papillomavirus type 16 in bowenoid papulosis and invasive carcinoma occurring in the same patient with a history of cervical carcinoma. *Arch Dermatol* 1988; 124:851.

105. Goette DK. Erythroplasia of Queyrat. *Arch Dermatol* 1974; 110:271.

105. Mikhail GR. Cancers, precancers, and pseudocancers on the male genitalia. *J Dermatol Surg Oncol* 1980; 6:1027.

106. Graham JH, Helwig EB. Erythroplasia of Queyrat. In: Graham JH, Johnson WP, Helwig EB, eds. *Dermal pathology.* Hagerstown, MD: Harper & Row, 1972; 597–606.

107. Aird I, Johnson HD, Lennox B, et al. Epithelioma cuniculatum—a variety of squamous cell carcinoma peculiar to the foot. *Br J Surg* 1954; 42:245.

108. McKee PH, Wilkinson JD, Corbett MF, et al. Carcinoma cuniculatum: a case metastasizing to skin and lymph nodes. *Clin Exp Derm* 1981; 6:613.

109. Schnur PL, Bozzo P. Metastasizing keratoacanthomas: the difficulties in differentiating keratoacanthomas from squamous cell carcinoma. *Plast Reconstr Surg* 1978; 62:258.

110. Smoller BR, Kwan TH, Said JW, et al. Keratoacanthoma and squamous cell carcinoma of the skin: Immunohistochemical localization of involucrin and keratin proteins. *J Am Acad Dermatol* 1986; 14:226.

111. Sanders GH, Miller TA. Are keratoacanthomas really squamous cell carcinomas? *Ann Plast Surg* 1982; 9:306.

112. Pickrell K, Villarreal-Rios A, Neale H. Giant keratoacanthoma. *Ann Plast Surg* 1979; 2:525.

113. Stranc MF, Robertson GA. Conservative treatment of keratoacanthoma. *Ann Plast Surg* 1979; 2:525.

114. Wolinsky S, Silvers DN, Kohn SR, et al. Spontaneous regression of a giant keratoacanthoma. Photographic documentation and histopathologic correlation. *J Dermatol Surg Oncol* 1981; 7:897.

115. Goette DK. Treatment of keratoacanthoma with topical flourouracil. *Arch Dermatol* 1983; 119:951.

116. Goette DK, Odom RB. Successful treatment of keratoacanthoma with intralesional fluorouracil. *J Am Acad Dermatol* 1980; 2:212.

117. Snider BL, Benjamin DR. Eruptive keratoacathoma with an internal malignant neoplasm. *Arch Dermatol* 1981; 117:788.

118. Sina B, Adrian RM. Multiple keratoacanthomas possibly induced by psoralens and ultraviolet A photochemotherapy. *J Am Acad Dermatol* 1983; 9:686.

119. Reid BJ, Cheesebrough MJ. Multiple keratoacanthoma. A unique case and review of the present classification. *Acta Derm Venereol* 1978; 58:169.

120. Majewski S, Jablonska S. Epidermodysplasia verruciformis as a model of human papillomavirus-induced genetic cancer of the skin. *Arch Dermatol l* 1995; 31:1312–1318.

121. Prawer SE, Pass F, Vance JC, et al. Depressive immune function in epidermodysplasia verruciformis. *Arch Dermatol* 1977; 113:495.

122. Ostrow RS, Manias D, Mitchell AJ, et al. Epidermodysplasia verruciformis. A case associated with primary lymphatic dysplasia, depressed cell-mediated immunity, and Bowen's disease containing human papillomavirus 16 DNA. *Arch Dermatol* 1987; 123:1511.

123. Fahmy A, Burgdorf WH, Schosser RH, et al. Muir-Torre syndrome: report of a case and reevaluation of the dermatopathologic features. *Cancer* 1983; 49:1898.

124. Finan MC, Connolly SM. Sebaceous gland tumors and systemic disease: a clinicopathologic analysis. *Medicine* 1984; 63:232.

125. Immerman SC, Scanlon EF, Christ M, et al. Recurrent squamous cell carcinoma of the the skin. *Cancer* 1983; 51:1537.

126. Robins P, Dzubow LM, Rigel DS. Squamous cell carcinoma treated by Mohs' surgery. An experience with 414 cases in a period of 15 years. *J Dermatol Surg Oncol* 1981; 7:800.

127. Levine N, Miller RC, Meyskens FL, Jr. Oral isotretinoin therapy. Use in a patient with multiple cutaneous squamous cell carcinomas and keratoacanthomas. *Arch Dermatol* 1984; 120:1215.

128. Lippman SM, Meyskens FL Jr. Treatment of advanced squamous cell carcinoma of the skin with isotretinoin. *Ann Intern Med* 1987; 107:499.

129. Naylor MF, Boyd A, Smith DW, et al. High sun protection factor sunscreens in the suppression of actinic neoplasia. *Arch Dermatol* 1995; 131:170–175.

130. Black HS, Herd A, Goldberg LN, et al. Effect of a low-fat diet on the incidence of actinic keratosis. *N Eng J Med* 1994; 330:1272–1275.

131. Boring CC, Squires TS, Tong T, et al. Cancer statistics, 1993. *CA Cancer J Clin* 1994; 44:7–26.

132. Roush GC, Schymura MJ, Holford TR. Patterns of invasive melanoma in the Connecticut tumor registry. Is the long tern increase real? *Cancer* 1988; 61:2586.

133. Lee JAH. Trends in melanoma incidence and mortality. *Clin Dermatol* 1992; 10:9–13.

134. Elwood JM, Gallagher RP, Hill GB, et al. Pigmentation and skin reaction to sun as risk factors for cutaneous melanoma: Western Canada melanoma study. *Br Med J* 1984; 288:99.

135. Horn-Ross PL, Holly EA, Brown SR, et al. Temporal trends in the incidence of cutaneous malignant melanoma among Caucasians in the San Francisco-Oakland MSA. *Cancer Causes Control* 1993; 4:93–100.

136. Deaths from melanoma—United States, 1973–1992. *MMWR* 1995; 44:337, 343–347.

137. Hartman AM. Melanoma of the skin. In: Miller BA, et al, eds. *Cancer statistics review: 1973–1989.* National Cancer Institute. NIH Publ No. 92-2789, 1992.

138. Friedman RJ, Rigel DS, Silverman MK, et al. Malignant melanoma in the 1990s: the continued importance of early detection. *CA Cancer J Clin* 1991; 41:201–226.

139. Silverberg E, Lubera JA. Cancer statistics, 1989. *Cancer* 1989; 39:3.

140. Doherty VR, MacKie RM. Experience of a public education program on early detection of cutaneous malignant melanoma. *Br Med J* 1988; 297:388.

141. Rigel DS, Friedman RJ, Kopf AW, et al. Importance of complete cutaneous examination for the detection of malignant melanoma. *J Am Acad Dermatol* 1986; 14:857.

142. Hardie IR, Strong RW, Hartley LC, et al. Skin cancer in Caucasian renal allograft recipients living in a subtropical climate. *Surgery* 1980; 87:177.

143. Tindall B, Finlayson R, Mutimer K, et al. Malignant melanoma associated with human immunodeficiency virus infection in three homosexual men. *J Am Acad Dermatol* 1989; 20:587.

144. McWhirter WR, Dobson C. Childhood melanoma in Australia. *World J Surg* 1995; 19:334–336.

145. Takebe H, Nishigori C, Tatsumi K. Melanoma and other skin cancers in xeroderma pigmentosum patients and mutations in their cells. *J Invest Dermatol* (suppl) 1989; 92:236.

146. Licata AG, Wilson LD, Braverman IM, et al. Malignant melanoma and other second cutaneous malignancies in cutaneous T-cell lymphoma. The influence of additional therapy after total skin electron beam radiation. *Arch Dermatol* 1995; 131:432–435.

147. Ross PM, Carter DM. Actinic DNA damage and the pathogenesis of cutaneous malignant melanoma *J Invest Dermatol* (suppl) 1989; 92:293.

148. Osterlind A, Tucker MA, Stone BJ, et al. The Danish case-control study of cutaneous malignant melanoma. II. Importance of UV light exposure. *Int J Cancer* 1988; 42:319.

149. Khlat M, Vail A, Parkin M, et al. Mortality from melanoma in migrants to Australia: variation by age at arrival and duration of stay. *Am J Epidemiol* 1992; 135:1103–1113.

150. Marghoob AA, Slade J, Salopek TG, et al. Basal cell and squamous cell carcinomas are important risk factors for cutaneous malignant melanoma. *Cancer* 1995; 75:707–714.

151. Tucker MA, Shields JA, Hartge P, et al. Sunlight exposure as risk factor for intraocular malignant melanoma. *N Engl J Med* 1985; 313:789.

152. Marks R, Whiteman D. Sunburn and melanoma—how strong is the evidence? *Br Med J* 1994; 308:75–76.

153. Mihm MC, Fitzpatrick TB, Lane-Brown MM, et al. Early detection of primary cutaneous malignant melanoma: a color atlas. *N Engl J Med* 1973; 289–989.

154. Anderson WK, Silvers DN. Melanoma? It can't be melanoma! *JAMA* 1991; 24:3463–3465.

155. Day CL, Mihm MC, Sober AJ, et al. Skin lesions suspected to be melanoma should be photographed. Gross morphological features of primary melanoma associated with metastases. *JAMA* 1982; 248:1077.

156. Sober AJ, Day CL, Kopf AW, et al. Detection of "thin" primary melanomas. *Cancer* 1983; 33:160.

157. Bondi EE, Elder DE, Guerry D, et al. Skin markings in malignant melanoma. *JAMA* 1983; 250:503.

158. Ridgeway CA, Hicken TJ, Ronan SG, et al. Acral lentiginous melanoma. *Arch Surg* 1995; 130:88–92.

159. Coleman WP, Gately LE, Krementz AB, et al. Nevi, lentigines and melanomas in blacks. *Arch Dermatol* 1980; 116:548.

160. Carlson JA, Dickersin GR, Sober AJ, et al. Desmoplastic Neurotropic Melanoma. *Cancer* 1995; 75:478–494.

161. Weinzweig N, Tuthill RJ, Yetman RJ. Desmoplastic malignant melanoma: a clinicohistopathologic review. *Plast Reconstr Surg* 1995; 95:548–555.

162. Brady MS, Kavolius JP, Quan SH. Anorectal melanoma. A 64-year experience at Memorial Sloan-Kettering Cancer Center. *Dis Colon Rectum* 1995; 38:146–151.

163. Scheistroen M, Trope C, Koern J, et al. Malignant melanoma of the vulva. Evaluation of prognostic factors with emphasis on DNA ploidy in 75 patients. *Cancer* 1995; 75:72–80.

164. Grin CM, Kopf AW, Welkovich B, et al. Accuracy in the clinical diagnosis of malignant melanoma. *Arch Dermatol* 1990; 126:763–766.

165. Binder M, Schwarz M, Winkler A, et al. Epiluminescence microscopy: a useful tool for diagnosis of pigmented skin lesions for formally trained dermatologists. *Arch Dermatol* 1995; 131:286–291.

166. Dummer W, Blaheta HJ, Bastian BC, et al. Preoperative characterization of pigmented skin lesions by epiluminescence microscopy and high-frequency ultrasound. *Arch Dermatol* 1995; 131:279–285.

167. Lederman JS, Sober AJ. Does biopsy type influence survival in clinical stage I cutaneous melanoma? *J Am Acad Dermatol* 1985; 13:983.

168. Elder DE, Greene MH, Bondi EE, et al. Acquired melanocytic nevi and melanoma. The dysplastic nevus syndrome. In: Ackerman AB, ed. *Pathology of malignant melanoma.* New York: Masson Publications, 1981; 185–215.

169. Rhodes AR. Pigmented birthmarks and precursor melanocytic lesions of cutaneous melanoma identifiable in childhood. *Pediatr Clin North Am* 1983; 30:435.

170. Weinstock MA, Colditz GA, Willett WC, et al. Moles and site-specific risk of nonfamilial cutaneous malignant melanoma in women. *JNCI* 1989; 81:948.

171. Osterlind A, Tucker MA, Hou-Jensen K, et al. The Danish case-control study of cutaneous malignant melanoma. I. Importance of host factors. *Int J Cancer* 1988; 42:200.

172. Holly EA, Kelly JW, Shpall SN, et al. Number of melanocytic nevi as a major risk factor for malignant melanoma. *J Am Acad Dermatol* 1987; 17:459.

173. Lorentzen M, Pers M, Bretteville-Jensen G. The incidence of malignant transformation in giant pigmented nevi. *Scand J Plast Surg* 1977; 11:163.

174. Trozak DJ, Rowland WD, Hu F. Metastatic malignant melanoma in prepubertal children. *Pediatrics* 1975; 55:191–204.

175. Trozak DJ, Rowland WD, HU F. Metastatic malignant melanoma in prepubertal children. *Pediatrics* 1975; 55:191.

176. Castilla EE, DaGraca-Dutra M, Orioli-Parreiras JM. Epidemiology of congenital pigmented nevi: incidence rate and relative frequencies. *Br J Dermatol* 1981; 104:307.

177. Rhodes AR, Sober AJ, Day CL, et al. The malignant potential of small congenital nevocullular nevi. *J Am Acad Dermatol* 1982; 6:230.

178. Greene MH, Clark WH, Tucker MA, et al. Acquired precursors of cutaneous malignant melanoma. The familial dysplastic nevus syndrome. *N Engl J Med* 1985; 312:91.

179. Kopf AW, Goldman RJ, Rivers JK, et al. Skin types in dysplastic nevus syndrome. *J Dermatol Surg Oncol* 1988; 14:827.

180. Clark WH, Reimer RR, Greene M, et al. Origin of familial malignant melanomas from heritable melanocytic lesions: the B-K mole syndrome. *Arch Dermatol* 1978; 114:732.

181. Carey WP, Thompson CJ, Synnestvedt M, et al. Dysplastic nevi as a melanoma risk factor in patients with familial melanoma. *Cancer* 1994; 74:3118–3125.

182. Meyer LJ, Zone JH. Genetics of cutaneous melanoma. *J Invest Dermatol* 1994; 103:112S–116S.

183. Elder DE, Goldman LI, Goldman SC, et al. Dysplastic nevus syndrome: a phenotypic association of sporadic cutaneous melanoma. *Cancer* 1980; 46:1787.

184. Mackie RM. Multiple melanoma and atypical melanocytic nevi—evidence of an activated and expanded melanocytic system. *Br J Dermatol* 1982; 107:621.

185. Roush GC, Nordlund JJ, Forget B, et al. Independence of dysplastic nevi from total nevi in determining risk for nonfamilial melanoma. *Prev Med* 1988; 17:273.

186. Rigel DS, Rivers DK, Kopf AW, et al. Dysplastic nevi. Markers for increased risk for melanoma. *Cancer* 1989; 63:389.

187. Mackie RM. Which moles matter? The association between melanocytic nevi and malignant melanomata. *Br J Dermatol* 1981; 105:607.

188. Raghavan D, Zalcberg JR, Grygiel JJ, et al. Multiple atypical nevi: a cutaneous marker of germ cell tumors. *J Clin Oncol* 1994; 12:2284–2287.

189. Goldstein AM, Fraser MC, Struewing JP, et al. Increased risk of pancreatic cancer in melanoma-prone kindreds with p16INK4 mutations. *N Engl J Med* 1995; 333:970–974.

190. Davis J, Pack GT, Higgins GK. Melanotic freckle of Hutchinson. *Am J Surg* 1967; 113:457.

191. Day CL, Mihm MC, Lew RE, et al. Cutaneous malignant melanoma: prognostic guidelines for physicians and patients. *Cancer* 1982; 32:113.

192. Garbe C, Buttner P, Bertz J, et al. Primary cutaneous melanoma. Identification of prognostic groups and estimation of individual prognosis for 5093 patients. *Cancer* 1995; 75:2484–2491.

193. Iscoe N, Kersey P, Gapski J, et al. Predictive value of staging investigations in patients with clinical stage I malignant melanoma. *Plast Reconstr Surg* 1987; 80:233.

194. Barth A, Wanek LA, Morton DL. Prognostic factors in 1521 melanoma patients with distant metastases. *J Am Coll Surg* 1995; 181:193–201.

195. Day CL, Sober AJ, Lew RA. Malignant melanoma patients with positive nodes and relatively good prognoses. *Cancer* 1981; 47:955.

196. Wanebo HJ, Cooper PH, Young DV, et al. Prognostic factors in head and neck melanoma. Effect of lesion location. *Cancer* 1988; 62:831.

197. Benmeir P, Baruchin A, Lusthaus S, et al. Melanoma of the scalp: the invisible killer. *Plast Reconstr Surg* 1995; 95:496–500.

198. Davidson T, Kissin M, Westburg G. Vulvo-vaginal melanoma. Should radical surgery be abandoned? *Br J Obstet Gynaecol* 1987; 94:473.

199. Ward MW, Romano G, Nicholls RJ. The surgical treatment of anorectal malignant melanoma. *Br J Surg* 1986; 73:68.

200. Garbe C, Buttner P, Bertz J, et al. Primary cutaneous melanoma. Prognostic classification of anatomic location. *Cancer* 1995; 75:2492–2498.

201. Day CL, Harrist TJ, Gorstein F, et al. Malignant melanoma. Prognostic significance of "microscopic satellites" in the reticular dermis and subcutaneous fat. *Ann Surg* 1981; 194:108.

202. Harrist TJ, Rigel DS, Day CL, et al. "Microscopic satellites" are more highly associated with regional lymph node metastases than is primary melanoma thickness. *Cancer* 1984; 53:2183.

203. Kelly JN, Sagebiel RW, Blois MS. Regression in malignant melanoma. A histologic feature without independent prognostic significance. *Cancer* 1985; 56:2287.

204. Slingluff CL, Vollmor RT, Reintgen DS, et al. Lethal "thin" melanoma. Identifying patients at risk. *Ann Surg* 1988; 208:150.

205. Cascinelli N, van der Esch EP, Breslow A, et al. Stage I melanoma of the skin: the problems of resection margins. *Eur J Cancer* 1980; 16:1079.

206. Schmoeckel C, Bockelbrink A, Bockelbrink H, et al. Is wide excision necessary in malignant melanoma? *J Invest Dermatol* 1981; 76:424.

207. Day CL, Lew RA. Malignant melanoma prognostic factors. III. Surgical margins. *J Dermatol Oncol Surg* 1983; 9:797.

208. Zeitels J, LaRossa D, Hamilton R, et al. A comparison of local recurrence and resection margins for stage I primary cutaneous malignant melanomas. *Plast Reconstr Surg* 1988; 81:688.

209. O'Rourke MG, Bourke C. Recommended width of excision for primary malignant melanoma. *World J Surg* 1995; 19:343–345.

210. Day CL, Mihm MC, Sober AJ, et al. Narrower margins for clinical Stage I malignant melanoma. *N Engl J Med* 1982; 306:479.

211. Breslow A. The surgical treatment of Stage I cutaneous melanoma. *Cancer Treat Rev* 1979; 5:195.

212. Balch CM, Murrad TM, Soong S, et al. Tumor thickness as a guide to surgical management of clinical Stage I melanoma patients. *Cancer* 1979; 43:883.

213. Veronesi U, Cascinelli N, Adamus J, et al. Thin stage I primary cutaneous malignant melanoma. Comparison of excision with margins of 1 or 3 cm. *N Engl J Med* 1988; 318:1159.

214. Karakousis C, More R, Holyoke E. Surgery in recurrent malignant melanoma. *Cancer* 52:1343.

215. Overett TK, Shiu MH. Surgical treatment of distant metastatic melanoma. Indications and results. *Cancer* 1985; 56:1222.

216. Burmeister BH, Smithers BM, Poulsen M, et al. Radiation therapy for nodal disease in malignant melanoma. *World J Surg* 1995; 19. 369–371.

217. Day CL, Lew RA, Mihm MC, et al. A multivariate analysis of prognostic factors for melanoma patients with lesions 3.65 millimeters in thickness. *Ann Surg* 1982; 195:44.

218. Day CL, Mihm MC, Lew RA, et al. Prognostic factors for patients with clinical stage I melanoma of intermediate thickness (1.51–3.99 millimeters). *Ann Surg* 1982; 195:35.

219. Veronesi U, Adamus J, Bandiera DC, et al. Inefficacy of immediate node dissection in stage I melanoma of the limbs. *N Engl J Med* 1977; 297:627.

220. Elder DE, Guerry D, Van Horn M, et al. The role of lymph node dissection for clinical stage I malignant melanoma of intermediate thickness (1.51–3.99 mm). *Cancer* 1985; 56:413.

221. Coates AS, Inguar CI, Petersen-Schaefer K, et al. Elective lymph node dissection in patients with primary melanoma of the trunk and limbs treated by the Sydney Melanoma Unit from 1960 to 1991. *J Am Coll Surg* 1995; 180:402–409.

222. Balch CM, Soong S, Murad T, et al. A multifactorial analysis of melanoma. II. Prognostic factors in patients with stage I (localized) melanoma. *Surgery* 1979; 86:343.

223. Sim FH, Taylor WF, Pritchard DJ, et al. Lymphadenectomy in the management of stage I malignant melanoma: a prospective randomized study. *Surg Gynecol Obstet* 1985; 161:575.

224. Sim FH, Taylor WF, Pritchard DJ, et al. Lymphadenopathy in management of stage I malignant melanoma: a prospective randomized study. *Mayo Clinic Proc* 1986; 61:697.

225. Stone CA, Goodacre TE. Surgical management of regional lymph nodes in primary cutaneous malignant melanoma. *Br J Surg* 1995; 82:1015–1022.

226. Reintgen D, Cruse CW, Wells K, et al. The orderly progression of melanoma nodal metastases. *Ann Surg* 1994; 220:759–767.

227. Eberback MA, Wahl RL, Argenta LC, et al. Utility of lymphoscintigraphy in directing surgical therapy for melanomas of the head, neck, and upper thorax. *Surgery* 1987; 102:433.

228. Krag DN, Meijer SJ, Weaver DL, et al. Minimal-access surgery for staging of malignant melanoma. *Arch Surg* 1995; 130:654–660.

229. Bryant PJ, Balderson GA, Mead P, et al. Hyperthermic isolated limb perfusion for malignant melanoma: response and survival. *World J Surg* 1995; 19:363–368.

230. DiFilippo F, Carlini S, Garinei R, et al. Local hyperthermia and systemic chemotherapy for treatment of recurrent melanoma. *World J Surg* 1995; 19:359–362.

231. Ghussen F, Kruger I, Groth W, et al. The role of regional hyperthermic cytostatic perfusion in the treatment of extremity melanoma. *Cancer* 1988; 61:654.

232. Franklin HR, Koops HS, Oldhoff J, et al. To perfuse or not to perfuse? A retrospective comparative study to evaluate the effect of adjuvant isolated regional perfusion in patients with clinical stage I extremity melanoma with a thickness of 1.5 mm or greater. *J Clin Oncol* 1988; 6:701.

233. Barth A, Morton DL. The role of adjuvant therapy in melanoma management. *Cancer* 1995; 75:726–734.

234. Legha SS. Current therapy for malignant melanoma. *Sem Oncol* 1989; 16(S1):34.

235. Miller K, Abeles G, Oratz R, et al. Improved survival of patients with melanoma with an antibody response to immunization to a polyvalent melanoma vaccine. *Cancer* 1995; 75:495–502.

236. Walsh P, Dorner A, Dulce RC. Macrophage colony-stimulating factor complementary DNA: a candidate for gene therapy in metastatic melanoma. *J Natl Cancer Inst* 1995; 87:809–816.

237. Slade J, Marghoob AA, Salopek TG, et al. Atypical-mole syndrome: risk for cutaneous malignant melanoma and implications for management. *J Am Acad Derm* 1995; 32:197–215.

238. Voigt H, Classen R. Topodermatographic image analysis for melanoma screening and the quantitative assessment of tumor dimension parameters of the skin. *Cancer* 1995; 75:981–988.

239. Rhodes AR, Wood WC, Sober AJ, et al. Nonepidermal origin of malignant melanoma associated with a giant congenital nevocellular nevus. *Plast Reconstr Surg* 1981; 67:782.

17

Benign Skin Tumors: Clinical Aspects and Histopathology

John C. Murray, M.D., Robin T. Vollmer, M.D., and Gregory S. Georgiade, M.D., F.A.C.S.

Benign tumors of the skin have varied characteristics as to size, shape, and color differentiation. These skin tumors fall naturally into five categories, depending on their tissue origin: tumors of the skin appendages, cysts, tumors of soft-tissue elements, keratosis of epidermis, and pigmented tumors (Table 17–1).

Skin Appendage Tumors

FOLLICULAR DIFFERENTIATION

Trichoepitheliomas

Trichoepitheliomas are flesh-colored papules of 2 to 8 mm, generally located on the face, and occurring in either multiple or solitary forms (1). The solitary form is more common and occurs sporadically. Lesions are usually less than 2 cm and occur in childhood or early adult life. The most common location is the face.

Multiple trichoepitheliomas are inherited as an autosomal dominant trait. The onset is adolescence, and lesions increase in size and numbers during adult life. The most common locations are the nose, nasolabial folds, and central face. Usually the lesions do not ulcerate, and larger lesions may have telangiectasias (Fig. 17–1).

Histologic examination reveals horn cyst with fully keratinized center surrounded by basaloid cells. The keratinization is complete, and a few layers of cells with eosinophilic cytoplasm and large pale nuclei are located between the basophilic cells and the horn cyst. Trichoepitheliomas also demonstrate tumor islands of basophilic cells similar to those in basal cell carcinomas. These cells may be arranged in a lacy network or in solid aggregates. These cell collections may have peripheral palisading and surrounding stroma with moderate fibroblasts (Fig. 17–2).

Treatment of solitary trichoepitheliomas includes surgical excision. Incomplete excision is frequently followed by recurrence. Multiple trichoepitheliomas have been treated by a variety of methods including laser surgery, curettage, surgical excision, electrosurgery, and cryosurgery.

Trichofolliculoma

Trichofolliculomas are generally solitary papules occurring in adults on the head and neck (2). The lesion is generally a small, flesh-colored papule with a central pore. From the central pore a collection of immature white hairs may emerge.

Histologic examination reveals a cystic space lined with squamous epithelium containing horny material and fragments of hair shaft. Secondary hair follicles may connect with the primary pore or primary hair follicle. The secondary hair follicles are connected by basaloid epithelial strands. Peripheral cell rows demonstrate palisading and large glycogen content (Fig. 17–3).

Trichilemmoma

Trichilemmoma may be single or multiple 3–8 mm papules usually occurring on the head and neck (3). Generally the lesions are flesh-colored and may resemble verrucae.

Histologically, the lesions are comprised of several lobules which descend into the dermis. The lobules are oriented around hair-containing follicle. Many clear cells with high glycogen content form these lobules and the periphery of the lobules contains palisading columnar cells with thickened basement membrane and features resembling the lower portion of normal hair follicles.

Multiple trichilemmomas have been described with Cowden syndrome, which is an inherited condition with fibroepithelial polyps of the oral mucosa, keratoses of the palms and soles, multiple trichilemmomas, and increased incidence of breast cancer in women (4). Generally the multiple trichilemmomas precede the development of breast cancer and other visceral malignancies have occasionally occurred in Cowden syndrome. In Cowden syndrome the multiple trichilemmomas are located on the face, generally around the mouth, nose, and ears. Biopsy of these lesions is helpful to distinguish trichilemmomas from verrucae and identify those patients who may possibly have Cowden syndrome.

Pilomatricoma

Pilomatricoma, or benign calcifying epithelioma of Malherbe, is a firm, deep-seeded nodule covered with normal epidermis. When the nodule is more superficial, the lesion may appear bluish-red. Pilomatricoma generally occurs as a solitary lesion on the face and upper extremities (5). Generally the lesion is 0.5 to 3 cm, but some lesions may be larger. The lesions may occur at any age, but 40% occur in children before 10 years of age. Several incidences of familial occurrence have been described, but pilomatricoma is not felt to be a hereditary condition. Pilomatricoma has been reported to be associated with myotonic dystrophy (Fig. 17–4).

Histologically, the tumor is sharply demarcated and surrounded by a connective-tissue capsule. The lesion is composed of a cellular stroma that contains islands of epithelial cells. Two types of epithelial cells present: basophilic and shadow. The basophilic cells have round or elongated ba-

Table 17–1.
Benign Tumors of Skin

Skin appendage tumors
    Follicular differentiation
    Sebaceous differentiation
    Eccrine differentiation
    Apocrine differentiation

Cysts

Soft tissue tumors
    Fibrous tissue tumors
    Fatty tissue tumors
    Smooth muscle tumor
    Neural tissue tumors
    Vascular tissue tumors
    Uncertain origin

Keratoses

Pigmented skin tumors

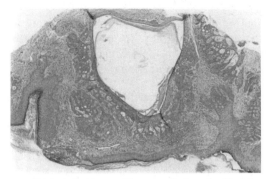

FIG. 17–3. Trichofolliculoma. Note cystic keratin-filled tumor with peripheral follicular-like buds.

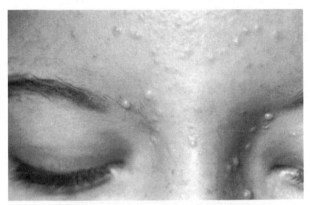

FIG. 17–1. Multiple tricoepitheliomas, an autosomal dominant inheritance, are shown involving skin of forehead, eyelid, and nasal areas.

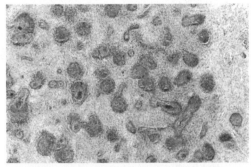

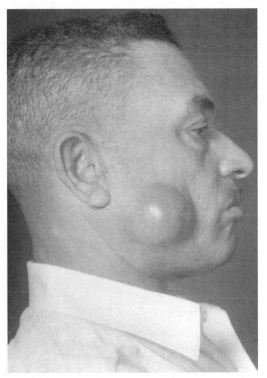

FIG. 17–4. A calcifying epithelioma of Malherbe of the cheek.

FIG. 17–2. Trichoepithelioma is composed of epithelial strands mimicking rudimentary follicule. The cellular connective tissue surrounding these is key for diagnosis.

sophilic nuclei and little if any cytoplasm; the nuclei appear packed together in these islands. The shadow cells have distinct borders and a central unstained area. Some keratinization occurs within areas of basophilic cells or shadow cells. About eighty percent of tumors have calcifications within shadow cells or as deposits replacing shadow cells (5). Surgical excision is the treatment of choice.

ECCRINE AND APOCRINE DIFFERENTIATION

Eccrine Poroma

Eccrine poromas are usually painful papules, most commonly occurring on the soles or side of the feet (6). Lesions may also occur on the hands and fingers, or less commonly on the neck, chest, or nose. Eccrine poromas are commonly seen in middle-aged patients as firm papules less than 2 cm in size. Lesions occasionally may be pedunculated or asymptomatic.

Histologically, eccrine poromas arise from the lower epidermis and consist of broad bands of uniformly small cuboidal cells connected by intracellular bridges. Tumor cells have a distinct appearance smaller than squamous cells and have a uniform cuboidal appearance with round basophilic nucleus. No tendency to keratinize appears in the tumor and the distinct border between the tumor and surrounding stroma contains no palisading. Tumor cells contain significant glycogen content.

Eccrine poromas are treated by surgical excision so that histologic examination may distinguish these lesions from basal cell carcinomas or other skin tumors.

Eccrine Spiradenoma

Eccrine spiradenomas are usually solitary intradermal nodules 1 to 2 cm in diameter that occur in early adulthood (7). These skin tumors occur anywhere and are generally tender or painful nodules. Lesions are usually flesh-colored or slightly bluish and may occur in multiple forms. Rare incidences of zosteriform or linear arrangements have been described.

Histologically, the tumor consists of lobules located in the dermis with deeply basophilic cells (8). The lobules contain intertwining cords with two cell types. One type contains small, dark nuclei and are located at the periphery of the cellular aggregates. The second type have large, pale nuclei and are located in the center around small luminae (Fig. 17–5).

The treatment of choice is surgical excision.

Clear Cell Hidradenoma

Clear cell hidradenomas are 0.5–2 cm nodules occurring in adults as solitary tumors. Lesions may occur anywhere and rarely ulcerate. Clear cell hidradenoma is an eccrine sweat gland tumor.

Histologically, the tumor is well circumscribed and consists of lobulated masses within the dermis. Multiple tubular luminae extend through the tumor, which also contains multiple cystic spaces that are often filled with faintly eosinophilic ma-

terial (9). The tubular luminae are lined by cuboidal ductal cells. The cystic spaces are lined by tumor cells showing degenerative changes. The cell types of the tumor are either polyhedral with rounded nucleus and slightly basophilic cytoplasm, or round with very clear cytoplasm. The treatment of choice is surgical excision (Fig. 17–6).

Syringoma

Syringomas are flesh-colored or yellow papules generally occurring in women in adolescence or early adult life. These tumors are often multiple and less than 3 mm in size. Lesions are often multiple and may be present in large numbers (10). They frequently may be limited to the lower eyelids but some patients may have widespread lesions over the face and trunk. Sites of predilection include the cheeks, axilla, and abdomen (Fig. 17–7). Histologically, the lesions are small ducts embedded in a fibrous stroma. The walls of the ducts are lined by rows of epithelial cells. Some epithelial cells may possess small commalike tails suggesting a tadpole appearance. Some solid strands of basophilic epithelial cells may be independent of the ducts. A variety of destructive techniques have been employed to remove these tumors, with variable success (Fig. 17–8).

SEBACEOUS DIFFERENTIATION

Nevus Sebaceous

Nevus sebaceous is generally located on the scalp or face as a single lesion. Usually the lesion is present at birth and

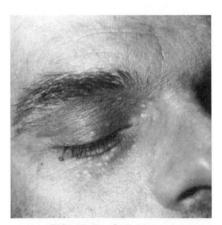

FIG. 17–7. Syringomas.

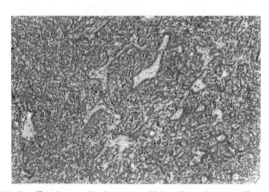

FIG. 17–5. Eccrine spiradenoma. Note the circumscribed round base of this tumor as well as the hints of ductular differentiation within the tumor.

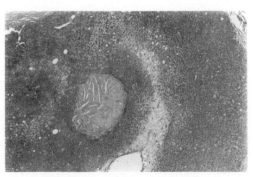

FIG. 17–6. Nodular hidradenoma.

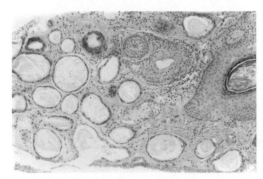

FIG. 17–8. Syringoma. Note the tumor comprised of multiple cystic structures filled with a clear appearing fluid.

appears as a hairless plaque of variable shape. At puberty the lesion may grow and become verrucous and nodular. This change represents hyperplasia of sebaceous glands and apocrine glands. Five to seven percent of nevus sebaceous may develop basal cell carcinomas (11). Other appendageal tumors (e.g., nodular hidradenoma, syringoma, and sebaceous epithelioma) may occur. Rarely, squamous cell carcinoma may develop within a nevus sebaceous (12) (Fig. 17–9).

Sebaceous glands within nevus sebaceous follow the normal development and pattern of sebaceous glands in other body sites. After puberty, histologic appearance of nevus sebaceous becomes diagnostic. These findings include large numbers of mature sebaceous glands and papillomatous hyperplasia of the epidermis.

Since nevus sebaceous may be associated with development of basal cell carcinoma and squamous cell carcinoma, complete surgical excision is generally recommended.

Sebaceous Hyperplasia

Sebaceous hyperplasia are 2–4 mm papules occurring on the face of middle-aged adults. Lesions are pale yellow with central umbilication and telangiectasias. Lesions appear stable and do not ulcerate (13).

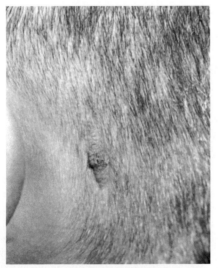

FIG. 17–9. An organoid nevus (nevus-sebaceous) is shown in the second stage.

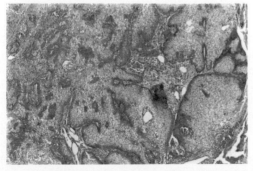

FIG. 17–10. Sebaceous adenoma. Note the nodule comprised of a mix of basaloid and sebaceous cells.

Histologically, the lesions are collections of sebaceous glands with enlarged lobules located around a central wide sebaceous duct. Often these same patients may have ectopic sebaceous glands on the vermilion borders of the lips and oral mucosa that are known as Fordyce spots.

Treatment of these lesions includes excisional biopsy and other destructive techniques such as cryotherapy, electrosurgery, or laser therapy.

Sebaceous Adenoma

Sebaceous adenomas are rare, small, flesh-colored papules without particular location predilection. Single lesions may occur on the face or scalp of older adults (13).

Histologically, the lesion is an incompletely differentiated sebaceous lobule with irregular size and shape. Lobules contain undifferentiated germinating sebaceous cells and more mature sebaceous cells. Simple excision is the preferred treatment choice (Fig. 17–10).

Multiple sebaceous adenomas may be seen in Muir Torre syndrome, which is associated with internal malignancy (14).

Sebaceous Epithelioma

Sebaceous epitheliomas may resemble basal cell epitheliomas as pale or yellow papules with ulceration. Lesions are usually single and located on the face or scalp. The surgeon should perform a biopsy of these lesions for histopathologic examination (13).

Histologically, sebaceous epitheliomas are not well circumscribed, but irregularly-shaped cell masses. Lesions are differentiated toward sebaceous cells, and most cells are undifferentiated and arranged in clusters with peripheral palisading. Mature sebaceous cells may be located in the center of most cell masses.

Cysts of the Skin

Epidermal Cysts

Epidermal cysts are the most common form of cysts; they can occur at any age and virtually any body location. Most commonly, they occur in areas of increased pilosebaceous activity on the head and upper trunk (Fig. 17–11). Epidermal cysts may be intradermal or subcutaneous tumors, and may grow to sizes ranging from 1 to 5 cm in diameter. The lesions are believed to arise from the infundibular portion of the pilosebaceous unit as epithelial cells become trapped and form a cystic lesion. Patients may have one or several lesions (Fig. 17–12). Some patients may have multiple epidermal cysts on the head and trunk, as can be seen in Gardner syndrome. Gardner syndrome has been described as associating multiple epidermal cysts with polyposis coli, osteomas of the jaw, and intestinal desmoid tumors (15).

Histologically, epidermal cysts are lined by true epidermis that forms a granular layer and keratin. The accumulated keratin forms the bulk of the tumor in laminated layers. The epidermal cyst may rupture and the extrusion of the keratin debris into the dermis or subcutaneous tissue may incite a foreign-body reaction. This phenomenon is clinically associated with intense pain, erythema, and drainage of purulent material (Fig. 17–13).

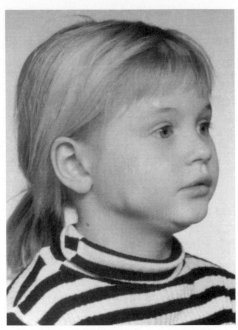

FIG. 17–11. A single epidermal cyst of the right cheek in a 5-year-old girl.

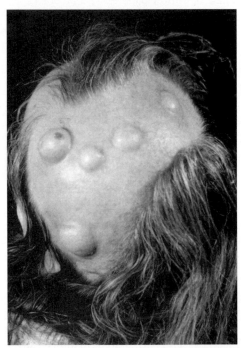

FIG. 17–12. Multiple epidermal cysts of the scalp.

Pilar Cysts

Pilar cysts are clinically similar to epidermal cysts. They occur most commonly on the scalp, but other locations include face, neck, and trunk. The clinical findings and course are similar for both types of cysts. Pilar cysts often may show an autosomal dominant inherence and occur as solitary lesions in only 30% of the cases. Approximately ten percent of patients may have more than ten cysts. Pilar cysts appear as firm and white-walled and may be easily enucleated (16).

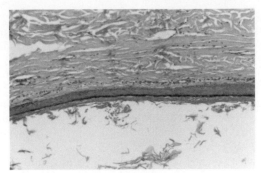

FIG. 17–13. Epidermoid cyst is lined by keratinocytes identical to those of the epidermis, and it is filled with keratin debris.

Histologically, pilar cysts are composed of epithelial cells without intercellular bridges. The innermost cells are not flattened; they appear swollen and are filled with pale cytoplasm. These cells do not form a granular layer and appear to keratinize abruptly. Occasional pilar cysts may calcify.

Milia

Milia are 1–2 mm papules that are white, superficial, firm lesions. They are superficial epidermal cysts, commonly occurring on the face. These lesions may occur following healing from blistering diseases or local trauma.

Histologically, milia are epidermal cysts varying only in size. These lesions are lined with mature epithelium with few cell layers and central keratin material.

Dermoid Cysts

Dermoid cysts are subcutaneous cysts that form along lines of embryologic effusion. Commonly, dermoid cysts are congenital and occur on the head, around the eyes, and occasionally on the neck. Dermoid cysts on the head may be located near the periosteum. Lesions may grow to 1 to 4 cm in size (Fig. 17–14).

Histologically, dermoid cysts are lined by epidermis and epidermal appendages. Usually the appendages are fully matured and contain hair follicles, sebaceous glands, eccrine glands, and infrequently apocrine glands.

Treatment of choice is surgical excision, which is performed to minimize the risk of infection or rupture and inflammation. Because some lesions in the nasal frontal region may extend through bone to the meninges, it is helpful to have perioperative assessment of lesion location before excision.

Steatocystoma Multiplex

Steatocystoma multiplex is an autosomal dominant inherited condition. Patients have cysts occurring on the trunk and scrotum in males and axillae and groin in females. Lesions are numerous, small, cystic nodules that measure 1 to 3 cm in diameter. When drained, the cysts may discharge a keratinaceous fluid or debris with hair.

Histologically, these cysts have complex walls with several layers of epithelial cells. Cyst walls also contain flattened sebaceous gland lobules within or close to the wall. Cyst invaginations may also have hair follicles with hairs extending into the lumen.

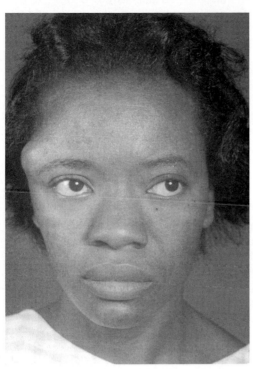

FIG. 17–14. A large dermoid cyst at the right frontotemporal suture line.

Often these lesions are too numerous to excise totally. Individual lesions may be incised and drained to help decrease the cyst load.

Thyroglossal Duct Cysts

Thyroglossal duct cysts usually occur on the anterior midline of the neck near the hyoid bone. These lesions are similar to bronchogenic cysts; characteristically the lesions are small, solitary lesions in the dermis or subcutaneous layer. Lesions appear shortly after birth and may be associated with a draining sinus. Histologically, thyroglossal duct cysts contain columnar epithelium and thyroid tissue in the cyst wall. Bronchogenic cysts contain mucosa with pseudostratified columnar epithelium and varying numbers of goblet cells and smooth muscle with mucous glands (see Chapter 46, Cervical Masses).

Hidrocystoma

Apocrine hidrocystoma is commonly a solitary cystic papule. The lesions vary from 3 to 15 mm and commonly present as a flesh-colored or bluish papule on the face. Multiple lesions are uncommon (17).

Histologically, the dermis has one or several cystic spaces lined with rows of secretory cells showing decapitation secretion suggesting apocrine secretion.

Eccrine hidrocystomas share similar characteristics, in that lesions are small, cystic papules 1 to 3 mm in size, with a bluish hue. Lesions may be solitary but some patient have numerous lesions, which may increase with warm weather. Commonly, eccrine hidrocystomas are found on the malar eminence (18).

Histologically, eccrine hidrocystomas demonstrate a single cystic cavity within the dermis. The cell wall is lined with two layers of small cuboidal epithelial cells.

Surgical excision is elective.

Tumors of Connective-Tissue Differentiation

FIBROUS TISSUE TUMORS

Dermatofibroma

Dermatofibromas are fibrous papules that commonly occur on the lower extremities of young adults. The lesions are firm papules measuring 2 to 30 mm in size. Commonly, lesions will dimple with lateral compression. The most common location is the lower extremities; patients will recount antecedent local trauma such as insect bite, shaving injury, or folliculitis. Although patients may commonly have only one lesion, some patients may have multiple lesions. Typically lesions are red-brown or even hyperpigmented. They tend to remain stable for years as discrete, solitary lesions (Fig. 17–15).

Histologically, dermatofibromas are mixtures of fibroblasts, collagen, capillaries, and histiocytes. Some lesions have predominantly fibrous reaction and are composed of fibroblasts and collagen, whereas cellular lesions contain histiocytes. Both fibrous and cellular types of dermatofibromas contain small capillaries with endothelial cells. Often, the overlying epidermis contains significant hyperplasia (Fig. 17–16).

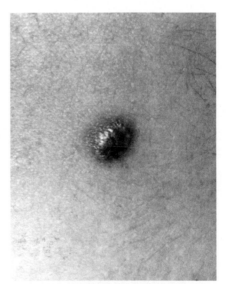

FIG. 17–15. Dermatofibroma.

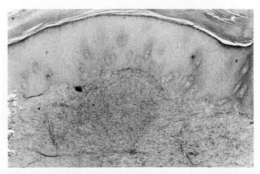

FIG. 17–16. Dermatofibroma. Note the nodule of cellular stroma in the mid dermis. The cellularity is most intense centrally and then falls gradually to the perimeter, where there are thickened collagen fibers.

Lesions are treated by surgical excision when atypia is suspected clinically.

Acrochordons

Acrochordons represent benign papules generally occurring on the neck, axilla, and upper chest of middle-aged adults. These lesions are usually flesh-colored or hyperpigmented. Lesions are asymptomatic and may become irritated. Commonly lesions are delicate, filiform papules that have a benign course except for possible irritation. A larger, solitary type of acrochordon is a pedunculated nodule that may occur on the trunk or extremities (Fig. 17–17).

Histologically, acrochordons contain hyperplastic epidermis with excessive dermal connective tissue. Solitary, soft fibromas or pedunculated lesions may have adipose tissue in the center.

Acrochordons are treated, when indicated, with local destructive techniques such as surgical excision, cryotherapy, electrosurgery, or laser surgery.

FATTY TISSUE TUMORS

Lipomas

Lipomas are dermal or subcutaneous collections of benign adipose tissue. Most lesions are solitary, discrete nodules that remain asymptomatic and occur over the trunk and extremities. Some patients may have an autosomal dominant inherited condition of multiple lipomatosis. A clinical variant that may be difficult to distinguish is angiolipomas. These lesions are uncommon, and generally are firmer and more painful (Fig. 17–18).

Histologically, these lesions are composed of mature adipose cells. Often lesions may have a fibrous capsule that can surround the collection of adipose cells. Angiolipomas contain numerous capillaries.

Surgical excision is the treatment of choice, when appropriate or desired. Lesions may be removed by liposuction or excised through a punch biopsy port.

Hypertrophic Scar and Keloids

The distinction between hypertrophic scars and keloids may be a difficult clinical challenge. Both lesions may be erythematous, raised, firm papules with a smooth surface. In general, hypertrophic scars remain within the confines of a wound and resolve spontaneously with time. Keloids extend beyond the original confines of the wound and persistently enlarge. Spontaneous resolution of keloids is unusual.

Histologically, hypertrophic scars and keloids are similar, in that both demonstrate whorls and collagen nodules. Hypertrophic scars demonstrate progressive flattening of these collagen nodules, whereas keloids have persistent disarray of these fibrous growths.

Treatment options depend upon identifying the difference between hypertrophic scars and keloids (if possible). Often, lesions may be treated with intralesional corticosteroid injection or surgical excision combined with other treatment to help minimize recurrence. Therapeutic intervention should be undertaken with caution to minimize the possibility of recurrence or untoward effect of a larger resulting lesion.

SMOOTH MUSCLE TUMORS

Leiomyomas

Leiomyomas are typically painful papules that may occur over the trunk or genitals. Lesions are typically erythematous papules of less than 6 mm.

Histologically, leiomyomas are composed of bundles of smooth-muscle fibers with varying amounts of collagen. Angioleiomyomas differ, in that they tend to be more encapsulated and contain numerous veins. In general, angioleiomyomas contain less collagen.

Surgical excision for appropriate lesions is the treatment of choice.

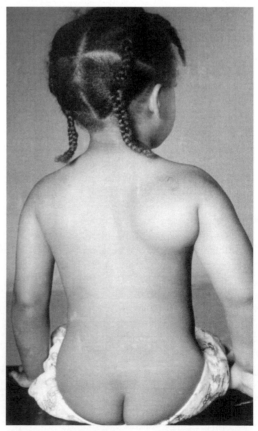

FIG. 17–18.   A large lipoma of the back in a 4-year-old girl.

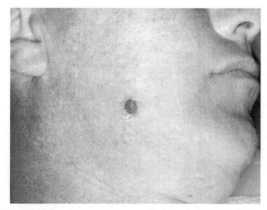

FIG. 17–17.   A squamous papilloma of the right cheek.

XANTHOMATOUS TUMORS

Xanthomas

Hyperlipoproteinemias are associated with cutaneous xanthomas. Multiple types of xanthomas have been described and recognized. Eruptive xanthomas are associated with hypertriglyceridemia and hyperlipemia. Lesions appear as 2–6 mm papules over the buttocks and extensor extremities. They are related to hypertriglyceridemia. Tuberous xanthomas are predominantly found with elevated beta-lipoproteins. These lesions are large plaques located commonly on the elbows, knees, fingers, and buttocks. Xanthelasma are slightly raised, yellowish plaques on the eyelids. Cutaneous xanthelasma are found in type IIA and type III hyperlipoproteinemia. Approximately two-thirds of patients with xanthelasma have normal serum lipid levels (Figs. 17–19, 17–20).

Histologically, xanthomas have characteristic foam cells that are macrophages filled with lipid droplets. Eruptive xanthomas contain mixtures of nonfoamy cells with lymphocytes, histiocytes, and neutrophils. Tuberous xanthomas contain foam cells along with nonfoamy cells, lymphocytes, histiocytes, and neutrophils. With more mature lesions, increased fibrosis will replace foam cells. Xanthelasma contain superficial foam cells and little if any fibrosis.

Treatment of these lesions involves investigation of the serum lipoprotein profile. Eruptive xanthomas will resolve with correction of the hypertriglyceridemia. Lesions not associated with hypertriglyceridemia may be excised or treated with various destructive means such as topical trichloroacetic peels, cryotherapy, or laser surgery.

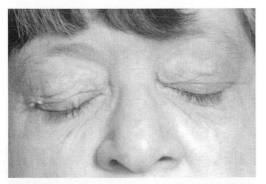

FIG. 17–19. Extensive xanthomatous plaques of the eyelids.

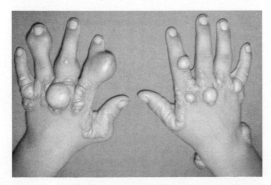

FIG. 17–20. Extensive xanthomatous nodules of the hands.

Atypical Fibroxanthomas

Atypical fibroxanthomas of the skin are nodular lesions in sun-exposed areas of the head and neck in elderly patients (19). An occasional lesion may occur on the trunk and extremities in younger patients. The surface of the tumor may be normal or, occasionally, eroded. The size of the lesion generally exceeds 2 cm in diameter. The clinical course is generally benign, but occasional metastasis to regional lymph nodes have been described; thus atypical fibroxanthoma may be a low-grade malignancy thought related to malignant fibrous histiocytoma.

Histologically, atypical fibroxanthoma demonstrates a highly cellular dermal infiltrate extending to the epidermis and occasionally to subcutaneous fat. The cellular infiltrate is pleomorphic, with hyperchromatic nuclei in irregular arrangement. Many mitoses are present.

Complete surgical excision is recommended as the treatment of choice.

Juvenile Xanthogranuloma

Juvenile xanthogranuloma are self-limited, benign papules that occur in early infancy (20). Some lesions may be present at birth. These red-to-yellow papules measure 0.5 cm to 1 cm and occur singly or as multiple lesions. Lesions generally involute spontaneously; they may be present up to 1 year or longer. Occasionally, lesions may involve the iris or the epibulbar area. Lesions of the iris may lead to glaucoma.

Histologically, these papules are accumulations of histiocytes with few lymphocytes and eosinophils. A granulomatous infiltrate may be present that contains foam cells, foreign-body giant cells, and Touton giant cells. The Touton giant cell is characteristic for juvenile xanthogranuloma.

This lesion may occur in adults and is identified by biopsy.

TUMORS OF NEURAL TISSUE

Neurofibromas

Neurofibromas may occur as solitary lesions without café-au-lait lesions or as other evidence of the neurocutaneous syndrome, von Recklinghausen, or as neurofibromatosis. Neurofibromatosis is an autosomal dominant inherited syndrome of multiple neurofibromas, café-au-lait spots, and other associated findings. In general, neurofibromatosis begins in childhood and progresses to adulthood. Neurofibromatosis may occur in bone, spinal root, and peripheral nerves, and neurofibromatosis may be associated with pheochromocytoma in 10% of cases. Neurofibromas are flesh-colored papules or nodules with soft consistency. Occasional lesions may be pedunculated (Fig. 17–21). The size varies considerably. Occasionally, in neurofibromatosis, large masses with numerous thickened nerves can be palpated; this finding is called plexiform neuroma (Fig. 17–22). Café-au-lait spots may occur at birth, but they may appear up to 1 year of age. They increase in number and size throughout adolescence. Generally the café-au-lait spots are lentigos that precede the onset of neurofibromas. The presence of six or more café-au-lait spots exceeding 1.5 cm suggests neurofibromatosis. Patients with neurofibromatosis often will have freckling in the axilla and may have Lisch nodules that can be seen on slit-lamp examination.

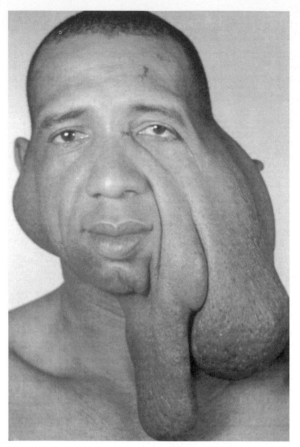

FIG. 17–21. An extensive pedunculated neurofibroma involving the face and neck.

Histologically, cutaneous neurofibromas reveal the same finding whether solitary neurofibromas or neurofibromatosis. Neurofibromas are well circumscribed but not encapsulated. Lesions are located within the dermis, and may extend to the subcutaneous fat. The lesion is a collection of wavy fibers collected in textured strands that extend in various directions. The wavy fibers contain large nuclei that are oval- to spindle shaped and uniform in size (Fig. 17–23). On electron microscopy, neurofibromas are felt to be aggregates of Schwann cells. Cutaneous neurofibromas have been described as developing neurofibrosarcomas or malignant schwannomas; this malignant transformation is uncommon. Neurofibromas may be excised for histopathologic confirmation. Some lesions may be removed for cosmetic reasons or to improve functional capability.

Neurilemmoma

Neurilemmomas are usually solitary tumors along a peripheral or cranial nerve. Generally neurilemmomas are located on the head and neck, and may involve the vestibular branch of the acoustic nerve. Lesions are 2 to 4 cm, and the nodule is located in the subcutaneous layer. Lesions are often painful; pain may radiate along the affected nerve (Fig. 17–24).

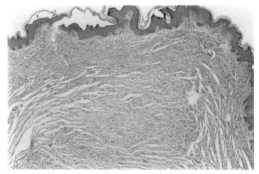

FIG. 17–23. Neurofibroma. This common skin tumor thickens the dermis and is comprised of a loose arrangement of spindle cells, capillaries and mast cells in a mucoid matrix.

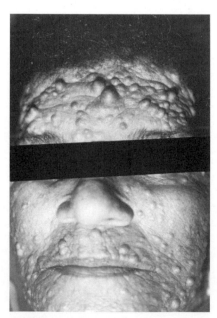

FIG. 17–22. Multiple neurofibromas involving extensive areas of the scalp and face in von Recklinghausen disease.

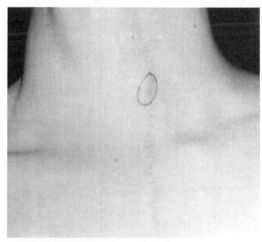

FIG. 17–24. A small neurolemmoma in the neck skin.

On histopathologic examination, neurilemmomas are well encapsulated and contain two types of tissue known as antony type A or B. Antony type A is composed of cells with elongated nuclei and tightly packed cellular arrangement. A characteristic feature is the arrangement of nuclei in two parallel rows enclosing an area of nearly homogeneous material. This formation is called verocay body. Antony type B tissue consists of edematous stroma with few cells. This tissue may contain fluid-filled cystic spaces and stroma may reveal mucoid changes.

Neurilemmomas may be surgically excised from the nerve, with preservation of the nerve when possible.

Granular Cell Tumor

Granular cell tumors are generally solitary tumors, found commonly on the tongue and in subcutaneous tissue (21). Multiple sites have been identified including esophagus, stomach, appendix, larynx bronchus, and pituitary gland. The lesion is an intradermal tumor that is well circumscribed and may vary in size from 0.5 to 3 cm. Symptoms are variable, including pain and pruritus. Occasionally the surface is verrucous.

Histologically, the cells are large and elongated. The cells have a distinct cellular membrane and pale cytoplasm with eosinophilic coarse granules. A characteristic feature is the arrangement of cells in clusters with strands that are surrounded by periodic acid-Schiff (PAS) positive, diastase-resistant membrane and strands of collagen fibers.

Lesions are surgically excised for diagnostic confirmation.

TUMORS OF THE EPIDERMIS

Keratoacanthoma

Keratoacanthoma is a common cutaneous neoplasm occurring more frequently in elderly men after the 6th decade. Generally, lesions are in sun-exposed areas and are believed to arise from hair follicles. The clinical course, with its rapid growth and histologic appearance, is suggestive of a carcinoma, but the tumor frequently regresses spontaneously and may be cured by curettage or simple excision. Keratoacanthoma is often well circumscribed with firm, round borders and an umbilicated keratotic center. This center has a keratin plug filled with crust. Typically the lesion grows rapidly over

4 to 8 weeks; this rapid growth is followed by a latent period of another 8 weeks, after which lesions may regress. Lesions may measure 1 to 2.5 cm, but larger sizes have been described (Fig. 17–25).

Histologically, keratoacanthomas can be difficult to distinguish from squamous cell carcinomas. A keratoacanthoma typically is composed of well-differentiated squamous epithelium showing little pleomorphism and excessive keratin formation. Keratoacanthomas generally have a smooth, well-demarcated infiltration of tumor into the dermis with limited depth that does not extend beyond the level of the hair follicles. Adequate biopsy is essential to provide sufficient tissue for proper clinical and histopathologic correlation. Keratoacanthomas may be single or multiple. Despite the number of lesions, keratoacanthomas share similar clinical and microscopic features as well as clinical course.

Although keratoacanthomas may regress spontaneously, the tumor should be surgically excised for histopathologic confirmation. Excising the lesion early will limit the resultant scar and avoid the atrophic scar that may occur with spontaneous regression. Excision will also afford histopathologic confirmation of keratoacanthoma and exclude the possibility of squamous cell carcinoma.

Seborrheic Keratoses

Seborrheic keratoses are common, benign keratoses seen on the trunk and face. In general, the lesions appear after the 4th decade and are brown, hyperpigmented, verrucous papules measuring from 3 mm to more than several cm. The lesions are discrete and well demarcated, and appear attached to the skin with a waxy, verrucous surface. The lesions may be occasionally irritated with trauma. They are not thought to be photo-induced (Fig. 17–26).

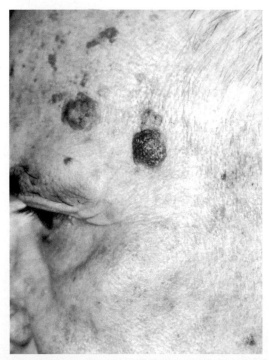

FIG. 17–26. Multiple raised, brown lesions of the skin typical of seborrheic keratoses.

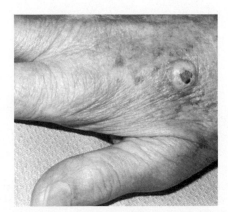

FIG. 17–25. Keratoacanthoma of the hand. Note resemblance to a squamous cell carcinoma.

Two variants of seborrheic keratoses have been described. These include dermatosis papulosa nigra (22) and stucco keratoses (23). Dermatosis papulosis nigra are keratotic papules, generally less than 3 mm, that often appear over the malar eminence in blacks. Stucco keratoses are flat, hyperkeratotic 2–5 mm verrucous papules commonly seen over the dorsal feet, wrists, and forearms of middle-aged adults.

Histologically, seborrheic keratoses have hyperkeratosis, acanthosis, and papillomatosis. The lower edge of the tumor is generally flat, with upward extension of either squamous cells or basaloid cells. The lesions may have entrapped dermal papillae and keratin debris (pseudocyst). Irritated lesions may demonstrate an inflammatory infiltrate that resembles lichen planus. Some seborrheic keratoses may undergo hyperplasia and squamous metaplasia (Fig. 17–27).

Lesions with atypical features should be examined by biopsy and sent for histopathologic diagnosis. Lesions may be removed by a variety of destructive techniques including excision, cryosurgery, or electrosurgery.

Actinic Keratoses

Actinic keratoses are premalignant keratotic papules seen in sun-exposed areas of middle-aged or elderly, fair-complexioned patients who have had significant sun exposure. These lesions occur over the scalp, forehead, and dorsum of the forearms and hands. The lesions are erythematous and keratotic, with ill-defined edges and generally flattened keratotic

scale. In general, patients have multiple lesions and other signs of dermatoheliosis including wrinkling, lentigos, colloid milium, atrophy, and skin fragility. Some actinic keratoses may have hyperpigmentation, suggesting a diagnosis of lentigo maligna. Occasionally, actinic keratoses may become hyperkeratotic and resemble cutaneous horns. Lesions on the lower lip are solar cheilitis and patients will describe scaling and erosions (Fig. 17–28).

A major concern of actinic keratoses is their transformation into squamous cell carcinomas. The rate of transformation is difficult to determine (24), but some estimates imply that 20% of patients with actinic keratoses will eventually develop squamous cell carcinomas from one of the keratoses (25). Keratotic lesions that persist, thicken, ulcerate, or grow rapidly should be considered potential candidates for transformation into squamous cell carcinomas.

Histologically, actinic keratoses demonstrate an atypical differentiation of keratinocytes with varying involvement of the epidermal layer. The epidermis is characterized by hyperkeratosis and parakeratosis. Atypical keratinocytes may be confined to the basal cell layer or extend throughout the epidermis and even into the superficial papillary dermis (Fig. 17–29).

Actinic keratoses are commonly treated with superficial destructive means such as cryotherapy, electrosurgery, curettage, shave excision, or chemical peels. Isolated, or few, lesions are best treated by local destructive means, whereas multiple or widespread lesions are best treated with chemical peels or topical 5-fluorouracil. Patients are instructed to continue sun protection with sunscreens and protective clothing and to maintain close follow-up in the event of transformation of actinic keratoses into squamous cell carcinomas.

Cylindroma

Cylindromas are variably sized tumors that commonly occur on the scalp (26). Lesions may be single or multiple. Multiple lesions are often dominantly inherited. Lesions are smooth papules and nodules that may cover the entire scalp. Lesions may be round and firm and are often flesh-colored or erythematous. Lesions generally occur in adulthood and increase in size and number with time. The size may vary from several millimeters to several centimeters. In some cases, lesions may appear on the face and even on the trunk or extremities (Fig. 17–30).

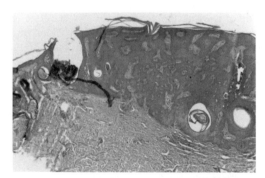

FIG. 17–27. Seborrheic keratosis. Note the thickened basaloid epidermis with keratin-filled pseudocysts.

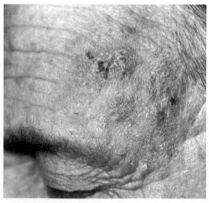

FIG. 17–28. Actinic keratosis characterized by scaly, encrusted lesions and skin pigmentary changes.

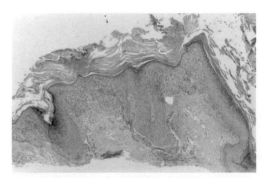

FIG. 17–29. Actinic (or solar) keratosis. Note the horn overlying the keratosis. Although there is a hyperplastic extension downward, there is no true invasion, but rather a hyperplastic thickening of the epidermis and with some altered maturation.

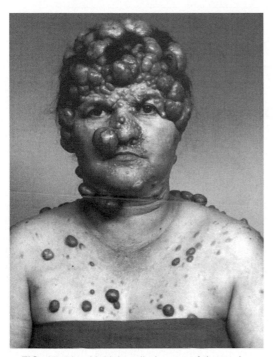

FIG. 17–30. Multiple cylindromas of the scalp.

The histopathologic examination reveals islands of epithelial cells. Cells vary in size and shape because islands are separated by hyaline sheath and narrow bands of collagen. This pattern of islands and bands may resemble pieces of a jigsaw puzzle. The islands are composed of two types of cells, one of which has a small, darkly stained nucleus that occurs predominantly at the periphery and often palisades. The other cell type has a large, lightly staining nuclei that lies in the center of the islands. Few cases of malignant degeneration have been reported. Surgical excision is the preferred treatment.

References

1. Gray HR, Helwig EB. Epithelioma adenoides cysticum and solitary trichoepithelioma. *Arch Dermatol* 1963; 87:102–114.
2. Gray HR, Helwig EB. Trichofolliculoma. *Arch Dermatol* 1962; 86:619–625.
3. Brownstein MH, Shapiro L. Trichilemmoma. *Arch Dermatol* 1973; 107:866–869.
4. Brownstein MH, Wolf M, Bikowski JB. Cowden's disease: a cutaneous marker of breast cancer. *Cancer* 1978; 41:2393–2398.
5. Forbis R Jr, Helwig EB. Pilomatrixoma (calcifying epithelioma). *Arch Dermatol* 1961; 83:606–618.
6. Hyman AB, Brownstein MH. Eccrine poroma: an analysis of 45 new cases. *Dermatologica* 1969; 138:29–38.
7. Mambo NC. Eccrine spiradenoma: clinical and pathological study of 49 tumors. *J Cutan Pathol* 1983; 10:312–320.
8. Kersting DW, Helwig EB. Eccrine spiradenoma. *Arch Dermatol* 1956; 73:199–227.
9. Winkelmann RK, Wolff K. Solid-cystic hidradenoma of the skin. *Arch Dermatol* 97:651, 1968.
10. Hashimoto K, DiBella RJ, Borsuk GM, Lever WF. Eruptive hidradenoma and syringoma. *Arch Dermatol* 1967; 96:500–519.
11. Greer KE, Bishop GF, Ober WC. Nevus sebaceous and syringocystadenoma papilliferum. *Arch Dermatol* 1976; 112:206–208.
12. Coskey RJ. The spectrum of organoid nevi. *Cutis* 1982; 29:290–294.
13. Mehregan AH, Rahbari H. Benign epithelial tumors of the skin. II. Benign sebaceous tumors. *Cutis* 1977; 19:317–320.
14. Housholder MS, Zeligman I. Sebaceous neoplasms associated with visceral carcinoma. *Arch Dermatol* 1980; 116:61–64.
15. Weary PE, Linthicum A, Cawley EP, et al. Gardner's syndrome. *Arch Dermatol* 1964; 90:20–30.
16. Headington JT. Tumors of the hair follicles. *Am J Pathol* 1976; 85:480.
17. Smith JD, Chernosky ME. Apocrine hidrocystoma (cystadenoma). *Arch Dermatol* 1974; 109:700–702.
18. Smith JD, Chernosky ME. Hidrocystomas. *Arch Dermatol* 1973; 108:676–679.
19. Fretzin DF, Helwig EB. Atypical fibroxanthoma of the skin: a clinicopathologic study of 140 cases. *Cancer* 1973; 31:1541.
20. Cohen BA, Hood AF. Xanthogranuloma: reports on clinical and histological findings in 64 patients. *Pediatr Dermatol* 1989; 6:262–266.
21. Apisarnthanarax P. Granular cell tumor (review). *J Am Acad Dermatol* 1981; 5:171–182.
22. Grimes PE, Arora S, Minus HR, et al. Dermatosis papulosa nigra. *Cutis* 1983; 32:385–392.
23. Willoughby C, Sater NA. Stucco keratosis. *Arch Dermatol* 1972; 105:859–861.
24. Montgomery H, Dorffel J. Verruca senilis and keratoma senile. *Arch Dermatol Syph* 1932; 166:286.
25. Moller R, Reymann F, Hon-Jensen K. Metastases in dermatological patients with squamous cell carcinoma. *Arch Dermatol* 1979; 115:703.
26. Crain RC, Helwig EB. Dermal cylindroma (dermal eccrine cylindroma). *Am J Clin Pathol* 1961; 35:504–515.

Suggested Reading

Demis DJ, ed. *Clinical dermatology.* Philadelphia: JB Lippincott, 1994.
Farmer ER, Hood AF. *Pathology of the skin.* East Norwalk, CN: Appleton and Lange, 1990.
Fitzpatrick TB, et al. *Dermatology in general medicine.* New York: McGraw-Hill, 1993.
Lever WF, Schaumburg-Lever G. *Histopathology of the skin.* Philadelphia: JB Lippincott, 1990.

18

Surgical Management of Cutaneous Melanoma

Hilliard F. Seigler, M.D., F.A.C.S.

The incidence of cutaneous melanoma is increasing. Historically, this malignancy comprised approximately three percent of all neoplastic diseases. Over the past decade, melanoma has increased in our population by more than 90%. A generation ago, melanoma occurred in 1 in 1500 Americans, whereas currently 1 in 100 are expected to develop the disease. It is predicted that by the turn of the century this will increase to 1 in 90 whites living in the Southern Hemisphere. The reconstructive surgeon is involved both with the management of primary disease and reconstructive procedures and with the surgical management of metastatic disease. Questions concerning biopsy procedures, operative management of the primary lesion, the role of regional lymphadnectomy, and the type of reconstruction depend on both clinical presentation and histopathologic features. The prognostic factors and indicators for cutaneous melanoma have been investigated thoroughly and are of utmost importance to the surgeon who is devising a comprehensive treatment plan for the patient.

Clinical and Pathologic Features

There are four histopathologic types of cutaneous melanoma: (a) lentigo maligna melanoma (Fig. 18–1); (b) superficial spreading melanoma (Fig. 18–2); (c) acral lentiginous melanoma (Fig. 18–3); and (d) nodular melanoma (Fig. 18–4). With the exception of nodular melanoma, all others demonstrate an intraepidermal component. In a clinical sense, the early-growth phase is in a radial direction, and only nodular melanoma exhibits vertical growth from its inception. If early diagnosis could be established for the first three types before vertical growth and involvement of the vascular structures took place, most could be cured by simple excision alone. Unfortunately, diagnosis is often delayed, and thus the prognosis is less favorable. Lentigo melanoma occurs most commonly in older people in sun-exposed areas of the body. These cutaneous areas demonstrate prominent solar elastosis. Superficial spreading melanoma is characterized by differing areas of pigmentation with irregular borders. Acral lentiginous melanomas occur in focal body sites and have a typical appearance. Nodular melanomas usually have homogenous pigmentation with well-circumscribed borders and pronounced vertical growth.

Adequate tissue representation obtained by a biopsy is the responsibility of the surgeon or dermatologist. The pathologist can be helpful only if the tissue received is representative of the most severe involvement of the primary tumor

process. Whenever possible, excisional biopsy is preferred. However, should the lesion be in a difficult location or be quite large, an incisional biopsy should be done in the area of the primary tumor that exhibits the most severe clinical involvement. The indications for biopsy are dictated by changes that have taken place in the pigmented lesions. These changes are characterized by (a) irregular surfaces, (b) irregular borders, and (c) changes in pigmentation. Scaling and ulceration are also important characteristics.

The pathologist should make careful notations concerning the depth of invasion, tumor thickness, tumor ulceration, type of primary, and presence or absence of satellitosis. Each of these histopathologic features is an important prognostic factor. The contributions of Clark and colleagues (1) on the importance of level of invasion is well recognized (Table 18–1). In terms of reproducibility and clinical correlation, tumor thickness as described by Breslow (2) carries with it a greater statistical significance (Fig. 18–5).

Balch and others (3) have reported the importance of tumor ulceration. If the tumor is confined to the epidermis and measures less than a millimeter in thickness, simple excision alone will cure more than 90% of the patients. For tumor thickness of 1 to 1.5 mm a margin of 1 cm is adequate. If the tumor is 1.5 mm in thickness or greater, the general recommendation is a margin of 2 cm. Only large, primary tumors with either microscopic or macroscopic satellitosis will require broader tissue margins.

Association of Pathologic Types with Clinical Presentation

Lentigo maligna melanoma has a tendency to occur in older individuals and is generally seen on sun-exposed areas of the body. The most common location is the head and neck; however, this type of melanoma can occur on the dorsum of the hands and feet. Its biologic behavior demonstrates a pro-

Table 18–1
Description of Tumor Invasion by Clark's Level

Clark Level	Description
1	All tumor cells above basement membrane
2	Invasion into loose connective tissue of papillary dermis
3	Tumor cells at junction of papillary and reticular dermis
4	Invasion into reticular dermis
5	Invasion into subcutaneous fat

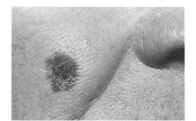

FIG. 18–1. Lentigo maligna melanoma of the right cheek.

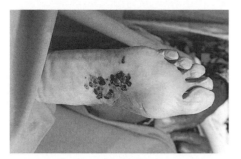

FIG. 18–3. Acral lentiginous melanoma.

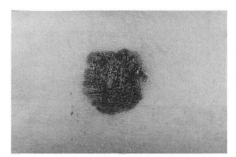

FIG. 18–2. Superficial spreading melanoma.

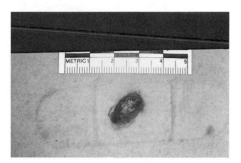

FIG. 18–4. Nodular melanoma.

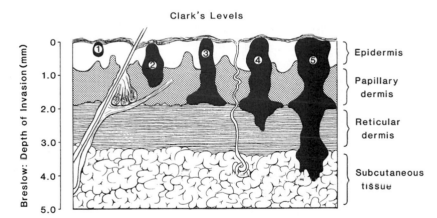

Clark's Levels

FIG. 18–5. Prognostic factors showing Clark's level of invasion and Breslow's depth of invasion.

longed radial-growth phase. The lesion has a tendency to exist for a number of years before undergoing rapid change that directs the patient to seek medical attention. If the lesion involves the dorsum of the hands and feet, excision and primary closure of small lesions is adequate, whereas larger lesions may require split-thickness skin grafting. If the lesion involves the skin of the face, excision and cosmetic grafting or flap coverage may be required. Overall, the prognosis of lentigo maligna is excellent.

Superficial spreading melanoma and nodular melanoma have a tendency to occur in similar areas of the body. Nodular melanomas can usually be excised and the wound closed primarily. If the primary lesion has extended secondary to delayed detection, skin grafts or flaps can usually be accomplished without undue difficulty. If the scalp is involved and the tumor is small, it is preferable to excise the primary lesion with flap coverage. If the lesion has a wide diameter, excision extending to the galea plus skin grafting is usually

necessary. Because of the rich lymphatic and vascular supply, scalp lesions have a tendency to recur locally if adequate borders are not accomplished by the surgeon. Lesions involving the ala of the nose and pinna of the ear are associated with a guarded prognosis and a high incidence of local recurrence and regional metastasis. We recommend partial amputation in these areas.

Reconstruction can be accomplished for nasal primaries using composite grafts, but standard reconstruction should be done if a large portion of the ear has been deleted in an effort to gain control of the primary (Fig. 18–6). Fortunately, eyelid primaries are extremely rare. If the lid is involved, excision with standard lid reconstruction is the recommended procedure for lesions greater than 1 mm in thickness. If lesion thickness is less than 1 mm, excision and thin split-thickness skin grafting can be accomplished.

Acral lentiginous melanomas occur in the subungual area, the palms, plantar surfaces, mucous membranes, and anorec-

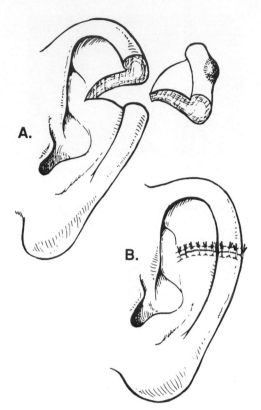

FIG. 18–6. Wedge excision of ear.

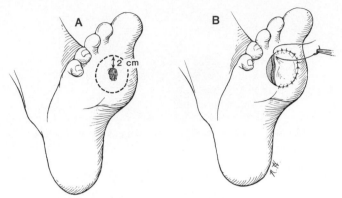

FIG. 18–7.   A, local excision of primary melanoma. Two-centimeter margins represent adequate measurement for excision. **B,** split-thickness skin grafting providing wound closure.

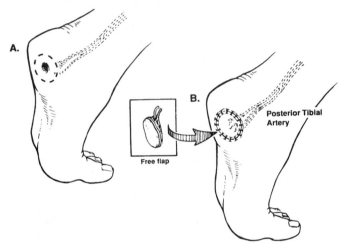

FIG. 18–8. Vascularized flap coverage.

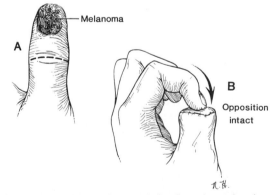

FIG. 18–9. A, partial thumb amputation for subungal melanoma. B, thumb amputation permits functional digital opposition.

tal junction. Palmer and plantar acral lentiginous primaries require wide local excision and either split thickness skin grafting or vascularized flap coverage (Figs. 18–7, 18–8). If the area of involvement is near the toe or web space, wide local excision, with toe amputation and a fillet flap, usually provides excellent coverage without functional disability.

Lesions involving mucous membranes often have a poor prognosis. Not only is local control difficult to achieve but the likelihood of systemic spread of the disease is also high. If the lesion is confined to the mucous membranes of the genital tract, excision with 2-cm margins should be planned. The type of closure will be dictated by the area of the primary lesion. If the glans penis or clitoris is involved, amputation is necessary.

Melanomas occurring in the mucous membranes of the nose and sinuses should be approached with the realization that the prognosis is poor. Local excision followed by irradiation and adjuvant systemic therapy is the usual recommended regimen.

Biopsies are done on pigmented lesions in the subungual position if they persist beyond 3–4 weeks. The procedure requires removal of the nail and wedge biopsy of the nail bed. It is necessary to amputate at the distal interphalangeal joint and no attempt at local control by excision and cross-digit flap should be entertained. If the lesion is quite large and advanced to the area of the distal joint, total deletion of the digit may be necessary. If the thumb is involved, the surgeon should attempt to preserve opposition (Fig. 18–9). A reasonably functional result can be realized if the amputation is done at the level of the interphalangeal joint.

FIRST-ORDER LYMPH NODES

Efficacy of elective lymph-node dissection in patients with melanoma has been argued over the years. Large series of patients followed for a number of years provide data suggesting that the benefit of elective lymph-node dissection is not statistically significant (4). Patients who have a tumor thickness of 1.5 mm or less only rarely demonstrate even occult micrometastasis to lymph nodes. Patients who have primary tumors of 4 mm or greater in thickness have a high probability of systemic disease that exceeds the potential therapeutic benefit of performing regional elective lymph-node dissection. Clinical trials are presently underway as to identification and removal of the sentinel node. Either vital dye or isotope is injected at the primary site and the dominant first-order lymph node identified and removed under local anesthesia. If the sentinel node is involved with metastatic disease, that lymph node basin is subjected to surgical lymphadenectomy. If the sentinel node is free from metastatic disease, the lymph node basin is left intact and followed clinically. Insufficient data exist to recommend this as a standard of care.

There is little argument of the prognostic value of lymphadenectomy. Patients with a single positive lymph node have a 60% risk of recurrent disease. Those with 2 to 4 positive lymph nodes have a 75% risk factor, and those with more than 4 positive lymph nodes are at greater than 90% risk of recurrent disease. If the lesion occurs on the lower extremity, a computed tomography (CT) scan of the pelvis and abdomen should be completed. If abnormal lymph nodes are not detected at the site of iliac lymph nodes and peri-aortic lymph nodes, then a superficial groin dissection is probably adequate. Removal of the deep iliac nodes adds to limb morbidity, and resection probably does not increase the disease-free interval. If the deep iliac nodes are involved, the probability of systemic disease usually dictates the eventual outcome, and more than 90% of patients die secondary to the disease. If the lesion occurs on the upper extremity, standard axillary dissection preserving the pectoralis major and minor muscles is recommended.

CHEMOTHERAPY

Chemotherapeutic drugs can be administered either systemically or by regional infusion. They can be given for an adjuvant effect in patients at high risk with no evidence of disease, or to those patients with obvious tumor burdens in a treatment modality. Adjuvant systemic chemotherapy, either with a single drug or multiple drugs in varying combinations, has proven to be of little significant clinical benefit in patients at high risk of developing recurrent disease. A number of studies report marginal benefit from adjuvant chemotherapy (5).

Patients with documented tumor burden have demonstrated therapeutic benefit from systemic chemotherapy. The two most beneficial combinations include DTIC, CCNU, Vincristine, and Bleomycin administered over a 5-day period every 6 weeks (6) or Cis-platin, DTIC, BCNU, and Tamoxifen administered monthly (7). The total-response rate of either regimen is 10%, while an additional 25 to 30% of patients will realize a partial response. Chemotherapy has been most useful for those patients with metastatic disease involving the skin, subcutaneous tissue, lymph nodes, and lungs. Anatomic areas of involvement associated with a poor response include brain, bone, liver, and the gastrointestinal tract (8).

Regional drug infusion, either at normothermic or hyperthermic temperatures, has undergone numerous clinical trials. Limb perfusion for high-risk patients in an adjuvant setting has shown clear benefit. Additionally, studies show limb perfusion has a significant therapeutic benefit in patients with local recurrent disease, in-transit lesions, or those with numerous metastatic lesions involving only the affected extremity (9,10). The major shortcoming of this technique is that patients are at high risk for the development of systemic disease. Failures in the regional form of therapy usually lead to the development of distant disease. For this reason, many oncologists recommend systemic combination chemotherapy for patients receiving regional perfusion. Morbidity following limb perfusion includes muscle compartment syndrome, major skin loss, and decrease in range of motion. These are significant side effects and must be weighed carefully when recommending regional therapy for patients treated in the adjuvant mode.

IMMUNOTHERAPY

In a classical sense, immunotherapy can be administered either passively or actively. Passive immunotherapy includes passive serotherapy and passive cellular therapy. Active immunotherapy includes nonspecific immunogens as well as a specific immunogen. Passive administration of specific monoclonal antibody alone, or of immunoconjugants, continues to be evaluated. A phase I clinical trial reported some clinical benefit (11) The passive administration of modified host lymphocytes has been under intensive investigation over the past few years. This technique has utilized lymphokine activated lymphocytes, expanded tumor infiltrating lymphocytes and specific cytotoxic T cells. Traditionally, the most efficient means of producing clinically relative immunity has been in the area of specific active immunization. Melanoma patients have been immunized, either with intact autologous or allogenic melanoma cells, or with a viral oncolysate prepared from such cells (12,13) The data suggests that statistically significant therapeutic benefit is produced in high-risk stage I and stage II patients treated in the adjuvant mode. At present, numerous gene therapy trials are underway. Most of the relevant interleukin genes have been cloned and can successfully be transduced into the cell gnome. Cytokines, including interleukin-1, interleukin-2, interleukin-4, interleukin-12, tumor necrosis factor, and G-CSF, are presently being evaluated in phase I and phase II trials. Melanoma tumor cells transduced with the gene for human ∞-interferon have up-regulated MHC antigens as well as tumor-associated antigens expressed in the context of these histocompatibility antigens. Experimentally, these tumor cells are far more immunogenic than tumor cells not genetically altered. Alteration of the immunogenecity of tumor cells by genetic manipulation is undergoing experimental and clinical trials at present (14).

Bibliography

1. Clark WH Jr, From L, Bernardino EA, et al. The histogenesis and biologic behavior of primary human malignant melanomas of the skin. *Cancer Res* 1969; 29:705.
2. Breslow A. Thickness cross-sectional areas of depth of invasion in the prognosis of cutaneous melanoma. *Ann Surg* 1970; 172:902.
3. Balch CM, Soong S, Murad TM, et al. A multifactorial analysis of melanoma. III. Prognostic factors in melanoma patients with lymph node metastases (stage II). *Ann Surg* 1981; 193:377.
4. Slingluff CL Jr, Stidham KR, Ricci WM, et al. Surgical management of regional lymph nodes in patients with melanoma: experience with 4,682 patients. *Ann Surg* 1995; 221:435.
5. Barth A, Morton DL. The role of adjuvant therapy in melanoma management (review). *Cancer* 1995; 75 (2 suppl): 726.

6. Seigler HF, Lucas VS, Pickett NJ, et al. DTIC, CCNU, Bleomycin and Vincristine (BOLD) in metastatic melanoma. *Cancer* 1980; 46: 2346.

7. McClay EF, Mastangelo MJ, et al. The importance of tamoxifen to a cisplatin-containing regimen in the treatment of metastatic melanoma. *Cancer* 1989; 63:1292.

8. Atzpodien J, Lopez HE, Kirchner H, et al. Chemoimmunotherapy of advanced malignant melanoma: sequential administration of subcutaneous interleukin-2 and interferon-alpha after intravenous dacarbazine and carboplatin or intravenous dacarbazine, cisplatin, carmustine and tamoxifen. *Eur J Cancer* 1995; 31A:876.

9. McBridge CM, Sugarbaker EV, Hickey RC. Prophylactic isolation-perfusion as the primary therapy for invasive malignant melanoma of the limbs. *Ann Surg* 1975; 182:316.

10. Stehlen JS, Smith JL, Jing B, et al. Melanomas of the extremities complicated by intransit metastases. *Surg Gynecol Obstet* 1966; 122:3.

11. Hougton AN, Mintzer D, et al. Mouse monoclonal 1g G3 antibody detecting GD3 ganglioside: a phase I trial in patients with malignant melanoma. *Proc Natl Acad Sci USA* 1985; 82:1242–1246.

12. Cassel WA, Murray DR, Phillips HS. A phase II study on the postsurgical management of stage II malignant melanoma with a Newcastle disease virus oncolysate. *Cancer* 1983; 52:856.

13. Seigler HF, Cos E, Mutzner F, et al. Specific active immunotherapy for melanoma. *Ann Surg* 1979; 190:366.

14. Lu C, Kerbel RS. Cytokines, growth factors and the loss of negative growth controls in the progression of human cutaneous malignant melanoma (review). *Curr Opin Oncol* 1994; 6:212.

19

Management of Benign and Malignant Primary Salivary-Gland Tumors

Mark S. Granick, M.D. F.A.C.S., Dwight C. Hanna, M.D. F.A.C.S., and Mark P. Solomon, M.D. F.A.C.S.

Primary neoplasms of the salivary glands are uncommon, comprising less than 3% of all head and neck tumors (1). Their diverse range of pathology, the complex interrelationships between the tumors, their location adjacent to various critical anatomic structures, and the variable biologic behavior of the different histopathologic tumor types all complicate their management.

Proper treatment begins with an accurate histopathologic diagnosis. Foote and Frazell (2) were the first to attempt a comprehensive pathologic classification of parotid tumors. Batsakis and colleagues (3) have redefined and clarified this categorization into the currently accepted standard (Table 19–1).

A number of large series have been published during the past 30 years, and in general the distribution and percentage of histopathologic types are similar. The larger glands have the most tumors and the highest percentage of benign tumors (Table 19–2). By far the most common benign tumor in all of the salivary glands is the pleomorphic adenoma (benign mixed tumor). Mucoepidermoid carcinoma is the most common parotid malignancy, while adenoid cystic carcinoma is the most common malignancy in the submandibular and minor salivary glands.

Preoperative Evaluation

The most common presentation is that of a painless mass (Fig. 19–1). A fluctuant or soft mass is most commonly associated with the benign Warthin tumor. A mass bulging behind the lateral oropharyngeal wall frequently represents a parotid deep lobe tumor. Associated symptoms may include pain or facial weakness, both of which are suggestive of underlying malignancies; but, even the most experienced examiners cannot reliably determine whether a mass is benign or malignant. Duration of symptoms is more than 1.5 years in 50% of patients (4,5).

Gallia and Johnson (6) demonstrated that as many as 85% of submandibular and 27% of parotid lesions treated by excision were inflammatory disorders. At least two-thirds of the patients with submandibular gland disease gave a history of recurrent postprandial pain, erythema, swelling, and purulent discharge. Examination of each patient should include careful attention to the oral cavity and oropharynx. Warthin and Stensen ducts and orifices must be viewed and palpated for signs of inflammation, tumor, scarring, sialolithiasis, and saliva flow. Lack of resolution with appropriate medical treatment of a mass suspected of being inflammatory demands histopathologic analysis.

The tonsillar fossa and soft palate must be examined for the presence of deep-lobe parotid involvement. Direct palpation of the individual glands must be done bimanually to appreciate intraglandular masses. Bilateral comparison of the glands is important to detect subtle abnormalities. The neck needs to be thoroughly examined for nodal involvement. In addition, potential primary sites that can metastasize to the salivary glands must be examined such as scalp, face, and distant sites (7-9).

Preoperative radiographic studies may delineate a mass lesion but are useless in deciding whether it is malignant (10). Imaging studies, however, are externally useful in assessing local tissue invasion and destruction, as well as the extent of tumor. Preoperative computed tomography (CT) or magnetic resonance (MR) imaging is recommended for invasive tumors, some recurrent tumors, and large oral tumors. Ultrasonic analysis is not clinically valuable at this time (11). Radionuclide imaging is only able to detect mass lesions greater than 1.5 cm in diameter (12). Warthin tumor and oncocytoma specifically concentrate technetium 99m, but this is not presently of clinical use.

BIOPSY

As a rule, all salivary gland tumors should be excised. The value of preliminary biopsy is controversial. Eneroth (13) and others (14) have advocated fine-needle aspiration, reporting a 74 to 92% accuracy. Fine-needle aspiration is particularly useful in identifying nonneoplastic masses that may respond to medication, tumor metastases to the parotid, and nonsurgical lymphomas (15). Almost all neoplasms should be excised regardless of the result of fine-needle biopsy since only positive diagnoses are significant (16).

Indications for large-core needle or incisional biopsy include differentiation of inflammatory from neoplastic masses and diagnosis of inflammatory masses. Frozen-section diagnosis of malignant salivary neoplasms is unreliable in some hands (17,18). In our experience, frozen-section analysis has been accurate and useful, particularly in those instances when we are debating the necessity of facial-nerve resection. Our accuracy rate of frozen section, based on 462 salivary tumors, is 95.7% (19).

STAGING

The current American Joint Committee on Cancer (20) clinical staging system for cancer of the salivary gland is based on five clinical variables that influence survival rates over a 10-year period. These variables include tumor size,

Table 19–1
Classification of Epithelial Salivary Gland Tumors[a]

Type of Lesion	Variations
Benign	Mixed tumor (pleomorphic adenoma)
	Papillary cystadenoma lymphomatosum (Warthin's tumor)
	Oncocystoma oncocytosis
	Monomorphic tumors
	Basal cell adenoma
	Glycogen-rich adenoma (?)
	Clear-cell adenoma (?)
	Membranous adenoma
	Myoepithelioma
	Sebaceous tumors
	Adenoma
	Lymphadenoma
	Papillary ductal adenoma (papilloma)
	Benign lymphoepithelial lesion
	Unclassified
Malignant	Carcinoma ex pleomorphic adenoma (carcinoma arising in a mixed tumor)
	Malignant mixed tumor (biphasic malignancy)
	Mucoepidermoid carcinoma
	Low grade
	Intermediate grade
	High grade
	Adenoid cystic carcinoma
	Adenocarcinoma
	Mucus-producing adenopapillary and nonpapillary carcinoma
	Salivary duct carcinoma (ductal carcinoma)
	Other adenocarcinomas
	Oncocytic cell carcinoma (malignant oncocytoma)
	Clear-cell carcinoma (nonmucinous and glycogen containing or non-glycogen containing)
	Primary squamous cell carcinoma
	Hybrid basal cell adenoma-adenoid cystic carcinoma
	Undifferentiated carcinoma
	Epithelial myoepithelial carcinoma of intercalated ducts
	Miscellaneous (includes sebaceous lesions, Stenson's duct lesions, melanoma, and carcinoma exlymphoepithelial lesions)
	Metastatic
	Unclassified

[a]From Batsakis JG, Regezi JA: The pathology of head and neck tumors: Salivary glands part 1. *Head Neck Surg* 1:59, 1978–1979.

Table 19–2
Distribution of Salivary Gland Tumors

Gland	% Salivary Gland Tumors	% Malignant Tumors
Parotid	80	25
Submandibular	15	35
Minor salivary glands	5	50

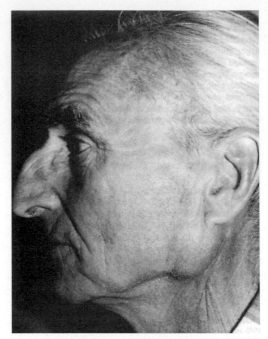

FIG. 19–1. Most salivary gland tumors present as a painless mass.

Table 19–3
Proposed Staging System for Major Salivary Gland Cancer (Parotid and Submandibular)[a]

Code	Criterion
T_0	No clinical evidence of primary tumor
T_1	Tumor less than 2.0 cm in diameter without significant local extension
T_2	Tumor 2.1–4.0 cm in diameter without significant local extension
T_3	Tumor 4.1–6.0 cm in diameter without significant local extension
T_{4a}	Tumor more than 6 cm in diameter without significant local extension
T_{4b}	Tumor of any size with significant local extension
N_0	No evidence of regional lymph node involvement (including palpable but not suspicious regional lymph nodes)
N_1	Evidence of regional lymph node involvement (including palpable and suspicious regional lymph ndes)
N_x	Regional lymph nodes not assessed
M_0	No distant metastases
M_1	Distant metastases such as to bone, lung, etc.
	Stage I $T_1N_0M_0$
	$T_2N_0M_0$
	Stage II $T_3N_0M_0$
	Stage III $T_1N_1M_0$
	$T_2N_1M_0$
	$T_{4a}N_0M_0$
	$T_{4b}N_0M_0$
	Stage IV $T_3N_1M_0$
	$T_{4a}N_1M_0$
	$T_{4b}N_1M_0$
	Any T, Any N, and M_1

[a]From Levitt SH, McHugh RB, Gomez-Martin O, et al: Clinical staging system for cancer of the salivary gland. A retrospective study. *Cancer* 47:2712, 1981.

Table 19–4
Stage Grouping in Salivary Gland Cancer (Using Five Clinical Variables)[a,b]

TNM Set	No. of Patients	5-year Survival Probability (%)	SE (%)
Stage I			
$T_1N_0M_0$	136	90.1	2.6
$T_2N_0M_0$	151	85.9	2.9
Overall	287	87.9	2.0
Stage II			
$T_3N_0M_0$	51	56.9	6.9
Overall	51	56.9	6.9
Stage III			
$T_1N_1M_0$	4		
$T_2N_1M_0$	16	0.0	0.0
$T_{4a}N_0M_0$	30	40.2	9.3
$T_{4b}N_0M_0$	106	45.2	4.9
Overall	156	39.4	4.0
Stage IV			
$T_3N_1M_0$	8		
$T_{4a}N_1M_0$	12	17.7	10.8
$T_{4b}N_1M_0$	38	7.9	4.4
Any T, Any N, and M_1	8		
Overall	66	9.1	3.5

[a]From Levitt SH, McHugh RB, Gomez-Martin O, et al: Clinical staging system for cancer of the salivary gland. A retrospective study. *Cancer* 47:2712, 1981.
[b]Combination of five variables: *primary tumor:* size, local extension; *regional lymph nodes:* palpability, suspicion; *motastasis:* distant metastasis.

local extension, presence of distant metastases, palpability of regional nodes, and "suspicion of metastatic carcinoma" in regional nodes (Table 19–3). Clinical stage and histologic grade have been reliable predictors of outcome for salivary gland cancers of different types and in varied locations (21-24).Five-year survival probabilities range from 85 to 90% for stage II and III tumors to 9% for stage IV tumors (Table 19–4).

Clinical Management

BENIGN PAROTID TUMORS

Pleomorphic Adenoma (Mixed Tumor)

Pleomorphic adenomas are the most common salivary-gland tumors. Rauch's (25) review of 4245 pleomorphic adenomas revealed that 84% of them occur in the parotid gland. In Spiro's evaluation of 2807 salivary gland tumors, 70% of the parotid and 45% of all tumors were benign mixed (16). Clinically, they appear as firm, discrete, gradually enlarging parotid masses. Rarely, pain or facial paralysis may occur. Grossly, the tumors appear to be solid and encapsulated. Histologicallly, however, the capsule is actually composed of compressed tumor cells. There are, in addition, multiple projections, and sometimes multicentric foci of tumor, in the gland (26). The cell types composing this tumor consist of a spectrum ranging from epithelial to myoepithelial cells (3).

When a pleomorphic adenoma recurs, the morbidity of the tumor and necessity of additional therapy increases dramatically. Recurrent benign mixed tumors are generally locally

aggressive and infiltrative. O'Dwyer and others (27) cited a 26% incidence of facial nerve sacrifice in recurrent tumor excisions, and claimed that the major morbidity associated with benign mixed tumors is related to skill in managing recurrence. Because of the high risk to the facial nerve as well as the aggressive nature of recurrent benign tumors, Piorkowski and Guillamondegui have advocated radiation treatment for these lesions (28).

Pleomorphic adenomas tend to recur if inadequately excised, and there is potential for malignancy in long standing tumors (29-32), dictating their management by generous excision. Lanier and colleagues (29) demonstrated that there was a 70% recurrence rate in enucleated tumors, whereas following superficial parotidectomy there was a 3.6% recurrence rate. Adequate surgical removal of pleomorphic adenoma consists of superficial or total parotidectomy. Dawson and Orr (32) demonstrated that irradiation was useful to prevent recurrences in difficult surgical situations such as in deep-lobe tumor, poor margins of resection, or tumor adjacent to the facial nerve.

Narvig and Soberg (33) followed 238 patients who underwent superficial parotidectomies for plemorphic adenoma for a mean of 18 years. Six (2.5%) developed recurrences between 7 and 18 years (mean, 11.8 years) postoperatively. Surprisingly, the patients who had intraoperative tumor spillage did not have a significantly increased rate of recurrence (8%). Some researchers advocate partial parotidectomy (34,35), claiming no recurrences between 1 and 5 years following surgery. A 5-year follow-up, however, is an inadequate period for evaluating the efficacy of surgery for plemorphic adenoma.

Warthin Tumor (Papillary Cystadenoma Lymphomatosum)

Warthin tumor is the second most common benign parotid neoplasm, accounting for 15% of all parotid tumors. It is a tumor of the salivary oncocyte, a cell that is thought to be an epithelial-cell mutant, rarely present in parotid tissues before 40 to 50 years of age (3). In addition, there is a lymphoid stroma in these lesions. The tumors are multicentric and/or bilateral in 10 to 15% of patients (36). Patients are generally middle-aged men who have a soft, cystic-feeling mass in the tail of the parotid. Adequate therapy consists of superficial parotidectomy. In spite of the apparent localization of the tumor in the tail of the parotid in many patients, the high incidence of multicentricity dictates against limited parotid resections.

MALIGNANT PAROTID TUMORS

The best staging parameters, the appropriate extent of surgery, the management of the facial nerve, the treatment of the clinically negative neck, and the use of adjuvant therapy are all issues of current concern in parotid cancer. Tumor histology is an important predictor of survival, with mucoepidermoid carcinoma and acinic cell carcinoma having the best survival statistics (37). Histologic grading is also a critical predictor, with low-grade tumors having a 90% 10-year survival, while high-grade tumors have a 25% 10-year survival (15). Interestingly, (TNM) staging also correlates with prognosis, the 10-year survivals being 90%, 65%, and 22% for stages I, II, and III tumors, respectively (16,22,23).

Adequacy of surgical treatment is also an independent predictor of outcome. In one series of patients with acinic cell carcinoma, a relatively low-grade malignancy, 6 of 7 patients treated with tumor enucleation recurred. One of eight patients undergoing parotidectomy recurred (38). In a similar recent series of acinic cell carcinomas (39), 9 of 20 patients recurred. Recurrence was correlated with inadequate surgical margins.

The best procedure, in terms of local tumor control, still consists of wide local excision. Superficial parotidectomy with facial-nerve preservation is the minimum treatment. The extent of surgery depends on the extent of disease rather than histology (16,37,40). The facial nerve should be excised if it is involved with malignant tumor. All additional tumor-involved tissue, including adjacent skin, bone, and muscle, should be similarly ablated. Some studies suggest elective neck dissection as a staging aid (41). The use of adjuvant irradiation to the primary site and ipsilateral neck for advanced, high-grade, or marginally resected tumors has provided significant improvement in locoregional control but has not improved long-term survival (37,42,48).

Mucoepidermoid Carcinoma

This malignant tumor accounts for 50% of parotid malignancies (37). It arises from interlobular and intralobular ductal epithelium and is mucin producing. There is a spectrum of biologic activity, with low-grade or well-differentiated types acting in an almost benign fashion. The intermediate-grade tumors are less differentiated and tend to be locally invasive. The high-grade or poorly differentiated tumors are very cellular and may be confused with squamous cell tumors. These lesions are very aggressive locally, have a high recurrence rate, and tend to metastasize. Patients usually present with a painless solitary parotid mass having been present for 1 year or less. As many as 20% of patients with high-grade tumors have facial-nerve dysfunction (49). Factors most influencing survival of these patients are the histologic grade of the tumor, the presence of clinically positive cervical nodes, and the clinical stage of the tumor.

Appropriate therapy consists of parotidectomy with excision and immediate nerve grafting of the facial nerve only if the tumor involves the nerve. Cervical lymphadenectomy is reserved for patients with palpable nodes. Radiation therapy to the primary site and lateral neck is advisable at 3 to 5 weeks postoperatively for moderate to high-grade tumors and advanced stage tumors.

In Pleomorphic Adenoma

Malignant tumors in pleomorphic adenomas comprise 10 to 20% of salivary malignancies. This neoplasm is highly malignant with a tendency to metastasize. In the series by Spiro and others (50), 25% of patients had cervical-node metastases and 32% had distant metastases to brain, bone, and lung. The presence of metastatic disease was usually associated with death within 1 year. Tortoledo and colleagues (51) demonstrated that survival was related to the degree of extension of malignant disease beyond the benign aspect of the tumor. Tumor extension greater than 8 mm was uniformly fatal, whereas those patients having less than 6 mm tumor extension all survived.

A malignant tumor in a pleomorphic adenoma is of controversial histopathologic origin (3). Six histologic subtypes

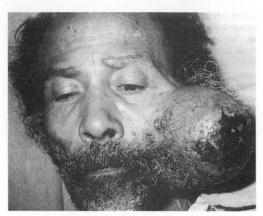

FIG. 19–2. This 67-year-old patient had a longstanding stable parotid mass that suddenly and rapidly began to enlarge. The pathology revealed malignant tumor in pleomorphic adenoma.

with differing prognoses have been identified (51). The common type occurs in long standing or recurrent benign mixed tumor (Fig. 19–2). Treatment includes total parotidectomy, resection and immediate grafting of the facial nerve if involved with tumor, and neck dissection if there are nodal metastases.

Adenoid Cystic Carcinoma

This lesion is relatively uncommon in the parotid (7 to 15% of malignancies) but is the most common malignant tumor of the submandibular and minor salivary glands (35%). Adenoid cystic carcinoma has a variable histologic pattern ranging from cellular to cystic even within the same tumor.

Early perineural invasion with local spread is common, and later distant metastases, especially to lung, contribute to long-term failure. Recurrences or metastases may occur after 20 or more disease-free years following initial treatment. Clinical staging is the only accurate predictor of survival (23).

The accepted form of treatment for this tumor is similar to other parotid malignant tumors. Particular attention must be paid to the facial nerve because of this tumor's tendency to spread perineurally. Postoperative radiation therapy has improved locoregional control, but not improved long-term survival owing to poor control of distant metastases Z (52-55). Our current preference is for wide local excision and radiation therapy for advanced tumors, and local excision for small lesions.

Other Malignant Parotid Tumors

There are a variety of less common cancers also occur in the parotid (see Table 19–1) (3,5,56-59). Acinic cell carcinoma is locally aggressive but rarely involves the facial nerve or metastasizes to the neck (38,39). Adenocarcinoma (54,60) and epidermoid carcinoma often require facial-nerve resection and cervical lymphadenectomy. Lymphoma may present in the parotid and is the only nonsurgically treated parotid cancer (61). Tumors that can metastasize to parotid include squamous cell carcinoma in the watershed area draining through the gland (62). Additional distant sources of metastases include lung, breast, kidney, colon, stomach, pancreas, prostate, and distant melanoma (9,62,63). A recently recognized source of parotid tumors is the lymphadenopathies related to acquired immunodeficiency syndrome (AIDS) (64,65).

STRATEGY FOR MANAGEMENT OF PAROTID TUMORS

Our guidelines include a number of basic concepts that are little changed from those proposed in 1975 (4), from which decisions can be formulated for the management of specific cases.

1. Excisional biopsy is accomplished by superficial or total parotidectomy.
   (a) Preliminary biopsy is rarely indicated.
   (b) Superficial parotidectomy is performed for all tumors.
   (c) Deep-lobe tumors require superficial parotidectomy for exposure of the facial nerve, followed by resection of the deep lobe.
   (d) Frozen-section analysis of the tumor is routinely performed as an aid in determining the extent of surgery.
2. Management of the facial nerve.
   (a) Possible facial nerve dysfunction following surgery is explained to all patients.
   (b) Sacrifice of the facial nerve trunk or branches is necessary only when malignant tumor invades or is directly adherent to the nerve.
   (c) Immediate nerve graft reconstruction is performed in all cases following nerve resection.
3. Management of malignant tumors.
   (a) Total parotidectomy with facial-nerve preservation is appropriate for most malignant tumors.
   (b) see 2(b).
   (c) Cervical lymphadenectomy is performed when there is palpable cervical adenopathy associated with a malignant neoplasm. Prophylactic node (NO) neck dissection is considered in patients with squamous cell carcinoma and highly undifferentiated malignancies.
   (d) Radical resection of all tumor-involved tissue is required if extraglandular spread has occurred.
   (e) Postoperative radiation therapy is advisable for all moderate to high-grade malignancies, and any stage II or greater malignancy.

SUBMANDIBULAR GLAND TUMORS

Submandibular gland tumors (Fig. 19–3) are less common than parotid tumors, but are more likely to be malignant (see Table 19–3). The histopathologic types are the same as parotid, but adenoid cystic carcinoma is the more common malignancy (66,67). Benign pleomorphic adenoma is by far the most common benign neoplasm. Total gland excision is the biopsy technique. In small tumors, this may be adequate treatment. If frozen-section diagnosis discloses malignancy, an upper neck dissection should be performed to assure adequate resection and to sample the upper neck nodes and nerves. Indicators of poor prognosis include extraglandular spread or cervical metastases (24).

STRATEGY FOR MANAGEMENT OF SUBMANDIBULAR GLAND TUMORS

1. Excisional biopsy is accomplished by total glandular excision.
   (a) Preliminary biopsy is not indicated.
   (b) Frozen-section analysis of the tumor is routinely performed as an aid in determining the extent of surgery.

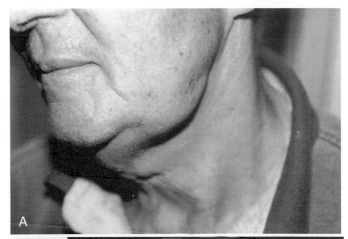

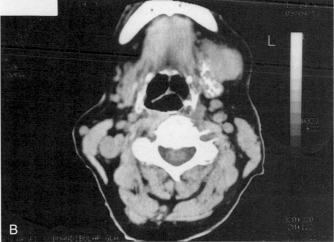

FIG. 19–3. **A,** this 60-year-old man presented with an asymptomatic mass in the region of the left submandibular gland. **B,** while we do not advocate routine imaging studies for submandibular tumors, this patient had a CT sialogram performed, demonstrating an intrinsic submandibular gland tumor. It was removed and found to be lymphoma.

2. Management of adjacent nerves.
   (a) Possible postoperative dysfunction of the marginal mandibular branch of the facial nerve, the hypoglossal nerve, and the lingual nerve, is explained to all patients.
   (b) Sacrifice of any of the adjacent nerves is performed only when malignant tumor invades or is directly adherent to a nerve.
   (c) Immediate nerve graft reconstruction should be performed if possible.
3. Management of malignant tumors.
   (a) Excision of the submandibular gland with submental and submandibular lymphadenectomy is appropriate for most malignant tumors.
   (b) see 2(b).
   (c) Cervical lymphadenectomy is performed when there is palpable cervical adenopathy associated with a malignant neoplasm and for high-grade, T_3 or T_4 malignant tumors.

(d) Radical resection of all tumor-involved tissue is performed if extracapsular spread has occurred.

(e) Postoperative radiation therapy is advisable for all stage II or greater malignancies.

MINOR SALIVARY-GLAND NEOPLASMS

Benign pleomorphic adenoma is the most common benign neoplasm of the minor salivary glands, but more than half of the neoplasms are malignant and most of these are adenoid cystic carcinoma (54). The palate is the most commonly involved site (Fig. 19–4) (55,68). These lesions generally present as firm smooth, asymptomatic submucosal masses. Neither the history nor the gross physical appearance of these tumors is predictive of their histopathology.

Necrotizing sialometaplasia, which commonly occurs as an ulcerated palatal mass, is a benign lesion but can be mistaken for mucoepidermoid or undifferentiated carcinoma on histologic examination. The histopathologic features that characterize this entity are squamous metaplasia of necrotic seromucinous glands with maintenance of lobular architecture, nonanaplastic nuclear morphology, and prominent acute

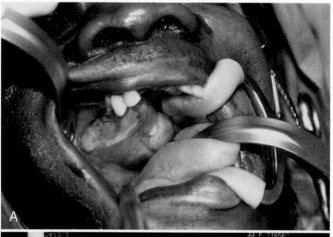

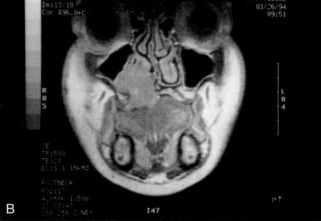

FIG. 19–4. A, this 52-year-old patient had an enormous palatal minor salivary gland tumor, an adenoid cystic carcinoma. **B,** CT scan demonstrates the local destruction associated with this tumor and the extent of disease. CT imaging is very helpful in tumors that involve deep-tissue invasion, or are inaccessible or difficult to examine.

and chronic inflammation (70). This lesion is a reactive metaplasia apparently related to local ischemia. Necrotizing sialometaplasia heals spontaneously and does not require excision (69-72).

STRATEGY FOR MANAGEMENT OF MINOR SALIVARY-GLAND TUMORS

1. Biopsy.
   (a) Excisional biopsy with a small margin of normal tissue is performed for most lesions less than 4 cm in diameter.
   (b) Preliminary incisional biopsy is advisable before definitive resection for lesions larger than 4 cm in diameter or for masses that are suspected of being necrotizing sialometaplasia.
   (c) Frozen-section analysis is routinely obtained as an aid in determining the extent of surgery and for control of the margins of resection.
2. Management of malignant tumors.
   (a) Local excision of the tumor with a small margin of adjacent normal tissue is appropriate for most malignancies.
   (b) Cervical metastases are rare and cervical lymphadenectomy should be performed only for palpable cervical adenopathy.
   (c) Immediate reconstruction of the excisional defect with local or distant tissue should be performed.
   (d) Postoperative radiation therapy should be considered for all moderate to high-grade malignancies, all malignant tumors larger than 4 cm, all tumors invading nonmucosal tissues, all cases of neural invasion, all cases associated with cervical metastases, and all instances of positive surgical margins.

PEDIATRIC SALIVARY TUMORS

Salivary-gland tumors in infants and children are rare and the topic is not widely covered in the literature. Mayo Clinic and M.D. Anderson (74) experiences showed a proportion of benign parotid lesions similar to adults, while the Iowa series had a 70% malignancy rate (75), and the Johns Hopkins experience demonstrated a 50% malignancy rate (76).

Benign pleomorphic adenoma was the most common benign tumor, followed by hemangioma, lymphangioma, and cystic hygroma (73,77). Mucoepidermoid carcinoma was the principle malignancy (74). A large survey of salivary-gland lesions in children revealed that 61% of 430 lesions were inflammatory (78). The evaluation of a child with a salivary-gland mass should be directed toward establishing whether the mass is inflammatory. If there is any doubt, or if the lesion is apparently a tumor, the treatment of choice is surgical excision.

Treatment

PAROTIDECTOMY: OPERATIVE TECHNIQUE

The key to parotidectomy is accurate, safe localization of the facial nerve. This has traditionally been performed by locating the main trunk of the nerve proximal to the parotid gland. We have found a distal nerve localization technique to be more expeditious in most cases (79,80). The consistent location of the distal facial-nerve branches allows them to be identified easily, and the majority of tumors overlie the main trunk, which makes nerve identification under that area more difficult. Additionally, the trunk is more difficult to identify proximally within its surrounding connective tissue than are the peripheral branches, which are surrounded by loose areolar-type tissue.

Preoperative planning should anticipate the possibility of total parotidectomy, facial-nerve grafting, temporal bone resection, mandibulectomy, or cervical lymphadenectomy. Usually, however, superficial parotidectomy is the operation performed.

The patient is placed in a supine position with the head of the table elevated. The head is turned away from the lesion so that the entire side of the face can be prepped into the operative field.

General endotracheal anesthesia is preferred, but local anesthesia may sometimes be used. Any interference with facial-nerve function makes its preservation more difficult. Facial-nerve activity is closely monitored during surgery by observing the movement of facial muscles. Therefore, muscle relaxants commonly used in anesthesia should be avoided except for short-acting agents during induction.

The incision begins at the helical insertion of the ear, continues inferiorly to below the earlobe and curves anteriorly, paralleling the angle of the jaw and approximately two centimeters below it. Sharp dissection is carried out anteriorly at the level of the superficial parotid fascia, with electrocautery of bleeding vessels. When this flap has been raised to the anterior border of the gland, it is sutured to the cheek, retracting it anteriorly (Fig. 19–5). Dissection continues posteriorly and inferiorly, exposing the remaining gland and the anterior border of the sternocleidomastoid muscle. At this point the great auricular nerve is identified and as much of it as possible is preserved. This nerve not only supplies sensation to the ear lobule, but is the best source for nerve graft should it be needed. When operating on recurrent tumors, the scar of the previous surgery should be excised in continuity with the deeper specimen. On rare occasions, a deep-lobe tumor may displace the facial nerve to a superficial position just below the lobule of the ear where it can be easily injured by the unwary surgeon. Normally, however, the nerve is deep within

the gland and becomes superficial only along the anterior border of the gland.

Actual dissection of the facial nerve begins peripherally. A straight hemostat is used bluntly to separate the overlying tissue from the nerve branches by inserting the jaws of the instrument along the path of the nerve and spreading them (Fig. 19–6). The surgeon extrapolates the direction and approximate location of the radiating nerve branches and proceeds along each branch in this fashion. This method of blunt dissection, when properly executed, should not injure normal nerve tissue. Stensen duct is dissected free, clamped, divided, and ligated. Early identification and division of the duct facilitates quick mobilization of the anterior portion of the gland. The peripheral branches of the nerve are easily located, lying on the temporalis muscle fascia superiorly, the masseter muscle fascia anteriorly, with the marginal branch found within the fibrofatty tissue of the upper neck overlying the facial vessels and submandibular gland (see Fig. 19–5). The temporal branch of the facial nerve crosses the superficial temporal vein and artery just below the level of the mandibular condyle (Fig. 19–7).

During dissection, care must be taken to manipulate the specimen as little as possible in order to prevent rupture of the tumor as well as stretching of the facial nerve. If dissec-

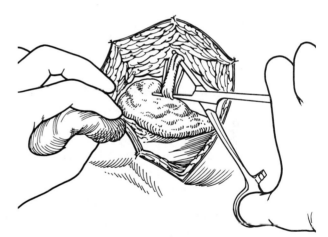

FIG. 19–6. The technique of dissection consists of bluntly separating the overlying parotid tissue from the branches of the facial nerve.

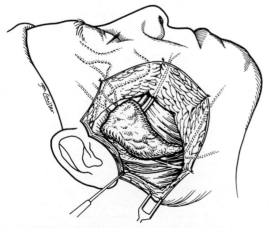

FIG. 19–5. This schematic shows complete exposure of the parotid gland and the peripheral branches of the facial nerve.

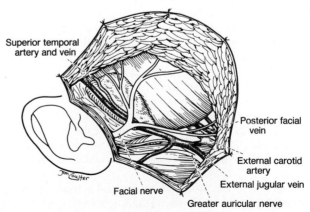

Superior temporal artery and vein

Posterior facial vein

External carotid artery

External jugular vein

Facial nerve

Greater auricular nerve

FIG. 19–7. This illustrates the vascular and neural anatomy in the operative field after removal of the superficial parotid lobe.

tion should become slow in one area, or if landmarks are unclear, it is always wise to progress to another location in which dissection is found to be easier and then return to the more difficult area.

When the tumor is located in the superficial portion of the gland, generally very little parotid tissue is found in the deep lobe. However, when the tumor is located in the deep portion of the gland, the facial nerve will be found stretched over the top of the tumor after the superficial portion has been removed. At this point the nerve should be teased carefully off of the tumor and the tumor removed from the fossa. On rare occasions, it has been necessary for us to divide the jaw just distal to the mental foramen in order to obtain enough exposure to remove the tumor.

Following the removal of the tumor, frozen-section diagnosis is obtained in order to confirm the adequacy of the procedure or to indicate the need for further action. The facial nerve is sacrificed only when malignant or recurrent tumor directly involves the nerve. If the nerve is divided during the procedure, microneurorrhaphy under no tension should yield a 60 to 90% return of function. Our experience has been that microsurgical nerve grafting using the greater auricular nerve should yield similar results.

When the bleeding has been controlled, the wound is carefully flushed with saline and closed with a suction drain brought out through a stab wound inferior to the incision. The external auditory canal is carefully flushed in order to remove any blood that may have entered the canal during the procedure. The use of a suction drain eliminates the need for a pressure dressing.

SUBMANDIBULECTOMY: OPERATIVE TECHNIQUE

The patient is placed supine on the operating table and general endotracheal anaesthesia is administered. Precautions similar to those for parotidectomy about the use of paralytic agents should be observed. The patients' head is turned and the entire neck and lower face is prepped and draped into the operative field.

The submandibular gland is approached through an incision along a line beginning at the level of the mastoid process and carried anteriorly 2 cm below the lower border of the mandible to the midline at the point of the chin. The actual incision is usually only 6 cm long overlying the gland but can be extended as necessary along this line, which also serves as the upper limb of a MacFee incision if a neck dissection is performed.

The incision is carried down through the platysma muscle, leaving the platysma attached to the skin flap unless there is adherence of the tumor to this tissue. As the flap is elevated, the marginal branch of the facial nerve will be found just deep to the platysma muscle, superficial to the facial vessels. The position of the nerve is variable in relation to the gland. The safest way to avoid nerve injury is to divide the posterior facial vein inferiorly and raise the flap in the plane just deep to this vessel. In this way it is possible to elevate the nerve still attached to the platysma muscle, and thus preserve its function.

Dissection of the submandibular gland is then begun at the level of the hyoid bone where the lower border of the gland can be visualized. Deep to the gland and just superior to the digastric muscle, the hypoglossal nerve and accompanying

ranine veins will be found. Dissection is continued superiorly until the facial artery is encountered exiting the gland anteriorly. The artery is clamped, divided, and ligated at this point. Retraction of the mylohyoid muscle anteriorly will reveal the lingual nerve pulled inferiorly by the submandibular ganglion and accompanying vessels attached to the gland. This pedicle must be divided and ligated carefully, in order to preserve the main trunk of the lingual nerve. Warthin duct will also be seen in this field and should be clamped, divided, and ligated. This allows for complete removal of the gland along with any adjacent lymph nodes that might be attached to it.

Following removal of the submandibular gland, the wound is flushed out with saline and a layered closure is performed along with placement of a suction drain; this eliminates the necessity for a compression dressing.

COMPLICATIONS OF SURGERY

The primary complication that all surgeons should try to avoid is tumor recurrence. This is, unfortunately, not always possible, even with excision that was considered adequate at the time of surgery. In our experience, locally recurrent tumor has been related almost exclusively to inadequate initial extirpation.

Several reports detail the surgical precautions necessary to prevent common intraoperative complications such as bleeding, injury to the ear canal, and poor exposure. Injury to the facial nerve is an avoidable complication if proper surgical technique is used; however, if the nerve is inadvertently divided, it should be repaired immediately under magnification (4,81,82).

Frey syndrome is a common complication following parotidectomy. This is manifested by a spectrum of symptoms from erythema related to eating to copious gustatory sweating. Its etiology is thought to be aberrant connection of the regenerating salivary parasympathetic fibers to the sweat glands of the overlying skin flap. Numerous treatment plans have been proposed: irradiation, division of the glossopharyngeal or auriculotemporal nerves, topical applications of atropinelike creams, and insertion of synthetic materials, fascial grafts, or vascularized tissue under the skin flap. Recent recommendations for minimizing the risk of Frey syndrome include raising a superficial musculoaponeurotic system (SMAS) flap at the time of surgery (83) or performing a selective parotidectomy (84).

Postoperative complications such as seroma, hematoma, salivary fistula, and wound-healing problems are uncommon. Temporary paralysis of all or a portion of the facial nerve is

Table 19–5
Salivary Gland Cancer Indications for Postoperative Radiation[a]

1. Highly malignant tumors
2. Extraglandular extension of tumor: neural, perineural, lymphatic invasion
3. Regional nodal metastases
4. After resection of recurrent tumor
5. Parotid deep lobe tumor
6. Tumor adjacent to facial nerve
7. Gross residual tumor after resection

[a]From Guillamondegui OM, Byers RM, Luna MA, et al: Aggressive surgery in treatment for parotid cancer: The role of adjunctive post-operative radiotherapy. *AJR* 123:49, 1975.

common, probably resulting from partial devascularization of the nerve, direct trauma to the nerve, or postoperative inflammation. Temporary paresis generally disappears within a few weeks but it may take as long as 6 months. Patients reconstructed with nerve grafts may develop inappropriate twitching or pain several years postoperatively.

Surgery of the submandibular gland exposes the hypoglossal nerve and the lingual nerve to potential injury. In addition, the mandibular branch of the facial nerve can be injured during the approach to the gland. The technique of submandibular gland excision is specifically designed to avoid unintentional injuries to these important structures.

Table 19–6
Comprehensive Treatment Plan for Salivary Gland Tumors

A. Parotid Gland Management					
Tumor Characteristics	Parotidectomy	Facial Nerve	Neck Dissection	Radiation	Chemotherapy
Benign tumors; T_1 + T_2 + low grade acinic cell or mucoepidermoid carcinomas	Superficial or total	Preservation	No	No	No
T_1 and T_2 moderate to high grade mucoepidermoid carcinoma; malignant mixed; adenocarcinoma; undifferentiated; epidermoid carcinoma	Total	Resection and immediate nerve graft only if nerve is involved by tumor	Yes, when there is palpable lymphadenopathy Consider neck dissection for N0 epidermoid or undifferentiated carcinoma	Yes	No
T_3; recurrent malignancy	Total	Resection and immediate nerve graft only if nerve is involved by tumor	Yes, when there is palpable lymphadenopathy	Yes	Possible
Any size tumor with extra-glandular spread or T_4	Radical with involved adjacent tissues	Resection and immediate nerve graft if nerve is involved by tumor	Yes, when there is palpable lymphadenopathy	Yes	Possible

B. Submandibular Gland Management			
Tumor Status	Surgery	Radiation	Chemotherapy
Benign tumors, T_1 and T_2 malignancies	Total gland excision; limited upper cervical lymphadenectomy for malignant tumors without palpable adenopathy and full cervical lymphadenectomy if palpable nodes	Yes, if moderate to high-grade malignancy or adenoid cystic carcinoma	No
Any size with extra-glandular spread, T_3, T_4	Radical gland excision; excision of involved adjacent tissue; cervical lymphadenectomy	Yes	Possible

C. Minor Salivary Gland Management			
Tumor Status	Surgery	Radiation	Chemotherapy
Benign tumors, T_1 and T_2	Local excision with clear margin	Possible, if moderate to high grade malignancy or adenoid cystic carcinoma	No
T_3 and T_4	Radical resection of all tumor involved tissues, immediate reconstruction after surgical margins are confirmed	Yes	Possible

RADIATION THERAPY

Surgical excision is the primary treatment of salivary neoplasms. Radiation therapy is a very useful adjunctive treatment modality following surgery (41-48). The improved locoregional control in patients receiving postoperative radiation demonstrates that small foci of residual tumor cells are radiosensitive. Indications for postoperative radiation depend on the tumor type and stage (Table19–5).

CHEMOTHERAPY

Chemotherapy should be reserved for advanced tumors that are not likely to benefit from surgery. Chemotherapy of recurrent, locally advanced, or metastatic tumor has not enjoyed a high response rate. Studies report partial responses in 35 to 50% of patients, but there has not been any survival advantage (85-88). Adenocarcinoma, mixed tumors, and acinic cell carcinomas responded better to adriamycin, cisplatinum and 5FU, while mucoepidermoid and squamous carcinoma respond better to methotrexate and cis-platinum (86,88).

SUMMARY OF TREATMENT PLAN (TABLE 19–6)

This treatment plan has been presented as a guideline. It cannot account for the many ideosyncratic social and physical factors that will influence the course of therapy for an individual patient.

Bibliography

1. Leegaard T, Lindeman H. Salivary gland tumors: clinical picture and treatment. *Acta Otolaryngol* 1970; 263:155.
2. Foote FW Jr, Frazell EL. Tumors of the major salivary glands. *Cancer* 1953; 6:1065.
3. Batsakis JG, Regezi JA, et al. The pathology of head and neck tumors: salivary glands, parts 1–4. *Head Neck Surg* 1978–1979; 1:59, 167, 260, 340.
4. Richardson GS, Dickason WL, Gaisford JC, et al. Tumors of salivary glands: an analysis of 752 cases. *Plast Reconstr Surg* 1975; 55:131.
5. Spiro RH, Huvos AA, Strong EW. Cancer of the parotid gland: a clinicopathologic study of 288 primary cases. *Am J Surg* 1975; 130:452.
6. Gallia LJ, Johnson JT. The incidence of neoplastic versus inflammatory disease in major salivary gland masses diagnosed by surgery. *Laryngoscope* 1981; 91:512.
7. Storm FK, Eilber FR, Sparks FC, et al. A prospective study of parotid metastases from head and neck cancer. *Am J Surg* 1977; 34:115.
8. Rees R, Maples M, Lynch JB. Malignant secondary parotid tumors. *South Med J* 1981; 74:1050.
9. Yarington CT. Metastatic malignant disease to the parotid gland. *Laryngoscope* 1981; 91:517.
10. Kushner DC, Weber AL. Sialography of salivary gland tumors with fluoroscopy and tomography. *Amer J Radiol* 1978; 130:941.
11. Baker SR, Krause CJ. Ultrasonic analysis of head and neck neoplasms correlation with surgical findings. *An Otol* 1981; 90:126.
12. Bladh WH, Rose JG. Nuclear medicine in diagnosis and treatment of diseases of the head and neck. 1. Salivary and parathyroid gland disease. *Head Neck Surg* 1981; 4:129.
13. Eneroth CM, Franzen S, Zajicek J. Aspiration biopsy of salivary gland tumors. A critical review of 910 biopsies. *Acta Cytol* 1967; 11:470.
14. Sismanis A, Merriam JM, Kline TS, et al. Diagnosis of salivary gland tumors by fine-needle biopsy. *Head Neck Surg* 1981; 3:482.
15. Cross DL, Gansler TS, Morris RC. Fine needle aspiration and frozen section of salivary gland lesions. *So Med J* 1990; 83:283.
16. Spiro RH. Salivary neoplasms: overview of 35 years' experience with 2807 patients. *Head and Neck Surg* 1986; 8:177.
17. Hillel AD, Fee WE Jr. Evaluation of frozen section in parotid gland surgery. *Arch Otolaryngol* 1983; 109:230.
18. Miller RH, Calcaterra TC, Paglia DE. Accuracy of frozen section diagnosis of parotid lesions. *Ann Otol* 1979; 88:573.
19. Granick MS, Erickson ER, Hanna DC. Accuracy of frozen section diagnosis in salivary gland lesions. *Head and Neck Surg* 1985; 7:465.
20. Levitt SH, McHugh RB, Gomez-Marin O, et al. Clinical staging system for cancer of the salivary gland. A retrospective study. *Cancer* 1981; 47:2712.
21. Clode AL, Fonseca I, Santos JR, et al. Mucoepidermoid carcinoma of the salivary glands: a reappraisal of the influence of tumor differentation on prognosis. *J Surg Oncol* 1991; 46:100.
22. Spiro RH, Thaler HT, Hicks WF, et al. The importance of clinical staging of minor salivary gland carcinoma. *Am J Surg* 1991; 162:330.
23. Spiro RH and Huvos AG. Stage means more than grade in adenoid cystic carcinoma. *Am J Surg* 1992; 164:623.
24. Weber RS, Byers RM, Petit B, et al. Submandibular gland tumors: adverse histologic factors and therapeutic implications. *Arch Otolaryngol* 1990; 116:1055.
25. Rauch S. *Die speicheldrusen des meuschen.* Stuttgart: Thieme, 1959.
26. Conley J, Clairmont AA. Facial nerve in recurrent benign pleomorphic adenoma. *Arch Otolaryngol* 1979; 105:247.
27. O'Dwyer PJ, Farrar WB, Finkelmeier WR, et al. Facial nerve sacrifice and tumor recurrence in primary and recurrent benign parotid tumor. *Am J Surg* 1986; 152:442.
28. Piorkowski RJ, Guillamondegui OM. Is aggressive surgical treatment indicated for recurrent benign mixed tumors of the parotid gland? *Amer J Surg* 1981; 142:434.
29. Lanier VC, McSwain B, Rosenfeld L. Mixed tumors of salivary glands: a 44-year study. *South Med J* 1972; 65:1485.
30. Judd ES. Development of cancer in mixed tumors of salivary glands. *Postgrad Med* 1952; 21:112.
31. Beahrs OH, Woolner LB, Kirklin JW, et al. Carcinomatous transformation of mixed tumors of the parotid gland. *Arch Surg* 1957; 75:605.
32. Dawson AK, Orr JA. Long-term results of local excision and radiation therapy in pleomorphic adenoma of the parotid. *Int J Radiat Oncol Biol Phys* 1985; 11:451.
33. Natvig K, Soberg, R. Relationship of intraoperative rupture of pleomorphic adeonomas to recurrence: an 11–25 year follow-up study. *Head & Neck* 1994; 16:213.
34. Yamashita T, Tomoda K, Kumazawa T. The usefulness of partial parotidectomy for benign parotid tumors. *Acta Otolaryngol* Suppl 1993; 500:113.
35. Yu LT, Hamilton R. Frey's syndrome: prevention with conservative parotidectomy and superficial musculoaponeurotic system preservation. *Ann Plast Surg* 1992; 29:217.
36. Lamelas J, Terry JH, Alfonso AE. Warthin's tumor: multicentricy and increasing incidence in women. *Amer J Surg* 1987; 154:347.
37. Tran L, Sadeghi A, Hanson D, et al. Major salivary gland tumors: treatment results and prognostic factors. *Laryngoscope* 1986; 96:1139.
38. Oliveira P, Fonseca I, Soares J. Acinic cell carcinoma of the salivary glands. A long-term follow-up of 15 cases. *Eur J Surg Oncol* 1992; 18:7.
39. Colmenero C, Parton M, Sierra I. Acinic cell carcinoma of the salivary glands. *J Cranio-Max-Fac Surg* 1991; 19:260.
40. Friedman M, Levin B, Grybauskas V, et al. Malignant tumors of the major salivary glands. *Otol Clin N Amer* 1986; 19:625.
41. Jackson GL, Luna MA, Byers RM. Results of surgery alone and surgery combined with postoperative radiotherapy in the treatment of cancer of the parotid gland. *Amer J Surg* 1983; 146:497.
42. Sullivan ZMR, Breslin K, McClatchey KD, et al. Malignant parotid gland tumors: a retrospective. *Otolaryngol—Head and Neck Surg* 1987; 97:529.
43. Reddy SP, Marks JE. Treatment of locally advanced high-grade malignant tumors of major salivary glands. *Laryngoscope* 1988; 98:450.
44. McNaney D, McNeese MD, Guillamondeguie OM, et al. Postoperative irradiation in malignant epithelial tumors of the parotid. *Int J Radiat Oncol Biol Phys* 1983; 9:1289.
45. Eapen LJ, Gerig LH, Catton GE. Impact of local radiation in the management of salivary gland carcinomas. *Head and Neck Surg* 1988; 10:239.
46. Harrison LB, Armstrong JG, Spiro RH, et al. Postoperative radiation therapy for major salivary gland malignancies. *J Surg Oncol* 1990; 45:52.
47. Sagegni E, Tran LM, Mark R, et al. Minor salivary gland tumors of the head and neck: treatment strategies and prognosis. *Am J Clin Oncol* 1993; 16:3.

48. Sakata K, Aoki Y, Karasawa K, et al. Radiation therapy for patients with malignant salivary gland tumors with positive surgical margins. *Stiahientherapie and Onkologie* 1994; 170:342.

49. Spiro RH, Huvos AG, Berk R, et al. Mucoepidermoid carcinoma of salivary gland origin: a clinopathologic study of 367 cases. *Am J Surg* 1978; 136:461.

50. Spiro RH, Huvos AF, Strong EW. Malignant mixed tumor of salivary origin. A clinicopathologic study of 146 cases. *Cancer* 1977; 39:388.

51. Tortoledo ME, Luna MA, Batsakis JG. Carcinomas ex pleomorphic adenoma and malignant mixed tumors. *Arch Otolaryngol* 1984; 110:172.

52. Matsuba HM, Spector GJ, Thawley SE, et al. Adenoid cystic salivary gland carcinoma. *Cancer* 1986; 57:519.

53. Nascimento AG, Amaral ALP, Prado LAF, et al. Adenoid cystic carcinoma of the salivary glands. *Cancer* 1986; 57:317.

54. Sadeghi A, Tran LM, Mark R, et al. Tumor salivary gland tumors of the head and neck: treatment strategies and prognosis. *Am J Oncol* 1993; 16:3.

55. Tran L, Sidrys J, Sadeghi A, et al. Salivary gland tumors of the oral cavity. *Intrl J Rad Oncol* 1990; 18:413.

56. Bardwil JM. Tumors of the parotid gland. *Am J Surg* 1967; 114:498.

57. Eneroth CM. Histopathological and clinical aspects of parotid tumors. *Acta Otolaryngol (Suppl)* 1964; 191:1.

58. Lambert JA. Parotid gland tumors. *Milit Med* 1971; 136:484.

59. Skolnick EM, Friedman M, Becker S, et al. Tumors of the major salivary glands. *Laryngoscope* 1977; 87:843.

60. Matsuba HM, Mauney M, Simpson JR, et al. Adenocarcinoma of the major and minor salivary gland origin: a histopathologic review of treatment failure patterns. *Laryngoscope* 1988; 98:784.

61. Schusterman MA, Granick MS, Erickson ER, et al. Lymphoma presenting as a salivary gland mass. *Head and Neck Surg* 1988; 10:411.

62. Kucan JO, Frank DH, Robson MC. Tumors metastatic to the parotid gland. *Br J Plast Surg* 1981; 34:299.

63. Batsakis JG, Bautina E. Metastases to major salivary glands. *Ann Otol Rhinol Laryngol* 1990; 99:501.

64. Ryan JR, Ioachim HL, Marmer J, et al. Acquired immune deficiency syndrome–related lymphadenopathies presenting in the salivary gland nodes. *Arch Otolaryngol* 1985; 111:554.

65. deVries EJ, Kapadia SB, Johnson JT, et al. Salivary gland lymphoproliferative disease in acquired immune disease. *Otolaryngol—Head and Neck Surg* 1988; 99:59.

66. Eneroth CM. Salivary gland tumors in the parotid gland, submandibular gland, and the palate region. *Cancer* 1971; 27:1415.

67. Spiro RH, Hajdu SI, Strong EW. Tumors of the submaxillary gland. *Am J Surg* 1976; 132:463.

68. Tran L, Sadeghi A, Hanson D, et al. Salivary gland tumors of the palate: the UCLA experience. *Laryngoscope* 1987; 97:1343.

69. Abrams AM, Melrose RJ, Howell FV. Necrotizing sialometaplasia. *Cancer* 1973; 32:130.

70. Granick MS, Pilch BZ. Necrotizing sialometaplasia in the setting of acute and chronic sinusitis. *Laryngoscope* 1981; 91:1532.

71. Gahhos F, Enriquez RE, Bahn SL, et al. Necrotizing sialometaplasia: report of five cases. *Plast Reconstr Surg* 1983; 71:650.

72. Granick MS, Solomon MP, Benadetto AV, et al. Necrotizing sialometaplasia masquerading as residual lip cancer. *Ann Plast Surg* 1988; 71:650.

73. Chong GC, Beahrs OH, Chen MLC, et al. Management of parotid gland tumors in infants and children. *May Clin Proc* 1975; 50:279.

74. Callender DL, Frankenthaler RA, Luna MA, et al. Salivary gland neoplasms in children. *Arch Otolaryngol—Head and Neck Surg* 1992; 118:472.

75. Schuller DC, McCabe BF. The firm salivary mass in children. *Laryngoscope* 1977; 87:1891.

76. Shikhani AH, Johns ME. Tumors of the major salivary glands in children. *Head and Neck Surg* 1988; 10:257.

77. Luna MA, Batsakis JG, el-Naggar, AK. Salivary gland tumors in children (review). *Ann Otol Rhinol Laryngol* 1991; 100:869.

78. Kroll SO, Trodahl JN, Byers RC. Salivary gland lesions in children: a study of 430 cases. *Cancer* 1972; 30:459.

79. Granick MS, Hanna DC. Salivary glands. In: Nora PF, ed. *Operative surgery.* Philadelphia: WB Saunders, 1990; 172.

80. Granick MS and Hanna DC. Surgical management of salivary gland disease. In: Granick MS and Hanna DC, eds. *Management of salivary gland lesions.* Baltimore: Williams & Wilkins, 1992; 145.

81. Gaisford JC, Hanna DC. Parotid tumor surgery. In: Goldwyn RM, ed. *The unfavorable result in plastic surgery.* Boston: Little, Brown, 1984; 419.

82. Rankow RM, Polayes IM. Complications of surgery of the salivary glands. In: Conley JJ, ed. *Complications of head and neck surgery.* Philadelphia: WB Saunders, 1979; 196.

83. Allison GR, Rappaport I. Prevention of Frey's syndrome with superficial aponeurotic system interposition. *Am J Surg* 1993; 166:407.

84. Zhao K, Qi DY, Wang LM. Functional superficial parotidectomy. *J Oral and Maxillo Surg* 1994; 52:1038.

85. Rentschler R, Burgess MA, Byers R. Chemotherapy of malignant major salivary gland neoplasms. *Cancer* 1976; 40:619.

86. Suen JY, Johns ME. Chemotherapy for salivary gland cancer. *Laryngoscope* 1982; 92:235.

87. Creagan ET, Woods JE, Rubin J, et al. Cisplatin-based chemotherapy for neoplasms arising from salivary glands and contiguous structures in the head and neck. *Cancer* 1988; 62:2313.

88. Kaplan MJ, Johns ME, Cantrell RW. Chemotherapy for salivary gland cancer. *Otolaryngol—Head and Neck Surg* 1986; 95:165.

20

Surgical Management of Soft-Tissue Sarcomas of the Extremities

Edmond F. Ritter, M.D. and John M. Harrelson, M.D.

There are an estimated 6,000 new cases of soft-tissue sarcoma in the United States each year that comprise less than 1% of all malignant disease. Fifty percent of these cases occur in the lower extremity, with the majority occurring in the thigh. The upper extremity accounts for 10% and the remaining 40% occur in the head, neck, truck, and retroperitoneum. Although these lesions are categorized histologically by their connective-tissue cell of origin (fat, muscle, fibrous tissue, vascular, neural, synovial), the specific cell type does not make a difference from the therapeutic standpoint because the biologic behavior of these lesions and their response to treatment is similar. The peak incidence of soft-tissue sarcoma is in the 5th and 6th decade of life with a slight male predominance (1,2).

BIOLOGIC BEHAVIOR

Local patterns of growth and mechanisms of metastatic spread govern the treatment of soft-tissue sarcomas. In addition to invading the structure of origin, these lesions expand centripetally, compressing normal tissues at their periphery. This expansile growth produces a pseudocapsule at the margins of the lesion that consists of compressed muscle and fascial structures. Neural, vascular, and osseous elements in the path of an expanding tumor may become embedded in the pseudocapsule. Both the pseudocapsule and the local vascular structures may be invaded by tumor. Satellite lesions develop external to the pseudocapsule and physically separate from the primary tumor by seeding within the venous drainage of the tumor. Lymphatic invasion and nodal metastasis are rare because muscle contains only sparse lymphatics (3).

The site of tumor origin governs to some extent the potential distribution of satellite lesions. Primary soft-tissue sarcomas may arise either within major anatomic compartments (intracompartmental) or within fascial planes separating major anatomic compartments (extracompartmental), or may arise within the subcutaneous tissue external to underlying fascia. Intracompartmental primary lesions place at risk all tissue within the anatomic compartment, with the likelihood of satellite lesions increasing with proximity to the primary tumor. Extracompartmental lesions expose the fascial plane of origin and all bordering structures to potential tumor spread. Subcutaneous primary lesions expose the subcutaneous tissues surrounding the lesion and have a greater likelihood of lymphatic spread. Usually, major fascial planes serve as a barrier to local invasion of sarcoma and penetration into adjacent compartments is rare (4).

CLINICAL PRESENTATION

Most patients with soft-tissue sarcoma present with complaints of a painless, slowly enlarging mass. Aching discomfort, with local tenderness, overlying venous distention, and local erythema may be present in longstanding lesions. Occasionally, patients may present with a history of the sudden appearance of a painful mass. Investigation usually reveals hemorrhage occurring in a previously unrecognized lesion. Symptoms of neural and vascular compression are rare unless the primary is of neural origin or is situated in the popliteal fossa, femoral triangle, or antecubital fossa where neurovascular structures are more easily compressed by an expanding tumor. Weight loss and other systemic symptoms are usually not present when the patient is first seen. Fever and chills may occasionally be observed in patients with large lesions in which central hemorrhage and necrosis have occurred.

STAGING

Staging provides a means for making treatment decisions, determining prognosis, and evaluating outcomes of treatment. Many staging systems have been described (5–7). We have used the system described by Enneking, which stages tumors by site, histology, and presence or absence of metastases (Table 20–1). Tumor size is also an important prognostic factor and is included in other staging systems.

Numerous schemes for histologic grading have been described (8,9). Most systems divide malignant lesions into at least four categories based on progressive pleomorphism and atypia. From a practical point of view, surgical decisions regarding soft-tissue sarcomas can be based on a knowledge of whether the lesion is low-grade or high-grade. Most soft-tissue sarcomas present as high-grade lesions.

In those patients presenting with an extremity mass, anatomic staging information regarding the lesion must be gathered before biopsy is undertaken. In addition to local physical examination, radiographic imaging studies aid in the determination of site, proximity to major neural and vascular structures, proximity to bone, and the vascularity of the lesion. All of these factors are of importance in planning the subsequent biopsy and surgical treatment. Routine radiographs of the tumor should be obtained but are of limited benefit. Only when the lesion contains calcium or has eroded adjacent bone will these studies be informative.

Magnetic resonance imaging (MRI) provides the best visualization of soft-tissue sarcomas. Standard T1 and T2 images will define the anatomic extent of the lesion and its relationship to neural and vascular structures. Image manipulation in various planes and imaging with gadolinium contrast provides maximum information and allows for optimum preoperative planning (Fig. 20–1). Magnetic resonance imaging has also proved useful in evaluating the effects of biopsy and of neoadjuvant therapy (10).

Table 20–1
Surgical Staging System[a]

Stage	Grade	Site	Metastases
IA	Low	Intracompartmental	None
IB	Low	Extracompartmental	None
IIA	High	Intracompartmental	None
IIB	High	Extracompartmental	None
III	Any	Any	Regional or distant

[a]Adapted from Enneking, et al. (7).

Computed tomography (CT) is of value in staging the chest, pelvis, and abdomen for metastatic disease, and may be helpful if there has been tumor erosion of adjacent bone. The role of CT scanning for primary soft-tissue lesions has diminished with the development of MRI (11).

Radionuclide imaging with technetium and gallium are useful adjuncts in the evaluation of soft-tissue sarcomas (12). Studies are performed in three phases with immediate scan following injection, a delayed blood pool image at 15 minutes, and a delayed bone scan in 3 hours. In this manner, the arterial supply of the lesion, the venous pooling within the lesion, and the effect of the lesion on adjacent osseous structures can be appreciated. Increased uptake in bone on the delayed scan indicates involvement of that bone with the pseudocapsule of the tumor (Fig. 20–2).

When tumor abuts a major vessel, angiography may be beneficial in surgical planning. The study should be performed in two planes in order to assess vessel displacement (13). Lymphangiography is not indicated as a primary stag-

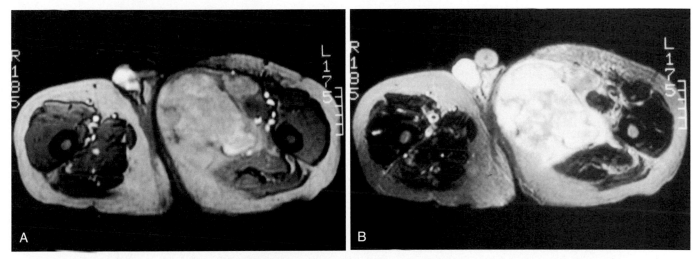

FIG. 20–1. **A,** T1 image of a large medial carcoma. The relationship to vessels is clearly shown. **B,** T2 image shows the extensive perineoplastic edema.

FIG. 20–2. **A,** CT scan shows a subcutaneous high-grade sarcoma immediately adjacent to the anterior tibia. **B,** an anterior radionuclide scan shows increased uptake in the right mid tibia. This indicates that the reactive capsule is involving bone.

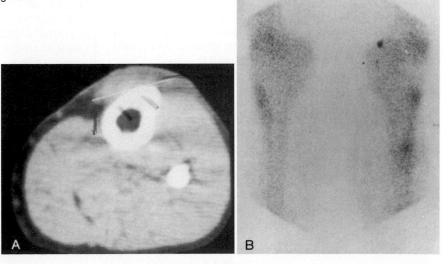

ing study. Although synovial sarcoma and some subcutaneous primaries have a predisposition for lymphatic spread, MRI and CT staging studies usually encompasses the lymphatic drainage of the primary lesion. If enlarged, suspicious nodes are observed, then lymphangiography may be considered (14).

Biopsy for diagnosis and histological grading is undertaken only after anatomic localization of the lesion has been accomplished. Biopsy is of equal importance to the definitive surgical procedure and must be planned carefully (15). Although direct local invasion and vascular penetration are the natural modes of tumor spread, tumor dissemination by biopsy is a common occurrence. Fine needle aspiration (FNA), core needle biopsy, and open biopsy are all suitable means of obtaining tissue. FNA with a 22-gauge needle (or smaller) has not been shown to produce tumor seeding. The study often does not provide a specific histologic diagnosis and there may not be adequate tissue for special stains.

Core needle biopsy and open biopsy introduced the risk of tumor seeding along the biopsy tract and by postbiopsy hemorrhage and hematoma. Therefore, the surgeon must consider what type of definitive surgical section is to be performed and place the biopsy incision in a location that will allow its complete extirpation at the time of definitive surgery. The biopsy should not expose neurovascular structures or bone and should be restricted to the compartment of origin when possible. Because virtually all tumor excision in the extremities is accomplished through longitudinal exposure, transverse incisions are to be avoided. Excision of a transverse biopsy is difficult and requires the sacrifice of more skin and soft tissue. Because hemorrhage from the biopsy tract may disseminate tumor cells in the hematoma, meticulous hemostasis is mandatory. It should be remembered that the placement of the biopsy incision and contamination resulting from the procedure may adversely affect the prognosis by increasing the extent of definitive surgery required and by increasing the chances of local recurrence. A potentially salvageable limb may require amputation if these factors are not considered (Fig. 20–3).

Using the imaging data to select an exposure for definitive resection, the biopsy incision is placed in line with a chosen resection incision and sharp dissection is used to expose the tumor. Care is taken not to undermine adjacent skin or to dissect within the tumor pseudocapsule, which provides an inviting plane through which to "shell out" the lesion. Only lesions of 3 cm or smaller are recommended for excisional biopsy. An adequate sample of tumor is removed and frozen section utilized to assure that vital diagnostic tissue has been obtained. Hemostasis is then achieved with electrocautery and, if necessary, local thrombotic agents. If definitive surgery is immediately to follow, with the biopsy based on frozen-section diagnosis, the wound is closed and dressed, the limb reprepped and draped, and new instruments, gowns and gloves used for the definitive resection (Fig. 20–4). If delayed resection is planned, a small suction drain is inserted in line with the biopsy incision, exiting the skin 1 to 2 cm from the end of the incision to avoid the accumulation of hematoma.

SURGICAL ALTERNATIVES

Historically, surgery has been considered the definitive treatment for soft-tissue sarcomas (16,17). Within the last decade,

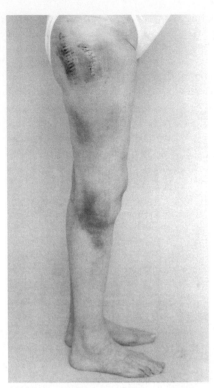

FIG. 20–3. This patient had a biopsy of a high-grade liposarcoma over the right greater trochanter 1 week earlier. Contaminated hematoma extends from the midcalf to above the iliac crest.

the role of surgery and adjunctive radiotherapy has been extensively evaluated. The accepted treatment of soft-tissue sarcomas today consists of wide surgical excision coupled with either neoadjuvant or adjuvant radiotherapy (18–23). It is important that the surgeon understand the definition of each surgical procedure and the potential for local recurrence with either of these procedures for both high-grade and low-grade lesions.

Marginal excision is defined as tumor removal through or adjacent to the reactive capsule at the pushing margin of the tumor. This "shelling out" of the lesion leaves microscopic tumor and, for high-grade lesions, results in predictable local recurrence. Marginal excision would therefore not be considered therapeutic in the treatment of soft-tissue sarcoma.

Wide excision is defined as removal of the lesion with a cuff of normal tissue, including the biopsy tract. The tumor is not visualized during the surgical procedure. The distance the surgeon must be from the tumor depends, to some extent, on local anatomic structures. It is acceptable to pass within a centimeter of the tumor if there is a major fascial plane between the tumor and the resection margin. Conversely, if the surgeon is transecting the anatomic compartment containing the tumor through the muscle fibers of that compartment, a distance of 5 cm or more would be desirable. For low-grade lesions and for subcutaneous sarcomas, wide excision results in less than 10% local recurrence. For high-grade lesions, in the absence of any adjunctive radiotherapy, wide excision results in up to 40% local recurrence. Lack of local control in this circumstance is most likely the result of satellite lesions within the compartment of origin or contamination by venous efflux from the tumor during surgery. When coupled with radiotherapy, wide excision results in less than 5% local recurrence.

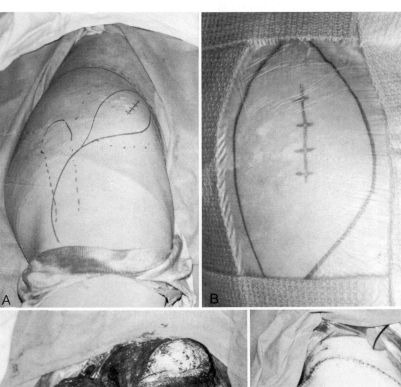

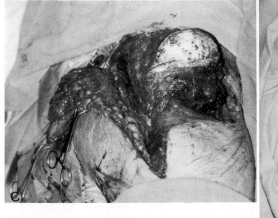

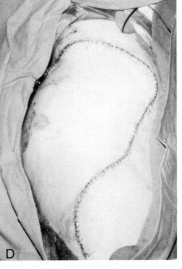

FIG. 20–4. **A,** sarcome of the tensor fascia femoris muscle. The femur is outlined with a dotted line; the biopsy incision is shown as a cross-hatched line with a major resection ellipsing the biopsy planned from the iliac crest above to the lateral femur below. **B,** the biopsy incision has been isolated with adhesive drapes. **C,** after frozen section, the biopsy incision has been closed and isolated with a sterile plastic drape. The major resection includes the biopsy site. **D,** wound closure from iliac crest to femur. Loss of muscle bulk allows tension-free skin closure despite biopsy ellipse.

Radical excision is defined as complete removal of the major anatomic compartment in which the tumor arises without violation of the major fascial boundaries of that compartment. For high-grade sarcomas, in the absence of adjuvant radiotherapy, radical excision results in less than 10% of local recurrence.

The importance of these definitions must be emphasized. Note that the question of amputation is not addressed by the definition of these surgical procedures. For example, above-knee amputation for a lesion of the quadriceps achieves only a wide margin because a portion of the anterior compartment remains. A radical margin for such a lesion would involve removal of the entire anterior compartment of the thigh, whether or not amputation was a part of that procedure. The major anatomic compartments in the upper extremity illustrated in Figure 20–5. The major anatomic compartments in the lower extremity are illustrated in Figure 20–6.

The combination of radiotherapy and wide surgical excision as a means of local tumor control have produced results equivalent to those achieved by radical compartmental excision (24–31). The results are the same whether the radiation

is given preoperatively as neoadjuvant therapy or postoperatively as brachytherapy or external-beam therapy.

The selection of a surgical procedure requires the analysis of many factors. Localization of the lesion to an anatomic compartment or extracompartmental site, the proximity of the pseudocapsule to bone, blood vessels and neural structures, and the histologic grade of the lesion are all considered. When the tumor is an untreated primary, radiation and wide excision should be the treatment of choice. When the tumor pseudocapsule is in contact with major neural or vascular structures or produces increased uptake on bone scan, any surgical procedure that spares these structures will result in a marginal excision and near-certain local recurrence. In some situations, it may be necessary to include the involved bone as a part of the resection (Fig. 20–7) or to resect the major vessel en bloc with the tumor and to perform vascular bypass. In general, procedures that require sacrifice of a major nerve (sciatic, median plus ulnar) produce a degree of disability equal to amputation, and limb salvage in such situations may not be advisable. This condition arises most frequently with extracompartmental tumors of the popliteal

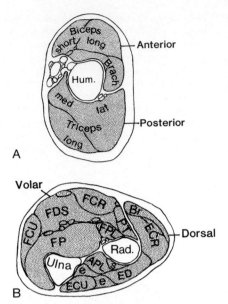

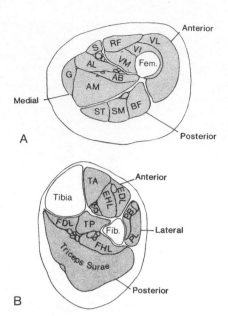

FIG. 20–5. A, major anatomic compartments in the upper arm. Brach, brachialis. **B,** major anatomic compartments in the forearm. Volar compartment: FCR, flexor carpi radialis; FCU, flexor carpi ulnaris; FDS, flexor digitorum superficialis; FP, flexor profundus; FPL, flexor pollicis longus; PT, pronator teres. Dorsal compartment: APL, abductor pollicis longus; Br, brachioradialis; ECR, extensor carpi radialis; ECU, extensor carpi ulnaris; ED, extensor digitorum.

FIG. 20–6. A, major anatomic compartments of the thigh. Anteror: RF, rectus femoris; VI, vastus intermedius; VL, vastus lateralis; VM, vastus medialis. Medial: AB, adductor brevis; AL, adductor longus; AM, adductor magnus; G, gracilis; S, sartorius. Posterior: BF, biceps femoris; SM, semimenbranosus; ST, semitendinosus. **B,** major anatomic compartents of the lower leg. Anterior: EDL, extensor digitorum longus; EHL, extensor hallucis longus; TA, tibialis anterior. Lateral: PB, peroneus brevis; PL, peroneus longus. Posterior: FDL, flexor digitorum longus; FHL, flexor hallucis longus; TP, tibialis posterior.

FIG. 20–7. A, planned resection of biopsy site and lesion shown in Figure 20–2. The anterior tibia is involved, according to the bone scan. **B,** resection includes the anterior tibial cortex. Closure is accomplished by gastrocnemius rotational flap and split-skin coverage.

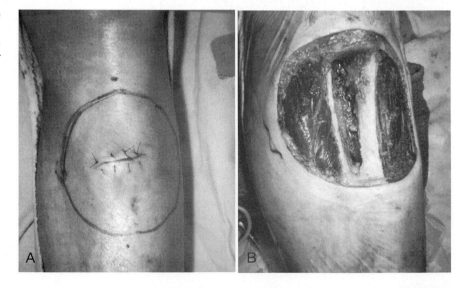

fossa, femoral triangle, axilla, and antecubital fossa. Soft-tissue sarcomas of the hands and feet are fortunately rare. In these locations, proximity to neural, osseous, and vascular structures may make salvage difficult. Sarcomas of the hands and feet usually result in amputation.

The patient should be apprised of the factors that govern the choice of surgical procedures as well as expected limb function after surgery. Contingency plans should be established preoperatively to deal with unexpected findings.

Transgression of the tumor or the presence of hematoma from the previous biopsy extending into the surgical field results in a contaminated wound and the equivalent of a marginal or intralesional excision. It may be necessary to abandon the attempt at resection and resort to more radical procedures or amputation at a higher level. Five-year disease-free survival following radiation and wide excision is approximately 65%. To date, no chemotherapy regimen has produced a significant increase in survivorship (32–37).

Reconstruction

The primary objective of operative treatment is eradication of local disease, while maximizing the quality of the patient's life. The primary goals of the reconstructive surgeon are to facilitate the ablative surgeons ability to perform an adequate resection by providing efficient, reliable wound closure with minimal morbidity and mortality (38).

Due to the complexity and magnitude of major resective and reconstructive procedures, it is often beneficial to divide the procedure between two teams, one performing the tumor resection and one performing the reconstruction. One of the advantages of such a team approach includes the possibility of simultaneous resection and flap harvesting (using separate sets of instruments).

Adequate preoperative planning facilitates efficient execution of these complex procedures. Selection of the method of wound closure should be individualized for each patient. Basic considerations include (a) replacing like tissue with like tissue, (b) minimizing donor-site morbidity; (c) consideration of the patient's medical fitness, (d) obtaining healthy well-vascularized tissue coverage of critical structures, including major nerves, vessels, and, when present, allografts. Methods of closure range from simple to complex. In general, the simplest adequate method is selected, because with unnecessary complexity, morbidity and mortality may increase. We favor immediate reconstruction when prudent.

Immediate closure of greatest importance when a resection leaves major neural or vascular structures exposed. However, it is also important to establish tumor-free surgical margins and, if margins are in question, delayed reconstruction after thorough histologic examination of specimen margins may be prudent. In such situations we have found placement of pigskin homograft for temporary wound coverage useful.

METHODS OF SOFT-TISSUE RECONSTRUCTION

Primary Closure

This is the simplest method, and it is applicable when adequate healthy skin subcutaneous and facial tissue remain for tension-free closure (Fig. 20–8). Unfortunately, in our experience primary closure of radiated wounds is associated with a 51% rate of major wound complications (defined as infection, wound dehiscence, or drainage requiring reoperation) (39). Many host and treatment factors predispose to major wound complications. A large volume of tumor resection, postoperative radiation boost (brachy therapy before postoperative day 5), diabetes, preoperative hyperthermia, smoking, extensive skin damage by radiation, moderate or greater tension in the wound closure may adversely affect wound healing. Sarcoma in the lower extremities has a significantly higher wound-complication rate than upper extremity tumors. Old age, greater than 1 liter of blood loss, long operative times, and the need for wide skin excisions may also increase complications (40–42). Of interest is the fact that adjuvant chemotherapy has been shown not to increase the rate of wound complications in these patients (43,44). We reserve primary closure for patients who have not been radiated or will have minimal wounds that close without tension and do not have critical neural or vascular structures in the wound. Patients who have very little physiologic reserve, and

who undergo resection that will not leave a vital structure exposed as a part of a wound complication, are sometimes reconstructed by primary closure. If primary closure fails, these patients receive hyperbaric oxygen therapy and secondary closure with skin graft or muscle flap (45).

Skin Graft

If resection leaves a healthy, well-vascularized tissue bed with no exposed critical structures, skin grafting is often an excellent reconstructive option. Subcutaneous sarcomas treated by wide excision leaving muscle as a deep margin can usually be treated by split-thickness skin grafting. However, when resection is performed around joints (popliteal fossa, antecubital fossa), joint function may be compromised by subsequent wound contracture after simple skin grafting. In these patients, consideration is given to transfer of a fasciocutaneous flap for closure. In some cases, skin graft placed on radiated muscle may not survive and a microvascular transfer of muscle or fasciocutaneous flap may be required as a secondary procedure.

Local Flap Closure

Local flap closure permits the importation of adjacent tissue for resurfacing tumor bed not amenable to primary closure or skin-graft closure. Usually the flap donor site can't be primarily closed and requires closure using a skin graft. Local flap closure is of little use in patients who have undergone radiation treatment, because transfer of radiated adjacent tissue is fraught with difficulties including partial flap loss and poor wound healing.

Distant Pedicle Flap Closure

This modality permits importation of well-vascularized tissue to the tumor bed with a high degree of reliability. Despite the fact that the flap pedicle is often in the radiation field, we have found this technique useful as long as the portion of the flap that is being transferred to close the wound has not received significant radiation dosage. The surgeon should avoid creating a donor-site defect that has been radiated because it would be at high risk for wound healing complications (Fig. 20–9).

The most common site of soft-tissue sarcomas is the anterior compartment of the thigh. When primary closure in this area is not possible or desirable, the surgeon is usually faced with a wound that cannot be skin-grafted (often because the femur forms the base of the wound). In this location, the use of the rectus abdominus muscle as an extended musculocutaneous flap has served well. The inferior epigastric artery, which supplies the flap, enters adjacent to the inguinal ligament from the external iliac artery.

Patients who smoke are at increased risk of partial loss of pedicled or local flaps (approximately 25% partial flap loss). The most commonly lost part of the flap is the distal portion, which is usually critical to the success of the reconstruction. Conversely, there is no increased rate of partial or complete flap loss for microsurgically planted tissue in smokers as compared to nonsmokers. These factors should be taken into consideration when choosing the best reconstructive option (46). A theoretical factor further mitigating against the use of local pedicled flaps for sarcoma reconstruction includes the fact that harvest and transfer require the extension of the tumor bed with possible contamination of unviolated tissue

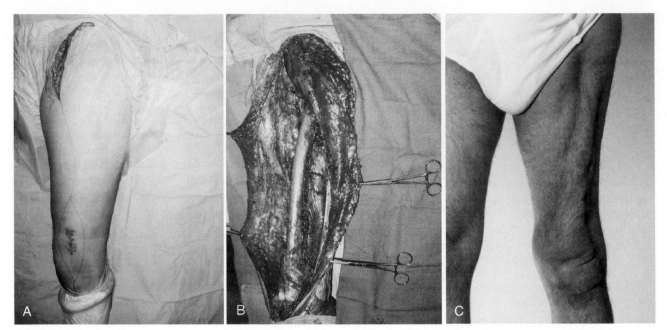

FIG. 20–8. **A,** planned resection of high-grade quadriceps sarcoma. The resection begins at the anterior superior iliac spine and ends at the patellar tendon, ellipsing the biopsy. **B,** the completed resection leaves the femur exposed from the femoral condyles to the lesser trochanter. The medial and lateral intermuscular septae have been excised. The bed of the wound consists of the femur, portions of the adductors, and the hamstring muscles. **C,** postoperative photo following compartmental excision.

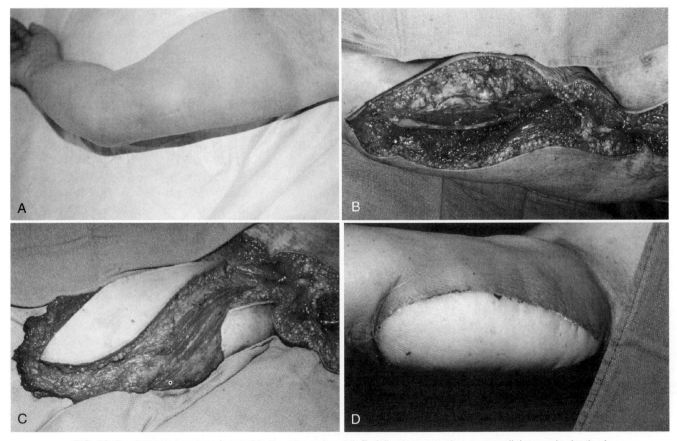

FIG. 20–9. **A,** large sarcoma located in the triceps brachii. **B,** following resection, note radial nerve in depth of wound. **C,** pedicle latissimus transfer provides excellent coverage. **D,** wound closure.

plane and compartments. Furthermore, distant pedicle flaps often result in enosculation of an already compromised extremity. Some of these theoretical and practical factors which may mitigate against the use of pedicle flaps as a reconstructive modality and lead us to a composite tissue transplantation from remote locations.

Microsurgical Composite Tissue Transplantation

When anatomic, aesthetic, or physiologic factors mitigate against simpler reconstructive modalities, current microsurgical techniques permit safe and efficient transfer of any tissue block with an adequate supplying artery and draining vein (47). Inclusion of a sensory or motor nerve coapted to an appropriate nerve at the recipient site permits reinnervation. Occasionally, simultaneous transfer of two separate blocks of tissue is required for optimal reconstructive results (e.g., fibula and latissimus dorsi transfer for a patient with a major bone and soft-tissue defect) (48). Preexpansion of a flap using a tissue expander can increase the size of the flap and lesion donor-site morbidity. The main limitation in this modality of reconstruction is acceptance of donor-site morbidity by the patient and surgeon (49,50).

Appreciation of the importance of meticulous construction and anastomosis to recipient vessels outside of the zone of injury together with improved technical skills of reconstructive surgery have led to a success rate of 95% at most institutions (59). We favor the use of large end-to-side anastomoses when possible, as advocated by Godina (52). Vein grafts are avoided, but an attempt is made to place them electively when needed (53). It is not possible in this review to cover all of the microvascular tissue transfers. Flaps have been described consisting of skin, fascia, muscle, bone, omentum and combinations of most of these (47). Some of the most useful flaps for reconstruction will be briefly enumerated.

SKIN FLAPS

Multiple skin flaps have been described. Most of these include the underlying fascia and subcutaneous vessels. Perforator flaps have been described which, although complicated to harvest, may decrease morbidity by avoidance of fascial harvesting. The free groin flap was particularly popular among early microsurgeons and still remain as an excellent donor site for a free or pedicle flap. Its use as a free-tissue transfer is less common today because of a small donor vascular pedicle of considerable anatomic variability. The radial forearm flap unfortunately requires sacrifice of one of the axial vessels to the hand, but in most patients does not produce objectionable morbidity. The periscapular flap and the scapular flap suffer from poor donor-site aesthetics and a somewhat tedious pedicle dissection. The pedicle of these flaps, however, are usually large, permitting reliable transfer (Fig. 20–10). The lateral arm flap is supplied by the radial collateral artery. Donor-site aesthetics are excellent, and there is a potential for sensibility. The dorsalis pedis flap is a useful part of the armamenterium but suffers from a high morbidity at its donor site.

FASCIAL FLAPS

Free fascial transfers are used when well-vascularized thin cover is required. The tempoparietal fascial flap has a reliable vascular pedicle of large caliber; this flap has many applications. Its major disadvantage is its unreliability when reelevated for secondary procedures (Fig. 20–11).

MUSCLE FLAPS

Skeletal muscle transfer is most commonly used in our sarcoma reconstructive practice. Donor morbidity is relatively low. The most frequently used muscle flaps in our practice are the latissimus dorsi, rectus abdominus, and serratus anterior. Muscles fill dead space well and usually assume an excellent contour. During the first year postoperatively, the noninnervated muscle shrinks by approximately 80% in volume. Muscle flaps are superior for resurfacing weight-bearing portions of the foot.

Muscle flaps may be transferred as a functional flap in patients who have lost muscle and tendon. Functional muscle transfer requires microvascular anastomoses of the artery and vein as well as reinnervation by microsurgical coaptation of the motor nerve in the transplanted muscle to a healthy viable motor nerve at the recipient site (54) (Fig. 20–12). The gracilis and latissimus dorsi muscles have achieved the greatest utility in our practice for functional muscle transplantation.

When transferring these muscles, it is particularly important to place them at their resting length. This is achieved by placing sutures at regular intervals before detaching the muscle from its origin insertion at its donor site. Once it is transferred, it is stretched out to length using the preplaced sutures at regular intervals for reference. Preservation or addition of a fascial extension is sometimes useful; this serves as a noveau tendon that can be woven into other tendons or secured to bone with a metallic anchor. The functional strength of a transplanted skeletal muscle is directly proportional to the cross-sectional area of the innervated, contracting muscle fibers. The range of muscle contraction is a factor of fiber length. Free muscle transplants can partly replace the lost function of muscle groups in the upper extremity (Fig. 20–13). Functional muscle transplantation may be an alternative to tendon transfer. It is somewhat difficult to obtain coverage as well as function from a transplanted muscle, and some patients require transplantation of one flap to provide coverage and a separate flap to provide function, though this is not an invariable but rather a relative requirement. Musculocutaneous flaps muscles can be transplanted with their overlying subcutaneous tissue and skin. The skin and subcutaneous tissues is largely supplied by perforating vessels. These flaps are particularly useful when it is necessary to import a large amount of soft tissue. They also should be considered when it is necessary to provide both coverage and functioning muscle. The disadvantage in many cases is that the flap is such a bulky nature that it does not provide for an aesthetic reconstruction.

OSSEOUS FLAPS

When tumor resection requires creation of an unstable skeletal defect, bone grafting may be required in reconstruction. When the native bone in the resection site has been irradiated, allografts and non-vascularized autografts heal slowly and unpredictably. Vascularized bone grafts are superior to nonvascularized autogenous bone grafts or allografts with regard to early incorporation, hypertrophy, and mechanical

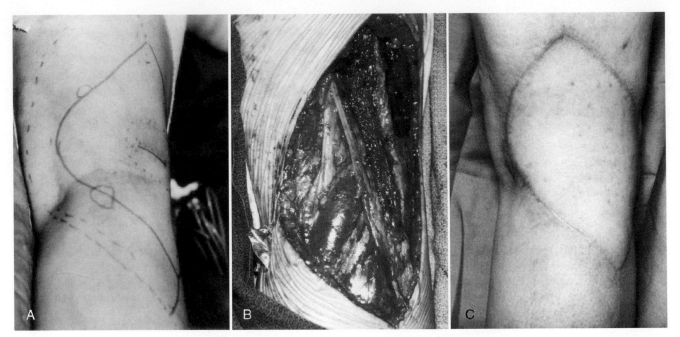

FIG. 20–10. **A,** popliteal subcutaneous sarcoma with biopsy through transverse incision. Dotted line surrounding incision indicates hematoma. Solid line indicates resection ellipse. **B,** completed re- section takes fascia as a deep margin, leaving exposed the posterior tibial and peroneal nerves. **C,** closure with free scapular flap provides excellent coverage.

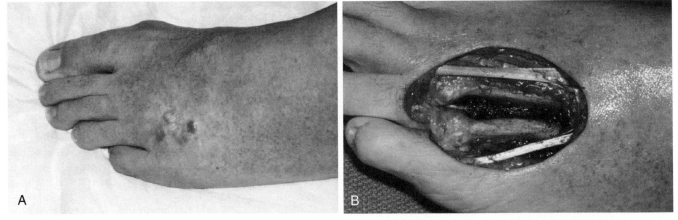

FIG. 20–11. **A,** dermatofibrosarcoma protuberans recurrent after marginal excision. **B,** wide excision exposes bone and tendon. Fascial flap allows coverage and STG without undesirable bulk.

FIG. 20–12. Excision of the dorsal forearm compartment with skin loss requires free-tissue transfer of a latissimus myocutaneous flap. The radial nerve is preserved proximally in the wound for anastomosis to the motor nerve of the latissimus.

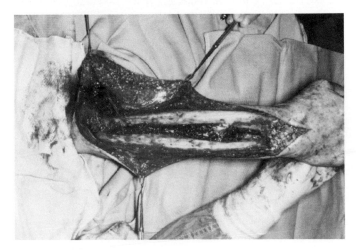

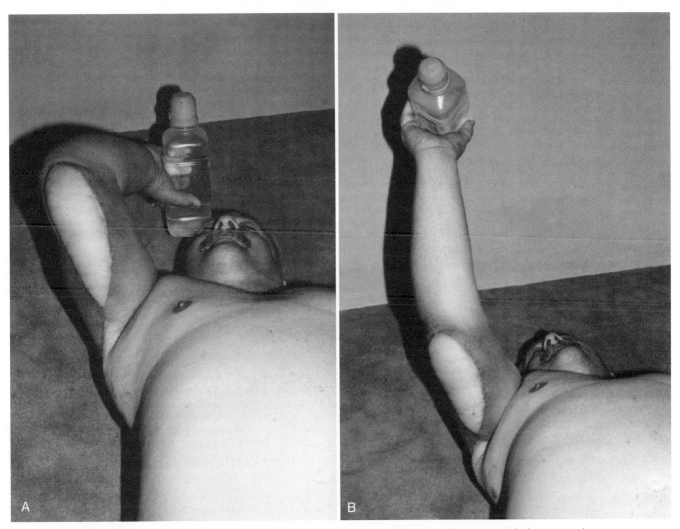

FIG. 20–13. A, B, patient following latissimus pedicle flap procedure to replace resected triceps muscle.

stress to failure for long bone defects over time (55). When bone defects are large, or the recipient is dysvascular, clinical evidence suggest that osteocyte survival is superior for free-vascularized bone grafts. The fibula, as well as vascularized ilium on the deep circumflex iliac vessels, are the two flaps that have achieved the greatest utility in modern reconstructive surgery. For most patients, the fibula provides an excellent vascularized bone graft with acceptable donor-site morbidity (56), or it can be harvested with a skin island. The fibulae soft-tissue coverage provides for monitoring (57). The popularization of the Ilizarov method of distraction osteogenesis has revolutionized reconstruction of bony defects. These techniques may be combined with the use of allografts or metallic prostheses. The performance of allograft may be improved by placement of a vascularized fibula through their center.

The improved success rates and the facility with which microvascular reconstruction may be performed, permitting optimal wound closure with well-vascularized tissue in one stage, led to an increased popularity of this technique. Distant donor site serves to provide large amounts of healthy tissue without further altering the functional status of an already-compromised limb. The use of this distant site also avoids extensive dissection in local tissue planes that could spread the local disease. Because of these advantages, microsurgical tissue transplantation has achieved a very important role in reconstruction of limb sparing procedures for the treatment of soft-tissue sarcoma (58).

VASCULAR RECONSTRUCTION

Tumor resection requiring sacrifice of a major vascular structure is not a contraindication to limb salvage. Critical arterial structures are replaced either with vein graft or vascular prostheses (Fig. 20–14). We do not attempt venous reconstruction because of the potential problems with patency and pulmonary emboli. When possible, we attempt to preserve large collateral veins. For example, if resection of the femoral vein is required, an attempt is made to preserve the saphenous vein.

TISSUE EXPANSION

Tissue expansion has been increasingly used in reconstructive operative procedures. This technique has been thought to produce more complications when used in the extremities. While there is a limited role for tissue expansion in resurfacing extremities that have not been irradiated, its role in sarcoma reconstruction remains limited.

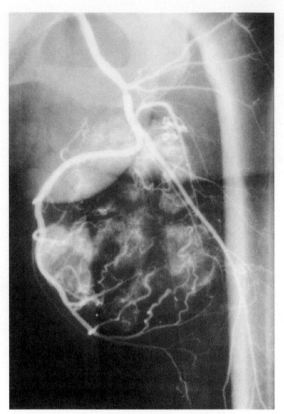

FIG. 20–14. Medial thigh sarcoma displacing femoral vessels. Resection required intercalary resection of involved vessel and vascular bypass.

Summary

Increasing advances in our understanding of the biology of soft-tissue sarcoma, coupled with objective review of the outcomes of various techniques of management, have resulted in improved management. Eighty percent of patients are appropriately treated by limb-sparing procedures. Immediate bony reconstruction with prosthetic implantation, or vascularized bone grafts preserve appendicular skeletal function. Microvascular transfer of tissue provides one-stage wound closure with large amounts of healthy well-vascularized tissue.

References

1. Enneking WF. *Musculoskeletal tumor surgery.* New York: Churchill Livingstone, 1983.
2. Wingo PA, Tong T, Bolden S. Cancer statistics: 1995 published erratum appears in CA Cancer J Clin CA 1995; 45:8–30.
3. Simon MA, Enneking WF. The management of soft-tissue sarcomas of the extremities. *J Bone Joint Surg* 1976; 58:317.
4. Enneking WF, Spanier SS, Malawer MM. The effect of the anatomic setting on the results of surgical procedures for soft parts sarcoma of the thigh. *Cancer* 1981; 47:1005.
5. American Joint Committee. *Manual for staging of cancer.* Chicago: American Joint Committee, 1977.
6. Enneking WF, Spanier SS, Goodman MA. Current concepts review: the surgical staging of musculoskeletal sarcoma. *J Bone Joint Surg* 1980; 62:1027.
7. Enneking WF, Spanier SS, Goodman MA. A system for the surgical staging of musculoskeletal sarcoma. *Clin Orthop* 1980; 153:106.
8. Broder AC. The microscopic grading of cancer. In: Pack GT, Arrel IM, eds. *Treatment of cancer and allied diseases.* New York: PB Hoeber, 1964.
9. Leyvarz S, Costa J. Histologic diagnosis and grading of soft-tissue sarcomas. *Seminars in Surgical Oncology* 1988; 4:3–6.
10. Dewhirst MW, Sostman HD, Leopold KA, et al. Soft-tissue sarcomas: MR imaging and MR spectroscopy for prognosis and therapy monitoring. *Radiology* 1990; 174:847–53.
11. Schumacher TM, Genant HK, Korobkin M, et al. Computed tomography. Its use in space-occupying lesions of the musculoskeletal system. *J Bone Joint Surg* 1978; 60:600.
12. Kirschner PT, Simon MA. The clinical value of bone and gallium scintigraphy for soft-tissue sarcomas of the extremities. *J Bone Joint Surg* 1984; 66:319.
13. Hudson TM, Haas G, Enneking WF, et al. Angiography in the management of musculoskeletal tumors. *Surgery* 1975; 141:11.
14. DeSantos LA, Wallace S, Finklestine JB. Angiography and lymphangiography in peripheral soft-tissue sarcomas. In: *Management of primary bone and soft-tissue tumors.* Chicago: Year Book, 1977; 235.
15. Mankin HJ, Lange TA, Spanier SS. The hazards of biopsy in patients with malignant primary bone and soft-tissue tumors. *J Bone Joint Surg* 1982; 64:1121.
16. Pack GT, Arrel IM. Principles of treatment of tumors of the soft somatic tissues. In: Pack GT, Arrel IM, eds. *Treatment of cancer and allied diseases.* New York, PB Hoeber, 1964.
17. Bowder L, Booher RJ. The principles and techniques of resection of soft parts for sarcoma. *Surgery* 1958; 44:963.
18. Eilber FR, Morton DL, Eckardt J, et al. Limb salvage for skeletal soft-tissue sarcomas. Multi-disciplinary preoperative therapy. *Cancer* 1984; 53:2579.
19. Eilber FR, Mirra JJ, Grant TT, et al. Is amputation necessary for sarcomas? A seven-year experience with limb salvage. *Ann Surg* 1980; 192:431.
20. Mantravadi RV, Trippon MJ, Patel MK, et al. Limb salvage in extremity soft-tissue sarcoma: combined modality therapy. *Radiology* 1984; 152:523.
21. Yang JC, Rosenburg SA. Surgery for adult patients with soft-tissue sarcoma. *Seminars in Oncology* 1989; 16:289–296.
22. Zelefsky MJ, Nori D, Shiu MH, et al. Limb salvage in soft-tissue sarcomas involving neurovascular structures using combined surgical resection and therapy. *Int J Radiation Oncology, Biology and Physics* 1990; 19:913–918.
23. Brant TA, Parsons JT, Marcus RB Jr., et al. Preoperative irradiation soft-tissue sarcomas of the trunk and extremities in adults. *Int J Radiation Oncology, Biology and Physics* 1990; 19:899–906.
24. Leopold KA, Harrelson JM, Prosnitz L, et al. Preoperative hyperthermia and radiation for soft-tissue sarcomas: vanish one versus two hyperthermia treatments per week. *Int J Radiation Oncology, Biology and Physics* 1989; 16:107–115.
25. Lindberg RD, Martin RG, Romsdahl MM, et al. Conservative surgery and postoperative radiotherapy in 300 adults with soft-tissue sarcomas. *Cancer* 1981; 47:2391–2397.
26. Tepper JE, Suit HD. Radiation therapy of soft-tissue sarcomas. *Cancer* 1985; 55:2273–2277.
27. Suit HD, Mankin HJ, Wood WC, et al. Preoperative, intraoperative, and postoperative radiation therapy in the treatment of primary soft-tissue sarcoma. *Cancer* 1985; 55:2659–2667.
28. Barkley HT Jr., Martin RG, Romsdahl MM, et al. Treatment of soft-tissue sarcomas by preoperative radiation and conservative surgical resection. *Int J Oncology, Biology and Physics* 1988; 14:693–699.
29. Pao WJ, Pilepich MV. Postoperative radiotherapy in the treatment of extremity soft-tissue sarcoma. *Int J Oncology, Biology and Physics* 1990; 19:901–911.
30. Oleson JR, Dewhirst MW, Harrelson JM, et al. Tumor temperature distributions predict hyperthermia effect. *Int J Oncology, Biology and Physics* 1988; 16:559–570.
31. Scully SP, Oleson JR, Leopold JA, et al. Clinical outcome after neoadjuvant thermoradiography in high-grade soft-tissue sarcomas. *Journal of Surgical Oncology* 1994; 57:143–151.
32. Antiman KH, Elias AD. Chemotherapy of advanced soft-tissue sarcomas. *Seminars in Oncology* 1988; 4:53–58.
33. Antiman KH, Eilber FR, Siu MH. Soft-tissue sarcomas: current trends and diagnosis and management. *Current Problems in Cancer* 1989; 340–367.
34. Bramwell V, Rouesse J, Steward W, et al. Adjuvant CYVADIC chemotherapy for adult soft-tissue sarcoma—reduced local recurrence but no improvement in survival. A study of the European Organization for Research and Treatment of Cancer Soft-tissue and Bone Sarcoma Group. *J Clin Oncol* 1994; 12:1137

35. Zalupski MM, Baker LH. Systemic adjuvant chemotherapy for soft-tissue sarcomas. *Hematol Oncol Clin North Am* 1995; 9:787–800.

36. Tierney JF, Mosseri V, Stewart LA, et al. Adjuvant chemotherapy for soft-tissue sarcoma: review and meta-analysis of the published results of randomized clinical trials. *Br J Cancer* 1995; 72:469–475.

37. McGrath PC, Sloan DA, Kenady DE. Adjuvant therapy for soft-tissue sarcomas. *Clin Plast Surg* 1995; 22:21–29.

38. Ormsby MV, Hilaris BS, Mori D, et al. Wound complications of adjuvant radiation therapy in patients with soft-tissue sarcomas. *Ann Surg* 1989; 210:93–99.

39. Barwick WJ, Goldberg JA, Scully SP, et al. Vascularized tissue transfer for closure of irradiated wounds after soft-tissue sarcoma resection. *Ann Surg* 1992; 216:591–595.

40. Peat BG, Bell RS, Davis A, et al. Wound-healing complications after soft-tissue sarcoma surgery. *Plast Reconstr Surg* 1994; 93:980–987.

41. Bujko K, Suit HD, Springfield DS, et al. Wound healing after preoperative radiation for sarcoma of soft tissues. *Surg Gynecol Obstet* 1993; 176:124–134.

42. O'Connor MI, Pritchard DJ, Gunderon LL. Integration of limb-sparing surgery, brachytherapy, and external-beam irradiation in the treatment of soft-tissue sarcomas. *Clin Orthop* 1993; 289:73–80.

43. Bertermann O, Marcove RC, Rosen G. Effect of intensive adjuvant chemotherapy on wound healing in 69 patients with osteogenic sarcomas of the lower extremities. *Recent Results Cancer Res* 1985; 98:135–141.

44. Arbeit JM, Hilaris BS, Brennan MF. Wound complications in the multimodality treatment of extremity and superficial truncal sarcomas. *J Clin Oncol* 1987; 5:480–488.

45. Kindwall EP. Hyperbaric oxygen's effect on radiation necrosis. *Clinics in Plastic Surgery* 1993; 20:473–483.

46. Mathes SJ, Clinical applications for muscle and musculocutaneous flaps. St. Louis: CV Mosby, 1982.

47. Serafin D, Atlas of microsurgical composite tissue transplantation. Philadelphia: WB Saunders, 1996.

48. Whitney TM, Buncke HJ, Lineaweaver WC, et al. Multiple microvascular transplants: a preliminary report of simultaneous versus sequential reconstruction. *Ann Plast Surg* 1989; 22:391.

49. Leighton WD, et al. Experimental pretransfer expansion of free-flap donor sites. 1. Flap viability and expansion characteristics. *Plast Reconstr Surg* 1988; 82:69.

50. Leighton WD, et al. Experimental pretransfer expansion of free-flap donor sites. 11. Physiology, histology, and clinical correlation. *Plast Reconstr Surg* 1988; 28:76.

51. Khouri RK. Avoid free-flap failure. *Clin Plast Surg* 1992; 19:773.

52. Godina M. Early microsurgical reconstruction of complex trauma of extremities. *Plast Reconstr Surg* 1986; 78:285.

53. Ritter EF, Anthony JP, Levin LS, et al. Microsurgical composite tissue transplantation at difficult recipient sites facilitated by preliminary installation of vein grafts as arteriovenous loops. *Journal of Reconstructive Microsurgery* 1996; 12:229–238.

54. Mankelow RT, Zuker RM, McKee NH. Functioning free muscle transplantation. *J Hand Surg* 1984; 9:32.

55. Taylor GI. The current status of free vascularized bone grafts. *Clin Plast Surg* 1983; 10:185.

56. Anthony JP, Rawnsley JD, Benahim P, et al. Donor leg morbidity and function after fibular free flap mandible reconstruction. *Plast and Reconstructive Surgery* 1995; 96:145–152.

57. Anthony JP, Ritter EF, Young DM, et al. Enhancing fibular free flap skin island reliability and versatility for mandibular reconstruction. *Ann Plast Surg* 1993; 31:106–111.

58. Drake DB. Reconstruction for limb-sparing procedures in soft-tissue sarcomas of the extremities. *Clinics in Plast Surg* 1995; 22:123–128.

21

Cutaneous Vascular Anomalies: Hemangiomas and Malformations

A.J. Burns, M.D., F.A.C.S., and J.B. Mulliken, M.D., F.A.C.S.

Cutaneous vascular anomalies all look rather alike: they are either flat or raised, in various shades of blue, red, and purple. These anomalies have been labeled by terms, often confusing, that are entrenched in medical parlance and literature. Vascular anomalies are pathogenetically heterogenous; although they often look similar, they are biologically different. Histologic terms for vascular anomalies, introduced during the mid-19th century, have only confused the field. Bewildering nomenclature and classification of superficial vascular anomalies continue to be responsible, in no small measure, for improper diagnosis, illogical treatment, and misdirected research efforts.

There is no effective classification without a proper definition of terms. The Greek nominative suffix -*oma* means "swelling" or "tumor." In moderate usage, however, -*oma* denotes a tumor, a lesion characterized by increased cellular turnover. This semantic refinement is crucial to a biologic classification of vascular anomalies.

A biologic classification proposed in 1982 defines the cellular features of vascular anomalies and correlates these with clinical presentation and natural history (1,2). According to this system, there are two main types of biologically different cutaneous vascular anomalies occurring in infants and children: hemangiomas and vascular malformations. Further studies confirm that this system of classification is based not only on cellular and clinical criteria but also on radiological, hemodynamic, and immunohistochemical characteristics (2,3,4). The nosology used in this chapter has the imprimatur of the International Society for the Study of Vascular Anomalies (ISSVA), which was founded in 1992.

Hemangioma is the most common benign tumor of infancy. In the past, it was variously labeled as "capillary," "strawberry," "immature" or "juvenile," or it was called "benign hemangioendothelioma." Hemangiomas exhibit remarkable proliferation during infancy, followed by invariable spontaneous regression during childhood. These tumors never appear in an adolescent or adult.

The term *cavernous hemangioma* has been used to delineate deeply located hemangiomas and/or venous malformations. The word *cavernous* should be mentioned only to be condemned, because it is confusing at best. Histologic examination of hemangiomas with both superficial and deep components reveals a remarkably consistent endothelial pattern throughout the depth of the tumor (2) (Fig. 21–1). Color variations of hemangiomas depend on the level to which the tumor has invaded the papillary dermis, (i.e., the red tones prevail, with progressively superficial location). There is no

such lesion as a "cavernous" hemangioma! The lesion is either a deep hemangioma or a venous malformation. Quite simply, hemangioma is hemangioma. No descriptive terminology is needed other than to describe its location as being superficial or deep, or to qualify whether it was first seen in the proliferating, involuting, or involuted phase.

Vascular malformations are errors of embryonic development. They are composed of dysmorphic channels lined by fat endothelium that exhibits a normal, exceedingly slow rate of cellular turnover. These anomalies grow proportionately with the child; however, some types can expand coincident with thrombosis, sepsis, hormonal alteration, trauma, or surgical intervention. Vascular malformations can be subcategorized according to rheology and channel morphology: slow-flow capillary, lymphatic, or venous, or fast-flow arterial or arteriovenous. There are also complex-combined vascular malformations, many of them known by eponyms.

In over 90% of cases, an accurate diagnosis can be made by history and physical examination, which spares the child expensive, painful, and unnecessary investigations. Radiologic imaging is rarely necessary to make a correct diagnosis.

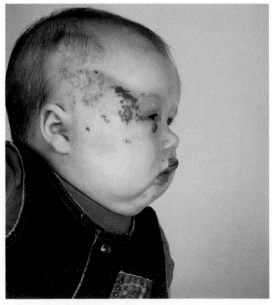

FIG. 21–1. Four-month-old white male with hemangioma of the right hemiface. The hemangioma has both a superficial and deep component.

Hemangioma

PATHOGENESIS

There are several theories as to the pathogenesis of hemangiomas; the etiology is not known. Folkman (5–9) proposes that hemangiomas are angiogenesis dependent. Takahashi and colleagues (4) used immunohistochemistry to distinguish the proliferating, involuting, and involuted phases of the hemangioma's life cycle. Hemangiomas in the rapid growth phase of infancy are defined by high expression of proliferating cell nuclear antigen, type IV, collagenase and growth factors, basic fibroblast growth factor (BFGF) and vascular endothelial growth factor (VEGF). Elevated expression of tissue inhibitor of metalloproteinase, TIMP-1 (an inhibitor of new blood vessel formation) is observed only in involutional lesions.

CLINICAL FEATURES

Hemangiomas occur in 8 to 12% of full-term white infants (10, 11) and up to 22% of preterm neonates who weigh less than 1000 gm (12). There is a female preponderance of 3 to 5:1 (13,14,15). A 1 to 2% incidence is noted among black newborns (16). Fourteen to twenty percent of affected infants have more than one hemangioma. The head and neck regions make up less than 14% of the total body surface, yet approximately 60% of all hemangiomas occur there.

There are examples, with a high female predilection, in which true hemangiomas are associated with dysmorphic anomalies (malformations) (17). Specifically, large cervicofacial hemangiomas are observed variously with sternal nonunion, supraumbilical raphe, absence of ipsilateral carotid/vertebral vessels, coarctation of a right-sided aortic arch, dilation of the carotid siphon, and Dandy-Walker malformation (18,19). Overlapping of these associated anomalies suggests a spectrum (19). Lumbosacral hemangioma is associated with occult spinal dysraphism (i.e., lipomeningocele, tethered cord, and diastematomyelia) (2).

There are two differing observations as to the evolution of the hemangioma. Some believe that a hemangioma starts at a focal point and spreads by proliferation, whereas others believe that hemangioma begins as a "field transformation" (20). Multiple tumors, in skin and other organs, appear concurrently. Most often, hemangioma manifests within the first few weeks of life. Premonitory signs are either a pale white spot (anemic nevus), a telangiectatic or macular red stain, or a blue ecchymotic patch mimicking a bruise (2). Rarely, a hemangioma can be present at birth, fully grown. These congenital (intrauterine) hemangiomas exhibit accelerated regression (21).

There are no known predictors of which hemangiomas will grow most rapidly; each hemangioma is unique. Hemangioma grows rapidly for the first 9 to 12 months, reaching a

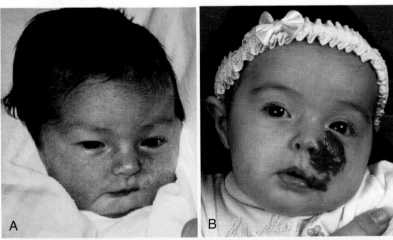
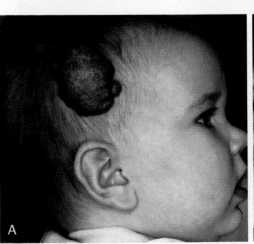
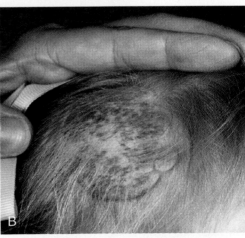

FIG. 21–2. **A,** 3-week-old newborn with faint macular patch in left superior nasolabial fold area. **B,** same child at 4 months, revealing hemangioma in proliferative phase.

FIG. 21–3. **A,** 6-month-old white female with hemangioma of the right scalp. Note central pallor and scattered "greying" areas, heralding the beginning of involution. **B,** same child at 2 years of age, showing more advanced stages of involution.

plateau (proliferation phase) followed by a slow phase of involution (Fig. 21–2). Stabilization and beginning involution are heralded by a central pallor and a fading of the bright crimson color to a dull purple or gray (Fig. 21–3). These changes should be pointed out to the parents to encourage them about the improvement of the hemangioma.

The involuting phase lasts 2 to 9 years. The rate of involution of a particular hemangioma cannot be predicted by

site, size, or appearance. Nearly normal skin results in about 50% of children with involuted hemangioma. Even after involution, especially in lesions that were once large, the skin evidences telangiectasia, yellowish hypoelastic patches, sagging, and scarring if ulceration occurred during proliferation. Fibrofatty residual "tumor" can persist as well (Fig. 21–4).

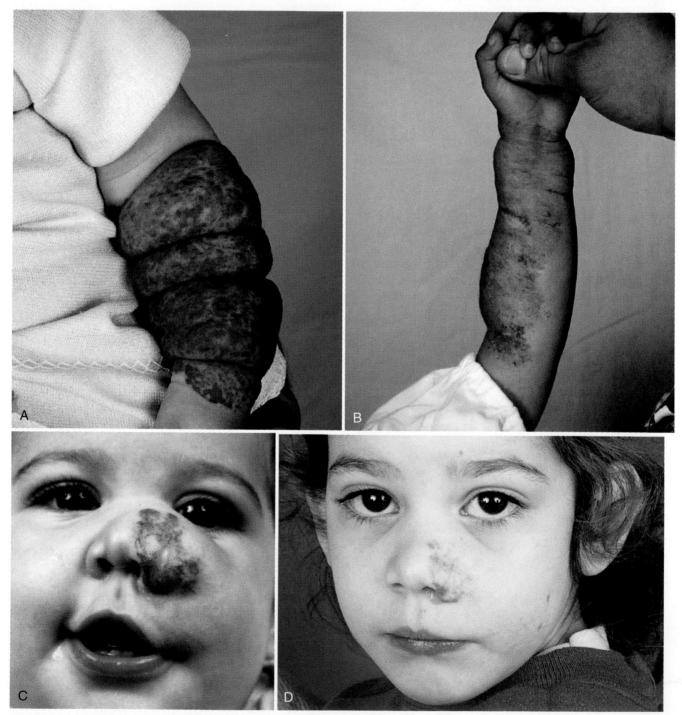

FIG. 21–4. A, 9-month-old white female with large bulky hemangioma of the left forearm. **B,** same child at 30 months, showing residual fibrofatty tumor and scattered telangiectasias. **C,** 4-month-old white female with hemangioma of the left nose. Note bulky hemangioma deep-seated under the left cheek, nose, and left upper lip. **D,** same child at 4 years of age, with resolving hemangioma in involutional stage. Note that the majority of the bulk has resolved; however, residual telangiectasia persists, and a scar in the left lateral alar base is unchanged as a result of previous ulceration.

DIFFERENTIAL DIAGNOSIS

Over 90% of hemangiomas can be accurately diagnosed within the 1st or 2nd office visit by history and physical examination alone. If the diagnosis is in question, repeated examination with careful photographic documentation of the growth usually confirms the nature of the lesion. Radiologic investigation helps establish the diagnosis in a deep subcutaneous or intramuscular tumor, or in the case of visceral hemangiomatosis (Fig. 21–5). Ultrasonography with color-flow imaging is the most cost-effective. It sometimes can be difficult for an ultrasonographer to distinguish proliferative hemangioma from arteriovenous malformation because both are high-flow lesions. Ultrasonography is very helpful in differentiating hemangiomas from low-flow lesions such as venous or lymphatic malformations. Ultrasonography does not, however, show clearly the relationship of the vascular lesion to adjacent structures.

Magnetic resonance imaging (MRI) is the gold standard for showing the extent of a vascular lesion and its relationship to adjacent structures. Hemangioma has a characteristic lobular, parenchymatous tissue appearance, with intermediate heterogeneous signal on T1-weighted sequences, that is brightly enhanced on T2-weighted sequences. Flow voids usually are seen on T1-weighted sequences, indicating the feeding arteries. Fatty tissue is seen in involuting hemangiomas. These MRI findings are distinctly different from lymphatic, venous, or arteriovenous malformations (3,18,22,23).

MANAGEMENT

The vast majority of hemangiomas do not require treatment. These lesions are not referred to a specialist if they are small in size or are not in a cosmetically sensitive location. Even the majority of infants referred to a specialist require only observation and reassurance to the parents. The physician must remain an advocate for the child and not succumb to pressures by well-meaning but emotionally distraught parents, family members, and friends. There are, however, definite indications for therapeutic intervention in proliferating phase hemangioma:

Obstruction
Deformation
Ulceration
Coagulopathy
Congestive heart failure

Large and/or strategically located hemangiomas can cause functional impairment and may have to be dealt with more aggressively. Relative indications for early treatment also include hemangiomas in anatomically troublesome locations that are prone to long-term deformity (e.g., nose, lips, or breast buds). Tumors that merit immediate or early intervention include hemangiomas causing functional obstruction of the visual axis, airway, or oropharynx. Lesions that are large or ulcerated with secondary hemorrhage or infection, or those associated with Kasabach-Merritt coagulopathy and/or congestive heart failure, must be treated as well.

Ulceration occurs in 5% of lesions, most commonly on the lips and genital areas (24). Punctate bleeding is unusual in hemangioma; it usually occurs in association with ulceration. Once there is ulceration, a scar inevitably results (Fig. 21–6). Some favor meticulous wound care to permit epithelialization. It should be kept in mind that laser therapy is more expensive than conventional local care. Nevertheless, there are reports of accelerated wound healing and lessening of pain using the pulse-dye laser (24). Laser therapy is particularly effective in healing ulcerated hemangiomas in intertriginous areas, particularly the perineum, with decreased pain. It should be noted that larger ulcerative lesions require a second treatment at 10 to 14 days.

Periorbital hemangiomas can cause visual axis obstruction with deprivation amblyopia and failure to develop binocular vision (25–28). Visual obstruction for 1 week or more between birth and 1 year of age is detrimental to subsequent vision (27). More insidious is the mass effect from a periorbital hemangioma that distorts the cornea, producing asymmetrical refractive errors (astigmatism or myopia) that, in turn, cause amblyopia. Children with periorbital hemangioma of any size, particularly those with tumors of the upper lid, should have an immediate ophthalmologic evaluation. Lower-eyelid hemangioma is much less prone to cause corneal deformation.

Periauricular and cervical hemangiomas are not infrequently accompanied by upper-airway lesions. Even small

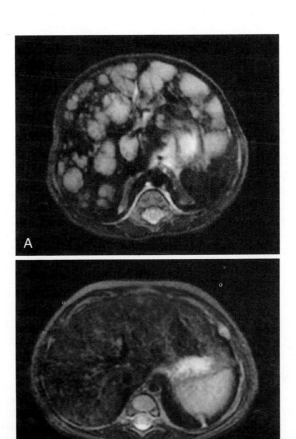

FIG. 21–5. **A,** axial MRI, 2-month-old girl with multiple cutaneous hemangiomas, hepatomegaly, anemia, and congestive heart failure. Fast spin-echo T2-weighted sequence with fat suppression shows multifocal hemangiomas throughout liver. **B,** axial MRI (same sequence) 1 year later, after 9 months of interferon alpha-2a therapy, liver hemangiomas virtually disappeared.

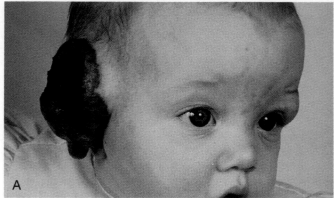

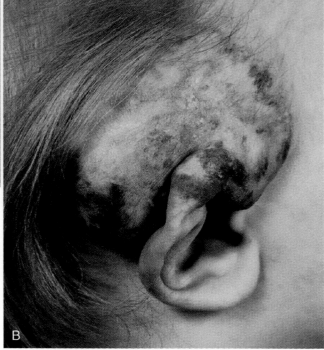

FIG. 21–6. A, 3-month-old white female with large ulcerative hemangioma of the right auricular region. **B,** same child 4 months later after three treatments with the pulsed-dye laser. Note the scarring that inevitably results from the ulceration in the central portion of the hemangioma. Note also hypopigmentation, not uncommon after laser therapy.

hemangiomas in the subglottic airway (18,29–33) are life threatening and should be treated aggressively. Clinical signs are biphasic stridor, often accompanied by laryngotracheitis and/or recurrent bouts of croup occasionally progressing to respiratory distress (34).

Any large cutaneous hemangioma, especially visceral hemangiomas, may be complicated by profound thrombocytopenia (Kasabach-Merritt phenomenon). Clinical signs include petechiae and ecchymoses or internal bleeding. Morbidity, even with aggressive pharmacologic therapy, is reported to be 30 to 40% (35).

Multiple cutaneous hemangiomas (neonatal hemangiomatosis), typically dome-shaped lesions, may indicate the presence of large visceral hemangiomas, particularly in the liver. This scenario presents as a triad of anemia, hepatomegaly, and congestive heart failure (2,36). The mortality rate of infants with multiple or diffuse hemangiomatosis is as high as 50%.

Pharmacologic Therapy

Corticosteroid

Systemic corticosteroid is the frontline drug for treatment of endangering, deforming, or life-threatening hemangioma. Prednisone or prednisolone is used: 2 mg/kg/day PO in the morning for 4 weeks, followed by a slow tapering dose over several months. For life-threatening tumors (e.g., Kasabach-Merritt coagulopathy, congestive heart failure, or subglottic location), longer treatment may be required. A sensitive hemangioma exhibits responsiveness within days or 1 to 2 weeks: softening, lightening of color, and diminished growth.

In general, the rate of response to systemic corticosteroids is 30%, demonstrating a dramatic sensitivity, usually within 2 to 3 weeks, and the hemangioma stops growing and begins to pale and shrink. Thirty percent fail to respond, even with increased steroid dosage, and 40% have an equivocal (stabilization) response (22) (Fig. 21–7).

Systemic complications are minimal with this regimen. The most common complication of steroids is a change in the growth curve, with either an increase or decrease in weight gain. This change in growth rate, however, is short-lived and, once the steroids are discontinued, gradual return to the pretreatment growth curve is noted.

Similar results are obtained with intralesional injections of triamcinolone for small lesions, particularly hemangiomas of the eyelid, cheeks, nasal tip, and periorbital area (37–39,48). In theory, the advantage of intralesional steroid instillation is to minimize systemic effects. However, studies show that the action of intralesional steroids can be systemic, with reported cases of adrenal suppression following intralesional steroid injection (39). Local complications of intralesional injections include temporary atrophy and, in the periorbital location, ptosis, third-nerve palsy, necrosis, and even blindness (secondary to embolic central retinal artery occlusion) have been reported (40–42).

Interferon Alpha-2a

Recombinant interferon alpha-2a is the second-line drug for large, endangering, or life-threatening hemangiomas, particularly for those tumors resistant to corticosteroids (see Fig. 21–5). The dosage is 3 million units subcutaneously daily. Six to twelve months of sustained therapy is usually required (43,44). Complications of interferon alpha-2a therapy are transient fever and neutropenia early on, as well as rare minor elevations of liver enzymes. The children appear to grow and gain weight normally, in contrast to those receiving prolonged corticosteroids (44). Anti-aggregating drugs, such as ticlopidine, aspirin, and/or pentoxifylline, have also proven successful in correcting Kasabach-Merritt thrombocytopenia.

Embolization

Embolization of hemangiomas with superselective arterial catheterization is considered if there is failure or slow response to pharmacologic therapy (47).

Laser

There is controversy regarding both the need for and efficacy of treating hemangioma with the FLPD. Pulse-dye laser penetrates from 0.7 mm to 1 mm at most; therefore, only the superficial layer of hemangioma is affected. Thus, treatment of bulky lesions is clearly not cost-effective and can even be dangerous; anesthesia is required. However, small flat lesions, noted in the first few weeks of life, can be treated effectively in one or two sessions with no anesthesia in an office environment for very little cost (Fig. 21–8). In these circumstances, the laser is a very cost-effective treatment for such superficial hemangiomas. Pulse-dye laser is also useful for telangiectasia that can persist in an involuted hemangioma.

Surgical Excision

Surgical resection has a role during all three phases of hemangioma life cycle: proliferating, involuting, and involuted. Indications for subtotal or total excision in infancy include: upper eyelid lesions that are unresponsive to pharmacologic therapy, pedunculated lesions with troublesome ulceration and/or bleeding, and CO_2 laser removal of subglottic tumor. Surgical removal should be considered during the preschool period for lesions in sensitive areas (e.g., the nasal tip, glabella, and cheek), especially if it is obvious that skin removal will be necessary in the future (Fig. 21–9). Most often, surgical endeavors should be carried out after involution is complete, at 4 or 5 years of age, just before entering school. (The child usually suffers no emotional consequences of the hemangioma and no morbidity until entering kindergarten or the 1st grade.) At this point, surgical excision and reconstruction should be carried out to achieve the optimum result. Optimally, if one can wait until completion of regression, blood loss is minimized and there is extra skin to achieve the best surgical result. In rare instances, there can be scarring and actual skin loss; thus, tissue expansion may be a surgical stratagem.

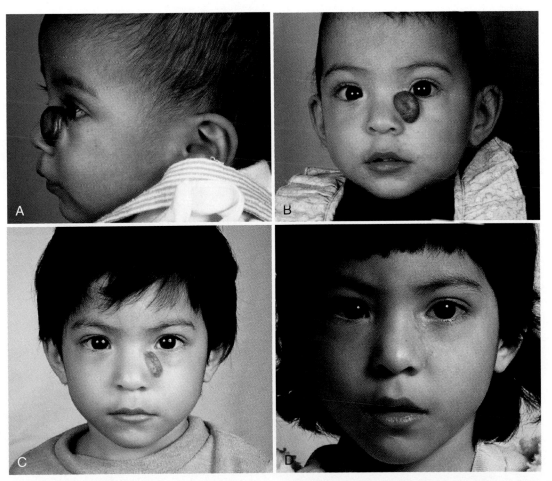

FIG. 21–7. **A,** 6-month-old white female with proliferative hemangioma enlarging, causing potential impairment of the visual axis. **B,** same child 2 months after steroid therapy begun. A subtle but distinctly noticeable difference is apparent with a greying of the lesion. On physical examination, the lesion has softened considerably (steroids). **C,** same child at 3 years of age, showing progressive natural involution of the lesion. **D,** same child 8 months postoperative resection of the left nasolabial hemangioma.

Vascular Malformations

PATHOGENESIS

Vascular malformations are structural abnormalities resulting from faulty embryonic morphogenesis. These lesions are present at birth (although not always obvious); they grow proportionately with the child, and they never regress (1). Vascular malformations are subcategorized based on rheology and channel morphology.

Low-flow malformations include capillary (CM), venous (VM), and lymphatic (LM). These lesions can be pure channel types of complex, combined with any of the three elements (i.e., CLM, CVM, LVM, CLVM).

High-flow malformations include arterial (aneurysm, 15 stenosis, ectasia), arteriovenous (AVM), and arteriovenous fistula (AVF). More than 90% of cutaneous vascular malformations in infants and children are easily diagnosed by clinical features (49); radiologic investigation is thus unnecessary to make the diagnosis. Nevertheless, imaging is usually indicated to delineate the vascular malformation, detect associated dysmorphogenic anomalies, and facilitate therapeutic considerations.

Capillary Malformation (CM)

CLINICAL PRESENTATION

Capillary malformation must be differentiated in infants from "salmon patch" (also known as "nevus flammeus neonatorum"), "angel kiss" for the forehead, and "stork bite" for the nuchal area. These fading macular patches occur in one-half of neonates; typically, they disappear in the facial region and are more apt to persist in the nape of the neck and the occiput (Fig. 21–10).

Port wine stains are intradermal capillary or venular malformations that are present at birth. The incidence rate in newborns is 0.3%. Two-thirds of these lesions darken in color over time and develop ectatic vessels that appear as progressively enlarging nodules, causing a pebbly or "cobblestone" appearance of the stain in adult life (50). Curiously, these hyperplastic skin changes occur in facial CM, but not in truncal or limb

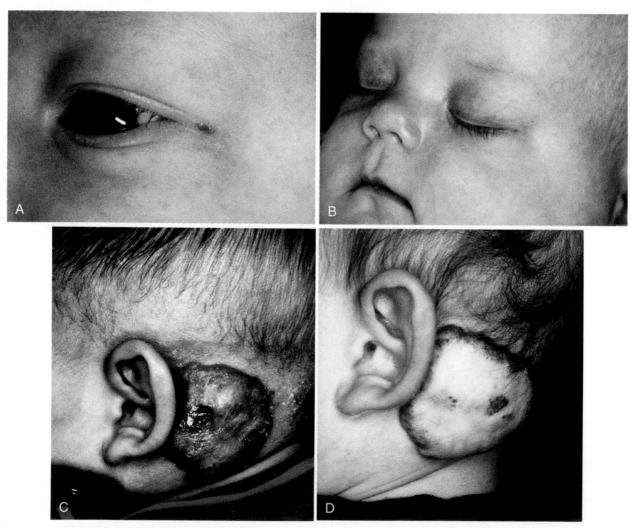

FIG. 21–8. **A,** 3-week-old infant with small macular hemangioma at left lateral canthal region. **B,** same child after one treatment with almost total resolution of the vascular lesion. This child required no further treatment with no evidence of growth or recurrence of the he-mangioma. **C,** ulcerative hemangioma in the postauricular region of a 3-month-old white male. **D,** results of laser treatment reveal healing of the ulceration; however, little change is present in the overall bulk of the large hemangioma and hypopigmentation of the skin.

CM. The most common locations in the face are along the distribution of the trigeminal nerve. Most port wine stains are isolated lesions. However, they can be a red flag for associated anomalies of vascular, skeletal, and soft tissues, and potential for overgrowth. Sturge-Weber syndrome is a complex cutaneous neuroectodermal malformation syndrome comprised of facial port-wine stain, ipsilateral ocular anomalies, and pial vascular malformations (Fig. 21–11).

All patients with Sturge-Weber syndrome have involvement of the first division of the trigeminal nerve (V1) (51). The risk of the Sturge-Weber syndrome is even higher if the port wine stain is found over both the V1 and V2 distributions and other facial locations (52). It should be emphasized that infants with port wine stains in the V2 and V3 distributions without V1 are not at increased risk for Sturge-Weber syndrome (Fig. 21–12). The ocular defects include glaucoma,

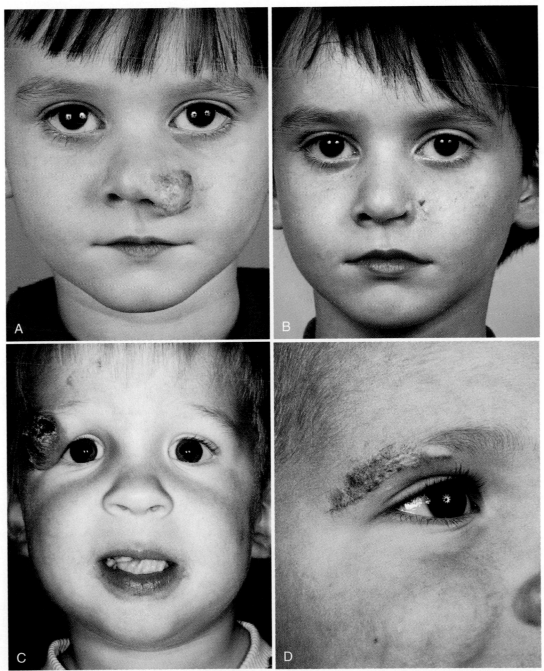

FIG. 21–9. **A,** 5-year-old, preschool child with involuted hemangioma that has been stable over 2 years. Surgical resection is warranted. **B,** 6 months' status postsurgical resection hemangioma of left nose. There is some residual notching and residual telangiectasia, but overall improvement. **C,** 15-month-old white male with hemangioma of right upper eyebrow. The lesion failed to respond to steroids and was a persistent nuisance for this child, indicating surgical intervention. **D,** same child after surgical resection sparing the lateral right eyebrow. This residual telangiectasia should respond well to natural involution or pulsed-dye laser.

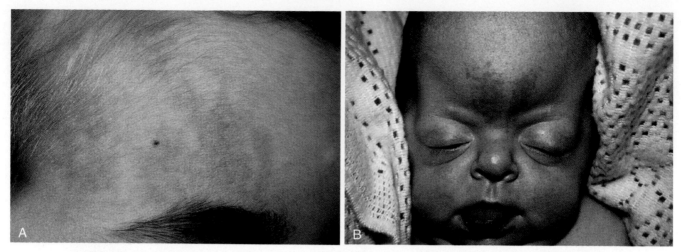

FIG. 21–10. **A,** example of macular patches that usually fade within the 1st year of life. **B,** macular patch known as angel's kiss, salmon patch, or nevus flammeus neonatorum.

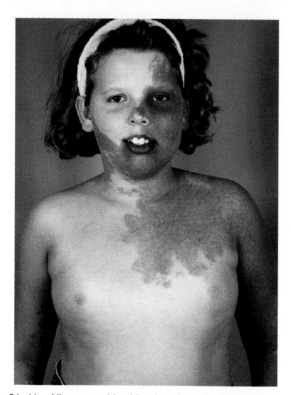

FIG. 21–11. Nine-year-old white female with Sturge-Weber syndrome. Notice the port wine stain involving V1, V2, V3 distribution of the face associated with left upper trunk and arm.

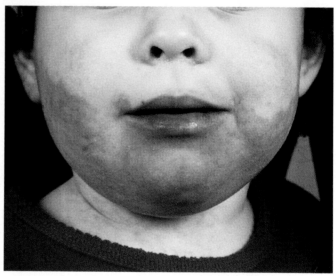

FIG. 21–12. Three-year-old with port wine stain and bilateral V3 distribution. Although the port wine stain is extensive, this child is not at increased risk for Sturge-Weber because there is no V1 or V2 involvement.

astigmatism, and choroidal vascular anomalies, even in the absence of a facial stain. Glaucoma is even more likely with the combined involvement of V1 and V2. Plastic surgeons involved in the evaluation of children with port wine stain must suggest ophthalmologic consultation. Ophthalmologic examination (visual study, funduscopic examination, eye-pressure measurement) must be done twice a year until puberty. It is necessary to use CT (with iodinated contrast) or MRI for every port wine–stain patient with V1 distribution, to rule out Sturge-Weber. This syndrome is a medical quasi-emergency. Prompt drug treatment of epilepsy prevents neuronal death and minimizes motor and psychomotor deterioration. The ma-

jority of patients with Sturge-Weber leptomeningeal involvement do not have seizures. It is recommended to follow carefully any patient with V1 and V2–distribution port wine stain, and if seizures occur promptly initiate the appropriate scans and begin control of the epilepsy.

TREATMENT

Treatment of a port wine stain is with yellow-light laser, specifically the flashlamp pulse-dye laser (FLPD), particularly early in childhood. Argon laser is used to treat port wine stains in adults (52). However, in children and patients younger than 18 years, argon laser therapy is less successful, producing unacceptable scars in up to 40% of patients (53). The FLPD represents the concept of "selective photothermolysis" targeting abnormal dilated vessels at a depth of up to 1 mm with less collateral damage. Scarring is extremely rare with the FLPD (54). Although 100% fading can occur in some instances (54), it is not usual. The surgeon can expect

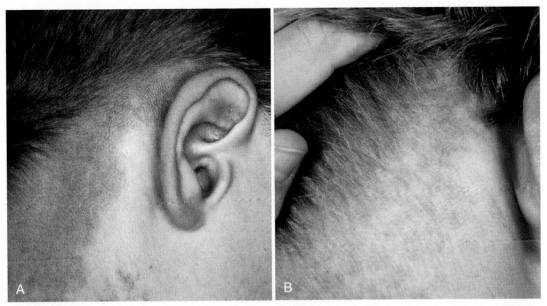

FIG. 21–13. **A,** postauricular port wine stain before treatment. **B,** postauricular port wine stain after one treatment.

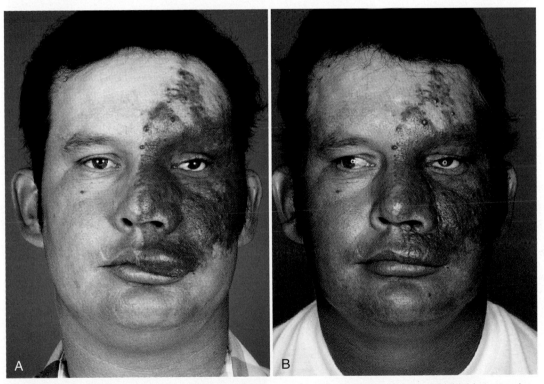

FIG. 21–14. **A,** adult with port wine stain showing progressive dilated ectatic lesions and labial hypertrophy. **B,** status post resection and partial debulking of left upper-lip port wine stain hypertrophy.

an average fade of 80% with eight treatments (55). The yellow-light lasers can also be used for mature port wine stains in adults, such as the argon ion or copper vapor laser; however, they must be used with scanners to achieve a reasonable safety risk, and even with scanners, the scarring is more likely than with pulse-dye laser (Fig. 21–13).

Surgical intervention may be necessary for glaucoma unresponsive to medication. Soft-tissue and skeletal hypertrophy also can require surgical therapy. Laser therapy cannot correct soft-tissue overgrowth; excision, split-thickness skin grafting, or tissue expansion may be necessary in some patients. Contour resection is particularly useful for labial hypertrophy (Fig. 21–14). These patients often develop malocclusion, tilting, and open bite; orthognathic correction is done at the completion of skeletal growth. Gingival hypertrophy is common; careful dental care and hygiene are important. "Pyogenic granuloma" of the skin or gingiva (epulis) requires excision and electrodesiccation.

Venous Malformation (VM)

CLINICAL PRESENTATION

Venous malformations are localized or extensive, minor or distorting, single or multiple, and located anywhere on the head, limbs, or trunk. Most VMs are sporadic; however, there are families with multiple VMs inherited in an autosomal dominant pattern. One chromosomal locus for familial VM (both cutaneous and mucosal) maps to 9p (54). Blue color, spongy compressible texture on palpation, a slow refill, and increased size with dependency are pathognomonic for venous malformation (Fig. 21–15). VMs enlarge with hormonal changes, during puberty and pregnancy. Histologically, VMs are composed of networks of various sizes of malformed channels that vary in size

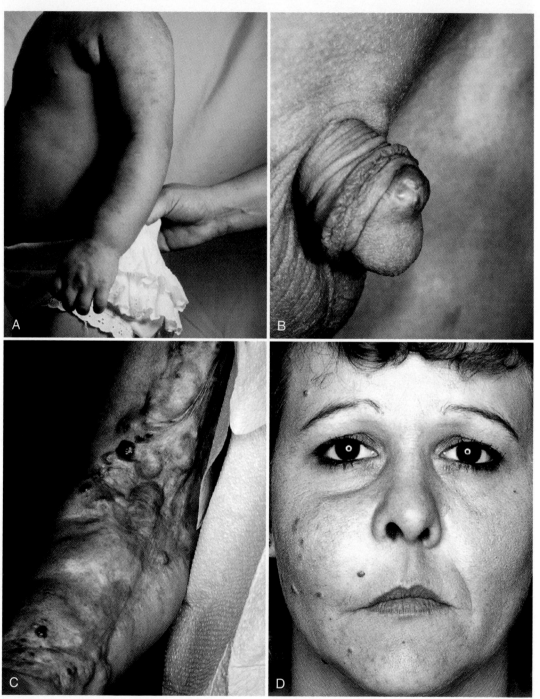

FIG. 21–15. **A,** 2-year-old white female with diffuse venous malformation of the left upper arm and shoulder region. **B,** isolated venous malformation of glans portion of the penis. **C,** venous malformation of the right upper arm in a 52-year-ol.d white female. Surgical resection had been attempted in the past. Note the spongy subcutaneous and cutaneous blebs pathognomonic of venous malformations. **D,** more subtle venous malformation deeply seated within the right cheek. Diagnosis was made in this patient by increase of the vascular mass upon recumbency and compressibility with slow refill.

from a fine, spongelike quality to large, tortuous ectatic vessels. The vessels are dysplastic and thin-walled, with a hypoplastic and clumped smooth-muscle layer.

VMs swell with exertion or when the area is dependent. The usual presenting symptom is pain that may or may not be associated with episodes of thrombosis. Thrombosis presents as a sudden hard swelling, with or without redness, usually associated with tenderness and acute discomfort. The acute swelling generally responds to warm packs and elevation. The clot may resolve totally or may become, in time, a phlebolith that is apparent on plain radiography or by palpation. Venous malformations can affect underlying bone, usually manifesting as either distortion, hypertrophy, or hypotrophy (57). Large craniofacial VMs often cause asymmetry of the facial features. Oral VMs typically cause dental misalignment and open bite. Intraorbital VM induces enlargement of the orbital cavity and can alter position of the globe. Pharyngeal VM commonly is associated with obstructive sleep apnea. Pure VM in the limbs is uncommon. VM can cause enlarged blue fingers/toes, limb overgrowth or undergrowth, and painful hemarthrosis with involvement of the synovium of the knee. Large VMs, particularly in the extremities, are associated with disseminated intravascular coagulopathy (DIC). Therefore, a coagulation profile should be obtained for any patient with a large venous malformation exhibiting a clotting disorder and/or a patient being considered for resection.

DIAGNOSIS

MRI is usually done only before treatment. MRI with spin-echo, T1- and T2-weighted sequences best delineate a VM. If functional/cosmetic deformity exists, the MRI is warranted to determine the extent of the lesion.

TREATMENT

Sclerotherapy is the primary treatment for VMs, although subsequent surgical resection is often needed. Ethibloc is used for percutaneous sclerotherapy in Europe (58), whereas 100% alcohol and sodium tetradecyl sulfate (Sotradecol) are the most common sclerosants in the United States (59). Sclerotherapy causes endothelial necrosis, resulting in thrombosis and shrinkage of the malformation (Fig. 21–16). Unfortunately, recurrence is common and multiple treatments are often required. However, there is no better alternative for extensive venous lesions. Ulceration is the most common complication of sclerotherapy, especially with superficial venous malformations; the patient must be well informed of this possibility. The patient must also be informed that surgical undermining of skin during debulking of a VM is likely to cause ischemia and possible skin loss. Usually these postsclerotherapy ulcers heal well by contraction; sometimes there is a need for skin grafting. Only tiny VMs respond to currently available lasers.

Lymphatic Malformation (LM)

CLINICAL PRESENTATION

"Lymphangioma" is a misnomer; the term should be discarded in favor of *lymphatic malformation*. The old terms "lymphangioma circumscriptum" and "cystic hygroma" are entrenched in the literature. LMs exhibit a normal rate of endothelial cell turnover. LMs can be described as microcystic, macrocystic, and combined lymphaticovenous (LVM) forms. Lymphatic anomalies present in a wide spectrum, from lymphedema to large cystic malformations. "Lymphangioma circumscriptum" is an old term to describe anomalous subcutaneous lymphatic cisterns communicating through dilated lymphatic channels with superficial and cutaneous vesicles (60). Well-circumscribed lesions are the exception rather than the rule. The superficial manifestations of dermal lymphatic malformations ("lymphangioma circumscriptum") are misleading, and the cutaneous vesicles are usually but the tip of the iceberg obscuring extensive intradermal and subcutaneous pathology. LMs are generally detected at birth or shortly thereafter, but they can present both in childhood and adulthood. LMs grow commensurately with the child. They can expand or contract, depending on the occurrence of either inflammation, infection, or intralesional bleeding.

In a series of 112 patients with lymphatic malformations, 65 (58%) of the malformations were present at birth, 80% were diagnosed by 1 year of age, and 90% had become evident by 2 years of age. Males and females were equally affected (9). Lymphatic malformations can affect all areas of the body, but most are located in the cervicofacial region and axilla. Seventy-five to ninety percent of cystic LMs ("cystic hygroma") occur in the cervical region, and the majority of these are in the posterior triangle. Lesions in the anterior cervical triangle are more problematic because they are often intertwined with complex vascular and neural structures. Approximately one-half percent of all neck masses are eventually diagnosed as cystic LM, and 10% of these have a mediastinal component (Fig. 21–17).

LMs are the most common cause of congenital tongue enlargement (macroglossia), lip enlargement (macrocheilia), and ear enlargement (macrotia). A vascular anomaly affecting some part of the skeleton is most likely an LM. Skeletal hypertrophy and distortion in 80% of cervicofacial LMs occur by 10 years of age (57). Typically, there is anterior distortion of the mandible or maxillary enlargement that results in prognathism, open bite, or other complex malocclusion. The mechanism for bone overgrowth is not known. One theory is that direct pressure on the bone by the expanding mass causes hypertrophy. Increased blood flow is not believed to cause the osseous changes. LM has also been found within the bone itself and may account for overgrowth (61).

DIFFERENTIAL DIAGNOSIS

Many LMs are diagnosed in utero by ultrasonography. Large cystic cervicofacial masses can be detected, and their characteristic features clearly identified as early as the 12th week of embryonic life. Large cystic LMs are brought to the physician's attention primarily because of their size and appearance. Although they generally grow proportionately with the child, sudden and rapid increases in the size of the lesions are common, usually following an upper-respiratory or soft-tissue infection.

There is a litany for differential diagnoses of neck masses in children. Inflammatory masses are most common, but the surgeon must keep in mind the possibility of a thyroglossal duct cyst (in the cervical midline), deep-seated hemangioma, and vascular malformations of nonlymphatic origin. Neuroblastoma is the 3rd most common tumor of childhood; therefore, it should be considered, as should teratoma, lymphoma,

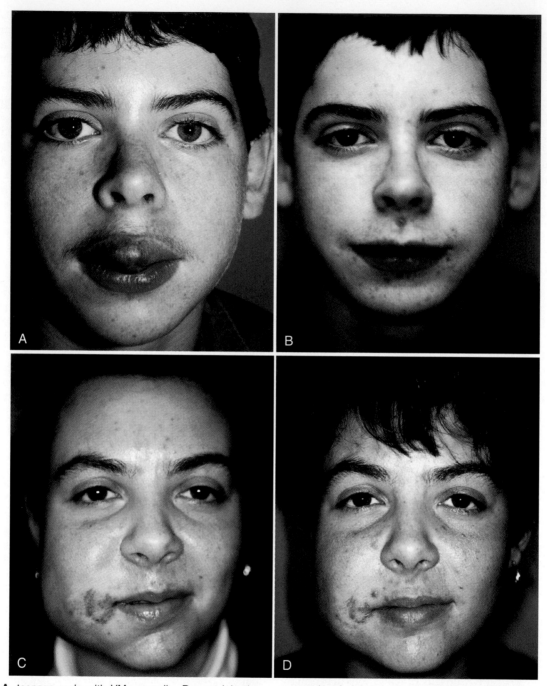

FIG. 21–16. A, teenage male with VM upper lip. **B,** post injection with sotradecol sulfate and ETOH and surgical resection. **C,** venous anomaly of right cheek, present since birth. **D,** same patient 5 months post ETOH sclerotherapy.

and infantile fibrosarcoma (62). Thyroid masses are typically in the midline, which is an unusual presentation for cystic LMs. Large cystic LMs are usually translucent and easily imaged by radiographic examination (49). Deep LM is difficult to diagnose in these instances. Ultrasonography with color Doppler or MRI is indicated. LMs usually have a characteristic tissue density on MRI, but they can sometimes be confused with lipomatous tissue (Fig. 21–18). The finding of multiple septa evidences their loculated cystic nature. LMs are typically hyperintense on T-2 images, with "rim" enhancement (the vessels in walls) (3).

TREATMENT

A newborn with a large cervicofacial LM may require emergent tracheostomy. Large cysts can be treated with aspiration of the lymphatic fluid followed by percutaneous (image-guided) intralesional injection of sclerosing agent. A number of agents have been used (Ethibloc, pure ethanol, bleomycin, sodium tetradecyl sulfate, and OK-432—a killed strain of group-A Streptococcus). Sclerotherapy is rarely successful in the long-term.

Sudden enlargement of an LM is usually the result of intralesional bleeding or cellulitis. Pain medication, rest, and

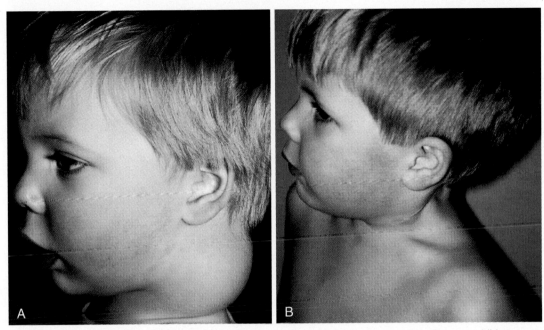

FIG. 21–17. **A,** 2-year-old boy with macrocystic LM of left posterior cervical triangle. **B,** same child, 1 year postresection; no evidence of persistence.

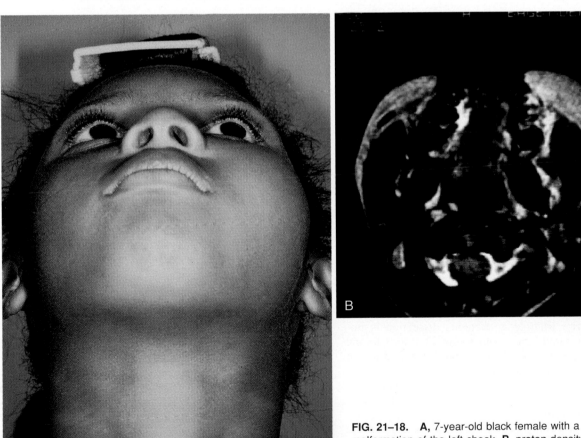

FIG. 21–18. **A,** 7-year-old black female with a subtle lymphatic malformation of the left cheek. **B,** proton density image shows thickened area of increased signal density characteristic of the increased interstitial fluid seen in lymphatic malformations.

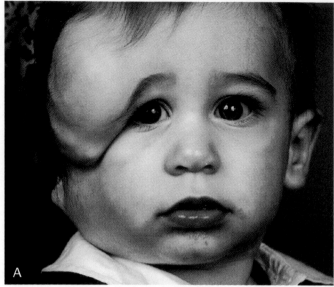
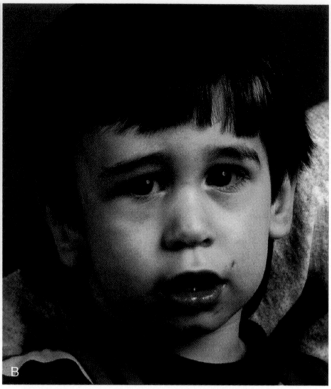

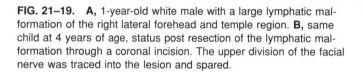
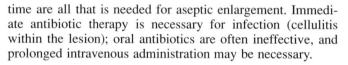

FIG. 21–19. **A,** 1-year-old white male with a large lymphatic malformation of the right lateral forehead and temple region. **B,** same child at 4 years of age, status post resection of the lymphatic malformation through a coronal incision. The upper division of the facial nerve was traced into the lesion and spared.

time are all that is needed for aseptic enlargement. Immediate antibiotic therapy is necessary for infection (cellulitis within the lesion); oral antibiotics are often ineffective, and prolonged intravenous administration may be necessary.

Surgical Resection

Surgical resection offers the only potential for cure of an LM. Anatomic restrictions and difficulty in dissecting normal from involved tissues often result in an incomplete resection or damage to normal structures. The surgical strategy is to remove as much of the LM as possible in a single anatomic region in a single operation. Staged excisions (perforce subtotal) are often necessary for extensive lesions.

Complete extirpation of the lesion is the objective, but unfortunately this goal is rarely achieved (Fig. 21–19). In well-demarcated, unilocular lesions (e.g., in the posterior cervical triangle), total excision can be carried out with relative ease, minimal morbidity, and a low recurrence rate. However, for larger or multiloculated masses, particularly those in the anterior triangle, meticulous dissection is imperative and care should be taken to avoid injury to the marginal mandibular branch of the facial nerve and to the greater auricular, spinal accessory, and phrenic nerves. In these lesions, it is often best to confine excision to one side of the neck and to stage resection of the opposite neck and ipsilateral chest or axilla.

Timing of the procedure depends on the location of the LM and on functional considerations. The older the child, the easier and safer the procedure will be (63). Some authors recommend waiting until 3 years of age; rarely, LMs shrink (64). Transient enlargement of the mass secondary to infection should not force the surgeon to operate unless the airway is compromised.

Sclerosis and Laser

In general, sclerosing injections are not met with enthusiasm in the literature, although the Japanese experience with sclerotherapy for large cervicofacial lymphatic malformations in children is favorable. Tanigawa and colleagues (65) report on their experience with bleomycin fat emulsion.

Intracystic injection of OK-432 has been used as another sclerosing agent for cystic hygroma in children in Japan (66). There are some reports of excellent response to OK-432 (67).

Percutaneous sclerotherapy with 100% ETOH and Ethibloc is being tried, but long-term results are not available.

CO_2 or YAG laser has been tried for the cutaneous vesicles of "lymphangioma circumscriptum"; however, this carries high recurrence rates and causes moderate to severe scarring. It is best reserved for those intradermal lymphatic anomalies that cannot be excised and/or for high-risk/elderly patients.

Complex-Combined Malformations

Lymphatic malformation is sometimes seen in combination with other vascular anomalies. The most common is Klippel-Trenaunay syndrome, which consists of a dermal capillary malformation (port wine stain) with an underlying lymphatic and venous malformation (CLVM), usually associated with bony overgrowth and limb hypertrophy. The syndrome is usually restricted to one lower extremity, but it may extend into the lower abdomen and trunk. A similar complex vascular anomaly can be seen in the upper limbs, either unilaterally or bilaterally, or the trunk.

A complex-combined anomaly of an extremity with all the findings of Klippel-Trenaunay syndrome, but with arteriovenous fistula(s), is known as Parkes-Weber syndrome. The

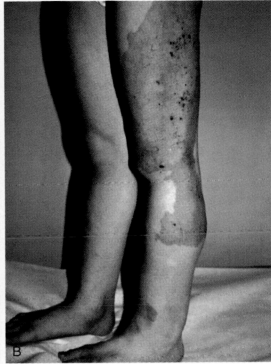

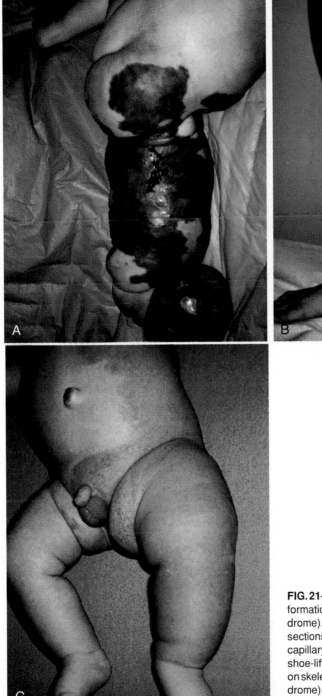

FIG. 21–20.   A, newborn boy with capillary-lymphatico-venous malformation and grotesque hypertrophy (CLVM = Klippel-Trenaunay syndrome). Underwent amputation of the foot and subsequent contour resections. **B,** CLVM left lower extremity; note geographic capillary-lymphatic cutaneous patch and hypertrophy. She wears right shoe-lift. Epiphyseal arrest will be necessary at appropriate age, based on skeletal growth. **C,** CLVM with AV shunting (Parkes-Weber syndrome); warm capillary stain of abdomen and left lower extremity with overgrowth in length/girth. Loud Doppler signal heard throughout.

possible presence of arteriovenous fistulas must be assessed in any patient with a complex-combined vascular malformation (Fig. 21–20).

Arteriovenous Malformation (AVM)

AVM is a high-flow vascular malformation comprised of micro- and macro-arteriovenous fistulas (AVFs). The epicenter, referred to as the "nidus," consists of dysplastic arterial feeders and enlarged veins. AVMs are present at birth, or they become evident in infancy or childhood.

Most patients present after a rapid increase in the size of a known pulsatile mass that has remained quiescent for several years. Occasionally, AVM presents in a young child; these tend to be extremely aggressive. On histology, AVM is poorly delineated and consists of elongated tortuous arteries and veins with thickened fibromuscular walls and a discontinuous elastic lamina.

AVM is often underappraised in childhood; it is often mistaken for hemangioma. Puberty and trauma appear to trigger expansion. The AVM evidences cutaneous signs of

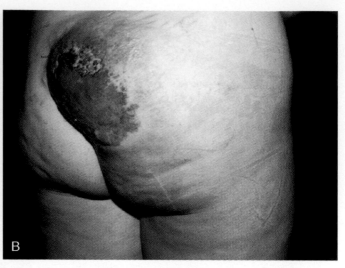

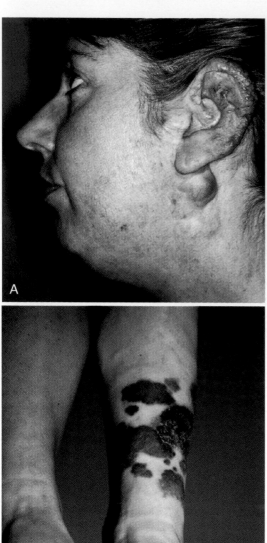

FIG. 21–21.   **A,** 35-year-old female with left cervicoauricular AVM, first appeared during pregnancy at age 21 years. Had ill-advised ligation of distal external carotid artery and laser therapy. She presents with episodic bleeding, pain, and annoying bruit. **B,** adolescent girl with ulcerated AVM right buttock; born with capillary blush, expansion began with pubertal growth. **C,** AVM left leg. Note pseudo-Kaposi skin changes and dilated veins.

its high-flow nature: skin becomes a deep red or violaceous color; a warm mass appears beneath the skin; and a thrill can be palpated, along with a bruit. A facial AVM causes asymmetric hypertrophy, and gingival hemorrhage can be the emergent presenting complaint. Dental extraction is perilous; it should be undertaken only after embolization. The end-stage of an AVM, whatever the anatomic site, is violaceous skin atrophy, ulceration, intractable pain, and intermittent bleeding. Pseudo-Kaposi sarcomatous skin changes commonly occur in association with an AVM of the lower limb (Fig. 21–21).

Diagnosis of an AVM is easily made by these physical findings; however, radiologic investigation is recommended as soon as AVM is suspected clinically. Ultrasonography, combined with gray-scale and color Doppler, documents AV

shunting. Pulsed Doppler quantitates arterial output, as compared to the normal side, and this is also a useful way to follow noninvasively the progress of AVM.

MRI is done first, used in conjunction with arteriography, to determine the extent of the lesion, which aids in determining the extent of resection. MRI of an AVM shows the characteristic flow-voids (corresponding to the high-flow vessels). There is no parenchymal staining (as seen in true hemangioma). Angiography plays an important role in defining the hemodynamics of the lesions as well, and is usually done concurrent with interventional embolotherapy.

MANAGEMENT

Treatment of an AVM is challenging, frustrating, and potentially as life-threatening as the lesion itself. Ligation of feed-

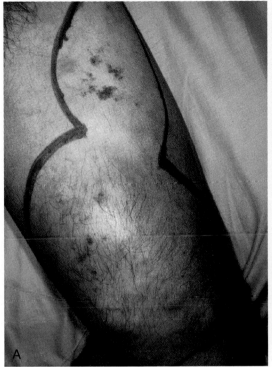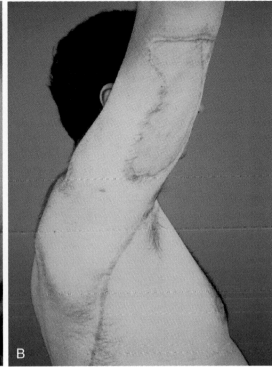

FIG. 21–22. **A,** 37-year-old white male with arteriovenous malformation of the right upper arm. AVM encircled with marker as area to be resected. **B,** 1-year status post resection of arteriovenous malformation with reconstruction using split-thickness skin graft. No recurrence is noted 9 years postoperatively.

ing vessels only worsens the problem, and should never be done. There follows a vascular recruitment phenomenon (collateralization) as small arteries expand from neighboring areas to supply the nidus. Furthermore, proximal ligation of feeding arteries impedes access for therapeutic embolization.

An AVM is usually not treated in its quiescent stage. Early combined embolization/surgical resection for an AVM in childhood is debatable; it should be considered if resection can be easily achieved. Intervention becomes necessary when signs and symptoms of evolution occur: ulceration, bleeding, pain, disfigurement, or cardiac failure (Fig. 21–22).

Superselective arterial embolization alone can be palliative for some AVMs, particularly when surgical resection would cause disfigurement or mutilation. Pain can be diminished, bleeding can stop, and ulcerations can heal. However, palliative embolization is only temporary; it cannot cure an AVM, unlike the case of embolization of a single direct AVF. Another interventional approach is direct intralesional sclerotherapy of the AVM using 100% ethanol.

The best stratagem for a symptomatic cutaneous AVM is combined embolization and surgical resection. Arterial embolization is done to temporarily occlude the nidus; this facilitates the surgical procedure done 24 to 72 hours later. Embolization minimizes intraoperative bleeding but does not diminish the limits of resection. The entire AVM nidus, and usually the skin as well, must be widely resected. Wound coverage is preferably done at the same time. Microsurgical free-flap transfer is often necessary to provide adequate reconstruction. Overlying skin is saved only if it is normal; if it is stained, then the chances for recurrence are

increased. After combined embolization/resection, the patient must be followed over many years by clinical examination, ultrasonography, and/or MRI. Definitive cures are uncommon.

Conclusion

No single practitioner or specialist has all the answers for patients with cutaneous vascular anomalies. As a result, many of these patients become "medical nomads," journeying from physician to physician. These patients need interdisciplinary care. Each major referral center should have a vascular anomalies team. The membership will differ depending on local enthusiasm. These patients rarely engender battles over turf. Because many of these problems seem to be insoluble, physicians are all too happy to send their patients for consultation. A vascular anomalies team will make the best decisions as to intervention, be less likely to cause iatrogenic complications, and provide a "critical mass" for clinical and basic research in this field.

References

1. Mulliken JB, Glowacki J. Hemangiomas and vascular malformations in infants and children: a classification based on endothelial characteristics. *Plast Reconstr Surg* 1982; 69:412–423.
2. Mulliken JB, Young AE. *Vascular birthmarks: hemangiomas and malformations.* Philadelphia: WB Saunders, 1988.
3. Meyer JS, Haffer FA, Barnes PD, et al. Biological classification of soft tissue vascular anomalies. *Am J Roentgenol* 1991; 157:559–564.
4. Takahashi K, Mulliken JB, Kozakewich HPW, et al. Cellular markers that distinguish the phases of hemangioma during infancy and childhood. *J Clin Invest* 1994; 93(6):2357–2364.

5. Folkman J. Proceedings: tumor angiogenesis factor. *Cancer Res* 1974; 34(8):2109.
6. Folkman J. The vascularization of tumors. *Sci Amer* 1976; 234 (5):58–64, 70–73.
7. Folkman J, Haudenschild C, Zetter BR. Long-term culture of capillary endothelial cells. Proceedings of the National Academy of Sciences of the United States of America, 1979; 76(10):5217–5221.
8. Folkman J, Haudenschild C. Angiogenesis in vitro. *Nature* 1980; 288(5791):551–556.
9. Folkman J, Klagsburn M. Angiogenic factors. *Science* 1987; 235 (4787):442–447.
10. Holmdahl K. Cutaneous hemangiomas in premature and mature infants. *Acta Paediat Upps* 1955; 44(4):370–379.
11. Bowers RE, Graham EA, Tomlinson KM. The natural history of the strawberry nevus. *AMA Arch Derm* 1960; 82:667–680.
12. Amir J, Metzker A, Krikler R, et al. Strawberry hemangioma in preterm infants. *Pediatr Dermatol* 1986; 3:131–132.
13. Brown SH, Neerhout RC, Fonkalsrud EW. Prednisone therapy in the management of large hemangiomas in infants and children. *Surgery.* 1972; 71:168–173.
14. Esterly N. The management of disseminated hemangiomatosis. *Pediatr Dermatol* 1984; 1:312–317.
15. Edgerton MT. The treatment of hemangiomas with special reference to the role of the steroid therapy. *Ann Surg* 1976; 183:517–532.
16. Pereyra R, Andrassy RJ, Mahour GH. Management of massive hepatic hemangiomas in infants and children: a review of 13 cases. *Pediatrics* 1982; 70:254–258.
17. Burns AJ, Kaplan LC, Mulliken JB. Is there an association between hemangioma and syndromes with dysmorphic features? *Pediatrics* 1991; 88(6):1257.
18. Reese V, Frieden IJ, Paller AS, et al. Associated of facial hemangiomas with Dandy Walker and the other posterior fossa malformations. *J Pediatr* 1993; 122:379–384.
19. Gorlin RJ, Kantaputra P, Aughton DJ, et al. Marked female predilection in some syndromes associated with facial hemangiomas. *Am J Med Genet* 1994; 52(2):130–135.
20. Mulliken JB. A plea for a biologic approach to hemangiomas of infancy (editorial). *Arch Dermatol* 1991; 127(2):243–244.
21. Boon LM, Enjolras O, Mulliken JB. Congenital hemangiomas: evidence for accelerated involution. *Pediatrics* 1996 (in press).
22. Enjolras O, Mulliken JB. Current management of vascular birthmarks. *Pediatr Dermatol* 1993; 10:311–333.
23. Esterly NB. Hemangiomas in infants and children, clinical observations. *Pediatr Dermatol* 1992; 9:353–355.
24. Margileth AM, Museles M. Cutaneous hemangiomas in children. Diagnosis and conservative management. *JAMA* 1965; 194(5):523–526.
25. Robb RM. Refractive errors associated with hemangiomas of the eyelids and orbits in infancy. *Am J Ophthalmol* 1977; 83(1):52–58.
26. Stigmar G, Crawford JS, Ward CM, et al. Ophthalmic sequelae of infantile hemangiomas of the eyelids and orbit. *Am J Ophthalmol* 1978; 85:806.
27. Thomson HG, Ward CM, Crawford JS, et al. Hemangiomas of the eyelid: visual complications and prophylactic concepts. *Plast Reconstr Surg* 1979; 63:641.
28. Haik BG, Karcioglu ZA, Gordon RA, et al. Capillary hemangioma (infantile periocular hemangioma). *Surv Ophthal* 1994; 38:399–426.
29. Cooper AG, Bolande RP. Multiple hemangiomas in an infant with cardiac hypertrophy. *Pediatrics* 1965; 35:27–33.
30. Ferguson CF, Flake CG. Subglottic hemangioma as a cause of respiratory obstruction in infants. *Ann Otol Rhinol Laryngol* 1961; 70: 1095–1112.
31. Larcher VF, Howard ER, Mowat AP. Hepatic haemangiomata: diagnosis and management. *Arch Dis Child* 1981; 56(1): 7–14.
32. Kasabach HH, Meritt KK. Capillary hemangioma with extensive purpura. *Am J Dis Child* 1940; 59:1063–1070.
33. Moroz B. The course of hemangiomas in children. In: Ryan TJ, Cheery GW, eds. *Vascular birthmarks: pathogenesis and management.* Oxford: Medical Publications, 1987; 55.
34. Sie KC, McGill T, Healy GB. Subglottic hemangioma: ten years' experience with the carbon dioxide laser. *Ann Oto Rhinol Laryngol* 1994; 103(3):167–172.
35. El-Dossouky M, Azmy AF, Raine PAM, et al. Kasabach-Merritt syndrome. *J Pediatr Surg* 1988; 23:109–111.
36. McLean RH, Moller JH, Warwick WJ, et al. Multinodular hemangiomatosis of the liver in infancy. *Pediatrics* 1972; 49(4):563–573.
37. Fost NC, Esterly NB. Successful treatment of juvenile hemangiomas with prednisone. *J Pediatr* 1968; 72(3):351–357.
38. Sloan GM, Reinisch JF, Nichter LS, et al. Intralesional corticosteroid therapy for infantile hemangiomas. *Plast Reconstr Surg* 1989; 83(3):459–467.
39. Edgerton MT. The treatment of hemangiomas: with special reference to the role of steroid therapy. *Ann Surg* 1976; 183:517.
40. Sutula FC, Glover AT. Eyelid necrosis following intralesional corticosteroid injection for capillary hemangioma. *Ophthalmol Surg* 1987; 18(2):103–105.
41. Shorr N, Seiff SR. Central retinal artery occlusion associated with periocular corticosteroid injection for juvenile hemangiomas. *Ophthalmol Surg* 1986; 17:229–231.
42. Droste PJ, Ellis FD, Sondhi N, et al. Linear subcutaneous fat atrophy after corticosteroid injection of periocular hemangiomas. *Am J Ophthalmol* 1988; 105(1):65–69.
43. White CW. Treatment of hemangiomatosis with recombinant interferon alpha. *Sem Hematol* 1990; 27(3 Suppl 4):15–22.
44. Ezekowitz RAB, Mulliken JB, Folkman J. Interferon alpha-2a therapy for life-threatening hemangiomas. *N Engl J Med* 1992; 326:1456–1463. Ibid, corrections 1994; 330:300. Ibid, additional corrections 1995; 333:395–396.
45. Morelli JG, Tan OT, Weston WL. Treatment of ulcerated hemangiomas with the pulsed tunable dye laser. *Am J Dis Child* 1991; 145 (9):1062–1064.
46. Achauer BM, VanderKam VM. Ulcerated anogenital hemangioma of infancy. *Plast Reconstr Surg* 1991; 87:861–866.
47. Burrows PE, Lasjaunias PL, Ter Brugge KG, et al. Urgent and emergent embolization of lesions of the head and neck in children: indications and results. *Pediatrics* 1987; 80(3):386–394.
48. Kushner BJ. The treatment of periorbital infantile hemangioma with intralesional corticosteroids. *Plast Reconstr Surg* 1985; 76:517–526.
49. Finn MC, Glowacke J, Mulliken JB. Congenital vascular lesions: clinical application of a new classification. *J Pediatr Surg* 1983; 18(6): 894–900.
50. Geronenus RG, Ashinoff R. The medical necessity of evaluation and treatment of port-wine stains. *J Dermatol Surg Oncol* 1991; 17:76–79.
51. Alexander JL. Sturge-Weber syndrome. *Handb Clin Neurol* 1972; 14:223–240.
52. Enjolras O, Riche MC, Merland JJ. Facial port-wine stains and Sturge-Weber syndrome. *Pediatrics* 1985; 76:48–51.
53. Abramson SJ, Lack EE, Teele RL. Benign vascular tumors of the liver in infants: sonographic appearance. *Am J Roentgenol* 1982; 138(4): 629–632.
54. Apfelberg DB, Maser MR, White DN, et al. Combination treatment for massive cavernous hemangioma of the face: YAG laser photocoagulation plus direct steroid injection followed by YAG laser resection with sapphire scalpel tips, aided by superselective embolization. *Lasers in Surgery and Medicine* 1990; 10(3):217–223.
55. Enjolras O, Riche MC, Merland JJ, et al. Management of alarming hemangiomas in infancy: a review of 25 cases. *Pediatrics* 1990; 85(4): 491–498.
56. Boon LM, Mulliken JB, Vikkula M, et al. Assignment of a locus of dominantly inherited venous malformations to chromosome 9. *Hum Mol Genet* 1994; 3:1583–587.
57. Boyd JB, Mulliken JB, Kaban LB, et al. Skeletal changes associated with vascular malformations. *Plast Reconstr Surg* 1984; 74(6):789–797.
58. Tegtmeyer CJ, Smith TH, Shaw A, et al. Renal infarction: a complication of gelfoam embolization of hemangioendothelioma of the liver. *Am J Roentgenol* 1977; 128(2):305–307.
59. Weber TR, Connors RH, Tracy TF Jr, et al. Complex hemangiomas of infants and children. Individualized management in 22 cases. *Arch Surg* 1990; 125(8):1017–1021.
60. Osburn K, Schosser RH, Everett MA. Congenital pigmented and vascular lesions in newborn infants. *J Am Acad Dermatol* 1987; 16(4):788–792.
61. Padwa BL, Hayward PG, Ferraro NF, et al. Cervicofacial lymphatic malformation: clinical course, surgical intervention, and pathogenesis of skeletal hypertrophy. *Plast Reconstr Surg* 1995; 95:951–960.
62. Hayward PG, Orgill DP, Mulliken JB, et al. Congenital fibrosarcoma masquerading as lymphatic malformation: report of two cases. *J Ped Surg* 1995; 30(1):84–88.

63. Little D, Said JW, Siegel RJ, et al. Endothelial cell markers in vascular neoplasms: an immunohistochemical study comparing factor VIII–related antigen, blood group–specific antigens, 6-keto-PGF1 alpha, and Ulex europaeus 1 lectin. *J Pathol* 1986; 149(2):89–95.

64. Grabb WC, Dingman RO, Oneal RM, et al. Facial hamartomas in children: neurofibroma, lymphangioma, and hemangioma. *Plast Reconstr Surg* 1980; 66:509–527.

65. Tanigawa N, Shimomatsuya T, Takahashi K, et al. Treatment of cystic hygroma and lymphangioma with use of bleomycin fat emulsion. *Cancer* 1987; 60(4):741–749.

66. Ogita S, Tsuto T, Tokiwa K, et al. Intracystic injection of OK-432: a new sclerosing therapy for cystic hygroma in children. *Br J Surg* 1987; 74(8):690–691.

67. Ogita S, Tsuto T, Deguchi E, et al. OK-432 therapy for unresectable lymphangiomas in children. *J Ped Surg* 1991; 26(3):263–268.

22

Burn Injury

Oktavijan P. Minanov, M.D., and H.D. Peterson, D.D.S., M.D., F.A.C.S.

Of all acute injuries, burns may be the most confounding for the physician to manage. Burn care has essentially evolved as a cottage industry. To paraphrase an old anecdote, three burn directors equal four opinions. The endless variety of approaches to burn care has led to an enormous amount of confusion among physicians. This chapter focuses on the initial management, triage, and disposition of a burn patient; these points are not as hotly debated.

The initial question posed to a primary care physician presented with thermal injury is, Where would the patient best be cared for? The American Burn Association recommends that "those patients with major burn injury" be triaged to a burn center whose specialized staff and facilities ensure optimal outcome. Generally, only 25% of all burns qualify for triage to a major burn center. Major burn injuries are described as (1):

1. Burns that involve more than 10% of the total body surface area in a patient younger than 10 and older than 50 years of age
2. Burns that involve more than 20% of the total body surface area in patients of intervening age
3. Significant burns of the face, hands, feet, genitalia, perineum, or major joints
4. Full-thickness burns that involve more than 5% of the total body surface area in a patient of any age
5. Significant electrical injury
6. Significant chemical injury

Inhalation injury, concomitant mechanical trauma, and significant preexisting medical disorders mandate burn center care for patients with lesser burns.

The initial thermal assault that resulted in the burn injury should not be viewed as a finite entity. Rather, thermal injury should be viewed as a trigger that initiates a cascade of events, which we are only now starting to understand and modulate. It is during these subsequent events that we have the greatest impact on morbidity and mortality. Major burn trauma has significant local and systemic effects. Local burn injury has been subdivided into three zones (2):

1. The *zone of coagulation* is the area closest to and most affected by the heat. Tissue in this area has no blood flow and is nonviable.
2. The *zone of stasis*. The initial thermal injury was not severe enough to result in permanent damage, but microvascular sludging and thrombosis of vessels soon results in progressive tissue necrosis. Over the first 72 hours the zone of stasis may become the zone of coagulation, making the initial burn deeper. This viable area is where appropriate early intervention can have the most profound effect in minimizing injury.
3. The outermost zone is the *zone of hyperemia,* which is entirely viable. This zone, however, contributes to the systemic consequences seen in patients with major burns.

Following a major burn injury a mediator cascade is initiated that peaks at day 5, but continues through day 7. These systemic effects are most characteristic of burns involving greater than 20% of the total body surface area (TBSA). In these larger burns, the immunological cascade disrupts every organ system in the body, leading to burn shock. Locally, the burn injury and the associated immunologic cascade cause cell-wall dysfunction with an increasing capillary leak. The subsequent influx of fluid into the 3rd space results in significant edema of tissue. In larger injuries, mediators result in similar changes throughout the body, even in unburned tissues, resulting in total-body edema. It is important to replace the intravascular volume lost to the 3rd space because as the intravascular volume is depleted, cardiac preload is reduced and cardiac output is compromised. Likewise, a drop in systemic vascular resistance caused by mediators in the immunologic cascade results in a decrease in tissue perfusion with associated oliguria, hypoxia, and confusion. The majority of burn patients in shock can be supported through this phase with adequate intravenous resuscitation.

The effect of burn injury however, is not limited to the cardiovascular system. The most profound sequelae of burns are the adverse effects on immune and respiratory systems. Burn injury causes deterioration of both the cellular and humeral immune responses. This general immune suppression is directly proportional to the burn size. Compounding this fact is the disruption of the skin barrier, which exposes the patient to a host of pathogens the body might otherwise be able to fend off.

The pulmonary system is also profoundly affected, and leads to most of the morbidity and mortality in a burn center. The lungs, unfortunately, are not spared the capillary leak that afflicts the entire body. This capillary leak predisposes the lungs to pneumonia, which may initiate an immunologic cascade, exacerbating local injury and possibly progressing to adult respiratory distress syndrome. Therefore, burn injury should be viewed as a profound initial injury, the results of which take weeks to materialize. If the patient is supported through this time without added injury, excellent results may be obtained.

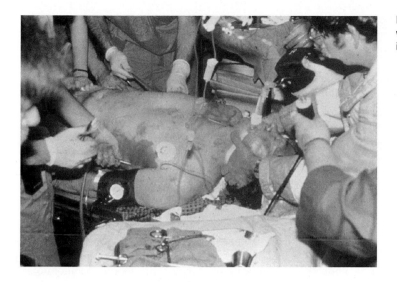

FIG. 22–1. Patient with 30% chest, back, and head burns, with associated intrathoracic and closed head injury from flaming automobile accident.

Initial emergency department care (Fig. 22–1) is as basic as the ABCs that are stressed in Advanced Trauma Life Support (ATLS) algorithms. The airway is of paramount importance, especially since patients with significant injuries may have to be transferred to other facilities. In a burn patient, the incompetence of the airway is not usually readily apparent since the patient may initially have no signs of respiratory distress. As total-body edema progresses and burn shock results in mental status changes, a patient's airway may become compromised, resulting in the patient's being transferred with a life-threatening problem. If a patient has any suggestion of an inhalation injury or upper-airway injury, or a burn of greater than 40% of the total body surface, it is best to intubate at the time of the initial evaluation. It is important to secure intravenous access early, before the development of extensive tissue edema. It is ideal to place intravenous lines through unburned tissue, though that may not always be possible. Likewise, both a Foley catheter and a nasogastric tube should be placed early, the first to monitor the adequacy of burn resuscitation, and the second to reduce the risk of aspiration secondary to the gastric ileus that is associated with burns involving greater than 20% of the total body surface. Ibuprofen should be given to help modify the local inflammatory response and to help prevent conversion of the zone of stasis to a deeper injury. Additionally, stress ulcer prophylaxis should be initiated and a tetanus booster given. If the patient is a child, streptococcal antibiotic coverage should be started. Initial wound treatment should only consist of saline-soaked gauze bandages until the patient is transferred to a burn center. At the burn center, a full evaluation can be carried out during a bath with mild soap and tepid water. Burn bullae should be lanced, since the transudate acts as a bacterial medium. However, the overlying skin should not be removed because it may still act as a biologic dressing and it is more comfortable for the patient.

Treatment of burn shock has led to the greatest strides in reducing acute burn morbidity. Resuscitating the patient primarily involves infusing enough balanced salt solution to replace the fluid losses from the vascular compartment following injury. Arriving at the appropriate volume of resuscitating fluid is of paramount importance. Inadequate volume will result in

burn shock with acute tubular necrosis and renal failure, and excessive volume results in both excessive peripheral and pulmonary edema. Increased peripheral edema results in an increased need for escharotomies. Pulmonary edema leads to higher rates of pneumonia and Acute Respiratory Distress Syndrome (ARDS). All burn resuscitation formulas rely heavily on accurate calculations of burned surface area. The "rule of nines" is adequate for an initial estimate for the extent of injury. This is done by assigning each portion of the adult body approximately 9% TBSA. That is, the head and two upper extremities are each worth 9% TBSA. The anterior and posterior trunk and each lower extremity each comprise 18% TBSA. A more accurate representation of the surface area injured can be obtained using a Lund-Browder chart (3) (Fig. 22–2). This chart takes into consideration the relative proportion of the extremities in each age group. It also subdivides the patients into smaller segments, and therefore arrives at a more accurate representation of the injured tissue. Numerous formulas have been proposed for calculating the appropriate amount of resuscitative volume. The most famous of these, the Parkland formula, uses 4 mls/kg/% TBSA burned as the total 24-hour resuscitative value. Half of this volume is given within the first 8 hours postburn and half is given over the final 16 hours. The reason for this is that a large volume is needed at first to compensate for the plasma lost into the burn wound and, since most of the loss has subsided after the first 12 hours, less volume is subsequently needed (4).

Lactated Ringer functions well as a resuscitative fluid, since large volumes can be used without causing electrolyte derangements. However, in an effort to reduce total-body edema, some centers advocate using hypertonic saline. The theory is that a smaller quantity of hypertonic saline will recruit a comparable amount of extravascular and intracellular fluid to fill the intravascular space. The margin of safety using this resuscitative regimen is low and requires extensive monitoring; furthermore, the clinical benefits have yet to be proven (5). Using colloid within the first 24 hours has not been shown to be beneficial; conversely, it has been shown to be rather destructive (6). The profound capillary leak previously described does not generally resolve until approximately 24 hours following injury. With such a capillary leak,

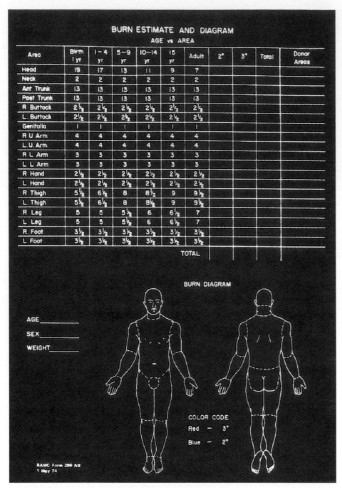

Area	Birth 1 yr	1-4 yr	5-9 yr	10-14 yr	15 yr	Adult	2°	3°	Total	Donor Areas
Head	19	17	13	11	9	7				
Neck	2	2	2	2	2	2				
Ant Trunk	13	13	13	13	13	13				
Post Trunk	13	13	13	13	13	13				
R Buttock	2½	2½	2½	2½	2½	2½				
L Buttock	2½	2½	2½	2½	2½	2½				
Genitalia	1	1	1	1	1	1				
R U Arm	4	4	4	4	4	4				
L U Arm	4	4	4	4	4	4				
R L Arm	3	3	3	3	3	3				
L L Arm	3	3	3	3	3	3				
R Hand	2½	2½	2½	2½	2½	2½				
L Hand	2½	2½	2½	2½	2½	2½				
R Thigh	5½	6½	8	8½	9	9½				
L Thigh	5½	6½	8	8½	9	9½				
R Leg	5	5	5½	6	6½	7				
L Leg	5	5	5½	6	6½	7				
R Foot	3½	3½	3½	3½	3½	3½				
L Foot	3½	3½	3½	3½	3½	3½				

TOTAL

BURN DIAGRAM

AGE _____

SEX _____

WEIGHT _____

COLOR CODE

Red — 3°

Blue — 2°

BAMC Form 296 NS
1 May 74

FIG. 22–2. The Lund-Browder diagram allows a more accurate estimate of the injured area.

the 3rd space sequesters the majority of the circulating serum proteins. Colloid, if given during this period, exacerbates rather than improves the total-body edema. Once the capillary leak resolves, the enormous amounts of resuscitative fluid are slowly recruited back into the vascular space. Therefore, the hallmark of the 2nd and 3rd day postburn is gentle diuresis. This is when colloid can be beneficial. There is generally a profound hypoproteinemia following the initial resuscitation, and extra intravenous albumin generally favors recruitment of interstitial fluid. During the 2nd day, 5% dextrose in water is the fluid of choice. At this point the patient has total-body salt overload and, as the vascular compartment recruits interstitial fluid, the patient is in danger of becoming profoundly hypernatremic. In addition, a further salt load would inhibit diuresis (7).

Adequacy of resuscitation can best be judged by following the patient's urine output. Urine volumes of 0.5 cc/kg/hr in adults and at least 1 cc/kg/hr in children are desired. Heart rate and blood pressure are also helpful indicators of the adequacy of the resuscitation. Neither is as specific as oliguria, since tachycardia is associated with hypermetabolism and pain, and bradycardia can be the result of heart disease. Should the patient become progressively oliguric, the patient's hourly intravenous rate should be increased.

Bolusing large amounts of intravenous fluid should be discouraged, since boluses of fluid only increase the patient's edema. Underlying medical conditions (e.g., inhalation injury, diuretic use, alcoholism, electrical injury, and escharotomies) can contribute to the need for far larger resuscitative volumes than those calculated based on weight and percentage of TBSA burned. Usually, if the patient is requiring more than 6 ml/kg/% TBSA burned to achieve adequate urine output, central venous pressure monitoring and splanchnic doses of Dopamine can be helpful in reestablishing an adequate urine output. Pulmonary arterial catheters are helpful only in elderly patients or patients where cardiac function is a concern. The vast majority of burn patients do not require central monitoring and generally resuscitate easily. The use of pulmonary artery catheters should be not be taken lightly, since the risks of line sepsis with invasive monitoring is especially high in burn patients and should only be used with specific indications. Glucosuria should be monitored throughout the resuscitative time so that an osmotic diuresis does not result in a spurious urine output. An osmotic diuresis does not adequately reflect resuscitation and contributes to a severely depleted intravascular volume. If significant glucosuria is diagnosed steps should be taken to correct this promptly. Generally all that needs to be done is to switch the patient's intravenous fluids over to glucose-free solutions. Insulin rarely needs to be used, except in diabetic patients. Generally, glucose-free solutions are used during the resuscitative period; however, children are an exception to this rule, since children have unusually low glycogen storages and are at risk for profound hypoglycemia.

Other than the adequacy of resuscitation and organ perfusion, the state of extremity perfusion is also critical to monitor during resuscitation. Circumferential burn injury, almost always full-thickness injury, will require escharotomies to maintain peripheral perfusion. The need for an escharotomy is generally not readily apparent at the time of injury, but after appropriate resuscitation has been instituted. Burned tissue is noncompliant, and as tissue edema increases secondary to resuscitation, compartment pressures increase, causing venous congestion and ultimately arterial insufficiency (8). The adequacy of peripheral perfusion can be determined by using an ultrasonic probe to assess peripheral pulses. If there is any confusion about the need for an escharotomy, a more objective method is to measure compartment pressures directly with a catheter (9). Once compartment pressures exceed capillary perfusion pressures, approximately 30 mm Hg, escharotomies are indicated. It should be noted that if escharotomies do not improve peripheral perfusion, sufficient edema in the underlying muscle compartment has occurred and fasciotomies are required. This rarely occurs in thermal injury alone, but is strongly associated with electrical injury. Before performing fasciotomies in a cutaneous burn, the surgeon should be certain that peripheral perfusion is not impaired secondary to hypothermia, hypovolemia, or peripheral vascular occlusive disease.

Escharotomies are best performed with electric cautery. Anesthesia is not required because full-thickness injury is insensate. The incision should be carried down through the dermis into the subcutaneous tissue. Extension of the escharotomy on the medial and lateral aspects of the upper extremities down to the thenar eminence is frequently bene-

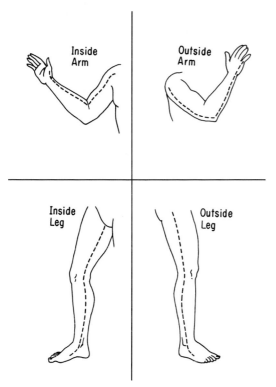

FIG. 22–3. Upper- and lower-extremity escharotomies of medial and lateral aspects of a limb.

ficial. On the lower extremities such extension is done on the medial and lateral aspects of the leg to below the malleolus (Fig. 22–3). Escharotomies on the chest become necessary when the static pulmonary compliance of a patient deteriorates to the point where ventilation is impaired. Full-thickness injury to the dorsum of a hand can best be decompressed with the aid of enzymatic débridement.

Inhalation injury is the largest contributor to mortality in the modern burn unit. The mortality rate for burns without inhalation is approximately 4.1%, but with inhalation injury the number skyrockets to approximately 56% (10). This significant difference in outcome highlights the importance of proper pulmonary support.

Inhalation injury can best be understood if subdivided into three postinsult phases: early (0 to 36 hours), postresuscitative (2 to 5 days), and inflammation-infection (usually 5 days to lung healing and burn wound closure) (11). Early injury is characterized by damage resulting from the initial thermal burn as well as damage to the pulmonary system secondary to inhaled noxious fumes. The resuscitative phase is characterized by increased lung weight secondary to pulmonary edema and resulting decreased lung compliance. The final phase occurs as the lung rebuilds its ciliated epithelium. However, until the epithelium is rebuilt, the lung is vulnerable because it is unable to clear secretions. The lungs are also taxed by increased work of breathing. The patient is hypermetabolic and there is a significant increase in the production of CO_2, which requires an increase in ventilation to keep metabolic parameters within normal limits. Consequently, this phase is associated with increased atelectasis and pneumonia. Once pneumonia is es-

tablished, it can quickly escalate pulmonary and systemic injury secondary to cytokine release. Sepsis, respiratory failure and ARDS follow.

Respiratory tract damage affects three different anatomic areas: the upper airway, the tracheobronchial airways, and the bronchioles and the alveoli (12). In the upper airway, the inflammatory response can cause significant edema and swelling with a corresponding decrease in upper airway diameter and resultant upper airway obstruction. Direct thermal injury is greatest in the upper airway, because most thermal energy dissipates before reaching the lower trachea. If the patient's inhalation injury is limited to the upper airway, the patient can usually be easily supported through this phase, because most of the edema subsides by day 3 to day 5. The use of steroids in an attempt to reduce the upper airway obstruction has been shown to be of no benefit and actually increases morbidity secondary to increased infectious complications. Heliox and racemic epinephrine have been shown to be effective in reducing postinjury upper airway stridor (13).

Inhalation injury involving the tracheobronchial tree and alveoli is associated with the highest mortality. Smoke exposure results in direct epithelial disruption and cellular sloughing into the airway lumen. Decreased ciliary clearance of the airway results in retained secretions and debris. The acute inflammatory response stimulates neutrophil sequestration, complement activation, and the release of tissue-degradation products and oxygen radicals. Damage at the bronchial level is caused by the incomplete products of combustion. Damage at the alveolar level is caused by capillary leak with transudation of proteins and subsequent interstitial edema. The interstitial alveolar edema increases alveolar atelectasis, V/Q mismatching, and pulmonary shunting, with resultant respiratory failure.

The treatment of inhalation injury primarily involves supportive care and limiting iatrogenic injury. Trying to prevent airway edema by limiting fluid resuscitation in an effort to keep the "lung dry," has only been shown to increase cardiopulmonary instability and patient mortality. Likewise, the use of corticosteroids in an effort to ameliorate the pulmonary consequences of the inhalation injury is associated with an increased risk of infection and death. Positive end expiratory pressure (PEEP) during this phase increases functional residual capacity, increases alveolar recruitment, and allows lower oxygen tensions to overcome intrapulmonary shunting (14). The largest treatment strides have occurred during the inflammation-infection period of pulmonary injury. Recently, the benefits of high-frequency percussive ventilation have been demonstrated (15). This modality requires lower inspired oxygen tensions, thus minimizing oxidant injury; requires lower peak inspiratory pressures, thus minimizing barotrauma; and is, furthermore, far better at pulmonary toilet than conventional volume ventilators. One study has shown high-frequency percussive ventilation to have decreased the incidence of pneumonia by nearly 50% (16). This is a significant stride because preventing pneumonia in burn patients ultimately prevents the most deadly complication, ARDS.

To diagnose inhalation injury, generally all that is necessary is to obtain a thorough history and perform a complete physical exam. However, fiberoptic bronchoscopy can be useful. In the history, it is important to determine the circumstances of the fire and whether the patient was trapped in an enclosed space, as prolonged extraction from burning cars or trailers are highly associated with profound pulmonary injury. Signs and symptoms of inhalation injury to note on physical exam include the presence of head and neck burns, the production of sooty sputum or a hoarse voice, and the auscultation of wheezes. Radiographs of the chest are uniformly not helpful in the initial assessment because the characteristic chest x ray associated with inhalation injury is normal. Subsequent daily radiographs are required however, to follow tube position and to monitor the evolution of pulmonary infiltrates. Xenon lung scans and pulmonary function tests have not been especially useful outside the research setting. Fiberoptic bronchoscopy has shown itself, however, to be useful as both a diagnostic and therapeutic modality. Diagnostically, the initial extent of upper-airway injury can be documented, and if significant injury has been appreciated the patient can be intubated nasopharyngeally over the bronchoscope (Fig. 22–4). This is beneficial, because significant upper-airway obstruction secondary to edema has not yet occurred. Concomitantly, mucus plugs and airway secretions can be suctioned away with the bronchoscope in an effort to reduce infectious complications.

Following initial resuscitation, management of the burn wound is the major focus of burn care. In the past, before topical antimicrobial agents and operative débridement, the wounds were bandaged with saline gauze to prevent wound dessication. Daily washings were used to reduce bacterial colonization, and the nonviable burned tissue was removed through bacterial digestion and daily débridements (Fig. 22–5). With the advent of topical antimicrobial agents, the bacterial counts of burn wounds were sharply reduced, to the point where the separation of the eschar from the underlying healthy tissue took considerably longer. Consequently, more aggressive daily débridements were needed to remove the nonviable tissue. These débridements significantly increased patient discomfort. Therefore, at present the approach to wound care is continued daily washing, application of topical agents, and operative débridement with skin grafting. This approach has reduced patient discomfort and reduced morbidity and mortality. The function of topical agents is not to sterilize the wound per se, but rather to keep bacterial colonization at levels that prevent pseudoeschar formation, severe desiccation, and invasive burn wound infection. Ultimately, débridement of the burned tissue and coverage with split-thickness autograft is desired (17).

Excision of burn tissue can be accomplished through two methods. The first method is tangential excision, removing burned tissue down to the dermis with a Goulian knife. The second method is removal of the burn to the fascial level. Tangential excision is preferred because it keeps the natural contour of the extremity; however, it results in greater blood loss and an intermediate level of graft take. Greater blood loss prevents extensive amounts of débridement to be carried out at one time; therefore, it is only appropriate for small burns. Excision to fascia is more deforming, but the operative blood loss is less and the take is nearly 100%; therefore, larger portions can be excised at one time and it is best used for large life-threatening burns. Blood loss can be kept to a minimum by using topical hemostatic agents such as Thrombin spray, as well as injecting the subcutaneous tissues of the patient with Neo-synephrine solution before excision.

Presently there are three topical antibacterial agents available for use. First is silver sulfadiazine (Silvadene). Sulfadiazine has efficacy against gram-negative organisms and yeast, has moderate eschar penetration, and is painless once applied (Figs. 22–6 and 22–7). It is applied daily following the patient's bath. Its shortcomings are that it has poor activity against pseudomonas and enterobacter, results in neutropenia, and cannot be used on patients allergic to sulfa. The next available agent is mafenide (Sulfamylon). It is active against gram-positive and gram-negative organisms, including pseudomonas and enterobacter. It also has rapid eschar penetration. Mafenide's shortcomings, however, are significant. First, it is painful when applied, especially on partial-

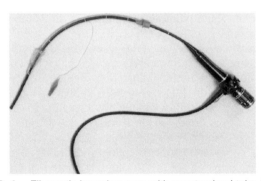

FIG. 22–4. Fiberoptic bronchoscope with nasotracheal tube in place preceding bronchoscopic examination. Tube can be inserted at the time of bronchoscopy if intubation is necessary.

FIG. 22–5. Freshly excised wound with mesh skin graft in place.

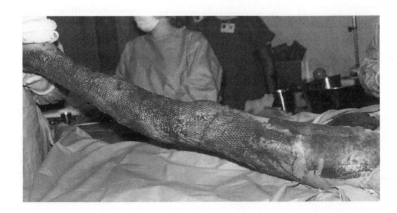

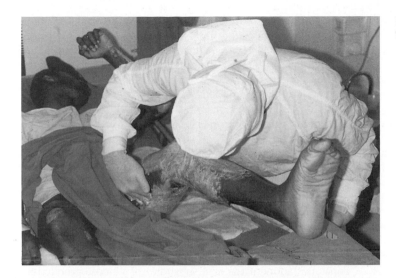

FIG. 22–6. Silvadene application to lower extremity following third-degree wound.

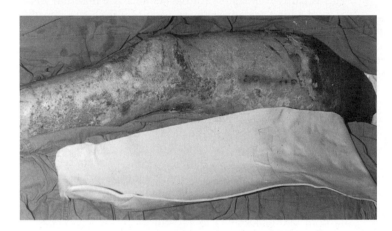

FIG. 22–7. Same wound after removal of Silvadene by gentle washing. The wound is carefully examined before each new application of topical cream to detect any evidence of burn wound sepsis.

thickness burns. Second, it has a profound carbonic anhydrase effect with resultant metabolic acidosis, and it has been associated with increased incidence of ARDS. Silver nitrate is the final agent. This is rarely used, being primarily indicated for patients with profound sulfa allergies. It too is effective against gram-positive organisms, gram-negative organisms, and yeast. Silver nitrate is inexpensive but it has no eschar penetration. Silver nitrate is markedly hypotonic, so it leeches potassium, sodium, and chloride from the wound, resulting in profound electrolyte abnormalities. Furthermore, it stains everything with which it comes into contact an unsightly black. Generally, Silvadene is the first agent of choice; it is applied daily following the patient's bath with a mild antimicrobial soap. It is dressed in a closed fashion with clean gauze. If the wound deteriorates and there is evidence of invasive burn wound infection, including development of a pseudoeschar, an increase in bacterial counts, and signs of patient deterioration, mafenide is then used. If there is a significant yeast component to the infection, a specific antifungal like Nystatin should be applied topically. If there is systemic fungal invasion, noted by positive blood cultures, then Amphotericin B is indicated.

The majority of burn patients succumb to infectious complications. These involve pneumonia, invasive burn wound sepsis, and septic thrombophlebitis. In the past, most pneumonias were caused by organisms spread hematogenously. Such pneumonias used to comprise about 67% of patients (18). Today, however, only about one-third of all pneumonias are caused by bloodborne organisms; the majority are caused by airborne pathogens. As might be expected, the causative pathogens have also changed; a profound increase in the number of staphlococcal pneumonias has been seen. This change in epidemiology coincides with the advent of powerful intravenous antibiotics, topical antimicrobial therapy, and more aggressive wound excision techniques.

The typical pattern for airborne pneumonias are fever, leukocytosis, purulent sputum, progressive ventilatory impairment, and worsening infiltrates. These tend to occur about postburn day 7. Pneumonias caused by airborne pathogens differ from hematogenous pneumonias in that the infiltrates tend to be more centrally located and tend to occur much earlier in the patient's course. Gram-negative organisms still tend to be the initial culprit, especially in the elderly and alcoholic population. Empiric antimicrobial coverage is indicated once a pneumonia is suspected. The agents of choice are generally an antipseudomonal penicillin with a concomitant aminoglycoside. Ten days of treatment is generally adequate. As was previously noted, however, staphylococcal pneumonias are of increasing predominance. If there is no clinical improvement within the first 2 days of treatment, Vancomycin should be initiated. Using empiric antibiotics before postburn day 6 or 7 is of no benefit. Treatment of bacterial colonization without evidence of clinical pneumonia does not prevent the patient from developing pneumonia. Furthermore, prophylactic antimicrobial administration can be detrimental, because it generally selects out resistent organisms. Ventilatory impairment before postburn day 7 is not the result of infectious complications, but rather the result of the pulmonary injury discussed earlier.

Hematogenous pneumonia is generally the result of bacteremia from nondébrided burn tissue or from invasive burn wound sepsis. In the past, prophylactic penicillin was given to decrease tissue bacterial counts in an effort to prevent streptococcal pneumonia. Again, this is not currently recommended, because it has been shown that this selects resistant organisms (19) and is of little to no help in reducing the bacterial counts of eschar. Eschar is nonviable tissue, and therefore lacks a blood supply. Parenteral antibiotics are, subsequently, not able to penetrate the eschar.

Invasive burn wound sepsis occurs in patients with large burns, is primarily an immunologic phenomenon, and is almost always caused by pseudomonas or yeast. Such loss of wound control occurs only in profoundly burned patients who do not have the systemic immunity to prevent bacterial invasion. Antimicrobial agents have reduced this phenomena, but have not eradicated it. Clinical signs include rapid eschar separation, bleeding, systemic sepsis, and dark, hemorrhagic discoloration of a previously normal burn wound. Histologically, the tissue shows increased bacterial counts and increased capillary thrombosis and necrosis. This occurrence is an indication for parenteral antibiotics, subeschar infusion of an antipseudomonal penicillin, and subsequent burn wound débridement. Fungal invasive burn wound infections have become far more common (20). This is most likely the result of our ability to "sterilize" the patients with enormous quantities of antibiotics. Invasive fungal wound infections are essentially a death sentence. The only treatment options involve extensive débridements of all nonviable tissue and extensive dosages of Amphotericin B.

Finally, suppurative thrombophlebitis is an infectious complication that can easily be overlooked. It is of paramount importance to ensure that a patient with a deteriorating clinical course does not have a septic source in a peripheral vein (or worse, a central vein). If a peripheral vein is located as a septic source, the only treatment available is complete excision of that vein. If a septic thrombophlebitis is associated with a central vein, little can be done except possibly lytic therapy. Both of these complications can be reduced by routine rotation of peripheral intravenous lines, exchanging central access lines, and limiting the use of parenteral nutrition.

Recent advances in our knowledge of the immunologic cascade associated with burn injury and how it correlates to patients' metabolic and nutritional requirements have aided our ability to reduce burn wound morbidity. Initially, there is an ebb phase in which there is a decrease in the patient's metabolic rate and cardiac output. Approximately 12 to 24 hours following injury this response changes to a hypermetabolic state, with a marked increase in metabolic energy expenditure and metabolic rates approaching twice normal (21). This increased rate of metabolism continues until the patient's wounds are healed. At one time it was hoped that

very early excision could reduce this hypermetabolic state; unfortunately, this is not the case (22).

Shortly after a burn occurs, the hypothalamic temperature setpoint is reset. This is exhibited by a marked increase in the skin and core temperatures. To support this increase in body temperature, the basal metabolic rate increases with a corresponding rise in plasma levels of stress hormones such as epinephine, glucagon, cortisol, and insulin. The glucagon/insulin ratio also increases with a resultant hyperglycemia. Interestingly, one of the most sensitive signs of impending sepsis is a further increase in this ratio and an increase in serum glucose levels. This occurs because the immunologic assault that is associated with sepsis, further promotes this hypermetabolic state with increased glycogenolysis and gluconeogenesis. The elevated glucose levels that occur, therefore, reflect increased glucose production, not decreased utilization. In addition, the increased rate of gluconeogenesis consumes amino acids as a substrate for glucose production. This is partly responsible for the net decrease in serum levels of most amino acids in the burn patient. It is also responsible for the obligatory muscle wasting associated with thermal injury. As a result of the increased level of catecholamines, there is also a significantly increased rate of lipolysis. Burn patients, however, have decreased rates of ketogenesis because the elevated levels of insulin hinder ketone production.

Beta oxidation is not the only system with increased activity, the cyclooxygenase system is more active as well, with a corresponding increase in the production of eicosanoids. It is hoped that the use of omega-3 fatty acids, which cannot be used as a substrate for the cyclooxygenase system, will aid in quelling this outpouring of immunologic mediators; however, the specifics remain to be determined.

Appropriate nutrition in burn patients is essential. They have an enormous level of protein turnover. It is essential, therefore, to avoid negative nitrogen balance. Determining caloric needs in the past was done by using the Harris-Bendict formula to calculate basal energy expenditure (BEE) and then estimate the resting energy expenditure (REE). In the past, it was estimated that the REE was approximately twice the BEE in burn patients. This method has proven to overestimate the actual REE by as much as 50% (23). With the advent of bedside indirect calorimetry, a machine can arrive at an accurate resting energy expenditure by measuring the difference in the concentrations of oxygen and carbon dioxide between inspired and expired air. An accurate representation of the patient's REE is important, because overfeeding patients has been shown to have detrimental consequences, namely, increased serum glucose and fat levels, which directly correlate with a decrease in immunologic function as well as an increase in mediator release (24).

There are two methods by which nutritional goals can be met: parenteral or enteral. Parenteral nutrition is fraught with complications and should only be used when absolutely necessary. Enteral nutrition has been conclusively shown to be of far greater benefit. Enteral feeds have numerous advantages and few disadvantages. The advantages rest primarily on maintaining the integrity of the gastrointestinal tract, thus avoiding serious complications (e.g., sepsis) resulting from gut translocation, stress ulceration resulting from the loss of the gastric mucosal barrier, and acalculous cholecystitis resulting from cholestasis. Furthermore, insulin secretion is also enhanced by enteral nutrition, and increased insulin levels enhanced protein anabolism. The only disadvantage of enteral nutrition is the physician's fear of aspiration pneumonitis that is usually unsubstantiated. Once the patient's gastric ileus resolves, most patients can be fed within 3 days of injury. Patients with smaller burns may even be fed earlier. Of note, however, is that feeding patients during the resuscitative phase should be avoided because of its high complication rate and its marginal benefit. Large burns, where patients will be intubated for long periods of time, are associated with prolonged gastric ileus. Fortunately, enteral feeds are still generally tolerated in this population and nutrition can usually be instilled through a small-bore nasoduodenal tube. Occasionally, prolonged post resuscitative ileus prevents gastric feeds. If this is the case, correctable causes of ileus (e.g., electrolyte abnormalities and overuse of narcotics) should be investigated. Prolonged ileus is also a hallmark of sepsis; therefore, any patient with a prolonged ileus should have a thorough sepsis work-up as well. In general, prepyloric feeds are preferred. They are more physiologic and are associated with reduced instances of diarrhea, stress gastritis, and theoretically cholecystitis, because the enterohepatic hormones are stimulated with gastric feeding. In patients with residual gastric ileus in whom there is an increased risk of aspiration pneumonitis with gastric feeds, nasoduodenal feeds are preferred. It should be noted that convalescent patients will rarely eat more than when they were healthy. To meet the increased nutritional goals, supplemental gastric tube feeds are necessary.

Burn patients also suffer from stress gastric ulceration and acalculous cholecystitis. Prevention of stress gastritis starts during the resuscitative phase, because loss of the protective mucosal barrier occurs with the initial splanchnic ischemia associated with burn shock (25). Adequate resuscitation aids in reducing, but does not remove, this complication. Therefore, gastric ulcer prophylaxis is always indicated. In the past, antacids and H_2 antagonists were used to reduce the erosive potential from the gastric secretions. It has recently been found, however, that reducing gastric acidity has contributed to gastric bacterial overgrowth and increased aspiration pneumonia (26). Therefore, cytoprotective agents such as sucralfate are currently recommended for ulcer prophylaxis. Sucralfate maintains the integrity of the mucosal barrier without changing gastric pH and without altering gastric flora. Furthermore, sucralfate is much less expensive than either H_2 antagonists or antacids and has virtually no side effects. However, if gastric emptying is severely compromised, parenteral H_2 antagonists are still the agent of choice, because in this setting sucralfate may accumulate in the stomach and cause a bezaar. No good pharmaceutical prophylaxis for acalculous cholecystitis exists. Pathophysiology of this complication appears to be biliary stasis with splanchnic ischemia. (27). As noted previously, though, enteral feeds appear to reduce this complication by stimulating the enteral biliary hormones, thus increasing biliary emptying.

Considering the level of immobilization burn patients are subjected to, thromboembolic complications are surprisingly rare. A 10-year review of more than 2000 burn patients states that significant pulmonary thrombosis occurred in only 1.2% of the patients, and in only 0.19% of patients was it felt that the pulmonary embolus contributed to their death (28). Con-

sidering the high rate of gastrointestinal bleeds in burn patients, the routine use of anticoagulants such as low-dose heparin or aspirin is contraindicated, because their benefit would certainly not outweigh their risk. Sequential compression stockings are not especially useful because most burn patients have extensive bulky dressings on their extremities. The best prevention of deep venous thrombosis is to avoid femoral access. In those instances in which femoral access is absolutely necessary, the routine rotation of these intravenous lines is mandatory.

Following the acute therapy, the long road to burn rehabilitation begins. This is an area where a host of dedicated physical and occupational therapists use specially designed physical exercises, splints, and elastic stockings to reduce scar formation. These activities help the patient regain use and mobility of burned extremities and help the patient relearn activities of daily living necessary to function in society.

In conclusion, care of the patient who has sustained a thermal injury is optimized when an organized team, with a thorough understanding of burn pathophysiology, develops and implements a plan to prevent further complications. A large stride in burn morbidity occurred when the benefits of resuscitation were appreciated. Later, improvements in topical antimicrobials and wound excision techniques further improved outcome. Some of the greatest advances today are occurring in mechanical ventilation, nutrition, and parenteral chemotherapy. As more is learned about the complications of burns and the body's response to such profound injury, outcomes will hopefully continue to improve.

References

1. Pruitt BA Jr, Goodwin CW Jr, and Pruitt SK. Burns: including cold, chemical and electrical injuries. In: Sabiston, DC, ed. *Textbook of surgery*. 14th ed. Philadelphia, WB Saunders, 1991.
2. Jackson DM. The diagnosis of the depth of burning. *Brit J Surg* 1953; 40:588.
3. Hammond JS, and Ward CG. Transfers from emergency room to burn center: errors in burn size estimate. *J Trauma* 1987; 27:1161.
4. Warden GD. Burn shock resuscitation. *World J Surg* 1992; 16:16.
5. Monafo WW, Halverson JD, Schechtman K. The role of concentrated sodium solutions in the resuscitation of patients with severe burns. *Surgery* 1984; 95:129.
6. Baxter CR, Shires T. Physiologic response to crystalloid resuscitation of severe burns. *Ann NY Acad Sci* 1968; 150:874.
7. Morehouse JD, Finklestein JL, et al. Resuscitation of the thermally injured patient. *Critical Care Clinics* 1992; 8:355.
8. Moyland J, Inge WW Jr, Pruitt BA Jr. Circulatory changes following circumferential extremity burns evaluted by the ultrasonic flow meter: An analysis of 60 thermally injured limbs. *J Trauma* 1971; 11:763.
9. Saffle JR, Zeluff GR, Warden GD. Intramuscular pressure in the burned arm: measurement and response to escharotomy. *Am J Surg* 1980; 140:25.
10. Thompson PB, Herndon DN, et al. Effect on mortality of inhalation injury. *J Trauma* 1986; 26:163.
11. Demling RH. Smoke inhalation injury. *New Horizons* 1993; 1:442.
12. Sharar SR, Heimbach DM. Inhalation injury: current concepts and controversies. *Advances in Trauma and Critical Care* 1991; 6:213.
13. Kempe KJ, Izenberg S, et al. Treatment of post extubation stridor in a pediatric patient with burns: the role of Heliox. *J Burn Care and Rehabilitation* 1990; 11:337.
14. Clark WR. Smoke inhalation: diagnosis and treatment. *World J Surg* 1992; 16:24.
15. Cioffi WG, Graves TA, et al. High vent frequency: percussive inhalation in patients with inhalation Injury. *J Trauma* 1989; 29:350.
16. Cioffi WG Jr, Rue LW III, et al. Prophylactic use of high-frequency percussive inhalation in patients with inhalation injury. *Ann Surg* 1991; 213:575.

17. Tompkins RG, Burke JF, et al. Prompt eschar excision: a treatment system contributing to reduced burn mortality: a statistical evaluation of burn care at the Massachussets General Hospital (1974–1984). *Ann Surg* 1986; 204:272.

18. Pruitt BA Jr, McManus AT. The changing epidemiology of infection in burn patients. *World J Surg* 1992; 16:57.

19. Mozingo DW, McManus AT, et al. Appropriate use of parenteral antibiotics in managing burns. *Surgical Infections: Index and Review* 1993; 1:16.

20. Becker WK, Cioffi WG Jr, et al. Fungal burn wound infection: a 10-year experience. *Arch Surg* 1991; 126:44.

21. Waymack JP, Herndon DN. Nutritional support of the burn patient. *World J Surg* 1992; 16:80.

22. Rutan TC, Herndon DN, et al. Metabolic rate alterations in early excision and grafting versus conservative treatment. *J Trauma* 1986; 26:140.

23. Saffle JR, Medina E, Raymond J, et al. Use of indirect calorimetry in the nutritional management of burned patients. *J Trauma* 1985; 25:32.

24. Ireton-Jones C, Baxter CR. Nutrition for adult burn patients: a review. *Nutrition in Clinical Practice* 1991; 6:3.

25. Rath T, Walzer LR, Meissl G. Preventive measures for stress ulcers in burn patients. *Burn Inc Therm Inj* 1988; 14:504.

26. Marino PL, Stress ulcers: gastric acid, friend or foe? In: Marino PL *The ICU Book*. Philadelphia: Lee and Febiger, 1991.

27. Mobermoh MW, Scudamor CH, Boileau LO, et al. Acalculous cholecystitis: its role as a complication of major burn injury. *Can J Surg* 1985; 28:527.

28. Rue LW III, Cioffi WG Jr, Rush R, et al. Thromboembolic complications in thermally injured patients. *World J Surg* 1992; 16:1151.

23

Principles and Management of Injuries from Chemical and Physical Agents

Anthony J. DeFranzo, M.D., F.A.C.S.

In any industrialized society, injuries from chemical and physical agents pose an ever-present hazard. Chemical products are commonly used in the home, in agriculture, in scientific laboratories, in industry, and in the military; more than 25,000 products capable of producing chemical injury are marketed today. Annually in the United States, accidental contact and/or criminal assault with chemicals produce more than 3000 deaths and 60,000 cases that require medical attention (1). Physical agents (e.g., high-voltage electricity) cause more than 1000 deaths per year in this country. Clinical outcomes for electrical injuries have not improved over the past 20 years (2). The pathophysiology of electrical trauma deserves special consideration later in the chapter.

Acid Injuries

In most acid burns, the moiety responsible for injury is the hydrogen ion. Strong acids in common use (e.g., sulfuric, nitric, hydrochloric, and trichloroacetic acid) produce similar injuries and require similar methods of treatment. The hydrogen ion produces an exothermic reaction, cellular dehydration, and precipitation of proteins, with coagulation necrosis the result. Fortunately, in acid burns the hydrogen ion appears to be neutralized at the point of initial tissue reaction (3). The injuries are proportional to the concentration of the acid and the length of time the acid is in contact with the tissue. Acid burns produce extreme and longlasting pain; it does not disappear until the neutralization of hydrogen ions has been completed (4). As in thermal burns, the appearance of the acid burn varies with the severity of the injury. Minor acid burns appear erythematous and soft in texture whereas major burns are gray, yellow brown, or black and leatherlike in texture.

Common acid injuries should be treated with copious water irrigation. Dilute solutions of sodium bicarbonate may follow as a neutralizing agent (3). Water irrigation should begin at once and the area of the acid injury should not be underestimated. Spills or splatters are the most frequent acid injuries and may involve several remote patches of skin. The immediate removal of all clothing that may contain acid and the use of a shower stall is most effective. Bromberg and colleagues (5) recommend hydrotherapy for several hours. Blisters and nonviable tissue are débrided and topical antibiotics are applied, as in thermal burns. Primary excision and grafting of severe but small localized burns is a time-and cost-effective treatment. Acid burns of the upper extremities, such as the dorsum of the hands, are common and lend themselves to the above management.

Systemic complications of common acid burns are not usually significant. However, hydrofluoric acid burns may result in severe systemic complications.

HYDROFLUORIC ACID BURNS

Hydrofluoric acid is one of the strongest of all inorganic acids (6). Its expanded uses have led to increased numbers of related injuries. The pathophysiology of hydrofluoric acid burns is different from all other acid burns. The hydrogen ion plays only a small part in the chemical burn (i.e., cellular dehydration, protein precipitation, and coagulation necrosis). The freely dissociable fluoride ion is chiefly responsible for the hydrofluoric acid injury. It quickly penetrates skin to reach the deep tissues, producing liquefaction necrosis and even decalcification and erosion of bone. The pain associated with tissue damage is excruciating, although with dilute concentrations the onset of pain may be delayed for many hours. Without proper treatment, the pain persists for several days. Klauder and coworkers (7) suggest that the excruciating pain is due to mobilization of calcium ions in the tissues, which leads to a shift of potassium ions and intense nerve stimulation.

The clinical appearance of hydrofluoric acid burns begins with simple erythematous, swollen, and painful areas similar to other acid burns. With concentrated solutions, or with neglected burns from more dilute solutions, progressive tissue destruction occurs. The affected area becomes firm, edematous, and pasty-white to yellow-white. Blisters form, containing a white caseous, necrotic material. Erythema surrounds this area of severe tissue destruction. Full-thickness tissue loss may occur with severe permanent scarring.

The hands and upper extremities are the most common sites of hydrofluoric acid burns (6,8). Untreated or improperly treated hand injuries may result in erosion of the distal phalanx and destruction of the nail bed. Gangrenous loss of a finger is not uncommon (9,10). Shewmake and Anderson (10) point out that hydrofluoric acid will easily pass through pinholes in protective rubber gloves and penetrate subungual tissues. This exposure may go unrecognized by the patient for 6 to 24 hours, until severe pain begins. Leather gloves offer no protection and cannot be decontaminated. they must be destroyed, or further burns may occur when they are worn again. Subungual burns are of particular concern because subungual tissue has no stratum corneum. The remainder of the hand, especially the palm, is much more resistant to acid penetration. Hydrofluoric acid rapidly penetrates the nail matrix and if allowed to progress will rapidly destroy the soft tissue and distal phalanx. Subungual tissue destruction causes intolerable pain that may seem out of proportion to the clinical impression of the inexperienced physician.

The effective treatment of a hydrofluoric acid burn differs from that of other acid burns because treatment must deactivate both the hydrogen ion and the powerful fluoride ion. In addition to initial dilution and neutralization of the acid with copious amounts of water or dilute solutions of sodium bicarbonate or alkaline soap, treatment must also be directed specifically toward the fluoride ion. Many salts are formed by hydrofluoric acid, but only calcium fluoride and magnesium fluoride are insoluble in tissue and therefore neutralizing (3). All other fluoride salts dissociate freely, allowing the destructive effects of the fluoride ion to continue.

Opinions differ as to the best method of neutralizing the fluoride ion. Topical agents include: magnesium oxide ointment; cold 25% magnesium sulfate soaks; cold Hyamine chloride soaks (this is an aquaternary ammonium compound that exchanges chloride for fluoride, producing a nonionized fluoride complex); cold Zephiran soaks (benzalkonium chloride, which has an action similar to that of Hyamine); calcium gluconate gel; and calcium carbonate gel (3,6,11,12). Cold itself is thought to decrease blood and lymph flow, hinder the development of edema, and slow the penetration of fluoride ions through the tissues. Calcium carbonate gel, made from 10-gm calcium carbonate tablets and 20 mL of K–Y jelly, is readily available. The calcium carbonate preparation is applied directly to burns of the hand and can also be poured into a surgeon's glove, which is put on the hand and changed every 4 hours (12).

In severe hydrofluoric acid burns, injectable agents are introduced directly into the burned tissue. Calcium gluconate, 5–10% solution, has been shown to be the most effective injectable agent, although 25% magnesium sulfate may be used (13). Treviño and others (14) believe calcium gluconate stronger than 5% causes severe pain and tissue damage and may itself cause severe scarring and keloids. Injections should be done within, under, and around the injured area using a 30-gauge needle (10). The injections should extend 0.5 cm beyond the area of obvious injury into uninjured tissue (15). Severe pain may be eliminated within 15 minutes and the tissue destruction abruptly halted. However, precautions must be taken, because overinjection in burn tissue will cause distention and subsequent necrosis. Inject only enough calcium gluconate to effectively stop the pain; the maximum safe amount to inject is 0.5 mL/cm^2 burn. Injections must be carefully controlled in the fingers and nail beds, which have little soft tissue. A local or regional block given before injection may prevent the pain experienced with calcium gluconate injection (6,10). However, pain is a valuable symptom to follow; if it recurs, reinjection is indicated immediately (6).

The severity of burns from hydrofluoric acid injury depends, as with any acid, on the concentration of the acid and the duration of the exposure. The decision simply to use topical therapy or inject calcium gluconate is made with knowledge of the concentration of the hydrofluoric acid causing the injury. The National Institute of Health has classified hydrofluoric acid burns on the basis of acid concentration. This can be useful in management and in the prediction of the clinical course of the burn (16) (Table 23–1). Determining the concentration may avoid undertreating the injury.

Table 23–1
Classification of Hydrofluoric Acid Burns Proposed by Division of Industrial Hygiene, National Institutes of Health

Concentration	Human Burn
0–20%	This burn manifests itself by pain and erythema as late as 24 h after burn.
20–50%	This burn becomes apparent 1–8 h after exposure to the acid.
>50%	This burn is felt immediately and tissue destruction is rapidly apparent.

Reproduced with permission from Dibbell DG, Iverson RE, Jones W, et al.[14]

There is general agreement that burns caused by hydrofluoric acid concentrations less than 20% can be treated safely with iced Zephiran or Hyamine chloride soaks for 1 to 4 hours (15). Calcium gluconate 2.5% gel or calcium carbonate gel may also be used. The patient, if treated as an outpatient, should be instructed to reapply the gel whenever pain returns to the burned area (14). Burns known to result from concentrations greater than 20% should be treated with calcium gluconate injections. If pain or skin changes become apparent with hydrofluoric acid exposures of concentrations less than 20%, calcium gluconate injections should also be used. Injections that could not be initiated until 36 hours following exposure have still provided prompt pain relief and arrest of tissue destruction (15). Following calcium gluconate injections, severely burned areas that are demarcated may be débrided under appropriate anesthesia. Routine topical antibiotic treatment should be initiated, and the burned area placed in a bulky dressing and elevated. Fingernails should be removed if subungal burns are present to facilitate rapid neutralization of hydrofluoric acid in the nail bed.

Intraarterial injection may also be considered for hydrofluoric acid burns of the upper extremity. Vance and colleagues have proposed intraarterial injection of calcium chloride or calcium gluconate for hydrofluoric acid burns of the hands (16). Calcium chloride is too irritating to tissue to allow direct injection but may be given intraarterially. Intraarterial injection is performed through the radial or brachial artery and has distinct advantages over tissue injection of calcium gluconate. A much greater amount of elemental calcium can be delivered with intraarterial injection, especially with calcium chloride. Furthermore the fluoride ion is more effectively neutralized with intraarterial injection, which is an important consideration in severe hydrofluoric acid burns. Calcium is more efficiently supplied to depleted cells and intraarterial infusion is much less painful. Fingernails do not have to be removed because the nail bed is well perfused. The disadvantage of intraarterial infusion is possible damage to, or spasm of, the artery cannulated. However, arterial cannulation complications are reported infrequently and there appears to be no direct toxic effect to the artery from calcium gluconate or calcium chloride (17).

If the total hydrofluoric acid burn area is greater than 50–100 square centimeters, hospitalization for optimal care is suggested. Burn areas greater than 100–150 square centimeters can cause systemic complications and require close monitoring in a burn unit or an intensive care unit (14). Systemic treatments must be directed specifically at pulmonary injuries and electrolyte imbalance that may result in cardiac dysfunction. Inhalation injuries should be treated immediately with 100% oxygen by face mask. A 2.5–3.0% calcium gluconate solution should be given by inhalation using a nebulizer or Intermittent positive pressure breathing (IPPB) machine (14). The patient should be watched expectantly for 24 to 48 hours for the development of severe upper airway edema and/or pulmonary edema. Intubation may become mandatory if pulmonary edema develops. Calcium gluconate should continue by inhalation in the intubated patient and positive end-expiratory pressure ventilation should be initiated (14). Systemic antibiotics and steroids may be helpful. The acute pulmonary injury from hydrofluoric acid continues for several weeks and dyspnea with moderate physical activity may last for 9 months. Steroid therapy every 3rd day for 3 months has been advocated after inhalation injury (14). Pulmonary function tests may reveal permanent damage in severe injuries. Electrolyte imbalance must be carefully monitored, with frequent serum calcium and magnesium levels. The fluoride ion rapidly penetrates tissue following severe hydrofluoric acid injuries to the skin or respiratory tree. Intravenous (IV) calcium gluconate therapy should maintain the calcium level at or above the normal upper limit. Continuous electrocardiograms (ECG), liver function, blood urea nitrogen (BUN), and creatinine must also be monitored. Hepatic and renal toxicity may develop rapidly in severe hydrofluoric acid exposures to the skin and respiratory tree. Hemodialysis may become mandatory.

Vapor or liquid hydrofluoric acid injuries to the face may severely damage the eye. Hydrofluoric acid vapor alone may cause extensive injury to the cornea and conjunctiva. A 1% calcium gluconate solution should be used to wash the eye as soon as possible (14). As in the management of all other significant injuries to the eye, an ophthalmologist should be consulted as soon as possible.

Alkali Injuries

The vast majority of alkali injuries occur during personal quarrels. Among 416 patients with reported alkali injuries, only 9 had been injured in industrial accidents (18). Strong alkalis such as caustic potash (KOH) and caustic soda (NaOH) are available in any supermarket. Alkalis can be fabricated into cheap disfiguring weapons referred to as "12-cent pistols (19)." The moiety responsible for alkali burns is the hydroxyl ion (OH^-). Erythema and epidermal bullae appear early in the wound and an eschar may form later. The wound is painful to palpation and is soapy and slippery to the touch. Alkali burns produced by common strong alkalis are more penetrating than burns produced by acids other than hydrofluoric acid and phenol. Whereas in common acid burns the hydrogen ion is inactivated immediately by its chemical reaction with tissue, in alkali burns the hydroxyl ion is not. Alkali proteinates, which are formed in alkali-tissue reactions, are soluble (3). Thus, the hydroxyl ion may continue to pass more deeply into tissue, denaturing one protein molecule after another. This penetrating injury has been called *liquefaction necrosis*. The total picture of alkali injury includes saponification of fats and cellular dehydration, resulting in cell death. *Saponification* is an exothermic reaction producing a significant amount of heat, which causes severe tissue damage. Destruction of fat allows an increase in water penetration of the alkali burn eschar, negating the natural water barrier that lipid provides (18). Untreated alkali injuries will often penetrate the full thickness of skin, destroying all ectodermal elements such as hair follicles and sweat glands. Regeneration of skin, therefore, can occur only from the edge of the wound because skin islands usually do not develop in the center of the wound. An eschar may form and if untreated may continue to harbor alkali, which may penetrate into and damage the tissue further (5).

In alkali injuries, there seems to be a significant latent period during which proper therapy can be administered advantageously (20). Progressive and immediate hydrotherapy is the best treatment, and serves the following purposes: (a) washing away or diluting the offending agent; (b) decreasing the rate of chemical reaction; (c) decreasing tissue metabolism and thus inflammatory reaction; (d) minimizing dehydration; and (e) restoring normal skin pH (5). Some heat is given off with dilution, making high water flow important. The length of time for hydrotherapy is another important consideration. Because the hydroxyl ion is soluble in tissue over long periods and may be quantitatively significant in the eschar, Bromberg and coworkers (5) have advocated prolonged water irrigation in a shower stall. In their study, patients underwent hydrotherapy from 6 hours to 6 days. The elapsed time between injury and beneficial initiation of hydrotherapy ranged from immediate to 12 hours. During and after hydrotherapy, nonviable tissue that may contain alkali should be débrided to prevent further penetration of alkali and to increase the effectiveness of hydrotherapy. Early excision of small full-thickness injuries with delayed closure or split-thickness skin grafting is advantageous. Open wounds should be treated with topical antibacterial agents. Sulfamylon is the agent of choice because it is bacteriostatic; it also combines with active alkali to form sodium acetate and sulfamylon radicals. These reactions give off no heat and the products are innocuous to the wound (18).

The penetrating nature of lye injuries has been associated with special complications, including tympanic membrane perforations, parotid fistulas, severe keloid formation, and the early development of Marjolin ulcers. Although the average time to development of a Marjolin ulcer in a thermal injury scar is 34 years, these ulcers occurred at 3, 7, and 9 years after injury in a series of lye burns reported by Wolfort and others (18).

Phosphorus Burns

Burns caused by white phosphorus, also called yellow phosphorus, deserve special attention. White phosphorus is used in the military as an incendiary or an ignitor for munitions, and is found in various weapons such as artillery shells, mines, hand grenades, and mortar rounds (13). In the military, human or mechanical errors as well as battlefield action account for a significant number of phosphorus burns (1). In civilian life, white phosphorus is used to manufacture munitions, insecticides, fertilizers, and rodent poisons (12). Industrial as well as military accidents may lead to explosions that cause injury.

White phosphorus burns are caused by both liquids and solids. When a weapon containing phosphorus explodes, it spreads flaming droplets of inorganic phosphorus, which become embedded in the skin (22). Phosphorus is highly lipid-soluble and may spread quickly beneath the dermis where it will continue to oxidize until removed by débridement or consumed by oxidation (21). The pain associated with burning white phosphorus is extreme. Tissue damage is due mainly to the heat of combustion. However, phosphorus pentoxide formed by oxidation of phosphorus is also damaging because it is intensely hygroscopic, and phosphoric acid (the end product of phosphorus combustion) is corrosive (22). In military injuries tissue is frequently damaged by shell fragments, with significant areas of 3rd-degree burns. Clinically, the burn wounds become necrotic and yellowish, and may fluoresce. The wound may give off a white vapor and has a characteristic garlicky smell (13).

A patient burned with phosphorus requires immediate treatment. All contaminated clothing should be removed to prevent further contact of phosphorus with the skin. The wound should be irrigated copiously with water and all identifiable particles of phosphorus removed. These particles must be placed under water to avoid their spontaneous ignition as they dry. A thick layer of wet gauze should be placed over the wound and the patient transported directly to an operating room, where definitive removal of all phosphorus must proceed meticulously.

Smoke may aid in the localization of embedded phosphorus, but phosphorus can burrow deeply and its detection may be difficult.

Copper sulfate solutions ranging in concentration from 0.5 to 5.0% have been advocated to aid in the identification of phosphorus particles (13,19,21,22). The chemicals react to form cupric phosphide, which is black. The formation of cupric phosphide may also slow the oxidation reaction of phosphorus. It must be pointed out however, that copper is toxic and may cause massive hemolysis, gastrointestinal disturbances, hepatic necrosis, and cardiorespiratory collapse. A 1% copper sulfate solution is sufficient to tag the phosphorus particles (3). Copper sulfate soaks or baths should not be employed. A brief irrigation of phosphorus burns with 1% copper sulfate should be followed by copious amounts of water to remove excess copper sulfate solution. More than one session of débridement may be required to removal all phosphorus particles. Small areas of full-thickness burns are treated effectively by primary excision with delayed-closure or split-thickness skin grafting. Subsequent management of the burn wound is like that of any other burn.

Systemic toxicity from phosphorus burns has been somewhat unpredictable and mysterious. In Vietnam there were reports of sudden unexpected deaths with phosphorus burns over only 10 to 15% of total body surface area (23). The literature does not report consistent systemic toxicity due to absorption of elemental phosphorus from the burn wound. However, toxicity due to ingestion or inhalation of this substance has been well documented. Ingestion has been known to induce generalized petechiae, seizures, electrocardiographic changes, hematuria, oliguria, icterus, and acute yellow atrophy of the liver (22). Massive hemolysis has been reported by Summerlin and others (22) in patients with phosphorus burns of 29%, 12.5%, and 7.5% of body surface. Whether hemolysis was due to systemic toxicity from phosphorus or from copper is not clear. All patients with phosphorus burns, therefore, should be monitored closely even if the burn surface area is small. The patient should be placed in an intensive care unit or well-equipped burn unit with particular attention being directed to electrocardiographic changes, calcium-phosphorus shifts, and precipitous fallen hematocrit due to hemolysis.

Electrical Injuries

Electricity causes two types of burns of interest to the plastic surgeon: those caused by electrical arc, or flash, and those caused by the passage of current through the patient's body. Male workers in the 3rd and 4th decades of life are most frequently injured. Electrical injuries are very complex, and despite the typical health and youth of the patient, the mortality rate from electrical injuries reaches 15%.

Basic terms and equations include:

- Voltage—electrical energy potential produced by a power source
- Amperage—current flow per unit of time
- Resistance—impedance to current flow measured in ohms

$$Resistance = \frac{Voltage}{Amperage}$$
$$Amperage = \frac{Voltage}{Resistance}$$

Most electrical injuries seen today are direct results of alternating current (24,25). This type of current has virtually replaced direct current, since it is inexpensive to produce and can be transformed into any required voltage. Use of direct current is limited to streetcars, subways, ships, metallurgy, and the chemical industries. Alternating current is produced with a cyclic change in the direction of electron pressure (voltage). The pressure pushes, then pulls, electrons, resulting in alternating current (26). The current frequency *hertz* (Hz) is the number of complete forward and reverse electron cycles in one second. For example, the typical 120-volt (v) wall outlet is 60-cycle current, exhibiting 60 forward flows and 60 reverse flows per second.

Alternating current is more dangerous than direct current at low voltages for two reasons: First, the skin offers lower resistance to alternating current than to direct current, and second, alternating current has a tetanizing effect on muscle, which increases the duration of contact. At high voltage, direct current is as dangerous as alternating current.

As the amperage progressively increases, the experience of contact changes from tingling to shock to a feeling of muscle contraction to an actual tetany of voluntary muscle contraction. These muscle contractions can be strong enough to cause fractures and dislocations. The point at which the muscle contractions are so severe that individuals grasping on the electrical conductor cannot let go is called the "let-go" threshold. Muscle contractions are most pronounced between the frequencies of 15 and 150 Hz. Household current at 60 Hz can therefore be dangerous. The let-go threshold at 60 Hz for men and women is 15.9 and 10.5 milliamperes (mamp), respectively (25). The inability to let go of the conductor is the main cause of prolonged heat buildup and tissue damage in low-tension accidents. If the alternating current increases above 20 mamp, there usually is a sustained contraction of the muscles of respiration, leading in time to respiratory asphyxiation and death. When the flow increases above 40 mamp, ventricular fibrillation may be induced.

The most common electrical injury seen today is caused by high-voltage alternating current. High-voltage injuries are classified as those injuries arising from a source of greater than 1000 v; low-voltage injuries from a source of less than 1000 v (27). Two types of injuries occur with high-voltage alternating current. First, high-tension electrical injuries are frequently associated with an arc, or flash of light, formed between the high-voltage power source and the body, which is usually grounded (28). The temperature of this arc may be as high as 4000° C, and the flash may ignite the victim's clothing and even melt bone. In high-tension accidents, the victim does not hold the conductor but is thrown away from it and may sustain traumatic injuries to the arms, head, or legs. Most injuries from high-tension contact are not caused by sustained contact because the circuit is completed by arcing before the victim even touches the voltage power source. For every 10,000 v, electrical current can arc 1 inch. The second type of high-tension electrical burn injury is caused by the passage of an electrical current between the power source and the patient's exit wound (i.e., within the patient's body) (28). Direct injury to cells from the current itself occurs in nerves, blood vessels, and muscle. In addition, tissue resistance to the passage of current causes the buildup of intense heat.

Skin represents an initial barrier to current and serves as a relatively good insulator, or resistor, against a low-voltage, but not a high-voltage, source. Skin resistance is related directly to skin moisture. A moist hand is 10 to 100 times less resistant than a dry hand. The production of heat as current enters the body through the skin produces necrosis of skin and underlying tissues. Once the resistance of the skin is overcome, the current enters the underlying tissues and flows through the body with negligible resistance except for when it encounters bone. In decreasing order, tissue resistance is as follows: bone, fat, tendon, skin, muscle, vessels, and nerve. A high-voltage current can produce temperatures greater than 1000° C along bone, causing bone destruction and deep tissue necrosis. Because almost all current is concentrated at the entrance to the body and again at the exit, more severe tissue damage occurs at those sites. Baxter (28) has pointed out that high-tension electrical entrance wounds are usually charred and centrally depressed with severe eschar; exit wounds are more likely to be exploded. Entrance wounds may show a central charred area surrounded by a grey-white zone, which in turn is surrounded by a red zone of coagulation. All three zones are full-thickness injuries. The amount and type of injury between the entrance and the exit wounds is difficult to determine. Almost every organ in the body can be injured by an electrical current.

High-tension injuries, unfortunately, have very severe sequelae. The patient must be hospitalized, have a Foley catheter inserted, and be treated aggressively. The condition of the entrance and exit wounds is a clue to the extent of local destruction of deeper tissues. Muscle necrosis within a compartment has severe systemic consequences. Myoglobin pigment from the damaged muscle cells and hemoglobin released from injured red cells rapidly enter the circulation. Thus, the kidney is exposed to significant pigment loads and the absorption of this pigment may lead to acute renal shutdown. Attempted prevention of renal shutdown by early fas-

ciotomy and débridement, even in a limb that may later require amputation, is most important (28). The presence of dark, tea-colored urine almost certainly indicates the presence of myoglobinuria. Mannitol has been used to enhance pigment excretion after adequate urine output has been established through volume replacement. Usually, the mannitol treatment consists of a 25-g loading dose followed by 12.5 g/hour for several hours. Baxter (28) reports that the duration of myoglobinuria can be used to predict morbidity from muscle necrosis. In his series of 19 patients with electrical injury who had myoglobinuria for longer than 6 hours, high amputation of one or more extremities or wider excision of trunk musculature was necessary. Detection of muscle necrosis is most important. Technetium-99m stannous pyrophosphate scintigraphy appears to be a sensitive and reliable tool for diagnosing muscle necrosis. This test can be performed in almost any hospital with a nuclear scanner. Increased uptake of this radioactive material identifies muscle damage but does not necessarily predict death. Areas with no uptake are devoid of blood supply and are thus necrotic.

Other problems associated with high-tension electrical burns may be classed as neurologic, cardiovascular, pulmonary, abdominal, and opthalmologic. Neurologic sequelae include unconsciousness (in approximately seventy percent of victims), headaches, and epilepsy. Hemiplegia or quadriplegia may develop immediately or within 2 to 3 days as a result of spinal cord damage. Signs suggestive of amyotropic lateral sclerosis and transverse myelitis can also be seen. Motor deficits are more common than sensory losses. Most experimental animal studies demonstrate that the electrical injury may cause hemorrhage around the myelin sheath, reactive gliosis, and neuronal sheath death. Common cardiovascular complications are sinus tachycardia and ST-T wave changes which may persist for several weeks. Myocardial infarction is uncommon but may occur as late as 36 hours after the electrical injury. A minimum of 3 to 4 days of constant heart monitoring is required. Abdominal complications include necrosis of the gallbladder and damage to segments of bowel. Gallstones have been reported several years after electrical injuries; they most likely result from large amounts of pigment mobilized from damaged muscle. Cataracts are an opthalmic complication when injury near the eye results from voltage higher than 220 v. Cataracts may become apparent from 3 weeks to 2 years following electrical injury.

A major problem of interest to the plastic surgeon is the treatment of severe electrical burns of the extremities. Large blood vessels within the extremity may remain patent, but damage to the intima and media may have occurred, leading to the formation of surface thrombi. Delayed hemorrhage and/or thrombosis can result. Segmental portions of the large vessels may remain patent. Microsurgical replacement of damaged vessel segments in the extremities has been described (29). Small blood vessels show severe vessel wall injury with complete thrombosis and necrosis. Muscle necrosis occurs owing to decreased inflow and direct heat damage from adjacent bone. After a few hours, this causes the interstitial pressure of the involved compartment to rise and exceed the capillary perfusion pressure. Ischemia then develops in the muscles and, after 6 hours, muscle damage is irreversible (28). Compartment pressure may be monitored for minor injuries. Most frequently, immediate fasciotomy and débridement is indicated.

The sequence of increased interstitial pressure, suppressed capillary perfusion pressure, and ischemia can be interrupted by early fasciotomy. Fasciotomy increases blood supply and limits ischemic injury. Most patients with a severe electrical injury to the arm should have fascial decompression of the forearm, hand, and carpal tunnel within the first 4 hours, and no later than the first 6 hours. Dead tissue should be débrided in the area as far as it can be seen. All visible devitalized tissue should be excised, and the débridements repeated at 2-to 3-day intervals until only viable tissue remains. Whether an electrical injury is progressive is still controversial. Robson and colleagues (30) suggest that increased production of arachidonic acid causes vasoactive substances such as thromboxane to be elevated. This, in turn, causes progressive necrosis and explains why the wound may need to be débrided every 2 to 3 days. Amputation of part or all of an upper extremity is not uncommon.

A few words about low-voltage injuries are in order. Most common low-voltage burns are exclusively of the contact type and are localized to the hands and the mouth. Local voltage burns of the hand are small but may be deep, involving blood vessels, tendons, and nerves. Burns of the lips and mouth are low-voltage injuries typical in children from 3 months to 3 years of age, most often in boys 1 to 2 years of age. Most are the result of a child's biting an electrical cord or an infant's sucking an electrical cord socket. The electrical injury thus sustained is believed to be a combination of a flash burn and a contact burn. The commissures are the most frequently damaged sites of entrance (in about 50% of children with electrical injuries). The injury is local and usually not accompanied by systemic side effects. Significant perioral edema occurs during the 1st week. In the 2nd and 3rd weeks after an oral electrical burn, tissue slough occurs. During this period, 20% of such patients bleed from the labial artery; parents must be warned of the possibility and instructed to apply firm digital pressure to control any hemorrhage that occurs. Most physicians now believe that a conservative surgical approach is indicated and that reconstructive surgical procedures should be delayed until the eschar has separated and the scar has softened and remodeled over 6 months or longer. Most advocate the use of intraoral prostheses that may later reduce the possibility of microstomia or labial alveolar adhesions (31). Splinting should be maintained for as long as 6 months.

Bibliography

1. Curreri PW, Asch MJ, Pruitt BA. The treatment of chemical burns: specialized diagnostic, therapeutic, and prognostic considerations. *J Trauma* 1970; 10:634.
2. Lee RC, Cravallio EG, Burke JF. Electrical trauma. New York: Cambridge University Press, 1992; 33.
3. Orcutt TJ, Pruitt BA. Chemical injuries of the upper extremity. *Major Probl Clin Surg* 1976; 19:84.
4. Artz CP, Moncrief JA. Chemical burns. In: Artz CP, Moncrief JA, ed. *The treatment of burns*. 2nd ed. Philadelphia: WB Saunders, 1969; 214.
5. Bromberg BE, Song IC, Walden RH. Hydrotherapy of chemical burns. *Plast Reconstr Surg* 1965; 35:85.
6. Iverson RE, Laub DR, Madison MS. Hydrofluoric acid burns. *Plast Reconstr Surg* 1971; 48:107.
7. Klauder JV, Shelanski L, Gabriel K. Industrial uses of compounds of fluorine and oxalic acid. Cutaneous reaction and calcium therapy. *Arch Indus Health* 1955; 12:412.
8. Blunt CP. Treatment of hydrofluoric acid skin burns by injection with calcium gluconate. *Indus Med Surg* 1964; 33:869.
9. Kleinert HE, Bronson JL. Hydrofluoric acid burns of the hand. *Medical Times* 1976; 104:75.
10. Shewmake SW, Anderson BG. Hydrofluoric acid burns. A report of a case and review of the literature. *Arch Dermatol* 1979; 115:593.
11. Reinhardt CF, Hume WG, Linch AL, et al. Hydrofluoric acid burn treatment. *J Chem Education* 1969; 46:A171.
12. Chick L, Borah G. Calcium carbonate gel therapy for hydrofluoric acid burns of the hand. *Plast Reconstr Surg* 1990; 86:935–940.
13. Ben-Hur N, Giladi A, Neuman Z, et al. Phosphorus burns—a pathophysiological study. *Br J Plast Surg* 1972; 25:238.
14. Treviño MA, Herrmann GH, Sprout WL. Treatment of severe hydrofluoric acid exposures. *J Occup Med* 1983; 25:861.
15. Dibbell DG, Iverson RE, Jones W, et al. Hydrofluoric acid burns of the hand. *J Bone Joint Surg* 1970; 52-A:931.
16. Division of Industrial Hygiene, National Institute of Health. Hydrofluoric acid burns. *Indus Med* 1943; 12:634.
17. Vance MV, Curry SC, Kunkel DB, et al. Digital hydrofluoric acid burns: treatment with intraarterial calcium infusion. *Ann Emer Med* 1986; 15:890.
18. Wolfort FG, DeMeester T, Knorr N, et al. Surgical management of cutaneous lye burns. *Surg Gynecol Obstet* 1970; 131:873.
19. Ben-Hur N, Giladi A, Applebaum J, et al. Phosphorus burns. The antidote: a new approach. *Br J Plast Surg* 1972; 25:245.
20. Davidson EC. The treatment of acid and alkali burns. An experimental study. *Ann Surg* 1927; 85:481.
21. Konjoyan TR. White phosphorus burns: case report and literature review. *Military Med* 1983; 148:881.
22. Summerlin WT, Walder AI, Moncrief JA. White phosphorus burns and massive hemolysis. *J Trauma* 1967; 7:476.
23. Bowen TE, Whelan TJ Jr, Nelson TG. Sudden death after phosphorus burns: experimental observations of hypocalcemia, hyperphosphatemia and electrocardiographic abnormalities following production of a standard white phosphorus burn. *Ann Surg* 1971; 174:779.
24. Skoog T. Electrical injuries. *J Trauma* 1970; 10:816.
25. Nichter LS, Bryant CA, Kenney JG, et al: Injuries due to commercial electric current. *J Burn Care Rehab* 1984; 5:124.
26. Langworthy OR. Necrosis of the spinal cord produced by electrical injuries. *Bul Johns Hopkins Hosp* 1932; 51:210.
27. Peterson RA, Gibney J. Electrical burns. In: Grabb WC, Smith JW, eds. *Plastic surgery*. 3rd ed. Boston: Little, Brown, 1979; 489–496.
28. Baxter CR. Present concepts in the management of major electrical injury. *Surg Clin North Am* 1970; 50:1401.
29. Xue-wei W, Yong hua S, Nai-ze W, et al. Early reconstructing blood circulation of wrist to prevent upper extremity necrosis after electrical injuries with the wrist as the injury center: a new surgical consideration. *Proc Am Burn Assoc* 1984; 16:47.
30. Robson MC, Murphy RC, Heggers JP. A new explanation for the progressive tissue loss in electrical injuries. *Plast Reconstr Surg* 1984; 73:431.
31. Colcleugh RG, Ryan JE. Splinting electrical burns of the mouth in 35 children. *Plast Reconstr Surg* 1976; 58:239.

THREE

Head and Neck

24

Embryology of the Head and Neck

Ellen Beatty, M.D.

In the 4th to the 8th weeks of fetal development the normalcy of the embryo's face and pharynx is determined by the timing and completeness of cell growth and migration. During the 4th week of embryonic development the human face and pharynx begin forming with closure of the anterior neuropore. This is the time that the ectodermal cells, known as the neural crest cells and located adjacent to the neural plate, will migrate peripherally. These neural crest cells are fully responsible for facial, muscular, and skeletal elements, in contrast to their lesser role in other areas (1,2). This chapter summarizes the development of the head and neck.

The brachial arches are the basic structures from which the face and pharynx develop. They can be recognized in an embryo at the 10-somite stage. They form in pairs flanking the stomodeum and pharynx (Fig. 24–1). The first and largest arch is known as the mandibular arch. This arch has a small superior portion that contributes to the maxilla and a larger inferior portion that will contribute to the mandible, malleus, and incus. The second, and only other named, arch is the hyoid arch. Its contribution is to the body of the hyoid, the stapes, and adjacent neck structures. The remaining arches are smaller, and the 5th and 6th arches are rudimentary. The hyoid arch will actually grow caudally over the 3rd and 4th arches, creating a temporary cervical sinus. Rarely, a persistence of this sinus communicates with the second pharyngeal pouch, providing a fistula that will track between the internal and external carotid to drain in the skin at the anterior border of the sternocleidomastoid (Fig. 24–2) (3).

These arches have a common structure (Fig. 24–3). Each arch is composed of internal and external walls of endoderm and ectoderm, respectively. The center of each arch is filled with mesoderm. At the time of migration, neural crest cells go from a compact collection to dispersed isolated cells when they arrive in the branchial arches. They travel between ectoderm and mesoderm initially and then proceed throughout the mesoderm, with the exception of the central mesodermal core, which they go around (2). The other components of the mesoderm of each arch include an artery, a nerve, a cartilaginous bar, somitic mesoderm for muscle formation, and a cranial nerve. The arches appear as definite ridges along the future neck early in the 4th week of embryonic development. By the end of the 4th week, there are four distinct arches and two rudimentary arches that make little future contribution.

Externally each arch is bounded by a groove, which eventually smoothes out to yield a normal neck contour. The internal surface of each arch is bounded by a pharyngeal pouch (Fig. 24–4). Each pouch follows an arch, making four

pouches and a last rudimentary pouch after the small final arch. The pouches provide recesses for vital pharyngeal structures (Fig. 24–5). The first pouch lengthens and includes the middle ear ossicles. The long channel will be known as the Eustachian tube. The distal end of the pouch will contribute to the tympanic membrane as it grows to meet the first branchial groove, which is concurrently forming the external auditory canal. The second pharyngeal pouch becomes the tonsillar fossa. Its endoderm will proliferate to cover the lymphoid tissue of the tonsil, which forms in the 5th month of development (4). The third pouch has elongated and lost its opening into the pharynx. The dorsal portion of this pouch will proliferate into the inferior parathyroid as the ventral pouch is obliterated by expanding thymic tissue forming there. The tissue of this pouch migrates caudally, and the inferior parathyroids will join the posterior thyroid while the thymus continues into the mediastinum. The 4th pharyngeal pouch allows the formation of the superior parathyroids. These glands also migrate caudally to a position on the posterior thyroid surface at a level above the 3rd pouch derivatives. The ventral portion of this 4th pouch will develop into the ultimobranchial bodies, which will join to the forming thyroid to provide the parafollicular cells of this gland (3). The 5th pouch coalesces with the 4th or disappears. Although the thyroid is not derived from a pharyngeal pouch, it does form in the 3rd week of development as a diverticulum in the pharyngeal floor (Fig. 24–6). These endodermal cells proliferate and migrate as the neck and pharynx mature and straighten to their usual position anterior to the trachea. The site of the early thyroid diverticulum will become the foramen cecum. Incomplete migration of any of these glandular cells formed in the pharyngeal pouches or diverticula will result in ectopic tissue located in the usual path of migration. In the case of the thyroid, the thyroglossal duct may remain patent with a trail of thyroid leading to the isthmus.

The cartilaginous bars in the branchial arches differentiate into the initial cartilages of the head and neck (Fig. 24–7). The dorsal portion of the 1st bar will ossify and become the malleus and incus. The ventral portion of the 1st bar is known as Meckel cartilage and will form the mandible by intramembranous ossification. The dorsal portion of the second bar will become known as Reichart cartilage and will ossify to form the stapes and styloid process. The lesser cornu and upper part of the hyoid body are formed from the ventral portion of the 2nd bar. The 3rd cartilaginous bar contributes its ventral portion, which ossifies to the greater cornu and lower body of the hyoid. A fusion of the ventral portions of the 4th

215

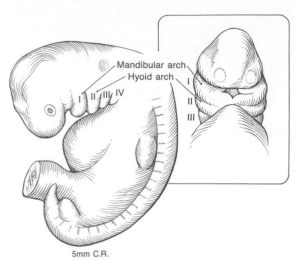

FIG. 24–1. Branchial arch differentiation in the early embryo. CR, crown-rump length. (Redrawn from embryo 6502 in the Carnegie Collection.)

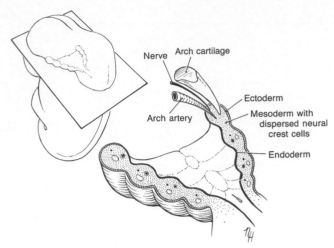

FIG. 24–3. Branchial arch structure in cross section.

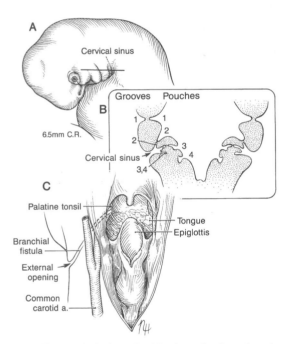

FIG. 24–2. The cervical sinus. **A,** side view of a 4-week embryo depicts location of cervical sinus. **B,** cross section of an embryo demonstrates overgrowth of the 3rd and 4th arches by hyoid arch. **C,** longitudinal section of neck shows persistent cervical sinus tracking between the internal and external carotid.

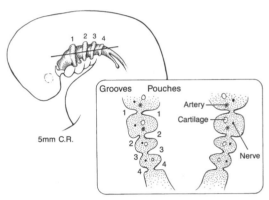

FIG. 24–4. Branchial pouches in 4-week embryo. (Modified from Patten BM, Ductless glands and pharyngeal derivatives. In: *Human embryology,* 3rd ed. New York: McGraw-Hill, 1968; 432.)

and 6th bars forms the laryngeal cartilages, except for the epiglottis. The epiglottis forms from mesenchyme derived from the 3rd and 4th branchial arches (3).

The branchial arches are each supplied by a cranial nerve (Table 24–1). The nerve to the 1st arch is the trigeminal, whose branches innervate the facial skin. The maxillary and mandibular branches supply the teeth, the mucous membranes of the oral and nasal cavities, and the tongue. The 2nd

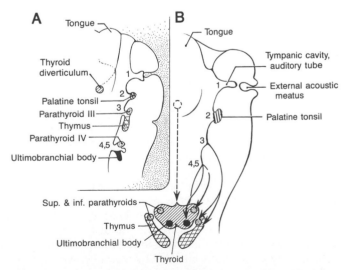

FIG. 24–5. Derivatives of the pharyngeal pouches. **A,** cross section. **B,** frontal view. (Modified from Moore KL, *The developing human.* Philadelphia: WB Saunders, 1977; 163.)

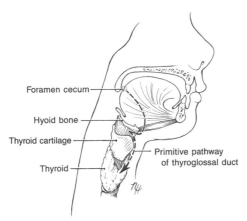

FIG. 24–6. The development of the thyroid involves migration of these endodermal cells from their origin in the foramen cecum to their destination in the neck.

arch is supplied by the facial nerve, which supplies the facial expression muscles. The glossopharyngeal nerve supplies the 3rd branchial arch. The 4th arch is supplied by the superior laryngeal branch of the vagus, and the recurrent laryngeal branch supplies the rudimentary 5th and 6th arches.

The musculature of the face and neck are derived from the somitic cells of the branchial arches' mesodermal core (see Table 24–1). The 1st arch will contribute the muscles of mastication, which include the temporalis, masseter, and medial and lateral pterygoids, along with the mylohyoid, anterior belly of the digastric, and the tensors veli palatini and tympani. The 2nd arch supplies the muscle cells for the facial expression muscles (orbicularis oris and oculi, frontalis, platysma, auricularis, and buccinator), the posterior belly of the digastric, stapedius, and stylohyoid. The sole muscle originating from the 3rd arch is the stylopharyngeus. The pharyngeal and laryngeal muscles are derivatives of the 4th and 6th arches.

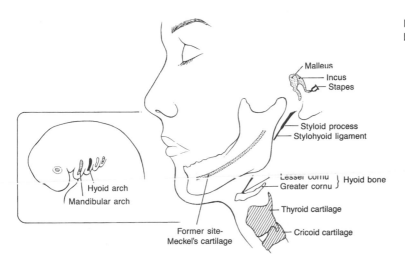

FIG. 24–7. Derivation of the cartilaginous component of the branchial arches.

Table 24–1
Derivatives of the Branchial Arches

Arch	Nerve	Muscles	Skeleton
First	Trigeminal (V)	Muscles of mastication Mylohyoid and anterior belly of digastric Tensor tympani Tensor veli palatine	Malleus Incus
Second	Facial (VII)	Muscles of facial expression Stapedius Stylohyoid Posterior belly of digastric	Stapes Styloid process Lesser cornu of hyoid Upper part of body of the hyoid bone
Third	Glossopharyngeal (IX)	Stylopharyngeus	Greater cornu of hyoid Lower part of body of the hyoid bone
Fourth and sixth	Superior laryngeal branch of vagus and recurrent laryngeal branch of vagus, respectively (X)	Pharyngeal and laryngeal	Laryngeal cartilages

Formation of the face begins in the 3rd week of development with the genesis of the brachial arches and growth of the frontonasal prominence (Fig. 24–8). Kissel and colleagues (1) described a streaming of neural crest cells into the mesoderm of the early facial and frontonasal prominences and laterally into the 1st and 2nd branchial arches, which will become the maxilla and mandible. These neural crest cells are believed to be responsible for the fusion of the facial prominences. The frontonasal prominence will contribute the philtrum and primary palate (Fig. 24–9) when it fuses with the maxillary prominences in the 6th to 7th weeks of development. The maxillary prominences are responsible for the lateral upper lip and maxilla and the secondary palate. The palate forms from two lateral palatine shelves that initially lie in a vertical plane adjacent to the tongue (Fig. 24–10). With differential growth of the face, the shelves are normally able to grow to the horizontal plane, allowing fusion of the shelves in the midline to form the secondary palate and fusion with the triangular primary palate anteriorly. The nasal septum will form from the fusing of the medial nasal prominences and grow downward to join the fused palatal shelves. This growth and fusion process should be complete by the 12th week of development.

While the facial prominences are developing, the remainder of the sense organs also form. The external auditory canal forms from the first branchial groove. The 1st and 2nd arches provide the mesoderm to form the auricle (Fig. 24–11). The 2nd arch contributes the major portion of the auricle, and the innervation will come from branches of the cervical plexus (3). The ear forms in the area of the branchial arches and grooves, but differential growth of the head will allow the auricle to move gradually from the neck to the level of the eye.

The eyes begin development in the 3rd week as grooves over optic vesicles from the forebrain. The retina, neurovascular bundle, and lens develop before the formation of eyelids in the late embryonic period. The lids form from ectodermal folds that grow and will fuse until the 6th month of fetal development (3).

This summary of normal head and neck development provides a basis for understanding the consequences of failed or incomplete formation. The clefts, pits, tags, sinuses, cysts, and asymmetries should be thought of in these terms before we attempt correction, in order to avoid overlooking a more serious, related anomaly.

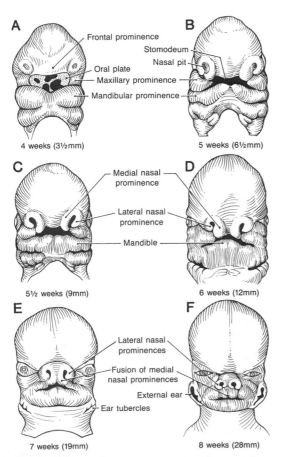

FIG. 24–8. Formation of facial features. (Modified from Patten BM. In Schaeffer JP, ed. *Morris' human anatomy,* 10th ed. Philadelphia: McGraw-Hill, Blakiston Division, 1942; 27.)

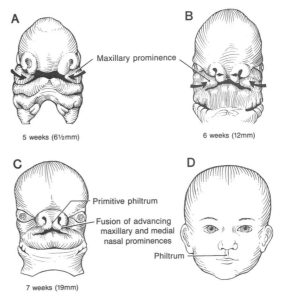

FIG. 24–9. Fusion of the facial prominences. (Modified from Patten BM. In Schaeffer JP, ed. *Morris' human anatomy,* 10th ed. Philadelphia: McGraw-Hill, Blakiston Division, 1942; 27.)

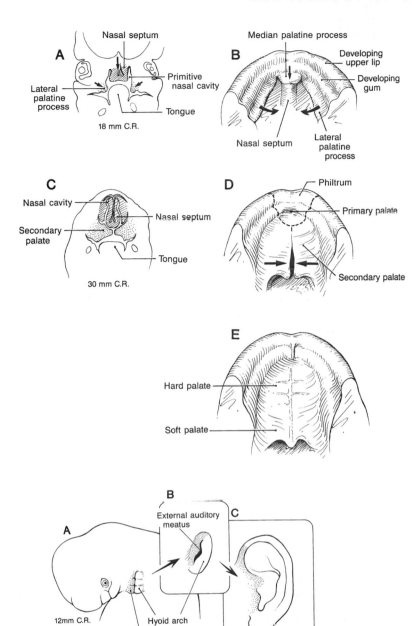

FIG. 24–10. The primary and secondary palate form by fusion of lateral palatine shelves with the median palatine process. (Modified from Moore KL, The brachial apparatus. In: *The developing human,* 2nd ed. Philadelphia: WB Saunders, 1977; 173.)

FIG. 24–11. The differentiation of the first and second branchial arches for the formation of the ear. (After Streeter GL, Development of the auricle in the human embryo. *Carnegie Contrib Embryol* 1922; 14:111.)

Bibliography

1. Kissel P, André JM, Jacquier A. *The neurocristopathies.* New York: Masson, 1981.
2. Moore KL. *The developing human.* Philadelphia: WB Saunders, 1977.
3. Slavkin HD. *Developmental craniofacial biology.* Philadelphia: Lea & Febiger, 1979.
4. Johnson MG, Sulik KK. Embryology of the head and neck. In: Serafin D, Georgiade NG, eds. *Pediatric plastic surgery.* St. Louis: CV Mosby, 1984; 184.

25

Unilateral Cleft Lip

Don LaRossa, M.D., F.A.C.S., F.A.A.P., and Peter Randall, M.D., F.A.C.S.

Cleft lip and cleft palate are the second most frequently occurring of the major congenital anomalies (1:750 to 1:1,000 live births), club foot being the most common. Racial and ethnic variations exist, with clefting occurring more commonly in Asians (1:1000) and less frequently in African-Americans (1:500), while whites are intermediate in occurrence (1:750) (1,2). Embryologically, clefts of the lip result from a failure of mesenchymal penetration and fusion of the nasofrontal and lateral facial processes of the developing face at 4 to 7 weeks of gestation. (3). The condition is expressed in those structures anterior to the incisive foramen: the prepalatal alveolus, maxilla, lip, and nasal structures, sometimes up to and including the lacrimal ducts. The degree of expression varies considerably: from the typical wide, gaping cleft of the alveolus and lip structures straddled by a stretched and flattened ala, to a mere "scar" of the minimal incomplete cleft (forme fruste) with the lip almost "healed by nature" to near normalcy. An absolute deficiency is seen in all tissues involved in the cleft: skin, muscles, mucous membranes, maxillary and nasal bones, and nasal cartilages. The quantitative differences vary with the severity of the cleft. It is up to the surgeon to evaluate how much tissue remains and to rearrange and augment the remnants to create near normal–appearing lip, nose, and alveolodental structures.

The term *cleft lip* often fails to describe fully the extent of the deformity. A more appropriate term might be "prepalatal cleft," or even "cleft lip, nose and maxillary complex," because the nose and alveolus are integral parts of the anomaly (4). Likewise, the maxilla should be included in the definition because the bony infrastructure of the cleft has a great impact on the appearance of the external soft tissues. Maxillary orthopedics and orthodontics, with or without bone grafting of the alveolar cleft, play an integral part in successful management of the cleft-lip patient, thus they are covered in later sections.

Fortunately, many anatomic landmarks and "clues" remain in the cleft structures to aid in the repair. Each lip cleft has unique features and is different from every other cleft, yet there are similarites that allow us to repair them using general types of surgical techniques (e.g., triangular flap, quadrangular flap, rotation advancement). Each lip cleft retains some anatomic features that can be incorporated into the repair, and each lends itself to repair by one of these general techniques or a variation of them. Just as there is no single approach to a rhinoplasty, but a spectrum of techniques and principles applied to each unique nose, so the cleft surgeon must be able to devise a procedure to address the specific requirements of each unique lip cleft. This begins with a careful assessment of the lip and an analysis of what it would take to duplicate the features of the normal side from the remnants on the cleft side.

Cardoso drew our attention to the existance of the Cupid's bow and led surgeons to preserve it in lip repair; formerly it was discarded, which resulted in a lip that was too tight. Millard offered us a repair design that placed incisions along the anatomic boundary of the philtral column. Mohler described a modification that permitted flexibility in duplicating the shape of the philtrum when it was more rectangular than shield-shaped (5–10). Others have offered their refinements of the skin repair to further enhance the results.

Fara (11) delineated the abnormal architecture of the orbicularis oris muscle in the cleft diverting the focus to lip function. Nicolau, Delaire, and others have further refined our understanding of the fine anatomy of the cleft and normal lip musculature, describing its deep and superficial components (12,13). Latham beautifully demonstrated the anatomic details of the philtral columns, describing the long and short fibers that criss-cross to create the complex anatomy of the philtrum (14). Schendel further described the histochemical abnormalities in the muscle at the cleft site, pointing out abnormalities in the mitochondria that seem to revert to normal following lip repair (15). Thus, muscle repair was incorporated into cleft lip surgery by Randall and colleagues, and others (16,17).

A cleft lip can be repaired at any time after birth in an otherwise healthy infant. Most surgeons adhere to the three pediatric surgical dictums of 10 weeks of age, 10 pounds in weight, and 10 grams of hemoglobin. General anesthesia is used because it allows the surgeon to work in a precise fashion. An uncuffed oral Rae tube (Rae preformed tracheal tube; NCC Division, Mallinckrodt Inc., Argyle, NY) is used. Care must be taken to tape it precisely in the midline, with the tape kept inferior to the commissures to minimize distortion of the lips.

The head and face remain accessible to the surgeon. Marking is conveniently done with methylene blue dye and a straight pen. Key points are tattooed into the skin with the pen point or a hypodermic needle to finalize the operative plan before injection with vasoconstrictive agents. Epinephrine 1:100,000 or 1:200,000 should be injected locally to reduce bleeding and to facilitate the accuracy of the repair. Commercial preparations of epinephrine mixed with 1% or 0.5% lidocaine provide the most convenient way to use these agents. Care is necessary because of the toxic effects of both drugs. The maximum dose of lidocaine is 7 mg/kg. Seven minutes, by the clock, are required for the full vasoconstrictive effect.

Anatomy of Repair

The markings begin with a careful and accurate identification of the normal and abnormal landmarks in the cleft lip (Fig. 25–1). The key points to identify are:

Point 1: The midline point of the arch of Cupid's bow.
Point 2: The peak of Cupid's bow on the non-cleft side.
Point 3: The proposed peak of Cupid's bow on the cleft side (distance from 1 to 2).
Point 4: The midline of the columella.
Points 5&6: The base of the columella laterally on the cleft side and noncleft sides.
Points 7&8: The points at which the alar bases insert into the nostril sill.
Point 9: A point on the vermilion-cutaneous roll that is in the same horizontal plane with the peak of cupid's bow on the noncleft side.

The difference in distance from the base of the columella to the peak of Cupid's bow on the cleft (3) and noncleft (2) side—measured in millimeters—is the lengthening that must be achieved to produce symmetry.

Techniques of Repair

Pool (18) noted that it is not the width of the cleft but the vertical height discrepancy between the cleft and noncleft sides that determines the difficulty of the repair. The surgeon must bring into balance the peak of Cupid's bow on the cleft and noncleft sides. The surgical principle involved in correcting the cleft lip defect is to lengthen the medial side of the cleft, so that it equals the vertical dimensions of the noncleft side. A tissue rearrangement is designed to borrow tissue from the lateral element of the cleft, where there is usually available tissue, and introduce it into the medial element, where tissue is deficient. Modern techniques of lip repair lengthen the medial side of the cleft by opening incisions in the medial lip element into which flaps from the lateral side of the cleft are introduced. The most commonly used flap designs can be broadly categorized as triangular, quadrangular, or rotation advancement types (19–22,8,9). The Rose-Thompson technique can be used in very minor or forme fruste clefts where very little height discrepancy exists (23,24). The success of the repair depends largely on the skill of the surgeon in assessing the abnormal anatomy, identifying remaining anatomic details and landmarks, and using these key points to recreate the missing or displaced lip structures.

TRIANGULAR FLAP TECHNIQUE (TENNISON-RANDALL)

Originally described by Tennison (20), the geometry of this technique was explained by Randall (22). It permits the surgeon relatively inexperienced with cleft lip to obtain reproducible results. Lips repaired by this method are sometimes slightly long on the cleft side. If this occurs, secondary revisions can be achieved by selective excisions in the horizontal limb of the triangular flap (Fig. 25–2). If recognized at the time of surgery, a small amount of tissue can be removed either from the triangular flap or from the tissue just above it on the medial side.

ROTATION ADVANCEMENT TECHNIQUE

Millard

Described as a "cut as you go" technique by Millard (8,9), this method places most of the scar in a more anatomically correct position along the philtral column (Fig. 25–3). It is not as easy as the triangular flap method for the beginner to

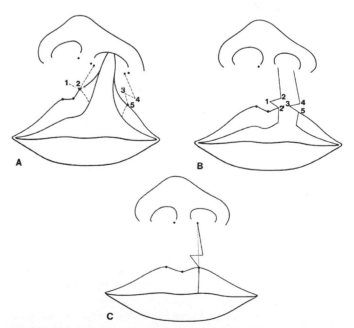

FIG. 25–2. Triangular flap technique. The medial lip element is lengthened by a back-cut (**1-2**) and a triangular flap (**3-5**) on the lateral lip element is introduced into it. The lengthening achieved is a little less than the base of the triangular flap (**4-5**) for practical purposes.

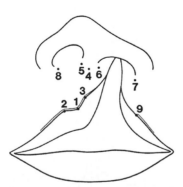

FIG. 25–1. Anatomy of the normal and unrepaired unilateral cleft lip indicating key points used for planning repair: **1,** lowest point in arch of Cupid's bow, midline of the lip; **2,** peak of Cupid's bow on the noncleft side; **3,** proposed peak of Cupid's bow; **4,** midpoint of the columella; **5, 6,** base of columella laterally; **7, 8,** inset of alar base into nostril sill; **9,** a point on the well developed vermilion cutaneous roll of the lateral lip and the same horizontal plane as the peak of Cupid's bow on the noncleft side.

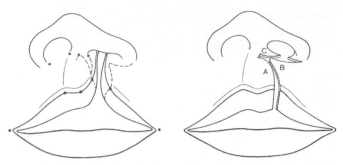

FIG. 25–3. Technique of rotation advancement. **A,** the flap on the medial lip element rotates downward to achieve the necessary lengthening. **B,** the flap from the lateral lip element advances into the defect. **C,** a small pennant-shaped medial flap can be used as needed to restore the nostril sill or to lengthen the columella. A backcut into the superior part of the philtral column on the noncleft side is often needed.

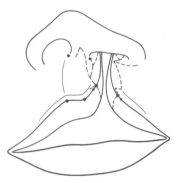

FIG. 25–4. Mohler repair. The incision for the rotation flap extends into the base of the columella. This method can be used when there is a rectangular shape to the philtrum.

master. Insufficient lengthening is sometimes a problem in the cleft lip, with a marked discrepancy in height between the cleft and noncleft sides. A small Z-plasty just above the white roll can be added at the time of the primary repair, or as a secondary procedure.

Mohler

Mohler pointed out that there is a variation in philtral shape in individuals he studied. He found three types: shield-shaped, low shield-shaped, and rectanglar-shaped philtrums. Based on this, and in an attempt to imitate more accurately the philtral anatomy in those infants who had a rectangular-shaped philtrum, he modified the rotation flap to extend into the base of the columella (10) (Fig. 25–4).

Helpful Details

1. Use the normal side as a guide to planning incisions on the cleft side. Draw on the normal side where the incision lines would lie in the intact lip and duplicate them on the cleft side using the key points as a guide.
2. Curved lines should be used in designing the advancement and rotation flaps to compensate for the outward pull of the orbicularis muscles. Careful analysis of the position of the philtral column reveals that it curves away from the midline, and the incision line for the rotation flap should be drawn to parallel it. Likewise, in the lateral lip

element, the incision line should curve gently away from the vertical to compensate for the lateral pull of the muscle (see Fig. 25–5A, B).

3. To gain a little extra length in a rotation advancement repair of the cleft with marked discrepancy of vertical height, the medial side of the cleft (point 3 in Fig. 25–1) can be moved 1 mm medially (Fig. 25–6).
4. Point 9 should be level with the Cupid's bow point on the noncleft side (point 2) and where the roll is well developed, rather than where it begins to disappear, in order to maintain the continuity of the roll in the repaired lip. It will also set the proper vertical height on the repaired side. The rotation flap can be adjusted to its dimensions. Conversely, if this dimension is not correct, increasing the amount of rotation of the rotation flap will not help achieve an adequate vertical lengthening. It is akin to the mainsail (rotation flap) adjusting to the mast (advancement flap) in a sailboat.
5. The distance from the commissure to the peak of Cupid's bow on each side need not be equal because of the differences in the tension of the orbicularis muscle in the unrepaired lip, which shortens these distances, making them unreliable for marking the lip.

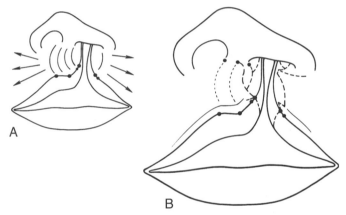

A

B

FIG. 25–5. **A,** in the unrepaired lip the orbicularis oris muscle pulls the philtral column and lip structures away from the cleft into a "family of curves." **B,** these can serve as a guide in the design of the incisions for the lip repair. A small (2-mm) triangular flap incorporating the vermilion cutaneous roll is designed into the lateral lip incision and a 2-mm backcut is incorporated in the medial incision. It is approximately 60° to the vermilion line and lies within the vermilion cutaneous roll.

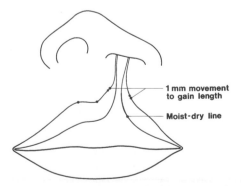

1 mm movement to gain length

Moist-dry line

FIG. 25–6. Double marks where the incisions cross the vermilion cutaneous junction aid in realignment during lip closure.

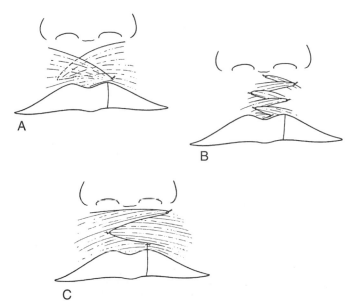

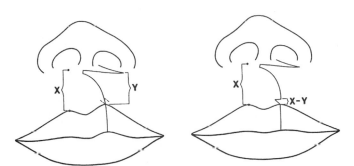

FIG. 25–7. **A,** Original technique is shown for reorientation of displaced or orbicularis oris muscle bundles at the time of primary lip repair. **B,** Division of the muscle bundle into three tails, which are interdigitated. The uppermost bundles are attached to dermis along the philtrum. The inferior two are sutured to each other to minimize tightness at the free border. **C,** Division of the muscle into an upper triangular portion and lower rectangular portion is shown. The triangular portions are interdigitated like a Z-plasty, lengthening the lip. The rectangular portions are sutured end-to-end. We have abandoned technique **A** and are using **B** and **C**.

FIG. 25–8. Most commonly seen after rotation advancement repairs, a Z-plasty can be used to lengthen the short scar. The Z should be introduced just above the vermilion cutaneous junction where it will help improve the profile of the lip in the region of the white roll.

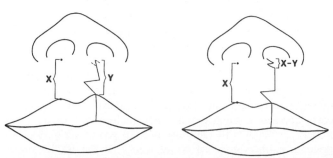

FIG. 25–9. When this deformity follows a triangular flap or quadrangular flap repair, a Z-plasty can be introduced at the upper end of the lip scar, or the triangular flap can be advanced further toward the midline.

6. Double marks can be made at points 2 and 3, leaving a tattoo mark adjacent to the incision to serve as a guide for accurate alignment of the vermilion cutaneous junction at the time of lip closure (see Fig. 25–5A).

7. In a rotation advancement repair, a 2-mm triangular flap from the lateral lip element can be introduced into a 2-mm backcut of the medial lip at the junction of skin and vermilion. This will add vertical height and emphasize the white roll as well as improve the lip profile. The triangular flap is equilateral in dimension and extends from the depression above the roll to the vermilion cutaneous border. The angle of the backcut is designed to place the end-

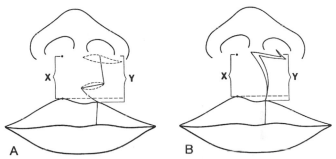

FIG. 25–10. **A,** Most commonly seen in triangular and quadrangular flap repairs, all or most of the repair may have to be redone, or an elliptical segment equal to about twice the amount of shortening desired can be excised from the transverse incision along the superior edge. **B,** In the rotation advancement technique, the flaps are recut and the amount of rotation reduced by trimming the lateral flap an appropriate amount.

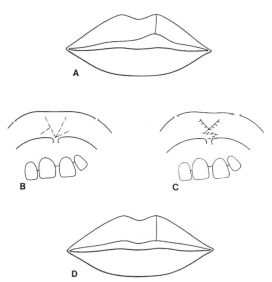

FIG. 25–11. The off-center, elevated vermilion-free border at the site of cleft repair is referred to as the whistling deformity because it simulates the configuration of the upper lip when whistling. In most instances, a V-Y advancement of mucosa can correct the deficiency of tissue. Incorporation of a Z-plasty in the verticle limb of the Y aids in preventing relapse. Care should be taken to include the mucous glands of the lip in the mucosal flaps to prevent the complications of a chronically dry, scaling lip. If a muscle dehiscence is present, it should be closed as well. For more severe defects, composite musculo-mucosal "pendulum flaps" bordering the area of depression can be brought together to restore an even, vermilion-free border (26).

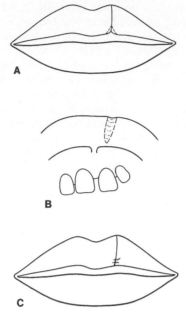

FIG. 25–12. **A–C,** Often an attempt to preserve too much tissue is made at the original operation, utilizing vermilion that does not have full thickness. The segment of excess vermilion may need to be excised to achieve an even, full vermilion.

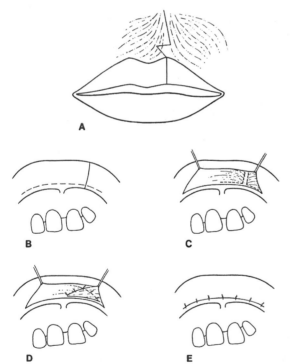

FIG. 25–13. The orbicularis bulge is often a major clue to the presence of a cleft, even in the most elegantly repaired lips. It is caused by the abnormal position and "bunching up" of the orbicularis oris muscle on the cleft side. The muscle can be detached and reoriented in a secondary procedure via a labial sulcus approach. **A,** Abnormal muscle position is shown in a cleft lip repaired without muscle reorientation. **B,** Buccal sulcus incision gives access to the orbicularis oris muscle. **C,** The muscle is detached from mucosa and skin is divided at the repair site. **D,** The muscle is reoriented from a vertical to a horizontal position. **E,** Mucosa is closed.

point in the high point of the vermilion-cutaneous roll (Fig. 25–6B).

8. The point on the lip where the moist and dry vermilion (red-line) meet should be lined up when possible (25; Fig. 25–6B). However, because of the shortened dimensions of the tissues in the medial lip element this may not be possible.

9. The nose and the lip should always be repaired from the inside out. The temptation to close the lip skin to assure that the repair will work should be avoided.

Reconstruction of the Orbicularis Muscle

In describing the anatomy of the orbicularis oris musculature in cleft lips, Fara (11) pointed out that the muscle fibers parallel the margin of the cleft in the vast majority of instances. If the margins of the cleft are pared and closed side to side, as was done in the early repairs of cleft lips, the abnormal attachments and orientation of the muscle persist. The result is a distortion of the motion of many repaired cleft lips during speaking, grimacing, smiling, and whistling. Detaching the muscle from its dermal and mucosal attachments and reorienting it has been advocated by many authors. The results have not been fully evaluated, and the proper method of muscle reconstruction has not fully evolved. Most results are displayed in still photographs, while videos will be needed to give a more accurate depiction of the function of the lip. Current techniques are shown in Figure 25–7.

Revisional Surgery of the Unilateral Cleft Lip

The timing of revisional procedures should be guided by the conspicuousness of the deformity. Once scar maturation has occurred, an accurate assessment of the deformity can be made, and a plan for correction and timing developed. As a general principle, contour and realignment should take precedence over scar, since scars can be camouflaged with cosmetics while contour cannot. Some of the more common defects after primary cleft-lip surgery are illustrated and described in Figures 25–8 through 25–13:

1. Lips that are "too short" (Figs. 25–8 and 25–9).
2. Lips that are "too long" (Fig. 25–10).
3. The "whistling deformity" (Figs. 25–11 and 25–12).
4. The "orbicularis bulge" (Fig. 25–13).

Cleft Effects on Nasal Cartilages and Bone

The cleft lip nasal distortion is a reflection of nasal cartilage and bone deformity and displacement. The reconstruction, therefore, depends on remodeling this infrastructure (Fig. 25–14). The timing of intervention remains controversial. Some repositioning of the distorted tip cartilages can be done at the time of primary lip closure, although it is frequently postponed and treated secondarily. Proponents of early correction suggest that early realignment of malpositioned cartilages will facilitate normal growth (27–29). Opponents express concern about injury to the fragile infant cartilages and subsequent interference with normal growth by surgical scar, making the eventual rhinoplasty more difficult (30–34).

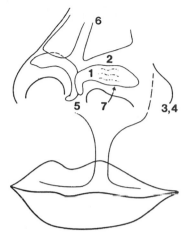

FIG. 25–14. The unilateral cleft lip nasal deformity: **(1)** hypoplastic alar cartilage with depressed dome; **(2)** loss of normal overlap of upper and lower lateral cartilages; **(3)** laterally displaced ala; **(4)** hypoplasia and retrusion of the bony platform at the pyriform aperture; **(5)** deviation of the nasal spine and caudal septum to the noncleft side; **(6)** flattening and displacement of the nasal bones and upper lateral cartilage; **(7)** buckling of the lateral crus of the lower lateral cartilage creating a web in the vestibule.

The deformity, as described by Huffman and Lierle (35) and others (36), consists of a flattened and splayed out alar cartilage, loss of the normal overlapping relationship of upper lateral and alar cartilages, lateral displacement of alar base, nasal septal deviation to the noncleft side, and retrodisplacement of pyriform aperture. After lip repair, a characteristically flattened and displaced nasal tip persists. Further, the alar rim hangs below the normal position, a ridge or fold projects into the nasal vestibule, and the deficient bony platform at the pyriform aperture causes an inward displacement of the alar base.

Principles involved in correction of the cleft lip nasal deformity (see Fig. 25–14) include:

1. Elevation of the medial crus and dome of the alar cartilage to parity, or to a slightly overcorrected position, relative to the noncleft side. Onlay grafts of auricular, septal, or contralateral alar cartilage on the depressed dome can be used.
2. Reestablishment of the overlap of the upper and lower lateral cartilages.
3. Medial repositioning of the laterally displaced alar base by V–Y advancement or Wier excision.
4. Forward advancement of the alar base by augmentation of the bony platform at the pyriform aperture with bone or cartilage grafts or artificial implants.
5. Straightening of the caudal portion of the nasal septum, which is typically deflected away from the cleft side.
6. Osteotomy of the bony pyramid when the dorsum is broad or displaced as a consequence of the cleft (rhinoplasty).
7. Reduction of the internal vestibular ridge or web, often with a Z-plasty in the vestibule.

Cleft-Lip Nasal Deformity

The management of the cleft-lip nasal deformity remains the most difficult, involved, and challenging aspect of cleft-lip surgery. The conservative approach of delaying nasal-tip surgery until more growth has occurred has withstood the test of time, but it is often not accepted by the growing child. Hence, many surgeons now advocate primary nasoplasty at the time of lip repair. Although this does not usually completely correct the problem, it often is successful in reducing the amount of distortion. (see Figs. 25–15 and 25–16) There is sufficient evidence that it does not interfere with nasal growth and it may lessen the burden of deformity in the growing and developing child (27–29).

PRIMARY NASOPLASTY

We have utilized a five-step technique for primary correction of the unilateral cleft-lip nasal deformity (37).

1. Wide undermining of the nasal tip cartilages. The medial and lateral crura of both alar cartilages are widely undermined between cartilage and overlying skin laterally and between medial crura medially through the medial lip incision at the base of the columella; the incision is used to release the attachment of the lateral lip element to the maxilla and to free their skin attachments. An intercartilaginous incision should be avoided because of the risk of nostril stenosis in the growing child.
2. Repositioning of the cleft lower lateral cartilage. The lateral crus dome and medial crus are pulled superiorly over the upper lateral cartilage to restore the normal overlap. The surgeon uses internal through-and-through absorbable mattress sutures along the ridge of overlap of the upper and lower alar cartilages (internal valve) and across the dome as a transfixion suture; alternately, external sutures on bolsters as described by McComb may be used to maintain the new anatomy during healing (27).
3. Alar base flap. A V-shaped flap incorporating the alar base helps to rotate it medially.
4. V–Y advancement flap closure of the nostril floor. This can help create a curved rather than a grooved floor and a narrow constricted nostril can theoretically be widened by moving the flaps apart in a secondary correction.
5. Muscle reconstruction. Muscle repair with attachment of the upper slips of the medial muscle near the alar base to help move it medially. The uppermost slips of the lateral muscle can be attached near the base of the columella, helping to move it medially.

A pennant-shaped mucosal flap of lateral lip vermilion, based in the lateral maxillary segment, can be introduced into the gap that results from release of the floor of the nose from the maxilla. This leaves a permanent fistula that requires secondary closure.

TECHNIQUES FOR SECONDARY CORRECTION

A Berkeley-type incision can be performed in the nasal tip; however, the external tip scar is a detractor and it is therefore rarely used (38).

A number of other surgical exposures and techniques have been proposed to achieve symmetry (39–41). The most useful of these is the open-tip technique, which permits direct visualization and manipulation of the affected lower lateral cartilage. Correction of the deviated caudal end of the nasal septum can also be done through this approach. The transcolumellar incision can be placed at the columellar–lip angle, incorporating the sill flap from a Millard rotation ad-

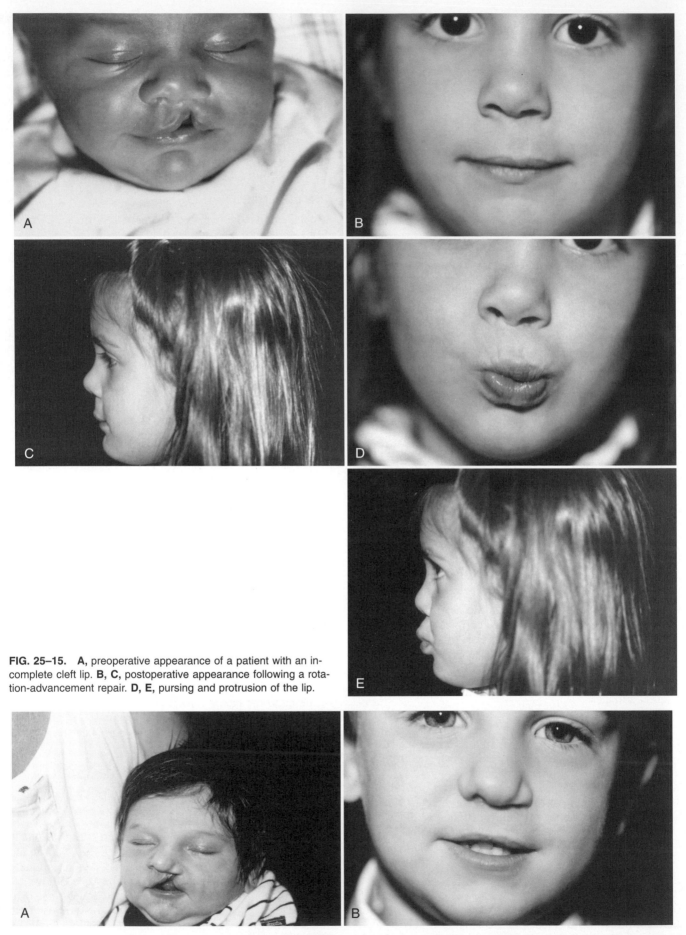

FIG. 25–15. **A,** preoperative appearance of a patient with an incomplete cleft lip. **B, C,** postoperative appearance following a rotation-advancement repair. **D, E,** pursing and protrusion of the lip.

FIG. 25–16. **A,** preoperative appearance of a patient with a complete unilateral cleft lip, exhibiting a rectangular shaped philtrum that lends itself to a Mohler-type repair. **B,** postoperative appearance following a modified Mohler repair.

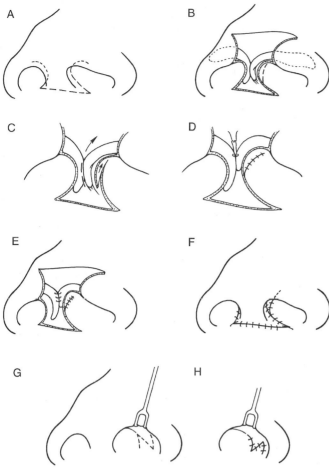

FIG. 25–17. A, incisions for the open-tip approach. The transverse incision can be at the columellar waist or at the base, incorporating the sill flap. **B,** undermining is carried over both alar domes, exposing the disparity between them. Dissection between them gives access to the caudal end of the septum. **C, D, E,** as described by Lewis, a V–Y composite flap of medial crus and adjacent vestibular lining helps to elevate the medial crus and dome (42). **F,** the completed closure. **G, H,** the intranasal web can be corrected with a Z-plasty.

vancement repair for columellar lengthening, although many surgeons prefer an incision at the columellar waist (Fig. 25–17). Lewis has described a V–Y composite advancement flap of the medial crus that is useful in achieving elevation of the dome and the shortened vestibular skin. Ortiz-Monasterio uses a similar flap of lateral crus for the same purpose (42,43) (see Fig. 25–13).

Maxillary Orthopedics and Orthodontics in the Management of Cleft Lip

CLEFT EFFECTS ON MAXILLA

The extent of maxillary clefting is proportional to the severity of the cleft-lip deformity. Clefts of the prepalatal structures can extend to the incisive foramen posteriorly and affect the nasal bones superiorly. Incomplete cleft lips may have minimal bony deficiency. When alveolar bone is involved, the lateral incisor tooth in the area of the cleft is usually malpositioned, malformed, or absent. It may be located

in the medial or lateral segment. The process of lip repair reestablishes the soft tissue and muscular forces on the displaced maxillary segments, forcing them together. Scar from dissection of the hard palate mucoperiosteum during palate repair may exacerbate the collapse. The result is displacement of the alveolus into cross-bite, and depression in the region of the pyriform aperture, maxilla, and zygoma on the cleft side. Marked displacement will result in maxillary collapse and a skeletal class III malocclusion, but this is not often seen in clefts of the lip alone; rather, it is seen with complete clefts of the lip and palate. The goals of management are to maintain or restore the position and bony continuity of the maxillary segments and the health and position of the teeth.

Early management may include presurgical orthopedics or lip adhesion procedures to facilitate the surgical repair of the lip and to restore alignment of the alveolar segments. The principle involves the use of external pressure on the displaced alveolar segments. This can be accomplished by use of a head cap and elastic traction across the lip, a technique more commonly used in complete bilateral clefts. Pool (44) has described the use of tape on the lip skin to bring the medial and lateral lip elements closer together facilitating surgical repair.

Lip adhesion procedures are a physiologic means to this end. Done early in infancy (0 to 3 months of age) under general or local anesthesia, this procedure restores tension across the cleft, helping to mold the maxillary segments, expand the soft tissues of the lip, and convert a complete cleft to an incomplete cleft, thereby facilitating the final repair (45).

The use of traction devices or lip adhesion is often combined with the use of intraoral orthopedic appliances to guide the movement of the maxillary segments into an ideal position. This can be done with a passive appliance as advocated by McNeil (46) and Burston (47), or by active traction as described by Georgiade and Latham (48), and others (49). This approach can facilitate eventual lip and palate closure, or can be used to prepare for early bone grafting.

Although it is still controversial, some proponents of early bone grafting have demonstrated minimal harmful effects from rib grafts inserted into the alveolar cleft only after minimal undermining of the alveolar mucoperiosteum (50,51). When more extensive undermining is done, severe growth disturbances have been described that caused disenchantment with the early bone grafting of alveolar clefts. (52–58). Secondary bone grafting during the period of mixed dentition (between 7 and 10 years of age) is now a well-accepted part of the management of the patient with a significant bone deficit of the alveolus (59,60).

Orthodontic and orthopedic methods are used to realign the teeth and alveolar segments. Rib, iliac cancellous, and cranial bone have been successfully used to replace the missing bone (61–64). The grafts fill the bony defect, stabilize the maxillary segments, and provide bone for the eruption, stabilization, and growth of the adjacent teeth. At the same time, onlay bone grafts can be used to augment the hypoplastic bone of the pyriform aperture, to help restore facial symmetry, and to reposition the alar base on the cleft side.

Nonsurgical methods involve orthodontic repositioning of malpositioned segments, orthodontic repositioning of teeth, and stabilization by fixed or removable bridgework. These appliances, fashioned by a prosthodontist, maintain and complete the functional and cosmetic dental restoration in the cleft patient. Their continued and ultimate success is dependent on maintenance of good dental health, since the stability is dependent on the presence of stable teeth in the maxillary segments.

For a minority of patients with severe problems, orthognathic surgical movement of displaced, hypoplastic, or hyperplastic dentoalveolar elements may be required. In some patients, these techniques provide the only solution to disordered dentoalveolar relationships. In particular, older patients with severe class III malocclusion, open-bite deformity, or prognathism (true or pseudo), will need orthognathic surgery to bring the facial profile into harmony. Such procedures are deferred until facial growth and tooth eruption is complete. It is sometime justified in patients at an earlier age when it can benefit the psychologic well being of the patient. Radiographs for bone age and dental age are helpful in determining when this has occurred. Orthognathic surgery is rarely needed in patients with cleft lip only.

It is clear from the foregoing that expertise from orthodontic and prosthodontic cleft-palate team members is essential throughout the entire treatment period in patients with clefts involving the maxilla.

References

1. Ivy RH. Modern concept of cleft lip and cleft palate management. *Plast Reconstr Surg* 1952; 9:121.
2. Fogh-Anderson P. *Inheritance of harelip and cleft palate.* Copenhagen: Ejuar Munksgaard Forlag, 1943.
3. Stark RB. The pathogenesis of harelip and cleft palate. *Plast Reconstr Surg* 1954; 13:20.
4. Stark RB. Embryology, pathogenesis and classification of cleft lip and cleft palate. In: Pruzansky S, ed. *Congenital anomalies of the face and associated structures.* Springfield, IL: Charles C Thomas, 1961.
5. Cardoso AD. A new technique for harelip. *Plast Reconstr Surg* 1952; 10:92.
6. Blair VP, Brown JB. Mirault operation for single harelip. *Surg Gynecol Obstet* 1930; 51:81.
7. Brown JB, McDowell F. Surgical repair of cleft lips. *Arch Surg* 1948; 56:750.
8. Millard DR. A primary camouflage of the unilateral harelip. In: *Transactions of the International Society of Plastic Surgeons,* First Congress, 1955. Baltimore: Williams & Wilkins, 1957; 160.
9. Millard DR Jr. Cleft craft: the evolution of its surgery. In: *The unilateral deformity.* Vol. 1. Boston: Little, Brown, 1976.
10. Mohler LR. Unilateral cleft lip repair. *Plast Reconstr Surg* 1987; 80:511.
11. Fara M. The importance of folding down muscle stumps in the operation of unilateral clefts of the lip. *Acta Chir Plast (Praha)* 1971; 13:162.
12. Delaire J, Fève JR, Chateau JP, et al. Anatomie et physiologie des muscles et du frein médian de la lèure supérieure. *Rev Stomatol Chir Maxillofac* 1977; 78:821.
13. Nicolau JP. The orbicularis muscle: a functional approach to its repair in the cleft lip. *Br J Plast Surg* 1983; 36:141.
14. Latham RA, Deaton TG. The structural basis of the philtrum and the contour of the vermilion border: a study of the musculature of the upper lip. *J Anat* 1976; 121:151.
15. Schendel SA, Pearl RM, DeArmond SJ. Pathophysiology of cleft lip muscles following the initial surgical repair. *Plast Reconstr Surg* 1991; 88:197.
16. Randall P, Whitaker LA, LaRossa, D. The importance of muscle reconstruction in primary and secondary cleft lip repair. *Plast Reconstr Surg* 1974; 54:316.
17. Kernahan DA, Bauer BS. Functional cleft lip repair: a sequential layered closure with orbicularis muscle realignment. *Plast Reconstr Surg* 1983; 72:459.
18. Pool R Jr. Analysis of the anatomy and geometry of the unilateral cleft lip. *Plast Reconstr Surg* 1959; 24:311.
19. LeMesurier AB. A method of cutting and suturing the lip in the treatment of complete unilateral clefts. *Plast Reconstr Surg* 1949; 4:1.
20. Tennison CW. The repair of the unilateral cleft lip by the stencil method. *Plast Reconstr Surg* 1952; 9:115.
21. Marcks KM, Travaskis AE, daCosta A. Further observations in cleft lip repair. *Plast Reconstr Surg* 1953; 12:392.
22. Randall P. A triangular flap operation for the primary repair of unilateral clefts of the lip. *Plast Reconstr Surg* 1951; 23:331.
23. Rose W. *Harelip and cleft palate.* London: HK Lewis, 1976.
24. Thompson JE. An artisitic and mathematically accurate method of repairing the defect in cases of harelip. *Surg Gynecol Obstet* 1912; 14:498.
25. Noordhoff MS. Reconstruction of vermilion in unilateral and bilateral cleft lips. *Plast Reconstr Surg* 1984; 73:52.
26. Kapetansky DI. Double pendulum flaps for whistling deformities in bilateral cleft lips. *Plast Reconstr Surg* 1971; 47:321.
27. McComb H. Primary correction of unilateral cleft lip nasal deformity. A 10-year review. *Plast Reconstr Surg* 1985; 75:791.
28. Salyer KF. Primary correction of the unilateral cleft lip nose: a 15-year experience. *Plast Reconstr Surg* 1986; 77:558.
29. Anderl H. Simultaneous repair of lip and nose in the unilateral cleft (a long-term report). In: Jackson IT, Sommerland B, eds. *Recent advances in plastic surgery.* Edinburgh: Churchill Livingstone, 1985; 1
30. Brown JB, McDowell F. Secondary repair of cleft lips and their nasal deformities. *Ann Surg* 1941; 114:101.
31. Peet EW, McDowell F. Secondary repair of cleft lips and their nasal deformities. *Ann Surg* 1941; 114:101.
32. Marcks KM, Travaskis AE, Berg EM, et al. Nasal defects associated with cleft lip nasal deformity. *Plast Reconstr Surg* 1964; 34:176.
33. Matthews D. The nose tip. *Br J Plast Surg* 1968; 21:153.
34. McIndoe AH. Correction of the alar deformity in cleft lip. *Lancet* 1938; 1:607.
35. Huffman WC, Leirle DM. Studies in the pathologic anatomy of the unilateral harelip nose. *Plast Reconstr Surg* 1949; 4:225.
36. Berkeley WT. The cleft lip nose. *Plast Reconstr Surg* 1959; 23:576.
37. LaRossa D, Donath G. Primary nasoplasty in unilateral and bilateral cleft lip nasal deformity. *Clin Plast Surg* 1993; 20:781.
38. Berkeley WT. Correction of secondary cleft-lip nasal deformities. *Plast Reconstr Surg* 1969; 44:234.
39. Millard DR. The unilateral cleft lip nose. *Plast Reconstr Surg* 1964; 34:169.
40. Rethi A. Reaccourissement dir nez trop long. *Rev Chir Plast* 1934; 2:85.
41. Anderl, H. Simultaneous repair of lip and nose in the unilateral cleft (a long-term report). In: Jackson IT, Sommerland B, eds. *Recent advances in plastic surgery.* Edinburgh: Churchill Livingstone, 1985; 1.
42. Lewis M. Personal communication.
43. Ortiz-Monasterio F. Personal communiation.
44. Pool R, Farnworth TK. Peroperative lip taping in the cleft lip. *Ann Plast Surg* 1994; 32:3, 243.
45. Randall P. A lip adhesion operation in cleft lip surgery. *Plast Reconstr Surg* 1965; 35:371.
46. McNeil CK. *Oral and facial deformity.* London: Pitman, 1954.
47. Burston WR. The early orthodontic treatment of cleft palate conditions. *Dental Pract (Bristol)* 1958; 9:41.
48. Georgiade NG, Latham RA. Maxillary arch alignment in the bilateral cleft lip and palate infant, using the pinned coaxial screw appliance. *Plast Reconstr Surg* 1975; 56:52.
49. Millard DR, Jr. Unilateral cleft lip deformity. In: McCarthy, ed. *Plastic surgery.* Vol. 4, 2627. Philadelphia: WB Saunders, 1990.
50. Rosenstein SW, Monroe CW, Kernahan DA, et al. The case of early bone grafting in cleft lip and cleft palate. *Plast Reconstr Surg* 1982; 70:297.
51. Sadove AM, Eppley BL. Timing of alveolar bone grafting. *Problems in Plast Surg* 1992; 2:39.
52. Schmid E. Die Aufbauende Kieferkammplastik. *Ost Z Stomat* 1954; 51.
53. Nordin K, Johanson B. Frei knochentransplantation bei defekten im alveolarkamm nack kieferortopadischer einstellug der maxilla bei Lippen-Kiefer-Gaumenspalten. In: Schuchart K, Wassmund M, eds. *Fortschritte der Kiefer- und Gesights-chirurgie.* Vol. 1. Stuttgart: Geor Thieme Verlag, 1955; 168–171.
54. Schrudde J, Stellmach R. Die primäre osteoplastik der defekte des kieferbogens bei Lippen-Kiefer-Gaumenspalten am Saugling. *Zentralbl Chir* 1958; 83:849.
55. Schuchardt K, Pfeifer G. Erfahrungen der primäre knochentransplantationen bei Lippen-Kiefer-Gaumenspalten. *Langenbecks Arch Klin Chir* 1960; 295:881.

56. Johanson B. Secondary osteoplastic completion of maxilla and palate. In: Schuchardt K, ed. Treatment of patients with clefts of the lip, alveolus and palate. Topic 10: Second Hamburg International Symposium, 1964. Stuttgart: Georg Theime Verlag, 1966.

57. Johanson B, Ohlsson A, Friede H, et al. A follow-up study of cleft lip and palate patients treated with orthodontics, secondary bone grafting and prosthetic rehabilitation. *Scand J Plast Reconstr Surg* 1974; 1974; 8:121.

58. Schmid E, Widmaier W, Reichert H, et al. The development of the cleft upper jaw following primary osteoplasty and orthodontic treatment. *J Maxillofac Surg* 1974; 2:92.

59. Boyne PJ, Sands NR. Secondary bone grafting of residual alveolar and palatal clefts. *J Oral Surg* 1972; 30:87.

60. Abyholm F, Bergland O, Semb G. Secondary bone grafting of alveolar clefts. *Scand J Plast Reconstr Surg* 1981; 15:127.

61. Sadove AM, Nelson CL, Eppley BL, et al. An evaluation of calavarial and iliac donor sites in alveolar cleft grafting. *Cleft Palate Jour* 1990; 27:3, 225.

62. Cohen M, Figueroa AA, Haviv Y, et al. Iliac versus cranial bone for secondary grafting of residual alveolar clefts. *Plast Reconstr Surg* 1991; 87:3, 423.

63. Wolfe SA, Berkowitz S. The use of cranial bone grafts in the closure of alveolar and anterior palatal clefts. *Plast Reconstr Surg* 1983; 72:5, 659.

64. LaRossa D, Buchman S, Rothkopf DM, et al. A comparison of iliac and cranial bone in secondary grafting of alveolar clefts. *Plast Reconstr Surg* 1995; 96:789.

26

Primary Repair of the Bilateral Cleft Lip and Nasal Deformity

John B. Mulliken, M.D., F.A.C.S.

Bilateral complete cleft lip may be the most challenging malformation within the purview of plastic surgeons. James Barrett Brown wrote that the bilateral cleft deformity is twice as difficult to repair as the unilateral cleft lip and, furthermore, the result is only half as good (1). Brown is also reputed to have remarked that cleft lip is a three-dimensional problem for a two-dimensional mind. Labial clefting, particularly the bilateral malformation, is a four-dimensional problem for a three-dimensional mind (2).

The Deformity: Primary and Secondary

An error of embryonic morphogenesis can be categorized simply as either a malformation, a deformation, or a disruption. The double cleft lip is the result of bilateral failed fusion and merging between the median nasal process and maxillary prominence. Consequently, there is insufficient mesodermal penetration of the lateral lip ectodermal envelopes. Furthermore, there is a total absence of muscle in the prolabial segment, resulting in abortive formation of the philtral dimple/columns/white ridge and the median tubercle (3–5).

Whereas cleft lip is a malformation, the accompanying nasal deformity is primarily a deformation of normal architectural elements. The alar genua are splayed, the tip is broad, and the alae nasi are flared, but the hallmark of the cleft nasal deformity is the short columella. There are also deformational distortions that result from the disjoined skeletal framework and abnormal muscular forces. There can be some degree of primary hypoplasia of the embryonic lateral nasal prominences, evidenced as underdeveloped alae nasi, and involving genua, lateral crura, accessory cartilages, and lobular fat.

Other anatomic stigmata of a child born with bilateral cleft lip may be iatrogenic, the consequences of well-intentioned surgical repair. The prolabium is typically bowed and abnormally wide; the distance between the Cupid's bow peaks is increased correspondingly. Often, the orbicularis oris bundles are not joined; this causes a bulge in the lateral lips that accentuates during labial contraction. The lateral lip elements are often too long and hang like swags, flanking a deficient median tubercle that is covered by chapped mucosa (2,5).

Labial repair typically aggravates the primary nasal deformity and often creates additional distortions (6). Conventional techniques pull the medial crura inferoposteriorly, buckle the slumped alar domes, and accentuate the splayed genua, flared nostrils, and the short columella. Usually there is a technical failure to narrow and properly position the alar bases and construct the nostril sills. If there are no amends

for the vertically long lateral lip elements, there will be an unnatural superior posture of the alae nasi that becomes more pronounced whenever the child smiles (6). By the time these nasal distortions are addressed at a second procedure, the alar cartilages are rigidly deformed/displaced and difficult to model and position.

Synchronous Repair of the Lip and Nose

Surgical correction of the bilateral cleft deformity has always focused on closure of the two sides of the lip. Staged repair, one side and then the other, has been superseded by simultaneous/symmetrical closure of both sides (2,7,8,9). The bilateral cleft nasal deformity either has been ignored or deferred. Earlier, surgeons were thwarted by the squatty columella. Sundry secondary "columellar lengthening" procedures were devised based on the observation that the columella is deficient and thus skin must be added to it (10). The best-known techniques involve either transferring tissue from the sides of the prolabium, the forked-flap procedure (7,11), or advancing local tissue from the nasal floors (12). These secondary procedures, for what are in large part secondary deformities, result in their own peculiar tertiary distortions (13,14). Most techniques introduce scar(s) at the columella-labial join; this causes the prolabium to bulge rather than have a normal concave configuration. If the columella–labial junction is violated, a crease forms during smiling. This deformity is probably impossible to correct, and it is unnecessary. Never incise the columella–labial junction (6).

Surgical history reveals that complex malformations once considered amenable only to staged repair can be corrected more successfully by a single procedure. Indeed, primary correction of the cleft lip nasal deformity is accepted practice for a unilateral cleft lip. In contrast, primary correction of the bilateral cleft nasal deformity is still evolving. The primary forked-flap procedure, introduced by Millard (15), was tried by McComb for 15 years (16,17), and then abandoned (14). McComb continues in the vanguard of primary correction of the bilateral cleft lip nasal deformity. He uses an open tip approach to the splayed alar cartilages, however, he delays definitive closure of the labial clefts (14,18). Other surgeons espouse *simultaneous* repair of the cleft nasal deformity and the bilateral cleft lip and describe their own technical variations on how to construct a normal-sized columella (19–23).Thus, the principle of primary nasal correction has gained a foothold. The next step is to re-analyze the anatomic abnormalities and plan surgical strategy.

DECEPTION OF A SHORT COLUMELLA

The columella is neither short nor deficient in the bilateral complete cleft lip deformity; it is only looks diminutive because of the malpositioned alar cartilages and abnormally draped soft tissue (6,23). The apparently missing columella is actually in the nose. McComb made the analogy: "The columella has been unzipped and its component parts lie within the broad nasal tip (14)." There is no shortage of investing skin and consequently no need to recruit tissue for the columella from the lip or from the sills. Nasal dissection of stillborn infants with bilateral labial clefting reveals the alar domes and upper medial crura are splayed and that the alar cartilages are rotated caudally, subluxed from their normal position overlying the upper lateral cartilages (6,17). Thus, primary correction of the bilateral cleft lip nasal deformity requires surgical modeling: (a) anatomic placement of the alar cartilages in relation to the upper lateral cartilages, (b) apposition of the genua, (c) trimming excess skin, and (d) draping the soft tissues (6,23).

A FINAL BRIEFING

This presentation focusses on the principles that are the foundation for simultaneous primary repair of the bilateral cleft lip and associated nasal deformities. Like all surgical principles, they have attained a certain permanence; yet, they continue to evolve and may need modification in the future. In contrast, the operative techniques presented in this chapter, perforce, can change depending on circumstances, ongoing analysis of outcome, and new methodologies.

Surgical craftsmanship in three-dimensions must take into account nasolabial variations in the fourth-dimension. Successful surgical repair of bilateral complete cleft lip, like perfection, is an asymptote. Tissue for a prominent central white roll, along the handle of the Cupid's bow, is often lacking. The philtral groove and flanking columns seem to be just beyond the surgeon's craft.

Textbooks of plastic surgery are replete with various techniques for primary repair of the bilateral complete cleft lip. The longest chapter, however, recounts numerous secondary procedures for persisting labial and nasal deformities. The surgical goal is primary repair of the primary palate. The degree of success in achieving this goal, is inversely proportional to the number of residual deformities, secondary operations, and textual pages devoted to stigmata.

Dentofacial Orthopedics

Correction of the protrusive and sometimes-rotated premaxilla sets the stage for labial closure, including the platform for primary nasal correction. Plaster models of the jaws are taken soon after the infant is first seen. The preferred technique is "active" premaxillary orthopedics, pioneered by Georgiade and Latham (24–26). With the infant under general anesthetic, the acrylic plates of the custom-made appliance are pinned to the maxillary shelves and a staple is passed transversely through the premaxilla, just anterior to the prevomerine suture. An elastic chain on each side is connected to the staple, looped around a pulley in the posterior section of the appliance, and attached to a hook on the anterior part of the acrylic plate (Fig. 26–1). The tension on the elastic chains is initially set at 90 grams (g); the chains

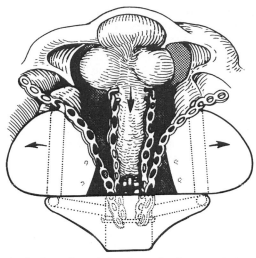

FIG. 26–1. Latham-Georgiade pin-retained presurgical orthopedic appliance. Vector arrows depict movement of premaxilla and palatal shelves as the screw is turned.

can be tightened at intervals during treatment. The parents are taught to turn the screw (daily) so as to expand the maxillary elements. The Georgiade-Latham device is most successful in correcting the premaxillary anterior-posterior dimension, secondly successful in amending rotation, and least successful in altering vertical elongation. It takes, on average, 1 to 2 months before the premaxilla is in optimal position. The infant is usually 4 to 5 months of age at time of nasolabial repair. In some instances, premaxillary retropositioning fails because the two pins of the staple gradually slip through the vomer.

"Passive" premaxillary orthopedics is recommended by those who are concerned about the potential deleterious effects of a pin-retained prosthesis that forces the segments into alignment. A custom-made semirigid plate is retained by undercuts. This plate is for stabilization; there is no expansion. It is designed to maintain posterior transverse dimension, relying on the forces of either external elastic traction or bilateral lip adhesion to mold the premaxilla. In the absence of muscle in the prolabial segment, lip adhesions for a bilateral complete cleft deformity are prone to dehiscence. Furthermore, preliminary adhesion can cause scarring in the precious vermilion-mucosal tissue of the lateral lip elements. Finally, either lip adhesions or an external elastic band tend to focus the pressure away from the fulcrum of the premaxilla, causing a tipping of the premaxilla and thus accentuating vertical elongation and lingual inclination.

Principles

Too often, one surgeon will ask of another "What technique do you use?" rather than more properly inquiring "What principles do you follow?" For without the proper principles, even the most skillfully accomplished cleft lip repair will fall short of expectations. Five principles guide this surgeon's hands in repair of bilateral complete cleft lip and nasal deformity (2,23).

I. *Symmetry.* This is the foremost principle of bilateral cleft lip repair. Staged closure of the lip cleft (one side and then the other) portends asymmetry. Even the smallest nasolabial dissimilarities on the two sides must be remedied during primary repair.

II. *Primary muscle continuity.* Orbicularis oris muscle bundles must be mobilized from the lateral lip elements and apposed, under minimal tension, throughout the vertical extent of the prolabium. Complete dissection of the orbicularis oris rectifies the muscle bulges in the lateral lip elements. Muscle repair allows normal forces to act on the premaxilla, maxillae, and alar bases, and permits normal labial movement.

III. *Proper prolabial size and shape.* The prolabium, once in continuity with the skin and muscle from the lateral elements, displays remarkable growth potential, and this growth must be envisioned in designing the configuration of the prolabium.

IV. *Formation of median tubercle from laterallLip vermilion-mucosa.* To obtain a central white ridge and a vermilion of sufficient vertical height and color match, the median tubercle should be constructed with white roll–vermilion-mucosal flaps from the lateral lip elements.

V. *Positioning alar cartilages to construct the nasal tip and columella.* The columella is concealed within the nasal tip of an infant with bilateral complete cleft lip. The surgical stratagem is anatomic positioning of the slumped and splayed alar cartilages with sculpturing/draping of the nasal soft tissues.

Technical Steps

MARKINGS

Markings are made with a sharp toothpick dipped in brilliant green (malachite) dye. Holding the nares upward with a double-ball retractor gives a symmetrical disposition of the nasolabial soft tissues. The midline vertical nasal incision and rim (marginal) incisions are drawn first. The prolabial flap is designed with slightly biconcave sides and a dart-shaped tip. The dimensions of the prolabial flap are chosen depending on the racial background, age of the infant, and predicted changes with growth. For a white infant, 3 to 6 months of age, suggested dimensions for the prolabial flap are: length, 6 to 8 mm; distance from peak-to-peak of Cupid's bow, 3–4 mm; and width across the base at the columella-labial junction, 2.0–2.5 mm. Redundant skin on each side of the prolabial flap is delineated for excision, leaving a tiny dart on each side of the columellar base (Fig. 26–2).

The Cupid's bow peak-points are carefully sighted on the lateral labial elements. The lateral position of the each peak-point is chosen to provide sufficient height of lateral lip vermilion to form the median tubercle and about three millimeters of lateral white roll. The vertical position of each peak-point is marked just at the top of the white roll that will become the handle of the Cupid's bow. A line is drawn medially from the Cupid's bow peak-point, atop the stripe of white roll and along the cutaneous–vermilion and cutaneous–mucosal junction. The alar base flaps and their junction with the lateral lips are drawn (see Fig. 26–2).

Critical anatomic points are tattooed using a 30-gauge needle dipped in dye: base and 3 points at the tip of the prolabial flap, Cupid's bow peaks, and the vermilion–mucosal (red line) junctions on each lateral labial element.

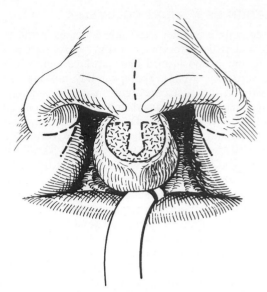

FIG. 26–2. Incisional markings for synchronous repair of complete bilateral cleft lip and nasal deformity. Alar incisions noted on inner side of rim margins. Prolabial flap dimensions vary slightly for each child. Note: dots at "red line" and short section of white roll carried atop the lateral vermilion–mucosal flaps that become the median tubercle.

DISSECTION

Labial

The nasolabial tissues are infiltrated with local anesthetic solution containing 1:200,000 epinephrine. All incisions are scored. The prolabial flap is incised and elevated, leaving all the subcutaneous fat on its underside. Thinning the prolabial flap is a futile effort to create a dimple and only jeopardizes the flap's blood supply. The surgeon excises the disposable lateral prolabial tissue. The alar base is separated from the piriform aperture by an incision at the mucosal–cutaneous junction; this incision extends in the labial sulcus to the premolar region. The alar bases are dissociated from the lateral labial elements. Each lateral lip complex is elevated from the anterior maxilla by supraperiosteal dissection, extending over the malar eminences. The white roll–vermilion-mucosal flaps are incised just inferior to the orbicularis oris layer. The orbicularis oris muscular bundle is carefully dissected within the lateral lip complex, in both the subdermal and submucosal planes. While holding the muscle bundle with a fine-toothed forceps, dissection extends laterally until the muscle bulge is eliminated (Fig. 26–3).

Nasal

The vertical nasal tip and rim incisions are deepened, and utilizing both approaches, a fine iris scissors is used to expose the anterior surface of the dislocated alar domes (Fig. 26–4). Fatty tissue, lying between the splayed alar genua, is elevated. The vestibular lining is left attached to the underside of the alar cartilages. Neither the distal lateral or the medial crura are displayed and care is taken not to disrupt attachments between the columella, septum, and medial footplates.

Alveolar

The surgeon elevates mucosal flaps from the lateral and medial sides of the cleft defect to construct the nasal floors. If

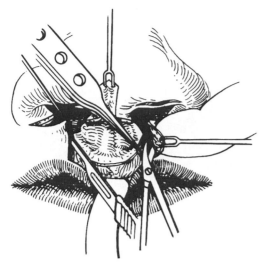

FIG. 26–3. Orbicularis oris muscle dissected within lateral lip elements. Scalpel used to incise dermal–muscular junction; scissors used to complete dissection in subdermal and submucosal planes.

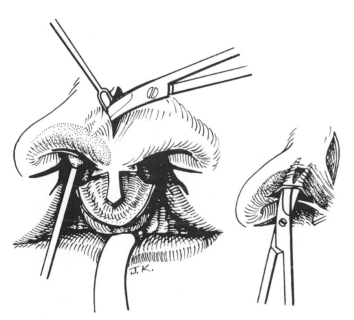

FIG. 26–4. Dissection of dislocated alar cartilages through tip and rim incisions. Cotton-tipped applicator stick supports alar cartilage during dissection.

the premaxillary and maxillary segments are well aligned, the gingivomucoperiosteal flaps are elevated.

CLOSURE

Alveolae, Muscle and Median Tubercle

The nasal floors are constructed first; then, if possible, the alveolar clefts are closed (gingivoperiosteoplasty). The prolabial vermilion and a strip of excess mucosa is trimmed from the premaxillary flap; the latter is sutured to the premaxillary periosteum to form the posterior wall of the gingivolabial sulcus (Fig. 26–5). The lateral labial elements are transposed medially, and the sulci are closed with interrupted chromic sutures. The bundles of the m. orbicularis

oris are apposed seriatim, inferiorly to superiorly, with vertical mattress sutures of polydioxanone. The vertical extent of muscular closure is the same as the vermilion-cutaneous height of the lip. The uppermost portion of the muscular closure is secured, with a polypropylene suture, to the periosteum at the junction of caudal septum and anterior nasal spine (Fig. 26–6, left). The lateral white roll–vermilion-mucosal flaps are held inferiorly and symmetrically, each with a tiny single hook, and sutured to one another to construct the median tubercle. After tying the sutures in the vermilion section of the median raphe, the redundant mucosa is excised from the leading edge of each lateral labial flap to construct a full tubercle, align the vermilion–mucosal junction, and close the anterior sulcus (Fig. 26–6, right).

Nasal

The alar cartilages are positioned prior to insetting the prolabial flap. Through the tip incision, the splayed genua are secured with polydioxanone suture on a one-half circle (5-mm diameter) reverse cutting needle; one or two mattress sutures are placed and left untied. Placement of the interdomal suture(s) is facilitated by elevation of the subluxed alar cartilages with a cotton-tipped applicator stick (Fig. 26–7, left). The next step is symmetric suspension of the superior border of each dome (lateral genu) to the ipsilateral upper lateral cartilage, near its junction with the septum. This is accomplished, under direct vision through the rim incision, using polydioxanone suture armed with a one-half circle (5-mm diameter) reverse cutting needle. Usually one, sometimes two, horizontal mattress sutures are sufficient, between the upper and lower lateral cartilages. The upper lateral-to-alar sutures are tied first, suspending the genua, and the interdomal suture(s) is tied next, apposing the genua (Fig. 26–7, right).

The alae nasi must be properly positioned in both the vertical and horizontal axes. The inferiolateral vestibular floor is closed as the alar base is transposed medially. A horizontal mattress polypropylene suture is placed from base to base, and this "cinch" suture is tied to reduce the transverse (interalar) width, which is 2.4 to 2.6 cm for a white infant (Fig. 26–8, left). The nostril sills are constructed by trimming the appropriate amount of tissue from each side of the columellar base and the tip of each alar flap (Fig. 26–8, right). The alae nasi are positioned inferiorly by a suture from the dermis of the alar base to the upper ipsilateral orbicularis oris muscle. This suture also forms the normal depression in the lateral nasal sill (Fig. 26–8, right).

Redundant skin in the nasal soft triangles becomes evident after the alar cartilages and bases are properly positioned. The surgeon trims a crescent-shaped section of excess skin from the superior side of each rim incision (Fig. 26–9, left). If the infratip region is too wide, a small strip of skin is excised from each edge of the lower portion of the vertical incision. The three nasal incisions are closed in two layers.

Usually a superiolateral mucocutaneous web appears along the intercartilaginous junction of each vestibule. This fold results from constriction of the expanded vestibular lining and superior traction, both due to positioning the alar cartilages and alar bases. A lenticular excision is done on the cutaneous side of this web with its axis along the intercartilaginous line. In closing the defect, the web is effaced (Fig. 26–9, inset right).

FIG. 26–5.   Closure of nasal floors and alveolar clefts (gingivoperiosteoplasty). Prolabial vermilion and excess mucosa excised before suturing premaxillary mucosa to periosteum.

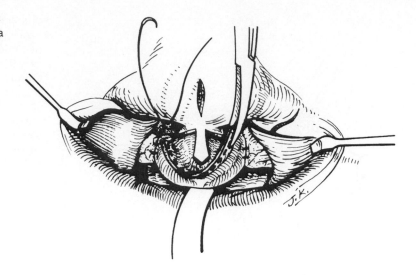

FIG. 26–6.   Apposition of orbicularis oris bundles (left). Uppermost suture, through periosteum at anterior nasal spine, secures the muscle and lateral lip elements relative to premaxilla and nose. Construction of median tubercle: trimming excess vermilion-muscle to form raphe (right).

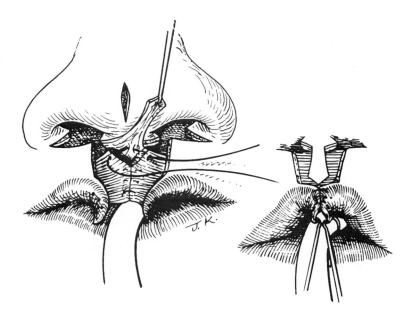

FIG. 26–7.   Apposition of splayed alars by interdomal mattress suture(s) (left). Elevation of subluxed alar cartilage to ipsilateral upper lateral cartilage (right).

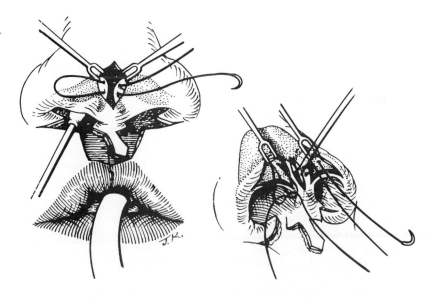

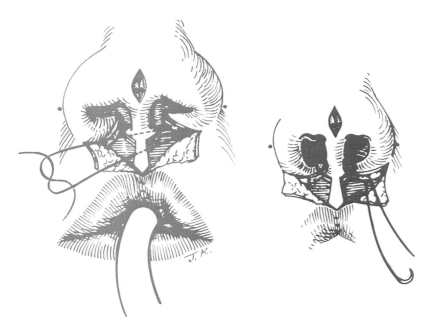

FIG. 26–8. Posturing alar bases: "cinch" suture adjusts horizontal (inter-alar) position (left). Construction of sills: columellar base flaps and alar base flaps are trimmed. Bases are sutured to underlying muscle to adjust vertical position and produce normal depression in lateral sill (right).

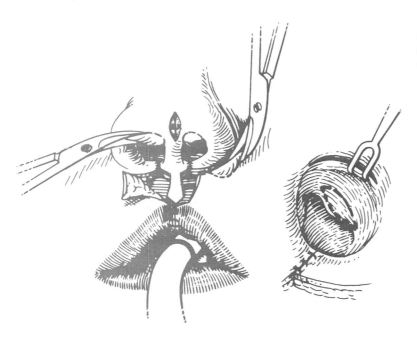

FIG. 26–9. Excision of redundant nasal skin in soft triangles and trimming superior margin of lateral labial flaps in shape of cyma (ogee) molding (left). Enlarged inset shows outline for excision of lateral web in left nostril vestibule (right).

Labial

Cutaneous closure is completed by insetting the tip of the prolabial flap into the notch at the top of the constructed median tubercle. The medial edge of the lateral labial flaps almost never requires trimming. The superior margin, however, must be trimmed, in a cymal (ogee) configuration (Fig. 26–9, left). This maneuver corrects for the tendency to position the alar bases too high and shortens the vertically long lateral labial elements. Closure of the nostril sill–labial junction begins laterally so that the "dog-ear" is placed medially, at the philtral column. The philtral and sill incisions are closed in two layers, with intradermal 6-0 dissolvable sutures and percutaneous 7-0 nylon sutures (Fig. 26–10).

Synchronous nasolabial repair is typically done at 3 to 5 months of age. At this stage, the infant can still be an obligatory nasal breather. For this reason, a vented plug is placed in each nostril, consisting of 1-cm Xeroform gauze wrapped around a short section of 19-gauge polyethylene catheter. These wrapped tubes permit nasal airflow, minimize intranasal swelling, and prevent nasal secretions from macerating the nasolabial wounds.

Postoperative Care

At the end of the procedure, beginning in the operating room, an iced-saline gauze sponge is placed on the repaired lip and held through the loops of a Logan bow. This moistened

to adulthood. Therefore, any surgeon who undertakes the care of infants born with a bilateral cleft deformity also has the obligation to analyze his own results periodically and to perpetually learn from his predecessors, colleagues, and patients.

An infant born with a bilateral labial cleft cannot afford to wait for the surgeon to learn from technical misadventures. Residual stigmata of bilateral cleft lip closure usually cannot be erased completely by revisionary operations. Repairing a cleft lip is analogous to cutting a diamond: A diamond lasts forever, a cleft lip repair affects a lifetime.

Bibliography

1. Brown JB, McDowell F, Byars LT. Double clefts of the lip. *Surg Gynecol Obstet* 1947; 85:20.
2. Mulliken JB. Principles and techniques of bilateral complete cleft lip repair. *Plast Reconstr Surg* 1985; 75:477.
3. Latham RA, Deaton TG. The structural basis of the philtrum and the contour of the vermilion border: a study of the musculature of the upper lip. *J Anat* 1976; 121:151.
4. Briedis J, Jackson IT. The anatomy of the philtrum: observations made on dissections in the normal lip. *Br J Plast Surg* 1981; 34:128.
5. Mulliken JB, Pensler JM, Kozakewich HPW. The anatomy of Cupid's bow in normal and cleft lip. *Plast Reconstr Surg* 1993; 92:395.
6. Mulliken JB. Correction of the bilateral cleft lip nasal deformity: evolution of a surgical concept. *Cleft Palate-Craniofac J* 1992; 29:540.
7. Millard DR Jr. *Cleft craft: bilateral and rare deformities.* Vol II. Boston: Little, Brown, 1977.
8. Black PW, Scheflan M. Bilateral cleft lip repair. "Putting it all together." *Ann Plast Surg* 1984; 12:118.
9. Noordhoff MS. Bilateral cleft lip reconstruction. *Plast Reconstr Surg* 1986; 78:45.
10. Cronin TD, Upton J. Lengthening of the short columella associated with bilateral cleft lip. *Ann Plast Surg* 1978; 1:75.
11. Millard DR Jr. Closure of bilateral cleft lip and elongation of columella by two operations in infancy. *Plast Reconstr Surg* 1971; 47:324.
12. Cronin TD. Lengthening of the columella by the use of skin from the nasal floor and alae. *Plast Reconstr Surg* 1958; 21:417.
13. Pigott RW. Aesthetic considerations related to repair of bilateral cleft lip nasal deformity. *Brit J Plast Surg* 1988; 41:593.
14. McComb H. Primary repair of the bilateral cleft lip nose: a 15-year review and a new treatment plan. *Plast Reconstr Surg* 1990; 86:882.
15. Millard DR Jr. Bilateral cleft lip and primary forked flap: a preliminary report. *Plast Reconstr Surg* 1967; 39:59.
16. McComb H. Primary repair of the bilateral cleft lip nose. *Brit J Plast Surg* 1975; 28:262.
17. McComb H. Primary repair of the bilateral cleft lip nose: a 10-year review. *Plast Reconstr Surg* 1986; 77:701.
18. McComb H. Primary repair of the bilateral cleft lip nose: a 4-year review. *Plast Reconstr Surg* 1994; 94:37.
19. Broadbent TR, Woolf RM. Cleft lip nasal deformity. *Ann Plast Surg* 1984; 12:216.
20. Nakajima T, Yoshimura Y, Nakanishi M, et al. Comprehensive treatment of bilateral cleft lip by multidisciplinary team approach. *Brit J Plast Surg* 1991; 44:486.
21. Cutting C, Grayson B. The prolabial unwinding flap method for one-stage repair of bilateral cleft lip, nose, and alveolus. *Plast Reconstr Surg* 1993; 91:37.
22. Trott JA, Mohan N. A preliminary report on one-stage open tip rhinoplasty at the time of lip repair in bilateral cleft lip and palate: the alor setar experience. *Brit J Plast Surg* 1993; 46:215.
23. Mulliken JB. Bilateral complete cleft lip and nasal deformity: an anthropometric analysis of staged to synchronous repair. *Plast Reconstr Surg* 1995; 96:9.
24. Georgiade NG, Latham RA. Maxillary arch alignment in bilateral cleft lip and palate infant, using the coaxial screw appliance. *Plast Reconstr Surg* 1975; 56:52.
25. Georgiade NG, Mason R, Riefkohl R, et al. Preoperative positioning of the protruding premaxilla in the bilateral cleft lip patient. *Plast Reconstr Surg* 1989; 83:32.
26. Millard DR Jr, Latham RA. Improved primary surgical and dental treatment of clefts. *Plast Reconstr Surg* 1990; 86:856.
27. Friede H, Pruzansky S. Longitudinal study of growth in bilateral cleft lip and palate from infancy to adolescence. *Plast Reconstr Surg* 1972; 49:392.
28. Vargevik K. Growth characteristics of the premaxilla and orthodontic principles in bilateral cleft lip and palate. *Cleft Palate J* 1983; 20:289.
29. Friede H, Pruzansky S. Long-term effects of premaxillary setback on facial skeletal profile in complete bilateral cleft lip and palate. *Cleft Palate J* 1985; 22:97.
30. Rodgers CM, Mulliken JB. De-epithelialized mucosal-submucosal flaps to correct the "whistling lip" deformity. *Cleft Palate J* 1989; 26:136.
31. Pensler JM, Mulliken JB. The cleft lip lower-lip deformity. *Plast Reconstr Surg* 1988; 82:602.
32. Farkas LG, Posnick JC, Hrenczko TM, et al. Growth patterns of the nasolabial region: a morphometric study. *Cleft Palate-Craniofac J* 1992; 29:318.

27

Cleft Palate

Bruce S. Bauer, M.D., F.A.C.S., F.A.A.P., and Pravin-Kumar K. Patel, M.D.

Under normal conditions, the palate functions in concert with the pharyngeal musculature to close the velopharyngeal valve. Clefting of the palate results in an absence of velopharyngeal closure and the inability to build up and sustain intraoral pressure. This has significant effects on both early feeding and the development of normal speech. In addition, the abnormal muscle anatomy present in cleft palate has an indirect effect on the function of the middle ear through the resultant anatomic disturbance present along the eustachian tube orifice from which the primary palatal muscles originate.

Before discussing the clinical aspects of cleft palate care and treatment, we will review the normal and abnormal embryology, classification, possible etiologies, incidence, genetics, and palatal anatomy of the condition.

Embryology

The embryonic and fetal growth processes active in the development of the human face and cranium are of considerable interest with respect to both normal and abnormal development. Much of what we know and understand of these processes comes from study of nonmammalian species; the basic mechanisms active in the formation of the facial structures are similar, and we continue to learn from the study of these models.

Normal development is dependent on mesodermal reinforcement of the two-layered ectodermal branchial membrane in the facial region (1,2). This facial mesenchyme has its origin in neuroectoderm bordering the neural tube and migrates in three directions: anteriorly over the developing brain and around either side of the developing stomodeum (3).

While recent studies of human embryos have raised questions as to whether both the frontonasal process and neural-crest cell migration exist in humans the way they do in other species (4,5), there is little doubt that facial development involves a complex interaction of cell proliferation, cell differentiation, cell movement, and cell death (2,4). The ultimate product of this complex balance of processes is the development of normal facial structures. If the balance is disrupted, facial structures may be cleft, malpositioned, or even absent. Our understanding of the pathogenesis of clefting is still rudimentary, but it is best viewed in relation to the normal development of both primary and secondary palates.

NORMAL DEVELOPMENT

Primary Palate

The cells of the anterior neural crest that give rise to the developing upper lip must arrive in their proper location at the appropriate time and in adequate numbers for the lip to develop normally. For the upper lip, these events occur between the 4th and 7th weeks of gestation (2,7).

At the 4th week, the oral plate ruptures to establish continuity between the oral cavity and the foregut. At the same time, the nasal placodes appear cephalad to the oral cavity. As mesoderm is heaped up on either side of the paired nasal structures forming the medial and lateral nasal processes, the nasal pits begin to burrow deeper to create the nasal airways. Simultaneously, neuroectoderm is migrating anteriorly around the head in both directions to reinforce the maxillary processes. The migration continues medially until mesoderm streams into the intermaxillary (premaxillary) segment at the midline. The two medial nasal processes ultimately join to form the single definitive nose and contribute to the development of the nasal septum, columella, premaxilla, and philtrum. The lateral nasal process gives rise to the nasal alae (5).

In the upper lip, the mesoderm arrives to fill out the bilamellar branchial membrane, first in the area of the incisive foramen. Additional mesoderm is then successively deposited, first anteriorly and then inferiorly, effecting closure of the nostril still, followed by the lip, down to and including the vermilion (2).

Once the mesoderm has completed its migration and reinforcement of the entire primary palate (all structures anterior to the incisive foramen), the early facial structures are refined by a process of ectodermal sculpting wherein cells proliferate, move into areas, carve furrows, dig cavities, and hollow tunnels. This sculpting is accomplished through a sequence of cell polarization, followed by further differentiation (and alignment) of those cells close enough to the basement membrane to be nourished by transudate, and cell death of those farthest from the source of nourishment. This sculpting separates the dental lamina within the developing alveolus from the lip, thereby creating the alveolar–labial sulcus. It is also responsible for the deepening of the nasal pits and the lateral rupture of the buccal pharyngeal membrane.

Finally, at the 7th week, after all essential mesoderm has been deposited, additional "late-arriving" mesoderm migrates from each lateral side and piles up in the center of the prolabium and thickens to form the parallel philtral ridges (2).

Secondary Palate

The formation of the secondary palate also involves a complex interaction of cell growth, differentiation, and movement. These processes occur during the 7th through 12th week of embryonic life and differ significantly from those that occur during earlier development of the lip.

The palatal shelves arise as outgrowths of the maxillary processes of the first branchial arch as migrating mesoderm bulges outward against the ectodermal surface. Initially, the palatal shelves lie caudally alongside the tongue (in the sagittal plane). This vertical orientation is maintained as long as the relatively large mass of developing tongue sits between the shelves in the small oral cavity.

With growth, the head begins to extend and the tongue drops downward, first posteriorly (at its base) an then progressively toward the horizontal (axial) plane above the tongue. The posterior shelves reach the horizontal position first, followed by the middle and finally the anterior portions adjacent to the incisive foramen (1,3).

Once the palatal shelves reach the horizontal plane, they begin to merge and fuse in the midline. This occurs through a true process of fusion, unlike the mesodermal penetration process occurring in the primary palate. Contact of the opposing shelves is followed by adherence and then ectodermal degeneration at the contact points. A new ectodermal layer is formed over the fused palatal midline, and mesoderm merges beneath it.

Although fusion occurs primarily from anterior to posterior, it begins initially at one-third of the way posterior, in the region of the hard palate, not at the incisive foramen. Fusion then proceeds up to the incisive foramen and back to the uvula. This may explain the rare findings of either a congenital fistula of the anterior hard palate or an epithelial cyst in a similar location.

PATHOGENESIS OF CLEFT LIP AND PALATE

Primary Palate

The normal development of the lip, as noted, is dependent on the maxillary processes and then progresses toward the midline, overgrowing the medial nasal contribution of the intermaxillary/frontonasal process. This reinforcement of the central lip requires mesoderm of sufficient quantity arriving at the appropriate time. When mesoderm is of insufficient quantity, the unreinforced bilamellar branchial membrane ruptures and a cleft results. If there is total failure of mesodermal penetration, there is a complete cleft extending back to the incisive foramen (complete cleft of the primary palate). If mesoderm is present but insufficient, partial clefting occurs. Minimal deficiency in quantity may result in notching of the vermilion, a subcutaneous furrow, or an isolated thinning of the nostril sill (2,7).

Because mesoderm is programmed to arrive in the area of the incisive foramen before the nostril sill, mid-lip, and vermilion, any event that slows mesodermal migration will affect the lower portions of the lip more than the area of the nostril floor. Failure of migration bilaterally will obviously result in a bilateral cleft, and asymmetrical clefts can be explained as a variable delay in medial migration of the reinforcing layer (2).

The fact that the fetal head is initially turned to the right, and the left side is dependent, may increase the time necessary to complete migration on the left side. This relative delay in left-sided migration may partly explain the greater incidence of left-sided clefts compared to right-sided clefts.

Finally, the process of ectodermal sculpting appears to be active late in the sequence of events leading to formation of a normal lip. Because it is dependent on the prior arrival of mesoderm, it will not occur in cases of complete clefting. Here, the mesodermal contribution to the premaxilla is absent. Therefore, in complete bilateral clefts, the refinement of an alveolar–labial sulcus and philtrum are absent.

Secondary Palate

Formation of the normal secondary palate is also dependent on sufficient mesoderm and precise timing of its movement in the palatal shelf. Even in the presence of sufficient mesoderm, the palatal shelves will not reach one another in the midline if the tongue fails to move out of the way. This simple mechanical obstruction appears to explain those clefts associated with an abnormally small mandible and malpositioned tongue mass (e.g., Pierre Robin sequence) (1).

When no obvious obstruction exists to prevent palatal shelf movement from the vertical to the horizontal plane, it appears that clefting results from a failure of fusion alone. Total failure of adherence and fusion will result in a complete cleft from the incisive foremen back to the uvula, and a lesser degree of failure will result in an incomplete cleft. Because fusion is apparently preceded by a transient adherence of the palatal shelves, rupture occurring immediately after adherence may explain the occasional appearance of epithelial pearls in the cleft margin.

Finally, because adherence and fusion are followed by a merging of mesoderm from the opposing shelves, the concept of fusion of the shelves without mesodermal merging appears to explain the origin of a submucous cleft palate. This cleft variant may likewise be explained on the basis of fusion occurring in normal sequence but with mesenchyme in short supply.

Classification

On the basis of the distinctive embryologic formation of the primary and secondary palate, clefts can be classified as shown in Table 27–1. For simplification in record keeping, clefts can be diagrammatically represented by the striped-Y logo shown in Figure 27–1 (8).

Etiology of Cleft Lip and Palate

In some 25% of cases, there is a family history of facial clefting, which does not follow either a normal recessive or dom-

Table 27–1
Classification of Cleft Palates

Clefts of first degree palate	Unilateral or bilateral, complete or incomplete
Clefts of second degree palate	Incomplete or complete
Clefts of first and second degree palate	Unilateral or bilateral, complete or incomplete

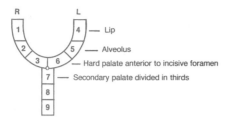

FIG. 27–1. Classification of cleft lip and palate.

inant pattern. The condition appears to be multifactorial. It has been suggested that some cases of clefting are due to an overall reduction in the volume of the facial mesenchyme, which leads to clefting by virtue of failure of mesodermal penetration. In some cases, clefting appears associated with increased facial width, either alone or in association with encephalocele, idiopathic hypertelorism, or the presence of a teratoma. The characteristic U-shaped cleft of the Pierre Robin anomaly is thought to be dependent upon a persistent high position of the tongue, perhaps associated with a failure or delay of neck extension. This prevents descent of the tongue, which in turn prevents elevation and a medial growth of the palatal shelves. Distortion of the facial processes or malposition resulting from oligohydramnios has been suggested as another possible etiological factor. The production of clefts of the secondary palate in experimental animals has frequently been accomplished by drug administration. The agents commonly used are steroids, anticonvulsants, diazepam, and aminopterin. There is some suggestion that phenytoin and diazepam may also be factors in causing clefting in humans. Infections during the first trimester of pregnancy, such as rubella or toxoplasmosis, have been associated with clefting.

Incidence

It would appear that some degree of clefting occurs in approximately 1:600 to 1:1000 live births in this country. Clefting is much more common in stillborns and abortuses.[9,10] The incidence of clefting varies with race. It is estimated to be 1:750 live births in whites, 1:2000 in blacks, and 1:5000 in Asians. Racial variation appears to be more marked in cleft lip without (CL) or with cleft palate (CL ± P) than in cleft palate (CP) alone.

Complete clefts of the primary and secondary palate are more common than clefts of the primary palate alone, in a ratio of 2:1. There are also significant differences in the incidence of CL ± P versus CP in the two sexes: CL ± P occurs twice as commonly in males as in females, whereas the exact reverse is true in clefts of the secondary palate, which occurs twice as frequently in females as in males.

Complete clefts of the lip and palate are twice as common on the left side as on the right, although there is no known reason for this difference. The comparative frequency of unilateral clefts on the left, versus unilateral clefts on the right, versus bilateral clefts, is 6:3:1. In a large cleft-palate population, the distribution of types of clefting has been reported as 21% CL, 46% CL ± P, and 33% CP.

Clefts may be considered as falling into one of three groups: genetic, environmental, and syndromic. A family history is twice as common in CL ± P as it is in CP. Cleft palate

appears to be more commonly environmental than hereditary. Other associated congenital anomalies are seen in 29% of cases of clefting. More commonly, these other anomalies are associated with isolated CP rather than with CL ± P. As an isolated deformity, CP occurs slightly more frequently than CL ± P, but the majority of cases of CL ± P are isolated deformities. There are more than 150 syndromes described in which clefting may be a feature. CP alone is more commonly associated with a syndrome than is CL ± P.

The incidence of short stature in cleft patients has been noted to be 40 times that of the general population. Possibly, the midline clefting is associated with a disturbance in development of the anterior pituitary from the Rathke pouch.

Some association has been found between low socioeconomic status and an increased incidence of facial clefting, and it has been suggested that this is possibly related to inadequate nutrition. However, environmentally, isolated cleft cases appear to be significantly associated with higher socioeconomic status.

Genetics

Once a child with a cleft is born into a family, the chance of clefting increases significantly for subsequent siblings. From the point of view of inheritance, it appears that CL ± P and CP follow different patterns (9–11). The figures for inheritance are given in Table 27–2. Recent investigations suggest that, if the initial form of clefting in the family is

Table 27–2
Cleft Lip and Cleft Palate Inheritance Risks

	Genetic Guidance
Cleft lip and palate (CL ± P)	
Normal parents and 1 child with CL ± P	4% risk of another child with CL ± P
Normal parents and 1 affected child and positive family history	4%
Normal parents and affected child and child with additional anomaly	2%
Normal parents and 2 affected children	4%
Parent with CL ± P and no affected children	4%
Parent with CL ± P and child with CL ± P	14–17%
Cleft Palate (CP)	
Normal parents and child with CP	2% risk of affected child
Normal parents and child with CP and positive family history	7%
Normal parents and child with CP and another anomaly	2%
Normal parents and 2 children with CP	1%
Parent with CP and no affected child	2–4%
Parent with CP and child with CP	15%

severe, the chance of further clefts appearing in subsequent family members is greater than when the initial degree of clefting is minor (11).

Van der Woude syndrome represents an important variation for the genetic guidelines listed in Table 27–2. It is an autosomal dominant disorder with lower lip pits in association with different degrees of lip and palatal clefting. There is a 70–80% risk of lip pits and a 40–50% change for clefting of the lip and/or palate in families with this syndrome. Absent other signs of overt clefts, submucous clefting of the palate should be looked for when detailing the pedigree of a family with Van der Woude syndrome.

Submucous cleft palate, nonsyndromal, has an incidence of approximately 1:1200 live births; however, only about ten percent of children with submucous clefts of the palate have speech problems. Thus the condition may go undetected throughout life and the incidence could, in fact, be higher.

Anatomy of the Palate in Clefting

The three muscles of the palate work in concert with the pharyngeal muscles to produce velopharyngeal closure. The tensor veli palatini muscles arise from the membranous wall of the eustachian tube. Their tendons pass around the hamular processes of the pterygoid and insert into the palatine aponeurosis. The levator veli palatini muscles also have their origin along the eustachian tube orifice. They meet in the midline in a slinglike fashion above and behind the aponeurosis. The musculus uvulae is a small midline muscle sitting above and behind the levator sling.

The vascular supply of the palate arises from the palatine vessels (greater and lesser) and from posterior septal contributions through the incisive foramen. Sensation is supplied by the maxillary division of the trigeminal nerve by way of the pterygopalatine and nasopalatine foramina. There is a dual motor innervation with motor branches of the trigeminal nerve to the tensor palatini and the vagus nerve through the pharyngeal plexus to the levator and musculus uvulae.

Functionally, the normal closure of the velopharyngeal valve is accomplished by the sphincter action of the levator sling, which pulls the palate upward and backward toward the posterior pharyngeal wall. The palatopharyngeus muscles (which also form a sling) and the superior constrictor muscles help in this action. The musculus uvulae also contracts during speech, adding bulk to the area of convexity on the upper surface of the soft palate.

Most important in the anatomy of the cleft palate is that the levator muscles, rather than running toward the midline, are directed anteriorly (longitudinally); they insert into the posterior border of the hard palate with their fibers parallel to the cleft margin. Several authors have emphasized this (12–14). This abnormal orientation also occurs in submucous cleft palate; in these cases, the dehiscence of muscle in the midline can be seen clearly on transillumination through the nose. The triad of signs of submucous cleft palate is completed by the bony notch in the posterior border of the hard palate and a bifid uvula.

Early Considerations in Cleft Palate Care

Randall (15) emphasized four points in the treatment of infants with clefts of the palate. These include: (a) feeding; (b) maintenance of an airway; (c) middle-ear disease; and (d) the possibility of other abnormalities.

FEEDING

Although a child with a cleft palate may make sucking movements with the mouth, the cleft prevents the child from developing adequate suction. In general, however, swallowing mechanisms are normal; therefore, if the milk or formula can be delivered to the back of the child's throat, the infant will feed effectively.

While many specialized types of nipples have been recommended for the child with cleft palate, we have found the use of a standard disposable nipple with an enlarged hole to be successful in almost all cases. We think it important that this allows the mother to use the same type of bottle and nipple as she would any other child and thus minimizes the feeling that the cleft child is different.

Breastfeeding is usually not successful, unless milk production is very abundant. If the mother insists on breastfeeding, the physician must monitor the infant's weight closely to assure sufficient intake.

AIRWAY

The infant with Pierre Robin anomaly or other conditions in which the cleft palate is seen in association with a micrognathia or retrognathic mandible may be particularly prone to upper airway obstruction. Treatment of these problems is beyond the scope of this chapter, but a logical management approach would be to attempt the simpler, more conservative techniques (e.g., prone positioning) before progressing to surgical intervention.

MIDDLE EAR DISEASE

As mentioned earlier, the disturbance in anatomy associated with cleft palate also affects the function of the eustachian tube orifices. Parents should be made aware of the increased possibility of middle ear infection so that the child will receive treatment promptly if symptoms arise. Careful follow-up, in collaboration with an audiologist and an otolaryngologist, including examination, myringotomy, and tube placement when necessary, will prevent long-term hearing deficits.

ASSOCIATED DEFORMITIES

The surgeon must always keep in mind that, in as many as 29% of cases, the child with cleft palate may have other anomalies. These may be more commonly associated with isolated CP than with CL ± P, but the inclusion of Pierre Robin cases in these figures makes that difference more apparent than real. High among the associated anomalies are those affecting the circulatory and skeletal systems.

Techniques of Palate Repair

The object of palate repair is the production of a competent velopharyngeal sphincter. It is not the purpose of this chapter to give a detailed description of all palate repair techniques, but to describe the more common techniques, the similarities and differences in technique, and some changing trends in repair.

The standard techniques of palate repair have changed little in recent years, with the two most common repairs being the V–Y (Veau-Wardill-Kilner) and the von Langenbeck repair. While various modifications can be combined with each of these repairs, the main difference between the two is that the V–Y repair, and its variations, involves elongation of the palate, while the von Langenbeck repair does not.

The von Langenbeck repair involves paring the margins of the cleft and closure in the midline with the use of lateral relaxing incisions to relieve tension on the repair. As the palatal flaps remain bipedicle, no elongation is accomplished. In the V–Y repair, elongation is accomplished, at least on the oral surface, by the well-known technique of V to Y advancement (Fig. 27–2). Other techniques to achieve palatal lengthening have been described by Dorrance (16), Cronin (17), Millard (18), and Manchester (19).

More recently Furlow (20), then Randall and colleagues (21), using Furlow's technique have gained additional soft-palate length with a double reversing Z-plasty (Fig. 27–3), but it is difficult to say if the speech results will be significantly better than the standard V–Y repair or von Langenbeck repair. The methods used to evaluate the latter two repairs and the reports in the literature of their speech results are difficult to interpret. Lindsay and coworkers (22) showed there was no difference in speech results between the two procedures. Although our results confirm these findings, we observed significantly better results with the V–Y repair when clefts involved both primary and secondary palates.

Brief comments are warranted about two other types of repair. First, although speech results may be very good after repairs incorporating a pharyngeal flap as a primary procedure, it would appear that most standard methods of palate repair achieve acceptable speech results in about 75% of cases with a single procedure carried out in infancy without a pharyngeal flap. Therefore, it seems that in 3 of 4 cases the primary pharyngeal flap is unnecessary. It may be even be contraindicated in children with a limited nasopharyngeal airway. Since recent reports based on long-term follow-up indicate that neither the objective of good speech nor the avoidance of maxillary collapse is achieved by the Schweckendiek procedure (delayed hard-palate repair), it will probably be relegated to history (23).

Finally, with the increasing emphasis on a functional repair in cleft lip and palate surgery, attention has been directed recently towards reconstruction of the levator sling or intravelar veloplasty. By detaching the levator muscles from their abnormal attachment to the hard palate and repairing them in the midline with the muscle fibers oriented more normally, velopharyngeal closure may be accomplished more easily (24). An alternative approach to the levator reconstruction is that described by Furlow (20) and modified by Randall and coworkers (21). Any of the above approaches to muscle reconstruction can be used in combination with traditional techniques for closure of the hard-palate cleft. The Furlow

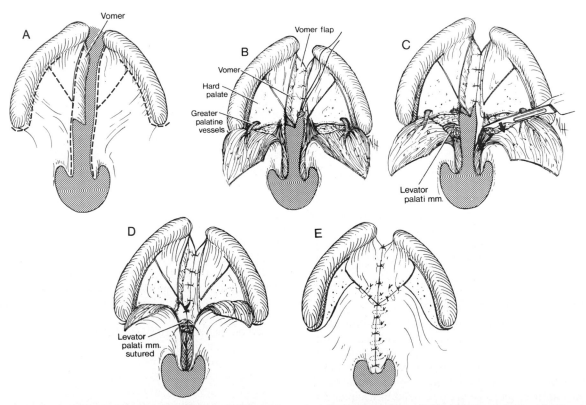

FIG. 27–2. The standard markings for the Wardill-Kilner V–Y palatal repair. The palatal flaps are elevated. Note that the vomer bone mucosa has been elevated and transferred laterally to create an anterior nasal floor closure. The palatine vessels can be further released from the flaps for greater movement of the flaps medially as needed in the wider palatal clefts. The levator muscles of the palate have been dissected from their abnormal longitudinal attachments along the hard palate and rotated into a cross-sectional position. The levator musculature has now been sutured across the midline to construct the sling mechanism, as in a normal palate. This is carried out after the closure of the palatal nasal mucosa. The palatal mucosa, in its new V–Y position, is closed with interrupted and mattress sutures of Dexon 3-0 or Vicryl 3-0.

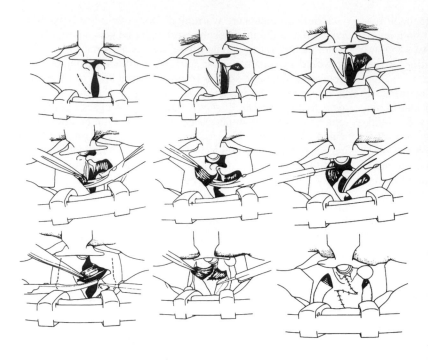

FIG. 27–3. Top left, the posteriorly based limb of the Z-plasty in the oral mucosa includes the levator muscle on that side. Top center, the anteriorly based limb of the Z-plasty contains only oral mucosa and is cut closer to an 80° than a 60° angle to keep the transposed levator muscle from being inserted close to the posterior edge of the palatine bone. Top right, the anteriorly based oral mucosal flap is dissected off the levator muscle. Center left, the levator muscle is detached from its abnormal insertion into the posterior edge of the palatine bone. The plane of dissection between the levator muscle and the nasal mucosa is easily determined by lifting the nasal mucosa off the palatine bone with a small elevator (not shown). Center, this dissection between the levator muscle and the nasal mucosa is very difficult because the nasal mucosa is so thin. Center right, the Z-plasty in the nasal mucosa is reversed. Here the anteriorly based flap contains only nasal mucosa. Bottom left, the posteriorly based flap contains levator muscle and nasal mucosa. The muscle usually extends well beyond the mucosal flap as it inserts on the palatine bone. Bottom center, closure of the nasal mucosa with the levator muscle from the right side allows shifting the muscle from its transverse orientation. Completion of the closure brings the left levator muscle into a transverse orientation overlapping the right levator muscle. Bottom right, relaxing incisions may or may not be needed. Because width is sacrificed for length, in a very wide cleft the Z-plasty cannot be made very large, although the muscle flaps will extend well beyond the mucosal flaps. (From Randall P, et al. Experience with the Furlow double-reversing Z-plasty for cleft palate repair. *Plast Reconstr Surg* 1986; 77:569.)

technique has the advantage of gaining additional soft-palate length without the need for raising or shifting large mucoperiosteal flaps from the hard palate. It can also be used in combination with a primary pharyngeal flap, should this be indicated, and can be adapted for early soft-palate closure (age 3 to 6 months) (21,25).

A closer look at the relationship between age at time of palate repair and speech has led toward a trend of early repair. While the average age of palate repair today is 12 to18 months, Dorf and Curtin (26) have pointed out that phoneme development is present as early as 6 months. Based on these studies, they carried out repairs in the first few months of life and showed significantly improved speech results. Randall and colleagues (25) have shown a marked reduction in the need for pharyngeal flaps.

SECONDARY PALATAL PROCEDURES

Secondary palatal surgery is directed at correction of two problem areas: the closure of palatal fistulas and the treatment of velopharyngeal incompetence. This requires close collaboration between a skilled speech pathologist and the surgeon. Techniques for the evaluation of fistulas and velopharyngeal incompetence are discussed in Chapter 30.

PALATAL FISTULAS

Palatal fistulas may allow the troublesome leakage of fluid or food particles through the nose. This can cause chronic nasal irritation and, on occasion, may contribute to articulation dis-

tortion during speech. In general, speech disturbances are only significant in the presence of a large fistula (26,27).

The closure of a palatal fistula can be among the most difficult of all surgical procedures and, in almost all cases, even small fistulas require the elevation of large palatal flaps. Whenever feasible, a two-layer (nasal and oral), tension-free closure should be accomplished. Without a completely tension-free repair, the recurrence rate is high, and the greater the number of attempts at closure, the higher the likelihood of failure with regional palatal tissue. Schultz (28) and Jackson (29,30) suggest the beneficial effect of simultaneous bone grafting at the time of anterior fistula closure. However, othodontic arch alignment should precede the closure of the defect.

In such cases of intractable oronasal fistula, posterior and anteriorly based dorsal tongue flaps have successfully closed large palatal fistulas when no other method seemed feasible (31–33). Recently, Pribaz (34) described a myomucosal flap based on the facial artery (FAMM flap) for the closure of the more difficult fistula. The flap can be based either superiorly with retrograde flow from the angular artery to reconstruct anterior palatal defects, or inferiorly with antegrade flow from the facial artery to reconstruct defects of the soft palate and posterior portion of the hard palate. Finally, distant tissue transfer always remains an alternative (35,36).

TREATMENT OF VELOPHARYNGEAL INCOMPETENCE

Despite anatomic restoration of the continuity of the palatal cleft, persistent velopharyngeal insufficiency (VPI) occurs.

Symptoms of VPI range from 5 to 35% in the literature (37), the difference depending not only on the type of palate repair but also on opinion as to what constitutes VPI and its cause (38). The assessment is made by the speech therapist, guided by findings on videofluoroscopy and nasoendoscopy. If significant improvement in speech cannot be demonstrated with speech therapy alone, then surgery for a structurally related cause of velopharyngeal incompetence is recommended. Numerous surgical techniques have been described; they can be broadly grouped into (a) posterior pharyngeal wall augmentation, (b) pharyngeal flap, (c) sphincter pharyngoplasty, and (d) palatal lengthening procedures.

When there is good mobility of the palate and a small discrepancy in the distance between the palate and the posterior pharynx, velopharyngeal augmentation techniques have been suggested. Implants introduced into the retropharyngeal space have limited usefulness (39–42). In cases with minimal velopharyngeal gap, palatal lengthening with either a V–Y push-back procedure or a Furlow double-opposing Z plasty should be considered when the initial palatal repair is judged to be inadequate (43,44).

When the soft palate is anatomically short or functionally immobile, the most common procedure has been the construction of a pharyngeal flap. The flap is developed from the posterior pharyngeal wall incorporating the superior constrictor muscle, turned anteriorly and inset into the soft palate by one of a number of variations (45–47). The superiorly based flaps have the advantage of drawing the palate in the direction favorable for velopharyngeal closure (48). The flap, as an isthmus of tissue joining the soft palate with the posterior pharynx, centrally decreases the cross-sectional area of the nasopharyngeal space. Success then relies on the degree to which the remaining lateral spaces or ports are occluded by the medial movement of the lateral pharyngeal walls during speech (49–51). In recent years major centers have increasingly considered sphincter pharyngoplasty as an alternative.

Hynes in 1950 first described the sphincter pharyngoplasty by approximating flaps developed from the lateral pharyngeal wall in a cross-over manner high on the posterior pharyngeal wall at the level of the Passavant ridge (52). While the initial description the flap incorporated only the salpingopharyngeus muscle, Hynes in 1953 included the posterior tonsillar pillar with the palatopharyngeus in the lateral flaps (53). In modifications proposed by Orticochea (54,55) and Jackson (56), only the palatopharyngeus of the posterior tonsillar pillar is used and the two lateral flaps are approximated end-to-end rather than overlapped, as in Hynes' description. Orticochea placed the sphincter below the level of the palatal plane, but as Jackson (57) and Riski and colleagues (58) have emphasized, placement of the sphincter at a higher level where the palate would come in contact with the posterior pharyngeal wall achieves a more satisfactory competence of velopharyngeal mechanism. Unlike the pharyngeal flap, the technique circumferentially decreases the nasopharyngeal orifice, and in theory there is the potential to function as a dynamic sphincter. In patients with poor lateral pharyngeal wall motion and good mobility of the palate, sphincter-type pharyngoplasty would be the obvious choice. The transposed flaps act to augment the posterior pharynx, decreasing the anterior–posterior diameter and allowing velopharyngeal closure.

No single technique can consistently accomplish (or substitute for) the complex mechanism involved in the normal velopharyngeal function during speech. We can hope that in time differential diagnosis of VPI will lead to differential surgical management (38) and—what is perhaps more important—the initial palatal repair, restoring the levator mechanism and gaining the soft palatal length and mobility (12,20,23).

Bibliography

1. Stark RB. Embryology of the oral cavity. In: Stark RB, ed. *Plastic surgery of the head and neck.* New York: Churchill Livingstone, 1986; 2:1277–1279.
2. Stark RB. Embryology of the lips and chin. In: Stark RB, ed. *Plastic surgery of the head and neck.* New York: Churchill Livingstone, 1986; 2:1167–1169.
3. Johnston MC. The neural crest in abnormalities of the face and brain. *Birth Defects* 1975; 11:1.
4. Vermeij-Keers CHR, Poelmann RE, Smiths-Van Prooije AE, et al. Hypertelorism and the median cleft face syndrome: An embryological analysis. *Ophthal Paediatr Genet* (Amsterdam) 1984; 4:97.
5. Sedano HO, Cohen MM Jr, Jirasek J, et al. Frontonasal dysplasia. *J Pediatr* 1970; 76:906.
6. Sulik KK. Craniofacial defects from genetic and teratogen-induced deficiencies in presomite embryos. *Birth Defects* 1984; 1:79.
7. Stark RB, Kaplan J. Development of the cleft lip and nose. *Plast Reconstr Surg* 1973; 51:413.
8. Kernahan DA, Stark RB. A new classification for cleft lip and cleft palate. *Plastic Reconstr Surg* 1958; 22:435.
9. Fogh-Anderson P. Vital statistics of cleft lip and palate—past, present, and future. *Acta Chir Plast* 1963; 5:169.
10. Fogh-Anderson P. *Inheritance of harelip and cleft palate.* Copenhagen: Nordisk, Forlag-Arnold Busch, 1942.
11. Lynch HT, Kimberling WJ. Genetic counseling in cleft lip and cleft palate. *Plast Reconstr Surg* 1981; 68:800.
12. Kriens OB. Anatomy of the velopharyngeal area in cleft palate. *Clin Plast Surg* 1975; 2:261.
13. Latham RA, Long RE Jr, Latham EA. Cleft palate velopharyngeal musculature in a 5-month-old infant: a three-dimensional histological reconstruction. *Cleft Palate J* 1980; 17:1.
14. Dickson DR, Dickson WM. Velopharyngeal anatomy. *J Speech Hear Res* 1972; 15:372.
15. Randall P. Cleft palate. In: Grabb WC, Smith JW, eds. *Plastic surgery.* Boston: Little, Brown, 1979; 205.
16. Dorrance GM. Lengthening of the soft palate operations. *Ann Surg* 1925; 82:208.
17. Cronin TD. Method of preventing raw area on the nasal surface of the hard palate in push-back surgery. *Plast Reconstr Surg* 1957; 20:474.
18. Millard DR Jr. The island flap in cleft palate surgery. *Surg Gynecol Obstet* 1963; 116:297.
19. Manchester WM. The repair of double cleft lip as part of an integrated program. *Plast Reconstr Surg* 1970; 45:207.
20. Furlow LT. Cleft palate repair by double opposing Z-plasty. *Plast Reconstr Surg* 1986; 78:724.
21. Randall P, LaRossa D, Solomon M, et al. Experience with the Furlow double-reversing Z-plasty for cleft palate repair. *Plast Reconstr Surg* 1986; 77:569.
22. Lindsay WK, LeMesurier AB, Farmer AW. A study of speech results of a large series of cleft palate patients. *Plast Reconstr Surg* 1962; 29:273.
23. Jackson IT, McLennan G, Scheker LR. Primary veloplasty or primary palatoplasty: some preliminary findings. *Plast Reconstr Surg* 1983; 72:153.
24. Braithwaite F. Cleft palate repair. In: Gibson T, ed. *Modern trends in plastic surgery.* London: Butterworth, 1964; 30–49.
25. Randall P, LaRossa DD, Fakhraee SM, et al. Cleft palate closure at 3 to 7 months of age: a preliminary report. *Plast Reconstr Surg* 1983; 71:624.
26. D'Antonio L, Barlow S, Warren D. Studies of oronasal fistulae: implications for speech motor control. Presented at the annual meeting, Speech-Language-Hearing Association, San Antonio, November 20, 1992. *ASHA* 1992; 34:28A.

27. Henningsson G, Isberg A. Oronasal fistulas and speech production. In: Bardach J, Morris HL, eds. *Multidisciplinary management of cleft lip and palate.* Philadelphia: WB Saunders, 1990; 787.

28. Schultz RC. Management and timing of cleft palate fistula repair. *Plast Reconstr Surg* 1986; 78:739.

29. Jackson IT. Closure of secondary palatal fistulae with intra-oral tissue and bone grafting. *Br J Plast Surg* 1972; 25:93.

30. Jackson MS, Jackson IT, Christie F. Improvement in speech following closure of anterior palatal fistulas with bone grafts. *Br J Plast Surg* 1976; 29:295.

31. Guerrero-Santos J, Altamirano JT. The use of lingual flaps in repair of fistulas of the hard palate. *Plast Reconstr Surg* 1966; 38:123.

32. Barone CM, Argamaso RV. Refinements of the tongue flap for closure of palatal fistulas. *J Craniofac Surg* 1993; 4:109.

33. Argamaso RV. The tongue flap: placement and fixation for closure of post-palatoplasty fistulae. *Cleft Palate J* 1990; 27:402.

34. Pribaz J, Stephens W, Crespo L, et al. A new intraoral flap: facial artery musculomucosal (FAMM) flap. *Plast Reconstr Surg* 1992; 90:421.

35. MacLeod AM, Morrison WA, McCann JJ, et al. The free radial forearm flap with and without bone for closure of large palatal fistulae. *Br J Plast Surg* 1987; 40:391.

36. Furnas DW. Temporal osteocutaneous island flaps for complete reconstruction of cleft palate defects. *Scand J Plast Reconstr Surg Hand Surg* 1987; 1987; 21:119.

37. Bardach J, Morris HL, eds. *Multidisciplinary management of cleft lip and palate.* Philadelphia: Saunders, 1990; 303–305.

38. Witt PD, D'Antonio LL. Velopharyngeal insufficiency and secondary palatal management: a new look at an old problem (review). *Clin Plast Surg* 1993; 20:707.

39. Denny AD, Marks SM, Oliff-Carneol S. Correction of velopharyngeal insufficiency by pharyngeal augmentation using autogenous cartilage: a preliminary report. *Cleft palate Craniofac J* 1993; 30:46.

40. Remacle M, Bertrand B, Eloy P, et al. The use of injectable collagen to correct velopharyngeal insufficiency. *Laryngoscope* 1990; 100:269.

41. Sturim HS, Jacob CT. Teflon pharyngoplasty. *Plast Reconstr Surg* 1972; 49:180.

42. Brauer RO. Retropharyngeal implantation of silicone gel pillows for velopharyngeal incompetence. *Plast Reconstr Surg* 1973; 51:254.

43. Dreyer TM, Trier WC. A comparison of palatoplasty techniques. *Cleft Palate J* 1984; 21:251.

44. Chen PK, Wu JT, Chen YR, et al. Correction of secondary velopharyngeal insufficiency in cleft palate patients with Furlow palatoplasty. *Plast Reconstr Surg* 1994; 94:933.

45. Sanvenero-Roselli G. Divisione palatine e sua cura chirurgica. Atti del Congresso Internazionale Stomatologia 1935; 36:391.

46. Johns DF, Cannito MP, Rohrich R, et al. The self-lined based pull-through velopharyngoplasty: plastic surgery–speech pathology interaction in the management of velopharyngeal insufficiency. *Plast Reconstr Surg* 1994; 94:436.

47. Fischer-Brandies E, Nejedlo I. A modification of the Sanvenero-Rosselli velopharyngoplasty. *J Craniomaxillofac Surg* 1993; 21:19.

48. Owsley JQ, Lawson LI, Miller ER, et al. Experience with high attached pharyngeal flap. *Plast Reconstr Surg* 1966; 38:232.

49. Skolnick ML, McCall GN. Velopharyngeal competence and incompetence following pharyngeal flap surgery: videofluoroscopic study in multiple projections. *Cleft Palate J* 1972; 9:1.

50. Shprintzen RJ, Lewin ML, Croft CB, et al. A comprehensive study of pharyngeal flap surgery: tailor-made flaps. *Cleft Palate J* 1979; 16:46.

51. Hogan VM. A biased approach to the treatment of velopharyngeal incompetence. *Clin Plast Surg* 1975; 2:319.

52. Hynes W. Pharyngoplasty by muscle transplantation. *Br J Plast Surg* 1950; 3:128.

53. Hynes W. Results of pharyngoplasty by muscle transplantation in "failed cleft palate" cases. *Ann R Coll Surg Engl* 1953; 13:17.

54. Orticochea M. A review of 236 cleft palate patients treated with dynamic muscle sphincter. *Plast Reconstr Surg* 1983; 73:180.

55. Orticochea M. Results of the dynamic muscle sphincter operation in cleft palates. *Br J Plast Surg* 1970; 23:108.

56. Jackson IT, Silverton JS. The sphincter pharyngoplasty as a secondary procedure in cleft palates. *Plast Reconstr Surg* 1977; 59:518.

57. Jackson IT. Sphincter pharyngoplasty. *Clin Plast Surg* 1985; 12:711.

58. Riski JR, Serafin D, Riefkohl R, et al. A rationale for modifying the site of insertion of the orticochea pharyngoplasty. *Plast Reconstr Surg* 1984; 73:882.

28

Secondary Deformities of Cleft Lip and Palate

Joseph G. McCarthy, M.D., F.A.C.S., and Court B. Cutting, M.D., F.A.C.S.

The variety of secondary facial deformities after cleft lip and palate repair is unending and usually reflects the surgical techniques and principles employed at the time of the primary repair. It is essential that all infants with a cleft of the lip and/or palate be enrolled with a multidisciplinary clinical team that can provide the judgment and clinical expertise to ensure an optimal result.

Secondary Lip Deformities

ANALYSIS OF THE PROBLEM

1. Full-thickness lip
   (a) Vertical excess
   (b) Vertical deficiency
   (c) Horizontal excess (including philtral)
   (d) Horizontal deficiency (including philtral)
2. Skin
   (a) Scars, stitch marks
   (b) Loss of philtral column
3. Vermilion–white line
   (a) Malalignment of white line
   (b) Loss of tubercle
   (c) Loss of Cupid's bow
   (d) Whistle deformity
4. Muscle
   (a) Incomplete union/malposition
5. Labiobuccal sulcus
   (a) Deficiency/obliteration

Full-Thickness Lip

The excessively long lip (vertical excess) (Fig. 28–1) is usually associated with certain types of primary lip repair. For example, the LeMesurier procedure has been generally abandoned because of this problem. Converse (1) described a technique of correcting the problem by excising the horizontal scar resulting from the closure. However, the excessively long lip is rarely seen after repair of a bilateral cleft lip.

Vertical deficiency (Fig. 28–2) in unilateral cleft lip is usually seen after a straight-line or Rose-Thompson repair. In such a situation, if the vertical deficiency is severe the cleft should be recreated by excising the surgical scar in a full-thickness fashion and lengthened using the procedure of Millard (2) or a Z-plasty technique. A vertical deficiency can be temporarily observed at the level of the vermilion or labial mucosa in the first year after the Millard repair.

The short (vertical) lip after repair of a bilateral cleft poses more of a problem, because lengthening of the lip is usually done at the expense of the horizontal lip dimension. For this reason, it is not uncommon to use an Abbé or cross-lip flap and recreate the entire philtrum. It is unlikely that simple Z-plasty techniques can correct this problem.

Horizontal excess is most commonly seen after bilateral cleft-lip repair when there is gradual widening of the philtrum. Correction of this deficiency is relatively straightforward and usually involves resection of sufficient lip tissue so that the resulting scars simulate the philtral columns. The excess lip tissue can be salvaged to lengthen the columella and elevate the nasal tip, as in the Millard forked-flap procedure (3; Fig. 28–3).

Horizontal deficiency (Fig. 28–4) is usually manifest as a tight upper lip resulting from excessive discarding of lip tissue at the time of the primary repair. On profile view, the lower lip usually projects more than the upper lip. The Abbé cross-lip flap is a satisfactory method of adding a significant amount of lip tissue to the midline of the upper lip and simulating the philtrum (Fig. 28–5). However, the appearance of the donor lower lip scar is not always satisfactory. In both the unilateral and bilateral cleft lip, it is preferable to place the Abbé flap in an upper midline incision (4). At a later date, the previous scars in the unilateral lip can be revised. In designing an Abbé flap, the surgeon should note that the width of the adult philtrum ranges from 8 to 12 mm at the vermilion border and from 6 to 9 mm at the base of the columella. The maximum length of the normal adult philtrum is 17 mm. These dimensions must be followed in designing the Abbé flap.

Skin

If the full-thickness dimensions of the upper lip are satisfactory and there are only superficial cutaneous irregularities such as scars and suture marks, simple excision and revision can be performed. While dermabrasion can be a helpful technique for improving the appearance of superficial irregularities, it is generally disappointing in treating lip scars.

The presence of the philtrum is an absolute requirement for an aesthetically satisfactory upper lip and is the main advantage of the Millard repair (2), because the resulting scar simulates the philtral columns. Techniques have been described for reconstructing the philtrum. The Abbé flap, when placed in the midline of the upper lip, simulates the philtrum (see Fig. 28–5). Cutaneous rotation flaps have been described by O'Connor and McGregor (5), and Neuner (6) used auricular cartilage grafts, placed subcutaneously, to reconstruct the philtral columns and dimple. Unfortunately, auricular cartilage reconstruction of the

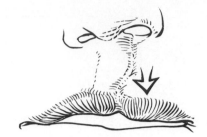

FIG. 28–1.   Vertical lip excess.

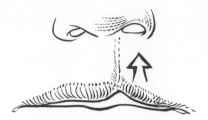

FIG. 28–2.   Vertical lip deficiency.

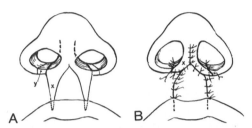

FIG. 28–3.   Forked flap technique of Millard (3). **A,** outline of incisions and wedge excisions from the nostril floor. **B,** closure after advancement of the lip flaps elevates the nasal tip and restores the Cupid's bow. (From Converse JM, et al. Secondary deformities of cleft lip, cleft lip and nose, and cleft palate. In: Converse JM, McCarthy JG, eds. *Reconstructive plastic surgery.* Philadelphia: WB Saunders, 1977; 4:2165.)

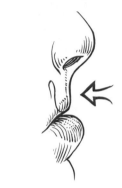

FIG. 28–4.   Horizontal lip deficiency.

FIG. 28–5.   Cross-lip flap reconstruction of a horizontal and verical lip deficiency. **A, B,** lower-lip donor flap and recipient incision. Note that the flap is placed midline to simulate the philtrum. The unilateral cleft lip scare can be revised at a later date. **C,** flap is prepared by applying the principles of the muscle shelf. The shelf fits snugly under the columella, producing an elevation of the columella and facilitating skin-to-skin approximation in the repair of the subnasal area. **D,** diagram shows the vascular supply. The flap is rotated on a small vascular pedicle that includes a mucosal bridge. **E,** shelving muscle flap is drawn under the columella by mattress sutures, which are tied over a small cotton bolster within the nostril. (From Converse JM, et al. Secondary deformities of cleft lip, cleft lip and nose, and cleft palate. In: Converse JM, McCarthy JG, eds. *Reconstructive plastic surgery.* Philadelphia: WB Saunders, 1977; 4:2165.)

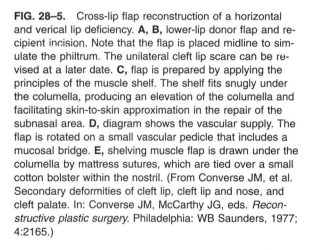

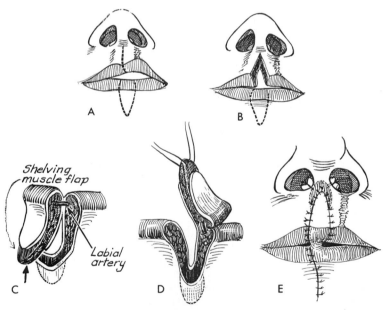

philtral column and dimple often looks satisfactory in a photograph but appears stiff and unnatural during facial animation. A more satisfactory reconstruction of the philtral column and dimple may be accomplished by the technique illustrated in Figure 28–6. At the time of cleft-lip revision, the medial skin edge is elevated away from the muscle of the lip. Care is taken not to dissect farther than the depth of the proposed philtral dimple. The muscle is then incised and overlapped over the medial muscle and sutured in place before skin repair. This type of "pants-over-vest" muscle repair exaggerates column projection and deepens the philtral dimple.

Vermilion–White Line

Malalignment at the level of the white line is not uncommon and has been referred to as the "red flare." It is usually corrected with an appropriately placed Z-plasty (Fig. 28–7).

The vermilion tubercle is also an essential aesthetic feature of the upper lip. Its absence is usually due to the fact that an excess of vermilion was sacrificed in the primary repair, or the orbicularis muscle was inadequately sutured at the cleft site. The correction usually requires that the inferior portion of the repair be reopened and flaps of vermilion and muscle advanced to the midline to simulate the tubercle.

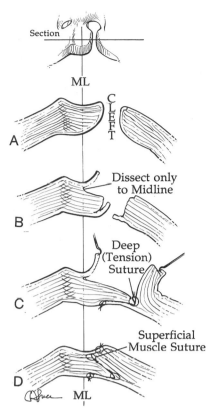

FIG. 28–6. Pants-over-vest closure to simulate the philtral column. **A,** unilateral cleft lip (ML, midline). **B,** elevation of medial skin flap to ML. **C,** posterior closure. **D,** completion of closure.

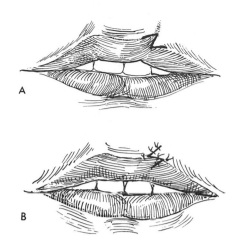

FIG. 28–7. Malalignment at the level of the white line of the upper lip. **A,** the Z-plasty is outlined. **B,** transposition of the flaps restores the white line. Secondary deformities of cleft lip, cleft lip and nose, and cleft palate. (From Converse JM, et al. Secondary deformities of cleft lip, cleft lip and nose, and cleft palate. In: Converse JM, McCarthy JG, eds. *Reconstructive plastic surgery.* Philadelphia: WB Saunders, 1977; 4:2165.)

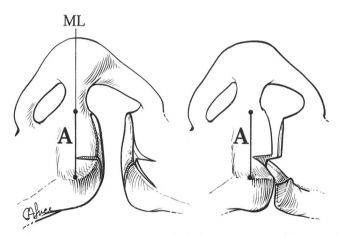

FIG. 28–8. Flattening of the Cupid's bow, as occurs with triangular cleft-lip repair. ML = midline; A = distance between depth of Cupid's bow and midpoint of columellor–lip junction. Note there is no increase in distance A.

The Cupid's bow is likewise a critical element of upper-lip aesthetics. The advantage of the Millard unilateral lip repair is that it preserves the Cupid's bow. The triangular repair, however, tends to flatten the Cupid's bow, as shown in Figure 28–8.

The Cupid's bow can be excessively wide in the bilateral cleft lip, and the excess can be incorporated into skin flaps and used in lengthening of the columella (see Fig. 28–3). If the lip scar is excised in a full-thickness fashion and the cleft recreated, the Millard rotation-advancement repair can be used, and a flap of orbicularis muscle from the lateral segment is advanced into a tunnel at the vermilion level of the medial portion of the lip.

The whistle deformity is characterized by a notching of the upper lip at the site of the lip repair. The incisors are usually exposed, and the patient lacks lip competence. The preferred repair includes the development of large bilateral rotation flaps with pedicles based on the vermilion border (Fig. 28–9). The flaps are then rotated toward the apex of the whistle deformity and closed in a V–Y fashion. It is essential that the flaps be broadly based. For less severe whistle deformities, a Z-plasty can be performed at the level of the vermilion and labial mucosa. A useful technique is the "unequal" Z-plasty (Fig. 28–10), in which one flap contains some of the underlying orbicularis muscle (7; see Fig. 28–8). Kapetansky (8) described double "pendulum" flaps of orbicularis muscle that are advanced into the whistle deformity defect. The addition of an autogenous fascial graft at the site of the defect has also been recommended (9).

Muscle

In cleft lip repair, it is important that particular emphasis be placed on restoring the orbicularis sphincter (10). Failure to do so at the time of the primary repair results in persistent bulging of the ununited muscle bundles at the alar base in the lateral segment and the columella in the medial segment of the unilateral cleft lip and at both alar bases of the bilateral cleft lip. Surgical correction (Fig. 28–11) involves full-thickness excision of the cleft lip scar, dissection of the muscle bundles, and division of the quadratus labii superioris muscle. The muscle flaps are then skeletonized and united at the cleft site in the unilateral cleft lip and in the prolabial segment of the bilateral cleft lip. The repair is completed by closure of the cutaneous, vermilion, and mucosal incisions.

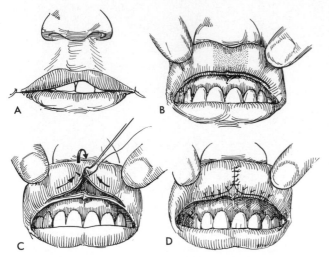

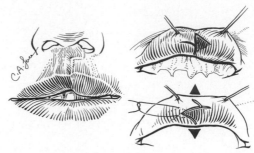

FIG. 28–10. "Unequal" Z-plasty is performed for correction of a mild whistle deformity. *Left,* lip incompetence with incisor exposure. *Right,* flaps are outlined. The central limb is aligned at the whistle deformity. The cross-hatched flap contains underlying orbicularis muscle. The flaps are transposed.

FIG. 28–9. Correction of the whistle deformity. **A,** at rest, the patient lacks complete lip competence, and the incisors are exposed. **B,** bilateral labial mucosal rotation flaps are outlined. **C,** rotation of the flaps lengthens the lip. **D,** incisions are closed in a V–Y fashion. (From Converse JM, et al. Secondary deformities of cleft lip, cleft lip and nose, and cleft palate. In: Converse JM, McCarthy JG, eds. *Reconstructive plastic surgery.* Philadelphia: WB Saunders, 1977; 4:2165.)

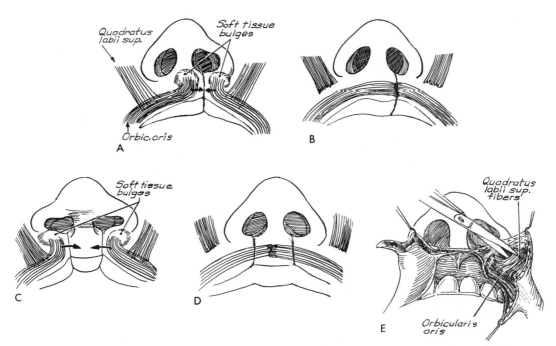

FIG. 28–11. **A,** orbicularis oris fibers are misdirected in the unilateral cleft lip, forming a bulge on each side of the cleft. **B,** after division of the fibers of the quadratus labii superioris muscle, the orbicularis oris muscle is redirected and sutured. **C,** a similar muscle malalignment is found in the complete bilateral cleft. **D,** the fibers of the orbicularis oris are redirected and introduced into the prolabial segment. **E,** sectioning of the quadratus labii superioris muscle allows redirection of the orbicularis oris muscle. (From Converse JM, et al. Secondary deformities of cleft lip, cleft lip and nose, and cleft palate. In: Converse JM, McCarthy JG, eds. *Reconstructive plastic surgery.* Philadelphia: WB Saunders, 1977; 4:2165.)

Labiobuccal Sulcus

For severe deficiencies involving obliteration of the labiobuccal sulcus, the Esser inlay technique, using either split-thickness skin graft or buccal mucosa, has been employed. However, a prosthesis usually must be constructed to achieve satisfactory inset of the graft, and also to prevent contracture of the sulcus in the year after surgery. The problem most often is seen at the junction of the prolabium and premaxilla after bilateral cleft lip repair. A variety of Z-plasty and V–Y advancement techniques have also been recommended for lesser deficiencies of the labiobuccal sulcus.

Deformities of the Alveolus, Maxilla, and Palate

ANALYSIS OF THE PROBLEM

1. Alveolus
   (a) Cleft, unilateral or bilateral ± lateral maxillary segment collapse
2. Maxilla
   (a) Pyriform aperture deficiency (class I occlusion)
   (b) Maxillary hypoplasia (class III malocclusion and anterior cross-bite)
3. Palate
   (a) Fistula
4. Combinations of the above

Alveolar Clefts

This discussion does not cover primary alveolar bone graft (performed as early as 3 months after the primary lip repair) but instead discusses secondary bone grafting of alveolar clefts performed before the eruption of the permanent canine teeth (7 to 12 years of age). There are numerous advantages associated with bone grafting of alveolar clefts at this age (11). If the erupting teeth can be brought into the bone-grafted space, the need for permanent dentures may be obviated. Moreover, the bone graft provides better periodontal support for teeth previously poorly encased in deficient alveolar bone at the site of the cleft. In addition, the bone grafts can also provide better support for the alar base and nasal platform. Bone grafting done in this region will also yield superior results in terms of simultaneous closure of associated oronasal fistulae.

In the repair of unilateral alveolar clefts, any lateral maxillary dentoalveolar segmental collapse is corrected orthodontically before the bone-grafting procedure. It is imperative that, at the time of surgery, the bone grafts are covered by adequate soft-tissue flaps on the nasal and oral sides (Fig. 28–12). In bilateral alveolar clefts, orthodontic therapy is usually required to expand the entire maxillary arch, and the orthodontic appliance must be kept in place at the time of surgery. Bone grafting in bilateral clefts requires careful attention to the maintenance of blood supply to the premaxilla. A variety of bone-graft donor sites are available; the most commonly used sites are the calvaria (cranium) and ilium.

Maxilla

The maxillary hypoplasia observed in the cleft-palate patient can take many forms. In some patients, the occlusion is satisfactory (class I), and the deficiency is restricted solely to the region of the pyriform aperture. In this situation, either autogenous septal cartilage (layered) or inner-table iliac or outer-table cranial bone grafts can be inserted through a buccal incision and carefully placed over the maxilla at the margin of the pyriform aperture (Fig. 28–13). In addition to improving maxillary contour, the technique also provides better support to the nasal platform.

The other type of maxillary hypoplasia observed in the cleft-palate patient is more generalized and involves the entire maxilla. An anterior cross-bite and class III malocclusion are observed. Preoperative orthodontic therapy is employed in order to expand the maxillary arch and to exaggerate the anterior cross-bite (12) in anticipation of a Le Fort I advancement osteotomy (Fig. 28–14). The latter is the ideal treatment for this type of maxillary hypoplasia. In addition to restoring the occlusion, the procedure affords considerable aesthetic improvement in lip posture and maxillary form. However, the patient with a repaired cleft palate is at risk for developing velopharyngeal incompetence after a Le Fort I advancement and must be forewarned preoperatively (13).

Posnick (14) has popularized concomitant closure of a residual alveolar cleft (13) by rotating the lateral maxillary segment to the midline at the time of the LeFort I osteotomy.

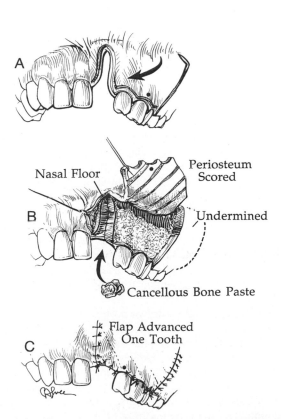

FIG. 28–12. Closure and bone grafting of an alveolar cleft. **A,** outline of gingival incisions. **B,** elevation of anterior flaps and closure of posterior flap. **C,** closure is complete. (From Converse JM, et al. Secondary deformities of cleft lip, cleft lip and nose, and cleft palate. In: Converse JM, McCarthy JG, eds. *Reconstructive plastic surgery.* Philadelphia: WB Saunders, 1977; 4:2165.)

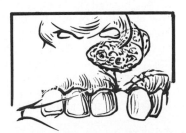

FIG. 28–13. Bone or cartilage grafting of the maxilla in the region of the pyriform aperture. (From Converse JM, et al. Secondary deformities of cleft lip, cleft lip and nose, and cleft palate. In: Converse JM, McCarthy JG, eds. *Reconstructive plastic surgery.* Philadelphia: WB Saunders, 1977; 4:2165.)

FIG. 28–14. Le Fort I advancement osteotomy. *Left,* maxillary hypoplasia, anterior cross-bite, and class III malocclusion are associated with repaired unilateral cleft lip/palate. *Center,* osteotomy and direction to advancement are outlined. *Right,* after advancement, the bone grafts are placed in the retromaxillary space and over the anterior maxilla. (From Converse JM, et al. Secondary deformities of cleft lip, cleft lip and nose, and cleft palate. In: Converse JM, McCarthy JG, eds. *Reconstructive plastic surgery.* Philadelphia: WB Saunders, 1977; 4:2165.)

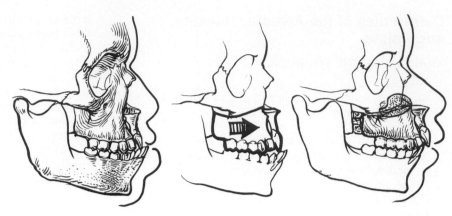

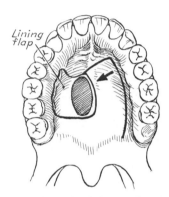

FIG. 28–15. Closure of a palatal fistula. The lining flap provides nasal closure, and a large papatal rotation flap is used for oral coverage. (From Converse JM, et al. Secondary deformities of cleft lip, cleft lip and nose, and cleft palate. In: Converse JM, McCarthy JG, eds. *Reconstructive plastic surgery.* Philadelphia: WB Saunders, 1977; 4:2165.)

Palate

Fistulae can be observed after cleft-palate repair, usually in the region of the incisive foramen or at the junction of the hard and soft palate. Small oronasal fistulae are amenable to surgical correction, provided there is adequate vascularization of the surrounding soft tissue to allow the mucoperiosteal flaps to provide coverage without tension. A basic principle in the repair of palatal fistulae is that the flaps are designed to be relatively large in size. The lining flaps are usually obtained from the nasal cavity or vomer. Alternatively, turnover flaps (Fig. 28–15) can provide nasal coverage. The oral coverage flap is usually obtained from the palatal mucoperiosteum. Closure of large palatal fistulae poses a greater problem because of the paucity of local tissue for their reconstruction. Tongue flaps, and even flaps from a distance, have been reported for successful closure. An obturator constructed by a prosthodontist is an alternative solution, but often this does not find patient favor.

Combination of the Above

The surgeon is often presented with a patient showing a combination of the above deformities: alveolar cleft, palatal fistula, deficiency in the region of the pyriform aperture, and unsatisfactory lip scar. In this situation, the technique illustrated in Figure 28–12 is indicated (15). In a single stage, the lip scar is excised and exposure of the alveolar cleft-oronasal fistula is gained. Nasal flaps in the region of the alveolus and turnover flaps are developed above the periphery of the oronasal (palatal) fistula in order to achieve nasal closure. Bone grafts, harvested either from the calvaria or ilium, are placed into the alveolar cleft and in the region of the pyriform aperture. A buccal vestibular flap is elevated and transposed across the alveolar flap in order to provide oral coverage in this area. Bilateral palatal mucoperiosteal flaps (Veau) are elevated in a subperiosteal plane and transposed over the palatal fistula. The lip revision is then accomplished as previously discussed.

Cleft Lip–Nose Deformity

DESCRIPTION

The surgical approach to the cleft nose deformity can be undertaken only after the surgeon gains an understanding of the anatomy and development of the deformity. The deformity may best be understood by reviewing Latham's (16) concept of cleft palate embryology. The premaxillary bony segment is connected to the base of the nasal septum by the "septopremaxillary ligament." As the nasal septum grows anteriorly and inferiorly, it carries the premaxilla with it by virtue of the attachment of this ligament. If the mesodermal streaming from the lateral premaxilla penetrates the epithelial bilayer and the premaxilla is joined to the lateral palatal shelves, the premaxilla is held somewhat posterior by this attachment, and the lateral palatal shelves are drawn anterior and held somewhat separated from one another by the premaxilla.

The premaxilla is then drawn posteriorly along the base of the nasal septum. As this process continues, a nasal columella gradually forms, and the base of the ala of the nose is brought further anteriorly. However, if fusion fails to occur, the premaxilla is placed anteriorly along the base of the nasal septum and the base of the ala is posteriorly placed. This anatomic arrangement has adverse effects on the shape and development of the growing nose (17).

Because of the anterior displacement of the premaxilla, which is especially pronounced in a bilateral deformity, the columellar skin does not elongate properly. A retracted nasal tip is usually associated with the short columella. The posterior position of the alar base with respect to the columella tends to pull the alar cartilage (and nostril rim) laterally and inferiorly, thus obliterating the soft triangle of the nose, pulling the domes apart, and producing a tendency to nasal-tip bifidity. The posterior distraction of the alar cartilage results in flattening of the dome on the cleft side.

The effects on the nasal septum of this process have been described by Hogan and Converse (4) as a "tilted tripod" (Fig. 28–16). The lateral aspects of the nose may be considered to be leaves of a tent with the nasal septum forming the tent pole in the middle. If one side is displaced posteriorly, there is a tendency of the tent pole (septum) to buckle in the midportion and shift its base, resulting in nasal septal deviation.

Aside from the simple positional aspects of the cleft lip–nasal deformity, one must also consider the mesodermal deficiency on the cleft side of the nose. Avery (18) studied the nasal capsule cartilage in the cleft deformity and documented a true deficiency in the nasal capsular cartilage. There is also an associated skeletal deficiency of the maxilla under the alar base and in the alveolus.

Because the cleft nasal deformity appears to arise from malposition and deficiency of tissue mass, surgical attempts to correct the problem must be tailored accordingly; efforts to correct the malposition alone are often inadequate. Grafting procedures under the alar base and in the nasal floor and pyriform aperture region are often required. We believe that the deficient soft-tissue matrix (i.e., nasal cutaneous and vestibular skin on the side of the cleft) poses the greatest challenge in the repair of the cleft lip–nose deformity.

Huffman and Lierle (19) described the unilateral cleft lip nose on the basis of their extensive clinical experience (Fig. 28–17). The nasal tip appears to be deviated to the noncleft side because of the flattening of the dome on the cleft side. The dorsally and caudally depressed dome on the cleft side obliterates the soft triangle of the nose and produces a flat dome. There is an obtuse angle between the medial and lateral groove of the cleft alar cartilage, and inward buckling of the cleft ala is also noted in the midposition of the lateral groove of the alar cartilage. There is usually a flattening or absence of the alar-facial groove. The bony platform under the cleft ala is deficient. Horizontal orientation of the nostril on the cleft side is present. It should also be noted that frequently the nostril is small. In association with the deviation of the septum, there is distortion of the columella, and the base of the columella is displaced to the noncleft side. The base of the medial crus is dorsally displaced on the cleft side. There is a vestibular web along the line of the upper edge of the lower lateral cartilage.

The above comments regarding the unilateral cleft-nose deformity are generally applicable to the bilateral deformity with several modifications. Because the premaxilla is anteriorly positioned along the base of the septum in the bilateral cleft nose, the columella skin is reduced in size. The anteriorly positioned premaxilla, in association with the posteriorly displaced alar bases, tends to produce tip bifidity, as described by Stenstrom and Oberg (17). There is often severe flattening in the dome area with bilateral absence of the soft triangle. The absence of projection of the tip further accentuates the skin envelope deficiency in the bilateral cleft lip.

REPAIR OF THE UNILATERAL CLEFT NASAL DEFORMITY

Reconstruction of the Nasal Tip

An "open" surgical approach is usually taken in reconstruction of the tip as part of the cleft rhinoplasty. Bilateral rim incisions, often connected across the columella, provide maximal exposure to the nasal tip. There are a number of suture suspension techniques that have been applied to the repositioning of the cleft ala to produce a more normal shape to the dome on the cleft side (Fig. 28–18). They usually involve suturing the surgically skeletonized ala to the upper lateral cartilages on the cleft and noncleft side, as well as suturing the cleft dome to the dome on the noncleft side. These maneuvers, performed under direct vision, mobilize the alar cartilage on the cleft side in a superior direction, reduce tip bifidity, and increase anterior projection of the cleft dome. Such a technique was described by Tajima and Maruyama (20). Potter (21) mobilized the entire cleft ala, including its mucosal

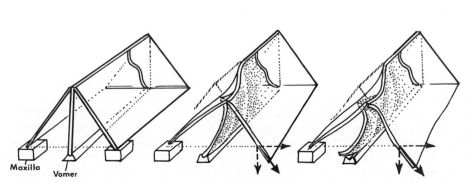

FIG. 28–16. The tilted tripod. **Left,** schematic of the nose illustrates the basic tripod nature of the nasal structures. The tripod consists of the dorsal portion of the septum and nasal bones and the two alar arms. **Middle,** the tilting effect results from maxillary hypoplasia with secondary deformity of the septum and cleft ala. **Right,** a more dramatic illustration of the convex deformity of the septum and the vertical bending of the septum posterior to the junction of the membranous and cartilaginous portions of the septum is evident. Restriction of the caudal border of the septum in its anterior thrust causes it to bend toward the normal nostril. If there is a more severe deformity of the vomer, the septum is displaced into the normal nostril. (After Hogan VM, Converse JM. Secondary deformities of unilateral cleft lip and nose. In: Grabb WC, Rosenstein SE, Bzoch KR, eds. *Cleft lip and palate.* Boston: Little, Brown, 1971.)

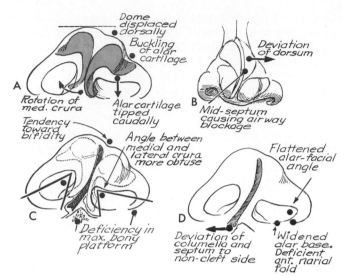

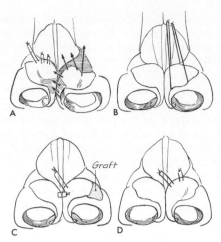

FIG. 28–17. Deformities of the unilateral cleft lip nose. **A,** deviation of the nasal tip is evident. **B,** deviation of the nasal dorsum. The alar cartilage is tipped caudally. **C,** the angle between the medial and lateral crura is more obtuse, and the dome is displaced dorsally. Note the buckling of the lateral crus and the deficiency of the maxillary bone platform. **D,** columella and caudal septum are deviated to the noncleft side. The septum on the convex side causes varying degress of obstruction and alss accentuates the tendency to bifidity. (From Converse JM, et al. Secondary deformities of cleft lip, cleft lip and nose, and cleft palate. In: Converse JM, McCarthy JG, eds. *Reconstructive plastic surgery.* Philadelphia: WB Saunders, 1977; 4:2165.)

FIG. 28–18. Suture fixation of the alar cartilage. **A,** the McIndoe and Rees (24) technique. **B,** the Stenstrom (23) technique. **C,** the method of repair by Rees et al. (39). **D,** the Reynolds and Horton (40) technique. (From Converse JM, et al. Secondary deformities of cleft lip, cleft lip and nose, and cleft palate. In: Converse JM, McCarthy JG, eds. *Reconstructive plastic surgery.* Philadelphia: WB Saunders, 1977; 4:2165.)

FIG. 28–19. Relocation of the alar cartilages. **A,** the Brown and McDowell (26) technique. **B,** the Erich (41) technique. **C,** the Humby (27) technique. **D,** Barsky's (28) method. **E,** the Whitlow and Constable (29) correction. (From Converse JM, et al. Secondary deformities of cleft lip, cleft lip and nose, and cleft palate. In: Converse JM, McCarthy JG, eds. *Reconstructive plastic surgery.* Philadelphia: WB Saunders, 1977; 4:2165.)

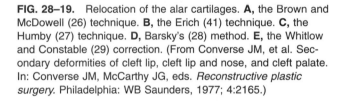

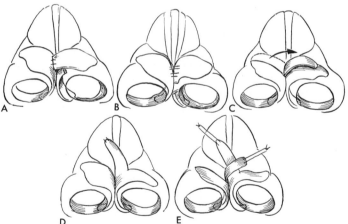

lining, advanced it into the dome region, and sutured it to the dome on the opposite side. This was performed in conjunction with a modified Rethi incision for external approach to the nasal tip. Spira and coworkers (22) and Stenstrom (23) advocated similar suture techniques. McIndoe and Rees (24) recommended mobilization of the cleft ala and suturing it to the upper lateral cartilage as well as the dome on the noncleft side. Similar sutures were used on the noncleft side to project the noncleft dome in a superior and anterior direction.

There are many techniques that mobilize one or both lower lateral (alar) cartilages, split them, and rearrange them in such a way as to obtain a satisfactory nasal tip (Fig. 28–19). Kazanjian (25) advocated sectioning of both lower lateral cartilages at approximately the middle of the lateral crus. The alar segments were then mobilized medially and sutured together. Brown and McDowell (26) sectioned the junction between the medial and lateral crura on the cleft side and mobilized the lateral crus superiorly and medially such that it overlapped the tip of the noncleft dome, to which it was sutured. Humby (27) divided the cephalic portion of the lateral crus on the noncleft side, leaving it attached on a medial pedicle. It was then mobilized and used to overlap the dome on the cleft side to gain tip projection. Barsky (28) divided the cephalic portion of the alar cartilage on the cleft side and mobilized it superiorly over the septum, suturing it in place. Whitlow and Constable (29) mod-

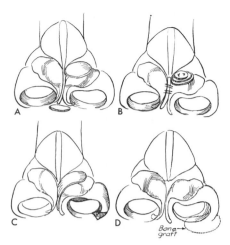

FIG. 28–20. Graft augmentation. **A,** the revision by Fomon et al. (30). **B,** the Musgrave and Dupertuis (42) technique. **C,** Millard's (43) method. **D,** the approach described by Farrior (44), Longacre et al. (45), and Hogan and Converse (4). (From Converse JM, et al. Secondary deformities of cleft lip, cleft lip and nose, and cleft palate. In: Converse JM, McCarthy JG, eds. *Reconstructive plastic surgery.* Philadelphia: WB Saunders, 1977; 4:2165.)

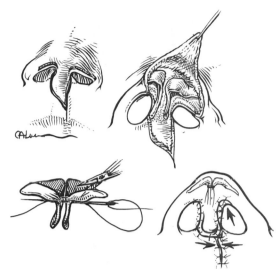

FIG. 28–21. Bardach technique (7) of the cleft rhioplasty. V–Y incision on the lip lengthens the skin of the columella. The external approach with complete mobilization of lateral crura allows recontouring of the cartilages with suture approximation, cartilage grafting, and precise control of tip shape.

ified the preceding techniques in such a way that the cephalic scrolls overlapped one another in the dome region to add projection to the nasal tip.

To avoid cartilage "irregularities," we prefer cartilage grafting techniques over relocation of the alar cartilages in the correction of the cleft nose deformity (Fig. 28–20). Fomon and associates (30) placed grafts under the base of the columella and over the cleft dome. Other surgeons have also written of placing auricular and septal cartilage grafts over the flattened cleft dome. Gorney and Falces (31) advocated placing a cartilage strut along the base of the septum to project the tip. Dibbell (32) sutured a rib cartilage graft in a pocket along the caudal border of the nasal septum from the anterior nasal spine area into the tip.

Shaping the Skin Envelope over the Tip

Thus far, the discussion has been restricted to techniques aimed at creating a cartilaginous skeleton to form a symmetrical nasal tip. While many of these techniques produce a satisfactory skeletal tip, the more difficult problem in cleft rhinoplasty involves the shape of the skin envelope that overlies the tip. The remainder of this section deals with various surgical techniques that have been used to address the problem of the deficiency of the skin envelope over the cleft nose.

Much attention has been directed at the inner vestibular web in cleft rhinoplasty. The shortage of lining within the vestibule tends to pull the tip inferiorly and produces a small inner nostril. Potter (21) advocated a V–Y correction of the vestibular web, leaving the mucoperichondrium attached to the alar cartilage. The alar cartilage is then completely mobilized and transposed to create a skeletal support for the tip. Other authors have suggested that the vestibular web should simply be incised and a secondary defect created—this defect to be grafted with mucosa or split-thickness skin. Millard (33) suggested management of the vestibular web at the

time of initial cleft-lip repair by using an "L flap" from the lateral cleft segment and inserting it into the vestibular mucosa to correct the deficiency in this region.

Cutaneous hooding in the region of the soft triangle of the nose on the cleft side presents the most difficult problem in managing the skin envelope in the cleft nose. The flattening of the cartilaginous dome on the cleft side is accompanied by a cutaneous hood at the apex of the nostril. The lower edge of the deformed alar cartilage lies just within the flattened nostril margin. After mobilizing the alar cartilage with any of the methods previously described, the problem of the cutaneous hood remains to be addressed.

External (cutaneous) approaches to cleft rhinoplasty offer several advantages. Rim incisions coupled with an incision across the base of the columella allow complete unroofing of the dome and structural framework. The complete exposure permits cartilaginous dome reconstruction under direct vision. The benefits of this approach must be balanced against the unfortunate necessity of an external, albeit minor, scar. Bardach (7) recognized the shortage of skin of the columella and recommended the addition of a V–Y advancement of the excess skin from the lip on the cleft side (Fig. 28–21). This technique allows the surgeon to place the external scar within the lines of the cleft-lip scar. Closure of the secondary defect in a V–Y fashion mobilizes the alar base on the cleft side medially. The tendency of the skin to "hood over" once again at the nostril apex may be reduced by suturing the rim incision at the nostril apex to the reconstructed nasal tip cartilage as just described.

If the skin on the cleft side of the columella is severely reduced in relation to that of the normal side, a more radical approach may be required. A vertical incision may be made in the columella between the medial crura. This incision is usually extended onto the dome to varying degrees and into the nostril floor. A superior advancement of the skin and the medial crus thus is achieved to augment the

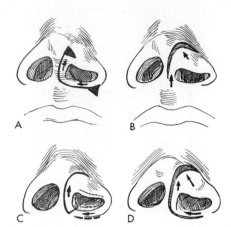

FIG. 28–22. Alar unit rotations. **A,** the Blair (34) approach. **B,** Joseph's (35) technique. **C,** the Gillies and Kilner (36) method. **D,** Berkeley's (46) correction. (From Converse JM, et al. Secondary deformities of cleft lip, cleft lip and nose, and cleft palate. In: Converse JM, McCarthy JG, eds. *Reconstructive plastic surgery.* Philadelphia: WB Saunders, 1977; 4:2165.)

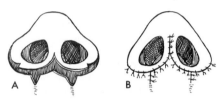

FIG. 28–23. The columella is lengthened using the method of correcting the flat nasal tip with short columella. **A,** bipedicle flaps of skin and subcutaneous tissue in the floor of the nostrils are based medially on the columella and laterally on the alae. A wedge of skin removed form the lower part of each ala diminishes the vertical length of the ala. **B,** freely mobilized flaps are advanced medially and sutured together in the midline to provide the desired increase in the length of the columella. Triangles of skin on the upper lip, as shown in **A,** have been resected because redundant skin is present on the lip when the alae are transferred medially. (From Converse JM, et al. Secondary deformities of cleft lip, cleft lip and nose, and cleft palate. In: Converse JM, McCarthy JG, eds. *Reconstructive plastic surgery.* Philadelphia: WB Saunders, 1977; 4:2165.)

dome region and to increase the length of the columella skin. While this approach is often the most satisfactory, for some patients the scars may be disappointing. Blair (34) advocated such a procedure, including small Burrow triangles in the region of the dome and the alar base on the cleft side (Fig. 28–22A). Using this incision, Joseph (35) excised ellipses of the skin in the dome region and advanced the flattened cleft dome superiorly and medially (Fig. 28–22B). Gillies and Kilner (36) advanced the columella–dome complex with a similar vertical incision along the length of the columella and mobilized a skin flap from the nasal floor to resurface the secondary defect created at the base of the columella (Fig. 28–22C). Berkeley (37) described what is probably the most widely used of these approaches (Fig. 28–22D). An incision is made around the base of the ala and extended along the nostril floor between the medial crura, then onto the dome. The entire cleft-dome–nostril complex is then rotated to increase projection of the tip and lengthen the columella.

Repair of the Bilateral Cleft Lip Nasal Deformity

In the bilateral cleft lip nasal deformity, many of the findings previously discussed are observed on both sides. In addition, the extreme anterior position of the premaxilla at the base of the septum results in a columella that is often short or absent. The posterior position of the alar bases causes the domes to be splayed apart, producing tip bifidity.

Any of the cartilaginous skeletal tip reconstruction techniques discussed in the repair of the unilateral cleft lip nose may be applied to the bilateral cleft lip nose. Because the deformity is bilateral and symmetrical, the surgical results are usually superior to those following unilateral (asymmetrical) cleft-lip rhinoplasty.

There are a number of approaches to the skin envelope problem. The short columella may be done in a number of ways and is one of the most difficult aspects of the correction of the bilateral cleft lip nasal deformity.

Columella lengthening can be the most difficult aspect of correction of the bilateral cleft lip nasal deformity. A fork-flap technique has been advocated (see Fig. 28–3) in which a bilateral V–Y advancement is accomplished. The excess tissue is derived from the wide prolabium along the lines of the previously created lip scar. The technique has the advantage that a new midline scar is not added to the lip. Furthermore, it allows the surgeon to revise the previous lip scars at the time of columella lengthening. However, closure of the fork-flap creates a midline scar at the base of the columella. Closure of the secondary deformities on the lip also tends to produce a slight weakening of the architecture of the Cupid's bow. Cronin (38) recommended lengthening the columella by extending an incision from the base of the columella just below the floor of the nose and onto the area around the alar base (Fig. 28–23). Rotation of the tissue anteriorly and medially is accomplished, producing a V–Y with the point of the Y being advanced to the middle of the columella. This technique has the added advantage of mobilizing the alar bases, which are usually flared, toward the midline.

References

1. Converse JM. Correction of the dropping lateral portion of the cleft lip following the LeMesurier repair. *Plast Reconstr Surg* 1975; 55:501.
2. Millard DR. A primary camouflage in the unilateral harelip. In: Skoog T, ed. *Transactions of the International Congress Plastic Surgery.* Baltimore: Williams & Wilkins, 1955; 160.
3. Millard DR. Columella lengthening by a forked flap. *Plast Reconstr Surg* 1958; 22:454.
4. Hogan VM, Converse JM. Secondary deformities of unilateral cleft lip and nose. In: Grabb WC, Rosenstein SE, Bzoch KR, eds. *Cleft lip and palate.* Boston: Little, Brown, 1971; 245.
5. O'Connor GB, McGregor MW. Surgical formation of the philtrum and the cutaneous upsweep. *Am J Surg* 1958; 95:227.
6. Neuner O. Secondary correction of cleft lip and palate. In: Sanvenero-Rosselli G, ed. *Transactions of the 4th International Congress of Plastic Surgery.* Amsterdam: Excerpta Medica, 1967; 390.
7. Bardach J. Rozszczepy wargi gornej podniebienig. *Panstwowy Zaklad Wydawnictw Lekarskich* (in Polish). Warsaw: Poland, 1967.
8. Kapetansky DI. Double pendulum flaps for whistling deformities in bilateral cleft lips. *Plast Reconstr Surg* 1971; 47:321.
9. Chen PK-T, Noordhoff S, Chen Y-R, et al. Augmentation of the free border of the lip in cleft lip patients using temporoparietal fascia. *Plast Reconstr Surg* 1995; 95:781.

10. Randall P, Whitaker L, LaRossa D. The importance of muscle reconstruction in primary and secondary cleft lip repair. *Plast Reconstr Surg* 1974; 54:316.
11. Wolfe SA, Berkowitz S. The use of cranial bone grafts in the closure of alveolar and anterior palatal clefts. *Plast Reconstr Surg* 1983; 72:659.
12. McCarthy JG, Grayson B, Zide B. The relationship between the surgeon and orthodontist in orthognatic surgery. *Clin Plast Surg* 1982; 9:423.
13. McCarthy JG, Coccaro PJ, Schwartz M, et al. Velopharyngeal function following maxillary advancement. *Plast Reconstr Surg* 1979; 64:180.
14. Posnick JC and Tompson B. Cleft-orthognathic surgery: complications and long-term results. *Plast Reconstr Surg* 1995; 96:255.
15. Jackson IA, Munro IR, Salyer KE, et al, eds. Secondary problems in cleft lip and palate. In: *Atlas of craniomaxillofacial surgery.* St. Louis: CV Mosby, 1982; 590.
16. Latham RA. The pathogenesis of the skeletal deformity associated with unilateral cleft lip and palate. *Cleft Palate J* 1969; 6:404.
17. Stenstrom SJ, Oberg TRH. The nasal deformity in unilateral cleft lip. *Plast Reconstr Surg* 1961; 28:295.
18. Avery JK. The nasal capsule in cleft palate. *Anat Anz* 1961; 109:722.
19. Huffman WC, Lierle DM. Studies on the pathologic anatomy of the unilateral harelip nose. *Plast Reconstr Surg* 1949; 4:225.
20. Tajima S, Maruyama M. Reverse-U incision for secondary repair of the cleft lip nose. *Plast Reconstr Surg* 1977; 60:256.
21. Potter J. Some nasal tip deformities due to alar cartilage abnormalities. *Plast Reconstr Surg* 1954, 13:358.
22. Spira M, Hardy SB, Gerow FJ. Correction of nasal deformities accompanying unilateral cleft lip. *Cleft Palate J* 1970; 7:112.
23. Stenstrom SJ. The alar cartilage and the nasal deformity in unilateral cleft lip. *Plast Reconstr Surg* 1966; 38:223.
24. McIndoe AH, Rees TD. Synchronous repair of secondary deformities in cleft lip and nose. *Plast Reconstr Surg* 1959; 24:150.
25. Kazanjian VH. Secondary deformities in cleft palate patients. *Ann Surg* 1939; 109:442.
26. Brown JB, McDowell F. Secondary repair of cleft lips and their nasal deformities. *Ann Surg* 1941; 114:101.
27. Humby G. The nostril in secondary harelip. *Lancet* 1938; 1:1275.
28. Barsky AJ. *Principles and practice of plastic surgery.* Baltimore: Williams & Wilkins, 1950; 243.
29. Whitlow DR, Constable JD: Crossed alar wing procedure for correction of late deformity in the unilateral cleft lip nose. *Plast Reconstr Surg* 1973; 52:38.
30. Fomon S, Bell JW, Syracuse VR. Harelip–nose revision. *Arch Otolaryngol* 1956; 64:14.
31. Gorney M, Falces E. Repair of post cleft nasal deformities with gull-wing cartilage graft. In: *Abstracts of the 2nd International Congress on Cleft Palate,* Copenhagen, 1973; 53.
32. Dibbell DG. A cartilaginous columellar strut in cleft lip rhinoplasties. *Br J Plast Surg* 1976; 29:247.
33. Millard DR. Earlier correction of the unilateral cleft lip nose. *Plast Reconstr Surg* 1982; 70:64.
34. Blair VP. Nasal deformities associated with congenital cleft of the lip. *JAMA* 1925; 84:185.
35. Joseph J. Nasenplastik und sonstige gesichtsplastik nebst einem anhang uber mammaplastik. *Und korperplastik.* Leipzig: Curt Kabitsch, 1931.
36. Gillies H, Kilner TP. Harelip: operations for the correction of secondary deformities of cleft lip. *Lancet* 1932; 2:1369.
37. Berkeley WT. The cleft lip nose. *Plast Reconstr Surg* 1959; 23:567.
38. Cronin TD. Lengthening of columella by use of skin from nasal floor and alae. *Plast Reconstr Surg* 1958; 21:417.
39. Rees TD, Guy CL, Converse JM. Repair of the cleft lip nose: addendum to the synchronous technique with full thickness skin grafting of the nasal vestibule. *Plast Reconstr Surg* 1966; 37:47.
40. Reynolds JR, Horton CE. An alar lift in cleft lip rhinoplasty. *Plast Reconstr Surg* 1965; 35:377.
41. Erich JB. A technique for correcting a flat nostril in cases of repaired harelip. *Plast Reconstr Surg* 1953; 12:320.
42. Musgrave RH, Dupertuis SM. Revision of the unilateral cleft lip nostril. *Plast Reconstr Surg* 1960; 25:223.
43. Millard DR. The unilateral cleft lip nose. *Plast Reconstr Surg* 1964; 34:169.
44. Farrior RT. The problem of the unilateral cleft lip nose. *Laryngoscope* 1962; 72:239.
45. Longacre JJ, Halak DB, Munick LH, et al. A new approach to the correction of the nasal deformity following cleft lip repair. *Plast Reconstr Surg* 1966; 38:555.
46. Berkeley WT. Correction of secondary cleft-lip nasal deformities. *Plast Reconstr Surg* 1969; 44:234.

29

Orthodontics and Cephalometrics

Robert M. Mason, Ph.D., D.M.D.

Orthodontics is a specialty area of dentistry that is concerned primarily with diagnosing and treating abnormalities of the dental arches (1). Many malrelationships between the dental arches, or malocclusions, are intrinsic problems of tooth eruption or position. Other malocclusions, however, relate to malposition of the jaws. Such conditions are skeletal malocclusions, denoting that the underlying problem in tooth position relates to an abnormal position of the jaw(s).

The teeth provide lip support; that is, the position of the lips at rest is determined in part by support from the anterior dentition. In determining whether extractions would compromise the profile, many orthodontists use the guideline of the "aesthetic line" (2). This is an imaginary line that connects the tip of the nose and the most prominent projection of the chin. For a well-balanced face, the lower lip should be within a few millimeters of approximating this line. The upper lip should be several millimeters behind this line. The diagnostic use of the aesthetic line should be tempered with a range of differences in various racial or ethnic groups, as well as the patient's desires for facial appearance.

Orthodontics for the Patient with Cleft Lip and Palate

The interaction between orthodontist and plastic surgeon for patients with cleft lip and palate is an ongoing one that begins at birth and ends at the completion of all treatment in adulthood. In infancy, the orthodontist may be called upon to assist the surgeon in providing an environment wherein the cleft can be successfully closed after some retraction of a protrusive premaxillary segment. A protrusive premaxilla can be retracted with extraoral traction of some type, or by intraoral appliances that pit the palatal shelves against the premaxillary-vomerine complex. In such instances, the orthodontist serves at the pleasure of the surgeon in providing such retractions in those cases in which some appliance or headgear is needed.

There is considerable variation in the activities and philosophies of orthodontists regarding the disposition of the dental arches in the growing child with a repaired cleft lip or palate (3–5). In all patients, a hypoplastic situation is involved, in that the cleft itself represents a loss of either soft tissue or bone to some extent.

Most children with a repaired cleft palate exhibit some form of collapse of the dental arch during development, especially between 3 and 8 years of age. Collapse of the upper dental arch results in a cross-bite condition, usually posterior to the cleft. A cross-bite is a condition in which one or a group of maxillary teeth are positioned lingual or palatal to their mandibular counterparts. In most children, whether clefted or not, a cross-bite represents a *condition* rather than a problem. Accordingly, it is now held that there is no need to correct a cross-bite just because it is there. A cross-bite corrected in the primary or mixed dentition period (when some baby and some permanent teeth are present) does not ensure that no treatment will be needed when the permanent teeth erupt.

Most orthodontists working with children who have clefts do not treat many conditions in the primary dentition. Exceptions to this are badly rotated incisor teeth that either interfere with mastication or create a cosmetic or psychologic problem for the child. The general guideline for treating a child with a cleft for orthodontic conditions before all permanent teeth have erupted is that, when indicated, work should be accomplished quickly and then be discontinued as expediently as possible. In this way, a child's cooperation is not severely compromised for a variety of orthodontic and surgical treatments that may be anticipated in the teenage years.

Expansion of the dental arch is an example of a procedure in orthodontics that may be considered from birth onward. Some infants may require expansion of the dental arch and palate to retroposition the premaxilla properly before lip repair. Such expansion would be done with an acrylic appliance either pinned into the palate or affixed using the undercuts of the palatal shelves (4).

In the period of primary or mixed dentition, expansion may be indicated for those patients who need a maxillary or alveolar crestal bone graft. A maxillary bone graft is usually placed in the line of the primary palatal cleft up at the area of the nasal floor. Such grafts serve to stabilize the dental arch of the maxilla and provide an improved contour and support for the base of the nose (6).

Alveolar crestal bone grafts, by contrast, are placed on the crest of the alveolar ridge in many patients. Such grafts provide an adequate bony bed from which permanent teeth erupt to find a normal place in the dental arch. A crestal graft also provides a more normal gingival contour to the maxillary dental arch. For mechanical support, a marrow graft seems most useful at the crest of the maxillary alveolus. The marrow is usually put through a bone mill and made into paste, and used at the crest of the maxillary alveolus. This procedure provides a means for a permanent tooth to erupt through the graft, unlike a cortical bone graft, which forms an obstacle for tooth eruption.

The use of an alveolar crestal bone graft in a cleft patient is usually accomplished at 6 or 11 years of age. These age preferences relate to the development of the permanent lateral incisor and canine, respectively. The optimal time to place an alveolar crestal graft is before the permanent tooth in the area has erupted, and when the root of the tooth is half-formed (6).

Many children with clefts grow appropriately in the early school-age years, only to become midfacially retrusive as they approach the teenage range. It is very difficult to identify these children in the early years of development. Orthodontic treatment to prepare a child for midfacial surgery differs significantly from that designed simply to match the upper dental arch to the lower. Accordingly, the identification of potential cases of midfacial retrusion should be accomplished as soon as possible. Because there are no universally applicable principles or observations that would separate out potential jaw surgery cases at an early age, most orthodontists minimize therapy efforts until the full extent of the skeletal situation can be properly assessed (7).

It is generally accepted in orthodontics that problems of jaw deficiency can be treated early either by surgery or reverse-pull headgear (such as in midface syndromes), while problems of jaw excess cannot be stopped and need to run their course before definitive surgical treatment (7–8).

Orthodontics for the Osteotomy Patient

Whether a patient has a history of cleft lip and palate or not, the appearance of a skeletal jaw dysplasia signals the need for treatment planning interactions between surgeon and orthodontist. It is uncommon for any patient to have surgery to reposition one of the jaws and dental arches without some orthodontic planning and treatment preoperatively and in the postsurgical stabilization period. Orthodontic treatment is a necessary part of the sequence of treatment for such patients because there are almost always dental compensations for the jaw variations seen. In the instance of a midfacial retrusion problem, for example, the upper incisor teeth usually flare forward, and the lower incisors are tipped lingually to maintain some contactual relationship in the presence of a skeletal malocclusion. Such positional changes of the teeth are not stable or desirable as the jaws are realigned surgically. Hence, orthodontic treatment preoperatively for the osteotomy patient involves decompensating the dentition; that is, realigning the teeth over each bone to which they are attached. The surgical correction of jaw position would then not only align the jaws but also place the teeth in a stable relationship, one jaw to the other (9).

An orthodontist working with an orthognathic surgery patient must know where the jaws are intended to be repositioned before planning any orthodontic treatment as a part of the total therapy. If the jaws are going to be tipped, impacted, rotated, or reduced in any way, the position of the teeth must be considered. One of the ways the orthodontist prepares the patient for orthodontics is to mimic the surgery on stone models set up on a metal articulator. This laboratory procedure can change the jaw position in the laboratory and can guide the orthodontist in determining the type and extent of orthodontic movement of the dentition before surgery.

Another role the orthodontist usually plays in planning jaw surgery is constructing an acrylic splint that is wired between the teeth during surgery to stabilize the surgically created repositioning of the jaw(s). The use of such a splint ensures that there is no guesswork in surgery as to the desired position of the jaws and teeth, or the proper position of the skeletal and dental midlines. Work done preoperatively in the orthodontic laboratory can provide the surgeon with important, specific information as to the amount of bone to be removed or added and the direction of movement of the jaw(s) (8,9).

For an optimal result from orthognathic surgery, a database should include dental study models, facial and intraoral photographs, a Panorex radiograph of the teeth, and a frontal and lateral cephalogram. In addition, a careful clinical examination and history are necessary for adequate planning (10). Overall, osteotomy procedures to mobilize one jaw or the other, or both, involve the combined efforts of several specialty areas, especially orthodontics and surgery.

Because of the problems of moving bone and soft tissues in patients with clefts, there is a general guideline in surgery that any movements of the maxilla over 8 mm should probably involve both jaws. That is, it is usually better to accomplish some movement of the maxilla and some in the opposite direction of the mandible rather than to risk the vascular and other problems (such as relapse) inherent in attempting to move a cleft maxilla a greater distance than 8 mm. While it may be possible safely to advance a cleft maxilla more than 8 mm, most clinicians would tend to agree that the 8-mm figure is a reasonable cutoff point for deciding to do two-jaw surgery in a well-controlled osteotomy procedure associated with maxillary and mandibular dysplasia.

Orthodontics and Cephalometrics

Cephalometric x-ray films provide a means of evaluating the interrelationships of cranial, facial and pharyngeal structures either on a longitudinal or a serial basis. Speech clinicians have utilized lateral single-exposure (static) x-ray head films to study the functions of the velopharyngeal mechanism. Such films are obtained while the patient sustains a phonation of "ah," "ee," or "s." These tasks are thought to assess the functional potential of the velopharyngeal apparatus to achieve velopharyngeal closure as seen in the two dimensions of the lateral cephalogram (11).

The dynamics of speech are better appreciated by moving picture x-ray techniques, such as videofluoroscopy. Other techniques, such as magnetic resonance imaging (MRI), may provide a noninvasive means of obtaining baseline information currently being assessed by a host of radiographic instruments and techniques.

The orthodontist continues to rely primarily on the lateral and frontal static headplate for most diagnostic information. This is associated with the standardization of patient position and a fixed, 5-foot distance between the anode of the x-ray source and the midsagittal plane of the head. Radiographs so obtained can be measured, and the resultant data can be compared to normative information. Most of the cephalometric database in orthodontics of interest to the plastic surgeon is associated with findings from the lateral, static x-ray film (12–14). Selected landmarks and normative data will be presented here (11).

UPPER FACE

The most common method of assessing the relative position of the maxilla is in relation to the cranial base. In the antero-posterior dimension, the angle formed by landmarks SNA provides this assessment (Fig. 29–1). The SN arm of the angle contributes the cranial component. The nasion (N) is the frontonasal suture, and sella (S) is the middle of the sella turcica. The line drawn from N to point A expresses the position of the maxilla. Point A is the most involuted portion of the anterior maxilla. This point is less variable than the anterior nasal spine (ANS), which is buried under the soft tissues of the nose. A normal SNA is 82 plus 4°. Therefore, an SNA of 70° would indicate midface retrusion and an SNA of 90° would indicate maxillary protrusion. There are, of course, exceptions to such findings. A low position of S would affect this angle and would have to be corrected to obtain an accurate estimate of the SNA significance.

There are no well-established cephalometric norms for the vertical dimensions of the maxilla. Upper facial height is usually measured from N to the ANS, and lower facial height from the ANS to the menton (lowest point on the chin). The normative data for upper facial height (N-ANS) in adult males is 60 plus 4 mm, and for females, 56 plus 3 mm. Caution is urged in the use of these norms, however, because upper facial height should be viewed as a proportion of total facial height (45%) rather than as an isolated finding.

Useful information about facial height can also be obtained by identifying the location of the ANS and the PNS (the posterior nasal spine). The palatal plane, as determined by a line extending from ANS to PNS, is usually parallel with the SN line and should extend posteriorly to the anterior tubercle of the atlas.

If the ANS if higher or lower than the PNS, this may signal a vertical discrepancy in the position of the maxilla. A "canted" maxillary plane, such as that with the PNS lower than the ANS, is often a sign of a skeletal dysplasia of the maxilla, such as posterior vertical maxillary excess. This situation would, incidentally, also create an anterior open-bite malocclusion.

LOWER FACE

The mandible is certainly an important structure to evaluate because it interrelates with the tongue, hyoid bone, and oropharyngeal area. The most frequently used measure of the horizontal position of the mandible is the angle SNB. Point B is the most involved portion of the anterior mandible (Fig. 29–2). This area is above the chin and below the alveolus and is known as supramentale. The measurement SNB expresses the horizontal position of the mandible with reference to the cranial base. The norm for SNB is 79 plus 3°. Comparing the SNB measurement to the SNA provides the clinician with a basis for determining whether the patient has a true or a pseudo prognathism. As one might expect, a normal SNB in combination with a diminished SNA might give the appearance of mandibular prognathism rather than of midfacial retrusion, which is often the real cause of the jaw discrepancy.

While SNA and SNB relate the maxilla and mandible to the cranial base area, the measurement ANB relates maxilla to mandible. An ANB of 3° is normal, with a range of 0° to 5°.

DENTITION

Of the many dental measurements utilized in orthodontics and other areas of dentistry, the most useful for describing the position of the teeth relative to the bones to which they are attached involves the incisors. The angulation of the upper incisors is measured by extending a line from the upper incisor tip, through the root of the incisor, to intersect a line from sella to nasion. The norm for upper incisor to NS is 104 plus 6°. For the lower incisor, the line from incisor tip through the root is extended to intersect a line that follows the mandibular plane. This is constructed by connecting a line from the mandibular angle (gonion) to the most an-

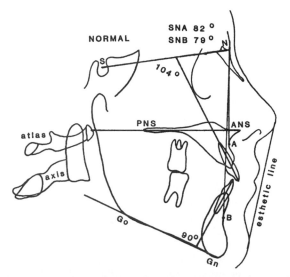

FIG. 29–1. Selected radiographic landmarks and angles express the position of maxilla and mandible compared to the base of the skull. SNA expresses the horizontal position of the maxilla. SNB expresses the horizontal position of the mandible. ANS-PNS shows the palatal plane, which is typically at the same vertical level as the atlas. The upper incisor to the SN plane is shown, and the lower incisor to the mandibular plane (Go-Gn) is demonstrated.

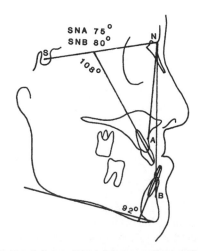

FIG. 29–2. Lateral x-ray film traces a patient with pseudoprognathism. The cephalometric measures indicate a normal mandible and a retruded maxilla in spite of the clinical appearance of a large mandible.

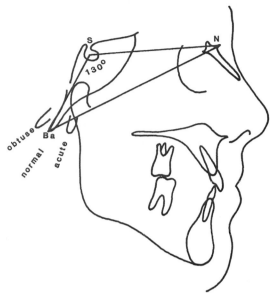

FIG. 29–3. X-ray film traces the cranial base area from nasion (N) to basion (Ba). The configuration of the cranial base is expressed by cranial base angle from nasion (N) to sella turcica (S) to basion (Ba). Variations in cranial base angle are shown.

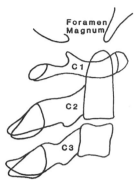

FIG. 29–4. Right lateral view of a normal cervical spine shows C1, C2, and C3 in relationship to the foramen magnum.

teroinferior point of the chin (gnathion). The norm for lower incisor to Go-Gn (the mandibular plane) is 95 plus 7°.

When the upper and lower incisor positions are considered, especially in comparison with the maxillary and mandibular positions (SNA and SNB), the clinician is provided with sufficient information to evaluate whether dental, skeletal, or a combination of variations is present.

CRANIAL BASE

Because the facial skeleton attaches onto the cranial base and is influenced in growth by the configuration of the base of the cranium, it is important to assess the cranial base area as part of a lateral cephalometric analysis. The landmarks, nasion (N) and basion (Ba), serve to separate the neurocranium from the facial skeleton (Fig. 29–3). The basion is the most anterior projection of the foramen magnum. Unfortunately, a straight line drawn from nasion to basion does not reveal much of value about the configuration of the cranial base. The addition of another landmark, sella (S), permits an angular measure to be made as an expression of the cranial base area and its relationship with the facial skeleton.

The cranial base angle is formed by connecting lines between the nasion, the middle of the sella turcica, and the basion. Normal cranial base angle (N-S-Ba) is 130° plus 10°. That means that a cranial base angle less than 120° would indicate an acute cranial base, while one greater than 140° would be considered an obtuse cranial base.

Cranial base angle does not change greatly from childhood to adult form. Some fluctuation in the S-Ba arm of the angle does occur, however. Nonetheless, an individual with an acute cranial base early on maintains this pattern over time.

An acute cranial base could contribute to reduction of the nasopharyngeal airspace, while also encouraging a forward growth tendency of the face. An obtuse cranial base angle, by contrast, would encourage a downward growth pattern of the face. This is because the temporomandibular joint area is positioned more posteriorly, as are other structures.

CERVICAL SPINE

The morphology of the cervical spine area is an important component of a lateral radiographic assessment. The upper vertebral column serves as an attachment for the muscles and soft tissues of the nasopharynx. If the cranial base angle is obtuse, for example, and the cervical spine is obliged to be positioned more posteriorly than normal because of the flexion of the cranial base, the bony or osseous depth of the nasopharynx is increased. This observation may be an especially important one if the patient is a candidate for adenoidectomy. Removal of the adenoid mass may lead to the development of hypernasal speech because of the increased osseous pharyngeal depth. In such situations, the adenoid mass is said to have masked a morphological problem that was there all along. The upper three cervical vertebrae are most appropriate to examine because they are located in the area where velopharyngeal and lingual activity is prominent. It is quite common that the area of velopharyngeal closure is adjacent to the first cervical vertebra (the atlas, or C1). The normal atlas, as seen in the lateral cephalometric projection (Fig. 29–4), has an anterior tubercle that extends about 2 to 3 mm anterior to the plane of the other cervical vertebrae. This is true whether the configuration of the cervical spine is straight (a "military" spine) or slightly curved (a lordotic cervical spine). In most adults, some normal lordosis is observed.

It is well known from cephalometric studies that a velopharyngeal gap of 3 mm is sufficient to create a hypernasal condition. Consequently, small variations in the configuration of the anterior tubercle of the atlas can potentially contribute in a significant way to the increased depth of the nasopharynx. The most common variations in the anterior tubercle of the atlas include flattening and superoposterior rotation (Fig. 29–5). These conditions are developmental variations that are not associated with any neurologic deficit. Consequently, a radiologist may not attach any special significance to such findings. While they are morphologic variations, they are common in the cleft palate population but not in a normal sample. Their appearance should alert the clinician to the possible deleterious consequences to normal nasal resonance balance (nasality) from a total adenoidectomy (15).

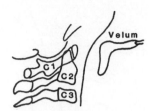

FIG. 29–5. Flattening and superoposterior rotation of the anterior tubercle of the atlas. This minor variation can contribute to an increased depth of the pharynx.

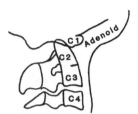

FIG. 29–6. An anomalous cervical spine is shown in a patient with a sub-mucous cleft palate deformity. The atlas is fused to the base of the skull (occipitalization of the atlas), and the spinous processes of C2 and C3 are fused. The odontoid process of C2 has invaginated into the foramen magnum, creating a potential hazard (see text for discussion).

The atlas can be positioned in a superior location, above the usual area for velopharyngeal closure, if the occipital condyles are flattened or hypoplastic. The epitome of this situation is where the atlas is fused to the base of the skull (Fig. 29–6). Occipitalization of the atlas, as this condition is called, can be potentially dangerous to the patient's health because the second cervical vertebra is also positioned superiorly. If the odontoid process of C2 is positioned within the confines of the foramen magnum, the space for the spinal cord is compromised. This situation is referred to as basilar invagination of the axis (C2) into the foramen magnum. Any suspicious instances of the odontoid appearing to invade the space of the foramen magnum should be referred to a radiologist for a definitive evaluation. Such a patient needs to be positioned very carefully for intubation if surgery is undertaken. Hyperextension of the head for intubation serves to bring forward the opisthion, the posterior margin of the foramen magnum. The spinal cord could potentially be damaged between the odontoid and opisthion.

Individuals with submucous cleft deformities have a relatively high incidence of cervical spine variations. In addition to the conditions mentioned above, fusion of the bodies or spinous processes of the 2nd and 3rd cervical vertebrae are common variations. Fusion of C1 and C2 is very rare. While cervical spine variations are more prominent in cleft than noncleft individuals, it appears that the frequency of occurrence in clefts increases as the severity of clefts decreases.

Cervical spine variations are also frequent in many syndromes, such as Klippel-Feil (short neck, low hairline, reduction in number of cervical vertebrae, or fusion of several vertebrae).

Altogether, the cervical spine area comprises one of the components of the osseous pharyngeal depth. Its configuration also contributes to the framework for the velopharyngeal portal. The anteroposterior location of the cervical spine is determined in large part by the configuration of the cranial base (15).

References

1. Graber TM. *Orthodontics.* 3rd ed. Philadelphia: WB Saunders, 1972.
2. Ricketts RM. Esthetics, environment, and the law of the lip relation. *Am J Orthod* 1968; 54:272.
3. Ross RB, Johnston MC. The effect of early orthodontic treatment on a facial growth in cleft lip and palate. *Cleft Palate J* 1967; 4:157.
4. Georgiade NG, Mason RM, Riefkohl R, et al. Preoperative positioning of the protruding premaxilla in the bilateral cleft lip patient. *Plast Reconstr Surg* 1989; 83:1, 32.
5. Mason RM. Is seeing believing? (guest editorial). *Cleft Palate–Craniofacial J* 1994; 31:3.
6. Waite DE, Kersten RB. Residual alveolar and palatal clefts. In: Bell WH, Profitt WR, White RP, eds. *Surgical correction of dentofacial deformities.* Philadelphia: WB Saunders, 1980; 1329.
7. Profitt WR, Epker BN. Treatment planning for dentofacial deformities. In: Bell WH, Profitt WR, White RP, eds. *Surgical correction of dentofacial deformities.* Philadelphia: WB Saunders, 1980; 155.
8. Bell WH, Profitt WR, White RP. *Surgical correction of dentofacial deformities.* Vols. I and II. Philadelphia: WB Saunders, 1980.
9. Epker BN, Woolford LM. *Dentofacial deformities: surgical-orthodontic corrections.* St. Louis: CV Mosby, 1980.
10. Profitt WR, Epker BN, Ackerman JL. Systematic description of dentofacial deformities: the database. In: Bell WF, Profitt WR, White RP, eds. *Surgical correction of dentofacial deformities.* Philadelphia: WB Saunders, 1980; 105.
11. Bateman HE, Mason RM. *Applied Anatomy and Physiology of the Speech and Hearing Mechanism.* Springfield, IL, Charles C Thomas Co, 1984.
12. Broadbent BH, Broadbent BH Jr, Golden WH. *Bolton standards of dentofacial developmental growth.* St. Louis: CV Mosby, 1975.
13. Riolo ML, Moyers RE, McNamara JA Jr, et al. *An atlas of craniofacial growth.* Monograph #2, craniofacial growth series. Ann Arbor: Center for Human Growth and Development, University of Michigan, 1974.
14. Zide B, Grayson B, McCarthy JG. Cephalometric analysis. I. *Plast Reconstr Surg* 1981; 68:5, 816.
15. Mason RM. The pharynx in clefts. *Oral and Maxillofacial Surgery Clinics of North America* 1991; 3:481.

30

Principles of Speech Pathology in the Cleft Lip and Palate Child

John E. Riski, Ph.D., F. A.S.H.A.

The numerous problems found in the child born with cleft lip and palate require the orchestrated efforts of a team of professionals. The plastic surgeon is frequently the conductor; nevertheless, the surgeon depends on the skills and expertise of other team members to help determine the necessity and timing of surgical procedures. The speech pathologist, for example, provides the plastic surgeon with information about speech and velopharyngeal function pertinent to surgical management. Speech pathologists enjoy many recent advances in imaging, microcomputer instrumental assessment, and research into velopharyngeal function. The purpose of this chapter is to describe the principles of evaluating and managing the speech and velopharyngeal function of patients with cleft palate.

Speech Sound System

ARTICULATION

Understanding the normal speech system is necessary to assess the outcome of treatment and to understand compensatory articulation. The consonant sound system of English is illustrated in Table 30–1. Consonants are described by their place of articulation (the location of articulators in the oral cavity) and by the manner of articulation (the way in which the sound is produced). Plosives are made by a brief interruption of the airstream. Fricatives are made by constricting the airstream. Some consonants are voiced and others are not. Some require intraoral air pressure and others do not. Intraoral air pressure requires appropriate coordination of velopharyngeal competency with adequate respiratory pressure and oral articulatory function. All vowels are voiced, and are described by the position of the tongue in the oral cavity (Table 30–2). The horizontal position is described as high, middle, or low. A high tongue carriage offers more resistance to sound energy as it exits the oral cavity. In the presence of even a small VPI, high vowels are more susceptible to hypernasal resonance than low vowels.

NASAL COUPLING

The terminology used to describe the characteristics of nasal coupling was established in 1979 by Riski and Millard (1). The resonance qualities are associated with the acoustic or voiced elements of speech, while nasal air emission is associated with the nonacoustic or unvoiced elements of speech.

Oral-nasal resonance is the balance of oral and nasal acoustic (voiced) energies. It is achieved by the appropriate coupling and isolation of the nasal cavity from the remainder of the vocal tract during speech by the movements of the velopharyngeal valve. Three English sounds require the nasal cavity to be coupled with the vocal tract (i.e., /m/, /n/, /ng/). All other sounds require the velopharyngeal valve to isolate the nasal cavity from the vocal tract. *Hypernasality* is the quality perceived by the listener that is caused by inappropriate nasal coupling with the vocal tract during speech. It is most easily perceived on vowel sounds. In contrast, *hyponasality* is perceived as inadequate coupling or obstruction of the nasal tract during production of those sounds normally associated with nasal energy. The obstruction may be posterior (e.g., hypertrophied adenoids) or anterior (e.g., hypertrophied turbinates). Further, a speaker may also demonstrate a mixed hyper-hyponasality when velopharyngeal closure is incomplete but the nasal cavity is occluded anteriorly.

Nasal air emission is the quality of the nonacoustic sounds and is mostly easily perceived on the unvoiced consonants. Nasal air emission may be inaudible in patients with patent nasal cavities. In these patients, the air passes through the nasal cavity without creating any audible turbulence. Oral pressure is required for the frication associated with the fricative consonants (e.g., /s/ and /f/) or the stop and release of pressure associated with the plosive consonants (e.g., /p/ and /t/). Oral pressure is often inversely related to nasal air emission, which represents the loss of pressure out the nose. Posterior nasal frication in association with attempts at oral air flow generally represents touch velopharyngeal contact; velopharyngeal closing force is not maintained and the air leak through the port creates the posterior nasal frication. Air flows simultaneously through the oral and nasal cavities.

COMPENSATORY ARTICULATION

Children born with cleft palate/lip often learn articulation compensatory to the loss of oral pressure or dental arch collapse. The classic compensatory misarticulations of glottal stops and pharyngeal fricatives have been expanded by Trost-Cardamone (2) to include:

1. *Pharyngeal stop.* Point of stop is tongue base to the posterior pharyngeal wall. Used as substitution for /k/ or /g/.
2. *Midpalatal stop.* Point of stop is midpalate, between position of /t/ and /k/. Used as substitution for /t/, /d/, /k/, or /g/.
3. *Posterior nasal fricative.* Point of frication is the velopharyngeal valve. The tongue stops the airstream. Nasal airflow is the only airflow. Used as a substitution for /s/, /z/.

Table 30–1.
Classification of American English Consonants by Place and Manner of Articulation.

	Manner									
	Pressure Sounds						Nonpressure Sounds			
	Plosive		Fricative		Affricate		Nasal		Semivowel	
Place	UV*	V*	UV*	V*	UV*	V*	UV*	V*	UV*	V*
Bilabial	p	b						m		w
	pie	boy						me		water
Labiodental			f	v						
			fan	van						
Interdental			th	th						
			thin	this						
Lingual-	t	d	s	z				n		l
Alveolar	tie	do	sun	zoo				no		love
Palatal			sh	zh	ch	dg				y
			shoe	vision	chair	jump				yes
Velar	k	g						ng		r
	cat	go						sing		run
Glottal	*MidPalatal*	*Glottal Stop*	h							
	Stop	uh huh	horse							
Pharyngeal	*Pharyngeal*		*Pharyngeal*							
	Stop		*Fricative*							
Velopharyngeal			*Posterior*							
			Nasal							
			Fricative							

The compensatory misarticulations unique to the dental arch and VPI of children with cleft palate have been added in *italics*. See text for further explanantion.

We might also consider the *anterior nasal fricative*. This is similar to the posterior nasal fricative but, the point of frication is the anterior nostrils. Nasal grimacing may accompany this substitution.

Table 30–2.
Classification of American English Vowels by Tongue Position Within the Oral Cavity.

High Back	**Mid**	**High Front**
Boot		Beat
Book		Bit
	But	
	Bird	
	Sofa	
Bought		Bet
Balm		Bat
Low Back		**Low Front**

Diphthongs are not listed. Diphthongs are vowel combinations in which the tongue (and mandible) move from a low position to a higher position. Examples are found in the words *bay, bye, boy,* and *ouch.*

Assessment of Velopharyngeal Function

The task of evaluating velopharyngeal function may be approached as a multilevel problem. The first level should include the perceptual evaluation of resonance, nasal air escape and articulation. The trained ear is still the gold standard of the evaluation. Resonance should be neither hypernasal nor hyponasal (3). The second level is the screening of velopharyngeal closure. This step uses inexpensive tools and is underutilized. Patients who fail these two steps should undergo the third step of objective assessment with computerized instruments for acoustic (4) and nonacoustic (5,6) velopharyngeal function. Finally, imaging should account for the three-dimensional nature of the velopharyngeal port and should include some combination of flexible fiberoptic nasendoscopy (7–10), radiography, or fluoroscopy (11–14) during speech. Articulation should be evaluated separately, with special attention to any compensatory misarticulations and the age-appropriateness of articulation.

Each technique has its advantages and disadvantages. No one instrument provides all necessary information. An ad hoc committee of the American Cleft Palate–Craniofacial Association suggested minimal standards for evaluation of velopharyngeal function. The standards included a perceptual evaluation of resonance and assessment using at least one instrument that provides evaluation during connected speech (i.e., fluoroscopy or pressure-flow) (15). More recently, consensus conference of 71 individuals experienced in the diagnosis and treatment of individuals with craniofacial anomalies developed the "Parameters for Evaluation and Treatment of Patients with Cleft Lip/Palate or Other Craniofacial Anomalies" (16).

Longitudinal study of velopharyngeal port function has demonstrated its instability in children as their phonologic system develops and craniofacial growth and adenoid involution occur (17, 18). Some children develop velopharyngeal incompetency as the adenoids involute (19,20). Some children eventually resolve the hypernasality that is identified immediately following palatoplasty (21). These studies demonstrate the need for longitudinal assessment of velopharyngeal function and the need to exercise some caution before performing a pharyngoplasty.

Velopharyngeal function impacts speech proficiency. However, speech proficiency is not an adequate measure of velopharyngeal function (22). The two areas should be evaluated separately. It is possible to have severely defective speech and a competent velopharyngeal mechanism. On the other hand, normal speech usually cannot be produced without a competent velopharyngeal mechanism.

NASOPHARYNGEAL PATENCY

Aerodynamic assessment has demonstrated the requirements of adequate nasal airway patency (23). Nasal deformities decrease nasal patency in the cleft palate population (24) and pharyngeal flap surgery further decreases nasal airway patency in children, but not in adults (25). Recent investigations revealed that both children and adults with cleft lip and palate demonstrate increased breathing compared to the noncleft population (15 to 30%) (26). Further, the minimal cross-section of the nose can be estimated from pressure-flow measures and has been reported for cleft and noncleft individuals (27). Surgeons have become so successful in managing hypernasality that *hyponasality* may now be a more frequent velopharyngeal dysfunction (28).

PERCEPTUAL EVALUATION OF VELOPHARYNGEAL FUNCTION

Observations made of a young child's speech can provide important information when the child will not cooperate as an active participant in the evaluation. The observation of accurately produced pressure sounds (especially /p/ and /b/) are good prognostic indicators of future velopharyngeal competency (29). Oral breath pressure behind the pressure consonants and nasal air emission should also be assessed. Oral breath pressure is that pressure which develops behind the oral articulators. For example, the breath pressure that develops behind the closed lips differentiates the /b/ from the /m/ sound. During conversation, listen to the force of the airstream behind the pressure consonants /p/, /b/, /t/, /d/, /k/, /g/, especially, and behind the other pressure consonants (see Table 30–1). The presence of grimacing is typically a positive indicator of VPI. Grimacing is an attempt to occlude the nasal airway anteriorly.

SCREENING VELOPHARYNGEAL CLOSURE

Numerous devices are available to screen velopharyngeal closure. Generally, anything that is sensitive to air flow can be used. The advantage of these devices is that they are inexpensive, portable, noninvasive, and very accurate for determining the presence of nasal air flow. Examples of these devices include the See Scape (30), nasal listening tube (1,31), nasal mirrors, and paper paddles. Nasal air flow is monitored during words, such as "puppy, puppy," that should be devoid of nasal air flow. The presence of any air flow indicates some degree of velopharyngeal opening and that further objective testing is warranted.

OBJECTIVE ASSESSMENT OF VELOPHARYNGEAL FUNCTION

Pressure flow evaluates nonvocalic elements and nasometry documents vocalic elements. The two measures are taken consecutively and correlations are in the 70% range. Powerful personal computers and improved multichannel software now allow simultaneous recording of the vocalic and nonvocalic elements (Fig. 30–1).

Pressure Flow

Pressure-flow instrumentation measures of the oral–nasal pressure differential and the volume–velocity of nasal air flow provide quantifiable data about velopharyngeal port

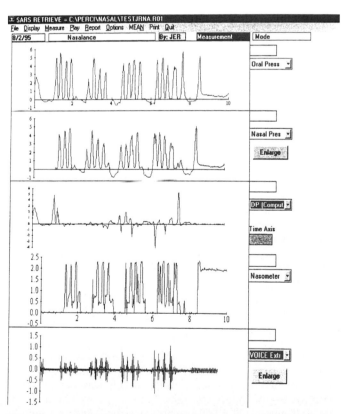

FIG. 30–1. Printout from Perci-SARS including: Oral Pressure (in cmH2O); Nasal Pressure (in cmH2O); (Calculated) Differential Pressure; Nasometry (in Volts) and Voice Waveform. Simultaneous recording of the vocalic and nonvocalic elements may improve our understanding of velopharyngeal function. The five "Oral Press(ure) peaks represent the plosives in the sentence "Papa piped up."

function for speech. The hydrokinetic equation has been modified by Warren and Dubois (5) for estimating velopharyngeal port orifice area. This modification of the hydrokinetic equation has stood up to vigorous study (32,33). Pressure-flow study is an objective and reliable method for repeated, noninvasive measures of velopharyngeal port function. The Perci-SARS (palatal efficiency rating computed instantaneously–Speech Aeromechanical Research System; MicroTronics Corp., Drawer 399, Carrboro, NC 27510) allows six channels of input including two pressure, two flow; a high-speed voice channel; and a low-speed DC channel. Software is included for velopharyngeal function, nasopharyngeal airway patency, laryngeal airway resistance, and several other voice analysis measures (34).

Acoustic Measures

The Nasometer (Kay Elemetrics Corp., 2 Bridgewater Lane, Lincoln Park, NJ, 07035-1488) has become a popular and useful instrument for evaluating the acoustic elements (i.e. hypernasality) of velopharyngeal function. The Nasometer provides an objective measure of nasality termed Nasalance. *Nasalance* is the ratio of nasal acoustic energy divided by nasal plus oral acoustic energy. Hardin and colleagues (35) reported 91% agreement of Nasalance with listener ratings of hypernasality. In addition, Nasalance values greater than 26% were correlated with hypernasality, values between 26 and 39% correlated with mild hypernasality, and values greater than 40% correlated with moderate to severe hypernasality. Dalston and coworkers (36) reported a sensitivity of 89%, specificity of 99%, for listeners ratings of mild hypernasality. Dalston and Warren (37) observed that Nasalance and velopharyngeal area estimates change in concert. Normative Nasalance values were reported by Adams and others (38). A completely oral passage ("Zoo Passage") yielded an average Nasalance of 15.53% (SD = 4.86). A mixed oral and nasal passage ("Rainbow Passage") yielded an average Nasalance of 35.69% (SD = 5.20). Nasal laden sentences yielded an average Nasalance of 61.06% (SD = 6.94).

Nasalance correlations with hyponasality have been reported also. Dalston, Warren, and Dalston (39) reported a sensitivity of 0.48 and a specificity of 79. The measure may have been influenced by nasal air escape in some patients, since the measures improved to 1.0 and 0.95, respectively, when patients with nasal air escape were eliminated. Hardin and colleagues (35) reported that the listener's perception of hyponasality was related to Nasalance scores less than 50% of the time.

IMAGING

Radiography and Fluoroscopy

Lateral still cephalometric radiographs and videofluoroscopy have been used for some time to assess velopharyngeal function. Sphincteric function during speech was demonstrated with the use of multiview videofluoroscopy by Skolnick and his colleagues (11,12,40), who described and labeled the velopharyngeal closure patterns: coronal, circular, and sagittal. A coronal pattern included active velar elevation with some simultaneous mesial movement of the lateral pharyngeal walls. Closure was in the coronal plane. A circular pattern was demonstrated by relatively greater lateral wall mo-

tion than velar movement. Finally, a sagittal pattern was characterized by lateral wall movement and contact with little velar elevation. These patterns are significant because pharyngoplasties have been designed and their success reviewed with reference type and amount of movement. Videofluoroscopy allows the assessment of velar function in its dynamic state for connected speech. Still radiographs often misrepresent velar function because of the limited speech sample that can be employed (14). In addition, shadows and the two-dimensional nature of the still radiograph can distort the true nature of velopharyngeal function.

Flexible Fiberoptic Nasendoscopy

Flexible fiberoptic nasal endoscopes are a popular tool for evaluating velopharyngeal function because there is no irradiation and because they allow direct observation of the portal during connected speech. There are both rigid and flexible endoscopes. Rigid scopes provide better optics, but flexible scopes are more comfortable for the patient. Each allows recording of the image using 35-mm or videotape formats. Each suffers from the disadvantage that younger patients are often difficult to scope successfully. Endoscopy provides information similar to that obtained by base view videofluoroscopy. It provides information about the mesial movement of the lateral pharyngeal walls that cannot be provided by lateral radiography.

Articulation Assessment

There have been numerous studies of articulation development in the cleft lip/palate population (41,42). There is a positive relationship between the extent of clefting and the articulation deficiency. Children of any one type of cleft demonstrate heterogeneous development of articulation skills (42). Recent investigation suggests that the type of cleft may affect the early sound development. Lohmander-Agerskov (43) found the noncleft and cleft palate–only children learned anteriorly placed sounds such as bilabial, dental, and alveolar sounds. In contrast, children with cleft lip and palate learned posteriorly placed sounds.

Under normal valving conditions, a fairly constant pressure is maintained along the vocal tract during speech articulation. The unique misarticulations associated with VPI (e.g. glottal stops and pharyngeal fricative sound substitutions) may then be attempts to maintain a constant resistance in the presence of a loss of pressure through the velopharyngeal port. It has been suggested that the vocal tract functions with the use of pressure-sensing regulators (44). Recent investigations suggest that some of the receptors needed for feedback may be in the oral mucosa valve (45).

In contrast to the errors compensatory to VPI, errors such as "tat/cat," "wabbit/rabbit," and "teef/teeth" are examples of normal developmental errors. Children are expected to outgrow these errors, although excessive errors (given the age of the child) should be treated with speech therapy.

When compensatory errors are concomitant with VPI, the course of management is two-pronged: (a) the VPI must be treated, and (b) the speech problem must be treated. In some cases, speech therapy can begin before the VPI is managed. In such cases, the nostrils can be occluded manually to direct the airstream orally. The child usually cannot employ newly learned sounds without holding his nose. Therapy before surgery can assist learning after surgery (46). Speech therapy has a limited role in treating velopharyngeal incompetence. Increasing oral air pressure increases muscular activity of the levators and may increase velopharyngeal movements (47), and continuous positive nasal airway pressure (CPAP) may be used to increase velopharyngeal closure (48). With these few exceptions, a review of velopharyngeal exercises demonstrates their ineffectiveness (49,50).

Special Concerns and Treatment Strategies

PALATOPLASTY

Children who have their palate closed early (before 1 year of age) often develop normal speech earlier and more easily than children who have the palate closed later (after 1 year) (51). The best timing of palatoplasty has not been defined, possibly because studies have controlled only for chronologic age and not for language age at the time of palatoplasty (52). The coordination of palatal closure to the development of babbling is intuitive. It is at this point in speech and language development that a child must learn to coordinate velopharyngeal function with respiratory pressure, laryngeal abduction and adduction, and oral articulation, to produce consonants. In short, the child's first "dada" is much more complicated than it appears.

The palatoplasty is usually successful in creating a competent velopharyngeal mechanism in 80% of children. This 80% success rate may or may not be influenced by the initial type of cleft (22,42,53). One report demonstrated that the dimensions of the unoperated nasopharynx vary within each type of cleft, and suggested the type and extent of palatoplasty should be tailored to the preoperative dimensions of the nasopharynx (54). Furlow (55) first described the double opposing Z-plasty for primary repair of cleft palate with good results.

ORONASAL FISTULA

The loss of air through an oronasal fistula can be detected and quantified with the assessment tools described earlier. It is wise to repeat these measures once with the fistula open and a second time with the fistula temporarily occluded with dental wax (56) or chewing gum. With the fistula successfully occluded, the velopharyngeal port function can also be adequately tested. Accurate assessment of air flow through the fistula is often confounded by obstructing turbinates or a deviated nasal septum. If the fistula is not patent for speech, surgical intervention may not be warranted. A patent fistula allows the loss of air for speech sounds produced anterior to its site. These are usually the /p/, /b/, /f/, /v/, /θ/ and ð/ sounds, although others may be affected, depending on the location of the fistula and the placement of the tongue. Fistulae should be managed when testing indicates air loss sufficient to undermine speech, or when there is a nasal hygiene problem from nasal regurgitation. Research suggests that only larger fistulae are capable of such air loss (57). Fistulae may be covered with a dental appliance or closed surgically. Surgical intervention might be delayed until after any planned maxillary arch expansion, because this might reopen any fistula closed under tension.

SUBMUCOUS CLEFT PALATE

Children with submucous cleft palate (SMCP) are unique in the cleft-palate population. Frequency is reported to be between 1:10,000 and 1:20,000. VPI is more common in the coronal-type closure pattern (58). Individuals with SMCP should be managed conservatively unless a VPI is diagnosed. A large percentage (44%) remain asymptomatic through adulthood (59).

READING DISABILITIES

Recent investigation of reading abilities revealed that children within the cleft lip/palate group displayed a prevalence for reading disabilities similar to the general population (9%). In contrast, children with cleft palate only demonstrated a much higher rate of reading disabilities (33%) (60).

Surgical Management of Velopharyngeal Incompetence

POSTERIOR PHARYNGEAL FLAP PHARYNGOPLASTY

The concept of a surgical procedure to manage VPI was first introduced by Passavant (61), who surgically tethered the uvula to the posterior pharyngeal wall in an attempt to restore a competent valving mechanism for speech. This was modified to the superiorly based flap by Bardenheur (62) and Sanvernero-Rosselli (63).

Postoperative studies of pharyngeal flap surgery using electromyographic analysis and endoscopic and videofluoroscopic imaging have suggested several methods by which the nasopharynx is obturated. The primary method of velopharyngeal closure is by active mesial movement of the lateral pharyngeal walls against the static, obturating flap (64). Secondarily, circumferential scar contracture narrows the pharynx. Finally, contracture of the flap itself elevates the velum into the pharynx, diminishing the anterior-posterior dimension. Crockett, Bumstead, and Van Demark (65) suggested that three variables should be controlled for successful pharyngeal flap surgery. These are: flap width, height or level of flap, and control of lateral port size. Strategies have been developed cope with these variables. The size of the lateral ports has been controlled (66) and the width of the pharyngeal flaps has been tailored to the amount of wall motion (67). Some have suggested that little strategy, if any, is needed for small VPI. Randall (68) observed that if the VPI is small any method should have a good result.

POSTERIOR PHARYNGEAL WALL AUGMENTATION AND MUSCLE TRANSPOSITION

An attempt to augment the posterior pharyngeal wall was first reported by Wardill (69,70). He created a permanent ridge of fibrous tissue on the posterior pharyngeal wall. This was created by making transverse incisions through the superior constrictor at the level of the Passavant ridge. The tissue was sutured vertically, creating a ridge for the elevated velum to contact. Hynes (71,72) and later Orticochea (73–75) advocated pharyngoplasties by muscle transposition that were similar in design, but differed in their intended function. Each procedure has undergone modification and refinement by the following: Jackson and Silverton (76), Huskie and Jackson (77), Pigott (78), Riski and others

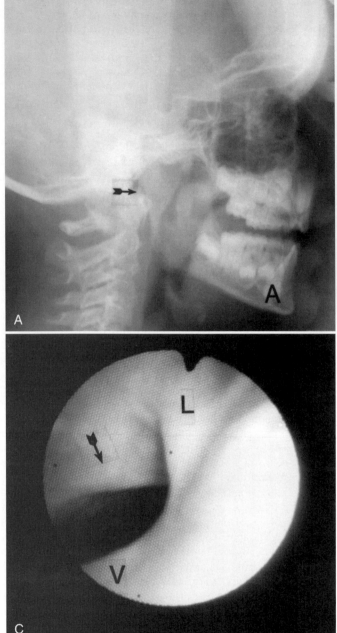

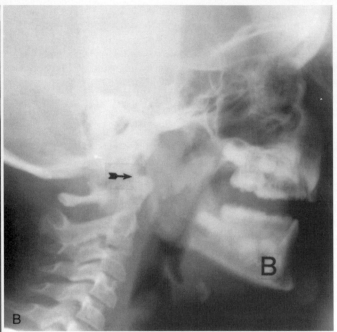

FIG. 30–2. **A,** preoperative phonation radiograph demonstrating velum elevated and failing to contact the adenoid pad. The attempted contact is just above the level of C1 (arrow). **B,** postoperative phonation radiograph demonstrating insertion of the sphincter pharyngoplasty at and just above the level of C1 (arrow). **C,** postoperative nasendoscopic view demonstrating the prominence of the sphincter pharyngoplasty on the posterior pharyngeal wall (arrow). The left lateral pharyngeal wall (L) and velum (V) are also labeled. (From Riski JE, Ruff GL, Georgiade GS, et al. Evaluation of failed sphincter pharyngoplasties. *Ann Plast Surg* 1992; 28:545–553.)

(79,80), Roberts and Brown (81), Stratoudakis and Bambace (82), Moss, Pigott, and Albery (83), and Mirrett, Riski, and Georgiade (84) (Figures 30–2 and 30–3).

The height of insertion for the sphincter pharyngoplasty on the posterior pharyngeal wall has been elevated from the low insertion recommended by Orticochea (73). Several have recommended elevating the insertion as high as possible (76,81). Riski and coworkers (79) offered a rationale for tailoring the height of flap insertion. The height of attempted velopharyngeal contact was identified relative to the anterior tubercle of the first cervical vertebra, the atlas. The atlas was identified by palpation at the time of surgery and the flaps

were surgically inset at that predetermined height. Success improved from 61 to 93% when the height of the flaps were elevated to the level of attempted velopharyngeal contact.

COMBINED PHARYNGOPLASTY AND PRIMARY PALATOPLASTY

Because the initial palatoplasty may not be completely successful, a number of investigators have incorporated a primary pharyngoplasty. The procedure remains controversial. Most report more patients with normal resonance than with palatoplasty alone (85–87), but not all (88). One study demonstrated 54% of the children receiving a combined pro-

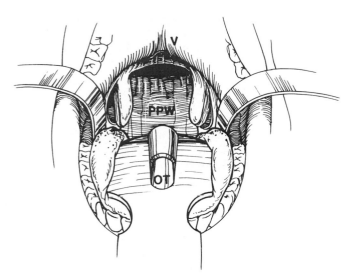

FIG. 30–3. The posterior pharyngeal wall is exposed by elevating the velum (V) with a catheter, inserted through the nose and sutured to the uvula. The transverse incision is made into the the posterior pharyngeal wall (PPW) at the radiographically determined height of attempted velopharyngeal contact. The lateral palatopharyngeus flaps are elevated and retain their superior attachment. The orotracheal tube (OT) is also labeled. (From Riski JE, Ruff GL, Georgiade GS, et al. Evaluation of the sphincter pharyngoplasty. *Cleft Palate J* 1992; 29:254-261.)

cedure did not require a pharyngoplasty (89). Mazaheri and colleagues (90) could not identify any differences in velar length or nasopharyngeal depth between one group of children with clefts who required pharyngeal flaps and a second group of children with clefts who did not. Although it is clear that some children born with cleft palate will require a pharyngoplasty, we cannot accurately identify those children at the time of palatoplasty.

FURLOW Z-PLASTY

Recently, Chen and colleagues (91) reported their results with the Furlow Z-plasty as a secondary procedure. They documented velopharyngeal closure in 16 of 18 patients. Furlow (92), in his review of the series, observed that retroposition of the levator muscle sling seemed the chief benefit of the procedure and any lengthening of the velum may be an incidental benefit.

COMPLICATIONS OF PHARYNGOPLASTY

Complications with pharyngoplasties are not uncommon. Some complications are immediate and some develop long term. Obstruction may be severe enough to warrant takedown of the flap, according to Caouette-Laberge and colleagues (93). Ren and associates (94) suggested that the loss of tongue-lip balance may be one factor causing midface retrusion. Kravath and others (95) reported three patients who developed obstructive sleep apnea (OSA) immediately following pharyngeal flap surgery. Thurston and coworkers (96) reported significant nasal obstruction in 8 of 85 patients post pharyngeal flap. Obstruction was often occult and identified only after careful questioning. Seven of the eight patients required surgical revision to relieve airway obstruction. Sturim (97) reported hemorrhaging from pharyngeal flap

surgery in two patients who previously had a teflon injection for VPI. Zaworski (98) reported anorexia nervosa in a 15-year-old female after pharyngeal flap surgery. Hoffman (99) reported the surgical revision followed by dilation and stenting with a dental prosthesis to prevent repeat contracture of a pharyngeal flap that stenosed. Drew, Tripathi, and Lehman (100) reported that 12 of 25 pharyngeal flap patients demonstrated elevated serum ADH levels, low serum osmolity, and hyponatremia in the postoperative period.

OBSTRUCTIVE SLEEP APNEA

Orr, Levine, and Buchanan (101) observed obstructive sleep apnea in 9 of 10 patients at 2 to 3 days postsurgery. Apnea resolved in 7 of 9 patients by 3 months. Shprintzen (102) identified OSA by polysomnography in 30 of 300 patients following pharyngeal flap surgery. OSA lasted longer than 6 months in three and resolved in the remaining patients. Narrow and wide flaps had the same incidence of OSA. These surgeons postulated that the causes of OSA were: obstruction of the portals by large tonsils, contraction of the nasopharynx around the flap, postoperative nasopharyngeal edema, or a sudden change in breathing pattern. Sirois and others (103) reported 14 of 40 (35%) patients with abnormal polysomnograms after pharyngeal flap surgery. Six had OSA, six had central sleep apnea, and two had both central and obstructive sleep apneas. Long-term follow-up demonstrated residual central apneas. Witsell, Drake, and Warren (104) showed decreased nasal patency in 5 of 7 patients after a pharyngeal flap.

Shprintzen and colleagues (105) modified pharyngeal flaps (shorter) for less contracture below the flap in an attempt to lessen airway obstruction. They also suggested using nasopharyngeal tubes for nasal respiration until the patient is awake and can breathe orally. The authors reported that the protocol reduced all complications. OSA was eliminated in all patients, snoring was reduced from 82 to 10.5%, and hospital stay reduced from 7 to 3 days.

SPEECH THERAPY

Before Palatal Closure

Parents are counseled regarding what to expect from their child's early speech attempts. Resonance will be hypernasal. The child will be able to say correctly words with nasal sounds, such as "mama," but will not correctly say words with pressure sounds, such as "dada." The parents are instructed in play activities that focus on verbal interaction between parent and child and in appropriate modeling of speech and language by the parents.

AFTER PALATAL CLOSURE

Speech and language stimulation should continue with age-appropriate games, vocabulary, and syntax. The parents are now asked to monitor the sounds that the child makes. If there are no confounding developmental problems, we expect the child to begin making crisp, pressure consonants such as /p/, /b/, /t/, /d/, /k/, and /g/. Often the parents are asked to occlude the child's nose manually while playing "sound games" such as repeating the syllable "ba ba ba ba." Occluding the nose prevents any nasal air flow and directs the air stream to the oral cavity. The parents are also asked to observe any signs of velopharyngeal dysfunction or oral-nasal fistulae. These include nasal reflux while eating or drinking, nasal air flow or facial grimacing, or the continued use of nasal sounds and the lack of pressure consonants while talking.

Speech therapy for the child with a cleft palate is unique because the child may present with unique misarticulations not found in the noncleft population (2). Unique speech therapy strategies and facilitating postures are used to correct misarticulations in the cleft lip/palate child. Moreover, exercises are generally unsuccessful in increasing velopharyngeal movements except in some very specific situations (106,107). Maximizing oral pressure for pressure consonants will maximize velopharyngeal elevation and may gain velopharyngeal closure for small VPIs. A unique therapy technique using continuous positive airway pressure to the nasal surface of the soft palate has been developed by Kuehn (48). Velar elevation for speech under the resistance of CPAP may improve velopharyngeal closure.

As soon as a VPI is diagnosed as adversely affecting speech or speech development, it should be managed. Articulation skills improve immediately following management of VPI (22). That patients with VPI make little or no progress in speech therapy until the VPI is managed was noted by Van Demark (108), Riski and DeLong (42), and Hardin (109). When a VPI is suspected or documented, speech therapy should be considered diagnostic and should be short-term. Referral to a cleft palate–craniofacial team is appropriate after no more than several weeks of ineffective speech therapy.

FUNCTIONAL VPI

The practicing clinician should also recognize that there are a small number of cleft (and noncleft) children with normal soft-palate function who use some form of nasal air emission as a sound substitution (110,111). This is termed a functional VPI or "sound-specific VPI." The characteristics include: normal resonance, sound-specific use of some form of nasal air escape (usually a posterior nasal fricative), normal velopharyngeal function for correctly produced sounds, and the ability to correctly produce the errored sound without nasal air escape. This patient presents a special diagnostic challenge, and the differential diagnosis of an organic VPI from a functional VPI is the key to appropriate management.

Summary

The child with a cleft lip/palate represents a special challenge. Successful management of the various problems requires special knowledge, special tools, and most importantly close communication among professionals. Instrumentation and imaging can provide the clinician with objective measures of velopharyngeal dynamics including the size, shape, and position of a velopharyngeal opening. Outcome is often improved by applying information obtained from preoperative imaging to patient selection and surgical procedure.

Despite some advances, success rates are not much better than those described in reviews more than 2 decades ago (112). This is especially disheartening, given the advances in computer instrumentation and imaging during the same time. Surgeons, or possibly teams, are slow to learn from the mistakes of others and appear more content to follow their own learning curve. There appears to be greater im-

provement in individual results over time than there is in the collective management of hypernasality. Further, a pharyngoplasty is not without risk to the patient. The benefits of pharyngoplasty should be weighed against possible complications.

A number of clinical-research challenges remain, including: early identification of those children who will require a pharyngoplasty, development of criteria for selecting a pharyngeal flap or a sphincter pharyngoplasty in individual situations, and management of VPI without creating hyponasality and obstruction. Hyponasality has been considered more socially acceptable than hypernasality, and many (including Crockett, Bumstead, and Van Demark; 65) consider hyponasality an improvement over hypernasality.

A pharyngoplasty should have a physiologic basis, and evaluation of velopharyngeal physiology has been the responsibility of the speech pathologist. The clinician is challenged to incorporate available instrumentation into the evaluation process. The clinician may be guided by experience and by the "Parameters for Evaluation and Treatment of Patients with Cleft Lip/Palate or Other Craniofacial Anomalies" (16). This peer reviewed document offers several recommendations for evaluation and treatment. The document recommends that "secondary palatal and pharyngeal surgery for velopharyngeal inadequacy should be performed only after evaluation of the velopharyngeal mechanism and review by the team," including: "in-depth analysis of articulatory performance, aerodynamic measures, videofluoroscopy, nasopharyngoscopy, and nasometric studies, all of which should be conducted with the participation of the team speech-language pathologist." It will be the task of today's clinical researchers to utilize the available instrumentation to better plan and conceive secondary management procedures and to learn from mistakes of the past—so as not to repeat them.

References

1. Riski JE, Millard RT. The process of speech evaluation and treatment. In: Cooper HK, et al., eds. *Cleft palate and cleft lip: a team approach to clinical management and rehabilitation of the patient.* Philadelphia: WB Saunders, 1979; 431–484.
2. Trost JE. Articulatory additions to the classical description of the speech of persons with cleft palate. *Cleft Palate J* 1981; 18:193.
3. Riski JE, Hoke JA, Dolan EA. The role of pressure-flow and endoscopic assessment in successful palatal obturator revision. *Cleft Palate J* 1989; 26:1.
4. Fletcher SC. *Diagnosing speech disorders from cleft palate.* New York: Grune & Stratton, 1978.
5. Warren DW, DuBois AB. A pressure flow technique for measuring velopharyngeal orifice area during continuous speech. *Cleft Palate J* 1964; 1:52.
6. Warren DW, Devereux JL. An analog study of cleft palate speech. *Cleft Palate J* 1966; 3:103.
7. Pigott RW. The results of nasopharyngoscopic assessment of pharyngoplasty. *Scand J Plast Surg* 1974; 8:148.
8. Gilbert STJ, Pigott RW. The feasibility of nasal pharyngoscopy using the 70 degrees Storz-Hopkins nasopharyngoscope. *Br J Plast Surg* 1982; 35:14.
9. Zwitman DH. Velopharyngeal physiology after pharyngeal flap surgery as assessed by oral endoscopy. *Cleft Palate J* 1982; 19:40.
10. Zwitman DH. Oral endoscopic comparison of velopharyngeal closure before and after pharyngeal flap. *Cleft Palate J* 1982; 19:40.
11. Skolnick ML. Videofluoroscopic examination of the velopharyngeal portal during phonation in lateral and base projections—a new technique for studying the mechanics of closure. *Cleft Palate J* 1970; 7:803.

12. Skolnick ML. Velopharyngeal function in cleft palate. *Clin Plast Surg* 1975; 2:285.
13. Williams WN. Radiological measures of abnormal speech physiology. In: Bzoch KR, ed. *Communicative disorders related to cleft lip and palate.* Boston: Little, Brown, 1979; 249–262.
14. Williams WN, Eisenbach OR. Assessing VP function: the lateral still technique vs. cinefluorography. *Cleft Palate J* 1981; 18:45.
15. Dalston RM, Marsh JL, Vig KW, et al. Minimal standards for reporting the results of surgery on patients with cleft lip, cleft palate, or both: a proposal. *Cleft Palate J* 1988; 25:3.
16. American Cleft Palate–Craniofacial Association. Parameters for evaluation and treatment of patients with cleft lip/palate or other craniofacial anomalies, March 1993.
17. Van Demark DR, Morris HL. Stability of velopharyngeal competency. *Cleft Palate J* 1983; 20:18.
18. Van Demark DR, Hardin MA, Morris HL. Assessment of velopharyngeal competence: a long-term process. *Cleft Palate J* 1988; 25:362.
19. Riski JE, Mason RM. Adenoid involution as a cause of velopharyngeal incompetence in children with cleft palate. Presentation at the annual meeting of the American Cleft Palate–Craniofacial Association, Toronto, 1994.
20. Mason RM, Warren DW. Adenoid involution and developing hypernasality in cleft palate. *J Speech Hear Dis* 1980; 45:469.
21. Fox DR, Lynch JI, Cronin TD. Change in nasal resonance over time: a clinical study. *Cleft Palate J* 1988; 25:245.
22. Riski JE. Articulation skills and oral-nasal resonance in children with pharyngeal flaps. *Cleft Palate J* 1979; 16:421.
23. Warren DW. A quantitative technique for assessing nasal airway impairment. *Am J Orthod* 1984; 86:306.
24. Warren DW, Duany LF, Fischer ND. Nasal pathway resistance in normal and cleft lip and cleft palate subjects. *Cleft Palate J* 1969; 6:134.
25. Warren DW, Trier WC, Bevin AG. Effect of restorative procedures on the nasopharyngeal airway in cleft palate. *Cleft Palate J* 1974; 11:367.
26. Hairfield WM, Warren DW, Seaton DL. Prevalence of mouthbreathing in cleft lip and palate. *Cleft Palate J* 1988; 25:135.
27. Warren DW, Drake AF, Davis JU. Nasal airway in breathing and speech. *Cleft Palate–Craniofacial J* 1992; 29:511–519.
28. Riski JE. Assessment of speech in adolescents with cleft palate. *Cleft Palate J* 1995; 32:109–113.
29. Van Demark DR. Predictability of velopharyngeal competency. *Cleft Palate J* 1979; 16:429.
30. See Scape: Pro-Ed, Austin, TX, 1995.
31. Blakeley RW. *The practice of speech pathology: a clinical diary.* Springfield, IL: Charles C Thomas, 1972.
32. Smith BE, Weinberg B. Prediction of velopharyngeal orifice size: a re-examination of model experimentation. *Cleft Palate J* 1980; 17:277.
33. Smith BE, Weinberg B. Prediction of modeled velopharyngeal orifice areas during steady flow conditions and during aerodynamic stimulation of voiceless stop consonants. *Cleft Palate J* 1982; 19:172.
34. Riski JE, Warren DW, Lutz RL, et al. Application of Perci-SARS for speech evaluation. Study session, American Cleft Palate–Craniofacial Association, Tampa, 1995.
35. Hardin MA, Van Demark DR, Morris HL, et al. Correspondence between nasalance scores and listener judgements of hypernasality and hyponasality. *Cleft Palate J* 1992; 29:346.
36. Dalston RM, Warren DW, Dalston ET. A preliminary investigation concerning the use of nasometry in identifying patients with hyponasality and/or nasal airway impairment. *J Speech Hear Res* 199; 34:11.
37. Dalston RM, Warren DW. Comparison of tonar II, pressure flow, and listener judgements of hypernasality in the assessment of velopharyngeal function. *Cleft Palate J* 1986; 23:108.
38. Adams L, Fletcher S, McCutcheon M. Cleft palate speech assessment through oral-nasal acoustic measures. In: Bzoch K, ed. *Communicative disorders related to cleft lip and palate.* Boston: College Hill Press, 1989.
39. Dalston RM, Warren DW, Dalston ET. Use of nasometry as a diagnostic tool for identifying patients with velopharyngeal impairment. *Cleft Palate J* 1991; 28:184.
40. Skolnick ML, McCall GN. Velopharyngeal competence and incompetence following pharyngeal flap surgery: Videofluoroscopic study in multiple projections. *Cleft Palate J* 1972; 9:1–12.
41. Van Demark DR, Morris HL, VandeHaar C. Patterns of articulation abilities in speakers with cleft palate. *Cleft Palate J* 1979; 16:230.
42. Riski JE, DeLong E. Articulation development in children with cleft lip/palate. *Cleft Palate J* 1984; 21:57.
43. Lohmander-Agerskov A, Söderpalm E, Friede H, et al. Pre-speech in children with cleft lip and palate or cleft palate only: phonetic analysis related to morphologic and functional factors. *Cleft Palate J* 1994; 31:271.
44. Warren DW. Compensatory speech behaviors in individuals with cleft palate: a regulation/control phenomenon? *Cleft Palate J* 1986; 23:251.
45. Furusawa K, Yamaoka M, Ichikawa N. Responsiveness of single afferents in the infraorbital nerve to oral air pressure generated by consonants. *Cleft Palate J* 1994; 31:161.
46. Riski JE, Kunze LH, Nailling KR, et al. Speech patterns and disturbances associated with clefts and craniofacial anomalies. In: Serafin D, Georgiade NG, eds. St. Louis: CV Mosby, 1984; 246.
47. Kuehn DP, Moon JB, Folkins JW. Levator veli palatini muscle activity in relation to intranasal air pressure variation. *Cleft Palate J* 1993; 30:361.
48. Kuehn DP. New therapy for treating hypernasal speech using continuous positive airway pressure (CPAP). *Plast Reconstr Surg* 1991; 88:959–966.
49. Ruscello DM. A selected review of palatal training procedures. *Cleft Palate J* 1982; 19:181.
50. Ruscello DM. Modifying velopharyngeal closure through training procedures. In: Bzoch K, ed. *Communicative disorders related to cleft lip and palate.* 3rd ed. Boston: College Hill Press, 1989.
51. Dorf DS, Curtin JW. Early cleft palate repair and speech outcome. *Plast Reconstr Surg* 1982; 70:74.
52. O'Gara MM, Logemann JA. Phonetic analyses of the speech development of babies with cleft palate. *Cleft Palate J* 1988; 25:122.
53. Karnell MP, Van Demark DR. Longitudinal speech performance in patients with cleft palate: comparisons based on secondary management. *Cleft Palate J* 1986; 23:278.
54. Komatsu Y, Genba R, Kohama G. Morphological studies of the velopharyngeal orifice in cleft palate. *Cleft Palate J* 1982; 19:275.
55. Furlow LT. Cleft palate repair by double opposing Z-plasty. *Plast Reconstr Surg* 1986; 78:724–738.
56. Bless DM, Ewanowski SJ, Dibbell DG. A technique for temporary obturation of fistulae—a clinical note. *Cleft Palate J* 1980; 17:297.
57. Shelton RL, Blank JL. Oronasal fistulas, intraoral air pressure, and nasal air flow during speech. *Cleft Palate J* 1984; 21:91.
58. Velasco MG, Ysunza A, Hernandez X, et al. Diagnosis and treatment of submucous cleft palate: a review of 108 cases. *Cleft Palate J* 1988; 25:171.
59. McWilliams BJ. Submucous clefts of the palate: how likely are they to be symptomatic? *Cleft Palate J* 1991; 28:247–248.
60. Richman LC, Eliason MJ, Lindgren SD. Reading disability in children with clefts. *Cleft Palate J* 1988; 25:21.
61. Passavant G. Ueber die operation der angeborenen spalten des harten gaumens und der damit complicirten hasenscharten. *Arch Ohr Nas Kehlkopfheilk* 1862; 3:193.
62. Bardenheur D. Vorschlage zu plastischen operationen bei chirurgischen eingriffen in der mundhohle. *Arch Klin Chir* 1892; 43:32.
63. Sanvernero-Rosselli G. Divisione palatina a sua aura chirugica alu congr. *Intl Stomat* 1935; 391.
64. Shprintzen RJ, McCall GN, Skolnick ML. The effect of pharyngeal flap surgery on the movements of the lateral pharyngeal walls. *Plast Reconstr Surg* 1980; 66:570–573.
65. Crockett DM, Bumstead RM, Van Demark DR. Experience with surgical management of velopharyngeal incompetence. *Otolaryngol Head Neck Surg* 1988; 99:1–9.
66. Hogan VM, Schwartz MF. Velopharyngeal incompetence. In: Converse JM, ed. *Reconstructive plastic surgery.* 4th ed. Philadelphia: WB Saunders, 1977; 4:2268–2283.
67. Shprintzen RJ, Lewin ML, Croft CB, et al. A comprehensive study of pharyngeal flap surgery: tailor-made flaps. *Cleft Palate J* 1979; 16:46–55.
68. Randall P, Whitaker LA, Noone RB, et al. The case for the inferiorly based posterior pharyngeal flap. *Cleft Palate J* 1978; 15:262–265.
69. Wardill WEM. Results of operation for cleft palate. *Br J Surg* 1928; 16:127.
70. Wardill WEM. Cleft palate. *Br J Surg* 1933; 21:347.
71. Hynes W. Pharyngoplasty by muscle transposition. *Br J Plast Surg* 1951; 3:128–135.

72. Hynes W. The results of pharyngoplasty by muscle transplantation in "failed cleft palate" cases, with special reference to the influence of the pharynx on voice production. *Ann R Coll Surg Engl* 1953; 13:17–35.

73. Orticochea M. Construction of a dynamic muscle sphincter in cleft palates. *Plast Reconstr Surg* 1968; 41:323–327.

74. Orticochea M. Results of the dynamic muscle sphincter operation in cleft palates. *Br J Plast Surg* 1970; 23:108–114.

75. Orticochea M. A review of 236 cleft palate patients treated with dynamic muscle sphincter. *Plast Reconstr Surg* 1983; 71:180–188.

76. Jackson IT, Silverton JS. The sphincter pharyngoplasty as a secondary procedure in cleft palates. *Plast Reconstr Surg* 1977; 59:518–524.

77. Huskie CF, Jackson IT. The sphincter pharyngoplasty—a new approach to the speech problem of velopharyngeal incompetence. *Br J Disord Commun* 1977; 12:31–35.

78. Pigott RW. The results of pharyngoplasty by muscle transplantation by Wilfred Hynes. *Br J Plast Surg* 1993; 46:440–442.

79. Riski JE, Serafin D, Riefkohl R, et al. A rationale for modifying the site of insertion of the orticochea pharyngoplasty. *Plast Reconstr Surg* 1984; 73:882–894.

80. Riski JE, Ruff GL, Georgiade GS, et al. Evaluation of the sphincter pharyngoplasty. *Cleft Palate J* 1992; 29:254–261.

81. Roberts TMF, Brown BSJ. Evaluation of a modified sphincter pharyngoplasty in the treatment of speech problems due to palatal insufficiency. *Ann Plast Surg* 1983; 10:209–213.

82. Stratoudakis AC, Bombace C. Sphincter pharyngoplasty for correction velopharyngeal incompetence. *Ann Plast Surg* 1984; 12:243–248.

83. Moss AL, Pigott RW, Albery EH. Hynes pharyngoplasty revisited. *Plast Reconstr Surg* 1987; 79:346–355.

84. Mirrett P, Georgiade GS, Riski JE. Annual meeting of the American Cleft Palate–Craniofacial Association, Pittsburgh, 1993.

85. Bingham HG, Suthunyara P, Richards S, et al.. Should the pharyngeal flap be used primarily with palatoplasty? *Cleft Palate J* 1972; 9:319.

86. Dalston RM, Stutteville OM. A clinical investigation of the efficacy of primary nasopalatal pharyngoplasty. *Cleft Palate J* 1975; 12:177.

87. Dorf DS, Curtin JW. Early cleft palate repair and speech outcome. *Plast Reconstr Surg* 1982; 70:74.

88. Morris HL. Velopharyngeal competence and primary cleft palate surgery, 1960–1971: a critical review. *Cleft Palate J* 1973; 10:62.

89. Riski JE, Georgiade NG, Serafin D, et al. The orticochea pharyngoplasty and primary palatoplasty: an evaluation. *Ann Plast Surg*

90. Mazaheri M, Athanasiou AE, Long RE. Comparison of velopharyngeal growth between cleft lip and/or palate patients requiring or not requiring pharyngeal flap surgery. *Cleft Palate J* 1994; 31:452–460.

91. Chen PK-T, Wu JTH, Chen YR, et al. Correction of velopharyngeal insufficiency in cleft palate patients with the Furlow palatoplasty. *Plast Reconstr Surg* 1994; 94:933–941.

92. Furlow LT. Discussion: correction of velopharyngeal insufficiency in cleft palate patients with the Furlow palatoplasty. *Plast Reconstr Surg* 1994; 94:942–943.

93. Caouette-Laberge L, Egerszegi EP, de Remont AM, et al. Long-term follow-up after division of a pharyngeal flap for severe nasal obstruction. *Cleft Palate–Craniofacial J* 1992; 29:27–31.

94. Ren YF, Isberg A, Henningsson G, et al. Tongue posture in cleft palate patients with a pharyngeal flap. *Scand J Plast Reconstr Surg Hand Surg* 1992; 26:307–312.

95. Kravath RE, Pollak CP, Borowiecki B, et al. Obstructive sleep apnea and death associated with surgical correction of velopharyngeal incompetence. *J Pediatrics* 1980; 96:645–648.

96. Thurston JB, Larson DL, Shanks JC, et al. Nasal obstruction as a complication of pharyngeal flap surgery. *Cleft Palate J* 1980; 17:148–154.

97. Sturim HS. Bleeding complications with pharyngeal flap construction in humans following teflon pharyngoplasty. *Cleft Palate J* 1974; 11:292–294.

98. Zaworski RE. Anorexia nervosa following a pharyngeal flap operation. *Cleft Palate J* 1981; 18:223–224.

99. Hoffman S. Correction of lateral port stenosis following a pharyngeal flap operation. *Cleft Palate J* 1985; 22:51–55.

100. Drew GS, Tripathi S, Lehman JA Jr. The syndrome of inappropriate secretion of antidiuretic hormone in the pharyngeal flap operation. *Cleft Palate J* 1985; 22:88–92.

101. Orr WC, Levine NS, Buchanan RT. Effect of cleft palate repair and pharyngeal flap surgery on upper airway obstruction during sleep. *Plast Reconstr Surg* 1987; 80:226–232.

102. Shprintzen RJ. Pharyngeal flap surgery and the pediatric upper airway. *Int Anesthes Clin* 1988; 26:79–88.

103. Sirois M, Caouette-Laberge L, Spier S, et al. Sleep apnea following pharyngeal flap: a feared complication. *Plast Reconstr Surg* 1994; 93:943–947.

104. Witsell DL, Drake AF, Warren DW. Preliminary data on the effect of pharyngeal flaps on the upper airway in children with velopharyngeal inadequacy. *Laryngoscope* 1994; 104:12–15.

105. Shprintzen RJ, Singer L, Sidoti EJ, et al. Pharyngeal flap surgery: postoperative complications. *Int Anesthes Clin* 1992; 30:115–124.

106. Ruscello DM. A selected review of palatal training procedures. *Cleft Palate J* 1982; 19:181.

107. Ruscello DM. Modifying velopharyngeal closure through training procedures. In: Bzoch K, ed. *Communicative disorders related to cleft lip and palate.* 3rd ed. Boston: College Hill Press, 1989.

108. Van Demark DR. A comparison of articulation abilities and velopharyngeal competence between Danish and Iowa children with cleft palate. *Cleft Palate J* 1974; 11:463.

109. Van Demark DR, Hardin MA. Longitudinal evaluation of articulation and velopharyngeal competence of patients with pharyngeal flaps. *Cleft Palate J* 1985; 22:163–172.

110. Peterson SJ. Nasal emission as a component of the misarticulation of sibilants and affricates. *J Speech Hear Disord* 1975; 40:106.

111. Riski JE. Functional velopharyngeal incompetence: diagnoses and management. In: Winitz H, ed. *Treating articulation disorders: for clinicians by clinicians.* Baltimore: University Park Press, 1984.

112. Yules RB, Chase RA. Secondary techniques for correction of palatopharyngeal incompetence. In: Bzoch K, et al., eds. *Cleft lip and palate.* Boston: Little, Brown, 1971.

31

Craniofacial Anomalies and Principles of Their Correction

Alexander C. Stratoudakis, M.D., F.A.C.S.

The classification and correction of craniofacial anomalies became possible in the sixties when Tessier (1) laid the foundations of modern craniofacial surgery by systematically describing the major facial osteotomies and proving their feasibility. For the first time, every part of the facial skeleton could be accessed, mobilized, and moved as needed. The principles on which craniofacial surgery is based are:

1. Wide dissection of the affected regions
2. Combined intra- and extra-cranial approach to carry out safely osteotomies and mobilization of bony segments
3. Extensive use of bone grafts to fill defects and establish skeletal continuity

Techniques learned from craniofacial (CRF) surgery have had a profound influence on (a) the treatment of facial trauma, which has been revolutionized by exposure of fracture sites, extensive use of rigid fixation, and immediate bone grafting of defects; (b) oncologic surgery, by allowing access to areas heretofore inaccessible for en bloc resection of tumors once considered unresectable, (c) cosmetic surgery, with the subperiosteal facelift, orbital reshaping, and use of cranial bone grafts.

The systematic use of specialized imaging techniques such as three-dimensional computed tomography (3DCT) and magnetic resonance imaging (MRI) has greatly enhanced our understanding of both the skeletal anomalies and the underlying central nervous system (CNS) pathology. As computer technology progresses rapidly, virtual surgery, which will allow optimization of surgical planning, is currently on the horizon. Although still expensive, model construction of rare anomalies from data obtained by 3DCT through photopolymerization of a liquid resin for model surgery has become readily available.

Long-term follow-up of craniofacial procedures has in many ways been a sobering experience. A result judged satisfactory in the early postoperative period does not necessarily remain so. Surgery may have had little effect on the deformity (2) and in fact produced secondary iatrogenic deformities that are difficult to correct. It is thus extremely important to develop treatment plans based soundly on the physiologic principles uncovered in the past 3 decades.

Despite ongoing research, basic questions continue to elude us. What is the etiology of craniosynostosis? Does the cause lie in the cranial base or in the sutures themselves? There are arguments for both. Are the effects of cranial expansion on intracranial hypertension (ICH) predictable? In simple single-suture synostosis, the incidence of ICH seems to be greater than previously realized, and early surgery is still recommended for relief as well as for aesthetic improvement. In syndromic synostoses matters are considerably more complex. Factors including cephalocranial disproportion, impaired Cerebral Spinal Fluid (CSF) circulation, venous hypertension, and airway obstruction are all associated with increased ICP. Intracranial pressure appears to be related to respiration. Acute rises in ICP were found to be related to altered breathing patterns associated with obstructive sleep apnea (3). The response of the central nervous system to cranial vault expansion is uncertain (4) Intracranial pressure is not necessarily reduced, and surgery and shunting may be ineffective in preventing hindbrain herniation. In fact, cranial vault expansion may actually trigger hindbrain herniation in cases of syndromic synostoses. Chronic tonsillar herniation seems to occur frequently in cases of syndromic craniosynostosis. In a well-conducted study it was observed on 25 out of 60 patients on MRI, and on 17 following surgery and 8 who had never been operated upon (5).

We now know that the genetic cause of Crouzon syndrome probably lies in the long arm of chromosome 10 (6), but the etiology of most anomalies is still obscure.

Enthusiasm about new methods fades as their drawbacks and limitations become apparent (e.g., the restriction of growth caused by rigid fixation, the inward migration of metal microplates and screws in the growing craniofacial skeleton) (7). Several prototypes of absorbable plate and screw systems are currently being developed and tested, but so far they have not gained general acceptance.

Finally, an interesting new trend has been the use of distraction osteogenesis in the treatment of craniofacial anomalies. Distraction osteogenesis is the spontaneous induction of intramembranous ossification across a gap between the surfaces of a low-energy osteotomy undergoing gradual distraction. The technique, pioneered by Ilizaroff as early as 1951 in orthopedic surgery, has recently been utilized for the elongation of the mandible, and to a lesser extent for the manipulation of other facial bones. A corticotomy is performed between the pins of an external fixator-distractor, and after a period of about one week gradual distraction of 1 mm daily in three 8-hour increments is started. When the desired length of bone is achieved, the distraction is discontinued and the fixation device is left in place for a consolidation period about double the time it took to achieve the distraction. The lengthening represents true new-bone formation and not just stretching of available bone. Soft-tissue adaptation to the lengthening has also been studied. Muscle fibres adapt by hypertrophy as well as by cellular regeneration (hyperplasia), arteries by reorientation of their smooth muscle fibres, capillaries by budding, and nerves by an initial degeneration followed by regeneration (8–10).

Craniostenoses

Craniostenosis is a general term encompassing a variety of developmental disorders characterized by inadequate capacity of the cranium to accommodate the growing brain, which results in compensatory deformities. The term, however, does not accurately describe the milder forms, in which there is cranial deformity without real restriction of the cranial capacity.

Craniosynostosis points to the premature closure of cranial sutures. Skull deformity may exist without premature sutural obliteration (11) and, conversely, premature sutural obliteration may occur without deformation of the calvaria. This has been pointed out by Huxley (quoted in Bolk), and confirmed by Bolk (12) and Tessier (13).

Craniostenoses can generally be divided into simple and syndromic forms. In simple synostoses the pathology is confined to the cranial suture system, although the deformities may involve facial features as well. It is generally agreed that single-sutural synostosis does not strictly exist, but that a "system" of sutures is involved. Seeger and Gabrielsen (14) have demonstrated in a radiographic study that the process of premature closure of the coronal suture frequently extends into the base of the skull to involve the frontosphenoidal and perhaps other sutures. In syndromic forms, the pathologic process involves the facial sutures as well, and frequently there arc limb and other systemic anomalies. Facial deformity may occur without concomitant cranial deformity. Delaire (15) has used the term "faciosynostosis."

The dura mater (inner periosteum) is considered the guiding tissue in the morphogenesis of the calvaria. It is attached anteriorly to the crista galli, anterolaterally to the lesser sphenoidal wings, and posterolaterally to the petrous ridges. These sites of attachment correspond to the major dural reflections that conform to the early recesses in the developing brain. Thus, a longitudinal dural reflection develops between the cerebral hemispheres to become the falx cerebri; a band of dura reflects off the sphenoid wing into the early insular sulcus between the major frontal and parietotemporal regions of brain outgrowth to become the major anterolateral dural band. The dural reflections off the petrous ridges develop between the cerebrum and cerebellum to become the tentorium cerebelli, the major posterolateral dural band. Between 12 and 16 weeks of gestation, intramembranous ossification progresses in the central zones between the major reflective bands of the dura. From these central points, the mineralization spreads centrifugally toward the major bands within the dura. By 16 weeks, the radiating centers of ossification have almost reached the sites of reflective bands in the dura. These latter sites remain unossified as regions of connective tissue between outspreading islands of membranous bone.

Smith and Tondury (16) studied brain malformations in which abnormal dural reflections were found to conform to the nature of the aberrant brain. They observed the cranial sutures to be related directly to the unusual sites of dural reflections. This confirmed and extended the concepts of Moss: that there is no genetic determination of the site of development of sutures, and that there is no basic impetus for growth in the calvaria or its sutures, but that they respond in a compensatory fashion to the interior forces that normally consist of the outgrowth of the brain (16) Doubt has been cast upon this last point, however, by more recent experimental work (17,18).

Separative motion of adjacent calvarial bones occurs in a direction perpendicular to the long axis of the intervening suture. Any functional ankylosis at a given sutural area will have two interrelated results: (a) inhibition of expansive growth in directions normal (perpendicular) to the suture line; and (b) consequent redirection of the growth vector of the neural mass (11). This observation was first made by Virchow (19). Redirection of the growth vector of the neural mass causes deformation either in the cranial vault (cranial dysmorphias) or in the weaker areas of the cranial base (greater sphenoidal wing and frontal bone exorbitism, or ethmoid prolapse of the cribriform plate and telorbitism) (13). Moss (20,21) has attributed premature sutural obliteration to dysmorphias of the cranial base, and the postmortem studies by Stewart and others (22), Kreiborg and others (23), and Ousterhout and Melsen (24) further localize the pathology in Apert disease in the cranial base. It appears to be a progressive disorder observed as an abnormality indicating decreased growth (short cranial base) in the bones of the cranial base in a 24- to 26-week-old embryo. An abnormality in the sutures and a histologically abnormal cranial base were observed at 22 months of age. In the 38-month-old specimen, there was synostosis of the sphenooccipital synchondrosis as well as synostosis of the vomer to the sphenoid and the maxilla.

Apart from the aesthetic disfigurement, craniosynostoses may cause functional disorders such as intracranial hypertension and hydrocephalus. This occurs more frequently in syndromic cases, although even in simple single-suture involvement the incidence is probably higher than was previously realized.

Signs of increased intracranial pressure include fundoscopic changes (papilledema, which may lead to visual loss), headaches, vomiting, or a beaten-silver appearance of the cranium on roentgenographic examination. Because these signs are frequently absent or difficult to detect in children, direct measurements should be carried out by means of an extradural transducer. Noninvasive monitors currently being developed will aid detection in children.

The terminology used in the description of cranial deformities is confusing. It is presented here as clearly as possible.

1. *Acrocephaly* is a term introduced by Lucea in 1847; it is generally used synonymously with the "tower skull" or oxycephaly of Virchow (see below). It describes a cranium the anterior part of which is higher than the posterior, the vault slanting in a front-to-back direction (Figs. 31–1 and 31–2).
2. *Oxycephaly* is a term used by Virchow in 1852 to describe a deformity characterized by extreme upward growth with reduction of the lateral and the anteroposterior (AP) diameters. The nasofrontal angle is usually too obtuse or absent. This deformity is usually caused by synostoses resulting in fusion of the coronal sutures in which growth occurs in the interfrontal and interparietal lines.

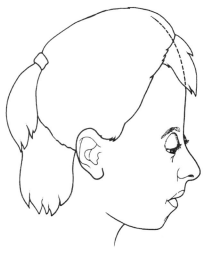

FIG. 31–1. Acrocephaly (oxycephaly).

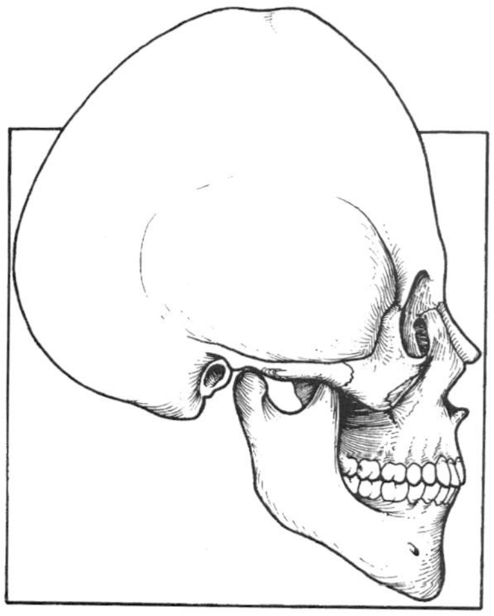

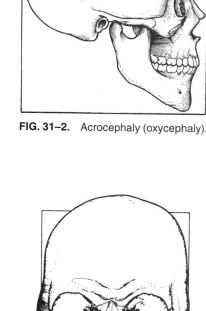

FIG. 31–2. Acrocephaly (oxycephaly).

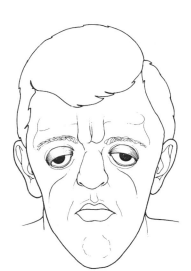

FIG. 31–3. Acrocephalosyndactyly (Apert syndrome) (turricephalic type).

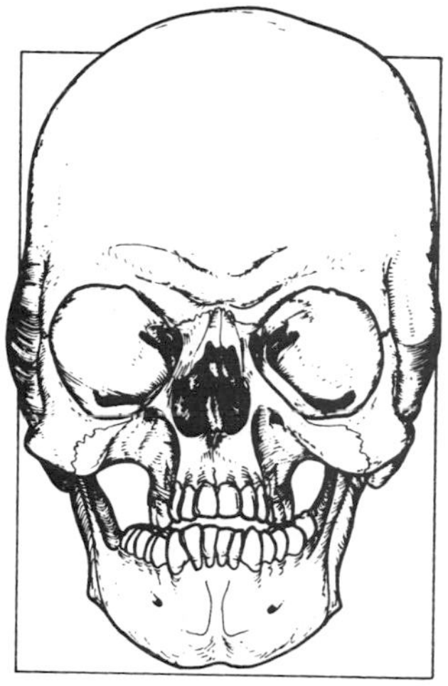

FIG. 31–4. Acrocephalosyndactyly (Apert syndrome) (turricephalic type).

3. *Turricephaly* describes a cranium with exaggerated upward growth caused by fusion of the frontoparietal sutures (Figs. 31–3 and 31–4).
4. *Scaphocephaly,* or hull-shaped cranium, is characterized by reduced cranial width with a compensatory increase in the AP length. It is seen with premature closure of the sagittal suture (Figs. 31–5 and 31–6).
5. *Trigonocephaly* is a cranial deformity in which the forehead is narrow and triangular, with a prominent ridge corresponding to the prematurely fused metopic suture (Fig. 31–7).
6. *Plagiocephaly* implies cranial asymmetry and may either be frontal, occipital, or hemicranial (25). Frontal plagiocephaly usually occurs with premature synostosis of the ipsilateral half of the coronal suture and frontosphenoidal suture and presents as a deformity involving both the cranium and the facial skeleton. The forehead is flattened on the affected side, with a backward and upward dis-

placement of the affected orbit. The lesser sphenoidal wing has a more vertical orientation than normal, while the greater sphenoidal wing is retracted medially, altering the angle of the lateral orbital wall. The calvaria may also be deformed, bulging in the contralateral parietal area. The deformity becomes less pronounced at the level of the maxilla. Even less pronounced is the mandibular asymmetry. The mandible, even though asymmetrical, functions symmetrically, possibly because of a lower and more anterior position of the ipsilateral glenoid fossa (Tessier, unpublished data) (Figs. 31–8 and 31–9). Occipital plagiocephaly is a rare condition caused by "synostosis" of the lambdoid suture and the region of the asterion. It presents with significant flattening of the parietooccipital region with compensatory bulging and projection of the opposite side. In fact, the suture is always open on radiographs and is accompanied by an adjacent sclerotic ridge. We have shown that, even though

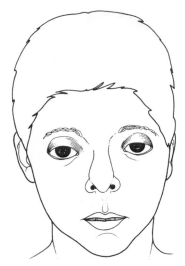

FIG. 31–15. Saethre-Chotzen syndrome.

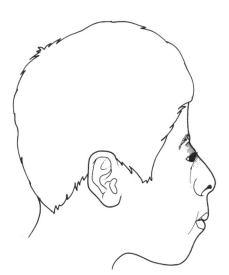

FIG. 31–16. Saethre-Chotzen syndrome.

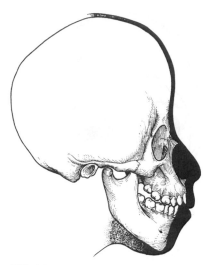

FIG. 31–17. Saethre-Chotzen syndrome.

dle cranial fossa); the posterior cranial fossa, which is also short, bulges downward. "The forehead is deformed in a peculiar fashion. The supraorbital margins protrude and above them is a transverse depression in the form of a concavity; above this concavity the superior part of the forehead forms a very prominent bulge, frequently more pronounced in the midline than laterally (32)." If telorbitism is present, it is generally of a mild degree. Midfacial retrusion is a constant feature, but the orbitostenosis and ocular proptosis are not as marked as in Crouzon syndrome (25). The maxillary sinuses are underdeveloped in contrast to the overdevelopment of the ethmoid cells and frontal sinus. The maxilla is deficient, and the dentition is abnormal, with crowded and impacted teeth. The incidence of cleft palate in this syndrome is reported to range from 11 to 30% (33). Low-set hairline, hypertrichosis of the eyebrows, and mild ptosis of the eyelids (particularly of their lateral aspect) may be present. The lower lip is well developed, while the oral commissures drop (see Figs. 31–3 and 31–4).

Hydrocephalus has been reported, but the frequency of this finding is uncertain. Mental retardation is occasionally present. Whether it is primary or caused by raised intracranial pressure is an unresolved question (25) (also Tessier, unpublished data).

Symmetrical syndactyly of all four limbs is characteristic, involving at least the three central digits, but frequently all five. The syndactyly involves the phalanges and nails as well as the soft tissues.

SAETHRE-CHOTZEN SYNDROME

This syndrome is characterized by a brachycephalic cranium with a variable degree of craniosynostosis (but not true craniostenosis), facial asymmetry, shallow orbits, telecanthus, nasal septal deviation, low-set hairline, and partial cutaneous syndactyly (which, however, is not a constant feature). Maxillary hypoplasia is not as pronounced as it is in Apert or in Crouzon syndromes (Figs. 31–15 to 31–17). Intelligence is frequently normal, but severe mental retardation has also been reported (25).

PFEIFFER SYNDROME

Described in 1964, this syndrome consists of craniosynostosis with cranial deformity of the brachy-turricephalic type, broad thumbs and great toes having deformed proximal phalanges, and occasionally partial soft-tissue syndactyly. Other skeletal anomalies have also been described. Faciostenosis with maxillary retrusion and exorbitism, or telorbitism, may be present. Hydrocephalus and intracranial hypertension have been reported (Figs. 31–18 and 31–19). Intelligence is usually normal, but mental retardation is possible (25).

CARPENTER SYNDROME

This syndrome was reported in 1901 and 1909 by Carpenter, a pediatrician, as a disorder of development in three (and probably four) siblings. It consists of cranial malformations of variable shape (scapho- or acro-cephalic) caused by various combinations of synostoses. The nasal bridge is flat, and the canthi are usually dystopic. There may be associated anomalies of the globe. The ears appear to be low-set, and preauricular fistulas have been reported.

Digital anomalies are an obligatory component of the syndrome. The hands are short with brachydactyly and variable soft-tissue syndactyly. The feet show accessory preaxial digits and soft-tissue syndactyly, which is usually extensive. Other skeletal findings have been reported.

Height is usually below the 25th percentile, but weight is often above average. Other visceral congenital anomalies may be present. Inheritance is autosomal recessive (25,29).

Craniofacial Clefts

The incidence of major facial clefts is significantly lower than that of the common CL ± P, and is estimated at 1.45 to 4.85 per 100,000 births (34) although the true incidence is probably higher. This is easily understood when one considers that: (a) conditions such as the Treacher Collins syndrome and hemifacial microsomia may be included among the clefting syndromes; (b) many conditions previously regarded as "hypoplasias" are, in reality, clefts (35); and (c)

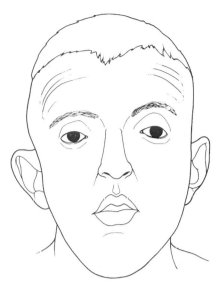

FIG. 31–18.   Pfeiffer syndrome.

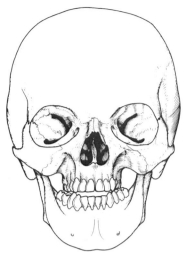

FIG. 31–19.   Pfeiffer syndrome.

formes frustes and incomplete forms may go unnoticed. There is no recognizable pattern of inheritance. Craniofacial clefts occur sporadically. Their etiology is unknown, and amniotic bands, which have been incriminated as being etiogenetic factors, can be blamed only in the rare case in which the cleft does not follow the "usual" pattern. Of the seven patients reported by Jones and colleagues (35), whose clefts were attributed to amniotic bands, six had encephaloceles of unusual pattern, and five (or six) had constriction rings or amputations of limbs. They may affect facial or cranial structures, or both, and they generally occur along axes following constant patterns. They do not necessarily involve all layers of tissue to the same extent. It seems that, from the midline to the infraorbital foramen, defects of the soft tissues are more severe than those of the bone, while from the infraorbital foramen to the temporal bone, the opposite holds.

Although several classifications of the major clefts have been proposed, the one put forward by Tessier has gained universal acceptance.

THE TESSIER CLASSIFICATION

In this classification the orbit is selected as the point of reference because it belongs both to the cranial and the facial skeleton. A numerical system was developed, numbering the axes of the various clefts around the orbit in a counter-clockwise direction. Numbering starts from the "southbound" facial clefts and continues with the "northbound" cranial clefts (Figs. 31–20 and 31–21).

This numerical system is one simply of topographic description; it describes neither the structures involved nor the severity of involvement of each structure. A cleft, for example, may spare the cheek and involve only the palpebral and labial structures. A "sclerodermic" patch of skin or an abnormal line of hair growth may be the only superficial indication of a cleft involving the deeper layers. Moore and coworkers (37) have also reported the frequent occurrence of "hairline indicators," or markers in the hairline, in cases of northbound clefts, pointing in the direction of the cleft.

Whereas not all hypoplasias are clefts, all clefts have hypoplastic edges. Clefts do not course through foramina or grooves of neurovascular bundles, although these may be involved in the hypoplasia of the cleft margins.

Northbound and southbound clefts frequently coexist, and when they do their axes often (but not always) follow the same direction. The cleft is then described by the dual number indicating each of the component clefts. Clefts may be bilateral and, when this is the case, they are frequently symmetrical (with regard to the axis of the cleft and not necessarily the severity of involvement of each side). Multiple clefts occasionally coexist, rendering the deformity even more complex and "unclassifiable."

The so-called clefts 0, 1, and 2 follow a course that is medial to the canthus and, therefore, they do not pass through and do not disrupt the orbit itself. Similarly, the so-called cleft 7 is a laterofacial cleft and does not have a course leading to or through the orbit. Clefts affecting the orbit frequently cause anomalies of the orbital contents (globe and extraocular muscles).

Cleft 0

Cleft 0, or median craniofacial dysrrhaphia, represents failure or delay in closure of the anterior neuropore. Its course is outlined from the anterior fontanelle through the frontal bone, crista galli, midline of the nose, columella, lip, and maxilla, and may actually involve the tongue, lower lip, and mandible. It may give rise to frontal, frontonasal, or frontoethmoidal encephaloceles, telorbitism, duplication of the nasal septum, and midline cleft of the lip. In its minor forms, it may present with minor telorbitism and a "flat" appearance in the area of the glabella. Nasal gliomata are frequent, representing sequestration of glial tissue after obliteration of the anterior neuropore. Its cranial extension is cleft 14 (Figs. 31–22 and 31–23).

Cleft 1

Cleft 1, or paramedian craniofacial dysrrhaphia, courses through the frontal bone and the olfactory groove of the rib-

FIG. 31–20. The Tessier classification of craniofacial clefts.

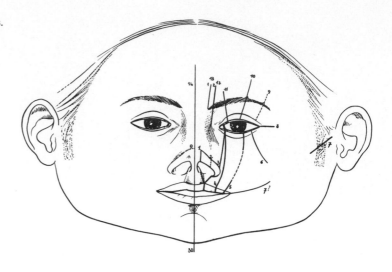

FIG. 31–21. The Tessier classification of craniofacial clefts.

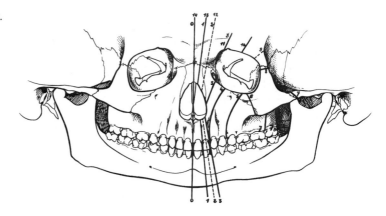

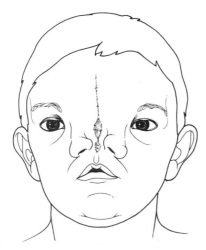

FIG. 31–22. Cleft 0–14 (median craniofacial dysrrhaphia).

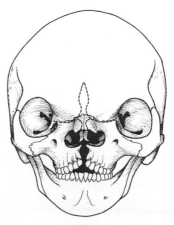

FIG. 31–23. Cleft 0–14 (median craniofacial dyssrhaphia).

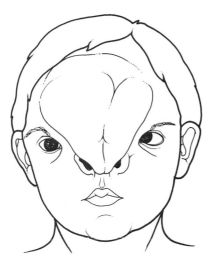

FIG. 31–24. Cleft 1-13 (bilateral).

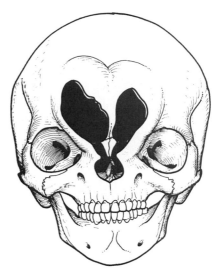

FIG. 31–25. Cleft 1-13 (bilateral).

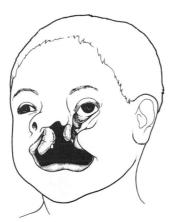

FIG. 31–26. Cleft 3.

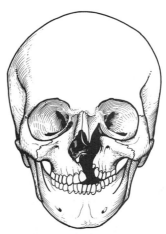

FIG. 31–27. Cleft 3.

riform plate, between the nasal bone and the frontal process of the maxilla, and through the maxilla between the central and lateral incisors. It may cause telorbitism with a deep invagination of the dura in the area of the cribriform plate defect, nasoorbital encephalocele (which could also be caused by cleft 0), notching of the nostril in the area of the alar dome, and occasionally a cleft lip. Its cranial extension is cleft 13 (Figs. 31–24 and 31–25).

Cleft 2

Cleft 2, or paranasal cleft, is similar to cleft 1, but it is slightly more lateral. Its cranial extension is cleft 12.

Cleft 3

Cleft 3, or oculonasal cleft, is a medial orbitomaxillary cleft. Its course runs through the lacrimal bone, the frontal process of the maxilla, and into the alveolus between the lateral incisor and the canine. There is absence of the inferomedial wall of the orbit and lack of pneumatization of the maxillary antrum with absence of the septum separating the nasal cavity from the antrum. As to the soft tissues, the medial canthus is displaced inferiorly. There is a coloboma of the lower eyelid, the conjunctiva and nasal mucosa being separated by a thin band of fibrous tissue. The lacrimal apparatus is invariably affected; the sac is either absent or present in the form of a mucocele. The lateral aspect of the nose is separated from the cheek, with considerable vertical shortness of the nose on the cleft side. The defect ends as a cleft lip. Its northbound continuation is cleft 11 (Figs. 31–26 and 31–27).

Cleft 4

Cleft 4, or oculofacial 1 cleft, is a central orbitomaxillary cleft. The upper portion of its course is similar to that of cleft 3. It courses medially to the infraorbital nerve and through the maxillary sinus, causing exstrophy of the antral mucosa. However, the septum between the nasal cavity and the antrum is present. It ends, as in cleft 3, between the lateral incisor and the canine. With respect to the soft tissues, the medial canthal, palpebral, and lacrimal problems are similar to those of cleft 3, while the clefting between the nose and cheek occurs more laterally, sparing the nostril. The lip clefting takes place lateral to the philtral crest (Figs. 31–28 and

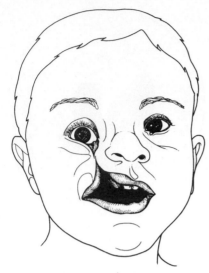

FIG. 31–28. Cleft 4.

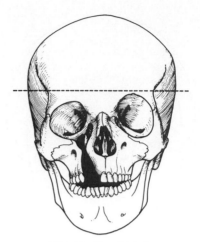

FIG. 31–29. Cleft 4.

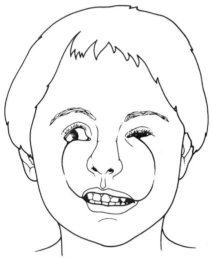

FIG. 31–30. Cleft 5 (bilateral).

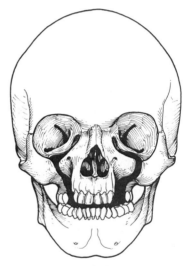

FIG. 31–31. Cleft 5 (bilateral).

31–29). In its bilateral form, there is considerable shortness of the central part of the face.

Cleft 5

Cleft 5, or oculofacial 2 cleft, is a very rare lateral orbito-maxillary cleft, the course of which runs through the orbital floor, lateral to the infraorbital nerve and the maxillary sinus, ending behind the canine in the premolar region. The soft tissue deformities consist of a coloboma of lateral third of the lower lid, ending as a cleft of the lip slightly medial to the commissure (Figs. 31–30 and 31–31).

Cleft 6

Cleft 6 separates the maxilla from the malar bone. The corresponding soft-tissue deformities consist of a coloboma of the lower lid and a "sclerodermic" furrow of skin from the coloboma to the angle of the mandible (Figs. 31–32 and 31–33).

Cleft 7

Cleft 7 courses between the malar and the temporal bones. The zygomatic arch is usually absent. The condyle, coronoid process, and mandibular ramus suffer various degrees of deformity. The temporal muscle is either absent or atrophic, forming a continuous temporomasseteric muscle. There may be an associated cleft of the scalp, or an abnormal pattern of hair growth may overlie the bony cleft. There are varying degrees of ear malformations. Cleft 7, however, may exist as pure macrostomia without any appreciable skeletal or ear deformity.

Cleft 8

Cleft 8 is a frontozygomatic cleft extending to the greater sphenoidal wing. In the soft tissues there may either be a true cleft of the lateral canthus or a notch of the lower eyelid close to the canthus with a dermatocele.

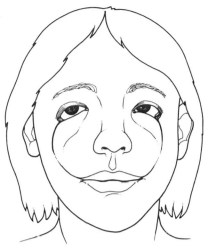

FIG. 31–32. Cleft 6 (pure form, bilateral).

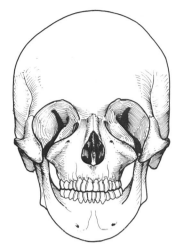

FIG. 31–33. Cleft 6 (pure form, bilateral).

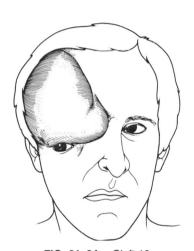

FIG. 31–34. Cleft 10.

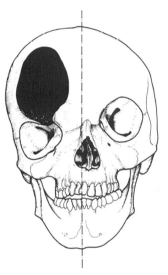

FIG. 31–35. Cleft 10.

Combinations of clefts 6, 7, and 8, in varying degrees of severity, constitute the Treacher Collins syndrome. With complete clefts 6, 7, and 8, the malar bone may be totally absent, or it may be present only as sesamoidlike bones in the temporo-masseteric fascia.

Cleft 9

Cleft 9 is an upper lateral orbital cleft of the superolateral orbital ridge-angle with a corresponding coloboma of the upper lid.

Cleft 10

Cleft 10 is an upper central orbital cleft of the frontal bone, supraorbital ridge, and orbital rod, which is lateral to the supraorbital neurovascular bundle, causing an encephalocele. It could be associated with a coloboma of the medial third of the upper lid and/or eyebrow (Figs. 31–34 and 31–35).

Cleft 11

Cleft 11 is an upper medial orbital cleft through the frontal bone, frontal sinus, and lateral mass of the ethmoid, which is medial to the supraorbital neurovascular bundle. The corresponding soft-tissue deformity is a coloboma of the medial third of the upper eyelid.

TELORBITISM OR ORBITAL HYPERTELORISM

The terms *orbital hypertelorism* and *telorbitism* were proposed by Tessier (38) and are used interchangeably. Telorbitism is usually a congenital condition, with the exception of cases caused by fibrous dysplasia (39). Tessier (35,38,40) considers that telorbitism is always secondary either to a cleft or to craniostenosis (16,48) (Figs. 31–36 and 31–37). A differing opinion is expressed by Van der Meulen and Vaandrager (51), who attribute it to a developmental arrest occurring between the 5th and 8th weeks of gestation (51).

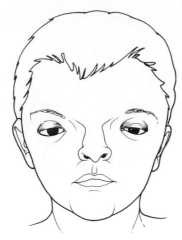

FIG. 31–36. Telorbitism (with brachycephaly).

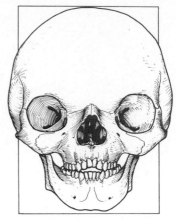

FIG. 31–37. Telorbitism (with brachycephaly).

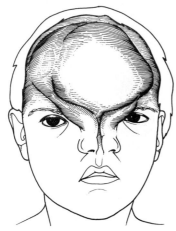

FIG. 31–38. Encephalomeningocele (secondary to cleft 0–14) may be accompanied by telorbitism.

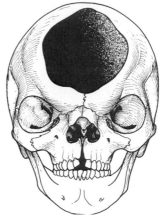

FIG. 31–39. Encephalomeningocele (secondary to cleft 0–14) deviates laterally, protruding through the medial orbital walls (46).

The interorbital distance is measured between the anterior lacrimal crests. This distance varies in women from 18.5 to 29.5 mm, and in men from 19.5 to 30.7 mm.

The classification into 1st-, 2nd-, and 3rd-degree hypertelorism is no longer being used because it serves no practical purpose. Up to 40 mm of interorbital distance, there is no true ocular malposition or deviation (except in cases associated with craniofacial dysostosis and exorbitism). It is noteworthy that, even in the more severe form—at least in those compatible with life and normal intellect, the malformations spare the sphenoid bone, leaving the distance between the inner rims of the optic canals normal or near-normal (1), making it possible for the "useful orbits (12)" to be brought closer together.

Severe forms of telorbitism are associated with lateralization of the orbits (i.e., with a lateral tilting of the orbital plane). A foreshortened distance between the lateral canthus and the external auditory meatus (38), a wider-than-90° angle between the lateral orbital walls on CT scan cuts, or increased distance of the lateral orbital walls as compared to the values of Johr (42) and Laestadius and coworkers (43) characterize lateralized orbits. Munro (44) pointed out that

true lateralization is always accompanied by displacement of the medial orbital walls.

Operative correction of telorbitism is undertaken both for functional reasons (restoration of binocular vision, if possible) and for obvious esthetic and psychologic purpose.

FRONTOETHMOIDAL ENCEPHALOMENINGOCELES

Meningoceles represent failure of the neural tube to close, with herniation of central nervous system tissue. They occur in the midline of the head and spine from the region of the nose to the occiput and spinal column. Encephalomeningoceles of the anterior part of the head are rare in Western Europe, America, Australia, Japan, China, and Southern India. They are most frequent in Southeast Asia and Russia. Their incidence is reported to be 1:6000 live births in Thailand (45).

Encephalomeningoceles may occur with a frontal bone defect in clefts 0 to 14 (Figs. 31–38 and 31–39) or 1 to 13 (see Figs. 31–24 and 31–25), in which they are associated with telorbitism. When they are not associated with a cleft, the deformity may consist in a telecanthus with displacement of the medial orbital walls and deformation of the orbits rather than with true telorbitism.

The basic defect occurs between the frontal and ethmoid bones, and they are divided into: (a) *nasofrontal,* when they project between the nasal and frontal bones into the arc of the glabella, pushing the nasal bones inferiorly and displacing the medial orbital walls laterally; (b) *nasoethmoidal,* in which the herniation protrudes under the nasal bones and over the upper lateral nasal cartilages, still remaining extranasal; and (c) *nasoorbital,* in which the herniation is located behind the nasal bones and then deviates laterally, protruding through the medial orbital walls (46).

The dura is attached to the circumference of the bony defect, while beyond that it may be attenuated or absent, whereas the mass may contain atrophied parts of the frontal lobe or may be lined with ependyma and filled with cerebrospinal fluid (Tessier, unpublished data).

Early repair is advised in order to prevent the possibility of rupture and ulceration with ensuing meningitis and to prevent the secondary deformities, which increase in severity with age (45,46).

Treatment generally consists of excision of the sac and its contents, obliteration of the dural and bony defects with pericranial and bone grafts, respectively, and in older individuals, correction of the secondary deformities as indicated.

There are other rare forms of meningoceles that exist through the base of the skull; however, the description of these is beyond the scope of this book (47,48).

OCULOMOTOR DISTURBANCES IN CRANIOFACIAL MALFORMATION

Craniofacial malformations are characterized by the frequent occurrence of oculomotor disturbances. Abnormal ocular alignment can be explained on the basis of:

1. Abnormal extraocular muscle vectors of action
2. Altered interorbital distance and angulation
3. Involvement of cranial nerves
4. Structural abnormality or absence of specific extraocular muscles (49)

Diamond and Whitaker (49) reported a 42% incidence of extraocular muscle anomalies in patients with strabismus due to craniofacial dysostosis, while pointing out that the true incidence is hard to estimate because only a small percentage of patients undergo exploration (49,50).

Ocular deviation may occur in either the vertical or horizontal plane. Overall, Morax (50) has observed more vertical than horizontal imbalance. The V syndrome is the most classical (exotropia on upward gaze, esotropia on lower gaze), representing weakness of one or both superior obliques and hyperactivity of one or both inferior obliques (51).

The effect of correction of the craniofacial anomaly on the extraocular muscle balance is unpredictable. A preexisting deviation may remain unaffected by the procedure, or it may improve or be converted into a different type of imbalance (52).

Patients undergoing sagittal advancement show little tendency to change in their postoperative horizontal oculomotor deviation, in contrast to patients with telorbitism. Because orbital translocation in these patients is often delayed, correction of their strabismus should be considered before orbital translocation. In contrast, patients with telorbitism show a definite trend toward esodeviation after medial orbital

translocation. The squint seems to stabilize about 6 months postoperatively, and Choy and colleagues (52) recommended that no orbital translocation be carried out in this group of patients until at least 6 months after the correction of telorbitism. Diamond and associates (49,53) also recommended early alignment of the ocular axis, without distinction between sagittal and medial orbital translocation.

Surgical Correction of Craniofacial Anomalies

CORRECTION OF SIMPLE SUTURAL SYNOSTOSES

The correction of simple sutural synostoses is undertaken in order to correct both functional (ICH) and aesthetic problems. It is generally accepted that strip craniectomies alone are ineffective in correcting an already established deformity. If, however, the affected parts of the cranial and facial skeleton are dissected, mobilized, brought to an optimal position, and fixed there, the improved form is likely to be maintained. If such a correction is carried out during infancy (there is disagreement about the age at which correction is undertaken; most people feel that 6 months of age is most appropriate), the surgeon can take advantage of the forward thrust of the growing brain to maintain normal growth, and bone regeneration will probably fill any bone defects resulting from the osteotomies and bony advancements.

A frontoorbital remodeling and advancement is the procedure of choice for correction of plagiocephaly (unilateral) (Figs. 31–40 through 31–43) and brachycephaly (bilateral). A bifrontal craniotomy is carried out, the anterior and front part of the middle cranial fossae, as well as the orbit on the involved side, are dissected, and the supraorbital bar is removed, given an appropriate curvature, and fixed in an advanced position. If the frontal bone is too deformed, a new bony forehead is fashioned from the parietal bones. If not, the frontal bone is replaced and wired into position. The dead space created by the advancement in the anterior cranial fossa is obliterated by the advancing brain in a matter of a few weeks. The literature is replete with variations on this surgical theme but detailed descriptions are beyond the scope of this book. In the majority of cases, growth continues unimpeded and satisfactory form is maintained. In a few instances, however, the deformity may recur (54) and operative correction has to be repeated.

It is on the same principle that correction of occipital plagiocephaly is carried out. The ankylosed lambdoid suture (radiographically, the affected lambdoid suture is usually open with a sclerotic ridge adjacent to it) and asterion are resected, and the deformed occipital bones are removed, fragmented and replaced as necessary, so that the shape of both parietooccipital regions is normalized.

CORRECTION OF SYNDROMIC SYNOSTOSES

Surgical correction of syndromic forms of craniosynostoses is a matter of significant complexity because of the many developmental and technical factors to be considered. In the older child with craniofacial dysostosis, simultaneous advancement of the forehead and the midface with a monoblock frontofacial osteotomy is usually the procedure of choice. It is the only operation that in combination with other smaller ancillary operations is likely to give a near-normal face.

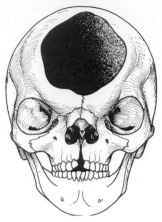

FIG. 31–40. Correction of unilateral coronal synostosis (plagio-cephaly) in infancy.

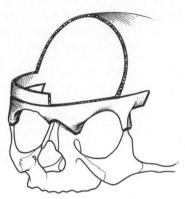

FIG. 31–41. Correction of unilateral coronal synostosis (plagio-cephaly) in infancy.

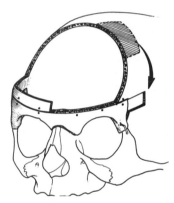

FIG. 31–42. Correction of unilateral coronal synostosis (plagio-cephaly) in infancy.

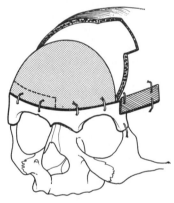

FIG. 31–43. Correction of unilateral coronal synostosis (plagio-cephaly) in infancy.

The procedure is performed via an intracranial approach. The entire dissection is carried out through a coronal and a vestibular incision. The craniotomy is designed preserving a frontal bone bar between the frontal bone segment and the orbits. The frontal lobes are retracted, giving access to the orbital roofs. The temporal muscles are dissected from the temporal fossae, and the orbits and zygomata are dissected in a subperiosteal plane. A horizontal osteotomy is carried out through the lower frontal bone. The orbital roofs are sectioned intracranially. The lateral and inferior orbital walls are sectioned, starting in the sphenomaxillary (inferior orbital) fissure, and the medial orbital walls are sectioned behind the posterior lacrimal crest. The zygomatic arches are sectioned. Through the vestibular incision, the maxilla is dissected, and a pteryomaxillary disjunction carried out. At this point, the frontofacial mass is mobilized with Rowe forceps, and the posterior portion of the nasal septum and the ethmoid are divided through the frontoethmoidal osteotomy. After advancement of the facial mass, the frontal bar is lengthened accordingly with a step osteotomy. Fixation is effected at the level of the forehead (to the frontal bar) and at the zygomatic arches (Figs. 31–44 and 31–45).

In the infant and young child this procedure is frought with considerable morbidity, and should be reserved for extreme cases in which there is both pronounced exorbitism jeopardizing the cornea and severe airway restriction. If intercranial hypertension has to be relieved, then a frontoorbital advancement (as described above) may be carried out and the midface dealt with later using a Le Fort III extracranial procedure. However, the results of this combined treatment have been disappointing aesthetically, and secondary deformities such as turricephaly may follow. Consideration has been given to relieving the raised intracranial pressure by carrying out a posterior, parietooccipital decompression (55).

In adults, the monoblock advancement may be followed by infection and bone sequestration because of the limited ability of the brain to expand and obliterate the dead space thus created in the anterior cranial fossa. Instead, the midfacial retrusion is corrected with a Le Fort III craniofacial disjunction. This procedure was pioneered by Tessier (56) and later modified by him. The transverse frontal crescent, the vertical frontal spur, and the semiopen method are all modifications of the same procedure designed to overcome specific problems (57) (Figs. 31–46 to 31–48).

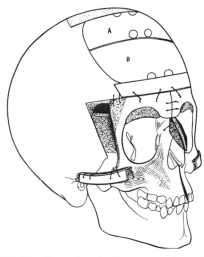

FIG. 31–44. Frontofacial advancement (monoblock).

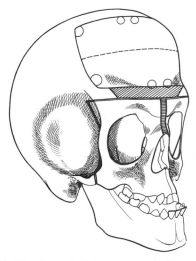

FIG. 31–45. Frontofacial advancement (monoblock).

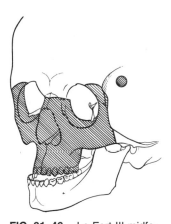

FIG. 31–46. Le Fort III midfacial advancement.

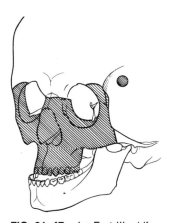

FIG. 31–47. Le Fort III midfacial advancement.

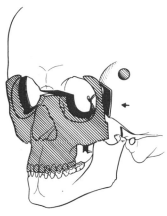

FIG. 31–48. Le Fort III midfacial advancement.

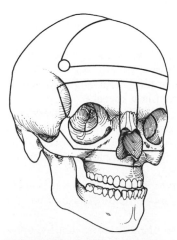

FIG. 31–49. Orbital osteotomies for correction of telorbitism, and Le Fort I maxillary osteotomy.

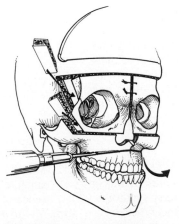

FIG. 31–50. Orbital osteotomies for correction of telorbitism, and Le Fort I maxillary osteotomy.

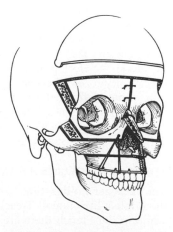

FIG. 31–51. Orbital osteotomies for correction of telorbitism, and Le Fort I maxillary osteotomy.

Aesthetic results are improved by individualizing the procedures to suit the particular needs of each case. Osteotomies can be combined for differential advancement of the upper and middle thirds of the face, and segments of bone can be removed from the interorbital region and anterior cranial fossa in combination with a frontofacial monoblock advancement when reduction of interorbital distance and maxillary expansion are required (facial bipartition).

Correction of telorbitism is based on the observation that the facial deformities stop at the level of the sphenoid and that the "useful orbits can be mobilized and approximated following resection of a central block of the floor of the anterior cranial fossa and frontal bone, including the ethmoid." Unfortunately, olfaction is sacrificed with resection of the ethmoid. Trying to overcome this drawback, Converse and others (58) modified the osteotomies. Subsequent experience, however, showed that it is not always possible (38). Sailer and Landolt resect the cribriform plate using the operative microscope in an effort to preserve olfaction (59).

The surgeon carries out the various osteotomies separating the entire bony orbit from the cranium and adjacent facial bones. The orbits are mobilized and brought toward the midline. A bilateral medial transnasal canthopexy is performed if the medial canthal tendons have been detached. The bony defects resulting from mobilization of the osteotomized segments are obliterated with bone grafts, while another bone graft is pegged into the frontal bone and wired to the frontal process of the maxilla to reconstruct and support the nasal bridge. A midline excision of skin is frequently necessary to eliminate the cutaneous redundancy, approximating the eyebrows and canthi and providing a more pleasing appearance (Figs. 31–49 to 31–51).

The subcranial method of correction (1,38) is no longer being used. Minor degrees of telorbitism can be camouflaged by burring the anterior lacrimal crests and performing a bilateral medial canthopexy (the intercanthal distance may be reduced up to 10 mm by this procedure). The intracranial route is used in all other cases.

Laterofacial Microsomias

Tessier has chosen this term to group together the following entities: Treacher Collins–Franceschetti complex, hemifacial microsomia, and the Goldenhar syndrome. He also includes Romberg disease, which will not be discussed in this chapter.

These entities may be grouped together for descriptive purposes because they represent combinations of the same group of lateral facial clefts (clefts 6, 7, and 8). Cleft 6 belongs specifically to the Treacher Collins and hemifacial microsomia, while cleft 8 belongs to both the Treacher Collins and Goldenhar syndromes. These clefts can occur either singly or in any combination with each other, and their phenotypes are varied and inconsistent (Figs. 31–52 to 31–58) (35).

TREACHER COLLINS–FRANCESCHETTI COMPLEX

The Treacher Collins–Franceschetti complex is referred to in the English literature as Treacher Collins or Berry syndrome, while in the French literature it is called Franceschetti syndrome. It is also referred to as mandibulofacial dysostosis.

The importance of Tessier's description of the Treacher Collins–Franceschetti complex (Figs. 31–59 to 31–64) is that it is based on operative findings rather than on simple de-

scription of surface characteristics. Tessier pointed out that the main characteristic of the complete forms is *a more or less total absence of the malar bone and of the zygomatic arch.* The bony deficits are between maxilla and zygoma, frontal bone and zygoma, or temporal bone and zygoma. The following malformations are observed:

1. *Eye.* Frequently strabismus and amblyopia are evident.
2. *Lower eyelid.* There is a notch between the lateral and middle thirds; along the edges the eyelashes are absent, and the tarsus is atrophic.
3. *Upper eyelids.* There is occasional microform of a coloboma.
4. *Eyebrow.* There is occasionally a notch or an ectropion of the lateral tail of the eyebrow.
5. *Lacrimal apparatus.* Frequent absence of the lower lacrimal punctum is apparent.
6. *Lateral canthus.* Deprived of a site of insertion, it is totally free, causing a brevity of the palpebral fissure.
7. *Nose.* It may be narrow, deviated, hooked, or kyphotic. Frequent choanal atresia, which is rarely complete, is due to the vertical shortness of the maxilla and to the height of the palate.
8. *Cheek.* A sclerodermic furrow extends from the lower eyelid notch toward the mandibular angle. On it are occasionally observed hairs, which represent ectopic eyelashes.
9. *Buccal commissure.* It is frequently enlarged by a rudimentary macrostomia.
10. *The orbit in general.* The sphenomaxillary fissure (inferior orbital fissure) is open anteriorly because of the absence of the malar bone. The maxillary hypoplasia renders the infraorbital canal short. The infraorbital neurovascular pedicle may exit the orbital cavity without any bony trajectory. The orbital floor may have an inclination of up to 45° toward the sphenomaxillary fissure. The orbital contents are engaged in a large deficit, corresponding to a vertical increase of the orbit and, consequently, a decrease of the transverse diameter. The supraorbital ridge and superolateral angle and the lateral process of the frontal bone develop inferiorly and medially because of absence of the frontal process of the malar bone; the lateral canthus, therefore, is displaced inferiorly. There is no real lateral orbital ridge. The greater sphenoid wing develops anteriorly because it does not encounter the zygomatic bone. The anterior portion of the greater wing is thin and irregular. It develops medially because the orbital contents sink in the inferolateral angle, which is widely open to the retromaxillary space.
11. *Alveolar bone and palate.* The dental arch is narrow, the palate is high. The maxillary tuberosity is elevated, as is the palate, causing a vertical atresia of the choanae. The narrowing of the maxilla is responsible for their transverse atresia.
12. *Maxilla and maxillary sinus.* The body of the maxilla is small, even though it appears normal, because of the absence of the malar bone.
13. *Malar bone.* The complete agenesis or severe hypoplasia of the malar bone is the characteristic malformation that explains all of the orbital anomalies. A rudimentary malar bone has been observed attached to the greater sphenoidal wing.

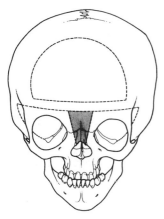

FIG. 31–52.   Facial bipartition.

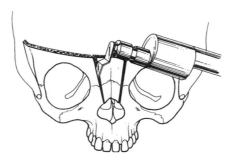

FIG. 31–53.   Facial bipartition.

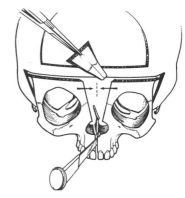

FIG. 31–54.   Facial bipartition.

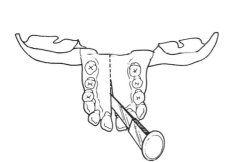

FIG. 31–55.   Facial bipartition.

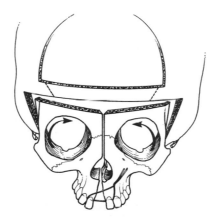

FIG. 31–56.   Facial bipartition.

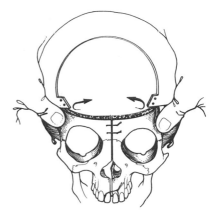

FIG. 31–57.   Facial bipartition.

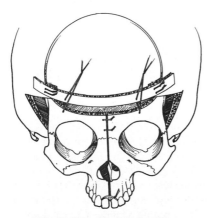

FIG. 31–58.   Facial bipartition.

14. *Temporal region and muscles.* In the majority of cases, one does not find even a small vestige of a zygomatic arch on the temporal bone. There might be one or more sesamoid bones in the normal course of the zygomatic arch. The absence of the zygomatic arch does not imply absence of the masseter because it inserts on the temporal fascia. This fascia belongs to both muscles, which become a common temporomasseteric muscle. The temporal muscle is usually atrophic.

15. *Temporomandibular joint.* The condyle and coronoid process are frequently hypoplastic.

16. *Mandible.* The ascending ramus is short. There is a prominent antegonial notch. The lower border of the mandibular body is hypoplastic.

17. *Chin.* Its retrusion and increase in height seem to be related to the vertical shortness of the ramus and to the cervical malformations.

18. *Ear and facial nerve.* Microtia and cryptotia are frequent. In the pure form of Treacher Collins–Franceschetti syndrome, there is no facial nerve palsy.

19. *Associated malformations.* Cleft palate and vertebral malformations may accompany this complex. Franceschetti and Klein pointed out that individuals afflicted by this condition have a strong, almost "familial" resemblance.

Treatment

Operative correction of the Treacher Collins–Franceschetti deformities is aimed at reconstructing the missing or deficient elements of the facial skeleton, generally in three or four stages. The soft tissues are usually dealt with after the skeletal reconstruction, with the exception of the notches or colobomas of the lower lids. These are repaired first because, when at a later stage the orbits are dissected and bone grafts placed, the tension on the soft tissues might not allow their effective closure (Tessier, personal communication, 1983).

The sequence of procedures depends on the degree of the maxillomandibular deformities. If the deformities are not very

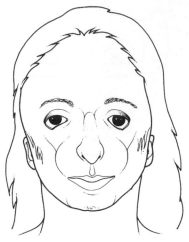

FIG. 31–59. Treacher Collins–Franceschetti syndrome.

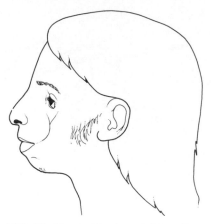

FIG. 31–60. A side view of deformities in the Treacher Collins–Franceschetti syndrome.

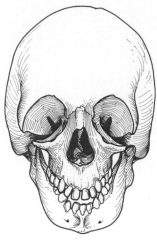

FIG. 31–61. Treacher Collins–Franceschetti syndrome.

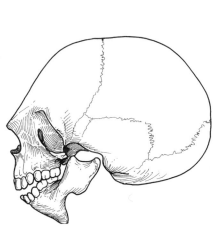

FIG. 31–62. Treacher Collins–Franceschetti syndrome.

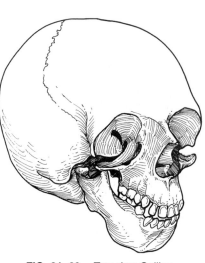

FIG. 31–63. Treacher Collins–Franceschetti syndrome.

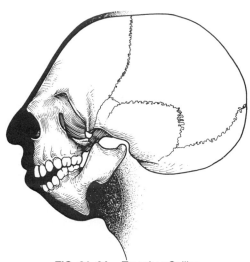

FIG. 31–64. Treacher Collins–Franceschetti syndrome.

severe, the first stage will consist in reconstruction of the orbits and zygomatic arches with bone grafts. Later, more appositional bone grafts may become necessary to build up further the areas of deficiency. Eventually, the maxillomandibular deformities are corrected as necessary. In cases with severe deformities, in which restriction of the airway is likely to exist because of a combination of maxillary atresia (restriction) and mandibular hypoplasia, Tessier has developed a procedure to which he has given the term *integrale* (integral-total procedure, indicating the performance simultaneously of midfacial and mandibular osteotomies). It consists in a midfacial osteotomy and forward "tilting" of the midface, with the area of the nasion as fulcrum, combined with a mandibular osteotomy to advance the mandible. The midfacial osteotomy is essentially a Le Fort II osteotomy because the zygomatic arches are absent and the sphenomaxillary (inferior orbital) fissures may be open anteriorly as a result of cleft 6.

The mandibular osteotomy is of the C or inverted-V type. The mobilized skeletal segments are stabilized with rigid fix-

ation and with cranial and iliac bone grafts. Excellent midfacial stability is essential in order for this combination of procedures to be successful. The integrale is a difficult, lengthy procedure involving hazardous dissection and requires a tracheostomy for airway control (Figs. 31–65 to 31–69). A safer approach might be to carry out the midfacial and mandibular osteotomies in separate stages. Complementary procedures (e.g., lateral canthopexy adjustments, rhinoplasty, genioplasty, and/or lengthening of the suprahyoidal region with a Z-plasty) are carried out after the major stages of reconstruction have been completed.

HEMIFACIAL MICROSOMIA

This term was first used by Gorlin and associates (60,61) to refer to patients with unilateral microtia, macrostomia, and failure of formation of the mandibular ramus and condyle. They have suggested that oculoauriculovertebral dysplasia (Goldenhar syndrome) is a variant of this complex characterized by vertebral anomalies, most often

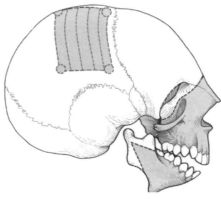

FIG. 31–65. Integrale (midfacial and mandibular osteotomies for correction of severe forms of Treacher Collins–Franceschetti syndrome).

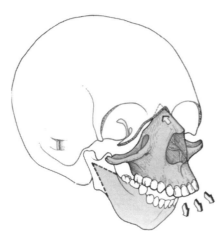

FIG. 31–66. Integrale (midfacial and mandibular osteotomies for correction of severe forms of Treacher Collins–Franceschetti syndrome).

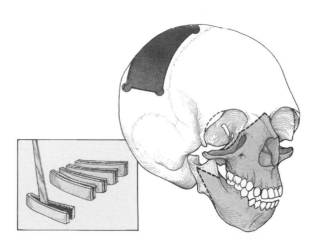

FIG. 31–67. Integrale (midfacial and mandibular osteotomies for correction of severe forms of Treacher Collins–Franceschetti syndrome).

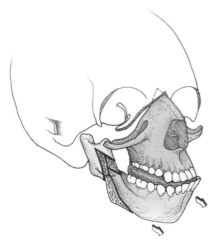

FIG. 31–68. Integrale (midfacial and mandibular osteotomies for correction of severe forms of Treacher Collins–Franceschetti syndrome).

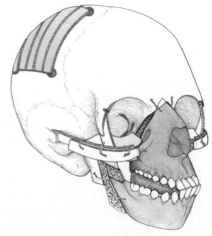

FIG. 31–69. Integrale (midfacial and mandibular osteotomies for correction of severe forms of Treacher Collins–Franceschetti syndrome).

hemivertebras, and epibulbar dermoids. Several other terms have been used to designate this condition: first and second branchial arch syndrome (62), otomandibular dystosis (63), craniofacial microsomia (64), lateral facial dysplasia (65), otomandibular syndrome (the term used in the French literature), and others. Furthermore, there have been several classifications into groups (62), types (66), and grades or types (67–69), which do not necessarily describe the same or similar phenotypes.

As previously mentioned, Tessier (35) considers this malformation to be a clefting syndrome—among the most complex ones affecting the cranium, the upper part of the face, and the mandible. It is, in contradistinction to the Treacher Collins–Franceschetti complex, an *asymmetrical malformation* for which no genetic background has been identified (70). Its incidence is estimated to be between 1:3500 (68) and 1:5642 births (71). Although it is described as a unilateral deformity, bilateral forms are not infrequent (65,66,69,71).

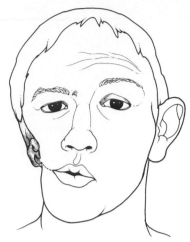

FIG. 31–70. Hemifacial microsomia.

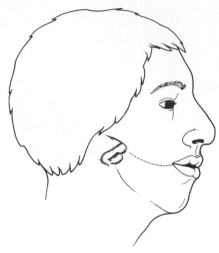

FIG. 31–71. Hemifacial microsomia.

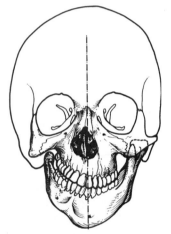

FIG. 31–72. Hemifacial microsomia.

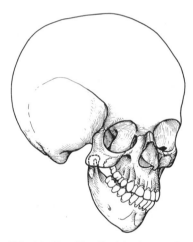

FIG. 31–73. Hemifacial microsomia.

Skeletal Deformities

Even though the orbit, zygoma, temporal bone, maxilla, and nose may be involved, the mandibular deformity is assumed to be the abnormal keystone. Asymmetrical mandibular growth is the earliest skeletal manifestation and seems to play a pivotal role in the progressive distortion of both ipsilateral and contralateral structures (71) with deviation toward the affected side. At birth, the defect often appears mild; with growth, asymmetry becomes more marked because of progressive development of the normal side. Only after full growth of the patient is the end-stage deformity evident (69) (Figs. 31–70 to 31–73).

The Mandible

Pruzansky's classification of the mandibular deformity in hemifacial microsomia into grades (67) has been adopted by other authors (64,69,71) because it provides a workable repository for cases with similar presentation. In grade I, the hypoplasia is minimal, and the difference with the assumed normal side is one of size. In grade II, there is a functioning but deformed temporomandibular joint that is usually displaced anteriorly and medially. The condyle, ramus, and sigmoid notch are distorted. In grade III, there is complete absence of the ramus and glenoid fossa. The mandibular body ends abruptly in the molar region.

The Maxilla

The maxilla is characterized by a transverse and vertical shortness. Its downward growth is impeded by the vertical mandibular deficiency, causing an increasing obliquity of the occlusal plane.

The Malar Bone

Variable degrees of hypoplasia are demonstrated (64). In severe cases, the temporal portion of the zygomatic arch is absent, while its malar portion is long with an inferior, posterior, and medial inclination toward the styloid. The orbit itself is retropositioned.

Soft Tissue Deformities

Facial soft tissues on the affected side may vary from normal to severely deficient. The skin, subcutaneous tissue, and facial musculature of expression may be affected. Hypoplasia of the parotid gland is not infrequent, placing the facial nerve in a vulnerable position (64).

The muscles of mastication may be underdeveloped or absent, especially in the grade III patient. In grade I defects, the muscles, although small, can usually be identified. Grade II patients exhibit combinations of these findings (69) Macrostomia (soft tissue component of cleft 7) of a variable degree may be present.

The external ear is characterized by a wide spectrum of anomalies, varying from a normal appearance to total absence.

Anomalies of the Nervous System

A wide variety of CNS anomalies have been described in conjunction with hemifacial microsomia (e.g., agenesis of the corpus callosum, hydrocephalus, unilateral hypoplasia of the brainstem and cerebellum, and others). Cranial nerve anomalies are also frequent. The most common cranial nerve anomaly is facial palsy. Converse and associates (64) provide an extensive bibliography on this subject.

GOLDENHAR SYNDROME

As in hemifacial microsomia, the Goldenhar syndrome consists of a cleft 7 but of lesser severity; it is also associated with a cleft 8 with oculopalpebral predominance that, contrary to the Treacher Collins-Franceschetti complex, only slightly affects the orbital cavity. The epibulbar dermoids are frequently in the inferolateral quadrant, along the axis of a cleft 6. It is frequently bilateral, but contrary to the Treacher Collins–Franceschetti complex, it is always very asymmetrical. Its anatomic characteristics are similar to those of hemifacial microsomia; however, characterization of this syndrome probably depends on the presence of oculopalpebral anomalies, particularly because Goldenhar's original paper (72) was focused on the association of anomalies of the eye and ear.

Treatment

The asymmetrical nature of these syndromes, their progressive character, the diminished growth potential of all tissues involved, and the three-dimensional distortion of anatomic structures, account for the difficulties in their treatment. It is evident that because of the tremendous variability with which they present their treatment will also vary greatly. General guidelines must be established as to the principles, timing, and rationale of the various procedures and the coordination of disciplines (jaw orthopedics, surgery, and orthodontics) that must be combined for optimal results.

The goal of treatment in patients with hemifacial microsomia is improved function and optimal facial symmetry when growth is completed (73). The principles of treatment are: (a) stimulation of existing musculoskeletal units so that maximum growth may be achieved; (b) prevention of secondary underdevelopment of structures; (c) augmentation of deficient osseous structures and construction of missing portions of the skeleton with autogenous bone grafts; and (d) reconstruction of soft tissue defects. It follows that treatment becomes more complex and the anticipated results less favorable as the deformity progresses from a grade (or type) I to a grade (or type) III.

The assessment and radiographic evaluation of patients with hemifacial microsomia and Goldenhar syndrome will not be discussed here. Detailed descriptions of this subject have been published elsewhere (71,74,75).

Clinical observation has shown that the use of orthopedic orthodontic appliances can stimulate mandibular growth. This has been confirmed experimentally by Petrovic and colleagues (76). Any jaw orthopedic appliance that causes forward positioning of the condylar process in a steady pattern will bring about remodeling and bone apposition on the condylar head (77,78).

When the temporomandibular joint is present, if only the condylar cartilage and disc are missing, and the joint functions without difficulty, the deficient growth may be successfully compensated with the use of an orthopedic appliance (activator).

Distraction osteogenesis will probably become the method of choice for correction of the mandibular asymmetry in grades I and II, carried out at a very early age. Experience so far is limited with this method but it appears that not only is the length of the ramus increased but the shape of the condyle itself also tends to improve (8,79,80). If this fails to establish the required symmetry, a mandibular osteotomy of the ramus on the affected side to elongate and rotate the mandible is usually carried out during the age of mixed dentition (6 to 12 years). An open bite is created on the affected side, allowing for vertical maxillary downgrowth and extrusion of the maxillary teeth in order to obtain a horizontal occlusal plane (69) The treatment becomes more complex if the patient is first seen as an adult. A compensatory osteotomy of the opposite ramus has to be performed, because the nonaffected condyle cannot remodel and a Le Fort I procedure is necessary to level the occlusal plane.

In seriously affected temporomandibular joints, severe growth restrictions must be anticipated (81). Treatment should probably be initiated with the use of an activator because it may improve mobility and prevent further tipping of the occlusal plane (81). Furthermore, the stretching effort on the skin and muscles is beneficial (69). Early surgery aimed at correcting the mandibular asymmetry in three planes must be anticipated. If the existing temporomandibular joint is in a relatively normal anatomic location, it is maintained, and the mandible is osteotomized and elongated, rotated, and advanced. If the temporomandibular joint is displaced medially or anteriorly, it is excised, and a new joint is constructed at a site symmetrical with the opposite side. A compensatory osteotomy of the opposite side is almost always required. A posterior open bite, deliberately created, will allow vertical growth on the maxilla and eruption of maxillary teeth. In the adults, a Le Fort I osteotomy becomes necessary to achieve a horizontal occlusal plane (69).

If the temporomandibular joint is ankylosed, the preliminary orthopedic treatment is eliminated because of the severe restriction of mobility, and surgical release becomes the first step of the treatment (82).

When the mandibular ramus is missing (type III deformity), a ramus and glenoid fossa must be constructed, as symmetrically as possible to the opposite side. The surgical procedure is carried out when the child has a full complement of deciduous teeth (69). The mandibular ramus may be constructed either with rib grafts or with cranial bone grafts. When carried out early, an osteotomy of the opposite ramus is usually not necessary.

Optimal position of the mandible is determined with bite registration splints, which are constructed on scale models preoperatively. Postoperatively, following the period of interdental fixation, the splint is wired to the maxilla, and the mandibular movements are controlled with rubber bands, which guide the mandible into proper occlusion in the splint. *A consistent pattern of jaw movements is considered essential for the strain distribution in the mandible and is a prerequisite for the remodeling of the bone graft.* Growth continues to be deficient on the affected side, and additional osteotomies are frequently necessary to reestablish symmetry (73).

Tessier has pointed out that not enough attention has been paid to the malformations of the orbit and the absence of the glenoid fossa and the zygomatic arch. The zygomatic arch is constructed, when absent, preferably with a cranial bone graft mortised into the temporal bone. The glenoid fossa may be constructed with iliac bone. The orbit is remodeled as needed. All these procedures are adapted, of course, to the patient's age.

Finally, onlay bone grafts to improve skeletal contour, soft-tissue augmentation, and reconstruction of the auricle (which is deferred until the skeletal reconstruction is completed and optimal symmetry attained) are carried out as needed.

Complications

The potential for complications in the domain of craniofacial surgery is high. This is hardly surprising when one considers the extent and duration of craniofacial procedures, the multiple structures involved (cranium, orbits, maxilla, and occasionally the mandible), the close proximity of somewhat septic cavities (nose, paranasal sinuses, oral cavity), the large amounts of grafted tissue, and the frequent creation of dead spaces (83). A significant complication rate can be expected even in the most experienced hands and best-organized centers, particularly in cases with complex pathology such as syndromic synostoses (84).

A review of the largest published series substantiates the logical assumption that the majority of lethal complications follow procedures in which the intracranial route was used. Reported causes of death include:

1. Inadequate or excessive replacement of blood volume (83,85,86)
2. Cerebral edema (83,85,86)
3. Respiratory obstruction (83,85,86)
4. Infection (meningitis) (83,85,86)
5. Pneumomediastinum (83); an explanation of the pathogenesis of this complication is provided in another report (87)
6. Sagittal sinus thrombosis (86)
7. Tracheoesophageal fistula (83)
8. Erosion of the vena cava of a central line placed through the femoral vein (83)
9. Pulmonary embolism (83)

Other nonlethal but nevertheless serious complications may also follow craniofacial procedures.

1. Infection may lead to soft-tissue loss, osteomyelitis, localized abscesses, and sequestration of bone grafts. This appears to be the most frequent complication in all major reported series. The highest infection rate occurs in patients undergoing intracranial procedures, particularly where a communication of the cranial cavity with the nose, paranasal sinuses, and oral cavity is created (85,86). In an effort to reduce the incidence of infection, Jackson and coworkers have described the use of a galeal frontalis myofascial flap to eliminate communication of the nasopharynx with the anterior cranial fossa (88). The occurrence of bacterial contamination was shown to be directly proportional to the duration of the operative procedure (89).
2. Complications related to the orbital cavity and its contents include: (a) blindness due to injury of the optic nerve (83,85,86); (b) hemianopsia (83); (c) diplopia (83,85); (d) corneal ulceration (83); (e) neurogenic oculomotor palsy (85); and (f) obstruction of the lacrimal sac or nasolacrimal duct (83). A distinction must be made between true complications and sequelae of an operative procedure, which are more or less predictable and will be corrected at a later stage (e.g., ptosis of the upper lid after correction of exophthalmia by midfacial advancement and enophthalmia after correction of telorbitism, caused by the increase in volume of the orbit brought about by the orbital translocation).
3. Resorption of bone grafts, other than the true septic sequestrations, is another complication. The incidence and degree of resorption is difficult to quantify (83).
4. Cerebrospinal fluid leaks, frequently self-limiting, may require treatment by shunting or application of a dural patch (83,85). When cerebrospinal fluid leakage occurred in conjunction with an intraoral procedure, the infection rate was 25% (18). Spontaneous subdural hygromas may occur after prolonged spinal drainage (90).
5. Velopharyngeal incompetence has been reported after facial advancement. Generally, however, the effect of such procedures on speech is beneficial because of improvement of the airway and of dental occlusion (83,85).
6. Canthal drift and displacement of skeletal segments from their position of fixation may occur, comprising the esthetic result.
7. Inappropriate antidiuretic hormone secretion has been reported to follow craniofacial procedures (91) and after cleft palate surgery (92). If it is not recognized and treated immediately, this condition may have grave consequences. Serum electrolytes and osmolality must be monitored very closely.
8. Seizures, occuring in the early postoperative, or in the follow-up period (84).

Acknowledgment

This chapter is dedicated to Paul Tessier, my respected teacher and friend, who has graciously allowed me the publication of his valuable collection of illustrations. Note: To preserve this original and unique collection of illustrations, skeletal fixation is shown as it was originally drawn, with wire, whereas today mini or micro plates and screws would be used in many instances.

References

1. Tessier P, Guiot G, Rougerie J, et al. Ostéotomies cranio-nasoorbito-faciales. Hypertélorisme. *Ann Chir Plast* 1967; 12:103.
2. Posnic JC, Lin KY, Jhawar BJ, et al. Crouzon syndrome: quantitative assessment of presenting deformity and surgical results based on CT scans. Presented at the 5th International Congress, International Society of Craniofacial Surgery, Oaxaca, Mexico, October 1993.

3. Hayward R, Gonzales S, Lane R, et al. Temporal relationship between changes in sleep state, intracranial pressure and upper airway obstruction in children with craniosynostosis. Presented at the 5th International Congress, International Society of Craniofacial Surgery, Oaxaca, Mexico, October 1993.

4. Spinelli HM, Irizarry D, McCarthy JG, et al. An analysis of extradural dead space after fronto-orbital surgery. *J Plast Reconstr Surg* 1994; 93:1372.

5. Thompson D. Information presented at the Meeting of the European Association of Craniofacial Surgery, Jerusalem, Israel, 1994.

6. Jones B. Presented at the meeting of the European Association of Craniofacial Surgeons, Jerusalem, Israel, 1994.

7. Fearon JA, Munro IR, and Bruce DA. Observations on the use of rigid fixation for craniofacial deformities in infants and young children. *Plast Reconstr Surg* 1995; 95:634.

8. Data presented at the Workshop on Distraction of the Craniofacial Skeketon, NYU Medical Center, March 1994.

9. Komuro Y, Takato T, Harii K, et al. The histologic analysis of distraction osteogenesis of the mandible. *Plast Reconstr Surg* 1994; 94:152.

10. Aronson J. Experimental and clinical experience with distraction osteogenesis. *Cleft Palate-Craniofacial J* 1994; 31:473.

11. Moss M. Functional anatomy of cranial synostosis. *Child's Brain* 1975; 1:22.

12. Bolk L. On the premature obliteration of sutures in the human skull. *Am J Anat* 1915; 17:495.

13. Tessier P. Relationship of craniostenoses to craniofacial dysostoses and to fasciostenoses. A study with therapeutic implications. *Plast Reconstr Surg* 1971; 48:224.

14. Seeger JF, Gabrielsen TO. Premature closure of the frontosphenoidal suture in synostosis of the coronal suture. *Radiology* 1971; 101:631.

15. Delaire J. Considerations sur les synostoses prematures et leurs consequences au crane et a la face. *Rev Stolmatol* 1963; 64:97.

16. Smith DW, Tondury G: Origin of the calvaria and its sutures. *Am J Dis Child* 1978; 132:662.

17. La Trenta GS, McCarthy JG, Cutting CB. The growth of vascularized onlay bone transfers. *Ann Plast Surg* 1987; 18:511.

18. Hirabayashi S, Harii K, Sakurai A, et al. An experimental study of craniofacial growth in a heterotopic rat head transplant. *Plast Reconstr Surg* 1988; 82:236.

19. Virchow R. Ueber den cretinismus, nametlich in franken und über pathologische schädelforamen. *Verhanl D Phvs-Med Gesellschin Wurzborg* 1851–1852; 2:230.

20. Moss ML. Premature synostosis of the frontal suture in the cleft palate skull. *Plast Reconstr Surg* 1957; 20:199.

21. Moss ML. The pathogenesis of premature cranial synostosis in man. *Acta Anat* 1959; 37:351.

22. Stewart RE, Dixon G, Cohen A. The pathogenesis of premature craniosynostosis in acrocephalosyndactyly (Apert's syndrome). A reconsideration. *Plast Reconstr Surg* 1977; 59:699.

23. Kreiborg S, Prydsoe U, Dahl E, et al. Calvarium and cranial base in Apert's syndrome. An autopsy report. *Cleft Palate J* 1976; 13:296.

24. Ousterhout D, Melsen B. Cranial base deformity in Apert's syndrome. *Plast Reconstr Surg* 1982; 69:254.

25. David JD, Poswillo D, Simpson D. *The craniosynostoses causes, natural history and management.* New York: Springer-Verlag, 1982; 153.

26. Stutzmann J, Petrovic A, Stratoudakis AC. Cytological features in craniosynostosis. Presented to the 67th Congress of the European Orthodontic Society, Copenhagen, June 1990.

27. Holtermueller K, Wiedemann HR. The clover leaf skull syndrome. *Med Monatsschr* 1960; 14:439.

28. Kokkich VG, Moffet BC, Cohen MM. The cloverleaf skull anomaly: an anatomic and histologic study of two specimens. *Cleft Palate J* 1982; 19:89.

29. Cohen MM. An etiologic and nosologic overview of craniosynostosis syndromes. *Birth Defects* 1975; 11:137.

30. Crouzon MO. Dysostose cranio-faciale hereditaire. *Bull Mém Soc Méd Hôp Paris* 1912; 33:545.

31. Schiller JG. Craniofacial dysostosis of Crouzon: a case report and pedigree with emphasis on heredity. *Pediatrics* 1959; 23:107.

32. Apert EE. De l'acrocéphalosyndactylie. *Bull Mém Soc Méd Hôp Paris* 1906; 23:1310.

33. Cohen MM. Craniosynostosis and syndromes with craniosynostosis: incidence, genetics, penetrance, variability, and new syndrome updating. *Birth Defects* 1979; 15(5B):13.

34. Kawamoto HK. The kaleidoscopic world of rare craniofacial clefts: Order out of chaos (Tessier classification). *Clin Plast Surg* 1976; 3:529.

35. Tessier P. Anatomical classification of facial, craniofacial, and laterofacial clefts. In: Tessier P, Callahan A, Mustardé JC, et al., eds. *Symposium on plastic surgery in the orbital region.* St. Louis: CV Mosby, 1976; 12:189.

36. Jones KL, Smith DW, Hall BD, et al. A pattern of craniofacial and limb defects secondary to abberant tissue bands. *J Pediatr* 1974; 84:90.

37. Moore MH, David JD, Cooter RD. Hairline indicators of craniofacial clefts. *Plast Reconstr Surg* 1988; 82:589.

38. Tessier P. Orbital hypertelorism. In: Tessier P, et al., eds. *Symposium on plastic surgery in the orbital region.* St. Louis: CV Mosby, 1976; 12:255.

39. Derome PJ, Visot A. La dysplasie fibreuse cranienne. *Neuro Chirurg* 1983; 29(Suppl 1):5, 67.

40. Tessier P, Guiot G, Derome P. Orbital hypertelorism. Definitive treatment of orbital hypertelorism (ORH) by craniofacial or by extracranial osteotomics. *Scand J Plast Reconstr Surg* 1983; 7:39.

41. Van der Meulen JCH, Vaandrager JM. Surgery related to the correction of hypertelorism. *Plast Reconstr Surg* 1983; 71:6.

42. Johr P. Valeurs moyennes et limites normales en fonction de l'âge, de quelques mésures de la tête et de la région orbitaire. *J Génét Hum* 1953; 2:247.

43. Laestadius ND, Aase JM, Smith DW. Normal inner canthal and outer orbital dimensions. *J Pediatr* 1969; 74:465.

44. Munro IR. Discussion of surgery related to the correction of hypertelorism by Van der Meulen JCH, Vaandrager JM (reference 26). *Plast Reconstr Surg* 1982; 7118.

45. Charoonsmith T. Review of 310 patients with frontoethmoidal encephalomeningocele with reference to plastic reconstruction. In: Williams B, ed. *Transactions of the 8th International Congress of Plastic Surgery,* Canadian Society of Plastic Surgeons, Montreal, 1983; 314.

46. David JD, Simpson D, White J. Fronto-nasal encephaloceles: morphology and treatment. In: Williams B, ed. *Transactions of the 8th International Congress of Plastic Surgery,* Canadian Society of Plastic Surgeons, Montreal, 1983; 311.

47. Suwanwela CN, Suwanwela A. A morphological classification of sincipital encephalomeningoceles. *J Neurosurg* 1972; 36:201.

48. Morris WMM, Locksen W, Le Roux PAJ. Sphenomaxillary meningoencephalocele. *J Cranio-Maxillofac Surg* 1989; 17:359.

49. Diamond GR, Whitaker L. Ocular motility in craniofacial reconstruction. *Plast Reconstr Surg* 1984; 73:31.

50. Morax S. Oculomotor disorders in craniofacial malformations. *J Maxillofac Surg* 1984; 12:1.

51. Ortiz-Monasterio F, Fuente del Campo A, Limon-Brown E. Mechanism and correction of V syndrome in craniofacial dysostosis. In: Tessier P, et al., eds. *Symposium on plastic surgery in the orbital region.* St. Louis: CV Mosby, 1976; 12:246.

52. Choy AE, Margolis S, Breinin GM, et al. Analysis of preoperative and postoperative extraocular muscle function in surgical translocation of bony orbits: a preliminary report. In: Converse JM, McCarthy J, Wood-Smith D, eds. *Symposium on diagnosis and treatment of craniofacial anomalies.* St. Louis: CV Mosby, 1979; 20:128.

53. Diamond G, Katowitz JA, Whitaker LH, et al. Ocular alignment after craniofacial reconstruction. *Am J Ophthalmol* 1980; 90:248.

54. Renier D, Sainte Rose G, and Marchac D. Recurrent craniosynostoses. When and why? Presented at the 5th International Congress, International Society of Craniofacial Surgery, Oaxaca, Mexico, October 1993.

55. Jones BM, Hayward RD, Harkness D, et al. The Influence of intracranial pressure monitoring on the staged surgical management of craniosunostosis. Presented at the 5th International Congress, International Society of Craniofacial Surgery, Oaxaca, Mexico, October 1993.

56. Tessier P. Ostéotomies totales de la face. Syndrome de Crouzon. Syndrome d'Apert. Oxycéphalies Scaphocéphalies Trurricéphalies. *Ann Chir Plast* 1967; 12:273.

57. Tessier P. Recent improvements in treatment of facial and cranial deformities of Crouzon's disease and Apert's syndrome. In: Tessier P, et al., eds. *Symposium on plastic surgery in the orbital region.* St. Louis: CV Mosby, 1976; 12:271.

58. Converse JM, Ransohoff J, Matthews ES, et al. Ocular hypertelorism and pseudohypertelorism. Advances in surgical treatment. *Plast Reconstr Surg* 1970; 45:1.

59. Sailer RF, Landolt RM. A new method for the correction of hypertelorism with preservation of the olfactory nerve filaments. *J Cranio-Maxillofac Surg* 1987; 15:122.

60. Gorlin RJ, Jue KL, Jacobsen U, et al. Oculoauriculovertebral dysplasia. *J Pediatr* 1963; 63:991.

61. Gorlin RJ, Pindborg JJ, Cohen MM. *Syndromes of the Head and Neck.* New York: McGraw-Hill, 1976.

62. Grabb WC. The first and second branchial arch syndrome. *Plast Reconstr Surg* 1965; 36:485.

63. Obwegeser HL. Correction of the skeletal anomalies of otomandibular dysostosis. *J Maxillofac Surg* 1974; 2:73.

64. Converse JM, McCarthy JG, Wood-Smith D, et al. Craniofacial microsomia. In: Converse JM, ed. *Reconstructive Plastic Surgery.* Philadelphia: WB Saunders, 1977; IV:2359–2400.

65. Ross RB. Lateral facial dysplasia (first and second branchial arch syndrome, hemifacial microsomia). *Birth Defects* 1975; 11:51.

66. Tenconi R, Hall BD. Hemifacial microsomia: phenotypic classification, clinical implications and genetic aspects. In: Harvold EP, ed. *Treatment of hemifacial microsomia.* New York: Alan R. Liss, 1983; 39–50.

67. Pruzansky S. Not all dwarfed mandibles are alike. *Birth Defects* 1969; 5:120.

68. Swanson LT, Murray JE. Asymmetries of the lower part of the face. In: Whitaker LA, Randall P, eds. *Symposium on reconstruction of jaw deformities.* St. Louis: CV Mosby, 1978; 171–211.

69. Murray JE, Kaban LB, Mulliken JB. Analysis and treatment of hemifacial microsomia. *Plast Reconstr Surg* 1984; 74:186.

70. Poswillo D. Otomandibular deformity: pathogenesis as a guide to reconstruction. *J Maxillofac Surg* 1974; 2:64.

71. Kaban LB, Mulliken JB, Murray JE. Three-dimensional approach to analysis and treatment of hemifacial microsomia. *Cleft Palate J* 1981; 18:90.

72. Goldenhar M. Associations malformations de l'oeil et de l'oreille, en particulier le syndrome dermoide épibulbaire appendices auriculaires-fistula auris congenita et ses relations avec la dysostose mandibulo-faciale. *J Génét Hum* 1952; 1:243.

73. Vargervik K. Sequence and timing of treatment phases in hemifacial microsomia. In: Harvold EP, ed. *Treatment of hemifacial microsomia.* New York: Alan R. Liss, 1983; 133–138.

74. Chierici, G. Radiologic assessment of facial asymmetry. In: Harvold EP, cd. *Treatment of hemifacial microsomia.* New York: Alan R. Liss, 1983; 57–88.

75. Vargervik K, Miller A. Assessment of facial and masticatory muscles in hemifacial microsomia. In: Harvold EP, ed. *Treatment of hemifacial microsomia.* New York: Alan R. Liss, 1983; 113–132.

76. Petrovic AG, Stutzmann JJ, Gasson N. The final length of the mandible: is it genetically predetermined? In: Carlson DS, ed. *Craniofacial biology monograph no. 10, craniofacial growth series.* Ann Arbor: Center for Human Growth and Development, University of Michigan, 1981.

77. Harvold EP. The theoretical basis for the treatment of hemifacial microsomia. In: Harvold EP, ed. *Treatment of hemifacial microsomia.* New York: Alan R. Liss, 1983; 1–38.

78. McNamara JA. Neuromuscular and skeletal adaptations to altered function in the orofacial region. *Am J Orthod* 1973; 64:578.

79. McCarthy JG. The role of distraction osteogenesis in the reconstruction of the mandible in unilateral craniofacial microsomia. *Clin Plast Surg* 1994; 21:625.

80. Losken HW, Patterson GT, Lazarou SA, et al. Planning mandibular distraction: preliminary report. *Cleft Palate-Craniofacial J* 1995; 32:71.

81. Vargervik K. Treatment of hemifacial microsomia in patients with abnormal but functioning temporomandibular articulation. In: Harvold EP, ed. *Treatment of hemifacial microsomia.* New York: Alan R. Liss, 1983; 179–206.

82. Vargervik K. Treatment of hemifacial microsomia in patients without a functioning temporomandibular articulation. In: Harvold EP, ed. *Treatment of hemifacial microsomia.* New York: Alan R. Liss, 1983; 207–242.

83. Tessier P. Fentes orbito-faciales verticales et obliques (Colobomas) completes et frustes. *Ann Chir Plast* 1969; 14:301.

84. McCarthy JG, Glasberg SB, and Cutting CB. Twenty year experience with early surgery for craniosynostosis: II pansynostosis and the craniofacial synostosis syndromes—results and unresolved problems. Presented at the 5th International Congress, International Society of Craniofacial Surgery, Oaxaca, Mexico, October 1993.

85. Whitaker LW, Munro IR, Salyer KE, et al. Combined report of problems and complications in 793 craniofacial operations. *Plast Reconstr Surg* 1979; 64:198.

86. Sabatier RE, Munro IR, Lauritzen CG. A review of two thousand craniomaxillofacial operations. In: Williams B, ed. *Transactions of the 8th International Congress of Plastic Surgery,* Montreal, Canadian Society of Plastic Surgeons, 1983; 318.

87. Diaz JH, Henling CE. Pneumoperitoneum and cardiac arrest during craniofacial reconstruction. *Anesth Analg* 1982; 61:146.

88. Jackson IT, Adham MN, March RW. Use of the galea frontalis myofascial flap in craniofacial surgery. *Plast Reconstr Surg* 1986; 77:905.

89. Cerisola JA, Rohwedder R. Bacteriological contamination of the operating field in craniofacial surgery. A new schedule of antibiotic prophylaxis. In: Williams B, ed. *Transactions of the 8th International Congress of Plastic Surgery,* Canadian Society of Plastic Surgeons, Montreal, 1983; 283.

90. Rosen HM, Simeone FR. Spontaneous subdural hygromas: a complication following craniofacial surgery. *Ann Plast Surg* 1987; 18:245.

91. Brones MF, Kawamoto HK, Renaudin J. Inappropriate antidiuretic hormone syndrome in craniofacial surgery. *Plast Reconstr Surg* 1983; 71:1.

92. Coleman JC III. The syndrome of inappropriate secretion of antidiuretic hormone associated with cleft palate: report of a case and review of the literature. *Ann Plast Surg* 1984; 12:207.

32

Facial Osteotomies

S. Anthony Wolfe, M.D., F.A.C.S., and Louis Bucky, M.D.

Webster defines the face as the front part of the human head, including the chin, mouth, cheeks, eyes, and usually the forehead. Osteotomies of the underlying facial skeleton can alter the form and function of all of these external soft-tissue structures.

Osteotomies That Alter Neither Form Nor Function

Osteotomies that do not alter form or function are *osteotomies for access,* and most of the earliest osteotomies performed on the facial skeleton fell into this category (1,2). They are still of great usefulness, and should not be forgotten when a difficult problem in surgical exposure presents itself (Fig. 32–1).

A frontal craniotomy is the most commonly used osteotomy for access, and is the first part of every intracranial neurosurgical intervention. Craniofacial surgery, a joint enterprise by a neurosurgeon and plastic surgeon, usually involves a frontal craniotomy to retract the frontal lobes so that facial osteotomies can be performed safely through the orbital cavities and midportion of the cranial base. Craniofacial surgery has been a catalyst for advances in both specialties, and each specialty has learned from the other. For neurosurgeons who have not had the opportunity to be part of a craniofacial team, we put forward the following respectful requests, so that any subsequent procedures will be easier.

1. Use a coronal (i.e., ear-to-ear) incision whenever possible. Almost all areas of the skull can be approached through it, and the same incision can be used again, if necessary, rather than making further scars. (There are coronal incisions and hemi-coronal incisions, but to say "bicoronal" is redundant and incorrect, as it implies two coronal incisions.) The incision should be kept at least 5 cm behind the anterior hairline, not at or near the scalp–hairline junction. The incision may be zig-zagged if desired, and should continue to a point above and behind the ear, then take a cutback aimed at the alar base but still remaining in the hair-bearing sideburn (Fig. 32–2).

2. The temporal muscle should be respected and preserved; it has innumerable uses to the reconstructive surgeon. If it requires elevation, leave a strip of muscle along the anterior temporal crest so that the main body of the muscle can be reattached under appropriate tension.

3. The frontal bone segment (it is not a "flap" unless it has preserved soft-tissue attachments providing blood supply), when replaced, should be rigidly fixed in place at its

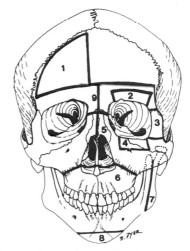

FIG. 32–1. Commonly used access osteotomies. **1,** frontal craniotomy; **2,** superior marginotomy; **3,** lateral orbitotomy (Krönlein); **4,** inferior marginotomy; **5,** extended across the orbital floor to 3-subcranial Le Fort III osteotomy; **6,** Le Fort I osteotomy; **7,** sagittal osteotomy of the mandibular ramus; **8,** horizontal osteotomy of the mandibular symphysis; **9,** transcranial facial bipartition.

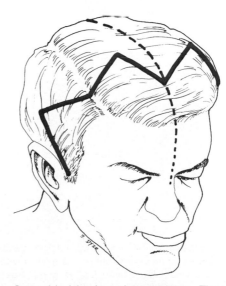

FIG. 32–2. Coronal incision in a zig-zag pattern. The zigs and the zags can be made shorter and closer together with somewhat better camouflaging of the incision, but operating time will also be a bit longer.

proper level (wires are sufficient, and using miniplates is an unnecessary expense), and gaps in the osteotomy lines should be filled in with bone slivers or bone paste from the craniotomy perforator. A "cookie cutter" can take a plug of inner-table bone to fit precisely into the burr holes, which also aids in stability (GC Lovaas, personal communication) (Case 32.1).

4. As much of the skull should be preserved as possible. Craniotomy by rongeur, with discarding of the bone removed, creates a defect and is often not necessary. Rongeuring away bone simply for exposure creates a defect that may require subsequent correction, and discards a valuable bone-graft donor source.

5. Bone grafts, if required, can be taken from the inner table of the removed frontal bone segment by ex vivo splitting after 3 or 4 years of age; if further bone is required, a full-thickness segment is removed from an area adjacent to the craniotomy after the dura is dissected, the bone is split, and the outer table replaced. Rarely in craniofacial surgical procedures is it now necessary to harvest bone from another part of the body (3).

6. Subsequent operations, as mentioned above, should use the same coronal incision and not make another incision several centimeters or inches away. If this is done, segments of the scalp may necrose. It has become standard practice not to shave the head for craniofacial procedures, but one should know precisely where any previous incisions are located.

Osteotomies for access to the orbital contents include the superior, lateral and inferior marginotomies, in which the segment is removed and replaced after the intraorbital work is done (4,5,6) (Case 32.2).

Another type of osteotomy, done not for access but for passage, would be the temporary removal of the zygomatic arch and a portion of the malar bone. This is performed for temporalis muscle transfers in maxillary reconstruction. If the temporal muscle is passed over the zygomatic arch it makes a fairly noticeable bulge, and the arc of rotation of the muscle is limited. Removal of the zygoma takes care of both problems, and after the muscle flap has been transposed to the place where it is needed the zygomatic arch/malar bone segment is replaced with a miniplate anteriorly and a single wire posteriorly (Case 32.3).

Le Fort I and extracranial Le Fort III osteotomies, coupled with midpalatal splits, provide access to the nasopharynx for

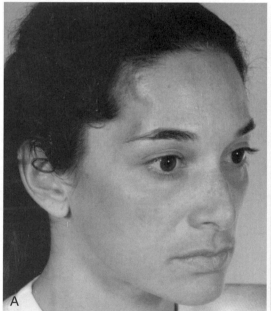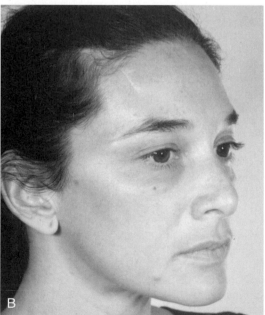

CASE 32–1. This woman had previously undergone a lifesaving operation to control a ruptured cerebral aneurysm. However, the neurosurgeon's access would have been just as good if use had been made of a coronal incision, which would have avoided the scar running down into her upper forehead. Also, the anterior half of the temporalis muscle was somehow lost, and the craniotomy flap reposi- tioned in a way that allowed it to sink inwardly. These defects, along with the visible burr holes, necessitated a secondary operation that should not have been necessary. She was treated by a large split cranial bone graft over the bony depression and advancement of the remaining temporalis muscle.

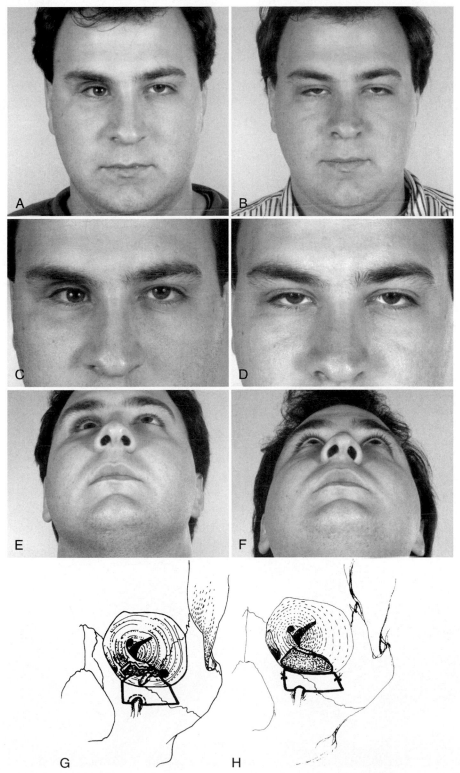

CASE 32–2, A–H. Patient with posttraumatic enophthalmos of the right eye treated by circumferential orbital dissection and cranial bone grafts to the defects of the orbital floor and medial orbital wall. When there is difficulty in removing orbital contents from the maxillary sinus, removal of the inferior orbital rim (as depicted) will be facilitating. Note that the incision for access to the orbital floor is made in a sub-tarsal crease and is still visible 1 month postoperatively. This incision is preferred to the subciliary incision as used for blepharoplasty, which can be associated with vertical eyelid retraction and does not give a better aesthetic result.

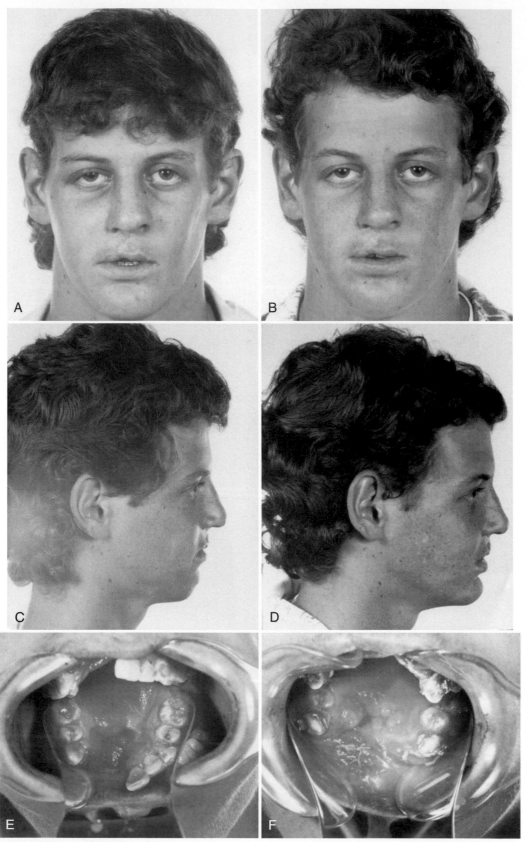

CASE 32–3, A–F. This 18-year-old patient had a cleft lip repair in infancy, followed by a palatal island flap to provide nasal tissue for maintenance of the push-back type palatal repair. In his midteens, he was operated on elsewhere and underwent a Le Fort I osteotomy. Unfortunately, the circulation through and beyond the donor areas of the island flap was inadequate, and he lost a portion of his anterior palate. Correction was obtained by performing another Le Fort I osteotomy and transposing temporal muscle down to the defect. Cranial bone grafting was used at the same time to fill in the alveolar defect. The patient underwent a genioplasty at the same surgery. The temporal muscle is a very useful tool in facial reconstructive surgery. When it is transposed to the lower face, removing the zygomatic arch temporarily permits the muscle to be brought below rather than over the arch, which has in the past been associated with an unsightly bulge. After the muscle transposition, the zygomatic arch is put back in place.

complex tumor removal (8). The osteotomies used for a monobloc frontofacial advancement with facial partition can be used to provide access to tumors of the cranial base and central midface (Case 32.4).

Luhr (7) has described the removal of the lateral cortical plate of the mandible to give access to difficult impacted 3rd molars. The segment is plated back in place after tooth removal (Case 32.5).

The mandible can be split in the midline or through the ramus to provide access to the floor of the mouth and the pterygopalatine fossa (9). When marginotomies are done on irradiated tissues or on the mandible, some soft-tissue attachments should be maintained if possible to provide blood supply. If bone segments are replaced into an irradiated field as free grafts, they are more likely to undergo necrosis. At the termination of an exposure osteotomy, the displaced segment is rigidly fixed back into its original position with wire or miniplate osteosyntheses.

When tumors involving the facial skeleton—particularly tumors of limited or no malignant potential, such as low-grade meningiomas or fibrous dysplasia—are removed, form and function are altered. Whenever possible, immediate reconstruction using autogenous bone grafts, usually cranial in origin, is performed with rigid fixation.

Osteotomies That Alter Form But Not Function

This type of "aesthetic facial sculpting" (10) includes osteotomies to advance or reduce the malar eminences (11), genioplasty, correction of masseteric hypertrophy, and recession of the anterior wall of the frontal sinus to reduce frontal bossing (12).

GENIOPLASTY

Although a genioplasty may provide some functional improvement with lip seal and improve certain patients with sleep apnea, it can still be regarded as an osteotomy performed largely to improve form rather than function. A genioplasty is the simplest and most commonly performed facial osteotomy and as such should be part of every plastic surgeon's repertoire. Chin implants are acceptable treatment for cases with minor degrees of retrogenia in which there are neither alterations in the vertical dimension of the chin nor lateral asymmetry. All other types of chin deformity require the ability to deal directly with the osseous malformation. The following types of genioplasty are commonly used (13):

1. *Sliding advancement.* A sliding advancement genioplasty is the most commonly performed variety, and all of the other types of genioplasty are variations on it. A lower labial sulcus incision is made, sparing the frenulum and developing a superior cuff that contains a small amount of muscle to aid in subsequent closure of the incision. A subperiosteal dissection of the symphysis is performed, and the mental nerves, located at the base of the 1st bicuspid or between the 1st and 2nd bicuspids, may be visualized. They do not need to be further dissected. A horizontal osteotomy is then performed with an oscillating saw, 7 to 10 mm above the lower border of the symphysis. The entire osteotomy should be performed with the saw, and in some cases a reciprocating saw is required to cut the posterior cortex laterally. The surgeon should avoid downfracturing the basilar segment before the bone has been completely cut with the saw, since a small lip of bone will remain on the upper portion of the symphysis that will act as an inter-

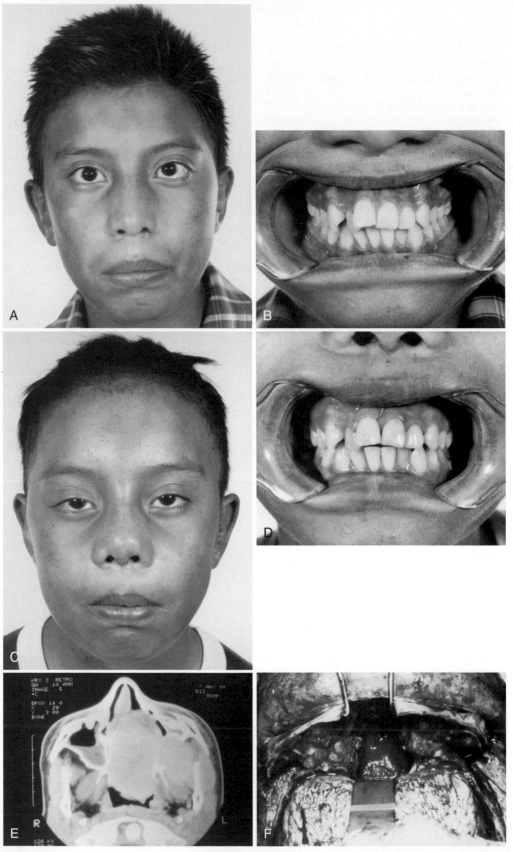

CASE 32–4, A–F. After being treated for some time for nosebleeds and "sinusitis," this young man eventually had a CT scan taken after he lost vision in the left eye. The CT scan showed a large tumor mass occupying the entire midportion of the anterior cranial base, and the interorbital space extending down to the palate. It was consistent in history and appearance with a juvenile angiofibroma. After preliminary embolization, the tumor was approached intracranially through a midfacial bipartition with similar osteotomy patterns to those used in the correction of orbital hypertelorism and Apert syndrome. Operative photographs show the approach to the cranial base with the facial halves and the brain retracted, and transposition of a portion of the temporalis muscle to seal off the cranial base from the nasopharynx. Postoperative CT scans show cranial bone grafts reconstructing the entire anterior cranial base. The approach allowed complete removal of the tumor, with return of vision in the left eye.

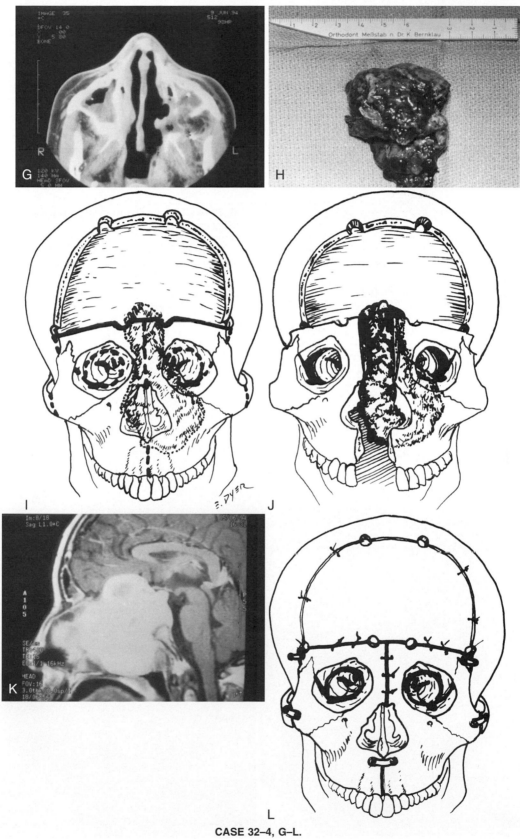

CASE 32–4, G–L.

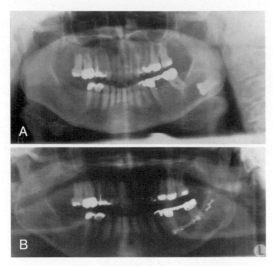

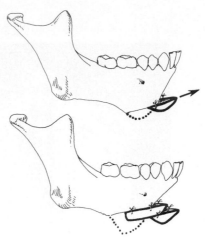

FIG. 32–3. Sliding advancement genioplasty (above) and two-tiered genioplasty (below).

CASE 32–5. A 70-year-old patient with a low impacted 3rd molar tooth. It had formed a dentigerous cyst, which then became infected. The lateral cortex of the mandible was removed by a modified sagittal split; both of the cuts were through the outer cortex, one midway up the ascending ramus and the other through the tooth space between the bicuspid and the remaining molar. The lateral cortical segment was maintained, with some of the masseteric fibers attached and retracted laterally. This provided exposure to remove the tooth and the entire cyst wall, and to visualize and preserve the infraorbital nerve over a distance of almost 5 cm. The lateral cortical segments were replaced with 1 miniplate and several small screws, and the patient went on to make an uneventful recovery. This is another example of an osteotomy for access.

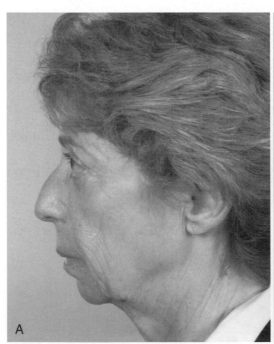

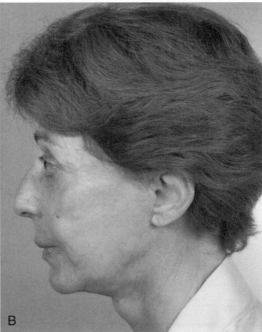

CASE 32–6. Patient shown before and after a sliding advancement genioplasty, performed along with a face lift. We prefer a genioplasty over a chin implant because it provides some tightening of the anterior neck muscles and obviates the need for an alloplastic material.

ference to proper advancement and will need to be burred down. If the osteotomy is carried beyond the mental foramen, it must remain 4 to 5 mm below it, because the mental nerve is lower in the mandible before it ascends to emerge through the mental foramen. The basilar segment, with its muscular attachments (geniohyoid, genioglossus, anterior belly of the digastric, and possibly some of the myelohyloid) is then advanced and fixed into its desired position. This osteosynthesis is rapidly and stably performed with three wires passed through the anterior cortex of the upper segment and the posterior cortex of the basilar segment. This can provide between 4 and 10 mm of advancement, depending upon where the drill holes are placed in the basilar segment and the angle at which the osteotomy was performed. Some surgeons perform the osteosynthesis with a miniplate, but we feel this is not necessary for stability in a standard sliding genioplasty, and is an unnecessary expense (Fig. 32–3) (Case 32.6).

2. *Centering genioplasty.* In a centering genioplasty, the basilar segment can be shifted from side to side, or cut obliquely and a triangular wedge of bone removed from the long side to be used as a bone graft on the short side (Fig. 32–4).

3. *Reduction genioplasty.* Reduction genioplasty is performed when the surgeon wishes to reduce the vertical dimension of the chin. A second horizontal osteotomy is performed parallel to the first osteotomy, and a segment of bone is removed. In cleft lip and palate patients, who often appear to have large chins, this bone segment can be used for maxillary needs, such as an onlay bone graft beneath a deficient alar base, or over the osteotomy lines of a Le Fort I osteotomy. The basilar segment is often advanced slightly to maintain a labiomental crease. One should not strip the muscles from the basilar segment, or burr down or resect the lower border to reduce a prominent chin; this will result in a flat-appearing chin with a sac of redundant skin hanging down beneath it (Fig. 32–5) (Case 32.7).

4. *Jumping genioplasty.* In a jumping genioplasty, the basilar segment is elevated on top of the upper symphysis. Thus it both increases chin projection (up to 10–15 mm) and shortens the vertical dimension of the chin by the height of the "jumped" segment. Fixation is more difficult than for a regular sliding genioplasty. The surgeon should use either countersunk Kirschner wires or screws, to offset the tendency of the attached musculature to tilt the basilar segment downward (Fig. 32–6) (Case 32.8).

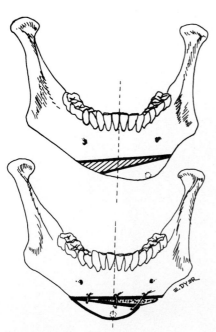

FIG. 32–4. Centering genioplasty.

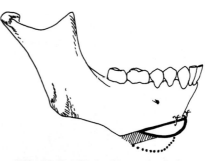

FIG. 32–5. Reduction genioplasty.

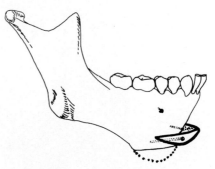

FIG. 32–6. Jumping genioplasty.

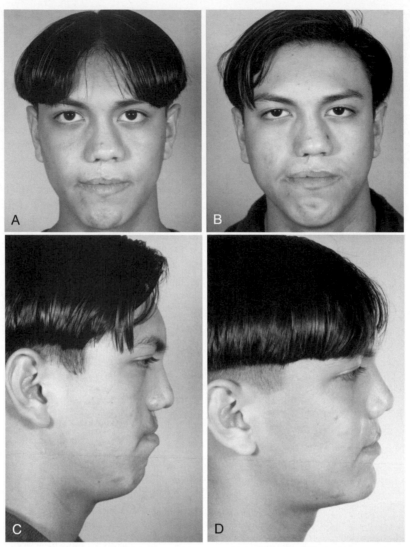

CASE 32–7. Patient with cleft lip and palate and class I occlusion, shown before and after a reduction/advancement genioplasty, onlay cranial bone grafting of the anterior maxilla, and anterior advancement of the upper buccal sulcus mucoperiosteum.

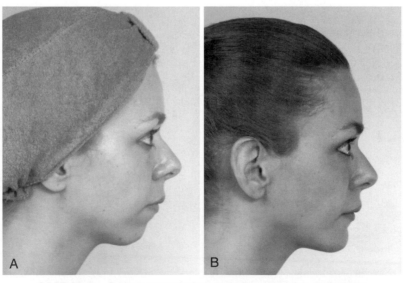

CASE 32–8. Patient shown before and after a jumping genioplasty.

5. *Lengthening genioplasty.* In a lengthening genioplasty, after the horizontal osteotomy, a bone graft of the desired dimension to lengthen the chin is fixed to the upper symphyseal segment with several miniplates. The surgeon can use iliac bone, but we find three outer-table cranial grafts, fixed together with several miniscrews, to be ideal. Once the bone graft has been fixed to the upper chin with good stability, the basilar segment can be fixed to the bone graft, with advancement if desired. The soft-tissue closure must be done with particular care in two layers if free bone grafts are used, and antibiotics are obligatory. In our opinion, there is no place for the use of alloplastic substances as an interpositional material, nor do we feel that a large gap between the bone segments should be left unsatisfied and ungrafted, relying on the miniplates to maintain the position of the basilar segment, and waiting for ossification to gradually take place between the two bone segments (Case 32.9).

6. *Staged serial genioplasty.* Patients with particularly severe microgenia may appear not to have any chin at all, but rather a straight line that runs from lower lip to the hyoid. These patients all have mandibular retrognathia (class 2 malocclusion) as well, and associated premaxillary protrusion and a steep occlusal plane are often present. A staged procedure might include a premaxillary setback (Wassmund procedure) and a jumping or lengthening genioplasty as the first stage, and then 6 months later a mandibular advancement and a sliding genioplasty through the old genioplasty (Case 32.10).

A genioplasty is often a complimentary procedure performed along with other aesthetic or reconstructive operations, and it can add substantially to the overall result.

Masseteric Hypertrophy

The condition of masseteric hypertrophy usually has two components: an increase in the bulk of the masseter muscle, and visible exostoses at the gonial angle. Dental occlusion is usually normal. Treatment consists of trimming the thickened muscle and removal of the excessive bone from the mandibular angle through an intraoral approach. Here the instrumentation used in the sagittal split procedure is indispensable.

Reduction of Frontal Bossing

Excessive frontal bossing is usually seen in men and, for this reason, examination of the frontal region is one of the methods used by physical anthropologists and forensic pathologists to establish the sex of a skull. Transsexual patients may seek to change a normal male frontal pattern to a softer, more female configuration.

In milder cases, it is sufficient to burr down the bony excess, stopping short of entering the frontal sinus. More pronounced cases are often associated with a hyperpneumatization of the frontal sinus, and the lateral extent of the sinus

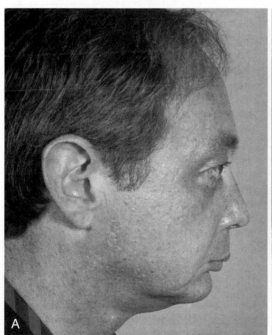 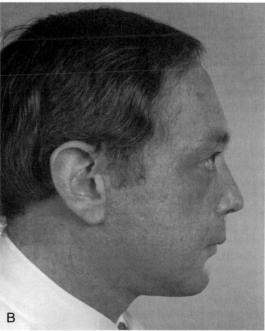

CASE 32–9. Patient shown before and after removal of a chin implant and a lengthening/advancing genioplasty with an interpositional cranial bone graft. A facelift was performed at the same surgery.

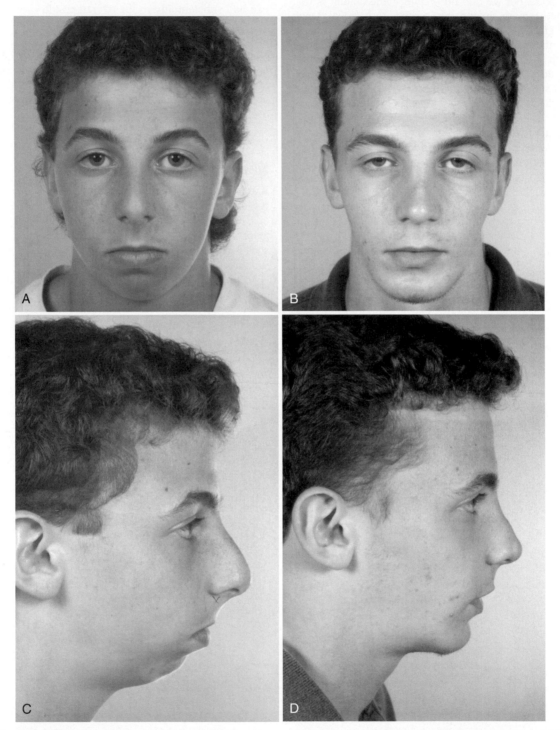

CASE 32–10. Patient with substantial microgenia treated by a Le Fort I impaction and a jumping genioplasty. Six months later, a sliding genioplasty was performed through the now-consolidated chin, giving a substantial improvement both in appearance and in lip seal. A rhinoplasty was also performed, and the patient declines revision of his slight dorsal irregularity.

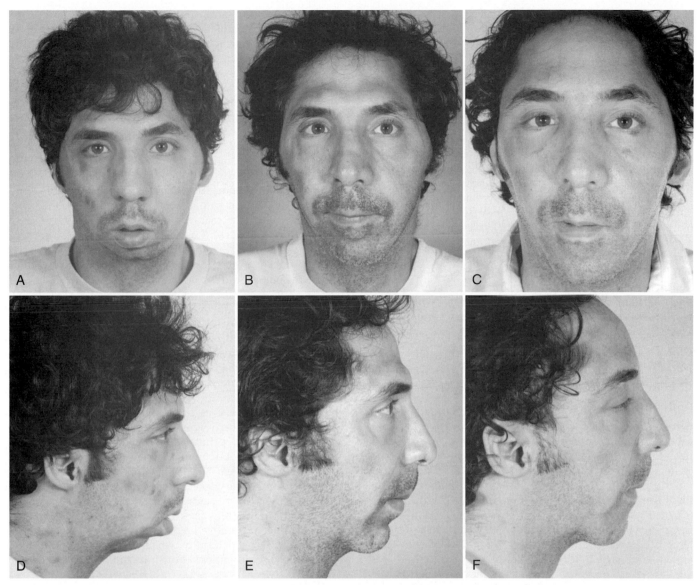

CASE 32–11. Patient shown in initial condition, after a jumping ge- nioplasty, reduction of the zygomatic arches, and recession of the an- terior wall of the frontal sinus to reduce frontal bossing. A subsequent staged genioplasty is planned, as was shown in the previous patient.

should be determined beforehand by radiography. A coronal incision is extended into an upper orbital dissection, and os- teotomies are made into the frontal sinus near its uppermost extent and across the orbital roof, avoiding intracranial pene- tration. The anterior wall of the frontal sinus is removed, and cortical supporting septae in the sinus are burred down until the anterior wall can be sufficiently recessed. The sinus is ir- rigated free of debris, and the anterior wall is replaced with stable osteosyntheses (wire is sufficient). Note that, if over- done, this procedure can be feminizing (Case 32.11).

Malar Osteotomies

Most malar augmentations are performed with alloplastic material (14), and osteotomies to increase malar projection are relatively unexplored territory. In Asia, however (particularly in Korea), malar reduction is a very common procedure; it is often coupled with a reduction of the gonial angles to convert a square face to a more oval one.

Onlay bone grafts to increase malar projection, even when rigidly fixed, are subject to varying degrees of resorption, and must be completely symmetrical to be successful. An oblique osteotomy of the malar bone, via an intraoral and often coronal approach, is carried beneath the malar prominence, avoiding entering the orbit or damaging the infraorbital nerve. Most of the masseteric attachments are left in place so, like a genioplasty, this is a "vascularized bone flap." The osteotomized segment is pivoted anteriorly with a rotation plane along the infraorbital rim, and interpositional cranial bone grafts are placed in the defect in the anterior maxilla. Several miniplates are used for precise stable fixation. The procedure can be combined with the "mask lift" or subperiosteal face-lift with lateral canthopexy, originally described by Tessier (15,16) (Case 32.12).

Osteotomies That Affect Form and Function

IN INFANCY AND CHILDHOOD

Frontoorbital advancement is performed as a unilateral procedure for plagiocephaly (unilateral coronal synostosis); or bilaterally for brachycephaly (bilateral coronal synostosis); or in the craniofacial dysostoses (Crouzon disease, Apert and a variety of other syndromes). These deformities, in which there is a premature sutural closure or lack of growth potential of the suture, are associated with restricted skull growth. Increased intracranial pressure and ventricular distortion have been observed in untreated patients, even with unilateral conditions (17) (Case 32.13).

The *monobloc frontofacial advancement* is a Le Fort III advancement that includes the orbital roof and frontal bone. It is a major surgical undertaking, and can give excellent functional results from the substantial increase in intracranial, orbital, and airway capacity. However, it has considerable risk in infancy and should be performed only when there are compelling functional reasons, such as severe exorbitism threatening vision, or airway inadequacy with documented oxygen desaturation and a likely need for tracheostomy. This procedure should be performed only by the most experienced craniofacial teams in a limited number of centers, but in the 4- to 10-year-old age group, we feel it is the procedure of choice for Crouzon disease in young children. When coupled with a facial bipartition, this is the only procedure that can remove all of the facial stigmata of Apert's syndrome (18) (Case 32.14).

Orbital dystopias, either transverse (hypertelorism, hypotelorism) or vertical, can be corrected near 2 years of age with satisfactory results, but better results will be obtained if the surgeon waits until 4 or 5 years of age. A nasal reconstruction, if carried out in childhood, will almost certainly require further work when the child has grown.

Osteotomies on the upper portion of the face (orbitocranial) can be performed in infancy and childhood with satisfactory, stable results. The brain and the eyes, as they grow, exert a "growth force" on surrounding osseous structures. Tooth-bearing structures may be shifted along with the orbitocranial structures, as in the monobloc frontofacial advancement; these early craniofacial procedures are *not* intended to effect a permanent correction of malocclusion. Instead, they provide functional relief in other areas, such as an increase in cranial and orbital capacity and an enlargement of the nasopharyngeal airway. Subsequent maxillofacial surgery on the tooth-bearing structures will almost certainly be required in the teens to provide satisfactory dental occlusion. In effect, a craniofacial deformity is converted to a simpler maxillofacial deformity, which is dealt with like other maxillofacial deformities. Growth of the orbital and cranial

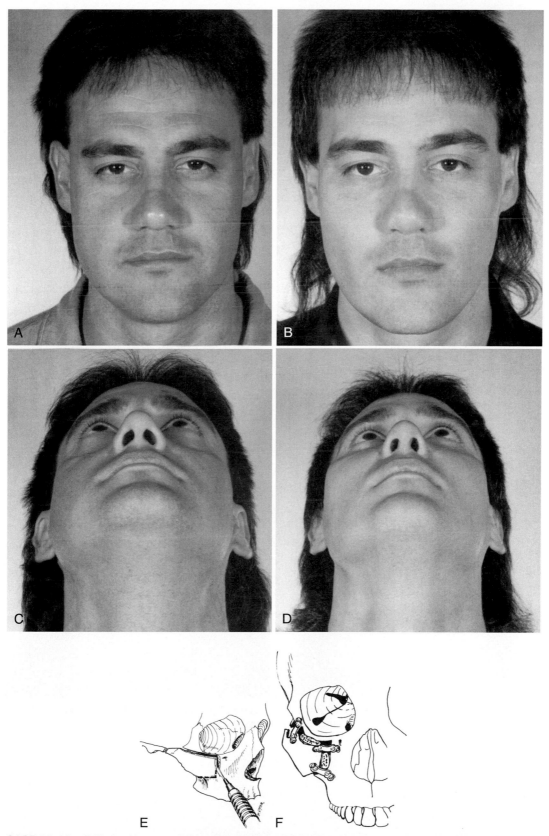

CASE 32–12. Patient with congenital hypoplasia of the infraorbital rims shown before and after rotational-advancement osteotomies of the malar bones.

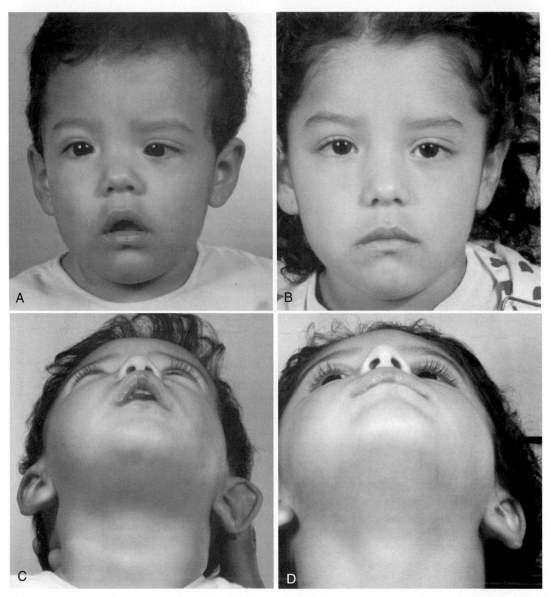

CASE 32–13. Patient with right unilateral coronal synostos shown before, and 3 years after, a right frontoorbital advancement, performed at 14 months of age. She also had correction of a left eso-tropia. The preferred age for plagiocephaly correction is about 6 months of age].

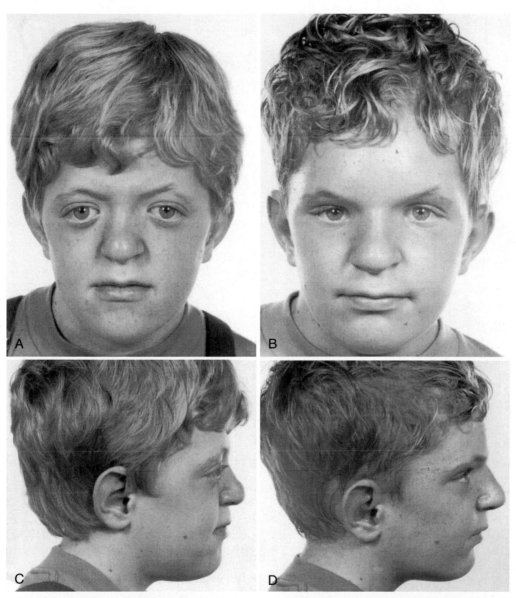

CASE 32–14. Eleven-year-old patient with Apert syndrome shown before and after a transcranial monobloc frontofacial advancement. This is a major surgical undertaking, but provides the best results for the craniofacial dysostoses of Crouzon and Apert. In particular, it can be coupled with correction of orbital hypertelorism by facial bipartition, frontofacial bending to provide more central projection, and orbital rotation to correct antimongoloid slanting of the orbits and palpebral fissures; this provides the only true correction of all of the facial stigmata of severe Apert deformity. The monobloc procedure is ideally done between 4 and 12 years of age, although it can be done earlier if there are compelling functional reasons such as airway obstruction. After the early teens, the complication rate may increase due to the lessened ability of the brain to expand into the retrofrontal dead space. For this reason, a relative contraindication to the monobloc procedure is the presence of a ventriculoperitoneal shunt (33).

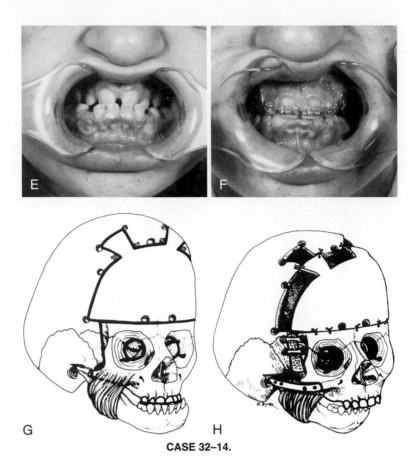

CASE 32–14.

areas is largely complete by 6 years of age, but the tooth-bearing structures do not reach their final growth, irrespective of what growth potential is present, until the midteens (Case 32. 15).

Distraction Osteogenesis

It was a logical step for plastic surgeons to apply to the facial skeleton the experience gained by orthopedic surgeons with the Ilizarov method (19) of distraction osteogenesis, which has proven its usefulness in lengthening the long bones. Following the initial reports by McCarthy (20) and Molina (21), the procedure is finding increasing use in a number of centers for gradual lengthening of the mandible, and it is also being used for maxillary advancement and expansion. The procedure may become the treatment of choice for children with hemi- and bilateral facial microsomia, particularly the severe forms of micrognathia where the patients are tracheostomy-dependent. The operative procedure is exceedingly simple, and consists of a corticotomy of about three-quarters of the mandibular circumference and application of percutaneous fixation pins. This can be an overnight, or even outpatient, procedure. Distraction begins on the 3rd or 4th day at a rate of 1 mm a day (0.5 mm, A.M. and P.M.), and is continued to a mild overcorrection. The fixation devices are then left in place for twice the length of time of the active distraction, to allow the new bone that has formed to consolidate. Distraction osteogenesis has been used for maxillary advancement (21), and other possibilities for its use, as in infants with severe craniofacial dysostoses, remain largely unexplored (Case 32.16).

After Reaching Dental Maturity

Most maxillary growth is complete by the age of 10 to 12 years, and the mandible continues to grow until 14 to 15 years in a female (onset of menarche), and 16 to 18 years in a male, under normal circumstances (12). Patients with various types of skeletal dysplasia can, of course, exhibit markedly abnormal growth patterns. It is acceptable in severe malformations to operate earlier than usual, and to accept the fact that the correction obtained will not be permanent and that further corrective surgery will be required to provide a good final result. For less severe deformities, however, it is often better to wait and perform the correction once. Certainly the psychologic impact of the deformity on the child and the family must be appreciated, and weighed against the choice of having one or two operations.

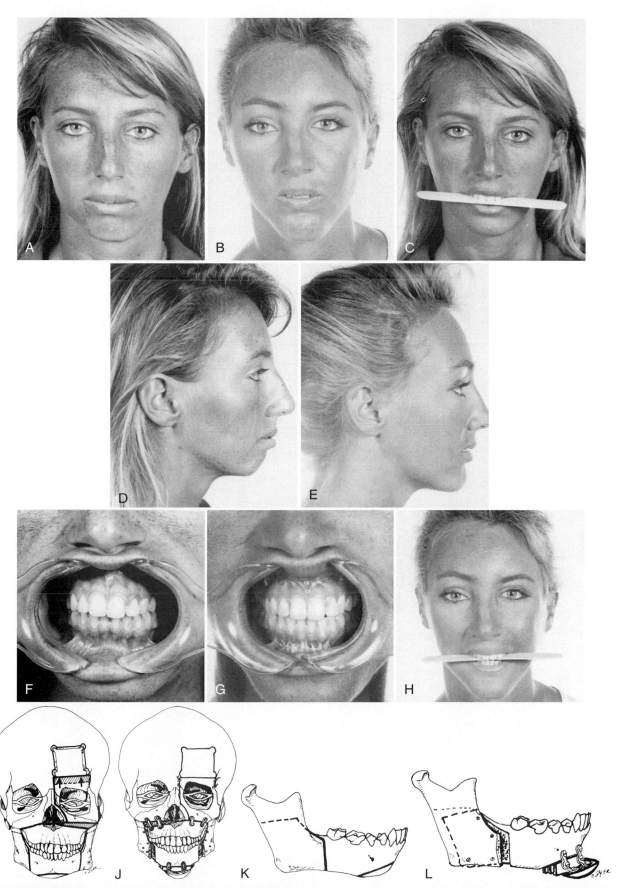

CASE 32–15, A–G. A 23-year-old patient shown before and after a transcranial elevation of the left orbital cavity to correct a left orbital dystopia (probably the result of torticollis). At the same time, a Le fort I maxiallary advancement, bilateral sagittal splits, and an advancement/lengthening genioplasty were performed. This was a one-stage procedure involving virtually all the areas of the facial skeleton. The drawings in **I–L** show one-stage correction of facial scoliosis by transcranial elevation of the left orbit, Le Fort I osteotomy and horizontalization of the maxillary occlusal plane, bilateral satgittal splitting to allow shifting of the mandible to the new midline, and horizontal osteotomy of the mandibular symphysis with an interpositional cranial bone graft.

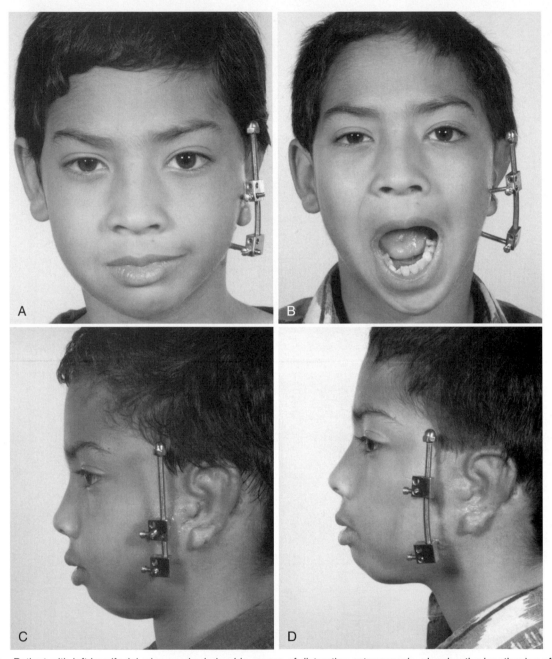

CASE 32–16. Patient with left hemifacial microsomia during his course of distraction osteogenesis, showing the lengthening of the mandible obtained by this relatively simple procedure.

Malocclusion

Malocclusion is defined as an abnormal relationship of the maxillary to the mandibular teeth. In certain types of malocclusion, the skeletal "platforms" of the maxilla and mandible are in good relationship to one another, and the malocclusion, which is dental only, can be corrected by orthodontic means alone, sometimes with extraction of teeth. In other situations, the skeletal platforms are *not* in a good relationship, and the jaws themselves will need to be moved before a good dental occlusion can be obtained. The following steps will allow the determination of where the problem lies, the institution of appropriate treatment, and the decision as to when treatment should be undertaken.

CLINICAL EXAMINATION

Very frequently, the diagnosis can be made by careful examination of the patient alone. Does the midface appear retrusive, with flatness in the malar and alar base regions? What portion of the maxillary incisors are in view in the rest position? Does the chin appear long, or short, and how is the labiomental crease? Are the gonial angles obtuse? How do the two jaws relate to the upper facial structures of the forehead, nose, and orbital cavities, and are these structures themselves normal?

DENTAL EXAMINATION

How does the upper dental arch relate to the lower dental arch? How are the individual teeth related? What is the occlusal plane, both in the vertical and horizontal dimensions? Edward Angle, considered to be the father of modern orthodontics, provided us with a classification of dental relationships that is used throughout the world (22) (Fig. 32–7):

1. *Class I* (a "normal" occlusal relationship). The mesiobuccal cusp of the first maxillary molar falls into the buccal groove of the first mandibular molar. The maxillary cuspid falls between the mandibular cuspid and first bicuspid. There is a normal overjet and overbite of the maxillary incisors in front of the mandibular incisors.
2. *Class II.* The maxillary teeth lie mesial (anterior, or toward the dental midline) to the class I relationship.
3. *Class III.* The maxillary teeth lie distal (posterior, or toward the end of the dental arch) to the class I relationship.

This occlusal classification relates exclusively to the relationship of the *teeth*. A patient can be class I and have both arches in an abnormal position relative to the cranial base, as in bimaxillary protrusion, or have a vertical maxillary excess or deficiency. A patient can be class II because of overdevelopment of the maxilla or underdevelopment of the mandible. A class III relationship can be the result of underdevelopment of the maxilla or overdevelopment of the mandible. Clinical examination gives the surgeon a good sense of where the problem lies. Confirmation of this impression is obtained by radiologic studies.

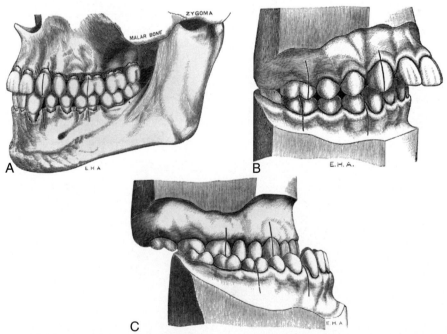

FIG. 32–7. Etchings made by Edward Hartley Angle, M.D., D.D.S., who is widely recognized as the father of American (and international) orthodontics. **A,** Fig. 2 represents normal occlusion (Angle class I) in which the mesiobuccal cusp of the maxillary first molar occludes into the buccal groove of the mandibular first molar. The maxillary cuspid falls on a line between the mandibular cuspid and first bicuspid. **B,** Fig. 22 shows class II malocclusion, in which the mesiobuccal cusp of the maxillary first molar occludes medial (more anterior) to the buccal groove. Note also the abnormal position of the maxillary cuspid in relation to the mandibular teeth. **C,** Fig. 3 shows class III malocclusion with the reverse situation, the mesiobuccal cusp of the maxillary first molar occluding distal (more posterior) to the buccal groove of the mandibular first molar. (From Angle EH. *Treatment of malocclusion of the teeth and fractures of the maxillae. Angle's system.* Philadelphia: SS White Dental Manufacturing System, 1990.)

CEPHALOMETRIC EVALUATION

A lateral cephalometric film is obtained with the patient's head in a headholder with a positioning prong in the external auditory meatus and another at the nasofrontal angle. The film is behind and parallel to the sagittal plane of the head, and the x-ray source is positioned 60 inches away from the midplane of the patient's head.

A number of methods of cephalometric analysis are available (23–28) and each orthodontist has a personal preference. Identifiable landmarks are found at the midpoint of the sella (point S), at the nasofrontal suture or nasion (point N), on the maxilla above the apices of the central incisors (point A), and at the level of the apices of the mandibular central incisors (point B). These points, along with many others, establish angular measurements that are compared with normative data largely derived from the Bolton standards. (It must be recognized that the Bolton standards were developed from serial films taken a number of years ago of faculty children at the University of Michigan; for this reason, they are representative only of a white population). Cephalometric analysis is of value in confirming a clinical impression as to which jaw structures should be moved. Note that treatment planning is not done from cephalometric evaluation alone; clinical and dental examination are of at least equal importance. Obtaining cephalometric values that are in the "normal" range should not be a goal, nor does it guarantee a good result. Cephalometric examination is even more limited in value for patients with major craniofacial malformations, in which there may be an abnormality of the cranial base or an absent or asymmetrically positioned ear canal. Perhaps the greatest value of cephalometry lies in following the growth patterns of patients with various abnormalities, and in evaluating the stability or relapse of altered jaw structures following surgery.

Orthognathic Surgery

All surgical procedures moving tooth-bearing structures in order to provide improved dental occlusion and better jaw/facial relationships *must* be coordinated with an orthodontist. A surgeon working without orthodontic input may end up with a patient who "looks good" but who has a disastrous occlusal result, which could be very difficult to correct orthodontically. Conversely, an orthodontist who is ignorant of the possibilities and indications for surgery may end up with a patient who *does not* look good, but whose teeth have, by long and laborious orthodontic treatment, often coupled with dental extractions, ended up with a reasonably good occlusal result. Unfortunately, this result is often obtained by inducing abnormal axial inclinations of the teeth, and therefore the dental result in fact may not be so satisfactory, or be particularly stable.

Surgery and Orthodontics versus Orthodontics Alone

Certain conditions, such as premaxillary or bimaxillary protrusion, can be treated satisfactorily by dental extractions and orthodontics alone. However, moving teeth through bone is a slow process, and sometimes an uncomfortable one, requiring 12 to 18 months or more until completion of the case. A surgical procedure such as a segmental maxillary osteotomy (Wassmund), in which several bicuspids are extracted and bone is removed to permit the premaxillary segment to be moved back surgically, may shorten the overall treatment time substantially. Intermaxillary fixation is not required, although an occlusal splint is generally fixed to the remaining stable maxillary teeth, and only relatively minor orthodontic adjustments are required to bring the case to completion. The decision as to which route to take should be made by the patient.

Once a diagnosis has been made that establishes the need for surgery to alter the position of the jaw bases (maxilla, mandible, or both), in the anteroposterior, vertical or horizontal planes (or all of them), the orthodontist should be the first involved.

INVOLVEMENT OF THE ORTHODONTIST IN ORTHOGNATHIC SURGERY (29)

1. The orthodontist aids in establishing the diagnosis and creating a treatment plan.
2. The orthodontist supervises dental treatment of caries and periodontal disease.
3. The orthodontist bands teeth and begins preliminary orthodontic treatment to remove dental interferences. These are nature's compensation to the deformity, and must be corrected before surgery. For example, in a patient with mandibular prognathism, partial compensation for the abnormal jaw position may be seen as a labial tilting of the maxillary incisors and a lingual tilting of the mandibular incisors. As a result of this, a discrepancy of only a few millimeters at the incisor level may exist. Surgery to move the jaw back only these few millimeters would be ill-advised, and the orthodontist should first bring the incisors into a proper axial relationship with supporting basal bone. This might increase the incisal gap to 8 to 10 mm, at which time surgery could appropriately be carried out.
4. Orthodontic treatment should provide two coherent dental arches that will fit together. If the bulk of the orthodontic treatment is done before surgery and the final arch form is obtained, the teeth may intercuspidate so well that a surgical occlusal splint is not required. Postoperative orthodontic treatment under these conditions may be minimal. This approach, however, makes no allowance for any postoperative shifts. Alternatively, the orthodontist may decide to remove only the gross dental interferences beforehand, and to make a splint that indicates to the surgeon where the jaw should be positioned at surgery. With the jaw in its desired new position, the orthodontist can then do most of the orthodontic alignment after surgery. Which approach to take depends on the preference of the individual team.
5. In two-jaw surgery, the orthodontist should take a face bow transfer to an articulated dental model, so that there can be some control of the occlusal plane and condylar position. During the stages of model surgery, an intermediate splint is made to establish the new position of the first jaw to be moved relative to the original position of the other jaw. The first jaw to be moved is then rigidly fixed in its new position using the intermediate splint. The other jaw is then moved to the position indicated by the

final splint. One hopes for as much precision in planning as possible, but the surgeon should also realize that a face bow transfer presumes that the center of mandibular rotation is at a point in front of the ear canal, which it rarely is (30). The surgeon must therefore be prepared to make necessary adjustments at the time of surgery, realizing that the three imperatives are (a) to have the midline of the jaws along the facial midline, (b) to have an appropriate show of the maxillary incisors, and (c) to have a proper occlusal relationship.

6. Before surgery, the orthodontist should apply a rigid arch wire with hooks to the orthodontic brackets to facilitate establishing intermaxillary fixation during surgery.

7. If intermaxillary fixation is maintained after surgery, it is necessary to obtain an orthopantomograph (Panorex) to be certain that the condyles are properly seated in the glenoid fossae. The use of rigid internal fixation has simplified this: the surgeon can be more certain about condylar position at the completion of the operation simply by checking passive jaw opening and closing, which should be done with the head in a somewhat flexed position. The goal is to avoid maintaining intermaxillary fixation after surgery whenever possible, both for patient comfort and safety. Most patients, even with two-jaw surgery, can be sent to the recovery room with only light elastic bands maintaining the teeth in the occlusal splint, and these can be removed to permit a soft diet.

8. After a short delay following surgery, the orthodontist can begin the final orthodontic alignment.

9. The orthodontist follows the patient postoperatively for signs of relapse. In some instances, if this is picked up early, it can be overcome by traction devices such as the Delaire headframe (31), which can be used after maxillary advancements.

Surgical Procedures on the Jaws to Correct Malocclusion

Once a proper diagnosis has been made and presurgical orthodontic preparation of the patient completed, most forms of malocclusion that do not involve the orbitocranial portion of the face can be corrected by using one or more of a relatively limited number of surgical procedures. With the capacity properly to perform a sagittal splitting procedure for the mandible, and a Le Fort I type osteotomy with its variations for the maxilla, a surgeon most likely would be able to deal with 80% or more of the patients presenting to him requiring orthognathic surgery. Technique, indubitably, is important for good results, but even the most flawlessly performed procedure will give a poor result if it is the wrong operation. Diagnosis, planning, and proper orthodontic preparation of the patient far overshadow the technical niceties of exactly how a cut in the bone is made.

Mandibular Osteotomies

SEGMENTAL OSTEOTOMIES

The Kole procedure can be used to correct an open bite that arises from a downward curve of the mandibular occlusal plane (the curve of Spee). If dental considerations permit, the two first bicuspids are removed, and a vertical osteotomy is carried down from the extraction sites to a level below the

apices of the teeth. If dental extractions are not to be done, the orthodontist should open up a space of 3 to 4 mm between the teeth to permit performing the osteotomy without injury to the dental roots. The two vertical osteotomies are connected by a horizontal osteotomy, and care is taken not to damage the posterior (labial) mucoperiosteum, which provides blood supply to the dentoalveolar segment. The tooth-bearing segment is then elevated to its desired position. An acrylic splint, which has been previously prepared on a sectioned dental model, is used both as a guide to the surgeon to the proper position for the dentoalveolar segment and as a means of stabilization of the segment. The splint is wired to stable posterior teeth and intermaxillary fixation is not required. A genioplasty can be performed at the same time, but care should be taken to maintain an intact strut of mandible between the horizontal osteotomy of the Kole procedure and the horizontal osteotomy of the genioplasty (Case 32.17).

SAGITTAL SPLIT PROCEDURE

With the increasing use of interfragment screws, and sometimes screws and plates, this has become the procedure of choice for movements of the entire tooth-bearing portion of the mandible. The other acceptable procedure for mandibular prognathism, the intraoral vertical osteotomy, has been largely superseded by the sagittal split, because intermaxillary fixation can be avoided with the rigidly fixed sagittal split. The extraoral vertical or oblique osteotomy should be considered extinct, since it makes an avoidable facial scar. The sagittal split is also the only procedure that can be used for correction of both mandibular prognathism and mandibular retrognathia, so it *must* be mastered by all surgeons planning to do orthognathic surgery (Fig. 32–8).

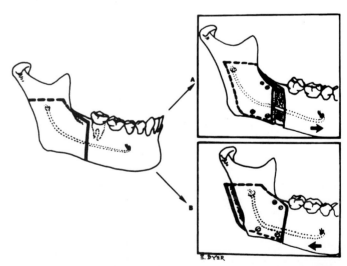

FIG. 32–8. The sagittal split procedure is the procedure of choice for most orthognathic surgery. The operation is performed entirely intraorally. It can be used both for retrognathia **(A)** and prognathia **(B)**. With the use of rigid internal fixation by small titanium screws (which can be placed either through a very small trocar or, in some cases, entirely transorally), intermaxillary fixation can be dispensed with in most cases. Two technically difficult parts of the operation are avoiding damage to the inferior alveolar nerve and properly positioning the condylar segment.

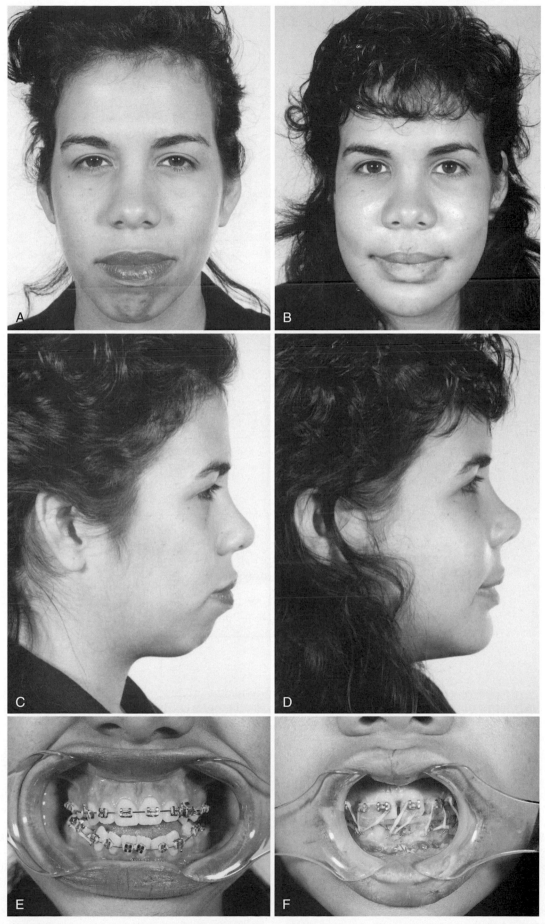

CASE 32–17. Patient shown before and after a Le Fort I osteotomy, extraction of two upper bicuspids, segmentation of the maxilla into four pieces, and vertical maxillary impaction, coupled with a lower anterior segmental osteotomy of the mandible and a jumping genioplasty. Note the relaxation of the perioral musculature that comes with the considerable improvement in lip seal.

FIG. 32–9. Variety of maxillary movements possible after a Le Fort I osteotomy.

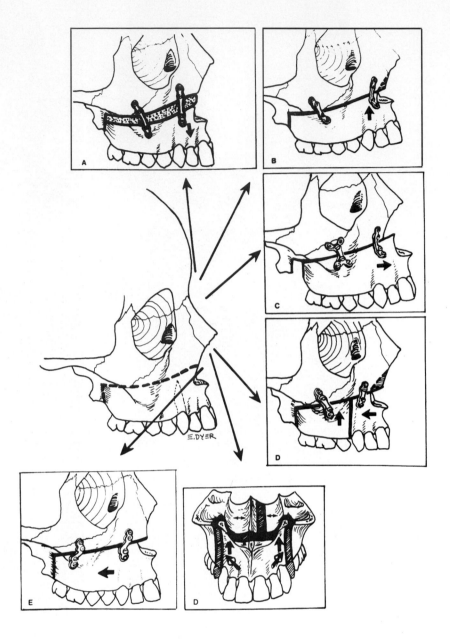

Technique

Incisions are made intraorally from the first molar, extending up the lateral aspect of the ascending ramus. This procedure cannot be properly performed without the special instruments designed specifically for this operation by Hugo Obwegeser. After subperiosteal dissection of the lateral aspect of the ramus and posterior border (stripping off the pterygomasseteric sling), the sigmoid notch is identified with a blunt nerve hook. A medial dissection is the performed about 11 to 15 mm below the sigmoid notch, well above the entry of the inferior alveolar nerve into the medial aspect of the ramus. With protective channel retractors in place (which are also used to bring the mandible anteriorly), a medial osteotomy is performed with a reciprocating saw or Lindemann side-cutting burr. This osteotomy should extend just through the medial cortex, and a bit more. A lateral osteotomy is then performed just through the cortex at about the level of the 2nd molar. A series of shallow drill holes are then made just

inside the external oblique ridge of the mandible, connecting the two previously made osteotomies. These holes are connected with a fissure burr that is carried just into bleeding cancellous bone. Then thin, slightly curved, Dautrey osteotomies are driven through the ramus, staying just beneath the lateral cortex to avoid injury to the inferior alveolar nerve.

When the split is completed, the lateral (condylar) segment should be freely mobile. The inferior alveolar nerve can often be seen coursing through the cancellous bone of the medial (tooth-bearing) segment. Once both osteotomies are done, the tooth-bearing segment is then either advanced or moved backwards, depending upon whether retrognathia or prognathia is being treated. One way to establish that the splits have been properly completed is to move the jaw more posteriorly than its original position. When the desired occlusal relationship of the tooth-bearing segment with the maxilla is established, usually by an occlusal splint, intermaxillary fix-

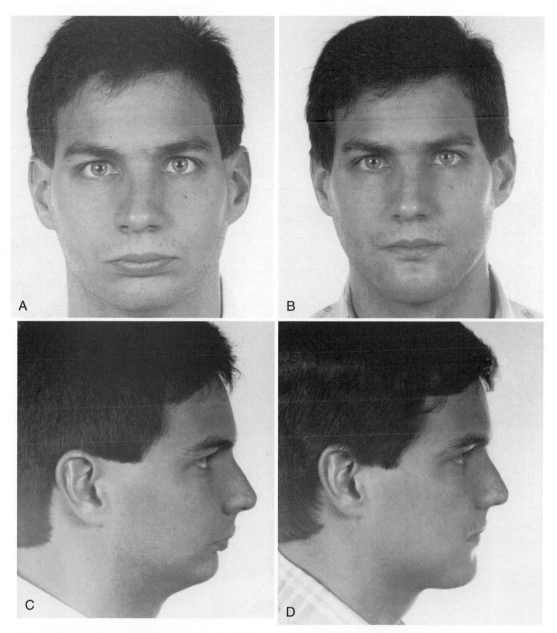

CASE 32–18, A–H A 25-year-old male shown before and after mandibular advancement by sagittal splitting and a lengthening genioplasty. Intermaxillary fixation was not employed. Note the improvement in the deep labiomental fold, which is obtained both by giving better dental support for the lower lip and by lengthening the chin.

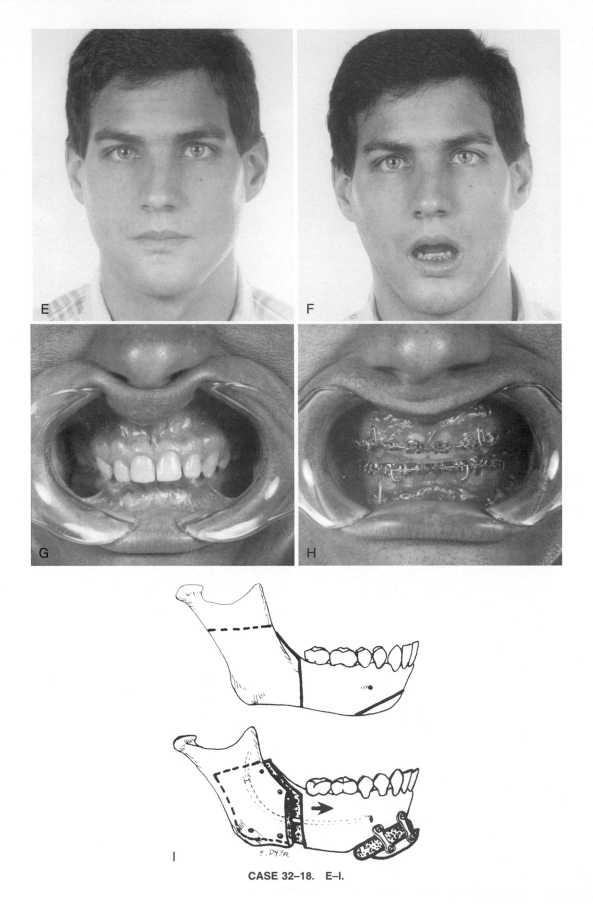

CASE 32–18.   E–I.

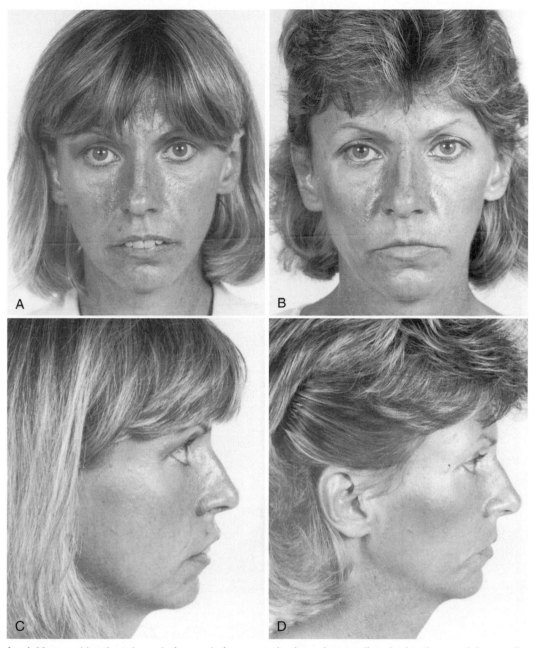

CASE 32–19, A–J. A 39-year-old patient shown before and after an anterior maxillary osteotomy (Wassmund), associated with the extraction of two first bicuspids. This type of anterior premaxillary set- back requires a splint wired to the remaining maxillary teeth but does not require intermaxillary fixation.

ation is temporarily established. The condylar segments are pushed gently backwards and upwards to seat the condyles in the glenoid fossae. In prognathism, a segment of the condylar segment just behind the lateral cut is resected, and in retrognathia, a gap will open up in this area corresponding to the extent of the mandibular advancement. Most surgeons are now using rigid fixation, which can done either with bicortical screws, passed either transorally or through the cheek using a guarded trochar, or with a miniplate. After completion of these osteosyntheses, the intermaxillary fixation is released, and the occlusal result is verified by passive movement of the mandible into the splint, with the patient's head flexed. The intraoral incisions are then closed with a running

absorbable suture. Some surgeons bring a hemovac drain either through the buccal mucosa or through the cheek, but we generally do not use drainage (Case 32.18).

Maxillary Osteotomies

SEGMENTAL OSTEOTOMIES

The premaxillary osteotomy, or Wassmund procedure, usually involves the extraction of the two first bicuspids. A vertical osteotomy is made from the extraction site to the level of the piriform rim, and a horizontal osteotomy is made through the premaxilla just below the nasal spine. Submucoperiosteal tunnels are dissected across the palate from the

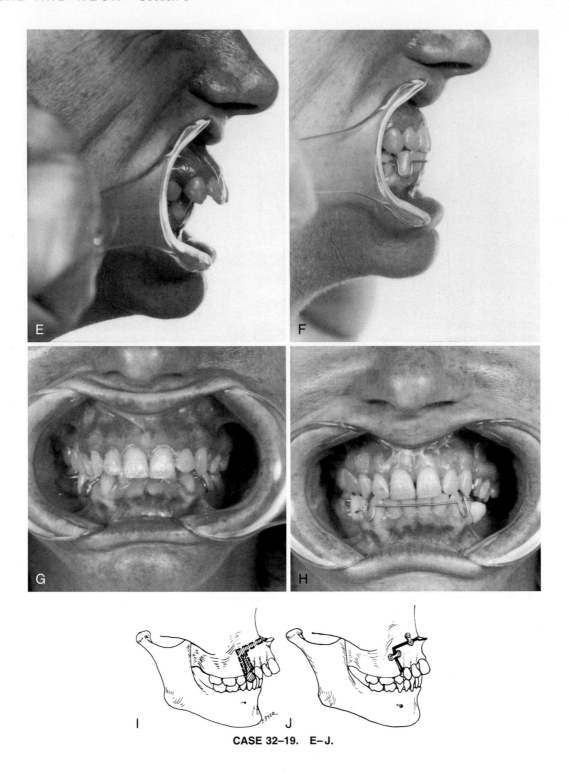

CASE 32–19. E–J.

dental extraction sites, and with one finger on the palatal mucosa to protect the vital blood supply, bone across the palate is removed with a burr. The premaxilla is then downfractured after several taps on an osteotomy directed from beneath the nasal spine towards the palatal surface, and further removal of bone is carried out under direct vision until the premaxillary segment can be moved back to its desired position, as determined by the occlusal splint. The splint is wired to the posterior teeth, and intermaxillary fixation is not required (Case 32.19).

The Schuchardt procedure is a segmental posterior osteotomy used to intrude the maxillary molar segments to close an anterior open bite, but it has been largely supplanted for this purpose by the Le Fort I osteotomy.

LE FORT I OSTEOTOMY

All Le Fort osteotomies received their name from the Le Fort fractures (I, II and III) described by the French anatomist René Le Fort at the turn of the century (32). The osteotomies used in orthognathic surgery differ from those fractures in

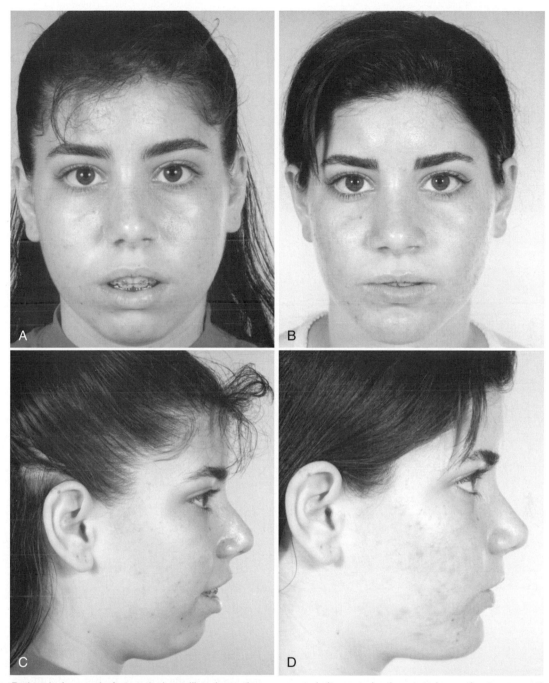

CASE 32–20. Patient before and after vertical maxillary impaction, genioplasty, and liposuction of the neck. The maxilla was elevated more in its posterior than anterior portion to correct the anterior open bite.

that the pterygoid plates are kept intact, and for this reason, strictly speaking, they should be called Le Fort I *type* osteotomies.

The Le Fort I osteotomy is the workhorse of maxillary surgery. After completion of the osteotomy and mobilization of the maxilla, the tooth-bearing segment can be moved upward, forward, down, side-to-side, backwards, or tilted and yawed in a variety of planes. Dental extractions may be combined with segmental osteotomies to shift multiple maxillary segments independently (Fig. 32–9).

A vertical measurement is taken at the beginning of the operation from a tattoo mark made on the medial canthal ten-

don to the edge of the lateral incisor. The amount of incisive show of the maxillary teeth should also be recorded preoperatively, with the patient sitting and the lips in the open rest position (patients will usually go into this position just after licking their lips). Normally, we see 2 to 3 mm (4 mm is acceptable for a female) of tooth below the vermillion border of the upper lip in the open rest position.

Technique

An upper buccal sulcus incision is made, preserving an adequate cuff of mucoperiosteum inferiorly for subsequent closure, and a subperiosteal dissection of the anterior maxilla is

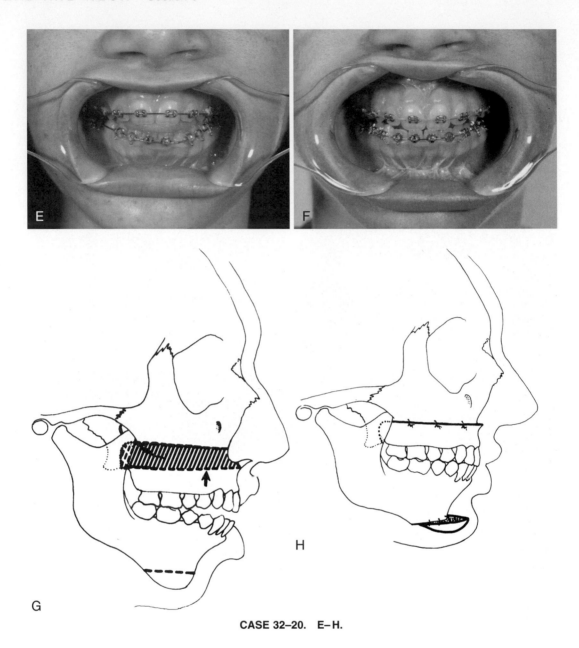

CASE 32–20. E–H.

performed, exposing the infraorbital nerves. The dissection is carried posteriorly into the pterygomaxillary space, and a dissection of the nasal mucosa is performed. A horizontal osteotomy with the reciprocating saw is then made from above the root of the cuspid at the piriform rim to beneath the malar prominence, as far back as the pterygomaxillary junction. The medial maxillary walls are also cut with the saw, and the septum is divided from the palate with a guarded osteotome. The final step of a Le Fort I type osteotomy is the insertion of a curved osteotome between the maxillary tuberosity and the pterygoid plate, and the cutting of the palatine bone, which is their only connection. The maxilla can generally be downfractured by downward finger pressure alone; in rare instances, the Rowe disimpaction forceps are required. Further mobilization of the maxilla is done with a blunt instrument behind the maxillary tuberosity, to lever the maxilla forward and complete the fracture of the posterior wall. In cleft patients with persistent alveolar clefts, the maxilla will be in two segments at this stage.

After the maxilla has been completely mobilized to the point that it can be easily moved in all directions with a tissue forceps, it can be placed in its desired position. Various possibilities are:

1. Resecting a portion of the superior maxilla and moving the tooth-bearing segment upward, to correct a vertical maxillary excess (long face) (Case 32.20).
2. Lengthening the maxilla with an interpositional bone graft (short face)
3. Advancing the maxilla. If the advancement is more than 6-8 mm., and in all cleft patients, a bone graft is used (Case 32.21).

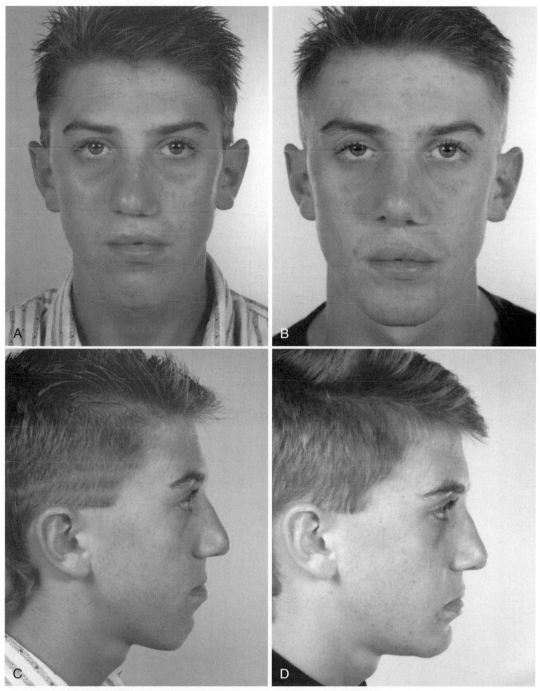

CASE 32–21. Patient with unilateral cleft lip and palate and class 3 malocclusion, treated by Le Fort I type osteotomy and maxillary advancement, and reduction genioplasty. It was possible to perform a rhinoplasty at the same sitting by having the anesthesiologist change from a nasotracheal to orotracheal intubation. Further minor work remains to be done on the free border of the upper lip and the left alar margin.

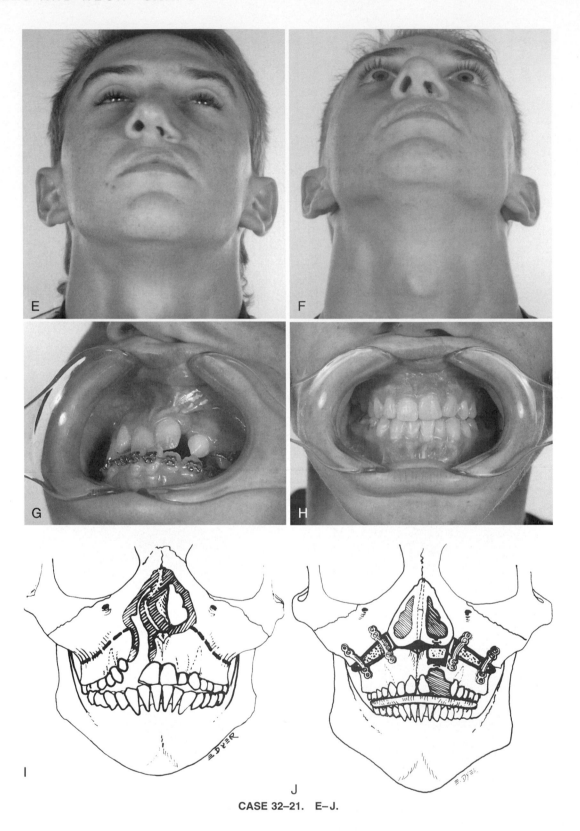

CASE 32–21. E–J.

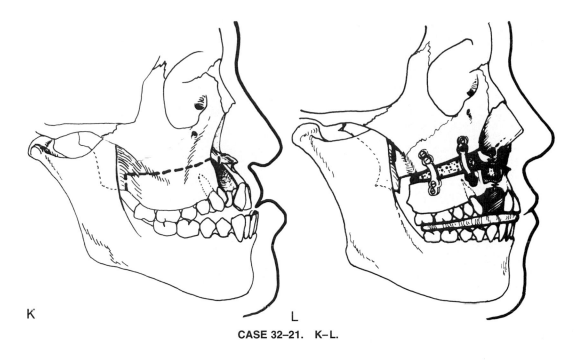

K   L

CASE 32–21.   K–L.

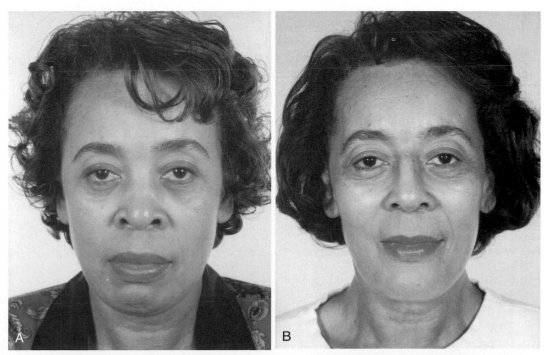

A   B

CASE 32–22.   Patient before and after Le Fort I osteotomy with removal of two bicuspids, anterior maxillary setback, and further setback of the entire maxilla by removal of the maxillary tuberosities and bone in the area where the third molars had been. An anterior seg-mental osteotomy of the mandible was performed, along with a reduction/advancement genioplasty. A cranial bone graft was placed over the nasal dorsum at a second operation.

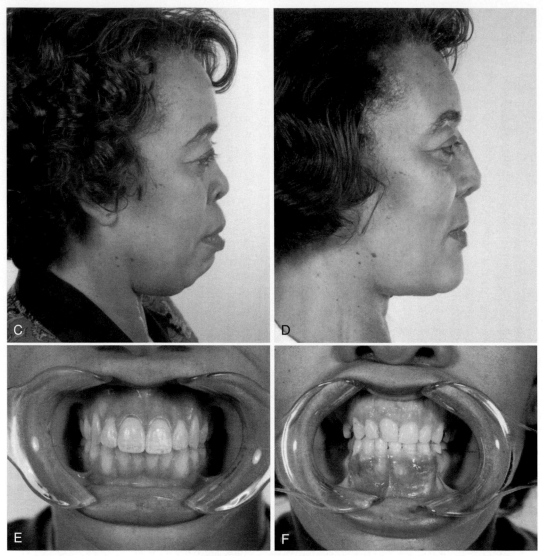

CASE 32–22. C–F.

4. Moving the maxilla posteriorly. This will require either dental extractions and segmentation, or removal of bone from the maxillary tuberosities and/or pterygoid plates (Case 32.22).
5. Tilting the maxilla up posteriorly (correction of an open bite), or tilting one side up or down (to straighten a canted occlusal plane)
6. Performing further segmentation, either a palatal split for palatal expansion, or various combinations of dental extractions with multiple maxillary osteotomies for complex maxillary deformities.

After the maxilla or the maxillary segments are fixed into the occlusal splint, the splint is brought into occlusion with the mandibular teeth, and the entire maxillomandibular complex is brought into its proper vertical relationship by using the measurements taken from the tattoo mark on the medial canthal tendon. The condyles are seated just as one would for mandibular surgery, one fixes the tooth-bearing segment of the maxilla to the stable upper maxilla with miniplates, and again one checks the passive movement of the mandible into the splint after removing the intermaxillary fixation.

Autogenous bone grafts, either cranial or iliac in origin, are placed in gaps such as those seen in lengthened or expanded maxillae, or in cleft patients.

In two-jaw surgery, the maxilla is usually done first, since it is easier to stabilize than the mandible. Sometimes, all of the sagittal split will be done except for the actual split itself, before moving to the maxillary procedure. The maxilla is moved to its desired position with the mandible in its old position, using a prefabricated occlusal splint. After the maxilla has been stabilized with miniplates, the mandibular osteotomies are completed, and the mandible is moved to its final position with the use of a second, final splint.

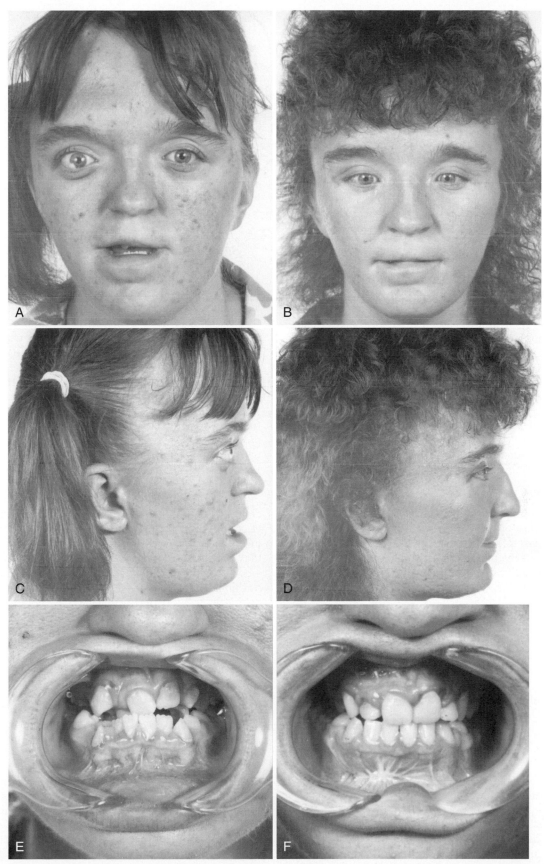

CASE 32–23. This 17-year-old patient with Apert syndrome underwent a one-stage extacranial Le Fort III maxillary advancement, genioplasty, and removal of a right epibulbar dermoid. The extracranial Le Fort III is preferred to the intracranial monobloc procedure in patients beyond the early teens, for reasons mentioned earlier in the text; however, it is evident that the extracranial procedure has still left this patient with some of the stigmata of Apert syndrome—a broad, flat face and forehead, and mild orbital hypertelorism, which could have been corrected by a monobloc and facial bipartition.

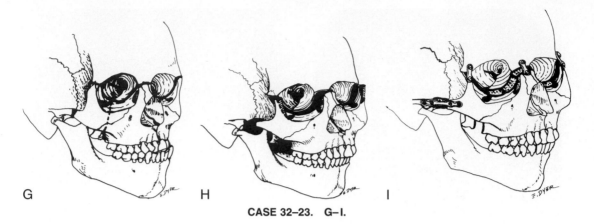

CASE 32–23.   G–I.

Two-jaw surgery is indicated when:

1. There is a major occlusal gap (12 mm. or more), and when cephalometric analysis shows that the deformity is shared by both the maxilla and the mandible.
2. There are horizontal abnormalities with a canted occlusal plane, such is in hemifacial microsomia.
3. A mandibular deformity is associated with an anterior open bite.

Rigid Internal Fixation

The advantages of rigid internal fixation in orthognathic surgery are that:

1. The occlusion can be checked on the operating table with functional opening and closing, even if two-jaw surgery is done.
2. Most often, intermaxillary fixation can be dispensed with altogether, or the period of intermaxillary fixation can be shortened. Post-operative airway control is safer, the patient can eat soft foods, and since hospital stays are shorter, use of the plates and screws is cost-effective.
3. With bones held by rigid osteosyntheses, there seems to be less swelling.

There are no disadvantages to the use of rigid fixation in the maxilla other than the cost of the plates and screws; in the mandible, the condyle may be torqued in the glenoid fossa, or the inferior alveolar nerve may be overly compressed. Both of these possibilities are avoidable with experience and a light touch.

If intermaxillary fixation is not used, the patient's occlusion must be followed carefully, because small shifts can occur even with the use of rigid internal fixation. Particular attention must be paid to dental midlines. If a slight shift is noted, several weeks of elastics in intermaxillary fixation will usually remedy the situation.

Miniplate systems

An acceptable miniplate system should be:

1. Relatively inexpensive.
2. Made of a metal that is soft enough that it can be bent, but hard enough to maintain rigid fixation (Vitallium, Titanium, and a number of other newer Titanium alloys are satisfactory).

3. Corrosion-proof (Titanium and Vitallium are acceptable; stainless steel is not).
4. Small enough, with flat screw heads, that the plates and screws cannot be felt through the skin.
5. Made with self-tapping (not requiring preliminary thread drilling) screws.
6. Provided with easy-to-load screwdrivers that are "scrub nurse" friendly, and hold the screws themselves.

Most of the commercially available systems fulfill these criteria, with the possible exception of number 1.

These plating systems are of obvious use in treating facial fractures in adults, although around the orbital cavity smaller profile plates can be used. For fixation of cranial segments, wire fixation is almost always adequate, and using plates and screws to replace a craniotomy segment is an unnecessary expense.

In pediatric facial fractures and elective pediatric craniofacial surgery in infants, we generally plan on removing plates after several months because they can cause localized growth disturbance; when used around the upper orbital framework, they have been noted to end up in an intracranial location when placed extracranially, probably by a mechanism of appositional bone growth in front of the plate and resorption behind it. In most plagiocephalies, we now use only Vicryl sutures, with somewhat more careful bone carpentry to obtain adequate stabilization. When small enough biodegradable plates become available, they will be of considerable use in children.

POWER SYSTEMS

Facial skeletal surgery developed as it has over the past two decades because of the availability of power systems having a variety of handpieces for cutting, drilling and burring bone.

The availability of thin saw blades has made it possible to split cranial bone segments through the diploic space in children as early as 3 or 4 years of age, and precision instruments make it possible to do precision surgery. We prefer an electrical system over ones driven by compressed air. Also desirable is a built-in irrigation system that can prevent heat build-up during cutting, thus avoiding burning or damaging bone. Primary bone healing occurs when the bone segments are placed in tight, close abutment (gaps less than 1 mm), when the bone is undamaged by heat from saws or burrs, and when there is adequate endosseous or periosteal blood sup-

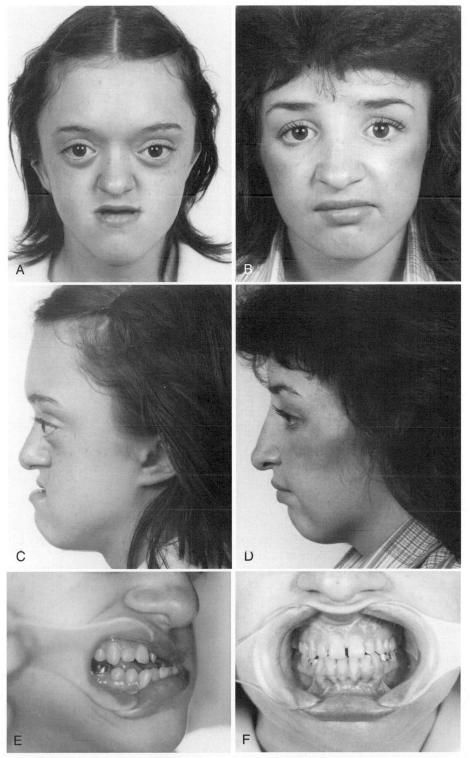

CASE 32–24. This patient was the first Le Fort III osteotomy performed for Crouzon disease by the senior author, in 1976, when the patient was 14. The patient is now approaching the 20th anniversary of her operation, and has had a completely stable result, both in terms of the exorbitism correction, and the correction of her class 3 malocclusion, with a Le Fort I osteotomy being performed in 1981 at age 19. The procedure lengthens the nose more than an intracranial would have done, but is still an indicated procedure in older patients. This was essentially the same as the landmark procedure first performed by Paul Tessier in the late 1960s, which opened the field of craniofacial surgery and rekindled the interest of plastic surgeons and others in facial skeletal surgery.

ply. Craftsmanship and precision are just as important in working with bone as in doing a primary cleft lip repair.

Higher Maxillary Osteotomies Requiring Extraoral Approaches

LE FORT II OSTEOTOMY

The indications for a Le Fort II osteotomy are fairly limited. It should be used in a case of severe midface retrusion *without* exorbitism, such as severe cleft lip and palate, a patient with Crouzon without exorbitism, or a case of hemifacial microsomia with a deviation of the nasoethmoid toward the short side of the face. The osteotomy is made across the nasal root as in a Le Fort III, avoiding damage to the cribriform plate, which is quite nearby, and carried either medial or lateral to the infraorbital foramen and then down the maxilla obliquely to continue posteriorly along the path of a Le Fort I osteotomy.

LE FORT III OSTEOTOMY

The subcranial Le Fort III osteotomy is indicated in patients who have major midface retrusion and exorbitism, such as Crouzon disease. In younger patients (<12–13 years of age) with Crouzon, Apert, and other craniofacial dysostoses, the monobloc frontofacial advancement, a transcranial approach, is often preferred to the subcranial procedure. The aesthetic result, in terms of maintaining the orbital framework, is better and there is less lengthening of the nose. Older patients do not seem to handle the retrofrontal dead space as well as younger ones, perhaps because the brain is less able to expand, and the complication rate is higher in terms of epidural abscess and infection of the frontal bone that requires bone removal. Patients with ventriculoperitoneal shunts in place also have higher complication rates after the monobloc advancement, and it may be better to treat them with an extracranial procedure, irrespective of age (33).

The subcranial Le Fort III can be performed through coronal and vestibular incisions alone. A transverse frontal crescent gives the best orbital contour, and is carried along the lateral orbital rim at its junction with the cranial base, extending to the inferior orbital fissure. The nasofrontal osteotomy is done in a keel-shaped fashion below the nasofrontal suture to avoid damaging the cribriform plate, and one should remain inferior (caudal) to the anterior ethmoidal vessels to avoid entering the anterior cranial fossa. This nasofrontal osteotomy, extended through the medial orbital walls behind the lacrimal fossa, almost connects with the lateral osteotomy extended into the inferior fissure. The surgeon should pass an osteotome into the nasofrontal osteotomy, directed at a finger on the posterior nasal spine at the back of the hard palate, and complete the sectioning of the vomer to prevent an avulsion of the cribriform plate. The nasotracheal tube should be avoided during this maneuver. The zygomatic arches are sectioned, and a pterygomaxillary disjunction is done as in a Le Fort I osteotomy. Frequently, however, more of the posterior maxilla needs to be sectioned from the pterygoid. This completes the osteotomies, and the midface can be mobilized with Rowe disimpaction forceps. The few remaining intact areas of the orbital floors are easily fractured during this maneuver. If there is a disproportion between the extent of the exorbitism and the retromaxillism, it is a very easy

matter to section the already-mobilized maxilla at the Le Fort I level to regulate the occlusion after the exorbitism has been corrected. The maxillary segments and the upper facial segment are fixed into their proper position with miniplates after establishing the desired occlusion, and cranial bone grafts are used in all bone gaps (Case 32.23) (Case 32.24).

Conclusion

The facial skeleton, in spite of the complexity of the soft-tissue structures of the face, is easily approached through coronal and intraoral incisions, and a large variety of osteotomies can be performed. Only a few have been shown; many others are possible, depending upon the anatomic problem encountered. Precise surgery, rigid fixation, and strict reliance on fresh autogenous bone grafts are important elements in a successful outcome, as is close collaboration with other specialists, particularly neurosurgeons and orthodontists.

References

1. Von Langenbeck B. *Deutsch Klin* 1861; 281.
2. Cheever DW. Displacement of the upper jaw. *Med Surg Rep Boston City Hosp* 1870; 1:156.
3. Kline RM, Wolfe SA. Complications associated with the harvesting of cranial bone grafts. *Plast Reconst Surg* 1995; 95(1):5–13.
4. Tessier P. Inferior orbitotomy: a new approach to the orbital floor. *Clin Plast Surg* 1982; 9:569.
5. Wolfe SA. A rationale for the surgical treatment of exophthalmos and exorbitism. *J Maxillofacial Surg* 1977; 5:249.
6. Sullivan W, Kawamoto HK Jr. Periorbital marginotomies: anatomy and applications. *J Craniomaxillofacial Surg* 1989; 17:206.
7. Luhr HG. Miniplates for the prevention of fractures in problem cases of dento-alveolar surgery. Presented at the Symposium on Rigid Fixation of the Craniomaxillofacial Skeleton, Toronto, September 1989.
8. Derome P. The transbasal approach to tumors involving the base of the skull. In: Schmidek HP, Sweet WH, eds. *Current techniques in operative neurosurgery.* New York: Grune & Stratton, 1977; 223.
9. Lore JM. *Atlas of head and neck surgery.* Philadelphia, WB Saunders, 1988.
10. Whitaker LA, Pertschuk M. Facial skeletal contouring for aesthetic purposes. *Plast Reconst Surg* 1982; 69:245.
11. Wolfe SA, Vitenas P Jr. Malar augmentation using autogenous material. *Clin Plast Surg* 1991; 18:39.
12. Wolfe SA, Berkowitz S. *Plastic surgery of the facial skeleton.* Boston: Little, Brown, 1989; 111–148, 198, 729–731.
13. This section on the chin abridged from Wolfe and Berkowitz, ibid., 111–148.
14. Whitaker LA. Aesthetic augmentation of the malar-midface structures. *Plast Reconst Surg* 1987; 80:337.
15. Tessier P. Face lifting and frontal rhytidectomy. In: *Transactions of the 7th International Congress of Plastic and Recontructive Surgeons,* Sao Paolo, 1979; 393.
16. Krastinova-Lolov D. Mask lift and facial aesthetic sculpturing. *Plast Reconst Surg* 1995; 95:21.
17. Marchac D, et al. Intracranial pressure in craniostenosis: 302 recordings. In: Marchac D, ed. *Craniofacial surgery.* New York: Springer-Verlag, 1987; 110.
18. Wolfe SA, Morrison G, Page L, et al. The monobloc frontofacial advancement: do the plusses outweigh the minuses? *Plast Reconst Surg* 1993; 91(6):977–987.
19. Ilizarov GA, Iryanov YM. The characteristics of osteogenesis under conditions of stretch tension. *Byul Eksper Biologii i Meditziny* 1991; 111(2):194–6.
20. McCarthy JG, Schreiber J, Karp N, et al. Lengthening the human mandible by gradual distraction. *Plast Reconst Surg* 1992; 89:1
21. Molina F. Presented at the New York University Bone Expansion Workshop, New York, March 1994. Also, Plastic Surgical Forum, San Diego, Vol. 17, 1994; 62–63.
22. Angle EW. *Treatment of malocclusion of the teeth and fractures of the mandible, Angle's system.* Philadelphia: SS White Publications, 1898.
23. Burstone DJ, James RB, Legan H, et al. Cephalometrics for orthognathic surgery. *J Oral Maxillofacial Surg* 1978; 36:269.

24. Downs UB. Variation in facial relationships: their significance in treatment and prognosis. *Am J Orthod Dentofac Orthoped* 1948; 34:812.

25. Steiner CC. The use of cephalometrics as an aid to planning and assessing orthodontic treatment. *Am J Orthodont Dentofacial Orthoped* 1960; 46:721.

26. Ricketts RM, Bench RW, et al. *Bioprogressive therapy.* Denver: Rocky Mountain Publications, 1979.

27. Jacobsen A. Re "WITS" appraisal of jaw disharmony. *Am J Orthodont Dentofac Orthoped* 1975; 67:125.

28. Wolford LM, Hilliard FW, Dugan DJ. *Surgical treatment objectives.* St. Louis: CV Mosby, 1985.

29. Berkowitz S. Analysis and treatment planning in patients with craniofacial anomalies. In: Wolfe SA, Berkowitz S, eds. *Plastic surgery of the facial skeleton.* Boston: Little, Brown, 1989; 39

30. Nattestad A, Vedtofte P. Mandibular autorotation in orthognathic surgery: a new method of locating the centre of mandibular rotation and determining its consequences in orthognathic surgery. *J Craniomaxillofac Surg* 1992; 20:163–170.

31. Delaire J. Ziele und ergebnisse extraoraler zuege in postero-anterorer richtung in anwendung eine orthopaedischen moske bei der behandlung von Faellen der klasse III. *Fortschr Kieferorthop* 1976; 37:247.

32. Le Fort, R. Étude experimental sur les fractures de la machoire superieure. *Rev Chir Paris* 1901; 23:214.

33. Kawamoto HK Jr. Complications following monobloc frontofacial advancement. Presented at the Annual Meeting of the American Association of Plastic Surgeons, Palm Beach, May 1988.

Suggested Readings

Bell WH, Profitt WR, White RP. *Surgical correction of dentofacial deformities.* Philadelphia: WB Saunders, 1980.

Bell WH. *Modern practice in orthognathic and reconstructive surgery.* Vols. I–III. Philadelphia: WB Saunders, 1992.

Epker BN, Fish LC. *Dentofacial deformities, integrated orthodontic and surgical correction.* St. Louis: CV Mosby, 1986.

Epker BN, Wolford LM. *Dentofacial deformities, surgical-orthodontic correction.* St. Louis: CV Mosby, 1980.

Wolfe SA, trans. Tessier P, et al. *Plastic surgery of the orbit and eyelids.* New York: Masson, 1981.

Wolfe SA, Berkowitz S. *Plastic surgery of the facial skeleton.* Boston: Little, Brown, 1989.

Yaremchuk MJ, Gruss JS, Manson PN. *Rigid fixation of the craniomaxillofacial skeleton.* Boston: Butterworth-Heinemann, 1992.

33

Principles in Management of Facial Injuries

Oleh Antonyshyn, M.D., F.R.C.S.(C.)

The management of facial trauma has evolved rapidly over the past decade. Multiple factors have contributed to these advances. Experimental studies have improved our appreciation of biomechanical principles and the pathophysiology of fracture healing. Developments in diagnostic imaging technology have facilitated accurate preoperative diagnosis and treatment planning. Technologic advances, particularly refinement in fixation devices and alloplastic implants, have made a significant impact on the range of treatment options. Most important, the adaptation of established craniomaxillofacial methods for exposure and bone manipulation, and the introduction of entirely new techniques (e.g., rigid skeletal fixation and primary bone grafting) have dramatically changed the scope and effectiveness of facial trauma management.

Etiology of Facial Trauma

Recent epidemiologic surveys reveal changing patterns of etiology. In the past, motor-vehicle accidents have been the leading cause of facial trauma (1–3). Interpersonal violence has now become the primary cause of facial trauma (4–7).

Associated Injuries

Facial injuries frequently present with associated multisystem trauma of varying complexity and severity.

Cervical spine injury has been documented in 1.3% of facial fractures (8) and up to 4% of facial injuries sustained in motor-vehicle accidents (9). Despite the low frequency, the severity and irreversibility of spinal cord trauma demands specific attention in the facial trauma patient, where intubation or fracture treatment may require neck manipulation and predispose to further injury.

Regional trauma to the head is more common. Loss of consciousness or posttrauma amnesia occurs in 55% of facial trauma patients (10), while more significant head injury, having CT evidence of intracranial damage, has been reported in 5.4% of cases (4). Associated skull-base fractures were noted in 25% of patients (11), predisposing to potentially serious complications including cerebrospinal fluid fistulae, risk of meningitis, and carotid artery injuries.

The incidence of ocular trauma associated with facial fractures varies from 25 to 29% (12,13). The documented frequency of blindness varies from 1.6 to 6% (14,12). Awareness of the possibility of ocular injury is particularly important at present, as the prognosis for visual recovery has improved significantly as the result of improved ophthalmologic surgical techniques.

Initial Management

PRIORITIES IN TREATMENT

The initial goals of treatment are to stabilize the patient and to rule out limb- or life-threatening injuries. Establishing a patent airway, ensuring adequate ventilation, control of hemorrhage, and the management of neurosurgical, thoracic, and abdominal trauma take precedence over the management of the facial injury.

SPECIAL CONSIDERATIONS

Airway Management

Patients with major facial injuries are at risk of developing upper airway obstruction. Blood clots, teeth, or fracture fragments may become displaced and occlude the airway. Mandibular or midface fractures frequently cause massive swelling in the pharynx and larynx. Comminuted unstable fractures of the mandible result in loss of support to the hyomandibular complex and consequent retroposition of the tongue.

Initial establishment and maintenance of an adequate airway is mandatory. Some form of artificial airway is indicated in the patient with respiratory obstruction, inability to clear secretions, or unconsciousness.

Concomitant injury to the cervical spine or cranial base complicates airway management. In the patient with a potentially unstable cervical spine, orotracheal intubation is generally avoided in favor of other techniques, including blind nasotracheal intubation and intubation over a flexible fiberoptic endoscope. Less commonly employed alternative techniques include percutaneous transtracheal ventilation, intubation using a lighted stylet, and retrograde intubation (15).

Intubation is further complicated in the patient with cranial-base fractures. Under these circumstances, blind nasotracheal intubation poses a risk of pyriform sinus perforation, epistaxis, and cribriform or sphenoid sinus penetration, as well as the possibility of entering the cranial cavity. Despite studies indicating that the complications associated with skull-base fractures are not markedly increased by attempted nasotracheal intubation (16), blind intubation is not attempted at our institution unless fingers can be positioned in the nasopharynx to guide the tube.

Massive Hemorrhage

Severe primary hemorrhage resulting from facial injuries is uncommon. Massive soft-tissue trauma, particularly scalp

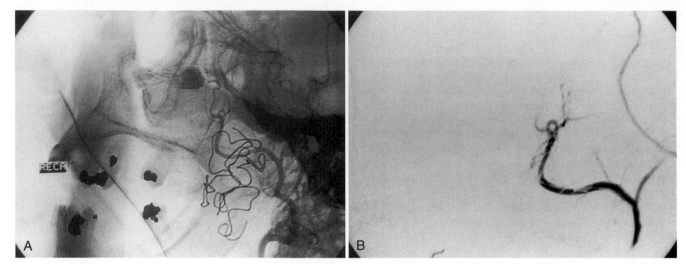

FIG. 33–1. Embolization for control of exsanguination associated with cranial base and midface fractures; bleeding persisted despite anterior and posterior nasal packing. **A,** lateral projection of a right external carotid artery injection, nonsubtracted view. Posterior nasal packing evident. Frank extravasation is seen arising from the infraor- bital branch of the 3rd portion of the internal maxillary artery. **B,** postembolization angiogram, subtracted view, demonstrating oc- clusion of the distal branches of the internal maxillary artery, includ- ing the greater palatine and infraorbital vessels. (Photos courtesy of RI Farb, Department of Radiology, Sunnybrook Hospital.)

avulsions, and direct penetrating injuries to vessels can lead to considerable blood loss. However, hemorrhage is usually effectively controlled by pressure or direct ligation of bleed- ing vessels.

Midfacial fractures can cause hemorrhage from sources that are less accessible and more difficult to control. Dis- placed midface fractures can cause lacerations and bleeding from the ethmoid branches of the ophthalmic artery or the pharyngeal branches of the maxillary artery, the vidian artery, the capsular branch of the internal carotid artery, and the as- cending pharyngeal artery.

Brisk epistaxis may respond to anterior and posterior nasal packing. Failure to control hemorrhage with these techniques is optimally managed by immediate angiography to detect the bleeding site and selective embolization (17) (Fig. 33–1).

OCULAR INJURY

Direct ocular injury must be ruled out in all patients with or- bital fractures and periorbital soft-tissue injuries. The sur- geon obtains brief history of the preinjury visual status and postinjury subjective visual status. The presence of pain, photophobia, decreased vision, or the appearance of spots be- fore the eyes are highly suggestive of ocular trauma. A screening ophthalmologic examination is performed in sys- tematic fashion to determine the visual acuity, pupillary re- sponses, visual fields, ocular motility, and appearance of the fundus. Injuries that may require immediate ophthalmologic treatment or result in permanent sequelae include corneal scleral lacerations, lens dislocation, major hyphema, acute glaucoma, and retinal detachment.

Globe rupture (Fig. 33–2) should be suspected, particu- larly if there is any physical evidence of penetrating trauma to the orbital region. Specific signs that suggest rupture include ec- centric or ovoid pupils, conjunctival or scleral lacerations, hy- phema, uveal exposure, or vitreal prolapse. Under these cir- cumstances, a protective shield should be applied to the eye and immediate ophthalmologic consultation obtained (18).

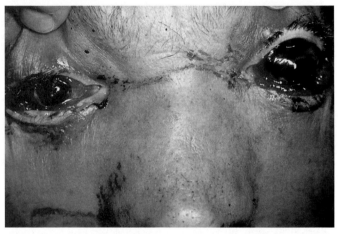

FIG. 33–2. Naso-orbital-ethmoid fracture associated with bilateral ocular globe rupture. Note telecanthus with intercanthal distance ex- ceeding palpebral fissure width bilaterally. Loss of vision, ovoid pupils, and scleral lacerations suggest globe disruption.

The presence of acutely decreased vision and afferent pupillary defect in an otherwise normal eye is indicative of a traumatic optic neuropathy (12). Ophthalmoplegia, upper- eyelid ptosis, fixed dilated pupil, and absence of sensation over the forehead are signs of a superior orbital fissure syn- drome (19). Direct traumatic neuropathies are caused by ac- tual compression of the optic nerve and/or the 3rd, 4th, and 6th cranial nerves by bone fragments, hematoma, or foreign body. Indirect neuropathy results in the same clinical findings but in the absence of any obvious radiographic evidence of pathology. In all patients presenting with these signs, imme- diate ophthalmologic consultation and CT evaluation of the orbit, optic canal, and superior orbital fissure are required. All patients are treated at the time of diagnosis with high- dose corticosteroids (1.0 mgs/kg dexamethasone loading, 0.5 mgs/kg q6h thereafter). In the presence of radiographic evidence of compression, surgical decompression should be considered.

CEREBROSPINAL FLUID RHINORRHEA

The discharge of cerebrospinal fluid (CSF) into the nasal cavity implies a defect in the arachnoid, dura, bone, and mucoperiosteum, resulting in a direct communication between the subarachnoid space and the external environment. Central midface and nasoethmoidal fractures, and craniofrontal and frontal sinus fractures, are commonly implicated. The resulting fracture lines extend to the posterior wall of the frontal sinus, the fovea ethmoidalis and cribriform plate, all of which are frequent sites of CSF fistulae.

Clinically, CSF leaks should be actively searched for in patients with craniofrontal or midfacial fractures. The presence of clear or serosanguineous nasal discharge, anosmia, or the ability to elicit a target sign are highly suggestive. The diagnosis is confirmed by collecting the nasal discharge and a concomitant blood sample and submitting both for laboratory investigation. CSF is differentiated from serum by its low protein concentration, and is further distinguished from normal nasal secretions by the presence of glucose ($\geq 50\%$ of serum glucose) but no mucus (20).

The site of CSF leakage should be accurately localized, particularly in situations where surgical closure of the breach is indicated. Attempts to show the site of leakage using intrathecal dyes and metrizamide cisternography may be unreliable because they depend on CSF leaking at the time of investigation. Recent studies (21,22) suggest that high-resolution CT scans in a coronal and axial plane are most effective in defining the site of CSF leakage.

Reduction and stabilization of facial fracture segments is effective in facilitating spontaneous closure of CSF fistulae. Therefore, we manage CSF fistulae by extracranial reduction and fixation of facial fractures. Dural defects are patched primarily only in those situations where craniotomy and intracranial exposure for craniofrontal fractures is indicated. Following the reduction of facial fractures, persistence of CSF leakage beyond the 1st postoperative week requires neurosurgical consultation and more aggressive investigation and treatment (20,23).

Clinical Assessment of the Face

Physical examination of the face begins with a thorough inspection and documentation of all lacerations and an assessment of facial nerve function.

CRANIOFRONTAL FRACTURES

The frontal bone is characterized by high-impact tolerance, and the majority of injuries result from direct high-velocity injury. Burst lacerations and periorbital ecchymoses are highly suggestive of underlying skeletal injury. Contour deformities resulting from displaced craniofrontal fractures are frequently masked by edema in the overlying soft tissues.

Central craniofrontal fractures involve the frontal sinus (Fig. 33-3). Disruption of the posterior wall of the sinus predisposes to intracranial injury and CSF rhinorrhea, while fractures of the floor of the sinus may obstruct nasofrontal duct drainage.

Displaced fractures of the orbital roof result in impingement on intraorbital structures and ocular globe displacement associated with volumetric changes of the orbit (Fig. 33-4).

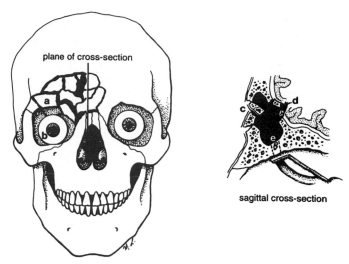

FIG. 33-3. Craniofrontal fractures, pathologic features. Displacement of frontal bone segments alters the surface contour of the forehead and eyebrow ridge (a), while displacement of supraorbital rim and roof fractures into the orbit (b) may cause globe ptosis or proptosis and impingement of the levator palpebrae or superior rectus muscles. The sagittal cross-section through the frontal sinus demonstrates sequelae of injury. Anterior wall fractures (c) alter central forehead contour, posterior wall fractures (d) potentially lacerate the dura, causing intracranial injury or CSF rhinorrhea, and floor fractures (e) may obstruct nasofrontal duct drainage, predisposing to mucocele or abscess formation.

Frequently associated signs include (24) ptosis of the upper eyelid, limitation of supraduction, and diplopia. Inferior displacement and proptosis of the affected ocular globe are the most common clinical manifestations, although enophthalmos may occur in the presence of outwardly displaced roof fractures or concomitant orbital floor fractures.

ORBITAL FRACTURES

An appreciation of orbital volumetric relationships is of primary importance to the understanding of orbital fractures and related treatment principles. Following orbital trauma, the position and projection of the ocular globe are determined by the precise anatomic location of volumetric change in relation to the axis of the globe. Pearl (25) first described a coronal plane that extends from the lateral orbital rim to the anterior lacrimal crest and bisects the globe into two equal halves (Fig. 33-5). Displaced orbital fractures located in this coronal plane (i.e., fractures of the orbital rim and anterior floor) result in globe displacement within the coronal plane and have no affect on ocular projection (26). Fractures posterior to this coronal plane (i.e., displaced fractures of the lateral orbital rim or posterior fractures of the inferomedial orbit) result in retrodisplacement of the globe and enophthalmos.

Displaced orbital fractures, regardless of whether they involve the rim or cavity, necessarily result in a volumetric change. Depending on the precise location of this volumetric change in relation to the globe axis, clinical features may include a change in ocular globe projection (Fig. 33-6) or position within the coronal plane.

The second common feature of orbital fracture is a restriction of ocular motility and diplopia. Muscle contusion is the principle mechanism for ocular motility imbalance.

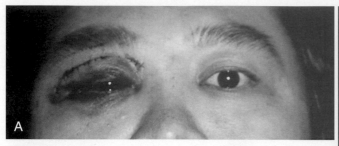

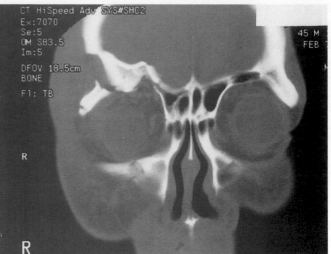

FIG. 33–4.   Right lateral craniofrontal fracture. **A,** frontal view of the face reveals subconjunctival hemorrhage, periorbital ecchymosis, burst laceration over the brow, upper-lid ptosis, and hypoglobus. **B,** coronal CT demonstrates displacement of the supraorbital rim and roof into the right orbit. Note impingement on the superior rectus and levator palpebrae superioris muscles and inferior displacement of the globe.

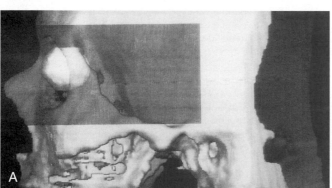

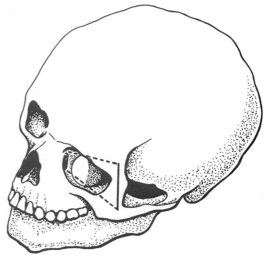

FIG. 33–5.   Coronal plane of the ocular globe. **A,** lateral 3DCT of the skull (semitransparent) with actual segmented ocular globe. Note that the equator of the globe in the coronal plane is aligned with the anterior margin of the lateral orbital rim. **B,** this coronal plane divides the orbital cavity into anterior and posterior segments. Volumetric alterations in the anterior segment affect globe position in the coronal plane, while displacements in the posterior segment affect globe projection.

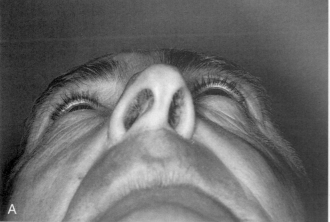

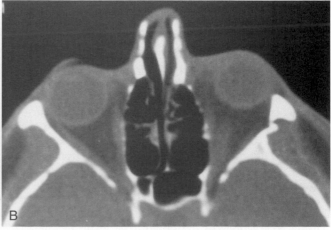

FIG. 33–6.   Left impure orbital blow-in fracture. **A,** acute proptosis of the left ocular globe. **B,** axial CT scan demonstrating intraorbital displacement of the lateral orbital rim and wall.

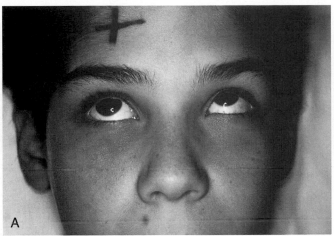

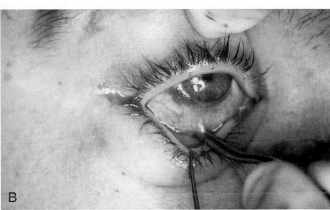

FIG. 33–7. Assessment of ocular motility. **A,** diplopia and abrupt restriction of the right globe on up gaze suggests inferior rectus or inferior oblique muscle contusion, incarceration, or fat entrapment. **B,** forced duction test confirms mechanical restriction.

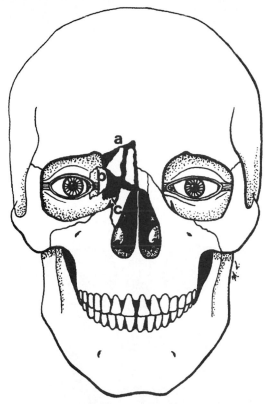

FIG. 33–8. Nasoethmoid fractures, pathologic features. Disruption of the nasal bones and nasomaxillary process (a) results in collapse of the nasal dorsum and potential extension of fractures into the cranial base or medial orbit. Displacement of the central segment bearing the medial canthal tendon insertion (b) causes telecanthus, diminished palpebral fissure width, and rounding of the medial canthus. Fractures circumscribing the lacrimal fossa and nasolacrimal duct (c) may cause obstruction and epiphora.

Other causes, in decreasing order of frequency, include entrapment of orbital fat with tethering of extraocular muscles via fibrous septa (Fig. 33–7), actual incarceration of muscles, or paresis as a result of traumatic neuropathy of cranial nerves 3, 4, and 6.

NASOETHMOID FRACTURES

The nasoethmoid complex constitutes the interorbital space and is circumscribed by the anterior cranial fossa superiorly, medial orbital walls laterally, and floor of the nose inferiorly. This delicate skeletal framework is buttressed anteriorly by the frontal processes of the maxilla, the nasal processes of the frontal bone, and the paired nasal bones. The central location of the nasoethmoid complex predisposes to concomitant injury of immediately adjacent structures. Nasoethmoid fractures potentially involve the cranial, orbital, and nasal cavities, as well as the lacrimal pathways.

Nasoethmoid fractures are characterized by disruption of the anterior abutments of the central midface (i.e., the nasomaxillary buttresses, nasal bones and septum) (Fig. 33–8). Disruption of the nasal bones and septum is clinically manifested by an exaggerated depth of the nasofrontal angle and decreased projection of the nasal dorsum, nasal airway obstruction, and epistaxis.

The nasomaxillary buttresses contain the lacrimal fossa and the insertion of the medial canthal tendon. Fracture and displacement of these buttresses therefore results in nasolacrimal duct obstruction and obvious changes in periorbital morphology featuring a rounding of the medial canthus, an increase in the intercanthal distance, and diminished palpebral fissure width (see Fig. 33–2). Once the anterior abutments are disrupted, there is no further resistance to applied impact forces. The medial orbital walls, bony septum, and cribriform plate comminute readily.

The degree of instability in the nasoethmoid complex and the integrity of the medial canthal tendons is tested actively (Fig. 33–9). Digital pressure on the nasal bones reveals the degree of support of the nasal dorsum. Collapse and prolapse of the distal nose into the pyriform aperture indicates gross disruption and implies the need for bone-graft reconstruction. The integrity of the medial canthal tendon attachment is tested by the eyelid traction test. Subtle fractures of the nasoethmoid skeleton are further confirmed using bimanual examination to evaluate the stability of the canthus-bearing bone.

ZYGOMATIC FRACTURES

The zygoma occupies a prominent position in the facial skeleton. Its spatial relationship to the adjacent skeleton de-

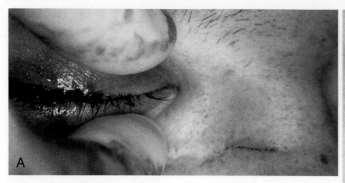

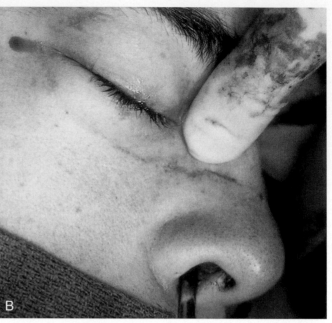

FIG. 33–9. Active tests of medial canthal integrity. **A,** eyelid traction test. Tension applied to the upper and lower eyelids causes puckering, provided that its insertion remains intact. Rounding and displacement of the canthus indicates avulsion. **B,** bimanual examination determines the stability of the central tendon-bearing segment. An elevator in the nasal cavity is used to exert pressure on the nasomaxillary buttress while instability is evaluated by external palpation.

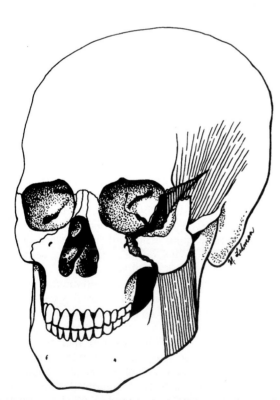

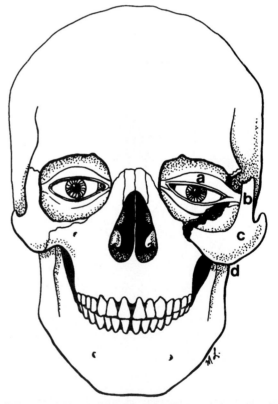

FIG. 33–10. Unstable zygoma fractures. Wide separation of the frontozygomatic fracture line at the lateral orbit rim implies gross disruption of the periosteum and deep temporal fascia. Loss of the superior soft-tissue supporting structures results in an unstable situation predisposing to unimpeded inferior distraction by the masseter muscle.

FIG. 33–11. Zygoma fractures, pathologic features. The zygoma contributes to the inferolateral orbital cavity. Displaced fractures are therefore necessarily associated with volumetric changes that affect the position and projection of the globe (a). The insertion of the lateral canthus into the Whitnall tubercle on the zygoma (b) results in alterations in the transverse dimension and obliquity of the palpebral fissure. The malar prominence is displaced (c), and impingement on the coronoid process (d) may cause trismus or mechanical restriction of jaw opening.

fines facial width, cheek prominence, and the transverse and vertical dimensions of the orbit. It further contributes to a significant portion of the inferior and lateral orbital walls.

Moderate impact forces applied to the zygoma are generally transmitted along the bony process, resulting in a disarticulation at the zygomaticotemporal and zygomaticomaxillary suture lines. More severe trauma further disrupts the insertion of the deep temporal fascia (Fig. 33–10), resulting in gross separation at the frontozygomatic fracture line and unresisted inferior displacement by the unopposed action of the masseter muscle (27).

The clinical manifestations of a zygomatic fracture are readily apparent: circumorbital tissues are swollen, subconjunctival hemorrhage is frequently present, and the patient reports decreased or abnormal sensation of the cheek, upper lip, and gingiva. The malar prominence may be depressed, and facial width increased.

Trismus or mechanical restriction of mandibular excursion are caused by impingement of the coronoid process of the mandible. This occurs in fractures of the zygomatic arch or in rotated body fractures and can be confirmed by intraoral palpation of the bony deformity in the upper buccal sulcus.

Deformities of the orbit must be actively searched for (Fig. 33–11). Displaced zygomatic fractures are necessarily associated with displacement of the lateral canthal position, alteration of palpebral fissure width and inclination, and commonly enophthalmos and hypoglobus. Extensive com-

minution of the orbital floor may further cause mechanical restriction of supraduction and diplopia.

MAXILLARY FRACTURES

The paired maxillae, united in the midline, comprise the major part of the midface and contribute to the formation of the inferomedial orbits, nasal cavity and palate. Functionally the maxilla is important in establishing the vertical height and projection of the midface in relation to the cranial base.

The midface is composed of transverse and vertical thickened buttresses interposed between areas of thinner bone of the orbits, nasal cavity, and perinasal sinuses (Fig. 33–12). These skeletal buttresses form a three-dimensional framework that reinforces the facial skeleton and dissipates applied impact forces. When applied forces exceed the impact resistance of these various buttresses (28), the adjacent weakened bone comminutes readily.

The pattern of midface fractures is primarily influenced by the magnitude and direction of the applied force in relation to the orientation and impact tolerance of the maxillary buttresses. The midfacial bones are considerably less resistant to horizontally directed forces as compared to vertically directed forces. Shearing across anatomically predisposed cleavage planes results in predictable patterns of maxillary fractures (Fig. 33–13). Extensive comminution, particularly in the weaker bone comprising the walls of the sinuses, causes instability and collapse of the maxillary skeleton.

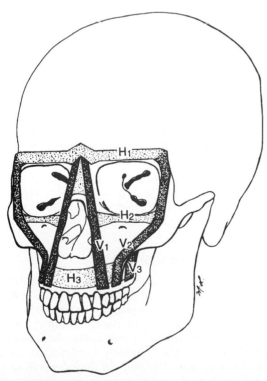

FIG. 33–12. Facial buttresses provide structural support to the facial skeleton. The principle vertical buttresses include the nasomaxillary or medial buttress (V_1), zygomaticomaxillary or lateral buttress (V_2), and pterygomaxillary buttress (V_3). The horizontal buttresses provide additional support by uniting the vertical buttresses. These consist of the supraorbital rim (H_1), infraorbital rim (H_2) and the nasal floor and palate (H_3).

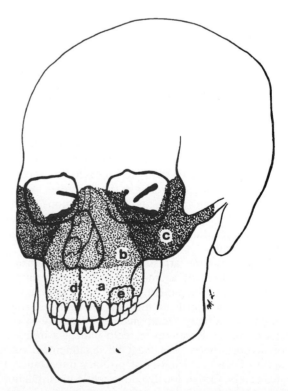

FIG. 33–13. Maxillary fractures, classification. Midface fractures are classified anatomically : (a) Le Fort I (transverse); (b) Le Fort II (pyramidal); (c) Le Fort III (craniofacial disjunction); (d) palatal split; and (e) dentoalveolar.

Periorbital and midface edema in the presence of subconjunctival hemorrhage suggests midface fracture. Gross disruption of midfacial bones results in posterior or inferior displacement characterized clinically by flattening or elongation of the face. More important, displacement of the maxillary dental arch necessarily results in a malocclusion. Epistaxis and nasal airway obstruction are commonly observed. Extension into the orbital cavity with LeFort II and III fractures alters globe position and projection and may result in visual disturbances, diplopia, and epiphora. Associated injury to the infraorbital and superior alveolar nerves results in altered sensation to the cheeks, upper lip, and maxillary dentition.

Active manipulation of the maxillary dental arch while sequentially palpating articulations at the root of the nose and inferior and lateral orbital rims, determines the degree of instability and level of fracture. Palatal fractures must be actively searched for, particularly in the presence of lacerations to the palatal vault and the presence of cross-bite.

MANDIBULAR FRACTURES

The mandible defines the projection and vertical height of the lower third of the face. It consists of a horseshoe-shaped arch extended at each end by vertically directed rami.

The pattern of fractures is influenced by the magnitude of the impact force and the anatomic predisposition at the site of injury. Mandibular bone is particularly susceptible to trauma at the condylar neck and the angle.

The configuration of the arch facilitates the transmission or distribution of applied forces to the entire mandible. In all fractures that disrupt the continuity of the arch, a second fracture line should be suspected and actively searched for in the contralateral aspect of the jaw.

Multiple factors determine the degree of displacement and instability in mandibular fractures. The precise location and direction of fracture lines in relation to attached muscle groups are important. In particular, fractures of the body of the mandible occur in the interval between the anterior and posterior muscle groups and are prone to distraction by the opposing actions of these muscles. The presence of teeth on either side of the fracture line minimize the extent of displacement in fractures of the anterior arch. Teeth act as occlusal stops, tending to realign the fractures where the mandible articulates with the maxillary dentition. Alternately, fractures that occur in the edentulous mandible or posterior to the mandibular dentition are predisposed to more significant displacement.

Mandibular fractures are suspected in the presence of ecchymosis, swelling, and asymmetry of the lower third of the face (Fig. 33–14). The patient complains of pain aggravated by any attempts at mastication or jaw movement. Dysphagia and pooling of salivary secretions are frequently associated. Anaesthesia in the lower lip or teeth indicates injury to the inferior alveolar nerve and must be documented. Accurate evaluation of the occlusion is of primary importance. Fracture sites can be further localized by gentle manipulation and palpation.

The frequency of condylar fractures occurring in association with other mandibular trauma demands specific examination of the temporomandibular joints. A limitation of

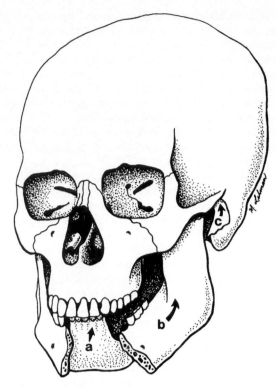

FIG. 33–14. Mandible fractures, pathologic features. Disruption of the dental arch (a) results in displacement in the direction of principle muscle pull and malocclusion. Displaced fractures of the condylar neck predispose to vertical collapse of vertical ramus of the mandible and open-bite deformity (b). Superior impaction of the condylar head (c) may result in injury to the glenoid fossa and external auditory canal.

mandibular excursion, deviation of the mandible upon opening, and a decrease in the vertical height of the vertical ramus with associated open-bite deformities suggest displaced condylar neck fractures. Examination of the external auditory canal is mandatory. Position of the condylar heads within the glenoid fossa should be palpated by inserting the examining fingers into the external auditory canals while the patient actively opens and closes the jaw. Failure in ability to palpate the condylar heads as they rotate and slide symmetrically within the joints indicates possible subluxation or dislocation.

Radiological Assessment

The ability simultaneously to display the facial skeleton, soft tissues, and sinuses make computed x-ray tomography the optimal modality for radiographic evaluation of facial trauma. Axial CT scans, comprising multiple 5-mm cuts from the skull to the mandible and 3-mm slices through the cranial base and orbits, are routinely employed for the evaluation of the craniofacial region. In the cooperative patient and in the absence of cervical spine injury, these images are supplemented with coronal CT scans to provide improved visualization of specific anatomic sites where indicated (i.e., the cranial base, the orbital cavities, and the temporomandibular joint regions). Where coronal imaging is contraindicated because of the patient's condition, reformatted multiplanar images are used. The sequence of images described above allows detailed evaluation of the facial fracture pattern and displacement, and the status of intracranial and intraorbital soft tissues.

The sequence of CT axial data acquisition also is sufficient to permit three-dimensional reconstructed images (3DCT). Three-dimensional images do not improve diagnostic accuracy (29) unless they are optimized by the application of submillimeter scanning thicknesses and sophisticated thresholding and segmentation algorithms (30). However, three-dimensional displays do provide a global view of the traumatized face from any angle. The size, rotation, and spatial relationship of bony fragments and their interrelationships can be assessed, facilitating perceptual evaluation of the trauma and presurgical planning for reduction and fixation.

Computed tomography has largely replaced conventional radiography for craniofacial assessment. However conventional radiographs are a useful modality in the lower third of the face. Mandibular views and panorex simply and effectively demonstrate mandibular fractures.

PRINCIPLES OF FACIAL FRACTURE AND SOFT TISSUE REPAIR

Treatment Goals

The overall objectives of facial trauma management are, first, to provide an accurate and stable three-dimensional reconstruction of the facial skeleton, and second, to ensure definitive repair and accurate redraping of all associated soft tissues. Over the past 20 years, surgical principles and techniques have evolved concomitantly to allow the practicing surgeon to meet the above objectives in an early single-stage repair.

Timing of Surgical Intervention

Primary one-stage reconstruction of facial fractures should ideally be performed in the first 24 to 48 hours following the injury. Early treatment facilitates both fracture reduction and repair. Even in the presence of extensive craniofrontal injuries where immediate craniotomy is indicated, combined intra- and extra-cranial approaches provide improved access to fractures, allowing single-stage repair with an acceptable rate of morbidity and an improved cosmetic and functional outcome (31).

A delay in facial reconstruction is indicated in patients who are unstable, in those with significant intracranial injury featuring a GCS score of less than 5, intracranial hemorrhage and/or midline cranial shift, or an ICP greater than 15 millimetres (32), and in patients with indirect traumatic optic neuropathy, or repaired intraocular injury that holds some promise of visual return. Under all these circumstances, surgery is deferred for up to 2 weeks. During this time, the patient's general condition is stabilized, the intracranial pressure is optimized, and sufficient time is allowed for intraorbital edema to resolve and potential vision to return.

Exposure

The first step in facial fracture reconstruction is to obtain wide exposure of the involved portions of the craniofacial skeleton. Exposure is obtained through standard "hidden" incisions and extended subperiosteal dissection. This minimizes the risk of inadvertent injury to soft tissue structures during fracture segment mobilization and permits direct visu-

alization of all fractures and their relation to adjacent intact segments of the facial skeleton.

The entire craniofacial skeleton can be visualized through four incisions. The coronal incision exposes the cranium, zygomatic arch, and superior portions of the orbits and nasoethmoid complex. The inferior half of the orbit and orbital rim are visualized through a transconjunctival or subciliary lower-lid incision. The upper gingivobuccal incision exposes the midface, while the lower gingivobuccal incision, in combination with submandibular or retromandibular incisions for specific indications, exposes the mandible.

RIGID INTERNAL FIXATION

Rigid fixation provides a surgeon with control over the spatial orientation and position of multiple fracture segments and thereby permits the sequential reduction of fractures to reestablish a stable, anatomically accurate facial skeleton in three dimensions. Rigid skeletal fixation relies on the provision of sufficient binding force at the fracture site to exceed functional forces acting on the bone. These functional forces are highly variable throughout the craniofacial skeleton. Forces generated in the upper facial skeleton resulting from tensions generated by CSF pulsations, eyelid movements via the canthal ligaments, and overlying soft tissues, particularly in the presence of edema or contracture, are minimal. In contrast, forces generated by mastication are considerable. The specific technical requirements for stability therefore vary according to anatomic site.

SEQUENCE OF FRACTURE REPAIR

Following exposure of all bone segments, fracture repair proceeds in an orderly fashion (Fig. 33–15). Premorbid occlusion is first reestablished and then maintained with interdental wiring and maxillomandibular fixation. In situations where the dental arches are grossly disrupted by palatal or dentoalveolar fractures, or in the presence of major edentulous segments, the use of acrylic splints or the patient's own dentures ensures proper relation of the maxillary and mandibular arches.

Attention is then directed to the mandible (33) or upper face (34) depending on personal preference. The underlying principle is to first identify stable uninjured regions of the craniofacial skeleton that provide reliable anatomic landmarks. The vertical and horizontal buttresses of the upper face are then reconstructed by sequential anatomic reduction and fixation of fracture segments, ensuring that the normal height, width, and projection of the face and functional spaces are reestablished.

Following reconstruction of the upper face (comprising the nasoethmoid and orbitozygomatic regions), the dental arches must be stabilized in their proper spatial relationship. The exact sequence of subsequent repair depends on the degree of disruption or comminution of the medial and lateral maxillary buttresses and the vertical rami or condylar necks of the mandible. Generally the medial and lateral maxillary buttresses are anatomically reduced and fixed first, followed by the mandible. Where the degree of maxillary comminution makes it impossible to reestablish lower facial height and projection accurately, condylar neck and mandible fractures are reconstructed first, followed by the maxillary buttresses.

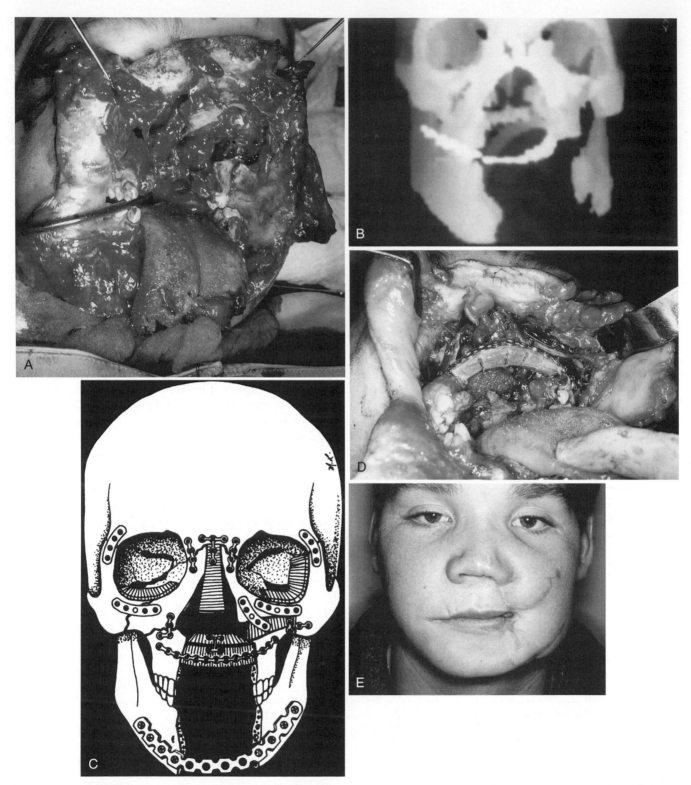

FIG. 33–15. A 15-year-old male with self-inflicted shotgun wound to the face. **A,** entry wound is submental, exiting through the nasoethmoid region and resulting in a large composite tissue defect. **B,** 3DCT, AP view, reveals nasoethmoid and orbitozygomatic fractures, and complete loss of bone in the central midface and mandible. (Reprinted with permission from *Can J Surg* 1993; 36(5):441–452.) **C,** schematic diagram, AP skull. Reconstruction was organized as follows: complete exposure maxillomandibular fixation, open reduction and fixa- tion of zygomatic and nasomaxillary fractures, plate stabilization of mandibular defect followed by primary bone grafts (stippled) to the anterior maxilla, palatal vault, orbital cavities, and cantilever strut to the nose. **D,** intraoral view demonstrating skeletal reconstruction of palate and anterior maxilla. A radial forearm free flap was used to resurface the oral cavity defect. (Reprinted with permission from *Can J Surg* 1993; 36(5):441–452.) **E,** result, 1 year postoperatively. (Reprinted with permission from *Can J Surg;* 1993; 36(5):441–452.)

PRIMARY BONE GRAFTING

The concept of employing free autogenous bone grafts in the primary reconstruction of facial fractures was introduced by Bonanno and Converse in 1975 (35). Gruss (36) and Manson (37) subsequently refined and developed the technique of primary bone grafting and firmly established it as a basic principle in immediate posttraumatic facial reconstruction.

The indications for primary bone grafting in trauma are as follows (see Fig. 33–15).

1. Reconstruction of both the vertical (38,39) and transverse (40,41) craniofacial buttresses. This preserves the structural integrity of the facial reconstruction in three dimensions. Bony defects in the supporting buttresses are replaced with onlay bone grafts using lag-screw fixation, or alternately with inlay bone grafts and miniplate fixation.
2. Restoring surface contour and maintaining soft-tissue expansion. Inadequate support for the overlying facial soft-tissues results in collapse and soft-tissue contracture with obvious external deformity. To prevent this, precisely shaped inlay bone grafts are used to restore bony continuity in the cranium and orbital-rim region. Cantilever bone grafts are further employed in the reconstruction of grossly comminuted nasoethmoid injuries to provide a supportive nasal framework.
3. Reconstruction of the orbital cavity. Skeletal defects within the orbit predispose to both enophthalmos and prolapse, with potential entrapment of extraocular muscles. Fixed or nonfixed grafts are used to obliterate defects and support the orbital soft-tissue contents.

Free autogenous bone grafts offer multiple advantages compared to other materials when used for the above indications. First, new bone formation is stimulated, both by surviving cellular elements in the graft and by the ability of the bone matrix to induce transformation of osteogenic precursors in the recipient site. Fracture healing can therefore be positively influenced, particularly in areas where bone gaps or significant comminution exists.

Cranial, rib, and iliac crest bone are the most commonly used bone-graft donor sites. Cranial bone is preferred in areas where rigidity is of primary importance (e.g., in the reconstruction of supporting buttresses). Iliac crest or rib grafts are malleable and more easily contoured, and are preferred in the reconstruction of the orbital cavity.

DEFINITIVE SOFT TISSUE REPAIR

Following reconstruction of facial skeleton, primary repair of all associated soft-tissue injuries is performed.

Débridement

Basic would management requires that all facial wounds be thoroughly irrigated, foreign materials removed, and clearly devitalized tissue excised regardless of its previous location or importance.

Repair of Lacerations

Lacerations range from simple ones resulting from penetrating trauma to undermined lacerations where soft tissues are avulsed in the plane of least resistance.

Injuries to underlying structures are addressed first. Parotid or nasolacrimal duct lacerations and injuries to the facial nerve or sensory nerve branches must be recognized and treated primarily where possible.

In repairing facial lacerations, particular care must be taken in returning displaced anatomic landmarks and structures to their original position. Landmarks are identified on either side of an irregular wound and precisely approximated. This facilitates the suturing of intervening wound edges in the position they occupied relative to one another before the injury. Irregularities in the lip margin, eyebrow, eyelid, or nostril can thus be avoided.

Tissue Loss

Once surviving tissues are replaced in their correct anatomic position, residual defects can be properly displayed and assessed in terms of tissue lost. The goals of reconstruction are then to resurface the wound without distorting adjacent anatomic structures and to provide adequate vascularized coverage in situations where bone or cartilage are exposed. Where the recipient site is adequately vascularized, application of skin grafts will promote rapid healing. However primary reconstruction with vascularized soft tissue is mandatory in situations where exposed bone or cartilage renders the recipient site unsuitable for grafting.

Traumatic composite defects pose the most significant challenge. These are characterized by a combined deficiency of multiple tissues including skin, muscle, fat, bone, and mucosal lining to varying degrees. Such defects most commonly are the result of facial gunshot wounds. Initial skeletal reconstruction frequently results in a situation where segments of the facial skeleton and bone grafts are exposed on multiple surfaces. Definitive resurfacing of both cutaneous and mucosal defects is mandatory to ensure fracture healing and bone graft consolidation (42,43) (see Fig. 33–15).

Controlled Soft-Tissue Redraping

The final results of facial trauma reconstruction are generally judged in terms of the accuracy with which premorbid surface morphology has been reestablished. Critical reviews of the long-term morphologic results of facial trauma reconstruction reveal deficiencies, disproportions, or asymmetries in facial surface anatomy despite accurate reconstruction of the facial skeleton. Deformities in surface morphology are particularly obvious in the periorbital region (where minor discrepancies result in canthal dystopias) and asymmetries in the height and width of the palpebral fissures (44).

Following completion of skeletal reconstruction, facial soft tissues are precisely repositioned and fixed to bone to ensure adequate redraping. This includes the use of external splints or bolsters in the nasoethmoid region, medial and lateral canthoplasties, and periosteal suspension of the lower eyelid and cheek (45).

Summary

These basic principles are generally applicable to virtually all patients with facial trauma. Systematic clinical and radiologic evaluation permits accurate diagnosis of the facial injury and formulation of an effective treatment plan. Surgical reconstruction then aims to reestablish facial skeletal anatomy and repair associated soft-tissue injuries in a single stage.

References

1. Luce EA, Tubb TD, Moore AM. Review of 1000 major facial fractures and associated injuries. *Plast Reconstr Surg* 1979; 63:26–30.
2. Van Hoof RF, Merkz CA, Stekelenburg EC. The different patterns of fractures of the facial skeleton in four European countries. *Int J Oral Surg* 1977; 6:3.
3. Afzelius LE, Rosen C. Facial fractures. A review of 368 cases. *Int J Oral Surg* 1980; 9:25.
4. Lim LH, Lam LK, Moore MH, et al. Associated injuries in facial fractures: review of 839 patients. *Brit J Plast Surg* 1993; 46:635–638.
5. Telfer MR, Jones GM, Shepherd JP. Trends in the aetiology of maxillofacial fractures in the United Kingdom (1977–1987). *Brit J Oral and Maxillofacial Surg* 1991; 29:250–255.
6. Vetter JD, Topazian RG, Goldberg MH, et al. Facial fractures occurring in a medium-sized metropolitan area: recent trends. *Int J Oral Maxillofacial Surg* 1991; 20:214–216.
7. Hussain K, Wijetunge DB, Grubnic S, et al. A comprehensive analysis of craniofacial trauma. *J Trauma* 1994; 36(1):34–47.
8. Davidson JS, Birdsell DC. Cervical spine injury in patients with facial skeletal trauma. *J Trauma* 1989; 29:1276–1278.
9. Shultz RC. Facial injuries from automobile accidents: a study of 400 consecutive cases. *Plast Reconstr Surg* 1967; 40:415–425.
10. Davidoff G, Jakubowski M, Thomas D, et al. The spectrum of closed-head injuries in facial trauma victims: incidence and impact. *Ann Emerg Med* 1988; 17:6–9.
11. Slupchynskyj OS, Berkower AS, Byrne DW, et al. Association of skull base and facial fractures. *Laryngoscope* 1992; 102:1247–1250.
12. Gossman MD, Roberts DM, Barr CC. Ophthalmic aspects of orbital injury: a comprehensive diagnostic and management approach. *Clin Plast Surg* 1992; 19(1):71–85.
13. Jabaley ME, Lerman M, Sanders HJ. Ocular injuries in orbital fractures: a review of 119 cases. *Plast Reconstr Surg* 1975; 56:410–418.
14. Kallela I, Hyrkas T, Paukku P, et al. Blindness after maxillofacial blunt trauma: evaluation of candidates for optic nerve decompression surgery. *J Craniomaxillofacial Surg* 1994; 22:220–225.
15. Kellman R. The cervical spine in maxillofacial trauma: assessment and airway management. *Otolaryngol Clin North America* 1991; 24(1):1–13.
16. Rhee KJ, Muntz CB, Donald PJ, et al. Does nasotracheal intubation increase complications in patients with skull base fractures? *Ann Emerg Med* 1993; 22:1145–1147.
17. Kurata A, Kitahara T, Miyasaka Y, et al. Superselective embolization for severe traumatic epistaxis caused by fracture of the skull base. *Am J Neuroradiology* 1993; 14:343–345.
18. Weisman RA, Savino PJ. Management of patients with facial trauma and associated ocular/orbital injuries. *Otolaryngol Clin North America* 1991; 24(1):37–57.
19. Kurzer A, Patel MP. Superior orbital fissure syndrome associated with fractures of the zygoma and orbit. *Plast Reconstr Surg* 1979; 64(5):715–719.
20. Marentette LJ, Valentino J. Traumatic anterior fossa cerebrospinal fluid fistulae and craniofacial considerations. *Otolaryngol Clin North America* 1991; 24(1)151–163.
21. Farrell VJ, Emby DJ. Meningitis following fractures of the paranasal sinuses: accurate, non-invasive localization of the dural defect by direct coronal computed tomography. *Surg Neurol* 1993; 37:378–382.
22. Lloyd MN, Kimber PM, Burrows EH. Post-traumatic cerebrospinal fluid rhinorrhea: modern high-definition computed tomography is all that is required for the effective demonstration of the site of leakage. *Clinical Radiology* 1994; 49:100–103.
23. Vrankovic D, Glavina K. Classification of frontal fossa fractures associated with cerebrospinal fluid rhinorrhea, pneumocephalus or meningitis. Indications and time for surgical treatment. *Neurochirurgia* 1993; 36:44–50.
24. Sullivan WG. Displaced orbital roof fractures: presentation and treatment. *Plast Reconstr Surg* 1991; 87:657.
25. Pearl RM. Surgical management of volumetric changes in the bony orbit. *Ann Plast Surg* 1987; 19:349–358.
26. Pearl RM: Treatment of enophthalmos. *Clin Plast Surg* 1992; 19(1):99–111.
27. Larsen OD, Thomsen M. Zygomatic fractures. I. A simplified classification of fracture use. *Scand J Plast Reconstr Surg* 1978; 12:55.
28. Nahum A. The biomechanics of maxillofacial trauma. *Clin Plast Surg* 1975; 2:59–64.
29. Broumand SR, Labs JD, Novelline RA, et al. The role of three-dimensional computed tomography in the evaluation of acute craniofacial trauma. *Ann Plast Surg* 1993; 31(6):488–494.
30. Levy RA, Edwards WT, Meyer JR, et al. Facial trauma and 3-D reconstructive imaging: insufficiencies and correctives. *Am J Neuroradiol* 1992; 13:885.
31. Benzil DL, Robotti E, Dagi TF, et al. Early single-stage repair of complex craniofacial trauma. *Neurosurgery* 1992; 30(2):166–171.
32. Derdeyn C, Persing JA, Broaddus WC, et al. Craniofacial trauma: an assessment of risk related to the timing of surgery. *Plast Reconstr Surg* 1990; 86:238–245.
33. Rohrich RJ, Shewmake KB. Evolving concepts of craniomaxillofacial fracture management. *Clin Plast Surg* 1992; 19(1):1–10.
34. Kelly KJ, Manson PN, Vander Kolk CA, et al. Sequencing Le Fort fracture treatment (organization of treatment for a panfacial fracture). *J Craniofac Surg* 1990; 1(4):168–178.
35. Bonanno PC, Converse JM. Primary bone grafting in management of facial fractures. *NY State J Med* 1975; 75:710.
36. Gruss JS, MacKinnon SE, Kassel E, et al. The role of primary bone grafting in complex craniomaxillofacial trauma. *Plast Reconstr Surg* 1985; 75:17.
37. Manson PN, Crawley WA, Yaremchuk MJ, et al. Midface fractures: advantages of immediate extended open reduction and bone grafting. *Plast Reconstr Surg* 1985; 76:1.
38. Manson PN, Hoopes JE, Su CT. Structural pillars of the facial skeleton: an approach to the management of Le Fort fractures. *Plast Reconstr Surg* 1980; 66:54.
39. Gruss JS, MacKinnon SE. Complex maxillary fractures: role of buttress reconstruction and immediate bone grafts. *Plast Reconstr Surg* 1986; 78:9.
40. Stanley RB, Nowak GM. Midfacial fractures: importance of angle impact to horizontal craniofacial buttresses. *Otolaryngol Head Neck Surg* 1985; 98:186–190.
41. Rimel F, Marentette LJ. Injuries of the hard palate and the horizontal buttress of the midface. *Otolaryngol Head Neck Surg* 1993; 109:499–505.
42. Gruss JS, Antonyshyn O, Phillips JH. Early definitive bone and soft-tissue reconstruction of major gunshot wounds of the face. *Plast Reconstr Surg* 1991; 87(3):436–450.
43. Antonyshyn O, Paletz JL, Wilson KL. Reconstruction of composite facial defects: the combined application of multiple reconstructive modalities. *Can J Surg* 1993; 36(5):441–452.
44. Dawar M, Antonyshyn O. Long-term results following immediate reconstruction of orbital fractures: a critical morphometric analysis. *Can J Plast Surg* 1993; 1:24–29.
45. Phillips JH, Gruss JS, Wells MD, et al. Periosteal suspension of the lower eyelid and cheek following subciliary exposure of facial fractures. *Plast Reconstr Surg* 1991; 88:145.

34

The Management of Midfacial and Frontal Bone Fractures

Paul N. Manson, M.D., F.A.C.S.

Management of Midfacial Fractures

The face and the frontal portion of the cranium are, by virtue of their exposed position, frequently injured in our society where sophisticated transportation and increased mobility permit a wide variety of accidents. In particular, the automobile and motorcycle, industrial accidents, fights, and falls account for the majority of etiological factors in facial trauma. The management of both bone and soft-tissue injury must be incorporated into a single diagnostic and treatment plan.

Patient Evaluation

Two-thirds of the patients with significant maxillofacial injuries will sustain injury to other organ systems (1,2). The brain and the cervical spine, because they are geographically near the face, must be suspected of simultaneous injury. The characteristic appearance of facial injuries will detract attention from cervical fractures and subtle brain injuries; therefore, the maxillofacial specialist must make sure that these injuries have been excluded. The plans for the maxillofacial injury must be coordinated with the activities of other specialists. A comprehensive plan for patient management should be coordinated by general surgeons specializing in trauma who supervise and direct the overall management of the patient and integrate the activities of all specialists. Initially, it is important that all organ systems be evaluated and then continuously monitored during the resuscitation and operative management of the multiply injured patient. Monitoring depends on placement of arterial and venous lines; urethral catheterization, diagnostic peritoneal lavage or abdominal CT; and pelvic, extremity, chest and spine radiographs. In the case of reduced Glasgow coma scores (Table 34–1), a brain CT is obtained. In some patients, intracranial monitoring would be appropriate whether or not operative intervention for facial injuries is to be undertaken.

The systematic examination of the patient with maxillofacial injuries begins with a complete physical examination. These data enable the examiner to determine priorities of treatment when multiple injuries are present. Individual treatment plans for the various organ systems must receive prioritization and integration into the general treatment plan.

The Emergency Treatment of Maxillofacial Injuries

There are three ways in which maxillofacial injuries may result in death: airway obstruction, hemorrhage, and aspiration.

AIRWAY OBSTRUCTION

Airway obstruction demands immediate attention and may be corrected with maneuvers as simple as repositioning the jaw or tongue or removal of obstructions created by fractured teeth, bridgework, or denture segments. Intubation provides the only safe control of the airway. An initial tracheostomy may be advisable in patients who demonstrate coma or chest injury, where the underlying neurologic or pulmonary processes are unlikely to be resolved in less than a week, as these patients are not able to be extubated in a short period of time. In other patients, an endotracheal or nasotracheal tube may be utilized to avoid a tracheostomy. The tube can be placed through the nose, through the mouth, or, in a case where intermaxillary fixation is necessary, be led through a gap in the dentition or placed behind the molar teeth. When rigid internal skeletal fixation is applied for fracture treatment, IMF may be released early or immediately following operative management of the facial injuries in selected cases. When the IMF is to be maintained on a prolonged basis postoperatively, a tracheostomy should be considered if airway management or patient cooperation are concerns. In general, tracheostomy is advisable in the following patients:

1. Patients who have head injuries and are comatose and not briskly purposeful. These patients will probably require management of their head injury over a prolonged period of time.
2. Head injury patients who are spastic, semi-purposeful, or rigid, who require IMF as a component of treatment for a jaw fracture. These patients are likely to be difficult management problems in terms of cooperation. Thus the airway cannot be guaranteed.
3. Patients with combined fractures of the maxilla and mandible, or combined nasal, maxillary, and mandibular fractures (panfacial injuries), who require intermaxillary fixation (IMF) and who present airway maintenance or cooperation problems.
4. Patients with combined midface and mandibular fractures, or combined midface, nasal and mandibular fractures, where unstable occlusal relationships make prolonged IMF desirable in the face of a tenuous airway (nasopharyngeal, floor of mouth, neck or tongue swelling).
5. Patients with massive soft-tissue swelling of the neck, or patients with facial burns, where reintubation might be difficult, especially if IMF is required as a component of fracture treatment.

Table 34–1.
Glasgow Coma Scale as Reprinted in Previous Chapter

Criteria	Points
Eyes open	5
Spontaneously	4
To speech	3
To pain	2
None	1
Best verbal response	
Oriented	5
Confused	4
Inappropriate	3
Incomprehensible	2
None	1
Best motor response	
Obey commands	5
Localized pain	4
Flexion to pain	3
Extension to pain	2
None	1

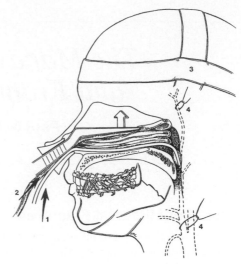

FIG. 34–1. Hemorrhage may be managed by anterior-posterior nasal packing, normal reduction of fractures (application of IMF), Barton bandage, and artery ligation. (From Maull, KI, ed. *Complications in trauma.* Philadelphia: WB Saunders, 1996.)

6. Patients with pulmonary injury who require prolonged intubation where early extubation is unlikely. It is difficult to confirm proper occlusal position in patients with indwelling orotracheal tubes. In addition, oral hygiene is difficult to maintain with the mouth taped or the endotracheal tube in place.

7. Patient with pharyngeal, laryngeal or tracheal injuries. Tracheostomies may be avoided in most other patients where airway access, swelling, the duration of rigid fixation, and the degree of patient cooperation permit management of the airway and maintenance of the occlusion without compromising respiration.

ASPIRATION

Pulmonary aspiration is perhaps the least appreciated mechanism of emergent deterioration in patients presenting with maxillofacial trauma. Patients with fractures of the jaws frequently have difficulty controlling their secretions, swallowing, and dealing with nasopharyngeal hemorrhage. Blood, saliva, or gastric contents may be aspirated. Aspirated material should be suctioned and a endotracheal tube placed to prevent further aspiration. If aspiration has resulted in hypoxia, employing intubation, positive end expiratory pressure (PEEP), broncodilators, antibiotics, and perhaps bronchoscopic aspiration may be advisable. In these patients, pulmonary compliance and oxygenation may be severely altered and operative procedures may need to be of limited duration.

HEMORRHAGE

Major hemorrhage from head and neck injury represents a life-threatening event. Hemorrhage may occur from cutaneous lacerations that involve major arteries; a partially lacerated artery is the most likely to continue bleeding. Hemorrhage may be controlled by direct pressure, clamp occlusion, pressure over the artery proximally, or perhaps bandages. The surgeon should take care when applying hemostats to avoid clamping facial nerve branches. When the source of bleeding is from the nose or mouth, the hemorrhage may not be easily controlled.

Nasopharyngeal hemorrhage that accompanies closed fractures of the midface usually presents from the nose and mouth. Occasionally, the source of nasopharyngeal hemorrhage may be a diffuse injury to the cranial base with lacerations of the carotid arterial system or dural venous sinuses. Otherwise, diffuse nasopharyngeal bleeding usually accompanies Le Fort maxillary fractures. Nasal bleeding can occur with any fracture of the nose, orbit or maxilla. Generally, most nasopharyngeal hemorrhage ceases spontaneously (>85%). Nasopharyngeal bleeding that requires control (<5%) is best managed with the following technique (Fig. 34–1):

1. *Anterior-posterior nasal packing.* A gauze pack or Foley balloon is led through each nostril in the posterior nasopharynx. This provides a "posterior obturator". The Foley balloon is placed in the pharynx by passing it through the nose, inflating it, and then drawing it against the posterior choanae. Antibiotic-impregnated gauze is then used to provide an "anterior" pack, pressing it into the recesses of the nasal cavity to provide pressure sufficient to result in tamponade of the bleeding. The posterior obturator keeps the anterior packing from falling into the pharynx.

2. *Maxillary fracture reduction.* Placing the teeth in IMF reapproximates the fractured walls of the maxilla, thus approximating fractures in the sinuses. Often, this reduces bleeding by reducing traction on lacerated veins and arteries.

3. *Coagulation of source arteries.* In hemorrhage uncontrolled by all of the above maneuvers, the surgeon can coagulate or ligate source arteries if specific bleeding points can be determined and are accessible. For the internal maxillary artery, access through the posterior wall of the maxillary sinus is one such option.

4. *External compression.* A multilayer facial occlusive bandage may be wrapped around the face in a "Barton" type dressing to provide light external pressure. This maneuver is generally not very effective.
5. *Angiography and embolization.*
6. *Bilateral, external carotid, and superficial temporal artery ligation.* In the face of generalized bleeding that is uncontrolled by all of the above maneuvers, the external carotid above the facial and superficial temporal on the ipsilateral side can be ligated. The occipital superficial temporal artery should also be ligated to prevent collateral flow. The multiple ligations of the branches of the external carotid trunk prevent collateral circulation. External carotid ligations are rarely required.

Persistent hemorrhage that does not respond to the above maneuvers requires an angiogram to identify the source of bleeding. Usually, bleeding occurs from fractures involving arteries and veins in the walls of sinuses; it can occur from the pterygoid area as well. The bleeding vessel may be embolized. There are small risks to the central nervous system with embolization.

It should be mentioned that patients with coagulopathies may continue to hemorrhage. In patients where severe bleeding is observed, coagulation factors should be monitored frequently and adequate replacement provided. It is well known, for instance, that patients with head injury display early coagulation abnormalities through depletion of clotting factors.

INJURIES TO THE HEAD AND NECK

Facial injuries often have a dramatic appearance and can distract attention from other injuries to the head and neck area. It is always important to exclude head injury and injury to the cervical spine in these patients.

CERVICAL SPINE AND SPINAL CORD INJURIES

Injuries to the cervical spine occur in 5 to 10% of patients with maxillofacial trauma. Conversely, 10 to 20% of patients with cervical spine injuries will have a maxillofacial injury of significance to bone or soft tissue (4). There is an association between injuries to the frontal bone and midface and cervical hyperextension injuries. There is also an association between injuries of the upper portion of the cervical spine and the mandible; therefore, mandibular fractures should prompt a careful examination of the cervical area. Injuries in the upper and lower portions of the cervical spine are the most difficult to demonstrate and thus the most commonly missed. C1, C2, and C7 lesions are the most difficult to visualize. Carefully taken cervical spine films with inferior traction on the shoulders usually demonstrates the entire cervical skeleton. Flexion-extension films and a cervical computed tomography (CT) scan should be obtained to confirm the presence of injury in specific cases. Pain is a reliable indication of cervical injury, but it is absent in those who are consciousness impaired. A neurologic examination is an essential part of any head and neck evaluation.

HEAD INJURY

Patients with presumed head injury (5) are assessed with a Glasgow Coma Scale evaluation (see Table 34–1), neuro-

logic examination, and craniofacial CT scan. The prognosis of head injuries is generally better for patients who are under 40 years of age. Patients who are in shock, who have abnormal posturing, who have pulmonary injury, and/or those whose Glasgow Coma Scale scores are less than 10, generally have a poorer prognosis (6–9). The Glasgow Coma Scale (see Table 34–1) uses a graded scale to evaluate eye-opening response, the ability to talk, the ability to move the extremities, and the ability to follow commands.

The presence of coma alone is not justification for postponing maxillofacial injury treatment. Often simple maneuvers, such as the placement of IMF, may accomplish reasonable reduction in a timely fashion. Many patients in coma will survive, improve, and ultimately be able to work and provide for their own needs. In fact, one-half of patients who are in coma for a period longer than 1 week are able to return to useful work (7–10). However, the presence of even short periods of unconsciousness does herald some minor disability and is associated with a "minor head injury" syndrome. These patients with minor head injuries may demonstrate difficulty with interpersonal relationships, memory, and irritability. The use of the Glasgow Coma Scale and the CT scan identifies patients who require intracranial pressure monitoring during anesthesia. This technique allows comatose patients to be safely monitored during prolonged operations. Blood loss and shock must especially be avoided, because they reduce cerebral circulation and contribute to increased cerebral edema through the mechanisms of ischemia and anoxia.

Intracranial pressures in excess of 25 mm Hg are accompanied by at least a 30% mortality rate. All routine maxillofacial injury management is postponed in the face of intracranial pressures above 15 mm Hg. The performance of intracranial neurosurgery and the necessity for removal of damaged cerebral cortex do not necessarily contraindicate maxillofacial injury repair. Many of these patients will have a relatively satisfactory prognosis despite the seriousness of their neurologic injury; therefore, it simply makes good sense and is a wise investment to achieve the best maxillofacial function and appearance.

EVALUATION OF MAXILLOFACIAL INJURIES

The evaluation of maxillofacial injuries consists of a thorough physical examination and appropriate radiographs. The physical examination begins with an accurate history and proceeds to a complete physical examination. Many trauma victims cannot provide an accurate history of the accident or relate details of their medical history; therefore, the physician must proceed to a complete physical examination. The complete examination involves the cranium, the face, and the neck, and is performed in a systematic manner progressing from either superior to inferior or inferior to superior. The evaluation begins by assessing appearance and symmetry, noting any contusions, lacerations, or bruises. The sequential palpation of all bony surfaces follows. Crepitance, bone contour discrepancies, symmetry of bone structure and areas of tenderness are noted. A sensory nerve evaluation detects sensory deficits. Motor evaluation, consisting of a survey of cranial nerve function, then completes the examination. A search for occult lacerations in the ear, including the ear canal, the scalp, the cavities of the nose or oral cavity, and the pharynx, should be completed. An evaluation follows of the patient's occlusion; excursion of the mandible; symmetry of the dental arches; presence of broken or fractured teeth; ability to bring the teeth into full intercuspation; presence of proper occlusion; and presence of intraoral lacerations, gaps, level discrepancies, tenderness, or movement of the occlusion should raise the possibility of fractures involving the teeth, or the upper and lower jaws. Bruising, lacerations, or ecchymosis in the palate, buccal sulcus, and gingiva suggest an underlying fracture.

The eye examination consists of visual acuity determination, pupillary response, extraocular motion, assessment of double vision, peripheral fields, intraocular pressure, and fundus examinations.

These data are collected during the initial resuscitation and complete the clinical evaluation. Additional records and studies may be obtained contingent upon the patient's presumed diagnosis and treatment needs.

Old photographs (wallet pictures, driver's license, the family) are helpful in demonstrating the preinjury structure of the patient's face. Facial asymmetry is sometimes not easily perceived during a clinical examination of a somewhat contused face. Study of preinjury photographs allows the surgeon to visualize the desired result of surgical reconstruction.

Plain x rays are of limited use in the diagnosis and treatment of most facial injuries; they have largely been replaced by the CT scans. The most prominent exception is the evaluation of mandible fractures by the Panorex examination, where additional information is provided. However, the Panorex examination must generally be obtained with a cooperative patient sitting or standing upright; therefore, it is not feasible in the evaluation of many mandibular and maxillary fractures. The multiply injured patient must not be sent unaccompanied or unmonitored to the radiology department for examinations. Generally, the combination of a physical examination and an appropriately obtained CT scan allows a detailed treatment plan to be constructed for any facial injury. Often, patients with cervical spine injuries are unable to cooperate for a coronal CT scan.

The craniofacial CT scan is an essential component in evaluating any midface injury. Generally, elective facial injury treatment should not proceed without a confirming CT scan that reenforces the clinical impressions from the physical examination. It should be obtained following the initial examination of the patient and stabilization of vital signs, and it is essential that the patient be generally stable before being sent unaccompanied to a CT scanner. In many patients who require a head CT scan, a short period of additional time can result in obtaining a facial scan, which can provide much additional information to the maxillofacial surgeon. The most helpful views include axial and coronal sets of images. Bone and soft-tissue windows are obtained to allow proper evaluation of the orbit and brain. In patients who are unable to be positioned for coronal examinations, reconstructed coronal images from the axial images may be performed by the computerized CT console (Fig. 34–2). CT scans completed at the time of cranial CT evaluations represent an extension of the head scan and are required on any patient to exclude frontal, basilar skull, frontal sinus, nasoethmoidal, orbital, zygomatic, and maxillary fractures. CT scans are even helpful in the diagnosis and treatment of nasal fractures, to confirm the

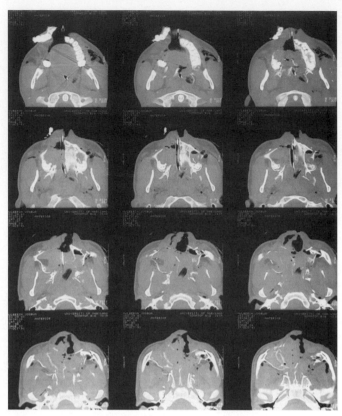

FIG. 34–2. A full axial and coronal CT scan with bones and soft-tissue windows and old pictures are necessary data to plan facial fracture reduction.

direction and degree of displacement of the nasal bones and the septum and to exclude injuries in adjacent portions of the facial skeleton.

Rarely, an arteriogram may be necessary to identify a source of bleeding. In penetrating injuries of the midface, arteriograms may be required to exclude damage to the internal carotid artery.

DENTAL RECORDS

Dental impressions and models provide an essential record of the occlusion. They are helpful in the construction of acrylic splints and other stabilizing devices that assist in the management of fractures involving the alveolar processes of the mandible and maxilla. Dental records will include taking impressions and making stone models. Previously obtained orthodontic records or models, earlier dental x rays, and other dental records provide clues to the preinjury occlusion (12). Patients who are partly dentulous often have abnormal dental relationships; they sometimes require splints as "occlusal stops" to supplement the missing occlusion. Patients who are edentulous should have their dentures present for fracture reduction as a positioning device. The fractured dentures may be repaired with acrylic cement, or splints substituting for the dentures may be made based on the dental impressions.

PNEUMOCEPHALUS AND CSF RHINORRHEA

The presence of cerebral spinal fluid (CSF) rhinorrhea or pneumocephalus may be seen with high maxillary and nasoethmoidal fractures. More commonly, CSF rhinorrhea and pneumocephalus accompany fractures of the frontal and basilar skull. One-fourth of the patients with Le Fort II and III fractures, especially if nasoethmoidal fractures are present, will demonstrate CSF rhinorrhea, in which cerebral spinal fluid leaks into the nose as a result of dural and arachnoid laceration. Air present intracranially may enter through a dural laceration and appear as pneumocephalus. Fifty to seventy-five percent of frontobasilar fractures will be accompanied by CSF rhinorrhea. It may be difficult to distinguish CSF rhinorrhea early in the presence of bloody nasal secretions. The double-ring sign, in which nasal discharge is absorbed onto a white paper towel, is sometimes helpful. A clear ring extending beyond a central blood-tinged spot is suggestive of blood-tinged cerebral spinal fluid. Dural fistulae, in the presence of displaced bone fractures, are usually managed by direct operative fistula repair and bone reduction.

In some cases, CSF fistulas are associated with nondisplaced fractures. These fistulas often cease spontaneously and may not require definitive repair. Many CSF fistulas existing with nondisplaced fractures will close within a short period of observation (15). In fact, most of these (75%) seal within several days.

Antibiotics are of limited effectiveness in sterilizing cerebral spinal fluid when employed over a prolonged period (16–18). An antibiotic selectively inhibits only the growth of suseptible organisms. Antibiotics are therefore only effective in preventing meningitis from bacteria suseptible to that antibiotic. In the presence of a prolonged CSF fistula, antibiotics will eventually select resistant organisms because the colonizing organism changes in response to the antibiotic. Resistant organisms are more difficult to treat. Thus, the prolonged treatment of a CSF leak with an antibiotic is not justified (19–21).

"Prophylactic antibiotics" are often employed for a short (48–72 hour) period around the time of fracture reduction or initial presentation of the CSF leak, especially if open injuries are present. Some believe that nasal packing and nasogastric tubes prevent free nasal drainage and contribute to local nasal infection. These physicians believe that the presence of local nasal infection increases the incidence of meningitis in patients with CSF fistula, and will avoid nasal packing and nasal gastric tubes to protect from bacterial growth.

Patients who have Le Fort fractures and CSF fistula should initially be placed in IMF. As a general principle, IMF stops movement of the maxilla and contributes to CSF leak closure. It is felt that the constant pumping action of a fractured displaced midface tends to wash organisms up toward the CSF fistula.

EARLY DEFINITIVE TREATMENT OF THE MIDFACE INJURY

Soft-tissue lacerations should be repaired as early as possible following the injury. The repair of soft-tissue injuries and the placement of the jaws in IMF represent two goals of midface injury treatment that can be accomplished immediately despite the condition of the patient through use of local anesthetics (12–14).

These soft-tissue repairs should *always* be accomplished. Further, dental impressions can be taken at this time for the construction of models and for dental records.

DETERMINING HOW MUCH DEFINITIVE TREATMENT CAN BE PERFORMED AT THE TIME OF THE INJURY

The amount of treatment to be administered on an early or immediate basis should be determined by an evaluation of the patient's general condition, by the severity of the maxillofacial injury, and by the need to establish reduction to prevent deformity. The patient's other injuries are evaluated by a thorough multisystem evaluation and in consultation with the general surgeon (4).

Theoretically, as much treatment as possible should be completed as early after the injury as the patient's condition permits. Treatment provided early is accomplished more easily, as the injury has done a portion of the dissection. Fragments are easily mobilized and soft tissue is pliable and flexible. Patients with multisystem injuries commonly suffer a number of septic complications that begin several days after the injury. These include systemic sepsis, pulmonary problems, and deterioration of liver and renal function. These complications preclude an early return to the operating room for definitive management of facial injuries.

The multiply injured patient is often in the best condition that he or she will be in for 1 or 2 weeks after the injury. The immediate postinjury period thus represents a desirable time for definitive maxillofacial treatment. In general, pulmonary instability, increased intracranial pressure, and coagulation problems represent the major contraindications to acute facial fracture management. In those who cannot immediately have complete management of their injury, some portion of the operative intervention may still be accomplished. Patients with open injuries (and all severe facial injuries) benefit from periodic return to the operating room for "wash outs" (i.e., cleansing of the intraoral area and sinuses, débridement of devitalized tissue, and confirmation that internal fixation is stable). These procedures greatly decrease the morbidly of major facial injuries, whether or not definitive reduction has been accomplished, and we routinely accomplish them pre and post operatively.

REGIONAL MANAGEMENT OF FACIAL FRACTURES

Nasal Fractures

The nose, because of it's prominent position, is one of the most commonly fractured bones of the facial skeleton. Additionally, its low resistance to impact makes it susceptible to fracture.

The nose consists of bone and cartilage. The bony nasal pyramid represents the proximal one-third and the cartilaginous nose the distal two-thirds. The septum is part bone and part cartilage. Nasal injuries always include injuries to the pyramid and the septum, and each structure must be assessed individually. In nasal fractures, displacement of the nasal pyramid is generally lateral and/or posterior. Combinations are the routine with more severe injuries; therefore, the surgeon must assess the degree of lateral and posterior displacement in order to plan treatment. Fractures with lateral displacement are frequently the result of an automobile mishap, altercation, or sporting accident. Injuries resulting in such insults vary from minimally depressed fractures isolated to the distal portion of the nasal skeleton to complex disruptions of the bony and cartilaginous components of the nose. The degree and type of displacement are confirmed by physical examinations, radiographs, and CT scans. Patients who demonstrate posterior displacement of the nose usually have widening of the nasal bridge. The symptoms of nasal fractures include edema, crepitus, periorbital ecchymosis, and epistaxis. External or internal lacerations are frequent and are usually minor. More severe nasal fractures have a through-and-through laceration that exposes portions of the internal nasal skeleton; these lacerations thereby provide access for treatment. A septal hematoma is always present around the septal fracture. It is usually small, but if large, it can produce pressure necrosis of the septum and require drainage. Tenderness and swelling are present over the areas of fracture. Partial or total airway obstruction may result from displaced bone, hematoma, swelling, or a combination of these problems. The nasal bones may be unstable, either laterally or bilaterally. Nasal fractures can be predominantly unilateral and, if so, sometimes require completion of the fracture on the opposite side for stability.

Laterally dislocated nasal fractures are managed by closed reduction under general or local anesthesia. The external nose is anesthetized by regional block. The internal nose is anesthetized by cocaine on 1:100,000 adrenalin-soaked pledgets. The nasal fractures are first "completed" by mobilization of the nasal pyramid bone segments and the septum. The instrumentation required is an elevator for the pyramid and an Asch forceps for the septum. Intranasal and external manipulation then mold the nasal pyramid back into its proper position; we believe the surgeon *must* mobilize the nasal bones and have them freely movable so as to position them with the expectation that their position will be maintained. Palpation and visualization confirm fracture reduction. There are some who believe it is difficult to confirm fracture reduction when edema and swelling are severe; therefore, some surgeons prefer to wait until edema has resolved to allow improved perception of proper fracture reduction. An external splint and internal nasal packing are used to support the fracture and septal reduction. Any significant septal hematoma is drained with a small incision to prevent cartilage necrosis. Soft, nonadherent antibiotic-soaked packing is used to approximate the mucoperichondrium to the septum.

Frontal-impact nasal injuries are characterized by posterior displacement of portions of the nasal skeleton (Fig. 34–3). Stranc and Robertson (22) categorize nasal fractures by separately identifying lateral and posterior displacement. Frontal-impact nasal injuries are divided into categories based on the degree on comminution and posterior displacement. Plane I, plane II, and plane III injuries (see Fig. 34–3) exist and vary with the force, comminution, and extent of the fracture involvement of the nasal skeleton. Plane I injuries present with edema and ecchymosis in the area of the distal nasal bridge and tip (see Fig. 34–3①). The force is concentrated predominantly on the cartilage structures of the septum and there is little comminution or displacement of the nasal bones. A fracture of the distal nasal bones, depressed unilaterally, is frequent. This fracture requires elevation and packing directly in the nasal fossa. The injury to the septum may be more severe than anticipated and result in some irregularity of the septum and loss of dorsal nasal height, with saddling of the nasal bridge. It is difficult to completely reduce these septal fractures, and patients are probably best managed by secondary septorhinoplasty, which may include

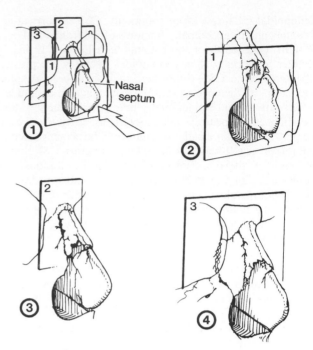

FIG. 34–3. ①, frontal-impact nasal injury in planes I, II, and III. ②, the pattern of disruption in Plane I frontal impact nasal injuries. ③, site of disruption in plane II frontal-impact nasal injuries. The nasal bones are comminuted. ④, site of disruption in plane III injuries. The frontal process of the maxilla (medial orbital rim) is comminuted. (Redrawn from Stranc MF, Robertson GA. A classification of internal injuries of the nasal skeleton. *Ann Plast Surg* 1979; 2:468.)

grafting. Plane I injuries should receive closed reduction and internal support.

Plane II injuries (see Fig. 34–3②) demonstrate increased comminution of the nasal pyramid and "saddling" of the nasal dorsum. The fractures are bilateral, usually worse on one side, and there is moderate edema, ecchymosis, and widening of the nasal bridge. Dorsal depression is easily identified. Most plane II fractures are managed by closed reduction. When the fracture involvement is severe, significant saddling of the dorsum may persist despite attempts at closed-reduction manipulation. Such patients may be managed with early or delayed bone or cartilage grafting to augment the height of the nose. When septal fractures are severe, initial repositioning may not guarantee nasal airway patency. Some warping of the nose occurs with healing, principally as a result of the deforming forces in injured cartilage. All patients with nasal fractures should be advised that they may require a nasal septal reconstruction some months after the injury, depending on the degree of cartilage deformation with healing.

Plane III nasal injuries (see Fig. 34–3③) result from severe frontal-impact forces. They demonstrate fractures extending outside the nasal skeleton and into the pyriform aperture and the medial orbital rim. Thus they are not really nasal injuries but nasoethmoidal orbital fractures; they represent the third category in the classification of Stranc (22) and should alert the practitioner that they require more treatment than a simple nasal fracture. They are in reality nasoethmoidal fractures, representing the first stage of nasoethmoidal orbital injury. Fractures of the pyriform aperture and frontal process of the maxilla characterize these injuries and distinguish between nasal fractures and nasoethmoidal orbital fractures. In these fractures, there is usually marked loss of nasal skeletal support and more comminution of the nasal bones, which can be detected on physical examination. If fractures surround the bone, providing insertion of the medial canthal ligament, unilateral or bilateral telecanthus is seen. Plane III injuries require open reduction and internal fixation of the frontal process of the maxilla and pyriform aperture, as well as transnasal reduction of medial canthal ligaments.

The frontal-impact nasal fracture should theoretically require bone or cartilage grafts for nasal support if reduction is not complete. In practice, most plane II injuries are not managed with immediate grafting; however, occasionally there is benefit from cartilage grafts. There is a technique of lateral nasal external compression where soft bolsters are connected to transnasal wires that are "walked" through the lower aspects of the nasal fracture on a large needle inserted percutaneously. These are used to slightly compress the nose. This bolster creates some nasal height and is an effective closed-reduction maneuver for plane II injuries. Plane III injuries require open reduction and bone or cartilage grafting. The plane III injury requires either lower-eyelid or gingival buccal sulcus incisions for injuries where the frontal process of the maxilla is depressed inferiorly (23). A full coronal incision [or perhaps in specific areas an external laceration or a horizontal incision from canthus to canthus—the horizontal limb alone of the "open sky" incision] is required for superior exposure. In severe nasal fractures, if bone and cartilage grafting are performed acutely, shortening and contraction of the soft tissue are prevented.

In the treatment of the common nasal fracture, the most frequent mistake is failure to complete the fracture thoroughly before stabilization. After adequate manipulation, the nasal bones are able to be freely deviated in either direction if the mobilization has been adequate. Adequate mobilization achieves additional postoperative stability. Occasionally, an osteotomy is necessary to complete a greenstick nasal fracture which is slightly deviated but not completely fractured. We emphasize that completion of septal fractures and repositioning by instrumentation with an Asch forcep allow replacement of the septum into a normal position. If the attachments of the upper or lower cartilages are torn, the dislocated cartilages should be repositioned by direct suturing techniques. Generally, such injuries are accompanied by external lacerations, so a precise repair is possible without making any incisions. Further, fractures of the nasal bones, if open, are ideally fixated with a microsystem. We also emphasize that involved cartilage can be subject to tension forces as the area heals. The cartilage warps, resulting in deviation. Therefore, the result of acute treatment or secondary surgery is not always predictable.

Certain nasal fractures exhibit depression of the nasal dorsum, principally in the cartilaginous section. These represent Stranc plane II (22) injuries, where loss of height and projection are identified. These fractures require either primary or secondary dorsal nasal bone or cartilage grafting. Open reductions utilize grafts and fixation of the bones with fine plates and screws, or small (#30) wires. A dorsal nasal bone graft (using either calvarial or rib graft sources) and a caudal cartilage strut are sometimes required to establish normal

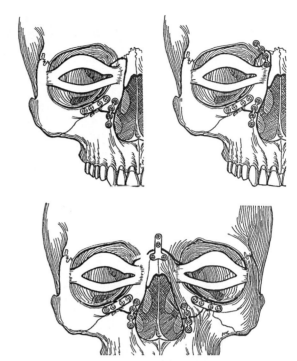

FIG. 34–4. Monobloc nasoethmoidal-orbital fractures. These fractures may be treated by junctional plate and screw fixation at the frontal bone, inferior orbital rims, and pyriform aperture. Fractures without superior dislocation may be treated by inferior approaches along with lower-eyelid and gingival buccal sulcus incisions.

skeletal dimensions in the face of plane II or plane III nasal injuries (see Fig. 34–3).

NASO-ETHMOIDAL-ORBITAL FRACTURES

Naso-ethmoidal-orbital fractures are in reality plane III nasal fractures extended to the frontal process of the maxilla. In two-thirds of cases, they are severe enough that other structures in the frontal or midface area are injured (e.g., the zygoma or frontal bone). They represent a frequent component of Le Fort fractures.

The sine qua non of the naso-ethmoid-orbital injury is a fracture involving the medial orbital rim (the frontal process of the maxilla) containing the attachment of the medial canthal ligament (24). Fractures that separate the frontal process of the maxilla and its canthal bearing tendon from adjacent bones permit the possibility of canthal displacement; this is the most precise definition of the naso-ethmoid injury (26,27) (Figs. 34–4, 34–5). The lower two-thirds of the medial orbital rim contains the area for attachment of the medial canthal ligament. Once this section of bone is fractured, the potential for canthal ligament displacement exists (23–27). Recent schemes of classification of naso-ethmoidal-orbital injuries classify this area as the "central fragment" of more complicated naso-ethmoidal-orbital injuries (23–25). Mobility of this fragment may be assessed with a direct digital pressure over the canthal ligament (26). Displacement, or a click on deep palpation, indicate mobility. Alternatively, a bimanual examination may be performed with a clamp inside the nose underneath the canthal ligament and an index fingertip palpating deeply over the medial orbital rim externally (26). Simultaneous internal and external pressure by clamp

FIG. 34–5. **A,** nasoethmoid orbital fracture demonstrating medial orbital rim and medial orbital wall fractures. **B,** the lower cut of the axial CT scan demonstrates the inferior orbital rim fracture. This fracture is a unilateral nasoethmoidal orbital fracture.

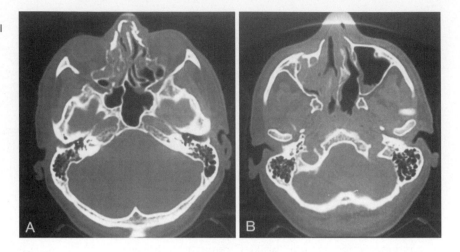

and digital manipulation allows the central fragment to move between the index finger and the clamp. Mobility or displacement indicates the need for an open reduction.

Minimal injures benefit from a high index of suspicion. About one-third of naso-ethmoidal-orbital fractures are unilateral. One-third are isolated to the central midface and two thirds are extended to other areas.

The symptoms of a naso-ethmoidal-orbital fracture include lacerations in the forehead or nasal area; the spectacle hematoma (a hematoma that extends to the insertion of the orbital septum); and the presence of a moderately displaced frontal-impact nasal fracture (with depression of the bridge and shortening of the nose) indicating the possibility of a naso-ethmoidal-orbital injury. The nose appears foreshortened, and has a dorsal depression and an obtuse nasolabial angle. Palpation of the nose reveals a lack of skeletal or cartilaginous support; sometimes the deficit is confined proximally, sometimes distally. Naso-ethmoidal-orbital fractures commonly are accompanied by nasal bleeding, and a CSF leak may be present. In the acute injury, the CSF leak may not be identifiable because of the presence of bloody nasal secretions.

Telecanthus is absolute evidence of a naso-ethmoidal-orbital fracture and represents the result of a complete fracture that has dislocated medial canthal ligament-bearing bone so that it can drift laterally. The degree of telecanthus depends of the degree of comminution of the fractures and the presence of intact periosteal attachments. Initially, the intercanthal distance may not appear increased, but it may increase with time and resolution of the swelling.

The radiographic diagnosis of naso-ethmoidal-orbital injuries is confirmed by fractures surrounding the central fragment on a CT scan (see Fig. 34–5). Fractures should involve the nose, the junction of the frontal process of the maxilla with the glabella, the inferior orbital rim, and the medial (ethmoidal) orbital wall. These four fractures define the central fragment as "free" and potentially able to displace. Medial orbital wall and floor fractures are seen universally with naso-ethmoidal-orbital injuries. There are fluid levels present in the ethmoid and maxillary sinuses.

Plain radiographs do not accurately confirm the naso-ethmoidal-orbital fracture. Axial and coronal CT scans with bone and soft-tissue windows provide precise capability for definition of the injury and for planning the reconstruction.

In particular, they are essential for developing a plan to restore the orbital component of the naso-ethmoidal-orbital injury. Frequently, they do not require treatment if displacement is minimal (23).

CT scans should be taken in the axial and coronal planes; if not, the frequency of sections should be reduced to 2 mm for clear reconstructions (see Fig. 34–5). The areas of the brain, frontal bone, and frontal sinus, as well as the entire maxilla, must be assessed because the injury extends inferiorly to the pyriform aperture. The examination must be complete in order to define extensions of naso-ethmoidal-orbital fractures that may occur either unilaterally or bilaterally. Naso-ethmoidal-orbital fractures commonly accompany unilateral orbital injuries (e.g., the supraorbital fracture or fracture dislocation of the zygoma). Bilateral injuries are often seen in craniofacial and Le Fort fractures.

FRACTURE PATTERNS OF NASO-ETHMOIDAL-ORBITAL INJURIES

Four generalized fracture patterns are seen with naso-ethmoidal-orbital fractures (see Fig. 34–5):

1. *Localized central midface injury.* This is an isolated naso-ethmoidal-orbital fracture that is usually observed bilaterally. The fracture may be confined to the naso-ethmoidal-orbital area, or it may extend into the zygomatic or frontal sinus region.
2. *Lateral orbital nasal injuries.* These fractures are unilateral and extend either superiorly into the frontal bone or inferiorly into the inferior orbital rim. Unilateral fractures occur with this injury.
3. *High Le Fort (II or III) fractures.* These injuries accompany Le Fort fractures and may be either unilateral or bilateral; they usually consist of large fragments.
4. *Craniofacial fractures.* The common pattern of a craniofacial fracture includes nasoethmoid and Le Fort III fracture on one side and a frontal bone fracture with involvement on the contralateral side.

The central fragment of the naso-ethmoidal-orbital injury consists of the lower two-thirds of the medial orbital rim, which includes the attached canthal ligament and the lacrimal fossa. Medial orbital rim fractures and fractures of the orbital floor, medial orbital wall, nose, frontal sinus, me-

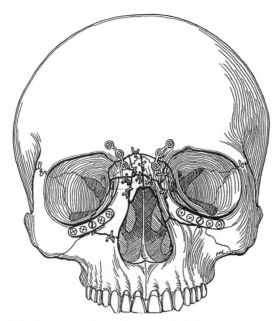

FIG. 34–6. Open reduction of the complete bilateral nasoethmoidal orbital fracture. After adequate exposure, all orbital rim and nasal bone fragments are linked within interfragment wires. The transnasal reduction of the medial orbital rims is the most important step in naso-ethmoidal-orbital fracture treatment and is performed posterior and superior to the medial canthal ligament and lacrimal fossa with a wire linking both bones. Dislocation of the central (canthal tendon–bearing) bone fragment anteriorly and laterally allows placement of drill holes posterior to the ligament. The wires are passed, then tightened. The assembled bone fragments are stabilized by junctional plate and screw fixation to the frontal bone and to the inferior orbital rims. When the comminuted fractures extend underneath the canthal ligaments, the canthal ligaments need to be stripped for fracture reduction. They must be reattached by transnasal wire reduction, posterior and superior to the lacrimal fossa. The canthal ligament in less comminuted fractures need not be detached, which avoids the step of canthal reattachment.

dial orbital rim, and medial superior maxilla are present with varying degrees of comminution.

The timing of treatment of naso-ethmoidal-orbital fractures is important because improved aesthetic results are more easily achieved when early open reduction is performed. Fractures are ideally treated soon after the injury, and it has been our experience that it becomes more difficult to obtain a good aesthetic result when reductions are performed more than 3 to 5 days after the fracture has occurred.

Closed treatment is not appropriate for significant naso-ethmoidal-orbital fractures. Open reduction must be performed; it consists of the following:

- A thorough exposure of all peripheral buttress attachments.
- Repositioning of the buttress attachments if large fragments are identified (type I or type II naso-ethmoidal-orbital fracture) (Fig. 34–6).
- Linking of fragments with interfragment with trans medial wires in type III injuries.
- Replacement with bone grafts of the bone gaps in the medial orbital wall, floor, and nose with autogenous bone graft material.

- Junctional (frontal bone and infraorbital rim) plate and screw fixation performed following internal open reduction with wires.

The central treatment maneuver for significant (i.e., type III or IV naso-ethmoidal-orbital fractures) includes a wire transnasal reduction of the frontal processes of the maxilla performed posterior and superior to the lacrimal fossa. This is the most essential component of naso-ethmoidal-orbital fracture treatment. The canthal ligament should not be detached in the reduction if it can be avoided, because the technique then precludes the tedious step of canthal reattachment.

SURGICAL EXPOSURE

Conceptionally, three incisions are required for visualization of all the peripheral buttresses and structure of a naso-ethmoidal-orbital injury. Occasionally an overlying laceration is suitable for superior exposure of a localized fracture. Lacerations should not be significantly extended; this generally results in additional deformity. There are two local incisions that can be appropriate in suitable cases (elderly or bald patients) for superior exposure in localized naso-ethmoidal-orbital fractures. One is a vertical midline incision over the root of the nose and the other is the horizontal limb alone of the previously described Converse "open sky" approach.

The standard superior surgical exposure of a naso-ethmoidal-orbital fracture involves a coronal incision. This exposes the orbital roofs, the medial orbital area, and the upper portion of the nasoethmoid injury.

The use of the subciliary incisions exposes the lower portion of the frontal process of the maxilla, as does the gingival buccal sulcus incision for the junction of the frontal process of the maxilla with the pyriform region. These lower incisions are required to expose inferior orbital rim and the vertical fronto-maxillary buttress of the naso-ethmoidal-orbital injury.

TECHNIQUE OF OPEN REDUCTION

The surgeon assesses the fracture pattern and determines the needs for exposure. The exposure is performed and dissection and mobilization of bone fragments completed. Thereafter, the entire orbital rims are linked with interfragment wires, as is the entire skeleton of the nose and frontal process of the maxilla. These are kept loose so the fragments may be mobilized. The surgeon then drills holes posterior and superior to the lacrimal fossa in the "central fragment" of the frontal process of the maxilla. Several sets of wires are passed transnasally at this level; one set is required for bone reduction; one to provide medial canthus reattachment; and one is provided to pass externally to a bolster to reapproximate the skin to the nasal skeleton. The bolster must be cushioned with soft material.

When all of the bone fragments have been assembled and transfixed with interfragment wires, the surgeon reassembles them into a nasoethmoidal unit. This unit may then be stabilized with peripheral buttress fixation (junctional rigid fixation), superiorly to the frontal bone and inferiorly to the infraorbital rim and pyriform margin of the maxilla. At this point, inspection of the medial and inferior orbit reveals the need for intraorbital bone grafts. A bone graft may also be required on the nasal dorsum to augment nasal height, smooth

FIG. 34–7. **A,** a patient with Le Fort III, nasoeth-moid, bilateral subcondylar, and mandibular body fractures is seen following injury. **B,** postoperative result following a single operation that included complete reduction and bone grafting.

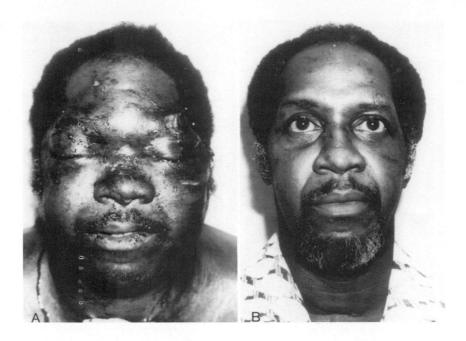

dorsal nasal contour, or increase projection. Similarly, the use of caudal bone or cartilage grafts is also required, as are wire reattachment of the septum to the anterior nasal spine.

MANAGEMENT OF THE NASO-ETHMOIDAL-ORBITAL FRACTURE WITHOUT DETACHMENT AT THE CANTHAL LIGAMENT

Ideally, the canthal ligament should not be detached from the frontal process of the maxilla in the reduction. This requires precise dissection. If the canthal ligament does require reattachment, it should be connected to an additional set of transnasal reduction wires that are passed posterior and superior to the lacrimal fossa; separate wires for bone stabilization and canthal ligament reduction are required. When the skeletal work is completed, the surgeon tightens two wire sets to reapproximate the canthal ligament to the bony nasal skeleton. Orbital bone grafting should be completed before the canthal reattachment is performed; otherwise, there is tendency to detach the canthus. If the canthal ligament has been partially detached, it should be completely detached and reattached. Partial detachment is common in dissection of the naso-ethmoidal-orbital injury. If detached, the lateral aspect of the canthal ligament is exposed externally with a 1 to 2 mm incision adjacent to the medial commissure of the eyelids. A suture of 2-0 or 3-0 material is passed two times through the canthal ligament, avoiding the lacrimal system. The surgeon then passes the suture internally through a small incision to the inner aspect of the coronal incision and connects it to the transnasal reduction wires. Tightening these wires is the last step in soft-tissue approximation; it provides accurate repositioning of the canthal ligament to the bony skeleton.

It is virtually impossible to overcorrect the inner canthal distance. The bony inner canthal distance in whites should be 16 to 23 mm, and an additional 5 to 7 mm per side of soft-tissue distance should be added for a total of 26 to 35 mm.

The use of soft-tissue bolsters helps approximate the skin (which has been dissected) to the bony nasoethmoidal skeleton. They help reestablish the "nasoorbital valley" of Converse, and prevent the accumulation of soft-tissue swelling or hematoma between the reconstructed skeleton and the skin.

Bolsters should be padded with orthopedic felt wrapped with xeroform gauze; they are removed 1 to 3 weeks after the surgery. These compression bolsters have no function in the maintenance of the inner canthal distance, which must be achieved with an internal open reduction (wire transnasal reduction of the medial orbital rims).

Dorsal nasal bone grafts are best positioned using a small maxillary adaption plate attached from the frontal bone to the posterior surface of the superior aspect of the dorsal nasal bone graft. This allows for adjustment of the projection of the dorsum of the nose. A patient treated with open reduction and bone grafting is seen in Figure 34–7. Occasionally, caudal cartilage grafts should be added to recreate the soft-tissue support for the caudal aspect of the nasal septum. The use of Doyle nasal splints helps to position the septum intranasally after a reduction.

INTERNAL ORBIT

The internal orbit is reconstructed by first positioning the fragments of the orbital rim. The location of the intact bone in the back of the orbit is determined. Bone grafts or artificial material may then be placed between the reconstructed rim and the posterior intact bone.

In the floor, an intact bone "ledge" is usually present 30 to 38 mm behind the anterior rim. Bone grafts may be structured to span the defect between the reconstructed anterior rim and the posterior ledge. Conceptually, intact bone all around the internal orbital defect must be identified as a guide to positioning of bone grafts.

In the medial orbit, the intact ledge of bone is usually present at, or just before, the posterior ethmoidal foramen. Bone grafts should be positioned from this area, extending anteriorly until the lacrimal system is identified. The normal contour of the medial orbit and of the orbital floor bulge inward toward the globe; this must be remembered in reconstructive techniques.

The lacrimal system is usually injured in the canalicular portion only by direct lacerations or in medial canthal ligament avulsion (27); neither of these conditions occurs often.

Most lacrimal system obstruction occurs in the "bony" lacrimal canal, and this is the most frequently compromised area. Repositioning the bone fragments provides the best functional integrity of the lacrimal system. Routine explorations of the lacrimal system, performed at the time of fracture repair in patients not having either direct lacerations or canthal ligament avulsion, have not been proven beneficial. Additionally, several studies have shown that the incidence of false passages is considerable when the lacrimal system is probed. Reenforcing these conclusions, at least two studies have shown that the lacrimal system functions best when the bone fragments are precisely reduced.

FRACTURES OF THE ZYGOMA

Fractures of the zygomatic area represent the second most frequent midfacial injury. The prominent position of the malar eminence and the importance of the zygoma in reconstruction of orbital volume places strong emphasis on its adequate reconstruction (28–35). Zygomatic fractures may occur either as an isolated injury or in combination with midfacial fracture such as the Le Fort (11). Frequently, the Le Fort fracture involves various subsegments, some of which are zygomatic fractures.

There are certain clinical findings that should suggest the presence of a zygomatic fracture. The most sensitive is the combination of a periorbital ecchymosis limited to the distribution of the orbital septum and a subconjunctival hematoma. Numbness in the distribution of the infraorbital nerve is usually present in a zygomatic fracture.

Depending on the amount of depression of the zygoma, the malar eminence is recessed and the lateral canthus is displaced inferiorly. The lateral canthus is attached to the Whitnall tubercle, a small rounded eminence on the internal surface of a frontal process of the zygoma. The cheek and the contents of the eye socket may be observed to be depressed following resolution of swelling. In significantly displaced fractures, there may be a palpable step deformity of the lateral and inferior orbital rim.

Unilateral epistaxis presents acutely because of the fractures involving the maxillary sinus. If extraocular muscles are contused or entrapped in the orbital floor component of the zygomatic fracture, diplopia may result. If the floor of the orbit is significantly depressed, the globe sinks backward and downward, producing enophthalmos and ocular dystopia. A hematoma may be observed in the upper buccal sulcus. If the zygomatic arch is depressed medially, it may impinge on the coronoid process of the mandible, restricting mandibular function. Numbness in the distribution of the infraorbital nerve is a reliable sign of zygomatic or orbital-floor fracture. The anesthesia or hypesthesia produced involves the upper anterior maxillary teeth and/or the soft tissue of the ipsilateral upper lip, cheek, and nose. Difficulty chewing, or a minor occlusal disturbance, may accompany zygomatic fractures in the presence of swelling involving the temporal region or when depression of the zygomatic arch is present. The mechanism involves interference with excursion of the coronoid process of the mandible.

The radiographic evaluation of a zygoma fracture was formerly accomplished with plain films (28–30), but now must include a CT scan (30–35). The plain films are unnecessary if a CT scan is taken. Plain films formerly utilized included the Waters', Caldwell, and submental vertex views. The Waters' view (Fig. 34–8A) identified the lateral wall of the maxillary antrum, the inferior orbital rim, and the orbital floor. The submental vertex view shows the zygomatic arch and the relationship of the malar eminence. The Caldwell view demonstrates distraction at the zygomaticofrontal suture.

In practice, a craniofacial CT scan with axial and coronal views and bone and soft-tissue windows most accurately demonstrates the injury. (Fig. 34–8B,C).

Isolated fractures of the zygomatic arch generally demonstrate medial displacement. Most frequently, a W-shaped deformity (with depression of lateral cheek just anterior to the glenoid fossa) is identified (Fig. 34–9). Sometimes the depression cannot be seen until the swelling resolves. If the medial displacement is sufficient, the arch interferes with the motion of the coronoid process of the mandible. Isolated fractures of the zygomatic arch may be reduced through a Gillies temporal approach (20). In this reduction maneuver, an incision is made in the temporal hair-bearing scalp until the deep temporal fascia is penetrated to expose the temporalis muscle. An elevator may be then passed directly underneath the arch. The surgeon then forces the arch laterally in a smooth, gentle maneuver to accomplish reduction. Usually, further support is not required because the arch has strong periosteal attachments that allow it to remain stable. Allegedly, there are those who have placed K-wires through it; some utilize packing beneath the arch to improve the stability of reduction; but generally these techniques are not necessary. Also, some surgeons place a protective guard over the arch, taping it to the skin in an effort to prevent postoperative displacement. The efficacy of this maneuver is open to question.

All zygomatic fractures should be evaluated with an axial and a coronal CT scan because of the orbital involvement. In patients who are not able to have true coronal images, axial images may be reconstructed coronally to provide a view of the orbital wall fragments. Zygomatic fractures should be analyzed by CT scans, both for confirmation of displacement and for analysis of the degree of fragmentation of the zygoma. Displaced fractures should be treated with an open reduction. About one-fourth of zygomatic fractures are so minimally displaced that an open reduction is not felt to be required as the disturbance in appearance will be minimal.

Reductions may utilize either anterior approaches (the combination of a lower-eyelid and gingival buccal sulcus incisions) or may require the use of a posterior incision (coronal). Fractures that demonstrate lateral displacement of the zygomatic arch or extreme comminution and posterior displacement of the zygomatic body are those that require both anterior and posterior incisions. The remainder of isolated zygoma fractures (> 90% of those seen) are able to be managed with anterior incisions alone. The extreme zygoma fracture can only be anatomically reduced, with a full visualization provided by both anterior incisions and posterior incisions. In the anterior incision technique, if the lateral canthus is detached, the lower-lid incision may be retracted upward to permit minimal visualization of the zygomaticofrontal suture, but enough for fixation and alignment. Otherwise, a zygomaticofrontal suture incision (either a local brow incision or the lateral limb of an upper-lid blepharoplasty) is utilized by those who do not prefer to detach the canthus. If the lateral canthus is detached, it requires reattachment. The peripheral buttresses of the zygoma require three incisions for visualization of all of the buttresses

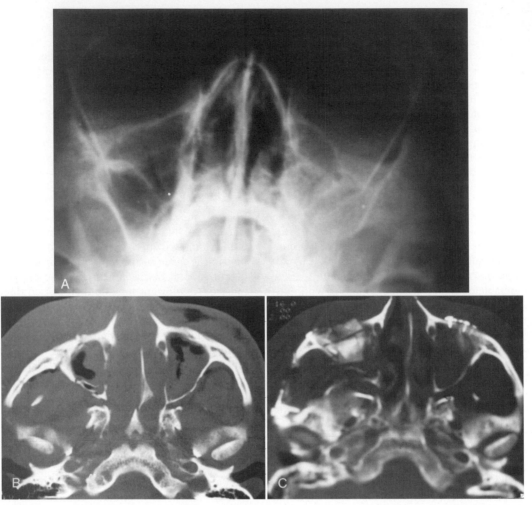

FIG. 34–8. **A,** a Waters' film demonstrates a left zygomatic fracture. Dislocation is seen at the frontal process of the zygoma, the inferior orbital rim, and the zygomatico maxillary buttress. **B,** CT scan demonstrates a complete zygomatic fracture with comminution of the malar body, posterior displacement of the inferior orbital rim, and lateral displacement and comminution of the zygomatic arch. This frac- ture would require open reduction of the arch. **C,** the result following internal orbital bone grafting and open reduction of the zygoma, in- cluding the arch. The patient actually has a bilateral Le Fort fracture. The symmetry of the arch has been reestablished. Three approaches were utilized: a coronal incision, a lower eyelid, and then gingival buccal sulcus exposure.

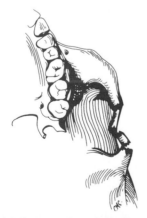

FIG. 34–9.   An isolated zygomatic arch fracture showing medial dis- placement in a W-shaped pattern. This fracture may be reduced by placing an elevator on the surface of the temporalis muscle and slid- ing it under the arch (the Gilles approach), then lifting the arch into re- duction. The arch is generally stable following this closed-reduction maneuver.

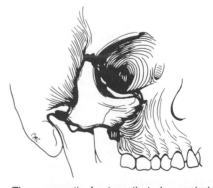

FIG. 34–10.   The zygomatic fracture that demonstrates complete dislocation at all anterior buttress articulations. Open reduction would be required and because the arch is not laterally displaced, anterior approaches alone are adequate. Anterior approaches consist of (a) a lower eyelid incision, and (b) an exposure through the gingival buccal sulcus. The zygomatico frontal sutures exposed by detaching the lat- eral canthal ligament and retracting the incision superiorly.

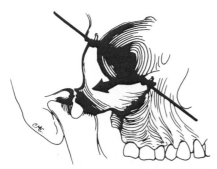

FIG. 34–11. Wire interfragment fixation of the zygoma at the inferior orbital rim and zygomatico frontal suture does not stabilize the zygoma against rotation. These wires merely create an axis about which rotation can occur. A similar deformity might be seen for plate-and-screw fixation of multiple fragment zygomatic fracture utilizing small malleable plates. In noncomminuted fractures the zygomaticofrontal suture, the inferior orbital rim, and the zygomaticomaxillary buttress may be used together, separately, or in combination. Many large-segment fractures are relatively stable and require fewer points of alignment and fixation. In comminuted injuries, all peripheral buttresses of the zygoma should be utilized for exposure and for fixation. An open reduction of the zygomatic arch is required in fractures with extreme posterior displacement or lateral displacement of the zygomatic arch.

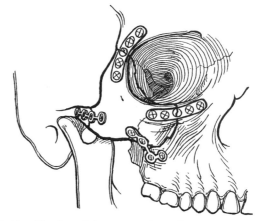

FIG. 34–12. Fixation of the zygoma is performed at its buttress articulations by an initial interfragment wire reduction at the zygomatico frontal suture, inferior orbital rim, and through the arch. The arch, and then the zygomaticomaxillary buttress, the inferior orbital rim, and the zygomaticofrontal suture are usually stabilized (in that order) with plate-and-screw fixation.

(Fig. 34–10). Since alignment of all of the buttress cannot be visualized simultaneously, it is essential to provide some kind of temporary positioning device, such as a wire, to provide provisional fixation. Initially, interfragment wires are placed in the zygomaticofrontal suture, at the inferior orbital rim and in the arch (Fig. 34–11). Final adjustments of bone position are then made and 2.0-mm maxillary adaption plates are placed in the arch and in the zygomaticomaxillary buttress region. (Fig. 34–12). The 1.0, 1.2 or 1.3 mm systems can be used at the infraorbital rim and at the Z-F suture (see Figs. 34–10, 34–11, 34–12). The strength of the plate required at the zygomaticofrontal suture depends upon the strength achieved by the other buttress reductions. Larger plates are visible in this area, but are sometimes required.

Zygomatic fractures, which are minimally displaced and only partially complete at the zygomaticofrontal suture, and may theoretically be managed by closed reduction. For a closed reduction to be stable, the fracture must be "greensticked" or incomplete at the zygomaticofrontal suture. The displaced portion of the fracture at the infraorbital rim is maneuvered back into position by a variety of reduction maneuvers that employ force, either directed within the maxillary sinus or beneath the malar eminence. The greenstick, or incomplete, component of the fracture then renders the fracture stable. Closed reductions are otherwise performed by wedging or interlocking of fracture edges. Closed reduction methods have disadvantages of increased malalignment as compared with open reductions. Also, they do not guarantee stability, but they have been successful when utilized by those with experience in zygomatic fracture treatment. Fractures should not be comminuted, and should be treated early if a closed reduction is to be selected. In practice, most people use closed reductions only for zygomatic arch fractures.

Conceptually, zygomatic fractures have five buttress articulations (see Fig. 34–10). Each buttress articulation might be utilized as a point of alignment or fixation. For most zygomatic injuries, one should provide both confirmation of alignment and fixation at three anterior sites: the zygomaticofrontal suture, the infraorbital rim, and the zygomaticomaxillary buttress. Exposure of these areas is obtained with two incisions: the lower-lid subciliary skin flap (36) and a gingival buccal sulcus incision. A conjunctival incision with a lateral canthotomy may substitute for a lower-lid skin muscle flap, or a mid-eyelid incision (subtarsal) may be utilized.

If a coronal incision is necessary, the arch should be carefully reduced (see Fig. 34–11). As the arch is brought into a flat reduction, the surgeon will notice that the greater wing of the sphenoid comes into alignment with the orbital process of the zygoma inside the orbit. This relationship is a sensitive guide to both malar projection and proper arch reduction and also reestablishes proper orbital volume.

FRONTAL BONE AND FRONTAL BASILAR FRACTURES

Trauma to the forehead may result in fractures of the frontal bone. Frontal-bone fractures may be divided into those that involve the supraorbital and temporal regions laterally and the frontal sinus centrally (37–42). Frequently, displaced fractures involve one or two areas of the frontal skull. Patients with forehead lacerations and periorbital ecchymosis should be thoroughly examined to exclude frontal fractures; a CT scan may be necessary. In these patients the neurologic status may be abnormal or surprisingly normal to examination. A high index of suspicion must therefore be present so that all fractures can be identified. Fractures of the posterior wall of the frontal sinus are especially important to exclude, because they imply the possibility of dural injury. The CT scan remains the best diagnostic evaluation of the frontal sinus and anterior cranial fossa components of the frontal basilar region. The frontal bone fractures generally require broad exposure (Fig. 34–13). Rarely, they may be treated through existing lacerations; however, existing lacerations provide no flexibility for dealing with hemorrhage or other complications. Conversion to a coronal incision should be prepared for, in case the local laceration proves inadequate.

scribed by Le Fort, in that multiple levels of fracture are simultaneously seen in the same patient and, the fracture is usually worse (or involves a higher Le Fort level) on one side as compared with the other (48–51). The Le Fort fracture levels do characterize the "weak areas" of the midfacial skeleton that are predisposed to fracture.

A *Le Fort I* fracture is a transverse (or horizontal) fracture that separates the maxillary alveolus from the superior midfacial skeleton. The fracture line runs above the base of the roots of maxillary teeth and across the lower aspect of the pyriform aperture. The pterygoid plate area is severed.

The *Le Fort II fracture* is a "pyramidal" fracture of the maxilla. It separates a central, pyramidally shaped nasomaxillary segment from the zygomatic and upper lateral aspect of the midfacial skeleton. The fragment bearing the occlusion is thus triangular in shape. The Le Fort II fracture may travel over the distal nose through its cartilaginous portion, entering the opposite orbit and crossing the inferior orbital rims to separate the zygoma from the medial aspect of the maxilla. The fracture lines may go beneath or above the canthal ligament insertion. As such, the fracture displays "low" and "high" varieties. Upper Le Fort II level fractures separate the frontal processes of the maxilla and the nasal bones from the glabellar region of the frontal bone.

The *Le Fort III fracture* represents the craniofacial disjunction. In this fracture, the cranium is completely separated from the facial bones (51–55). The fracture begins at the zygomatico-frontal junction and transverses the lateral, inferior, and medial orbit, traveling at the junction of the frontal process of the maxilla with the internal angular process of the frontal bone separating the nasal bones, midface, and zygomas from the cranium. Generally, pure Le Fort fractures that are bilaterally equal are not seen. The fracture is usually one level higher on the most injured side. The Le Fort III superior level fracture, for instance, is commonly accompanied by a Le Fort II superior level fracture on the opposite side. The surgeon will generally see a Le Fort I or II segment bearing the occlusion in this injury. Multiple fracture levels are usually observed simultaneously in the same patient. Thus, the fracture levels represent "lines of weakness" through which comminuted fractures occur, rather than the fractures occurring as single, pure segments. The Le Fort III level fracture, therefore, usually contains separate zygomatic segments and separate Le Fort I and Le Fort II maxillary segments. Occasionally, a single-fragment Le Fort III fracture will exist; it usually presents with bilateral periorbital ecchymosis and little or no maxillary mobility. These fractures are minimally displaced and present with a very slight occlusal disturbance that is easy to miss if the surgeon is not aware that this entity can exist. Bilateral eyelid ecchymoses are invariably present. Air fluid levels are seen in the maxillary and ethmoid sinuses on CT scan.

The Le Fort IV level fracture was not described by Le Fort (65–72). The designation of the frontal bone as the Le Fort IV level refers to the concept that frontobasilar injuries often accompany Le Fort fractures. Fractures that consist of the frontal bone, frontal sinus, superior orbital rims, and anterior cranial base therefore represent an extension of midface fractures both in concept and in treatment. Many Le Fort fractures extend into the frontal bone; these may conceptually be considered "Le Fort IV" level fractures.

The principle symptoms of a maxillary fracture are maxillary mobility and malocclusion. In the Le Fort II and Le Fort III level fractures, bilateral eyelid ecchymosis will also be present. Nasopharyngeal bleeding is routine, and may be profuse in some patients, depending on the severity of the fracture. Facial edema and deformity are present. As the maxilla drops downward and posteriorly, the midface appears to be retruded. One sees an elongated and retruded midface with anterior open bite in untreated injuries, as the midface lengthens posteriorly. Cerebral spinal fluid fistulae occur in 25 to 50% of upper (Le Fort II and III) fractures. Signs of zygomatic, naso-ethmoidal-orbital, orbital floor, and medial orbital fractures are present, depending on the level and extent of the fracture. Occasionally, a Le Fort fracture is displaced and impacted, and therefore displays no maxillary mobility. Malocclusion is the likely diagnosis in these cases.

The CT scan in patients with Le Fort fractures demonstrates fractures through at least the posterior walls of the maxillary sinuses and, in most injuries, fractures of the lower pterygoid plate region. Incomplete Le Fort fractures have no pterygoid plate fractures. The type and distribution of fractures therefore depends on the variety and pattern observed.

Treatment of Le Fort Fractures

Mobilization of the fragments is accomplished to reproduce a normal occlusal pattern (61–72). It is important that the maxilla be fully mobilized, so that the mandible is not tracted out of the glenoid fossa in order to meet a displaced but impacted maxillary fracture. The occlusion must be stable with the patient in relaxed mandibular position. IMF is the principle treatment utilized to restore the projection of the lower midface by placing the patient into proper occlusion (Fig. 34–16). The entire maxilla below the Le Fort I level is therefore related to the lower face, and depends on the presence of an intact or reconstructed mandible for proper position. IMF should be applied as soon as possible after the injury; there is literally no patient who is too sick to undergo IMF under local anesthesia. The use of IMF minimizes fracture displacement. In patients who have not had IMF, the maxilla tends to lengthen, and with late attempts at maxillary repositioning it may be difficult to overcome this lengthening, especially at the posterior (pterygoid) buttress of the maxilla. The stability and projection of the midface are restored by open reduction and rigid internal fixation utilizing the intact or reconstructed frontal bone as a guide. Bone grafts span bone defects where appropriate. Exposure of the lower portion of the Le Fort fracture is obtained through bilateral gingival buccal sulcus incisions which expose the entire Le Fort I level. In Le Fort II, III, and IV fractures, the use of coronal and lower-eyelid incisions provide exposure to the superior portion of the maxillofacial skeleton.

In the treatment of Le Fort fractures, the nasomaxillary and zygomatomaxillary buttresses are stabilized using plate-and-screw fixation. Bone grafts are added when bone defects occur or when it is necessary to strengthen the bone at a fractured area. These conditions are generally observed in patients with edentulous Le Fort fractures or in comminuted fractures. The coronal incision provides exposure for the zygomaticofrontal suture, the zygomatic arch, the orbital roof, the nasal frontal area, and the nasoethmoidal region. The lower portion of the orbit and zygoma are visualized through

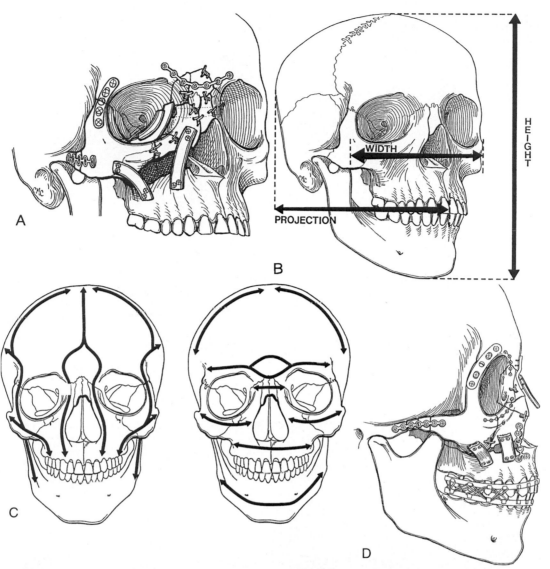

FIG. 34–16. **A,** buttress of the facial skeleton are reassembled utilizing bone grafts where required. The initial inter fragment wiring is stabilized with rigid fixation. **B,** the face must be reassembled and stabilized in its three dimensions of height, width, and projection. **C,** buttresses of the midfacial skeleton. **D,** open reduction of Le Fort fracture with bone grafting. The initial step must be IMF.

lower-eyelid incisions. The zygomatic arch is visualized by a coronal incision after incising the anterior layer of the deep temporal fascia.

Patients managed with rigid fixation may have IMF discontinued after fracture reduction if sufficient stability is obtained. In comminuted midfacial fractures, or those accompanied by fractures of the mandible, it is our practice to maintain IMF for 2 weeks or more. The patient is then allowed to function and take a soft diet, but must have his occlusion observed twice weekly. The length of IMF must be determined by the comminution of the fracture and the stability obtained by an open reduction. In patients released from IMF, at least biweekly observation of the occlusion is necessary to exclude postoperative displacement. Displacement may be observed in spite of performing open reduction with rigid internal fixation, because midface bones are thin and the buttress stability is limited. Brief elastic traction or reinstitution of IMF generally restores the occlusion in these cases.

Conceptually, maxillary fractures can be restored by reconstructing the horizontal and vertical buttress system of the facial skeleton. The maxilla lacks good "sagittal" buttresses (see Fig. 34–16); therefore, relating the upper midface to the frontal bone and the lower midface to the mandible provides strong sagittal buttresses for support.

Bone defects of the orbit and those over the maxillary sinus are bone grafted.

Late treatment of Le Fort fractures requires mobilization of the fracture segments (70–73) and repositioning the fracture fragments into proper anatomic relationships. In fractures treated late, the entire area of the skeleton must be degloved in an attempt to mobilize malpositioned bone. Early treatment is therefore preferred, because it necessitates less manipulation and dissection.

In edentulous Le Fort fractures, buttress bone grafting should be utilized in addition to rigid internal fixation. The surgeon should not omit use of dental splints or dentures to

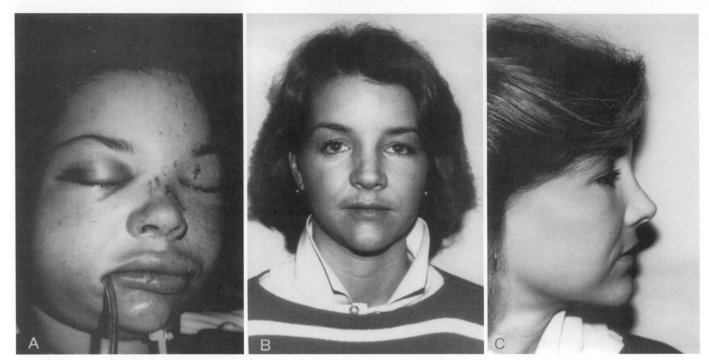

FIG. 34–17. **A,** patient demonstrating comminuted Le Fort, nasoethmoidal and bilateral mandibular fractures. **B,** frontal postoperative view. **C,** lateral postoperative view. These results demonstrate that early treatment with extended open reduction and bone grafting restores the appearance of the craniofacial skeleton.

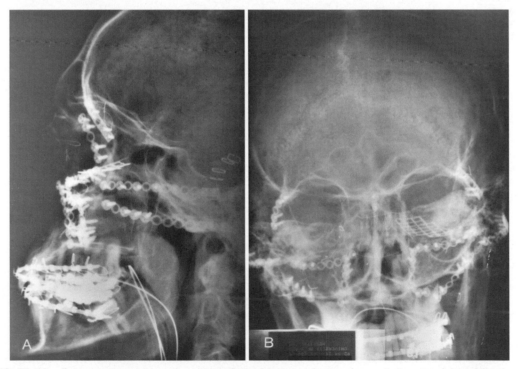

FIG. 34–18. Postoperative radiographs of a panfacial fracture reduction demonstrate extension stabilization of the facial buttresses by titanium plate-and-screw fixation. **A,** lateral view. **B,** frontal view.

line up the maxilla with the mandible as a component of intraoperative alignment. Intermaxillary fixation through dentures is a key step in obtaining proper projection of the lower maxilla. The use of IMF and splints may be discontinued after the application of rigid internal fixation if sufficient stability has been obtained. The dentures may be secured either with screws to the alveolus or by the use of wires that extend from the dental splint up over a stable point such as the maxillary alveolus, zygomatic arch, pyriform aperture, or the inferior orbital rim. In practice, it is much easier to use screws (Figs. 34–17, 34–18) than wires.

When comminuted fractures involve the maxilla and mandible, it is necessary to stabilize the mandible in both its vertical and horizontal components as a sagittal buttress for maxillary fracture reduction. The midface reduction cannot support a fractured mandible. When fractures of the frontal bone exist with comminuted midfacial fractures, the frontal-bone stabilization and any intracranial neurosurgery are completed first. Segments of the orbital rims are initially linked with wires and then stabilized with plate-and-screw fixation.

In stabilizing a zygoma, it is necessary to correct midfacial width, which tends to have widened in patients with high-energy zygoma fractures, as they displaced the zygomatic arch laterally (65–72). The zygomatic arch should first be reconstructed following wire interfragment orbital rim fixation, and the reconstruction should be as flat as possible, because it represents the first point of rigid fixation of the zygoma after linking the fragments with wires. The remainder of the zygoma may then be stabilized, and generally the inferior orbital rim and zygomatico-maxillary buttress are stabilized

next. The zygomaticofrontal suture is usually stabilized last.

Rigid fixation as a treatment for midface fractures has, for the most part, eliminated the use of suspension wires, head frames, and acrylic dental splints.

RE-FIXATION OF THE SOFT TISSUE OF THE CRANIOFACIAL SKELETON

When craniofacial exposures are employed for fracture stabilization, the bone is often widely degloved of its soft tissue (65–72). The soft tissue may drift to a lower location unless specific steps are obtained to (a) close the periosteal incisions to realign the soft tissue, and (b) *then* reattach the periosteum at appropriate locations. Periosteal closure should occur at the lateral orbital rim, the inferior orbital rim, the deep temporal fascia, the periosteum over the zygomaticofrontal suture, and the musculo-periosteal layers of the gingival buccal

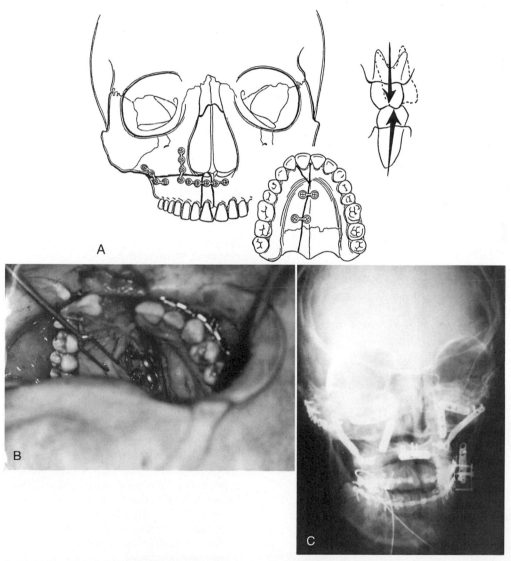

FIG. 34–19. **A,** the sagittal fracture of the maxilla requires precise open reduction spanning the fractures of the palate and alveolus. Exposure of the fracture in the roof of the mouth allows stabilization with plate-and-screw fixation. Open reduction and internal fixation are performed on the anterior face of the maxilla. **B,** plate-and-screw fixation is seen at the Le Fort I buttresses on the right and across the fracture at the pyriform aperture which divides the maxilla between the incisor and cuspid dentition. The diagram at the right demonstrates open reduction and internal fixation of a hemi–Le Fort fracture. It should be emphasized that arch bars are used as initial alignment technique prior to plate-and-screw fixation. **C,** postoperative radiograph demonstrates plate-and-screw fixation of the Le Fort buttresses and at the roof of the mouth. A mandibular angle fracture had been stabilized with miniplate fixation (photographs).

sulcus and mandibular incisions. Specifically designed ginigival buccal sulcus incisions are used so that a cuff of muscle (e.g., mentalis) is present to reattach the soft tissue of the chin to the mandible. If these areas are totally stripped, mentalis muscle attachment may be lost; the soft tissue then readheres inferiorly, which generates lower-lip ectropion.

The periosteum is reattached at the medial and lateral canthi, and at the inferior orbital rim.

SAGITTAL FRACTURES OF THE MAXILLA AND PALATE

The maxillary alveolus may be divided sagittally or transversely (65–72). In fractures that divide the maxilla and palate sagittally, two varieties exist that cleave large segments of the alveolus and therefore may be amendable to open reduction (74,75). The buttress system of the maxillary alveolus is visualized in Figures 34–16 and 34–19. It is necessary to stabilize the alveolus *before* IMF is accomplished (Fig. 34–20). The maxillary alveolus is made of a single fragment by reconstruction; it then can be utilized as in previously described Le Fort fracture schemes of treatment. Eight percent of Le Fort fractures have a split palate. Large segment, sagittally oriented fractures of the maxilla are amendable to open reduction. These fractures travel either adjacent to the midline or adjacent to the alveolus. In younger individuals, usually adolescents, the fracture may truly separate the palate in the midline. The palatal suture closes by 30 years of age and midline fractures are less frequently observed in older individuals. Sagittal fractures of the maxilla usually exit anteriorly between the bicuspid dentition. The type of displacement observed in the lateral maxillary segment is anterior, lateral, and superior. The fracture is diagnosed by abnormal mobility of the bicuspid and molar dentition. Frequently, a lip, gingival, and palatal laceration accompany these fractures, and lacerations should serve as clues to the possible presence of the fracture. These fractures benefit from stabilization with open reduction techniques. Previously, a dental acrylic splint was utilized, and it may still be necessary in some cases for fine adjustment of the occlusion. The use of internal fixation for sagit-

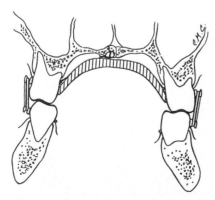

FIG. 34–20. The use of an acrylic palatal splint is helpful in some cases of dental alveolar fractures to stabilize the dentition. The acrylic splint, placed on the palatal surface of the teeth, stabilizes the teeth against rotation in the face of intermaxillary elastic traction. (From Manson PN, et al, eds. *Plastic Reconstructive Surgery Journal.* Vol 72. 1983.)

tal fractures of the maxilla involves stabilization in the roof of the mouth and at the pyriform aperture with screws of the 2.0-mm system. Either the palatal laceration or a longitudinal incision over the fracture in the palate (parallel to the greater palatine artery) is used for fixation. The palatal roof open reduction stabilizes the transverse width of the maxillary arch, and then the use of a pyriform aperture plate further unites the maxillary segments into a single unit.

The use of a dental acrylic splint is sometimes necessary to provide fine occlusal adjustment of the dentition (74). The dental splint is placed on the palatal surface of the maxillary teeth and covers a portion of the roof of the mouth. It prevents rotation of the maxillary dental segments. The dental splint can often avoided if adequate fixation is achieved by plate-and-screw fixation. The dental splint is assembled from dental models that are first sectioned at the areas of the fracture and then reassembled into a proper occlusal relationship. The dental splint may be ligated to molar and bicuspid teeth or fixed by the use of palatal screw or circumpalatal wire. Occasionally, small segments of the maxilla representing the postero-lateral or anterior teeth will be fractured. These segments can be stabilized with an acrylated arch bar, with a dental acrylic splint, or with dental bonding techniques. Alveolar fractures and sagittal fractures of the maxilla may require a longer period of healing. In contrast to the usual maxillary fracture, which is healed 6 to 8 weeks from the time of the injury, alveolar and sagittal fractures of the maxilla may require 12 to 16 weeks to fully consolidate. In practice, all patients must be observed throughout the period of healing to exclude the possibility of postoperative displacement. Observation of the occlusion at weekly or biweekly intervals for 12 to 16 weeks is therefore suggested for all patients.

ORBITAL FRACTURES

The symptoms of an orbital floor or medial orbital wall fracture are periorbital ecchymosis and subconjunctival hemorrhage. Frequently, hypesthesia or anesthesia are present in the distribution of the infraorbital nerve in orbital floor fractures. Epistaxis and orbital emphysema are common in fractures of the medial orbital wall. Depending on the extent of fracture and the damage to extraocular muscles, horizontal or vertical eye-muscle imbalances (diplopia) may be present (77–90). If the displacement of the wall is sufficient to allow the globe to migrate, orbital dystopia may be present or the globe may be noticed to have a medial position (82–90). If the fractures involve both the medial orbit and the orbital floor, the defect is large enough to produce substantial enophthalmos, or recession of the globe into the orbit. The expansion of the bony orbital volume (blow-out fracture) allows the soft tissue to descend into the space of increased volume. A medially displaced zygoma fracture contracts orbital volume and is termed a "blow-in" fracture; the orbital volume is constricted and the globe may be displaced forward (exophthalmos).

Fractures may therefore be confined only to the thin middle section of the orbit (pure orbital fracture) or they may be "impure," involving both the rim and the internal portions of the orbit (82–90). Obviously, impure fractures have substantially greater potential for increasing orbital volume and for orbital deformity. Commonly, pure orbital fractures involve the lower medial orbital wall and floor of the orbit simultaneously. Isolated fractures of the medial wall usually present with extensive subcutaneous emphysema, epistaxis, horizontal diplopia, and enophthalmos.

Only very rarely do medial wall fractures incarcerate extraocular muscles. In contrast, fractures of the orbital floor commonly incarcerate fat and, by virtue of their connections to the inferior rectus muscle, diplopia looking either superiorly or inferiorly may occur. Inferior diplopia is usually much more incapacitating than superior diplopia because it affects the down gaze (reading position). Rarely, the inferior rectus muscle itself may be incarcerated in an orbital floor fracture; we believe this situation represents a true emergency as it is imperative to relieve the obstruction to circulation that travels longitudinally within the muscle.

The mechanism of orbital floor fractures involves both a "hydraulic force" (77) created by soft-tissue compression, and a blow to the orbital rim that creates a "buckling force" (78), with displacement of the orbital floor accompanied by bending and fracture, often without a simultaneous fracture of the rim (77–81). The buckling occurs in the thin area of the orbital floor and, if sufficient, results in a fracture. The rim may or may not be fractured because its stronger structure makes it capable of some displacement without fracture. Soft-tissue pressure produced by the hydraulic compression of the tissue then forces extraocular fat (and perhaps an extraocular muscle) into the fracture site. Since the bone recoils before the soft

tissue, the result is incarceration of orbital soft tissue in the fracture, with impaired movement. Koorneef and Manson (83) have both described the fine ligament system that extends throughout all orbital soft tissue and, by virtue of these connections, may account for tethering of extraocular muscle by fat incarceration. When periorbital fat is incarcerated in an orbital fracture, the excursion of an eye muscle may be tethered because of these defined ligament connections, despite the fact that the muscle itself is not physically incarcerated. The fine ligament system explains how this limitation of movement occurs by diffuse interconnections.

All patients with orbital fractures deserve a careful clinical evaluation of the visual system. Visual acuity, speed of pupillary reaction, and asymmetry of pupillary reactivity provide evidence of optic nerve integrity. Confrontation fields, intraocular pressure, and funduscopic examination must also be performed.

Orbital fractures are evaluated radiographically by axial and coronal CT scan sections. In patients unable to cooperate for coronal sections, the axial sections are reconstructed into a coronal format. Although orbital fractures may be visualized on plain films, the lack of diagnostic detail provided for both bone and soft tissue makes them of little value.

A CT examination with axial and coronal views and bone and soft-tissue windows is required for the proper evaluation of the volume changes within the orbit and for the diagnosis of muscle incarceration versus muscle contusion (Fig. 34–21). The need for surgery in orbital-floor fractures is

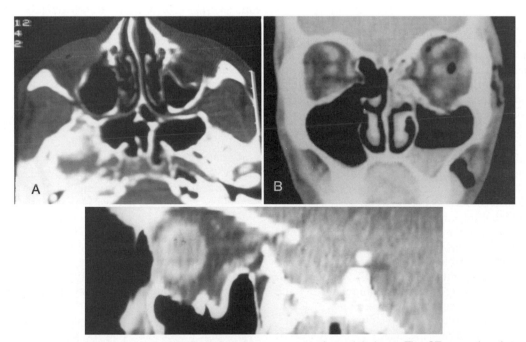

FIG. 34–21. A, a "blow-out" fracture of the orbital floor demonstrated on an axial CT scan. A fragment of bone is seen depressed in the right maxillary antrum. Little precise evaluation of fracture displacement is possible in the axial CT scan. **B,** coronal CT scan allows precise determination of the extent of displacement of the floor and medial wall fragment. The relationship of the inferior oblique and medial rectus muscles to the fracture site is identified in this scan emphasizing bone soft-tissue relationships. The amount of soft tissue incarcerated in the fracture may be quantified. There is a relationship between the volume of displaced tissue and the subsequent development of enophthalmos. The CT scan, therefore, permits accurate prediction of patients who benefit from operation for either release of muscle incarceration (diplopia) or volume correction (enophthalmos). **C,** CT scan taken in longitudinal orbital projection (after Marsh) demonstrates a blow-out fracture. Inferior displacement of the floor of the orbit is noted. The orbital contents are herniated downward into the maxillary sinus. The intact "ledge" bone is seen in the orbit posteriorly, and it is here that the reconstruction of the orbital floor must begin.

based on two considerations (81,83,85): (a) the need to correct a volume change of the orbit, and (b) the need to release incarcerated orbital soft tissue in the presence of functionally limiting diplopia. The following are indications for operative intervention:

1. Entrapment of an extraocular muscle or orbital fat with diplopia in a primary field of gaze. A positive-force duction examination is usually present, as is CT scan evidence of incarceration of orbital soft tissue. Peripheral field diplopia may or may not be incapacitating enough to justify surgery.
2. Enophthalmos or exophthalmos exceeding 2 to 3 mm as a result of fracture displacement and volumetric change within the orbit. More than 2 to 3 cc of orbital volume change begins to produce globe positional change.
3. Vertical or horizontal globe positional changes that are aesthetically undesirable.
4. Infraorbital sensory nerve deficit in the face of an orbital rim fracture that compresses the infraorbital nerve foramen.

Entrapment of the movement of an extraocular muscle or of its adjacent fat, may tether muscle excursion by virtue of ligament connections. These symptoms are a good indication for open reduction. It was formerly suggested that these cases should be allowed to heal for 10 days to 2 weeks to see if binocular vision was restored spontaneously. In practice, we believe those with visual limitation in a functional field of gaze should be operated early because of the more favorable anatomic situation created by early release of entrapped tissue. A forced duction examination, using a drop of a local anesthetic agent, is performed by grasping the insertion of the extraocular muscle just peripheral to the corneal limbus. The globe is rotated and compared with the other side. The absence of full rotation or increased tension indicates possible muscle incarceration. A stiff, forced duction examination may be the result of contusion, fibrosis or edema. It also may be owing to incarceration of the orbital soft tissue. The "force generation test" is performed by grasping the insertion of a muscle and asking the patient to voluntarily rotate the globe, noting the force generated. It is said (and this test is really of much more limited clinical usefulness) that the patient with a true incarceration is unable to generate force because of the functional impairment of the muscle.

More sophisticated examinations, such as saccadic velocities (80), to differentiate the rate of acceleration of ocular movements, are said to be able to differentiate not only muscle entrapment but also paralysis and contusion. Contusion may produce a positive-force duction examination by the production of edema and scarring. Most diplopia is due to contusion and may resolve almost completely spontaneously. Therefore, many internal orbital fractures that will not result in significant enophthalmos do not benefit from operative intervention. Obviously, muscle contusion and nerve deficits will not be benefited by surgical procedures. Superior and inferior muscle inbalances and double vision are more often due to muscle contusion than fat and fascial entrapment. This explains the popularity of the conservative (nonoperative) approach to orbital fractures that involve only the internal portion of the orbit and have mild symptoms likely to resolve

spontaneously. True muscle incarceration is quite uncommon, but should be released immediately, as has been pointed out previously.

The goal of treatment is to obtain functional (orthophoric) vision in the primary field of gaze and not necessarily fully normal movement without diplopia. This goal can be accomplished with nonoperative treatment in many limited orbital-floor fractures, a fact which was emphasized and popularized by Puterman and others (81,83,85).

Surgical treatment of orbital fractures is indicated for muscle or fat incarceration that produces visually handicapping diplopia. Likewise, when orbital volume changes will result in cosmetically deforming globe positional change, such as exophthalmos or enophthalmos, surgery is indicated (87–90). We believe early definitive surgery in the face of muscle restriction improves final range of motion, but this has yet to be proven by clinical outcome studies. The most disabling double vision is that which is present inferiorly in the down gaze or reading position. Paralysis of the superior rectus muscle may mimic a trapped inferior rectus muscle. A careful examination of the entire orbit with CT scans is mandatory, and formal visual fields are suggested. Vertical dystopia of the globe is corrected by orbital reconstruction of the walls of the orbit (73). The sensory deficit accompanying orbital-floor fractures usually resolves almost completely spontaneously unless the rim is involved. Any fracture that compresses the infraorbital nerve foramen should be decompressed; thus, hypesthesia or anesthesia is usually not an indication for operative intervention in fractures of the internal orbital walls. If rim fractures are explored, an infraorbital nerve decompression should be a specific component of operative intervention. The constriction of the foramen may be documented on CT scan. Patients with sensory deficits following orbital fractures may occasionally be improved by late nerve decompression or neurolysis. The disabling nature of some symptoms also improves spontaneously.

Supraorbital fractures involve the supraorbital rim and orbital roof. They are usually displaced inferiorly and posteriorly and create a downward and outward projection of the globe (Fig. 34–22). Lid closure may be incomplete, and, if so, corneal exposure is common. Early fracture reduction should be considered in these patients if the lids cannot close. Supraorbital fractures often involve the frontal sinus, and the potential for a dural fistula also exists. Supraorbital fractures should be managed by restoring the proper volume and contour of the orbital rim and orbit.

The lateral orbit (greater wing of the sphenoid) is often fractured in fractures of the zygoma. Lateral orbital fractures may only be a linear fracture of the junction of the orbital process of the zygoma and the greater wing of the sphenoid, or the area may be comminuted, extending into the greater wing of the sphenoid and enlarging the orbit in this location.

The weakest area of the orbital wall is the medial wall of the orbit over the ethmoid sinuses, which represents the lamina papyracea. The next weakest area is the orbital floor. The orbital floor fractures more commonly than the medial orbit because it is more often involved in trauma. The section of the orbital floor that fractures most commonly is the medial

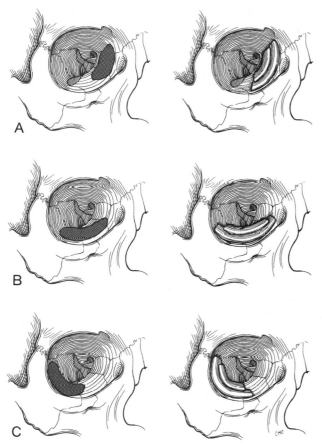

A

B

C

FIG. 34–22. **A,** a medial orbital wall fracture is managed by split rib or calvarial bone grafting. The intact bone posteriorly and laterally are utilized as guides to reconstruction. Posteriorly, intact bone is often present at the level of the posterior ethmoid foramen medially, and inferiorly adjacent to a ledge about 1 cm from the optic nerve at the back of the maxillary sinus. **B,** the usual location of an inferior medial or blow-out fracture. The area has been dissected and intact bone is identified around all the edges of the entire orbital defect. Bone grafts may then be placed to cover the defect. **C,** an inferior-lateral defect over the inferior orbital fissure is managed with a split rib or calvarial bone graft. This defect would usually accompany a zygoma fracture. (Copyright Johns Hopkins University, Art as Applied to Medicine.)

section, where it is inclined at a 30° angle as it extends posteriorly. The plane of the orbital floor also inclines superiorly at a 45° angle to reach the ethmoidal area. The inclined inferomedial section is the usual area "blown out" in internal orbital fractures; it is located medial to the groove and canal for the infraorbital nerve. In inferior medial orbital fractures, the postbulbar orbital constriction is lost; the orbital volume increases, allowing the globe to sink downward, backward, and medially.

Fractures of the orbital floor are exposed through a subciliary skin muscle flap, a lower-eyelid incision, or a conjunctival incision with or without lateral canthotomy, depending on the needs for exposure. The lower half of the medial orbital wall may be explored by lateral and superior displacement of the globe using a lower-lid incision. If the upper half of the medial orbital wall needs to be explored, a local incision in

the canthal area, a medial upper-lid incision, or a coronal incision is required.

The lateral orbit may also be explored through a subciliary incision by detaching the canthal ligament. If the greater wing of the sphenoid is fractured, exposure through a coronal incision is preferred. The orbital roof and superior orbital rim are explored via either a laceration or a coronal incision.

Safe exploration of the orbit is performed only with a knowledge of the location of the superior and inferior orbital fissures, the optic foramen, and their contents (see Figs. 34–21, 34–22). The exact location of the optic nerve should be kept in mind. The optic foramen is located 40 to 45 mm posterior to the inferior orbital rim and is superior and medial to the usual extent of floor dissection. The usual orbital blow-out fracture involves dissection to 35 to 38 mm behind the rim. As a guide to reconstruction, the entire area of an orbital bone defect should be visualized and the ledge of intact bone identified all around the orbit. The bone graft is then spanned between the ledge and the intact or reconstructed orbital rim. Either bone grafts or alloplastic material should be utilized. Currently, Medpor is the preferred material for isolated orbital floor alloplastic reconstruction, because it can be contoured similar to bone, has some tissue ingrowth, and resists infection because of its vascularity. Both the bone graft and the artificial material should be secured by screw fixation of the implant to the orbital floor. A forced duction examination should be performed before any dissection commences, and again after dissection has been completed. These forced duction examinations should be compared to an examination performed *after* the bone graft has been inserted to document that the reconstruction has not impinged an extraocular muscle. If any doubt exists, the bone graft should be removed, the duction examination repeated, and the bone graft then reinserted, with care being taken to avoid any impingement of the extraocular muscle system. The sequence of reconstruction, when orbital rim fractures coexist with fractures of the internal orbit, is that the rim segments should initially be linked with wires and then stabilized in anatomic position by further adjustment before plate-and-screw fixation. The entire orbital defect should have been dissected to identify intact posterior medial and lateral bone before reconstruction. Bone grafts or alloplastic materials are then used to span the area of the defect.

In simple, internal orbital fractures, alloplastic material (e.g., 0.8-mm Supramid, or 1.5- or 0.8-mm Medpor) is often employed, with a low (2%) long-term risk of infection. The implant must be contoured to avoid any pressure on the globe or orbital soft tissue; in particular, the implant should not be extended beyond the area visualized, so that it places no pressure on the optic nerve. In the reconstruction of medial orbital wall defects, the optic nerve is often directly posterior to the intact ledge of bone, which is usually in the area of the posterior ethmoidal foramen. Again, care must be taken so that medial implants do not impinge upon the area of the optic nerve. Sources for bone graft materials include split calvarium, rib, and iliac crest.

Complications from orbital surgery occur in 10 to 15% of all cases (91,92). The most common complications include eyelid deformities, such as scleral show and ectropion. Other

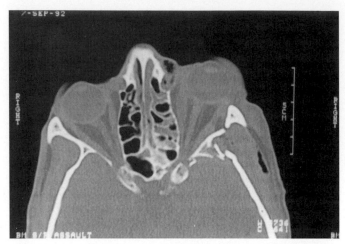

FIG. 34–23. Fractures of the posterior third of the orbit are seen which produce the superior orbital fissure syndrome. When blindness accompanies the superior orbital fissure syndrome, the combined condition is called the "orbital apex" syndrome.

problems include damage to extraocular muscles, with the production of diplopia. Careful attention to hemostasis and accurate dissection minimize these problems. Blindness can occur as a result reflex spasm of circulation, retrobulbar hematoma, or fractures of the optic canal, which alter blood flow to the optic nerve. Blindness has been associated with blind packing of the maxillary antrum without simultaneous visualization of the orbital floor. The use of large orbital-floor implants, vigorous zygomatic fracture mobilization with extension of fractures to the orbital apex, trauma to the globe, retrobulbar hemorrhage, retinal detachment, and edema are also related to visual loss. Late evolution or detection of an ocular injury such as a retinal detachment may be responsible for visual loss. It is important, therefore, that the surgeon document and note visual acuity and pupillary activity *before* the surgery, because these findings provide clues to preexisting optic nerve impairment. Optic nerve impairment that is not documented preoperatively may falsely be assumed to be secondary to the operative manipulation. Any significant postoperative hematoma should be evacuated.

In fractures that extend into the posterior third of the orbit, the superior orbital fissure syndrome may occur (Fig. 34–23). This consists of ophthalmoplegia (paralysis of cranial nerves IV, V, and/or VI), anesthesia in the first division of the trigeminal nerve (forehead), ptosis, and proptosis. When blindness is present in addition to these symptoms, the syndrome is called "orbital apex syndrome." Some superior orbital fissure syndromes can be partial; some recovery usually occurs, but recovery also may be partial (92). Both syndromes are managed initially with high-dose steroids, with surgical decompression reserved for those who do not respond.

Many simple orbital fractures can be managed with observation alone (if enophthalmos is not a consideration) because much of the diplopia resolves spontaneously because it is the result of muscle contusion. In the absence of any muscle or fat incarceration, or a positive forced duction test, the patient should simply be observed if the orbital defect is not sufficient that cosmetically deforming enophthalmos will occur.

Contraindications to orbital surgery include globe rupture, retinal detachment, hyphema, and internal globe injury. On the other hand, patients with significant orbital volume changes, who would develop cosmetically unacceptable enophthalmos if the fractures were untreated, or those with incarceration of the musculofibrous ligament system, are better treated with primary surgery.

The goal in midface and frontal fractures is to restore function and aesthetics. Nowhere in the face are the stakes so high, the rewards so great, and the necessity for immediate definitive treatment more important.

References

1. Gwyn PP, Carraway JH, Horton CE, et al. Facial fractures associated injuries and complications. *Plast Reconstr Surg* 1971; 47:225.
2. Schultz RC. Facila injuries from automobile accidents: a study of 400 consecutive cases. *Plast Reconstr Surg* 1967; 40:415.
3. Kaufman HH, Hui KS, Mattson KC, et al. Clincopathological correlations of disseminated intravascular coagulation in patients with head injury. *Neurosurgery* 1984; 15:34.
4. Dunham C, Cowley RA. *Shock trauma/critical care manual.* Baltimore: University Park Press, 1982.
5. Georgiade N, Nash T. An external cranial fixation apparatus for severe maxillofacial injuries. *Plast Reconstr Surg* 1966; 38:142.
6. Becker DP, Miller JD, Ward JD, et al. The outcome from severe head injury with early diagnosis and intensive management. *J. Neurosurgery* 1977; 47:491.
7. Lewin W, Marshall TF, Roberts AH. Long-term outcome after severe head injury. *Br Med J* 1979; 2:1533.
8. Klauber MR, Marshall LE, Barett-Conner E, et al. Prospective study of patients hospitalized with head injury in San Diego County, 1978. *Neurosurgery* 1981; 9:236.
9. McDonald JV. The surgical management of severe open brain injuries with consideration of the long-term results. *J Trauma* 1980; 20:842.
10. Mcktubjian SR. Operative policy in severe facial trauma in combination with other severe injuries. *J Maxillofacial Surg* 1982; 10:14.
11. Markowitz B, Manson PN, Mirvis S. Toward CT based facial fracture treatment. *Plast Reconstr Surg* 1990; 85:202.
12. Manson PN. Management of facial fractures. *Perspect Plastic Surg* 1988; 1:1.
13. Manson PN. The fourth dimension in facial injury treatment. In: *Proceedings of the Walter Reed Bone Symposium.* Washington: U.S. Government Printing Office, 1989.
14. Manson PN, Crawley WA, Yaremchuk MJ, et al. Midface fractures: advantages of extended open reduction and immediate bone grafting. *Plast Reconstr Surg* 1985; 76:1.
15. Leech P, Patterson A. Conservative and operative management of cerebrospinal leakage after closed head injury. *Lance* 1973; 1:1013.
16. Haines SJ. Systemic antibiotic prophylaxis in neurological surgery. *Neurosurgery* 1980; 6:355.
17. Hoff JT, Brewin AU. Antibiotics for basilar skull fractures. *J Newsurg* 1976; 44:649.
18. Klastersky J, Sadeghi M, Brihaye J. Antimicrobial prophylaxis in patient with rhinorrhea and otorrhea: a double blind study. *Surg Neurol* 1976; 6:111.
19. Gruss JS, MacKinnon SE. Complex maxillary fractures: the role of buttress stabilization and immediate bone grafting. *Plast Reconstr Surg* 1985; 75:303.
20. Gruss JE, MacKinnon SE, Kassek E, et al. The role of primary bone grafting in complex craniomaxillofacial trauma. *Plast Reconstr Surg* 1985; 75:17.
21. Irby WB, Rast WC. Extracranial fixation of the facial skeleton: Review and report of case. *J Oral Surg* 1969; 27:900.
22. Stranc MF, Robertson GA. A classification of internal injuries of the nasal skeleton. *Ann Plast Surg* 1979; 2:468.
23. Markowitz B, Manson PN, Sargent L, et al. Management of the medial canthal tendon in nasoethmoid-orbital fractures: the importance of the central fragment in treatment and classification. *Plast Reconstr Surg* 1991; 87:843.
24. Zide B, McCarthy J. The medial canthus revisited: An anatomical basis for canthopexy. *Ann Plast Surg* 1983; 9:1.

25. Gruss JS. Naso-ethmoid-orbital fractures: classification and role of primary bone grafting. *Plast Reconstr Surg* 1985; 75:303.

26. Pasker JP, Manson PN. The bimanual examination for assessing instability in naso-ethmoidal orbital injuries. *Plast Reconstr Surg* 1989; 83:165.

27. Gruss JS, Hurwitz JJ, Nik NA, et al. The pattern and incidence of nasolacrimal injury in naso-orbito-ethmoid fractures: the role of delayed assessment and dacryocystorhinostomy. *Br J Plast Surg* 1985; 38:116.

28. Gillies HD, Kilner TP, Stone D. Fractures of the malar-zygomatic compound: with a description of a new x-ray position. *Br J Surg* 1927; 14:651.

29. Knight JS, North JF. The classification of malar fractures: an analysis of displacement as a guide to treatment. *Br J Plast Surg* 1961; 13:325.

30. Yanagisawa B. Pitfalls in the management of zygomatic fractures. *Laryngoscope* 1973; 83:527.

31. Covington DS, Wainwright DJ, Teichgraeber JF, et al. Changing patterns in the epidemiology and treatment of zygoma fractures: a 10-year review. *J Trauma* 1994; 37:243.

32. Reinhart GC, Marsh JL, Hemmer KM, et al. Internal fixation of malar fractures: an experimental biophysical study. *Plast Reconstr Surg* 1989; 84:21.

33. Davidson J, Nickerson D, Nickerson B. Zygomatic fractures: comparison of methods of internal fixation. *Plast Reconstr Surg* 1990; 80:1.

34. Dal Santo F, Ellis E, Throckmorton GS. The effects of zygomatic complex fracture on masseteric muscle force. *J Oral Maxillofac Surg* 50:791.

35. Bahr W, Bagambisa FB, Schlegel G, et al. Comparison of transcutaneous incisions used for exposure of the infraorbital rim and orbital floor: a retrospective study. *Plast Reconstr Surg* 1992; 90:858.

36. Manson PN, Ruas E, Illif N, et al. Single lower-eyelid incision for exposure of the zygomatic bone and orbital reconstruction. *Plast Reconstr Surg* 1987; 79:210.

37. Manson PN. Frontobasilar fractures. I. Experimental mechanism and classification. II. Clinical management. (Submitted for publication.)

38. Heckler FR. Discussion of Luce EA: Frontal sinus fractures: Guidelines to management. *Plast Reconstr Surg* 1987; 80:509.

39. Mervill LC, Derome P. Concomitant dislocations of the face and skull. *J Maxillofacial Surg* 1978; 6:2.

40. Newman MH, Travis LW. Frontal sinus fractures. *Laryngoscope* 1973; 83:1281.

41. Pollak K, Payne E. Fractures of the frontal sinus. *Otolaryngol Clin North Am* 1976; 9:517.

42. Stanley R. Fractures of the frontal sinus. *Clin Plast Surg* 1989; 16:115.

43. Schenck NL. Frontal sinus disease. III. Experimental and clinical factors in failure of the frontal osteoplastic operation. *Laryngoscope* 1975; 85:76.

44. Wolfe SA, Johnson P. Frontal sinus injuries: primary care and management of late complications. *Plast Reconstr Surg* 1988; 92:78.

45. Nadell J, Kline DG. Primary reconstruction of depressed frontal skull fractures including those involving the sinus, orbit and cribriform plate. *J Neurosurg* 1974; 41:200.

46. Schultz RC. Supraorbital and glabellar fractures. Presented before the American College of Surgeons, Chicago, 1982.

47. Larrabee WF, Travis LW, Tabb HG. Frontal sinus fractures—their suppurative complications and surgical management. *Laryngoscope* 1980; 90:1810.

48. Le Fort R. Étude experimental sur les fracturs de la Machoire superieure. Partis I, II, III. *Rev Chir Paris* 1901; 23:208, 360, 479.

49. Manson PN. Some thoughts on the classification and treatment of Le Fort fractures. *Ann Plast Surg* 1986; 17:356.

50. Rudderman R, Mullen R. Biomechanics of the facial skeleton. *Clin Plast Surg* 1995; 19:11–30.

51. Sturla F, Absi D, Buquet J. Anatomic and mechanical considerations of craniofacial fractures: an experimental study. *Plast Reconstr Surg* 1980; 66:815.

52. Stanley RB Jr. Reconstruction of midface vertical dimension following Le Fort fractures. *Arch Otorhinolaryngol* 1984; 110:571.

53. Manson PN, Romano J, Crawley W, et al. Incomplete Le Fort fractures. *Plast Reconstr Surg* 1990; 85:355.

54. Salyer R, Jackson I, Whittaker L, et al. *Atlas of cranial-maxillofacial Surgery.* St. Louis: CV Mosby, 1980.

55. Manson PN, Hoopes JE, Su CT. Structural pillars of the facial skeleton: an approach to the management of Le Fort fractures. *Plast Reconstr Surg* 1980; 64:54.

56. Sofferman RA, Danielson PA, Quatela V, et al. Retrospective analysis of surgically treated Le Fort fractures. *Arch Otolaryngol* 1983; 109:466.

57. Stanley RB, Nowak GM. Midfacial fractures: the importance of angle of impact to horizontal craniofacial buttresses. *Otolaryngol Head Neck Surg* 1985; 93:186.

58. Row LD, Brandt-Zawadski M. Spacial analysis of midfacial fractures with multidirectional and computed tomography: clinipathologic correlates in 44 cases. *Otolaryngol Head Neck Surg* 1982; 90:651.

59. Gruss JS, Miacinnon SE, Kassel EE, et al. The role of primary bone grafting in complex cranio-maxillofacial trauma. *Plast Reconstr Surg* 1985; 75:17–24.

60. Manson P. Facial bone healing and grafts: a review of clinical physiology. *Clin Plast Surg* 1994; 21:331–348.

61. Gruss JS, Pollock RS, Phillips JH, et al. Combined injuries of the cranium and face. *Br J Plast Surg* 1989; 42:385–398.

62. Manson PN, Markowitz B, Mirvis S, et al. Toward CT-based facial fracture treatment. *Plast Reconstr Surg* 1990; 85:202.

63. Stanley RB. The zygomatic arch as a guide to reconstruction of comminuted malar fractures. *Arch Otolaryngol* 1989; 115:1459.

64. Yaremchuk MJ, Kim W-K. Soft tissue alterations associated with acute, extended open reduction and internal fixation of orbital fractures. *J Craniofac Surg* 1992; 3:134–140.

65. Phillips JH, Gruss JS, Wells MD, et al. Periosteal suspension of the lower eyelid and cheek following subciliary exposure of facial fractures. *Plast Reconstr Surg* 1991; 88:145.

66. Kelly K, Manson PN, Vander Kolk C, et al. Sequencing Le Fort fracture treatment. *J Craniofac Surg* 1990; 1:168–178.

67. Gruss JS, Van-Wyck L, Phillips JH, et al. The importance of the zygomatic arch in complex midfacial fracture repair and correction of post traumatic orbito-zygomatic deformities. *Plast Reconstr Surg* 1990; 85(6):878–890.

68. Gruss J, Bubak PJ, Egbert M. Craniofacial fractures: an algorithm to optimize results. *Clin Plast Surg* 1992; 19:195–206.

69. Manson PN. Reoperative facial fracture surgery. In: Grotting J, ed. *Reoperative plastic surgery.* St. Louis: Quality Medical Publishing, 1995.

70. Manson P, Clark N, Robertson B, et al. Comprehensive management of pan facial fractures. *J Craniofacial Trauma* 1995; 1:43–56.

71. Gruss J. Advances in craniofacial fracture repair. *Scan J Plast Reconstr Hand Surg (Suppl)* 1995; 27:67–81.

72. Gruss J. Craniofacial osteotomies and rigid fixation of post traumatic craniofacial deformities. *Scan J Plast Reconstr Hand Surg (Suppl)* 1995; 27:83–95.

73. Lacey M, Antonyshyn, O MacGregor, JA Temporal Contour Deformity after Cranial Flap Elevation—an anatomical study. *J Cranio Surg* 1994, 5:223–227.

74. Manson PN, Shack RB, Leonard LG, et al. Sagittal fractures of the maxilla and palate. *Plast Reconstr Surg* 1983; 72:484.

75. Manson P, Glassman D, Vander Kolk C, et al. Rigid stabilization of sagittal fractures of the maxilla and palate. *Plast Reconstr Surg* 1990; 85:711–716.

76. Irby W. *Facial Trauma and Concomitant Problems.* 2nd ed. St. Louis: CV Mosby, 1984.

77. Converse JM, Smith B, O'Bear MF, et al. Orbital blowout fractures: a 10-year survey. *Plast Reconstr Surg* 1967; 39:20.

78. Fujino T, Makino K. Entrapment mechanism and ocular injury in orbital blowout fracture. *Plast Reconstr Surg* 1980; 65:571.

79. Manson PN, Clifford CM, Su CT, et al. Mechanisms of global support and post-traumatic enohthalmos: (1) anatomy of the ligament sling and its relation to intramuscular cone orbital fat. *Plast Reconstr Surg* 1985; 77:193.

80. Metz HS, Scott WE, Madson E. Saccadic velocity and active force studies in blowout fractures of the orbit. *Am J Ophthalmol* 1975; 78:665.

81. Putterman AM, Steens T, Vrist MF. Nonsurgical management of blowout fractures of the orbital floor. *Am J Ophthalmol* 1974; 77:232.

82. Kawamoto HK Jr. Late post traumatic enophthalmos: a correctable deformity? *Plast Reconstr Surg* 1982; 69:423–432.

83. Manson PN, Illif N. Management of blow-out fractures of the orbital floor. II. Early repair for selected injuries. *Surv Ophthalmol* 1991; 35:280–292.

84. Antonyshyn O, Gruss JS, Kassell EE. Blow-in fractures of the orbit. *Plast Reconstr Surg* 1989; 84:10–20.

85. Putterman AM. Management of blow-out fractures of the orbital floor. III. The conservative approach. *Surv Ophthalmol* 1991; 35:292–298.

86. Messinger A, Radkowski MA, Greenwald MJ, et al. Orbital roof fractures in the pediatric population. *Plast Reconstr Surg* 1989; 84:213–218.

87. Hammerschlag SB, Hughes S, O'Reilly GV, et al. Blow-out fractures of the orbit: a comparison of computed tomography and conventional radiography with anatomical correlation. *Radiology* 1982; 143: 487–492.

88. Gilbard SM, Mafee MF, Lagouros PA, et al. Orbital blowout fractures. The prognostic significance of computed tomography. *Ophthalmology* 1985; 92:1523–1528.

89. Godoy J, Mathog RH. Malar fractures associated with exophthalmos. *Arch Otolaryngol* 1985; 111:174–747.

90. Mathog RH, Archer KF, Nesi FA. Posttraumatic enophthalmos and diplopia. *Otolaryngol Head Neck Surg* 1986; 94:69–77.

91. Schultz RC. Supraorbital and glabellar fractures. *Plast Reconstr Surg* 1970; 45:227.

92. Hedstrom J, Parsons J, Maloney J, et al. Superior orbital fissure syndrome: report of a case. *J Oral Surg* 1974; 32:198.

35

Mandibular Fractures

Norman Clark, M.D., D.M.D.

Mandibular form and function, the articulation of the mandible with the cranial base, and the mandible's support of the mobile portion of the occlusion are all unique. The mandible, the aesthetic as well as functional foundation of the lower face, is essential for many of the activities of daily living. With the prominence of the mandible, and its structure, mandibular fractures are common.

Goals in the management of mandibular fractures, include: restoration of the pre-injury form, function, and occlusion, or as close to the pre-injury condition as possible; achieving bony union reliably with the most cost-effective treatment available; and avoidance or minimization of the morbidity of the injury and of its treatment. Effective, safe management of mandibular fractures requires a thorough understanding of mandibular anatomy, and of the anatomy and function of the teeth and occlusion, as well as an adequate understanding of the enveloping soft tissues.

HISTORY

World War II was a period of major advances in the treatment of war injuries. A major development was the use of internal skeletal fixation of maxillary injuries and suspension techniques introduced by Milton Adams (1). Intramedullary pinning of maxillofacial fractures was first advocated by Major in 1938, with one or more 2-mm-diameter Kirschner wires being driven across the fracture. Such techniques did not adequately stabilize fractures, and maxillomandibular stabilization was also required (2). John Converse, treating British soldiers' mandibular fractures, adapted Roger Anderson's orthopedic external pin fixation to provide fracture stabilization without maxillomandibular stabilization (3). Numerous modifications have been made, most effectively a design by Joe Hall Morris, which remains in wide use today (4).

Robert Danis, a Belgian and a pupil of the Lambotte's (5–7), probably has made the greatest contributions to the field of internal fixation of fractures of any single individual. In 1949 he published *Theorie et Pratique de l'Ostéosynthéses* (8), which reported his vast experience in orthopedics, and put forth three requirements for internal fixation. First, he believed that no skeletal unit should be immobilized after fracture reduction. Such immobilization resulted in degenerative changes in the effected joints, bones, ligaments, and muscles ("fracture disease"). Danis so strongly believed in early mobilization that he espoused that internal fixation was indicated even in fractures that were not dislocated or that were easily reducible, so that the limb could be mobilized (8).

Pauwels published his investigations in tension/compression zone concept of bone biomechanics (9). He found that fixation devices should be placed where there is greatest force of tension from muscle forces and weight bearing, rather than in areas of surgical convenience. In 1958, Bagby and Jones reported a simple modification of a conventional noncompressive plate that allowed the induction of interfragmentary compression (10).

In Switzerland, a group led by Maurice Müller, who had spent time with Danis, adopted and expanded the principles of Danis. The group became known as the *Arbeitsgemeinschaft für Ostéosynthésefragen* (AO, or Association for Osteosynthesis) or Association for the Study of Internal Fixation (ASIF). The AO/ASIF group established four principles of fracture treatment that included: anatomic reduction, rigid internal fixation, atraumatic technique on bone and soft tissues, and early pain-free active mobilization during the first 10 postoperative days.

Advances in internal fracture fixation were applied somewhat more slowly to repair of maxillofacial fractures. Luhr published his development and use of a vitallium compression plate with self-tapping screws for mandible fractures in 1968 (11). Mittelmeir also reported the use of a compression plate for fracture treatment in 1968 (12). Also working in the late 1960s and early 1970s, Spiessl adapted the AO/ASIF principles and armamentarium to the treatment of mandibular fractures (13). The lag-screw technique was first introduced to maxillofacial surgery by Brons in 1970 (14). In 1973, Michelet reported the use of smaller, more easily adaptable, noncompression plates, placed transorally and affixed with unicortical screws for mandibular fracture treatments (15). In France, Champy's group has done extensive investigation of the use of miniplates for mandibular fracture treatment (16). Titanium, and titanium alloys, have essentially supplanted the use of stainless steel in maxillofacial skeletal fixation, though vitallium remains a useful implant alloy.

ETIOLOGY

Mandible fractures result when a sufficient force impacts on the lower face. An understanding of the mechanism of the injury underscores the importance of considering possible synchronous injuries (e.g., CNS, thoracic) that frequently accompany mandibular fractures.

Interpersonal violence, including blunt trauma (e.g., fist fights, assaults with blunt objects) and penetrating trauma (e.g., gunshot wounds), continues to be common causes of

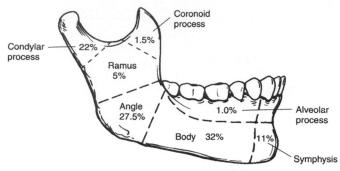

FIG. 35–1. The anatomic regions of the mandible with the percentages of frequency of fractures.

mandibular fractures, accounting for over 50% of mandibular fractures, several in series (17–20). This seems more often to do with males participating in interpersonal violence and other activity-related mechanisms of injury. Another form of interpersonal violence, the physical abuse of women and children, is probably significantly underreported, but may represent a common cause of mandibular fractures for some of these groups. In modern society, motor-vehicle accidents remain a frequent cause of mandibular fractures (23% [21], 25% [22]). Children have a lower overall frequency of mandibular fractures than adults, for several reasons (e.g., young children's bones are more resilient than adult bones, and less likely to fracture).

FREQUENCY

Mandibular fractures are the second most common facial fractures (after nasal fractures), accounting for between 10 and 25% of all facial fractures.

In compiling a number of series (17,18,19,22) for a combined total of 5451 patients with 8795 mandibular fractures, regional fracture frequencies were: body 31.9%, angle 27.5%, condyle 23.8%, parasymphysis 11.6%, symphysis 5.8%, ramus 2.5%, coronoid 1.8%, and alveolus 1.0% (Fig. 35–1). In children 10 years of age or younger, about two-thirds of mandibular fractures are of the condyle.

Basic Treatment Considerations

BIOMECHANICAL ASPECTS OF BONE HEALING

Strength and rigidity are the requisite qualities for bone function. Fractures disrupt bone continuity, altering load transmission, and disrupting bone's function.

Microanatomy of Bone

Bone is composed of inorganic mineral, organic matrix, and cells. The major component of bone (65%) is inorganic calcium phosphate crystals deposited as hydroxyapatite. The organic matrix, composing 35% of bone, consists of 95% collagen and 5% proteoglycans, and low-molecular-weight proteins. The cellular component of bone (less than 1%), consists of osteoblasts, osteocytes, and osteoclasts.

Osteoblasts differentiate from mesenchymal precursors and form osteoid, the organic precursor of bone. After deposition, the osteoid undergoes a sequence of maturation over a 10-day period prior to calcification. After maturation, the osteoid is mineralized along the calcification front. Two conditions are necessary for bone formation and mineralization: these include an ample vascular supply and stability.

Osteocytes, the cell type that osteoblasts mature into, are surrounded by the bone they have deposited. They still take part in calcium regulation (exchange of calcium between bone and body fluids), but do not form new osteoid or multiply.

Osteoclasts are multinucleated giant cells, thought to arise from the fusion of macrophages. These cells secrete hydrochloric acid from within the Howship lacuna (small subcellular organelles), dissolving the mineral component of bone. The organic matrix is degraded by collagenases and proteases. Osteoclastic activity is also requisite in bone maintenance, remodeling (adapting to changing stresses), and fracture healing.

Fracture Healing and Treatment

During fracture healing, there is an orderly evolution of various tissue types that develop or are induced during healing by the injury and by the conditions that prevail during healing. Elongation at rupture (the amount of elongation at the point of rupture) is a measure of the tolerance of tissues to tensile deformation (distraction). Granulation tissue, relatively elastic, tolerates elongation up to twice its original length before rupturing. However, granulation tissue has little strength to resist deformation (0.01 kg/mm^2 (i.e., little force is required to deform it). Other tissues (e.g., cartilage, 1.5 kg/mm^2; and bone, 12 kg/mm^2) are stronger—more resistant to strain (elongation)—but are progressively less tolerant of deformation. Successive tissues, increasingly stiff, form in and around the fracture, creating the stability necessary for bone formation and healing (i.e., fracture healing cascade [FHC] = hematoma→granulation tissue→fibrous tissue→cartilage→bone). Only those tissues that can tolerate the strain present across the interfragmentary gap can form in the fracture gap. As a tissue forms in the gap, it in turn decreases motion across the fracture, reducing interfragmentary strain. This reduction in strain allows, and perhaps promotes, the formation of the next tissue in the fracture healing cascade (23).

Other mechanisms also act at fracture sites to improve stability. Even with relatively stable fractures, there is resorption of fragment ends, and widening the interfragmentary gap, reducing interfragmentary strain per unit volume for a given amount of motion. Callous formation, by increasing the cross-sectional area of increasingly stiff tissues, increases resistance to deformation (24).

In practice, even the "anatomic" reduction results in interfragmentary areas of microscopic bony contact and areas of interfragmentary gapping. In the areas of bony contact, healing occurs, with osteons forming directly across the fracture. In the areas of microscopic gapping, the initial hematoma is replaced with sagittal bone (lamellar bone not formed about a central vascular supply), and secondarily remodeled with new osteons formed across the fracture, through the sagittal bone.

Therefore, in the circumstances of sufficient interfragmentary stability (rigid fixation), direct bone healing (contact and gap healing) occurs. In the circumstance of limited, relative, interfragmentary motion, indirect bony healing occurs. This is an orderly evolution of increasing rigid (and decreasingly strain tolerant) tissues in and around the fracture. Callous formation is an indication of indirect bone healing. In the circumstance of interfragmentary motion that exceeds the strain tolerance of the healing tissue forming within the fracture, indirect healing arrests, and nonunion occurs. Appropriate fracture management then consists of realignment of bony fragments to positions of optimal form and function ("anatomic reduction"), and techniques of stabilization to decrease or eliminate interfragmentary motion during healing ("adequate fixation," absolute or relative rigidity).

Traditional treatment of mandibular fractures with maxillomandibular stabilization (MMS) effectively removes or reduces active biomechanical considerations, though the muscles of mastication are never without some degree of activity and tone. Modern techniques of fracture treatment aim to achieve fracture union reliably, with minimal morbidity and enough stability to allow earlier return to function.

Placement of bicortical affixed plates on the inferio-lateral margin with unicortically affixed plates at the superior margin may reasonably be expected to effect an adequate result. Similarly, a combination of smaller miniplates for fixation may be adequate in the parasymphyseal region, based on smaller tensile and torsional forces being generated anteriorly. These may provide adequate fixation in regions where there is low probability of compressive loading.

Ellis (25) has measured bite forces in patients with mandibular fractures and found a significant reduction in bite forces for at least 6 weeks after fracture treatment. Therefore, at least initially, the fixation system used to reconstruct mandibular fractures may not be subjected to full, normal functional loading.

The fixation systems available today for rigid internal fixation will work reliably if they are properly instrumented and appropriate plates are selected for each specific fracture situation. If the physician is interested in simple solutions, more conservative treatment (i.e., larger palates, bicortical screws, longer periods of maxillomandibular stabilization) should be used. Understanding the stress distribution of the intact and fractured facial skeleton will aid in fracture management, ideally promoting optimal treatment with reproducible results.

In most metallic implants designed for fixation of maxillofacial fractures, the implants are made of alloys. (Alloys are mixtures of crystals of differing metals or compounds, intermixed microscopically into separate but contiguous phases.) Many of the implant alloys in use today, such as commercially pure titanium, are relatively resistant to corrosion.

ANATOMIC CONSIDERATIONS

The Mandible

Form follows (derives from) function, and both mandibular form and function are unique. For the purpose of mandibular fracture management, the mandible has been classified into several anatomic regions. The mandible may be considered as having two major divisions. The horizontal (anterior) portion supports the dentition, forming a U-shaped arch that connects the two vertical segments. The vertical (posterior) portions serve as the insertion for the muscles of mastication and forms the articulation of the mandible with the skull. The posterior vertical segments, the rami and condyles, oriented somewhat obliquely to the horizontal segment, create leverage with significant mechanical advantage for the development of chewing forces by the muscles of mastication.

The horizontal portion of the mandible may be divided into the alveolus and basilar bone. The alveolus supports the dental roots. The basilar bone may be further subdivided into the anterior parasymphysis region (which we will consider to include the symphysis mentalis), and the two lateral body regions. The parasymphysis supports the anterior alveolar segment containing the mandibular incisors. The body segments support the alveolar segments containing the premolar and molar teeth. Blood supply to the mandible is partly provided by the inferior alveolar artery. However, significant vascularity also is contributed through the insertions of muscles onto the mandible, and by a plexus of vessels in the mucogingival insertions onto the mandible. An appreciation of this multiple blood supply to the mandible allows safe surgical access and application of internal fixation of mandibular fractures.

The vertical portion of the mandible may also be subdivided into several regions: the angle, the ramus, the coronoid, and the condyle. The mandibular angle region is worthy of its own subdivision because of the concentration of stresses between the horizontal and vertical segments of the mandible and the propensity towards fracture healing problems. The angles are thin in the mediolateral aspect, with less surface area in fractures for bony buttressing and screw placement. This thinness and concavity of the angle region, especially when the roots of a horizontally impacted 3rd molar also encroaches into the angle region, significantly weaken the region.

Nerve Anatomy

There are two nerves that are most relevant to mandibular fracture repair: the mandibular division of the trigeminal nerve and the facial nerve (especially the marginal mandibular branch).

The main trunk of the sensory portion of the mandibular nerve continues inferiorly from foramen ovale and divides into the lingual nerve and inferior alveolar nerve, medial to the mandibular ramus. The lingual nerve passes anteriorly into the lateral tongue. The inferior alveolar nerve enters the medial aspect of the mandible through the mandibular foramen, at roughly the height of the occlusal plan of the posterior teeth (1.5 to 2 cm below the sigmoid notch). The nerve transverses the angle and body regions of the mandible within the mandibular canal. The canal dips inferiorly, usually well below the level of the mandibular and mental foramens, sometimes coming to within a centimeter or less of the inferior border of the mandible. The canal also comes to lie somewhat closer to the lateral surface of the mandible than to the lingual aspect. Therefore, in these regions, the only safe place for bicortical screws is along the inferior border of the mandible. The zone over the mandibular canal is unsafe for even unicortical screws. Safe placement of unicortical screws is below the apices of the dental roots, (usually no more than twice the length of the crown) and above the mandibular canal.

Another craniofacial nerve of relevance to surgical access to the mandible is cranial nerve VII, the facial nerve. It is primarily a motor nerve, innervating the muscles of facial expression, as well as the posterior belly of the digastric muscle and the stylohyoid muscle. The nerve exits the skull via the stylomastoid foramen, and promptly enters the substance of the parotid gland. Within the gland, the nerve most commonly divides into upper (temporofacial) and low (cervicofacial) divisions. Within the gland, the nerve further subdivides into five or more branches; however, there are multiple anastomoses between the branches and highly variable patterns of branching. The branches are named (temporal, zygomatic, buccal, marginal mandibular, and cervical), but these are their regions of distribution rather than individual branches. After branching within the gland, the terminal branches distribute to the mimetic muscles within the tissue plane deep to the platysma muscle and the superiorly contiguous superficial musculoaponeurotic layer.

The main nerve and temporofacial division are at risk during the preauricular approach to the temporomandibular joint and condyle. The safest approach is to identify the nerve during the dissection. Proximacy to the nerve can be best identified with the use of a nerve stimulator, so long as the patient has not been administered a muscle relaxant (the current, conducted along the nerve, stimulates the mimetic muscles). The temporal branch or branches (frequently two) cross over the lateral aspect of the zygomatic arch a variable distance (anywhere from 8 to 33 mm, and typically 20 mm) anterior to the external auditory canal. Therefore, the temporal branches can be protected by incision through skin, superficial fascia, and periosteum no more than 8 mm anterior to the external ear canal. This route of dissection should also leave the auriculotemporal nerve in the anterior soft-tissue flap, where it may be preserved. For more generous access to the condyle, the main nerve trunk may be identified by dissecting along the anterior aspect of the tragal cartilage. The nerve can be identified about 2 cm deep to the skin, before it enters the parotid gland, posterior and perhaps deep to the posterior border of the ramus and condyle. Access to the joint and condyle must begin superioposterior to the temporofacial and temporal branches of the nerve. Once access to the condyle has been obtained, subperiosteal dissection may be safely performed deep to the parotid and branches of the nerve.

External approaches to the angle region, sub and post mandibular incisions, place the inferior branches of the nerve (especially the cervicofacial trunk and its branches, the marginal mandibular, and cervical branches) at risk. The nerves are within the substance of the parotid, or more distally, deep to the platysma muscle. Dingman and Grabb found there was a single marginal mandibular nerve in 21% of their specimens. More commonly, there were more than one branch (67% had two branches, 9% had three branches, and 3% had four branches) (26).

Therefore, it is recommended that the submandibular incision be placed at least 1.5 cm below the border of the mandible in the angle region. It is also recommended to confirm the location of the nerve in the superior flap with a nerve stimulator.

In the (post) retromandibular approach, the cervicofacial division courses, anteroinferior and somewhat lateral, through the parotid gland to become more superficial than the posterior border of the ramus and angle. The marginal mandibular nerve may cross the angle before dipping below the inferior border of the mandible. Access to the mandible may be gained between the buccal and mandibular branches of the facial nerve. However, this places important nerve branches on either side of the incision and, as noted before, there is a highly variable pattern of branching of the mandibular branch. An approach between the mandibular and cervical branches may be safer, though this approach places the incision more or less over the retromandibular vein, which is located deep to the terminal branches of the nerve.

The external carotid artery ascends the upper neck deep to the mandible, on a course roughly paralleling the posterior border of the ramus. The superficial temporal artery is given off and passes laterally, posterior to the mandible, through the parotid towards the temporal scalp.

Deep to the angle-ramus area, the internal maxillary artery curves anteriorly. The facial artery (external maxillary artery) descends over the submandibular salivary gland, curving around the inferior border of the mandible in the body region, becoming superficial to the mandible. The facial artery then ascends over the lateral aspect of the mandible deep to the branches of the facial nerve.

Another important branch of the maxillary artery is the inferior alveolar branch that enters the mandible through the mandibular foramen with the inferior alveolar nerve. This branch represents an important vascular supply to the mandible and mandibular teeth.

Musculature

It is important to understand the direction of pull of the muscles inserting directly on the mandible. These forces acting on a fracture site must be anticipated and compensated for when the fracture is reduced and fixated. Several groups of muscles attach to, and effect the stability of, mandible fractures. The muscles of mastication, all attached posterior to the dentition, serve to elevate or protrude the mandible. The elevators (Fig. 35–2) (masseter, medial pterygoid, and temporalis muscles) can generate 50 lb/in (27) of biting force at the occlusal surfaces of the posterior teeth. The temporalis muscle originates in the temporal fossa on the skull and inserts onto the coronoid process and the superior aspect of the external oblique line. The masseter inserts on the lateral aspect of the mandibular angle and originates from the zygoma. The medial pterygoid inserts on the medial aspect of the angle, arising from the medial aspect of the lateral pterygoid plate and pyramidal process of the palatine bone. The two muscles effectively form a sling supporting the mandibular angle. The inferior belly of the lateral pterygoid originates from the lateral pterygoid plate and inserts onto the scaphoid fossa of the condyle and joint capsule. The lateral pterygoid produces protrusion of the mandible when contracting—either unilaterally, allowing mandibular deviation to the side opposite the contraction, or bilaterally, to produce protrusion. The superior belly of the lateral pterygoid originates from the sphenoid bone and inserts on the fibrous capsule and meniscus of the temporomandibular joint (TMJ), coordinating the position of the meniscus during condylar and jaw movement. In condylar neck fractures, the effect of the lateral pterygoid tends to displace the condyle medially and anteriorly, and to displace the meniscus anteriorly (see Fig. 35–2).

Some orientations of fractures are considered "favorable" or "unfavorable," depending on whether the predominant muscle forces tend to reduce or to distract the fracture site. The superiorly directed force of the masseter, medial pterygoid, and temporalis muscles (elevating muscles) may cause

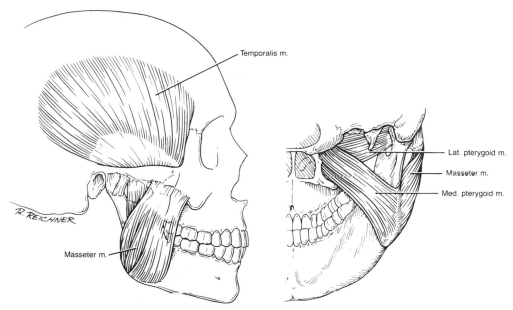

FIG. 35–2. The muscles of mastication.

a decrease in height of the posterior mandible with fractures of the vertical mandible, resulting in occlusal prematurities and an anterior open-bite deformity. When the line of the fracture goes through the mandibular angle, there may be enough of the masseter-medial pterygoid muscle sling on each side of the fracture site to tend to stabilize the fragments (Figs. 35–3, 35–4). However, with improved understanding of the biomechanics of mandibular fractures, and with routine postoperative radiologic evaluation of treatment results, the favorability or unfavorability of the fracture orientation, relative to these muscle forces, has become much less important in the appropriate treatment planning.

Muscles other than the muscles of mastication also can affect fracture stability. Segmental fractures of the body may be medially displaced by tension from the mylohyoid muscles, and in a bilateral parasymphyscal fracture, the anterior mandible may be posteriorly displaced by the geniohyoid and digastric muscles (Figs. 35–5, 35–6, 35–7, 35–8).

Temporomandibular Joint (TMJ)

The temporomandibular joints, the only ginglymoarthrodial joints (capable of both rotation [hinge joint], and translation [gliding joint]), must always work together in a coordinated pair to allow the complex movements of chewing, speech, and so on. The TMJ is a compound joint, with two synovial joints separated by a fibrous articular disc, the meniscus. When the normal condyle-disc-temporal relationships are disrupted, an internal derangement of the joint occurs that results in dysfunction, such as TMJ pain, clicking, locking, limited motion, and articular or disk degeneration. The joint is surrounded by a strong capsule, thickened laterally into the temporomandibular ligament.

Dentoalveolar Anatomy

The requisite basis for evaluation and treatment of dentoalveolar trauma is a working knowledge of dental anatomy and occlusion. There are 20 teeth in the primary (deciduous) dentition: maxillary and mandibular central and lateral in-

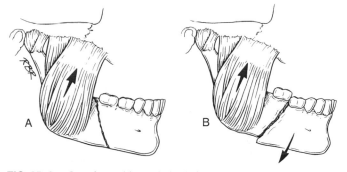

FIG. 35–3. **A,** unfavorable angle-body fracture. **B,** favorable fracture.

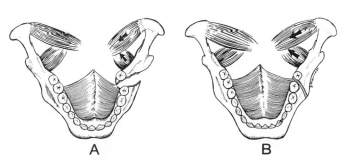

FIG. 35–4. **A,** unfavorable angle, and **B,** favorable fracture location.

cisors, canines, and 1st and 2nd molars. The adult secondary (permanent) dentition is composed of 32 teeth: maxillary central and lateral incisors, canines (cuspids), 1st and 2nd premolars (bicuspids), and 1st, 2nd, and 3rd molars.

Both sets of dentition begin development in utero. The deciduous teeth begin erupting during the 1st year of life, and eruption is usually complete by 3 years of age. The permanent dentition begins erupting by about 6 years of age, with the central incisors replacing the deciduous central incisors, and the permanent 1st molars erupting distal (posterior) to the deciduous 2nd molars. The remaining deciduous teeth are

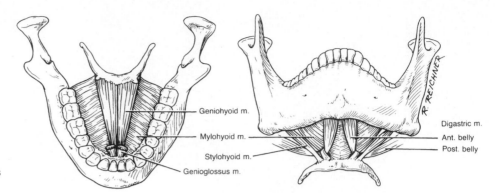

FIG. 35–5. Muscles of the floor of the mouth and suprahyoid region depressors of the mandible.

Geniohyoid m.
Mylohyoid m.
Stylohyoid m.
Genioglossus m.

Digastric m.
Ant. belly
Post. belly

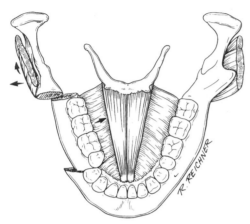

FIG. 35–6. Segmental fractures of the mandibular body displaced medially by the action of the mylohyoid musculature.

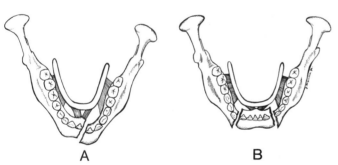

A   B

FIG. 35–7. A, a unilateral fracture in the mandibular midline will be displaced lingually by the action of the geniohyoid and mylohyoid musculature. **B,** the mechanism of pull of the geniohyoid and mylohyoid musculature.

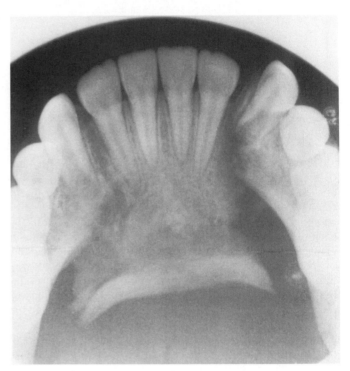

FIG. 35–8. Bilateral symphyseal mandibular fracture shown on an intraoral inferior-superior oblique projection. The teeth, alveolar process, and inferior border of the mandible are fractured as a unit, with displacement lingually by the genihyoid and mylohyoid muscle.

replaced by their secondary counterparts by 12 or 13 years of age. The permanent premolars replace the deciduous molars.

The occlusal relationship of the maxillary to mandibular teeth in the patient's habitual position of maximal intercuspation is classified into three groups by angle, based on the relative positions of the first molars and canine teeth. Class I occlusion (normoocclusion) has the mandibular teeth slightly mesial (anterior) to the corresponding maxillary teeth. Specifically, the mesiobuccal cusp of the maxillary first molar fits into the mesiobuccal groove of the mandibular 1st molar. The cusp of the maxillary canine fits over the groove between the mandibular canine and first premolar. Class II occlusion (distoocclusion) has the mandibular teeth positioned more posteriorly than in Class I occlusion. The mesiobuccal cusp of the maxillary 1st molar fits into the groove between the mandibular 2nd premolar and the 1st molar. The cusp of the maxillary cuspid is anterior to the cusp of the mandibular cuspid. Class III occlusion (mesioocclusion) is a relative anterior position of the mandibular teeth compared to the maxillary teeth. The mesiobuccal cusp of the maxillary 1st molar fits into the distobuccal groove of the mandibular 1st molar, and the cusp of the maxillary cuspid fits into the groove between the 1st and 2nd mandibular premolars. Often, there is also a cross-bite of the mandibular incisors anterior to the maxillary incisors.

The horizontal mandible is composed of the thick corticocancellous (basilar) bone, forming a foundation for the alveolar process. The alveolar process abuts along the superior

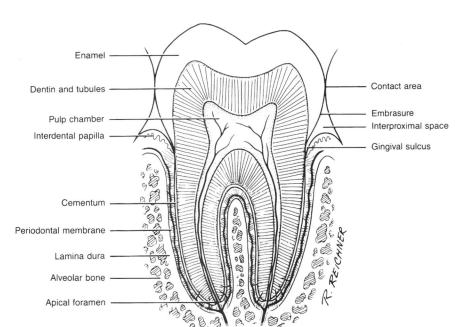

Enamel

Dentin and tubules

Pulp chamber

Interdental papilla

Cementum

Periodontal membrane

Lamina dura

Alveolar bone

Apical foramen

Contact area

Embrasure

Interproximal space

Gingival sulcus

FIG. 35–9. The anatomy of a molar tooth surrounded by alveolar bone. Note that blood supply to the pulp chamber in the molar is via the apex of the root.

border of the basilar horizontal mandible, and supports the teeth. Each tooth is supported in a socket, the remnant of the developmental crypt from which the tooth developed. The alveolus is formed of moderately thick cortical bone that varies in thickness overlaying the tooth sockets (6 to 8 mm posteriorly, and less than 1 mm anteriorly). Cancellous bone fills between the cortices and around the tooth sockets. Each tooth socket is lined with a thin but strong sheath of cortical bone, the lamina dura. The dental roots are suspended within the alveolar sockets by the periodontal ligaments (Fig. 35–9). The root-to-crown length ratio of most teeth is 2:1. The mandibular molars have two roots (mesial and distal), and the premolars usually have one or two partially fused roots (facial and lingual).

The strength of the periodontal ligament allows some degree of control of the attached bony segments. The incisor teeth have single, conical roots that are not routinely useful for circumdental ligatures to an arch bar, even if the teeth are uninjured, because of the tendency to extrude them from their sockets. Also, the length and location of the roots affects safe screw placement for fixation.

ACCESS TO THE MANDIBLE

Success in the operative management of facial fractures, including those of the mandible, depends on adequate access to and exposure of the involved skeleton. The primary factor in incision placement is not usually surgical convenience, but facial aesthetics; thus, techniques have been developed to place surgical incisions for access to the facial skeleton in inconspicuous areas, sometimes distant from the underlying skeletal condition being treated. For example, placement of incisions through the oral mucosa allows superb access of much of the facial skeleton and results in a completely hidden scar.

A factor that differentiates facial surgery from other skeletal surgery is the location and proximity of nerves (especially the facial nerve) and the muscles of facial expression. These muscles are subcutaneous structures, and the facial nerve supplying them can be easily traumatized if incisions are placed across their path.

Another factor important in facial surgery is the presence of many important sensory nerves traversing the facial skeleton at multiple locations. The facial soft tissues have more sensory input per unit area then soft tissues anywhere else in the body. Loss of this sensory input can be a great inconvenience for the individual.

Transoral Access

The mandibular vestibular approach is useful for surgical access to the parasymphyseal, as well as anterior, body regions; however, extension allows a relatively safe access to the entire facial surface of the mandible from condyle to symphysis. One advantage of this technique is the ability constantly to assess the dental occlusion during surgery. Of great benefit for aesthetic outcome is that the scar is hidden intraorally. Complications from the access are relatively few, but include mental nerve damage and lip malposition, both of which can be minimized with proper technique. Atraumatic technique with rigid fixation makes the approach safe, with acceptable low rates of wound infection, not different from extraoral approaches.

Incisions should be placed in the alveolar or buccal mucosa, and not through the gingiva. In the premolar region, the mental nerve should be identified and preserved. Anteriorly, the mentalis muscle is elevated inferiorly to provide access to the parasymphyseal region. After reduction and fixation, the mentalis muscle should be resuspended in its original position to avoid postoperative deformity. Closure is in two or more layers: muscle/fascia, and mucosa.

Transbuccal Access (Trocar Technique)

Transbuccal access is actually a combined intraoral and extraoral access (albeit very limited extraoral access). The access requires trocars, and instrumentation to fit through the trocars.

By working through the separate site, drilling and screwing can be done more perpendicular to plate and bone surface. Sufficient access must still be provided for fracture reduction, plate adaptation, and positioning the plate over the reduced fracture—usually a routine intra or extra oral incision.

Once the plate is positioned, it is usually fixed in place through the standard access incision. The accessory incisions are located roughly over the plate and up to several plate holes. Skin and subcutaneous incision may be down to the platysma, then blunt direction by spreading with a fine hemostat or with the penetrating tip of the trocar. Once placed through the overlaying soft tissues, many of the trocar system have some method of retention to help retract the soft tissues and to avoid accidental withdrawal of the trocar. After screw placement and trocar removal, the accessory incision may be closed in layers at the dermis and skin.

Transcutaneous Access

A number of surgical exposures may provide access to much of the mandible. Though leaving an apparent scar, such access avoids heavy inoculation of the fracture site with oral fluids and microbes. Judiciously placed incisions usually heal quite inconspicuously, while providing adequate access for reduction and fixation.

Submental Approach

Access to the inferior aspect of the mandible can be provided through the submental incision. Even a limited incision of a few centimeters provides access to the parasymphyseal and anterior body regions. The incision may be extended posterolaterally beneath the body of the mandible to gain access to the more posterior body and angle regions. However, this external scar is more apparent, as it does not follow typical rhytids or the lines of minimal skin tension.

This access has the advantage of not requiring the complete division of the mentalis muscle origin from the mandible. Also, the mental nerves are well protected during this exposure.

Submandibular (Modified Risdon) Approach

The modified Risdon incision is a curved incision placed on the lateral neck below the mandibular angle, extending 2 to 4 cm in length. It provides access from the ramus-sigmoid notch area to the midbody region. With anterior extension, the anterior body region can be approached. The curved incision, for access of the angle, is started 2 cm below the angle, to avoid the marginal mandibular branch of the facial nerve. If possible, the incision is placed in a neck rhytid or along lines of minimal skin tension. As the marginal mandibular nerve is located beneath the platysma muscle, the incision may be taken rapidly through the muscle. However, because of anatomic variation in the location of the nerve in relationship to the inferior mandibular border, muscle relaxants should be avoided for anesthesia, so that a nerve stimulator can be used to identify the location of the nerve during dissection in order to expose the mandible. At the subplatysmal level, until the course of the nerve is identified relative to the incision, the dissection proceeds by blunt spreading dissection towards the mandibular border, which should be easily palpable. When the inferior or posterior border of the mandible is exposed, the periosteum is incised and elevated. The broad insertion of the masseter muscle may be quite tenacious. Enough elevation should be done to expose the fracture adequately for reduction and fixation.

Postmandibular Approach

The incision is made 1 to 2 cm posterior to the border of the mandible, in a rhytid or along lines of minimal skin tension. The inferior branches of the facial nerve are anterior to this plane. Skin is incised deep to (through) the platysma muscle. With care, the great auricular nerve can be identified and preserved, being reflected posteriorly. Usually a plane of dissection can be developed between the auricular nerve and the posterior border of the parotid. Branches of the external jugular vein may be encountered, and can be ligated. A plane is developed over the sternocleidonastoid muscle (SCM) and deep to the parotid, anteriorly to the palpable border of the mandible.

The incision provides good access to the angle, ramus, and posterior body regions. Access to the condyle neck and coronoid process are gained by extensive elevation of the masseter and periosteum. Dissecting subperiosteally over the lateral aspect of the mandible will be safe for the facial nerve within the parotid gland.

Preauricular Approach

The preauricular access provides exposure of the lateral condyle and TMJ, through an anatomically busy area. It is important to avoid injury, during exposure of the TMJ, to the facial nerve (27). The facial nerve, shortly after exiting the skull through the stylomastoid foramen, enters the substance of the parotid gland. Within the gland the nerve subdivides, usually in to two trunks (temporofacial and cervicofacial), and then into five or more peripheral branches (temporal, zygomatic, buccal, marginal mandibular, and cervical). When extensive access to the condyle and temporomandibular joint is required, it is best to identify the nerve. This may best be done with a nerve stimulator. The main nerve may be found, about 2 cm to the skin, by following the anterior aspect of the tragal cartilage with blunt dissection. The temporofacial or temporal branches may be found crossing the zygomatic arch from 8 to 30 mm (usually about 20 mm) anterior to the meatus. So, dissection may be rapid over the posterior arch, with excision of the periosteum posterior to the facial nerve branches identified with a nerve stimulator (27).

Management of Mandibular Fractures

Management of mandibular fractures is directed towards restoration of the preinjury relationships between jaws and dentition, achieving a stable bone union of fracture fragments, and maintaining or restoring facial proportion and symmetry, while avoiding complications of the injury and treatment.

EVALUATION

History

A thorough history should be obtained, with attention to how and when the injury was sustained, and if there was any previous treatment. The patient should also be questioned about previous facial injuries, dental hygiene, tooth or periodontal disease, preinjury malocclusion and orthodontic treatment, and any TMJ symptoms.

Physical Examination

After carefully obtaining what history is available, the patient's symptoms should be elicited and a physical examination done to observe signs of injury. Subjective symptoms are reported by the patient, and for a mandibular injury may include pain, tenderness, loss of function, and an altered relationship of the teeth and occlusion. Objective signs of mandibular injuries include: deformity, abnormal mobility, malocclusion, crepitus, and swelling (28).

Airway and Overall Patient Evaluation

Even isolated mandibular injuries may contribute to potentially life-threatening conditions. Bleeding, dentures, or broken teeth can obstruct the airway or cause aspiration. Bilateral condylar and symphysis fractures may result in a "flail" mandible, allowing posterior displacement of the tongue and soft tissues and possible upper-airway obstruction. Mandibular fractures commonly have associated concurrent injuries of the head, spine, thorax, or abdomen. An essential first step is to rule out any of these conditions and any threat of airway interference. It is also necessary to undertake an overall evaluation of the patient, before the patient is taken for radiographs or to the operating room, again because of the frequency of associated injuries that may become life-threatening.

Oral and Dental Evaluation

Visual inspection should be done both externally and intraorally for asymmetry, malocclusion, lacerations, ecchymosis, fractured or displaced teeth, and restrictions or deviations in opening, closing, or protrusion. Intraoral ecchymosis or hematoma may indicate an underlying fracture. Careful external and internal palpation of the mandible will reveal areas of tenderness and bony step-off or crepitance. The condylar region may be palpated in the preauricular area and by placing the fingers in the external auditory canals.

A careful assessment of the dentition should be made, including an examination for any missing teeth (preinjury vs. acute), stability of remaining teeth and alveolus, and any intraoral wounds that may communicate with the fracture. Also, the degree of displacement of the dental arches, and their instability, should be assessed. The maxillary and mandibular teeth should be occluded to assess the nature of the posttraumatic occlusal relationship, and if possible to analyze the pretraumatic occlusion (analysis of wear facettes). Models made from dental impressions are useful in diagnosing malocclusion, as well as allowing a lingual view that is impossible in the patient.

Lacerations and Compound Fracture Assessment

Displaced fractures of the horizontal mandible usually lacerate the gingiva, and are compound fractures. Fractures extending through a tooth socket should also be considered compound. Any extraoral wounds should be carefully assessed for potential communication with the mandible and fracture.

Peripheral Nerve Evaluation

Two of the cranial nerves are commonly involved in mandibular fractures, the mandibular division of the trigeminal nerve, and the cervical and marginal mandibular branches of the facial nerve. Fractures of the horizontal mandible frequently compromise the mandibular canal. Often, the inferior alveolar branch of the mandibular division of the trigeminal nerve will be injured (usually contused). However, if a fracture interrupts the inferior alveolar nerve, there will be anesthesia of the mandibular teeth distal (anterior) to the fracture; this may also be true in the chin and lip if the fracture disrupts the nerve posterior to the mental foramen. If the branches of the facial nerve are injured, there will be weakness or paralysis of the innervated muscles of facial expression. Most often, the marginal mandibular branch is involved, resulting in weakness of the lower lip depressors. Any such deficiencies should be documented preoperatively.

Radiological Examination

Suspected mandibular fractures must be evaluated radiographically. Adequate radiologic evaluation of facial fractures is requisite for accurate efficient treatment planning and fracture treatment, as well as for thorough postoperative evaluation of treatment.

Different parts of the mandible may be seen better in each of these radiographic studies, but it is the panoramic view (pantograph) that may be the most informative, because it shows the entire mandible and allows evaluation of the state of dental health. The pantograph is a nonlinear tomogram, designed to take a curved "cut" through the lower face (through the jaws). A diagnostic quality pantograph will demonstrate the TMJs, the entire mandible and lower maxilla, as well as the dentition; all but the most subtle, nondisplaced root fractures should be visualized with this study. However, artifact (superimposition of the vertebral bodies) in the anterior symphysial region may obscure definition, and a fracture in this area may go undetected. Most pantograph machines require the patient to hold still during exposure, and to be seated upright, though some will accept a supine patient. Special film and equipment are necessary, and they are seldom available in the emergency room or the operating room.

The mandibular series usually includes a posterior-anterior (PA) view, Townes view, and right and left lateral oblique views. These views may be modified for the severely injured patient who must remain supine. To a large extent, this plain x-ray series has been superseded by the pantograph and computed tomograms (CTs). A mandibular series is a poor substitute for other radiographic studies. The chief advantage of this technique is that no special film or equipment is necessary, and little patient cooperation is required.

Dental (intraoral) periapical x rays are effective for showing detailed root and alveolar anatomy; preinjury dental disease can also be diagnosed. However, special films, processing, and x-ray equipment are required. The intraoral dental mandibular occlusal x-ray is very effective at showing the horizontal mandible's facial and lingual cortices, but again special film and equipment are necessary.

Computed tomography (CT) is the other essential study in the thorough evaluation of the mandible. An axial series of scans will visualize the horizontal mandible and condyles well, as fractures or displacements of these regions tend to be out of the plane of the scan. However, alveolar and root fractures may fall into the plane of the scan and be poorly visualized. Fractures of the thinner aspects of the horizontal mandible (angle, ramus, coronoid, and condyle neck), which often closely parallel the plane of the scan, may not be well visualized if not significantly displaced. Coronal scans and sagittal reconstructions are of benefit for subtle fractures of this region. Computed tomography is also an excellent tool for postoperative radiologic evaluation of the accuracy of the reconstruction. Computed tomography requires specialized equipment, generally widely available. Computed tomographic scans are relatively expensive, and the patient receives a moderate radiation dose.

INITIAL MANAGEMENT

Mechanisms of injury that inflict mandibular fractures commonly inflict other injuries as well. Other maxillofacial fractures (49%) frequently accompany mandibular fractures (29). Other potentially life-threatening injuries that may accompany mandibular fractures includes head injury, spinal cord injury, airway obstruction, hemorrhage, infection, blunt thoracic and abdominal injury, and long bone fracture. Such patients should receive the trauma resuscitation ABCs—a quick but systematic evaluation of major systems searching for associated injuries. The airway must be expectantly controlled, if the patient is unable to do so from impaired mental status, from injury, or from substance intoxication. Foreign bodies (e.g., blood clot, fractured or avulsed teeth) should be removed from the upper aerodigestive tract to preclude possible aspiration. Hemorrhage should be controlled, which often can be obtained with pressure (e.g., nasal packing for nose bleeds). Hemorrhage associated with unstable facial fractures usually decreases with stabilization of the fractures (e.g., MMS).

Because many mandibular fractures are open fractures, either to the skin or to the mouth, perioperative antibiotics are indicated. Fractures that involve tooth roots or alveolar sockets should be considered open fractures and treated accordingly; coverage should be tailored as specifically as possible. Penicillin remains a very inexpensive and therapeutically effective antibiotic. Clindamycin also has good gram-positive and anerobic coverage. Frequently, displaced fractures of the horizontal mandible will cause lacerations of the mucosa of the alveolus and floor of the mouth, wounds that may go unrecognized. Even if definitive fracture treatment is deferred, prompt care of facial wounds is necessary to reduce rates of infection. Such wounds, whether intraoral or extraoral, should be débrided of foreign material, copiously irrigated to reduce the microbiologic inoculum, and closed in an adequate fashion. Fractures should also be reduced and stabilized with interarch ligatures (MMS).

Mandibular fractures should be reduced as soon as possible after injury to minimize pain and decrease the risk of infection. Displaced, unstabilized fractures move, with increased injury, pain, and edema to the surrounding tissue. Over several days, soft-tissue edema transforms into tissue induration, with soft-tissue handling more difficult. Intraorally compounded fractures pump oral secretions into the fracture site with speech, swallowing, and other mandibular motions. Microbes multiply, causing infection. Hematoma organizes within the fracture, impairing reduction. Even after a few days of wound inflammation, fragment ends begin resorption, complicating reduction. Definitive care may be delayed for a few days without dire consequences; however, outcome is not improved by delay.

Some patients present some time after their injury, frequently with infected fractures. Infected wounds require débridement and antibiotics. Control of the infection may require delay of definitive fracture treatment. However, even such wounds, with adequate débridement, may be safely internally fixated if absolute rigidity is created; generally, a rigidly fixated foreign body placed in a surgically clean wound will not become infected. On the other hand, even without a preexisting infection, a *loose* foreign body is likely to become infected.

CHOICE OF FRACTURE TREATMENT

A very few mandibular fractures—those nondisplaced, stable, or incomplete—may be successfully treated with reduced function (soft diet), and expectant observation of the occlusion and mandible. The occlusion should be and remain stable, and the fracture site should become nontender. At least weekly observation of the dentition, occlusion, and fracture site is necessary for the first month, or longer. If the mandible becomes unstable and the occlusion changes, the treatment plan must be modified to allow reduction and greater stabilization.

Splints

Splints remain a useful technique of mandibular fracture treatment, as well as a useful adjunct to other management techniques. These include occlusal, lingual, and Gunning splints. Dental splints may stabilize loose teeth and alveolar fractures and provide occlusal stops when the patient is partially or fully edentulous. Gunning splints, or the patient's modified dentures, if they have adequate fit to the edentulous alveolar arches, are quite useful to stabilize edentulous mandibular fractures and to restore occlusal relationships with the maxilla.

Fabrication of mandibular splints requires models made from dental impressions of the patient. Taking of impressions of the maxilla and mandible entails the use of dental alginate and impression trays. For patients with multiple facial fractures, or other multiple injuries, impressions may need to be taken under general anesthesia. Taking impressions of the orally intubated patient can be challenging. The alginate is mixed to a paste consistency, loaded into the impression tray, and placed in the patient's mouth. The alginate takes a few minutes to set, and then is removed. After rinsing off blood and mucus, dental stone or plaster is mixed and poured into these impressions and allowed to set, creating models of the dental arches. If the fractures have not been reduced, or cannot be held in reduction at the time of impression taking (e.g., the impression is taken with interfragmentary malpositioning), the models may be cut and the individual segments aligned ("model surgery") for proper occlusion with sticky wax, so that they fit with the opposing model.

With the corrected models, a lingual or occlusal splint is made with the models mounted into an articulator. The stone models must be lubricated, or a separating medium used to prevent sticking of the acrylic, and a roll of partially set acrylic is placed between the models. For lingual splints, the acrylic roll is adapted to the lingual surfaces of the mandibular model with finger pressure. For an occlusal splint, the models are mounted into an articulator, with the roll of acrylic placed over the occlusal surfaces, and the models closed into the acrylic. The articulator should be set to leave a minimal residual opening between the teeth of 1 to 2 mm. After setting of the acrylic, the splint is then trimmed, and holes may be made along its edge to allow for the passage of wires. The lingual splint must be trimmed so as not to interfere with maximal intercuspation. Preparation of the models and splints takes some time, so after the splint is prepared the patient may be taken back to surgery and placed into maxillomandibular occlusion with the splint guiding the teeth into their proper positions. Circumdental ligatures, passing through the splint, stabilize the teeth against the splint.

Gunning splints are made for the edentulous mandible or maxilla, similar in construction to full dentures. Gunning splints may require stabilization to the mandible with circummandibular ligatures; maxillary Gunning splints require stabilization with suspension wires to the pyriform rim, orbital rim, or zygomatic arch. If the patient has adequately fitting dentures, these can be modified by the attachment of arch bars or by placing hooks or holes in the lateral surfaces for the passage of maxillomandibular wires. The anterior region of the splints or dentures may also be removed to permit eating and drinking, with the splints wired into place (Figs. 35–10, 35–11).

Interdental Ligatures and Arch Bars

Isolated dentoalveolar fractures, in which the teeth remain securely affixed in their sockets, can be treated by reduction and stabilization with interdental ligatures or an arch bar (Fig. 35–12). Such buccal or labial splinting methods may not adequately stabilize the fracture segments, and may be supplemented with a lingual splint, especially if one or more teeth are loose, adding stability and helping to prevent any vertical extrusion of the teeth by the arch bar. Mandibular fractures can be reduced, at least to some extent, by interdental ligatures, including teeth on either side of the fracture (bridle wire).

Many types of maxillomandibular stabilization (intermaxillary fixation) are available, but the arch bar is most commonly used. Regardless of the specific technique of interdental ligation, wires will be passed around and between the teeth. Such wires should be placed apical to the heights of contour of the teeth, and apical to the contact points of adjacent teeth, in order to be stable on the teeth. However, care should be taken to avoid injury to the gingiva—especially the interdental papilla. Careless passing of the circumdental ligatures, strangling or piercing the papilla, just serves to create soft-tissue wounds in proximity to the most virulent oral flora, increasing the risk of soft-tissue infection. Also, the twisted ends of the wires, as well as exposed ends of arch bars, should be carefully positioned to avoid exposed sharp ends that can inflict painful wounds on the patient's mucosa, an additional potential sources of infection; these sharp ends can also inoculate the unwary surgeon with the patient's blood, saliva, and dental plaque.

A number of loop interdental ligatures have been developed for fracture stabilization. The chief advantage of such

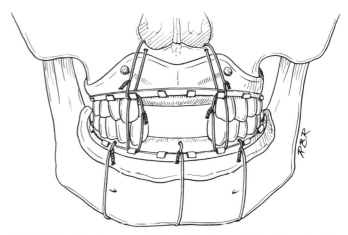

FIG. 35–10. Dentures modified as Gunning splints. Note: Fixation is by circummandibular wires for the lower splint and by pyriform aperature and/or transalveolar screws or wires into the maxilla. The incisor teeth have been removed from the dentures to allow an adequate airway.

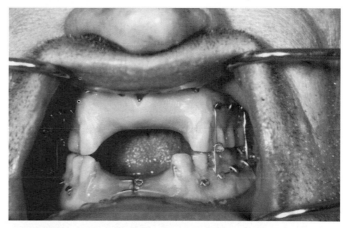

FIG. 35–11. A patient's dentures converted to a modified Gunning-type splint. K-wires were used to stabilize the maxillary dentures.

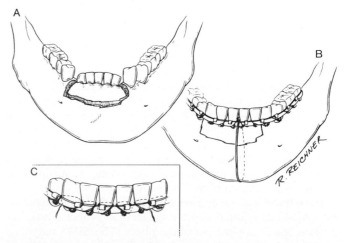

FIG. 35–12. A, segmental dentoalveolar mandibular fracture. **B,** an arch bar has been placed across the fracture sites. An additional circummandibular 25-gauge stainless-steel wire had been placed to further stabilize the fractured segment. **C,** the wiring technique.

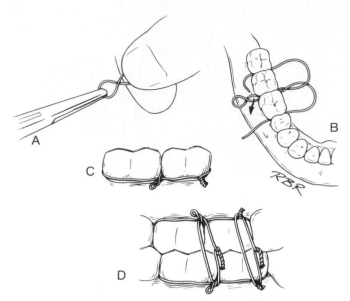

FIG. 35–13.   Techniques of continuous loop wire fixation.

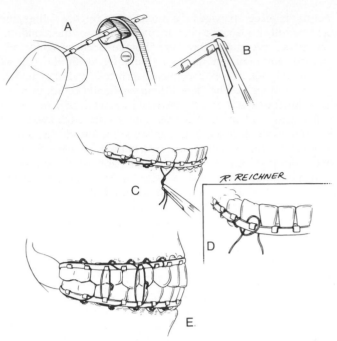

FIG. 35–14.   The technique for Ivy eyelet interdental wiring. Individual intermaxillary wiring can be applied easily. **A,** the appropriate length of the arch bar is cut. **B,** the arch is then contoured with the edges turned inward to prevent trauma to the buccal mucosa. **C,D,** the molars and bicuspids are the most suitable. The anterior teeth can be wired with care. **E,** the intermaxillary wiring should not include the incisor teeth.

methods is the minimal amount of equipment and supplies necessary to stabilize dentate facial fractures. Such methods are less stable than arch bars, but may be rapidly applied at bedside. One such method is maxillomandibular stabilization with interarch wires or elastics (Fig. 35–13).

Maxillomandibular Stabilization (MMS)

Maxillomandibular stabilization is the term used in this chapter to describe the wiring together of the maxillary and mandibular teeth, with or without arch bars. The Erich arch bar is the most frequently used of the many types available. If not properly secured, the arch bar may contribute to malocclusion, malunion, or nonunion, as well as inflict injury to the teeth and gingiva.

The period of immobilization required for clinical adequacy of fracture stability (no palpable motion of fracture site, nontender on opening against resistance), varies with patient age. Rowe and Killey (30,31) published their guidelines for MMS immobilization: 4 weeks for children, 6 weeks for adults, and 8 weeks for the elderly. However, more current studies indicate a shorter period of immobilization is required for many mandibular fractures. Juniper and Awty (32) suggest that 3 to 4 weeks of MMS immobilization is sufficient for about 80 % of mandibular fractures.

After the period of MMS, if the fracture site seems stable and nontender, the jaws may be released. If there is no pain or motion at the fracture site after a few days to a week of a soft diet, and if the occlusion is maintained, the arch bars and ligatures may be removed. This period of interarch wire stabilization may be supplemented with elastic stabilization or elastic guidance into centric occlusion.

Even those patients treated with techniques of internal fixation, MMS is required to place the teeth in proper centric occlusion before application of the plates. The MMS may then be released either at the completion of surgery or soon thereafter. This approach minimizes the risk of airway compromise and aspiration in the immediate postoperative period. However, many of these patients benefit from a brief postoperative

period of maxillomandibular stabilization for a up to a few days so as to place the soft tissues and fractures at rest.

The arch bar is cut to length to allow circumdental ligatures around the posterior teeth with centric stops (usually 4 teeth on each side of the dental arch, including the canines, premolars, and 1st molars). The arch bar should not extend posteriorly beyond the last tooth included in ligation to the arch bar. If some of these teeth are missing, or additionally stability is required, the 2nd molar is included as an abutment for the arch bar. The bar is secured with 24- or 26-gauge stainless steel wire, circumdentally with constant tension during twisting, directed toward the roots of the teeth. The twisted ends are then formed into a small loop, not extending beyond the mucogingival junction, and with no sharp contours exposed to wound the buccal mucosa or surgeon. The height of contour of the canine is on the lingual aspect, low at the cingulum. When tightening the canine circumdental ligature, an instrument (wire ligature passer, band pusher, or elevator) should be used to keep the wire apical to the cingulum. The immobility of the arch bar should then be tested, and the circumdental wires tightened further, if necessary. With the maxillary arch bar applied in the same fashion, the teeth may be put into centric occlusion, and the mandibular and maxillary stabilized in maximal intercuspation with interarch wire (24- or 26-gauge). To aid in reduction, these wires may be oriented in a direction to produce traction in a desired vector. For closed-reduction cases, if maximal intercuspation is not easily achieved, interarch elastics for 24 to 48 hours often further reduces the fracture alignment, allowing the elastics to be replaced with wires (Fig. 35–14).

Generally, the arch bar should not be ligated to the incisor teeth. These single, conical rooted teeth, without centric stops, are easily extruded from their sockets. If it is necessary to stabilize anterior dentoalveolar fractures, 26- or 28-gauge wire should be used, and interarch elastics not used. If interarch elastics or ligatures are necessary, the anterior portion of the mandibular arch bar should be stabilized with one or more circummandibular ligatures to avoid the tendency to displace coronally, extruding the incisors. The maxillary arch bar can be similarly supported with suspension wires to the pyriform rim or anterior nasal spine.

The arch bar may be used to help reduce multiple segments of the mandible, but the teeth should be placed into centric occlusion when doing the final tightening of the circumdental wires, so the preinjury centric occlusion is correctly reconstructed. A dental splint will improve the stability of this technique.

Maxillomandibular stabilization is not completely benign. Obviously, the upper aerodigestive tract is significantly impaired. Nutrition may be significantly compromised, with weight losses of 15 or more pounds during a 6-week period of MMS not uncommon. Especially during emergence from general anesthesia, MMS is associated with impairment of respiratory mechanics, which may contribute to aspiration and respiratory or cardiac arrest (33). Williams (34) found a significant decrease in pulmonary function with the teeth occluded (equivalent to MMS) in healthy individuals. There was a significant decrease (52%) in mean expiratory flow (50) and a drop in forced expiratory volume percent (48%), which according to the American Thoracic Society is a moderate impairment of pulmonary function. The decreased expiratory flows decrease effectiveness of expiration, which may be significant in patients with bronchitis, cystic fibrosis, pneumonia, for example. There was also a decrease in inspiratory flows, that would impair the delivery of inhaled bronchodilators.

Therefore, in patients with compromised pulmonary function, the treatment plan for management of mandibular fractures should take into consideration the effect of postoperative MMS on pulmonary function. Maxillomandibular stabilization should also be minimized or avoided in patients with reduced respiratory reserve, such as patients with chronic obstructive pulmonary disease.

Even a period of a few weeks of MMS has deleterious effects on the masticatory system (35,36). Immobilization of an extremity has long been known to induce muscle atrophy. Though the exact mechanism for this atrophy remains elusive, there is loss of both contractile and metabolic proteins from the muscle cells that begins within hours of immobilization (37). The amount of protein loss is dependent to some extent on position. Stretching a muscle while immobilization it induces some protein synthesis, which somewhat offsets the immobilization-induced protein loss. On the other hand, immobilization of a shortened muscle induces a greater protein loss. The contractile properties of the involved muscles parallel the changes in protein content; a more severe loss of contractile force accompanies immobilization of a shortened muscle.

Immobilization of synovial joints also has deleterious effects, especially if the articular surfaces are in contact, under compression. Areas of compression undergo pressure necro-

sis, liquefaction of the articular cartilage, and the formation of intracartilaginous cysts. Also with joint immobilization there is a progressive contracture of the joint capsule and pericapsular structures that increase over time. The amount of synovial joint degeneration and contracture induced by immobilization seems directly related to duration and frequency of immobilization. Mandibular immobilization also has deleterious effects on the soft-tissue envelope surrounding the fracture. Reparative collagen is laid down in a more disorganized, haphazard pattern when the area is immobilized than when the forming scar is exposed to functional stimulation early on.

Finally MMS imparts orthodontically significant forces to the dentition. Oral hygiene is also severely compromised, and many patients are quite uncomfortable from the arch bars and wire ligatures.

OPEN REDUCTION AND MMS

Rarely, a fracture cannot be acceptably reduced by closed reduction, but once reduced would be stable enough that internal fixation is not required. In such unusual cases, a limited open exposure of the fracture may allow accurate reduction, and then the fracture may be adequately stabilized with MMS for 6 weeks. However, in the vast majority of cases, if open reduction is required, some form of internal fixation is warranted.

EXTERNAL FIXATION

External fixators for treatment of mandibular fractures have limited indications. Two of the most common indications are the severely infected wound (to avoid placement of a foreign body within the infected wound), and the wound without adequate soft tissues to cover an internal fixation device (38,39). With significant soft-tissue damage and segmental loss of bone secondary to the initial trauma or subsequent infection, this approach allows soft tissues to heal without the impedance of an internal foreign body and avoids the necessity of prolonged MMS, so that motion may be resumed in the immediate postoperative period. Disadvantages include external scarring at the pin holes, potential infection via the pin tracts, and the cumbersome nature of the appliance.

After placing the patient into MMS, threaded bone pins, a pair on either side of the fracture (usually well away from the fracture), are placed percutaneously. The pins must be placed to avoid the mandibular canal and dental roots. This is accomplished by making small stab incisions over the lateral inferior border of the mandible, no deeper than the platysma, and bluntly dissecting down to bone. An trocar or small pediatric nasal speculum may be used for exposure and to prevent damage to the soft tissues. Appropriate-sized drill holes are then created below the mandibular canal, and the pins (or 3.6- or 4.0-mm threaded Steinmann pins, usually easily available) are screwed through both cortices. The external ends of the pins should be roughly on the same plane, and a slight amount of divergence is preferable. Then the pins are linked together, either with monophasic and biphasic techniques (3,8).

Once the pins are in place, a large-diameter (no. 10, or larger) endotracheal tube is placed over the outer ends of the pins by cutting holes in the tube to go over the end of each pin. Once the tube is in place, the fracture is held in a reduced, well-aligned position, and the mixed acrylic is injected into the end of the tube with a large syringe. The tube is held in place until the acrylic hardens. The pins and tube may be coated with petroleum ointment before injecting the acrylic so that the excess acrylic may be easily removed from these areas when it is in the doughy stage. Alternately, a quick-setting acrylic can be poured it into a long, rectangular metal tray, and allowed to become doughy. When the acrylic is doughy to the touch, it is transferred to the ends of the four pins, and then the nuts are screwed on the ends. The acrylic is held in position while it hardens so that it is far enough away from the skin to allow cleaning of the pins.

Antibacterial ointment is placed around the pins at the skin. Daily care of these pin sites is needed (e.g., cleansing with half-strength hydrogen peroxide, then dressing with an antibiotic ointment). Removal of these external fixators is a simple task of cutting the acrylic and removing the bone pins.

INTERNAL FIXATION

A vast number of internal fixation methods and devices have been developed for the stabilization of mandibular fractures. Each has its own advantages and disadvantages. Sound surgical judgment is required to pick the best method of management for the presenting circumstances. No one method is the best for all cases, and sometimes a change in treatment is necessary if healing does not proceed as planned.

Wire Osteosynthesis

Interfragmentary wire fixation has been developed in a number of patterns to impose improved stability on mandibular fractures. Wire stabilization of fractures during plate adaption and fixation remains a useful technique to aid reduction; however, wire stabilization of fractures, even when combined with MMS, is not adequately stable for many fractures. Interfragmentary wires have little bone contact, and poorly resist torsion and compression. Wire osteosynthesis allows significant fragment "micromotion" which, when combined with the inoculation of the wound from compounded fractures or even skin incisions, has a higher rate of wound infection than rigid methods of internal fixation.

A common pattern of wire osteosynthesis is a simple wire ligature, passed through a pair of holes placed one on either side of the fracture, and either unicortical or bicortical. The teeth must be in centric occlusion as the interfragmentary wire is tightened, but it may be easier to place the interfragmentary wires before MMS. Another common pattern of wire osteosynthesis is also placed through a pair of holes on either side of the fracture, but then the wire is criss-crossed beneath the inferior border of the mandible and twisted tight. There is no role for circumferential cerclage wires in the treatment of mandibular fractures.

Wire osteosynthesis may be stable enough for pediatric fractures, especially of younger children, as their fractures tend to heal rapidly, their fractures are often incomplete ("greenstick fractures"), and their functional loading of the mandible is less than in the adult (Fig. 35–15).

The chief advantages of wire stabilization are the minimal equipment an instrumentation required, the minimal expense involved, and the minimal exposure necessary to apply. However, the disadvantages include poor stabilization of most fractures, increased rates of wound infections, and the

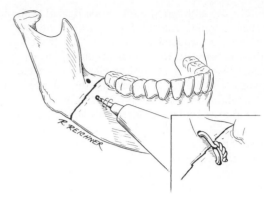

FIG. 35–15. The technique of simple wire fixation placed through an intraoral approach at the mandibular angle. Note: The patient must be in intermaxillary fixation before tightening this wire fixator.

inability of wire osteosynthesis to hold complex three-dimensions shapes of comminuted fractures. Wire fixation should be reserved for simple, relative stable fractures, and combined with stable MMS for up to 6 weeks, or until the fracture becomes clinically and radiographically stable.

Open reduction and wire osteosynthesis is associated with higher rates of infection and a greater number of other complication than either closed reduction or open reduction with rigid internal fixation methods (40).

Metal Plate and Screw Fixation

Many mandibular plating devices and systems have been developed that incorporate similar principles and remain in current usage. The systems are usually classified on the basis of the diameter of the screw that fits into the plate (i.e., a 2.0-mm miniplate accepts 2-mm screws; a 2.7-mm plate accepts 2.7-mm screws). The size specified for the system usually does not denote any measurement of the plate itself. The systems made of titanium or vitallium have such excellent tissue compatibility that the hardware does not routinely need to be removed. Fixation hardware should be removed from the growing child to avoid potential growth impairment, and in patients for whom it was used to stabilize a defect that has been bone grafted so that functional stress may be reestablished through the bone graft to allow stress-induced remodeling.

Metallic implants of differing composition should not be used together in the same wound, because dissimilar metals in close proximity in an electrolytic solution give rise to galvanic currents that cause corrosion; this leads to weakening of the fixation and solubilization of potentially toxic metallic ions, and possible demineralization. The type of implants placed should be recorded, to facilitate having the proper instrumentation available if the implants must be removed later.

Most of the currently available systems have self-tapping screws—screws with cutting flutes that cut their own treads in bone as the screws are driven. Some systems require a tapping step before screw insertion. Whatever system is used, the appropriate instrumentation, including appropriately sized drill bits, drill guides, and screwdriver bits must be used. It is also essential that sharp drill bits be used at slow speeds, not exceeding the manufacture's recommendations, with plenty of cooling irrigation to minimize frictional heat damage to bone viability.

With plate-and-screw fixation, the plate must be adapted perfectly to conform passively to the reduced surface of the mandible, while maintaining the preinjury centric occlusion. If the plate does not conform accurately, when the screws are tightened the bone will be drawn to the plate, altering the reduction and possibly disturbing the occlusion.

Nonrigid Plate-and-Screw Osteosynthesis

Unicortical miniplate osteosyntheses has been popularized for the treatment of mandibular fractures. This technique is based on concepts of fracture stabilization and theories of mandibular fracture behavior radically different from those of the rigid, bicortical fixation techniques (i.e., AO/ASIF techniques). Basically, one or two miniplates (2.0-mm screws) are fixed with unicortical screws to the lateral cortex of the mandible along idealized neutrality or tension (distraction). Anatomic reduction is stressed in the technique, as is placement of the plates to avoid injury of teeth or the inferior alveolar neurovascular bundle. These techniques are based on assumptions of concentration of tensile forces along the superior border of the horizontal mandible, and compressive forces along the inferior border. The miniplate is placed over the superior portion of the mandible, below the apices of the to resist distraction of the fracture. In the anterior region, a second plate is placed inferiorly to resist torsion. The superior plate cannot contribute significantly to resistance of inferior border compression, and the system depends on bony buttressing of the fracture edges to resist compression. The system also is unable to provide significant resistance to distraction (tension) of the inferior border. Maxillomandibular stabilization is not required to stabilize the repaired fracture, and early function is one goal of the technique.

These techniques of fracture treatment are best applied to simple fractures (no comminution or bone loss) with orientations that provide for solid bony buttressing (i.e., fractures roughly perpendicular to the bone surface and fixation plate). Sharply oblique fractures, and comminuted fractures are less suited for this technique. Fractures with bone loss, or limited bone contact (e.g., fractures with a significant butterfly fragment of the inferior border) should not be treated by this method.

This technique does have the advantages of limited required access, ease of plate adaptation, and low plate profile (less palpable). However, the technique imposes less resistance to fracture displacement (the strength of the reconstructed mandible is closer to the critical limit of failure than with rigid bicortical techniques), therefore appropriate patient selection is important.

Rigid Plate and/or Screw Osteosynthesis

Rigid internal fixation (RIF) is based on the premise that optimal bone healing can be reliably achieved with a degree of stability that prevents micromotion across the fracture. Rigidity is assured by the use of larger plates (2.3-mm to 2.7-mm screw sizes). These larger plates are affixed to the inferior aspect of the mandible with bicortical screws, usually at least three screws at each end of the fracture. The plates are usually applied along the lateral-inferior border of the mandible to avoid the mandibular canal and roots of the teeth. The plate must include enough holes on either side of the fracture to allow the inner pair of holes to be in sound bone, yet far enough away from the fracture line (of both cortices) so that the area is not further fractured with the application of the screws. The actual relationship of the fracture lines relative to the facial and lingual cortices may be determined by evaluation of computed tomograms and direct inspection. Appropriate-length screws should be used to obtain maximal holding power, as determined by the use of the appropriate depth gauge. Excessively long screws (>2–3 mm beyond the lingual cortex of bone), may become problematic, creating hardware exposure and difficulty with denture wear.

With such strong plates, it is essential that the plates be accurately adapted to the restored mandibular contours. Malleable bending templates facilitate obtaining the requisite accuracy of form. The rigidity of the fracture fixation is improved with a smaller, unicortical tension band (2.0-mm) plate at the superior aspect of the mandible.

If the inferior border plate is placed with compression from the plate and screws, the rigidity of fixation will be enhanced, though the accuracy of the reduction must not be compromised. However, compression applied to the lateral inferior cortex will tend to cause distraction of the lingual cortex and at the superior border. The superiorly placed tension band (especially if placed with the fracture reduced by a compressive preload supplied with a reduction forceps) will resist the tendency for superior border distraction. Distraction of the lingual cortex can be resisted with the plate overbending technique. The plate is accurately adapted to the outer cortex of the inferior border region. As the last step before fixation into place, the region of plate directly over the fracture is slightly overbent (made more concave) by 1 to 2 mm. This imparts a small angulation to the screws on either side of the fracture. As a pair of screws are placed, one on either side of the fracture, the bone will be drawn to the plate. Because of the overbending, the lingual cortices will come into contact before the facial cortices. With further tightening, the overbend will be reduced (flattened), bringing the facial cortices into approximation, and imparting a small degree of compression (mainly at the lingual cortex) to the fracture.

The advantages of RIF are the reliable fracture healing obtained, with rates of complication that compare favorable with other fixation techniques. Another advantage of rigid techniques is that the patient may be immediately released from MMS, so that there is less potential compromise of the airway during emergence from anesthesia. The weight loss commonly associated with 6 weeks of MMS may also be avoided. With concomitant fractures in the condylar region, early mobilization and physiotherapy may be instituted to optimize treatment in that area. The techniques of rigid internal fixation are widely adaptable to many patterns of mandibular fracture. The techniques are especially adaptable to more complex patterns of fracture, and should be the treatment of choice for difficult fractures (i.e., comminuted or bone-loss fractures).

Disadvantages include the technical sensitivity of the method. As the reconstruction is rigid, fracture malalignment or malocclusion are rigid mistakes, not amenable to correction with MMS and elastics. There is a steep learning curve but, once learned, these technique are widely adaptable to many mandibular fracture types. Assael (41), evaluating the models produced in various plating courses, found 76% of fractures overall had been treated "anatomically" satisfactorily, according to AO/ASIF principles and techniques.

Noncompression Technique. Rigid fixation techniques without interfragmentary compression have become widely used, probably more widely used than compressive techniques. Interfragmentary compression does increase fracture stability; however, interfragmentary compression is a very technique sensitive, and should not be used on some patterns of fracture. As interfragmentary compression depends on bony buttressing, comminuted and bone-loss fractures cannot be compressed (compression only produces foreshortening). Compression should also be used with caution on oblique fractures (relative to the plate), because of the tendency to telescope the fragments. It may also be difficult to apply plate compression of the fracture without distorting the reduction. Applying compression to the lateral cortex at the inferior border of the mandible, tends to distract the superior border (and the teeth and occlusion) and the lingual cortex. A compression plate (i.e., a plate with eccentric holes designed to cause lateral plate motion with the full insertion of a screw) may be used in neutral mode by placing the screws centered within the holes. A small degree of interfragmentary compression may be developed by the use of bone reduction forceps before placement of the noncompression plate. Also, the technique of overbending, described in the previous section, will develop a small degree of compression of the lingual cortex.

Basically, the rigid, noncompression fixation techniques employ robust plates (2.3-mm to 2.7-mm) accurately adapted to the precisely reduced fractures. An adequate number of screws are placed bicortical on either side of the fracture (for simple fractures, usually three screws on each side). The fixation may also be made more rigid by the use of a tension band plate.

Compression Plate Fixation. Compression is a technique of fracture fixation that can tremendously increase the rigidity of fracture fixation. Compression requires contact of the fractures surfaces of bone to achieve bony buttressing. Compression puts a compressive preload across the fracture that, with the microscopic interdigitation of the irregular fragment surfaces, increases the fraction between the fragments and therefore the resistance to shear and torsional displacements (42). The compressive preload must also be overcome, before tensional stresses can distract the fragments. Under compression, the fixation plate bears less of any compressive or torsional stresses acting across the fracture, because some of the load is born by the contacting bone fragments.

Compression plates have one or more of the screw holes made excentrically with an inclined plane along the edge of the screw hole away from the fracture line. As the compression screw is tightened into the plate, if the plate is affixed to the opposite fracture fragment, it engages the inclined plane, forcing the plate to slide away from the fracture relative to the compression screw (Fig. 35–16). Compression, with the mandibular plating systems currently available, requires a plate with an eccentric compression screw hole and a pair of screws, one on either side of the fracture. The remaining screws are placed in a neutral position within the plate's screw holes. Attempting to place more eccentric screws only creates strain within the fragment between the screws, and does not increase compression across the fracture.

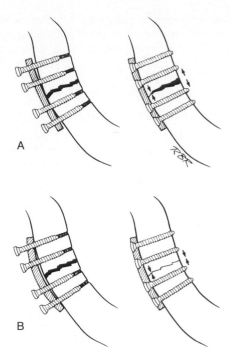

FIG. 35–16. Application of compression plates to the mandible. **A,** it is important that the plate be well adapted to the fracture site because a straight plate will cause distraction at the lingual cortex. **B,** overbending of the plate as depicted will allow for compression at the lingual cortex.

Compression requires fragment contact; it cannot be applied across a bone gap or comminuted region. If it is applied across a comminuted fracture, unless each fragment is affixed to the plate, compression will just displace fragments. For compression plate technique, the best relationship of plate to fracture is perpendicular. Oblique fractures may be telescoped, or driven to override by compression.

Compression tends to compress the fracture edges immediately adjacent to the plate. Such a plate applied to the lateral inferior border of the mandible will tend to distract the superior border and the lingual cortex, as noted above, unless these tendencies are counteracted. The tendency for the distraction of the superior border can compensated for by placement of a tension band (arch bar or second plate) near the superior border, before activation of the compression, or by preloading the fracture with reduction forceps. The tendency to distract the lingual cortex can be counteracted by overbending of the plate, creating "lingual compression."

Another potential complication arising from compression is the entrapment of the inferior alveolar nerve between the fracture segments, with injury to the nerve.

Compression (Lag) Screw Fixation. The lag-screw technique is a powerful compression technique. The lag-screw principle involves placing one or more screws through fragments so that the threads of the screw take hold only in the far or deep cortical bone (relative to the head of the screw). The proximal or near cortex is overdrilled, so that the threads of the screw slide through without holding. As the screw is tightened, it screws into the distal cortex, eventually pulling the head of the screw against the proximal cortex. The proximal fragment is then compressed between the head of the screw and the distal cortex. Usually, the bone around the entrance of the proximal cortex is countersunk to match the shape of the screw head, spreading the stress caused by the screw head. Because of the relationship of the screw and bony fragments, lag-screw technique is best applied to oblique fractures. The most compression will be created by placing the screw perpendicular to the fracture. However, the strongest interaction of the screw head and proximal cortex is when the screw is placed perpendicular to the surface of the bone. In practice, the screw is placed between these two orientations, typically bisecting the angle between the perpendicular to the fracture, and perpendicular to the bone surface. A single lag screw provides strong compression, but little resistance to rotation about the screw. So, a minimum of two screws are necessary to fixate most fractures that have the appropriate pattern (Fig. 35–17).

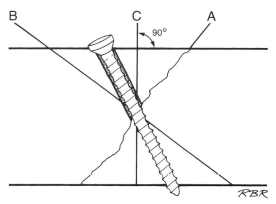

FIG. 35–17. Most of the compression is created by placing the screws perpendicular to the fracture. A minimum of two screws is necessary to fixate most fractures.

TREATMENT CONSIDERATIONS BY FRACTURE PATTERN AND LOCATION

Regional Considerations

Although the techniques of fracture stabilization have been discussed, certain regional considerations also require attention.

Alveolar Process and Teeth

Maxillofacial trauma is frequently associated with significant injuries of the teeth and their supporting structures. While the treatment of such injuries must be appropriately prioritized in the context of the patient's overall condition and other injuries, all too frequently significant dental injuries go unrecognized or are simply ignored until (or after) the time of hospital discharge. Along with considerations of the effect of the presence or absence of teeth associated with the fracture on the fracture treatment and healing, the prognosis of the involved teeth must also be taken into account (43). Consideration must also include the overall status and state of development of the dentition (e.g., deciduous or primary dentition, transitional dentition—mixed primary and secondary dentition—and permanent or secondary dentition), and of the involved teeth (degree of root formation and apex closure).

Because the (severely) multiply injured patient is treated in the hospital emergency room or operating room and not the dental office, specialized dental radiographic equipment and instrumentation are not commonly available. The appropriate dental treatment for these injuries is beyond the scope of this chapter. However, the initial treating surgeon should have a basic familiarity with the anatomy of the teeth and supporting structures, understand the significance of commonly occurring patterns of dental injury, and know some practical dental treatments for these injuries (or work closely with a hospital-based restorative dentist who has access to these patients) (44).

Often, alveolar fractures will remain viable through the vascularity of their attached mucosa. If these segments are to be salvaged, the mucosal attachment should not be further reduced, which may preclude any form of internal fixation. These fractured segments should be reduced and immobilized with interdental fixation, a composite resin orthodontic splint, and possibly a dental acrylic splint. Some of these teeth may require endodontic treatment or extraction at a later date if

they prove to be devitalized. If a segment of alveolar process has been avulsed to the point of being grossly devitalized, removal of this bone and contained teeth is indicated. Completely avulsed teeth may be salvaged if promptly placed back into their sockets and appropriately stabilized. If this is not done before reimplantation, such teeth will need root canal therapy and possibly restorative dentistry at a later time. Appropriate timely intervention in many of these dentoalveolar injuries will permit salvage of teeth that otherwise might be lost, decreasing pain and potential morbidity, as well as retaining functional teeth, or preserving the teeth as abutments for prosthetic oral rehabilitation.

Some of the sequelae of dentoalveolar injuries, such as tooth hypermobility, root resorption, and pulp necrosis may not become clinically apparent for a year or more, and require expectant dental observation and management. Teeth associated with mandibular fracture may subsequently undergo pulp necrosis, pulp obliteration, root resorption, and loss of alveolar bone support (45). Such teeth need to be followed for some time, a year or longer, to detect these changes (43,45,46). Dental follow-up is suggested at 1 week, 2 weeks, 1 month, 3 months, 6 months, and 12 months (47).

Dentoalveolar injuries may be classified on the basis of the tissues involved. Included are injuries confined to the teeth, the periodontal ligament, and the supporting alveolus, or various combinations of these structures.

Deciduous and permanent teeth may be impacted (intruded), luxated (displaced, with some degree of disruption of the periodontal ligament), or avulsed (complete luxation).

Crown Fractures. Preservation of these teeth may be of mechanical advantage, for control of the attached bony fragments as well as providing the foundation for dental restoration and decreasing resorption of the alveolar bone. Teeth with fractured crowns and pulpal exposure require prompt treatment to reseal the pulp from the oral environment. The exposed pulp may be cleansed with saline, the tooth dried, and the pulp "capped" with an application of calcium hydroxide paste. For extensive pulp exposures, or those unable to be treated promptly, the tooth will require root cancel therapy, or extraction. If available, a barbed dental broach should be used to extirpate the pulp and thus lessen the patient's pain from that tooth. In the setting of severe maxillofacial injuries or multiple trauma, care of pulpal exposures may be deferred. However, without the required dental treatment, such teeth may be quite painful for the patient, developing pulpal necrosis or infection, and root resorption; they may best be treated with extraction during fracture treatment. Successful salvage of coronally fractured teeth may be expensive and require multiple dental visits (i.e., root canal, preparation and insertion of crown). Many patients will not have the resources or the will to undertake such treatment, and would be best served by extraction.

Root Fractures.   Many teeth with root fractures, even if the fracture is subosseous, may be salvaged, at least as abutments for crowns or other prosthesis. However, such efforts are rarely indicated in the setting of severe maxillofacial injuries or in the multiple trauma patient. Generally, root fractures are and indication for the extraction of the involved tooth or teeth. The root fragments should be completely removed to reduce risk of infection and to promote healing of the site.

Periodontal Injury.   The periodontium (i.e., the tissues supporting the teeth—gingiva, periodontal ligament, and alveolar bone) are frequently injured with fractures of the jaws. The periodontal ligament (PDL), a series of highly organized collagen fibers, attached at either end to the cementum of the tooth root and to the lamina dura for the socket, suspends the tooth in the alveolar socket. Trauma of the teeth and jaws may partially or completely disrupt the PDL. A partial tearing of the PDL (luxation) results in increased mobility. Such traumatized teeth may be salvaged by avoiding further trauma to the tooth, specifically, assuring the tooth is not occlusally stressed (taken out of occlusion).

Intrusion of the deciduous teeth may not require treatment beyond observation. If the tooth is partially intruded, it may be left to reerupt. If it does not do so over several months, the root probably has undergone ankylosis to alveolar bone, and the tooth will require surgical extraction. For more complete intrusions, the deciduous tooth may have caused injury to the underlying developing permanent tooth in its developmental crypt. The deciduous tooth should then be gently removed to minimize chances for the later impairment of the development and eruption of the permanent tooth. For permanent teeth, the anterior, single-rooted teeth are more commonly impacted, though this injury is uncommon in adults. If the degree of impaction is less than one-half of the crown, the tooth may be observed over several months as it reerupts. If the tooth is impacted more than half the crown height, an orthodontic bracket or hook can be bonded onto the crown and elastics used to gently direct the tooth into position. Whether primary or secondary, intruded teeth usually have disrupted the pulpal pedical at the apex of the root, which may lead to internal resorption and discoloration. Secondary teeth will require root canal therapy.

Teeth may also be partially extruded from the socket, with varying degrees of disruption of the PDL. Such teeth should be reduced to normal position, stabilized, and taken out of occlusion. Teeth may also be completely avulsed from their sockets. Even these teeth may be salvaged by prompt reinsertion into the socket and stabilization, if this can be done within 30 minutes of injury. The rate of survival decreases at approximately 1% per minute delay in reimplantation after 30 minutes (45). Trauma sufficient to injure the PDL may also injure the neurovascular pedical that enters the apex of each root. Such teeth may become nonvital, as the pulpal tissues necrose, and the teeth do not respond normally to pulp testing. However, such teeth may be salvaged if the periodontal attachment of the teeth is preserved or restored. These teeth will require root canal therapy.

The splinting cannot be rigid, such as that provided by an arch bar, but must allow small "physiologic" strains in the healing periodontal ligament to minimize ankylosis. Orthodontic bonding composite resin with a monofilament (i.e., 2-0 nylon) or a small-gauge stainless wire (28 gauge) provides the necessary stability, with occlusal adjustments to avoid traumatic occlusion.

Anderson suggests that an avulsed tooth should be reimplanted promptly, preferably within 30 minutes of avulsion. During transportation, the best storage place for the tooth is within the buccal vestibule (47), bathed in saliva, but obviously not if the patient's condition (impaired mentation or aerodigestive tract function and coordination) contraindicates. Milk is the second-best storage medium, and is commonly available. Tap water (hypoosmotic) is detrimental to periodontal ligament cells. The root surface should be handled as little as possible, with any contaminants gently washed off with a stream of saline.

Symphysis and Parasymphysis

Isolated midline mandibular symphysis fractures are uncommon. When they occur, such fractures are frequently associated with condyle fractures. Symphyseal fractures are usually not stable enough to treat by closed means, especially when associated with condyle fractures. In this case, there is a marked tendency for the distance between the mandibular angles to widen, with the posterior segments flaring lateralward. Maxillomandibular stabilization may worsen this tendency. It is essential to understand the pattern of fracture, especially the relationship of the facial and lingual cortical fractures. These fractures may be poorly imaged on pantographs because of the artifact of the superimposed cervical spine. However, axial computed tomograms usually image these fractures well. With an appreciation of the line of fracture, which often has some degree of obliquity, all screws should be angulated to be in sound cortical bone. For the bicortical technique, all screws should engage both cortices without causing fragmentation near either fracture line. With the anterior curvature of the mandible, the lag-screw technique is often useful to treat these fractures.

Parasymphyseal fractures are more common, and like the symphyseal fractures, are frequently associated with fractures of the contralateral mandible, either angle or condyle. Parasymphyseal fractures may be treated much like symphyseal fractures. Care must be taken to avoid injury to the mental nerve. Often a fixation plate will have to be placed both anterior and posterior to the nerve. This can be done with careful intraoral exposure and retraction of the nerve; the extraoral, submental approach avoids the nerve as well. The contours in this region can be quite difficult to read accurately for plate adaption, and bending templates are helpful. Also, the severe changes in convexity and concavity that occur in the inferior-superior dimension over the anterior mandible may be simplified by slight flattening with a bur or osteotome. The outer cortex is not removed, but the change of contour lessened. This maneuver also lessens the plate profile.

Body

The body region may be approached intraorally, extraorally, or by a combination of the two. The intraoral access requires working around the mental nerve. There are both relatively flat contours and an adequate thickness of mandible for good screw holding and bony buttressing. Anatomically, the area is made somewhat difficult because of the variable path of the mandibular canal, which dips below the level of the mental foramen. Bicortically fixed plates must be placed below the canal. The bone overlaying the canal and roots of the teeth also varies in thickness.

Angle

Mandibular angle fractures are common, and may be associated with contralateral condyle or other contralateral mandible fractures. Exposure may be intraoral, extraoral, or (rarely) a combination of the two.

Angle fractures seem to have a disproportional rate of complications, including malunion, nonunion, and infection. The higher rates of complication, even when using rigid fixation techniques, are related to the mandibular anatomy (thinness of the width of the mandible, with reduced bony buttressing), the common involvement of 3rd molar teeth, the concentration of displacing stress in this transition between the horizontal and vertical portions of the mandible, and the difficulty of working through inadequate surgical access.

Patients with nondisplaced fractures may be treated with MMS alone. Displaced fractures are difficult to reduce closed, and the proximal (posterior) edentulous fragment is not controlled with MMS. Such fractures require open reduction and internal rigid fixation.

The presence of a 3rd molar makes the mandibular angle particularly prone to fracture, especially from a lateral impact. The fracture line often extends through the socket of this molar, making it an open fracture. The management of teeth in the line of fracture was discussed in detail earlier. Fractures involving partially erupted 3rd molars still partly covered with a gingival operculum, are particularly prone to infection. The anaerobic environments of the deep gingival pockets are populated with particularly virulent flora. Usually, if the fracture propagates through a tooth socket without fracturing the tooth root, the tooth and its roots will aid in the accurate reduction of the fracture and may aid in stability (by increasing the contact area between the fragments). If such teeth require extraction, doing so after fracture reduction and fixation may be helpful. However, sometimes the presence of exposed roots in the fracture prevents an accurate reduction of the fracture, necessitating the extraction of the tooth before reduction and fixation. In either case of extraction, the entire tooth should be removed, including root tips, and diseased granulation tissue removed from the socket. Normally, such extraction sockets are not closed. However, a watertight mucosal closure should be obtained when the socket is associated with a fracture to reduce rates of wound infection.

Ramus

Fractures of the ramus are uncommon and rarely displaced because of the splinting effect of the masseter-medial pterygoid muscle sling. Unless displacement causes vertical shortening, these fractures are generally immobilized with MMS.

If open reduction and internal rigid fixation are needed, an intraoral approach may be used, with the help of percutaneous drilling and screwing or right-angled instruments. An external incision may be made if further exposure is needed.

Coronoid Process

Isolated fractures of the coronoid process are rare, and the possibility of concomitant fractures should be investigated. Distraction of the fractured coronoid is seldom found, because the tendinous attachments from the temporalis muscle extend onto the anterior border of the vertical ramus. These isolated fractures are usually treated without any type of fixation, and the patient is placed on a soft diet until the pain resolves. Patients with complaints of severe pain may benefit from short-term MMS in order to alleviate this problem. Early motion is desirable to reduce or avoid the tendency to ankylose the coronoid fragment to both the adjacent maxilla or zygoma.

Condyle

The condylar process of the mandible is a common site of fracture because of the relative structural weakness of the condylar head and neck (48). Classification of the location of the fracture is important both diagnostically and prognostically. The fracture may occur within the joint capsule, either involving or sparing the articular surface of the condylar head. In either case, the vascularity of the proximal fragment is severely compromised, and may then undergo avascular necrosis. Osteoarthritis is a common outcome from intraarticular fractures. Little is known about the fate of the articular disk in such fractures. Forces sufficient to fracture the condylar head may also lacerate or avulse the disk from the head fragment or the lateral pterygoid muscle. At a minimum, there will be hemarthrosis of the lower joint compartment, which may undergo organization and scarring of the disk, or cause progressive joint inflammation and degeneration. Intraarticular fractures are exceeding difficult to reduce in the confines of the joint, and opening the joint capsule further compromises the vascularity of the fragments. Such fractures are all but impossible to fixate stably, because of the thin cortical bone available for screw or pin placement.

Condylar fractures in children have such a remarkable potential for healing, remodeling, or even reforming a condyle, that the vast majority of these fractures should be observed, with early motion.

Frequently such fractures do not alter the occlusion, and treatment should be early limited function and expectant observation. If the intracapsular condylar fracture alters the occlusion, usually from a loss of posterior vertical height with an ipsilateral occlusal prematurity and a contralateral open bite, the patient should be placed into MMS. Maxillomandibular stabilization should be brief—perhaps wire MMS for 1 to 2 weeks, with guiding elastics for up to 2 additional weeks. This period of MMS would be followed by progressive physical therapy to maximize opening and protrusion of the mandible (48,49). The occlusion should be followed expectantly for recurrence of the malocclusion.

Condylar fractures may also occur through the condylar neck, outside of the joint capsule. Such fractures may not be significantly displaced or angulated because of the support of the joint capsule. However, usually the lateral pterygoid muscle will tend to displace or angulate the proximal condyle fragment anteromedially. Presumably with such displacements there will be discoordination between the positions of the condylar head and the joint meniscus. Frequently such fractures do well with only MMS for up to 6 weeks. However these low condylar neck fractures may also be associated with disruptions of the joint capsule, with more severe angulations or displacements of the proximal fragments. Lateral displacement, or severe anteromedial angulation of more than 45° with dislocation of the head from the glenoid fossa, suggests disruption of the joint capsule, and such fractures may benefit from open reduction and internal fixation.

Most of these fractures do exceedingly well with conservative treatment—closed reduction (50) and MMS for 2 to 3 weeks—and, if there is a tendency for poster vertical collapse, interarch elastic guidance into centric occlusion for several months. This is especially true when the condylar head is still in the glenoid fossa. Indications for open reduction of condylar fractures include: the condyle is displaced into the middle cranial fossa; there is lateral extracapsular displacement of the condyle; the displaced condyle functionally blocks opening or closing of the mandible; or severe anteromedial angulation of more than 45° to 90° with dislocation of the head from the glenoid fossa; and a posterior vertical shortening of the mandible with an open-bite deformity persists after a 2-week trial period of MMS. Relative indications include bilateral condylar fractures associated with comminuted, unstable midfacial fractures; and bilateral condylar fractures in an edentulous patient when a splint is unavailable or impossible because of alveolar ridge atrophy.

Many methods of stabilization have been described, including: rigid plating, interosseous wiring, K-wire or pin fixation, and replacement of the condyle with a prosthesis (the placement of a threaded Steinmann pin from below into the fractured condylar neck and its fixation into a trough cut into the vertical ramus and angle). Exposure of the condylar region may require both a submandibular and preauricular approach, depending on the exact position of the fracture. If necessary, the condylar head may be removed in order to apply appropriate screws and plates and then replaced as a bone graft with rigid fixation, though this technique frequently results in avascular necrosis of the head.

Late sequelae of both closed and open reductions include avascular necrosis of the condylar head, TMJ pain, arthritic changes in the TMJ, and decreased motion. These are also the late sequelae of conservatively treated condylar fractures.

Management of Teeth In/Near Fracture

Traumatic forces sufficient to inflict fractures of the maxillofacial skeleton are also sufficient to inflict dental injuries. Appropriate treatment of the dental as well as maxillofacial injuries requires at least a basic understanding of the prognosis of the teeth injured, and of the likelihood of the involved teeth affecting the treatment of the mandibular fracture or fractures. The goal for treating mandibular fractures is the restoration of the preinjury form and function, including the occlusion. Of course this includes healing of the fracture, but it also includes the salvage of sound teeth.

Fractures of the horizontal mandible often involve the dental sockets or roots. Any fracture passing through the socket of a tooth should be considered to be compounded intra-orally, even if the fracture is nondisplaced and the tooth firm in the socket. Such fractures with involved teeth potentially may have higher incidences of infection (osteomyelitis), nonunion, delayed healing, and severe dental pain (51,52).

Treatment of otherwise sound teeth (i.e., the teeth are clinically intact) must be individualized to the circumstances of the patient, but generally such teeth can be maintained. While it may be technically possible to salvage many teeth involved with mandibular fractures, doing so may not be in the best interest of the patient. The salvage of some teeth associated with mandibular fractures will require appropriate dental treatment, in addition to the fracture treatment. Many patients do not have the financial resources to undertake such treatment, and such treatment is increasingly not covered by government insurance programs.

There are a number of indications to extract teeth involved with mandibular fractures. Loose or avulsed teeth that present a danger of aspiration should be débrided promptly. If a tooth or teeth are attached to a nonviable alveolar segment, the nonviable segment (and tooth or teeth) should be débrided. Teeth with advanced preexisting dental disease (caries and periodontal disease) involved in the line of fracture should be considered for extraction. Retention of such teeth increases the risk of fracture infection. Partially erupted 3rd molars should also be considered for extraction when involved in the line of fracture. The microbiologic flora associated with the deep, anaerobic soft-tissue pockets (operculum) of these teeth is particularly virulent and prone to causing infection.

Teeth that have had two-thirds or more of the circumference of their bony sockets disrupted and are in the line of fracture should be extracted, especially if gingival injuries are associated with the alveolar fractures. Such teeth usually have been devitalized (nerve and vascular supply to the dental pulp disrupted). The significant periodontal ligament disruption, often associated with a gingival disruption, especially with the impairment of oral hygiene associated with arch bars and MMS, decreases the chance of healing the complex wound (i.e., gingiva, alveolar bone, periodontal ligament) and increases the risk of infection.

Multirooted teeth that have one or more of their roots disrupted from their sockets should be considered for extraction. Though exposure of one of the root apicis does not completely devitalize the tooth, some of the pulp is devitalized, and with the apex inoculated with oral fluids, the risk is increased for infecting the tooth (retrograde pulpitis). At the least, such teeth will require early root canal therapy.

Full-thickness mucosal wounds overlying root surfaces (facial or lingula cortex lost) will usually be unable to heal over the root. The root surface is not an adequate wound bed for the mucosa to heal over, and overlying repairs will probably dehisce. These teeth may be stable and useful for the occlusion. Good periodontal care may be able to restore nominal periodontal relationships. However, if the mucosal wound is associated directly with a mandibular fracture line, especially if more than half of the root length has been exposed or the socket has also been disrupted, the tooth should be considered for extraction.

Relative contraindications for dental extractions include teeth that are necessary to achieve anatomic reductions of fractures (i.e., the bone contact of angle fractures, especially superiorly is minimal, the fit of a retained 3rd molar into the residual socket on the opposite fragment may significantly improve the accuracy of the reduction). Teeth that provide essential occlusal stops should be retained at least during the reduction and fixation. Teeth in children, if at all stable, should be retained, though they will require dental evaluation and possible treatment. Deciduous teeth with over one-half of their roots resorbed by the erupting secondary tooth, will often be hypermobile and unsuitable for aiding stabilization with circumdental ligatures and arch bars. However, the deciduous teeth help to maintain dental spacing to allow the orderly eruption of the permanent dentition.

Simple Fracture Treatment

Simple mandibular fractures may be successfully treated by a number of methods. Treatment choices should be individualized to the specific circumstances of the case at hand. Reliable, compliant patients who elect conservative management do well with the necessary follow-up. In noncompliant patients, even simple fractures may benefit from rigid internal fixation that requires little or no effort on the part of the patient. Often simple fractures, if not severely displaced, may be treated successfully by closed reduction and MMS, or with one of the nonrigid (miniplate) techniques of osteosynthesis.

Complex Fractures

Fractures in Children

In Rowe's study (30,31) of 550 facial fractures, there was only a 1.2% incidence of mandibular fractures in children 5 years of age and younger, and a 4.4% incidence in the 6- to 12-year-old group. Children's mandibular fractures result from falls, athletic activities, and bicycle and automobile accidents.

Mandibular fractures in children have several additional considerations that must be factored into management schemes. Pediatric bones heal rapidly, so these fractures should be rapidly reduced to avoid malunion. Also, periods of immobilization may be reduced, often to as little as 2 weeks. Most pediatric mandibular fractures can be treated with closed reduction, and a limited period of immobilization (53,54).

Deciduous teeth have a conical shape that is less retentive for circumdental ligatures, making application of arch bars more difficult and less stable. Arch bars may be secured with 28-gauge circumdental ligatures, supplemented with circummandibular ligatures. Also, bonded orthodontic brackets may be useful. If there are sufficient stable erupted teeth, deciduous or permanent, MMS with interarch elastics provides adequate fracture stabilization in most cases. In the transitional dentition or the neglected mouth, there may be too few stable, noncarious teeth in occlusion for such stabilization. In this situation, a lingual acrylic splint, secured with circumdental and circummandibular wires is necessary.

Because of the great healing potential of pediatric mandibular fractures, open reduction with internal fixation is rarely indicated. A single arch, arch bar, or lingual splint will sufficiently stabilize the mandible in most cases, while allowing for mandibular motion. The presence of numerous tooth buds, the position of the mandibular canal, and the potential for growth disturbance makes internal fixation riskier, and therefore it is used only when absolutely necessary. Indications for internal fixation include unstable fractures not amenable to closed treatment, and bilateral fractures with gross instability. When indicated, unicortical affixed microplates or miniplates should be placed at the very inferior border of the mandible. Because of the potential for growth disturbance, or translocation into the mandible, internal fixation hardware should generally be removed by 6 to 8 weeks.

For the first few years of life, the condylar head consists of a very delicate vascular spongelike tissue with a thin cortical shell. The condyle is a growth center for the mandible. A significant injury, either traumatic or surgical, at this early age can result in disruption of the condyle, with hemarthrosis, and possible growth disturbance, arthritis, mobility disturbance, and ankylosis. Also, children's condyles have tremendous potential for remodeling. Pediatric condylar fractures should be managed by closed techniques, avoiding open techniques in almost all cases. Intracapsular fractures that do not alter the centric occlusion should not be immobilized, to avoid ankylosis. Ankylosis may occur late, more than 6 to 12 months after injury, and requires aggressive management. Unilateral condylar fractures, with alteration of centric occlusion, are treated with arch bars or lingual splints and elastic interarch stabilization, allowing for limited mandibular motion for a period as short as about 1 week. Displaced bilateral condyle fractures, with posterior vertical collapse and anterior open-bite deformity, require closed reduction and MMS for up to 3 to 4 weeks.

Fractures in the Edentulous Patient

Fractures of the edentulous mandible are generally managed similar to other mandibular fractures. Fractures of the severely atrophic mandible can be difficult to manage. After the loss of teeth, there is resorption of the alveolar bone, and the vertical height of the area is significantly reduced. The atrophied edentulous mandible becomes osteopenic and weaker, with thin cortical plates. There is an earlier incidence of atherosclerosis of the inferior alveolar vessels. Bradly (55) found that the artery was affected about 15 years earlier than the carotid arteries. The blood supply derives mainly from periosteal vessels. These factors contribute to a decreased healing potential, resulting in a 20% incidence of nonunion (56).

Simple undisplaced fractures can often be managed with puréed diet and observation. Unstable fractures may be openly reduced and immobilized with interosseous wires or, preferably, with rigid plate-and-screw fixation. Primary bone grafting should be considered. In the severely atrophied jaw, the periosteum may be left on the bone to maximize blood supply, and the plate placed over the periosteum.

Many edentulous patients with fractured mandibles may also be treated by splinting of the fracture with the patient's own dentures or a Gunning-type splint, as previously described. These are secured to the mandible on each side of the fracture with circummandibular wires. Adequate immobilization is sometimes difficult with this method because the denture or splint may not sit well on the mobile soft tissues usually present and cannot be secured too tightly to the mandible without causing soft-tissue necrosis.

Infected Fractures (Delay of Treatment)

Many fractures that present infected, present some time after infliction of the fracture. The delay between injury and presentation may come from the time required for transportation from some distant site, or (more commonly in the United

States) from the patients' neglect of their condition. Infected wounds and fractures usually have intense inflammation around the fracture site, and may have abscess formation. Many will have spontaneously decompressed, and present with a draining tract.

The usual examination and radiographic workup need to be accomplished, with the patient receiving antibiotics (penicillin, clindamycin, cephalosporin + metronidazole). Occasionally, the infection will have spread into the floor of the mouth and potential spaces of the neck, and may severely impair the upper aerodigestive tract. This subgroup needs expectant management of airways and prompt incision and drainage of infected spaces and tissue planes. Generally, active infection does not preclude definitive treatment of mandibular fractures.

After adequate workup, the infected wound needs thorough débridement of the infected wound and fracture. Frequently a tooth, or teeth, will be involved in the infection and should be extracted. Occasionally, a preliminary débridement will be necessary before the final débridement and definitive fracture treatment. Usually, with an adequate débridement, including any nonviable bone, definitive reconstruction with rigid fixation is indicated (57). Nonrigid methods of fixation or stabilization will prolong wound healing and compromise control of the infection. Because of the usual degree of fragment end resorption, these fractures become gap defects, and must be treated with rigid (large) plates and at least four screws per major fragment. Bone grafting will generally be required for bony union. Primary bone grafting may be done with an adequate débridement and control of infection, or may be done in a delayed fashion. For extreme cases with soft-tissue coverage deficiencies (i.e., unable to provide reliable coverage of any plates and the fracture wound), an external fixator may be a useful interim treatment to restore mandibular alignment and motion.

Multiple or Segmental Fracture

Many mandibular injuries, perhaps most, involve more than one fracture. Multiple fractures are much more difficult to treat, as any small errors at each fracture site tend to multiply the overall errors of the reduction. Also, either more extended exposure or multiple sites of exposure are necessary, increasing chance of wound healing problems and iatrogenic injury. Careful technical judgment is necessary to determine the sequence of repair. Often, even distant fractures must be simultaneously treated for the best accuracy of reduction. Generally, bone fragments are large enough to allow routine exposure and fixation techniques. It may be useful to simplify the multiple fragment situation by at least rough alignment with interosseous wires or rarely temporary plates.

Bilateral Fracture of Each Hemimandible. Bilateral fractures often require a simultaneous reduction of both sites. Any small discrepancy at the first reduction will be magnified at the second site, possible precluding an accurate reduction of the second site. The accuracy of the lingual cortical reduction is especially critical. This region may be difficult to directly visualize. Underreduction (lingual gaping) at one or both fractures all but precludes an accurate restoration of the occlusion.

With widely separated fractures, once accurately reduced, each fracture may be plated separately (separate plates or

techniques). Because of increased weakening of the mandible, more rigid techniques of fixation are indicated. It is uncommon that closed techniques will be successful for these cases. Arch bars and MMS may actually increase the tendency to widen the posterior segments, and to incline the molar teeth lingually.

Anterior Fracture with One or Both Condyles Fractured. With a condyle fracture, and a more anterior second fracture, there is a tremendous tendency for the interposed segment to be flared laterally, widening the mandibular arch. Maxillomandibular stabilization may only worsen this tendency, because of the lateral off-axis forces created by the interarch ligatures. If there is difficulty in controlling this lateral flaring of the inferior border of the posterior body and angle regions, consideration should be given to open reduction and internal fixation of the condyle(s). Once the freedom of displacement or angulation has been controlled at the condyle(s), the anterior fracture may be more accurately treated by rigid techniques. Again the principle of simplifying a multiple fracture situation is useful.

Unilateral Segmental Fracture in One Hemimandible. Multiple fractures within one side of the mandible may be treated as an area of comminution. As before, any inaccuracy at one fracture site will make the second reduction more difficult. Fortunately, it is often the case that all of the fragments are large enough to accept an adequate number of screws for rigid fixation. If the fractures are relatively close together, a long spanning plate may be used, fixating both fractures. Longer plates may be much more difficult to adapt accurately at both fracture sites simultaneously. Bending templates are a useful aid. Also, the complex multiple fracture situation may be simplified with interosseous wire stabilization, and perhaps with application of superior tension band plates, before the adaption and application of the major spanning plate. Access will need to be more generous, often with multiple incisions, or use of the trocar (transbuccal) technique and instrumentation.

Comminuted Fracture. With higher-energy wounding mechanisms, multiple fractures of the mandible become more common. The severe end of this spectrum of injury is the comminuted fracture. Comminuted fractures are more difficult to expose because of the wide zone of involvement and the likelihood of devitalizing small fragments from soft-tissue stripping. Comminuted fractures are more difficult to reduce accurately because of the multiple fragments involved (something akin to building a ship in a bottle—an opaque bottle with fluids frequently obscuring the access to the ship). Smaller fragments may not contain teeth to aid in reduction and stabilization. These fragments may not be large enough to accept screws, or be favorably positioned to accept screws through the limited number of holes in the plate. Additionally, some fragments may be missing, or require débridement.

Comminuted fractures of the mandible require rigid fixation with large spanning plates, and four or more sound screws in the major fragments at either end of the zone of comminution. Generally, larger reconstruction plates will be required. If there has not been extensive bone loss or devitalization, bone union will occur. Occasionally, mainly because of soft-tissue considerations, or perhaps because the patient's condition has deferred definitive treatment, temporary treatment with an external fixator is necessary. When the patient improves, or the soft tissues allow, the external fixation can be converted to definitive internal fixation. With extensive bone loss, bone grafting may be necessary, usually as a secondary procedure.

If a comminuted fracture has become infected prior to treatment, extensive débridement of small bone fragments is necessary. With adequate débridement, definitive reconstruction with a spanning reconstruction type plate may be undertaken. If infection develops after adequate stable fixation has been placed, usually a foreign body will be the source (either a bony sequestrum or a loose screw). These must be débrided to control the infection.

Fracture with Bone Defect. Mandibular fractures with a segmental bone loss generally benefit from rigid fixation with spanning reconstruction-type plates. These plates will carry all stresses across the defect, and so must be large, with an adequate number of screws (four or more per fragment) to insure stability. Because of the defect, the mandible cannot bear some of the stress, and will not regain continuity. However, even the larger reconstruction plates will eventually fail, with an increasing incidence of plate fracture after 5 to 10 years. Some time before this, the defect should be reconstructed with a bone graft or flap.

Avulsive wounds with loss of both soft tissues and mandible require treatment of the soft-tissue deficit, and of the bone deficit. Such reconstruction may be simultaneous (e.g., free-tissue transfer of osteocutaneous flap such as fibular flap) or, more commonly, sequential. Sequentially, first the soft tissues are controlled (one or more débridements) and reconstructed or repaired. During this interval, the mandibular fragment may be controlled with MMS or with an external fixator, trying to avoid scar contracture of the remaining soft tissues and malposition of the mandibular fragments. After control of the soft tissues and, if necessary, soft-tissue reconstruction, the bone deficit is reconstructed. With an adequate soft-tissue envelope, this may be a bone graft, or a spanning reconstruction plate with secondary bone grafting. For truly massive avulsive wounds, a careful staged reconstructive treatment plan must be developed for optimal reconstruction. Treatment may require many months to several years.

Postoperative Care

As treatment is concluding for mandibular fractures, the MMS should be released and centric occlusion and condylar position and motion confirmed. If malocclusion is noted at this time, the reduction and fixation must be revised. If centric occlusion has been restored accurately and adequate rigid fixation assured, the patient may be left out of MMS, which improves the safety of emergence from anesthesia. However, even with adequately rigid fixation, many patients benefit from a brief period (up to several days) of MMS for "tissue rest."

Perioperative antibiotics are clearly of benefit for mandibular fractures compounded to the skin or oral mucosa, covering either or both skin flora and oral flora. The benefit of postoperative antibiotics is less well established, and usually based empirically, or on the surgeon's experience or training (58).

Airway control is critical for the patient in MMS, especially during emergence from anesthesia, when protective re-

flexes may be impaired. Prior to extubation, the stomach should be aspirated with a nasogastric or orogastric tube, to minimize risk of emesis and aspiration. A head-raised position helps with secretion control and with swallowing. Facial swelling may be quite impressive after open management of mandibular, as well as other, facial fractures. Cold compresses and ice packs, as well as the head-elevated position will aid in minimizing and resolving edema. Patients should be extubated when alert enough to have protective reflexes restored. Wire cutters and adequate suction must be kept with the patient at all times, to allow release of MMS in case need arises for emergent airway access.

Ice chips and clear liquids may be begun, once the patient is alert enough to swallow and protect the airway. Early liquids allows the patient to learn to swallow with MMS. However, it is common for facial fracture patients, especially those in MMS, to have inadequate oral intake to maintain adequate hydration, much less adequate nutrition, for several days. Intravenous hydration should be maintained until oral intake is adequate. After 1 to 2 days, the diet should be advanced to full liquids, and may be extended to include puréed items. Those patients not expected to regain swallowing rapidly (e.g., those with impaired consciousness, tracheostomy) should have small-diameter flexible feeding tubes placed, to ensure prompt resumption of an adequate nutrition. Many patients benefit from dietary counseling, as weight loss during MMS may exceed 10 to 15 pounds.

Oral hygiene should be strongly encouraged, especially in patients with compound oral wounds or intraoral lacerations. Oral plaque, the bacterial film that rapidly grows over oral surfaces, becomes increasing anaerobic and virulent as it matures. Soft pediatric toothbrushes and mouthwashes mixed with hydrogen peroxide will be helpful, but often uncomfortable (i.e., there may be poor patient compliance), and, when in MMS, most oral mucosa and tooth surfaces are not accessible to the tooth brush. If the airway is protected (i.e., patient alert, or endotracheal cuff on tracheostomy or endotracheal tube inflated) oral rinses with antimicrobial mouthwash and peroxide, or other solutions (i.e., chlorhexidine) can cleanse the inaccessible surfaces. If there are no intraoral wounds or incisions, oral irrigators (i.e., Water Pik) will improve oral hygiene further. However, even the relatively low pressure of such irrigators may disrupt delicate mucosal repairs or dissect into incisions. Many patients are bothered by the numerous sharp edges of arch bars and wire ligatures. They benefit by the application of soft dental wax over the sharp points. The wax should be removed at least once a day to permit oral hygiene.

Complications of Mandibular Fractures

MALOCCLUSION

Causation

Malocclusion is the most common complication after mandibular fractures; it arises from a great many diverse factors, including the original injury, patient compliance, and factors growing out of the treatment of such fractures. Malocclusion must also result from malalignment of one or more fracture fragments. Restoration of the "normal" (preinjury) centric occlusion includes restoration of the preinjury maximal intercuspation (centric occlusion), preservation of temporomandibular joint function and range of motion, and preservation of the complex neuromotor function of the muscles of mastication. Minor malocclusions may often be corrected with selective occlusal adjustments of the dentition, or perhaps orthodontia. Early malocclusions in nonrigidly fixated cases may respond to "orthodontic" elastic MMS. However, it is unclear if the malocclusion is reduced by fragment motion or orthodontic tooth movement. Significant malocclusions require reoperation.

Patient lack of compliance may contribute to malocclusion. Patients have released themselves from MMS and have removed their arch bars. Patients have also failed to participate for adequate follow-up, occasionally presenting a year or more after initial treatment for arch bar removal.

However, a more common cause of malocclusion in treated mandibular fractures is failure to restore the preinjury centric occlusion, or failure to adequately stabilize the restored occlusion during fracture healing. Assessing the centric occlusion may be subtle, especially in fracture cases (with patient cooperation often compromised) or if the upper aerodigestive tract is occupied with endotracheal and nasogastric tubes. Furthermore, some treatment options may contribute to malocclusion, such as the tendency for MMS to cause a lingual open bite or to cause "orthodontic" tooth movement.

Malocclusion can occur even with techniques of rigid internal fixation. One such cause is the improper use of compression for mandibular fracture fixation. Compression applied to the lateral cortex of the inferior border of the horizontal mandible, even with bicortical screws, tends to distract the lingual cortex and the superior border. This tendency should be compensated for with other techniques: plate overbending, preloading the fracture with reduction forceps, and application of a superior border plate before applying the inferior border plate with compression. It is also possible to misuse compression. Compression should not be used with comminuted or segmental loss fracture patterns. Of course, an improperly contoured plate will distort fracture fragments, as the bone will be drawn to the maladapted plate, and not the plate to the properly reduced bone.

One entirely unnecessary cause of malocclusion is the failure to place the patient into centric occlusion with MMS before open methods of fracture reduction. Use of MMS, at least intraoperatively, is necessary to restore centric occlusion; it also reduces the freedom of displacement of unstable fractures, and aids in the overall reduction of the mandibular fragments. The arch bar also acts a tension band helping to stabilize the mandibular fracture.

Occasionally, because the arch bars are usually placed before the fractures are opened, the mandibular arch bar will be placed incorrectly, inaccurately restoring the length ("circumference") of the mandibular alveolar arch, typically when teeth are missing. The arch bar will then prevent the accurate reduction of the fragments, or prevent the restoration of maximal intercuspation. The arch bar can be cut into two separate components, or the circumdental ligatures from one side of the fracture can be removed, the bar adjusted, and the ligatures reapplied.

Another cause of malocclusion is the misreading of the preinjury occlusion. Many patients have malocclusions before they sustain facial fractures. Careful examination of wear facettes, and of the dental models, can indicate the

proper position of maximal intercuspation for that patient. It is also difficult to restore centric occlusion when most or all of the centric stops have been lost on one or both sides of the dentition. In this situation, dental splints with circummandibular wires may be the only way to restore centric occlusion with MMS.

Other potential causes of malocclusion include the failure to diagnosis a separate fracture (or fractures) that also affect the occlusion (i.e., a condylar neck fracture, with loss of posterior vertical height), and placing the dental arches into MMS, but to a maxilla that is not properly related to the cranial base. In either case, the treated mandibular fracture may be anatomically reduced (interfragmentary alignment correct), but malocclusion still occurs because the whole occlusion (the correct relationship of the mandible and maxilla to each other, to the muscles of mastication, and to the cranial base), has not been restored. This is likely to happen with incomplete maxillary Le Fort fractures with impaction of the maxilla. The maxilla may clinically feel stable, but has altered its relationship to the cranial base. If the mandible is placed into MMS against the displaced maxilla, before the maxilla is disimpacted and reduced, one or both TMJs will be distorted as long as the patient is in MMS. However, when the patient is released from MMS, the condyles will tend to return to their physiologic position, with the mandible changing its relationship to the maxilla, and malocclusion results.

Treatment and Prevention

The best treatment for posttreatment malocclusion is accurate restoration of the preinjury occlusion in the first place. For many patients, their preinjury status can be readily determined from a careful examination of the dentition for the apparent maximal intercuspation and wear facettes. Some patients will have had significant preinjury malocclusions that may be difficult to diagnose after injury. Dental models are helpful in assessing the occlusion, and provides a lingual view of the dentition that cannot be obtained from the patient. Models also allow the fabrication of splints and occlusal stints that may be helpful in mandibular fracture treatment.

Maxillomandibular stabilization is essential during the treatment of mandibular fractures, and the period of stabilization depends on the technique of fracture fixation. Especially with tooth or bony loss, the mandibular arch bar may be placed improperly, inaccurately restoring the mandibular arch length. It may be necessary to adjust or divide the arch bar into two segments to allow placing the dentition into maximal intercuspation.

Instability (Delayed Union/Nonunion)

Causation

With adequate stabilization, the fracture healing cascade will result in bony union quite predictably. In orthopedics, fractures not healed within 4 months are considered delayed unions, and fractures not healed by 6 months are considered nonunions (or pseudoarthroses) (59). However, maxillofacial fractures heal more rapidly. Facial fractures not clinically stable by 6 weeks should be considered delayed unions; nonunions are fractures not clinically stable after 10 weeks of treatment.

Delayed union or nonunion of mandibular fractures results from failure to provide adequate stability to allow the fracture healing cascade to achieve full bony union. Delayed or nonunion results represent an arrest or interruption of the fracture healing cascade, possibly because of infection, inadequate stabilization, or both; or, in rarely, because of inadequate vascularity. Most commonly, delayed unions and nonunions result from inadequate stability. Occasionally, this will result from patient noncompliance, as when the patient removes MMS or arch bars prematurely. However, most commonly inadequate stability of treated fractures results from inappropriate treatment selection, or poor fixation techniques (e.g., too few screws, too small a plate, screw stripping).

As fixation systems have been progressively downsized, the difference between the stability of the fixation system and the stability required to promote fracture healing decreases. Nonrigid techniques of fracture stabilization may require supplementation with MMS and reduced function to avoid disruption of the fracture healing cascade. Even techniques of rigid fixation require appropriate application techniques to insure adequate fracture fixation during the fracture healing cascade (e.g., improper screw placement technique, with inadequate irrigation, may result in premature screw loosening and fixation compromise).

Rarely, the fixation system itself will fail, with breakage of plate or screws. This has become more common with the downsizing of fixation plates towards the critical minimum necessary to stabilize mandible fractures. It also may result from improper plate contouring, especially with repetitive bending and unbending of a plate. Plates can also be damaged by the improper use of bending instruments, so that the plates are nicked or deformed.

Another cause of nonunion is fracture infection. Infected nonunions result from inadequate fracture stabilization accompanied by inflammation with microbial inoculation. There are several causations for inadequate fixation contributing to infected nonunions. Improper screw placement, with damage of the bone holding the screw, will contribute to early loosening of the screw and reduced stability of the fixation. Loose screws (bone stripping) must be removed. One of the most common errors of internal fixation techniques is to allow a loose foreign body to remain in the wound. Loose screws do not contribute to fracture fixation stability. Such screws must be removed and replaced with an emergency screw or left out; or, the plate may be repositioned. Another common problem with fracture infection and resultant nonunion is the inadequate management of teeth associated with the fracture. Teeth both tend to weaken the mandible and act as a potential portal for oral flora and dental plaque to gain access to the fracture wound.

Treatment and Prevention

Again, the best treatment of nonunion is to prevent it by making the appropriate choice of fracture management. However, once nonunion is present, a change in management is necessary to assure progression through the fracture healing cascade to union. Occasionally, nonrigid stabilization techniques may lead to fracture healing with resumption or extension of MMS, but at a cost of increased fracture end resorption, worsened TMJ motion, and chondromalacia. The required treatment for nonunion is absolute stability, almost always by techniques of rigid internal fixation. When bone resorption, or resection of interfragmentary inflammation tissues, results in a significant bony defect, bone grafting will also be necessary.

The patient should be placed into MMS and centric occlusion. To accomplish this, it may be necessary to open the fracture and remove the fibrous scar tissue or previous fixation that is preventing the realignment of the bony fragments. Once centric occlusion is restored (if not required in the previous step), the fibrous tissue occupying the fracture should be removed. Next, rigid fixation is applied, which, with fragment end resorption and removal of scar tissue, must be a fracture-bridging plate (reconstruction plate). If, after accurate reduction, a significant bone gap remains (>1–2 mm) consideration should be given to bone grafting.

MALPOSITION (MALUNION)

Causation

Malposition of treated fractures results either from an inaccuracy of the initial reduction, or from inadequate stabilization. Untreated fractures typically heal malaligned. In either case, the fracture may heal with a fibrous (nonbony) scar, or with bony union in malalignment. Small malalignments, especially posterior to the occlusion, may be tolerated without malocclusion or apparent deformity. Usually, however, a significant malocclusion will accompany the malunion, and treatment is indicated to restore the occlusion.

Generally, malposition should be treated early to avoid deleterious effects on the TMJs and changes of the dentition (supereruption of unopposed teeth). If nonrigid or rigid internal fixation has been used, there is little hope of correcting the malalignment with MMS or elastics.

Treatment and Prevention

If malposition has occurred, and is significant enough to warrant treatment, generally the fracture must be addressed open, with a more stable degree of fixation, usually rigid fixation. For fibrous malunions, the patient is placed into MMS, if possible; however, the malalignment may be so severe as to preclude placing the patient into centric occlusion. In this case, the arch bars are applied, and then the fracture accessed and the intervening fibrous scar removed to allow a better reduction and achieve centric occlusion. If there has been bony union with significant malalignment, an osteotomy will have to be made to allow reduction. Often, the osteotomy will be made at the original fracture site. However, for some fractures (i.e., body fractures) the location of the mandibular nerve may prevent a safe osteotomy through the original fracture (assuming a degree of nerve function). The osteotomy may be more safely made elsewhere, such as in the parasymphyseal region or in the posterior mandible (i.e., sagittal split osteotomy).

In the case of fibrous union, and in many osteotomy cases, a bone gap will result, and must be treated rigidly with a spanning plate and bone grafting.

Infection

Causation

Many factors involved with mandibular fractures may contribute to infection. Many mandibular fractures of the horizontal mandible are compounded through skin or, more commonly, the oral mucosa. Also, many of these horizontal mandibular fractures involve teeth or their sockets, which have various stages of preexisting dental disease. Many patients delay presenting for care for mandible fractures from hours to days, weeks, and even months after initial injury. Often when delayed presentation is made it is because of the severity of the progression of their complaints of malocclusion, pain, and established infection.

Multiple investigators have shown that the incidence of infection is directly related to the stability of the bone fragments, and that rigid fixation decreases infection rates. Stone and colleagues (40) found a significant difference in rates of infection between groups treated by open reduction and wire osteosynthesis (20%) and by open reduction and rigid fixation (6.3%). Poor patient compliance was a component of the high rate of infection in the wire osteosynthesis group, in that nearly all of the 20% of this group that developed infections had removed themselves from intermaxillary fixation before fracture healing was complete.

In fact, the increased risk, or presence, of infection in mandibular fractures, which are amenable to internal rigid fixation, is an indication for the use of compression plates or screws (60,61).

Treatment and Prevention

Regardless of whether there is infection of the fracture, osteomyelitis around the fracture gap, or an infected nonunion, absolute stabilization of the fracture ends must be the overriding concern (57). Basic treatment of fracture associated infections includes: (a) culture-specific antibiotic therapy; (b) stable, rigid fixation of fractures with adequately rigid plates and screws; (c) drainage of the area for several days; (d) with adequate débridement and soft-tissue coverage, autologous cancellous bone grafting as necessary.

EXPOSED OR LOOSE HARDWARE

Causation

Fixation hardware may become exposed, usually intraorally, with inadequate soft-tissue management (i.e., inappropriate placement of incisions), or with protracted tissue inflammation, either from infection or inadequate fixation. Exposures can also develop from wound or tissue contracture, or from the wearing of a dental prosthesis over the hardware.

Hardware, mainly screws (if stripped or improperly inserted with thermal damage to the bone from drilling) may become loose. Such loose hardware may become palpable, visible, or be found on a follow-up x ray. If not found early, loose hardware will often become infected and develop a sinus tract.

Treatment and Prevention

Avoidance of exposure by appropriate selection of technique and application is best. If the exposure is minor, and not associated with infection, the hardware may be left in place until the fracture has healed, and then be removed. If the exposure is major, or the fracture develops significant exposure before healing, or infection develops, usually the offending hardware must be removed, and a more stable form of fixation employed. If the exposure results from denture wear, the prosthesis should not be used until the fracture heals, and then the hardware can be removed. After healing of the incision, the prosthesis can be adjusted and worn.

Loose hardware, not yet infected, may be briefly observed until fracture healing. However, if union becomes delayed, infection intervenes, or fixation becomes unstable, the loose hardware should be removed and replaced.

Hardware Failure

Causation

Generally, modern internal fixation devices are well made and, when used as intended by the manufacturer, will not fail in normal usage. An unfavorable outcome resulting from the fixation hardware is almost always the result of the plate's not being used as intended, or of poor technique. The internal fixation devices have been carefully designed to preform in specific usages. Usage other than intended by the manufacture may exceed the design parameters of the plate and be a cause of failure. Improper technique includes improper bending of the plate. Using the improper instruments, or the proper instruments in an improper fashion, may nick or deform the plate, weakening it or impairing the fit of one or more screws into it. A common error is to ignore the supplied bending templates and repeatedly bend and unbend the actual implant. Repetitive bending causes work hardening of the plate and weakens it.

Another common cause of fixation failure is the use of too few screws. A plate and a pair of screws with one on either side of the fracture will hold the fragments together, but rotation about the screws is possible. The pair of screws adjacent to the fracture experiences over 90% of the strain across the fracture. A second screw on each side of the fracture will resist the potential to rotate, and bear a small percentage of the strain across the fracture. However, if any of the screws loosen, perhaps because of poor drilling technique that caused thermal damage of the bone, the fixation will fail. So, if two screws are used on either side of the fracture, all must be placed with optimal technique in sound bone to retain stability of the fixation. It is useful to use at least three screws on either side of the fracture for simple fractures, to assure that at least two screws are sound enough to provide stability during fracture healing. At least four screws should be used in the major fragments on either end of a comminuted fracture or segmental defect.

Loose or stripped screws must be removed, to be replaced with larger-diameter emergency screws, left out, or repositioned. Loose screws not only do not contribute to the stability of the fixation but also severely increase the risk of infection and healing failure. Additionally, if motion occurs between a screw and its plate, fritting will occur, with abrasion of the plate and screw. Fritting weakens the plate and screw, and finely grinds flakes of the plate and screw, increasing corrosion and release of metallic ions.

Even properly applied plates used as the manufacture recommends may fail. The large reconstruction plates are used for the spanning of bone defects in mandibular reconstruction. These largest plates cannot indefinitely withstand functional load the way living bone can. There seems to be a concentration of strain in the plate in the region of the border between gap and bone end. Work hardening occurs over time, with the plate becoming brittle, which can lead to eventual fracture of the plate. Such bone gap defects should be bone grafted, so that living bone can adapt to the strains developed across the defect.

Treatment and Prevention

When fracture fixation is determined to have failed, it is generally because of a complication such as delayed union or nonunion, or perhaps a wound infection. To obtain successful fracture healing, it is usually necessary to remove the inadequate fixation hardware, rereduce the fracture, and provide a more stable method of fixation, such as rigid internal fixation.

Fixation failures can be minimized by the selection of an appropriately stable form of fixation for the pattern of fracture, properly applied as suggested by the manufacture, with appropriate techniques. It is essential to have, and to use, the appropriate instrumentation for the set being used. The use of bending templates will minimize the working of a plate. Plates overworked or significantly nicked or deformed should be discarded, and a new plate adapted.

IATROGENIC INJURIES

Teeth

Teeth and their supporting structures may be injured in a number of ways during the treatment of mandibular fractures. The application of interdental ligatures and arch bars may inflict significant injury to the gingiva, periodontal ligament, and the teeth themselves, or just worsen existing periodontal disease. The wires necessary for such stabilization, if sloppily applied, will damage the gingiva. Even if applied carefully, the mere presence of the wires and arch bars severely impairs oral hygiene. Maxillomandibular stabilization makes at least seven-eighths of the tooth surfaces and most of the oral mucosa inaccessible for routine methods of oral hygiene.

Dental roots may be easily injured during the steps of screw placement, even from unicortical screws. Generally, screws in the mandible should be placed beneath the apices of the teeth. If it is recognized during fixation that a root may have been injured, the screw should be removed. If the injury is only to periodontal ligament, cementum, or dentin, usually the tooth may remain viable. If the dental pulp is injured, the tooth may become nonviable, or internal resorption may be initiated. Both conditions may require endodontic therapy or extraction.

Sensorimotor Disturbances

Temporary sensorimotor disturbances are a common sequelae after mandibular fractures, regardless of method of treatment. There is also great potential for iatrogenic injury of sensory and motor nerves, which may have permanent impairment.

Sensor disturbances involve the branches of the trigeminal nerve—usually in the inferior alveolar nerve or the mental nerve distributions because of the pathway of the inferior alveolar nerve through the mandibular canal. However, the mental nerve may be directly injured during fracture exposure, or from traction applied during plate insertion and fixation. Nerve injury may also result from drilling through the mandibular canal during screw placement. The inferior alveolar neurovascular bundle may be injured by too-severe motion of fragments during reduction, or by entrapment of the nerve between the fragments (especially with compression techniques of fixation).

Motor injuries usually involve the marginal mandibular branch of the facial nerve or, much more rarely, the trigeminal innervation of the muscles of mastication. Facial nerve injury may result from lacerations across the course of the branches of the facial nerve. If a nerve stimulator is not used to locate the nerve, iatrogenic injury of the nerve during extraoral access to the angle region is likely because of the degree of anatomic variability in the course of the nerve. Even with identification of the nerve, retraction may inflict a neuropraxia, with temporary weakness of the lip depressors.

In colder climates, some patients complain of hypersensitivity to cold, most often when the larger plates have been implanted, especially in areas near the skin. Though the plate is at body temperature, it is more thermally conductive than the surrounding soft tissues, so the patient perceives the plate as being cold. Such sensations subside after plate removal.

Temporomandibular Joint (TMJ) Pain

Temporomandibular joint pain and dysfunction are common sequelae of mandibular fractures, and may also result from the treatment of the fractures. Maxillomandibular stabilization for as little as 4 to 6 weeks causes some degree of capsular contracture, as well as changes in the articular cartilage of the condylar head (35). The longer the period of immobilization, the more severe the changes. Some changes begin within hours of immobilization. Usually these changes will be minimal, and essentially full recovery made with appropriate physical therapy. However, these sequelae may arise from the treatment of even simple fractures, and if unrecognized or untreated may result in significant disability.

Another potential cause of joint pain is to have wired the patient into maximal intercuspation, with a midface fracture and the maxilla malpositioned relative to the cranial base. In this case, the teeth will appear to be in proper occlusion, but the condylar head in not in a physiologic position within the joint. When the MMS is released, the occlusion will appear correct for a few hours to days, but shortly the condyle will seek its physiologic position, resulting in an early malocclusion and possible joint pain. This discrepancy will not correct itself. Most likely, the maxilla will have to be repositioned correctly.

Little is understood about the fate of the articular disk in cases of mandibular fractures. In cases of condylar fractures, the fine coordinated function between the two heads of the lateral pterygoid muscle, one inserting on the head, and one on the disk and capsule, may be disrupted. The muscle may be in spasm and acting to displace or angulate the head fragment anteromedially, altering its relationship to the disk and glenoid fossa and temporal articular eminence. Even without a condylar fracture, little is known about the effect on the disk of MMS.

Exacerbation of Dental Disease

Preexisting dental disease, caries, and periodontal disease will often be worsened by the impairment of oral hygiene imposed by MMS. Fracture treatment, such as MMS, may also worsen periodontal disease directly by imposing pathologic forces on the involved teeth. With advanced periodontal disease, less stability from MMS can be depended on, and a more stable form of internal fixation must be used. Fractured teeth with pulpal exposures may rapidly develop periapical inflammation and abscesses.

Conclusion

For a number of reasons, treatment of mandibular fractures remains challenging. Optimal treatment of the sometimes bewildering patterns and complexity of mandibular fractures is based on the understanding and application of a relative few principles: biology of bone and fracture healing, anatomy of the mandible, dentition, occlusion, and enveloping soft tissues, and techniques of fracture fixation. The proficient surgeon treating such fractures needs a number of techniques in his surgical armamentarium, as well as to be adept with the instrumentation required for these techniques. Postoperative imaging is essential to assess the accuracy of the reduction. Most orthopedic surgeons would consider it negligence if postreduction confirmatory x rays were not taken; maxillofacial surgeons should not accept less.

Optimal outcomes can be reliably obtained by adherence to time-tested principles. However, methods and materials continue to evolve, which should continue to improve patient care and outcome. Today, a good result for mandibular fracture treatment should be considered nothing less than uneventful bony union, with a full recovery of function, including a stable functional occlusion, as well as full TMJ stability with a normal range of motion. Facial sensibility and motor function should be intact, and the patient should have no disfiguring scars that resulted from treatment.

References

1. Adams WM. Internal wiring fixation of facial fractures. *Surgery* 1932; 12:523 (25:909).
2. Vero D. Jaw injuries: the use of Kirschner wires to supplement fixation. *Br J Oral Surg* 1968; 6:18.
3. Converse JM, Waknitz FW. External skeletal fixation of the mandibular angle. *J Bone Joint Surg (Am)* 1942; 24:154.
4. Morris JH. Biphasic connector, external skeletal splint for reduction and fixation of mandible fractures. *Oral Surg* 1949; 2:1382.
5. Lambotte A. *L'traitement des fractures.* Paris: Verlag Masson, 1907.
6. Lambotte A. Technique and indications for buried prosthesis in the treatment of fractures. *Presse Med* 1909; 17:321.
7. Lambotte A. *Chirugie opératoire des fractures.* Paris: Masson, 1913.
8. Danis R. *Theorie et pratique de l'ostéosynthèses.* Paris: Libraries de L'Academie de Medicine, 1949.
9. Pauwels F. Grundriss einer biomechanik der frankturheilung. *Ver Dtsch Ges Othop* 1940; 34:62.
10. Bagby GW, Janes JM. The effect of compression on the rate of fracture healing using a special plate. *Am J Surg* 1958; 95:761.
11. Luhr HG. Zur stabilen ostésynthèse bei unterkieferfrakturen. *Dtsch Zahnarztl Z* 1968; 23:754.
12. Mittlemeier H. Drukosteosynthese mit selbstspannended Platten (technik und erfahrungsbericht). Homberg/Saar: Saarl Westplfälz Orthopädentretten, 1968.
13. Spiessl B. Rigid internal fixation of fractures of the lower jaw. *Reconstr Surg Traumatel* 1972; 13:124.
14. Brons R, Goering G. Fractures of the mandibular body treated by stable internal fixation: a preliminary report. *J Oral Maxillofac Surg* 1970; 28:407.
15. Michelet FX, Deymes J, Dessus B. Osteosynthesis with minaturized screwed plates in maxillofacial surgery. *J Maxillofac Surg* 1973; 1:79.
16. Champy M, Loddé JP, Schmitt R, et al. Mandibular osteosynthesis by minature screwed plates via buccal approach. *J Maxillofac Surg* 1978; 6:14.
17. Busuito MJ, Smith DJ Jr, Robson MD. Mandibular fractures in an urban trauma center. *J Trauma* 1986; 26:826.
18. Ellis E III, Moos KF, El-Attar A. Ten years of mandibular fractures: an analysis of 2137 cases. *Oral Surg* 1985; 59:120.
19. James RB, Fredrickson C, Kent JN. Prospective study of mandibular fractures. *J Oral Surg* 1981; 39:275–281.
20. Larsen OD, Nielsen A. Mandibular fractures—an analysis of their etiology and location in 286 patients. *Scand J Plast Reconstr Surg* 1976; 10:213.
21. Gilmer TL. Fractures of the inferior maxilla. *Ill St Dent Soc Trans* 1881; 67:67.
22. Hagan EH, Huelke DF. An analysis of 319 case report of mandibular fractues. *J Oral Surg* 1961; 19:93.
23. Schenk RK, Willenegger H. Morphological findings in primary fracture healing. *Sump Biol Hung* 1967; 7:75.
24. Reitzik M, Schoorl W. Bone repair in the mandible. *J Oral Maxillofac Surg* 1983; 41:215.
25. Sinn DP. Unpublished data from Parkland Memorial Hospital, Dallas, Texas, 1989, as reported in Selected Readings in Plastic Surgery 1989; 25(26):4.
26. Dingman RO, Grabb WC. Surgical anatomy of the mandibular ramus of the facial nerve based on the dissection of 100 facial halves. *Plast Reconstr Surg* 1962; 29:266.
27. Al-Kayat A, Bramley P. A modified pre-auricular approach to the temporomandibular joint and malar arch. *Br J Oral Maxillofac Surg* 1979; 17:91.
28. Lyons CJ. *A practical treatise on fractures and dislocations of the jaws.* Toledo: Ransom & Randolph, 1919.
29. Gilmer TL. A case of fracture of the lower jaw with remarks on treatment. *Arch Dent* 1887; 4:388.
30. Rowe NL. Fractures of the facial skeleton in children. *J Oral Surg* 1968; 26:505.
31. Rowe NL. Fractures of the jaws in children. *J Oral Surg* 1969; 27:497.
32. Juniper RP, Awty MD. The immobilization period for fractures of the mandible body. *Oral Surg* 1973; 36:159.
33. Fischer SE. Respiratory/cardiac arrest complicating intermaxillary fixation. *Br J Oral Surg* 1982; 20:192.
34. Williams JG, Cawood JI. Effect of intermaxillary fixation on pulmonary function. *JOMS* 1990; 19:76–78.
35. Ellis E III, Carlson DS. The effects of mandibular immoblization on the masticatory system. A review. *Clin Plast Surg* 1989; 16(1):133–146.
36. Mayo KH, Ellis E III, Carlson DS. Histochemical characteristics of masseter and temporalis muscles after five weeks of maxillomandibular fixation. An investigation in Macaca mulatta. *Oral Surg* 1988; 66:421.
37. Jokl P, Konstadt S. The effect of limb immobilization on muscle function and protein composition. *Clin Orthop* 1983; 174:222.
38. Waite DE. External biphase pin method for fixation of mandible. *Mayo Clin Proc* 1967; 42:294.
39. Wessberg GA, Schendel S, Epker BN. Monophase extraskeletal fixation. *Oral Surg* 1979; 37:892.
40. Stone IE, Dodson TB, Bays RA. Risk factors for infection following operative treatment of mandibular fractures: a multivariate analysis. *PRS* 1993; 91:64–68.
41. Assael LA. Evaluation of rigid internal fixation of mandible fractures performed in the teaching laboratory. *J Oral Maxillofac Surg* 1993; 51:1315–1319.
42. Tu HK, Tenhulzen D. Compression osteosynthesis of mandibular fractures: a retrospective study. *J Oral Maxillofac Surg* 1985; 43:585.
43. Roed-Peterson B, Anderson JO. Prognosis of permanent teeth involved in jaw fractures. A clinical and radiographic follow-up study. *Scand J Dent Res* 1970; 78:343–352.
44. Magee WP Jr. Dental principles applied to management of mandibular fractures. In: Schultz RC, ed. *Facial injuries.* 3rd ed. Chicago: Year Book Medical Publishers, 1988.
45. Amaratunga NA. The relation of age to immobilization period required for healing of mandibular fractures. *Oral Maxillofac Surg* 1987; 45:111–113.
46. Coccia CT. A clinical investigation of root resorption rates and reimplanted permanent incisors: A five-year study. *J. Endodontics* 1980; 6:413.
47. Tan PM, Zweig BE. Clinical management of dentoalveolar trauma: a discussion of current philosophy and methodology and a review of a case. *Military Medicine* 1989; 154:518–521.
48. Russell D, Nosti JC, Reavis C. Treatment of fractures of the mandibular condyle. *J Trauma* 1972; 12:704.
49. Zide MF, Kent JN. Indication for open reduction of mandibular condyle fractures. *J Oral Maxillofac Surg* 1983; 41:89.
50. Beekler DM, Walker RV. Condyle fractures. *J Oral Surg* 1969; 27:563.
51. Schneider SS, Stern M. Teeth in the line of mandibular fracture. *J Oral Surg* 1971; 29:107–109.
52. Neal DC, Wagner WF, Alpert B. Morbidity associated with teeth in the line of mandibular fractures. *J Oral Surg* 1978; 36:859–862.
53. König F. Operative chirurgie der knochenbüche. 1 Bd: operationen am frischen und verschleppten knochenbrüch. Berlin: Springer, 1931.

54. Ludinghausen MV, Meister P, Probst J. Metallosus after osteosynthesis. *Path Eur* 1970; 5:307.
55. Bradley JC. Radiological investigation into the age changes of the inferior dental artery. *Br J Oral Surg* 1975; 13:82.
56. Bruce RA, Strachan DS. Fractures of the edentulous mandible. The Chalmers J. Lyons Academy study. *J Oral Surg* 1976; 34:973.
57. Prein J, Beyer M. Management of infection and nonunion in mandibular fractures. *Oral and Maxillofacial/Surgery Clinics of North America* 1990; 2:187–194.
58. Zallen RD, Curry JT. A study of antibiotic usage in compound mandibular fractures. *J Oral Surg* 1975; 33:431.
59. Müller ME, Allgöwer M, Willenegger H. *Manual of internal fixation.* 2nd ed. Berlin: Springer, 1977; 335.
60. Becker HL. Treatment of initially infected mandibular fractures with bone plates. *J Oral Surg* 1979; 37:310.
61. Coleman RF, Herrington J, Scales JT. Concentration of wear products in hair, blood, and urine after total hip replacement. *British Med J* 1973; 1:527.

36

Benign and Malignant Tumors of the Oral Cavity

Mark S. Granick, M.D., F.A.C.S., Mark P. Solomon, M.D., F.A.C.S., and Dwight C. Hanna, M.D., F.A.C.S.

Anatomy

Tumors of the oral cavity are classified according to their size and location within the oral cavity. The classification and staging of these lesions aid in determining the proper treatment program and in prognosis. Consequently, a clear understanding of the various anatomic zones within the oral cavity is necessary to precisely define the extent and location of tumor growth. In addition, it is important to understand the anatomy of the remaining portions of the upper aerodigestive tract because some tumors extend beyond the oral cavity and, in some instances, there are synchronous or metachronous tumors.

The oral cavity (Fig. 36–1) begins at the cutaneous–vermilion border and extends to the level of the tonsillar pillars. Included within the oral cavity are the lips, the buccal surfaces, the buccal sulci, the alveolus and teeth, the hard palate, the floor of the mouth, the mobile portion of the tongue (anterior two-thirds of the tongue, anterior to the circumvallate papillae), and the retromolar trigone.

Other areas of relevance include the oropharynx, the hypopharynx, and the larynx; the nasopharynx must also be considered. The nasopharynx includes the nasal side of the soft palate and the area posterior to the choana, extending to the level of the posterior pharyngeal wall where the soft palate makes contact. The oropharynx includes the tonsils, the posterior tonsillar pillars, and the lateral and posterior pharyngeal walls to the level of the hyoid. Also included within the oropharynx is the sessile portion of the tongue posterior to the circumvallate papillae, known as the base of the tongue, and the valleculae. The hypopharynx is the area inferior to the hyoid to the level of the esophageal inlet. This includes the pyriform sinuses and the pharyngeal walls. The larynx includes the epiglottis and all of the structures leading into the larynx, as well as the glottis and the area immediately below the glottis and above the trachea. The larynx is subclassified into the supraglottic, glottic, and subglottic regions.

Examination

Patients who have tumors of the oral cavity require complete head and neck examinations. This examination is relatively simple to perform, but it should be done systematically each time to avoid overlooking pathology.

The first portion of the examination consists of a gross inspection of the patient's habitus, including personal hygiene, nutritional status, and affect. Personal factors are very important in deciding the appropriate course of therapy in patients with head and neck cancer. The next area of concern is inspection of the external ears, the external auditory canal, and the tympanic membranes. Tumors of the external auditory canal can metastasize to the neck, and alterations in middle-ear physiology can actually represent lesions obstructing the eustachian orifice in the nasopharynx. Many patients with oral tumors will present with ear pain, and it is important to rule out otological pathology in their evaluation.

The examination then proceeds to the nose, and an intranasal examination is performed. In order to do this examination properly, a coaxial light source is required. This will allow direct visualization of all of the areas of the nasal cavity. The nondominant hand should hold the nasal specula, which is placed in the nostril and opened in a longitudinal direction to avoid impact on the nasal septum. When the nasal speculum is opened against the nasal septum, it is quite irritating for the patient. Care must be taken not to overlook evaluation of the nasal vestibule, which can easily be covered by the nasal speculum during the intranasal examination. If the patient has congested nasal mucosa, it is necessary to spray the nasal membranes with a vasoconstrictor.

Examination of the oral cavity commences with a look at the lips. Then, using two tongue depressors, the lips are retracted, and the buccal sulci and membranes are directly viewed. The teeth and alveolus are examined. Loose teeth without evidence of periodontal disease or infection are early warning signs of cancer. The floor of the mouth is next examined, and it is necessary to retract the tongue using a tongue blade to view the floor of the mouth fully. Function of the submandibular gland is assessed by milking the submandibular gland and observing the orifice of the Wharton duct. The entire tongue is then checked, starting at the root, where the frenulum attaches to the floor of the mouth, then the lateral surfaces, and finally the dorsal portion of the tongue. The retromolar trigone is then inspected by retracting the tongue medially and looking at the inner surface of the mandible inferior and posterior to the level of the molars. This mucosally lined surface is easily overlooked unless it is directly examined. The hard and soft palates are then visualized. After completion of this thorough visual inspection of the oral cavity, the oropharynx is similarly examined. The tonsils, soft palate, sessile tongue, and pharyngeal walls are checked. After completion of the visual examination, it is necessary to palpate the mucosal surfaces and the teeth. This is done with a gloved finger in the mouth and a hand placed externally so as to bimanually palpate the structures in the floor of the mouth and cheek.

Anatomy of the Oral Cavity

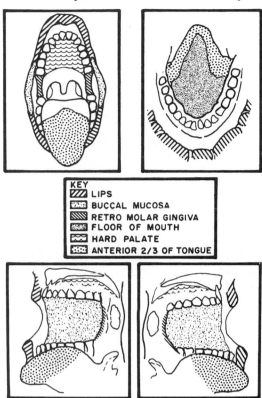

KEY
🗌 LIPS
🗌 BUCCAL MUCOSA
🗌 RETRO MOLAR GINGIVA
🗌 FLOOR OF MOUTH
🗌 HARD PALATE
🗌 ANTERIOR 2/3 OF TONGUE

FIG. 36–1. Anatomy of the oral cavity. (From Granick MS, Larson DL. Management of head and neck cancer. In: Russell R, ed. *PSEF: instructional courses.* II. St. Louis: CV Mosby, 1989.

An indirect laryngoscopy is then performed on all patients. This consists of retracting the tongue with one hand and using the coaxial light source to illuminate the larynx indirectly by means of a laryngeal mirror. This technique is used to visualize the laryngeal structures. In patients with pathology involving any of the upper aerodigestive tract, fiberoptic laryngoscopy is then performed.

The examination is completed by a thorough palpation of the neck. Each of the different areas of the neck is palpated individually and gently. A light touch is optimally effective in discerning subcutaneous and deeper lesions. It is easiest to stand behind the seated patient and palpate the neck by starting cephalad, gradually working downward using both hands on either side of the neck so that the two sides can be compared to each other. The thyroid is then palpated by having the patient swallow while the examiner feels the thyroid lobes.

It is necessary to carefully document any and all abnormal findings on a pictorial record. Anatomic charts of the head and neck are available through The American Cancer Society and through many publishers. On one of these charts, the size and precise location of each lesion should be carefully documented. This information is critical in staging the patient and as an accurate record for comparison in the future.

At this time, biopsies should be performed on any suspicious lesions in the oral cavity. Normally, biopsy can be done under local anesthesia or without anesthesia in the office with a simple biopsy punch. In patients who are extremely anxious or who have a hyperactive gag reflex, it may be necessary to perform a more thorough examination and biopsy under anesthesia. Certainly, if there are any lesions elsewhere in the upper aerodigestive tract, it is necessary to perform a direct laryngoscopy under general anesthesia.

SALIVARY GLAND LESIONS

Minor salivary glands are found throughout the oral mucosa. These glands produce a seromucinous secretion. Obstruction or rupture of the ducts of these glands can lead to formation of mucous cyst (mucocele) (Fig. 36–2). The cystic lesions involving the sublingual glands are called ranulae (Fig. 36–3). A ranula can occupy a large area in the floor of the mouth and can plunge deep into the anterior neck structures. Treatment of these lesions consists of simple excision or marsupialization of larger cysts. Plunging ranulae require removal of the submandibular gland for access.

Salivary duct stones can be found in the Wharton duct and can be palpated as hard submucosal masses in the floor of the mouth. Frequently, the presence of sialolithiasis causes symptoms of swelling and pain in the submandibular gland associated with eating. Stones can be removed transorally if they are in the distal portions of the duct. Stones located in the hilar area of the gland need to be removed through an ex-

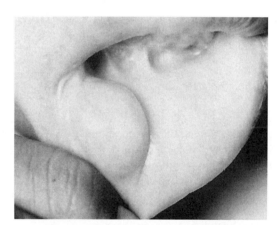

FIG. 36–2. A mucocele of the lower lip.

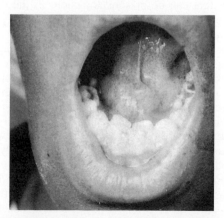

FIG. 36–3. A ranula in the floor of the mouth.

ternal approach in the neck in connection with removal of the submandibular gland. Attempted removal of hilar stones through the floor of the mouth can lead to injury of the lingual artery and nerve.

Benign tumors of the minor salivary glands can occur anywhere that minor salivary glands are present. The most common of these lesions is a benign mixed tumor (pleomorphic adenoma). These are typically firm, slow-growing, mobile, and submucosal. Approximately fifty percent of minor salivary gland tumors are malignant. Malignant tumors may be clinically indistinguishable from benign tumors. This necessitates a local excision, with a margin of normal tissue, of any small salivary gland tumor in the oral cavity. Larger lesions that cannot be simply removed should undergo an incisional biopsy.

Necrotizing sialometaplasia is a benign tumor that is most commonly present on the palate. It usually occurs as a spontaneously forming mass with ulceration. It can also be present secondary to surgery, trauma, or infection, and can occur anywhere within the oral cavity. This tumor is benign but can be mistaken for a malignancy (see Chapter 19).

OTHER BENIGN LESIONS

Dermoid cysts can occur in the floor of the mouth near the midline. They can also occur at the base of the tongue. They are slow growing and generally present with swelling in the submental area and the floor of the mouth. Dermoid cysts require excision of the cyst and cyst wall and are unlikely to recur.

Bony exostoses of the mandible or palate are bony masses attached to the skeletal structures and covered by a thin layer of mucosa. They present functional problems in patients who need to be fitted for prostheses or dentures. In those settings, they can be removed by simple excision (Fig. 36–4).

Reparative giant cell granulomas (epulides) are reddish-brown, friable tumors that occur along the alveolar ridge. They are frequently present between incisor and canine teeth (Fig. 36–5). Histologically, they resemble the brown tumor associated with hyperparathyroidism. Consequently, patients who have these lesions should have their serum calcium level evaluated. Treatment of giant cell granulomas consists of wide local excision.

Granular cell myoblastomas are well-circumscribed, firm lesions that are frequently found within the muscle of the tongue but that can be present anywhere in the oral cavity. These lesions are derived from the neural crest cells, are benign, and are adequately treated by local excision.

Vascular malformations, including hemangiomas and lymphangiomas, can occur in the oral cavity and are most frequent in children. In the absence of ulceration, bleeding, or functional disabilities associated with these tumors, no treatment is necessary. When these tumors are growing rapidly or are symptomatic, they can be treated by local excision, high-dose short-term steroids, laser vaporization, or low-dose external beam irradiation (Fig. 36–6). Mucosal polyps and fibromas can occur in areas of mucosal trauma. These are usually found on the buccal mucosa along the bite plane where mucosa can be caught between the teeth. Median rhomboid glossitis is a raised reddish area, usually on the central raphe of the dorsal surface of the tongue. It is another

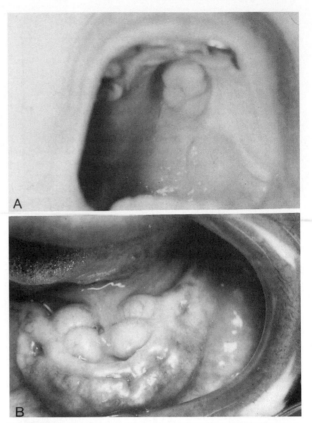

FIG. 36–4.   **A,** bony exostoses of the palate and **B,** mandible.

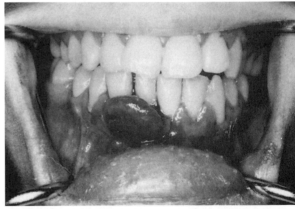

FIG. 36–5.   A reparative granuloma (epulis) of the lower jaw.

benign condition that can be treated with local excision or simply observed.

Aphthous ulcers (canker sores) are painful ulcerations that occur in the oral cavity. These are generally of short duration. They can occur in a cyclical fashion in some patients. In general, these lesions have a white base and an erythematous rim. They resolve without treatment.

Tuberculous granulomas can occur in the oral cavity and can appear quite similar to squamous cell carcinoma. These need to be distinguished from squamous cell carcinoma by histologic examination of a biopsy specimen. Treatment consists of antituberculous medications using established protocols over prolonged periods of time.

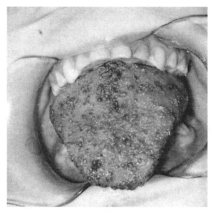

FIG. 36–6. The tongue is infiltrated with hemangioma.

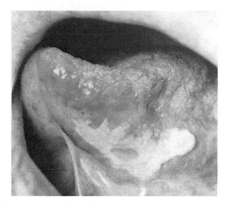

FIG. 36–7. Leukoplakia of the tongue is seen as a white patch.

PREMALIGNANT TUMORS

Leukoplakia (Fig. 36–7) refers to any white patch on the oral mucosa. Leukoplakia is generally associated with hyperkeratosis. Most leukoplakias are found in patients who smoke. They can be directly related to the type of smoking. For instance, patients who use chewing tobacco will frequently have leukoplakia in the buccal sulcus, whereas patients who smoke cheroots (small cigars with square-cut ends) are predisposed to developing leukoplakia on the ventral surface of the tongue. There is considerable disagreement in the literature as to the degree of malignant transformation in oral leukoplakia (1). This is because many studies are based on the appearance of the lesions rather than their histologic evaluation. The best indicator for likely malignant degeneration of a white oral lesion is the presence of dysplasia or carcinoma in situ on histologic evaluation.

The treatment of oral leukoplakia involves histologic confirmation of the nature of the lesion, followed by removal of the etiological factor responsible for its formation. The most effective means to resolve leukoplakia is cessation of smoking. In lesions that demonstrate dysplasia or carcinoma in situ, surgical excision is necessary.

Erythroplakia is a bright red, velvety lesion that occurs anywhere in the oral cavity. This is a dangerous lesion because it is almost always associated with dysplasia, carcinoma in situ, or invasive carcinoma (2). Any red lesion of the oral cavity requires histologic evaluation. Treatment generally consists of excision. Patients must be warned about the risk of continued tobacco and alcohol use.

MALIGNANT TUMORS

The vast majority of malignancies occurring in the oral cavity are squamous cell carcinomas (SCC). Most of the remaining tumors are of salivary gland origin and were discussed in detail in Chapter 19; consequently, this chapter will focus entirely on SCC.

Chronic exposure to a variety of irritants in susceptible people initiates the development of SCC. Tobacco use in any form is the major irritant responsible for its development. The effect of tobacco works synergistically with alcohol, although alcohol alone does not appear to be carcinogenic. A variety of other environmental irritants, including occupational exposure to chemicals and nutritional factors, appear to influence the development of SCC. Several potentially premalignant conditions have been identified and are thought to sensitize individuals to become more susceptible to carcinogenic agents. These disorders include Plummer-Vinson syndrome, lichen planus, tertiary syphilis, and discoid lupus erythematosus (1). In addition, there are several hereditary syndromes associated with the development of SCC (e.g., basal cell nevus syndrome and xeroderma pigmentosum). There has been an association between the Epstein-Barr virus and carcinoma of the nasopharynx, as well as an association between herpes simplex virus and carcinoma of the oral cavity. Finally, poor oral hygiene, with chronic gingivitis, periodontitis, and poor dental care, is frequently associated in patients who present with SCC of the oral cavity. Another known etiological factor is the effect of ultraviolet radiation from sunlight, which influences the development of SCC on the vermilion portion of the lip.

Histopathology

Squamous cell carcinoma consists of a tumor with nests and columns of malignant epithelial cells that infiltrate into the subepithelial layers. Nuclear pleomorphism is typical. Tumors can be graded from well differentiated to poorly differentiated. In well-differentiated tumors, the malignant cells produce keratin, and keratin pearls can be identified. Under oil-immersion views, intercellular bridging can be seen. As the tumors become less well differentiated, the nuclear differentiation degenerates, and the density of mitotic figures increases. The histologic pattern of SCC can usually be reliably identified on frozen-section analysis. This enables the pathologist to perform an accurate intraoperative assessment of the excised tissue.

Tumor Classification

Classification of SCC is currently based on a "TNM" system, which considers several descriptors in characterizing the tumor. The first descriptor is T, which refers to two-dimensional tumor size. The N descriptor refers to the nodal status in the cervical region. The final descriptor, M, refers to metastatic disease beyond the cervical lymph nodes (Table 36–1). The TNM classification is based on the clinical evaluation of the patient, not the pathologic evaluation. Once a TNM status is derived, the tumor can be staged (Table 36–2).

Table 36–1
TNM Classification of Head and Neck Tumors

TIS	Tumor in situ
T_1	0.1–2.0 cm
T_2	2.1–4.0 cm
T_3	4.1–6.0 cm
T_4	< 6.1 cm or invading adjacent structures
N_0	No regional adenopathy
N_1	Ipsilateral adenopathy < 3 cm
N_2	Single ipsilateral node 3–6 cm or multiple ipsilateral nodes < 6 cm
N_3	Massive ipsilateral or contralateral nodes
M_0	No evidence of metastases
M_I	Metastases beyond the cervical lymph nodes

Table 36–2
Clinical Staging of Oral Cancer

Stage I	$T_1 N_0 M_0$
Stage II	$T_2 N_0 M_0$
Stage III	$T_3 N_0 M_0$
	$T_1, T_2, T_3 N_I M_0$
Stage IV	$T_4 N_0, N_I M_0$
	ANY T, $N_2, N_3 M_0$
	ANY T, ANY N, MI

The widely used TNM system allows the surgeon to classify a patient's lesion in such a way that appropriate therapy for a given tumor can be selected and prognosis of outcome can be made fairly accurately. The system does have some limitations. The primary limitation is the use of two-dimensional tumor size as the basis for the T classification. Recently, attempts have been made to modify the classification system by examining tumor depth as a variable in oral carcinoma. In fact, tumor depth beyond 5 mm has been shown to be associated with a highly increased risk of loco-regional failure and cervical metastases (3–5). As studies of this nature emerge, the classification system of oral cancer will undoubtedly be modified.

Patient Considerations

Once a patient has been diagnosed as having SCC of the oral cavity, the surgeon must review a variety of considerations having to do with the patient's habits, social setting, and physiologic state before developing a comprehensive treatment plan. There are numerous ways to treat any of these tumors, and the goal of therapy is to benefit the patient. Consequently, therapy needs to be adapted to the individual.

The first important aspect of the evaluation is to determine whether the index tumor site is, in fact, the only involved area of the upper aerodigestive tract. In approximately ten percent of these patients, there is a synchronous second primary tumor (6). It is imperative to examine the patient thoroughly to rule out the possibility of a second primary. This assessment requires a detailed physical examination and, usually, a laryngoscopy under anesthesia. A laryngoscopy can be combined with the initial diagnostic biopsy if a patient is unable to cooperate with an office biopsy technique. Otherwise, if a second lesion is suspected or a suspicious

area is noted, the laryngoscopy can be performed as a separate procedure. If the patient has been thoroughly evaluated in the office with a fiberoptic endoscope and an indirect examination and there is no evidence of a secondary primary, a laryngoscopy can be performed prior to definitive surgery at the same setting.

In evaluating the patient for a second primary, the examiner should realize that the possibility of metastatic disease also exists. In general, SCC metastasizes first to the lymph nodes of the neck; beyond that point, it tends to spread to the lung. An extensive metastatic workup is not indicated. A plain chest radiograph and liver function studies are the only tests required. If additional studies are needed to develop a treatment plan or to further evaluate an abnormal result on the basic screen, they can be ordered as indicated. Arteriography is useful in patients who have vascular tumors, but it is rarely necessary in patients with squamous cell carcinoma. Radionuclide scanning has little use in these patients. In the head and neck, radionuclide scanning is primarily useful in evaluating thyroid tumors. Fine-needle aspiration has a role in evaluating an undiagnosed mass in the neck that is not associated with any evident oral tumor. The accuracy of a fine-needle aspiration is largely dependent on the pathologist's experience with cytologic interpretation.

The patient's dental status is critical to the outcome of treatment. Patients who have poor oral hygiene are more prone to complications of infection and wound healing after surgery. During the course of treatment with radiotherapy, dental caries and periodontitis will increase the risk of osteoradionecrosis of the mandible and maxilla. Each patient, before undergoing any treatment for oral cancer, needs a dental evaluation and prophylactic treatment.

The patient's nutritional needs must also be addressed. Many patients have sustained significant weight loss and are malnourished at the time of presentation. Dietary supplementation—either orally, by nasogastric tube, or by percutaneous endoscopic gastrostomy—is indicated before initiating a definitive treatment plan in most patients with oral tumors.

Certain patient habits, such as smoking and alcohol abuse, are critical factors in the patient's survival outcome. Patients who continue to smoke and drink have a 40% risk of developing a second primary SCC in the upper aerodigestive tract after treatment of their first lesion. This very high risk level can be considerably reduced by cessation of smoking. Alcoholic patients are difficult to treaty by any modality. However, radiation therapy requires long-term compliance. Outside of a protected setting, patients who are alcoholic are unlikely to participate adequately in the full course of radiation therapy. Consequently, we find that definitive surgery is the preferred treatment modality in alcoholics.

The patient's physiologic status is also a critical factor. In this regard, age is a consideration. Young patients who develop SCC tend to have more aggressive tumors and a worse prognosis than middle-aged or older patients (7). The metabolic status of the patient who presents with SCC is often poor because of personal abuse and nutritional deficiencies. The metabolic status of patients should be corrected with nutritional supplementation and metabolic support prior to surgery. Most unfavorable metabolic states can be reversed before surgery with proper medical care.

Treatment of Oral Squamous Cell[11,12] Carcinoma (SCC)

PREDICTING OUTCOMES

Treatment of SCC in the oral cavity is predicated on the presumed aggressiveness of the tumor. The most favorable indicator of outcome is a small T size (8–10) and thickness (3–5). The presence of cervical metastases, particularly N_3, is a strong indicator of loco-regional failure (11,12). TNM classification has thus been used as the basis for formulating treatment plans.

A variety of laboratory analyses hold promise as potential indicators of tumor aggressiveness, and may at some point be useful as planning aids. Tumor angiogenesis is correlated with patient outcome (13) and regional recurrence (14) and can be assessed by a simple immunofluorescent stain. Tumor necrosis factor (15), thrombospondin receptor (13), E-calherin (16), and other molecules (17,18), are expressed by SCC and may have prognostic importance.

SURGERY

Surgery is still the preferred method of treatment for most cancers of the oral cavity. Surgical therapy consists of precise removal of tumor and a margin of normal-appearing tissue around the tumor. Frozen-section analysis at the time of surgery is used to confirm that the tumor has been removed with adequate margins. Patients who are in good metabolic shape generally tolerate these surgical procedures well. In most instances, surgical therapy provides the best opportunity for cure.

There are, however, disadvantages to the surgical approach to these tumors. A primary disadvantage is the functional problems with speech and swallowing that can result from ablation of structures in the oral cavity. In addition, surgery leads to aesthetic alterations, which can be devastating to a patient. Reconstructive options that can minimize these problems are currently available. Another disadvantage of surgery is its inability to eliminate precisely foci of microscopic disease. For this reason, adjuvant radiotherapy and, potentially, chemotherapy are useful adjuncts in the treatment of patients with advanced disease. Finally, surgical procedures in the oral cavity have a relatively high incidence of complications. In the head and neck region, postoperative infection and the development of orocutaneous fistulae are always worrisome and problematic. However, these complications are rarely fatal.

RADIOTHERAPY

Radiation therapy offers the distinct advantage of minimal aesthetic and functional alterations following treatment. Radiation also has the ability to sterilize microscopic tumor deposits. The limitations of radiation therapy are the considerable acute and progressive chronic morbidity, as well as the ineffectiveness of radiation to ablate large tumor volumes. Acute morbidity associated with radiation therapy consists of mucositis, odynophagia, swelling, and a general feeling of malaise. The long-term effects of radiation therapy include lost of taste, a chronically irritated and dry mouth, the risk of osteonecrosis of the mandible and temporal bone (which can be a disastrous occurrence), and permanent alteration in the healing abilities of the tissues that have been treated.

ADDITIONAL TREATMENT MODALITIES

Chemotherapy is at this time an unreliable adjunct in the treatment of head and neck cancer. Some patients respond dramatically to chemotherapy treatments, but the effects are usually short lived, and regrowth of the tumor usually occurs in 3 to 6 months.

As an adjuvant in treating massive or potentially unresectable tumors, however, there is a definite place for chemotherapy in today's treatment armamentarium. If a patient is pretreated with chemotherapy, tumor size is often reduced to the point where surgical ablation of the tumor is feasible. The appropriate extent of surgery after a tumor has been pretreated is an issue that is presently unresolved. A variety of multicenter protocols are currently evaluating the impact that chemotherapy pretreatment has on the extent of surgical ablation (19,20).

Heat has been considered a potentially worthwhile adjunct to chemotherapy and radiation. By heating a tumor to 43° C, the effect of the chemotherapy and radiation seems to be potentiated. Difficulties with these methods include the techniques available for delivery of the heat and the level of discomfort to the patient during the treatment.

Cryotherapy and electrocautery have been used as destructive techniques to palliate massive tumors, and to that extent they are acceptable therapies. Photodynamic therapy consists of laser activation of a photosensitizing dye, which concentrates in the tumor. As of this time, it does not have a clear role in tumor management.

Tumors by Site

LIP

Lip cancers are the most common form of oral SCC. Approximately ninety-five percent of lip cancers are SCC. A history of smoking and sun exposure are typical. Basal cell carcinomas occur less frequently and usually appear on the upper lip, often as a direct extension of a cutaneous lesion.

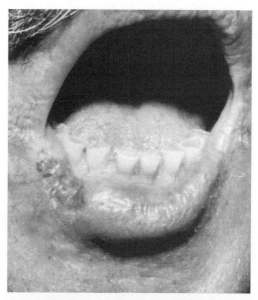

FIG. 36–8. A SCC on the lower lip.

Lip cancer usually presents as an ulceration (Fig. 36–8). Induration around the base of the tumor is a common clinical finding and helps to delineate the extent of tumor infiltration. Leukoplakia often is present adjacent to the tumor.

While most of the patients with lip cancer have a relatively benign course, approximately ten percent of these tumors become extremely aggressive and are lethal (21). Ominous clinical findings are the presence of cervical lymphadenopathy and evidence of perineural invasion. Nerve involvement is noted by anesthesia in the distribution of the mental nerve and by an enlarged mental foramen on Panorex.

The treatment of lip cancer is surgical. A margin of 1 cm circumferentially around the tumor should be obtained. All specimens should be checked by frozen section before reconstructing the defect. Adjacent leukoplakia needs to be removed with a lip-shave procedure. Tumors that present with anesthesia along the mental nerve should be carefully checked for adequacy of margins. Squamous cell carcinoma can spread perineurally, and cancers of the lip can involve the mental nerve, which travels through the mandible. Tumors of the lip usually do not present with clinically positive cervical nodes; however, these tumors can metastasize to the neck. Neck dissection is reserved for patients with clinically evident disease in the neck or those with very advanced tumors of the lip. Primary radiation treatment is an alternative.

Reconstruction of the ablative lip defect depends on the size and location of the wound. Tumors measuring less than one-quarter of the lip length can be closed primarily after removing them as a wedge. Larger tumor defects require flap closure. There are a number of flaps available for closing the lip, and these are described in Chapter 41.

Survival of patients with lip carcinoma is 95% at 5 years. These patients clearly do better than patients with other oral tumors; however, this can be a fatal disease, and they must be monitored regularly during the 5 years after initial treatment.

ORAL TONGUE

The oral tongue consists of the mobile portion of the tongue distal to the circumvallate papillae. This is the next most frequent site of oral carcinoma. The vast majority of tongue tumors are SCC (Fig. 36–9). The lateral surface of the tongue is the most common location of primary tongue cancer. Tumors are detected earlier in the oral tongue than in the base of the tongue because the base is more posterior and hidden from easy examination. Patients with tongue tumors present with either exophytic or invasive tumors. Palpation of the tumor is an accurate means of assessing the extent of the lesion. Tongue tumors tend to be painful and can interfere with eating. Advanced tumors of the tongue are usually associated with severe nutritional deficits. Referred otalgia is a common presenting symptom. Tongue cancers tend to metastasize early and commonly spread to the upper and mid-jugular nodal chains.

Treatment of tongue tumors consists of a partial glossectomy that includes the hemitongue distal to the circumvallate papillae (22–24). T_1 lesions can be removed by wedge resection. Treatment of the neck is a controversial issue. The current trend in treating SCC of the oral tongue includes the increased use of elective neck dissection, mandible sparing surgery, and adjuvant postoperative radiotherapy for advanced lesions (25). This treatment paradigm improved the overall 5-year survival from 56 to 65% at Memorial Sloan-Kettering Hospital (25,26). Clearly, in patients with clinically evident nodal disease, lymphadenectomy is appropriate. In patients with clinically negative necks, elective neck dissection reveals histologic evidence of tumor in 25% of patients. Consequently, in patients with T_2 or greater lesions, elective neck dissection is appropriate. Since cervical metastases appear in a predictable anatomic sequence, the use of limited neck dissections in N_O necks is gaining acceptance as a staging procedure (27).

Radiation treatment of tongue lesions, including external beam or implantation, yields survival rates comparable to those following surgery (28). The long-term and short-term complications of irradiation, however, are much more severe than those of surgery, and we prefer to use radiation therapy as an adjunctive treatment in more advanced tumors.

FLOOR OF THE MOUTH

Carcinoma of the floor of the mouth (Fig. 36–10) is a disease of older patients. This is a relatively quiet area of the mouth, and symptoms are generally present only with advanced disease. The usual complaints are local or referred pain to the ear caused by involvement of the lingual nerve. The pattern

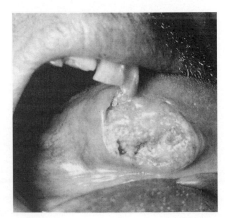

FIG. 36–9. This SCC is located on the lateral mobile tongue.

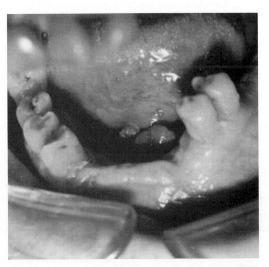

FIG. 36–10. The floor of this mouth contains a SCC.

of nodal metastases is to the submental and submandibular lymph nodes.

Treatment of these lesions (29) consists of local excision with a skin graft or local flap reconstruction in T_1 lesions. T_2 lesions require more aggressive resection. A close inspection of the status of the mandible is important. (31,32) Mandibular involvement can usually be treated by marginal mandibulectomy if the tumor encroaches on the alveolar aspect of the mandible (32–34). For very large advanced tumors with gross mandibular involvement, composite resection is necessary. Resulting surgical defects require elaborate reconstructive procedures. Treatment of the neck necessitates lymphadenectomy in clinically positive necks (35). Tumor thickness is found to be highly predictive of neck metastases in floor-of-the-mouth tumors (36). For lesions thicker than 1.5 mm, there is a 60% risk of neck metastases, and cervical lymphadenectomy is appropriate (37). Radiation therapy plays a distinct role in these tumors, particularly as a postsurgical adjunct, although primary irradiation or brachytherapy can be used (38).

BUCCAL MUCOSA

Buccal carcinomas are primarily associated with the use of oral tobacco (1). These tumors account for less than 10% of oral tumors. With the increasing incidence of snuff dipping in the United States, there has been a higher incidence of these tumors in the past several years, with increasing occurrence of these lesions in younger patients (39). Buccal carcinomas are frequently of a verrucous nature, and these have a slightly better prognosis than other forms of SCC found in the oral cavity. However, approximately twenty percent of the verrucous carcinomas have foci of SCC, and these have a more aggressive course, like the usual SCC (40). Metastases to the submandibular and jugular lymph nodes are typical, and the incidence of cervical metastases is 40%.

Surgical treatment of buccal carcinoma is more effective than primary radiation treatment (40,41). For improved local control of tumors, postoperative adjuvant radiation therapy is advantageous, particularly in advanced tumors and in those hybrid tumors with foci of SCC. Because of the high incidence of metastases to the neck, elective neck dissection is appropriate. Reconstruction of the defect depends on the extent of excision. Split-thickness skin grafts are appropriate for mucosal defects. Musculocutaneous or microvascular flaps are better suited for repairing composite tissue losses.

PALATE

Carcinomas of the superior alveolus and hard palate are unusual tumors in the United States. They are more common in other areas of the world, where reverse smoking (smoking with the lit end of the cigarette in the mouth) is a common practice. In the United States, the majority of palatal tumors arise from the minor salivary gland (42) (see Chapter 19). Treatment of tumors of the palate consists of local excision with removal of bone where indicated. Reconstruction of this area can be performed by using distant pedicle flaps or microvascular tissue transfers. It is not always necessary to replace bone that has been removed from the palate. The primary goal of reconstruction is to achieve oronasal separation that will allow speech and eating to continue with minimal disruption. Postoperative radiation yields a 11-year disease free survival of 77% (42).

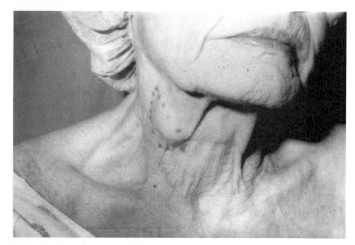

FIG. 36–11. Any unexplained neck mass in an adult is cancer until proven otherwise.

UNKNOWN PRIMARY

Unknown primary tumors in the neck are metastatic SCC with no known source of the primary tumor. An adult who presents with a mass (Fig. 36–11) in the upper two-thirds of the neck is considered to have SCC until proven otherwise. In the Memorial Sloan-Kettering (43) series, 73 patients were evaluated. Most of them (83%) were treated with surgery and adjuvant irradiation. The 5-year follow-up revealed primary tumors in only 9 of 73 (12%) patients. One primary tumor was from lung, the other 8 were upper aerodigestive tract.

Appropriate workup of these patient consists of a complete physical examination, laryngoscopy, and an aspiration needle biopsy. Random biopsies of normal appearing mucosa are not productive. Imaging studies, such as CT or MRI scans are rarely useful (44). The treatment of these patients consists of a thorough neck dissection. In a patient with N_1 disease and no histologic evidence of extracapsular spread, irradiation is probably not warranted. In patients with N_2–N_3, or a worsened pathologic stage compared to a clinical N_1, adjuvant radiation treatment should be given (44). These patients should be followed carefully for the remainder of their lives.

NECK DISSECTION

Crile described the basic technique of radical neck dissection in 1906 (45). His operation consisted of an en bloc removal of all of the contents of the lateral neck, including the cervical lymphatics, jugular vein, sternocleidomastoid muscle, and any nerves that were present. In 1951, Martin and coworkers (46) outlined the indications, technique, and complications of radical neck dissection, and their work has remained the oncological standard. In the 1960s, various forms of less radical neck dissections were introduced. Functional (modified or conservative) neck dissections have proven to be comparable to radical neck dissections in terms of outcome. Survival outcome following functional neck dissection is similar to that of the classic radical neck dissection. In addition, some function is preserved by removing only the lymph nodal groups at risk and not the remaining structures of the neck (47).

The approach to treatment of SCC metastatic to the neck is controversial to this day. It is fairly well agreed that patients who have clinically positive neck disease at or subsequent to the time of presentation with their tumor require cervical lymphadenectomy. The issue of elective or "prophylactic" neck dissection is where the controversy exists. One approach is to perform elective neck dissections in patients who have tumors that are at high risk for having occult metastases or for developing metastatic disease at some future date (25,26,48,49). The alternative approach is to perform a staging neck dissection: the first echelon of lymphatic tissue is removed, and if this is pathologically negative the lymphadenectomy is halted (27,50). If the first echelon nodes are histologically involved, the lymphadenectomy can be extended. The next option is to observe the patient without performing lymphadenectomy and to operate on the neck only if clinically evident disease appears (51). There is a real risk of poor follow-up in some of these pa-

tients, but patients who have late lymph-node dissections do comparably well. One final option is to irradiate clinically negative necks in patients with high-risk primary tumors (52). Because aggressive, high-risk primary tumors are generally treated with adjunctive radiation, it is a relatively straightforward matter to include the ipsilateral neck within the treatment portal at little additional morbidity or risk to the patient. Occasionally, there are midline tumors in the oral cavity with metastatic disease to both sides of the neck. In these cases, it is best either to stage the neck dissections, if the internal jugular is to be removed, or to perform bilateral simultaneous neck dissections using the functional jugular-vein preservation techniques.

Access to the neck is best obtained with a MacFee incision (Fig. 36–12). There are many options for gaining access to the

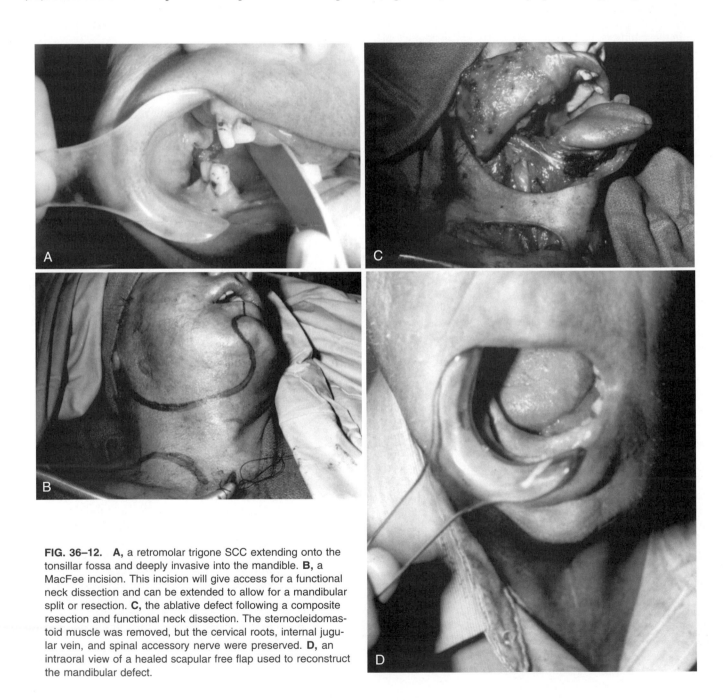

FIG. 36–12. A, a retromolar trigone SCC extending onto the tonsillar fossa and deeply invasive into the mandible. **B,** a MacFee incision. This incision will give access for a functional neck dissection and can be extended to allow for a mandibular split or resection. **C,** the ablative defect following a composite resection and functional neck dissection. The sternocleidomastoid muscle was removed, but the cervical roots, internal jugular vein, and spinal accessory nerve were preserved. **D,** an intraoral view of a healed scapular free flap used to reconstruct the mandibular defect.

neck structures, but the MacFee incision affords consistent wound healing with minimal risk of exposure to the underlying vessels of the neck. The upper incision is made from the mastoid tip to the contralateral submental area. It is carried approximately 2.5 cm below the mandibular border. The lower incision is made approximately 3.0 cm above the clavicle in a curvilinear fashion from the midline anteriorly to the border of the trapezius posteriorly. The incisions are carried through skin and subcutaneous tissue and then through the platysma. The superior flap is raised carefully, and the marginal mandibular branch of the facial nerve is identified and preserved. The nerve is usually found immediately below the platysma, crossing the posterior facial vein. This is retracted along with the cheek flap superiorly. The inferior incision is raised below the level of the platysma. Both flaps are sutured for retraction during the remainder of the procedure. The central skin flap is raised in the subplatysmal plane. A 1-inch Penrose drain is then passed around the central flap and used for retraction of this tissue during various parts of the neck dissection.

The classical radical neck dissection involves removal of the sternocleidomastoid muscle, the internal jugular vein, the spinal accessory nerve, and all of the remaining tissue. Borders of the dissection are the trapezius posteriorly, the clavicle inferiorly, the midline of the neck medially, and the marginal rim of the mandible superiorly. First, the inferior heads

of the sternocleidomastoid muscle are divided at their insertions. The individual structures of the carotid sheath are identified and cleaned of fascia. The internal jugular vein is divided and suture ligated. The fascial carpet of the neck is identified and left intact, and the posterior triangle contents are divided to the level of the trapezius muscle. The contents of the neck are then swept superiorly and medially, dividing the cervical nerves along the way. Care is taken to prevent injury to the vagus, phrenic, and branchial plexus structures. The omohyoid muscle is divided as it crosses the scalene muscles. The central skin flap is carefully retracted during this procedure, and the contents of the neck can be brought out through the upper pole of the incision for better exposure once the inferior attachments are divided.

As the dissection proceeds superiorly, the hypoglossal nerve, which is located deep to the posterior belly of the digastric muscle crossing above the carotid bifurcation, is carefully preserved. The omohyoid muscle is divided. The insertion of the sternocleidomastoid muscle is divided. The tail of the parotid is divided from the remaining portion of the parotid gland. The underlying digastric and stylohyoid muscles are divided as well. The contents of the submandibular triangle are then dissected with care to preserve the lingual nerve as well as the previously identified and protected branch of the facial nerve. The jugular vein is di-

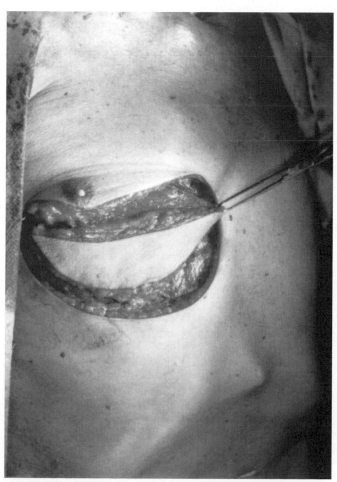

FIG. 36–13. Shin paddle overlying the distal pectoralis major muscle. This flap was used to reconstruct a defect in the pharynx.

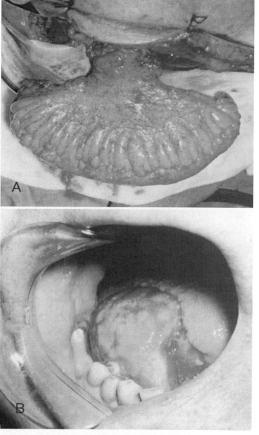

FIG. 36–14. **A,** a jejunal segment has been connected to the neck by microvascular anastomoses. **B,** the flap is used to reconstruct a hemiglossectomy defect.

vided below the skull base and suture-ligated. After assuring complete hemostasis and checking for the absence of chylous leakage, two suction catheters are introduced through inferior stab incisions, placed in the wound, and the skin flaps are closed in layers.

Following Martin's (46) standardization of the classic radical neck dissection, little variation took place until the 1980s. At that time, Bocca and colleagues (47) popularized a variation of the classical radical neck dissection by removing the fascial envelope containing the lymphatics of the neck and preserving the contents of the submandibular triangle and the spinal accessory nerve. As the literature began to support the oncological validity of this approach, many variations were performed. The most universally accepted aspect of functional neck dissection is the preserva-

tion of the spinal accessory nerve in cases in which this nerve is not directly involved with tumor. The most widely performed functional neck dissection preserves not only the spinal accessory nerve but also the cervical roots, the sternocleidomastoid muscle, and the internal jugular vein (see Fig. 36–12C). All of the areolar tissue surrounding the carotid sheath, as well as all of the lymphatic-bearing tissue of the neck from the rim of the mandible down to the clavicle, is removed. In recent years, limited regional dissections of the neck have been popularized. The rationale for regional neck resection is that tumors of the oral cavity generally spread in a predictable fashion (53). Thus, by removing the first echelon of involved nodes the surgeon can make a reliable prediction as to the involvement of more distal lymphatics. If the tumor can be arrested at the first

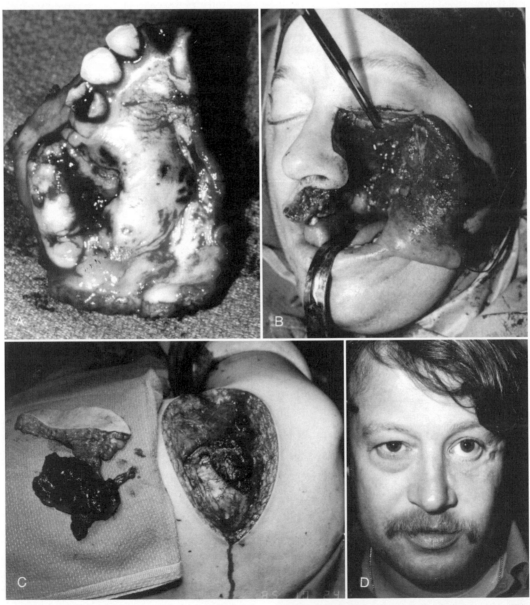

FIG. 36–15. A, a total maxillectomy specimen. **B,** the maxillectomy defect consists of loss of bony support of the eye and full-thickness hard palate. **C,** a composite scapula free flap is harvested. The bone segment will support the eye and facial tissues. The skin will line the palate. The fat will obliterate the sinus. **D,** the patient, 1 year postoperatively.

echelon of nodes, it is necessary only to extend the dissection to the next echelon of nodes without risking incomplete removal of involved lymphatics.

Reconstruction

The principles of reconstructive surgery in the head and neck region are identical to those elsewhere in the body. The difficulty with head and neck reconstructive surgery is the need for improvement in the patient's function, structure, and appearance. Failure to provide satisfactory improvements in any of these areas is considered a poor result (54). Many defects can be closed by simply reapproximating tissues or by applying a simple skin graft, such as the resection of a lesion of the floor of the mouth. Occasionally, skin grafts can be used in conjunction with a prosthesis to achieve a satisfactory result for the patient with minimal reconstructive effort. The complexity arises when there is need for composite tissue restoration or restoration of the integrity of the oral cavity.

Skin grafts are easily applied to the intraoral structures. The grafts are usually meshed at 1.5 to 1 and are then sutured in place with chromic catgut sutures. The graft is quilted to the underlying bed to prevent it from shearing during the motion of the residual oral tissues. A bolster consisting of a single piece of cotton gauze immersed in balsam of Peru is applied over the graft. This mixture has the unique ability to not adhere to the underlying skin graft and to suppress bacterial growth within the bolster. After 1 week, the bolster is removed, and a program of local hygiene is instituted.

Larger defects require more sophisticated reconstruction using a variety of local, regional, or distant flaps, depending on the specific needs of the patient. The major workhorse pedicled flaps for the head and neck remain the pectoralis myocutaneous flap (55), latissimus dorsi myocutaneous flap (56), and the trapezius myocutaneous flap (57,58). Each of these three flaps has a consistent and dependable vascular pedicle, is easily accessed, and is easily dissected. The donor sites can usually be closed primarily, and the functional losses from the rotation of the donor muscles are minimal. The advantage of the use of the pectoralis muscle over the trapezius and latissimus muscles is the availability of this flap on the anterior chest wall, which eliminates the need to reposition the patient intraoperatively (Fig. 36–13). The advent of a diverse group of microvascular tissue transfers that are reliable and particularly well suited for head and neck reconstruction has largely supplanted the classic forms of head and neck reconstruction. The use of free flaps has, in fact, led to fewer complications, decreased length of stay, and fewer procedures per patient (59). Free bowel transfers are well suited for lining the pharynx, oral cavity, or cervical esophagus with mucosal tissue (60) (Fig. 36–14). Radial forearm (61), dorsalis pedis (62), and scapular (63,64) flaps have become the standard for lining the oral cavity with thin, hairless tissue. The vascularized bone accompanying the iliac crest and groin flap combination (65), the scapular flap, the dorsalis pedis flap along with the metatarsal bone, the fibula (66), the radial bone in association with skin islands, and other composite tissues, have vastly improved the options for reconstructing extensive mandibular and maxillary defects (Fig. 36–15). All of these flaps can be revascularized by anastomoses either directly to the remaining vessels in the neck or via vein grafts to the contralateral neck. When properly designed and executed, these flaps are robust and withstand irradiation postoperatively quite satisfactorily. The level of sophistication in reconstructing head and neck tumor defects continues to improve. The available donor tissues must be individualized for the specific needs of the patient before selecting a reconstructive technique.

The surgeon's first objective in approaching a patient with oral cancer is eliminating the tumor. A variety of reconstructive options are kept in mind, but the final choice of the reconstructive technique must wait until the tumor is adequately removed. One final caution is to avoid predetermining the reconstruction before completing the ablation. The primary goal in operating on patients with head and neck cancer is to cure the cancer. While the reconstructive aspect of head and neck surgery is challenging and gratifying, it plays a secondary role to the management of the cancer. The vast array of reconstructive options should act as a support to the oncological surgeon and allow an aggressive, complete tumor resection with the knowledge that residual defects can almost always be satisfactorily restored. The final point to emphasize is the necessity to maintain long-term follow-up in these patients (67), who are at risk for recurrences and metachronous primary tumors.

Bibliography

1. Pindborg JJ. Premalignant and malignant lesions of the oral mucosa. In: Ariyan SE, ed. *Cancer of the head and neck.* St. Louis: CV Mosby, 1987; 163.
2. Shafer WG, Waldron CA. Erythoplakias of the oral cavity. *Cancer* 1975; 36:1021.
3. Spiro RH, Huvos AG, Wong GY, et al. Predictive value of tumor thickness in SCC confined to the tongue and floor of the mouth. *Am J Surg* 1986; 152:345.
4. Jones KR, Lodge-Rigal RD, Reddick RL, et al. Prognostic factors in the recurrence of stage I and II squamous cell cancer of the oral cavity. *Arch Otol head neck surg* 1992; 118:483–485.
5. Akine Y, Tokita N, Ogino T, et al. Stage I–II carcinoma of the anterior two-thirds of the tongue treated with different modalities. *Radiation Oncol* 1991; 21:24.
6. Leipzig B, Zellmer JE, Klug D. The role of endoscopy in evaluating patients with head and neck cancer. *Arch Otolaryngol* 1985; 111:589.
7. Sarkaria JN, Harari PM. Oral tongue cancer in young adults less than 40 years of age: rationale for aggressive therapy. *Head and Neck* 1994; 16:107.
8. Pernot M, Malissard L, Hoffstetter S, et al. The study of tumoral, radiobiological, and general health factors that influence results and complication in a series of 448 oral tongue carcinomas treated exclusively by irradiation. *Int J Rad Oncol Biol Phys* 1994; 29:673.
9. Rodgers LW Jr, Stringer SP, Mendenhall WM. Management of squamous cell carcinoma of the floor of the mouth. *Head and Neck* 1993; 15:16.
10. Cherian T, Sebastian P, Ahamed MI, et al. Evaluation of salvage surgery in heavily irradiated cancer of the buccal mucosa. *Cancer* 1991; 68:295.
11. Ho CM, Lam KH, Wei WI, Lau WF. Treatment of neck nodes in oral cancer. *Surg Oncol* 192; 1:73.
12. Mitchell R, Crighton LE. The management of patients with carcinoma of the tongue. *Brit J Oral Max Surg* 1993; 31:304.
13. Arnoletti JP, Albo D, Jhala N, et al. Computer-assisted image analysis of tumor sections for a new thrombospondin receptor. *Am J Surg* 1994; 168:433.
14. Williams JK, Carlson GW, Cohen C, et al. Tumor angiogenesis as a prognostic factor in oral cavity tumors. *Am J Surg* 1994; 168:373.
15. Von Biberstein SE, Lindquist R, Spiro J, et al. Enhanced tumor cell expression of tumor necrosis factor receptors in head and neck squamous cell carcinoma. Presented at Society of Head Neck Surgeons, Boston, May 1995.
16. Schipper JH, Frixen UH, Behrens J, et al. E-cadherin expression in squamous cell carcinomas of the head and neck. *Cancer Res* 1991; 51:6328.

17. Ishitoya J, Toriyama M, Oguchi N, et al. Gene amplification and over-expression of EGF receptors in squamous cell carcinomas of the head and neck. *Brit J Cancer* 1989; 59:559.
18. Das SN, Khanna NN, Khanna S, et al. Cell surface antigens in squamous cell carcinoma of the oral cavity. *J Surg Oncol* 1986; 31:166.
19. Dobrowsky W, Dobrowsky E, Strassel H, et al. Combined modality treatment of advanced cancers of the oral cavity and oropharynx. *Int J Rad Oncol Biol Phys* 1991; 20:239.
20. Depondt J, Gehanno P, Martin M, et al. Neoadjuvant chemotherapy with carboplatin/5-fluorouracil in head and neck cancer. *Oncol* 1993; 50(Suppl 2):23.
21. Cerezo L, Liu FF, Tsang R, Payne D. Squamous cell carcinoma of the lip: analysis of the Princess Margaret Hospital experience. *Rad Oncol* 1993; 28:142.
22. Ferraro J, Beaver BL, Young D, et al. Primary procedure in carcinoma of the tongue: local resection versus combined local resection and radial neck dissection. *J Surg Oncol* 1982; 21:245.
23. Ildstad ST, Bigelow ME, Remensnyder JP. Squamous cell carcinoma of the mobile tongue. *Am J Surg* 1983; 145:443.
24. Leipzig B, Cummings CW, Chung CT, et al. Carcinoma of the anterior tongue. *Ann Otol* 1982; 91:94.
25. Franceschi D, Gupta R, Spiro RH, Shah JP. Improved survival in the treatment of squamous carcinoma of the oral tongue. *Am J Surg* 1993; 166:360.
26. Callery CD, Spiro RH, Strong EW. Changing trends in the management of squamous cell carcinoma of the tongue. *Am J Surg* 1984; 148:449.
27. Manni JJ, Van Den Hoogen FJA. Supraomohyoid neck dissection with frozen section biopsy as a staging procedure in the clinically node-negative neck in carcinoma of the oral cavity. *Am J Surg* 1991; 162:373.
28. Leung TW, Lee AW, Chan DK. Definitive radiotherapy for carcinoma of the oral tongue. *Acta Oncol* 1993; 32:559.
29. Applebaum EL, Collins WL, Bytell DE. Carcinoma of the floor of the mouth. *Arch Otolaryngol* 1980; 106:419.
30. O'Brien CJ, Carter RL, Soo KC, et al. Invasion of the mandible by squamous carcinoma of the oral cavity and oropharynx. *Head Neck Surg* 1986; 8:247.
31. Gilbert S, Tzadik A, Leonard G. Mandibular involvement by oral squamous cell carcinoma. *Laryngoscope* 1986; 96:96.
32. Dubner S, Heller KS. Local control of squamous cell carcinoma following marginal and segmental mandibulectomy. *Head and Neck* 1993; 15:29.
33. Marchetta FC, Sako K, Murphy JB. The periosteum of the mandible and intraoral carcinoma. *Am J Surg* 1971; 122:711.
34. Barttelbort SW, Ariyan S. Mandible preservation with oral cavity carcinoma: rim mandibulectomy versus sagittal mandibulectomy. *Am J Surg* 1993; 166:411.
35. Patterson HC, Dobie RA, Cummings GW. Treatment of clinically negative necks in floor of mouth carcinoma. *Laryngoscope* 1984; 94:820.
36. Crossman JD, Gluckman J, Whiteley J, et al. Squamous cell carcinoma of the floor of the mouth. *Head Neck Surg* 1980; 3:2.
37. Mohit-Tabatabi MA, Sobel HJ, Rush BF, et al. Relation of thickness of floor of mouth stage I and stage II cancers to regional metastases. *Am J Surg* 1986; 152:351.
38. Cole DA, Patel PM, Matar JR et al. Floor of the mouth cancer. *Arch Otolaryngol* 1994; 120:260.
39. Greer RO, Poulson TC. Oral tissue alterations associated with the use of smokeless tobacco by teenagers. I. Clinical findings. *Oral Surg* 1983; 56:275.
40. Medina JE, Dichtel W, Luna MA. Verrucous-squamous carcinomas of the oral cavity: clinicopathologic study of 104 cases. *Arch Otolaryngol* 1984; 110:437.
41. Ildstad ST, Bigelow ME, Remensnyder JP. Clinical behavior and results of current therapeutic modalities for squamous cell carcinoma of the buccal mucosa. *Surg Gynecol Obstet* 1985; 160:254.
42. Kovalic JJ, Simpson JR. Carcinoma of the hard palate. *J Otolaryngol* 1993; 22:118.
43. Davidson BJ, Spiro RH, Patel S, et al. Cervical metastases of occult origin: the impact of combined modality therapy. *Am J Surg* 1995; 168:395.
44. Larson DL. Management of cervical metastases of occult origin: an update. *Plast Surg Outlook* 1995; 9(2):1.
45. Crile G Sr. Excision of cancer of the head and neck with special reference to the plan of dissection based on 132 operations. *JAMA* 1906; 47:1780.
46. Martin H, Del Valle B, Ehrlich H, et al. Neck dissection. *Cancer* 1951; 4:441.
47. Bocca E, Pignataro O, Oldini C, et al. Functional neck dissection: evaluation and review of 843 cases. *Laryngoscope* 1984; 94:942.
48. Jesse RH. The philosophy of treatment of neck nodes. *Ear Nose Throat J* 1977; 56:125.
49. Lydiatt DD, Robbins KT, Byers RM, Wolf PF. Treatment of stage I and II oral cancer. *Head and Neck* 1993; 15:308–312.
50. Van Den Hoogen FJ, and Manni JJ. Value of the supraomohyoid neck dissection with frozen section analysis as a staging procedure in the clinically negative neck in squamous cell carcinoma of the oral cavity. *Eur Tech Oto-Rhino-Laryngol* 1992; 249:144.
51. Vandenbrouck G, Sancho-Garmer H, Chassagne D, et al. Elective versus therapeutic neck dissection in epidermoid carcinoma of the oral cavity: results of a randomized clinical trial. *Cancer* 1980; 46:386.
52. Spaulding CA, Korb LJ, Constable WC, et al. The influence of extent of neck treatment upon control of cervical lymphadenopathy in cancers of the oral tongue. *Int J Rad Oncol Biol Phys* 1991; 21:577.
53. Lindberg R. Distribution of cervical lymph node metastases from squamous cell carcinoma of the upper respiratory and digestive tracts. *Cancer* 1972; 29:1446.
54. Langius A, Bjorvell H, Lind MG. Functional status and coping in patients with oral and pharyngeal cancer before and after surgery. *Head and Neck* 1994; 16:559.
55. Ariyan S. The pectoralis major myocutaneous flap: a versatile flap for reconstruction in the head and neck. *Plast Reconstr Surg* 1979; 63:73.
56. Quillen CG. Latissimus dorsi myocutaneous flaps in head and neck reconstruction. *Plast Reconstr Surg* 1979; 63:664.
57. Demergasso F, Piazza MV. Trapezius myocutaneous flap in reconstructive surgery for head and neck cancer: an original technique. *Am J Surg* 1979; 138:533.
58. Nichter LS, Morgan RF, Harman DM, et al. The trapezius musculocutaneous flap in head and neck reconstruction: potential pitfalls. *Head Neck Surg* 1984; 7:129.
59. O'Brien CJ, Nettle WJ, Lee KK. Changing trends in the management of carcinoma of the oral cavity and oropharynx. *Austr and N Zealand J Surg* 1993; 63:270–274.
60. Hester JR, McConnell FMS, Nahai F, et al. Reconstruction of cervical esophagus, hypopharynx, and oral cavity using the free jejunal transfer. *Am J Surg* 1980; 140:487.
61. Soutar DS, Scheker LR, Tanner NSB, et al. The radial forearm flap: a versatile method for intraoral reconstruction. *Br J Plast Surg* 1983; 36:1.
62. Man D, Acland RD. The microarterial anatomy of the dorsalis pedis flap and its clinical applications. *Plast Reconstr Surg* 1980; 64:419.
63. Silverberg B, Banis JC, Acland RD. Mandibular reconstruction with bone transfer. *Am J Surg* 1985; 150:440.
64. Granick MS, Newton ED, Hanna DC. Scapular free flap for repair of massive lower facial defects. *Head Neck Surg* 1986; 8:436.
65. Taylor GI. Reconstruction of the mandible with free composite iliac bone grafts. *Ann Plast Surg* 1982; 9:361.
66. Hidalgo DA. Fibula free flap: a new method of mandible reconstruction. *Plast Reconstr Surg* 1989; 84:71.
67. De Vissher AV, Manni JJ. Routine long-term follow-up in patients treated with curative intent for squamous cell carcinoma of the larynx, pharynx, and oral cavity. Does it make sense? *Arch Otolaryngol Head Neck Surg* 1994; 120:934.

37

Chemotherapy in the Treatment of Head and Neck Cancer

Mary E. Albers, M.D., and Andrew T. Huang, M.D.

Surgical resection and radiotherapy are effective treatment modalities for locoregional disease of head and neck cancer. Because of the high propensity for advanced stage disease to recur locally and to disseminate, chemotherapy was introduced as an adjunctive treatment to improve locoregional and systemic control of the disease.

Chemotherapy was initiated in head and neck cancer over 30 years ago for the treatment of patients with recurrent or metastatic disease. It can also enhance the effect of radiation, when both modalities of treatment are given simultaneously, and result in better control of the primary or recurrent disease. Therefore, chemotherapy has been integrated into the therapeutic strategy for primary treatment of advanced-stage tumors of the head and neck in an effort to improve both local control and overall survival. Furthermore, chemotherapy has become increasingly important now that disfiguring surgery is less desirable and organ preservation can be a goal of therapy. Despite the accepted practice of a multimodality treatment approach in locally advanced head and neck tumors, many questions regarding the use of chemotherapy remain unanswered. The optimal number of drugs, their dosage, schedule, and sequence within a treatment plan are but a few of those questions currently under investigation in clinical trial.

This chapter will review antineoplastic agents that demonstrate activity against squamous cell cancer (SCC) of the head, neck, and nasopharynx, and the use of those agents in primary therapy for locally advanced disease and recurrent or metastatic disease. Other histologic subtypes of malignancy such as lymphoma, sarcoma, melanoma, and adenoid cystic tumors are not covered in this chapter.

Antineoplastic Agents with Activity in Head and Neck Cancer

PHARMACOLOGY

The number of antineoplastic agents that have clearly demonstrated clinical activity against squamous cell cancer of the head and neck is limited (Table 37–1). Currently, those drugs with well-known activity belong to three different classes of chemotherapeutic agents: antimetabolites, alkylating agents, and antitumor antibiotics. These classes of chemotherapeutic agents differ significantly with regard to molecular structure, mechanism of action, and toxicity.

The antimetabolite drugs that are active against SCC of the head and neck include an antifolate, methotrexate, and a fluoropyrimidine, 5-fluorouracil (5-FU). The mechanisms of these two drugs are biochemically related, because they both result in inhibition of DNA synthesis. Methotrexate inhibits the enzyme, dihydrofolate reductase; this results in cellular accumulation of precursor folates and subsequent decrease in thymidylate and DNA synthesis. 5-Fluorouracil is a synthetic uracil analogue. After ribosylation and phosphorylation, it binds and inhibits thymidylate synthase. Antimetabolites require that cells sensitive to the cytotoxic effect be actively dividing, and thus "cell cycle–specific" agents. These agents are also most effective when cells are in the cell cycle phase (the "S phase"), during which DNA synthesis occurs.

Like many other antineoplastic agents, the toxicity associated with the antimetabolites is myriad. However, because of cell cycle specificity, the most frequently observed toxicity occurs in rapidly proliferating tissues such as bone marrow and gastrointestinal epithelium. Clinically, this results in myelosuppression and mucositis. Methotrexate is also associated with hepatotoxicity and pneumonitis. The use of 5-FU may result in severe diarrhea with life-threatening dehydration, as well as cutaneous and neurologic side effects. A syndrome of chest pain and elevation of cardiac enzymes suggesting cardiac ischemia is increasingly recognized with the use of 5-FU by protracted infusion.

Unlike the antimetabolites, the alkylating agents are not cell cycle–specific but do have increased activity in rapidly dividing cells. In general, these compounds chemically interact with DNA. The alkyl groups form covalent bonds with the guanine moiety of nucleic acids; this results in single- or double-strand DNA breaks, inhibition of DNA and RNA synthesis, and misreading of the DNA code. The heavy-metal compound, cisplatin (i.e., cis-diamminedichloroplatinum, or CDDP), is an alkylating agent with a unique molecular structure and pharmacologic characteristics. The activated complex attaches nucleophilic sites to DNA, RNA, and proteins, forming covalent links with these compounds. The dose limiting toxicity is nephrotoxicity, however nausea and vomiting may be moderately severe. Myelosuppression is mild, but may be problematic with cumulative and higher doses of CDDP. Ototoxicity is also observed. Neuropathy, which is typically peripheral and sensory, is not always reversible. Carboplatin, a synthetic analogue of CDDP, is less emetogenic and may be given as a bolus infusion without copious hydration as required for CDDP. It does cause significant myelosuppression, particularly thrombocytopenia.

Bleomycin is classified as an antitumor antibiotic. The compound is a group of peptides with two binding sites isolated from the fungus *Streptomyces verticallus*. Bleomycin

DNA-damaging effects of radiation therapy. It also has a cell synchronizing effect and blocks cells from leaving the radiosensitive G_1 phase (11).

Synergistic activity between 5-fluorouracil and radiation therapy has also been described (12). 5-Fluorouracil is converted to fluorodeoxyuridine monophosphate (FdUMP), the active nucleotide form that inhibits thymidylate synthase. Radiation-induced DNA damage is not repaired, because thymidylate synthase-mediated synthesis of thymidylate is required.

The potential interaction of platinum coordinates (CDDP or carboplatin) and radiation has been reviewed elsewhere in detail (13). Preclinical work suggests that free-radical generation and the inhibition of recovery from radiation-induced damage are two mechanisms through which radiopotentiation occurs.

CDDP displays antitumor activity in SCC of the head and neck and also enhances radiotherapy by inhibition of repair of sublethal radiation-induced damage. As mentioned previously, not only is the 5-fluorouracil and CDDP combination synergistic with respect to antitumor activity but each agent also has radiosensitizing properties. Therefore, the potential to enhance the overall tumor kill by combining radiation with different chemotherapeutic approaches, including biochemical modulation and/or the interaction of a number of effective antineoplastic agents, is substantial and should be explored further.

Concomitant Single-Drug Chemotherapy and Radiation Trials

The use of concomitant chemotherapy and radiation therapy has been investigated for nearly 30 years. Early clinical trials used single-agent chemotherapy in conjunction with radiation for patients with advanced-stage head and neck cancer. Several phase I/II trials have investigated single agents such as methotrexate, bleomycin, hydroxyurea, CDDP and 5-FU given concurrently with definitive radiotherapy.

The Northern California Oncology Group (NCOG) randomized patients to either radiation alone or radiation with concomitant bleomycin (14). This study also used maintenance chemotherapy in the experimental arm, which precluded a clear comparison between concomitant chemoradiation and radiation alone. Nonetheless, the group reported a significant increase in locoregional control in the combined therapy group, albeit with significant toxicity and poor patient compliance. In similar studies, poor results were observed with bleomycin, hydroxyurea, and 5-FU that were attributed to toxicity or lack of improved locoregional control.

5-FU has been studied more extensively as a radiosensitizer in head and neck cancer as well as in other solid tumors. In the only randomized trial, Lo and colleagues (15) at the University of Wisconsin reported superior local control and survival benefit with concomitant 5-FU and radiation therapy. A phase I/II trial reported a complete response rate of 75% in stage IV patients with radiotherapy and 5-day continuous infusion 5-FU; mucositis was also the dose limiting toxicity in this study (16). CDDP is potentially an ideal agent to use simultaneously with radiation for the treatment of SCC of the head and neck. It is a radiation potentiator, and has single-agent activity, and nonoverlapping toxicity. Therefore, it is not likely to enhance mucositis like 5-FU. A high complete response (CR) rate was reported from an early trial in which stage IV patients were treated with CDDP and concomitant radiation. However, the disease-free interval was short and a significant number of patients developed nephrotoxicity (17). The RTOG 8117 trial used a different schedule of CDDP every 3 weeks with radiation to treat advanced stage patients; following surgical salvage, a CR rate of over 70% was achieved (18). Of note, this particular study included favorable sites such as the nasopharynx and a higher proportion of patients with good performance status. However, when patients with nasopharyngeal carcinoma (NPC) were excluded, the locoregional control and survival rates were still better than a comparable patient group in the RTOG database. In a similar study, Memorial Sloan-Kettering treated all stage IV patients with CDDP every 3 weeks during the period of radiation (19). They also observed a high complete response rate; with surgical salvage, the CR rate increased from 64 to 73%. The only randomized trial, conducted by the Head and Neck Intergroup, has published interim results of treatment with weekly low-dose CDDP and radiation (20). The complete response rates were much lower than those reported in the earlier ECOG pilot study. And finally, the CDDP analogue, carboplatin, has been investigated with concomitant radiation therapy in stage IV patients by two different schedules in a pilot study (21). Similar CR rates were attained with milder toxicity on the weekly schedule.

In conclusion, studies investigating single-agent chemotherapy with radiation result in very high response rates (including CR rates of >70%) and improved local control. The best responses occur with either CDDP or 5-FU and radiation.

Concomitant Multiagent Chemotherapy and Radiation Trials

Early investigation of combination chemotherapy and radiation employed antineoplastic agents with suboptimal activity and treatment schedules. With the advent of the highly active CDDP and 5-FU combination, investigative pursuits have focused on the synergism of radiation with the radiosensitizing and cytotoxic properties of these two agents (Table 37–3). Taylor and coworkers (22) designed a treatment plan in which concomitant CDDP and 5-FU and radiation was repeated every other week for 7 weeks in inoperable stage III and IV patients. Follow-up at 51 months demonstrated that over 70% of patients had successful locoregional control, and median survival was 3 years. Median survival was improved when compared to the RTOG patient database, in which the median survival was 1 year.

In addition to different schedules and administration of chemotherapy, variations in the delivery of radiotherapy have been studied in an attempt to improve locoregional control and survival. In a pilot trial, Brizel and colleagues (23) used hyperfractionated (twice daily) radiation with concomitant CDDP and 5-FU, followed by surgery (for persistent disease) and two subsequent cycles of chemotherapy to treat advanced-stage patients. The 2-year locoregional control rate was over 70%, with the distant disease-free survival rate at nearly 90%. Wendt and others (24) used accelerated radiotherapy with CDDP, 5-FU, and leucovorin. Results were very similar at 2.5 years, with an overall locoregional control rate of 76% and distant relapse rate of 10%.

Table 37–3
Phase I/II Studies with Concomitant Chemotherapy and Radiation

Group	n	Treatment Plan	Locoregional Control		Distant Relapse
Taylor, 1989[22]	53	CDDP/5FU+RT		73%	15%
Brizel, 1993[23]	46	CDDP/5FU+RT→± Surg→CDDP/5FU × 2		72% (24 mo)	12% (24 mo)
Wendt, 1989[24]	62	CDDP/5FU/L+RT		76% (24 mo)	10% (24 mo)
Vokes, 1992[25]	64	PBM or PFL × 2→± Surg→RT+FHL	PBM	70%	24%
			PFL	74%	3%

CDDP, cis-diamminedichloroplatinum; 5FU, 5-fluorouracil; RT, radiation therapy; L, leucovorin; P, platinum (i.e., CDDP); B, bleomycin; F, 5-fluorouracil (i.e., 5-FU); H, hydroxyurea

The group at the University of Chicago has integrated chemotherapy into an aggressive treatment plan with curative intent for advanced head and neck cancer patients. Induction chemotherapy with either CDDP, bleomycin and methotrexate (PBM), or CDDP, 5-FU, and leucovorin (PFL), was followed by reevaluation for possible resection; inoperable/unresectable patients were treated immediately with concomitant radiation and 5-FU, hydroxyurea, and leucovorin. Not only does this combination provide radiosensitization, but the single-agent activity is also "biomodulated" to enhance tumor kill (25).

In summary, these studies show that an aggressive multimodality approach with concomitant chemoradiotherapy is feasible, with increased but tolerable toxicity. In poor-prognosis patients with advanced disease, intense treatment has resulted in very high complete response rates and a decrease in distant metastasis. This approach is very promising for both locoregional disease control and survival and should be pursued in clinical trial.

ADJUVANT (MAINTENANCE) CHEMOTHERAPY

Adjuvant or maintenance chemotherapy is given following primary local therapy when macroscopic disease is absent and the tumor burden is assumed to be low. The purpose of adjuvant chemotherapy is to consolidate local therapy response and eradicate microscopic local or distant metastasis. In head and neck cancer, adjuvant chemotherapy is not well studied. Both nonrandomized and randomized controlled trials published in the mid-1980s failed to demonstrate significant differences in either disease-free survival or overall survival. These trials frequently included induction courses of chemotherapy and therefore the addition of maintenance therapy alone was not adequately tested. Furthermore, the antineoplastic agents used are less active than combinations used in current regimens.

Two large, prospective randomized trials deserve mention. The Head and Neck Contracts Program randomized 462 resectable stage III and IV patients into one of three arms: (a) standard local therapy, (b) induction chemotherapy followed by standard local therapy, or (c) induction chemotherapy followed by standard local therapy and maintenance chemotherapy for 6 cycles (26). Of note, only 10% of the patients received all the chemotherapy as planned. At approximately 5 years, there was no significant difference in overall survival or disease-free survival among the three treatment arms. However, a decrease in the distant metastasis rate and an increase in time for first distant metastasis occurred in the maintenance arm. A subset analysis of this study showed that patients with oral-cavity lesions and patients with N1 or N2 disease had improved disease-free survival (27).

The second large cooperative group study, Intergroup 0034, also investigated 442 operable patients (28). Following surgery, patients were randomized to CDDP plus 5-FU for three cycles before radiotherapy, versus radiotherapy alone. At a 4-year follow-up, there was no significant difference in disease-free survival between the two groups. Locoregional failure rates were similar, but the distant failure rate in the chemotherapy group was significantly less.

More recently, SWOG reported interim data from a pilot feasibility trial in which 61 evaluable patients were treated with concomitant CDDP and radiation followed by CDDP plus 5-FU for three cycles (29). Less than 50% of the study subjects completed therapy as planned. The primary reason for noncompliance with chemotherapy was patient refusal.

In summary, there is inadequate data to support a definitive opinion about the role of chemotherapy in the adjuvant setting of head and neck cancer. However, observations made from secondary outcome measurements in the larger trials suggest that certain subsets of head and neck cancer patients may benefit from maintenance therapy. By lowering the rate of distant metastases, systemic chemotherapy demonstrates activity in this disease; however, this is at the cost of greater toxicity and difficulty with patient compliance.

OPTIMAL SEQUENCE OF MULTIMODALITY THERAPY

As discussed above, chemotherapy has been integrated into the primary treatment plan as either induction (sequential) chemotherapy with radiation ± surgery, or concomitant (simultaneous) with radiation ± surgery. The optimal timing of chemotherapy within the multimodality approach in head and neck cancer is not yet defined but continues to be explored in clinical trial. The South-East Cooperative Oncology Group prospectively randomized 277 stage III or IV patients to receive synchronous or sequential chemotherapy and radiation (30). Study subjects were further randomized to receive either vinblastine, bleomycin, or methotrexate (VBM), or VBM + 5-fluorouracil as the combination chemotherapy regimen. The overall survival was similar between the two arms, however, disease-free survival (DFS) was slightly better for the synchronous arm and significantly increased with the addition of 5-FU. In a smaller study, Adelstein and others (31) randomized 48 stage III and IV patients between simultaneous and sequential schedules of CDDP and 5-FU and radiation. Consistent with other studies, the overall survival was not significantly different, but relapse-free survival was significantly better in the simultaneous arm.

The Italian National Institute of Cancer Research used a different combination of chemotherapy in their randomized study of sequential versus simultaneous chemotherapy (32). In the sequential approach, VBM was given before radiotherapy and was compared to the simultaneous arm of VBM alternating with radiation in a "sandwiched" fashion. The complete response rate, disease-free survival, and 4-year survival rates were significantly better in the simultaneous arm at 5 years.

Finally, Taylor and others (33) randomized 215 unresectable stage III and IV patients to induction CDDP and 5-FU for three cycles, followed by radiation or CDDP-5-FU every other week given concomitantly with radiation. Although the overall response was significantly greater in the concomitant arm compared to the sequential arm, complete responses were similar between the two groups and there were no significant differences in survival.

In summary, data from studies comparing sequential versus simultaneous use of CDDP-based chemotherapy with radiation in head and neck cancer does show superiority in response and survival rates with the simultaneous approach in the majority of studies.

Nasopharyngeal Carcinoma

Nasopharyngeal carcinoma (NPC) is a distinct entity from other squamous cell carcinomas of the head and neck region. While NPC is a very rare tumor in North America, it accounts for approximately 20% of all malignant tumors in the Chinese population. All types of NPC are associated with the Epstein-Barr virus. Over the past decade it has become evident that NPC is biologically different from other SCC of the head and neck region with regard to both natural history of the disease and response to therapy. NPC has a higher rate of distant metastasis and is frequently unresectable because of both extent of disease and location of the tumor within the bony skull. Unlike SCC of other sites in the head and neck, the rate of distant metastasis is high, approaching 60 to 80% in N3 disease. Nonetheless, durable remissions and even cures may be achieved in patients with advanced disease.

In general, multiagent chemotherapy results in high overall response rates of 30 to 100%, with complete responses ranging from 25 to 30%. With this level of chemosensitivity, antineoplastic agents have been integrated into the primary treatment of NPC patients who have advanced disease and poor prognosis. Multiagent chemotherapy when used as induction before definitive radiotherapy has attained high response rates in patients with advanced disease (34). Preliminary results of an international phase III trial demonstrates a significant increase in disease free survival in patients treated with chemotherapy followed by radiotherapy compared to radiotherapy alone (35).

The Radiation Therapy Oncology Group (RTOG 8117) reported very high responses in stage IV NPC patients treated with concomitant chemotherapy and radiation (36). CDDP given every 3 weeks for three cycles during radiation resulted in nearly 90% complete responses; disease-free survival and overall survival rates are 49% and 63%, respec-

tively, at a 3-year follow-up. On the other hand, results from a large, multicenter randomized study showed adjuvant/maintenance chemotherapy administered following definitive radiotherapy in NPC has not resulted in improved disease-free survival (37).

In summary, NPC responds well to both radiation and chemotherapy. Concomitant combination treatment of both modalities offer good results that have surpassed any previous attempts with radiation only. It seems likely that some variation of concomitant chemotherapy and radiation will result in both higher complete-response rates and long-term survival in this disease. Future studies should also focus on the use of maintenance chemotherapy in the hope of controlling distant disease with the use of optimal drugs.

Treatment of Recurrent or Metastatic Disease

SINGLE AGENT

When first introduced in the treatment of head and neck cancer in the early 1960s, chemotherapy was used for the palliation of recurrent or metastatic disease. Expected response to single agents ranges from 15 to 60%, depending on both patient and tumor factors. Performance status is the most important predictive patient factor for response. Methotrexate, administered intravenous weekly, demonstrates an average partial response rate of 30% with 2- to 6-month duration of response. High doses of intravenous methotrexate with leucovorin rescue have not clearly shown benefit over standard dose methotrexate.

Cisplatin given every 3 to 4 weeks has similar response rates to intravenous methotrexate, although there have been some reports of complete responses. Changes in schedule of drug administration have not significantly impacted on response rates; however, the side-effect profile may be ameliorated when CDDP is given by protracted infusion. Carboplatin, a CDDP analogue that may be given intravenous bolus in an outpatient setting, appears to have similar activity as a single agent, although experience with this agent is less than with methotrexate or CDDP. Some studies report lower response rates; however, interpatient variability in clearance of the drug may be important. In conclusion, weekly intravenous methotrexate is frequently offered to patients for attempt at palliation because of its ease of administration, lower cost, and milder side-effect profile. There is inadequate data regarding cross-resistance among single agents in this setting; however, with disease progression, 2nd and 3rd line treatment with single agents results in an extremely low probability of response.

COMBINATION THERAPY

Rationale

By far, the vast majority of tumors are treated successfully not with single-agent therapy but with combination chemotherapy. Improved efficacy of multiagent therapy is based on: (a) prevention of drug resistance (Goldie-Coleman hypothesis), and (b) increased tumor-cell kill. The use of combination therapy is guided primarily by the principles that effective combinations include drugs with single-agent activity and that the drugs have nonoverlapping toxicity. There are numerous sources that review these concepts in detail. As mentioned above, the single agents known to have activity in SCC of the head and neck have different mechanisms of action and different side-effect profiles. This allows for multiple permutations of combination of drugs in an attempt to improve therapeutic efficacy over single-agent treatment; extensive clinical testing over the past decade has addressed this very question. The body of clinical investigational work is considerable and may be easily summarized: combination chemotherapy may result in higher response rates, but there is no evidence for increased survival in recurrent or metastatic SCC of the head and neck.

Randomized Clinical Trials

Table 37–4 includes selected randomized, controlled studies that compare active single agents to combinations of those agents in the treatment of recurrent or metastatic SCC of the head and neck. While there is some heterogeneity within the patient population as a whole, the vast majority of subjects who entered these studies had recurrent disease following surgery and/or radiation therapy. A small fraction of patients from several studies presented with metastatic disease and had not received any local therapy.

The earliest trials that studied multiagent therapy frequently combined those agents thought to be most active in SCC of the head and neck: CDDP, bleomycin, and methotrexate. After the synergistic activity of the combination of CDDP and 5-FU was described, the Wayne State group investigated the combination in a pilot study and reported an overall response rate of 70% and a complete response rate of 27% in patients with recurrent head and neck cancer (1). Given these remarkably high response rates, the CDDP and 5-FU combination continues to be the most frequently used combination in this population of patients. However, as is frequently the case, results from larger, randomized controlled studies fail to reproduce the higher response rates that

are seen in smaller, uncontrolled trials. As was shown in Table 37–4, the overall response rate to single agent therapy ranges from 10 to 35%. The overall response rate to multiagent therapy ranges from 21 to 48%. The median survival times reported for treatment with single agent or combination chemotherapy are remarkably similar, ranging from 3 months to 7 months. Acceptable toxicity is described in nearly all multiagent regimens compared to single-agent therapy with mild-to-moderate mucositis and myelosuppression occurring in the CDDP-based regimens.

In conclusion, while individual studies may report higher response rates with multiagent chemotherapy compared to single-agent therapy, this has not translated into improved survival. Furthermore, median response rates of single-agent therapy compared to multiagent therapy are not significantly different. Is there any benefit in treating patients who have recurrent or metastatic disease with multiagent therapy? If one looks at the data provided by stratification of patient characteristics, certain patients may indeed have a better response. For example, those patients with a better performance status and lower tumor burden appear to experience higher response rates with multiagent chemotherapy (42). Furthermore, as will be discussed later, tumor responses and survival should not be considered the only measurements of potential therapeutic benefit. Quality-of-life studies are still lacking in this population of patients. We should use quality-of-life data to help measure our efforts to palliate disease we cannot cure. It would not be unreasonable to expect that, with acceptable toxicity, higher response rates result in improved quality of life.

Summary and Future Directions

Cumulative data supports a role for chemotherapy not only for palliation in recurrent or metastatic disease but also as a component of the multimodality approach for primary treatment. Problems inherent to the head and neck cancer patients in most studies generally attenuate the apparent impact

Table 37–4
Selected Randomized Controlled Trials Comparing Single-Agent to Multiagent Regimens in Recurrent/Metastatic Head and Neck Cancer

Group	Regimen	n	Response Rates	Median Survival	Ref
NCOG,[†] 1983	CDDP vs CDDP/M	79	18 vs 33%	6.2 vs 6.9 mo	38
ECOG,[‡] 1985	M vs CDDP/M/B	163	35 vs 48%	5.6 vs 5.6 mo	39
SECSG,[#] 1986	M vs CDDP/VBL/B	191	16 vs 24%	7.8 vs 7.3 mo	40
Liverpool, 1990	M vs CDDP vs CDDP/M vs CDDP/5FU	200	12 vs 28 vs 22 vs 24%	NSD*	41
Jacobs, 1992	CDDP vs 5FU vs CDDP/5FU	245	17 vs 13 vs 32%	5.7 mo (all)	42
SWOG[¥,] 1992	M vs CDDP/5FU vs CBDCA/5FU	261	10 vs 32 vs 21%	5.6 vs 6.6 vs 5.0 mo	43

[†]NCOG, Northern California Oncology Group
[‡]ECOG, Eastern Cooperative Oncology Group
[#]SECSG, Southeastern Cancer Study Group
[¥]SWOG, Southwest Oncology Group
*NSD, no significant difference
CDDP, cisdiamminedichloroplatinum; M, methotrexate; VBL, vinblastine; B, bleomycin; VCR, vincristine; 5-FU, 5-fluorouracil; CBDCA, carboplatin

chemotherapy has made in the treatment of this disease. It is well recognized that the study population is heterogeneous with regard to factors such as anatomic location of the tumor in the head and neck, tumor burden, nutrition, and prior treatment. Moreover, the majority of published clinical trials have inadequate sample size and lack enough power to detect differences in survival rates. Perhaps a more important issue when investigating therapy in this disease is to better understand the background of these patients. That is to say, patients with head and neck cancer often have a history of tobacco and alcohol abuse and therefore they have other highly significant comorbid medical conditions such as cardiovascular and pulmonary disease, malnutrition, and poor performance status, among other problems. Ultimately, this same patient population is at high risk to die of a second malignancy or a catastrophic cardiovascular or pulmonary illness. Therefore, specific disease-free survival may be more clinically relevant and meaningful than overall survival in this population. Furthermore, the use of chemotherapy in recurrent or metastatic disease should be studied in concert with quality-of-life analysis. While improvement in survival rates remains our preeminent goal, high response rates with acceptable toxicity may very well correlate with improved quality of life and patient benefit. The future holds promise for continued development of drugs with greater activity and a wider therapeutic margin. Other exciting avenues of investigation include the use of biologic modifiers, differentiation agents and tumor biology for response to chemotherapy. Finally, extensive work has taken place in the laboratory in an effort to predict who might benefit from chemotherapy. DNA content parameters that predict for sensitivity to CDDP-based chemotherapy include aneuploidy and the absence of keratin (44). Numerous immunologic determinants have been analyzed for correlation to prognosis and response to therapy. C1q binding activity levels were found to be predictive; however, the mechanism for this correlation remains to be elucidated (45).

The future for improved therapeutic endeavors in SCC of the head and neck appears promising. As we learn more about the biology of the tumor and are able to predict response to different treatment modalities, we will make significant inroads in the treatment of this disease. In particular, concomitant therapy may be a better treatment approach for advanced-stage or unresectable patients. Quality-of-life issues are becoming of equal importance and must be considered in treatment planning.

References

1. Kish JA, Ensley JF, Jacobs J, et al. A randomized trial of cisplatin (CACP) + 5-fluorouracil (5-FU) infusion and CACP + 5-FU bolus for recurrent and advanced squamous cell carcinoma of the head and neck. *Cancer* 1985; 56:2740–2744.
2. Uen W, Huang AT, Mennel R, et al. A phase II study of piritrexim in patients with advanced squamous head and neck cancer. *Cancer* 1992; 69:1008–1011.
3. Schornagel JH, Verweij J, Cognetti F, et al. A randomized phase III trial of methotrexate (MTX) vs 10-ethyl-10-deazaaminopterin (10-Edam) in patients with advanced and/or metastatic squamous cell carcinoma of the head and neck (abstract). *Eur J Cancer* 1991; 27(suppl 2):S138.
4. Robert F. Trimetrexate as a single agent in patients with advanced head and neck cancer. *Seminars in Oncology* 1988; 15:22–26.
5. Braakhuis BJ, van Dongen GA, Vermorken JB, et al. Preclinical in vivo activity of 2′,2′-difluorodeoxycytidine (Gemcitabine) against human head and neck cancer. *Cancer Res* 1991; 51:211–214.
6. Rooney M, Kish J, Jacobs J, et al. Improved complete response rate and survival in advanced head and neck cancer after three-course induction therapy with 120-hour 5-FU infusion and cisplatin. *Cancer* 1985; 55: 1123–1128.
7. Schuller DE, Metch B, Stein DW, et al. Preoperative chemotherapy in advanced resectable head and neck cancer: final report of the Southwest Oncology Group. *Laryngoscope* 1988; 98:1205–1211.
8. Paccagnella A, Orlando A, Marchiori C, et al. Phase III trial of initial chemotherapy in stage III or IV head and neck cancers: a study by the gruppo di studio sui tumori della testa e del collo. *J Natl Canc Inst* 1994; 86:265–272.
9. Department of Veterans Affairs Laryngeal Cancer Study Group. Induction chemotherapy plus radiation compared with surgery plus radiation in patients with advanced laryngeal cancer. *NEJM* 1991;324: 1685–1690.
10. Steel GG, Peckham MJ. Exploitable mechanisms in combined radiotherapy-chemotherapy: the concept of additivity. *Int J Radiat Oncol Biol Phys* 1979; 5:85–91.
11. Sinclair WK. The combined effect of hydroxyurea and x rays on Chinese hamster cells in vitro. *Cancer Res* 1968; 28:198–206.
12. Byfield JE, Calabro-Jones P, Klisak I, et al. Pharmacologic requirements for obtaining sensitization of human tumor cells in vitro to combined 5-fluorouracil or ftorafur and x-rays. *Int J Radiat Oncol Biol Phys* 1982; 8:1923–1933.
13. Coughlin CT, Richmond RC. Biologic and clinical developments of cisplatin combined with radiation: concepts, utility, projections for new trials, and the emergence of carboplatin. *Seminars in Oncology* 1989; 16:31–43.
14. Fu KK, Phillips TL, Silverberg IJ, et al. Combined radiotherapy and chemotherapy with bleomycin and methotrexate for advanced inoperable head and neck cancer: Update of a Northern California Oncology Group randomized trial. *J Clin Oncol* 1987; 5:1410–1418.
15. Lo TC, Wiley AL, Ansfield FJ, et al. Combined radiation therapy and 5-Fluorouracil for advanced squamous cell carcinoma of the oral cavity and oropharynx: a randomized study. *Am J of Roentgenol* 1976; 126:229–235.
16. Byfield JE, Sharp TR, Frankel SS, et al. Phase I and II trial of 5-day infused 5-flurouracil and radiation in advanced cancer of the head and neck. *J Clin Oncol* 1984; 2:406–413.
17. Snyderman NL, Wetmore SJ, and Suen JY. Cisplatin sensitization to radiotherapy in stage IV squamous cell carcinoma of the head and neck. *Arch Otolaryngol Head and Neck Surg* 1986; 112:1147–1150.
18. Marcial VA, Pajak TF, Mohiuddin M, et al. Concomitant cisplatin chemotherapy and radiotherapy in advanced mucosal squamous cell carcinoma of the head and neck: long-term results of the Radiation Therapy Oncology Group Study 81-17. *Cancer* 1990; 66:1861–1868.
19. Harrison LB, Pfister DG, Fass DE, et al. Concomitant chemotherapy-radiation therapy followed by hyperfractionated radiation therapy for advanced unresectable head and neck cancer. *Int J Radiat Oncol Biol Phys* 1991; 21:703–708.
20. Haselow RE, Warshaw MG, Oken MM, et al. Radiation alone versus radiation with weekly low dose cis-platinum in unresectable cancer of the head and neck. In: Fee WE, et al, eds. *Head and neck cancer*. Philadelphia: B.C. Decker, 1990; 279–281.
21. Eisenberger M, and Jacobs M. Simultaneous treatment with single-agent chemotherapy and radiation for locally advanced cancer of the head and neck. *Review Semin in Oncol* 1992; 19:41–46.
22. Taylor SG IV, Murthy AK, Caldarelli DD, et al. Combined simultaneous cisplatin/fluorouracil chemotherapy and split course radiation in head and neck cancer. *J Clin Oncol* 1989; 7:846–856.
23. Brizel DM, Leopold KA, Fisher SR et al. A phase I/II trial of twice daily irradiation and concurrent chemotherapy for locally advanced squamous cell carcinoma of the head and neck. *Int J Radiat Oncol Biol Phys* 1993; 28:213–220.
24. Wendt TG, Hartenstein RC, Wustrow TP, et al. Cisplatin, fluorouracil with leucovorin calcium enhancement, and synchronous accelerated radiotherapy in the management of locally advanced head and neck cancer: a phase II study. *J Clin Oncol* 1989; 7:471–476.
25. Vokes EE, Weichselbaum RR, Mick R, et al. Favorable long-term survival following induction chemotherapy with cisplatin, fluorouracil, and leucovorin and concomitant chemoradiotherapy for locally advanced head and neck cancer. *JNCI* 1992; 84:877–882.
26. Adjuvant chemotherapy for advanced head and neck squamous carcinoma. Final report of the Head and Neck Contracts Program. *Cancer* 1987; 60:301–311.

27. Jacobs C, and Makuch R. Efficacy of adjuvant chemotherapy for patients with resectable head and neck cancer: a subset analysis of the head and neck contracts program. *J Clin Oncol* 1990; 8:838–847.

28. Laramore GE, Scott CB, al-Sarraf M, et al. Neck adjuvant chemotherapy for resectable squamous cell carcinomas of the head and neck: report on Intergroup Study 0034. *Int J Radiation Oncology Biol Phys* 1992; 23:705–713.

29. Kish JA, Ensley J, Benedetti J, et al. Postoperative adjuvant treatment of advanced head and neck cancer: Wayne State University experience and Southwest Oncology Group feasibility trial. *Proceedings of ASCO* 1993; 12:285.

30. A randomized trial of combined multidrug chemotherapy and radiotherapy in advanced squamous cell carcinoma of the head and neck. An interim report from the SECOG participants. *Europ J Surg Oncol* 1986; 12:289–295.

31. Adelstein DJ, Sharan VM, Earle AS, et al. Simultaneous versus sequential combined technique therapy for squamous cell head and neck cancer. *Cancer* 1990; 65:1685–1691.

32. Merlano M, Corvo R, Margarino G, et al. Combined chemotherapy and radiation therapy in advanced inoperable squamous cell carcinoma of the head and neck. Final report of a randomized trial. *Cancer* 1991; 67:915–921.

33. Taylor SG IV, Murthy AK, Vannetzel JM, et al. Randomized comparison of neoadjuvant cisplatin and fluorouracil infusion followed by radiation versus concomitant treatment in advanced head and neck cancer. *J Clin Oncol* 1994; 12:385–395.

34. Dimery IW, Peters LJ, Goepfert H, et al. Effectiveness of combined induction chemotherapy and radiotherapy in advanced nasopharyngeal carcinoma. *J Clin Oncol* 1993; 11:1919–1928.

35. Cvitkovic E, for the Int. Nasopharynx Study Group. Neoadjuvant chemotherapy with epirubicin, cisplatin, bleomycin in undifferentiated nasopharyngeal cancer: preliminary results of an international phase III Trial. *Proceedings of ASCO,* 1994; 13:283.

36. Al-Sarraf M, Pajak TF, Cooper JS, et al. Chemo-radiotherapy in patients with locally advanced nasopharyngeal carcinoma: a radiation therapy oncology study. *J Clin Oncol* 1990; 8:1342–1351.

37. Rossi A, Molinari R, Boracchi P, et al. Adjuvant chemotherapy with vincristine, cyclophosphamide, and doxorubicin after radiotherapy in local-regional nasopharyngeal cancer: results of a 4-year multicenter randomized study. *J Clin Oncol* 1988, 6:1401–1410.

38. Jacobs C, Meyers F, Hendrickson C, et al. Randomized phase III study of cisplatin with or without methotrexate for recurrent squamous cell carcinoma of the head and neck. A Northern California Oncology Group study. *Cancer* 1983; 52:1563–1569.

39. Vogl SE, Schoenfeld DA, Kaplan BH, et al. A randomized prospective comparison of methotrexate with a combination of methotrexate, bleomycin, and cisplatin in head and neck cancer. *Cancer* 1985; 56:432–442.

40. Williams SD, Velez-Garcia E, Essessee I, et al. Chemotherapy for head and neck cancer. Comparison of cisplatin + vinblastine + bleomycin versus methotrexate. *Cancer* 1986; 57:18–23.

41. A phase III randomised trial of cisplatinum, methotrexate, cisplatinum + methotrexate and cisplatinum + 5-FU in end stage squamous carcinoma of the head and neck. The Liverpool Head and Neck Oncology Group. *Br J Cancer* 1990; 61:311–315.

42. Jacobs C, Lyman G, Velez-Garcia E, et al. A phase III randomized study comparing cisplatin and fluorouracil as single agents and in combination for advanced squamous cell carcinoma of the head and neck. *J Clin Oncol* 1992; 10:257–263.

43. Forastiere AA, Metch B, Schuller DE, et al. Randomized comparison of cisplatin plus fluorouracil and carboplatin plus fluorouracil versus methotrexate in advanced squamous cell carcinoma of the head and neck: a Southwest Oncology Group study. *J Clin Oncol* 1992; 10:1245–1251.

44. Crissman JD, Pajak TF, Zarbo RJ, et al. Improved response and survival to combined cisplatin and radiation in non-keratinizing squamous cell carcinomas of the head and neck. An RTOG study of 114 advanced stage tumors. *Cancer* 1987; 59:1391–1397.

45. Schantz SP, Savage HE, Racz T, et al. Immunologic determinants of head and neck cancer response to induction chemotherapy. *J Clin Oncol* 1989; 7:857–864.

Suggested Reading

Vokes EE, Weichselbaum RR, Lippman SM, and Hong WK. Head and Neck Cancer. *NEJM* 1993; 328:184–194.

Schilsky RL. Biochemical pharmacology of chemotherapeutic drugs used as radiation enhancers. *Seminars in Oncology* 1992; 19:2–7.

Fandi A, Altun M, Azli N, Armand JP, et al. Nasopharyngeal cancer: epidemiology, staging and treatment. *Seminars in Oncology* 1994; 21:382–397.

38

Basic Principles of
Radiation Oncology

David M. Brizel, M.D., and Leonard R. Prosnitz, M.D.

The field of radiation oncology has undergone rapid growth since entering the "supervoltage" era in the early 1960s. The speciality, then referred to as "therapeutic radiology," formally separated from radiology in 1974. Because of its increasing involvement with cancer patients, the speciality was formally renamed *radiation oncology* in 1986.

The previous 3 decades have brought increasing levels of sophistication in radiobiology, physics, and treatment-related equipment. These factors, along with expanding clinical experience in the use of radiation, both by itself and combined with other therapeutic modalities, has led the speciality into a prominent position in the care of patients with cancer.

The estimated incidence of cancer in the United States is 1 million new cases (excluding nonmelanoma skin cancers and carcinoma in situ) in 1992 (1). Radiation is used in 50 to 60% of these patients (2). Because radiation is increasingly being employed earlier in patient's therapy, often with curative intent, and because patients often live longer after being treated with radiation, there are increasing numbers of patients who have undergone treatment with radiation who are also seen by other specialists. This is particularly true of the plastic surgeon, who might be called on to assist in the care of the chronic or delayed soft-tissue complications and other possible problems of long-term survivors who have been irradiated for their cancer. This chapter provides an overview of the field of radiation oncology, emphasizing aspects potentially important to the plastic surgeon.

Radiotherapy Equipment

Treatment of tumors with x-rays was first performed only 1 month after the discovery of x-rays by Roentgen in January 1896 (3). Treatment with radium was used shortly after its discovery by the Curies in 1898 (3). Advances followed slowly in the next several decades. These included more reliable tubes (Coolidge, 1913), the ionization chamber for output measurement (Szilard, 1914), and the use of fractionated radiation (Regaud, Coutard, Baclesse, 1920s) (4).

Major and rapid advances in radiotherapy were largely a result of the development of radioactive cobalt (CO_{60}) machines and linear accelerators in the decades following World War II. These machines produced "megavoltage" (or supervoltage) radiation that resulted in greater penetration into tissue and relative skin sparing (see radiation physics section). High photon output was obtained from this equipment, which allowed for the placement of energy sources at a much greater distance than was previously possible (typically 80 to 100 cm from the patient). This further aided delivery of relatively higher radia-

tion doses at depth, as well as allowing for placement of the machine on a gantry that could rotate 360° about the patient. These factors combined to allow relatively good delivery of radiation energy well inside the patient (where tumors are typically located), as well as timely, accurate, and reproducible patient setup and treatment (multifield treatments generally take 10 to 15 minutes per patient). Over the years, linear accelerators (Linacs) have largely replaced Cobalt-60 machines because of their improved delivery of radiation at depth and their sharper field edges (i.e., less radiation given to tissues outside of the desired target), radiation safety concerns, and the ability of Linacs to produce superficially penetrating electrons (see radiation physics section).

Modern radiation oncology departments have a number of other essential pieces of equipment. The vast majority of patients presently undergo a treatment simulation. The treatment simulator is a diagnostic/fluoroscopic x-ray machine designed with the same geometry as the Linac. This allows for appropriate radiation field placement because diagnostic quality radiographs may be taken to verify field placement. Simulator films are also used as templates for customized radiation blocks that allow field shaping to minimize radiation delivery to normal tissues. Specialized immobilization devices are frequently used to enhance reproducibility of field setup from treatment to patient.

Most patients undergo computerized treatment planning to determine the best field arrangement that will deliver a homogenous dose to the tumor and minimize the normal-tissue dose. Newer treatment planning techniques offer the potential for viewing dose distribution in three dimensions and from varying angles.

All radiation oncology departments have, or have available to them, a variety of radioisotopes useful in "implant" or brachytherapy. This technique has the advantage of concentrating the radiation dose in the tumor to a much greater extent than is possible with external beam therapy. In this setting, material-emitting radiation is placed on or within a tumor; commonly used isotopes include Cesium 137, Iridium 192, Gold 198, and Iodine 125.

Modern radiation oncology facilities are set up for a variety of clinical situations including head and neck and gynecologic examinations. Fiberoptic instruments and sophisticated photograph equipment are available as well.

Radiobiologic Principles

The fundamental radiobiologic principles that underlie clinical radiation therapy were largely elucidated after fundamental clinical radiotherapeutic practices were established on an empiric basis. Nonetheless, an understanding of these principles is of considerable importance both for the radiation oncologist and the surgeon because they provide a rationale basis by which to select radiotherapy or alternate treatments in particular clinical situations. They also enable the physician to plan combinations of radiation therapy, surgery, and chemotherapy in a scientific fashion. Finally, knowledge of radiobiology enables the oncologist to undertake new investigative approaches to improve management techniques for various types of cancer.

The essence of cancer therapy is to deprive tumor cells of their clonogenicity (i.e., their ability to replicate). This can be accomplished by their removal (surgery) or by cellular damage in situ. Radiation deprives cells of the clonogenicity via DNA damage. This comes about as a result of the ionizing effect of high-energy radiation. Interaction of any particular photon or particle of radiation with the material at which it is aimed is an all-or-none phenomenon. If there is an interaction, high-energy radiation has the ability to displace electrons from their normal orbits. These energetic electrons may interact directly with DNA, or they may interact with nearby bimolecules (such as water) to create highly reactive free radicals that may subsequently damage DNA. The type and extent of DNA damage is variable, ranging from nucleoside base changes to double-strand chain breaks. The ability of the cell to repair damage is dependent on the type and extent of changes as well as the integrity of repair mechanisms (5).

Attempts to understand the cellular effects of radiation have led investigators to irradiate cells in vitro. A typical radiation-cell survival curve is shown in Figure 38–1 (6). The data are derived from exposing cells in tissue culture to single doses of radiation. The logarithm of the fraction of cells that survive radiation is plotted on the y-axis against the dose of radiation, which is plotted linearly on the x-axis.

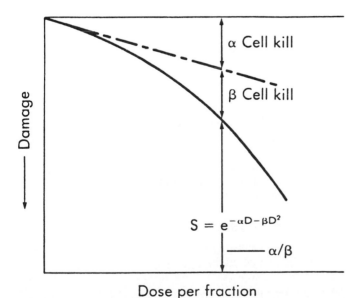

Dose per fraction

FIG. 38–1. Dose-response curves for mammalian cells are adequately fitted by the linear quadratic relationship, at least over the range of doses of concern in radiotherapy. The form of the equation is $S = e^{-}(\alpha D + \beta D^2)$, where S is the fraction of surviving cells per dose (d) and α and β are constants.

For the first several logs of survival, the survival curve can be described by a linear quadratic equation: $S = e^{-}(\alpha D + \beta D^2)$ where S is the fraction of surviving cells for a given dose (D) of irradiation. Alpha (α) and beta (β) are constants. The linear (α) component dominates at lower doses per fraction, while the quadratic (β) component exerts a greater influence as the fraction size increases. As a general rule, in tumors and acute responding normal tissues (oral mucosa, skin), the linear component of cell killing predominates. In other words, these tissues have high α:β ratios and will not be significantly affected by changes in fraction size. Conversely, the survival for late-responding normal tissues (e.g., bone, CNS, subcutaneous tissues) is controlled mainly by the β component (low α:β ratio). Their survival curves are "curvier," and the effect of radiation on these tissues is very much fraction-size dependent. The low α:β ratios for late-responding normal tissues is quite consistent with the clinical observation that late complications of radiation (e.g., fibrosis and osteonecrosis) are reduced when the fraction size is decreased (vide infra).

A number of clinically relevant conclusions can be made based on a consideration of the cell-survival curve. Because cell killing is proportional to the logarithm of the number of cells irradiated, smaller numbers of cells require lesser doses of radiation. This has led to the so-called shrinking field technique and the concept of subclinical disease in which doses in the range of 4500 to 5000 cGy are adequate to control potential microscopic foci of disease, but doses in the neighborhood of 6500 to 7500 cGy will be required for the control of gross disease (8). Conversely, we can appreciate that a reduction in tumor volume by approximately 90% by some surgical procedure is only a 1-log reduction (e.g. a reduction from 10^9 cells to 10^8 cells) in the number of cells being irradiated and has minimal influence on the overall radiation dose necessary for tumor control.

Cell survival-curve considerations lend further insight into the meaning of a clinical response. The average tumor contains approximately 10^9 cells per cm^3; thus, a tumor containing 10^{11} cells would be quite large and a reduction by any treatment from 10^{11} to 10^8 cells would constitute a visually impressive partial response, but would fall far short of the kind of cell kill required for local control. It is generally accepted that tumors containing 10^7 or fewer cells are not clinically detectable. Therefore, a "complete response" might involve death of all of the tumor cells in question but might also only represent a reduction to 10^7 or 10^6 viable cells. It is apparent that complete response as a measure of tumor cure is a very primitive assessment of treatment efficacy, and at the present time it is not a substitute for long-term observation.

Oxygen Effect

The inherent radiosensitivity of most tumors and normal tissues is nearly the same for well-oxygenated tissues. The situation is substantially altered in the setting of tissue hypoxia. Hypoxic cells (Po$_2$ = 1–2 mm Hg) in tissue culture, as well as in animal tumors, are 2.5 to 3.0 times more resistant to the lethal effects of radiation than well-oxygenated cells (Po$_2$ > 10 mm Hg). Tumor hypoxia has been demonstrated in human tumors in situ and is thought to have a major influence on the effectiveness of radiation therapy (8–11).

The problem of hypoxic cells has powerfully influenced the thinking of radiation oncologists and the entire direction of radiation oncology research. Many efforts in the field have been directed towards overcoming this problem. They have included the use of hyperbaric oxygen, electron affinic compounds that selectively sensitize hypoxic cells, and densely ionizing high-linear-energy transfer radiation, such as neutrons or pymazons whose biologic effect is not influenced by the lack of oxygen. Also, radiation-dose fractionation schedules can be altered in order to facilitate reoxygenation between fractions. Finally, the use of hyperthermia, which is known to sensitize cells to the action of radiation, and which is thought to be preferentially toxic to hypoxic cells in tissues, has been tried in an attempt to eliminate the effects of hypoxia (12).

Alterations in Radiation Dose Fractionation Schedules

The cell-survival curve shown in Figure 38–2 is derived from examining the lethal effect of graded single doses of irradiation. If two doses of radiation are given, at least 6 hours a part, a curve of the type shown in Figure 38–2 is obtained. The shoulder portion of the curve is repeated before the curve again becomes exponential. It can be readily seen from an examination of this figure that a larger dose of radiation is required to produce the same biologic effect if it is given in two increments rather than one. A certain amount of repair of radiation damage has taken place between the fractions.

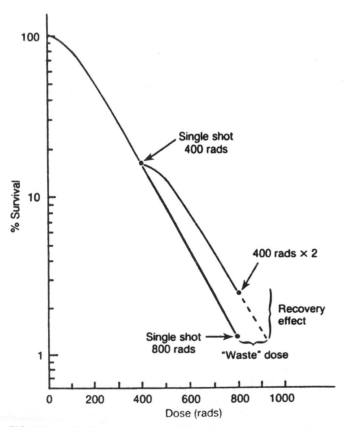

FIG. 38–2. Radiation cell-survival curve for two doses of 400 rad, each illustrating repair of radiation damage in the interval between the two treatments.

Long before this phenomenon was quantitatively explored by radiation biologists, fractionated radiation was used by clinicians because, empirically, this seemed to be the best way of delivering a tumoricidal dose without excessive damage to normal tissues. All radiation-dose schedules must be described in terms of the total number of rads or grays (1 Gy = 100 rad) delivered, the number of grays per fraction, and the overall treatment time period. It is clear that longer treatment times and smaller-sized fractions require a greater total dose in Gy for the same biologic effect. There is no simple formula, however, to relate different fractionation schedules. A variety of schedules have been tried empirically; the "traditional" schedule is 2 Gy per day, 5 fractions per week. The optimal schedule, however, remains unresolved for the great majority of human tumors (13).

Tumor Regression

The rate of growth of a tumor depends on numerous factors including cell-cycle time, the fraction of cells that are actively proliferating (growth fraction) and the rate at which dead cells of their breakdown products are removed from the tumor (cell-loss factor) (14). These factors also effect the rate at which a tumor regresses after irradiation. Volume changes in an irradiated tumor eventually reflect the extent of tumor-cell kill but may proceed with a variable rate.

The cellular target of ionizing irradiation is believed to be DNA, and the meaningful biologic endpoint is the loss of cellular reproductive capability (clonogenicity). Although the molecular effects of radiation are very rapid, occurring within seconds, the time to cell death is quite variable. Cell death typically occurs during mitosis (14), and there may be a number of mitotic cycles before a faulty division takes place. The time to mitosis depends on cell-cycle time and growth fraction. Once the cells are dead, their breakdown products must be removed from the tumor, and this time course can vary considerably. These factors make it difficult to base clinical decisions on the observed rate of the tumor response to irradiation (15,16). The only reliable guide to determining treatment perimeters remains observations of long-term results in large numbers of patients. The rationale for avoiding treatment decisions for a given patient, based largely on the clinical response, also applies to decision making based on histopathologic response. For the reason cited above, histopathologic response to radiation may be delayed by weeks to months, especially if the tissue in question has a long cell-cycle time or small growth fraction. Conversely, the absence of microscopic evidence of intact tumor cells in the biopsy specimen does not preclude the presence of intact tumor cells in situ.

Radiation Physics

A few basic concepts in radiation physics must be understood to appreciate radiation therapy adequately. In most situations, high-energy photons (x-rays) are used in radiation treatments. These photons are produced for clinical use in two ways. In the first, electrons are accelerated in linear accelerators and directed to impinge upon metallic targets. This interaction produces x-ray photons by interaction. The photons have a range of energies, the highest corresponding to the incident electrons energy. By convention, the beams energy is referred to by this peak energy. Most linear accelerators in clinical use today range in energy from 4 to 20 million electron volts (MeV). High-energy photons have alternately been obtained from the nuclear decay of CO_{60}. This decay yields to gamma-ray photons with energies of 1.7 and 1.33 MV. Whichever photon production method is used, the beams are subsequently filtered to give a homogenous dose throughout the treatment field and collimated to give a well-defined field edge.

Photons can interact with matter in a number of ways, depending upon the energy of the photons. In the range of energies used for therapy, absorption is largely dependent on the electron density of the irradiated material (Compton effect), as opposed to diagnostic x-rays in which absorption is dependent on the cube of the atomic number (photoelectric effect) and thus provides the well-recognized contrast patterns. This allows for more homogeneous distribution and less bone absorption, unlike the older orthovoltage and kilovoltage machines. When ionizing photons interact with matter, they give up their energy to electrons. The secondary electrons then interact with surrounding tissue to produce the biologic effects of radiation. At low-photon energies (kilovoltage and orthovoltage), these electrons are omitted through 360°; thus, the skin receives a full dose. With increasing energies (megavoltage), electrons tend to be omitted in more forward directions. Accordingly, the skin receives a relatively lower dose with increasing photon energies. The skin-sparing effect is a fundamental advantage of megavoltage irradiation over kilovoltage or orthovoltage.

The probability of high-energy photon interaction with matter decreases with increasing energy. This translates into higher dose at depth (better penetration for higher-energy beams). Greater depth dose is another important advantage of megavoltage radiation. Attempts are generally made to keep the dose delivered inside the tumor to within 10% of the prescribed dose (< 10% in homogeneity). This can rarely be done with a single treatment field; consequently, two or more fields are generally utilized. The dose at any point is found by summing the contributions from each field. Today this is done almost exclusively via computer (computerized dosimetry). Customized field shaping can be performed by inserting individually cut lead-based blocks in the path of the beam. Wedge-shaped blocks and tissue-compensation blocks can also be used to improve the homogeneity of dose.

Electrons are often used to treat skin or superficial lesions. Electrons have the advantage of relatively higher skin and superficial dose, and more abrupt decrease in dose at depth, than high-energy photons. Thus far, the discussion has concerned radiation beams generated at a distance of 80 to 100 cm from the patient. By virtue of this relatively long distance, these "external" beam treatments are able to deliver greater dose at depth. This is related to the $1/R^2$ phenomenon. The number of rays passing through any region at a distance R_1 from a source is related to the number of rays at distance R_2 by the inverse of the ratio of the squares of the distance $[1/(R_2^2/R_1^2)]$. In other words, the dose declines by the square of the distance from the source. Thus, without taking into account weakening of the beam and tissue by absorption (attenuation), the beam would be weaker at a depth because of the increased distance from the beam's origin.

Although the $1/R^2$ effect is an obstacle to be overcome in external beam treatment, it can be used to advantage in brachytherapy. In brachytherapy, radioactive material is placed *on* (with plaques or intracavitary devices), or *within* (with catheters or needles) tumors. If the entire volume can be adequately covered with such devices, there is a much higher dose of radiation delivered to the tumor than to surrounding tissue, predominantly as a result of $1/R^2$ effect.

General Clinical Principles

Radiation therapy, like surgery, is in general a local regional treatment modality. As such, its curative potential for any disease is limited by the incidence of distant metastases. The importance of local regional control cannot be overemphasized, however (17). The morbidity from local regional tumor extension in a variety of sites is well known to medical personnel who treat cancer patients. Cure obviously is impossible without local regional control, and systemic therapies such as chemotherapy are least effective at sites of clinically detectable (bulk) disease (18). Finally, as systemic therapy has become more effective and patients live longer, morbidity from local regional tumor extension will increase.

As with surgery, radiation therapy has its inherent risks and complications. It is incumbent upon the radiation oncologist to know the potential risks and benefits of irradiation, to devise a treatment plan that yields the best therapeutic ratio, and to know when other modalities are more appropriate than radiotherapy. The radiation oncologist must decide how much tissue to treat, what dose to use, and what physical perimeters to use. Tumor site and extent, patterns of spread, and the patient's tolerance of treatment and possible side effects (as influenced by age and nutritional status, for example) must be considered. The impact of therapy upon psychosocial factors such as sexual function and voice quality also must be weighed.

In general, the probabilities of both tumor sterilization and treatment complication rise with dose. The risk of these events occurring for a given dose is generally considered to follow a bell-shaped curve. If the cumulative probability of these events is thus plotted against dose, the result is a sigmoid-shaped curve (Fig. 38–3). It can be seen that, in the steep portion of the curve, small increases in dose can lead to large increases in both tumor control and complications. The optimal situation occurs when the probability of tumor sterilization is high with low doses, such as with small tumors or very radiosensitive tumors, and the probability of unacceptable complication is low with high doses, such as with small irradiated volumes or volumes devoid of vital structures.

Numerous strategies have been developed in attempts to improve the therapeutic gain ratio (TGR). The most important of these is the shrinking field concept popularized in the 1950s by Fletcher and colleagues at the MD Anderson Hospital (7). Both in theory and in practice, higher doses of radiation are needed to sterilize regions of great tumor burden. Accordingly, regions of clinically detectable disease should receive a higher dose than regions of presumed microscopic or occult disease. Fletcher advocated initial fields encompassing both known disease and suspected regions of extension, followed by smaller fields (boost or "coned down"

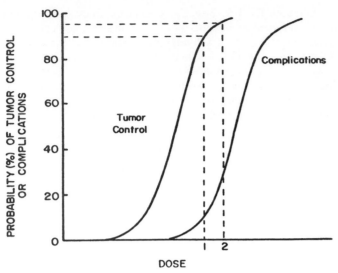

FIG. 38–3. Dose-response curves for control of a hypothetical tumor and for normal tissue damage. Treatment to dose level 1 results in a 90% probability of cure and 10% probability of complications. Because of the shape of the sigmoid response curves, if the dose is increased to level 2, the control rate increases by only 5% but the rate of complications increases more dramatically to 28%. By manipulation of factors other than total dose (time, fraction size, treatment volume), the actual separation between the two curves may also be varied. For some treatment regimens or tumor types, the complication curve lies to the left of the control curve, so that for any chosen dose the complication rate exceeds the cure rate.

fields) taken to higher doses in regions of greater tumor involvement.

Dosages will vary from case to case. In general, for solid tumors in patient treatments with curative intent, dosages for subclinical disease will range from 40 to 60 Gy (4000 to 6000 cGy) and for gross disease from 60 to 80 Gy, given in "conventional" fractionation (2 Gy per fraction, 5 fractions per week). It can theoretically be shown that if one part of the tumor receives a lesser dose than the rest, the probability of sterilization and cure is dependent on the dose to this region. Accordingly, the dosages usually prescribed to the portion of tumor that will receive the smallest dose (i.e., tumor minimum dose).

At times, in order to cover all points of tumor involvement, overlying critical structures may receive an unacceptably high dose. This dilemma can often be rectified by the use of angled and/or multiple fields. Such fields effectively lower the dose to any nontarget tissues.

ALTERED FRACTIONATION

Modification of the daily-dose fractionation is another method of improving TGR. Two such schemes are hyperfractionation (HF) and accelerated fractionation (AF). Both use multiple daily fractions instead of the single 2-Gy daily treatment. Accelerated fractionation aims to exploit the fact that tumor cells are proliferating more rapidly than normal tissues; AF uses dose fraction sizes that are only mildly reduced from those used with single daily fractionation. Consequently, the total treatment time is reduced significantly, which thus provides less time for tumor-cell repair between treatments than occurs with once-daily therapy (see Fig. 38–2) (19).

Hyperfractionation exploits the radiobiologic differences between tumors and slowly responding normal tissues that are responsible for radiation-related, long-term complications (i.e., in small blood vessels, bone, and connective tissue). The radiation survival curves of normal tissues are "curvier" (low α:β ratio) than those of tumors (high α:β ratio). Consequently, by significantly reducing the dose per fraction (1.1 to 1.2 Gy per fraction), HF reduces the overall amount of damage to normal tissues (risk of complication) relative to damage to tumor for a given total dose of irradiation. Conversely, by reducing the fraction size, the total dose can be raised above that given with once-daily therapy while holding the risk of long-term complications constant. The total time for a course of pure hyperfractionation is the same as for a course of once-daily treatment. A prospective randomized trial has confirmed the superiority of hyperfractionation to standard fractionation in patients with squamous cell carcinoma of the oropharynx (20).

HIGH LINEAR ENERGY TRANSFER RADIATION

High linear energy transfer (LET) radiation beams include neutrons, pi mesons, and a variety of other heavy particles, all of which are densely ionizing. This type of radiation alters the shape of the survival curve; the shoulder (repair) region is either reduced or absent, presumably because densely ionizing beams result in DNA damage that cannot be repaired. Because of the high density of the damage produced by this type of radiation, there is relatively little influence of oxygen on the process. This has been the area of impotence for the development of high LET radiation sources for use in clinical radiotherapy. To date, such efforts have been hampered by technical complexity and the expense of developing equipment. The most commonly studied type is neutron-beam irradiation. The most promising clinical results thus far have come in the treatment of unresectable or recurrent salivary-gland malignancies of the head and neck, where the use of neutron irradiation has resulted in better long-term local regional tumor control than conventional ionizing irradiation (21).

Multimodality Therapy

Tumors are often so extensive that attempts at cure with any single treatment modality have a very low probability of success. However, by combining modalities, each with its own toxicity, greater probability of tumor control can be achieved with lower probability of prohibitive toxicity. The added cost of such regimens is generally either more acute toxicity or additional types of non-life-threatening morbidity. For instance, attempted cure of advanced head and neck cancer may be undertaken with either radiation or surgery alone, leading to a high probability of radionecrosis or functional deficit, respectively. Alternatively, a higher probability of tumor control might be obtainable by combining the two approaches. In this case, the patient will be left with some xerostomia and radiation fibrosis and some functional impairment from resection.

SURGERY AND RADIATION THERAPY

Large tumors often necessitate unacceptably high doses of radiation or unacceptably extensive surgery to obtain reasonable chances of local regional control. In this context, resection may be used for extirpation of gross disease, with radiation to follow to irradicate microscopic extension. As a general principle, however, debulking surgery that does not remove all gross tumor is inadvisable because it does not reduce the dose of radiation required and in some instances may even increase the dose required, with consequent increase in risk of complication. Combined radiation and surgery is considered standard treatment in many situations, including head and neck cancer, breast cancer, rectal cancer, gynecologic cancer, and soft-tissue sarcoma.

Advocates exist for both preoperative and postoperative irradiation. Preoperative irradiation offers the advantage of undisturbed vascular (presumably resulting in less hypoxia in regions of microscopic extension), initial treatment of all presumed sites of disease, treatment of smaller volumes (all surgically manipulated tissue is at risk for dissemination postoperatively), and theoretically decreased risk of intraoperative tumor seeding of viable cells. The advantages of postoperative treatment include a lower risk of healing problems, avoiding inadequate resection secondary to tumor regression and unnecessary radiation of patients with very early or disseminated disease detected at the time of surgery. A randomized trial has shown no difference in overall efficacy for preoperative versus postoperative irradiation in head and neck cancer (22).

CHEMOTHERAPY AND RADIATION THERAPY

Although surgery and radiotherapy are both local treatments, the use of chemotherapy and radiation in combination may convey both systemic and local benefits. Frequently, all three modalities may be used in combination. Two general approaches to the interdigitation of chemotherapy and radiation have been used. One is sequential treatment, which allows for full doses of each modality. The hope is that the additive effects will render the patient disease free. The negative aspects to this approach are the possibility that cells that are resistant to chemotherapy might repopulate the tumor before radiation is given and that the patient will experience the full spectrum of long-term toxicities. Alternatively, simultaneous chemotherapy and radiation may be used. Here, tumor repopulation is less of an issue, and the two modalities might act synergistically within the irradiated volume. Also, because the required doses of each modality might be less, long-term toxicities could be lower. The negative aspects of concurrent therapy are increased acute toxicity and perhaps lower tolerability of chemotherapy, with a consequent reduction in the impact on occult distant disease (14).

HYPERTHERMIA AND RADIATION THERAPY

Heat is a potent cytotoxic agent, especially when combined with radiation (12). Radiation cell kill will be increased by several orders of magnitude when combined with temperatures of at least 42.5° C for about 1 hour. The combination of radiation and heat is theoretically appealing, because heat is most effective in those tumor populations in which radiation is least effective (hypoxic regions) (12). Heat is also more effective against cells in the S-phase of the cell cycle. Radiation is least effective on S-phase cells and most effective against cells undergoing mitosis. Furthermore, studies have shown that heat can potentiate radiation damage, probably through interference with repair mechanisms. Most tumors

are less able to dissipate heat than normal tissues because of abnormal tumor vasculature (absence of vasodilating arterials); this allows for the preferential heating of tumors. The actual heating of human tumors in situ, particularly those at a distance from the body surface, remains a formidable problem, however. Equipment is still very much in a developmental stage. Furthermore, the optimal thermal dose remains to be defined. This is an area of extensive research presently (12).

Radiation Complications

Radiation complications are generally divided into three temporal categories: acute, subacute, and chronic. In large part, this is a function of the cellular turnover rate of a given tissue or organ, as radiation damage is not expressed until cells attempt division. Tissues falling into the acutely reacting category include mucosa, hematopoietic lines, and germ cells. Late-reacting tissues include neural structures, muscle, bone, and endothelium. Radiation-induced skin changes vary with respect to time as a function of the turnover rates of the various skin tissues. In general, the latency period and degree of changes are dose-per-fraction and total-dose dependent. With conventionally fractionated, moderate-dose radiation, the first reaction is erythema of the skin surface, followed by flaking or peeling (dry desquamation). These changes are consequences of radiation effects on the epithelial stem cells. With higher doses to the skin, enough basal cells might be kill to cause denudation (moist desquamation). These acute reactions generally begin 10 to 20 days after initiation of therapy and spontaneously heal 10 to 20 days after completion.

With modern supervoltage radiotherapy, late skin changes are unusual unless a deliberate effort is made to treat the skin or the skin receives high doses from "tangential" beams. Skin at high risk for tumor involvement includes areas involved with tumor, surgical scars at risk for seeding, and areas of possible dermal lymphatic involvement (as in skin over the chest wall following mastectomy in patients with multiple nodal involvement or lymphatic vessel involvement). When the skin receives high radiation doses, epidermal atrophy and telangiectasias (from small blood vessel loss in the dermis), alopecia (hair follicle loss), dryness (sebaceous and sweat gland loss), and hypopigmentation (melanocyte loss) occur. Wounds heal poorly, and infections occur more readily and are harder to control secondary to poorer vasculature. These changes are usually first noticeable 6 to 12 months after treatment, and may be progressive with time.

Radiation fibrosis of the subcutaneous layer follows a similar temporal pattern. This is seen to some degree in practically all irradiated patients.

SURGERY FOLLOWING RADIATION THERAPY

Surgical procedures must be performed with caution in previously irradiated tissue (23). Tissues will be harder to manipulate secondary to subcutaneous fibrosis. Wound healing and infectious complications will be more prevalent because of depletion of the microvasculature. Not infrequently, myocutaneous or pedicle grafts are required to cover these regions adequately. In patients who have undergone surgical procedures, attempts should be made to avoid radiation to the wound for at least 6 to 10 days. During this proliferative stage of healing, the wound has a large number of macrophages and replicating fibroblasts that are quite sensitive to radiation. Loss of these elements will delay healing and, together with the loss of polynuclear leukocytes, will predispose to infection (24). However, when immediate tumor regression is required to alleviate morbid or life-threatening situations (major airway compression or spinal-cord compression), radiation therapy should be started immediately and appropriate wound care given as needed.

Specific Disease Sites

HEAD AND NECK CANCER

Radiation or surgery alone is sufficient for many small tumors without nodal involvement. As a general rule, surgery alone should not be used in large tumors (T4, and many T3s) (25), in any size tumor showing aggressive tendencies (high-grade, lymphatic and/or blood vessel involvement), or in situations in which more than one lymph node is involved with cancer or there is extracapsular extension of disease (25–27).

Heroic efforts using surgical procedures that are functionally debilitating in patients with extensive cancers are usually rewarded with tumor recurrence in addition to debilitating surgical defects (25). Such patients are almost invariably better treated primarily with radiation. Recent studies suggest that concurrent chemotherapy and/or hyperfractionation should be used (28).

BREAST CANCER

Numerous studies, both prospective and retrospective, have proven that local regional control and overall cure of breast cancer with excisional biopsy (lumpectomy) and radiation are at least as good as with modified radical or radical mastectomy (29,30). Few women with early-stage (I/II) breast cancer should be advised to undergo mastectomy because it is "better treatment," "safer," or "more likely to get rid of the cancer." Additionally, many effective ways exist to interdigitate radiation with chemotherapy (31), and this should not be used as an argument against lumpectomy and radiation. It is also worth noting that patients with multiple nodal metastases, extensive blood vessel and/or lymphatic vessel involvement, or involvement of the pectoral fascia, should generally be treated with a course of postmastectomy irradiation requiring nearly the same time commitment (6 weeks) as primary radiation therapy (32).

When good radiation technique is utilized, breast cosmesis is essentially a function of the operative procedure performed. Although negative tumor margins should be sought, the removal of large portions of the breast (including quadrantectomy) is usually unnecessary. Most radiation oncologists will boost doses to the tumor bed to a level that should be sufficient to sterilize any microscopic disease. The placement of radiopaque clips in the tumor bed will facilitate such boost treatments. Curvilinear incisions directly over the lesion generally lead to best results. Axillary lymph-node dissections should be performed through a separate incision (31).

The entire breast is included in the first course of radiation in order to treat any occult distinct foci of disease. The dose to the breast is usually 45 to 50 Gy, often with a boost dose to the tumor bed itself to bring that region's dose to a total of 60 to 64 Gy (31). Lymph-node-bearing regions are variably treated, depending on the clinical situation. After axillary node dissection, the supraclavicular fossa should be irradiated if the nodes are positive. It is usually unnecessary to irradiate the axilla itself after an axillary dissection (33).

SKIN CANCERS

Nonmelanoma skin cancers can usually be effectively treated with a number of methods including simple excision or cryosurgery. The use of the Mohs technique also has a strong theoretical and clinical basis. Radiation therapy is another very effective treatment modality for basal cell and squamous cell carcinomas of the skin. It should be strongly considered in areas where resection would entail extensive reconstruction (e.g., the nose, periorbital regions, and ears). Similar arguments pertain to squamous cell carcinomas of the lip when lesions are over 1.5 to 2.0 cm or involve a commissure. Should lesions involve cartilage, however, surgery is usually the preferred treatment, because radionecrosis of the cartilage is a distinct possibility. Using appropriately fractionated treatment, long-term cosmesis is excellent, and local control is over 90% (34,35).

References

1. Boring CC, Squires TS, Tong T. Cancer statistics. *Cancer* 1992; 42:19.
2. *Radiation oncology in integrated cancer management.* Report of the Inter-Society Council for Radiation Oncology, 1986.
3. Glasser O. *Wilhelm Conrad Roentgen and the early history of the Roentgen ray.* London: John Bale, 1933.
4. Coutard H. Principles of x-ray therapy of malignant disease. *Lancet* 1934; 2:1.
5. Stewart FA. Modification of normal tissue response to radiotherapy and chemotherapy. *Int J Radiat Oncol Biol Phys* 1989; 16:1195.
6. Cox JD. *Moss' radiation oncology: rationale, technique, results.* 7th ed. St. Louis: CV Mosby, ;13.
7. Fletcher GH. The evolution of the basic concepts underlying the practice of radiotherapy from 1949–1977. *Radiology* 1978; 127:3.
8. Andrews JR. *The radiobiology of human cancer radiotherapy.* 2nd ed. Baltimore: University Park Press, 1978.
9. Brizel DM, Rosner GL, Harrelson J, et al. Pretreatment oxygenation profiles of human soft-tissue sarcomas. *Int J Radiat Oncol Biol Phys* 1994; 30:635–642.
10. Gatenby RA, Kessler HB, Rosenblum JS, et al. Oxygen distribution in squamous cell carcinoma metastases and its relationship to outcome of radiation therapy. *Int J Radiat Oncol Biol Phys* 1988; 14:831–838.
11. Hockel M, Knoop C, Schlenger K, et al. Intratumoral PO_2 predicts survival in advanced cancer of the uterine cervix. *Radiotherapy and Oncology* 1993; 26:45–50.
12. Oleson JR, Calderwood SK, Coughlin CT, et al. Biological and clinical aspects of hyperthermia in cancer therapy. *Am J Clin Oncol* 1988; 11:368.
13. Peschel RE, Fischer JJ. Optimization of the time dose relationship. *Semin Oncol* 1981; 8:38.
14. Suit HD. Radiation biology: the conceptual and practical impact on radiation therapy. *Radiat Res* 1983; 94:10.
15. Suit HD, Walker AM. Assessment of the response of tumors to radiation: clinical and experimental studies. *Br J Cancer* 1980; 41 (suppl 4):1.
16. Dische S, Bennett MH, Saunders MI, et al. Tumor regression as a guide to prognosis: a clinical study. *Br J Radiol* 1980; 53:454.
17. Suit HD, Westgate SJ. Impact of local control on survival. *Int J Radiat Oncol Biol Phys* 1986;12:453.
18. DeVita VT Jr. Principles of chemotherapy. In: DeVita VT Jr, Hellman S, Rosenberg SA, eds. *Principles and practice of oncology.* 4th ed. Philadelphia: JB Lippincott, 1993.
19. Withers HR, Taylor LMJ, Maciejewski B. The hazard of accelerated tumor clonogen repopulation during radiotherapy. *Acta Oncol* 1988; 27:131.

20. Horiot JC, LeFur R, N'Guyen T, et al. Hyperfractionated compared with conventional radiotherapy in oropharyngeal carcinoma: an EORTC randomized trial. *Eur J Cancer* 1990; 26:779–780.
21. Griffin TW, Pajak TF, Laramore GE, et al. Neutron vs. photon irradiation of inoperable salivary gland tumors: results of an RTOG-MRC cooperative study. *Int J Radiat Oncol Biol Phys* 1988; 15:1085–1090.
22. Kramer S, Gelber RD, Snow JB, et al. Combined radiation therapy and surgery in the management of advanced head and neck cancer: final report of study 73-03 of the radiation therapy oncology group. *Head and Neck Surgery* 1987; 19–27.
23. Robinson DW. The hazards of surgery in irradiated tissue. *Ann Plastic Surg* 1983; 11:74.
24. Shamberger R. Effect of chemotherapy and radiotherapy on wound healing: experimental studies. *Recent Results Cancer Res* 1985; 98:17.
25. Million RM, Cassisi NJ. General principles for treatment of cancers in the head and neck: combining surgery and radiation therapy. In: Million RM, Cassisi NJ, *Management of head and neck cancer: a multidisciplinary approach.* 2nd ed. Philadelphia: JB Lippincott, 1994. 61.
26. Soo K-C, Carter R, Berr L, et al. Prognostic implications of perineural spread in squamous carcinomas of the head and neck. *Laryngoscope* 1986; 96:1145.
27. Carter R, Bliss J, Soo K-C, et al. Radical neck dissections for squamous cell carcinomas: pathological findings and their clinical implications with particular reference to transcapsular spread. *Int J Radiat Oncol Biol Phys* 1987; 13:825.
28. Brizel DB, Leopold KA, Fisher SR, et al. A phase I/II trial of twice daily irradiation and concurrent chemotherapy for locally advanced squamous cell carcinoma of the head and neck. *Int J Radiat Oncol Biol Phys* 1993; 28:213–220.
29. Fisher B, Redmond C, Poisson R, et al. Eight-year results of a randomized clinical trial comparing total mastectomy and lumpectomy with or without irradiation in the treatment of breast cancer. *N Engl J Med* 1989; 320:822.
30. Kurtz J, Amalric R, Brandone H, et al. Local recurrence after breast-conserving surgery and radiotherapy: frequency, time course, and prognosis. *Cancer* 1989; 63:1912.
31. Recht A, Connolly JL, Schnitt SJ, et al. Conservative surgery and radiation therapy for early breast cancer: results, controversies and unsolved problems. *Semin Oncol* 1986; 13:434.
32. Edland RW. Presidential address: does adjuvant radiotherapy have a role in postmastectomy management of patients with operable breast cancer—revisited. *Int J Radiat Oncol Biol Phys* 1988; 15:519.
33. Donegan WL, Stine SB, Samter TG. Implications of extracapsular nodal metastases for treatment and prognosis of breast cancer. *Cancer* 1993; 72:778–782.
34. Million RM, Cassisi NJ, Mancuso AA. Oral cavity. In: Million RM, Cassisi NJ, *Management of head and neck cancer: a multidisciplinary approach.* 2nd ed. Philadelphia: JB Lippincott, 1994: 321.
35. Brady LW, Binnick SA, Fitzpatrick PJ. Skin cancer. In: Perez CA, Brady LW, eds. *Principles and practice of radiation oncology.* Philadelphia: JB Lippincott, 1992.

39

Solid and Cystic Tumors of the Jaw

Nicholas G. Georgiade, D.D.S., M.D., F.A.C.S., Thomas A. McGraw, D.M.D., and Gregory S. Georgiade, M.D., F.A.C.S.

This chapter presents a broad overview of tumors in the mandible and maxilla. These tumors include cystic, inflammatory, developmental, and posttraumatic masses that should be considered in any differential diagnosis. Radiologic evaluation encompasses tumor tissues that are radiopaque, radiolucent, or combinations of varying densities. The final diagnosis or a presenting mass usually requires histologic interpretation. Characteristically, benign cysts and tumors expand the bone, but they do not invade the cortex (1–4).

Cysts

Cysts of the mandible and maxilla of odontogenic origin arise from an alteration of the enamel organ and include those discussed below. Odontogenic cysts can therefore arise from an array of epithelial and mesenchymal cysts during embryonic tooth development (5,6).

PERIAPICAL (RADICULAR) CYSTS

The periapical cyst is the most common cyst of the jawbones. It may arise at any age and affect any tooth (Fig. 39–1). The cyst usually occurs at the apex of a nonvital tooth as a sequela of chronic inflammation that stimulates the rests of Malassez to proliferate. This cyst is associated with degeneration of the pulp and may result in low-grade apical infection, appearing as a well-circumscribed periapical radiolucency. Because this process is thought to initiate the growth of the epithelial component, radicular cysts may be classified as inflammatory. These cysts may also be referred to as apical, periodontal, radiculodental, and/or root cysts. Like other odontogenic cysts, this variant may have cholesterol crystals in the liquid aspirant. Management of small periapical cysts is usually conservative, with nonsurgical root-canal therapy. Radicular cysts with radiolucencies over 2 cm in diameter may indicate the need for apical curettage and more extensive root resection. In cases in which restoration of dentition is not facilitated, extraction of the offending tooth may be the alternative of choice.

DENTIGEROUS CYSTS

The dentigerous cyst is the second most frequently occurring odontogenic cyst and is seen surrounding the crown of an unerupted tooth (Fig. 39–2). It is thought to arise as a result of reduction in the enamel-forming epithelium after the crown is completely formed. Typically, the cyst will have an epithelial lining and may vary from 2 cm in diameter to extensive expansion of the jaw. Dentigerous cysts are not usually painful in the absence of infection and rarely will expand so rapidly that discomfort results from pressure on a sensory nerve. The posterior area of the mandible is the most common site of dentigerous cysts, and the 3rd molar is the tooth most frequently involved. Signs and symptoms include delayed eruption of a tooth, swelling, and asymmetry. Smaller cysts may be managed successfully with enucleation and primary closure. When the dentigerous cyst is large, treatment alternatives (e.g., decompression, marsupialization) may be used to advantage, particularly in tooth-bearing areas of children when the tooth is not impacted and is ready to erupt once it is relieved of the cyst. These pericoronal lesions may recur as a cyst or as an ameloblastoma.

PRIMORDIAL (FOLLICULAR) CYSTS

A primordial cyst is a relatively rare type of odontogenic cyst that develops before calcified enamel or dentine is formed (Fig. 39–3). It is found in place of a tooth and is characterized by the absence of any dentition within the cyst. Such cysts usually occur as an abnormal formation of the enamel organ and present as a well-circumscribed, radiolucent area with a multilocular appearance. On microscopic examination, about one-half have proven to be filled with keratin, resulting in a radiolucent, hazy appearance. Primordial cysts are found most frequently between the ages of 10 and 30 years, and the mandibular molar region represents the most common site of development. Management is similar to that of other odontogenic cysts, although the high rate or recurrence of follicular cysts requires more vigorous curettement and postsurgical follow-up with radiographs to ensure resolution.

Nonodontogenic Developmental Cysts

Cysts of nonodontogenic origin of the mandible and maxilla are thought to derived from epithelium entrapped in the lines of fusion of the body process that form the jaws and face. These cysts may be lined with stratified squamous epithelium, respiratory epithelium, or a combination of the two.

NASOPALATINE (INCISIVE CANAL) CYSTS

The median cyst is formed as a result of "trapping" tissue during fusion of the palatine process with the premaxilla and is an uncommon bony cyst (Fig. 39–4). The type of epithelium found in the cyst will vary depending on its location.

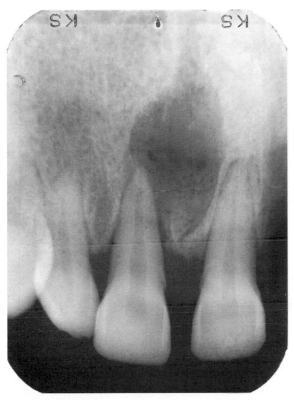

FIG. 39–1. Radicular cyst at the apex of the central incisor tooth. Note the thickened periodontal membrane and irregular walls of this low-grade inflammatory cyst.

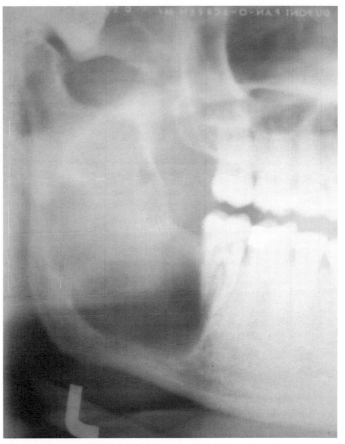

FIG. 39–3. Follicular (primordial) cyst is characterized by absence of embedded dentition; it is otherwise similar to a dentigerous cyst on the radiograph.

FIG. 39–2. Dentigerous cyst.

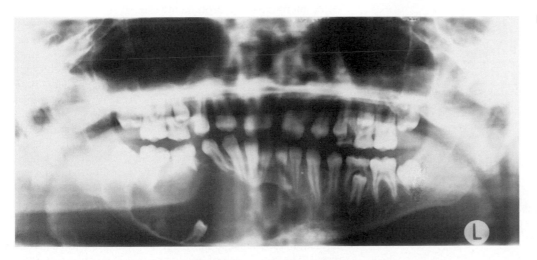

Cysts in the incisive canal area contain stratified squamous epithelium, whereas the posteriorly located cysts have cuboidal or respiratory epithelium. With increasing cyst size, patients may report a painless bulging in the roof of the mouth, and on inspection the mucosa may appear more glossy than usual. Unilocular radiolucency is seen in the midline of the palate. After surgical excision (with a mucoperiosteal flap raised from the anterior to ensure good access and permit total removal, clinical and radiographic follow-up is essential (7).

GLOBULOMAXILLARY CYSTS

The globulomaxillary cyst is a fissural cyst arising at the junction of the globular portion of the medial nasal process and the maxillary process, usually between the maxillary lateral incisor and the canine tooth, with no loss of pulp vi-

FIG. 39–4. Nasopalatine cyst. An incisive canal lesion is shown in the characteristic palatal midline area. Typically, these cysts do not increase remarkably; note the well-circumscribed cortical prominence of the cyst wall.

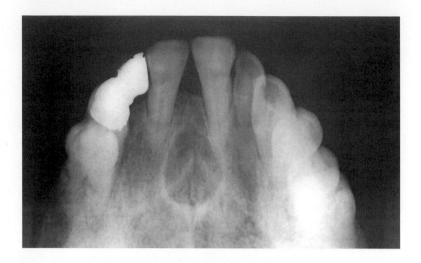

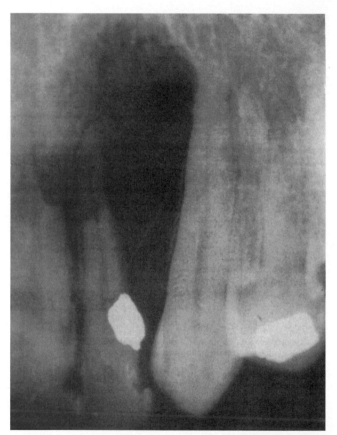

FIG. 39–5. A globulomaxillary cyst in its typical location between the lateral and canine tooth. Note the marked divergence of the root apices.

tality (Fig. 39–5). On the radiograph, it appears as a well-defined radiolucency between the roots and is shaped like an inverted tear. The amber-colored fluid on aspiration is a useful sign in differential diagnosis. It is probable that such cysts form as a result of entrapment of epithelial remnants in the region of the incisive suture; however, the origin of the epithelial nests is still a matter of dispute. Globulomax-

illary cysts are often asymptomatic until they become enlarged or expand, at which time complaints of swelling and pain may be reported. The latter are usually indicative of secondary infection. Surgical excision is the treatment modality, and care must be taken not to devitalize the adjacent teeth during the procedure. Radiographic follow-up is important to assure that the defect has resolved and there is no recurrence.

Nonodontogenic and Nondevelopmental Cysts

ANEURYSMAL BONE CYSTS

An aneurysmal bone cyst is characterized by numerous capillaries intermixed with prominent vascular spaces and the presence of multinucleated giant cells. It is sometimes referred to as a false cyst because it has no epithelial lining. In most instances, it expands the cortical plates but does not destroy them. Radiographs occasionally will reveal an irregular area of destruction of the cortical plate of the mandible and "scalloping." The histologic picture of the tissue reveals a cellular, fibrous pattern. Cysts of this variety are slow growing and affect the mandible considerably more often than the maxilla. These entities usually develop in young people under the age of 20 years. Aneurysmal bone cysts may be somewhat tender, and teeth may be displaced or missing (Fig. 39–6). On inspection, the cyst is reddish-brown in color, owing to its rich blood supply, and resembles a sponge. Management consists of aspiration to avoid the unexpected and dangerous entrance into a hemangioma or arteriovenous shunt. Treatment is then by surgical curettement; hemorrhage is moderate and easily arrested. The recurrence of an aneurysmal bone cyst is rare (8).

TRAUMATIC BONE CYSTS

In cases of traumatic bone cyst, the "cystic" area in the mandible results from a traumatic episode and is devoid of an epithelial lining, although it usually will have a thin area of connective tissue (Fig. 39–7). It is often found unexpectedly on routine radiographs and appears round to oval, with a scalloped superior margin produced by its molding around the roots of mandibular premolars or molars. As with cemen-

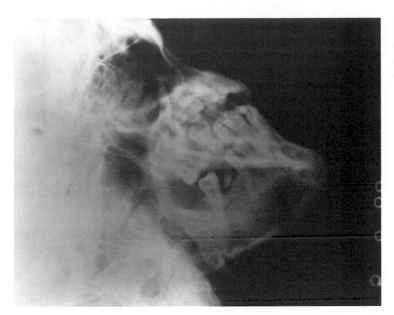

FIG. 39–6. An aneurysmal bone cyst (nonepithelial) simulates a developmental cyst but displays a sparse connective tissue lining (rather than an epithelial one). It is seen as a solid area of radiolucency with an irregular outline of the cyst wall.

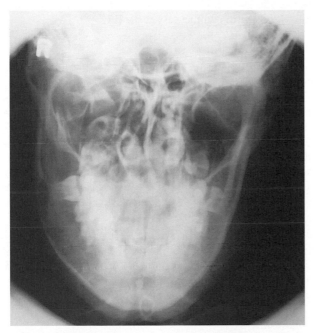

FIG. 39–7. A traumatic bone cyst is characterized by the absence of epithelial tissue, a scalloped superior margin molding around the roots of the premolars and molars, and regional expansion of the jaw (right).

toma, the tooth pulp is usually vital. The maxilla is seldom involved, and traumatic bone cyst is uncommon in those over 25 years of age. Infrequently, the jaw will reveal regional expansion, and typically there is no aspirant. Management includes surgical exploration to ensure a correct diagnosis (radiographic imaging and the usual clinical features are not sufficient). Subsequent enucleation and curettage, which produce hemorrhage into the cavity, will typically provide regression and obliteration by bone. During the healing period, close radiographic observation is recommended.

Tumors of Odontogenic Epithelium

AMELOBLASTOMA

The ameloblastoma originates from ectodermal epithelium with differentiation into ameloblasts, the enamel-forming cells. It may develop from any of the epithelial elements (e.g., dentigerous cysts, enamel organ, periodontal membranes). The picture will vary on the radiograph; it may closely resemble a dentigerous cyst, or it may represent a multilocular cyst with a bubblelike or honeycomb appearance. The predominant site is the posterior mandible. Destruction of the cortex and root apices is a usual finding in larger cystic masses. Ameloblastomas have their onset in adulthood, usually between the ages of 20 and 50 years.

Because of the propensity of ameloblastomas to recur, radical surgical management is an option, to be followed by regular reexamination. However, treatment modalities may range from conservative incision to wide block resection and bone graft. The latter approach has been most effective in precluding recurrence.

Microscopically, a true ameloblastoma may be one of several histologic types. The acanthomatous histologic type is more aggressive, and metastases have been seen in our series of patient with this cytological pattern (Fig. 39–8). The acanthomatous histologic picture is characteristic of squamous metaplasia with islands of keratinizing squamous epithelium. The most common histologic finding is the follicular ameloblastoma, which as the typical tall, columnar, deepstaining cells (the ameloblasts) that resemble stellate reticulum of the enamel organ (Fig. 39–9). The flexiform type of ameloblastoma will have irregular strands of epithelial cells interspaced with ameloblastoma cells.

The ameloblastic fibroma may mimic the ameloblastoma, and care must be taken to differentiate this asymptomatic, slowly expanding benign tumor. Histologically, it is characterized by proliferation of epithelial cells and mesenchymal elements with cords and islands of epithelial cells. This is a tumor of the young and it responds well to conservative curettage (9,10).

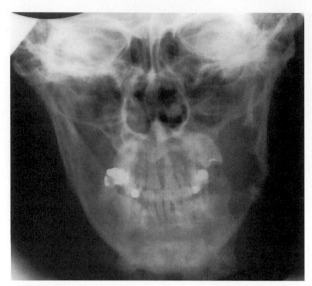

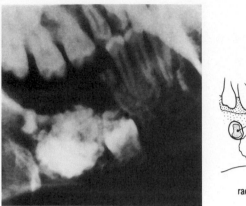

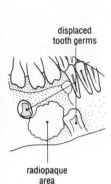

FIG. 39–10. Complex odontoma composed of aberrant dental tissue. Note the irregular, varying opaque mass.

FIG. 39–8. Mixed acanthoma and follicular ameloblastoma. Note irregular resorption of the mandible with expansion and destruction of the lingual and buccal cortical plates.

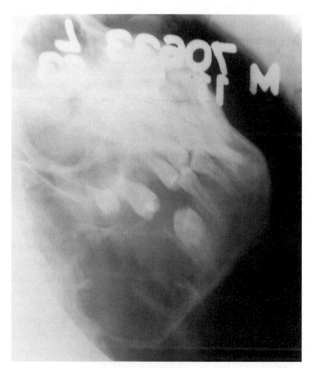

FIG. 39–9. Cystic ameloblastoma (follicular) revealed as a large multilocular cystic area of the mandible.

Tumors of Odontogenic Epithelium and Mesenchyme

COMPLEX, COMPOUND, AND MIX ODONTOMAS

Complex Odontoma

A complex odontoma is composed of aberrant tissue of all the dental elements. On the radiograph, there is an irregular opaque mass, usually in close proximity to a mandibular molar or pre-

molar tooth. The calcified dental tissues have no morphological similarity even to rudimentary teeth (Fig. 39–10).

Compound Odontoma

A compound odontoma develops independently of a tooth follicle but contains normal enamel, dentine, and cementum relationships (i.e., normal composition of a toothlike structure). It is observed more frequently than the complex odontoma. As a congregation of misshapen small teeth, the compound odontoma is easily recognized on radiographs as a radiopaque, irregular formation with varying numbers of small conical teeth present. The maxilla is the most common site of this odontoma (although it may occur in the mandible), with a predilection for the incisor-canine region.

Mixed Odontoma

Some tumors are a combination of both types discussed above. The mixed odontoma is constituted of calcified masses of dental tissue in random arrangement as well as multiple toothlike structures.

Cementoma

The cementoma has its origin from the periodontal ligament of an erupted tooth. It undergoes a transformation from an initial appearance of replacing the medullary bone to that of a fibrous matrix resembling an ossifying fibroma. This tumor occurs as a continuation of the periodontal membrane, usually of a mandibular premolar or molar tooth. The area is gradually replaced with scattered spicules of bone, and in the mature phase the entire original area of radiolucency will become calcified and appear as a well-defined, radiopaque lesion with fibrous tissue at the periphery (Fig. 39–11). The transformation requires at least 6 years. Over the course of this process, the involved tooth (or teeth) remains vital and no resorption of tooth apices occurs, as opposed to the tooth with a radicular cyst or granuloma. The surgeon performs a biopsy to establish the diagnosis, then follows with excision and curettement. Benign fibroosseous lesions originating in a periodontal ligament tend not to recur.

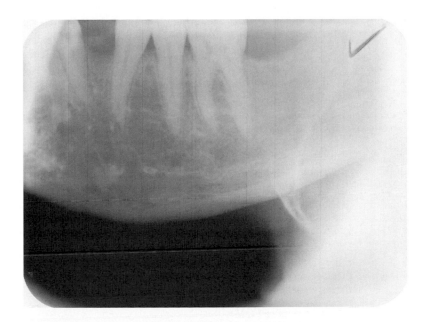

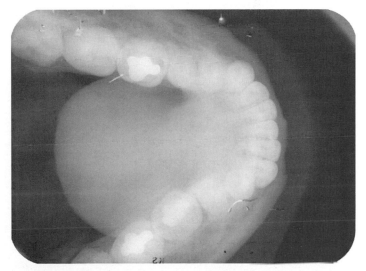

FIG. 39–11. Cementoma presents with a characteristic area of calcification shown surrounded by an irregular area of radiolucency.

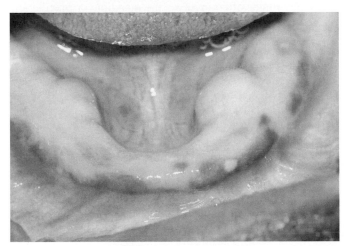

FIG. 39–12. Torus mandibularis.

FIG. 39–13. Osteomas are characterized by the presence of very dense bone with extensive radiopaque appearance.

Tumors of Nonodontogenic Origin

Nonodontogenic tumors of the mandible and maxilla encompass a large variety of benign and malignant lesions. This section presents those tumors most likely to be seen; there is no attempt to cover those only infrequently seen.

BONY EXOSTOSES (TORI)

The most common of the benign tumors are the bony exostoses usually found in the palate (torus palatinus), in the mandible (torus mandibularis) (Fig. 39–12), or on the buccal surfaces of either mandibular or maxillary dentition. They are thought to be hereditary in origin. Bony exostoses are slow-growing, painless, bony protrusions and cause mechanical and oral problems because of their progressive enlargement. Treatment is by surgical removal.

OSTEOMAS

These bony tumors are found in the mandible, the maxilla, or other facial bones. They are derived from osteoblastic activ-

ity and may be single or multiple. On the radiograph, they characteristically appear as irregular, very radiopaque masses (Fig. 39–13). Multiple osteomas, but no pigmented macules, occur in Gardner syndrome, which is a familial condition. This syndrome is manifested by multiple osteomas and by the presence of multiple polyps in the colon, epidermoid cysts, and desmoid tumors (1,2).

GIANT CELL REPARATIVE GRANULOMA

Clinically, the giant-cell reparative granuloma is characterized by a slowly expanding mass, with the most usual site of involvement in the mandible anterior to the 2nd molar teeth. It usually occurs in children or teenagers and is frequently noticed when there is displacement of dentition. Radiographs reveal an irregular, osteolytic area with migration of teeth (Fig. 39–14). There may also be an area that can be multi-locular in character. The differential diagnosis may be ob-

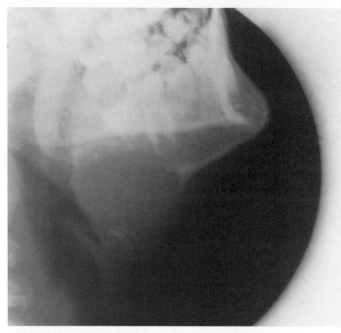

FIG. 39–14. Giant cell tumor. Irregular expanding translucent area at the angle of mandible in a 9-year-old child; haziness is typical of this semisolid tumor mass.

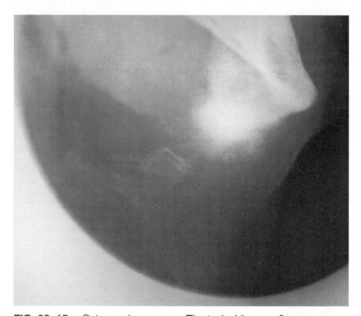

FIG. 39–15. Osteogenic sarcoma. The typical "sun ray" appearance can be seen in rapidly progressive tumor at the right angle of the mandible.

scured because of the similarity in appearance between this lesion and a benign cyst or ameloblastoma. Treatment is conservative, and curettage of the involved area is usually sufficient to yield a favorable response.

HEMANGIOMA

An infrequent occurrence in the mandible and even less frequent in the maxilla, the hemangioma may be of congenital or traumatic origin. It is composed of variously sized thin-walled vessels scattered throughout the bony trabeculae. Clinical find-

ings are of a firm, painless mass increasing in size. On the radiograph, a honeycomb, multiple cystic area is seen. The first clinical sign may be loosening of dentition or gingival bleeding. Treatment of a hemangioma may be by surgery, sclerosing solutions, or both. Angiograms are useful to determine the size before treatment, because what is observed radiographically may only be a minor portion of the lesion (11).

OSTEOGENIC SARCOMA

Osteogenic sarcoma is a highly malignant mass of the bone originating from connective tissue, forming osteoid and bone. It occurs in younger people (10 to 40 years, peaking at about age 27), and appears in the mandible more often than in the maxilla. The radiologic appearance will vary from an irregular, poorly defined lytic lesion to one with a preponderance of bony formation with characteristic bony spicules giving a "sun ray" appearance (Figs. 39–15, 39–16, 39–17). The prognosis is better in the mandible. Resection and radiation therapy is the treatment of choice.

MULTIPLE MYELOMA

This bony tumor often involves the mandible or maxilla and arises from plasmalike cells in the marrow (Fig. 39–18). The presence of multiple bone lesions is noted in older individuals. An early myeloma may appear as multiple osteolytic, radiolucent areas on the radiograph. In the latest stages, larger and more widespread areas of bony destruction are observed. Diagnosis is made based on the presence of hyperglobulinemia with a reversal of the serum albumin–globulin ratio and the presence of Bence Jones protein in the urine. Treatment includes alkylating agents, systemic steroids, and local irradiation for painful lesions (12).

METASTATIC TUMORS

Metastatic tumors involving the mandible and maxilla are more commonly from squamous cell carcinoma of the sur-

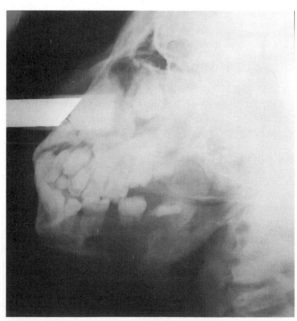

FIG. 39–16. Ewing sarcoma. Extensive irregular destruction of the mandible with apical tooth resorption and cortical bone loss in a 12-year-old patient.

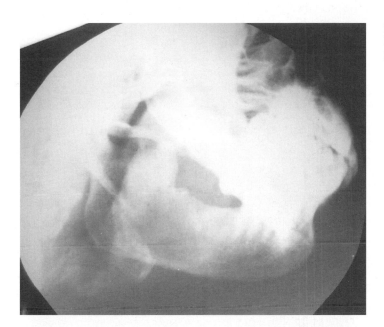

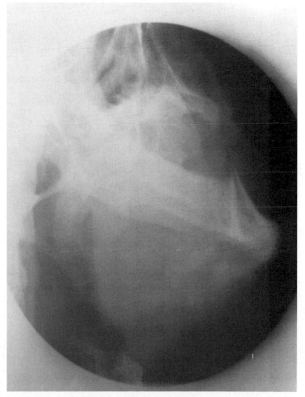

FIG. 39–17. Angiosarcoma. The scattered granular radiolucent lesion affects large areas of the mandible; areas of irregularly dispersed calcification are visualized.

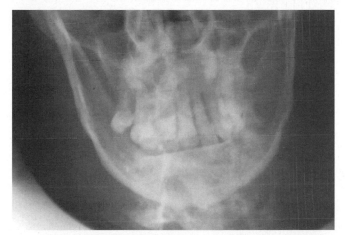

FIG. 39–18. Myeloma. Large radiolucent area at the angle and ramus of the mandible is at the typical site; multiple radiolucent ("punched out") areas are not uncommon.

rounding oral tissue (e.g., the lip, tongue, buccal, and alveolar areas). The mandible is the most common site of metastasis, and older people tend to be affected most often. However, some metastatic tumors of the jaw have a high incident in children. Primary tumors of the breast, uterus, lung, and thyroid will metastasize to the mandible. Radiographic evaluation reveals a singular osteolytic lesion centrally located in the mandible (Fig. 39–19). The varying areas of bone destruction may resemble osteomyelitis. In many instances, the differential diagnosis can only be made by tissue diagnosis (13). (Fig. 39–20).

FIBROUS DYSPLASIA

Fibrous dysplasia is found in the membranous facial bones of younger individuals and usually becomes less active with maturity. In this group, the proportion of fibrous tissue to osseous metaplasia is greater. The characteristic clinical picture is one of an increasing firm mass, presenting in either the maxilla or mandible. The area of fibrous dysplasia can man-

FIG. 39–19. Metastatic cancer. Moderately radiopaque, large diffuse mass in the mandible of a 70-year-old male with metastases from the prostate.

ifest as a single fibroosseous mass, or it may have multiple areas of involvement, most commonly occurring in the maxilla (Fig. 39–21).

The radiographic appearance will vary, depending on the amount of fibrous tissue in relation to osseous tissue. The radiograph may be one of a cystic-like appearance. However, magnification will usually reveal a pattern of diffuse areas of calcification (Fig. 39–22). A preponderance of osseous tissue

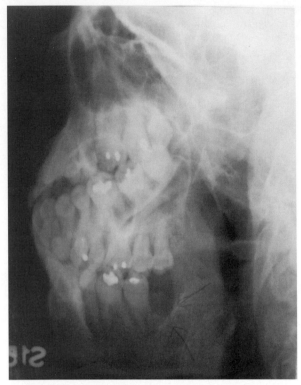

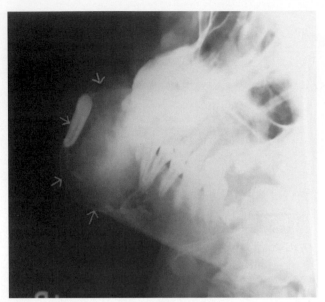

FIG. 39–22. Ossifying fibroma. A larger osseous lesion with fibrous elements expands the anterior mandible; marked displacement of the canine tooth with irregular erosion of the inferior cortical plate can be seen.

FIG. 39–20. Metastatic carcinoma. The irregular area of cortical loss in the retromolar area of the mandible represents metastasis of a uterine carcinoma in a 42-year-old female.

FIG. 39–21. Ossifying fibroma. A large radiopaque mass involving the right maxilla, orbital floor, and zygoma can be seen; the "ground glass" appearance is characteristic of mixed fibrous and osseous elements seen with fibrous dysplasia.

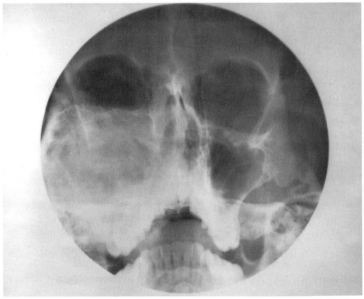

will be seen in more mature tumors, often being referred to as ossifying fibromas at this stage. Larger bony tumors should be evaluated with a computed tomography (CT) scan because of possible involvement of the orbital areas and base of the skull. Conservative surgical curettement via an intraoral approach will usually be sufficient in managing the tumor. There may be surges in growth during hormonal changes that require close clinical and radiographic observation. However, if growth continues, it is not uncommon to re-

peat this procedure a few years later. Radiation therapy is not generally recommended.

PAGET DISEASE (OSTEITIS DEFORMANS)

Paget's disease resembles an ossifying fibroma on radiographic and histologic evaluation. However, it occurs in the older age group and appears in multiple areas of the mandible and maxilla. The maxilla is the predominant jaw of involvement. In contrast, fibrous dysplasia occurs as a single

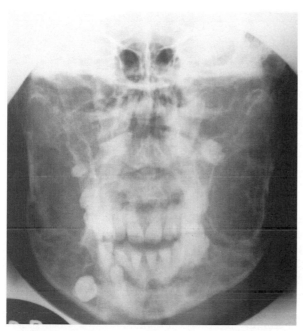

FIG. 39–23. Familial fibrous dysplasia (cherubism). Extensive multi-loculated, slightly radiopaque cystic expansile areas throughout the mandible and other facial bones; disrupted dentition can be seen surrounding these areas in a 14-year-old with painless masses that have been increasing gradually over a 10-year period. Notice the thinning of the cortex with irregular fine septa.

lesion and is seen more frequently in younger individuals. Paget's disease will also appear in other areas of the skull and skeleton. An elevated serum phosphatase level is another distinguishing feature.

FAMILIAL FIBROUS DYSPLASIA (CHERUBISM)

Familial fibrous dysplasia is characterized by multiple areas of fibrous dysplasia in the maxilla and mandible, occurring as early as 1 year of age (Fig. 39–23). As a variant of fibrous dysplasia, this is an inherited genetic disorder. The usual period of rapid growth precedes puberty. Radiographic appearance reveals multiple cystic areas in all regions of the mandible and maxilla with expansion of the bones. Treatment is conservative via an intraoral approach with multiple curettement procedures spaced as indicated over a number of years (1,14,15).

Bibliography

1. Lichtenstein L. *Bone tumors.* 5th ed. St. Louis: CV Mosby, 1977.
2. Shafer WG, Hine MK, Levy BM. *A textbook of oral pathology.* 4th ed. Philadelphia: WB Saunders, 1983.
3. Wood NK, Goaz PW. *Differential diagnosis of oral lesions.* 2nd ed. St. Louis: CV Mosby, 1980.
4. Gorlin RJ, Chaudhry AP, Pindborg JJ: Odontogenic tumors: classification, histopathology and clinical behavior in man and domesticated animals. *Cancer* 1961; 14:73.
5. Girod SC, Gerlach KL, et al. Cysts associated with long-standing impacted third molars. *J Oral Maxillofac Surg* 1993; 22:110–112.
6. Kreidler JR, Raubenheimer EJ, et al. A retrospective analysis of 367 cystic lesions of the jaw: the ulm experience. *J Craniomaxillofac Surg* 1993; 21:339–341.
7. Swanson KS, Kaugars GE, et al. Nasopalatine duct cyst: an analysis of 334 cases. *J Oral Maxillofac Surg* 1991; 49:268–271.
8. Montamedi MHK, Yazdi E. Aneurysmal bone cyst of the jaw: analysis of 11 cases. *J Oral Maxillofac Surg* 1994; 52:471–475.
9. Olaitan AA, Adeola DS, et al. Ameloblastoma: clinical features and management of 315 cases from Kaduna, Nigeria. *J Craniomaxillofac Surg* 1993; 21351–355.
10. Williams TP. Management of ameloblastoma: a changing perspective. *J Oral Maxillofac Surg* 1993; 51:1064–1070.
11. Jackson IT, Carreno R, et al. Hemangiomas, vascular malformations, and lymphovenous malformations: classification and methods of treatment. *Plast Reconstr Surg* 1993; 91:1216 1230.
12. Furutani M, Ohnishi M, et al. Mandibular involvement in patients with multiple myeloma. *J Oral Maxillofac Surg* 1994; 52:23–25.
13. Pogrel MA. Malignant tumors of the maxillofacial region. Oral and Maxillofac Surg Clin of North America 1993;
14. Lichtenstein L, Jaffe H. Fibrous dysplasia of bone. *Arch Pathol* 1942; 33:777.
15. Geschichter CF, Copeland MM. *Tumors of bone.* Philadelphia: Lippincott, 1949.

40

Craniofacial Tumors

Ian T. Jackson, M.D., D.Sc (Hon), F.R.C.S., F.A.C.S, F.R.A.C.S. (Hon)

It is important to state at the outset that craniofacial tumors are tumors of the base of the skull. In the past, because of difficulties in exposure, they have frequently been excised piecemeal or incompletely, if at all. Recurrences are frequent. Total resection is associated with significant complications, especially extradural abscesses and meningitis (1,2). Application of techniques adapted from the correction of congenital craniofacial anomalies has given us excellent ways of access and have allowed more en bloc resections with greatly decreased morbidity. The use of vascularized tissue either as a local flap or free-tissue transfer has greatly reduced the significant complications previously associated with this type of surgery. It is hoped that the cure rate will also be improved with this more aggressive approach.

These tumors may be untreated at the time of referral, but frequently there have been previous attempts at therapy—surgical, radiotherapeutic, or chemotherapeutic. The pathology varies from nonmalignant to malignant; the latter are carcinoma and frequently, in younger patients, sarcoma (Table 40–1). In the vast majority of cases, excisional surgery is the therapeutic modality of choice, followed by radiotherapy and/or chemotherapy as indicated. Only in rhabdomyosarcoma of the orbit in children is this regime not used. In these cases, the surgeon performs a biopsy on the lesion to confirm the diagnosis, and the definitive treatment is with radiotherapy and chemotherapy. The consensus is that this therapeutic regimen gives cure rates superior to those of surgical resection (3–6).

Anatomic Division of the Skull Base

Until recently there was no attempt to introduce order into skull base tumors. Currently it is useful surgically to divide the cranial base into segments and apportion the tumors to these segments (Table 40–2) (7,8).

The basic division is into an anterior and a posterior area; the former is the anterior cranial fossa, and the latter is a composite of the middle and posterior cranial fossae. The posterior area can be further subdivided into anterior, central, and posterior segments. The anterior surface segment lies between the orbit and the anterior surface of the petrous bone; the central segment is the petrous bone itself; and the posterior segment is bounded by the posterior face of the petrous bone anteriorly and the midline posteriorly.

These areas contain foramina, which are important because they allow escape of intracranial tumors and entry of extracranial tumors into the cranial cavity (Table 40–3). Knowledge of the contents and position of these foramina is mandatory in skull base surgery. It should also be appreciated that the intracranial end of the foreamen may lie in a different position from the extracranial end. This is important particularly in the resection of tumors involving the petrous bone, through which the tortuous carotid canal courses.

ANTERIOR AREA (ANTERIOR CRANIAL FOSSA)

Any tumors involving the frontal bone, frontal or ethmoid sinuses, orbit or its contents, or nasopharynx can directly in-

Table 40–1.
Tumors Involving Anterior Cranial Fossa

Malignant
  Squamous carcinoma
  Basal cell carcinoma
  Melanoma
  Adenocystic carcinoma
  Chondrosarcoma
  Osteogenic sarcoma
  Neuroblastoma
  Neurofibrosarcoma
  Liposarcoma
  Malignant hemangiopericytoma
  Adenocarcinoma
  Mucoepidermoid carcinoma
  Esthesioneuroblastoma

Nonmalignant
  Neurofibroma
  Osteoma
  Meningioma
  Pleomorphic salivary adenoma
  Intradiploic dermoid

Table 40–2.
Classification of Skull Base for Tumor Resection

Anterior area	Anterior cranial fossa
Posterior area	Middle and posterior cranial fossa, subdivided as follows:
	Anterior segment: anterior wall of middle cranial fossa to anterior border of petrous temporal bone
	Central segment: petrous temporal bone
	Posterior segment: posterior border of petrous temporal bone to midline of posterior cranial fossa

446

Table 40–3.
Foramina of the Posterior Area of the Skull Base

Anterior segment	Foramen rotundum—maxillary nerve
	Foramen ovale—mandibular nerve
	Foramen lacerum—internal carotid artery
	Foramen spinosum—middle meningeal artery
Central segment	Internal acoustic meatus
	Internal carotid canal
Posterior segment	Jugular foramen—internal jugular vein
	Foramen magnum

vade the anterior cranial fossa. Tumors arising in the brain or meninges can similarly involve the skull base. Indirect involvement may result from skin, maxilla, or muscle; this invasion uses the structures mentioned above as avenues for entry into the cranium.

When this is appreciated, the surgeon will tend to suspect intracranial involvement and order computed tomography (CT) scans and magnetic resonance imaging (MRI). Angiography and/or magnetic resonance angiography (MRA) may be necessary in vascular tumors. Any suggestion of this calls for a neurosurgical consultation before surgery. As a result of this, the neurosurgeon may plan to be involved or, if the invasion is not definite, be on call at the time of surgery.

Nonmalignant Tumors

There are few nonmalignant tumors, mainly bony in type (e.g., osteoma), although an intradiploic dermoid occasionally is seen. The best example, albeit not pathologically a true tumor, is fibrous dysplasia. It behaves like a tumor and is treated like one, using total resection and (because it is

nonmalignant) immediate reconstruction (9,10). The presenting problems are deformity and, occasionally, diminishing visual acuity owing to involvement of the optic foramen, although hemiparesis has been seen on one occasion as a result of space-occupying effect.

The frontoorbital region is affected most frequently; thus, the coronal flap approach is used. If possible, a complete intracranial and extracranial resection is performed, with removal of all affected bone (Fig. 40–1). This frequently means resection of frontal bone, orbital roof, and medial and lateral orbital walls. Reconstruction is performed using split-skull grafts and split-rib grafts. The former are a spinoff from the surgery of congenital defects and are now extensively and variously used (11,12). After this procedure there is little or no tendency for recurrence; the cosmetic defect is corrected and, if it has been necessary to decompress the optic nerve, deterioration of visual acuity may be halted.

Complications should be few if the appropriate antibiotics are given and surgery is performed with due care. A lesson learned from congenital craniofacial procedures is the importance of closing any connections between the extradural space and the nasopharynx. Failure to do this will result in possible extradural abscess and meningitis. Closure of this area can be effected in various ways, and these will be presented in the relevant sections. The most useful technique in the situation described here is the galeal-frontalis muscle flap (13). This flap is raised based on the supraorbital and supratrochlear vessels, and it can be made the length of the coronal flap, but if it is used entirely the distal end can be unreliable (14). After being elevated, it can be turned down and packed and sutured into the defect. This has proved to be most effective in dealing with this potentially disastrous situation.

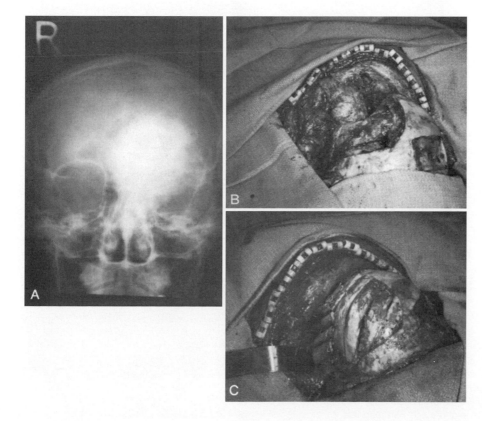

FIG. 40–1. **A,** radiograph shows left frontonasoorbital fibrous dysplasia. **B,** resection of left orbit to the floor together with the involved frontal and nasal regions. **C,** reconstruction is performed with split-skull and split-rib grafts.

MALIGNANT TUMORS

Frequently, malignant tumors recur, or have a potential for recurrence, after surgery, radiotherapy, and chemotherapy; thus, only limited reconstruction is performed. Covering up such a situation with a complex reconstruction may lead to a lethal delay in diagnosis of recurrence. We will discuss this later.

PENETRATING MIDFACE TUMORS

These tumors (Fig. 40–2) are usually recurrent basal cell carcinomas, occasionally squamous cell carcinomas (SCC), and much less frequently adenocystic or mucoepidermoid carcinomas, adenocarcinomas, sarcomas, or esthesioneuroblastomas. It is important to note that the basal and squamous cell carcinomas can frequently gain access intracranially by intraneural spread—facial and trigeminal. Resection is performed with frozen-section control. This encompasses removal of all involved facial areas (e.g., the nose or its remnants; varying parts of the orbit, perhaps exenteration; the palate; a varying amount of the nasopharynx; the central anterior cranial fossa base and the overlying dura; and the ethmoid and sphenoid sinuses.) A dural repair is performed using stored dura, fascia, or periosteum. This is exposed to the nasopharynx and must be protected by viable tissue. This

can be effected by suturing in an extended glabellar flap (15), a midline forehead flap (16,17), or a galeal frontalis flap (18) to the skull base and the posterior wall of the sphenoid sinus through drill holes (19).

Reconstruction is provided by an external prosthesis. These patients must be followed up with frequent visits, at least annual CT scans, and biopsies if any suspicious area appears in the field of resection. Using this regimen, we have had one local recurrence in 15 cases over a period of 4 years.

ETHMOID CARCINOMA

Any tumor arising in or invading the ethmoids should be treated as an anterior cranial-base tumor (Fig. 40–3). It should be approached using frontal scalp flap and a frontal bone flap. The surgeon outlines the oid block intra- and excranially and resects it; if skin is involved, it is included in the resection. Orbital involvement calls for orbitectomy, maxillary involvement for maxillectomy. Again, it is important to close the defect down into the nasopharynx with leal-frontalis flap or an extended glabellar flap. If there has been skin involvement, the skin defect is usually not reconstructed and is handled with an external prosthesis. Reconstruction can be undertaken at a later date.

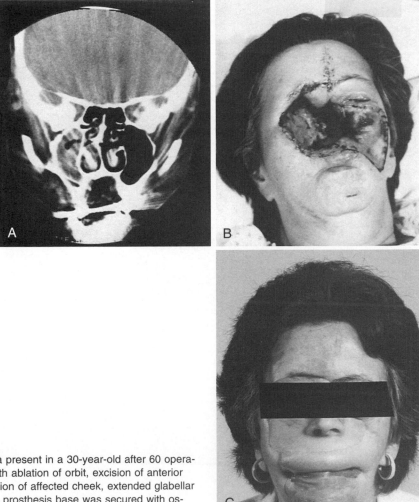

FIG. 40–2. **A,** recurrent midface basal cell carcinoma present in a 30-year-old after 60 operative procedures. **B,** extensive craniofacial resection with ablation of orbit, excision of anterior cranial fossa to posterior wall of sphenoid sinus, excision of affected cheek, extended glabellar flap was performed to reconstruct the cranial base. **C,** prosthesis base was secured with osteointegrated titanium pins. The prosthesis was held in place with magnets.

MIDFACE SARCOMA

These sarcomas (Fig. 40–4) frequently arise in the nasal septum; if they are far posterior, they defy early diagnosis because their main symptom is increasing nasal stuffiness. The nasal mucosa may be congested, and the patient is treated for allergy. The diagnosis is made on tomography, CT scan, and nasendoscopy. Because of the difficulty in early diagnosis, the tumors are frequently advanced by the time they present. In the past, these midface sarcomas gave great problems in exposure; consequently, complete resection was difficult, if not impossible in some cases.

The currently preferred approach is through a coronal flap and frontal bone flap with a face-splitting incision. A new concept in craniofacial approaches has been that of osteotomy for exposure with subsequent replacement (20). With this tumor, this approach makes all the difference to exposure after the frontal craniotomy. The bony midface, as required (e.g., glabella, nasal bones, orbit, maxilla sparing the teeth), is re-moved as a block. This exposes the base of the skull and the tumor. It is now possible to resect the tumor in one piece with good margins. This may not be possible in some cases; however, we have not yet encountered the situation.

The bony segment is replaced but is now exposed to the nasopharynx. This can, again, be covered with a galeal-frontalis flap. A split-skin graft is applied to this and held in place with sutures and a pack. The pack can be withdrawn through the nose in a few days' time. In this way, primary healing is achieved and the area can be observed for recurrence using the nasendoscope.

ORBITAL TUMORS

Orbital tumors (Fig. 40–5) can be exposed through a craniofacial approach; this is the approach of choice for tumors lying in the superior and posterior orbital area.

A coronal scalp flap and a frontal bone flap are used. The surgeon osteotomizes the orbital roof and supraorbital rim as

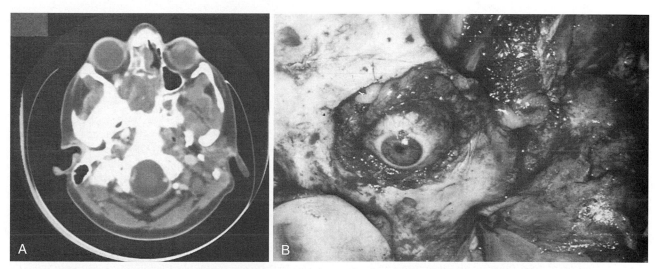

FIG. 40–3. **A,** extensive left ethmoid squamous carcinoma involves the nasopharynx, orbit, maxilla, and sphenoid. **B,** block resection of the central base of skull, left ethmoid sinus, sphenoid sinus, orbit, and maxilla.

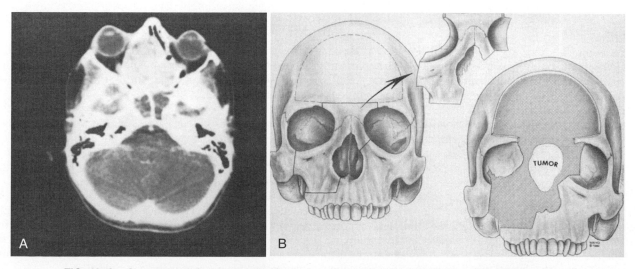

FIG. 40–4. **A,** a young patient presents with nasal septal and anterior cranial base chondrosarcoma well seen on the axial CT scan. **B,** midface osteotomy was performed to obtain tumor exposure.

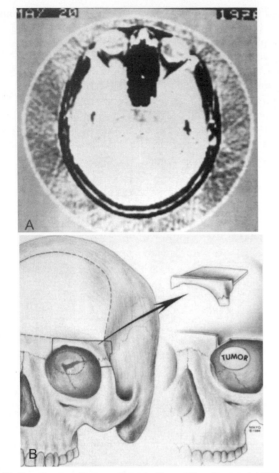

FIG. 40–5.   A, neurofibroma deep in the orbit well on axial CT scan. **B,** osteotomy is performed for exposure.

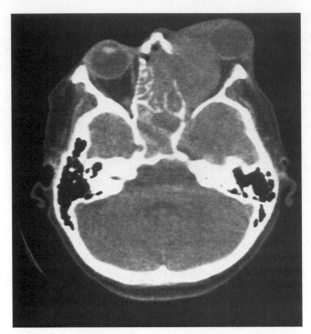

FIG. 40–6.   Recurrent aesthesioneuroblastoma of the right orbit maxilla, nose, and anterior cranial fossa, seen well on the axial CT scan.

a block and removes them. Exposure of the tumor is excellent. It can be removed en bloc under direct vision, then the osteotomy wired back into place. This resection can be accomplished without causing any cosmetic deformity or external facial scars.

An approach like this is also used for malignant tumors that are localized and can be resected with a margin of soft tissue.

PARTIAL ORBITECTOMY

When the tumor involves the orbital wall, a partial orbitectomy and exenteration may be necessary. The decision for an intracranial approach is made by tumor position. Any malignant osteoinvasive tumor in the posterosuperior position should be approached in this way. These may be tumors arising in the orbit, invading the bone from within, or extraorbital tumors invading from without. The amount of orbit removed is that which will give total tumor removal. This was well illustrated in Figure 40–3.

TOTAL ORBITECTOMY

Very rarely, extensive tumors (Fig. 40–6) or tumors known to be aggressive occurring in or around the orbit will require total resection of the orbit and its contents. The osteotomy is that which is used for hypertelorism, with bony cuts across the orbital roof, down the lateral wall, horizontally across the

maxilla below the infraorbital nerve, and vertically up the medial wall. In cases in which the tumor is situated far posteriorly in the orbit, the optic nerve is divided within the dura to allow for complete resection. The nasopharynx is closed off with a galeal-frontalis flap, and skin cover is achieved with a forehead or chest flap (e.g., pectoralis major, deltopectoral).

Middle Cranial Fossa (Posterior Area, Anterior Segment)

NONMALIGNANT TUMORS

The two most commonly encountered nonmalignant tumors here are partly orbital, partly middle fossa, tumors. These are orbital neurofibroma and fibrous dysplasia. These can be classified by severity of involvement, and the treatment can be planned accordingly (21).

NEUROFIBROMA

Only the advanced cases (Fig. 40–7) will be considered. The less severe cases call for surgery to the eyelid, recession of the globe (which is still functional), and reconstruction of any bony defects (22,23).

The problem case is that which presents with eyelid involvement so gross that the lids appear very edematous and cannot open; they may hang down onto the cheek. The eye is proptotic, pulsates, and is blind. There is neurofibroma present in the temple. The symptoms are pain and epiphora, and the patient usually wears a patch over the eye.

Radiologic examination and CT scans show the orbit to be enlarged and egg-shaped, with an absence of the greater wing of the sphenoid. This, in turn, causes a large defect in the posterior wall of the orbit (anterior wall of the middle cranial fossa), through which the temporal lobe herniates. This accounts for the eye protrusion and pulsation.

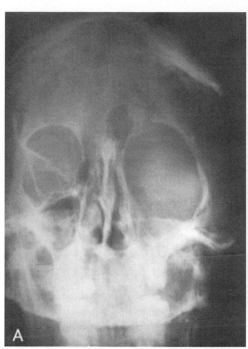
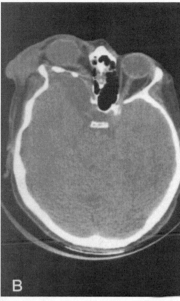

FIG. 40–7. A, radiograph shows enlarged orbit and absence of greater sphenoid wing due to neurofibroma. **B,** axial CT scan shows protrusion of the temporal lobe.

The approach to this problem is varied. It has been suggested that the bone defect be reconstructed, the orbit enlarged by an osteotomy, and some debunking of the neurofibroma undertaken with resulting recession of the globe. The eyelids are then trimmed in such a way as to thin them and leave the fissure permanently open. The result obtained using this technique is generally poor.

It has been found more satisfactory to remove the orbit contents completely, together with the involved temporal area. The eyelid skin is preserved, inasmuch as this is never involved by the neurofibroma. The bony posterior orbital defect is reconstructed with split-rib grafts or split-skull grafts; these are wired into position to give a solid closure of the defect. The orbit is then reduced in size using an ostectomy and osteotomies; any contour defects are made up with bone grafts (24).

The whole area is now covered with the eyelids; the edges are sutured together and the skin is pushed into the orbital cavity and held there with a pack. Once healing is achieved, the patient is fitted with an external prosthesis of eye and lids, masked by spectacles.

This technique may seem an admission of surgical defect, but it has resulted in satisfied patients having a good aesthetic result and complete relief of symptoms.

FIBROUS DYSPLASIA

This process (Fig. 40–8) may involve the posterolateral area of the orbit and the middle cranial fossa. The main reason for operating is proptosis and occasionally progressive diminution of visual acuity.

The area is approached using a coronal flap and a frontotemporal bone flap. The orbital contents and the temporalis muscle are dissected subperiosteally to expose the tumor in the temporal fossa and the orbit. An orbitomaxillary osteotomy is performed to further enhance exposure. The frontal and temporal lobes are elevated, and the involved area is resected with a margin of nonaffected bone. If the latter is not possible, a subtotal resection is done. Reconstruction is achieved using split-skull grafts wired in position, the osteotomies and craniotomies are replaced, and the scalp is sutured.

SUPERIOR INFRATEMPORAL FOSSA TUMORS

These are frequently meningiomas that appear in the orbit and the temporal area. This causes proptosis of the involved eye and the bulging above the zygomatic arch. There is often blindness or severe diminution of visual acuity.

CT scan shows the position of the lesion and the very considerable stretching of the optic nerve and extraocular muscles. The extent of the meningioma in the middle cranial fossa is clearly seen.

The surgical approach is similar to that described for fibrous dysplasia (Fig. 40–9); frequently the osteotomy must be more extensive. The supraorbital rim and roof, lateral orbital wall, a portion of the zygoma, and the zygomatic arch will give adequate exposure for removal of the extracranial portion of the tumor. The intracranial resection proceeds as indicated by the size and position of the tumor. Reconstruction is performed using split-skull grafts. The osteotomy and craniotomy segments are repositioned.

It must be realized that many of these meningiomas are recurrent and the chances of total resection are not high. However, even with subtotal removal, one can buy considerable time for the patient and alleviate the deformity to some degree.

LOW INFRATEMPORAL FOSSA TUMORS

These, again, may be meningiomas but may also be neurofibromas. Extracranial tumors invading this area include squamous carcinomas, adenocarcinomas, adenocystic carcinomas, and various types of sarcomas. There are two main approaches to this region: the microdrilling technique of Fisch and coworkers (25) and the combined intracranial and

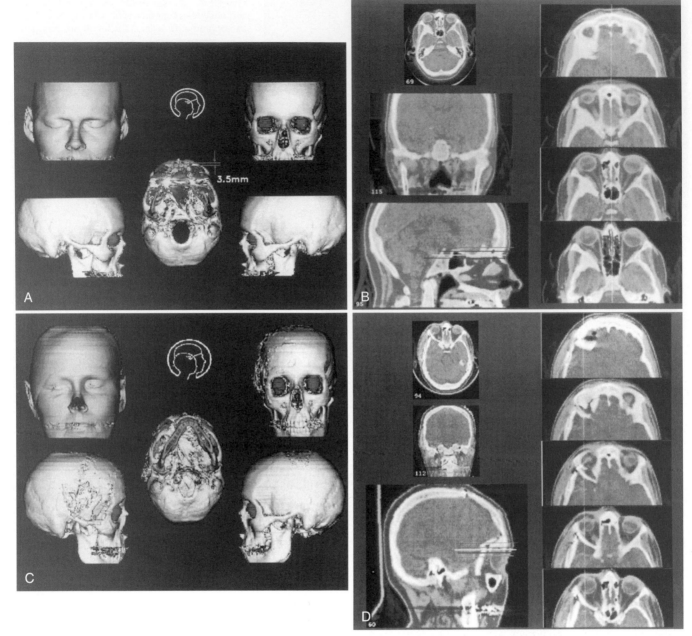

FIG. 40–8. **A,** 3-D CT scan showing fibrous dysplasia of the greater wing of the sphenoid involving the right orbit and resulting in enophthalmos. **B,** images produced from reformatted 3-D CT scan. Both orbits in exactly the same position and comparable. **C** and **D,** postoperative result, exactly comparable with preoperative situation.

extracranial technique (26,27). The former, of which we have no experience, is largely used by ear, nose, and throat surgeons. It is the combined intracranial and extracranial approach that will be described (Fig. 40–10).

The skin incision begins in the scalp and is taken down in front of the ear, as for a facelift, and continues into the neck as indicated. This large scalp, face, and neck flap is elevated to give exposure to the frontotemporal, zygomatic, and mandibular areas. A temporal craniotomy is performed and the temporal lobe elevated until the tumor comes into view. The chances of excision can be assessed at this point. If resection is considered possible, the operation proceeds. If the tumor is extensive and there is displacement or suggested in-

volvement of the carotid, or if there are palpable neck nodes, a neck dissection is performed. This has a twofold advantage: When the nodes are involved, they are removed; also, the external carotid artery and internal jugular vein are identified and can be followed up to the skull base, which makes the skull base resection much safer.

In order to clear the exposure to the base of the middle cranial fossa, certain structures must be removed (e.g., the total parotid, with facial nerve preservation (28); the zygomatic arch (29); and the ascending ramus of the mandible.) A dissection is performed extracranially to visualize the dimensions of the tumor. The skull base is now removed until the involved foramen is reached. The tumor can now be dis-

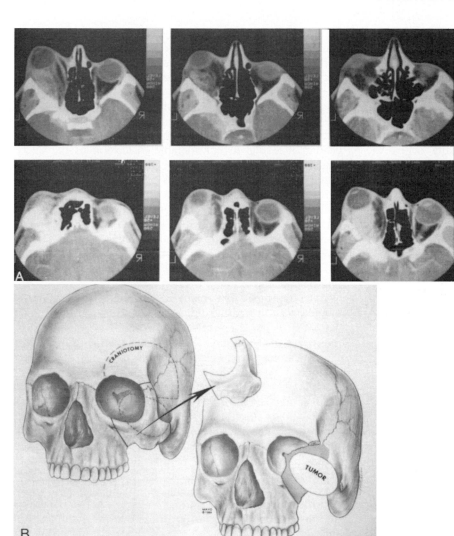

FIG. 40–9. **A,** recurrent meningioma of left middle cranial fossa, invading the orbit and upper infratemporal fossa shows well on axial CT scans.

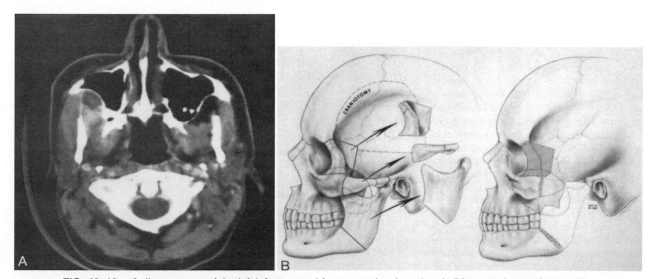

FIG. 40–10. **A,** liposarcoma of the left infratemporal fossa area involves the skull base and posterior maxilla; this is well seen on the axial CT scan. **B,** osteotomies are used for exposure.

sected out and removed under direction vision, with or without bone as indicated.

The temporal bone flap is replaced and the skull base is reconstructed with a split-skull graft (30). The zygomatic arch and, occasionally, the ascending ramus are replaced. The problem with this latter procedure is its potential for causing trismus. The skin incision is closed with drainage.

Occasionally in extensive tumors an orbital osteotomy may be necessary. In others, situated medially behind the maxilla, an anterior approach using the Weber-Ferguson incision and incorporating a partial maxillectomy in the procedure may be indicated.

Facial Disassembly

In some tumors, because of their position (e.g., cavernous sinus), it is necessary to carry out a very extensive facial disassembly. This may involve removal of several portions of skull; for example, the frontal temporoparietal and the orbit—either as an osteotomy to shift the orbit or in order to remove segments of the whole of the orbit. When even greater exposure is required, then osteotomies such as a hemi–LeFort III or bilateral hemi–LeFort III may be performed in order to move the bony segments of the face laterally and so gain central exposure. This allows the neurosurgeon to move into the area of the cavernous sinus with the microscope and so dissect the relevant structures in a more satisfactory fashion, remove the tumor, and obviate many of the serious complications that can result from operating in that area (31) (Fig. 40–11).

To reduce operating time and so minimize complications, it is common to reassemble as much as possible of the disassembled face on a side table while the resection is going on. This allows the reassembled segment of the face to be placed back into the defect and to be stabilized very quickly, thus shortening the operation time.

Central Segment

Tumors of the central segment are (a) external ear carcinomas, squamous or basal, involving the petrous bone; (b) parotid tumors, often recurrent, having had surgery and radiation therapy and now extending deeply into the ear cleft. These are adenocystic, mucoepidermoid, squamous, and undifferentiated carcinomas; and (c) squamous carcinomas arising in the middle ear. It is usually necessary to sacrifice the external ear.

Partial petrosectomy does not involve entry into the cranial cavity and will not be considered in this chapter. It is sufficient to say that in these cases cover is obtained with a temporal muscle transposition and split-skin graft. The radical petrosectomy will be presented here (26,32,33).

The incision curves over the temporoparietal area down in front, or around the ear if it is to be included in the resection. It continues in a vertical curvilinear fashion to give exposure in the neck. The external ear may, in some cases, be preserved; it is lifted with the posterior flap, the ear canal is transected. A temporal craniotomy is performed and the cranial aspect of the petrous bone exposed. This is necessary in order to assess resectability. Frequently there may be tumor extension into the temporal lobe dura; this is an ominous prognostic sign in middle ear cancer. The apex of the petrous bone is inspected; extension beyond this into the cavernous sinus may well preclude curative resection.

If the tumor is judged to be resectable, exposure from the neck is begun. Primary or recurrent parotid tumors necessitate total parotidectomy. A total or partial neck dissection is used to locate, particularly, the internal carotid artery as it enters the base of the skull. Care is taken to preserve intact the internal jugular vein. If this vein is tied off early in the procedure, it results in considerable distension of the lateral sinus. This increases the technical difficulties of the procedure because of increased venous oozing and can result in severe bleeding if the sinus is broached. As soft tissue is dissected from the skull anterior and posterior to the meatus, further extension of tumor may be noted and a wider resection executed. It is not unusual to remove the ascending ramus of the mandible and a portion of the zygomatic arch. No attempt is made to preserve the facial nerve because it will be sacrificed in the resection.

Osteotomies are now made downward from the temporal craniotomy to reach to skull base behind and in front of the ear canal; the position of the osteotomies is determined by the extent of the tumor. The temporal lobe is retracted and the osteotomies continue medially in the skull base. These extend until the most medial part of the tumor has been passed. Using an air drill from above and below, the carotid artery is freed from its bony canal. It should now be possible to access the petrous bone medially and, by a series of gentle rocking movements, free and remove it. At this point, the main concern is the disruption of the internal carotid artery. If possible, some indication of cross flow should be obtained before surgery. This can be done by compression during angiography, cross-clamping, and EEG evaluation over a time period, or by blood flow estimation using radioactive tracers during surgery with occlusion of the internal carotid on the side of surgery. Although these methods are not absolutely accurate, they can be most helpful to indicate which case may have the vessel sacrificed and subsequently maintain the patients neurologic status intact.

If dura has been sacrificed, a repair is performed. There may be no skin defect, and the ear is returned to its former position and sutured. Where a defect is present, it may be closed with a scalp rotation flap or, if it is more extensive, a pectoralis myocutaneous flap is ideal. Latissimus dorsi and trapezius myocutaneous flaps have been used, but these involve turning the patient and are not recommended. It is now more common to use a free transfer, and the rectus abdominis is the flap of choice.

This is technically a very difficult procedure and unfortunately the results are not always satisfactory. In penetrating external basal cell or squamous cell carcinoma, the results are usually good if the resection is adequate. Middle-ear carcinomas are rarely cured even with postoperative radiotherapy. Recurrent parotid tumors give mixed results, particularly types of adenocystic carcinoma that may recur long after the original resection. The complications of this procedure are deafness, facial palsy, a potential for severe hemorrhage during surgery and hemiplegia. Entry into the cavernous sinus may cause, at worst, blindness and, at best, an immobile eye. Perhaps the most troublesome postoperative problem is vertigo; fortunately, it tends to pass with time. Postoperative

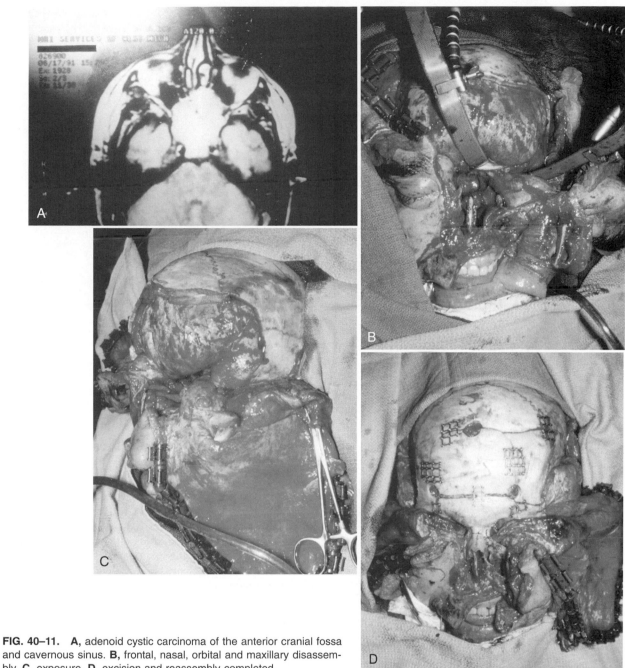

FIG. 40–11.   A, adenoid cystic carcinoma of the anterior cranial fossa and cavernous sinus. **B,** frontal, nasal, orbital and maxillary disassembly. **C,** exposure. **D,** excision and reassembly completed.

radiotherapy will aggravate this problem and make it more longlasting.

Posterior Segment

Tumors of the posterior cranial fossa rarely involve the plastic surgeon. These are usually acoustic neuromas, neurofibromas, or meningiomas; fibrous dysplasia may also occur in this region. Fortunately, these will usually cause intracranial symptoms such as headache or dizziness, and thus the patient is directed to the neurologist or neurosurgeon. Because of the

tumor position in relation to the cerebellar pontine region, the last four cranial nerves are compressed, resulting in some typical signs. There is wasting and weakness of the trapezius and sternomastoid muscles, wasting of the tongue, hoarseness, and occasionally dysphagia. The tumor escapes from the jugular foremen and can present as a deep lobe of parotid tumor. On basal tomography and CT scans, the jugular foramen is often seen to be much enlarged as compared to the noninvolved side (Fig. 40–12). There may be anterior displacement of the carotid vessels when the tumor extends into the neck.

FIG. 40–12. **A,** neurofibroma of the posterior cranial fossa exits into the neck through the jugular foramen, producing "parotid" swelling and wasting of trapezius and sternomastoid muscles. Coronal CT scan shows enlarged jugular foramen. **B,** carotid angiogram illustrates anterior displacement of the vessels by the tumor in the neck.

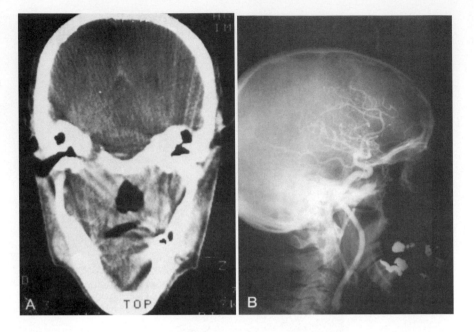

Exposure is by a posterior scalp flap based inferiorly; on the side of the tumor the anterior edge of the incision is carried forward and downward to deal with any tumor extension into the neck. The scalp flap is tedious to raise, because several layers of muscle must be stripped off the skull in the occipital area. The transverse processes of the atlas and axis are reached and the vertebral artery is preserved.

The jugular foramen is isolated by dissection from the neck. The facial nerve may have to be dissected away from the tumor. An occipital craniotomy is performed to view the intracranial aspect of the tumor. It is now usually possible to perform the resection under good vision. No reconstructive measures are necessary, apart from a dural repair if there has been dural damage or involvement.

Recent Developments

FREE-TISSUE TRANSFER IN CRANIOFACIAL SURGERY

Increasingly, when there are soft-tissue and hard-tissue defects in the skull base area, free-tissue transfer is used. This can be to prevent infection, treat infection, or fill a dead space. Most frequently the rectus abdominis muscle has been used in all of these situations—although undoubtedly when there is infection present, and also to some extent where there is a dead space in the anterior cranial fossa with impending infection, the omentum is an excellent material for filling every nook and cranny that is either harboring infection or providing a potential space for infection. Undoubtedly this type of reconstruction will be performed more routinely in the future. In fact, composite reconstruction with soft tissue and bone may well become the norm in many of these patients (34).

Radiation Following Free-Tissue Transfer

In patients who have had irradiation with or without surgery and have a recurrent tumor, a dilemma arises as to course of action if there is any suspicion of earlier incomplete resection or tumor spill. The radiation therapists believe they must not give further radiation and have tried to use radon seeds or af-terloading cannulae. This problem has been solved to some extent by using free-tissue transfer. In the resected area, the surgeon places a muscular or myocutaneous flap; a further full-tumor dose of radiation can then be delivered through the flap. This has proved to be effective in a small number of cases but awaits further evaluation (Fig. 40–13).

Cardiac Bypass in Skull Base Tumors

Some skull base tumors are so vascular (e.g., extensive, infiltrative angiofibroma) that conventional surgery cannot be performed, and it has been advocated that these be treated with radiation, chemotherapy, or a combination of the two (35). However, in these cases the patient can be placed on cardiac bypass with hypothermia either in a no-flow or low-flow situation. Usually the main part of the dissection is carried out before the patient is placed on bypass because in the no-flow situation it is safe to operate for only a limited amount of time (e.g., 20 minutes). The patient can then be warmed and, following the establishment of circulation, a further cooling can allow 20 minutes more for resection. In the low-flow situation, it is possible to operate for up to 2 hours. Low-flow is preferable, but there can be considerable bleeding over 2 hours. In both cases there is a significant problem with bleeding when the patient is being warmed and is still heparinized. To prepare for this, large amounts of blood should be made available. Using this technique it has been possible to resect otherwise unresectable tumors. The technique can be combined with extensive facial osteotomies and disassembly. This allows the surgical procedure to be carried out safely because of the extra exposure provided.

In some patients it will not be possible to stop the bleeding, so the facial defect has to be packed and a return to the area planned for 2 to 5 days later. It is hoped that bleeding will have stopped by then and the reconstruction can be carried out. If indicated, a free-tissue transfer can be carried out concurrently or soon afterwards. Remember that there may be portions of the tumor left behind or there may be seeding, and if possible these patients should be followed up by radi-

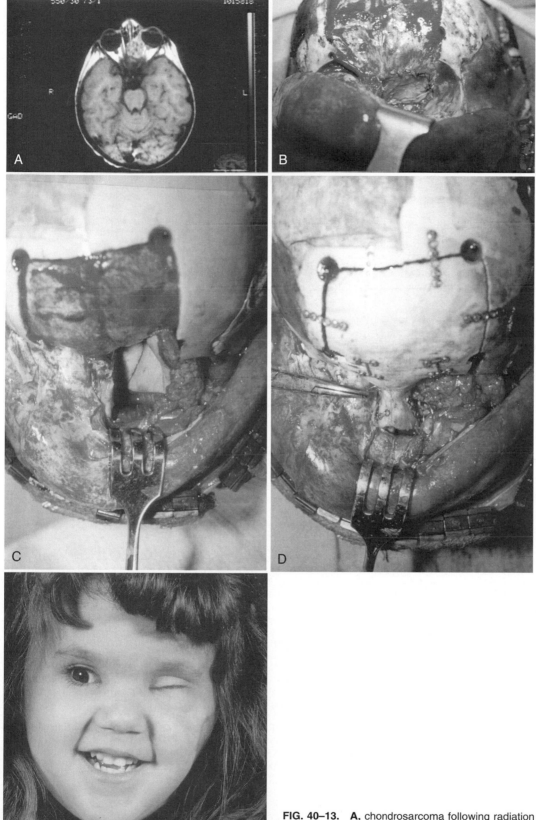

FIG. 40–13. A, chondrosarcoma following radiation for retinoblastoma. **B,** craniofacial resection. Note resection of portion of left frontal lobe and dura. **C,** reconstruction with free rectus abdominis flap. **D,** bony framework replaced. **E,** two years after second radiation treatment (total 12,000 rads).

ation therapy or chemotherapy or a combination of both. This surgical approach is only advised for tumors that in the past have been considered unresectable because of the potential for uncontrollable bleeding.

Conclusion

The adaptation of techniques used in craniofacial deformity correction to skull base tumor resection has greatly improved the lot of both patient and surgeon. Resections are carried out under good vision with good exposure, giving the opportunity for improved results. Areas of bone are removed for exposure and subsequently replaced, minimizing the eventual deformity. This makes the decision to proceed with surgery somewhat easier for all concerned. New methods of external prosthesis fitting make life more tolerable after these large procedures. Osteointegrated titanium pegs allow the establishment of an external framework onto which the prosthesis may be attached using magnets (see Fig. 40–2C,D).

Preoperative assessment is more sophisticated. All patients have CT and MR scans and may have angiography. It is unwise to proceed to excise skull base tumor without knowing the position of the carotid vessels. In some cases, three-dimensional imaging is used; this may be utilized more frequently in the future. With the advent of free-tissue transfer, using microvascular techniques, reconstruction has become and will become more sophisticated in time. However, enthusiasm must be tempered by knowledge of tumor biology. Reconstruction must be delayed until all chance of tumor recurrence appears to have receded. To have a method available is not a reason for using it!

Above all, this type of surgery is a cooperative effort. Neurosurgeon, plastic surgeon, anesthesiologist, oncologist, and radiotherapist must integrate their work smoothly. If this is done, the surgery should have low mortality and an improved cure rate can be expected.

References

1. Ketcham AS, Wilkins RH, VanBuren JM, et al. A combined intracranial facial approach to the paranasal sinuses. *Am J Surg* 1963; 106:698.
2. Ketcham AS, Hoye RD, Van Buren JM, et al. Complications of intracranial facial resection of tumors of the paranasal sinuses. *Am J Surg* 1966; 112:591.
3. Schuller DE, Lawrence TL, Newton WA Jr, et al. The role of combined chemotherapy in the treatment of rhabdomyosarcoma of the head and neck. *Arch Otolaryngol* 1979; 105:689.
4. Heyn RM, Holland R, Newton WA Jr, et al. The role of combined chemotherapy in the treatment of rhabdomyosarcoma in children. *Cancer* 1974; 34:2128.
5. Ghavimi F, Exelby PR, D'Angio GE, et al. Multi-disciplinary treatment of embryonal rhabdomyosarcoma in children. *Cancer* 1975; 35:677.
6. Healy GB, Jaffe N, Cassady JR. Rhabdomyosarcoma of the head and neck: diagnosis and management. *Head Neck Surg* 1979; 1:334.
7. Jackson IT, Hide TAH. Further extensions of craniofacial surgery. In: Jackson IT, ed. *Recent advances in plastic surgery*. Vol. 2. Edinburgh: Churchill Livingstone, 1981; 241–259.
8. Jackson IT, Hide TAH. A systematic approach to tumors of the base of the skull. *J Maxillofac Surg* 1982; 10:92.
9. Jackson IT, Hide TAH, Gomuwka PK, et al. Treatment of cranioorbital fibrous dysplasia. *J Maxillofac Surg* 1982; 10:138.
10. Munro IT, Chen YR. Radical treatment for frontoorbital fibrous dysplasia: the chain-link fence. *Plast Reconstr Surg* 1981; 67:719.
11. Tessier P. Autogenous bone grafts from the calvarium for facial and cranial applications. *Clin Plas Surg* 1982; 9:531.
12. Jackson IT, Pellett CC, Smith JM. The skull as bone graft donor site. *Ann Plast Surg* 1983; 11:527.
13. Jackson IT, Marsh WR, Hide TAH. Treatment of tumors involving the anterior cranial fossa. *Head Neck Surg* 1984; 6:901.
14. Fukuta K, Potparic Z, Sugihara T, et al. A cadaver investigation of the blood supply of the galeal frontalis flap. *Plast Reconstr Surg* 1994; 94:794.
15. Jackson IT, Laws ER, Martin RD. A craniofacial approach to advanced recurrent cancer of the central face. *Head Neck Surg* 1983; 5:474.
16. Ketcham AS, Chretien PB, Schour L, et al. Surgical treatment of patients with advanced cancer of the paranasal sinuses. In: *Neoplasia of the head and neck*. Chicago: Year Book, 1974; 187–209.
17. Ousterhout DK, Tessier P. Closure of large cribriform defects with a forehead flap. *J Maxillofac Surg* 1981; 9:7.
18. Bridger GP. Radical surgery for ethmoid cancer. *Arch Otolaryngol* 1980; 106:630.
19. Jackson IT, Adham MN, Marsh WR. Use of galeo-frontalis myofascial flap in craniofacial surgery. *Plast Reconstr Surg* 1986; 77:905.
20. Jackson IT, Marsh WR, Bite U, et al. Craniofacial osteotomies to facilitate skull base tumor resection. *Br J Plast Surg* 1986; 39:153.
21. Jackson I. Neurofibromatosis of the skull base. Clinics in plastic surgery. *Clin Plast Surg* 1995; 22:3, 513–530.
22. van der Meulen JC, Moscona AR, Vandrachen M, et al. Management of orbitofacial neurofibromatosis. *Ann Plast Surg* 1982; 8:213.
23. Marchac D. Intracranial management of the orbital cavity and palpebra remodeling for orbitopalpebral neurofibromatosis. *Plast Reconstr Surg* 1981; 73:534.
24. Jackson IT, Laws ER Jr, Martin RD. The surgical management of orbital neurofibromatosis. *Plast Reconstr Surg* 1981; 73:534.
25. Fisch U, Pillsbury HC, Sasaki CT. Infratemporal approach to the skull base. In: Sasaki CT, McCabe BF, Kirchner JA, eds. *Surgery of the skull base*. Philadelphia: JB Lippincott, 1984; 141–160.
26. Jackson IT, Munro IR, Salyer KE, et al. *Atlas of craniomaxillofacial surgery*. St. Louis: CV Mosby, 1982.
27. Donald PJ. Infratemporal fossa and skull base. In: Donald PG, ed. *Head and neck cancer management of the difficult case*. Philadelphia: WB Saunders, 1984; 277–312.
28. McCabe BF, Work WP. Parotidectomy with special reference to the facial nerve. Ch. 63. In: English GM, ed. *Otolaryngology*. Vol 3. Hagerstown, MD: Harper & Row, 1984.
29. Fisch U, Pillsbury HC. Infratemporal fossa approach to lesions in the temporal bone and base of the skull. *Arch Otolaryngol* 1979; 105:99.
30. Jackson IT, Smith J, Mixter RC. Nasal bone grafting using split skull grafts. *Ann Plast Surg* 1983; 11:533.
31. Janecka IP. Selected surgical approaches to the skull base. Procedures in Cranial Base Surgery. Problems in Plastic and Reconstructive Surgery 1993; 3:224–244.
32. Campbell E, Volk BM, Burklund CW. Total resection of the temporal bone for malignancy of the middle ear. *Ann Surg* 1951; 134:397.
33. Parsons H, Lewis JS. Subtotal resection of the temporal bone for cancer of the ear. *Cancer* 1954; 7:995.
34. Edington H, Ramasastry S. Microvascular flap transfer in cranial base surgery. Procedures in cranial base surgery. Problems in Plastic and Reconstructive Surgery 1993; 3:207–223.
35. Goepfert H, Cangir A, Lee Y-Y: Chemotherapy for aggressive juvenile nasopharyngeal angiofibroma. Arch Otolaryngol 111:285–289, 1985.

41

Basic Principles of Reconstruction of the Lip, Oral Commissure, and Cheek

Mark R. Sultan, M.D., F.A.C.S., and Norman E. Hugo, M.D., F.A.C.S.

The face and notably the lips and cheeks are important structures not only of aesthetic value but also for expression, vibrancy, and vitality. As such, both functional and aesthetic restoration of deformed parts receive high priority. The aims of reconstruction in the lips and cheeks are the restoration of appearance and reinstitution of function. Often, this involves the repair of several layers of missing tissues, and these need to be supplied in order to attain a superior result. This chapter will deal sequentially with deformities of the lips and then deformities of the cheeks. With the advent of newer approaches, many of the older procedures are no longer used. Such advances as musculocutaneous and free flaps have allowed us greater imagination and magnitude in reconstruction and, as a consequence, achieved superior results.

Lips

The lips are composed of three layers—skin, muscle, and buccal mucosa. Their principle muscle, the orbicularis oris, is circumferential and plays a primary role in oral competence. Other factors necessary for competence include sensation and an adequate buccal sulcus. Many other muscles of facial expression converge on the orbicularis oris, just lateral to the commissure, at a point called the modiolus (Fig. 41–1). The orbicularis oris and elevators of the lips are innervated by the buccal branches, while the depressors are innervated by the marginal mandibular nerve. Sensory innervation is provided by the infraorbital and mental branches of the trigeminal nerve. The superior and inferior labial arteries, branches at the facial artery, are the main vascular supply of the lips. There are no corresponding labial veins. Instead, the lips are drained by a series of tiny tributaries that eventually coalesce into the facial veins. The lymphatic drainage of the lips is rich and leads to the submental and submandibular nodal basins.

The choice of reconstructive procedure for a given lip defect must be based upon a series of considerations about the wound and the patient in whom it exists. The age and gender of the patient are assessed first. Older patients have more inherent laxity in their lips than do young patients, allowing primary closure of more extensive wounds without creating microstomia or distortion. Male patients require the use of hair-bearing tissue for upper lip wounds, while females with upper-lip, or either gender with lower-lip, defects do not. Next, the size, depth, and location of each wound must be carefully studied. Each of the three layers of the lip, with proper innervation, must be repaired or replaced to achieve the optimal result. Therefore, wounds that involve the cutaneous layer only are approached differently from those that involve muscle or muscle and mucosa. Finally, the proper balance between the upper and lower lip should be restored whenever possible.

It is axiomatic in the repair of cheek and lip defects that the best source of donor material is similar tissue. If the lip can be reconstructed with lip tissue, this is ideal. Similarly, if one can use tissues from the head and neck area in juxtaposition to the cheek for its reconstruction, the results are usually felicitous. Although it is not always possible, the surgeon should think of these donor areas primarily. While distant pedicled flaps and free flaps are more dramatic, their color and thickness often make them less desirable for repair in those areas.

VERMILION REPAIR

For patients with severe leukoplakia, or multiple superficial carcinomas from prolonged smoking and exposure to the elements, the procedure of choice is a lip shave. This is done by excising the mucosa from the vermilion border backward until the unaffected area is reached. The mucosa is excised down to the muscle. Bilateral relaxing incisions are made laterally at each corner of the mouth downward into the deep sulcus and the entire mucosa is elevated and advanced forward to cover the area (1). The mucosa will become keratinized after exposure (Fig. 41–2). The cosmetic result is quite acceptable and the recurrence rate minimal in properly selected patients (2). The procedure can also be performed in conjunction with wedge excisions of invasive carcinomas.

When the defect includes a discrete segment of the vermilion or a portion of the vermilion with its underlying orbicularis oris muscle, the remaining vermilion myocutaneous units may be utilized as flaps for reconstruction (3). These flaps include the labial arteries and sensory nerves and are developed by incising the lip along the vermilion border to allow their advancement toward the midline. The flaps can generally be stretched to twice their original length. For wide defects of the vermilion it is sometimes necessary to excise mental skin, thereby narrowing the defect before advancing the vermilion myocutaneous flaps to achieve wound closure (Fig. 41–3).

COMMISSURE REPAIR

After a traumatic insult (e.g., an electrical burn to the commissure) in which the vermilion and a portion of the skin and muscle are destroyed, the resultant cicatricial healing obliterates the normal sharp angle of the mouth and reduces the aperture. Previous methods of repair have called for creation

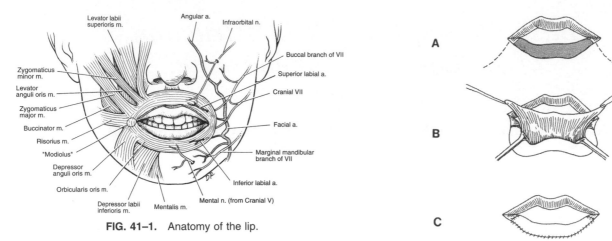

FIG. 41–1. Anatomy of the lip.

FIG. 41–2. An artist's sketch of lip shave. **A,** resection of mucosa and lower lip is diagrammed. **B,** advancement of intraoral labial mucosa. **C,** mucosa is sutured into place. Keratinization occurs with exposure.

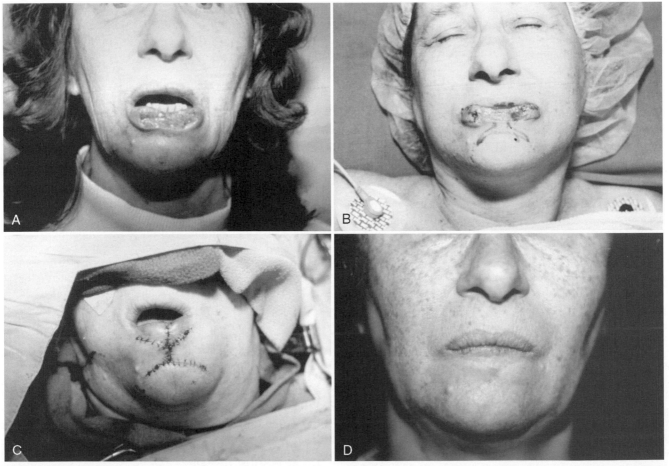

FIG. 41–3. **A,** defect of vermilion and obicularis oris following Mohs for squamous cell carcinoma of the lip. **B,** design of vermilion myocutaneous flaps and of central "flared W" excision of central lip skin to narrow defect. **C,** immediately following repair. **D,** 6 weeks following repair.

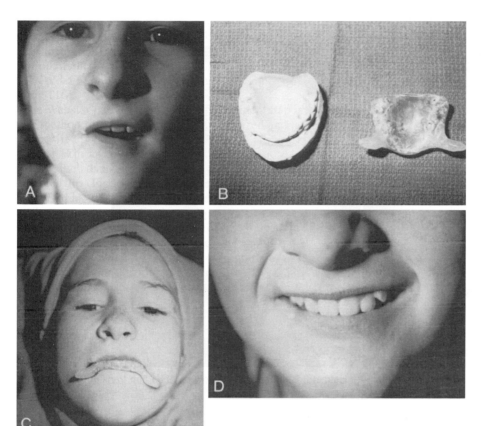

FIG. 41–4.   A, infiltrating morphea-type basal cell carcinoma with vermillion retraction. **B,** defect after Moh's chemosurgery. **C and D,** immediate repair is performed with Abbé-Estlander flap.

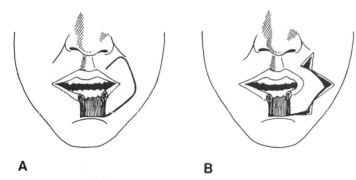

A   **B**

FIG. 41–5.   An artist's sketch of the fan flap. **A,** construction of the fan flap is performed by through-and-through incisions. **B,** the entire segment is rotated medially to close defect. Rounding of commissure occurs.

of small flaps in which either the upper or the lower lip is repaired and then mucosa advanced to cover the donor defect (4,5). This has resulted in adequate repair but usually a rounded commissure. A simpler method with better results is incision to restore the oral aperture and a hook to prevent reapproximation of the raw surfaces (6). With subsequent epithelialization, and maintaining the hook until scarring subsides, good results are obtained (Fig. 41–4).

When the commissure defect results from a tumor resection, the cheek skin, muscle, and mucosa are generally advanced medially as a unit to replace those tissues lost. This is done by excising vertical crescents of skin from the nasolabial fold above and below the commissure to allow the cheek transposition into the modiolus and commissure position (7).

PRIMARY CLOSURE OF THE LIP

Approximately one-third of the lip may be sacrificed and the lip closed directly without undue changes. This rule of thumb is slightly less applicable to young patients and there is a greater range with older patients, some of whom can have 40% of the lip removed and primary closure done (8,9). When planning an excision and primary closure of the lip, the vermilion border should be marked with indelible ink before excision to allow its meticulous reapproximation. Incision across the vermilion should be at right angle to the border whenever possible.

FAN FLAP

The fan flap (10) is based on the labial artery. A large, superiorly based flap is constructed by through-and-through incision of the lateral portions of the upper lip and the remaining portions of the lower lip. After complete mobilization, the flap is swung toward the midline of the lower lip to reconstruct the defect (Fig. 41–5). As a matter of practical import, the flap is well suited for large defects but the tip of this flap has a tendency to necrose—and again, it tends to round the commissures. Interestingly, both the fan flap and the Abbé-Estlander flap are capable of motor and sensory reinnervation (11).

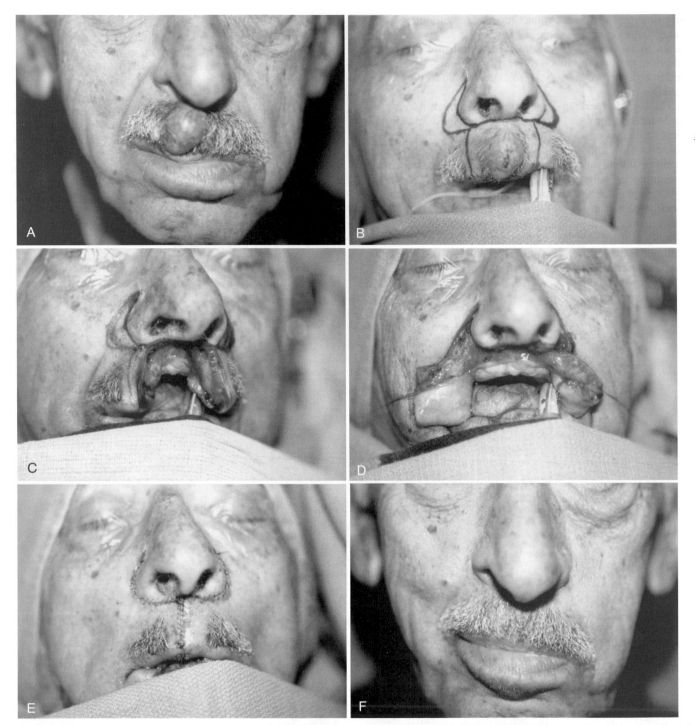

FIG. 41–9. **A,** sebaceous gland carcinoma of upper lip. **B,** bilateral crescentic advancement flap designed. **C,** extent of full-thickness defect of lip. **D,** elevation of flaps (note extent and location of mucosal-releasing incisions). **E,** immediately following flap advancement and closure. **F,** postoperative result.

or when the patient has previously received radiation therapy to the area. In these instances it may be necessary to import vascularized tissue from a distant site. Delayed bipedicle neck flaps (19), sternocleidomastoid myocutaneous flaps (20), and deltopectoral flaps (21) have all been described for this purpose with fair results. Another option is the free radial forearm flap (22). The advantage of this microsurgical method is its potential for reinnervation by the approximation of the mental nerve to the cutaneous nerve within the flap. Also, the flap may be designed to include vascularized palmaris longus tendon to suspend the flap from the cheeks in an effort to prevent drooling. However, the poor color match of the light forearm skin to the facial skin remains a significant disadvantage. These distant flaps may be used in

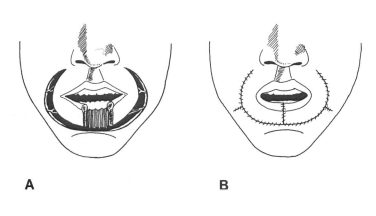

FIG. 41–10. An artist's sketch of Karapandzic repair. **A,** innervated and vascularized orbicularis oris myocutaneous flap is separated from the muscles of expression. **B,** closure with some microstomia is evident.

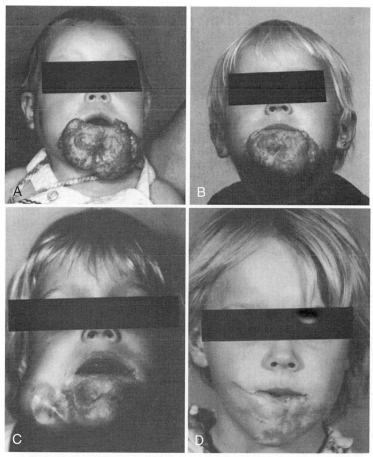

FIG. 41–11. **A,** a massive hemangioma of the lower lip. **B,** degree of involution after several years. **C,** tissue expander is used in the right cheek. The expander in left cheek had extruded. **D,** after resection of lip and chin, expanded tissue is advanced.

conjunction with staged tongue flaps to reconstruct the vermilion. More recently, tattooing of the free border of the imported flap has been reported to simulate the vermilion (23).

TISSUE EXPANSION

With the use of tissue expanders, the local recruitment of tissue for areas around the face is substantial (Fig. 41–11). It is done under the same principles that govern tissue expansion in any other area of the body. Large amounts of skin can be recruited and have substantially good blood supply (24). It is well known that the area becomes highly vascular, actually making the tissues look poor initially, with a great deal of redness and telangiectases (25). However, after it has been moved and sutured into place, this resolves and the area achieves normal facial color again. Its inherent advantage is the recruitment of large areas of tissue similar to that of the area that requires reconstruction.

Cheek

The anatomy of the medial and lateral cheek differ significantly. The medial cheek is similar to the lip in that it has three layers—skin, muscle, and oral mucosa. The lateral cheek houses the parotid gland and the main divisions of the facial nerve. The major muscle of the entire cheek is the buccinator. It originates from the maxilla, mandible, and pterygomandibular raphe and inserts at the commissure deep to the other lip musculature. In the region of the 3rd molar the muscle is pierced by the parotid duct. It is innervated by the buccal branch of the facial nerve and its main action is compression of the cheek. It thereby contributes both to facial expression and to mastication.

Several important factors must be considered when assessing defects of the cheek. As with wounds of the lips, assessment must begin with the patient (e.g., age, health, history of smoking or radiation therapy). The wound itself is then studied to determine its size, location, and depth. Small- and medium sized superficial defects of the cheek can often be closed primarily after undermining of the adjacent skin. This is especially true of the older patient with lax skin. Occasionally, Limberg-type (rhomboid) flaps are helpful for this purpose. For larger defects that are not through and through the cheek, alternatives include skin grafts and local flaps. Flaps generally provide superior color and contour match. The recent improvement in tissue-expansion techniques has led to another strategy, the temporary use of skin grafts to achieve wound closure followed by their excision and replacement by the expanded cheek and neck flaps. This may be particularly applicable to young patients where the morbidity of local flaps can be significant. Large full-thickness defects of the medial cheek that include buccal mucosa and extend into the oral cavity, and large deep wounds of the lateral cheek that expose facial nerve branches or bone, most often require distant flaps for reconstruction. The pedicle flaps generally originate from the temporal scalp or from the trunk, while the free microvas-

cular flaps may be chosen from any appropriate remote donor site. Multi-staged, delayed random flaps such as Zovickian flaps (26) are now largely of only historical interest.

SKIN GRAFTS

Skin grafts may be either a temporary or a permanent cover. Of course, they are restricted to partial-thickness defects. A temporary cover might be employed while evaluating the area for cancer recurrence in a particularly difficult case. Later, the graft can be removed and definitive reconstruction accomplished by local or expanded flaps. When the graft is large, or believed to be the permanent reconstructive method, the aesthetic unit principle of the cheek should be followed (27) (Fig. 41–12).

LOCAL FLAPS

Local flaps used in cheek reconstruction are basically Mustardé-type flaps (28). Grouped under the heading of cervicofacial flaps, a number of designs have been advocated (29). All rotate intact lateral cheek skin into medial cheek defects. The flaps incorporate the facial artery and vein but have random components as well. Some authors advocate raising the flap in the subplatysma plane (30). When the Mustardé flap itself is chosen, a high arc in the temporal region must be used to insure adequate height of the flap so as to reach the superomedial aspect of the defect. Also, the flap should be

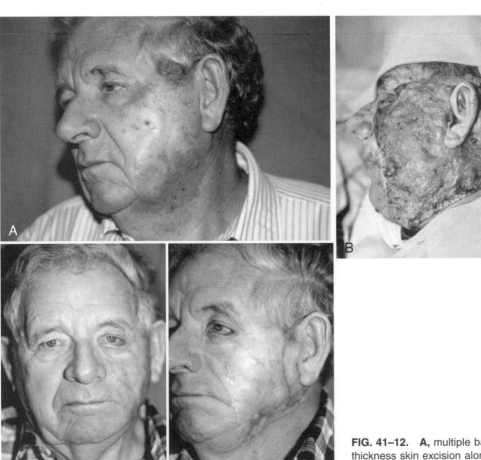

FIG. 41–12. A, multiple basal cell carcinoma of left cheek. **B,** full-thickness skin excision along cheek aesthetic units. **C, D,** reconstruction following full-thickness skin graft (ectropion repaired by subsequent revision).

anchored to periosteum superiorly to prevent the formation of a postoperative ectropion (31) (Fig. 41–13).

The cervicopectoral flap may be thought of as an extension of the cervicofacial flaps. It may be used to reconstruct extensive defects of the cheek. Its superior design and harvesting begins in a fashion similar to the cervicofacial flaps. The incision then continues inferiorly along the anterior border of the trapezius to include skin over the neck and upper chest (32). The flap includes the platysma and its vasculature as well as the first two or three perforators from the internal mammary artery, giving it a reliable blood supply. It provides thin tissue that is an excellent color match for the cheek, because the tissue used for coverage is recruited from the head and neck area (Fig. 41–14). In some cases the flap may lack the necessary bulk to restore proper cheek contour.

DISTANT FLAPS

Flap of the Temporal Region

Several flaps are available for transposition from the temporal region to the cheek. The scalping flap described and popularized by Converse is a variant of the forehead flap (33,34). It carries skin from the entire forehead on the superficial temporal vessels ipsilateral to the cheek defect. A skin graft may be applied to the intraoral surface of the flap to complete reconstruction of through-and-through defects. This is at least a two-stage procedure with potentially significant donor morbidity, in that the forehead often requires a skin graft for closure. For this reason, the scalping flap has been supplanted by single-stage myocutaneous, fascial, and free flaps for the reconstruction of extensive cheek defects. Similarly, the Washio flap (35), which provides thin, nonhair-bearing retroauricular skin based on the superficial temporal vessels, is a two-stage method that is no longer much used in cheek reconstruction. However, it may remain a viable option in specific instances (e.g., in young women where hidden donor-site incisions may outweigh other considerations).

The temporoparietal fascial flap is also based on the superficial temporal vessels. Lying immediately below the temporal scalp, this flap is broad and well vascularized. It is normally harvested as a fascial flap alone and covered with a skin graft, although hair-bearing scalp may also be included. Because of the ease of its harvest and transposition, it has become a common method for single-stage reconstruction of the ear and orbit as well as the cheek (36,37). It is particularly applicable for coverage of defects of the parotid bed following composite parotidectomy to cover and protect exposed facial nerve branches when the superficial temporal vessels are intact (38). Finally, the temporalis muscle may also be transposed to fill cheek defects (39). It is vascularized by temporal branches of the internal maxillary artery. It is generally chosen when the cheek defect requires a bulky flap; however, its transposition leaves a significant hollow of the temporal fossa that often de-

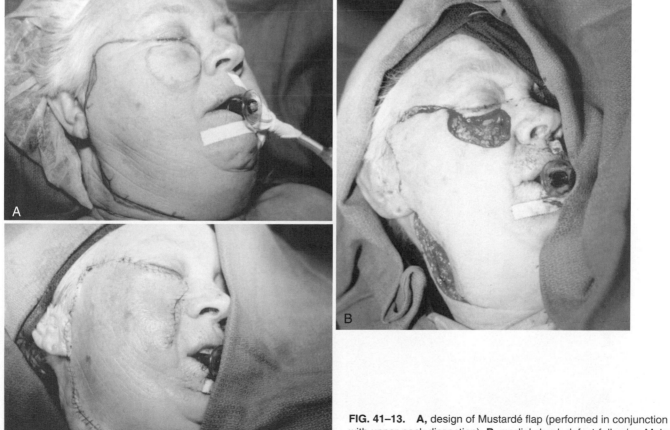

FIG. 41–13. **A,** design of Mustardé flap (performed in conjunction with upper-neck dissection). **B,** medial cheek defect following Mohs surgery for malignant melanoma. **C,** following repair by Mustarde flap.

FIG. 41–14. **A,** a squamous cell carcinoma in cyst. **B,** the defect after inadequate resection. **C,** a cervicopectoral flap is raised. **D,** the final result.

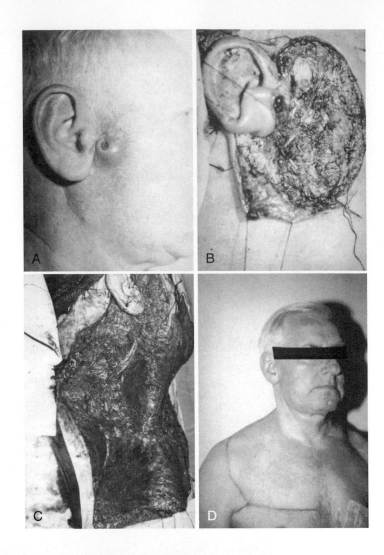

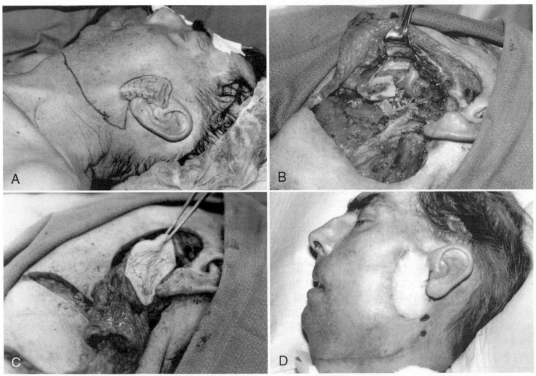

FIG. 41–15. **A,** planned incisions for radical parotidectomy and neck dissection for recurrent carcinoma of parotid. **B,** defect following radical parotidectomy and neck dissection. **C,** transposition of pectoralis major myocutaneous flap into defect. **D,** appearance following reconstruction.

mands secondary reconstruction. It is more often used in cases of facial reanimation than for coverage.

Pectoralis Major Myocutaneous Flap

The pectoralis major myocutaneous flap has supplanted the deltopectoral flap as a workhorse for head and neck reconstruction. This is because of its constant, reliable blood supply (thoracoacromial artery), proximity to the head and neck, and convenience of harvesting the flap with the patient in the supine position (40). It is utilized for many types of defects of the head and neck, including extensive cheek wounds. Its skin paddle is generally designed over the inferomedial aspect of the pectoralis major muscle (i.e., inferomedial to the nipple. The arc of rotation and vascularity reliably allows coverage of defects only as high as the zygomatic arch (Fig. 41–15), although its use in orbital reconstruction has also been described (41). When used for full-thickness defects of the medial cheek, the skin paddle is usually the intraoral component. The cutaneous coverage is then achieved by a skin graft applied to the pectoralis mus-

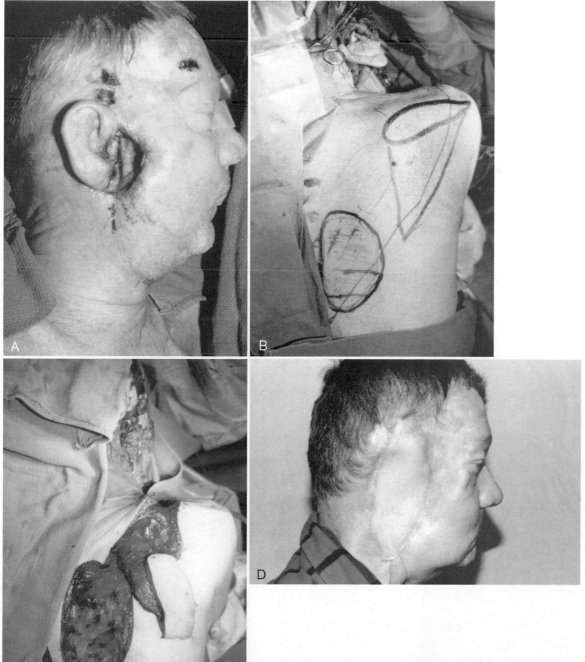

FIG. 41–16. **A,** recurrent carcinoma of parotid following prior resection and radiation therapy. Required radical parotidectomy and anterior skull base resection. **B,** design of trapezius myocutaneous flap. **C,** harvest of trapezius myocutaneous flap (note mobilization of muscle pedicle into root of neck). **D,** appearance following reconstruction.

cle itself or by a second flap such as a simultaneous ipsilateral deltopectoral flap.

Trapezius Flap

The blood supply of the trapezius myocutaneous flap is the transverse cervical artery. The skin paddle of the vertical flap is designed between the medial border of the scapula and the spine, no more than 5 cm below the scapular tip (42). It is generally used for lateral cheek defects when bulk as well as coverage are needed (Fig. 41–16). Full mobilization of the flap requires transection of the transverse fibers of the trapezius

above the spine of the scapula, leading to a shoulder drop. The transversese cervical artery allows the harvest of transversely oriented flap across the shoulder, during which muscle is included only in the proximal portion of the flap (43). With this variant, trapezius function can be preserved and the neck and lower cheek reconstructed with thin, well-vascularized skin.

Sternomastoid Flap

The sternomastoid myocutaneous flap was one of the first myocutaneous flaps described, but it was unrecognized as such at first presentation in 1949 (44). Its blood supply has

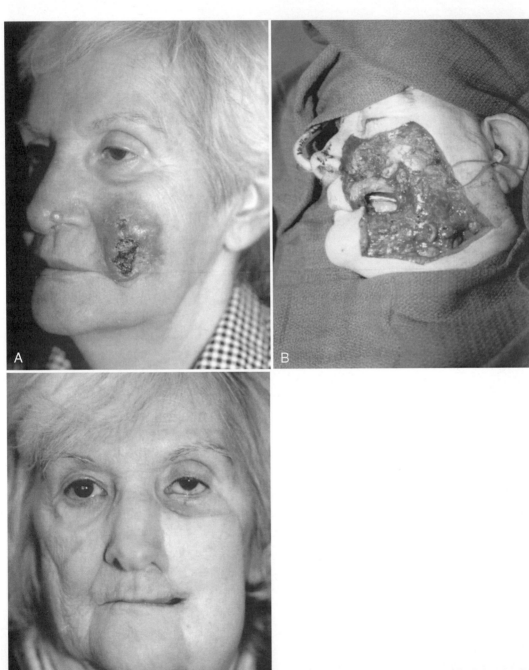

FIG. 41–17. **A,** squamous cell carcinoma involving full thickness of left cheek. **B,** following resection including commissure and oral mucosa. **C,** postoperative result following reconstruction with parascapular free flap (intra-oral portion of flap was covered with a skin graft to restore oral lining).

been documented by Jabaley and colleagues (45). It is not a first choice for soft-tissue repair of the cheek.

Platysma Flap

This flap is well described (46) and can be employed for coverage near the commissure or intraorally over the jaw. For these purposes, it is based superiorly upon the facial vessels and can provide a significant amount of well-vascularized skin for medial cheek reconstruction.

Free (Microvascular) Flaps

Despite the need for microsurgical techniques, free flaps often represent the best choice for the reconstruction of extensive defects of the cheek. Examples include wounds that require the importation of vascularized bone, muscle, or nerve in addition to cutaneous coverage, or wounds with complex three-dimensional requirements such as those of the midface. In these cases, free flaps may offer the best opportunity for definitive repair. In addition, in some patients free flaps may be necessary to salvage earlier failures with pedicled-flap techniques. Finally, in many instances free flaps offer less donor-site morbidity than local or distant pedicled flaps. When available, the facial artery and external jugular vein are most often first choice as recipient vessels. Commonly used free flaps in cheek reconstruction include the radial forearm flap for moderate-sized cutaneous defects (47), subscapular system free flaps for extensive cutaneous (Fig. 41–17) or complex midface defects (48) and free rectus abdominus muscle flaps (49) for full-thickness defects of the cheek. One drawback shared by all is the distinct color disparity between most distant flaps, which are light in color when compared to the reddish-hued cheek.

Acknowledgement

Surgery illustrated in Figures 41–13, 41–15, and 41–16 was performed under the direction of John C. Coleman III.

Bibliography

1. Spira M, Hardy SB. Vermilionectomy: review of cases with variations is techniques. *Plast Reconstr Surg* 1964; 33:39.
2. Birt BD. The "lip shave" operation for premalignant conditions and microinvasive carcinoma of the lower lip. *J Otolaryngol* 1977; 6:407.
3. Goldstein MH. A tissue-expanding vermilion myocutaneous flap for lip repair. *Plast Reconstr Surg* 1984; 73:768.
4. Kazanjian VH, Roopenian A. The treatment of lip deformities resulting from electric burns. *Am J Surg* 1954; 88:884.
5. Converse JM. Technique of elongation of the oral fissure and restoration of the angle of the mouth. In: Kazanjian VH, Converse JM, eds. *The surgical treatment of facial injuries.* Baltimore: Williams & Wilkins, 1959; 795.
6. Czerepak CS. Oral splint therapy to manage electrical burns of the mouth in children. *Clin Plast Surg* 1984; 11:685.
7. Zisser G. A contribution to the primary reconstruction of the upper lip and labial commissure following tumor excision. *J Maxillofac Surg* 1975; 3:211.
8. Fries R. Advantage of a basic concept in lip reconstruction after tumor resection. *J Maxillofac Surg* 1973; 1:13.
9. Madden JJ Jr, Erhardt WL Jr, Franklin JD, et al. Reconstruction of the upper and lower lip using a modified Bernard-Burrow technique. *Ann Plast Surg* 1980; 5:100.
10. Gillies H, Millard DR Jr. *The principles and art of plastic surgery.* Boston: Little, Brown, 1959; 117.
11. Rea JL, Davis WE, Rittenhouse LK. Reinnervation of an Abbé-Estlander and a Gillies fan flap of the lower lip. *Arch Otolaryngol* 1978; 104:294.
12. Kawamoto HK Jr. Correction of major defects of the vermilion with a cross-lip vermilion flap. *Plast Reconstr Surg* 1979; 64:315.
13. Abbé R. A new plastic operation for the relief of deformity due to double harelip. Med Rec 1898; 53:477.
14. Fukuta K, Potparic Z, Sugihara T, et al. A cadaver investigation of the blood supply of the galeal frontalis flap. *Plast Reconstr Surg* 1994; 94:794.
15. Burget GC, Menick FJ. Aesthetic restoration of one half the upper lip. *Plast Reconstr Surg* 1986; 78:583.
16. Meyer R, Abul Failat AS. *New concepts in lower lip reconstruction. Head Neck Surg* 1982; 4:240.
17. Webster JP. Crescentic peri-alar cheek excision for upper lip flap advancement with a short history of upper lip repair. *Plast Reconstr Surg* 1955; 16:434.
18. Jabaley ME, Clement RL, and Orcutt TW. Myocutaneous flaps in lip reconstruction: applications of the Karapandzic principle. *Plast Reconstr Surg* 1977; 59:680.
19. Jackson IT, Adham MN, Marsh WR. Use of galeo-frontalis myofascial flap in craniofacial surgery. *Plast Reconstr Surg* 1986; 77:905.
20. Jackson IT, Marsh WR, Bite U, et al. Craniofacial osteotomies to facilitate skull base tumor resection. *Br J Plast Surg* 1986; 39:153.
21. Jackson IT. Neurofibromatosis of the skull base. In: John Persing, ed. *Clinics in plastic surgery,* Vol. 22, No. 3. 1995; 513–530.
22. Sakai S, Soeda S, Endo T, et al. A compound radial artery forearm flap for the reconstruction of lip and chin defects. *Br J Plast Surg* 1989; 42:337.
23. Furuta S, Hataya Y, Watanabe T. Vermilionplasty using medical tattooing after radial forearm flap reconstruction of the lower lip. *Br J Plast Surg* 1994; 47:422.
24. Sasaki GH, Pang CY. Pathophysiology of skin flaps raised on expanded pig skin. *Plast Reconstr Surg* 1984; 74:59.
25. Manders EK, Schenden MJ, Furrey JA, et al. Soft-tissue expansion: concepts and complications. *Plast Reconstr Surg* 1984; 74:493.
26. Zovickian A. Pharyngeal fistulas: repair and prevention using mastoid-occiput based–shoulder flaps. *Plast Reconstr Surg* 1957; 19:355.
27. Gonzalez-Ulloa M, et al. Preliminary study of the total restoration of the facial skin. *Plast Reconstr Surg* 1954; 13:151.
28. Mustardé JC. *Repair and reconstruction in the orbital region. A practical guide.* Baltimore: Williams & Wilkins, 1966.
29. Juri J and Juri C. Advancement and rotation of a large cervicofacial flap for cheek repairs. *Plast Reconstr Surg* 1979; 64:692.
30. Crow ML and Crow FJ. Resurfacing large cheek defects with rotation flaps from the neck. *Plast Reconstr Surg* 1976; 58:196.
31. Janecka IP. Selected surgical approaches to the skull base. Procedures in cranial base surgery. *Problems in Plastic and Reconstructive Surgery* 1993; 3:224–244.
32. Becker DW. A cervicopectoral rotation flap for cheek coverage. *Plast Reconstr Surg* 1978; 61:868.
33. Converse JM. New forehead flap for nasal reconstruction. *Proc R Soc Med* 1942; 35:811.
34. Edington H, Ramasastry S. Microvascular flap transfer in cranial base surgery. Procedures in cranial base surgery. *Problems in Plastic and Reconstructive Surgery* 1993; 3:207–223.
35. Goepfert H, Cangir A, Lee Y-Y. Chemotherapy for aggressive juvenile nasopharyngeal aniofibroma. *Arch Otolaryngol* 1985; 111:285–289.
36. Avelar JM, Psillakis J. The use of galea flaps in craniofacial deformities. *Ann Plastic Surg* 1981; 6:464.
37. Horowitz JH, Persing JA, Nichter LS, et al. Galeal–pericranial flaps in head and neck reconstruction: anatomy and application. *Am J Surg* 1984; 148:489.
38. Sultan MR, Wider TM, Hugo NE. Frey syndrome: prevention with temporoparietal fascial flap interposition. *Ann Plast Surg* 1995; 34:292.
39. McGregor IA, Reid WH. The use of the temporal flap in primary repair of full-thickness defects of the cheek. *Plast Reconstr Surg* 1966; 38:1.
40. Ariyan S. The pectoralis major myocutaneous flap: a versatile flap for reconstruction in head and neck. *Plast Reconstr Surg* 1979; 63:73.
41. Ariyan S. The pectoralis major for single stage reconstruction of the difficult wound of the orbit and paryngoesophagus. *Plast Reconstr Surg* 1983; 72:468.
42. McGraw JB, Magee WP, Kalwaic H. Use of the trapezius and sternomastoid myocutaneous flaps in head and neck surgery. *Plast Reconstr Surg* 1979; 63:49.

43. Guillamondegui OM, Larson DL. The lateral trapezius musculocutaneous flap: its use in head and neck reconstruction. *Plast Reconstr Surg* 1981; 67:143.

44. Owens N. A compound neck pedicle designed for the repair of massive facial defects: formation, development, and application. *Plast Reconstr Surg* 1955; 15:369.

45. Jabaley ME, Heckler FR, Wallace WH, et al. Sternocleidomastoid regional flaps, a new look at an old concept. *Br J Plast Surg* 1979; 32:106.

46. Coleman JJ III, Jurkiewicz MJ, Nahai F, et al. The platysma musculocutaneous flap: experience with 24 cases. *Plast Reconstr Surg* 1983; 72:315.

47. Furuta S, Sakaguchi Y, Iwasawa M, et al. Reconstruction of the lips, oral commissure, and full-thickness cheek with a composite radial forearm palmaris longus free flap. *Ann Plast Surg* 1994; 33:544.

48. Coleman JJ III, Sultan MR. The bipedicled osteocutaneous scapula flap: a new subscapular system free flap. *Plast Reconstr Surg* 1991; 87:682.

49. Meland NB, Fisher J, Irons GB, et al. Experience with 80 rectus abdominus free-tissue transfers. *Plast Reconstr Surg* 1989; 83:482.

42

Reconstruction of the Nose

Frederick J. Menick, M.D.

Anatomically, the nose is covered by a thin vascular skin envelope which matches the face in color and texture. It is supported by a delicate three-dimensional framework of hard and soft tissues that are nourished by highly vascularized cover and lining layers. It is lined by thin and supple stratified squamous epithelium and mucous membrane. Visually, the nose is a highly contoured three-dimensional landmark in the central face. Seen in all facial views, the nose is normally balanced and symmetric. If part is missing, the remaining contralateral normal stands as a critical comparison to surgical reconstruction.

Historically, the reconstructive emphasis has been on the replacement of tissue loss in anatomic layers (cover, lining, and support) and on the technical aspects of tissue transfers (grafts or flaps) (1,2,3). Unfortunately, the final result often appeared as a patch outlined by constricting scar, neither blending into the residual nose nor matching the contralateral normal side. The subtle three-dimensional landmarks of the normal nose were rarely recreated. Multiple late revisions were often planned, but rarely undertaken or, if undertaken, successful.

Well vascularized and lying adjacent to the nose, the forehead has been acknowledged as the best donor site for nasal reconstruction because of its superb color and texture match (4). The earliest reconstructions used an unlined forehead flap to rebuild the nose. The classic Indian flap carried midline tissue on paired supraorbital and supratrochlear vessels. However, its base lay at or above the eyebrows, shortening its reach and limiting its length. Until recently there has been a trend away from the midline forehead flap. Because surgeons used it for both cover and lining (by folding its distal end onto itself, thus creating its own inside and outside) or employed forehead skin not only for nasal reconstruction but also for adjacent cheek and lip defects, many felt that the midline forehead flap was inadequate for major reconstructions. A number of variations were designed solely to provide additional length. Perhaps the most widely employed was the Converse "scalping" flap, which transferred lateral forehead skin on a long pedicle of hair-bearing scalp (5,6). Unfortunately, the transfer of greater amounts of forehead skin did not necessarily improve the results of nasal reconstruction, but it did worsen the forehead deformity. Despite poor skin color and quality, some surgeons transferred distant tissue in stages, or by microvascular anastomosis for nasal cover (7,8). Others used tissue expansion to increase the quantity of available forehead skin (9,10). This changed the skin texture and thickness and added unpredictable skin shrinkage to the reconstructive problem.

Traditionally, lining had been supplied by folding the distal covering flap upon itself, by hinging over adjacent skin based on scar along the wound edge, by the use of a secondary flap (a second forehead flap or a nasolabial flap), or by the preliminary placement of a chondrocutaneous or chondromucosal graft (11–13). Unfortunately, each method provided lining that was thick, stiff, and avascular. The external nasal shape became distorted and the airway crowded.

It also became obvious that without a skeletal framework, the soft tissue of lining and cover collapsed, impairing the airway and limiting projection. A rigid skeleton was needed to provide support and nasal contour (14). However, most lining methods precluded its placement because of the risk of necrosis, infection, and extrusion. Bulky and shapeless support grafts were sometimes placed secondarily. However, once gravity and the contractual effects of the healing process had distorted the nasal contour, the constricted and stiff covering skin was fixed by a scar. Multiple late revisions were required to sculpt subcutaneous tissue in an attempt to improve the result.

Principles of Aesthetic Nasal Restoration

REGIONAL FACIAL UNITS

The face can be divided into adjacent regions, each with its own characteristic skin color, texture, skin thickness, hair quality, and surface contour (15–18). The surface of the nose is made up of concave and convex surfaces separated from one another by ridges and valleys. The nose is a major facial unit and its smaller parts can be considered topographic subunits (Fig. 42–1). The surface of the nose, separated by slightly convex or concave surfaces, can be divided into the subunits of the tip, dorsum, paired sidewalls, alar lobules, and soft triangles. Nasal units are covered by skin with specific color, texture, and thickness. Each unit has specific contours determined by underlying soft and hard tissue. If a part of the nose is missing, the unique characteristics of the subunit must be restored (19,20). An aesthetic subunit reconstruction emphasizes:

1. The replacement of missing cover with skin that matches the nose in quality and is replaced in exact dimension. The nose is resurfaced precisely in quality and quantity.
2. A subsurface architecture of primary cartilage grafts is positioned to reestablish a nasal shape, to support the soft tissues, and to brace the reconstruction against the contractile effects of wound healing.

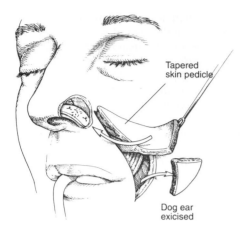

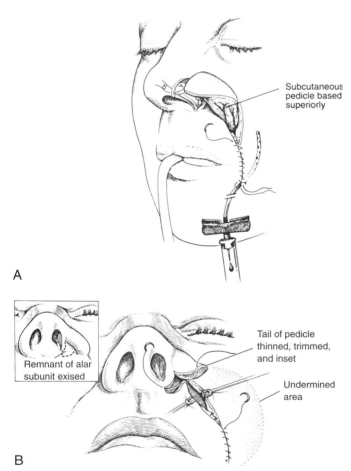

FIG. 42–3. Design of the two-stage nasolabial flap for subunit alar reconstruction. (From Burget GC, Menick FJ. *Aesthetic reconstruction of the nose.* St. Louis: Mosby–Year Book, 1994).

A three-dimensional pattern of the surface defect is used as a template for a two-dimensional design for the forehead flap. Most often the defect will be enlarged so that the skin loss conforms to a regional topographic subunit. This may require discarding residual normal adjacent skin. The contralateral normal nose, or the ideal, is used to design the pattern. The missing skin is replaced exactly. The pattern is flattened and placed at the hairline directly above the medial eyebrow frown crease, which overlies the branches of the supratrochlear vessels. The proximal two-thirds of the flap and its base are narrow, while the upper third rapidly widens to encompass the exact pattern of the missing subunits. The base of the flap is only 1.2 to 1.5 cm wide. The arc of rotation can be increased by extending the base inferiorly across the supraorbital rim or by positioning the distal columella replacement superiorly within the hair bearing skin of the scalp. Distally, the flap is elevated superficial to the frontalis muscle, allowing individual hair follicles to be coagulated and clipped from behind. Proximally, the frontalis muscle is included with the pedicle to protect the axial vessels. This thin flap is sutured over the nasal cartilage framework and will exactly replace the nasal tip, dorsum, and alar skin, as needed.

The forehead donor site is closed by undermining laterally at the subfrontalis level and advancing tissues medially. The lower forehead is easily approximated in layers, but a defect may remain below the hairline. If a gap remains superiorly, it is left to heal secondarily. At 3 weeks the pedicle is transected. The proximal stump is thinned and inset as a small inverted V just medial to the eyebrow. The flap inset is reelevated to within 1.5 to 2 cm of the alar rim. Excessive frontalis muscle, subcutaneous tissue and scar is then excised, sculpting a nasal shape, and the distal flap is trimmed to fit the defect and inset.

In some major nasal reconstructions, because wound contraction can cause unpredictable contour changes or shifting of cartilage grafts, it is useful to delay final pedicle division. In these cases, once the forehead flap, cartilage framework, and lining flaps become stable after 3 weeks, the forehead flap can be lifted from most of its inset except along the ala rim and columella. The underlying subcutaneous tissue, frontalis muscle, and scar is sculpted and additional cartilage grafts added as needed. The flap is then sutured back to its bed and its pedicle finally divided after an additional 3 weeks (6 weeks after beginning the reconstruction). Such early soft-tissue sculpturing helps create the aesthetic contour of the alar crease and nasal sidewall, and greatly lessens the need for multiple late operative revisions. This intermediate operation to sculpt the reconstruction is especially useful in smokers.

Nasal Support: Primary Cartilage Grafts

The reestablishment of a nasal framework recreates support, nasal projection, airway patency, and the expected nasal contours (44,45). Primary cartilage grafts should be positioned to replace missing tip, lateral sidewall, and septal support. Additionally a strip of cartilage must be placed along a new nostril margin, even though the alar lobule normally contains no cartilage. This braces the ala rim, preventing constriction, contraction, and collapse during the healing phase.

Cartilage grafts depend on lining for vascularization; lining depends on a cartilage graft for support and contour.

across the superior orbital rim near the midline of the forehead. They lie deep within the frontalis and corrugator muscles and then rapidly enter the subcutaneous tissue until they lie below the dermis within the subcutaneous fat near the hairline. This permits the flap to be thinned to the thickness of the nasal skin.

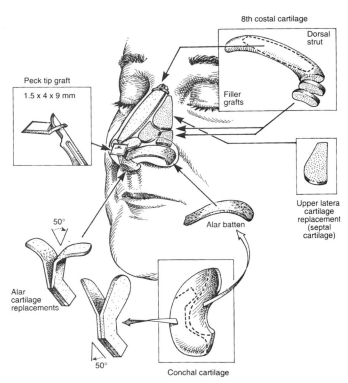

FIG. 42–4. Subunit subsurface primary support grafts. (From Burget GC, Menick FJ. *Aesthetic reconstruction of the nose.* St. Louis: Mosby–Year Book, 1994).

They should be used simultaneously. Nasal support is best supplied at the time of soft-tissue lining and cover construction. Secondary replacement never regains what has been lost to soft-tissue scarring. Septal or conchal cartilage, rib osseo-cartilaginous or cartilage grafts, or occasionally cranial bone can be shaped to reform a replacement for the alar cartilages, upper lateral cartilage, or dorsal support. A batten of cartilage should be fastened along the cartilage of the lining sleeve from the alar base to the nostril apex. This fixes the new ala rim in position and creates a normal bulging contour to the alar lobule (Fig. 42–4).

Restoration of Nasal Lining

In the past, lining has been provided by (a) turning in flaps of local nasal skin hinged on scar along the wound margin, (b) folding the end of a cover flap so that it lines itself, (c) using a second flap for lining (a nasolabial flap or a second forehead flap), or (d) grafting a cover flap on the forehead before transfer (46–53). Unfortunately such techniques do not provide a lining vascular reliable enough to support primary cartilage grafts. They are also thick and stiff, and rarely allow the recreation of a nasal shape. Only lining flap from intranasal donor sites (i.e., the vestibule, the middle vault, and the septum) are thin and supple. They are also vascular enough to nourish primary cartilage grafts and soft enough to conform to the shape of a cartilage framework.

The Septal Flap

The arterial supply of the nasal septum arrives anterior-superior from the ethmoid artery and anterior-inferior through the upper lip. Arising from the facial artery, the superior labial

artery winds through the orbicularis oris muscle at the level of the vermillion border and then ascends lateral to the philtrum to give off the septal branch that enters the nasal septum lateral to the nasal spine. A unilateral or bilateral flap of septal mucoperichondrium with or without a cartilage component will survive if based on a 1.3-mm pedicle located between the anterior plane of the upper lip and the lower edge of the pyriform aperture (38). Such septal flaps may extend from the nasal floor below to the level of medial canthi above and posteriorly beyond the ethmoid perpendicular plate. A unilateral mucoperichondrial flap based either on the right or left superior labial artery can be transposed laterally to replace missing lining for the vestibule or lateral sidewall. It can be used in combination with a bipedicle flap of vestibular skin, based medially on the nasal septum and laterally on the nasal floor. It may also be used in combination with the contralateral mucoperichondrial flap based on the dorsum of the septum, which is hinged laterally to line the sidewall of the mid and upper vault (Kazanjian technique). The entire septum may also be used as a composite chondro mucosal flap lined by the two leaves of septal mucous membrane and based on the septal branches of both the right and left labial arteries. This composite flap of lining and support can be pivoted anteriorly to supply support and lining to the vestibule, tip, and columella; for the middle and upper vaults; or for the entire nasal dorsum in cases of total nasal reconstruction (Fig. 42–5).

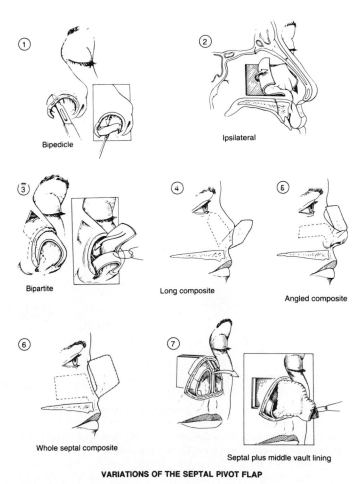

VARIATIONS OF THE SEPTAL PIVOT FLAP

FIG. 42–5. Intranasal lining options. (From Burget GC, Menick FJ. *Aesthetic reconstruction of the nose.* St. Louis: Mosby–Year Book, 1994).

Replacement of Ala and Lateral Sidewall Lining

When full-thickness defects occupy the nostril margin, vestibular skin and mucous membrane remain above the upper border of the defect. Such tissue is available as a bipedicle flap of vestibular skin or nasal mucosa 7 to 10 mm wide, designed just superior to the defect. The flap is based medially on the nasal septum and laterally on the nasal floor. If residual elements of alar cartilage remain, it may be necessary to incise the junction of the median and lateral crus so that the flap of vestibular skin and alar cartilage can move caudally to the level of the new nostril margin. A secondary lining defect persists above the nostril margin flap. The ipsilateral septum mucoperichondrium in incised as an inverted L and reflected. Septal cartilage and bone are removed as an in a submucous resection (SMR) and are used for cartilage graft material. An L-shaped septal strut is preserved. The contralateral mucosa is incised along three sides, but kept intact dorsally. It is transposed laterally across the airway to line the upper vault and is sutured inferiorly to the vestibular flap. The ipsilateral septal mucosal flap is repositioned to restore the septal partition, but frequently a fistula persists. Alternatively, the sidewall lining defect can be supplied by an ipsilateral septal mucous membrane flap. The mucoperichondrium of the ipsilateral septum is elevated. It is incised on all three borders, but left attached by a pedicle based on the zone of the superior labial artery in the region of the nasal spine. The ipsilateral septal flap is bent laterally and sutured to the remaining lining defect in the lateral midvault above the bipedicle vestibular flap.

HEMINASAL DEFECTS

In heminasal defects, the tissue loss extends superiorly towards the nasal bone (Fig. 42–6A-K). Residual vestibular skin is not available, so a bipedicle flap cannot be employed. In such cases an ipsilateral septal mucous membrane flap

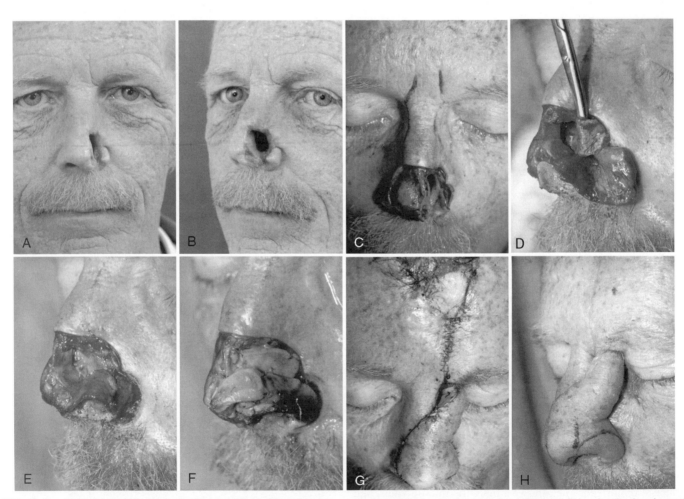

FIG. 42–6.   A, B, preoperative defect of the tip, left ala, and sidewall after tumor excision. **C,** residual normal skin within the left ala and tip are discarded to recreate a subunit defect of the entire tip and ala. **D,** an ipsilateral septal flap based on the septal branch of the superior labial artery is elevated to line the reconstructed ala. A contralateral septal flap based on the dorsal branch of the anterior ethmoid artery is swung across the airway to line the superior defect in the sidewall area. **E,** the ipsilateral and contralateral flaps are sutured together to create a highly supple, vascular, intranasal lining for the hemi nasal defect. **F,** primary cartilage grafts of ear and septal cartilage are fabricated to shape and support the ala, tip, and sidewall. **G,** a paramedian forehead flap is elevated to resurface the tip, left ala, and sidewall. The superior gap in the forehead, which remained after partial closure, was covered with Vaseline gauze and allowed to heal secondarily. **H,** three weeks later, the outline of expected subunits is drawn.

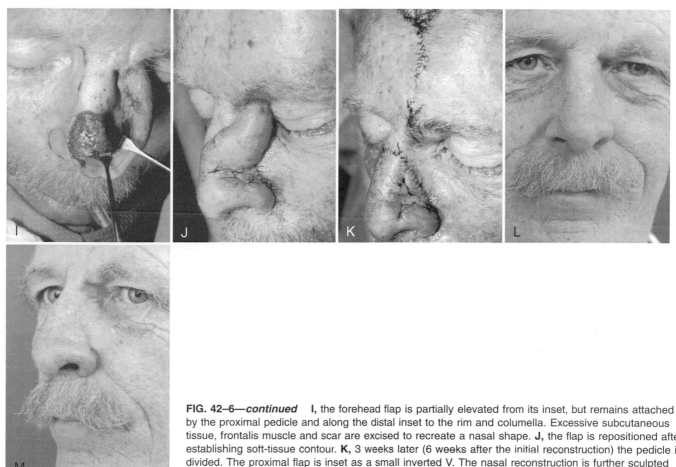

FIG. 42–6—*continued* **I,** the forehead flap is partially elevated from its inset, but remains attached by the proximal pedicle and along the distal inset to the rim and columella. Excessive subcutaneous tissue, frontalis muscle and scar are excised to recreate a nasal shape. **J,** the flap is repositioned after establishing soft-tissue contour. **K,** 3 weeks later (6 weeks after the initial reconstruction) the pedicle is divided. The proximal flap is inset as a small inverted V. The nasal reconstruction is further sculpted and the flap inset completed. **L,** the result at 6 months without further revision.

based on the ipsilateral superior labial artery can be transposed laterally to provide lining to the proposed ala rim. The sidewall defect that exists above this first flap is filled with a contralateral septal mucous membrane flap, vascularized dorsally on the anterior ethmoid vessels. A permanent septal fistula remains. This is usually asymptomatic.

CENTRAL NASAL DEFECTS

In central nasal defects when the tip and dorsum are missing, residual septal lining and support usually remains available within the residual septum in the pyriform aperture. A long, full-thickness septal flap can be incised along three borders and pivoted from the septal donor site to provide support and lining for the columella and tip of the nose. Its base is centered in the region of the nasal spine and upper lip, containing the septal branches of both superior labial arteries. Such a flap may extend from the nasal floor below to the medial canthi above and posteriorly behind the ethmoid perpendicular plate. Depending on the requirements of the defect, it may be used to reconstruct the tip or the entire dorsum. To allow easy rotation, the septal leaves must be gently separated above the nasal spine and the mucoperichondrium elevated with a Freer elevator. A strip of septal cartilage a few millimeters wide is then resected from the cartilaginous base of the flap between the soft-tissue perichondrial flap. This permits the flap to rotate up and out.

Vascularity through the soft tissues of the mucoperichondrium remains unaltered.

In all cases, septal, conchal or rib cartilage is harvested and fabricated into the necessary components of struts, buttresses, battens, and braces required to reconstruct nasal support and shape. Once the lining is positioned and sutured together, cartilage grafts are sutured to the underlying raw surface of the lining flaps. The lining flaps vascularize the primary cartilage grafts while the cartilage grafts give shape and support to the underlying lining flaps. A forehead flap supplies covering skin (54).

Bibliography

1. McDowell F, Valone JA, Brown JB. Bibliography and historical note on plastic surgery of the nose. *Plast Reconstr Surg* 1952; 10:149.
2. Gillies HD. Plastic surgery of the face. London: Oxford University Press, 1920; 224.
3. Gillies HD, Millard DR Jr. The principles and art of plastic surgery. Boston: Little, Brown, 1957; 576.
4. Converse JM, ed. Reconstructive plastic surgery. 2nd ed. Philadelphia: Saunders, 1977.
5. Converse JM. Reconstruction of the nose by the scalping flap technique. *Surg Clin North Am* 1959; 39:335.
6. Converse JM. Clinical applications of the scalping flap in reconstruction of the nose. *Plast Reconstr Surg* 1969; 43:247.
7. Miller TA. The Tagliacozzi flap as a method of nasal and palatal reconstruction. *Plast Reconstr Surg* 1985; 76:870.
8. Washio H. Retroauricular temporal flap. *Plast Reconstr Surg* 1969; 43:162.

9. Kroll SS. Forehead flap nasal reconstruction with tissue expansion and delayed pedicle separation. *Laryngoscope* 1989; 99:448.

10. Adamson JE. Nasal reconstruction with the expanded forehead flap. *Plast Reconstr Surg* 1988; 81:12.

11. Converse JM. Composite graft from the septum in nasal reconstruction. *Trans Lat Am Congr Plast Surg* 1956; 8:281.

12. Barton FE Jr. Aesthetic aspects of nasal reconstruction. *Clin Plast Surg* 1988; 15:155–166.

13. Barton FE. Aesthetic aspects of partial nasal reconstruction. *Clin Plast Surg* 1981; 8:177.

14. Wheeler ES, Kawamoto HK, Zarem HA. Bone grafts for nasal reconstruction. *Plast Reconstr Surg* 1982; 69:9.

15. Gonzalez-Ulloa M. Restoration of the face covering by means of selected skin in regional aesthetic units. *Br J Plast Surg* 1956; 9:212.

16. Burget GC, Menick FJ. Subunit principle in nasal reconstruction. *Plastic Reconstr Surg* 1985; 76:239.

17. Burget GC, Menick FJ. Restoration of nasal defects: an aesthetic viewpoint. In: Jurkiewicz M, Krizek T, eds. Plastic surgery: principles and practice. St. Louis: Mosby–Year Book, 1990.

18. Get GC, Menick FJ. Restoration of the nose after skin cancer. In: Reilly T, ed. Plastic surgery educational foundation: instructional courses. Vol 1. St. Louis: Mosby–Year Book, 1988.

19. Menick F. Artistry in facial surgery: aesthetic perceptions and the subunit principle. In: Furnas D, ed. Clinics in plastic surgery. Vol 14. Philadelphia: WB Saunders, 1987.

20. Menick FJ. Aesthetic restoration of the face. In: Cohen M, ed. Problems in general surgery. Philadelphia: JB Lippincott, 1989.

21. Menick FJ. Principles of head and neck reconstruction. In: Cohen M, ed.

22. Menick FJ, Burget GC. Aesthetic reconstruction of the nose. In: Cohen M, ed. Mastery of plastic and reconstructive surgery. Boston: Little, Brown, 1994.

23. Menick FJ, Burget GC. Nasal reconstruction: creating a visual illusion. In: Habal M, ed. Advances in Plastic Surgery. Vol. 6. St. Louis: Mosby–Year Book, 1989.

24. McGregor JC, Soutar DS. A critical assessment of the bilobed flap. *Br J Plast Surg* 1981; 34:197.

25. Zimany A. The bilobed flap. *Plast Reconstr Surg* 1953; 11:424.

26. Zitelli JA. The bilobed flap for nasal reconstruction. *Arch Dermatol* 1989; 125:957.

27. Lister GO, Gibson T. Closure of rhomboid skin defects: the flaps of Limberg and Dufourmentel. *Br J Plast Surg* 1972; 25:300.

28. Rieger RA. A local flap for repair of the nasal tip. *Plast Reconstr Surg* 1967; 40:147.

29. Lipshutz H, Penrod DS. Use of complete transverse nasal flap in repair of small defects of the nose. *Plast Reconstr Surg* 1972; 49:629.

30. Rigg BM. The dorsal nasal flap. *Plast Reconstr Surg* 1973; 52:361.

31. Marchac D, Toth B. The axial frontonasal flap revisited. *Plast Reconstr Surg* 1985; 76:686.

32. Rieger RA. A local flap for repair of the nasal tip. *Plast Reconstr Surg* 1967; 40:147.

33. Elliott RA Jr. Rotation flaps of the nose. *Plast Reconstr Surg* 1956; 17:444.

34. Staahl TE. Nasalis myocutaneous flap for nasal reconstruction. *Arch Otolaryngol Head Neck Surg* 1986; 112:302.

35. Rybka FJ. Reconstruction of the nasal tip using nasalis myocutaneous sliding flaps. *Plast Reconstr Surg* 1983; 71:40.

36. Spear SL, Kroll SS, Romm S. A new twist to the nasolabial flap for reconstruction of lateral alar defects. *Plast Reconstr Surg* 1987; 79:915.

37. Barton FE Jr. The nasolabial flap. *Perspect Plast Surg* 1990; 3(2):69

38. Burget GC, Menick FJ. Aesthetic reconstruction of the nose. St. Louis: Mosby–Year Book, 1994.

39. Kazanjian VH. The repair of nasal defects with the median forehead flap: primary closure of forehead wound. *Surg Gynecol Obstet* 1946; 983:37.

40. Millard DR Jr. Hemirhinoplasty. *Plast Reconstr Surg* 1967; 40:440.

41. Millard DR Jr. Reconstructive rhinoplasty for the lower half of a nose. *Plast Reconstr Surg* 1974; 53:133.

42. Millard DR Jr. Reconstructive rhinoplasty for the lower two-thirds of the nose. *Plast Reconstr Surg* 1976; 57:722.

43. McCarthy JG, Lorenc PZ, Cutting C, et al. The median forehead flap revisited: the blood supply. *Plast Reconstr Surg* 1985; 76:866–869.

44. Burget GC, Menick FJ. Nasal reconstruction: seeking a fourth dimension. *Plastic Reconstr Surg* 1986; 78:145.

45. Burget GC, Menick FJ. Nasal support and lining: the marriage of beauty and blood supply. *Plastic Reconstr Surg* 1989; 84:189.

46. Barton FE Jr. Aesthetic aspects of partial nasal reconstruction. *Clin Plast Surg* 1981; 8:177.

47. Millard DR Jr. Aesthetic reconstructive rhinoplasty. *Clin Plastic Surg* 1981; 8:169.

48. Argamaso RV. An ideal donor site for the auricular composite graft. *Br J Plast Surg* 1975; 28:219.

49. Millard DR Jr. Various uses of the septum in rhinoplasty. *Plast Reconstr Surg* 1988; 81:112.

50. Millard DR. Hemirhinoplasty. *Plast Reconstr Surg* 1967; 40:440–445.

51. Millard DR. Total reconstructive rhinoplasty and a missing link. *Plast Reconstr Surg* 1966; 37:167.

52. Millard DR. Alar margin sculpturing. *Plast Reconstr Surg* 1967; 40:337–342.

53. Millard DR. Aesthetic reconstructive rhinoplasty. *Clin Plastic Surg* 1981; 8:169.

54. Menick FJ. The aesthetic use of the forehead for nasal reconstruction—the paramedian forehead flaps. In: Tobin G, ed. *Clinics in plastic surgery*. Philadelphia: WB Saunders, 1990.

43

Reconstruction of Eyelid Deformities

James H. Carraway, M.D., F.A.C.S., Michael P. Vincent, M.D., F.A.C.S., and Craig Rubinstein, M.B.M.S., F.R.A.C.S.

Aims of Reconstruction

The eyelids frame the eyes, the focal points of the face. Their primary function is to protect the fragile and sensitive underlying conjunctiva and sclera of the globe. Protection is from injury, including abrasion and desiccation, both awake and asleep. Reconstruction of the eyelids is therefore subject to both functional and aesthetic considerations.

Each lid is a complex, multilayered skin fold highly adapted to its function. The broader upper lid is mobile to provide retractable opaque coverage to the globe. The shorter lower lid is relatively rigid and less mobile to provide fixed protection to the lower globe.

Normal motion of the upper eyelid is responsible for wetting of the cornea. Tears secreted from the lacrimal gland mix with secretions from the accessory lacrimal glands of Zeis and Moll and the meibomian glands. This mixture lubricates the cornea with each blink of the upper lid. The lower lid also facilitates tear drainage into the inferior punctum. It acts as a funnel to the lacus lacrimalis in the medial canthal area and, with each blink, negative pressure in the canaliculi draws the tears from the eye into the lacrimal system. The inferior canalicular system serves as the primary source of drainage. In paralyzed or reconstructed eyelids, this pumping mechanism may be lost, resulting in epiphora (1).

In terms of reconstruction, the eyelids comprise three functional layers:

1. The outermost layer is composed of skin with scant subcutaneous tissue and, deep to this, the circularly oriented, striated, orbicularis muscle.
2. The middle lamella consists of the relatively rigid tarsus with enclosed meibomian glands.
3. The inner lining consists of thin, smooth, conjunctival epithelium.

Pathologic Etiology of Adult Eyelid Defects

Extensive tissue defects in the orbital and periorbital region can result from congenital disorders, radiation, tumor resection, or trauma. In the adult, eyelid reconstruction is usually secondary to tumor resection or trauma.

Malignant tumors are relatively uncommon, but may present a challenge in reconstruction after their ablation. Adequate primary excision of the tumor is imperative, particularly with regard to recurrent tumors. Adequate resection must be monitored by proficient pathologic evaluation of the resection specimen. Delayed reconstruction or the Moh technique may be indicated for difficult tumors.

Primary, well-defined basal cell carcinoma may be resected with a surgical margin of 1 to 2 mm, whereas a basal cell carcinoma that recurs after irradiation, cautery, or inadequate surgical excision must be more widely excised. Squamous cell carcinoma, melanoma, and other eyelid malignancies are far less common than basal cell carcinoma. These tumors may present a problem in determining how extensive the resection must be and, consequently, the requisite reconstruction. Judgment must be balanced between assuring surgical excision with adequate margins and the desire to conserve eyelid tissue. Considerations may also include the tumor's level of invasion, aggressiveness, and extent, and the patient's requests, medical condition, and age.

Benign tumors are usually less complicated in their removal and reconstruction.

General and Aesthetic Considerations

Considerations in eyelid reconstruction include the following principles:

1. Cosmetic considerations should not compromise the functional requirements.
2. The shape, level, symmetry, and motion of the lid need to be as close to normal as possible, even at the expense of some scarring. When they are not corrected it is obvious even at a distance, while scars are usually visible only at relatively close range.
3. The medial and lateral canthi should be symmetrical with the contralateral side. The lateral canthus is usually located just above the horizontal line, as drawn through the medial canthus.
4. The lower lid should be without notching or ectropion.
5. Scars should be placed in natural lid crease lines, or laterally in the crows' feet. Vertical scar lines may later contract, detracting from the aesthetic result by causing notching or ectropion. In the medial canthal area, horizontal incisions result in better scars than do vertical ones.
6. The skin used for reconstruction should match as closely as possible the thin and delicate eyelid skin. Skin grafts and flaps are therefore chosen based on close proximity, texture, and color match.
7. Excessive hollowing of the upper eyelid, bulging of the lower lid fat pad, or marked asymmetry in relation to the opposite lid, should also be corrected.
8. In addition to being functional and aesthetically acceptable, the reconstructed lid must be durable. If the stiff tarsal plate is missing or the orbicularis muscle is paralyzed or absent, then the lid quickly loses its stability.

These components must be incorporated into the reconstructed lid as muscle continuity or facial support for replacement of the orbicularis. Cartilage can be employed as a "stiffener" for replacement of the tarsal plate.

Tissue Loss

LACERATIONS WITH MINIMAL LOSS

Simple lacerations of the eyelid are common. Where there is minimal tissue loss, management the tissue edges should be minimally débrided and closed primarily without tension. Closure should be with accurate, layered alignment.

Primary closure can be used for defects of up to one-third of the original lid margin, especially in older patients with greater tissue laxity. Closure is performed by placing a 6-0 silk suture at the gray line, matching up the lid edge. An absorbable suture is used to close the tarsus, which brings the conjunctival edges together. If there is excessive tension, a lateral canthotomy may provide the necessary relaxation to allow closure. An incision is made horizontally from the lateral canthal angle, and dissection is carried down to the periosteum of the lateral orbital rim, severing the inferior crura of the lateral canthal tendon. Medial canthotomy is to be avoided because of risk to the lacrimal apparatus and risk of producing a telecanthus.

PARTIAL- OR FULL-THICKNESS LOSS

Replacing Skin: Skin Grafting

Skin grafting of the lower lid may be used to replace a skin deficit and may be combined with other techniques (e.g., a local flap) to replace complex defects. It is the most common method of reconstruction because it is relatively simple technically and there are numerous potential donor sites.

Selection of the proper donor site to match color and thickness is important. The most frequently selected donor sites are postauricular, upper eyelid, supraclavicular, and occasionally preauricular skin.

Postauricular skin is thin and supple, provides a good color match, and also gives relatively good support where needed (2). It is also sufficient in size to reconstruct a full lower eyelid. The total amount of this skin may be taken, including the entire hairless area (approximately 6 × 8 cm), and the donor site is covered by a split-thickness graft.

Upper eyelid skin is very thin and supple and is an excellent color match, but is limited in quantity and does not have the thickness to give good support. The donor area is limited if primary closure of the donor site is desired.

Grafts taken below the clavicle are generally a poor color match and are rarely used.

If the full-thickness graft is used on part of the upper lid as a patch or to cover a round defect, it is best to do a zigzag incision to prevent pin-cushioning. When reconstructing partial-thickness defects of the upper lid, remember that the pretarsal orbicularis muscle is responsible for lid closure and is preserved if possible.

Grafting an entire unit usually gives a better aesthetic result than a patchy-appearing graft. Unit grafting can be used to an even greater advantage in the lower eyelid by carrying the end of the graft in a sling fashion beyond the medial and lateral canthi.

The scar contraction of burns requires special mention. Overcorrection of the ectropion by 15 to 20% is preferred (3), to avoid recurrent ectropion that may occur with wound contraction (Fig. 43–1).

The upper lid, with its increased mobility and thinner skin, is less amenable to skin graft reconstruction than the lower lid. The contralateral upper eyelid skin is the most suitable donor area, followed by split-thickness grafts (full-thickness skin grafts from all other donor sites are often too bulky).

To prevent underestimating the amount of skin graft required, the size of the defect must be measured with the lid in fully closed position. Coverage of the entire upper lid is aesthetically desirable. Because of the mobility of the upper lid, bolus dressings should be maintained at least 6 to 7 days to minimize graft loss or wrinkling. During this time, an intermarginal tarsorrhaphy suture may be indicated. In the case of ectropion from scarring, or skin loss when the tarsal margin is stretched and excessive in length, a wedge tarsectomy

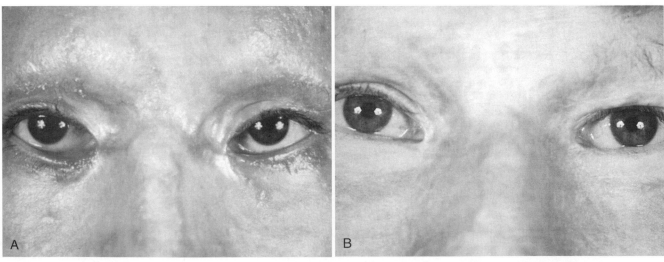

FIG. 43–1. **A,** bilateral burn scar ectropion and upper lid skin defect. **B,** postoperative resolution of skin shortage by full-thickness graft to lower and upper eyelids.

in addition to a full-thickness graft may be performed. A graft may then be placed directly over the suture line.

Technique

Tarsal resection is performed by placing a perpendicular cut in the tarsus approximately five millimeters from the lateral canthus. The two cut edges are overlapped to estimate the amount of lid resection necessary, and another perpendicular cut placed at the determined point of resection. Closure is performed by approximating the gray line with 6-0 silk and closing the tarsus with 6-0 chromic sutures. The muscle layer is then approximated with 6-0 chromic catgut.

Replacing Supporting Cartilage

It is unusual to require only supporting cartilage without mucosal coverage. A cartilage deficit nearly always implies a conjunctival deficit or a full-thickness deficit. These, respectively, require composite graft or flap reconstruction (see below). On the occasion that only supporting cartilage is needed without mucosal coverage, cartilage may be taken from the nasal septum in the same way a submucous resection is performed. Alternately, conchal cartilage may be used (4). The cartilage may then be thinned to an appropriate thickness so as to allow a subtle curvature. Once prepared, the cartilage graft is then sandwiched between the orbicularis muscle and the conjunctiva.

Replacing Conjunctival Lining

Defects less than 25% of the lid usually do not require formal conjunctival reconstruction, because they will epithelialize from adjacent conjunctiva. For other small defects of conjunctival lining, coverage may be restored by advancement of conjunctiva from the sulcus.

Defects larger than 25% of the lid usually require a free graft to make up for the loss of specialized tissue.

Conjunctiva harvested from another lid is the ideal match but is thin, difficult to handle, has a tendency to contract, and can only be harvested sparingly to avoid interfering with the donor fornices.

Oral mucosa is abundant and simple to remove but tends to contract.

Nasal mucosa is comparatively thick, easier to handle, and with minimal contraction need be only about one-sixth greater in size than the defect to be filled (5).

Skin should never be used to replace conjunctiva in the nonenucleated socket because the squamous epidermis and the tiny hairs irritate the sensitive cornea, provoking a troublesome discharge (6).

Composite Partial-Thickness Loss

Composite partial-thickness lid defects may be due to loss of lining and its supporting tarsus or to loss of the skin, orbicularis, and tarsus. When the defect is too large for primary closure, replacement of both the lining and supporting layer must be undertaken. This may be with either a composite free graft or a composite flap that uses local flaps in conjunction with mucosal lining and middle lamella support (7).

Composite Grafts

Composite grafts for eyelid reconstruction have the advantage of providing support, but their main disadvantage is the risk of partial or complete graft failure with subsequent shrinkage and scarring (8). For reconstruction of tarsal-conjunctival deficits up to 2×3 cm, the septal chondromucosal graft is easy to harvest and conforms well to the globe after thinning. Graft success approximates 100%, and the donor area usually heals uneventfully.

Technique

A template is made of the defect with, for example, cut suture-packet, then the pattern laid on the nasal septum. A Weir incision may be used for more exposure. Hemostasis is enhanced by infiltration of the septum with adrenalin solution and topical cocaine. After 10 to 15 minutes delay for hemostasis, an incision is made through the mucosa and cartilage to the perichondrium of the opposite side. After undermining the mucoperichondrium, the cartilage edges are cut, either with a scalpel or sharp dissector, leaving the opposite septal mucosa intact. Once the graft is removed, any exposed cartilage that remains in the defect is removed. Gelfoam (Upjohn) is cut to size and placed in the defect, the septum packed with Vaseline gauze, and the alar base incision closed. The cartilage graft is shaved on its exposed surface to help it conform to the round surface of the globe. A small (1.5-mm) cuff of mucosa is left on the upper border to suture to the covering flap. The graft is then sutured into place with either absorbable suture or a pull-out monofilament suture.

For replacement of skin and tarsus, a composite skin-perichondral graft harvested from the anterior concha of the ear may be ideal. It is thin and rigid enough to replace the support of the tarsal layer. Skin-cartilage composite grafts taken from the ear are usually too thick.

A deficit of one-third of the lid margin may be reconstructed with a composite full-thickness graft (skin, tarsus, and conjunctiva) from one of the three other eyelids. In upper-eyelid reconstruction, the superior portion of the graft should be sutured to the levator. Graft "take" may be maximized by excising all orbicularis fibers from the graft. Iced saline compresses may decrease metabolic requirements of the graft in the postoperative period, further increasing the likelihood of a successful take.

Local Flaps

Local flaps, with their independent blood supply, have the advantage of less contracture and potentially better color and texture match than grafts. Their disadvantages are increased thickness and potential donor-site scarring and deformity.

NASOLABIAL FLAP

The nasolabial flap is a commonly used, reliable, relatively simple and versatile method of reconstruction of the lower lid. The chief advantages of this flap are its rich blood supply, from the superior part of the angular artery and from the supratrochlear collaterals, and the good support this thicker skin can provide to the lower lid (9). If there is a shortage of tissue in the infraorbital area, particularly after trauma, atrophy, or scarring, then subcutaneous fat may be carried with the flap. The chief disadvantage of the nasolabial flap is that the thick skin gives an abnormal appearance because it lacks the supple and delicate attributes of eyelid skin. Technical considerations include raising a flap of properly measured size and

FIG. 43–2.   Nasolabial flap may be employed in cases in which full-thickness skin is needed in lower-lid reconstruction.

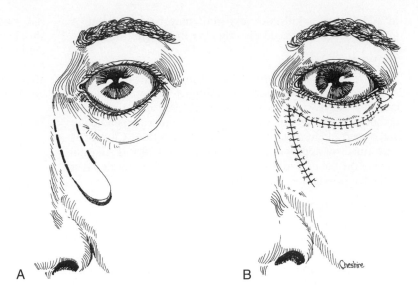

taking care to maintain a relatively thick base to preserve the blood supply. The usable portion of the flap may be thinned. The tip of the flap may be anchored into the lateral canthal tendon or the periosteum, giving added support to the lower lid. This flap will also support a cartilage–mucosa composite graft if indicated. The flap may require secondary thinning, as this tissue tends to be thicker than is desirable (Fig. 43–2).

V–Y ADVANCEMENT FLAP

A V–Y advancement flap in the periorbital area is useful. It may be relatively large, to replace a part of the lower lid, or small, in the case of a small wound that cannot be directly closed (10). The sides are cut, leaving the base of the pedicle intact with subcutaneous tissue attachments. Skin hooks are used to pull the flap in the direction of the defect. Strands of subcutaneous tissue that prevent adequate mobilization are freed by blunt or sharp dissection. The flap is then advanced into the defect and the donor area closed (Fig. 43–3).

LATERAL CHEEK FLAP

The lateral cheek flap is indicated for defects of the lower and upper eyelids that cannot be closed even after lateral canthotomy. The viability of this random flap is ensured by the rich subdermal facial plexus. In the age group that presents most commonly with eyelid malignancies, there is usually sufficient laxity of the skin that this flap is available to reconstruct the entire lower lid. With large lower-lid defects (>50%), a cheek flap may be combined with a septal chondromucosal graft. Complications include hematoma, infection, or flap necrosis, early in the postoperative course. Late complications include ectropion or lateral canthal distortion (Fig. 43–4).

Technique

Design of the cheek flap is important, with the curvilinear lateral incision rising from the lateral canthus laterally into the temporal area, then descending to the preauricular area as far down as the lobule. The medial incision should be made as close to the nasomaxillary line as possible so that, when the incision is closed, the sturdier dermal attachments on the side of the nose will support the sutured cheek skin. Undermining should be at the level of dermal subcutaneous tissue

interface, leaving about 0.5 to 1.0 mm of fat on the undersurface of the flap to protect the subdermal plexus. Extensive undermining is usually necessary to mobilize the flap completely so that there is no tension in its new position. With the flap in position, the upper border of the flap, at the point where it becomes the new lower lid, is sutured to the periosteum with a permanent suture to prevent later ectropion. The triangular defect is then closed with deep and superficial sutures. When a composite chondromucosal graft is to be included, it is sutured in the conjunctival defect before insetting the flap. Once the flap is inset, its upper edge is sutured to a cuff of mucosa overhanging the top of the chondromucosal graft. To prevent a dog-ear just medial to the nose with rotation of the flap, a triangle of skin medial to the flap (i.e., lateral to the nose and base up) may need to be excised.

For defects up to two-thirds of the lower lid, a useful semicircular flap similar in principle to the lateral cheek flap has been described by Tenzel (11,12).

Technique

A semicircular incision, commencing at the lateral canthus, is exaggerated superiorly and continued laterally to the level of the inferior continuation of the eyebrow. The inferior crus of the lateral canthal tendon is released and the flap is undermined beneath the orbicularis muscle until a tension-free closure of the defect can be accomplished.

TEMPORAL ADVANCEMENT FLAP TO THE UPPER LID

A temporal skin flap may be used to reconstruct defects of greater than one-half of the upper lid. The technique differs from that of the lower lid only in that (a) the lateral incision is straighter and is not carried out to the preauricular area, and (b) care is taken not to dissect too deep laterally because this can damage the facial nerve branches to the forehead (Fig. 43–5).

Technique

The skin is undermined, commencing beneath the orbicularis muscle, and a determination is made as to how much cheek skin will be needed. If a small amount of relaxation is needed, then simple undermining and advancement may be done. If a larger amount of skin is needed, then a back-cut

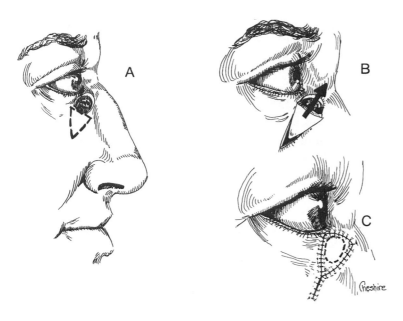

FIG. 43–3. A V–Y advancement flap may be used for coverage of medial canthal defects.

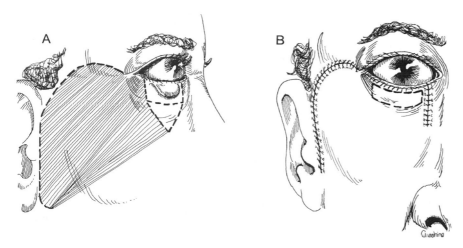

FIG. 43–4. A Mustardé cheek flap may be used with a chrondromucosal graft for reconstruction of large defects.

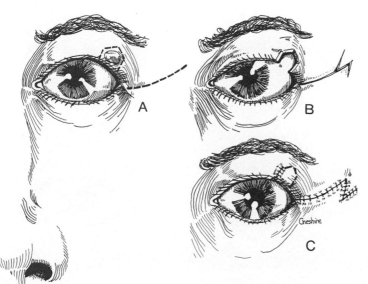

FIG. 43–5. The upper lid may be reconstructed in a similar fashion by an advancement flap and possibly a chondromucosal graft (dashed lines).

may be performed to allow better mobility. This is closed with a Z-plasty from adjacent tissue, thus filling in the defect created from the back-cut. This approach also gives the lateral incision an upward sweep, enhancing the support of the lower lid. It may be combined with a composite graft. In this case, the graft is first sutured in place, with careful approximation and no sutures visible on the mucosal side that could rub the cornea and cause abrasion or ulceration. The undermined temporal skin is then brought over for cover. The lateral incision is sutured so that there is minimal tension on the vertical suture line. Postoperatively the eye is protected for a few days with antibacterial ophthalmic ointment and a patch.

McGregor (13) has advocated a modification of the cheek advancement principle that adds a lateral Z-plasty for defects of less than 60% of the lower lid. The lateral Z-plasty technique incorporates the high lateral arch necessary to avoid sagging and does not interfere with the natural temporal hairline.

BIPEDICLE TRIPIER FLAP

The Tripier flap is indicated for reconstruction of horizontal defects of the lower lid. The viability of each pedicle of the flap decreases past the midline of the upper lid, but as a bipedicled flap it is capable of resurfacing the entire lower lid. It also avoids obvious facial scars. Although a flap from upper to lower lid is excellent, the reverse is generally not feasible (Fig. 43–6).

Technique

The defect in the lower lid is created and a flap of corresponding size is elevated from the upper lid. Preseptal orbicularis muscle should be included to ensure vascularity. In most cases, especially when the lateral canthus is to be elevated, the lower-lid incision joins the lower incision of the pedicle and the flap is inset directly. If the pedicle is not directly inset, it can be divided and contoured after 10 to 14 days. The upper-lid defect is simply closed by approximation of the skin. This flap may also be combined with a chondromucosal graft where tarsus needs to be replaced.

The eye is covered with ophthalmic ointment and covered for a few days, after which it may be left open. Where necessary the pedicles are divided and contoured at 10 to 14 days. When reconstruction is performed for paralytic ectropion, the bilateral pedicles may be left undivided to act as a sling for supporting the lax lower eyelid (14).

FULL-THICKNESS, SINGLE PEDICLE FLAP (CROSS LID)

An upper-lid defect of the tarsal margin too large to be closed even after lateral canthotomy may be reconstructed with a full-thickness lower-lid flap. This is pedicled on the marginal arcade located between the orbicularis muscle and tarsal plate. As a defect, up to 25% of the upper lid can be closed primarily; the size of the lower-lid flap need only be the size of the defect minus 25% the length of the upper lid. This technique permits reconstruction of any size upper-lid defect from one-third to total loss. The usual outcome is a natural upper lid that functions well. When it is necessary to mobilize cheek skin, the vascularity of the flap when based medially is better than when based laterally, and thus is preferable (Fig. 43–7).

Technique

To allow for rotation, the pedicle of the flap should be just lateral to the defect of the upper lid. Once the flap is measured and cut, the tarsal plate is completely divided, leaving the musculocutaneous pedicle intact for vascular support. The flap is rotated into place and the uppermost portion is attached to the levator aponeurosis, with the tarsal margins approximated as precisely as possible. The lower-lid defect may then be carefully closed in layers.

SINGLE PEDICLE FLAP, LOWER-LID DEFECT

Single pedicle flaps from the upper eyelid to the lower eyelid are easy to mobilize and are generally reliable. These flaps may be designed with as much as a 5:1 length ratio.

Technique

When designing the flap, a deep base should be included, with muscle to enhance vascularity. These flaps may be used to cover partial-thickness loss of the lids. If a concomitant cartilage graft is needed for tarsal and conjunctival layers, this flap is usually capable of nourishing this graft (Fig. 43–8).

FIG. 43–6. A combination of a chondromucosal graft with a bipedicle Tripier flap can be used for lower-lid reconstruction.

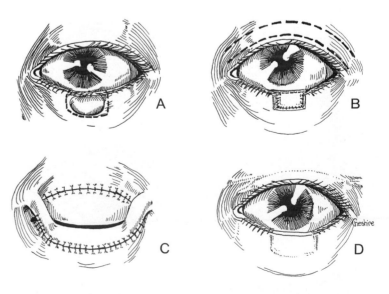

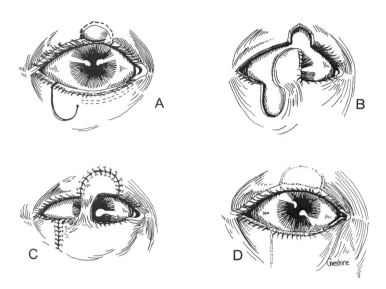

FIG. 43–7. A Mustardé cross-lid pedicle flap may be used for upper eyelid reconstruction. **D** shows detachment of the pedicle at about 10 days.

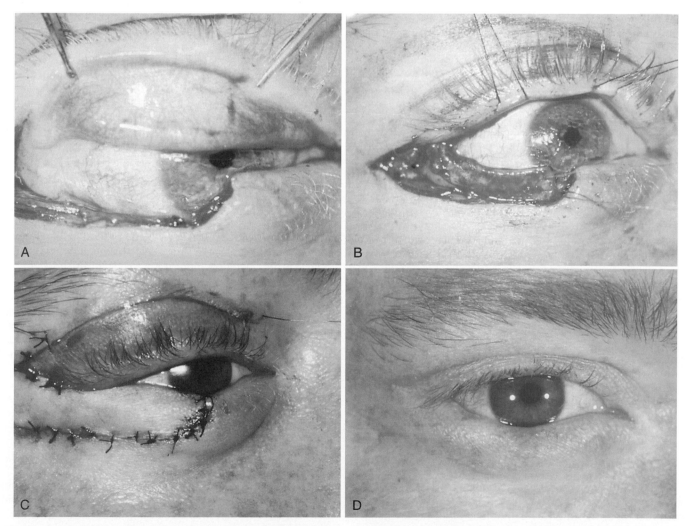

FIG. 43–8.   A, surgical defect after excision, tumor of two-thirds lateral lower lid, upper eyelid everted to reveal donor site for tarsoconjunctival graft. **B,** tarsoconjunctival graft from upper eyelid lying adjacent to globe to fill defect. **C,** myocutaneous pedicle flap from upper eyelid to cover graft. **D,** completed reconstruction including conjunctival lining, stiff tarsal plate, and external coverage.

GLABELLAR FLAP

A glabellar flap or median forehead flap based on the supra-trochlear vessels can be used to reconstruct the lids or defects in the medial canthal area. The skin in this location is thicker than eyelid skin and should be used only if other procedures are not feasible. These flaps usually require thinning at the time of the insetting as well as secondary thinning.

LID-SHARING TECHNIQUES

Lid-sharing procedures, such as the Hughes flap for horizontal defects of the lower lid, can be used to reconstruct upper eyelid defects (15). A tarsoconjunctival flap is detached from the upper lid and sutured into the lower-lid defect. This can be covered with either a full-thickness skin graft or advancement of the cheek skin. Care should be taken to leave the caudal 4 mm of the upper lid tarsus intact to prevent entropion formation of the upper lid. The flap is divided after 6 to 8 weeks to allow for stretching of the tarsoconjunctival flap and to ensure its vascularity. The disadvantages of this technique are that it requires two stages and occludes the visual axis for 6 to 8 weeks.

A Cutler-Beard flap may be used for upper-lid defects (16). This involves creating a full-thickness pedicle of the lower lid just caudal to the marginal arcade and suturing it into the defect after advancement. It must be sutured to the levator to provide for upward excursion of the lid. Separation is carried out 8 weeks later.

The lower-lid switch flap introduced by Esser in 1919 is based on the marginal artery. The flap is rotated 180° into the upper eyelid, similar to the Estlander Abbé principle of lip reconstruction. The main advantage of the switch flap procedure is that wide horizontal upper-lid defects with a significant vertical component can be repaired with full-thickness tissue at the expense of the lower lid. In addition, transfer of the lower-lid margin affords an incontinuity margin for the upper lid. The cross-lid pedicle can be divided 2 to 4 weeks after transfer, minimizing the occlusal period. Disadvantages of the technique are the deliberate sacrifice of lower-eyelid tissues that in turn may require simultaneous reconstruction with adjacent cheek tissue (17).

The lower lid–switch flap procedure was popularized by Mustardé for the repair of partial or total upper-eyelid defects. His standard operation involving a lower-lid switch flap with simultaneous lower-lid reconstruction has been recently modified. Mustardé now endorses a two-stage procedure. There is an initial lower-lid switch to the upper eyelid followed by a second-stage division and inset of the lower lid switch flap. Simultaneously, the lower-eyelid secondary defect is reconstructed with a cheek advancement flap and nasal chondromucosal graft (18). The chondromucosal graft is used to ensure long-term support of the lower eyelid.

Lower Eyelid Reconstruction

PARTIAL- AND FULL-THICKNESS DEFECTS

The general techniques for reconstruction of partial- and full-thickness loss have been described earlier. Specific for reconstruction of the lower eyelid include all of the techniques and principles that have been discussed except two: the temporal advancement flap and the cross-lid flap, both of which are used for upper-lid reconstruction.

For the lower lid, considerations include the size and composition of the defect and also whether the defect is mainly horizontal along the tarsal margin or is wider with a significant vertical loss of tissue. Even though the horizontal width of the defect may be the same, reconstruction is often different in these two differing circumstances. For example, in the horizontal-width case a nasal chondromucosal graft with a Tripier flap might be ideal, while in the vertical-loss case a nasal chondromucosal graft with a rotation cheek flap may be needed.

For small defects not involving the lid margin, the surgeon can choose V–Y advancement flaps and full-thickness, single-pedicle flaps from the upper lid to the lower lid. If there is an associated tarsal defect in the lateral or medial area, a lid-sharing procedure or a chondromucosal graft may be combined with this single-pedicle flap.

For more extensive defects where there is a problem with the cheek as a donor area, a nasolabial flap or glabellar midline forehead flap can be used. In both of these circumstances, the skin is quite thick and may not be an ideal color and texture match. The match may, however, be improved by selecting patients with a ruddy complexion and many actinic changes rather than patients with thin, delicate skin. Additionally, the distal flap may be thinned by defatting.

In our experience, the most useful method of reconstruction of the lower lid has been with advancement of the lateral eyelid skin. With a defect involving more than 25% of the lower lid that cannot be closed primarily, the two edges can be drawn together to judge the amount of lateral tissues release required. A lateral canthotomy may be performed by incision in the lateral fissure, with release of the lower limb of the lateral canthal tendon. This allows the external lid, the lower part of the lateral canthus, and the conjunctiva to rotate medially so that careful three-layer closure (tarsus, orbicularis muscle) can then be performed. If excessive tension still exists, further undermining of the cheek along with a small back-cut may be helpful. After the back-cut is made, a Z-plasty limb from the upper side of the incision can be used to fill in the back-cut. This can be made in the lateral temporal area; the postoperative healing is usually excellent, with minimal scarring. After rotation of the lower lid to allow closure of the defect, there may be a deficiency of tarsus along the lateral border of the newly reconstructed lid. If this defect is greater than 20 to 25% of the lower-lid margin, it is best to put in a supportive graft of cartilage and mucosa to prevent entropion or retraction of the lid margin. The cartilage graft can be obtained from the ear cartilage, nasal septum, or upper lateral area of the nose.

The whole lower eyelid may be reconstructed with a cheek rotation flap and a large nasal-septal, chondromucosal graft. To maintain good support to the lower eyelid, the graft's vertical height should be at least 1.5 to 2 cm to allow it to rest on the orbital rim inferiorly. The medial and lateral portions of this chondromucosal graft should also be attached to the remnants of the medial and lateral canthal tendons.

A large horizontal defect of the lower lid might occur from excision of an upper-cheek lesion adjacent to the lower lid that does not involve the lid margin or pretarsal orbicularis muscle. In this instance, the nasolabial flap is capable of providing a reasonable color match for the cheek area and furnishing tissue for reconstruction of this area. If the lower-lid defect also involves the medial canthal area, a thinned glabellar may be useful. In this case it is important to anchor the under-surface of the glabellar flap to the canthal tendon to prevent bulging.

For reconstruction, lid-sharing techniques from the upper to lower lid should be confined to smaller defects or situations where there is a narrow full-thickness loss that can be covered by a thin strip of upper-lid tarsus. If too much tarsus is taken, the normal anatomy of the upper lid may be disrupted, resulting in entropion and trichiasis.

The most common difficulty with lower-lid reconstruction is providing long-term support. Scar contracture and gravity work to displace the lower-lid position downward, resulting in lid retraction or ectropion. A wide chondromucosal graft at the time of reconstruction provides long-term support of the lid margin by resting on the infraorbital rim. Where the reconstruction has not provided support, a fascial sling support, hooked in from the medial to lateral canthal tendon, may be needed to prevent or correct the downward displacement.

Upper Eyelid Reconstruction

PARTIAL-THICKNESS DEFECTS

Partial-thickness defects of the eyelid are usually easier to treat than full-thickness defects. Where closure is not possible, the simplest method of skin replacement is a full-thickness graft from either or both of the upper lids. Many of the patients in the tumor age group have redundant skin due to dermachalasis, and a large graft may be obtained as part of a blepharoplasty. This graft may be a composite of skin and orbicularis muscle, and generally the segments of grafted muscle take and continue to function.

In cases where upper-eyelid skin is not available, postauricular skin is an alternative. It must be thinned down, but it makes the best graft over the pretarsal area. Outside the pretarsal area, postauricular skin is too thick and will never duplicate the original delicate upper eyelid skin. Split-thickness skin grafts can be harvested from the inner upper arm. They are homogenous but do not furnish a good color match and tend to contract.

After tumor resection, occasionally a small marginal defect may be combined with a larger partial-thickness skin defect. In this case, the marginal defect should be repaired first with, for example, an advancement of the lateral lid skin combined with canthotomy or temporal advancement. The remaining skin defect can then be treated as a simple partial-thickness defect.

When attempting to reconstruct the lid crease to achieve symmetry, the grafts should be sutured to the aponeurosis at the level of the lid crease. This crease is often difficult to reconstruct and the tendency to place it too high needs to be avoided.

FULL-THICKNESS DEFECTS

The reconstructed upper lid must provide coverage of the cornea and scleral conjunctiva and must move smoothly over the cornea without irritation. Therefore, the under-surface of any lid reconstruction must be free of sutures or knots, edges of cartilage, roughened portions of thick scar, or other irregularities that could rub the cornea. Excessive tightness of the upper lid in a horizontal plane should also be avoided, be-

cause this prevents elevation and closure of the lid. The simplest method of upper-lid reconstruction is closure after full-thickness defect. If tumor resection of one-fourth to one-third of the upper eyelid is performed, it is generally necessary to make parallel incisions in the tarsal plate to convert the defect to a pentagon, so that the whole segment will close without notching. Similarly, when the defect involves only the caudal part of the tarsal plate, the cranial part of the tarsal plate for the width of the defect may also need to be excised to allow closure. Sutures in the tarsal plate should only be placed through the superficial side, and may be interrupted, continuous, absorbable, or nonabsorbable (18).

Where the defect is too wide to close primarily, a lateral canthotomy may be performed. To prevent blunting of the lateral fissure, the lower limb of the lateral canthal tendon should be preserved. When the defect is larger than one-quarter of the horizontal lid length, either nasal or palatal mucosa may be used in the reconstruction of the eyelid lining. Both are easy to obtain and usually are not necessary in smaller defects, although larger defects have more stability if a chondromucosal graft is put into place. The advanced lateral temporal skin is anchored to the lateral canthal area and the graft is sutured underneath this area with sutures that are directed away from the conjunctival surface.

With a defect greater than one-half of the upper lid, the temporal advancement flap may be used. Once the flap has been mobilized, it will be necessary to place a chondromucosal graft to stabilize the lid margin. The cartilage graft should be thinned so that its curvature conforms to the globe. The lateral aspect of the cartilage is anchored to the lateral canthal tendon area, whereas the medial aspect is anchored to the tarsal segment. With the skin flap inset over this, graft take is assured along with a stable lid margin.

For segmental loss involving a horizontal defect with a small vertical height, it is possible to place a chondromucosal graft or a tarsal graft from the contralateral upper lid into the defect. A segment of tarsus from the contralateral lid several millimeters wide and up to 7 or 8 mm long can be obtained as a window excision from the donor lid. This can be taken without fear of damage to the contralateral upper lid and the segment may be used as a tarsal segment along with lid margin. Once inset, it is covered with a small rotation pedicle flap including skin and muscle from the adjacent tissue. These segmental reconstructions do very well and graft loss would be extremely unusual when covered by a local pedicle flap. If additional skin is needed for a defect in the medial or lateral canthal area, either a thinned glabellar flap or a single-pedicle temporal skin flap may be used. The temporal skin flap is a good color match and the take of this graft is usually excellent.

Lid-sharing procedures from the lower lid allows reconstruction of narrow marginal upper-lid defects by a simple method without obtaining graft material from a remote source. The Cutler-Beard flap involves horizontal incision through the substance of the lower lid, preservation of a cranial horizontal strip of tarsus including the marginal artery, and movement of this flap up and under the strip into the defect of the upper lid. Because the width of the lower-lid tarsus is usually 5 or 6 mm, only a small segment of tarsus can be removed. When this has been in place for several weeks however, the skin stretches, providing sufficient skin for both the upper-lid defect and the remaining secondary lower-lid defect. Several weeks, or even months, later when the flap is divided, the remaining flap is sutured to the under-surface of the transverse tarsal strip, allowing reconstruction of the lower lid to be completed. Careful preservation of the segment of tarsus will likely prevent secondary complications of the lower lid.

Another approach to segmental defects of the upper lid involves the use of full-thickness rotation pedicle flaps from the lower lid, including skin and muscle with tarsal conjunctival lining. In the case of defects of the upper lid, one-fourth of the width of the defect may be subtracted from this width since there is usually that much elasticity in the lid, enough to allow primary closure. Therefore, if one-half of the upper lid is involved, a pedicle flap only one-quarter of the width of the upper lid needs to be rotated from the lower lid. In rotation of these flaps from the lower lid, it is preferable to have the pedicle based medially and consisting mostly of orbicularis muscle and skin. Full transection of the tarsus is necessary to allow good rotation of this pedicle. The remaining bridge of orbicularis muscle and skin may be cut in about 2 weeks to allow full mobility of the upper lid. If the defect involves most of the upper lid, the whole lower lid may be used in its reconstruction. Transection of the medial tarsal area, with elevation of the whole lower lid attached to a lateral orbicularis and skin pedicle, can be used. The tarsus must be sutured to the upper lid aponeurosis to retain lid movement, and sutures should be used to repair continuity of the orbicularis muscle as well as the skin. Having reconstructed the upper lid, there is now total loss of the lower lid. This in turn necessitates reconstruction from a rotation cheek flap lined with a chondromucosal graft. When the cheek flap is mobilized and moved medially, it still retains the pedicle of the upper lid; therefore, blood supply of this newly reconstructed lid is dependent on the cheek flap itself.

Lateral Canthal Reconstruction

Assessment of the true defect of the lateral canthal area is of primary importance because reconstruction of this area is influenced by the etiology. In trauma, all of the component parts may be present, but the bone and tendon as well as soft tissues

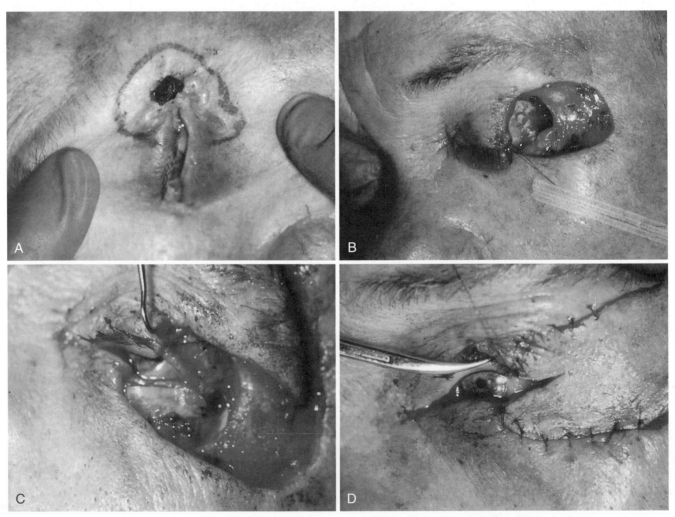

FIG. 43–9. **A,** recurrent basal cell carcinoma involving upper and lower eyelids and lateral canthus. **B,** wide excision of tumor left lateral canthal area and full-thickness lids. **C,** lining of conjunctival defect with chrondromucosal graft from nasal area. **D,** pedicle flap coverage from temporal area using lateral-based flap.

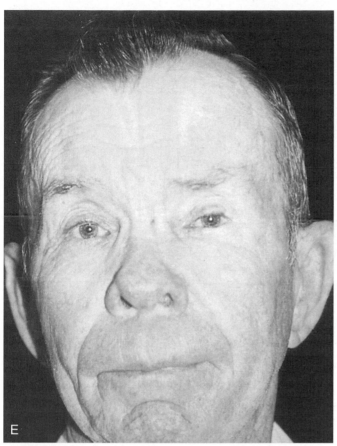

FIG. 43–9—*continued.*   E, postoperative result of pedicle flap coverage lateral canthal area.

may be disrupted or displaced. In tumor surgery all or some of these elements may be missing. In congenital problems these tissues may be weakened or partially absent. The underlying bony framework, the attachment of the upper and lower eyelids by the lateral canthal tendon, and the soft tissue—as well as lateral fissure adjacent to the lateral canthal tendon—are important structures to consider for reconstruction.

Assessment of the bone is best done by CT scan or MRI. Where bone is missing, it is difficult to reconstruct the soft tissue with normal contour. Bone grafts or alloplastic reconstruction may be necessary. Fixation of the lids may then be necessary, with a reconstructed lateral canthal tendon of fascia attached to the tarsal margin and then wired into place in the lateral orbital rim so that a good solid attachment is achieved. In cases where there is a soft-tissue defect, this fascia graft for reconstruction of the lateral canthal tendon can be combined with a mucosal graft and a local pedicle flap, which will furnish vascularity to both of the grafts.

In the lateral canthus the fornix extends several millimeters beyond the lateral fissure. Therefore, for larger defects involving the lateral canthus, there must be lining beyond the lateral fissure to allow mobility of the lateral conjunctival tissue and movement of the globe. The first consideration in full-thickness defects is lining, preferably from mucosal grafts of nasal or oral origin. Most often these grafts are put in place, sometimes in conjunction with associated cartilage for support of either the upper or lower lid, and then covered

with a pedicle flap. It is not possible to obtain healing when placing a graft on top of a graft, but if either surface is vascularized as a pedicle flap and that vascular supply is adequate, the graft will experience a good take in most circumstances.

One of the best flaps for an extensive defect of the lateral canthal area is the single-pedicle temporal skin transposition flap. This flap is capable of rotating from the temporal area on a moderate-sized base and is thin enough that it contours nicely to the lateral canthal area. Additionally, it has sufficient vasculature to support a graft of chondromucosa or oral mucosa. Other flaps for the lateral canthal area include a rotation cheek flap from the lateral temporal and cheek area. A superiorly based, inferiorly directed transposition flap is also a possibility if the cheek skin is relaxed enough. Lateral canthal reconstructions can usually be a one-stage procedure, since the local donor flaps along with mucosal lining give excellent reconstruction. Additional touch-ups may still be necessary. (Fig. 43–9).

Lateral canthopexy and tarsal-strip procedures must be mentioned in any discussion of reconstruction of the lateral canthus. When a lower lid and lateral canthal area have been dragged downward by scarring or edema, sometimes a tarsal-strip procedure or canthopexy is indicated in order to regain position of the lateral canthal area. If the lower lid is lax and the lateral part of the tarsal margin is not in continuity with the lateral orbital rim, a small fascia graft can be used to suspend that tarsal segment to the lateral canthal area. If there is simply traumatic ectropion, a small segment of tarsal strip can be dissected away from the lower lid and sutured into position, thereby tightening the lid margin. If the whole lateral canthus is disrupted and downward due to trauma, the lateral canthal tendon can be grasped and reattached to the lateral orbital rim in a more upward position (Figs. 43–10, 43–11).

Medial Canthal Reconstruction

Medial canthal defects can usually be closed by grafting, with upper lid or postauricular skin grafts as the donor areas of choice. After excision of the tumor, the medial canthal tendon often remains, but the graft takes well with the help of the "bridging" phenomenon. If there is bone in the base of the defect, the graft may also take, provided that no more than a few millimeters need to be covered. Once the defect is closed with the graft, a bolus of cotton or Vaseline gauze is held in place with the long sutures tied over the bolus. If there is more exposed bone, then a local flap is probably indicated.

Successful reconstruction of the medial canthal area is dependent on adequate positioning of the medial canthal complex to maintain proper intercanthal distance and apposition of the lids to the orbital globe. Reconstruction of the medial part of the upper lid requires special attention because of the presence of the lacrimal excretory system and the important medial canthal tendon. In addition, defects involving the medial canthal aspect of the upper eyelid are very prone to mechanical ptosis, owing to tethering of the more mobile central part of the levator complex to the fixed point of the canthal ligament. When eyelid tissue must be replaced in this area, reconstructive alternatives are the lower-lid switch with lateral cheek advancement flap and the upper-lid tarsoconjunc-

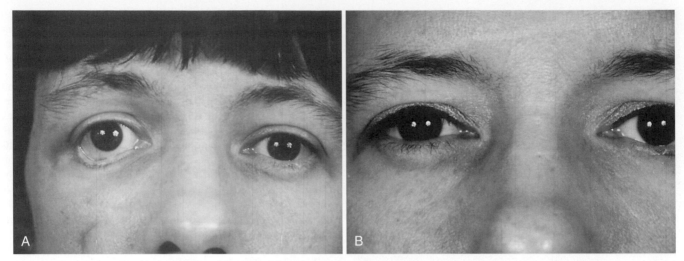

FIG. 43–10. **A,** posttraumatic ectropion, right lower lid. **B,** postoperative resolution of ectropion after lateral canthal suspension and release of scar tissue of capsulopalpebral area.

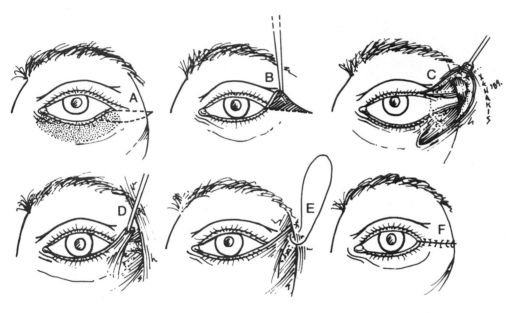

FIG. 43–11. The lateral tarsal flap canthoplasty involves release of the inferior crura, release of any underlying adhesions, deepithelialization of a lateral tarsodermal strip, and attachment to the superomedial aspect of the lateral orbital rim.

tival flap. If additional lid tissue is not required, soft-tissue coverage may be obtained by grafts (free full-thickness skin grafts) or by flaps from the glabellar area of the forehead if there is a large area of exposed bone.

Reasonable results may also be expected when the defect is allowed to heal secondarily, particularly when the wounds are in the medial half of the lower lid and 5 mm or less in diameter (19,20). Defects in the exact medial canthus typically heal satisfactorily without surgical closure, making spontaneous repair the preferred method over standard flaps and grafts when the medial canthal tendon complex is intact. As the medial canthal defect extends onto the side of the nose, there is an increasing tendency for the spontaneously reformed canthus to lie higher than the normal one and the lids to pull away from the globe. Accordingly, it seems reasonable to limit spontaneous repair of those defects in the immediate vicinity of the lid in its medial sector. Other methods of reconstruction should be considered when the defect extends into the parapalpebral tissues (21,22). Bilobed flaps from the nasal dorsum can take advantage of the good local color match and can be used for the reconstruction. Although the scars often heal very well, the thickness of the tissue may require secondary debulking.

A medial canthopexy should be performed when repairing inner canthus defects to avoid telecanthus. Medial canthoplasty involves suturing the medial ends of the upper- and lower-lid tarsus to the nasal periosteum. The point of fixation should be well posterior to the lacrimal fossa.

Telecanthus can occur as a traumatic deformity, as part of the blepharophimosis syndrome (in conjunction with epicanthus and ptosis), or in isolation without any bony abnormalities. If telecanthus is associated with the epicanthus, the repair of the telecanthus may also correct the epicanthus. In the mildest form of the deformity, correction involves simple plication of the medial canthal tendon. In the reconstruction of more severe problems, transnasal wire techniques are employed.

Technique

Nonabsorbable sutures or wires are passed through the medial canthus in a figure-eight fashion, while the other end is passed transnasally at a point posterior to the anterior lacrimal crest. These wires are then tightened to approximate the two medial canthal ligaments. Other techniques use either a Nelson stainless-steel screw (piton) or microplate fixation to anchor the tendons into the proper alignment (23,24).

Posttraumatic Reconstruction

Eyelid trauma must be considered in the context of possible trauma to the rest of the body. In the management of eyelid injuries, the patient must first be fully evaluated and treated according to all other more significant injuries, while remembering that penetrating orbital injuries are also emergencies.

During the period of initial assessment, the orbit should be assessed and desiccation or further injury prevented. Ophthalmologic assessment is indicated, with testing of visual acuity, visual fields, and inspection of the cornea. Fluorescein staining may be indicated to test corneal abrasion and radiographic imaging, including CT scanning, may be indicated with suspicion of an intraocular foreign body, such as windshield glass. Facial radiography for facial fractures may also be indicated. With the patient fully assessed and stabilized, reconstruction of the eyelid may proceed.

Eyelid trauma often results in a complex injury pattern that may include a combination of bone and soft-tissue damage and segmental loss. There is likely to be contamination, and there is an increased likelihood of later scar formation, because trauma usually does not respect surgical principles like incising along lines of minimal tension. This scarring may complicate secondary reconstructive procedures because the scar may limit the extent of dissection or the use of local flaps that would be available in a surgically created wound (e.g., after tumor excision).

During sleep, the cornea is protected by the Bell phenomena of upward rotation of the globe under the eyelid. It is estimated that 5 to 10% of the general population have a poor to absent Bell reflex, which makes them more susceptible to corneal irritation with an incompetent upper eyelid. An inadequate Bell reflex may necessitate more aggressive protection of the globe from drying, indicating both the necessity for earlier eyelid reconstruction and careful postoperative management.

PRIMARY RECONSTRUCTION

In the fully assessed and stabilized patient, once having managed any ophthalmologic emergencies, primary reconstruction may commence. After copious gentle irrigation, débridement with fine sharp scissors and atraumatic fine forceps must be thorough; usually it requires only a very small amount of tissue resection. This is because of the excellent eyelid vasculature that is nearly always at least partly intact, and means that any tissue not obviously nonviable will usually survive as long as the frankly nonviable tissue is removed and the remaining tissue does not desiccate or get infected. Because of the vascularity, infection is also extremely rare.

Since injuries to the periorbital and eyelid area often cross lines of tension and areas of vascular support, the stage is set for more difficult reconstruction than in the primary excision for tumor with subsequent reconstruction. The nature of reconstruction is often more difficult, and the results may be less successful than could be expected for other conditions that cause loss of tissue.

TIMING

Timing of reconstruction in posttraumatic complex injuries is not always easy or obvious. The first priority is to see that the cornea is covered, that the visual axis is preserved, and that there is potential for closure and opening of the upper lid. If the upper lid is partially or completely disrupted, or missing secondary to the injury, priority goes to immediate reconstruction of the upper lid to cover the cornea. Primary grafting of nasal mucosa as a substitute lining for conjunctiva is an acceptable approach. Grafts to reline conjunctiva need vascularization from an external source such as a local flap. If the cornea is left exposed, then corneal irritation or ulceration may occur.

In treating posttraumatic injuries, a comprehensive plan for all stages of reconstruction must be made. Optimal donor sites for both lining and external coverage are always limited in size and, where the zone of injury is extensive, local flaps may be excluded if the injuries have damaged them directly or transected their vascular pedicles. All available donors should be used in a way that allows the best reconstructive procedures without wastage or "burning bridges" for later stages of reconstruction. With limited reconstructive options, it may be best in some instances to delay reconstruction until healing has occurred and a definite plan for long-term reconstruction can be established. Primary bone grafts to the orbital area in the case of bony loss are usually not indicated because the potential for infection in the initial wound of injury is too high.

Upper-lid reconstruction is generally more complex than lower-lid reconstruction, because of the upper lid's mobility. In addition, mobility makes graft take more difficult. Primary repair is usually preferable when there is exposure of the cornea. In this case, immediate reconstruction with a mucosal graft and a local pedicle flap would likely be the best choice. If it is not possible to reconstruct the upper lid immediately, then the eyelids should be sutured with temporary tarsorrhaphy so that corneal exposure is limited and corneal drying and ulceration prevented. Sutures and knots must never lie on the conjunctival side and must have no contact with the cornea whatsoever. In the upper lid, with the constant movement of blinking, any rough or irregular area on the inner lid scratches and irritates the cornea, which may cause abrasion, infection, or perforation of the cornea. The tarsal closure is usually performed with 6-0 chromic gut with knots tied on the orbicularis side. As in the lower lid, a silk suture is placed into the gray line on the lid margin and left long so that it may be taped to the cheek for postoperative traction and immobilization of the upper lid. With traumatic injuries, it is important to make a perpendicular cut at the lid margin so that closure results in an even lid margin. If tissue is missing from the upper lid, full-thickness grafts from the contralateral upper lid or postauricular area may be the procedure of choice.

Lower-lid injuries that include partial or total loss are not as urgent as upper-lid injuries. There are cases reported where the upper lid had not been injured and the lower lid

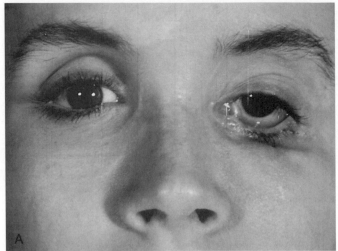

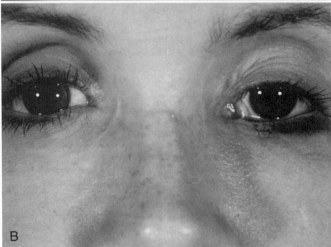

FIG. 43–12. **A,** posttraumatic deformity, left lower eyelid and lateral canthus, young female. **B,** postoperatively after lateral canthal suspension and lower lid dermal fat graft to improve soft-tissue defect.

was totally missing and the patient went on for years without serious damage to the cornea or scleral tissues. But this is aesthetically unacceptable, and reconstruction must still be planned because there can still be some corneal drying, discomfort, and epiphora secondary to the loss of the tear film on the lower part of the eye. Whilst lower-lid injuries can be reconstructed immediately, it is important not to use up the potential sources for reconstruction if, with the zone of injury not yet clarified, there is a significant chance for failure due to associated crush injury or infection (Fig. 43–12).

Reconstruction of Extensive Tissue Defects

In reconstruction of extensive tissue defects, the temporalis muscle flap is the most commonly used local flap, but more extensive defects require other options. With the advances in microvascular techniques, several alternatives are available to replace extensive or deep defects. Careful design of the musculocutaneous and osteocutaneous free flaps can provide the restoration of bulk, contour, bony architecture, and skin coverage. The capacity of microvascular flaps to provide im-

mediate coverage after extensive resections of orbital and periorbital tumors has greatly facilitated these radical extirpative procedures. Free-flap coverage is essential when local soft-tissue flaps are either not available secondary to previous surgery or radiation or when the volume of tissue required exceeds that locally available.

The choices most often used for free-flap coverage are the latissimus dorsi, parascapular, temporalis fascia—or the radial forearm free flaps for extensive defects, because they allow multiple skin islands to be designed and transferred independently on the underlying muscle, providing the restoration of both external coverage and internal lining when required. The tensor fascia lata myocutaneous flap provides a very large skin paddle with underlying muscle and/or fascia for the reconstruction of large defects. Temporalis fascial flaps can provide a much thinner flap, which can be skin grafted when a smaller amount of tissue is required. The deep circumflex, scapula, or trapezius osteomyocutaneous flaps are good choices if bone and soft-tissue lining is needed. The ability of microvascular flaps to provide immediate coverage after extensive resections of orbital and periorbital tumors has greatly facilitated these radical extirpative procedures.

Socket Reconstruction after Exenteration

After exenteration, the socket is usually covered with a split-thickness skin graft. There is generally excellent take of this graft, even though a moderately large area of membranous bone may constitute part of the defect. The size of the defect may be estimated by summing the measurements of the depth of the socket and the size of the defect at the base. As with other grafts, sutures are left long to tie over a bolus placed in the socket over the skin graft. The bolus must be left in place about 7 days. Healing is usually excellent, but spotty areas of crusting may remain for 1 to 2 months in some cases (Figs. 43–13, 43–14).

Complications

Complications may occur in eyelid reconstruction but they are not frequent, owing to the precise nature of reconstruction of these small parts and the rich blood supply around the orbit. Postoperative swelling is common, and is exacerbated by inadequate hemostasis; therefore, an absolutely dry field must be achieved in all cases. Steroids may be given postoperatively, along with head elevation and salt restriction. A hematoma may occur and it must be evacuated in order to achieve the best healing with diminished swelling and scarring. This complication can be serious if it occurs under a cheek flap and leads to partial necrosis of the flap. There is a higher incidence of necrosis in cheek flaps in patients who have had radiation therapy to this area. Loss of part or all of a flap should be treated by early débridement in most cases, and secondary coverage can be provided with a skin graft.

Corneal problems may occur, especially if a suture line is placed directly over the cornea. The surgeon should examine the deep surface of the lid to identify any suture fragments impinging on the cornea. A significant incidence of corneal problems occur after eyelid reconstruction, and frequent slit-lamp examinations may be indicated. Patching the eye, or placing a temporary intermarginal tarsorrhaphy, will help reduce the lid motion.

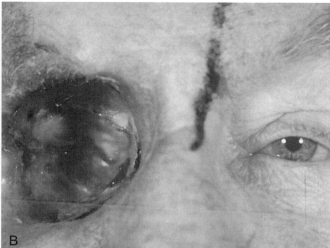

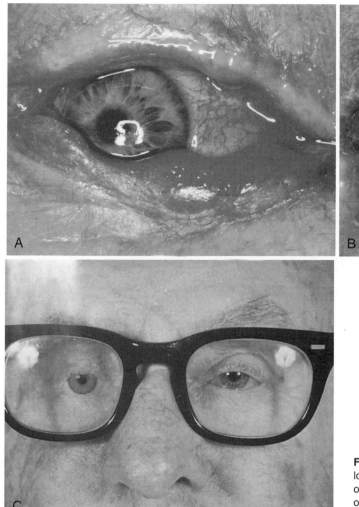

FIG. 43–13. **A,** invasive squamous cell carcinoma, upper and lower eyelids. **B,** post exenteration of lids and globe for treatment of squamous carcinoma. Split thickness skin graft used for lining of orbital socket. **C,** prosthetic device suspended on glasses to camouflage orbital deformity.

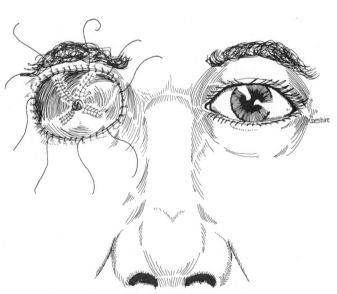

FIG. 43–14. Split-thickness grafts can be utilized for socket coverage after enucleation.

Notching of the lid margin at the area of closure may be excised as a secondary procedure or improved by Z-plasty technique. Irregularity of a lid margin can be reduced by opening the area over the cartilage and shaving the edge back to normal. Asymmetry of one lid may be present, usually as excess eyelid skin on the unoperated side compared to the operated side. Further revisions, including a blepharoplasty, may help in achieving symmetry of the lids.

Sagging of the lateral lid margin after reconstruction with a small or large cheek flap may be corrected by a small, laterally based flap from the upper lid. The base of this flap is superior to the lateral canthus and gives additional support to the sagging lid margin. If sagging is associated with a loose tarsal margin, removal of a tarsal wedge, in addition to a small flap or graft, aids in positioning the lid against the globe.

Postoperative edema caused by inadequate venous or lymphatic drainage may also be seen after cheek flap reconstruction. Although rare, these cases can be difficult to manage. Patience is critical, and staged revision can be beneficial.

Lid-sharing procedures have the inherent risk of postoperative scarring in the donor lid. If the lid margin is unstable after serving as a donor area in a lid-sharing procedure, entropion and trichiasis may occur over a period of time. Some degree of lagophthalmus or retraction of the upper eyelid may occur with the Hughes or Cutler-Bear procedures. In addition, instability of the lid can be produced unless at least 3 mm of the marginal tarsal plate is preserved. Their major disadvantage, however, is that two procedures are required and the eye remains closed for many weeks.

In general, it is extremely important to give careful attention to detail and undertake meticulous reconstruction of any part of the lid that comes in contact with the cornea.

References

1. Jelks G, Smith E. Reconstruction of the eyelids and associated structures. In: McCarthy JG, ed. *Plastic surgery.* Philadelphia: WB Saunders, 1990; 1671.
2. Mustardé JC. *Repair and reconstruction in the orbital region.* 2nd ed. Edinburgh: Churchill Livingstone, 1980; 133–147.
3. Grabb WC, Smith JW. *Plastic surgery.* Boston: Little, Brown, 1979; 431.
4. Matsuo K, Hirose T, Takahashi N, et al. Lower eyelid reconstruction with a conchal cartilage graft. *Plast Reconstr Surg* 1987; 80:547.
5. Van der Meulen JC. The use of mucosa-lined flaps in eyelid reconstruction: a new approach. *Plast Reconstr Surg* 1982; 70:139.
6. Jackson IT. *Local flaps in head and neck reconstruction.* St. Louis: CV Mosby, 1985; 273.
7. Callahan A. Free composite lid graft. *Arch Ophthalmol* 1954; 45:539.
8. Putterman AM. Viable composite grafting in eyelid reconstruction. *Am J Ophthalmol* 1978; 85:237.
9. Palletta FX. Lower eyelid reconstruction. *Plast Reconstr Surg* 1973; 51:653.
10. Price NM. Closure of surgical wounds using contiguous island flaps (double V to Y procedure). *Ann Plast Surg* 1979; 3:321.
11. Tenzel RR: Eyelid reconstruction by the semicircle flap technique. *Ophthalmology* 1978; 85:1164.
12. Tenzel RR. Lid reconstruction. In: Della Rocca RC, Nesi FA, Lisman RD, eds. *Ophthalmic plastic and reconstructive surgery.* St. Louis: CV Mosby, 1987; 771.
13. McGregor I. Eyelid reconstruction following subtotal resection of upper or lower lid. *Br J Plast Surg* 1973; 26:346.
14. Hughes WL. A new method for rebuilding a lower lid. Report of a case. *Arch Ophthalmol* 1937; 17:1008.
15. Hughes WL. *Reconstructive surgery of eyelids.* St. Louis: CV Mosby, 1959.
16. Cutler NL, Beard C. Method for partial and total upper lid reconstruction. *Am J Ophthalmol* 1955; 39:1.
17. Mustardé JC. The use of flaps in the orbital region. *Plast Reconstr Surg* 1978; 62:1.
18. Mustardé JC. Major reconstruction of the eyelids: functional and aesthetic considerations. *Clin Plast Surg* 1981; 8:227.
19. Fox SA, Beard C. Spontaneous lid repair. *Am J Ophthalmol* 1964; 50:947.
20. Mehta HK. Spontaneous reformation of lower eyelid. *Br J Ophthalmol* 1981; 65:202.
21. Smith B, English FP. Techniques available in reconstructive surgery of the eyelid. *Br J Ophthalmol* 1970; 54:450.
22. Wolfe SA. Eyelid reconstruction. *Clin Plast Surg* 1978; 5:525.
23. Flowers RS. Discussion: surgical treatment of the epicanthal fold. *Plast Reconstr Surg* 1984; 73:571.
24. Zide BM, McCarthy JG. The medial canthus revisited: an anatomical basis for canthopexy. *Ann Plast Surg* 1983; 11:1.

44

Ear Reconstruction

David C. Leber, M.D., F.A.C.S.

Reconstruction of a deformed ear, whether of congenital or traumatic origin, presents meticulous and aesthetic challenges. Advancements in technique and alternative approaches have resulted in the achievement of favorable outcomes that are gratifying to both patient and physician. This chapter presents methods of ear reconstruction that have been tested and proven reliable. Emphasis is placed on the use of autologous rib cartilage, with procurement and carving for the ear framework described in detail. Coverage in this chapter is in no sense definitive; the appended bibliography may be of assistance for particular ear reconstruction problems.

Congenital Ear Deformities

The most severe congenital deformities of the ear include anotia and microtia, in which there is complete or nearly complete absence of the external ear. Lesser deformities are those of hypoplasia of the middle third of the ear and hypoplasia of the superior third (i.e., the cup ear, lop ear, cryptotia, and cockleshell ear deformities) (1,2). The least severe deformity, that of prominent ears, is discussed in Chapter 55.

TOTAL EAR RECONSTRUCTION

In 1920 Gillies (3) was the first to describe total ear reconstruction with the use of carved cartilage placed under the scalp skin. The greatest advance in ear reconstruction came through the work of Tanzer in his classic description of the staged method of ear reconstruction using costocartilage as the framework (4,5). Brent (6–8) further improved these techniques into what is now considered a state-of-the-art procedure for total ear reconstruction.

Other methods for total ear reconstruction are available, including use of local tissues and use of cartilage from the opposite ear, but the most common technique involves ready-made frameworks of silicone (9) and, more recently, Medpor Surgical Implant (manufactured by Porex Surgical, Inc., College Park GA, 303-49-2417) (10). These techniques will be discussed later.

Some plastic surgeons suggest that reconstruction of a congenitally deformed ear be done at 6 years of age to avoid the psychologic trauma associated with the deformity. Others, including myself, prefer to wait until 8 to 10 years of age. Deferring surgery a few years allows the costocartilage to grow to a size that obviates the need for fragmentary or gradual fabrication of the framework (11,12).

The number of operations will vary depending on physical findings and patient preference for concha or tragus construction. At least two procedures are needed, and sometimes four or five can be anticipated.

Lobule formation may be done separately at an early age (4 to 6 years) or in combination with fabrication and insertion of the cartilage framework. The lobule also can be rotated into position after insertion of the framework.

PREOPERATIVE PLANNING

Though it is impossible to reconstruct an ear that appears exactly like the opposite ear, it is essential that the new ear be the correct size and in the proper position. Although many of the finely sculptured details are lost in a reconstructed ear because of a thicker skin cover, it is impressive how much detail will show through. The anatomy of a normal ear must be well understood (Fig. 44–1). Further, characteristics of the patient's intact ear should be noted and, where possible, incorporated into the planning and carving of the framework for the new ear.

Detailed preoperative planning is essential to achieve the above goals. If the lobule is rotated as a preliminary step, its exact desired location must be determined with as much accuracy as is needed for insertion of the cartilage framework. Precise measurements of size and position of the opposite ear are recorded (Fig. 44–2). The angle of inclination of the long axis of the ear usually falls between 10° and 30° in males, and 2° and 20° in females (13).

Clear x-ray film is helpful in determining the correct position for the reconstructed ear (Fig. 44–3). If there are problems with asymmetry of the face, as seen in hemifacial microsomia, location of the fabricated ear will need to be adjusted in proportion to the degree of facial hypoplasia. Patterns of the normal ear are drawn on clear x-ray film to determine the shape of the cartilage framework (Fig. 44–4). The patterns so devised are sterilized for use in the operating room during the carving process. Parallel strips of cardboard (Fig. 44–5) are helpful in checking the correct vertical position of the ear pattern (6,8). Acrylic models of the normal ear and microtic ear provide an excellent three-dimensional record of their size and shape and can be used in the operating room as a visual aid when carving the cartilage framework. These models are made from alginate molds of the ear and dental acrylic materials.

The most important preoperative aid is practice in carving an ear framework similar to the one planned for an individual patient. This helps the surgeon become familiar with the form and greatly decreases the amount of time required to carve the implant during actual surgery. If cadaver cartilage

FIG. 44–8. Carving cartilage framework. **A,** framework pattern is fixed to cartilage with two pins. Because of grain characteristics of cartilage, knife cuts are made with the grain (in the direction of the arrows). There is no need to draw an outline on cartilage. **B,** outline is cut with a no. 10 blade. Inside curve of antihelix is quickly removed with a 3/8-inch U X-ACTOR gouge. Cuts are perpendicular to surface. **C,** anterior surface is flattened by shaving the curved portion with a no. 10 blade (note that the synchondrosis is preserved). **D,** inside edge of the helical rim and triangular fossa are marked out with methylene blue. A checking cut 3 mm deep is made around the helical rim; this helps prevent accidental removal of the rim in subsequent steps. **E,** excavation of the scapula is done with a 3/32-inch U X-ACTOR gouge. **F,** successive cuts are made with the narrow gouge until the cartilage is removed through to the back surface in the area of the triangular fossa and posterior scapha. Holes through the framework permit better fixation of overlying skin, thus preventing loss of detail. The triangular fossa is completed with the 3/8-inch gouge. **G,** tail of the helical rim is thinned from the anterior surface. This allows the tail and lobular support to curve posteriorly as a result of uneven forces exerted within the cartilage (19). The antihelix is further refined with a no. 10 blade, rounding off the contours. **H,** anterior aspect of the helical rim is reduced in height to receive the added strip of cartilage that forms the root of the helix. Edges of the lobule, antitragus, and antihelix are carefully rounded to final shape. **I,** turning the framework over, the posterior margin of the helical rim is rounded off so that a more normal appearance is created when the ear is lifted away from the side of the head.

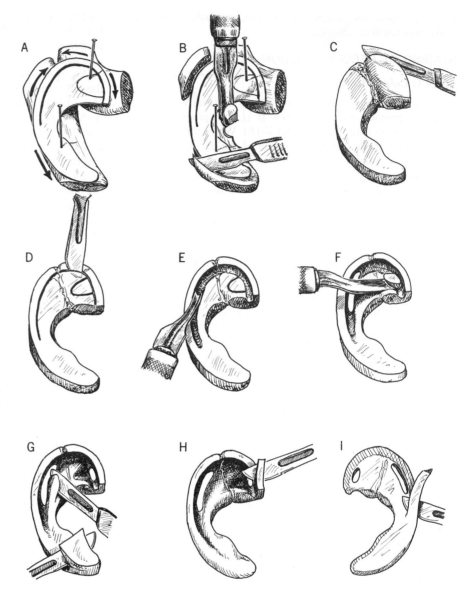

with interrupted 4-0 nylon. With appropriate care, there should be little concern about necrosis of the skin from excessive pressure and tension. The suction drain is tied off at 48 hours. The stents are kept in place for 2 to 3 weeks to keep the skin tightly applied to the underlying cartilage framework.

When there is insufficient skin to close the incision, a full-thickness skin graft is placed in the floor of the concha. The use of expanders has been fraught with many complications and I have not relied on them for additional skin cover. Upon completion of the procedure, the ear is dressed with cotton, fluffed 4 × 4 gauze, and soft pads, and wrapped with a conforming gauze dressing.

Stage III: Elevation of Ear and Creation of Postauricular Sulcus

If there is sufficient height of the ear and a postauricular sulcus is not desired by the patient, this stage can be eliminated (6). Most patients, however, do prefer to have the ear ele-

vated (Fig. 44–11). This procedure involves undermining the cartilage graft through a periauricular incision (taking care not to expose the cartilage framework). The banked piece of cartilage that had been placed under the scalp skin is removed, and the scalp skin is undermined and advanced anteriorly. A pocket is created under the ear framework and the ear is supported away from the head with the banked cartilage. The skin defect is then covered with a full-thickness skin graft. This procedure can be done 4 to 6 months after the framework was implanted.

Concha and Tragus Formation

When definition of the conchal floor and the tragus is lacking, the floor can be deepened while advancing a skin flap around the tragal cartilage support (Fig. 44–12). The conchal floor is than covered with a full-thickness skin graft (20). This graft can be taken from the postauricular sulcus of the normal ear while performing a setback of the normal ear when symmetry is indicated.

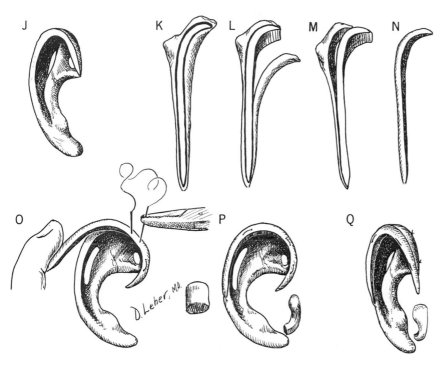

FIG. 44–9. Carving cartilage framework (continued). **J,** three-quarter view of completed framework base. Note undermining of helical rim. **K,** pattern for helical rim is drawn on 8th rib (note preformed curve in superior aspect). This will form the extension of the root of the helix. **L,** to prevent warpage, an equal amount of cartilage is removed from each side; removing the concave side first prevents accidental breakage of the narrow strip. **M,** completion of profile cuts. **N,** strip is also thinned on top and bottom. Outside edge is rounded, while inside edge is hollowed to increase overhang and detail of the helical rim. **O,** helical rim piece is easily fixed in position using 5-0 Ethilon (Ethicon, Inc.) clear monofilament nylon suture double armed with Ethicon ST-4 straight taper-point needles. The needles fix the cartilage until the suture is pulled through and tied posteriorly. When required, more flexibility of the rim can be achieved by small cuts around the outside edge. **P,** Four or five sutures complete the ear framework, which is now ready for implantation. Two additional pieces of cartilage are prepared for implantation. An extension for the tragus is carved, and a block 1 × 1 cm will be banked under the scalp for future support when lifting the ear away from the side of the head. **Q,** three-quarter view of completed cartilage framework.

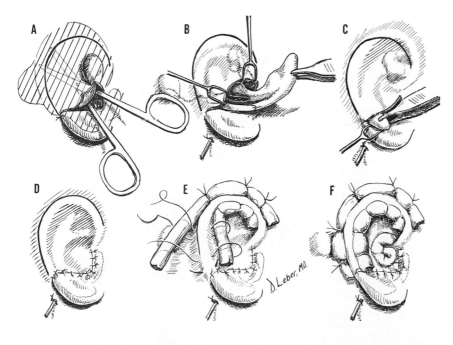

FIG. 44–10. Cartilage framework is implanted. **A,** subcutaneous pocket can be made through the incision of first-stage lobule transfer. If the lobule is being transferred at the same time as the cartilage implantation, even greater exposure is available. The thin skin is carefully dissected off the rudimentary ear cartilage in the upper pole, and the deformed cartilage removed. The pocket is dissected into the lobule to receive the tail of the helix and continued 1 cm beyond the planned ear outline. An extended pocket is dissected under the scalp in the postauricular area to receive a piece of banked cartilage, and another small pocket is created in the anterior aspect to receive the tragal cartilage. **B,** the banked cartilage is first placed in the scalp pocket. The framework is then inserted and rotated into position. A small silicone suction drain tube is placed into the pocket through a stab wound below the ear. **C,** the tail of the helix is then inserted into the lobule. **D,** the tragal cartilage is placed in its separate pocket. The incision is closed with 5-0 nylon. If there is insufficient skin to line the conchal floor, a full-thickness skin graft can be inserted. **E,** stents made of rolled petrolatum gauze are sutured into position with 4-0 nylon, snug enough to hold the skin into the undermined helical rim but not so tightly as to cause circulatory compromise. **F,** conchal floor is kept in place with a separate roll of gauze, which is held by a bulky soft-pressure dressing.

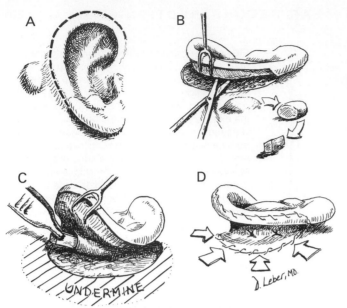

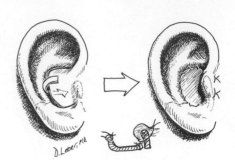

FIG. 44–12. The concha is deepened, and the tragus is formed.

FIG. 44–11. The auricle is elevated. **A,** a skin incision is made just outside the helical rim. **B,** the ear is lifted away from the scalp, and the sulcus is carefully dissected, avoiding exposure of the cartilage graft. The banked cartilage is removed from under the scalp and carved into a wedge 4–6 mm high and 10 mm long. **C,** a small pocket is developed under the fascia beneath the scapha and framework. The cartilage wedge is placed in the pocket to keep the ear in an anterior projection. The wedge must be covered with fascia so that the skin graft will survive. The scalp skin is undermined to permit advancement of the skin edge, thus reducing the size of the defect, hiding the graft behind the ear. **D,** the advanced scalp skin is sutured to underlying fascia, and the remaining defect is covered with a full-thickness skin graft. The ear is covered with a bulky pressure dressing and a wedge of foam rubber is placed in the sulcus.

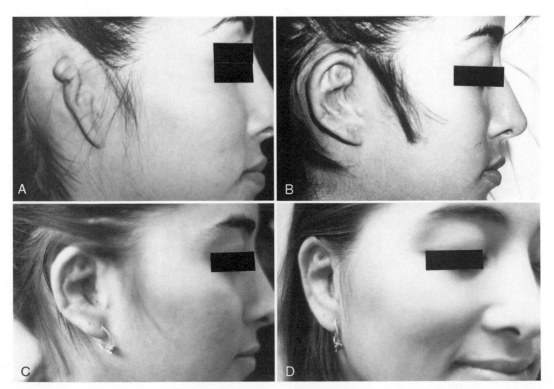

FIG. 44–13. Results using the previously described techniques. **A,** microtia, preoperative findings. **B,** result after first operation. **C, D,** final result after ear elevation, postauricular skin graft, conchal deepening, and tragus formation.

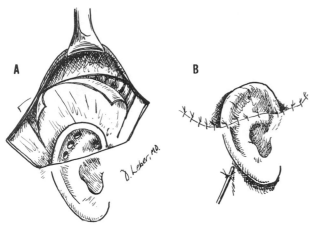

FIG. 44–14. A temporalis fascia "fan flap." **A,** temporalis fascia and periosteum are exposed and elevated. **B,** flap is draped over the exposed implant and covered with a split-thickness skin graft, while the skin flap is sutured behind the ear framework. (Redrawn from Fox JW, Edgerton MT. The fan flap: an adjunct to ear reconstruction. *Plast Reconstr Surg* 1976; 58:664.

Figure 44–13 shows preoperative and postoperative results using the previously described techniques.

ALTERNATIVE METHODS OF TOTAL EAR RECONSTRUCTION

When rib cartilage is of inadequate size, an expansible framework of cartilage may be indicated (21). Problems with loss of detail have been avoided by using Dacron backing on the cartilage framework (22). A method of ear reconstruction has been described that places emphasis on formation of the concha (23), using the expansile principle. With better understanding of the skin circulation, thinner flaps have been employed in a one-stage total ear reconstruction procedure (24). The advantages and disadvantages of this method should be evaluated carefully before discarding time-proven procedures. A bipedicle postauricular tubed flap has been used for less severe forms of microtia (25).

Preformed silicone frameworks have been the most commonly used implants in total ear construction when cartilage is not available, or used (9,26,27). The major disadvantage of this procedure is a high incidence of complications, such as infection and exposure of the implant. A new framework, Medpor Surgical Implant is a porous polyethylene material that has advantages over the silicone framework because of vascularization and ingrowth of tissue into the implant (10). Both silicone and Medpor implants are much more reliable when covered with either a temporal fascia "fan flap" (28,29) (Fig. 44–14) or temporoparietal fascia (30) (Fig. 44–15), followed by skin grafting. These flaps are also useful where good skin coverage is not available, such as in burn injuries (31).

PARTIAL EAR RECONSTRUCTION

Upper Third

Severe constriction and hypoplasia of the upper third of the ear is expressed in the cockleshell ear deformity (Fig. 44–16).

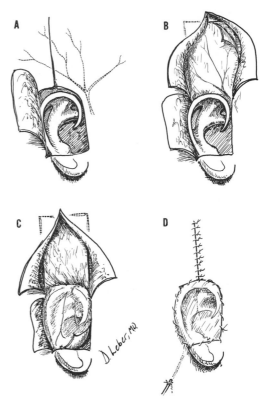

FIG. 44–15. The temporoparietalis fascia flap. **A,** skin incisions with posteriorly based flap for lining postauricular sulcus. **B,** scalp skin is carefully elevated just below the level of the hair follicles while avoiding injury to superficial temporal vessels. The parietal fascia flap is then elevated off the underlying temporalis fascia. **C,** fascial flap is draped over the ear implant and sutured in place with 5-0 absorbable sutures. **D,** suction is applied through small catheter to hold flap in place. A medium thickness skin graft from the suprascapular area is placed over the fascia flap. (Redrawn from Tegtmeier RE, Gooding RA. The use of a fascial flap in ear reconstruction. *Plast Reconstr Surg* 1977; 60:407.)

Reconstruction is accomplished by unfurling the ear and insetting it into the scalp. After several months, a cartilage graft is carved to correspond to the defect, buried under the scalp, and then later lifted away from the side of the head (7,32,33).

Middle Third

Hypoplasia of the middle third of the ear (Fig. 44–17) can be corrected by opening and expanding the ear in the midportion and insetting the cut edges into the scalp. An appropriately shaped cartilage graft is placed under the mature skin. The ear is lifted away from the scalp after several months and the postauricular sulcus is covered with a skin graft (34,35).

Lower Third or Lobule Construction

A number of methods have been suggested for lobule construction using local soft-tissue flaps (34–39). A representation of one of these methods (40) is presented in Figure 44–18. Lobule reconstruction can be very disappointing if there is no internal support, such as cartilage. In the absence of support, considerable atrophy of the new lobule will occur.

FIG. 44–16. Cockleshell ear deformity. **A,** typical deformity of cockleshell ear showing outline of the desired position of the ear. **B,** anterior superior portion of the constricted ear is separated from its attachment to the side of the head and unfurled, revealing the missing anterior superior one-third of the ear. Existing tissue is inserted into the scalp at this position. **C,** several months later, a cartilage graft is carved from costocartilage and buried under the scalp skin. **D,** three months later, the superior pole is lifted away from the head, and the sulcus is lined with a skin graft.

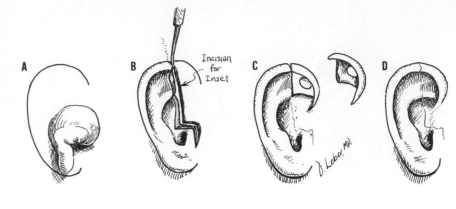

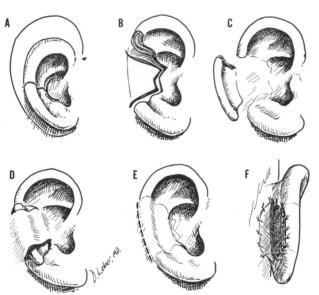

FIG. 44–17. Reconstruction of the middle one-third of the ear. **A,** severely constricted ear showing outline for the desired size and incision for expansion. **B,** posteriorly based scalp flap is incised. Posterior ear skin is sutured to outside margins of scalp incision. Anterior ear skin is sutured to inside flap margins. **C,** several months later, an appropriate costocartilage graft is carved to fill the central one-third of the defect. **D,** graft is inserted into tunnel through two small incisions. **E,** after incisions have matured, the ear is lifted from the side of the head through an incision along the posterior helical margin. Care is taken not to expose the cartilage graft. **F,** full-thickness skin graft covers the postauricular defect. (After Webster (34).)

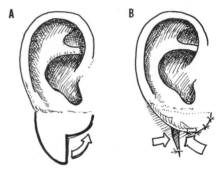

FIG. 44–18. The lobule is reconstructed. **A,** incisions for new lobule show that the inferior portion of the flap will be folded under the upper portion of the flap to provide double thickness. **B,** The anterior and posterior neck skin is undermined, advanced, and closed without need for a skin graft. (After Zentenio (40).)

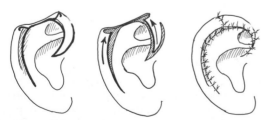

FIG. 44–19. Small acquired defects of the superior aspect of the ear can be corrected by advancing anterior and posterior skin and cartilage flaps. Incisions are made along heavy lines, and the flaps advanced superiorly and sutured. (After Antia and Buch (49).)

Acquired Ear Deformities

Acquired ear deformities include partial and complete traumatic amputations of the ear, burns, and tumors of the ear. Accidental loss of portions, or complete amputation, of the external ear is not common. Methods for treating such injuries have improved considerably. Simple replantation of the entire ear or parts of the ear has been successfully accomplished (41–44); however, the results are not dependable. Safer techniques such as the "pocket principle" (45,46) and microsurgical anastomoses of small blood vessels (47) have improved the success rate of ear replantation.

The pocket principle requires dermabrasion of the anterior skin of the amputated part, removal of the posterior skin, fenestration of the cartilage (48), and burying the part under a scalp flap while carefully suturing the part to its original point of attachment. Two weeks later, the buried part is exteriorized and allowed to epithelialize. A graft is then used to re-cover the postauricular surface.

When small portions of the ear are missing, local advancement flaps (Fig. 44–19) can be used to improve the contour (49,50). If larger portions of the ear are absent, the "tunnel procedure" of Converse (35) is useful (Fig. 44–20).

Other adjuncts in correcting partial defects due to trauma or losses due to tumor resection include the use of small

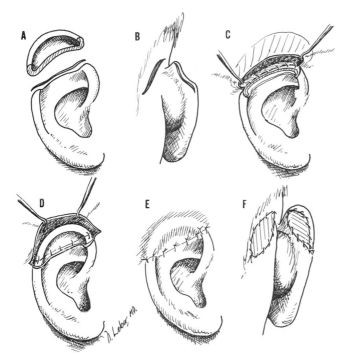

FIG. 44–20. The upper third of the ear (tunnel procedure) is reconstructed. **A,** size and shape of the lost ear part can be determined by placing a pattern of the opposite ear over the injured ear. A cartilage framework is then carved from costal cartilage corresponding to the missing part. **B,** incisions are made along the margin of the ear defect and over the corresponding scalp skin when the ear is pressed against the scalp. **C,** a pocket is dissected under the scalp skin. **D,** the carved cartilage framework is placed under the pocket and sutured to the margin of the remaining ear cartilage. **E,** scalp skin is then brought over the graft and sutured to the anterior ear skin margin. The scalp skin is held against the framework either with bolsters, as in Figure 44–10, or with suction. **F,** 3 to 6 months later the ear is separated from the scalp, and full-thickness skin grafts are used to cover the defects on the scalp and postauricular sulcus. (After Converse (35).)

tubed pedicle flaps, skin grafts, and composite grafts from the opposite ear (51).

Full-thickness burns of the ear present a difficult challenge in reconstruction. Frameworks of cartilage are preferred (21). Skin cover seems to be best provided with either the temporalis fascia flap or the temporoparietal fascia flap covered with a skin graft (29–31) (see Figs. 44–14 and 44–15). A thin cervical myocutaneous flap has also been used to cover exposed ear cartilage after burn injuries (52).

In the process of repairing defects of the ear, a slightly smaller ear may be the end result. If the difference is significant, symmetry of both ears can be obtained by a reduction in size of the normal ear (52,55).

Complications

The most significant complication of ear reconstruction is exposure of the implant. The causes of exposure are usually local trauma, infection, or too much tension of the skin cover leading to necrosis of the skin. When the ear framework is of silicone, the problems are more severe and may require removal of the implant. Salvage can be accomplished at times

with use of temporal fascia flaps (29–31). Exposure of a cartilage graft can usually be treated conservatively by preventing desiccation of the exposed cartilage, trimming the edges, and allowing the skin edges to grow over the defect. Rotation flaps may be needed for larger defects (56). Prevention of exposure requires attention to many details. These include absence of tension on the skin cover, avoidance of peripheral incisions in the area of the helical rim, and great care in dissecting the pocket for implant insertion so that skin circulation is not interrupted.

Bibliography

1. Rogers B. Microtia, lop, cup and protruding ears: four directly inheritable deformities? *Plast Reconstr Surg* 1968; 41:208.
2. Tanzer RC. The constricted (cup and lop) ear. *Plast Reconstr Surg* 1975; 5:406.
3. Gillies H. *Plastic surgery of the face.* London: H Frowde, Hodder and Stoughton, 1920.
4. Tanzer RC. Total reconstruction of the external ear. *Plast Reconstr Surg* 1959; 23:1.
5. Tanzer RC. Total reconstruction of the auricle. The evolution of a plan of treatment. *Plast Reconstr Surg* 1971; 47:523.
6. Brent B. The correction of microtia with autogenous cartilage grafts: I. The classic deformity. *Plast Reconstr Surg* 1980; 66:1.
7. Brent B. The correction of microtia with autogenous cartilage grafts: II. Atypical and complex deformities. *Plast Reconstr Surg* 1980; 66:13.
8. Brent B. A personal approach to total auricular construction. *Clin Plast Surg* 1981; 8:211.
9. Cronin TD. Use of a Silastic frame for total and subtotal reconstruction of the external ear: preliminary report. *Plast Reconstr Surg* 1966; 37:399.
10. Wellisz T. Reconstruction of the burned ear. *Plast Surg Techniques* 1995; 1:35.
11. Baurinka L. Congenital malformations of the auricle and their reconstruction by a new method. *Acta Chir Plast* 1966; 8:53.
12. Fukuda O, Yamada A. Reconstruction of the microtic ear with autogenous cartilage. *Clin Plast Surg* 1978; 5:351.
13. Farkas LG. Growth of normal and reconstructed auricles. In: Tanzer RC, Edgerton MT, eds. *Symposium on reconstruction of the auricle.* St. Louis: CV Mosby, 1974; 24.
14. Tanzer RC. Reconstruction of the auricle in four stages. In: *Transactions of the 5th International Congress of Plastic and Reconstructive Surgery.* Melbourne: Butterworth, 1971; 445.
15. Tanzer RC, Rueckert F. Reconstruction of the ear. In: Tanzer RC, Edgerton MT, eds. *Symposium on reconstruction of the auricle.* St. Louis; CV Mosby, 1974; 46.
16. Tanzer RC. Congenital deformities of the auricle. In: Converse JM, ed. *Reconstructive plastic surgery.* Philadelphia: WB Saunders, 1977; 1671.
17. Tanzer RC, Rueckert F. Reconstruction of the ear. In: Grabb WC, Smith JW, eds. *Plastic surgery, a concise guide to clinical practice.* 2nd ed. Boston: Little, Brown, 1973; 494.
18. Tanzer RC. Total reconstruction of the external ear. *Ann Plast Surg* 1983; 10:76.
19. Gibson T, Davis WB. The distortion of autogenous cartilage grafts: its cause and prevention. *Br J Plast Surg* 1958; 10:257.
20. Kirkham HJD. The use of preserved cartilage in ear reconstruction. *Ann Surg* 1940; 111:896.
21. Brent B. Reconstruction of ear, eyebrow, and sideburn in the burned patient. *Plast Reconstr Surg* 1975; 55:312.
22. McGibbon B. Use of Dacron backing on the cartilage framework in the construction of ears. *Plast Reconstr Surg* 1977; 60:262.
23. Matsumoto K. A new method of reconstruction in microtia with emphasis on conchal creation. *Ann Plast Surg* 1980; 5:51.
24. Song Y, Song Y. An improved one-stage total ear reconstruction procedure. *Plast Reconstr Surg* 1983; 71:615.
25. Sarig A, Ben-Bassat M, Taube E, et al. Reconstruction of the auricle in microtia by bipedicle postauricular tubed flap. *Ann Plast Surg* 1982; 8:221.
26. Cronin TD. Reconstruction of the external ear with a Silastic frame. *Transactions of the 5th International Congress of Plastic and Reconstructive Surgery.* Melbourne: Butterworth, 1971; 452.

27. Cronin TD. Use of a silastic frame for reconstruction of the auricle. In: Tanzer RC, Edgerton MT, eds. *Symposium on reconstruction of the auricle.* St. Louis: CV Mosby, 1974; 33.

28. Edgerton MT, Bacchetta C. Principles in the use and salvage of implants in ear reconstruction. In: Tanzer RC, Edgerton MT, eds. *Symposium on reconstruction of the auricle.* St. Louis: CV Mosby, 1974; 58.

29. Fox JW, Edgerton MT. The fan flap: an adjunct to ear reconstruction. *Plast Reconstr Surg* 1976; 58:663.

30. Tegtmeier RE, Gooding RA. The use of a fascial flap in ear reconstruction. *Plast Reconstr Surg* 1977; 60:406.

31. Cotlar SW. Reconstruction of the burned ear using a temporalis fascial flap. *Plast Reconstr Surg* 1983; 71:45.

32. Davis J. Repair of severe cup ear deformities. In: Tanzer RC, Edgerton MT, eds. *Symposium on reconstruction of the auricle.* St. Louis: CV Mosby, 1974; 134.

33. Cramer LM. Personal communication.

34. Webster JP. Some procedures for the correction of ear deformities. *Transactions of the 13th Annual Meeting of the American Society for Plastic and Reconstructive Surgery* 1944; 123.

35. Converse JM. Reconstruction of the auricle. *Plast Reconstr Surg* 1958; 22:150.

36. Davis J. Repair of traumatic defects of the auricle. In: Tanzer RC, Edgerton MT, eds. *Symposium on reconstruction of the auricle.* St. Louis: CV Mosby, 1974; 247.

37. Kazanjian VH, Converse JM. *The surgical treatment of facial injuries.* 2nd ed. Baltimore: Williams & Wilkins, 1959; 1013.

38. Subba Rao YV, Venkatesware Roa P. A quick technique for earlobe reconstruction. *Plast Reconstr Surg* 1968; 41:13.

39. Brent B. Earlobe reconstruction with an auriculomastoid flap. *Plast Reconstr Surg* 1976; 57:389.

40. Zentenio AS. A new method for earlobe reconstruction. *Plast Reconstr Surg* 1970; 45:254.

41. McDowell F. Successful replantation of a severed half ear. *Plast Reconstr Surg* 1971; 48:281.

42. Larsen J, Pless J. Replantation of severed ear parts. *Plast Reconstr Surg* 1976; 57:176.

43. Lewis EC, Fowler JR. Two replantations of severed ear parts. *Plast Reconstr Surg* 1979; 64:703.

44. Salyapongse A, Maun LP, Suthunyarat P. Successful replantation of a totally severed ear. *Plast Reconstr Surg* 1979; 64:706.

45. Mladick RA, Horton CE, Adamson JE, et al. The pocket principle: a new technique for reattachment of severed ear part. *Plast Reconstr Surg* 1971; 48:219.

46. Mladick RA, Carraway JH. Ear reattachment by modified pocket principle. *Plast Reconstr Surg* 1973; 51:584.

47. Pennington DG, Lai MF, Pelly AD. Successful replantation of a completely avulsed ear by microvascular anastomosis. *Plast Reconstr Surg* 1980; 65:820.

48. Converse JM, Brent B. Acquired deformities of the auricle. In: Converse JM, ed. *Reconstructive plastic surgery,* 2nd ed. Philadelphia: WB Saunders, 1977; 1724.

49. Antia NH, Buch VI. Chondrocutaneous advancement flap for the marginal defect of the ear. *Plast Reconstr Surg* 1967; 39:472.

50. Renard A. Post auricular flap based on a dermal pedicle for ear reconstruction. *Plast Reconstr Surg* 1981; 68:159.

51. Brent B. The acquired auricular deformity: a systemic approach to its analysis and reconstruction. *Plast Reconstr Surg* 1977; 59:475.

52. McGrath MH, Ariyan S. Immediate reconstruction of full-thickness burn of the ear with an undelayed myocutaneous flap. *Plast Reconstr Surg* 1978; 62:618.

53. Peer LA, Walker JC. Total reconstruction of the ear. *J Int Coll Surg* 1957; 27:290.

54. Furnas DW. Problems in planning reconstruction in microtia. In: Tanzer RC, Edgerton MT, eds. *Symposium on reconstruction of the auricle.* St Louis: CV Mosby, 1974; 93.

55. Tipton JB. A simple technique for reduction of the ear. *Plast Reconstr Surg* 1980; 66:630.

56. Tanzer RC. Reconstruction of the auricle. In: Goldwyn RM, ed. *The unfavorable result in plastic surgery.* Boston: Little, Brown, 1972; 147.

45

Facial Paralysis: Principles and Treatment

Ralph T. Manktelow, M.D., F.R.C.S.(C.), and Nancy Van Laeken, M.D., F.R.C.S.(C.)

The patient with facial paralysis experiences a very severe functional and cosmetic deformity. This deformity is related both to the muscular inactivity on the affected side and to apparent overactivity on the normal side. Treatment goals are patient-specific and are influenced by the aesthetic and functional deficits that bother the patient. It is important to create an individualized patient treatment plan to fit the particular concerns of the patient.

A careful history will identify what is most bothersome to the patient, and a detailed physical examination will reveal the anatomic abnormalities that concern the patient. From this the surgeon can review the treatment modalities available for the presenting functional and aesthetic problems and select the most appropriate procedures.

Most patients are hurt emotionally by the paralysis. It significantly affects their body image and thus their self-esteem. In the early years following the paralysis, patients are likely to be devastated by the appearance of their face and the stress of having to deal with friends and the public. With time, some patients learn to cope and adjust to their problem. However, most never completely adjust to it or accept it without ongoing emotional trauma. These patients are most appreciative of any improvements that the surgeon can provide to bring their faces closer to normal. Nevertheless, it is important that the surgeon develop realistic expectations in patients or their satisfaction with the procedure will be diminished.

Treatment options are influenced by the age of the patient, the duration of the facial paralysis, the status of the nerve trunk, and the state of the facial musculature and soft tissues (1,2).

Reconstructive goals are both functional and aesthetic. For the eye, functional rest recovery takes priority, as salvage of vision is the highest priority. Eye complications resulting from exposure and drying of the eye can lead to corneal ulceration and loss of vision.

Other goals of reconstruction are to provide symmetry at rest between the paralyzed and normal side and between voluntary and involuntary motion. The ultimate goal is to restore involuntary, independent, and spontaneous facial expression. Clearly, this is very difficult and cannot always be accomplished.

When it has been established that recovery will not take place spontaneously, timely reconstruction should be planned to minimize the patient's emotional stress and to take maximum benefit from the condition of the facial tissues (Fig. 45–1). Patients who have sustained a Bell palsy subsequent to an acoustic neuroma resection or injuries to the facial nerve (either intra- or extra-temporal) will usually show significant signs of recovery within 6 months or, at the most, 1 year. If useful recovery has not taken place at 1 year, the surgeon can be confident that it will not likely happen and proceed with plans for reconstruction.

Early Reconstruction (Table 45–1)

Suture of Divided Facial Nerve Ends

When possible, early direct suture of divided facial nerve ends will offer the best chance for functional recovery (3). "Early" reconstruction involves reinnervating the paralyzed musculature, and should be done as soon as possible, before significant muscle degeneration occurs (preferably < 6 months).

The nerve stumps should be realigned in fascicular groups without tension (4,5). The repair is epineural and is performed with the aid of a microscope (6). If the nerve laceration is to a single branch and is anterior to the parotid, nerve repair is not necessary because there is overlapping function of distal branches. If multiple branches are damaged, as is usually the case, nerve repair becomes necessary.

Nerve Graft

To avoid tension and overcome gaps, it may be necessary to use a nerve graft (7). The best results are achieved using a nerve graft of similar cross-sectional diameter (e.g., a split sural nerve, the greater auricular nerve), depending on the level of nerve injury.

The results of nerve grafting are dependent upon the ability of the axons to pass through the nerve coaptation, the state of the muscles once the axons have reached the myoneural junction, and the appropriateness of the reinnervation (7–11). A major problem in the patient who obtains reinnervation through direct nerve repair, and especially through nerve grafting in the proximal portion of the facial nerve, is synkinesis. Synkinesis is the involuntary movement of muscles of facial expression simultaneous with the voluntary contraction of other muscles (eg. elevation of the lip during voluntary eye closure). If the orbicularis oris contracts simultaneously with the lip elevators, the patient appears to be grimacing instead of smiling.

CROSS-FACIAL NERVE GRAFTS

In situations where it is not possible to do a direct nerve repair, VIIth nerve axons may be directed to the distal end(s) of the facial nerve by cross-facial nerve grafts from the nonparalyzed side.

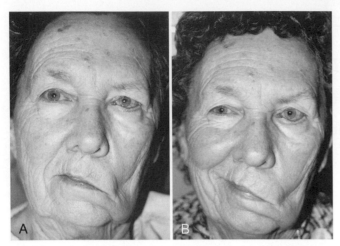

FIG. 45–1.   A, elderly patient with complete facial paralysis at rest. Note the marked asymmetry of the face with the paralyzed left side drooping and being drawn to the right side by the unopposed facial tone on the normal side. **B,** with smiling, the face becomes even more asymmetrical and deformed in appearance.

Table 45–1
Early Treatment of Facial Paralysis

Restore nerve continuity by:
   Primary nerve repair
   Nerve grafting (to overcome gaps)
   Cross-facial nerve grafting
   Nerve transfers
      Hypoglossal to facial (XII)
      Spinal accessory to facial (XI)
      Phrenic to facial (X)
   Muscular/neural neurotization of paralyzed facial muscles

The technique of cross-facial nerve grafting has been described by Smith and colleagues (9,12,13). The technique involves using a sural nerve graft to connect the functioning nerve fibers from the normal side to those on the paralyzed side. The fibers that are utilized on the normal side vary in location and number. Baker and Conley (10) grafted the entire lower division of the nerve from the normal side onto the main trunk of the nerve on the involved side. Other authors, including Anderl and Fisch, used several more peripheral nerve branches in the normal side for insertion of the nerve graft (Fig. 45–2). It is possible to sacrifice approximately one-half of the branches that supply any particular function without affecting function on that side. Anderl advocated a two-stage reconstruction. In the first stage, the sural nerve grafts are sutured to selected facial nerve branches on the nonparalyzed side. Four to nine months later, when it is believed that the axons have grown through the nerve graft, the nerve graft is sutured on the paralyzed side to the corresponding branches of the facial nerve. The proposed advantages of the two-stage procedure are reduced operative time and the ability to perform the 2nd nerve repair with axons crossing the repair shortly after its completion, rather than 6 months later when scar tissue may obstruct their path.

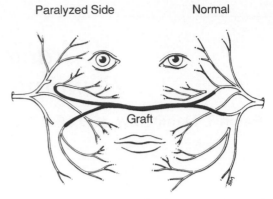

FIG. 45–2.   Cross-facial nerve graft using the sural nerve between branches of the facial nerve that supply the eye and mouth. The graft is attached to proximal branches of the face on the normal side and distal branches on the paralyzed side. Multiple grafts may be inserted, including separate grafts to the eye and separate grafts to the mouth.

The results of cross-facial nerve grafting have often been disappointing. These poor results are probably due to poor axonal regrowth and muscle degeneration (15–18). Presently we believe that cross-facial nerve grafting has a modest place in young patients if done within 6 months of paralysis. Tone, and some spontaneous movement, will occur in some patients providing symmetry at rest and spontaneous facial expression. Synkinesis can be expected.

Nerve Transfers

Nerve transfers have been used extensively to reinnervate the paralyzed nerve trunk. They should be done as quickly as possible after paralysis, preferably in less than 6 months. It is interesting (and fortunate) that patients will occasionally develop the ability to use the nerve transfer without conscious awareness. The hypoglossal-to-facial nerve transfer has been used most often (18–20). The optimal result that can be expected is symmetrical resting tone with an onset at 4 to 6 months and maximum at 12 months. Following transfer, the patient must learn to push the tongue against the incisors or palate in order to activate the facial muscles.

Hypoglossal transfer usually produces satisfactory orbicularis occuli tone and provides adequate eye function. This is a major value with this procedure. Another strength of the procedure is the resting muscle tone in the lower face. This produces good facial symmetry at rest for both the mouth and the cheek. Further procedures will usually be required to produce a satisfactory smile. The patient rarely develops good facial movement because there is a mass firing into all of the facial nerves at once, producing synkinesis.

There are several other major disadvantages of the hypoglossal transfer technique. They include excessive resting tone of the facial paralysis and atrophy of the ipsilateral tongue. Uncoordinated mass movements of the affected side of the face occur with eating, chewing, and talking. Tongue paralysis results in catching of food in the vestibule on the affected side and difficulty in clear articulation and swallowing. The creation of a smile is limited by simultaneous contraction of the orbicularis oris and the lip elevators and depressors, which produces a grimacelike movement of the face.

An alternative nerve transfer has been cranial nerve XI (spinal accessory) to facial (21). This transfer can provide good resting tone, but the patient must elevate the shoulder to produce facial movement. A significant problem is the severe shoulder droop, which is both a cosmetic and functional deficit, if the entire nerve is used. Partial nerve transfer may obviate this problem.

The phrenic nerve has also been used if both nerves XI and XII are unavailable (22). A smile can be produced while the patient is taking a deep breath. It is complicated by facial twitches and asymmetry with coughing and laughing.

An alternative to nerve transfer is the transference of functioning motor endplates to denervated muscle via a neuromuscular pedicle graft (21). This has not been very successful in the clinical setting (23–25). Conley (26) performed neurotization of the denervated muscle by placing the split surface of the masseter muscle into an area of paralyzed facial muscle. Axonal ingrowth into the adjacent empty neural tubules does occur and extends beyond the immediate contact surfaces (27). With this technique, Conley was able to achieve adequate physical support to the cheek and lip, as well as some voluntary movement of the lower face, including a simulated smile. It did not produce spontaneous emotional expression. Because of muscle atrophy, this technique cannot be used in cases of longstanding paralysis. An alternative neurotization procedure is the ansa hypoglossal transfer. It is designed to produce neurotization of the paralyzed face musculature by transfer of the nerve and a small piece of musculature directly to the paralyzed facial muscle. Few surgeons have duplicated the initial successful reports.

Late Reconstruction

In cases in which the patient is not suitable for muscle reinnervation because of longstanding paralysis and subsequent atrophy of myoneural junctions, reconstruction is achieved using static clings, dynamic slings, and free muscle transfers. Treatment is directed toward the eye, periorbital tissue, mouth, and cheeks.

MANAGEMENT OF THE MOUTH

There are a number of aesthetic and functional problems experienced by the patient with a facial paralysis (Table 45–2). Asymmetry at rest and the inability to smile are the two features that most bother the patient. Other problems associated with paralysis of the oral musculature are drooling and difficulties with speech and articulation. The flaccid lip and cheek soft tissues also lead to some difficulties with chewing food, cheek biting, and pocketing of food in the cheek and buccal sulcus. The surgical solutions should be selected to solve each patient's specific problems.

Static Slings

Early techniques included a circumoral tendon graft, which should not be used because it prevents wide opening of the mouth (e.g., for dental care).

Fascial suspension is used to achieve symmetry at rest without providing animation. It can be used alone or as an adjunct to nerve grafting or free muscle transfer to provide

immediate support while awaiting muscle reinnervation (26–30; Fig. 45–3). Autologous or synthetic material may be used (31,32). Fascial strips harvested from the thigh (tensor fasciae latae) or temporalis muscle fascia have been used most frequently. Gore-Tex, a substance used extensively in

Table 45–2
Reconstruction of the Mouth

Static slings
    Autologous materials
        Fasciae lata
        Temporalis fascia
        Tendon grafts
    Synthetic materials
        Silastic rods
        Mesh
        Gore-Tex

Dynamic transfers
    Temporalis muscle transfer
    Masseter transfer
        Split masseter transfer
        Complete masseter transfer
        Digastric transfer
    Free functioning muscle transfer
        Gracilis
        Extensor digitorum brevis
        Pectoralis minor
        Serratus anterior
        Latissimus dorsi
        Extensor carpi radialis brevis

Soft-tissue procedures to improve symmetry
    Rhytidectomy
    Excision of redundant intraoral mucosa

Procedures for drooling
    Wilkie procedure
    Submandibular gland resection with parotid duct ligation

Modification of normal side to improve symmetry
    Neurectomy
    Myectomy

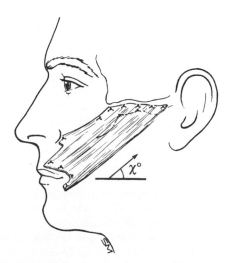

FIG. 45–3. Static slings provide good symmetry at rest and are particularly useful in elderly patients. Fasciae latae is a reliable material.

vascular surgery, has recently been employed to provide support. Its major advantages include its soft pliable texture, ready availability, strength, and, most important, resistance to stretching with time. The Gore-Tex used is available in a flat sheet of 0.6-mm thickness. In our experience, the inflammatory response produced by Gore-Tex and its susceptibility to infection detracts from its usefulness.

To insert the sling, a segment of the suspensory material is cut to the appropriate length and width to span the gap from the oral commissure to the body of the zygoma and temporal fascia. It is maintained in position with multiple permanent sutures. The sutures are strategically placed in the orbicularis oris around the corner of the mouth and in the upper lip, as directed by the patient's deformity. When tension is applied, the force is distributed evenly, reproducing the resting position that is noted on the normal side. Significant overcorrection is advised to allow for some suture relaxation. Even with significant overcorrection, there will be drooping (particularly in the 1st year) that will often require an adjustment. The sling is attached laterally to the periosteum over the body of the zygoma and to the temporalis fascia. The position can be checked by sitting the patient partly upright in the operating room.

Dynamic Slings

Regional muscle transfers have been used extensively for many years to achieve static support of the mouth and to produce a smile (33–38). The most frequently used muscles are the temporalis and the masseter. The digastric, platysma, and sternocleidomastoid muscles have also been used to reconstruct the depressor anguli oris (39,40).

Baker and Conley (41) have described in detail the technique of transposing the masseter muscle to the skin around the mouth for oral movement. They advocate using the entire muscle, splitting it in its most distal portion for insertion around the mouth into the upper and lower lip. Other authors recommend separating the most anterior half of the muscle only and transposing it to the upper and lower lip. The surgeon must be cautious during the splitting dissection to avoid injury to the masseteric nerve, a branch of the trigeminal that supplies the muscle, by entering the deep surface of the muscle in its midportion.

The patient maintains voluntary control over the muscle and can activate it by clenching the teeth. Good static control of the mouth can be achieved with this technique, but the muscle does not contract with sufficient force to allow for symmetry when smiling. There is also inadequate excursion to produce a full smile and the movement produced is too oblique for most faces. Removal of the masseter may leave a hollow above the angle of the mandible and produce a bulge in the cheek in the region of the transfer.

A more effective and versatile muscle for transfer is the temporalis (42). The temporalis muscle is harvested from its bed in the temporal fossa and turned over the zygomatic arch to extend to the oral commissure. It may be necessary to dissect the fascia off the muscle, leaving it attached superiorly so that it reaches the oral commissure (Fig. 45–4). Baker and Conley (41) recommended leaving a portion of the temporalis muscle anterior to the hairline to avoid an unsightly temporal hollow. The hollow can also be filled with a Silastic implant to improve the contour. Another aesthetic disad-

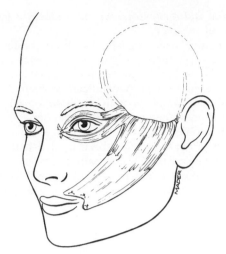

FIG. 45–4. Temporalis transfer over the arch of the zygoma for smile reconstruction and eye closure.

vantage of the temporalis transfer is the bulge of muscle present where the muscle passes over the arch of the zygoma. To avoid these complications, McLaughlin (43) used an intraoral incision. By detaching the coronoid process, he was able to attach the temporalis muscle insertion into the angle of the mouth with fascial strips.

The temporalis provides excellent static positioning as well as voluntary activity. It is capable of producing a more vertical lift to the mouth and greater movement than the masseter transfer. The muscle is also supplied by the trigeminal nerve; therefore, it is activated by the voluntary action of clenching the teeth.

To achieve a proper direction of pull, the patient's smile should be analyzed. If the major direction of pull is superior and lateral, a temporalis muscle transfer would provide the most appropriate movement. If the smile is more horizontal, then a masseter transposition would be the most appropriate.

Both muscles may be transferred together; this has been popularized by Rubin (44). He prefers the temporalis to provide motion to the nasolabial fold in the upper lip and the masseter to control the position and movement at the corner of the mouth and the lateral aspect of the lower lip. Patients receive a therapy program to teach them how to activate the muscles and provide the desired movement (44).

Freilinger (45) presented a novel concept that combines a cross-facial nerve graft and a temporalis transfer. This provides the reliable contractile force of the temporalis muscle without the need for more complex transfers and provides the potential for voluntary and involuntary motion being innervated by the opposite normal side of the face. This has not become popular, likely due to the popularity of microvascular transfers.

Free Muscle Transfer

The only techniques currently available to restore both voluntary and involuntary facial movement plus symmetry at rest require the use of the VIIth nerve. This nerve is most easily utilized when combined with a free functioning muscle transfer.

It is not possible to restore complete symmetry of movement of all facial muscles because of the complexity and the number of facial muscles involved (46–48). There are 18 separate muscles of facial expression. At present, it is possible to transfer only one or two functioning muscles in an attempt to produce some movement. The movement that is most appropriately created is the smile, because it is the deficit found to be the most distressing to the patient. In addition to providing active motion, muscle transplantation can also provide a symmetrical appearance to the mouth at rest. If the facial nerve is used to reinnervate the transferred muscle, then smile and laughter will be spontaneous. When other nerves are used (e.g., V, XI or XII), teeth clenching or other movements are required to activate the smile.

Preoperative Planning

A vascularized, innervated muscle transfer will be successful only if certain criteria are met. The basic requirement is muscle survival, and this is dependent upon patency of the microvascular anastomoses (49,50). Muscle function then requires appropriate reinnervation. To provide adequate movement in the proper direction, the muscle size, its attachment to the origin and insertion, and its tension must be carefully calculated. Analysis of facial movement, particularly direction and type of smile on the normal side, is essential to help determine the required movement on the paralyzed side.

Muscle Selection

Various muscles have been used to reanimate the paralyzed face. These include the gracilis, latissimus dorsi, serratus anterior, pectoralis minor, extensor digitorum brevis, extensor carpi radialis brevis, and rectus abdominis (51). The specific muscle used is probably not as important as its placement in the face and its functional anatomy (52). A muscle with a contractile capability of 1.0 to 1.5 cm, and sufficient strength to move the facial soft tissues effectively, is required. A constant vascular pedicle and nerve supply are needed to allow reliable microvascular transfer.

The muscle selected should leave no functional deficit. If two separate functions (e.g., eye closure and mouth movement) are required, it is desirable to choose one muscle that has two separately functioning neuromuscular units, one for the mouth and one for the eye (53). The pectoralis minor, serratus anterior, and gracilis have this anatomic capability. Nevertheless, a transfer that attempts to reconstruct the eye as well as the mouth does not produce a satisfactory eye closure.

Mayou and coworkers (54), O'Brien and colleagues (55), and Tolhurst and Bos (56) have reported their experience with the use of the extensor digitorum brevis muscle transplant to reconstruct facial paralysis. This reconstruction was done in conjunction with a cross-facial nerve graft. In follow-up, they noted that the power and excursion of the muscle are inadequate to provide consistently symmetrical facial movement.

Several authors have described the use of the pectoralis minor muscle for the treatment of unilateral facial palsy (57–59). It has the advantages of easy elevation from the anterior chest wall and a good size for insertion into the face. Disadvantages include a vascular pedicle of short length and innervation by nerve branches that support both pectoralis major and minor. The location of the muscle close to the

neck also makes simultaneous face and muscle dissection difficult, prolonging the procedure. Harrison (57) described the vascular pedicle as a separate artery and vein coming directly from the axillary artery and vein. Terzis and Manktelow (58) noted that the dominant pedicle is usually a branch of the thoracodorsal artery and accompanying vein. Harrison reported good results with this muscle; Terzis believes that this is a good muscle for children, but too bulky for adults.

The gracilis muscle is an excellent donor for muscle transplantation and is our preferred muscle (60). It leaves no functional deficit and easy access to it is provided by a small medial thigh incision. It has a reliable vascular pedicle that is a branch of the profunda femoris artery and enters the muscle approximately 9 cm from the muscle origin. The artery is an adequate size (1.2 to 2.0 mm) and is accompanied by a pair of venae comitantes of size suitable for anastomosis. It is supplied by a single motor nerve, a branch of the obturator nerve that enters the muscle obliquely just proximal to the dominant pedicle. The fascicles can be separated and individually stimulated to produce two longitudinal, separately functioning neuromuscular territories in the majority of muscles. The muscle can be cut transversely and longitudinally to produce the desired size of muscle for a transfer (Fig. 45–5). The amount of muscle that is transferred varies with the patient's face and the size of the gracilis muscle.

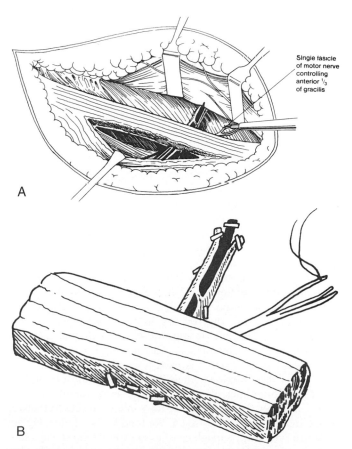

FIG. 45–5. A portion of the gracilis muscle is transferred. **A,** the portion is based on the dominant, proximal vascular pedicle. **B,** the motor nerve may be divided into separate fascicles and the portion of the muscle controlled by one fascicle is separated from the rest of the muscle.

We have used the extensor carpi radialis brevis for smile reconstruction. It has the advantage of having tendon or fascia at each end of the muscle for secure fixation. It has reliable but short neurovascular structures. The muscle is usually transferred by trimming some of the superficial and deep portions and leaving the central part attached to the tendon of origin and fascia of insertion. This provides a piece of muscle that has a fiber length of 6 to 7 cm that is ideal for insertion in the cheek. The disadvantage of this procedure is that the scar on the forearm may be visible and the patient may have some weakness of grip strength. This muscle has been used in twelve procedures. We feel that the place of this muscle is still being worked out but that it may be most useful for the older person who has a lot of sagging of the face—for whom the muscle needs to be very securely attached and in whom a forearm scar is not as visible (61).

Jiang and colleagues (62) have used the abductor hallucis muscle as a one-stage muscle transfer. They indicate that the muscle is the appropriate size and shape for smile reconstruction, has a reliable neurovascular anatomy, and its removal does not affect foot function.

In skeletal musculature, the force of muscle contraction is directly proportional to the cross-sectional area of the muscle fibers that are contracting. The range of excursion or the degree of shortening is directly proportional to the muscle-fiber length. Clinically, we have found that the more muscle is put in, the more excursion results, and this includes both length and cross-sectional area. There are limitations to both of these measurements. If too much bulk of muscle is inserted, there will be visible swelling on the face. Presently, our procedure is to remove some fat in the face in the region where the muscle is lying. It is important that this does not include too much fat under the skin, or the muscle, if it becomes stuck to the dermis, will wrinkle the skin in a very undesirable fashion. This buffering layer of fat between the muscle and the skin is important, or the skin will appear tethered, as has been previously described. The length of the zygomaticus major is approximately 6 cm and the muscle extends from the commissure to the body of the zygoma. If a longer segment of muscle is used, a larger excursion is produced, particularly if a cross-facial nerve graft does not provide as much innervation drive as an ipsilateral nerve. To put in a longer segment of muscle it is necessary to place the muscle more obliquely just lateral to the body of the zygoma and attach it to the arch of the zygoma and temporalis fascia. If the muscle passes over top of the arch of the zygoma it may produce an undesirable bulge. If the muscle is spread thinly, and there is some defatting, this bulge may not be noticeable. The amount of wasting that occurs in facial paralysis muscle transfers is remarkable; it appears to at least equal that of a completely denervated muscle. This finding is the opposite of the one when the gracilis is used to repower the extremities (e.g., for finger flexion) when the return of muscle bulk is good and sometimes becomes as large as it was in the thigh before transfer. The question of how much muscle to transfer is one that no one has resolved. We tend to do a balancing act between providing enough muscle to provide good excursion without providing too much bulk. Some surgeons do secondary procedures to debulk the muscle; we do very few, possibly because we use a relatively small piece of muscle in the first place.

Muscle Innervation

The choice of nerve for muscle reinnervation includes ipsilateral and contralateral facial nerve, as well as the hypoglossal, trigeminal, and accessory nerves (63). The facial nerve is the preferred source of innervation because it is the only source of nerve impulses that normally produce facial expression. Using the facial nerve is the only means of obtaining involuntary facial movements and spontaneous expression.

If facial nerve stumps leading to the mouth are present on the paralyzed side, they are the preferred source of innervation. However, their function is usually unknown and it is often difficult to determine which ones carry smile messages and which ones purse the lips.

If there are no suitable nerve stumps available on the paralyzed side, the preferred source of neurotization is the opposite facial nerve. A long nerve graft is placed from the normal to the paralyzed side, as originally described by Anderl and Smith. At least 50% of the normal peripheral facial nerve branches that elevate the lip are divided and attached to the cross-facial nerve graft on the normal side (Fig. 45–6). There will not be any functional deficit on the normal side. A single-stage transfer that avoids a nerve graft may be done by taking a long motor nerve on the muscle and joining it directly to branches of the facial nerve on the normal side (62,64).

The cross-facial graft is done 9 to 12 months before muscle transplantation (Fig. 45–7). The distal end of the nerve graft is banked in front of the ear in preparation for muscle transplantation. When reinnervation of the graft has occurred, tapping over the end of the graft on the paralyzed side will elicit a Tinel sign, which is referred to the normal side in the region of the zygoma. The Tinel sign localizes to the musculature supplied by the previously divided facial nerve branches. A buzzing sensation is noted as a positive Tinel sign. This indicates that some nerve regeneration has taken place and it is time for the muscle transplantation, which can be carried out a few months later.

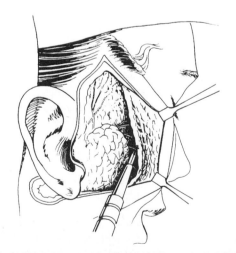

FIG. 45–6.   Staged muscle transfer for smile reconstruction is begun with a cross-facial nerve graft. This requires identification of the appropriate branches of the facial nerve that produce smile on the normal side. (From Manktelow RT. *Microvascular reconstruction.* Heidelberg, Springer-Verlag, 1986; 133.)

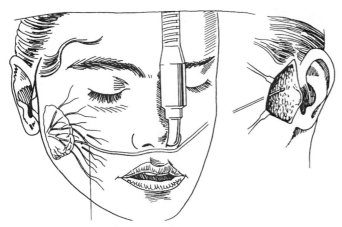

FIG. 45–7. The cross-facial nerve graft placed across the upper lip with the end banked in front of the ear on the paralyzed side. (From Manktelow RT. *Microvascular reconstruction.* Heidelberg, Springer-Verlag, 1986; 133.)

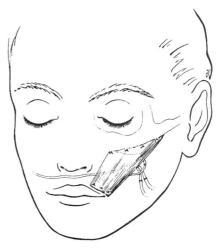

FIG. 45–8. Attachment of the muscle to the lip, maxilla, and zygoma, and appropriate repairs to the cross-facial nerve graft and facial artery and vein.

In patients with bilateral facial paralysis (e.g., Moebius syndrome), with no VIIth nerve source for neurotization, either the hypoglossal nerve or the motor branches of the trigeminal nerve can be used. The hypoglossal nerve can be split and only one-half used, in order to avoid loss of tongue function (59). The motor branch to the masseter can be sacrificed with little functional deficit. The disadvantages of using these two nerves include the retraining the patients must undergo to smile consciously, the likelihood that they will never develop a spontaneous smile, and the undesirable contraction of the muscle with eating.

Techniques

The procedure of facial reanimation with functioning muscle transfer usually proceeds through two stages (46).

If a cross-facial nerve graft is required, the sural nerve is the usual donor nerve. This nerve is harvested through a longitudinal incision with direct exposure of the nerve, or through multiple small transverse incisions and gentle avulsion of the nerve.

The nerve graft is placed through a subcutaneous tunnel from the paralyzed side to the normal side of the face using a face-lift incision that allows exposure and functional evaluation of the branches of the normal facial nerve (see Fig. 45–6). The normal facial nerve is dissected medial to the parotid gland and nerve stimulation is used to identify the function of the branches. Approximately one-half of the buccal branches will provide pure levator function. The others carry orbicularis oris function and well as levator or depressor function and should not be used, or the muscle will contract when the lips are pursed. It is not possible to assess nerve function accurately with anything less than a micro bipolar electrical probe attached to a stimulator source that allows variable voltage control and frequency; the disposable stimulators that are used to identify the presence of motor nerves do not provide a reliable controlled contracture of muscles that will allow you to palpate and identify what is contracting. For reinnervation of the nerve graft, facial nerve branches that, when stimulated, produce a smile and no other movement are selected.

One-half of the nerve branches that produce a smile are divided, and their proximal ends are sutured to the nerve graft using a fascicular repair with 11-0 nylon. The nerve graft is secured with a large silk suture in the preauricular area on the paralyzed side so that it can be found easily at the time of muscle transplantation.

The second stage is the muscle transfer which is done 9 to 12 months later. Preoperative markings outline the desired location of the muscle as determined by smile analysis; the correct placement of the transplanted muscle is determined by analysis of the shape of the smile on the nonparalyzed side of the face. The soft tissues are assessed for skin creases at rest and while smiling. The shape of the oral commissure varies between individuals. The amount of lip eversion also varies. The direction of the upper lip and commissure movement can be measured on the patient using a goniometer. Preoperative markings are used to aid proper muscle placement and direction of pull. Smile analysis is an important part of the preoperative planning.

Attaching the muscle to the mouth is a critical part of the procedure. It is usually inserted into the fibers of the orbicularis oris above and below the commissure and along the upper lip. The points of insertion are determined by intraoperative traction on the orbicularis oris while observing the movement of the mouth. The location and position of the traction are changed until the appropriate shape is achieved. The direction of movement of the commissure is determined by the origin of the muscle. It is determined preoperatively by smile analysis. The origin is usually placed along the anterior maxilla and body and the arch of the zygoma (Figs. 45–8, 45–9, 45–10). To produce greater excursion, it may be placed over the zygoma and attached to the temporal fascia allowing use of a longer piece of muscle.

Adjunctive Procedures for Static Support

There are many additional procedures available to provide improved facial symmetry in the patient who is not a candidate for reanimation or static slings. In certain cases the long duration of paralysis has produced severe facial muscle atro-

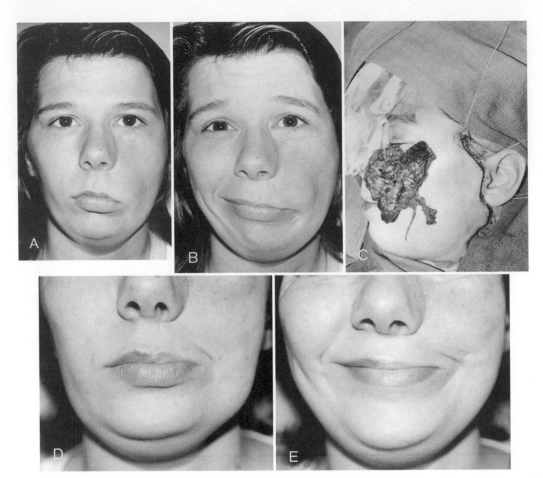

FIG. 45–9.   A, patient seen 3 years after resection of an angiosarcoma with facial paralysis involving the lower portion of the left face and a significant soft-tissue defect. **B,** paralysis is observed with smiling. **C,** patient had a lipomuscular transfer of a portion of the gracilis muscle using microneurovascular techniques. The motor nerve of the muscle is sutured to a branch of the facial nerve. **D,** transfer provides good contour reconstruction and symmetrical position of the lips at rest. **E,** patient has a spontaneous natural smile and good facial symmetry.

phy, associated skin laxity, and drooping of the face on the involved side. Procedures directed at altering the areas of skin redundancy can be of some benefit.

These procedures usually involve suspension and repositioning of the lax structures. This will include rhytidectomy with or without SMAS plication or suspension. In the older patient with a heavy drooping face, it may be useful to insert a static fascia lata sling as well as a functioning muscle to provide adequate support to the mouth and cheek at rest.

Treatment of Oral Incontinence

Chronic drooling can be a problem associated with facial paralysis. A lower-lip ectropion secondary to paralysis of the orbicularis oris can lead to oral incontinence and drooling. Usually repositioning of the mouth with static or dynamic procedures will correct this problem. There are several surgical procedures available to alleviate this problem if static and dynamic slings are not adequate.

One is redirection of the salivary flow using the Wilkie procedure. This involves creation of mucosal flaps around the orifice of the parotid duct. These flaps are tubed and then tunneled into the tonsillar fossa to divert saliva from the mouth directly into the oral pharynx. This procedure may be done in conjunction with submandibular gland resection. An alternative approach is submandibular gland resection with bilateral parotid duct ligation. Brundage and coworkers (60) have recently reported great success with this procedure. Both procedures alleviate the problems of drooling. Parotid duct ligation is considered to be a technically easier surgical procedure and it has less postoperative morbidity and a reduced duration of hospitalization.

Redundant intraoral mucosa may develop following long-standing paralysis. This mucosa is prone to being bitten by the molars and can be excised to prevent constant irritation. Eversion of the paralyzed lip can be corrected by an elliptical excision of the excessive mucosa.

The Mouth: Control of Antagonistic Muscle

In a patient with a complete unilateral nerve palsy, a portion of the disfigurement occurs secondary to overactivity or unrestrained activity of muscles on the normal side. With contraction, these unopposed muscles draw the paralyzed side toward the normal side, resulting in a deformity that worsens with smiling. This leads to exaggerated movement on the normal side and displacement of the atonic muscle groups to that side (see Fig. 45–1). One approach to this problem is to divide nerve or muscle on the normal side to decrease muscle activity (66–68).

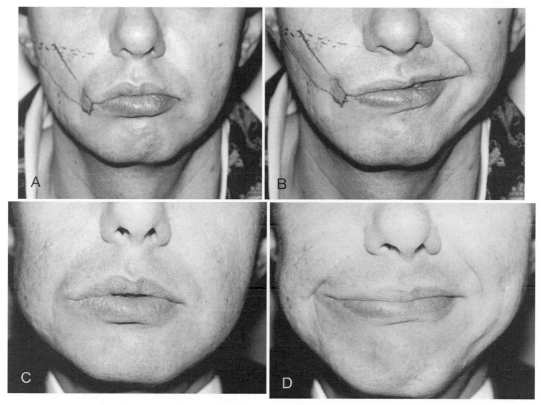

FIG. 45–10. **A,** patient with near-complete congenital paralysis. Deformity is minimal at rest. **B,** deformity is significant with smiling. Cross-facial nerve graft is dotted on cheek. It was attached by upper lip as well as commissure. **C,** following a staged cross-facial nerve graft and microneurovascular muscle transfer, the patient has good movement of the upper lip. **D,** smiling motion is spontaneous with reasonable symmetry.

Distortions and disfigurement result from overactivity of the levator labii superioris or inferioris, depressor anguli oris, or zygomaticus major. Attempts to improve symmetry have been made by denervation of the appropriate muscle or a reduction in muscle bulk. Myectomy of the depressor labia inferioris through an intraoral approach is particularly useful. This is a beneficial procedure for the person with lower-lip asymmetry resulting from hyperactivity of this muscle. A more normal appearance to the lower lip results.

Symmetry about the mouth is difficult to achieve with neurotomies because either over- or under-correction frequently occurs. A neurectomy of the frontal branch is sometimes carried out to obliterate unilateral forehead wrinkles. This is an excellent way to obliterate wrinkles on one side of the forehead and provide forehead symmetry. There may now be significant brow ptosis on both sides that will require brow lift procedures.

How to Select the Appropriate Reconstruction for the Mouth

The most suitable reconstruction will depend on the surgeon's experience and the patient's requirements. It is very important to listen to each patient carefully in order to identify which aspects of the paralysis are most troublesome. If the patient is disturbed about his or her appearance at rest and is not particularly interested in smiling, a static sling may be the most suitable procedure. For the older patient with a lot of sagging of the cheek and mouth, this is a satisfactory procedure.

A patient who wishes to be able to smile and to have better oral function will require a muscle transfer, either a free-functioning muscle transfer or a local muscle transfer (e.g., a temporalis transfer). The advantages of the temporalis transfer are timing and reliability: the results usually occur within a few months after surgery and most patients will get some motion and some improvement in the contour of the face at rest. A free-functioning muscle transfer may be most appropriate for the person who smiles a lot and wishes to do so spontaneously without having to think of biting to produce a smile. A socially active individual who frequently eats with others may be quite upset with a temporalis transfer because of the continual cheek motion while chewing.

Free-functioning muscle transfers using microneurovascular techniques are relatively new. When there is an appropriate branch of the VIIth nerve available on the side of paralysis, as may be the case following a tumor resection of the face or following facial injury, then reinnervation is more reliable and the final result of muscle transplantation is obtained within 1 year of the procedure. If there are no branches of the facial nerve available for muscle reinnervation, a preliminary cross-facial nerve graft is required. The disadvantages of these transfers are the time that it takes until a final result is obtained, the need for reinnervation to produce movement, the fact that reinnervation is not as strong with a cross-facial nerve compared with an ipsilateral nerve, and the relative complexity of the procedures. However, the advantages are the spontaneity of movement of the face that results from the fact that the muscle is governed by the VIIth nerve and the flexibility of the reconstruction technique that allows customization of the smile reconstruction.

It is generally recognized that reinnervation does not occur as well with older individuals. However, there is no clear definition of what is "old" in terms of muscle reinnervation. It is our practice to be cautious about doing functioning muscle transfers for individuals over 50 years of age, although there is no hard data to substantiate this. Our own results clearly show better reinnervation in the pediatric age group when compared with adults. Even though this procedure is still evolving in our hands, it is superior to local muscle transfers for smile reconstruction.

MANAGEMENT OF THE EYE

The treatment of eye problems in a facial palsy patient is directed toward preservation of function, alleviation of symptoms, and improvement in appearance (Table 45–3). Prevention of eye complications in a patient with facial paralysis is a primary goal of treatment. Inactivity of the orbicularis oculi combined with a relative overactivity of the levator palpebrae superioris produces a situation of chronic corneal exposure. This can lead to corneal erosions, corneal infections, and occasionally perforation and blindness. This problem is exacerbated if there is lacrimal gland dysfunction and/or loss of corneal sensation.

Loss of the lacrimal pumping mechanism leads to inadequate drainage of tears. The tear flow mechanism is disturbed for several reasons. The orbicularis oculi muscle in a patient with a VIIth nerve palsy is not capable of producing eye closure with the upper and lower lids. It is normally the movement of the lower lid that creates a vacuum in the lacrimal system and aids in drawing tears into the punctum. The lower-lid paralysis also leads to lower-lid laxity and ectropion, which is aggravated by constant wiping, and to secondary corneal irritation, which then produces reflex hypersecretion of tears.

The three major functional areas of concern are, therefore, lagophthalmos with chronic corneal exposure, epiphora, and ectropion.

Patients are often greatly disturbed by the aesthetic appearance of the eye on the paralyzed side. The primary aesthetic concern is the wide open, staring eye that is unable to show emotion. The unopposed activity of the levator palpebrae superioris produces elevation of the upper lid. The hypotonicity of the orbicularis oris produces depression of the lower lid. The eye appears larger than that on the normal side, with scleral show and a staring appearance.

Corneal Protection

Protection of the cornea can be provided by various ophthalmic solutions such as artificial tears, lubricants, and ophthalmic ointments. Forced blinking, lid taping, and patching have been tried. The cornea can also be protected by the use of soft contact lenses and bubble-type moisture chambers. Temporary eye closure can be provided by lid gluing or suturing.

Lateral tarsorrhaphy has been the mainstay of the emergency treatment for lagophthalmos and lid laxity and ectropion. The McLaughlin lateral tarsorrhaphy with preservation of eyelashes for camouflage is a popular technique. The pro-

Table 45–3
Reconstruction of the Eye

Early management
  Artificial tears
  Ophthalmic ointment
  Patching
  Moisture chambers
  Lip taping
  Forced blinking
  Contact lenses
  Lid suturing
  Tarsorrhaphy, medial/lateral

Late management
  Upper lid
    Lid weights
    Lid magnets
    Springs
    Blepharoplasty
  Lower lid
    Conchal cartilage
    Dermal flap
    Kuntz-Szymanowski lid-shortening procedure
    Static slings
  Both lids
    Silicon encircling band (Arion)
    Pedicled muscle transfer
    Free muscle transfer

Soft-tissue procedures for improved symmetry
  Blepharoplasty
  Brow lift

cedure consists of attaching the opposing surfaces of the upper and lower lid at the lateral margin. A wedge of skin, cilia, and orbicularis oculi muscle from the lower lid is excised as well as a wedge of tarsus and conjunctiva from the upper lid. The two raw surfaces are then approximated.

By decreasing the horizontal lid length, this procedure allows for an adequate eye coverage during sleep and approximates the upper and lower lids throughout their length. It may also prolong the effectiveness of the precorneal tear film. Most patients find the shorter lid aperture and the lower placement of the lateral canthus aesthetically undesirable. There is a permanent deformity of both upper and lower lids secondary to tissue loss. It is, however, the safest procedure for the patient who has a dry eye and/or an anesthetic cornea.

Lower Lid Procedures

There are many techniques available to correct lower-lid laxity and ectropion. The treatment can be directed to the medial and lateral canthal area.

In medial ectropion with punctal eversion, the lower lid can be repositioned against the globe by direct excision of a tarsoconjunctival ellipse, which causes a vertical shortening of the inner aspect of the lower lid. This helps reposition the punctum against the globe. Medial canthoplasty will also support the punctum. Combinations of vertical elevation and horizontal shortening of the medial eyelid are effective in more severe cases. Propping up the lid with a full-thickness skin graft with or without a cartilage graft may also be effective.

For lateral and central ectropion, a horizontal lid-shortening (e.g., the modified Kuntz-Szymanowski) procedure with or without a tarsorrhaphy or canthoplasty is an effective way to correct the lower eyelid position and maintain proper tear flow. The lateral canthoplasty can be done by mobilization of the lateral canthal tendon or by a deepithelialized dermal flap attached to the superolateral orbital margin.

Lower-lid ectropion can also be supported by the insertion of a Silastic sheet or conchal cartilage in the lower eyelid (70). A piece of cartilage or Silastic is cut to the shape of the lower lid, positioned deep to the orbicularis oculi, and attached to the inferior orbital margin by sutures placed through the periosteum or bone. It sits in the lower eyelid and projects the lid upward, advancing the lower margin of the lid. Our experience with these propping-up procedures is poor. We find that the cartilage tends to assume a more horizontal rather than vertical position and to project the skin forward, leaving a visible bulge.

Static support of the lower eyelid can also be supplied by a sling of fascia. The sling is placed subcutaneously in the lower-lid margin from the medial canthus to the lateral orbital margin. This sling provides good elevation of the lower eyelid. The problem lies in obtaining adequate tension. The sling often has to be revised because it loosens in time, but when the appropriate tension is present it is very satisfactory. It is important that the sling be placed right within the lid margin. If this is not done, there will be an eversion of the lid margin over top of the sling with loss of contact with the globe and a visible exposed rim of conjunctiva. In order to place the fascia accurately, it is passed on a curved Keith needle subcutaneously along the margin of the eyelid. The fascia is wrapped around and securely fixed to the medial canthal ligament. Laterally, the fascia is attached to the orbital margin either through a hole or through a flap of periosteum and doubled back on itself. Frequently we will use a small piece of the palmaris longus for this sling.

Our most satisfactory lower-lid procedures are the Kuntz-Szymanowski and the static sling. The Kuntz-Szymanowski should be used if there seems to be excessive or redundant lower eyelid tissue. If there is eversion and relatively tight lower eyelid skin and tissue, then a sling is the preferred procedure.

The Upper Eyelid

In addition to static support for the lower eyelid, there have been many attempts to provide dynamic eye closure by modification of the upper lids. These modifications are directed toward overcoming the unopposed action of the levator palpebrae superioris.

Lid loading with weights is the most popular and simplest technique (72–74). Twenty-four carat gold is the preferred substance because of its good colour match, high specific gravity, and relative nonreactivity. The appropriate weight is determined by taping or gluing a trial prosthesis to the upper lid over the tarsal plate with the patient awake. The weight is fixed in a subcutaneous position to the tarsal plate. This is a good procedure for lagophthalmos and provides good eye closure when the patient is upright or reclining. Patients may complain of the lump on the upper lid; however, this is rarely visible to the patient because it can only be seen when the eyes are closed. Complications include extrusion, a visible mass in the upper lid, and irritation of the eye; they are usually related to having selected too large a weight (75). The weight may be placed along the lid margin or above. If the weight is placed in higher positions, so that the weight covers only the upper half of the tarsal plate, it is less visible to the patient and less likely to extrude. Care must be taken that the attachment of the levator to the tarsal plate is left intact. Initial experience with 1.2–1.4 gram weights resulted in more patient complaints than with the lighter weights. We have found that 0.8 to 1.0 grams provide adequate improvement in eye closure and give the patient a comfortable eye without weight-related problems. It is not necessary to obtain complete closure for the patient to obtain eye comfort.

An alternative is the insertion of two small, permanently magnetized rods into the upper and lower lid. Mühlbauer (76) reported good initial results in 61% of patients. This procedure is used infrequently now because of the high rate of extrusion of the magnets. Currently Mühlbauer believes that, although the rods will remain permanently in some patients without extrusion, the best indication is for the patient who will likely recover from the paralysis and needs a short-term solution.

Dynamic closure of the upper and lower lid may be accomplished by a number of different procedures. One technique for eyelid closure is the palpebral spring described by Morel-Fatio (77). Problems with malpositioning of the spring, spring breakage, and skin erosion, which necessitate spring removal, have prevented widespread utilization of these springs. The Arion silicon encircling band, attached at the medial canthal ligament and lateral orbital rim, has also been used. Adjustment of the proper tension allows dynamic eyelid closure. As with the other foreign materials inserted into the eyelids, usually erosion of the Silastic band through the skin necessitates removal.

Temporalis muscle transfer with fascial strips passed through the upper and lower eyelids and sutured to the medial canthal ligament has been successful in supplying dynamic eyelid closure using autologous tissue (69–78). The fascia extension of the transferred temporalis muscle is tunneled through each eyelid close to the eyelid margin. Laterally, the orbicularis oculi is attached to the temporalis muscle. The patient must learn to clench the teeth to produce eyelid closure.

The major problem with this technique is fascial stretching, which results in loss of effective eyelid movement, and fascial adherence, which prevents motion. With muscle contraction, the lid aperture changes from an oval to a slit shape. There may also be distortion of the palpebral aperture through lateral displacement of the eyelids, skin wrinkling over the lateral orbital margin, and a bulge at the lateral orbital margin. Nevertheless, this procedure usually provides an excellent static support and provides some eye closure on command. Movement of the eye while chewing may be a disturbing feature for the patient.

Other dynamic procedures include microvascular muscle transfer to the eyelid. This has been done in combination with a transfer to the face. One muscle is used to provide both smile and orbicularis oris function—by splitting the muscle into strips, as when the gracilis is used, or using the pectoralis minor and placing one slip in the upper and one in the lower eyelid. With this procedure it is difficult to obtain finesse, because a single muscle serves the entire face.

Terzis (50) has had some success with procedures primarily to transfer small pieces of functioning muscle to the face. The frontalis muscle from the nonparalyzed side has been pediculed across the bridge of the nose and inserted into the upper and lower lids. Another procedure that is in its infancy but has met with some success is the microneurovascular transfer of the platysma muscle (79). The platysma is a thin, flat sheet of muscle that is admirably suited to insertion in the lower and upper eyelids. It is done as a microvascular transfer, revascularizing with the superficial temporal artery and vein, and reinnervation is accomplished with a cross-facial nerve graft. This is a tedious and complex procedure and should be reserved for patients for whom simpler techniques are unsuccessful in providing comfort and aesthetic reconstruction.

Ancillary Procedures: The Eye

Soft-tissue asymmetry can be corrected in several ways. Blepharoplasty may bring benefit through removal of lax skin from the paralyzed side in both upper and lower lid. Extreme caution must be used in doing a lower-lid blepharoplasty to avoid producing a lower-lid ectropion in an already hypotonic lid. Lagophthalmos may be produced by excessive resection of upper-lid skin.

Selecting the Appropriate Reconstruction for the Eye

Selection of the most appropriate procedures for the paralyzed eye is a difficult process; it depends on the patient's particular complaints and physical findings. The choice is between static and dynamic procedures. The static procedure is often adequate and gives good cosmesis. However, static procedures may not prevent epiphora, which in some patients requires a dynamic reconstruction. Reconstruction with a temporalis transfer can provide a dynamic movement; however, the transfer may become adherent and function primarily as a static sling. With dynamic motion, the disadvantages are the distortion of the lateral portion of the eye and a bulge that is sometimes present over the lateral orbital margin. Free-functioning muscle transfers using platysma or frontalis are still in the early stage of development and it is not yet possible to predict whether they are going to play major role. All of the variables that affect free muscle transfers for reconstruction of the mouth are present with the eye. In addition, there is the requirement of a very thin slip of muscle. To date, it has been difficult to transplant a muscle without producing some increase in bulk in the eye.

Most surgeons would agree that procedures that do not employ the VIIth nerve for reanimation of either the eye or the mouth will not likely provide an ideal solution. Only transfers that use the VIIth nerve have the potential for producing a spontaneous reanimation, and our reconstructive efforts should be directed toward using this nerve.

THE FOREHEAD

Asymmetry and distortion can occur in the upper face as a result of apparent overactivity of muscles. Overactivity of the frontalis muscle can lead to permanent forehead wrinkling with deep furrows on the normal side. This also produces a significant discrepancy in the height of the two eyebrows.

The problem can be treated by elevation of the paralyzed brow or weakening of the normal frontalis and elevation of both brows. The frontalis may be weakened by transection of the frontal branch on the normal side or resection of strips of frontalis muscle to paralyze or weaken the brow.

A brow lift is useful to correct asymmetrical eyebrow positions. It can be a direct lid-lift via an incision placed directly above the eyebrow or it can be done through a coronal approach. The brow lift can be further supported by suspension from the temporalis fascia or frontal periosteum (80,81). The simplest technique for doing a brow lift is to do it directly at the level of the upper margin of the eyebrow. This involves an incision of the appropriate width of skin above the eyebrow. Frontalis may also be removed to provide a more permanent elevation of the brow. Frontalis or subcutaneous tissue may be tacked to the frontal periosteum to provide more secure and longlasting fixation of the brow position.

The problem with doing a brow lift is that it is essentially a static procedure and tends to stretch over time. Thus it is usually best to slightly overcorrect the position of the brow initially because there will be some drooping soon after surgery and then a very slow progression of drooping over the years to come that will usually be faster than that on the normally innervated side. The other problem with the brow lift is that, because it is static and the opposite side moves, the height of the normal side will vary with emotional expression and also with the time of day. It is thus difficult, if not impossible, to get a position of the brow that is always symmetrical.

THE NOSE

The dilator alae nasi muscle plays an important role in maintaining airway patency. This is most important in the patient with unilateral facial paralysis, in which absence of dilator muscle function leads to airway collapse and malfunction of the nasal valve with each inspiration. Lack of lip and cheek elevators allows further collapse of this lateral nasal wall. Correction of airway collapse is best accomplished by static support of the nasal base with fascia and by upper-lip elevation procedures. Occasionally a septoplasty will provide an improvement in airway patency.

SUMMARY

There are a variety of treatment modalities available for the patient with a VIIth nerve palsy. The treatment goals are directed to the presenting functional and cosmetic deficits and are individualized to suit the patient's needs. Multiple factors are considered during the decision-making process including patient's age, duration of palsy, extent of palsy, and functional problems.

The first goal is to prevent eye complications secondary to corneal exposure. The second goal is to provide functional and cosmetic restoration of the forehead, eye, nose, and mouth. These procedures should provide static and dynamic symmetry to the face and allow the patient spontaneous facial animation.

References

1. Berger A, Bargmann HJ. Functional reconstruction after facial paralysis. *World J Surg* 1990; 14:748.

2. House JW. Facial nerve grading systems. *Laryngoscope* 1983; 93:1056.
3. Sade J. Facial nerve reconstruction and its prognosis. *Ann Otolaryngol* 1975; 84:695.
4. Kempe LG. Topical organization of the distal portion of the facial nerve. *J Neurosurg* 1980; 52:671.
5. May M. Muscle of the facial nerve (spatial orientation of fibres in the temporal bone). *Laryngoscope* 1973; 83:1311.
6. Millesi H. Nerve suture and grafting to restore extratemporal facial nerve. *Clin Plast Surg* 1979; 6:333.
7. McCabe BF. Facial nerve grafting. *Plast Reconstr Surg* 1970; 45:70.
8. Fisch U. Facial nerve grafting. *Otolaryngol Clin North Am* 1974; 7:517.
9. Scaramella L. On the repair of the injured facial nerve. *Ear Nose Throat J* 1979; 58:45.
10. Baker DC, Conley J. Facial nerve grafting: a thirty-year retrospective review. *Clin Plast Surg* 1979; 6:343.
11. Salimben-Ughi G. Evaluation of results in 36 cases of facial palsy treated with nerve grafts. *Ann Plast Surg* 1982; 33:195.
12. Smith JW. A new technique of facial reanimation. In: Hueston JW, ed. Transactions of the 5th International Congress of Plastic and Reconstructive Surgery. Melbourne: Butterworth, 1971.
13. Anderl H. Reconstruction of the face through cross face nerve transplantation in facial paralysis. *Chir Plast* 1973; 2:17.
14. Anderl H. Cross face nerve transplant. *Clin Plast Surg* 1979; 6:433.
15. Gary-Bobo A, Fuentes JM, Guerrier B. Cross facial nerve anastomosis in the treatment of facial paralysis: a preliminary report on 10 cases. *Br J Plast Surg* 1980; 33:195.
16. Ferrari CM. Cross facial nerve grafting. *Clin Plast Surg* 1984; 11:211.
17. Miehlke A, Stennert E. New techniques for optimum reconstruction of the facial nerve in its extratemporal course. *Acta Otolaryngol* 1981; 91:497.
18. Gary-Bobo A, Fuentes JM. Long-term follow-up report on cross facial nerve grafting in the treatment of facial paralysis. *Br J Plast Surg* 1983; 36:48.
19. Evans DM. Hypoglossal facial anastomosis in the treatment of facial palsy. *Br J Plast Surg* 1974; 27:251.
20. Conley J, Baker DC. Hypoglossal facial anastomosis for reinnervation of the paralysed face. *Plast Reconstr Surg* 1979; 63:66.
21. Bret P. Anastomosis of the spinal accessory or hypoglossal nerve to the facial nerve following cerebellopontine angle surgery. *Int J Microsurg* 1980; 2:44.
22. Tucker HM. Restoration of selective facial nerve function by the nerve muscle pedicle technique. *Clin Plast Surg* 1979; 6:293.
23. May M. Facial nerve disorders. Update 1982. *Am J Otol* 1982; 4:77.
24. Freilinger G. A new technique to correct facial paralysis. *Plast Reconstr Surg* 1975; 56:44.
25. Nicolai JP, Vingerhoets HM, Notermans SLH. Our experience with Freilinger's method for dynamic correction of facial paralysis. *Br J Plast Surg* 1982; 35:483.
26. Conley J. Mimetic neurotization from masseter muscle. *Ann Plast Surg* 1983; 10:273.
27. Frey M, Gruber H, Holle J, et al. An experimental comparison of the different kinds of muscle reinnervation: nerve suture, nerve implantation and muscular neurotization. *Plast Reconstr Surg* 1982; 69:656.
28. Anonsen CK, Duckert LG, Cummings CW. Preliminary observations after facial rehabilitation with the ansa hypoglossi pedicle transfer. *Otolaryngology—Head and Neck Surgery* 1986; 94:302.
29. Backdahl M, D'Alessio E. Experience with static reconstruction in cases of facial paralysis. *Plast Reconstr Surg* 1958; 21:211.
30. Freeman BS. An immediate combined approach for rehabilitation of the patient with facial paralysis. *Plast Reconstr Surg* 1966; 37:341.
31. Freeman BS. Review of long term results in supportive treatment of facial paralysis. *Plast Reconstr Surg* 1979; 63:214.
32. Freeman BS. Late reconstruction of the lax oral sphincter in facial paralysis. *Plast Reconstr Surg* 1973; 51:144.
33. Collier J. Reanimation in facial paralysis. *Br J Plast Surg* 1952; 5:243.
34. Battle RJV. A technique for reanimation of the face after paralysis of the seventh nerve. *Br J Plast Surg* 1952; 5:247.
35. Conway H. Muscle plastic operations for facial paralysis. *Ann Surg* 1958; 147:541.
36. Edgerton MT. Surgical correction of facial paralysis: a plea for better reconstruction. *Ann Surg* 1967; 165:986.
37. Correia PC, Zani R. Masseter muscle rotation in the treatment of inferior facial paralysis. *Plast Reconstr Surg* 1958; 21:214.
38. Ragnell A. A method for dynamic reconstruction in cases of facial paralysis. *Plast Reconstr Surg* 1958; 21:214.
39. Matthews DN. Reanimation in facial palsy. *Br J Plast Surg* 1952; 5:253.
40. Conley J, Baker DC, Selfe RE. Paralysis of the mandibular branch of the facial nerve. *Plast Reconstr Surg* 1982; 70:569.
41. Baker DC, Conley J. Regional muscle transposition for rehabilitation of the paralysed face. *Clin Plast Surg* 1979; 6:317.
42. May M. Muscle transposition for facial reanimation. *Arch Otolaryngol* 1984; 110:184.
43. McLaughlin CH. Permanent facial paralysis. *Lancet* 1952; 2:647.
44. Rubin LR. The paralysed face, ch. 22: Reanimation of total unilateral facial paralysis by the contiguous facial muscle technique. St. Louis: CV Mosby, 1991.
45. Freilinger G. A new technique to correct facial paralysis. *Plast Reconstr Surg* 1975; 56:44.
46. Manktelow RT. Microvascular reconstruction: anatomy, applications and surgical technique. Heidelberg: Springer-Verlag, 1986.
47. Freilinger G, Gruber H, Happak W, et al. Surgical anatomy of the mimic muscle system and the facial nerve: importance for reconstructive and aesthetic surgery. *Plast Reconstr Surg* 1987; 80:686.
48. Rubin LR. The anatomy of a smile: its importance in the treatment of facial paralysis. *Plast Reconstr Surg* 1974; 53:384.
49. Harelius L. Transplantation of free autogenous muscle in the treatment of facial paralysis. *Scand J Plast Reconstr Surg* 1974; 8:220.
50. Terzis JK, Sweet RD, Dykes RW, et al. Recovery of function in free-muscle transplants using microneurovascular anastomosis. *J Hand Surg* 1978; 3:37.
51. Hamilton SGl, Terzis JK. Surgical anatomy of donor sites for free muscle transplantation to the paralysed face. *Clin Plast Surg* 1984; 11:197.
52. Frey M, Gruber H, Freilinger G. The importance of the correct resting tension in muscle transplantation: experimental and clinical aspects. *Plast Reconstr Surg* 1983; 71:510.
53. Manktelow RT, Zuker RM. Muscle transplantation by fascicular territory. *Plast Reconstr Surg* 1984; 73:751.
54. Mayou BJ, Watson JS, Harrison DH, et al. Free microvascular and microneural transfer of the extensor digitorum brevis muscle for the treatment of unilateral facial palsy *Br J Plast Surg* 1981; 34:362.
55. O'Brien BM, Franklin JD, Morrison WA. Cross facial nerve grafts and micro-neurovascular free muscle transfer for long established facial palsy. *Br J Plast Surg* 1980; 33:202.
56. Tolhurst DE, Bos KE. Free revascularized muscle grafts in facial palsy. *Plast Reconstr Surg* 1982; 69:760.
57. Harrison DH. The pectoralis minor vascularized muscle graft for the treatment of unilateral facial palsy. *Plast Reconstr Surg* 1985; 75:206.
58. Terzis JK, Manktelow RT. Pectoralis minor: a new concept in facial reanimation. *Plastic Reconstructive Surgery Forum,* May 1982.
59. Manktelow RT. Free muscle transplantation for facial paralysis. *Clin Plast Surg* 1984; 11:215.
60. Harii K, Ohmoi Y, Torii T. Free gracilis muscle transplantation with microneurovascular anastomosis for the treatment of facial paralysis. *Plast Reconstr Surg* 1976; 57:133.
61. Binhammer P, Manktelow RT, Haswell T. Microsurgical and muscle fiber anatomy of the extensor carpi radialis brevis. 3rd Vienna Muscle Symposium. Freilinger G, ed. Deutinger: M. Blackwell–MZV, 1992; 326.
62. Jiang H, Guo E, Ji Z, et al. One-stage microneurovascular free abductor hallucis muscle transplantation for reanimation of facial paralysis. *Plast Reconstr Surg* 1995; 96:78.
63. Zuker RM, Manktelow RT. A smile for the Moebius syndrome patient. *Ann Plast Surg* 1989; 22:188.
64. Kumar PAV. Cross-face reanimation of the paralysed face with a single stage microneurovascular gracilis transfer without nerve graft: a preliminary report. *Br J Plast Surg* 1995; 48:83.
65. Brundage SR, Moore WD. Submandibular gland resection and bilateral parotid duct ligation as a management for chronic drooling in cerebral palsy. *Plast Reconstr Surg* 1989; 83:443.
66. Clodius L. Selective neurectomies to achieve symmetry in partial and complete facial paralysis. *Br J Plast Surg* 1976; 29:43.
67. Niklison J. Contribution to the subject of facial paralysis. *Plast Reconstr Surg* 1956; 17:276.
68. Niklison J. Facial paralysis: moderation of non-paralysed muscles. *Br J Plast Surg* 1965; 43:397.
69. Jelks GW, Smith B, Bosniak S. The evaluation and management of the eye in facial palsy. *Clin Plast Surg* 1979; 6:397.

70. Anderl H. A simple method for correcting ectropion. *Plast Reconstr Surg* 1972; 49:156.

71. Carroway J. Personal communication.

72. Nicolai JPA, deKoomen H, Van Leeuwen JBS, et al. Gold weights in upper eyelids for the correction of paralytic lagophthalmos. *Eur J Plast Surg* 1986; 9:66.

73. Jobe RP. A technique for lid loading in the management of the lagophthalmos of facial palsy. *Plast Reconstr Surg* 1974; 53:29.

74. Neuman AR, Weinberg A, Sela M, et al. The correction of 70 nerve palsies with gold lid load (16 years experience). *Ann Plast Surg* 1989; 22:142.

75. Pickford MA, Scamp T, Harrison DH. Morbidity after gold weight insertion into the upper eyelid in facial palsy. *Br J Plast Surg* 1992; 48:460.

76. Mühlbauer WD, Segeth H, Viessman A. Restoration of lid function in facial palsy with permanent magnets. *Chir Plastica* 1973; 1:295.

77. Morgan LR, Rich AM. Four years' experience with the Morel-Fatio palpebral spring. *Plast Reconstr Surg* 1974; 53:404.

78. Johnson HA. A modification of the Gillies treatment of lagophthalmos in leprosy. *Plast Reconstr Surg* 1962; 30:378.

79. Lee KK, Terzis JK. Reanimation of the eye sphincter in facial nerve. In: Portmann M. , ed. Proceedings of the Fifth International Symposium on the Facial Nerve (Bordeaux Sept 3–6, 1984). USA: Masson Pub. Distributed by Yearbook Medical Publishers, Masson, 1985; 119.

80. Castanares S. Forehead wrinkles, glabella frown and ptosis of the eyebrows. *Plast Reconstr Surg* 1964; 34:406.

81. Veda K, Harii K, Yamada A. Longterm follow-up study of browlift for treatment of facial paralysis. *Ann Plast Surg* 1994; 32:166.

46

Cervical Masses

Gregory S. Georgiade, M.D., F.A.C.S., and Nicholas G. Georgiade, D.D.S., M.D., F.A.C.S.

Cervical masses should be evaluated by their location in relation to anatomic landmarks (i.e., the submaxillary gland, trachea, hyoid bone, and thyroid gland). To make an adequate diagnosis a complete history is necessary, including the initial appearance, tenderness and duration of the mass, possible systemic problems, age of the patient and location of the mass. In younger patients, a frequent cause of cervical masses is inflammation and infection (i.e., otitis media, tonsillitis, dental and scalp infections). Visual inspection of the oral cavity, mirror laryngoscopy, and manual and bimanual palpation are of value in appraising masses in the upper cervical area.

A fine-needle aspiration biopsy is useful. If this is inconclusive, an open biopsy or excisional biopsy can be carried out. However, in the case of a parotid mass, total excison of the mass is mandatory to minimize the possibility of "seeding" with its high rate of local recurrence (1,2).

Evaluation of neck masses can be carried out using computed tomography (CT scan), ultrasonography (US), and magnetic resonance imaging (MRI). In obtaining a final diagnosis, the cost of these studies must be taken into consideration (3,4).

Three classifications, according to area(s) of neck involvement, are useful in diagnosing cervical masses: (a) lateral neck masses, (b) midcervical neck masses, (c) masses that may appear any place in the neck, either as single or multiple nodules (512; Table 46–1).

Lateral Neck Masses

The masses that appear most frequently in the lateral aspect of the neck are presented next.

BRANCHIAL CLEFT ANOMALIES

These developmental anomalies are the most frequently occurring masses of the lateral neck. They appear as soft, nontender, smooth, round lesions along the border of the sternocleidomastoid muscle, usually deep to the muscle. They may be located in sites extending from the region of the external auditory canal to the midclavicular area (Fig. 46–1A,B). The tract along which they occur may extend into the lateral pharyngeal area (the Rosenmuller pouch). These lateral neck masses are usually present by 8 years of age but have also been reported in patients in the 3rd decade of life.

Embryonically, branchial cleft anomalies and/or sinus tracts occur because of a failure of the 1st or 2nd branchial arch to attain maturity. The residual remnant is trapped in the neck tissue. Anomalies may be manifest (a) in the preauricu-

lar area, (b) posterior to the angle of the mandible, and (c) in the upper cervical area with extension into the bony and cartilaginous auditory canal in close proximity to the facial nerve. Anomalies of the 2nd branchial arch are manifested as fistulae, cysts, or sinuses in the lower mid-third of the sternocleidomastoid muscle. The cystic mass and its tract, if present, may extend through the platysma muscle and follow superiorly along the carotid sheath extending deep to the posterior belly of the digastric muscle and superficial to the hypoglossal nerve, below the hyoid bone with its internal opening at the base of the tonsillar fossa or lateral pharyngeal area (Fig. 46–1A,B II).

The 2nd branchial cleft anomaly will present as a cyst or fistula close to the 2nd branchial anomaly. The tract follows superiorly under the glossopharyngeal nerve and enters the pharynx at the level of the pyriform sinus (Fig. 46–1A, B III).

The 4th branchial cleft anomaly extends deep to the platysma muscle posterior to the internal carotid artery and along the hypoglossal nerve, and then descends beneath the subclavian artery on the right and aortic arch on the left with its internal opening in the region of the upper esophagus or pyriform sinus.

Histologically, the cyst and cystic tract are typically lined with stratified squamous or low columnar epithelium. Treatment consists of surgical excision with care being taken to keep the cervical incision small. A "stepladder" approach can be executed in the crease lines, tunneling the initial tract superiorly as high as possible before the next incision is made. Anatomic landmarks (noted above) must be identified carefully because of the close proximity of the carotid vessels to the facial nerve in the superior portion of the neck (12,13) (Fig. 46–2).

CYSTIC HYGROMA

Cystic hygroma usually presents in a newborn or in early infancy. It appears as a soft, cystic, lobulated mass that is displaced laterally. Often, the cystic hygroma extends to the midline of the neck and beyond. The mass will transilluminate and is soft to palpation.

A cystic hygroma is essentially a lymphangioma that arises as a developmental anomaly of the lymphatic channels. Displaced embryonic tissue results in the development of large endothelial-lined spaces from the venous system. These may be found along the branches of the jugular vein around the esophagus and larynx. The cystic hygroma interdigitates with cervical vessels, nerves, and muscle, rendering surgical removal both arduous and difficult. The size of the

Table 46–1
Classification of Cervical Masses by Location

Lateral neck masses
  Branchial cleft anomalies
  Cystic hygroma
  Hemangioma
  Lipoma
  Neurilemmoma
  Carotid body tumor
  Salivary gland (parotid)
    Adenoma
    Warthin tumor
  Other
    Thyroid or parathyroid
    Adenomas
    Sebaceous cysts
    Myomas
Midline neck masses
  Aberrant thyroid tissue
  Thyroglossal duct or sinus tract cysts
  Thyroid adenomas
  Delphian node
  Dermoid cyst
Single or multiple masses in one or more locations of the neck
  Suppuration in neck of dental or tonsillar origin
  Metastatic tumors
  Masses of lymphatic origin
    Lymphoma
    Hodgkins disease
    Lymphoepithelioma
  Inflammatory masses
    Tubercular
    Actinomycotic
    Blastomycosis
    Sporotrichotic
  Teratomas (congenital)

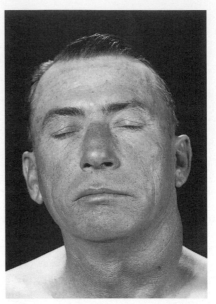

FIG. 46–2. Patient with a branchial cyst at the anterior border of the sternocleidomastoid muscle.

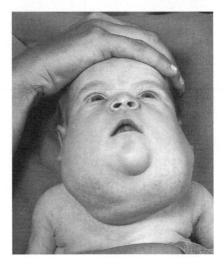

FIG. 46–3. Cystic hygroma in infant.

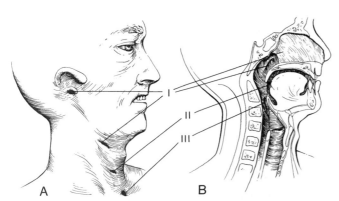

FIG. 46–1. Potential sites of branchial cleft anomalies with remnant trappings: I, preauricular; II, posterior to angle of mandible; III, upper cervical area.

mass may cause respiratory difficulty. Aspiration of the yellow fluid contents may be undertaken for temporary decompression. Lymphangioma tissue may be found extending into the axillary area and inferiorly into the mediastinum. Treatment is by surgical excision, and the initial procedure should maximize removal of the tumor mass for the best long-term result (15) (Fig. 46–3).

HEMANGIOMA

The cavernous hemangioma seen in infants or children represents a vascular developmental anomaly. Histologically, it is characterized by extensive proliferation of endothelial cells with resultant large vascular spaces that fill with blood. The cavernous hemangioma appears as a soft, round, collapsible mass. A distinctive diagnostic feature is the bluish tone of the skin overlying the mass.

The management plan must include ruling out the presence of an extensive vascular abnormality. Should there be any question about the extensiveness of the tumor, further vascular studies are indicated, including a CT scan and/or MRI.

A single hemangiomatous mass can usually be excised surgically without difficulty. Care must be taken to maintain dissection in the plane around the hemangioma to minimize bleeding from the blood-filled mass (see Chapter 21).

LIPOMA

Lipomas are often confused with branchial cleft cysts because of their relatively similar appearance, location, and softness. Treatment consists of surgical excision, which is usually accomplished easily by dissecting the lipoma free from surrounding tissue (Fig. 46–4).

NEURILEMMOMA

In contrast to previously described lateral neck masses, the neurilemmoma is more solid in consistency and deeper on palpation. The clinical picture is one of a slow-growing, painless mass presenting in the mature patient. It is frequently found in association with von Recklinghausen disease. When the growth rate is rapid, more pain and discomfort is experienced, and the proportion of malignancies is also higher. When a neurilemmoma is involved with the sympathetic nerve chain, Horner syndrome may occur.

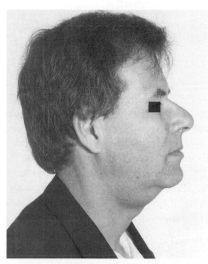

FIG. 46–4. Lipoma of the cervical area in an adult male patient.

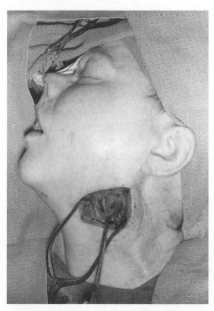

FIG. 46–5. Neurilemmoma as an encapsulated mass in an adult female patient.

Palpation of the deep-seated, encapsulated mass will allow some lateral and anterior movement. Because of the attached nerve sheath, which courses in a superior–inferior direction, no movement occurs in this vector. Treatment of the neurilemmoma consists of meticulous dissection from the encompassing nerve and usually results in no disability (16) (Figs. 46–5, 46–6).

CAROTID BODY TUMORS

The carotid body tumor is characterized by its slow, painless growth. It is located at the bifurcation of the carotid artery and can be moved laterally but not vertically. Carotid tumors may attain such size as to cause difficulty in swallowing, speaking, and breathing. They are usually found in patients over 50 years of age, and removal is quite hazardous. An open biopsy should be performed to rule out a malignancy, which occurs in slightly over 10% of patients. If the mass is nonmalignant and slow growing, it should probably be left in place because of the hazards of excision. Morbidity accompanying removal is usually high because excision of a portion of the involved common carotid artery is included. Should surgery be a treatment of choice, extirpation of this tumor should be planned. Preoperative compression of the carotid artery against the vertebra for 15 to 20 minutes four or five times a day for a 2-week period before surgery is recommended because of the high incidence of hemiplegia after ligation of the common carotid artery.

Histologically, the carotid body tumor is composed of sheets of polyhedral and epitheloid cells with large, pale-staining nuclei and pale-staining cytoplasm. These cells occur in cords or sheets of cells with an interspersion of fibrous tissue, vessels, and large numbers of neural elements (17).

SALIVARY GLAND MASSES

Parotid

Occasionally, an adenoma or Warthin tumor may present in the upper neck. Although it may be mistaken for a separate tumor mass, it is actually associated with the caudad portion of the parotid gland (Fig. 46–7). Tumors in this area are usually benign and are easily distinguished from other neck masses at the time of surgery.

Submaxillary gland tumors occur in the upper midneck and midsubmandibular area. They will present as firm, nonmobile masses that are somewhat painful on palpation. This mass is usually a benign adenoma, or it may manifest as a large calculus in the submaxillary gland. There is associated pain and tenderness, particularly when chewing and ingesting food. Surgical extirpation of the entire gland is necessary. Diagnostic differentiation between an adenoma and salivary

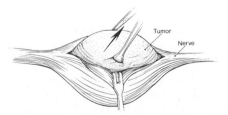

FIG. 46–6. Typical location of a neurilemmoma encapsulated in a nerve sheath.

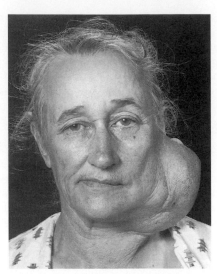

FIG. 46–7. Warthin tumor in the intramandibular area of the lateral neck.

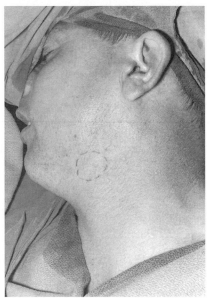

FIG. 46–8. Patient with a submaxillary gland tumor of the parotid in the midsubmandibular area.

calculus can be made by obtaining a suitable intraoral radiograph of the floor of the mouth. Orthopan radiography of the area will often reveal the presence of a calcified mass in the submaxillary gland (Fig. 46–8).

MISCELLANEOUS LATERAL MASSES

Occasionally, an aberrant thyroid or parathyroid adenoma will present in the lower lateral neck as a small, mobile mass in the region of the thyroid gland. Sebaceous cysts can appear in any area of the neck and are characterized by their ovoid appearance, ease of palpation, and close proximity to the skin surface. Myomas rarely occur in the lateral neck. When present, they are usually within the sternocleidomastoid muscle and are firm, ovoid, fixed masses that are painless.

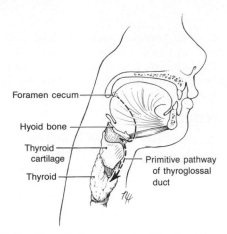

FIG. 46–9. The primitive pathway of the thyroglossal duct.

Midline Neck Masses

Primary masses of the midcervical area include those described below.

ABERRANT THYROID TISSUE

The presence of displaced thyroid tissue, cysts, or sinus tract is a result of the epithelial lining failing to disappear. It is present during the downward progression of the thyroid tissue from the foramen cecum linguae, through the hyoid bone, to its final position in the lower midneck.

Lingual thyroid is characterized by a supralingual protruding mass in the posterior area of the tongue at the foramen cecum linguae. The aberrant thyroid tissue may be located in any position from the foramen cecum linguae to the thyroid gland proper, including the thyroid isthmus.

THYROGLOSSAL DUCT OR SINUS TRACT CYSTS

These masses appear at a midline site anywhere from the thyroid isthmus to the foramen cecum linguae. The sinus tract usually appears in the region of the hyoid bone and thyroid isthmus. Duct cysts occur more frequently in children (Fig. 46–9). The histopathologic composition of the cyst tract is characteristically squamous cell epithelium together with some thyroid tissue. Treatment consists of horizontal excision of the initial sinus tract opening with dissection of the tract from the surrounding tissue. Traction is maintained to identify the tract better (Fig. 46–10A, B). The midportion of the hyoid bone is included in the resection (Fig. 46–10C). The tract is dissected superiorly to the base of the tongue. Intraoral digital pressure at the midline position of the foramen cecum linguae is beneficial in the superior dissection and in identifying the superior portion of the tract at the position of the posterior tongue (foramen cecum) (Figs. 46–10D, 46–11, and 46–12).

THYROID ADENOMA

This benign mass will occasionally present as an easily palpable, somewhat mobile mass.

DELPHIAN NODE

Delphian node is characterized as a firm mass that may be confused with an adenoma. It is attached to the fascia of the thyroid isthmus and may be diagnostic of a thyroid disease process or a malignancy involving the thyroid gland.

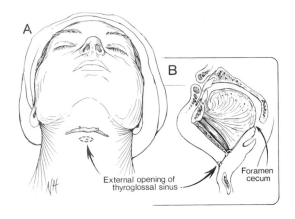

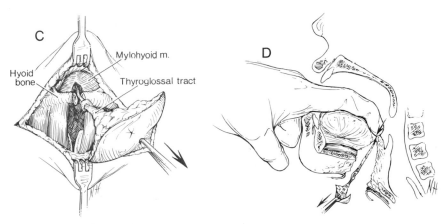

FIG. 46–10. Horizontal excision of initial sinus tract opening. **A,** external opening. **B,** anteroposterior view of foramen cecum and sinus tract. **C,** sinus tract cyst is dissected. Anterior view shows the hyoid bone combined in the surgical procedure. **D,** intraoral digital pressure at the midline position of the foramen cecum is of assistance in identifying the superior portion of sinus tract cyst in the dissection.

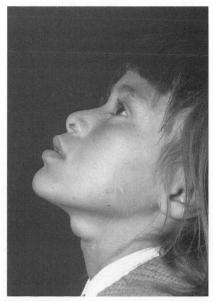

FIG. 46–11. Profile of a sinus tract cyst in an 8-year-old patient.

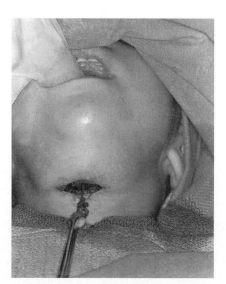

FIG. 46–12. Anterior view of duct cyst opening in an adult patient.

DERMOID CYST

The dermoid cyst is derived from remnants of epithelial cells remaining during fusion at the midline in the embryonic stage and may contain hair follicles, sebaceous glands, and other glandular elements. The characteristic dermoid cyst appears as an intraoral mass in children, usually up to 5 years of age, and is located intraorally above the geniohyoid muscle. It may also occur in the submental area, and in this position it is inferior to the geniohyoid muscle (Fig. 46–13A,B). Surgery can be carried out either intraorally or through the small submental incision, depending on the location of the presenting mass (17).

FIG. 46–13. Frontal (**A**) and profile (**B**) views of a dermoid cyst involving the geniohyoid muscle.

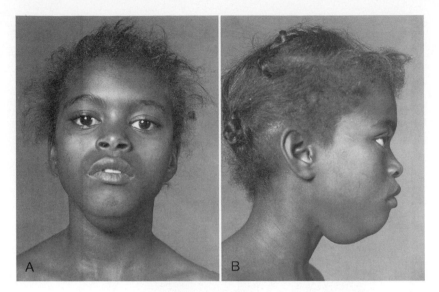

Single or Multiple Masses in One or More Neck Locations

Masses that occur in one or more locations of the neck and may appear as single or multiple nodules include those described below.

SUPPURATION IN THE NECK

An area of suppuration in the neck is most commonly of dental origin (Fig. 46–14). Infections related to the tonsillar area are another source. Usually, the mass is of recent origin, painful, and located at a site directly in the submandibular area. An orthopan radiograph of the entire mandible will usually reveal the primary source as a periapical dental infection that has eroded through the cortex of the mandible into the underlying soft tissues. A neck infection of tonsillar origin will extend into the parapharyngeal space with involvement of the cervical region. Extension of the infection along the fascial space will further complicate the clinical picture. Involvement of the cervical sympathetic chain with resultant Horner syndrome or even vagal involvement and vocal cord paralysis may occur. This condition is treated by incision and adequate drainage, with removal of the offending tooth. Suitable antibiotics are prescribed (11).

METASTATIC TUMORS

Metastatic tumors may occur in the neck and are usually from primary carcinomas of the oral cavity, pharynx, and nasal pharynx (Figs. 46–15A,B and 46–16). A small group of metastatic masses occur in the lower neck and will originate from primary sites below the clavicle, including lungs, esophagus, gastrointestinal tract, or even locations such as the prostate, kidneys, or uterus.

LYMPHATIC MASSES

Neck masses of lymphatic origin, such as lymphoma, Hodgkin disease (Fig. 46–17), and lymphoepithelioma, may appear anywhere in the neck, usually in clusters, and present as firm mobile, and painless. Treatment, once a diagnosis is made, is usually with chemotherapy and radiation therapy.

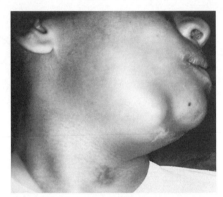

FIG. 46–14. Patient with an infection of dental origin.

INFLAMMATORY NECK MASSES

Inflammatory neck masses may occur occasionally as a result of tuberculosis, actinomycosis, blastomycosis, and sporotrichosis. Cat scratch fever is an inflammatory disease of viral origin usually seen in children. This disease will characteristically present as discrete neck masses that are firm and matted when palpated and are typically present for a number of weeks. A history of involvement with cats, dogs, and other animals is usual, as is intermittent low-grade fever. The disease is transmitted via a scratch, saliva, or excretia from animals (usually cats) to humans (usually children). Examination reveals moderate to tender, freely movable lymph nodes, which may often be suppurative. With exclusion of the animal, disappearance of the masses is the usual course. No antibiotics or other treatment is thought to be necessary. A skin-test antigen can be used.

TERATOMAS

Teratomas of the neck can appear at any location in the cervical region, are present at birth, and may attain considerable size. A teratoma presents as a large, irregular mass that, by virtue of its size, will cause tracheal compression and respiratory difficulties as a rule. The histologic appearance reveals a mixture of sebaceous squamous cell clusters

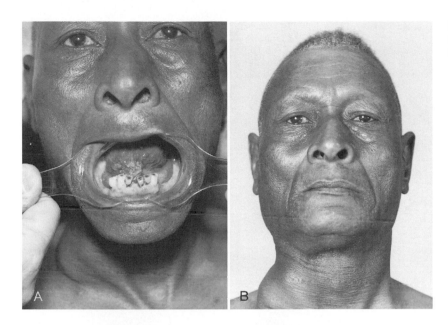

FIG. 46–15.   A, primary carcinoma of the oral cavity (sublingual) in an adult male patient. **B,** metastasis to the lateral neck is evident.

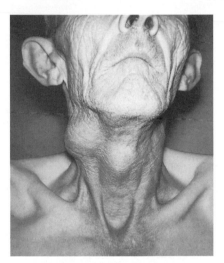

FIG. 46–16.   Metastatic tumor in the lateral neck of a patient in late maturity.

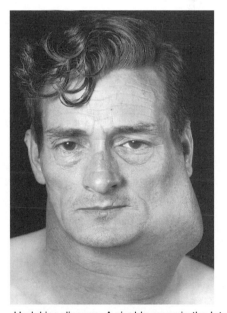

FIG. 46–17.   Hodgkins disease. A sizable mass in the lateral neck of an adult male patient.

and cysts containing respiratory or gastrointestinal epithelium. Teeth, neural tissues, cartilage, brain, and other tissues resulting from the presence of ectodermal, mesodermal, and entodermal germinal layers are usually present. Treatment is by surgical excision, which provides excellent long-term results if there has been careful excision of the entire mass (18).

Summary

Neck masses can appear at any age and in any location. About 50% occur in adults over 50 years of age. A significant number of neck masses appear in infants and children, and this dictates the need for careful evaluation and treatment. The physical examination and a complete history, including duration of symptoms, are central in determining further studies to be undertaken and subsequent management.

References

1. Beenken SW, Maddox WA, Marshall MU. Workup of a patient with a mass in the neck. *Adv Surg* St. Louis: CV Mosby, 1995; 28:371.
2. Burton DM, Pransky SM. Practical aspects of managing non-malignant lumps of the neck. *P Otolaryngol* 1998; 21:398.
3. Vazquez MD, Goya E, Castellote A, et al. US, CT, and MR imaging of neck lesions in children. *Radiographics* 1995; 15:105.
4. Fenwick JR, Kitch RD. Evaluation of the neck mass. *J SC Med Assoc* 1991; 90:513.
5. Bergman Kerry S, Harris Burton H. Scalp and neck masses. *Pediatric Surg* 1993; 401151.
6. Cady B. Differential diagnosis of tumors of the neck. *Compr Ther* 1983; 9:33.

7. Hogan D, Wilkinson RD, Williams A. Congenital anomalies of the head and neck. *Int J Dermatol* 1980; 19:479.

8. Rood SW, Johnson J. Examination for cervical masses. *Postgrad Med* 1982; 71:189.

9. Moloy P. How to (and how not to) manage the patient with a lump in the neck. *Primary Care* 1982; 9:269.

10. Simpson OT. The evaluation and management of neck masses of unknown etiology. *Otolaryngol Clin North Am* 1980; 13:489.

11. Weymuller EA. Problems in family practice: evaluation of neck masses. *J Fam Pract* 1980; 11:1099.

12. Shockley W, Pillsbury H. The neck: diagnosis and surgery. St. Louis: CV Mosby, 1994.

13. Chandler JR, Mitchell B. Brachial cleft cysts, sinuses, and fistulas. *Otolaryngol Clin North Am* 1981; 14:175.

14. New GB, Erich JB. Dermoid cysts of the head and neck. *Surg Gynecol Obstet* 1937; 65:48.

15. Karmody CS, Forston JK, Calcaterra VE. Lymphangiomas of the head and neck in adults. *Otolaryngol Head Neck Surg* 1982; 90:283.

16. Sharaki MM, Talaat M, Hamam SM. Schwannoma of the neck. *Clin Otolaryngol Allied Sci* 1982; 7:245.

17. Padberg FT, Cady B, Persson AV. Carotid body tumor. *Am J Surg* 1983; 145:526.

18. McGoon DC. Teratomas of the neck. *Surg Clin North Am* 1952; 32:1389.

47

Microvascular Reconstruction for Head and Neck Cancer Defects

Mark A. Schusterman, M.D., F.A.C.S.

The value of microvascular free-tissue transfer for reconstruction for head and neck cancer–related defects was recognized two decades ago. This is evidenced by two case reports of free-flap reconstruction of the oral cavity in 1976, only 2 years after the first free flap was transferred (1–3). Since then, microvascular surgery has been slowly accepted as the state-of-the-art for head and neck reconstruction. One of the factors preventing earlier acceptance was concern about the reliability of microvascular reconstructions. Patients with head and neck cancer, in general, are in poor health and have a limited life span (4,5). Thus, any surgical modality, particularly a reconstructive technique, needs to be reliable and associated with minimal complications. Fistulae, and infection, if they occur, can extend the hospitalization period or even shorten the lives of patients with an already limited life span. Therefore, for microvascular surgery to be accepted, its reliability needed to be proved. Over the last 20 years, numerous large series have been published demonstrating a greater than 90 to 95% success rate (6–8). Other studies have shown that free flaps compare favorably in terms of morbidity to more traditional pedicle techniques (9,10). In addition, free flaps allow one-stage, immediate reconstruction for cancer defects. It is for these reasons that, paradoxically, the most complicated technique has become the standard for reconstruction of head and neck cancer defects.

Soft-Tissue Reconstruction of the Oral Cavity

Cancer of the oral cavity occurs most commonly in the tongue and floor of the mouth (11). The redundancy of the tongue allows for primary closure after cancer resection in a number of cases. However, when the tongue is used to close the defect, function may be severely impaired because the tongue is immobilized and impedes speech and swallowing (12,13) (Fig. 47–1). For this reason, it is imperative to employ a reconstructive strategy that maximizes tongue function in order to provide the highest quality of life for the head and neck cancer patient.

PARTIAL GLOSSECTOMY DEFECTS

The goal for partial glossectomy defects is to maximize tongue mobility. A thick, bulky flap may adequately fill the defect, but it will prevent adequate mobility. Tongue function is enhanced with a thin, pliable flap. Several such flaps have been advocated and described, including the dorsalis pedis flap, the latissimus dorsi flap, the lateral arm flap, and the ulnar artery flap (14–18), but the free flap that has achieved the highest level of success for partial glossectomy defects has been the radial forearm flap (9,19–23).

First described by Song and Song in 1980 (19), the radial forearm flap is frequently used by reconstructive microsurgeons, owing to the ease of elevation of the flap and the large caliber of the vessels, making the flap highly reliable, and coupled with minimal donor-site morbidity. The flap is based on the radial vessels and the cephalic vein. One may use the cephalic vein or the venae comitantes of the radial artery as the donor veins, but the cephalic vein is of larger caliber and easier to anastomose (Fig. 47–2).

In addition to tongue defects, the radial forearm flap can be used to reconstruct defects involving the floor of mouth, buccal mucosa, or retromolar trigone. Its thin, pliable nature allows easy conformation of the flap to the contours of the oral cavity, and thus also facilitates dental restoration (Fig. 47–3).

The addition of the lateral antebrachial cutaneous nerve allow for creation of a neurotized flap, which has been advocated by some investigators (24,25). While the presence of sensory return has been documented in these cases, its actual functional effects (e.g., the possible enhancement of speech and swallowing) has not been established. Neurotized flaps may be of benefit in reconstruction of oropharyngeal defects, where protective sensation could prevent aspiration. At this juncture, however, the concept has still to demonstrate a clear functional advantage.

TOTAL AND SUBTOTAL GLOSSECTOMY DEFECTS

Resection of the majority of the mobile tongue is often required for advanced tumors of the tongue. Once this occurs, protection of the larynx is lost, and aspiration can be a problem. In contrast are pharyngeal defects, where a critical sensation is needed and a thin flap provides good contour and a low profile. In these cases, a bulky flap may be needed to prevent aspiration. Additionally, with T4 lesions of this area, the posterior mandible, including the ascending ramus, angle, and posterior body, is frequently resected to facilitate tumor removal and access to the posterior tongue. Under these circumstances, a large soft-tissue flap often suffices to obliterate the dead space, replace the missing tissues, provide bulk to the tongue, and prevent shifting of the mandible from scar contracture and contracture of the dead space.

Although many flaps have been described for use in this setting, we have found that the rectus abdominis myocutaneous flap, either vertical or transverse, provides a reliable

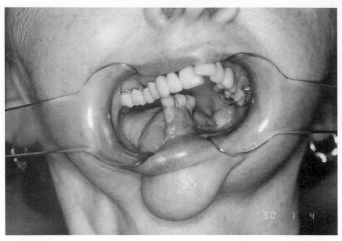

FIG. 47–1. Postoperative view of patient after partial glossectomy reconstructed with primary closure. Note the significant binding of the tongue and deviation of the mandible, which are severely limiting the functional and aesthetic outcomes in this patient.

mechanism for bulky reconstruction of the tongue (26–29) (Fig. 47–4). The rectus abdominis flap is based on perforators from the rectus abdominis muscle, which receives its blood supply from the deep inferior epigastric vessels. Use of this flap facilitates a two-team approach, with the ablative team at the head and the reconstructive team elevating the flap at the abdomen. Once the flap has been elevated, the recipient vessels are prepared, the flap is transferred and inset, and the vessels are then anastomosed to the recipient vessels in the neck. When this reconstruction is performed, it is important to overcorrect the defect by putting excess bulk in the oral cavity because atrophy will occur, particularly if postoperative radiation is given.

Mandibular Reconstruction

Restoration of the mandible is one of the more challenging head and neck reconstructions. Although the mandible itself is bone, cancer-related mandibular defects are often accompanied by large soft-tissue defects, since the majority of cancers of the oral cavity are squamous cell carcinomas that

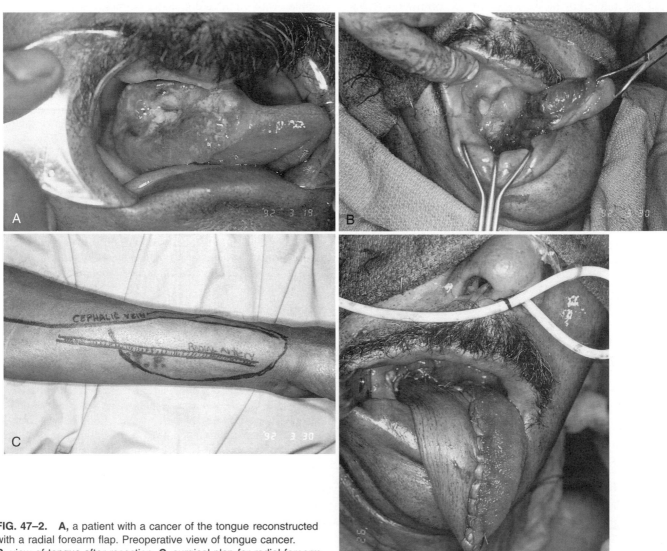

FIG. 47–2.   A, a patient with a cancer of the tongue reconstructed with a radial forearm flap. Preoperative view of tongue cancer. **B,** view of tongue after resection. **C,** surgical plan for radial forearm flap. **D,** patient after flap sutured into recipient site.

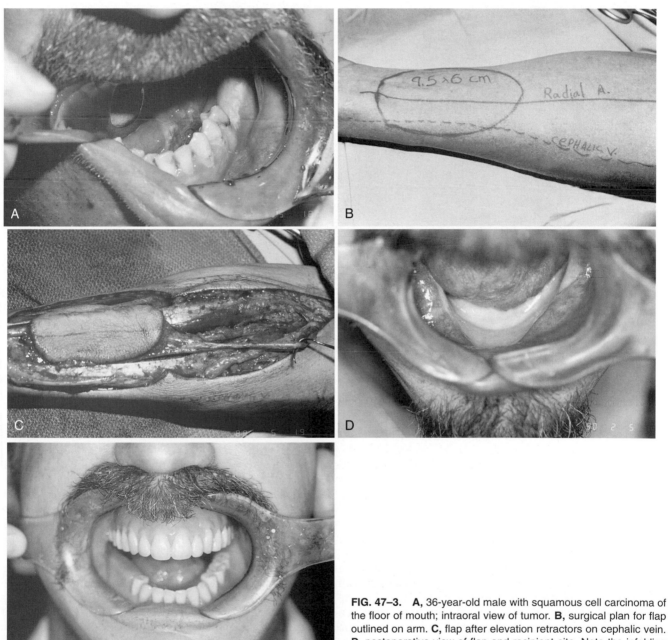

FIG. 47–3. **A,** 36-year-old male with squamous cell carcinoma of the floor of mouth; intraoral view of tumor. **B,** surgical plan for flap outlined on arm. **C,** flap after elevation retractors on cephalic vein. **D,** postoperative view of flap and recipient site. Note the infolding of the flap to follow the soft-tissue contours. **E,** dental restoration.

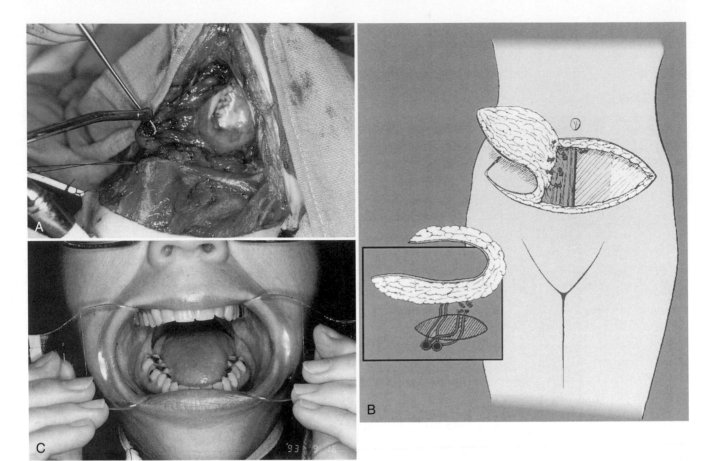

FIG. 47–4.   A, patient with advanced, recurrent squamous cell carcinoma requiring subtotal glossectomy. Intraoperative view from below through the glossectomy and floor of mouth defect. Note that the hard palate is visible through the defect. The retractor is on the remaining tongue musculature. **B,** schematic diagram of TRAM flap elevation. **C,** postoperative view of reconstructed tongue.

arise initially from the oral mucosa. By the time the tumor invades bone, there is often a large component of soft-tissue destruction as well. In this regard, there must be a strategy for reconstructing not only the osseous portion of the defect but also the soft-tissue component. A composite reconstruction of bone and soft tissue is generally required for repair of oral cavity defects involving bone. Although numerous types of bone flaps have been developed, including metatarsal and rib (30,31), by far the four most commonly utilized flaps in this setting are the free radial forearm osteocutaneous flap, the deep circumflex iliac artery/iliac crest osseomyocutaneous flap, the scapular osteocutaneous flap, and the fibular osteocutaneous flap (32–38).

The radial forearm osteocutaneous flap is an adaptation of the radial forearm flap incorporating a segment of the radius. This flap is very reliable and provides thin, pliable tissue for repair of the floor of the mouth or partial glossectomy defects. The principle limitation of this flap is the small segment of bone that is available. In addition, partial resection of the radius increases the donor-site morbidity of the procedure, resulting in a high incidence of diaphyseal fractures of the radius (32,39,40). Although techniques have been developed to help avert this complication, it must be a consideration if this flap is used. Perhaps the best application for the radial forearm

osteocutaneous flap is an infected nonunion of the mandible after radiation therapy, when only a small segment of bone is required, particularly if soft-tissue restoration provides a major component of the reconstructive strategy. When utilizing the free radial forearm osteocutaneous flap, it is imperative to immobilize the forearm and wrist in a short arm cast postoperatively for a minimum of 6 weeks.

The scapular osteocutaneous flap was popularized for use in the mandible by Swartz (34). It has a number qualities that make its use advantageous. The flap has three separate pedicles: two skin paddles and one bone paddle. Because of the design of the flap, it is easy to use one skin paddle for lining and one for coverage with the bone interposed between, thus making this an ideal flap for through-and-through defects. The pedicle is long and consistent and the donor site morbidity is well tolerated. The main problem with this flap is that the patient needs to be turned during the procedure to facilitate the dissection, thus making a long procedure even longer. Still, in patients with through-and-through defects, this flap provides a straightforward, one-stage method for reconstruction (41) (Fig. 47–5).

The deep circumflex iliac artery/iliac crest osseomyocutaneous flap consists of a portion of the iliac crest supplied by the blood vessel for which the flap is named. First de-

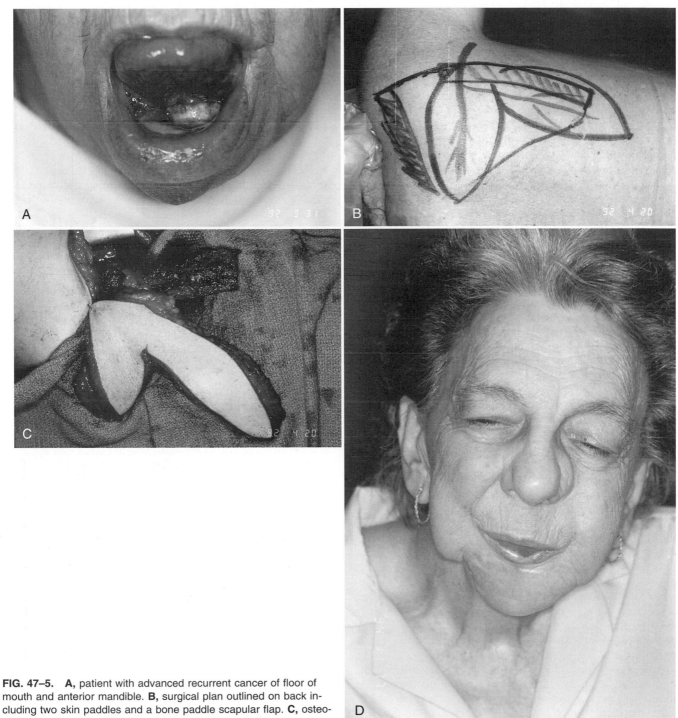

FIG. 47–5. **A,** patient with advanced recurrent cancer of floor of mouth and anterior mandible. **B,** surgical plan outlined on back including two skin paddles and a bone paddle scapular flap. **C,** osteocutaneous flap after elevation. **D,** postoperative result.

scribed by Taylor in 1979 (35,42) and popularized by Urken (43), this was the first flap described for osseous reconstruction of the mandible. The problems with this flap include the short vascular pedicle, the high donor-site morbidity, and an unreliable skin paddle. In addition, the skin paddle tends to be bulky, which in partial glossectomy defects can be a problem. However, the bone stock is excellent and provides a stable foundation for placement of osseointegrated implants.

The fibular osteocutaneous flap has achieved a high level of acceptance since its description by Hidalgo in 1989 (38). Anterior defects are the greatest challenges in mandible reconstruction, and the free fibula flap has become the flap of choice for these defects. This is due to the length of the bone and the segmental periosteal blood supply, which allows multiple osteotomies facilitating creation of an exact replica of the lost mandible. The bone stock is excellent, and osseointegrated implants can be used in this flap without difficulty. There has been some controversy about the reliability of the skin paddle in the originally described version of this flap (38). We therefore studied the vascular supply to the skin paddle in eighty cadavers, and found that the majority of the perforators came either from the muscle or were so adherent to the muscle that they could be considered myocutaneous perforators. For this reason, we started harvesting the skin with a small cuff of muscle, which has enhanced the skin survival rate (44). Thus, the fibular osteocutaneous flap has become a highly reliable composite flap, which makes it ideal for repair of anterior mandible and floor-of-mouth defects (Fig. 47–6).

In mandibular reconstruction, the location of the defect is an important factor in determining the reconstructive modality. An unrepaired anterior defect involving the arch of the mandible is by far the most functionally limiting and cosmetically appalling. It is therefore crucial to repair these defects with the most reliable method available. Posterior defects, on the other hand, are less sensitive both cosmetically and functionally, and a simple soft-tissue flap will often suffice. A simpler cutaneous flap with a reconstruction plate alone (without bone) can often be utilized to reconstruct patients with advanced disease in whom a complex osteocutaneous flap is not desired or required.

A reconstruction plate is useful for fixation of vascularized bone. In certain circumstances, a plate can be used alone (without the inclusion of bone), but it is advisable only for lateral and posterior defects of the mandible. When such a plate is used for anterior defects, the extrusion rate is prohibitive (45). A vascularized flap is therefore required for anterior defects, even in the presence of advanced disease. In such a setting, the scapular osteocutaneous flap is useful because it provides a one-stage reconstruction for a very large defect.

The surgeon should always strive to reconstruct the mandible immediately. If the wound is closed temporarily and allowed to heal, the soft tissues contract and become fibrotic, particularly if postoperative radiation is used. This makes subsequent reconstruction much more difficult. In reconstructions of the posterior mandible, the facial nerve is often involved in this fibrotic wound and needs to be dissected free before the reconstruction. This may result in temporary, and sometimes permanent, paresis. Definitive mandibular reconstruction at the time of tumor reconstruction is deferred, however, if there is any uncertainty as to the adequacy of the margins of resection, particularly in a bone tumor. A temporary reconstruction plate with adequate soft-tissue coverage can be used in the interim and bony reconstruction completed within 7 to 14 days after ensuring that the final surgical margins are free of disease.

Pharynx

Tumors involving the pharynx and larynx that require circumferential excision of the upper aerodigestive tract are formidable defects to repair. A lack of continuity of the upper gastrointestinal tract is, in most people's estimation, an unacceptable quality of life. Because the survival rate of these patients is poor (11), a reliable one-stage procedure is needed. Two reconstructive methods have emerged as the dominant choices at this time: the gastric pull-up and the free jejunal microvascular transfer.

The free jejunal transfer has become the method of choice at our institution. Free jejunal transfer is a single-stage technique that is not hampered by pedicle location or length. Transfer of the jejunum was one of the first free-tissue transfers described, first by Seidenberg in 1959 and then by Jurkiewicz in 1965 (46,47). Numerous series have been published demonstrating a high success rate, approaching 96% (48) (Table 47–1).

The location of the lesion determines the reconstructive strategy for pharyngoesophageal tumors. Defects caused by low-lying lesions may be better repaired with a gastric pull-up, particularly if the chest needs to be opened for resection of the lesion. Free jejunal transfer should be reserved for more proximal lesions, for which a gastric pull-up would not be an appropriate reconstructive choice (49).

In a free jejunal transfer, the abdomen is explored through a periumbilical incision while the ablative team is removing the tumor (Fig. 47–7). A loop of intestine approximately 20 to 30 cm distal from the ligament of Treitz is selected for use, and the mesentery is transilluminated to identify an appropriate vascular arcade. The vascular arcade should be located as close as possible to the proximal end of the bowel since the recipient vessels lie adjacent to the proximal enteric anastomosis. The vessels are dissected at the root of the mesentery to ascertain their suitability. The mesentery is then divided in a pie-shaped pattern and the bowel isolated using a gastrointestinal stapler. Once the ablative surgery is completed and the recipient vessels have been prepared, the flap is transferred. The proximal anastomosis is performed first, using a two-layer technique, and then the flap is revascularized. Once the flap is revascularized, it is easier to pull to length, an important step to avoid dysphagia from redundant folds of bowel. Excess flap tissue is trimmed, but left attached to the lower end of the mesentery for use as a monitoring segment (see Fig. 47–7). The distal anastomosis is then performed in an end-to-end spatulated fashion in one layer so as to prevent stricture. The flap is monitored for 7 days, and then the monitoring segment is removed in the clinic by ligating the mesentery. The function of the jejunal segment is determined by a barium-swallow x-ray series, usually postoperatively on day 7. Oral intake is begun, provided no structure or fistula is present. In patients who have had previous radiation, the surgeon should wait 10 to 14 days before assessing function of the flap and initiating oral intake for the patient.

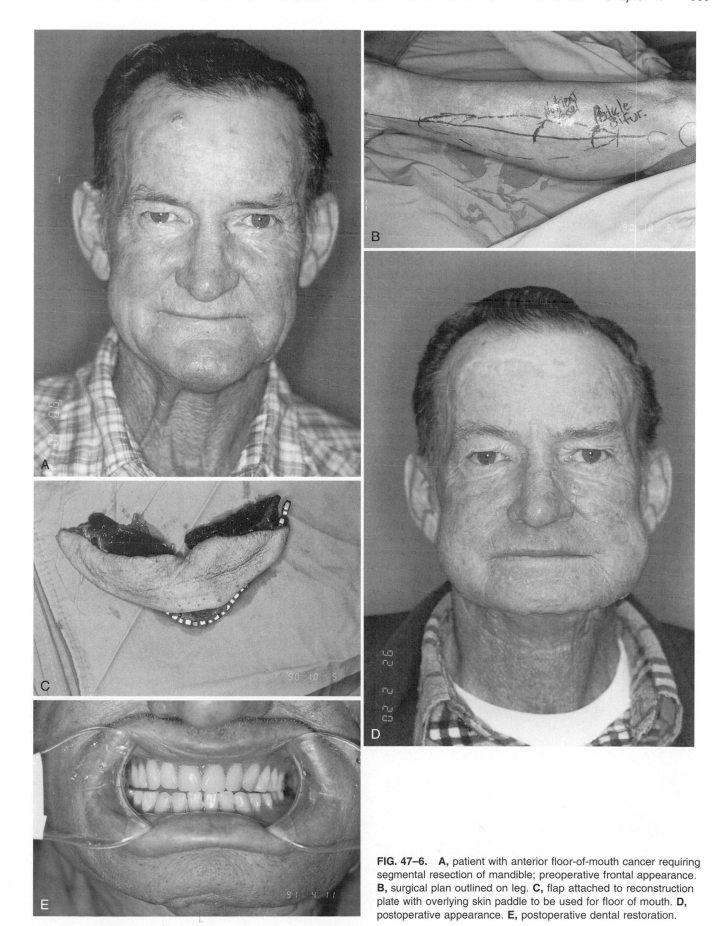

FIG. 47–6.   A, patient with anterior floor-of-mouth cancer requiring segmental resection of mandible; preoperative frontal appearance. **B,** surgical plan outlined on leg. **C,** flap attached to reconstruction plate with overlying skin paddle to be used for floor of mouth. **D,** postoperative appearance. **E,** postoperative dental restoration.

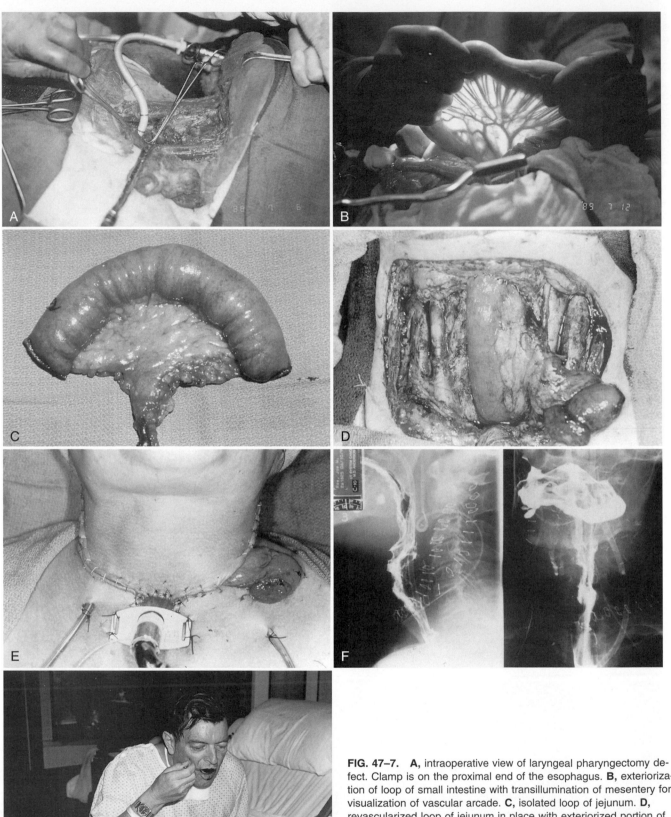

FIG. 47–7. **A,** intraoperative view of laryngeal pharyngectomy defect. Clamp is on the proximal end of the esophagus. **B,** exteriorization of loop of small intestine with transillumination of mesentery for visualization of vascular arcade. **C,** isolated loop of jejunum. **D,** revascularized loop of jejunum in place with exteriorized portion of jejunum for monitor. **E,** postoperative appearance of incision site with exteriorized loop of the jejunum for monitoring purposes. **F,** postoperative barium swallow illustrating continuity of reestablishment of continuity of GI tract. **G,** resumption of oral intake by patient on postoperative day 10.

Table 47–1
Series of Free Jejunal Transfer (FJT) Reconstructions: 1982 to 1992

Principal Author/Year	No. Patients/FJTs	C/F	FJT Survival Rate (%)	Functional Success Rate (%)	Operative Mortality (%)	Complication Rate (%)	Fistula Rate (%)	Stricture Rate (%)
Gluckman[13]/1982	17/17	17/0	68	81*	0	47	6	24
Tabah[38]/1984	12/12	12/0*	100	N/S	N/S	N/S	N/S	N/S
Deane[8]1985	17/17	13/4	82	88*	0	53	18	N/S
Fisher[11]/1985	40/43	43/0*	80	100*	10	68	8	20
Biel[3]/1987	17/18	18/0*	83	88	17	N/S	35	17
Schecter[29]/1987	17/17	13/4*	82	N/S	N/S	N/S	N/S	6*
Coleman[6]/1987	88/96	83/13	86	79	6	68	32	7
Ferguson[16]/1988	18/18	18/0	94	100	6	67	33	11
Schusterman[30]/1990	48/50	50/0*	94	88	2	N/S	16	22
Carlson[6]/1992	25/26	26.0	96	80	0	N/S	20	16

*Best interpretation of data
C/P = circumferential patch defect: N/S = not stated

If a fistula is present on barium swallow, or develops subsequently, treatment should include adequate drainage, avoidance of oral intake, use of antibiotics, and adequate débridement. Most fistulas will close spontaneously without surgical intervention, but in some patients who have received radiation, particularly neutron-beam radiation, inset of a vascularized flap may be necessary to close the fistula (50). If the patient develops a stricture, this is usually transient and may be due to edema from either the surgery or radiation. Dilatation with Maloney dilators usually is adequate to break the stricture. Dysphagia is often functional and can be due to xerostomia from the radiation. The jejunal flap tolerates radiation well, but intermittent periods of dysphagia are common during radiotherapy. A feeding tube should be maintained until the radiation is completed. We use a gastrostomy tube, which is placed at the time the abdominal enteric repair is performed and the belly closed. The surgeon must take care to ascertain the exact cause of dysphagia before embarking on nonsurgical dilation or surgical repair of a suspected stricture. Dysphagia can also arise from too long a jejunal segment, with foldings of the jejunum. This can be best avoided at the time of surgery by stretching the jejunum to length and using the shortest segment allowable for the repair.

Speech rehabilitation after free jejunal transfer is possible, but the quality of speech is poor. This is because the peristalsis and secretions of the jejunum cause a varied pitch and moist quality to the voice. If a patient strongly desires a high-quality voice restoration or has a contraindication to abdominal surgery, such as cirrhosis and ascites, the surgeon should consider utilizing the free radial forearm flap for pharyngeal reconstruction.

The free radial forearm flap has been well documented in floor-of-mouth and tongue reconstruction. It is also a useful flap for pharyngeal reconstruction in selected cases. In patients with small segments of missing pharynx, a free radial forearm flap can be the flap of choice. The benefits of utilizing this flap are that it avoids intraabdominal surgery and the flap has a firmer consistency, without peristalsis or secretions. The free radial forearm flap also provides a better resonating chamber for voice restoration using tracheoesophageal puncture techniques. To reconstruct the pharyngoesophagus, a tube is created by suturing the flap to itself, creating a long vertical suture line. The main disadvantage of the free radial forearm flap is the long vertical suture line, which increases the risk of fistula formation. Despite that, the voice quality with this reconstruction has been excellent, and the free radial forearm flap should be considered in certain patients (50).

Craniofacial Reconstruction

There are three basic areas in which microvascular surgery is helpful in reconstruction of craniofacial defects. The first is in surgery of the base of the skull. Resection of base-of-skull tumors often leaves a defect that brings the central nervous system (CNS) into communication with the upper aerodigestive tract. It is imperative under these circumstances to seal off the cranial cavity in order to prevent infection and morbidity. The flap of choice for these circumstances has routinely been a rectus abdominis muscle flap, which may be packed around the cranial defect, effectively obliterating the space. This technique has been described by several authors, most notably Jones (51,52).

Microvascular reconstruction has been successfully utilized for scalp and external cranial defects. It is often necessary to use a flap with a long pedicle because of the distance from the crown of the scalp to the recipient vessels in the neck. We have found that the latissimus dorsi flap is an excellent choice in these circumstances; it is broad and flat, useful for covering large deficiencies of scalp (Fig. 47–8). The rectus abdominis flap can be used for reconstruction of smaller defects. It is preferable to perform any necessary bony reconstruction such as bone grafts or cranioplasty in a separate stage in order to secure adequate soft-tissue coverage first. This is particularly important if the bone has been irradiated.

Perhaps the most useful role for free-tissue transfers is in reconstruction of midface defects (53–57). Extended resections of the maxilla often involve the orbit and can cross the midline. The traditional method of repairing these defects has been to utilize maxillofacial prosthetics. However, as the defects increase in size, the stability and utility of these devices diminish. The role of the reconstructive surgeon is not to replace maxillofacial prostheses but simply to aid their function by providing a stable platform for fixation (57). The two areas of the midface that most commonly require reconstructive surgery are the periorbital region and the palate. These defects

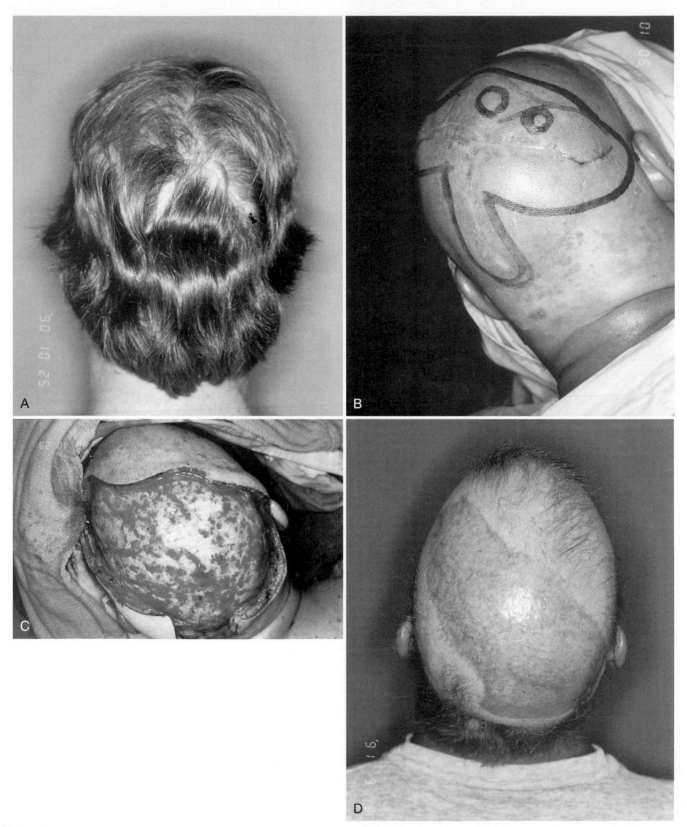

FIG. 47–8. **A,** preoperative view of scalp with recurrent dermatofibrosarcoma protuberans. **B,** operative plan for resection. **C,** defect
after surgical resection. **D,** postoperative result after latissimus dorsi
flap reconstruction with postoperative radiation.

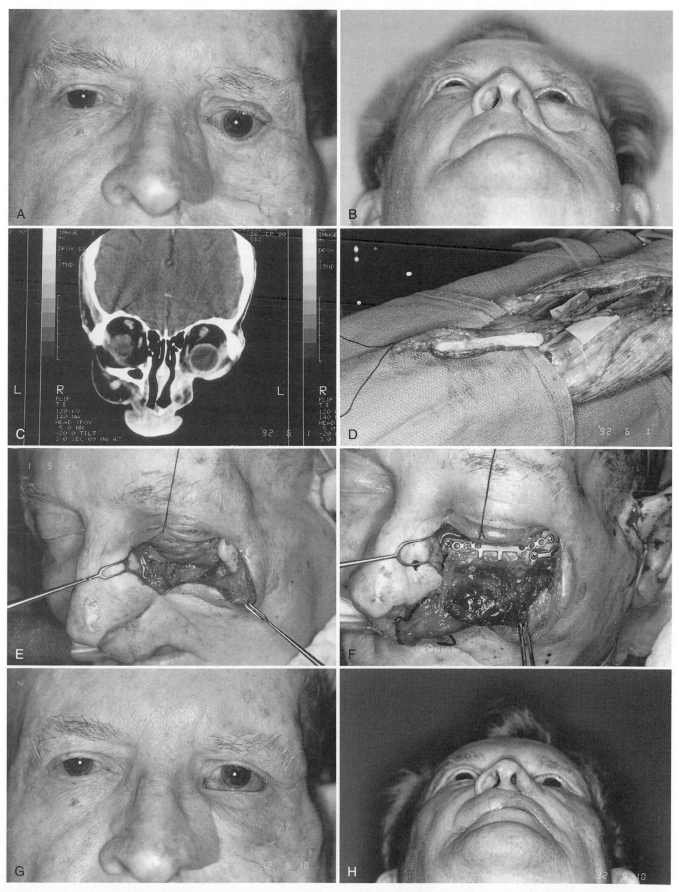

FIG. 47–9. **A,** patient with left orbital dystopia after radical maxillectomy; preoperative frontal view. **B,** preoperative worm's eye view. **C,** CT scan demonstrating lack of orbital floor. **D,** elevated osteocutaneous radial forearm flap in situ. **E,** exposed recipient site. **F,** flap inset with orbital reconstruction plate. **G,** postoperative frontal view. **H,** postoperative worm's eye view.

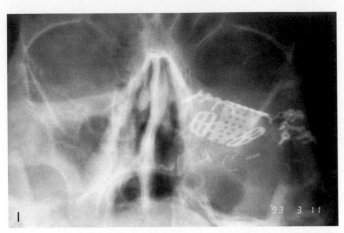

FIG. 47–9—*continued*. **I,** Waters view radiogram of reconstructed orbit with orbital reconstruction plate in place.

are most often due to the removal of the floor of the orbit during radical maxillectomy and extended resection of the maxilla that precludes adequate retention of a palatal prosthesis. Repair of defects of the orbit is most often accomplished by use of the radial forearm osteocutaneous flap (Fig. 47–9). While the morbidity of this flap cannot be ignored, the thin bone and small size of this flap are ideal for soft-tissue paddle replacing the orbit and relining the maxillary cavity. It is critical to support the orbital floor when reconstructing the orbital rim. An orbital-floor reconstruction plate can be suspended from the vascularized bone used for the orbital rim; such a device can serve both as a fixation device for the bone and a support device for the orbit (Fig. 47–9).

When attempting to reconstruct the maxilla, one should turn to larger flaps, particularly the scapular flap or the fibular osteocutaneous flap. It is not critical to completely obliterate an antral fistula; it is enough to secure a vascularized segment of bone that, with the help of osseointegrated implants, can serve as a foundation for maxillofacial prosthetics.

Complications

The most feared complication of microvascular surgery of the head and neck is vascular thrombosis and flap loss. Despite the high success rate enjoyed by most centers, this complication can prove disastrous for the patient, particularly if a fistula and subsequent infection ensue. These complications can cause prolonged hospitalization, thus negating the benefits of a one-stage immediate reconstruction. Flap loss can be minimized by utilizing safe, reliable flaps (such as those described in this chapter) with large-caliber vessels. One should also use the largest recipient vessels available. We routinely use the internal jugular vein and external carotid artery in head and neck reconstructions. These vessels provide a high inflow and outflow so that vascular thrombosis is minimized. The vessels are anastomosed in an end-to-side fashion, which also helps prevent vascular thrombosis. If vascular compromise is recognized early, the patient should be taken back to surgery immediately so that the flap can be reexplored, thrombectomized, and salvaged if possible. Several studies have shown that early vascular exploration can salvage a significant number of flaps (58).

Monitoring devices for flaps include the hand-held ultrasonic Doppler, the implantable 20-MHZ ultrasonic Doppler, and the laser Doppler probes (59,60). These devices have been reported to have variable success rates. It is more important to have a highly trained, experienced, and qualified nurse check the flap on an hourly basis to assess it for vascular compromise. If there is any hint of vascular compromise in a free flap, it is imperative that the flap be explored immediately, since that is usually the only chance for salvage.

Fistula formation in flaps used intraorally occurs in approximately 10% of cases (6). This can be avoided by meticulous attention to detail in approximating the flap to the native oral mucosa. With skin flaps, we utilize a vertical mattress technique, separating the sutures by no more than 0.5 cm. Despite this, in patients who have had radiation therapy the chance for fistula remains relatively high.

In our last series of 300 flaps, hematoma and infection occurred in approximately six percent of the cases (6).

Summary

Free-tissue transfer has revolutionized our ability to repair defects occurring after ablation of head and neck cancer. Soft-tissue defects can readily be addressed using either the free radial forearm flap for smaller defects or the rectus abdominis myocutaneous flap for larger defects. The free fibular flap has become the flap of choice for mandibular reconstruction, but the scapular, radial forearm, and iliac crest osteocutaneous flaps are also appropriate for selected cases. Muscle flaps such as the rectus abdominis and latissimus dorsi are useful for craniofacial and scalp defects. Midface defects and deformities after maxillectomy are best addressed using an osteocutaneous flap, which serves as a platform to stabilize maxillofacial prosthetics. Use of free flaps has achieved a 95% success rate in head and neck reconstruction, thus creating the paradox that the more complex procedure is actually the most reliable and therefore the first modality to consider in reconstruction for these difficult defects.

References

1. Daniel RK, Taylor GI. Distant transfer of an island flap by microvascular anastomses. *Plast Reconstr Surg* 1973; 52:111–117.
2. Harashina T, Fujino T, Aoyagi F. Reconstruction of the oral cavity with a free flap. *Plast Reconstr Surg* 1976; 58:412–414.
3. Panje W, Bardach J, Krause C. Reconstruction of the oral cavity with a free flap. *Plast Reconstr Surg* 1976; 58:415–418.
4. Martin HE, Munster H, Sugarbaker E. Cancer of the tongue. *Arch Surg* 1940; 41:888–936.
5. Martin HE. The history of lingual cancer. *Am J Surg* 1940; 48:703–716.
6. Schusterman MA, Miller MJ, Reece GP, et al. A single center's experience with 308 free flaps for repair of head and neck cancer defects. *Plast Reconstr Surg* 1994; 93(3):472–478.
7. Urken ML, Weinberg H, Buchbinder D, et al. Microvascular free flaps in head and neck reconstruction. Report of 200 cases and review of complications. *Arch Otolaryng Head Neck Surg* 1994; 120:633–640.
8. Shestak KC, Myers EN, Ramasastry SS, Jones NF, Johnson JT. Vascularized free-tissue transfer in head and neck surgery [review]. *Am J Otolaryg* 1993; 14:148–154.
9. Schusterman MA, Kroll SS, Weber RS, et al. Intraoral soft tissue reconstruction after cancer ablation: A comparison of the pectoralis major flap and the free radial forearm flap. *Am J Surg* 1991; 162:397–399.
10. Uthoff K, Zehr KJ, Lee PC, et al. Neutrophil modulation results in improved pulmonary function after 12 and 24 hours of preservation. *Ann Thorac Surg* 1995; 59:7–12; discussion 12–3X.
11. Blair EA, Callender DL. Head and neck cancer: the problem. In: Schusterman MA, ed. *Clinics in plastic surgery.* Philadelphia: WB Saunders, 1994; 1–7.

12. Conley JJ. The crippled oral cavity. *Plast Reconstr Surg* 1962; 30:469–478.
13. McGregor IA, McGregor RM. *Cancer of the face and mouth.* Edinburgh: Churchill Livingstone, 1986; 448.
14. Banis JC Jr. Thin cutaneous flap for intra oral reconstruction: the dorsalis pedis free flap revisited. *Microsurgery* 1988; 9:132–140.
15. Barton FE, Spicer TE, Byrd HS. Head and neck reconstruction with the latissimus dorsi myocutaneous flap: anatomic observations of 60 cases. *Plast Reconstr Surg* 1983; 71:199–204.
16. Sabatier RE, Bakamjian VY. Transaxillary latissimus dorsi flap reconstruction in head and neck cancer. Limitations and refinements in 56 cases. *Am J Surg* 1985; 150:427–434.
17. Katsaros J, Schusterman MA, Beppu M, et al. The lateral upper arm flap: anatomy and clinical applications. *Ann Plast Surg* 1984; 12:489–500.
18. Christie DRH, Duncan GM, Glasson DW. The ulnar artery free flap: the first 7 years. *Plast Reconstr Surg* 1994; 93(3):547–551.
19. Song R, Gao Y, Song Y, et al. The forearm flap. *Clin Plast Surg* 1982; 91:21–26.
20. Soutar DS, McGregor IA. The radial forearm flap in intraoral reconstruction: the experience of 60 consecutive cases. *Plast Reconstr Surg* 1986; 78:1–8.
21. Matthews RN, Hodge RA, Eyre J, et al. Radial forearm flap for floor of mouth reconstruction. *Brit J Surg* 1985; 72:561–564.
22. Lind MG, Arnander C, Gylbert L, et al. Reconstruction in the head and neck regions with free radial forearm flaps and split-rib bone grafts. *Am J Surg* 1987; 154:459–462.
23. Evans GR, Schusterman MA, Kroll SS, et al. The radial forearm free flap for head and neck reconstruction: a review. *Am J Surg* 1994; 168:446–450.
24. Dubner S, Heller KS. Reinnervated radial forearm free flaps in head and neck reconstruction. *J Reconstructive Microsurgery* 1992; 8:467–468.
25. Boyd B, Mulholland S, Gullane P, et al. Reinnervated lateral antebrachial cutaneous neurosome flaps in oral reconstruction: are we making sense? *Plast Reconstr Surg* 1994; 93:1350–1359; discussion 1360–13622.
26. Kroll SS, Baldwin BJ. Head and neck reconstruction with the rectus abdominis free flap [review]. *Clin Plast Surg* 1994; 21:97–105.
27. Urken ML, Weinberg H, Vickery C, et al. The rectus abdominis free flap in head and neck reconstruction. *Arch Otolaryngol Head Neck Surg* 1991; 117:857–866.
28. Nakatsuka T, Harii K, Yamada A, et al. Versatility of a free inferior rectus abdominis flap for head and neck reconstruction: analysis of 200 cases. *Plast Reconstr Surg* 1994; 93(4):762–769.
29. Kroll SS, Reece GP, Miller MJ, et al. Comparison of the rectus abdominis free flap with the pectoralis major myocutaneous flap for reconstructions in the head and neck. *Am J Surg* 1992; 164:615–618.
30. Serafin D, Riefkohl R, Thomas I, et al. Vascularized rib-periosteal and osteocutaneous reconstruction of the maxilla and mandible: an assessment. *Plast Reconstr Surg* 1980; 66:718–727.
31. Macleod AM. Vascularized metatarsal transfer in mandibular reconstruction. *Microsurgery* 1994; 15:257–261.
32. Soutar DS, Widdowson WP. Immediate reconstruction of the mandible using a vascularized segment of radius. *Head Neck Surg* 1986; 8:232–246.
33. Corrigan AM, O'Neill TJ. The use of the compound radial forearm flap in oro-mandibular reconstruction. *Br J Oral Maxillofac Surg* 1986; 24:86–95.
34. Swartz WM, Banis JC, Newton ED, et al. The osteocutaneous scapular flap for mandibular and maxillary reconstruction. *Plast Reconstr Surg* 1986; 77:530–545.
35. Taylor GI, Townsend P, Corlett R. Superiority of the deep circumflex iliac vessels as the supply for free groin flaps. Clinical work. *Plast Reconstr Surg* 1979; 64:745–759.
36. David DJ, Tan E, Katsaros J, et al. Mandibular reconstruction with vascularized iliac crest: a 10-year experience. *Plast Reconstr Surg* 1988; 82:792–801.
37. Beppu M, Hanel DP, Johnston GHF, et al. The osteocutaneous fibula flap: an anatomic study. *J Reconstr Microsurg* 1992; 8:215–223.
38. Hidalgo DA. Fibula free flap: a new method of mandible reconstruction. *Plast Reconstr Surg* 1989; 84:71–79.
39. Smith AA, Bowen CV, Rabczak T, et al. Donor site deficit of the osteocutaneous radial forearm flap. *Ann Plast Surg* 1994; 32:372–376.
40. Meland NB, Maki S, Chao EY, et al. The radial forearm flap: a biomechanical study of donor-site morbidity utilizing sheep tibia. *Plast Reconstr Surg* 1992; 90:763–773.
41. Boyd JB, Morris S, Rosen IB, et al. The through-and-through oromandibular defect: rationale for aggressive reconstruction. *Plast Reconstr Surg* 1994; 93:44–53.
42. Taylor GI, Townsend P, Corlett R. Superiority of the deep circumflex iliac vessels as the supply for free groin flaps. Experimental work. *Plast Reconstr Surg* 1979; 64:595–604.
43. Urken ML, Vickery C, Weinberg H, et al. The internal oblique–iliac crest osseomyocutaneous microvascular free flap in head and neck reconstruction. *J Reconstr Microsurg* 1989; 5:203 14; discussion, 215–216.
44. Schusterman MA, Reece GP, Miller MJ, et al. The osteocutaneous free fibula flap: is the skin paddle reliable? *Plast Reconstr Surg* 1992; 90:787–793.
45. Schusterman MA, Reece GP, Kroll SS, et al. Use of the AO plate for immediate mandibular reconstruction in cancer patients. *Plast Reconstr Surg* 1991; 88:588–593.
46. Seidenberg B, Rosenak SS, Hurwitt ES, et al. Immediate reconstruction of the cervical esophagus by a revascularized isolated jejunal segment. *Ann Surg* 1959; 149:162–171.
47. Jurkiewicz MJ. Vascularized intestinal graft for reconstruction of the cervical esophagus and pharynx. *Plast Reconstr Surg* 1965; 36:509–517.
48. Reece GP, Bengtson BP, Schusterman MA. Reconstruction of the pharynx and cervical esophagus using free jejunal transfer [review]. *Clin Plast Surg* 1994; 21:125–136.
49. Schusterman MA, Shestak KC, deVries EJ, et al. Reconstruction of the cervical esophagus: free jejunal transfer versus gastric pull-up. *Plast Reconstr Surg* 1990; 85:16–21.
50. Robb GL, Swartz WM. Pharyngocutaneous fistulas: management with one-stage lap reconstruction. *Ann Plast Surg* 1986; 16:125–135.
51. Jones NF, Schramm VL, Sekhar LN. Reconstruction of the cranial base following tumour resection. *Brit J Plast Surg* 1987; 40:155–162.
52. Jones NF, Sekhar LN, Schramm VL. Free rectus abdominis muscle flap reconstruction of the middle and posterior cranial base. *Plast Reconstr Surg* 1986; 78:471–479.
53. Jones NF. The contribution of microsurgical reconstruction to craniofacial surgery. *World J Surg* 1989; 13:454–464.
54. Jones NF, Hardesty RA, Swartz WM, et al. Extensive and complex defects of the scalp, middle third of the face, and palate: the role of microsurgical reconstruction. *Plast Reconstr Surg* 1988; 82:937–952.
55. Shestak KC, Schusterman MA, Jones NF, et al. Immediate microvascular reconstruction of combined palatal and midfacial defects using soft tissue only. *Microsurgery* 1988; 9:128–131.
56. Fisher J, Jackson IT. Microvascular surgery as an adjunct to craniomaxillofacial reconstruction. *Br J Plast Surg* 1989; 42:146–154.
57. Schusterman MA, Reece GP, Miller MJ. Osseous free flaps for orbit and midface reconstruction. *Am J Surg* 1993; 166:341–345.
58. Hidalgo DA, Jones CS. The role of emergent exploration in free-tissue transfer: a review of 150 consective cases. *Plast Reconstr Surg* 1990; 86:492–498.
59. Lowdon IMR, Ecker JO, Seaber AV, et al. Comparison of laser Doppler flow and cutaneous temperature recordings in postoperative monitoring of upper limb replatations and revascularizations. *Plast Reconstr Surg* 1988; 23.
60. Swartz WM, Izquierdo R, Miller MJ. Implantable venous doppler microvascular monitoring: laboratory investigation and clinical results. *Plast Reconstr Surg* 1994; 93:152–163.

48

Omentum, Stomach and Jejunum in Head and Neck Reconstruction

T.M.B. de Chalain, M.D., F.C.S. (SA) and M.J. Jurkiewicz, D.D.S., M.D., F.A.C.S.

While the advances in head and neck surgery have perhaps not been as dramatic as advances in other areas of surgery, they have been deceptively steady. For example, the craniofacial and skull-base procedures that are today almost commonplace, were virtually unheard of a brief two decades ago. Today, thanks to the evolution of surgical technique and expertise, there are few lesions that cannot be surgically addressed. But extirpation of a lesion is only half the battle; as the size and complexity of surgical excisions increases, so does the demand for more sophisticated, reliable, and imaginative surgical reconstruction. Beyond the limitations of local and regional flaps, the use of intraabdominal organs greatly expands the surgeon's ability to solve successfully those problems of reconstruction that are frequently encountered in the head and neck.

The development of microsurgical techniques permits reconstruction at a distance from the area of need. Plastic surgeons have found the peritoneal cavity a reservoir for several organs useful in reconstructive surgery—most notably, the stomach, omentum, and the bowel. Each has unique characteristics that suits it for specific purposes. The volume, texture, and pliability of the omentum makes it an admirable choice for coverage of large areas of soft-tissue loss as well as restoration of contour. The stomach, jejunum, and colon, possessing a mucosal surface, are suitable for the restoration of losses in lining of the alimentary tract of the oropharynx and replacement of the cervical esophagus.

The Omentum

For many years, local transfer of the omentum has facilitated its use in reconstructive surgery. Its pliability and rich lymphatic network make it ideal to fill cavities and combat infection. When transferred to the head and neck region as a free flap, it is used primarily for restoration of large areas of soft-tissue loss and to restore contour. Putatively, it retains its antimicrobial properties when transferred in this manner (1).

ANATOMY

The omentum is a syncitium of blood vessels, fat, and lymphatics (2). It hangs as a drape from the greater curvature of the stomach, supplied by the right and left gastroepiploic arteries (Fig. 48–1) and can be reliably based on either (1,3,4).

Generally, the right gastroepiploic vessels are preferred, since they are larger and dissection in the vicinity of the spleen is avoided. These arteries together form several arcades (5) that provide blood supply to the entire omentum. Several patterns to this system of arcades have been identi-

fied (5). These arcades allow surgical partitioning of the omentum (Fig. 48–2) that enhance its reconstructive versatility (1,5,6) and allows placement of discrete parcels, or fingers, of the omentum into individual areas of tissue deficiency.

The omentum, which is composed of a double layer of peritoneum folded on itself to form a richly vascularized, four-layered structure impregnated with varying amounts of fat, is pliable and easily shapes itself to irregularities. When skin covering or lining is needed, the omentum will easily support a skin or mucosal graft (1,3,7). Furthermore, because of its rich lymphatic network and reservoir of macrophages, the omentum aids in control of wound infection (1,2). A bone graft buried in or wrapped by omentum can be nutritionally supported (1).

SURGICAL TECHNIQUES

Open Method

Conventionally, the abdomen is opened through an upper midline incision, although routine vertical or transverse celiotomies have also been advocated (1). The omentum is freed from its areolar attachments to the transverse colon by sharp dissection until it hangs freely from the greater curvature of the stomach. This should be a relatively bloodless maneuver, but on occasion hemocoagulation with the electrocautery may be required. Occasionally there may be more difficulty separating the omentum from the transverse mesocolon. The plane of dissection between the omentum and mesocolon is more easily identified toward the splenic flexure. For technical ease, the omentum is usually based on the right gastroepiploic artery, although vascular support is satisfactory when based on the left gastroepiploic artery. The omentum is divided from the peripheral margin toward the gastroepiploic arcade at a point that would leave a suitable volume, based on the right gastroepiploic vessels. The short gastric vessels are clamped, divided, and ligated immediately, as the dissection proceeds from left to right (Figs. 48–3, 48–4).

The resultant pedicle is long and the vessels are adequate for microvascular anastomosis, averaging 1.5 to 2.5mm in diameter. After preparation of suitable recipient vessels, the omentum is transferred to the area of need in the head and neck region. Branches of the external carotid system most frequently serve as donor blood supply. The superficial temporal, superior thyroid, lingual, and facial arteries have all been used; surgeons have individual preferences, and the exigencies of each specific clinical case will largely dictate

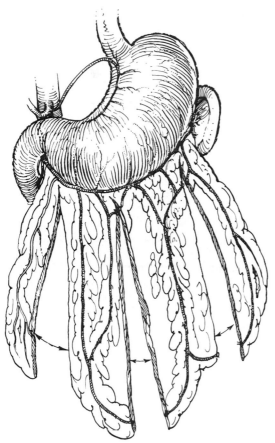

FIG. 48–1. The greater omentum, depending from the greater curvature of the stomach. In the region of the pylorus, the gastroduodenal artery is depicted by dotted lines, as is the splenic artery. The left and right gastroepiploic vessels, which supply the omentum, are shown, as are potential lines of omental division.

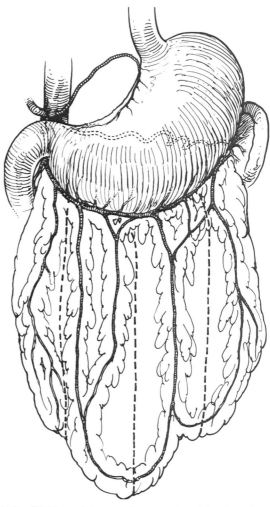

FIG. 48–2. Division of the greater omentum into discrete components, each of which is axially supplied by branches of the gastroepiploic vasculature. Note that the anastomosis between the left and right gastroepiploic arteries is often attenuated—and, on occasion, may be absent.

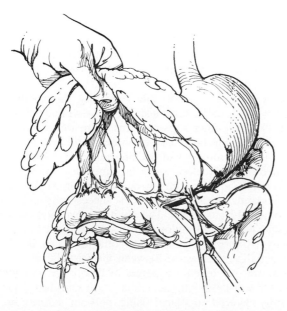

FIG. 48–3. Harvest of the omentum commences with careful, sharp dissection of the filmy omental attachments to the transverse colon.

which vessels should be used for anastomosis; but, it is probably true to say that in the elderly patient, with or without peripheral vascular disease, the superficial temporal vessels ought not to be the first choice. Venous drainage is directed into any convenient tributary of the deep or superficial jugular systems. Anastomoses of the artery and a single vein are usually sufficient although, when two veins are available, venous drainage may be enhanced by dual anastomosis. Vein grafts are seldom necessary because of the generous length of the pedicle.

A nasogastric tube is inserted for 24 to 48 hrs after the operation to decompress the stomach. This prevents gastric distention that, among other things, might dislodge any of the vascular ligations along the greater curvature. One report (8) advocates suturing the greater curvature to the transverse mesocolon to prevent the once-reported complication of cecal volvulus, but this is probably unnecessary on a regular basis. The abdomen is closed in routine fashion.

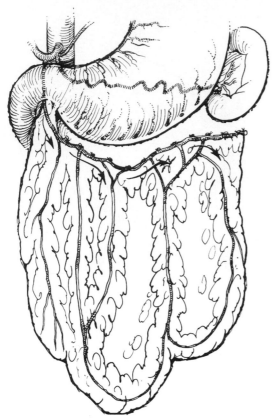

FIG. 48–4. Based on the right gastroepiploic vessels, an extensive omental flap can be developed, with a pedicle suitable for local transposition or free transplantation. Careful dissection and suture ligation of the short gastric vessels is tedious, but vital.

Closed (Endoscopic) Method

Over the past decade, endoscopic techniques have revolutionized the practice of general and gynecologic surgery. Plastic and reconstructive surgery is starting to feel the impact of this technology. Insofar as endoscopic techniques greatly reduce the morbidity of such intraabdominal operations as cholecystectomy, the idea of using endoscopy to aid in the harvest of intraabdominal organs such as the omentum is innately appealing. There has been only a single clinical case report of endoscopic omental harvest; this in 1993 was from Saltz and colleagues (9), reporting on the use of a laparoscope to aid in the harvest of an omentum for lower limb reconstruction. In this instance, the omentum was explored using the laparoscope, and was then exteriorized for dissection. In 1994 Miller and others (10) reported on the state of the art concerning endoscopic omental harvest. This team, working at the M.D. Anderson Cancer Center, had not, at the time of writing, applied their method clinically. Using a large-animal model, a team of three surgeons performs the harvest by making five access port incisions: Two in the left upper quadrant, two in the right upper quadrant, and one at midline incision beneath the umbilicus. The upper incisions were all placed lateral to the rectus abdominis. The technique proceeds by mobilization of the omentum from inferiorly, in order to allow visualization of the greater curvature of the

stomach and transverse colon. While minimal adhesions may be taken down endoscopically, significant adhesions that tether and distort the omentum probably demand conversion to an open technique. The single major problem remains a safe, reliable, and easily applied technique for rapidly controlling the many bleeding points exposed in an omental harvest. Failure to achieve adequate control of bleeding rapidly leads to formation of expansile hematomata in the compliant omentum, which makes further dissection difficult.

As with conventional harvest, the dissection proceeds from left to right, clipping and cutting the short gastric vessels, until the organ has been isolated to its right gastroepiploic vessels. These are then clipped and cut in turn, and the omentum is removed from the abdomen. On occasion, if the size of the omentum is too great to allow its passage through one of the existing ports, a separate Pfannensteil incision may have to be made.

At this juncture, the extreme mobility and vascularity of the omentum make its harvest technically difficult. However, endoscopic technology and instrumentation is evolving at a rapid pace and, while it is not yet clinically practical, it is certainly feasible that routine, laparoscopic harvest of the omentum will move from the laboratory to the operating room in the near future. Critics of the technique ask whether, if the primary motivation for developing minimally invasive techniques is to reduce morbidity, an endoscopic procedure that calls for five and possibly six access port incisions is really less invasive and less morbid than an upper midline laparotomy.

SPECIFIC USES

The revascularized omentum can be spread to cover large surface areas, which will provide skin coverage when a skin graft is applied (1,3,11,12). Alternately, the tissue is pliable and can be folded on itself to increase bulk and fill deeper depressions (1,3,4). Any contour problems are solvable provided the unit is large enough. The entire calvarium has been covered by spreading the microvascularly transferred omentum over the defect and covering this with a skin graft (11). Conversely, the omentum has been folded and packed into the exenterated and radiated orbit or the frontal sinus to obliterate dead space (1), and we have used it to fill dead space and revascularize bone in a devastating shotgun-blast injury of the forearm.

Because of its reliability and versatility, the omentum is a good choice of tissue for transfer to close wounds of the head and neck when other flaps or forms of treatment have failed. The omentum has been used to obliterate the draining frontal sinus where curettage and packing failed (1). The bulk and antimicrobial characteristics of the omentum contribute to its effectiveness in management of such wounds. An exposed and jeopardized carotid has been successfully covered by free omental transfer (1). The ability to partition the omentum was popularly employed in the treatment of hemifacial atrophy (Romberg disease). The omentum can be divided with viability maintained between the vascular arcades (4). This allows placement of parcels of this tissue into separate areas for soft-tissue augmentation. Each partitioned piece is carefully sutured in place, using pull-out sutures brought through the skin. The sutures are left in place for approxi-

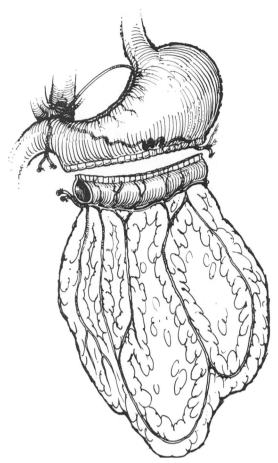

FIG. 48–5. In raising a gastroomental flap, a stapling device is used to fashion the greater curvature of the stomach into a tubular conduit. This is then used for pharyngoesophageal reconstruction, while the attached omentum is used to provide coverage, or to fill dead space. Note that this flap is best based on the right gastroepiploic vascular pedicle, with blood supply to the gastric conduit via the short gastric vessels. Great care must be taken, in harvesting this flap, not to obstruct or occlude the pylorus.

mately 5 days until the omentum has become adequately adherent to the surrounding tissues. Direct suturing has been advocated as a way of holding the tissue in the intended position. Soft-tissue deficiency can be precisely corrected by placement of parcels of omentum in the areas of need. This technique enjoyed historic primacy, and is still useful in selected cases. It is today less commonly used, largely because no reliable method has yet been found to fix the omentum in position and such reconstructions tend to droop and sag under the influence of gravity and time. In our experience, all free flaps sag with time when used to ameliorate the effects of hemifacial atrophy. The atrophic skin envelope, with its intrinsic loss of elasticity, remains a major problem.

The microscopically revascularized omentum has a rich blood supply and is capable of supporting a bone graft (1,2,13). In patients with facial skeletal loss due to trauma or neoplasm, bony contour can be reestablished by a bone graft wrapped with omentum. In this way, the bony architecture of the facial skeleton can be restored. If soft-tissue deficiencies are also present, any excess omentum can be used to correct this.

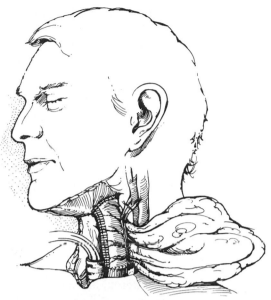

FIG. 48–6. This shows how a gastroomental flap might be used for hypopharyngeal reconstruction. It is apparent that after recreating the orogastric conduit, the attached omentum is readily available for coverage of the flap, or for filling dead space.

COMPOSITE FLAPS OF OMENTUM AND STOMACH

Baudet (14) is credited with the first description of a gastroomental flap, per se, in 1979, although Heibert and Cummings (15) reported in 1961 a case of successful cervical oesophageal reconstruction, with a free transplantation of gastric antrum that contained some omentum, along the greater gastric curvature. Since these beginnings, there have been sporadic reports of gastroomental flap utilization (16), the most recent being a series of 48 patients, from Guedon and coworkers in 1994 (17).

In essence, these flaps use the greater curvature of the stomach, harvested by means of a staple-suturing device, to form a tube or patch whose principal use is to replace pharyngeal defects; the omentum, left attached to the gastric flap by means of the short gastric vessels, is similarly harvested, the whole composite flap pedicled on the right gastroepiploic vessels. The primary application for this flap is in reconstructing defects of the pharynx or hypopharynx in which there has been associated skin loss—as in the resection of a pharyngeal tumour that has invaded overlying skin. Because of the long pedicle available, this flap may be sutured either to the neck vessels or, where these are unavailable, to the thoracodorsal vessels. Typically, the flap is divided once the recipient vessels have been prepared. The preformed gastric tube is then inset into the pharyngeal defect, and the microvascular anastomoses performed. Once the flap is perfusing well, the omentum is tailored, sutured into place in the defect and covered with a split-skin graft, or left to granulate (Figs. 48–5, 48–6).

The procedure is described as being no more morbid than jejunal free-flap reconstructions, and the postoperative course is similar, with a reasonably rapid return to oral alimentation. The fistula rate is low and the majority of these heal spontaneously. Fistulas are actively sought by means of a barium swallow, between postoperative days 7 and 10. In 1990 Mixter and others (16) reported some problems with omental sag, noting that care must be taken to protect the tracheostomy site from occlusion.

PROBLEMS AND COMPLICATIONS

While the problems associated with laparotomy for omental harvest have been minimal, this is still a potentially morbid procedure. For example:

1. There has been one case of reported cecal volvulus (8).
2. Bleeding from divided vessels along the greater curvature of the stomach or injured spleen is possible, but has not been reported.
3. Small bowel obstruction may result from the laparotomy and subsequent adhesions.
4. The procedure does demand a laparotomy and, therefore, a scar on the abdomen.

Major problems with transferred omentum have been uncommon but technical difficulties still exist. For example:

1. Failure of the free flap is rare, occuring less than 5% of the time (1).
2. The effect of gravity in displacing the tissue from its intended position has been a significant difficulty when the omentum is used to restore facial contour. This problem requires surgical repositioning of the omentum, often on a repeated basis. Extensive direct suturing of the omentum has been advocated as a way of combatting this, but its long-term efficacy has not been established (18).
3. The omentum, of course, has not restored any lost facial movement.
4. The amount of omentum available to the reconstructive surgeon cannot be ascertained before a laparotomy. Body habitus does not necessarily correlate with the size of the omentum (1,4). This can be a definite problem in children, and in cases in which a large amount of tissue is required. Potentially, the use of a scouting laparoscopy to assess size of the omentum in such cases could conceivably reduce morbidity by obviating the need for a laparotomy in cases where the omentum is endoscopically seen to be inadequate.

SUMMARY

The omentum has been found to be a useful organ to replace soft-tissue loss in the head and neck region. Its large area permits coverage of extensive open defects, such as full-thickness scalp loss over the calvarium. Its bulk can be used to restore volume. The nature of its blood supply allows its surgical partitioning for use in several different discrete areas of need. The transfer is technically easy to perform, but at this juncture it still requires a laparotomy. The main technical problem remains the effect of gravity on the transplanted tissue causing it to sag and requiring periodic revision.

The Jejunum

Major losses of alimentary tract lining in the head and neck by trauma such as caustic ingestion or extirpative cancer surgery commonly create reconstructive problems. In these cases, reconstruction can be accomplished by the direct suture of remaining local lining tissues; the mobilization of regional skin and muscle flaps, which introduce new lining in the form of skin islands; or the importation of new tissues by free-tissue transfer.

When large amounts of lining are lost, primary closure and local flaps result in stricture or tethering of mobile structures such as the tongue, which can be functionally devastating (19). Fistulas are frequent complications because of tension on the suture line.

Regional flaps avoid some of these problems but introduce new ones. Frequently, the procedures are performed in stages, necessitating obligatory alimentary tract cutaneous fistulas for a period of time. Size requirements are difficult to meet, with the operations tailored to the requirements of safe tissue transfer rather than specific tissue needs in the recipient area. Where lining is restored by skin rather than mucosa, these skin paddles lack secretory function and contribute nothing

FIG. 48–7. Use of a jejunal free flap for pharyngeal reconstruction. Starting at the top left, and moving counterclockwise, a suitable segment of jejunum is selected and harvested. A portion of this jejunum, based on the same pedicle of supply, is isolated and mobilized as shown. This segment may then be used in several ways. At bottom left, it is brought out through the skin incision as a monitoring segment. Since it is based on the same vascular pedicle as the major segment used in reconstructing the pharynx, it allows the viability of the occult reconstruction to be determined at a glance. Alternatively, as is shown at bottom right, the monitoring segment may be split along the antemesenteric border, demucosalized, and used to fill dead space, or skin grafted and used as a patch to close skin defects, as shown at top right.

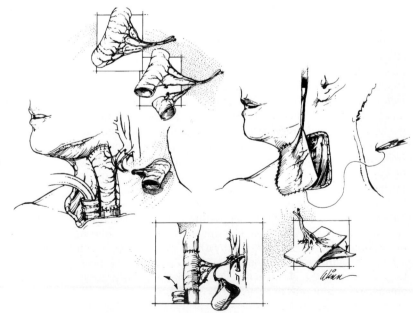

to the correction of xerostomia in irradiated patients. Furthermore, they shed epidermis and can grow hair, creating bothersome aesthetic and hygiene problems. Cicatricial stenosis at the sites of skin–mucosa coaptation is common.

Microsurgical transfer of bowel allows replacement of lining and is thus better tailored to the needs of the deficient recipient area. The transferred bowel retains secretory ability (20), which has proven an important boon in radiated patients. Furthermore, creative techniques have evolved, allowing for the use of bowel subcomponents to provide coverage and bulk, as well as simply lining (Carlson et al, in press) (Fig. 48–7). Because reconstruction is complete in one stage, convalescence has been shortened appreciably by this method (21).

Theoretically, any segment of bowel can be used in alimentary reconstruction. When a total esophagectomy is required, gastric transposition is the method of choice. It is reliable, and calls for only a single enteric anastomosis. The morbidity of such a procedure is high, combining abdominal, thoracic, and cervical operations, which are associated with a high operative mortality and frequent gastric reflux (22). Colon interposition, usually as a segment of the left colon, pedicled on the middle colic vessels, is an alternative, when gastric transposition is precluded by previous stomach surgery. Again, the combination of cervical, thoracic, and abdominal approaches, plus the necessity for one cervical and two abdominal bowel anastomoses, leads to considerable morbidity and a high complication rate (22).

When total esophagectomy is not required, free jejunal transfer is the method of choice for reconstruction of the hypopharynx and the cervical esophagus, because of its favorable position, vascular pedicle length and diameter, and bowel lumen caliber (which is well suited for cervical esophageal replacement). Operative morbidity is low and, in experienced hands, the technique offers a low complication rate and rapid return of oral intake. Right colon may be used on occasion when a larger area of replacement lining is needed. While its pedicle is long and the diameter of bowel greater than that of jejunum, the paracolonic vascular plexus does not provide the plethoric communications to the bowel wall seen in the jejunum. Thus, compared with jejunum, free transfers of colon are not as reliable.

ANATOMY

The duodenal flexure, leading to the jejunum is located to the left of the aorta, at the level of the superior border of the second lumbar vertebra (L2). The ligament of Treitz, a fibrous band, fixes the flexure to the right diaphragmatic crus, adjacent to the right side of the esophagus. The jejunum, some 4 cm in diameter, makes up the first 40% of the 7 meters of small bowel, which, in turn, is defined as that portion of the bowel between the splenic flexure and the ileocecal valve. The mesentery is a fan-shaped structure that supports the small bowel and transmits arterial supply and venous and lymphatic drainage. It is some 15 cm wide at the vertebral root, which lies along an oblique line running from the left side of L2 to the right sacroiliac joint, across the posterior abdominal wall. The length, from the vertebral to the intestinal border, averages about 20 cm, but it is greatest in the center.

The small bowel receives its nutrient blood flow via vascular arcades in the mesentery that derive from the superior

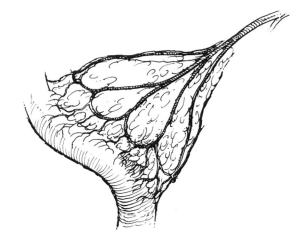

FIG. 48–8. The typical arcade structure of the blood supply to the jejunum is based on a series of branches of the superior mesenteric artery. As such, the jejunum lends itself to harvest for free-flap reconstructions, and the most popular choice is the second arcade. With care, a pedicle 36 cm in length can be obtained; this will contain a single artery and vein, of some 3.5 and 5 mm in diameter, respectively. This second arcade will typically supply a segment of jejunum up to 53 cm in length (From Strauch B, Yu H-L. *Atlas of microvascular surgery: anatomy and operative approaches.* New York: Thieme, 1993).

mesenteric artery. The arcades liberally interconnect with one another along the mesenteric side of the bowel (Fig. 48–8). On average, there are five jejunal branches from the superior mesenteric artery, with a total of 12 to 15 branches to the jejunum and ileum (23). A segment of bowel 10 to 20 cm in length can be perfused by such an arterial arcade and its accompanying vein(s). Surgical isolation of this arcade can provide a pedicle as long as 20 cm. The caliber of the vein and artery range from 1.5 to 3.0 mm (24). The length and caliber of the pedicle are ideal for microsurgical transfer.

SURGICAL TECHNIQUE

Open Method

The bowel is harvested through an upper midline incision. A suitable segment of jejunum is identified at a convenient working distance from the ligament of Treitz. The first intestinal branch from the superior mesenteric to the jejunum is usually not selected as the pedicle of choice: not only is it apt to be high and deeply situated, making dissection needlessly difficult, but also it often has a common stem with the inferior pancreatico-duodenal artery (22). Usually, the 2nd, 3rd, or 4th intestinal branch is selected. The pedicle is located in the mesenteric leaf by inspection or palpation. The vein and artery are surgically isolated and mobilized from the arborization of the vascular system near the wall of the bowel toward the root of the mesentery. The length should be generous, and can exceed 20 cm in some cases.

The segment of bowel supplied by the pedicle is isolated between bowel clamps and divided. It is maintained on its vascular pedicle until the head and neck region is prepared for the reception of the segment. This period of observation determines whether or not the entire segment of harvested bowel is viable on its vascular pedicle (21,25). The remaining intraabdominal bowel is anastomosed. Placement of a feeding jejunostomy is strongly indicated in most patients, ensuring adequate enternal alimentation until the patient can meet nutritional requirements by mouth. Likewise, a naso-gastric tube is a useful means of preventing gastric distension and emesis.

Branches of the external carotid system are most frequently used as donor arteries. Tributaries of the superficial or deep jugular system receive venous drainage. In cases where the external system has been sacrificed or irradiated, anastomosis to the contralateral neck vessels, the ipsilateral common carotid, or the subclavian vessels is performed. If the common carotid serves as a donor artery, the anastomosis is created end to side. This demands partial occlusion of the carotid while the anastamosis is accomplished. The contralateral carotid must be patent. This technique should be avoided in those patients with significant atherosclerotic disease of the carotid. With these precautions, neither transient ischemic attacks nor strokes have been reported (25). The bowel is tailored in size and partially secured before microvascular reconstruction (21). This guarantees appropriate vascular pedicle length and position. If the bowel is used to replace a segment of cervical esophagus, the entire proximal anastomosis is performed be-fore revascularization. The proximal repair is technically harder and demands manipulation of the bowel (and thus, the pedicle) in all directions to ensure proper placement of su-tures. The bowel anastomosis is performed with interrupted 4-0 or 3-0 absorbable suture and should be completed within 30 minutes. After revascularization the distal anastomosis is completed, again with interrupted absorbable suture. By com-parison, it is technically simple.

After revascularization, the bowel immediately becomes pink and peristalsis is apparent. In segmental esophageal re-placement, the jejunal segment should be isoperistaltic (19,21). Commonly, mucorrhea develops within minutes and may persist for several days up to 3 weeks. Its duration and magnitude seem to be related to the small-bowel ischemia time (20). Because copious amounts of mucus can be se-creted, any major replacement of lining can contribute to pul-monary toilet problems. If a tracheostomy is not present, or part of the procedure for other reasons, a temporary tra-cheostomy may be necessary to protect the patient until the mucorrhea spontaneously abates (24).

Monitoring of the flap after replantation is by direct visu-alization of the mucosa by oral examination, by construction of a small window through the neck incisions that will allow visualization of the serosa, or by placing a meshed split-thickness skin graft on a portion of the serosa (21,25). Split-thickness skin grafts heal well on transplanted bowel serosa. The thin skin coverage has created no long-term problems. A technique of monitoring that has been found to be very help-ful is to bring a segment of the jejunum, vascularized by ar-borizations of the same intestinal-branch pedicle, out through the neck incision, where it is protected from desiccation by a xeroform gauze dressing. Not only does this permit monitor-ing of vascularity, but also of the degree of mucorrhoea and swelling. Furthermore, in complicated cases, where a skin defect overlying the cervical oesophageal reconstruction needs to be made good, a similar segment of jejunum, split lengthways along the antemesenteric border and stripped of its mucosa, will provide a fairly generous surface area of ro-bust, well-vascularized tissue, which readily accepts a skin graft. If the free jejunum is to develop problems it usually

will do so within the first 48 hours (25). Close observation during this period is mandatory.

Postoperatively, the patient is maintained NPO for 5 to 7 days. A barium swallow is obtained to document any leak through the bowel anastomosis. Small sinuses are treated ex-pectantly with universal success. Larger fistulas often close, but on occasion may require revision, especially if the neck has been previously irradiated.

Closed or Endoscopic Method

Endoscopic harvest of jejunum has recently become a clini-cal reality. It has passed beyond the laboratory and is now performed in operating rooms across the country. The fol-lowing method is based on the clinical protocol in use at the M.D. Anderson Cancer Center (10).

Before commencing, a nasogastric tube and a Foley catheter are passed in order to ensure decompression of the stomach and bladder. First, an access port is placed in the right upper quadrant. This consists of a 3-cm transverse inci-sion, centered on the lateral edge of the rectus abdominis and 2 cm below the costal margin. This incision is carried down to the peritoneum, direct vision ensuring safe entry into the abdominal cavity. A hasson cannula is placed and sutured to the deep fascia. This cannula has a flap valve that allows the entry and removal of instruments without losing the insuf-flated CO_2 pressure; this is of critical importance, because it is this insufflated gas that provides the optical cavity without which visualization would not be possible. Having placed the cannula, the insufflation port is connected to the CO_2 hose and gas is forced into the abdominal cavity until a pressure of 12 cm H_2O is reached. At this point, the video camera is in-troduced through the Hasson camera and the abdominal cav-ity can be inspected. The next procedure is placement of three cannulas, under indirect videoscopic vision. Two are placed on the right, lateral to the rectus sheath, and a third is placed on the left lower abdomen, lateral to the midline. These cannulas are pushed through the abdominal wall, using a spring-loaded trocar that sharply penetrates the wall. As the trocar enters the peritoneal cavity, a protective guard is auto-matically advanced to shield the sharp tip and protect the vis-cera. Penetration of the abdominal wall, and tip guarding are observed from within the abdomen by the surgeon. Having secured penetration, the sharp trocar is withdrawn and the gas-tight cuff advanced into the tissues to secure the cannula in position.

With instruments in place, the abdomen well-insufflated with gas, and good visualization secured, the jejunal harvest may be begun. First the abdominal cavity is visually ex-plored and filmy adhesions gently taken down. Placing the patient in Trendelenburg position facilitates the superior mo-bilization of the omentum and transverse colon. The small bowel is followed proximally in order to locate the ligament of Treitz. A suitable segment of jejunum, together with its vascular pedicle, is then selected for harvest. This is usually some 40 cm below the duodeno–jejunal flexure. In order to dissect the mesentery, the selected segment of jejunum must be suspended from the anterior abdominal wall. This is done with 2-0 nylon sutures on straight Keith needles, which are pushed directly through the abdominal wall, through the an-temesenteric border of the jejunal segment, and back out through the abdominal wall, where a hemostat is used to secure the suture under the correct tension. Up to six such sutures may be needed to secure the jejunal segment adequately for dissection. At this juncture, if the mesentery is deemed too thick for adequate visualization, the procedure should be converted to an open one. With the jejunal segment well suspended, the vascular arcades can be dissected with relative ease. A second light source behind the segment provides transillumination, which facilitates identification and mobilization of vessels. Minimal use of electrocautery, sharp dissection, and ligature clips allows safe dissection of a 12- to 18-cm segment of jejunum, pedicled on a single vascular leash. As far proximally as possible, this pedicle is doubly clipped and divided. A Babcock clamp is then passed through the Hasson cannula and the midportion of the isolated loop of bowel is grasped. The suspension sutures are released and the Cannula, plus Babcock, are withdrawn from the abdomen, delivering the loop of bowel to the skin surface. As the cannula is withdrawn, the insufflated gas is lost; this allows deflation, which in turn increases the amount of bowel that can be delivered through the access incision. With the loop of bowel exteriorized, the proximal and distal limits of the segment to be resected are clamped and divided, using a gastrointestinal stapling device.

At this point, the isolated segment of jejunum is passed to the cervical recipient site for immediate insetting and anastomosis, since the length of ischemic time to which the jejunum is subjected materially affects such events as postoperative swelling and mucorrhea. Management of the bowel donor site is thus either deferred or becomes the responsibility of a second team of surgeons. The two ends of the jejunum at the donor site are anastomosed using conventional techniques, care being taken to ensure that they are adequately vascularized. The two edges of the divided mesentery are tacked together, and a jejunal feeding tube is placed before the bowel is returned to the abdominal cavity. A gastrostomy tube may be placed in lieu of a nasogastric tube, if desired, and the small fascial and skin defects are repaired to prevent herniation. The patient is left with four small skin incisions, the longest of which is approximately 3 cm, rather than a single long, midline incision. Early experience with this technique suggests that it takes some 3 hours to perform, and is thus much longer than the equivalent open harvest. This figure ought to diminish with the surgeon's increasing experience.

SPECIFIC USES

Microvascular transfer of jejunum allows replacement of lining in the upper alimentary tract. These transfers have been used for small oral patches as well as large segmental defects of cervical esophagus. The thickness of the bowel is well suited to reconstructive needs and excess bulk, often a drawback of musculocutaneous flaps, is avoided. The flaps retain their histologic and physiologic properties, which are more compatible lining substitutes than skin flaps or grafts.

The mesentery in some instances can provide a leaf of vascularized tissue that can be used to correct contour deficits (24). If appropriately located, it can cover the carotid or be used to cover a portion of the implanted bowel. With its mucosa stripped, and covered with a split-thickness skin graft, it has been used to provide coverage and, as such, satisfy local skin defects.

When a portion of the cervical esophagus remains, the jejunum can be sutured as a patch to close a fistula or to increase the caliber of the esophageal lumen. This can simplify the dissection, particularly in the radiated neck. Large patch grafts on the esophagus, however, should be avoided because of the excessively long suture line. Here, segmental replacement with a discrete cylinder of free jejunum, employing two separate suture lines, is preferred.

For the sake of completeness, it should be noted that, in specifically selected patients, where there is a need to shorten operating time because of the patient's instability, or where a successful microvascular anastomosis cannot be performed, it is possible to perform free jejunal grafting without revascularization. Panje and Hetherington (26) reported in 1994 on this technique and emphasize the importance of a well-vascularized recipient bed with no dead spaces between the jejunal muscularis (all serosa must be stripped from the graft) and the bed. They also recommend stenting of the graft and warn of delayed wound healing, possible fistula formation, and delayed initiation of oral intake, often leading to a prolonged need for tube feeding. They emphasize the importance of meticulously isolating the great vessels from the graft by means of a local flap (e.g., sternocleidomastoid muscle), and reiterate that this is not a method applicable to all comers. We would endorse the latter point wholeheartedly: This method is a last resort, to be employed only when no more attractive alternatives exist. When successfully employed, however, it does offer the advantages of a one-stage solution with reduced operating time that leads to a lining of thin, flat, moist mucosal tissue.

PROBLEMS AND COMPLICATIONS

As stated earlier, postrevascularization mucorrhea can complicate the maintenance of a clean airway. Appropriate measures, such as tracheostomy, should be employed to prevent aspiration. Mucorrhea is a self-limiting phenomenon, with resolution anticipated within 2 weeks.

The transplanted jejunum is not innervated and, therefore, lacks sensibility. In the pharynx, this area of anesthesia can lead to aspiration as the patient begins to attempt eating again. Suitable care must therefore be taken when initiating eating. On occasion, the patient must be retrained in deglutition, in order to prevent the development of chronic aspiration.

Anastomotic problems have been infrequent. Small sinuses observed on barium swallow have all closed without reoperation. Liquids can be given by mouth until a follow-up barium swallow demonstrates a closing or closed sinus. Oropharyngeal cutaneous fistulas occur infrequently and have been successfully treated in all cases. Almost all will close with expectant treatment if the neck has not been irradiated; the few that require reexploration and surgical closure are seen almost exclusively in the irradiated neck. Donor site complications occur in 5 to 10% of cases. No anastomotic leaks or feeding jejunostomy problems have yet been reported. Bowel obstruction has been reported (19). Disruption of the abdominal closure occurs infrequently, but is remedied by careful resuturing. The fascial problems seen in these patients are greatly influenced by their nutritional status. It is common to find that a patient who presents with a cancer of the oral cavity, pharynx, or hypopharynx has been unwilling or unable to eat adequately for some time; hence, the majority of these patients are malnourished at the time of presentation. If possible, nutritional deficiencies should be corrected before the procedure.

Summary

The use of jejunum to reconstruct lining deficiency in the head and neck is reliable and safe in the hands of an experienced microsurgeon. Many problems associated with older techniques have been solved by this free-tissue transfer. The problems with microsurgical transfer have been primarily technical and appear to be, for the most part, correctable. A laparotomy is usually required, but it has created major complications in only a few patients; the advent of endoscopic harvest may further reduce this morbidity. As experience increases, free bowel transfer will play an ever-increasing role in management of oropharyngeal and upper esophageal reconstructive problems.

References

1. Jurkiewicz MJ, Nahai F. The omentum: its use as a free vascularized graft for reconstruction of the head and neck *Ann Surg* 1982; 195:756.
2. Brown RG, Nahai F, Silverton JS. The omentum in facial reconstruction. *Br J Plast Surg* 1978; 31:58.
3. Harrii K. Clinical application of free omental flap transfer. *Clin Plast Surg* 1978; 5:273.
4. Alday ES, Goldsmith HS. Surgical technique for omental lengthening based on arterial anatomy. *Surg Gynecol Obstet* 1972; 135:103.
5. Upton J, Mulliken JB, Hicks PD, et al. Restoration of facial contour using free vascularized omental transfer. *Plast Reconstr Surg* 1980; 66:650.
6. Das SK. The size of the human omentum and methods of lengthening it for transplantation. *Br J Plast Surg* 1976; 29:170.
7. Harashina T, Imai T, Wada M. The omental sandwich reconstruction for a full-thickness cheek graft. *Plast Reconstr Surg* 1979; 29:411.
8. Hakelius L. Fatal complication after use of greater omentum for reconstruction of the chest wall. Case report. *Plast Recon Surg* 1978; 62:796.
9. Saltz R, Stowers R, Smith M, et al. Laparoscopically harvested omental free flap to cover a large soft-tissue defect. *Ann Surg* 1994; 21:149–159.
10. Miller MJ, Robb GL, Staley CA. Harvest of jejunum, rectus abdominis and omentum. In: Bostwick J, Eaves F, Nahai F, eds. *Endoscopic plastic surgery.* St. Louis: Quality Medical Publishing, 1995.
11. Ikuta Y. Autotransplant of omentum to cover large denudation of scalp. *Plast Reconstr Surg* 1975; 55:490.
12. McLean DH, Bunke HJ. Auto transplantation of omentum to a large scalp defect with microsurgical revascularization. *Plast Reconstr Surg* 1972; 49:268.
13. Arnold PG, Irons GB. The greater omentum extensions in transposition and free transfer. *Plast Reconstr Surg* 1981; 67:169.
14. Baudet J. Reconstruction of the pharyngeal wall by transfer of the greater omentum and stomach. *Int J Microsurg* 1979; 1:53.
15. Heibert CA, Cummings GO. Successful replacement of the cervical oesophagus by transplantation and revascularization of a free graft of gastric antrum. *Ann Surg* 1961; 154:103–106.
16. Heibert CA, Cummings GO. Successful replacement of the cervical oesophagus by transplantation and revascularization of a free graft of gastric antrum. *Ann Surg* 1961; 154:103–106.
17. Guedon CE, Marmuse JP, Gehanno P, et al. The use of gastro-omental free flaps in major neck defects. Presented at the Society of Head and Neck Surgeons Conference May 25–28, Paris, France.
18. Walinshaw M, Caffee HH, Wolfe SA. Vascularized omentum for facial contour restoration. *Ann Plast Surg* 1983; 10:292.
19. Sasaki TM, Baker HW, McConnell DB, et al. Free jejunal graft reconstruction after extensive head and neck surgery. *Am J Surg* 1980; 139:650.
20. Reuther JF, Steinau H, Wagner R. Reconstruction of large defects in the oropharynx with a revascularized intestinal graft: an experimental and clinical report. *Plast Reconstr Surg* 1984; 73:345.
21. McConnel FM, Hester TR, Nahai F, et al. Free jejunal grafts for reconstruction of pharynx and cervical esophagus. *Arch Otolaryngol* 1981; 107:476.
22. Carlson GW, Coleman JJ, Jurkiewicz MJ. Reconstruction of the hypopharynx and cervical esophagus. *Curr Prob in Surg* 1993; 30:425–480.
23. Strauch B, Yu H-L. *Atlas of microvascular surgery: anatomy and operative approaches.* New York: Thieme, 1993.
24. Sasaki TM, Baker HW, McConnell DB, et al. Free jejeunal mucosal patch graft reconstruction of the oropharynx *Arch Surg* 1982; 117:459.
25. Hester TR, McConnell F, Nahai F, et al. Pharyngo-esophagal stricture and fistula: treatment by free jejunal graft. *Ann Surg* 1984; 199:762.
26. Panje WR, Hetherington HE. Jejunal graft reconstruction of pharyngoesophageal defects without microvascular anastomoses. *Ann Otol Rhinol Laryngol* 1994; 103:693–698.

FOUR

Aesthetic Surgery

49

Aesthetic Surgery of the Brow, Face, and Neck

Joseph M. Pober, M.D., F.A.C.S., and Sherrell J. Aston, M.D., F.A.C.S.

Psychologic Considerations for Cervicofacioplasty

Many plastic surgeons concur with the results of psychiatric studies, which have demonstrated that 50% of patients receive definite psychologic benefit from rhytidectomy (1).

Some patients seek cosmetic surgery at a time of recent loss or significant change in their lives. A face-lift should usually be postponed for a period sufficient to allow psychologic adjustment, because the surgery will not replace the "loss."

One of the most important aspects of the psychologic profile of the face-lift patient is that, unlike patients seeking most other procedures, those desiring classical face-lifts are not principally disturbed by their basic body structure (2).

The prospective study by Goin and colleagues (3) of 50 face-lift patients indicated that patients often harbor secret or unconscious motivations for undergoing surgery. Sixty percent of the patients postoperatively stated different reasons for wanting the operation compared to their reasons stated preoperatively. Many who before surgery gave practical or "acceptable" reasons, such as wanting to look younger in order to get a better job, stated after the operation that they actually feared their age might lead to abandonment by spouses and friends, or hoped that the results of surgery might provide dramatic improvement in their sex lives, or could make them a "different person" (1).

While there are no clear-cut criteria that contraindicate a face-lift, several psychosocial "red flags" have been suggested. These include difficulty in delineating or isolating the anatomic alterations desired and lack of correlation between the degree of the deformity and the degree of personal inadequacy or misfortune ascribed to the deformity (4–6).

Over the past three years, endoscopy and superficial tumescent liposculpture have further minimized incisions required for aesthetic facial surgery. Consequently, the patient population seeking such surgery is rapidly expanding to include younger and more scar-conscious patients. Unlike older patients, younger patients frequently are seeking facial recontouring to improve their facial structure and self-image.

Preoperative Evaluation

PERTINENT PATIENT HISTORY AND LABORATORY EVALUATION

The patient interview for cervicofacioplasty or brow-lift should include a complete medical history, thorough physical examination, and pertinent laboratory investigation; frequently this is performed by a specialist in internal medicine who would also provide clearance for general anesthesia or sedation. The preoperative evaluation relevant to preventing complications should concentrate on factors that may predispose to bleeding, skin and hair loss, or facial nerve dysfunction (7–15).

PREOPERATIVE EXAMINATION

The ideal face-lift patient for the classical rejuvenation techniques is between 45 and 55 years old, is normal in weight, and has good bone structure, a thin neck, and a deep cervicomental angle.

The skin of the middle and lower thirds of the face is palpated for thickness, elasticity, and mobility. Severe texture changes, such as the crepe paper–like skin from actinic damage or surface irregularities along the lower lip and chin from muscular contractions, are noted because they remain unaffected by face-lift surgery. The malar area is observed for contour and symmetry. High cheekbones are a benefit in obtaining a favorable result. Flat malar areas are often associated with significant midface laxity, manifested by malar nasojugal grooves, infraorbital malar crescents, malar fat pad ptosis, and prominent nasolabial folds (Figs. 49–1 and 49–2). "Malar pouches" (fluid accumulations in the fatty tissue over the malar area) are not corrected by facioplasty. Grazer has indicated that suction-assisted lipectomy may be of benefit in improving this otherwise difficult problem. Nasolabial creases (Fig. 49–3) anchor the superficial musculoaponeurotic system (SMAS) and upper lip levators (levator labii superioris, levator anguli oris, zygomaticus minor and zygomaticus major), and are reportedly formed by the gravitational descent of the lipodystrophic fascial-fatty layer or malar fat pad, with overlying skin redundancy lateral to the crease, lipodystrophy of fat indigenous to the nasolabial fold region, atrophy of the adjacent medial lip subcutaneous tissue deep to the crease, and laxity of the zygomatic ligament (which appears to suspend the malar fat pad and medial cheek) (16,18). An idea of the improvement anticipated by lifting the face is obtained by gentle fingertip lifting of the facial skin with the fingers placed in the malar and temporal areas. However, classical face-lift surgery will not flatten the nasolabial folds to the degree that is possible with fingertip lifting. The nasolabial crease, which is engraved in the skin, will not be eliminated.

To minimize the nasolabial crease and fold (Fig. 49–3A), every component of the deformity must be surgically ad-

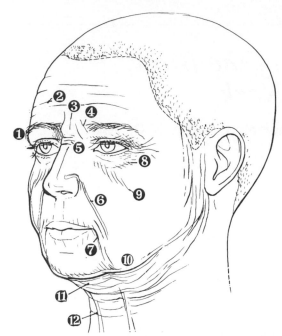

FIG. 49–1. Late signs of brow and cervicofacial aging. **1,** medial, arch and lateral brow ptosis. **2,** deep transverse forehead lines. **3,** marked vertical and **4,** oblique glabellar "frown" lines. **5,** severe transverse nasion lines. **6,** prominent nasolabial crease and fold. **7,** multiple labiomental creases and folds. **8,** deep malar crescent. **9,** severe nasojugal groove. **10,** marked jowl. **11,** neck obesity or **12,** platysmal severe laxity and banding. Significant skin excess and poor skin tone is evident, especially in the neck.

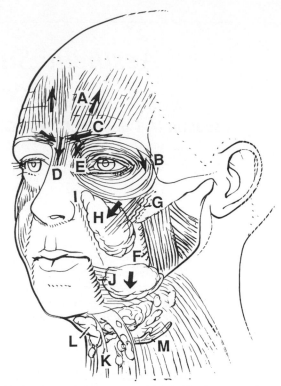

FIG. 49–2. Deep to the excess wrinkled skin, the anatomic bases of late signs of brow and cervicofacial aging include imbalance between brow elevator: **A,** frontalis and brow depressors; **B,** lateral orbicularis oculi; **C,** corrugator; **D,** procerus; and **E,** medial orbicularis oculi (depressor supercilii). **F,** lax masseteric cutaneous ligament weakly suspending ptotic SMAS-platysma muscle with overlying lipodystrophic fat (jowl). **G,** lax zygomatic ligaments weakly suspending ptotic lipodystrophic (**H**) malar fat pad, with a nasojugal groove at its posterior edge and malar crescent with sagging orbicularis oculi at its superior edge. **I,** levator alae nasi muscle contraction dynamically accentuating the medial nasolabial fold. **J,** medial platysma jowl border attached to mandibular ligaments adherent to prejowl mandibular sulcus. **K,** platysma band that lost support from its attenuated deep cervical fascia, accentuated by hypertrophy. **L,** lipodystrophy of preplatysmal and subplatsymal fat. **M,** low hyoid bone.

dressed. Currently advocated approaches include debulking any residual lipodystrophy in the fold after repositioning the ptotic midfacial malar fat pad, wide subcutaneous undermining (of about 3 cm centered on the crease) to release the SMAS and muscular attachments especially medial to the crease, prevention of their reattachment by interposing fat grafts superficial to the muscular/SMAS level, superficial soft and deep hard-tissue elevation of the crease, and redraping/excising excess skin to reduce cutaneous redundancy and subcutaneous ptosis (17–20).

The modiolus and "medial platysmal jowl border" (labiomandibular fold, labiomental furrows, or marionnette lines) are treated by SMAS platysma rotation flap techniques, occasionally benefited further by release of the investing SMAS from the lateral border of the zygomaticus major muscle (17–21) (see Figs. 49–1 to 49–3).

The jawline and jowl areas are examined for contour, fullness, and laxity. Gently lifting the skin along the posterior border of the face and just above the angle of the mandible will give an idea of the anticipated improvement in the lower one-third of the face. The need for resecting fat from the jowl area and SMAS lifting with release of the lax masseteric cutaneous ligament is determined at this time. A largely vertical vector lift is required to correct the jowl. The lower jawline and neck are inspected for submental and submandibular fat deposits, submaxillary gland ptosis and mandibular contour—especially pre-jowl mandibular erosion, position of the larynx, depth of the cervicomental angle, and platysma mus-

cle anatomy. Voluntary platysma animation helps demonstrate the platysma and its contribution to the presenting clinical appearance, as well as the presence of subplatysmal fat (see Figs. 49–1 and 49–2).

The surgeon should routinely reevaluate physical findings at surgery. In patients with bilateral vertical platysma bands, or "turkey gobbler" deformity, inspection usually suggests a lack of decussation of the medial platysma borders. However, at surgery, the platysma sometimes is observed to decussate across the midline above the hyoid, and bands are formed from folds of paramedian platysma muscle lateral to the decussation. Similarly, in patients with oblique cervicomental angles, palpation of a firm upper neck suggests a low-lying hyoid bone. However, occasionally at surgery, excessive subplatysma fat (that tensely bulges the superficial neck fascia and platysma anteriorly) is found, while the hyoid bone is in a normal position. Such subplatysma fat may be removed. An anterior larynx prevents formation of a deep cervical angle (see Figs. 49–1 and 49–2).

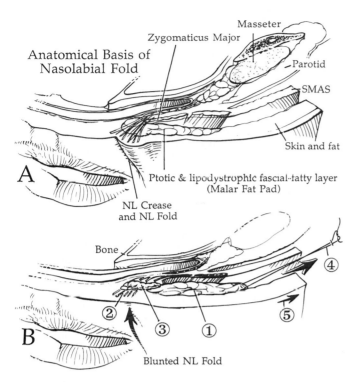

Anatomical Basis of Nasolabial Fold

Specific Component Approach

FIG. 49–3. A, nasolabial fold formed by ptotic and lipodystrophic superficial fascial-fatty layer (malar fat pad) with overlying redundant skin sagging anteroinferiorly from lax zygomatic ligaments against a fixed nasolabial crease demarcating fixation of the SMAS and upper lip elevators. **B,** surgical supraSMAS/supramuscular approaches treating specific anatomic components of the nasolabial fold: **(1)** debulk excess fat of fold; **(2)** wide subcutaneous undermining (for 2–3 cm, centered on crease, especially medially) from tethering SMAS and lip elevators attached to dermis. **(3)** Fat graft deep to crease to prevent reattachment of muscle to dermis. **(4)** Suture suspension of malar fat pad to reposition residual ptotic fat of fold. **(5)** Skin redraping.

The perioral area is examined for rhytidics and lax skin. The lax skin is corrected with the cervicofacioplasty, while the residual imprinted creases can be improved with dermabrasion, a range of chemical peels, or laser abrasion.

The patient's hair is examined in all areas for texture, thickness, and hairline contour. Incisions are planned to achieve maximal lift and camouflage with minimal hairline change. The temporal scalp posterior to the planned incision is examined for vertical laxity, which may be tightened by triangular scalp excision. A horizontal incision beneath the sideburn is often necessary to prevent too high an elevation of the sideburn. Hair that is brittle from excessive coloring will have a tendency to break off in the areas along the incision. This is an indication to attempt endoscopic and other "minimal incision" approaches to facial and brow rejuvention.

PREOPERATIVE PATIENT INSTRUCTIONS

In addition to the preoperative consultation, the surgeon should provide the patient with written information concerning the planned procedure. Vitamin E, aspirin, and estrogen compounds are forbidden for at least 10 days preoperatively. Vitamin C (1 g orally every day) is recommended for a 3-week period in an attempt to improve wound heal-

ing. Any planned weight reduction is to completed before surgery. Cigarette smoking is forbidden for 2 weeks preoperatively and 1 week postoperatively. To help thicken the dermis and improve circulation, especially in the smoker who has temporarily stopped smoking, skin care regimens are advised for 4 to 6 weeks preoperatively and the 4–6 week regimen is repeated, usually 2 weeks postoperatively. Currently, before face-lifts, dermabrasions, and chemical peels, the following topical skin care regimen is suggested: 0.05–0.1% Retin-A or 10% glycolic acid, every evening; 3–4% (up to 8%) hydroquinone (Solaquin Forte), twice daily; and 1–2% hydrocortisone cream (Hytone), twice daily (22). Photographs, preferably taken by a medical photographer, are obtained preoperatively.

PREOPERATIVE HOSPITAL ORDERS

A preoperative facial wash and shampoo with hexachlorophene (Phisohex) is ordered for the night before surgery (23–24). In recent years, with more extensive dissection and potential contamination from the hair and oral cavity, prophylactic antibiotics in the perioperative period have been used.

PREOPERATIVE MEDICATION

For procedures performed under general endotracheal or standby intravenous neuroleptic anesthesia, the anesthesiologist also evaluates the patient and selects the preanesthetic medications. The selection of preoperative medications must balance the desired effects of sedation and amnesia with undesirable effects such as cardiorespiratory depression. A thorough knowledge of each agent's beneficial effects and the management of any adverse reactions to the drugs are vital for the prescribing physician.

Anesthesia

Anesthesia for face-lifting can either be local, with IV sedation, or general endotracheal anesthesia.

Surgical Techniques

CLASSICAL RHYTIDECTOMY

The indications for the classical subcutaneous face-lift dissection are ptosis and redundancy of the skin of the face and neck. For several decades, the classical rhytidectomy has been shown to be effective and remains the standard for comparison. However, it does not attempt to correct the effect of the generalized aging process and the force of gravity on the tissues and structures below the skin. In addition, the procedure varies little from patient to patient, and it fails to accommodate the great variations in anatomic deformities with which patients present.

Operative Technique of the Skin Dissection Face-Lift

The cervical area and right side of the face are infiltrated with local anesthetic (lidocaine 0.5% with 1:200,000 epinephrine). During the 8 to 10 minutes required for the vasoconstrictive effect of epinephrine to become maximum, the patient is prepped and draped for the operation.

The face-lift incision begins in the temporal scalp and curves down gently toward the superior root of the helix, follows the curve of the crus of the helix into the incisura anterior, then curves slightly anteriorly around the tragus and continues downward into the natural skin crease to curve around the earlobe. Alternately, a posttragal or postauricular upper-hairline approach can be used (Fig. 49–4). The retrotragal incision courses anteromedial to the tragal margin until the infratragal level, where it courses directly anteriorly, preserving natural definition to the lower tragus.

The rhytidectomy provides permanent benefit because the resected skin and fat never return. Often in secondary lifts the skin is repositioned to a more superior position without much resection. The benefit derives from undermining and flap advancement. Excessive masklike tension must be avoided.

When the scalp posterior to the temporal incision is excessively loose, a triangle of scalp above the ear is outlined and excised in continuity with the temporal scalp incision.

The postauricular skin incision is carried 2 to 3 mm onto the posterior surface of the concha. The superior extent is usually made high near the level of the superior root of the helix. When there is excessive cervical cutaneous redundancy that will create a significant step-off in the mastoid scalp, the incision may slant along the hairline for 3 to 4 cm, and then extend posteriorly. Adding a parallel incision along the hairline to define a 2-mm strip of skin facilitates scissor deepithelializion, sparing deep hair follicles below a thin dermal cover. With a postauricular deepithelialized "strip" hairline approach, one anticipates that hair will grow through and anterior to the hairline scar.

Cervicofacial skin flap dissection begins in the temporal area where the plane of dissection may be subcutaneous or deep to the temporoparietal fascia. A transition to a subcutaneous plane of dissection is made at approximately the level of the lateral canthus.

A two-plane dissection leaves intact a subcutaneous pedicle of the superficial temporal fascia fusion line, or "mesotemporalis" (25), which is frequently divided to about three centimeters of the lateral canthal area to permit maximal rotation of the temporal skin flap, while preserving the more medial frontal branch of the facial nerve.

Scalpel dissection is performed in the preauricular, postauricular, and mastoid areas where the skin attachments are dense. The remaining dissection throughout the cheek and neck is performed under direct vision by the "spread-and-cut" scissor technique. When the premasseteric region is approached, a fiberoptic retractor is used to lift the flap gently and provide illumination for scissor division of the masseteric cutaneous ligaments between the SMAS and the dermis (16).

Subcutaneous undermining must extend beyond the area of cervicofacial cutaneous redundancy. In younger patients with minimal jowls and slight cervicofacial laxity, less undermining is required. In patients with deep nasolabial folds and extensive cervicofacial redundancy, dissection must extend medial to the folds for maximal improvement. Suction-assisted (26) or direct subcutaneous (27) lipectomy of the nasolabial fold followed by posterior cheek skin-flap advancement appears to help flatten many folds.

The limits of dissection usually extend to 1 cm posterior to the lateral orbital rim, across the malar area, beyond the nasolabial folds approaching the commissure of the mouth, and inferiorly from the nasolabial fold across the submandibular region to the level of the thyroid cartilage or, rarely, to the clavicle. To permit maximal superior advancement of the facial skin flap, this dissection carefully releases the retaining dermal zygomatic and mandibular ligaments (16,28).

Care is taken to avoid the greater auricular nerve, which pierces the superficial cervical fascia and is usually seen through the fascia, to pass at 6.5 cm below the bony external auditory canal (29). Trauma to the temporal branch of the facial nerve is avoided by maintaining a superficial plane of dissection at the anterior one-third of the temporal fusion line; trauma to the marginal mandibular branch of the facial nerve is avoided by remaining superficial anterior to the facial artery in the cervical mandibular region.

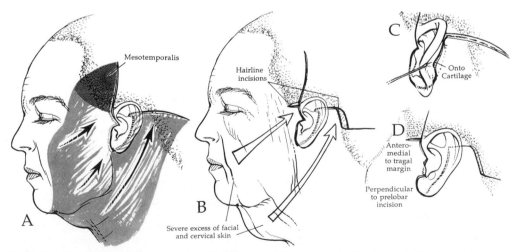

FIG. 49–4. **A,** the classical face-lift incision and area of subcutaneous infrazygomatic, cervicofacial, and temporal undermining, with details of the placement of preauricular, submental and postauricular incisions, as well as biplane temporal dissection. **B,** anterior sideburn wedge excision and posterior "strip" deepithelialized upper hairline incision limits hairline distortion when redraping excess cervicofacial skin. **C,** postauricular incision 3 mm onto cartilage. **D,** retrotragal approach coursing perpendicular to prelobular incision to enhance definition of lower tragus.

The skin flap is advanced at the cheek and rotated at the neck around an axis at the zygoma in a posterosuperior direction and redraped over the underlying soft- and hard-tissue foundation. In males, it is advisable to spare as much width of the sideburns as possible. This may limit the posterior traction, but most male patients prefer this compromise. Excessive elevation of the temporal hairline is very unnatural for both sexes and commits the patient to a camouflaging hairstyle. The need for excision of a triangle of skin below the temporal sideburn at the level of the superior root of the helix is now determined. The cervicofacial skin flap is fixed into its new position with two fixation sutures, one in the temporal scalp and the second at the apex of the postauricular incision. The overlapped skin is excised in the temporal area, and the wounds are approximated with surgical staples in the hair-bearing area.

In the mastoid area, the overlapped triangle of excess skin is excised in a straight line entirely or partially curving along the hairline. A flat vacuum suction drain (typically a 7-mm Jackson Pratt) is placed. The overlapped skin in the preauricular area is excised to fit the skin incision without tension and is sutured.

SMAS-PLATYSMA CERVICOFACIOPLASTY

The classical rhytidectomy (subcutaneous dissection and skin flap advancement) is effective for the ideal face-lift candidate. However, deeper soft-tissue defects (i.e., platysma bands; jowls; labiomandibular folds; excess submental, submandibular and subplatysma fat deposits; microgenia; an obtuse cervicomental angle; and asymmetries) produce various deformities that require a more aggressive approach if maximal benefit is to be provided.

Some patients do not need major platysma alteration. However, selective platysma surgery in the neck and SMAS tightening in the cheeks appear to benefit most patients. The platysma surgery indicated depends on a number of factors. These include the anatomy of the platysma muscle; the anatomy of the mandible and neck including the position of the hyoid and the size of thyroid cartilage; and the amount of submental, submandibular, or subplatysma fat. Excision of excess fat is more important than platysma surgery for some patients. Structural deformities such as malar atrophy may require cheek enhancement with silicone implants or injections with hydroxyapatite (HA) or autologous fat, and microgenia may require ancillary procedures such as a silicone chin implant or mandibular osteotomy to obtain the greatest improvement in contour. SMAS dissection and advancement in continuity with the platysma is almost always performed with the muscle techniques (30). As the various platysma procedures are discussed below, this point should be kept in mind.

The relationship between platysma anatomy and clinically presenting deformities must be appreciated if techniques to correct various neck deformities are to be used to the best advantage (31–37) (see Figs. 49–3 and 49–4).

Platysma Techniques

Aesthetic surgery of the neck (skin, platysma, and fat) attempts to reestablish a youthful appearance. This has been characterized by distinct skeletal (inferior mandibular border, hyoid), cartilaginous (thyroid bulge), and lateral muscu-

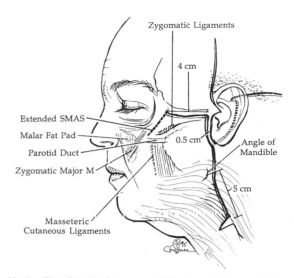

FIG. 49–5. The SMAS-platysma unit is elevated in continuity. The "extended SMAS" dissection also divides the upper masseteric cutaneous ligaments (deep to SMAS above level of parotid duct in an effort to further elevate the jowl).

lar (sternocleidomastoid) borders, and a cervicomental angle between that involves partial transection of the lateral border or vertical (or wedge) resection of the medial border of the muscle, with or without midline plication, to provide a more youthful, defined neck contour. Occasionally, full-width transection or no division is performed. All techniques require adequate SMAS platysma dissection and advancement (Fig. 49–5).

Operative Technique of the SMAS-Platysma Cervicofacioplasty

Cervicofacial skin flap dissection is performed as above for the classic face-lift operation. When a submental skin incision is indicated, this incision is made first. The anterior cervical flap is dissected in the subcutaneous plane. Lateral-to-medial facial flap dissection establishes continuity with the cervical flap such that the face and neck are completely dissected (Fig. 49–6). Thus, the upper platysma muscle with superficial and, occasionally, deep fat is exposed on the anterior and lateral neck. If present, excess fat is dissected from the surface of the platysma muscle and the submental area to give complete exposure to the platysma muscle. Care should be taken to leave a 3–4 cm wide strip of fat along the inferior border of the mandible; this will be advanced posterosuperiorly in connection with the SMAS-platysma flap. The medial platysma borders are altered (Fig. 49–7), as indicated by the anatomy of the individual patient. (Usually, the platysma muscle is approximated anteriorly from the mentum extending inferiorly to cover the entire thyroid cartilage for a thin female neck. Then an anterior wedge resection is performed inferior to the plication, usually at the cricoid cartilage level. The wedge resection extends laterally so that the inferior cut edge of the platysma muscle can blend with the sternocleidomastoid anterior border.)

Lateral SMAS-platysma dissection is performed as follows (see Fig. 49–5). The lateral border of the platysma muscle is identified by being cleared of overlying fat using a sin-

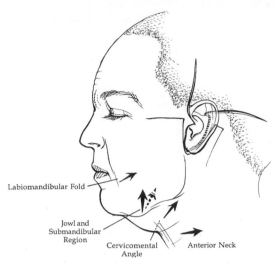

Labiomandibular Fold

Jowl and
Submandibular
Region

Cervicomental
Angle

Anterior Neck

FIG. 49–6. SMAS-platysma rotation flap creates multiple deep vector pulls. Jowls and submandibular region are pulled superiorly/cephaloposteriorly; labiomandibular folds and cervicomental angle are pulled cephaloposteriorly; and anterior neck is pulled posteriorly.

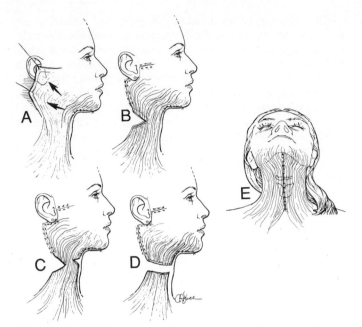

FIG. 49–7. SMAS-platysma techniques. **A,** elevation and advancement of the lateral borders. **B,** partial lateral width platysma transection and flap suspension. **C,** partial lateral width platysma flap transection and suspension with midline approximation and anterior (medial) wedge resection. **D,** full-width platysma muscle transection and flap suspension. **E,** corset platysmaplasty.

gle-lumen liposuction cannula starting 5 cm below angle of the mandible anterior to the sternocleidomastoid muscle. It is grasped with tissue forceps and pulled laterally. This places tension on the platysma muscle, making it easier to pass scissor tips between the anterior border of the sternocleido mastoid muscle (where the greater auricular nerve safely wraps deeply toward the parotid, deep to the SMAS) and the posterior surface of the platysma muscle. The scissor blades are directed inferior and anteriorly to pass just superficial to the external jugular vein. This establishes the inferior lateral border of platysma flap to within 5 to 9 cm below angle of the mandible.

Traditional SMAS dissection is begun with a 3–4 cm transverse incision through the SMAS that is placed at a level 1 cm below the inferior border of the zygomatic arch. The 1-cm cuff of SMAS along the zygomatic arch provides an anchor to which the surgeon can later secure the advanced flap without tension on the ear. An attempt is made to go just through the SMAS, sparing the parotidomasseteric fascia. A vertical incision through the SMAS is then made approximately one-half centimeter anterior to the auricle. It extends inferiorly from the transverse SMAS incision to continue posterior to the mandibular angle in order to develop a lateral SMAS flap border in continuity with the previously defined lateral margin of the platysma muscle. The SMAS is elevated from the parotidomasseteric fascia by scalpel dissection over the parotid. The SMAS-platysma flap dissection frequently extends bluntly with finger dissection beyond the anterior border of the parotid gland, superficial to the deep fascia of the masseter muscle in an areolar plane. Occasionally, when the SMAS is thin, the SMAS and parotid fascia are dissected together. The parotid fascia dissection has not resulted in complications and has been recommended by some authors (42). Traction on the SMAS alone or on the SMAS-parotid fascia unit serves the same function. The SMAS flap is developed until it can freely pull the anterior cheek and jowl without restraint from released attachments to the parotid gland, the zygoma, and the fascia of the zygomatic major

muscle. The masseteric cutaneous ligaments may be divided at a subSMAS level (see Fig. 49–5) as indicated to elevate the jowl fat. The masseteric cutaneous ligaments are divided in the subcutaneous level during skin flap elevation to the commisure (see Fig. 49–4). The platysma flap dissection is usually carried anteriorly to about the extent of the anterior parotid border.

The SMAS and platysma are mobilized as a continuous, single flap; each is important in its relationship to the other, and thus in determining the final result. Buccal and marginal mandibular nerve branches are frequently seen deep to both the parotidomasseteric fascia and the overlying SMAS anterior to the parotid gland.

When the desired dissection of the SMAS-platysma flap is completed, the flap is rotated in a cephaloposterior direction. More specifically, the dissected lateral SMAS-platysma border is grasped with two Allis clamps, one at the level of the transverse SMAS cut and another at a level 4 to 5 cm below the angle of the mandible (see Figs. 49–6 and 49–7). Cephaloposterior traction produces tension on the platysma muscle and lifts the jawline and lower one-third of the face. The lateral border of the platysma muscle can be altered (advanced and partially or fully transected) as indicated by the specific anatomy present. The SMAS-platysma flap can be secured in the lifted position without further altering the platysma muscle. When platysma division (partial- or full-width) is indicated, the scissor tips are used to cut the muscle fibers under direct vision. The muscle transection is at least 6 cm below the angle of the mandible and traverses the neck near the midcervical crease on a line parallel to the border of the mandible.

To tighten the anterior neck, deepen the cervicomental angle, and contour the jawline, the first buried horizontal mattress sutures of 4-0 white Mersilene or Gore-Tex or 3-0 PDS secures the lateral platysma border to the mastoid fascia. This creates a vector of pull parallel to the mandibular border.

Then, while exerting a cephaloposterior vector force, a triangle of redundant rotated SMAS is excised at the level of the zygomatic arch. It can, alternatively, be folded under the remaining SMAS flap for cheek augmentation or regrafted to fill a distant contour deficit (43). The resultant transverse defect is repaired by suturing the superior border of the SMAS-platysma flap to the cuff of SMAS left anchored to the zygomatic arch, using two or three simple buried or "figure-of-8" stitches of 4-0 white Mersilene or Gore-Tex or 3-0 PDS. A cephaloposterior pull is secured with suture fixation of the superior SMAS near the tragus to correct the labiomandibular fold. Additional vertical vector suture fixation of the superior SMAS secures the elevation of the jowl and submental area. Several more buried sutures complete the fixation of the lateral SMAS to the preauricular cuff to further lift the labiomandibular fold. Completing the fixation of the platysma to the upper sternocleidomastoid fascia defines the anterior neck further (see Fig. 49–6).

The edges of the SMAS and platysma are feathered to blend into the underlying fascia. Scissors or suction cannula are also used for final contouring, under direct vision, of the strip of fat deliberately left along the inferior border of the mandible. The cerviofacial skin flap repositioning, tailoring, and closure is performed as described for the classic face-lift operation.

SUBMENTAL AND SUBMANDIBULAR LIPECTOMY

Recently, there has been an increasing demand for cervical contouring in young patients with double-chin deformities. These patients have little or no excess cervicofacial skin to justify a face-lift incision. In fact, additional cervical skin is needed when an obtuse cervicomental angle is converted into a right angle. More extensive submental and submandibular lipectomies have produced satisfying results in some young patients (42). This can be performed through a small submental incision, using either sharp dissection or suction-assisted lipectomy. Patients with advanced senile skin changes overlying a fat neck are not candidates for such a selective approach. The older skin, which is needed to drape into the concavity created by cervical fat excision, does not possess the ability to spontaneously contract down and snugly fit the newly sculpted submental and submandibular region. These patients are treated best by combined submental lipectomy and cervicofacioplasty. Extensive undermining permits cephaloposterior skin advancement and resection of the excess skin laterally. Infrequently, patients require elliptical resection of submental skin excess.

Operative Technique for Submental Lipectomy

In patients who require submental lipectomy and/or surgery on the medial borders of the platysma muscle, the cervicofacioplasty is begun with a submental incision. The incision is made in the submental crease in males, where an incision may produce a scar that bears no hair. In females, the incision is made slightly anterior to the crease to help offset the submental crease. The neck is hyperextended to tighten the anterior neck skin, facilitating scissor flap dissection. A layer of subcutaneous fat 2 to 3 mm thick is maintained on the anterior cervical flap. The remaining fat is resected down to the surface of the platysma muscle. Medial subplatysma fat is resected if there is a subplatysma bulge. Care is taken not to cause a depression in the midline by fat resection. The corset platysmoplasty technique may be used to recruit sufficient platysma bulk to help correct this deformity. Fat resection laterally must be tapered if the lipectomy is being performed as an isolated procedure. However, if lipectomy is performed as part of a cervicofacioplasty within continuity dissection of cervical and facial flaps, a smooth, level cuff of fat is left intact at the inferior mandibular border. The fat on the surface of the platysma is resected or suctioned lateral to medial to join the defatted submental area. The defatting extends to below the level of the hyoid with an intact intervening cuff at the jawline. Final jawline fat contouring is made only after platysma SMAS flaps are secured in their final position. Failure to preserve a cuff of fat may lead to a step-off deformity at the juncture between the facial fat and the defatted muscle when the platysma flap is securely positioned. Fat remaining on the surface of the platysma near the mandibular border may be accentuated by platysma transection, which decreases the circumference of the neck below the transected muscle edge.

Frequently, the patient presenting with facial aging suffers from ptosis of the soft tissue of the chin, or "witch's chin" deformity. This deformity may discourage submental incision and submental defatting unless the condition can also be improved. The correction of the cleft between the drooping chin and the cervical region requires soft tissue to fill the defect. No single method has consistently succeeded in correcting this problem. External triangular or elliptical excisions have been proposed (44,45), as well as internal shifting of the medial raphe (46).

In our experience, the best methods involve advancement of dermal fat flaps. For the chin with adequate vertical height and anterior projection, anterior advancement and anchoring to the mentum of a posteriorly based elliptical dermis-fat flap is advised. If the chin lacks vertical height and anterior projection, then distributing the drooping chin by posterior advancement of an anteriorly based dermis-fat flap to the underlying platysma with augmentation mentoplasty is suggested (47). If the chin displays excess vertical height and lacks projection, a horizontal ostectomy, which leaves the inferior soft tissue and muscle attachments intact, reduces the bony height. Advancing and elevating the chin segment with the attached soft tissue may also redistribute the drooping chin to improve its contours.

ANCILLARY PROCEDURES

Aesthetic surgery of the face has been extended beyond resuspension of lax skin to deeper soft-tissue facial contouring by utilizing the principles of suction-assisted lipectomy, craniofacial surgery, and platysma surgery (48,49,50,53). The current one- and two-layer face-lift technique corrects most dramatically and primarily the lateral and lower portions of the face as well as neck contour. The forehead-lift corrects the upper one-third of the face, including the eyebrows. In the past, efforts to smooth the nasolabial fold have generally consisted of skin cheek flap advancement perpendicular to the crease, direct excision of the nasolabial skin, or defatting of the attached crescent of fat bordering the crease left attached to the classical cervicofacial skin flap, as well as collagen and autologous fat injection. Many new approaches to aesthetic enhancement of the mid-face have evolved over the past couple of years.

THE SUBPERIOSTEAL "MASK" FACELIFT

Further remodeling and rejuvenation to the central part of the face, particularly the sagging cheek folds and prominent nasolabial folds, has involved extending the craniofacial technique of subperiosteal dissection in the zygomatic area (50–53) and medially up to the lateral nasal area (54). Using a forehead-lift bicoronal approach, the subperiosteal dissection extends from the supraorbital rims to the nasolabial sulcus. It releases the bulk of the central facial muscle attachments to the upper and mid facial skeleton and frees the external canthal ligaments together with the attached overlying fibrofatty tissue of the central SMAS. They are resecured under increased tension largely to the deep temporal muscle fascia, thereby transmitting superior and lateral pull to the anterior central soft tissues of the cheek, jowls, and nasolabial fold. The customary SMAS cervicofacioplasty is performed concurrently through the usual preauricular incision. By combining the forehead-lift, subperiosteal central face-lift, and standard SMAS face-lift procedures, the lax soft tissues of the scalp to the neck are treated continuously. The mask lift also allows augmentation (with cranial bone grafts) and reduction of facial bone (by burring of prominences of the forehead, orbital, malar and chin regions) (55). Further study is required to demonstrate that subperiosteal face-lift provides longer lasting and/or improved results in flattening the nasolabial fold. To reduce the incidence of temporal frontal nerve paralysis, subperiosteal dissection is usually restricted to the medial one-third of the zygomatic arch.

Further extension of craniofacial technique to help correct the slack neck associated with microgenia is obtained by simple horizontal mandibular osteotomy and chin advancement.

The advancement of the inferior mandible segment as a bone-muscle flap produces an anterior pull on the attached anterior belly of the digastric, mylohyoid, and geniohyoid neck muscles. This parallels the effect of the posterior pull on the SMAS platysma unit. Chin advancements, as well as silicone chin implants, also aid in correcting the obtuse cervicomental angle, especially when the hyoid lies in an anterior and inferior position in a patient with microgenia. In younger patients with fatty necks, excellent results have been reported using a submental incision alone to perform both extensive submandibular defatting and midline platysma modifications (39).

THE FAME MIDFACE LIFT

Over the past few years, other approaches have been advanced to attack the central midface, including the composite face-lift (56), the extended SMAS (see Fig. 49–5) (57), and the famed-assisted malar elevation (FAME) midface lift procedure. These approaches are directed to correcting the malar soft-tissue descent that creates a parenthesis deformity against the nasolabial crease and the so-called nasojugal oblique depression, which is a parallel hollowing of the anterior malar region, presumably due to stretching or laxity of the zygomatic ligaments (16). A standard SMAS treatment will correct the laxity of the jawline, primarily the jowl. It complements the neck-lift with platysma muscle modification and cervical liposculpture, when indicated. It is currently performed in conjunction with the FAME midface lift for total facial rejuvenation.

The FAME procedure frees the zygomatic ligaments and lifts the malar soft-tissue fat pad, forming the parenthesis deformity, or nasolabial fold. The fat pad is fixed near the malar region, where it provides a pleasing prominence (Figs. 49–8 and 49–9).

The conventional platysma–SMAS flap elevation (about 1.5 cm anterior to the parotid, over halfway down the jawline and onto the neck) is almost in continuity with the deep plane of dissection of the FAME midface malar fat pad elevation. The discontinuous area is thin and flimsy. This bridge is partly transected in FAME II just at the corner (about 1 cm), still sparing the nerve to the orbicularis oculi.

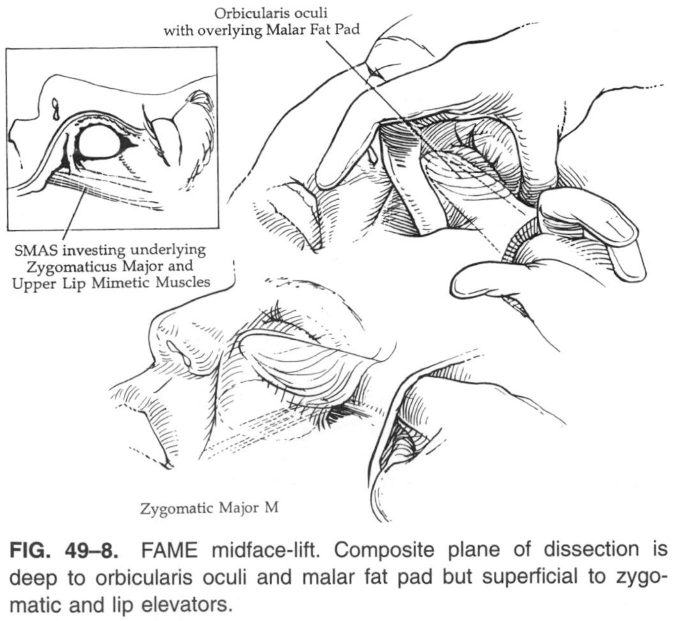

Orbicularis oculi
with overlying Malar Fat Pad

SMAS investing underlying
Zygomaticus Major and
Upper Lip Mimetic Muscles

Zygomatic Major M

FIG. 49–8. FAME midface-lift. Composite plane of dissection is deep to orbicularis oculi and malar fat pad but superficial to zygomatic and lip elevators.

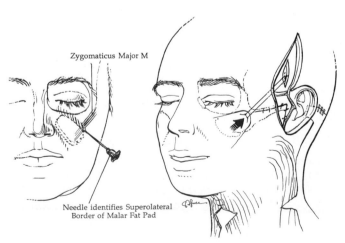

Zygomaticus Major M

Needle identifies Superolateral
Border of Malar Fat Pad

FIG. 49–9. FAME midface-lift. Superolateral border of the malar fat pad is resuspended.

The zygomatic ligaments are sufficiently freed in elevating the FAME I flap so the nose, lip, and cheek move when one pulls on the composite cutaneous flap incorporating the malar fat pad, the suborbicularis oculi fat (SOOF) (58) and the orbicularis oculi muscle. By blunt dissection of a composite orbicularis muscle–cutaneous flap, leaving a soft-tissue bridge overlying the zygomaticus major and inferiorly, caudad innervation is retained to the orbicularis. Similarly, blood supply to the malar fat pad and composite face-lift flap is retained from the central midface. Only the blunt entry point may have violated a small nerve branch to the deep surface of the orbicularis oculi, where it is elevated laterally off the zygomatic bone. With the extended SMAS (16), there is no repositioning of the orbicularis muscle or SOOF, there is greater risk to the facial nerves to the upper lip elevators, thinner cutaneous flaps, and reliance on unpredictable thickness of the extended portion of the SMAS to elevate the malar fat pad. Similar to the subperiosteal face-lift, the FAME malar fat pad elevation includes the SOOF. Also, similar to the composite facelift (56) the FAME malar fat pad remains attached to the skin flap (see Fig. 49–8).

At this time, the simplest, most effective, and safest midfacial surgical maneuver to lift the malar fat pad and improve the nasolabial fold is the FAME midface lift.

Operative Technique for the FAME Midface Lift

Wide standard subcutaneous cervicofacial flap elevation of a thick skin flap in the cheek is accomplished with scissor dissection and fiberoptic retraction, but only to the level of the zygomatic major (ZM), or from 2 cm lateral to the lateral canthus to 1 cm lateral to the commissure of the lips. The temporal area inferior to the mesotemporalis is dissected just to the lateral extreme of orbicularis oculi muscle, so that it can be raised with the subcutaneous flap as a composite orbicularis oculi musculocutaneous flap (see Fig. 49–4).

To accomplish the FAME midfacelift dissection (see Fig. 49–8), the index finger is passed under the thick subcutaneous face-lift flap to go deeper toward the periosteum of the zygomatic bone (just superior to the juncture of the lateral orbital rim and the zygomatic arch) and peel the inferolateral edge of the orbicularis oculi muscle, suborbicularis oculi fat, and overlying midface malar fat pad off the lateral zygomatic bone, the ZM, zygomaticus minor, infraorbital nerve, and lip elevators. After the digit establishes the supraperiosteal plane by peeling off the the orbicularis oculi muscle with the composite flap, an inferiorly sweeping motion separates the fat pad from the midfacial muscles. The subcutaneous flap therefore incorporates the orbicularis oculi muscle and the entire malar fat pad medial to the ZM, so that the composite flap with the orbicularis oculi muscle and malar fat pad can be grasped between the index and thumb while the thumb rests on the periosteum and lip elevators. To prevent dividing the facial nerve to the ZM, dissection must remain superficial to the ZM (see Fig. 49–8).

The platysma, and then the SMAS, are elevated in the routine fashion and treated as indicated. Then the mastoid cutaneous scalp flap is tailored and secured into position with staples.

To reposition the malar fat pad and smooth out or resuspend the nasolabial fold fat attached to the thick cutaneous face-lift flap, the FAME midface malar fat pad elevation is now performed. To place the fixation suture, feel the lateral border of the malar fat pad and define it with a transcutaneous needle. Through the digitally created tunnel, a 3-0 PDS suture is sewn from the cutaneous flap at the lateral border of the malar pad (defined by a needle percutaneously placed) to the deep temporalis fascia about 2 cm above and 1 cm in front of the ear, until there is slight dimpling to ensure there is maximal elevation of the malar fat pad while traction is placed on the skin flap. This shifts the fat pad superiorly and posteriorly to its original anatomic location or one where it enhances the facial contour (see Fig. 49–9).

The temporal cutaneous flap is then pulled superiorly, appropriately tailored, and fixed into position with several staples. The surgeon completes periauricular tailoring and closure and places a drain.

OTHER ANCILLARY MEASURES FOR MIDFACE ENHANCEMENT

The central malar soft-tissue laxity combined with nasojugal groove may be improved by rolling the SMAS layer upon itself for contouring. This serves to augment the zygomatic area and helps to elevate the hanging central facial soft tissues.

The midface of some patients may, as an alternative, be recontoured by augmenting a depressed malar region with an implant. This can be accomplished from an intraoral, subciliary, or face-lift approach. The intraoral approach is versatile and preferred.

A 1–2 cm incision is made in the upper buccal mucosa perpendicular to the upper first premolar. It is carried through the periosteum of the inferior margin of the zygomatic prominence. A subperiosteal pocket is made to just fit the implant, which is sculpted to augment the bone deficit. Dissection in this region must be cautious. Direct visualization and/or palpation of the infraorbital foramen and nerve is necessary.

Many sizes and shapes of implants have been designed specifically to address various zones and severities of deficiency in the midface, both individually and in combination (including zygomatic arch, malar, submalar, infraorbital crescent, and/or paranasal implants) and must be carefully selected to achieve optimal results (59,60).

FACIAL LIPOSCULPTURE/LIPOSTRUCTURE

Removal of the buccal fat pad may further enhance the angularity of the zygomatic prominence and moderately reduce the fullness of the cheeks in both old and young patients (50). The approach is through either an intraoral or a face-lift incision. The intraoral incision begins at the first molar and extends posteriorly for 1 cm, leaving a generous cuff of cheek mucosa parallel to the upper buccal sulcus, remaining superior to the parotid duct papilla (opposite the second molar). The fibers of the buccinator are separated by blunt dissection. Gentle digital pressure aids traction with forceps to draw the aesthetically appropriate amount of fat pad into the oral cavity. Small vessels in the pedicle are clamped and electrocoagulated before excising the fat pad. The oral mucosa is approximated with absorbable sutures. Postoperatively there is usually moderate trismus, which spontaneously disappears in a few days.

The round (or "fat") face is a poor indication for a classical face-lift. In children or adults with good skin elasticity and tissue turgor, unwanted facial fat deposits may be contoured by suction-assisted lipectomy (SAL) alone. Utilizing SAL, "fat face" problems such as cherubism, "chipmunk cheeks," and the "moon face" maybe corrected.

Cannula access for facial liposuction (Fig. 49–10) is gained via hidden sites such as the lateral nasal vestibule (to approach the nasolabial fold, labiomental fold, jowl, and upper cheek), the posterior earlobe (to approach the parotid, carotid triangle, jowl, and submandibular region), the submental crease (to approach the submental, submandibular, jowl, and subplatysma), and the hair-bearing temporal area (to approach the submalar and parotid). It may also be performed before, during, and after a face-lift procedure. SAL poses minimal risk for facial nerve injury (49,61–64). Introduction of tumescent local anesthetic infiltration has facilitated syringe liposculpture of the face and neck, primarily by increasing the target volume and dramatically decreasing blood loss (65–68).

Utilizing these advances, facial fat is sculpted to produce the appearance of a contoured malar eminence and jawline from a fatty face. After selective resection of the buccal fat pad to begin to define a submalar hollow, typically liposculpture is performed along a line transecting the submalar hollow, extending from the superior helix to about 2 cm lateral from the labial commissure. The nasolabial fold is also sculpted to a thinness of no less than 0.5 cm (utilizing a 1.5-mm spatula or Mercedes cannula and 10-cc syringe, with plunger only partly withdrawn successively for continuous minimal suction). Gentle uniform suction also mimimizes neuropraxia, which may especially occur with aggressive jowl liposuction. The submandibular and cervical regions are liposuctioned to a uniform thickness of no less than 1 cm (utilizing 1.5–3 mm Mercedes cannula). Liposculpture deliberately shapes the regional fat left behind so that the thickness of the malar and jawline fat layer can be retained while

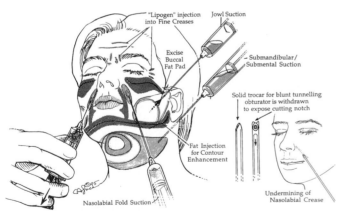

FIG. 49–10. Lipocontour/lipostructure/liporestructure. Liposuction reduces the submental/submandibular regions to a uniform thickness. For a fatty full face, the submalar, jowl, and nasolabial regions are differentially suctioned or liposculptured to define a malar eminence and a jawline, frequently along with buccal fat pad contouring. In contrast, for the thin face, multilevel microfilamentious fat grafting may be performed for further facial contouring (lipo-restructure) and correction of deep folds. (shaded areas)
Detail of release of corrugator and procerus, with fat grafting deep to glabellar creases. Detail of selective sharp release of residual musculoaponeurotic attachments to the nasolabial crease, following blunt liposculpture debulking and undermining the nasolabial region.

submalar hollows can be further contoured by selective liposculpture (see Fig. 49–10). Skin retraction of the neck is generally good. A low hyoid bone, platysmal bands and significant laxity limit the success of liposculpture alone and require cervicoplasty for better results.

When aging leads to atrophy of the facial substructure (69), in addition to a variety of exogenous materials and implants, simple "scarless" injections of autogenous fat and collagen have been offered with renewed interest over the past several years, with the increasing popularity of detailed tumescent liposculpture.

Autogenous fat grafts have been relatively safe. Long-term efficacy is slowly becoming established. Multilevel grafting (especially into muscle and subcutaneous fatty tissue) of microfilamentous threads of fat droplets are increasingly reported to provide enduring long-term volumetric enhancement for over 4 years in well-vascularized areas of relative nonmotion, such as the malar and chin regions (70,70A,71) (see Fig. 49–10). During a face-lift, autologous fat grafting may be performed for volume enhancement at the supraperiosteal and intramuscular levels deep to the classical subcutaneous and SMAS-platysmal planes of dissection and in the subcutaneous level in areas outside the field of subcutaneous flap elevation.

Today fat comes close to the ideal filling substance for microfilamentous grafting to help correct deep wrinkles and folds around the mouth (nasolabial folds) and forehead (frown lines), fill in sunken cheeks, and create fuller lips. A patient's fat is typically harvested from the thighs, abdomen, or double chin area. After creating a tunnel with a 1.5-mm blunt cannula or other dissector (freeing any adhesions or fibrous anchors of the crease or depression), the fat can be introduced, like a thread, with a 1.5-mm blunt cannula to where it would be most helpful soon after removal.

Patients are advised that properly performed fat grafts may rarely undergo an unpredictable amount of resorption, particularly in areas of relative motion with creases producing pressure necrosis or shearing forces on the graft. It is important to emphasize that in most cases following the basic principles of grafting a substantial portion of the fat graft is used to provide permanent volume enhancement. Therefore, the best permanent enhancements are expected in large, well-vascularized defects such as sunken cheeks, atrophic jawlines, and other flat areas that are not subject to pressure and motion.

In general, 10 to 30% overcorrection is recommended to account for immediate recipient-site edema and fluid-carrier volume injected along with the fat cells, as well as long-term partial fat resorption. However, in the facial area overcorrection may lead to significant edema, precluding early return to work and social activities. Consequently, many patients prefer several sessions to produce a gradual correction, usually 2 to 3 over 6 months, which may also create a longer-lasting result.

Postoperatively, the donor area is taped with elastic tape for 2 days. The treated area is left undisturbed, or paper tape–casted in areas of motion for further molding and graft immobilization. Usual preoperative precautions for surgery are advised, including refraining from aspirin for 2 weeks before and after grafting. On the same or following day after minimal overcorrection, patients usually return to work and can use their customary facial makeup, creams and hygiene routines, being careful to avoid the pinhole access sites for

36 hours. To prevent infection, the area to be treated and the donor site is cleansed preoperatively with PhisoHex and antibiotics are maintained perioperatively for several days.

Areas of temporary benefit include wrinkle lines around the mouth, such as the nasolabial and labiomental creases, where repeated motion causes folds, which crush the grafted fat deep to the crease, but spare fat flanking the crease. In these areas, successful fat grafts may appear as bulges that are minimally but noticeably displaced by the crease. Rigid surface immobilization is attempted, with paper or microfoam taping applied across the crease in bulk, and maintained for 1 to 2 weeks. This appears to deter creases from reforming, especially when combined with wide undermining, releasing attachments to the crease.

Further research may lead to increased survival of adipose grafts and a better understanding of the recipient tissue response, in order to optimize predictability of permanent contouring by volume enhancement with fat grafts.

Unlike fat injections, which can last for years and can be injected in large quantities, collagen injections consistently disappear within 3 to 12 months, and can be injected only in relatively small quantities. Currently, exogenous collagen (Zyderm I, Zyderm II, Zyplast) is less commonly used than "lipogen" (a natural collagenlike substance extracted from harvested fat) (70). While complications with fat grafting are rare, bovine collagen introduces, in addition to the usual risks of infection and bleeding, the possibility of allergic reactions.

Grafting of fat is combined with the injection of endogenous lipogen for correction of the etched, fine wrinkles (such as around the eyes and mouth) that remain after fat injection or even a face-lift. Attempted correction by face-lift techniques alone may produce the "permanent smile" or "masklike" facies. Instead, lipogen may be injected through a 23-gauge needle into the subdermis and deep dermis, to plump up the marionette lines and nasolabial creases. The patient is apprised that the effect will last as long as bovine collagen (Zyderm, Zyplast), or 3 to 12 months, but without the risk for an allergic reaction posed by foreign (bovine) collagen. As for bovine collagen, usually three injections are required at 2–4 week intervals for optimal correction.

The remaining lipogen is stored in the freezer in 1-cc tuberculin syringes, for convenient future use for up to 6 months to obviate the need for additional harvesting and processing.

Other techniques to correct fine marionnette creases include dermabrasion, chemical peels, and laser abrasion.

Routine Postoperative Management Following Cervicofacioplatsy

Antibiotics are continued. Alcohol intake and cigarette smoking are prohibited for 2 weeks postoperatively. A clear liquid diet is advanced to full liquids as tolerated by the 2nd postoperative day.

The head is elevated and ambulation is limited for the first 24 hours, after which the patient may resume light activities. The patient may be discharged either on the day of surgery or by the 2nd postoperative day.

Hair care is begun on the 2nd postoperative day. Males are permitted to shave (using an electric razor) on the 3rd postoperative day. Women are advised against wearing large earrings to avoid disruption of the incision around the earlobe. Sun ex-

posure is to be avoided for 1 month; subsequently, sunscreens and wide-brimmed hats are advised for bright sunlight for the next 3 months. Facial massage is avoided for 2 months.

On the 1st or 2nd postoperative day, the nonpressure dressing and the drains are removed. A scarf may be worn directly over the sutures. Preauricular and submental sutures are removed on the 5th to 6th postoperative day. Some facial swelling and cervical ecchymosis may still be evident. On day 9 or 10, all remaining postauricular and temporal sutures and staples are removed. Postoperatively, patients are reassured about the presence of edema, ecchymosis, and numbness about the neck and face, which may last up to 2 or 3 months. A mild depression is not uncommon in the early postoperative period. After 2 weeks, the patient without complications generally is able to attend social functions.

Complications of Rhytidectomy

The complicatin of rhytidectomy have been previously covered exhaustively. These include hematoma (72–76), allopecia (78,79), skin slough (10,72,78), and nerve injury (15,34,72,80–82).

COMPLICATIONS OF THE SMAS-PLATYSMA CERVICOFACIOPLASTY

The extensive dissection in the SMAS-platysma cervicofacioplasty has produced dramatic improvements over the classical rhytidectomy for some patients. However, there are sequelae and complications associated with the procedures (75). These include excessive and inadequate cervicofacial defatting, recurrent platysma muscle banding, inappropriate level of platysma muscle transection, cervical contour irregularities, tightness of the neck, and muscle–skin adhesions.

Forehead/Brow-Lifting

Forehead/brow-lifting is the most important procedure in facial rejuvenation for many patients. The indications for endoscopic or traditional forehead/brow-lifting are position-related:

1. A major indication is ptotic brow (medial, arch, and/or lateral) characterized by a pupil-to-hairbearing brow distance of less than 2.5 cm and the eyebrow *at* (in females) or *below* (in males) supraorbital rim (SOR) (98).
2. Lesser indications are:
   (a) an unattractive brow configuration (expressing sadness, anger, exhaustion).
   (b) brow ptosis, producing lateral upper-lid pseudoptosis, upper-lid fullness and crowding.
   (c) glabellar ptosis with associated upper nasal fullness and nasal tip droop.
   (d) lax lateral forehead, canthal, and temporal regions.
3. Other minor indications are related to muscle overactivity, including:
   (a) transverse forehead rhytides.
   (b) oblique and vertical glabellar "frown" lines.
   (c) transverse nasion rhytides.

Traditional forehead/brow-lifting can be employed to treat any and all of these indications, but with the advent of endoscopy it has increasingly been reserved for major indications, such as severe brow ptosis or extensive, deep transverse forehead folds. Endoscopic brow lift is usually the technique of first choice for any and all the indications, while more limited (upper blepharoplasty muscle resection/supra-orbital rim burr recontouring) incisions are only recommended to disrupt isolated muscle overactivity for selected patients. Some patients who request upper blepharoplasty have upper eyelid fullness or upper lid pseudoptosis that is largely owing to brow ptosis or congenitally asymmetric low forehead and eyebrows. Upper eyelid blepharoplasty does not correct this problem.

EXAMINATION

As always, the surgeon must address all the patient's complaints individually. The patient is examined in an upright position, face forward. The upper eyelids are observed for skin excess, fat deposits, and position of the eyebrows relative to the orbital rim and eyelid. The position of the medial, middle, and lateral portion of the eyebrows is observed. Many variations are seen in patients. If the medial or lateral brow or the entire brow is ptotic, the planned operation must be specifically aimed to correct the anatomic problem. Thus, some patients need more effort concentrated on lifting the medial brow, others on the lateral brow, and still others on the entire brow (Fig. 49–11).

The change that can be anticipated by forehead/brow-lifting is seen by manually lifting the eyebrow to the desired position above the orbital rim and observing the change in brow contour and the upper eyelid. This improvement is not possible to obtain with blepharoplasty.

With the brow manually elevated, the upper eyelid skin is evaluated for excess. The amount of skin to be removed with

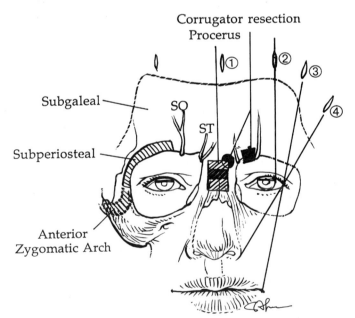

Corrugator resection
Procerus

Subgaleal

SO

ST

Subperiosteal

Anterior
Zygomatic Arch

FIG. 49–11. Deep-tissue modification for forehead rejuvenation. Addresses lower midforehead wrinkles with procerus subperiosteal release or resection, corrugator resection, and medial orbicularis oculi transection. Brow ptosis is approached by severing the superolateral attachments of the galea from the orbital rims and occasionally the anterior zygomatic arches. Fixation of the brow is achieved at points 1 and 2 for vertical lift, while 3 and 4 allow for additional lateral brow expansion.

an upper-lid blepharoplasty is lessened, and the lateral extent of the upper lid incision is shortened, by lifting the brow upward. For a few patients, upper-lid blepharoplasty is not needed if the forehead/brow-lift is performed.

Frequently, the brow ptosis is asymmetric because of underlying asymmetric bony architecture that cannot be addressed without another (upper blepharoplasty) incision and supraorbital rim burring.

If an upper-eyelid blepharoplasty is performed with wide excision of upper-eyelid skin and significant brow ptosis is present, the resultant scar will be poorly positioned, and the brow will be pulled further down.

The Westmore model provides guidelines for the ideal aesthetic eyebrow arch configuration and position (87). In this model, the medial and lateral boundaries of the ideal eyebrow arch are defined by two lines extending from the nasal ala and passing, respectively, through the medial and lateral canthi. Both of these extremes fall on a horizontal line that appears to be situated 1 cm above the supratarsal fold when brow ptosis is absent. The highest point of the ideal eyebrow arch lies above the temporal limits of the iris and, on average, is 4 cm from the midline. Traction at the midline along a coronal incision elevates the medial extreme of the eyebrow, and traction laterally along the coronal incision elevates the lateral extreme of the eyebrow.

After the relationship between eyebrow and eyelid sag is determined, attention is given to the glabella and the root of the nose (see Fig. 49–11), as discussed earlier. Corrugator excision and transection of the medial orbicularis oculi significantly reduces glabellar frown lines. Transverse nasion wrinkles, ptosis, and fullness at the root of the nose are usual findings of forehead/brow ptosis. Resection or release of the procerus muscle will reduce bulk and creases at the nasal root. Simple manual lifting of the midforehead can demonstrate the anticipated result in this area. The width of the soft tissue at the root of the nose is often significantly lessened by elevating the forehead. In older patients who have loose skin across the nasal framework and slight drooping of the tip, forehead/brow-lifting can lift the tip of the nose a few degrees.

Transverse forehead wrinkles that are due to frontalis muscle contraction are examined for depth and length. Frontalis muscle excision will reduce these transverse lines. However, by removing (myectomy) or releasing (myotomy, transection) the hairbearing eyebrow depressors, the frontalis may become more relaxed and transverse wrinkling may also be reduced. Moreover, posterior scalp dissection in the endoscopic forehead lift allows contraction of the epicranius posteriorally, following release of the frontalis muscle insertion at the brow level and removal of brow depressors. Therefore, direct attack at the frontalis by excision is infrequently performed so as to limit irregularities of the forehead and maintain dynamic brow elevation. Frontalis muscle and galea scoring horizontally (25), or vertically and horizontally (88), or circumferentially around deep transverse creases may be added, but at least the lateral extent of the brow elevator should be left intact to prevent early recurrence of ptosis. The scalp resection ratios with (2:1) and without (3:1) intact galea/frontalis are not constants because soft-tissue elasticity and reattachment to the periosteum is variable. Resection of galea and frontalis should always be individualized during surgery from response of traction on the scalp. Patients must be advised that minor facial asymmetry is common and perfect postoperative symmetry is impossible, due to preoperative asymmetry and/or unpredictable tissue response. However, significant brow asymmetries can frequently be modified.

The hairline, general pattern of hair growth, and hair texture and thickness are examined when anticipating the incision. Traditionally, a bicoronal incision 7 cm posterior to the anterior hairline has been used. A high forehead (if the frontal hairline is >5 cm from the brow) may be an indication for a partial anterior hairline incision that curves laterally into the temporal area. This technique only minimally changes the temporal hairline.

OPERATIVE TECHNIQUE OF CORONAL BROW-LIFT

The surgical technique and the associated complications for the traditional coronal brow-lift have been well described (89–94). As already mentioned, this technique has been largely supplanted by the endoscopic forehead/brow-lift.

The sequelae and complications of the coronal brow-lift have usually been quite acceptable to the patient and may be minimized with the endoscopic approach.

SEQUELAE AND COMPLICATIONS OF THE CORONAL BROW-LIFT

The sequaelae of the coronal brow-lift include some predictable scalp and forehead numbness, and usually the return of sensation is associated with pruritus and paresthesias, frontal headaches, elevation of the frontal hairline, and alteration of forehead expression. The minor complications reported include spot necrosis and hair loss, minor hematoma,

widened scars, temporal forehead lag, surface irregularities, and unaesthetic brow elevation (89). Major complications include excruciatingly painful large hematomas, lagophthalmos, and infection, all of which have a low incidence.

ENDOSCOPIC AESTHETIC SURGERY OF THE BROW, FACE, AND NECK

Endoscopy has allowed more patients—especially the younger ones who have indications for standard forehead or facial rejuvenation—to be acceptable candidates for surgery. Classical rejuvenation surgery was once discouraging to the scar-conscious patient, as well as to patients of both sexes in their thirties and forties, thin-haired patients, and especially balding patients. These patients were reluctant to proceed primarily due to their concern over a potentially detectable ear-to-ear or temple-to-mastoid periauricular scar associated with traditional open forehead-lift or face-lift techniques. These scars were associated with facial surgery for older patients, because classical rejuvenation techniques once centered on treating excess skin and wrinkles. After age 50, excess skin of the neck and face produces folds or wrinkles, usually requiring excision of facial and cervical skin (69). In contrast, anatomic studies have revealed that one of the earliest signs of facial aging is deepening of the nasolabial groove at about age 30, followed by magnification of the nasolabial fold by age 40, along with wrinkling of the glabella and forehead (69).

The causes of these signs of early facial aging are deep to the skin and may be addressed by endoscopic "minimal incision" surgery (16,20,54,56). More specifically, the following vectors of deep-tissue descent are reported to produce early signs of facial aging (Figs. 49–12 and 49–13). Just deep to

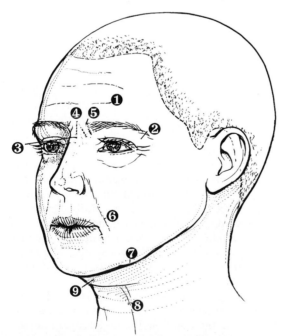

FIG. 49–12. Early signs of facial aging: **(1)** Mild transverse forehead creases. **(2)** Mild ptosis of eyebrow. **(3)** Mild transverse nasion creases. **(4)** Glabellar vertical and **(5)** oblique frown lines. **(6)** Nasolabial fold with malar fat pad ptosis. **(7)** Early jowls. **(8)** Lax bilateral early platysma bands. **(9)** Neck Fullness. No significant skin excess. Good skin elasticity.

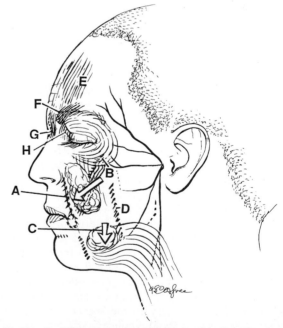

FIG. 49–13. Probable deep anatomic basis of early facial aging with soft-tissue vectors of descent. **A,** lipodystrophic ptotic malar fat pad (nasolabial fold), from **B,** lax zygomatic ligament, and **C,** ptotic SMAS-platsyma muscle with overlying lipodystrophic fat (jowl), from **D,** lax masseteric ligaments. Early brow ptosis and wrinkles from imbalance between elevator **E,** frontalis, and depressors **F,** corrugator, **G,** procerus. and **H,** orbicularis oculi.

the skin in the midface, aging is ascribed to zygomatic os-seous ligament laxity associated with early cheek or malar fat pad ptosis (supraSMAS, anteroinferior vector of descent). This contributes to a nasojugal groove with the bulging descent of the fat pad contributing to the nasolabial fold against the fixed nasolabial crease. Also, a bulky ptotic fat pad or anterior cheek fat excess may magnify the parenthesis deformity or "chipmunk" nasolabial bulge. At a deeper level in the lower face, SMAS platysma ptosis (SMAS level, largely vertical vector of descent) with overlying lower-cheek fat excess and/or ptosis contributes to "jowls." Similarly, in the neck deep to the skin, unaesthetic contour and aging is characterized by submental and submandibular subcutaneous/sub-platysmal fat excess accumulation and platysmal ptosis with band or turkey-gobbler deformity (SMAS-platysma level, largely vertical vector of descent). In the brow, aging is reflected by gravity and muscle imbalance. Excessive corrugator, procerus, and orbicularis oculi inferior pull leads to deep-tissue descent with eyebrow ptosis. Muscle overactivity leads to lower midforehead creases.

Many advances in open facial surgery have addressed these anatomic changes. Repositioning by resuspension of, and modification by, resection or transection of offending tissues (fat, muscle, fascia/SMAS) deep to the skin has achieved facial and forehead aesthetic recontouring and rejuvenation. With minimal (2 to 3 cm) access incision(s), endoscopic surgery permits similar repositioning and modification of fat, muscle, and fascia deep to the skin. In endoscopic surgery, the skin cover itself is not altered by excision. Instead, it is allowed to redrape over the changed underlying contour, much as in rhinoplasty and superficial liposculpture surgery, where some spontaneous skin retraction and contraction is anticipated.

For optimal results, ideal candidates for purely endoscopic surgery must possess elastic, tight, thick skin. Full classical skin excision, or some segmental skin excision, is currently still required in patients with excess forehead, facial, and/or neck skin. Chemical peels and additional ancillary procedures are employed to further correct other facial characteristics associated with aging, as with traditional techniques.

ENDOSCOPIC FOREHEAD/BROW-LIFTING

Our current endoscopic operative approach to forehead/brow-lifting is in an early stage and anticipates future progress. The traditional open brow-lift elevates the brow by scalp flap resection following scalp advancement as well as correction of muscle imbalance. Our endoscopic brow-lift reproduces the standard brow-lift muscle modification, but is performed through limited incisions, and substitutes scalp repositioning and contraction (redraping) for skin excision. Internal scalp fixation is substituted for flap reapproximation. It employs an endoscope to provide magnified (improved) visualization during primarily corrugator and procerus muscle modification to avoid injury to the supraorbital and supratrochlear nerves and to avoid a concavity.

Only three additional instruments are principally utilized: (a) a blunt curved soft-tissue elevator with integrated suction port, (b) an insulated soft-tissue biting forceps (Takahashi) or curved grasper with coagulation, and (c) a 4 or 5 mm, 30° down-angled endoscope with irrigation, suction, and a retracting sheath (Fig. 49–14).

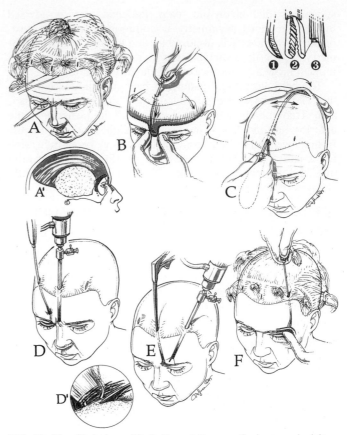

FIG. 49–14. Endo-brow lift. **A,** three 1.5-cm vertical access incisions in the scalp. **B,** subgaleal forehead dissection. **C,** subgaleal posterior scalp dissection. **D,** endoscopic resection of procerus and corrugator, with transection of medial orbicularis oculi. **E,** similar to **D** on the contralateral side. **F,** subperiosteal release of galea from lateral supraorbital rim, lateral orbit rim and, occasionally, zygomatic arch. Detail of basic instruments: **(1)** elevator, **(2)** biting forceps, and **(3)** endoscope with retracting sheath.

An appropriate candidate for endoscopic forehead surgery requires good skin elasticity, little skin excess, and a frontal hairline <5 cm from the eyebrow (95). In most cases, endoscopic forehead/brow elevation can selectively or concurrently treat any one or all of the mentioned indications for the traditional brow-lift with minimal scarring. Unlike the face and neck, there is minimal skin excess in the forehead to require skin resection. If the frontal hairline is >6 cm from the brow (high forehead), a semi-open anterior hairline skin resection is recommended to advance the hairline anteriorly.

It appears prudent at this juncture to aim for minimal overcorrection, especially medially, where the surgically unapposed elevation of the intact frontalis may provide further spontaneous elevation.

Multiple facial procedures may be performed in sequence. We prefer to complete dissection of the upper and lower blepharoplasty and the traditional or endoscopic midface lift or cervicofacioplasty before performing the endoscopic brow-lift. The browlift absorbs the laxity created by facial lifting. The lower-lid incision may be left open to facilitate elevation of the composite orbicularis oculi midface-lift flap. Similarly, the upper blepharoplasty incision may be left open to allow another approach for myectomy of the corrugator and pro-

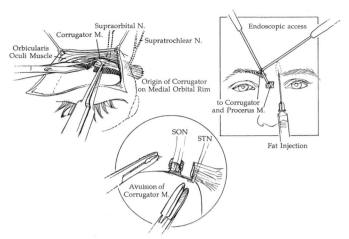

FIG. 49–15. Transblepharoplasty and endoscopic approach to modification of the forehead muscles addressing the glabellar creases by transecting the procerus and resecting the corrugators.

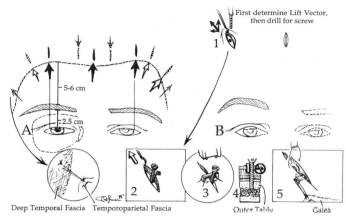

FIG. 49–16. A, B. (1-4), external screw and staple fixation, and **(5),** internal screw and suture fixation with detail of temporal internal suture fixation.

cerus (96) (Fig. 49–15). This approach may be used when isolated muscle modification without brow elevation is indicated for excessive glabellar wrinkling without brow ptosis. Alternatively, the corrugator and procerus muscle resections and release may be performed by placing both the endoscope and grasping/biting forceps through only one midline incision. The temporal incision is routinely left open to facilitate the endoscopic brow surgery or to permit segmental excision of excess temporal skin.

In overview, the endoscopic approach must minimize incisions while addressing all the patient's complaints in an individualized fashion. The usual goals of the endoscopic forehead lift are to elevate the entire brow aesthetically by soft-tissue release from the supraorbital, lateral orbital, and occasionaly anterior zygomatic arch, at the subperiosteal level. It may also rarely be used to reduce activity of the only brow elevator, the frontalis, if there are excessive deep transverse forehead creases. In the past, transverse and vertical incisions or partial resection of frontalis muscle between the supraorbital nerves limited the frontalis contraction, which relieved the transverse forehead creases but weakened brow elevation. More commonly today, resection or transection of the depressors (procerus, corrugator, and orbicularis oculi) allows unrestrained frontalis muscle elevation of the brow, relaxing forehead creases (97).

CURRENT OPERATIVE TECHNIQUE OF THE TOTAL SUBGALEAL ENDOSCOPIC FOREHEAD LIFT

The location of the markings is as described for the open technique. Preoperatively, with the patient sitting, the current location of the supraorbital rim (SOR) is marked on the forehead with the brow in repose and ptotic (medial, arch, and lateral) dots mark the SOR at or above the ptotic hairbearing eyebrow). Then the brow is elevated to the necessary anatomic level and the location of the SOR is re-marked on the upper-eyelid skin—the new location of SOR is re-marked *at* (males) or *below* (females) the anatomically lifted hairbearing eyebrow). With the brow maintained at the desired new level, the excess skin of the upper lid is conservatively marked, as are the transverse

forehead and nasion wrinkles and vertical glabellar wrinkles. The areas of corrugator and procerus muscle resection and orbicularis oculi transection are also marked, as are the locations of the temporal, supraorbital, and supratrochlear nerves (see Fig. 49–11).

However, no coronal incision is made. Typically, three 1.5-cm vertical access incisions are marked at least 1 cm posterior to the hairline: one in the midline, and two others laterally to provide vector forces aesthetically elevating the arch of the brow as individually desired by each patient. (Usually the lateral scalp incisions are along a line from the lateral canthus upward from the commisure or nasal ala for lateral brow expansion, or vertically upward from the lateral limbus for controlled isolated arch elevation, depending on the aesthetic objective. If the incision falls lateral to the anterior temporal crest, internal suture fixation between the deep temporal and the temporoparietal fascias is readily employed (Fig. 49–16).

With the patient in the supine position, the head is elevated slightly and allowed to project beyond the operating-room table while the patient is under general anesthesia or intravenous sedation. The scalp hair, face, and neck are prepped and draped so the neck to the occiput is fully exposed, with hair parted with elastic bands exposing planned incisions and extent of dissection (see Fig. 49–14A).

The supraorbital and supratrochlear neurovascular bundles, lateral orbit and dorsum of the nose, as well as the three (to six) vertical scalp access incisions are blocked with 0.5% lidocaine and 1:200,000 epinephrine in the standard fashion. Then the entire subgaleal anterior forehead and posterior scalp plane of dissection is infiltrated with 0.25% lidocaine and 1:400,000 epinephrine, achieving a ring scalp block and facilitating subgaleal dissection.

The subgaleal plane is defined by four 2-0 nylon traction sutures in the forehead flap, two placed through the galea over the corrugator muscles at the level between the supraorbital (2.7 cm from the midline) and supratrochlear nerves (1.7 cm from the midline), and two similarly flanking the midline near the hairline. These sutures allow for orientation and flap elevation for visualization.

The three marked vertical access incisions are made. The essential endoscopic work is dissecting the nerves from the muscles and the flap. The incisions are placed to replicate the views of an open approach (and to direct the forces for later internal screw/suture retention).

A blunt curved elevator in the midline (see Fig. 49–14B) begins the forehead subgaleal dissection to create the midline optical cavity, down to the root of the nose and laterally, remaining 3 cm superior to the SOR, similar to the open approach. The posterior scalp is elevated in the subgaleal plane (see Fig. 49–14C) to the level of the occiput.

If the lateral incisions do not overlie the temporoparietal fascia, an additional incision is made superior to the auricle to allow blunt digital temporal pocket dissection. Sweeping the blunt elevator over the deep temporal fascia toward the central scalp pocket disrupts the conjoined fascia. This tends to avoid trauma to the overlying frontal branch of the facial nerve. The frontal nerve lies on the undersurface of or within the temporoparietal fascia, which is superficially penetrated as the frontal branch passes more superficially to approach the deep surface of the frontalis muscle 1.5 cm above the lateral brow (see Fig. 49–14C).

The 4 to 5 mm, 30° down-angled endoscope with suction/irrigation is introduced with the left hand through the central incision, while the small blunt curved elevator with a suction aperture is introduced through the right lateral incision (see Fig. 49–14D).

Under video-direct visualization, the subgaleal dissection easily exposes the thinner procerus muscle in the midline, guided by the traction sutures and direct digital elevation of the flap. A coagulating biting forcep is introduced through the lateral port and is used for myectomy to tease out or avulse the body of the procerus in the midline in order to correct the nasion wrinkles and encourage medial brow elevation. Care must be taken to minimize deepening of the nasofrontal contour when it is not desired, as cut ends of procerus may retract cephalically and caudally. Alternatively, a blunt elevator is introduced for myotomy to simply detach the procerus from its deep nasal origins, when the muscle is not bulky and minimal wrinkling is present. The subgaleal dissection also eases the detection of the supratrochlear and supraorbital nerves (the periosteum need not be split at this point). To correct vertical and oblique glabellar frown lines, the corrugator and medial obicularis oculi are treated. Especially if there is significant muscle bulge preoperatively, corrugator is avulsed piecemeal, with coagulating biting forceps, between the two sensory nerves and medial to the supratrochlear nerve, beveling at the extremes of resection to avoid a step-off deformity. Patients must be cautioned that aggressive frown-line treatment by excessive resection of the corrugator may produce undesirable brow divergence. When there is minimal glabellar frowning, subperiosteal release of corrugator origin may be advised. To further allow brow elevation and correct oblique glabellar creases, the orbicularis oculi muscle may be transected near the lateral nasal wall just inferior to the brow, so that any retraction bulges under the hairbearing brow. Then the endoscope is introduced into the left lateral port and the elevator into the central port (see Fig. 49–14E). After again identifying the supratrochlear and supraorbital nerves, the contralateral orbicularis oculi and corrugator are treated as determined by their anatomy.

Avulsion myectomy instead of sharp muscle resection appears to produce less bleeding. Avulsion resection must be aggressive for deep creases or bulky muscles, while being careful to taper laterally and medially. Small bites are taken to prevent avulsion of subcutaneous fat, which produces a contour depression with dermal injury. Dermal or fascial grafting is usually unnecessary, even if immediate depression is evident. Immediate depression is usually because of local infiltration that distends the soft tissue. Myotomy or subperiosteal release of the muscle does not appear to provide as lasting a correction of the rhytides, but discourages undesirable position changes of the brow.

After all required muscle modification is performed in the subgaleal plane, sparing the supraorbital and supratrochlear nerves, the lateral supraorbital periosteum is transected above the level of the arcus marginalis (see Fig. 49–14F). More specifically, with the finger on the supraorbital nerve, the sharp curved periosteal elevator is pressed onto the bone along the lateral supraorbital rim, thereby cutting into the periosteum and changing the plane of dissection from subgaleal to subperiosteal. Scraping off the periosteum from the SOR and the lateral orbital rim frees the overlying soft tissue. Occasionally, release from the anterior zygomatic arch is required for total brow release. The temporal scalp is pulled superiorly and laterally. Visual inspection demonstrates that the forehead and brow move up and out readily for repositioning, by freeing the periosteum from the SOR to the zygomatic arch.

For maximum protection of the frontal nerve, the temporal dissection may be performed beneath the superficial or deep layers of the temporal fascia overlying the temporalis muscle. The dissection sweeps medially to elevate the periosteum off the superficial aspect of the anterior zygomatic arch as well as the lateral and superior orbital rim. Either deeper dissection can be connected to the subgaleal frontal dissection by sweeping from lateral to medial, cutting through the periosteum at the anterior temporal crest.

Screw fixation of the forehead flap to bone is currently used to secure aesthetic shaping and elevation of the brow, allowing the patient earlier freedom for hair care (Fig. 49–16). Concealed cortical screws (7 mm) attach galea by a 2-0 prolene anterior suture loop. Alternately, externally visible screws (12 mm) retain the scalp in position by abutting posteriorly placed skin staples, with optional galeal anterior suture loop fixation. To increase control of individual brow shaping and elevation, two scalp fixation screws may be used: one for the medial head and one for the arch elevation. To further correct the lateral brow ptosis, additional 2-0 PDS fixation sutures may elevate galea and temporoparietal fascia higher onto the deep temporal fascia. The forehead feels tense and stiff when the brow is elevated. No drains are typically used. Rarely, a 7-mm Jackson Pratt drain may be inserted.

No external dressing is routinely required. However, if desired to reduce stress on the fixation method, a dressing of microfoam tape is applied to the forehead, followed by circumferential Coban wrap. An elasticized tennis headband may be used for camouflage and further compression.

Routine Postoperative Management Following Endoscopic Brow-Forehead Lift

Antibiotics, soft diet, and limited activity are advised. Head elevation and ice compresses are recommended for 24 hours. On the 1st postoperative day the drain (rarely used) is removed. Gentle scalp shampoo is allowed on the 2nd post-operative day. By the 10th postoperative day, the dressing, internal fixation, and staples are removed. An elasticized tennis headband may be continued at night for an additional 2 to 3 weeks (to help maintain brow elevation, while continued reattachment of galea to periosteum, and periosteum to bone, occur at the desired level).

POSTOPERATIVE COMPLICATIONS

Preliminary results over the past 3 years with the endoscopic brow lift appear to be comparable to the traditional coronal brow lift (89,90,93,94) and offer decreased morbidity and lower incidence of the same complications (less alopecia, fewer sensory changes limited to the incision site). All patients are advised that conversion to a partial or total open approach may be required occasionally to avert complications (improve control of hemostasis) or achieve the desired results.

ENDOSCOPIC CERVICOFACIALPLASTY

The application of endoscopy to cervicofacioplasty is being explored at the cutting edge. Early reports suggest utility in correcting the ptotic deep structures of the face that are responsible for early signs of aging (see Figs. 49–12 and 49–13). When combined with liposculpture, excessive facial and neck fat may also be contoured using suction or scissor technique. Endoscopic cervicofacioplasty commonly requires a concomitant endobrow lift.

The indications for endoscopic cervicofacioplasty are limited but are evolving quickly; they currently include (see Figs. 49–12 and 49–13):

1. Excess submandibular/submental fat (neck fullness).
2. Loose platysma with early platysmal bands, early jowls, and slight labiomandibular fold.
3. Midface laxity with malar fat pad ptosis associated with early nasolabial folds and slight nasojugal groove.

Major advantages of endoscopy stem from the minimal scars. Consequently, there is better vascularity to the flaps,

less sensory change, less pain, quicker wound closure, and usually quicker recovery (98).

Prevailing candidates with indications for endoscopic forehead and facial surgery are in their late thirties, forties, and fifties, with relatively tight skin that is elastic and thick.

Endoscopic cervicofacioplasty currently is directed to modifying and repositioning the deeper tissues. It enables the application of deep-tissue vectors of repair in a direction opposite to the direction of deep-tissue (80) descent in aging, without "pulling the skin cover tightly" and excising excess skin. The younger patient may only require facial and neck fat contouring, which can be performed with closed liposculpture techniques alone or with endoscopically assisted scissor resection or semiopen liposuction (Fig. 49–17). If early platysmal bands are evident, the neck can be recontoured through the 2–3 cm submental incision by endoscopically assisted platysma plication/imbrication in the midline (Fig. 49–18). For further jawline contouring, an incision in the mastoid scalp may provide access for endoscopically assisted lateral cervical platysmal plication. In addition, through limited temporal incisions (2 to 5 cm) the SMAS-platysma unit may be plicated to help correct mild jowling, and the supramuscular malar fat pad/orbicularis oculi muscle may be suspended to help correct the nasolabial fold and nasojugal midfacial groove (99).

Currently, additional procedures and potentially longer incisions are required when the patient has the following clinical conditions:

1. Inelastic, thin skin with multiple fine wrinkles.
2. Visible facial (nasolabial, preauricular) and cervical skin excess (>2-cm fold).
3. Visible muscle activity translating through thin, fine skin.
4. Paucity of subcutaneous tissue.
5. Skin with severe degenerative cigarette smoking/solar damage.
6. Skeletal deficiency, especially in the malar or jawline region.

To mitigate these conditions, ancillary procedures are incorporated into the endoscopic approach, as for the standard

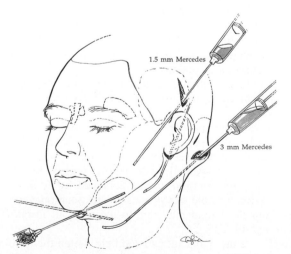

FIG. 49–17. Tumescent liposculpture of lateral cheek, jowl, submental/submandibular region and, occasionally, the nasolabial fold of round fatty face.

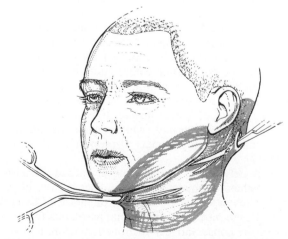

FIG. 49–18. Dissection of cervical subcutaneous flap and platysma modification.

SMAS-platysma rhytidoplasty. Facial augmentation with synthetic implants or natural bone/fat/fascia/dermal grafts for the malar region, chin, jawline, and lips—as well as facial volumetric reduction/contouring with procedures such as buccal fat pad excision, masseteric muscle reduction, and chin prominence (bony and soft tissue) reduction, may be indicated. Surface techniques, such as chemical peels and pretreatment with Retin A, may also be required of the surgeon to enable delivery of the expected, harmonious rejuvenation of the total face.

Skin redraping and retraction/contraction is anticipated to absorb spontaneously some excess skin, especially the preauricular redundancy (100). Uniform subdermal scar retraction/contracture in the subdermal plane reportedly occurs from defatting by using subdermal superficial liposculpture and is reportedly enhanced by all-layer liposuction (67,68,101).

Redraping and contraction may be guided by subcutaneous skin plication to the underlying fascia. At key points these plication sutures may be placed to elevate the nasolabial area, temples, and neck. Temporary (2–3 week) suture plication of a 3-fingerbreadth-wide skin roll, in the mastoid and temporal scalp, pulls resulting minimal (<2 cm) excess neck and temple skin posterosuperiorly. Furthermore, if indicated, isolated areas of excess skin can be segmentally addressed with open, segmental neck or temporal lifts or a traditional face-lift/brow-lift skin resection.

The future holds great promise for improved endoscopic approaches to facial rejuvenation and recontouring. New technology, surgical concepts, and methods of postoperative management are rapidly being advanced and evaluated. It is conceivable that, with these constant advances, some of the techniques to be described here may already have been superceded by newer, perhaps better techniques.

CURRENT OPERATIVE TECHNIQUE OF THE ENDOSCOPIC FAME COMPOSITE MIDFACE LIFT, SMAS-PLATYSMA CERVICOFACIOPLASTY COMBINED WITH THE ENDOBROW-LIFT AND FACIAL LIPOSCULPTURE

The facial endoscopic techniques described are actively evolving. One logical approach to endoscopic facioplasty that is currently being explored is as follows.

With the patient in reverse Trendelenberg's position, the brow, face, and neck are blocked (with supraorbital, supratrochlear, infraorbital, mental, and greater auricular nerve blocks). If indicated in an extremely fatty face, the areas of proposed liposculpture (submental region, lower third of the cheek, nasolabial fold) are infiltrated with modified tumescent solution in a 2:1 (submental) to 10:1 (cheek, nasolabial fold) ratio (using 200 cc of Ringer lactate, 10 cc 1% lidocaine, and 1 cc of 1:1000 epinephrine), while smaller traditional volumes are infiltrated in the areas of proposed flap dissection (Fig. 49–17).

For extremely fatty faces, the buccal fat pad is excised to form an aesthetic submalar concavity. Then regions of excess fat present (even with repositioning of the deep tissues) in the neck (>2 cm pinch test), jowls and nasolabial fold (>1 cm pinch test) are conservatively suctioned. A 1.5-mm Mercedes or flat double-slotted cannula and 10-cc or 60-cc syringe are used while the suctioned area is placed under tension.

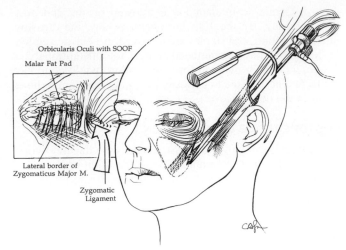

FIG. 49–19. Dissection of malar fat pad composite flap commencing at lateral border of zygomatic major.

To correct platysma bands, a 3-cm submental incision is made and the cervical flap elevated with face-lift scissors. Hemostatic control is achieved with insulated graspers and the endoscope. The medial platysma muscle borders are modified as indicated by the anatomy of the individual patient, as for the open technique (Fig. 49–18).

To prepare to correct malar fat pad ptosis and jowling, the lateral facial skin flap is then developed through the 2–5 cm temporal incision, using face-lift scissors, under endoscopic assist (Fig. 49–19). The lateral cheek subcutaneous dissection is superficial to SMAS and concludes at the lateral margin of the zygomatic major muscle. Then dissection deep to the orbicularis oculi and superficial to the lip elevators is performed to elevate the malar fat pad and orbicularis oculi in continuity with the lateral face-lift flap. This dissection is digitally assisted from the temporal incision in the fashion described for the open technique (see Fig. 49–8). Endoscopy may confirm the proper level of dissection. As indicated by the deformity, further subcutaneous cheek flap elevation is performed, lateral and inferior to the course of the zygomatic major. Dissection is performed at a superficial subcutaneous layer in the lower third of the cheek, allowing the jowl fat to stay attached to the SMAS-platysma unit. Any excess jowl fat above the mandibular border may be excised or suctioned under endoscopic visualization.

Once the cervicofacial cutaneous flaps are developed, the large optical cavity is inspected and hemostatic control is assured.

To elevate the jowl and tighten the jawline, the SMAS may then be plicated, usually with one to several 3-0 PDS vector sutures as required, from 1 cm inferior to the posterior zygomatic arch toward the lateral jowl region. In addition, SMAS-platysma rotation can be achieved by adding a 3–4 cm posterior mastoid scalp incision, to position vector sutures from the lateral platysma to the mastoid fascia (Figs. 49–19 and 49–20).

To elevate the malar fat pad and help flatten the nasolabial fold, a 2-0 PDS vector suture is placed into the superolateral malar pad identified with a percutaneous needle (see Fig. 49–9). Appropriate suture position is confirmed by suture

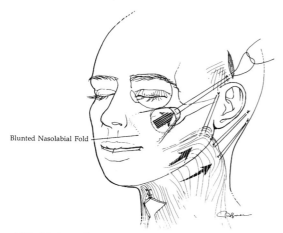

Blunted Nasolabial Fold

FIG. 49–20. Superolateral fixation of malar fat pad.

traction to demonstrate the desired improvement in the naso-jugal groove and nasolabial fold. The vector suture is then connected to the deep temporal fascia at the appropriate site near the incision (for ease of tying) and under sufficient tension just to create minimal dimpling of the skin. Alternately, especially if the skin flap is thin, the suture may be fixed directly to the fascia over the zygoma just anterolateral to the inferior orbital rim (see Fig. 49–20).

Ancillary procedures, such as the standard or endoscopically assisted malar and extended chin augmentation, may be performed as previously described. Also, if the nasolabial crease (see Fig. 49–3) remains deeply depressed, the 1.5-mm liposuction cannula may be used to elevate a skin flap deep to the crease and 1.5 cm medially and laterally to it. To elevate the crease and to prevent reattachment, a dermis fat graft may be placed or fat may be injected (superficially in the medial 1.5-cm dissection and in multiple layers deep to the crease), being careful not to allow fat to reach the lateral dissection by digital compression. Occasionally, the musculoaponeurotic attachments to the crease must be sharply released (e.g., with a 1.5-mm bi-pronged elevator) (see Figs. 49–20 and 49–l0).

Any submental and postauricular mastoid incisions are closed.

To absorb excess temporal and lateral canthal skin repositioned superolaterally, a subgaleal endoscopic brow lift is performed, as previously described, by the addition of one midforehead (vertical) incision. The already-open bilateral temporal scalp incision may be extended to 5 cm to excise an ellipse of possible excess temporal skin, if required. To absorb excess neck skin, 3-fingerbreadth-wide, bipedicle, postauricular scalp-skin rolls are developed and sutured to the occipital and mastoid fascia with at least 3 fingerbreadths of undermining posterior to the skin roll to allow the excess skin to redrape and shrink further (see Fig. 49–20).

The dressing for the forehead is as previously described. If fat was grafted to treat the nasolabial crease or to augment the malar region, a paper-tape molding "cast" may be applied to the medial cheeks and malar region followed by Micro-foam tape for immobilization. If liposculpturing was performed, strips of 1-inch elastoplast followed by paper tape may be applied to help reinforce the desired suctioned facial cheek contours. Drains may be used. A cervical compression garment with ¼-inch thick sponge contoured to the submental region may be secured, if submandibular suction was performed.

POSTOPERATIVE CARE

The current regimen emphasizes soft diet and minimal talking/facial movement to prevent suture pull-through. The face-lift and forehead-lift dressing is removed the next day, leaving the facial paper cast, forehead fixation, and cervicofacial compression garment intact for a total of up to 10 days. Antibiotics, and pain medications are prescribed for 3 to 5 days. Scalp sutures, if used, remain in place for 2 weeks.

COMPLICATIONS

When compared to the traditional face-lift for the same patient population, the endoscopic face-lift appears to provide comparable early benefits with decreased morbidity as a result of increased vascularity and lower incidence of some complications owing to minimal incisions (e.g., less alopecia and fewer sensory changes). However, additional studies are required to assess the long-term benefits and risks for this rapidly evolving technique. As with the endoscopic brow-lift, all patients are advised that conversion to a partial or total open approach may be required to avert complications or achieve the desired results.

References

1. Goin J, Goin MK. Facelift. In: Goin J, Goin MK. *Changing the body: psychological aspects of plastic surgery.* Baltimore: Williams & Wilkins, 1981; 145.
2. Butler RN. Psychiatry and psychology of the middle aged. In: Freedman AM, et al., eds. *Modern synopsis of comprehensive textbook of psychiatry.* 2nd ed. Baltimore, Williams & Wilkins, 1975; 2390.
3. Goin MK, Burgoyne RW, Goin JM, et al. A prospective psychological study of 50 female facelift patients. *Plast Reconstr Surg* 1980; 65:436.
4. Gifford S. Cosmetic surgery and personality change: a review of some clinical observations. In: Goldwyn RM, ed. *Unfavorable results in plastic surgery.* Boston: Little, Brown, 1972; 11.
5. Schweitzer I, Hirschfeld JJ. Postrhytidectomy psychosis: a rare complication. *Plast Reconstr Surg* 1984; 74:419.
6. Reich J. Factors influencing patient satisfaction with the results of aesthetic plastic surgery. *Plast Reconstr Surg* 1975; 55:5.
7. Mielke CH. Aspirin prolongation of template bleeding time: influence of venostasis and direction of incision. *Blood* 1982; 601139.
8. Rees TD. Preoperative preparation. Aesthetic surgery of the neck and face. In: Rees TD, ed. *Aesthetic plastic surgery.* Philadelphia: WB Saunders, 1980; 596.
9. Haut MJ, Cowan DH. The effect of ethanol on hemostatic properties of human blood platelets. *Am J Med* 1974; 56:22.
10. Rees RD, Liverett DM, Guy CL. The effect of cigarette smoking of skin flap survival in the facelift patient. *Plast Reconstr Surg* 1984; 73:911.
11. Zalla JA. Werner's syndrome. *Cutis* 1980; 25:275.
12. Beighton P, Bull JC. Plastic surgery in the Ehlers-Danlos syndrome. *Plast Reconstr Surg* 1970; 45:606.
13. Beighton P, Bull JC, Edgerton MT. Plastic surgery in cutis laxa. *Br J Plast Surg* 1970; 23:285.
14. Pope FM. Two types of autosomal recessive pseudo-xanthoma elasticum. *Arch Dermatol* 1974; 110:209.
15. Castanares S. Facial nerve parlysis coincident with or subsequent to rhytidectomy. *Plast Reconstr Surg* 1974; 54:637.
16. Stuzin JM, Baker TJ and Gordon HL. The relationships of the superficial and deep facial fascias: relevance to rhytidectomy and aging. *Plast Reconstr Surg* 1992; 89:441.
17. Barton FE Jr. Rhytidectomy and the nasolabial fold. *Plast Reconstr Surg* 1992; 90:601.

18. Guyuron B, Michelow B. The nasolabial fold: a challenge, a solution. *Plast Reconstr Surg* 1994; 93:522. Also, discussion by Young VL, Nemecek JR. *Plast Reconstr Surg* 1994; 93:530.

19. Aston SJ. Facelift with FAME midfacelift, browlift, and chin implant. Presented at Manhattan Eye, Ear and Throat Hospital's Aesthetic Surgery of the Aging Face, New York, l994.

20. Owsley JQ. Lifting the malar fat pad for correction of prominent nasolabial folds. *Plast Reconstr Surg* 1993; 91:463.

21. Owsley JQ. SMAS-platysma facelift. *Plast Reconstr Surg* 1983; 71:573.

22. Hoefflin S. Innovative procedures and new technologies: skin care regimens. Submitted for publication.

23. Harvey SC. Antiseptics and disinfectants; fungicides; ectoparasiticides. In: Goodman LS, Gilman A, eds. *The pharmacological basis of therapeutics.* New York: MacMillan, 1980; 964.

24. Cohn I, Bornside GH. Infections. In: Schwartz SI, ed. *Principles of surgery.* 3rd ed. New York: McGraw-Hill, 1979; 185.

25. Marino H. The forehead lift: some hints to secure better results. *Aesthetic Plast Surg,* 1977; 1:251.

26. Teimourian B. Face and neck suction-assisted lipectomy associated with rhytidectomy. *Plast Reconstr Surg* 1983; 72:627.

27. Millard DR Jr, Wyan RTW, Devine JW Jr. A challenge to the undefeated nasolabial fold. *Plast Reconstr Surg* 1987; 80:37.

28. Furnas DW. The retaining ligaments of the cheek. *Plast Reconstr Surg* 1989; 83:11.

29. McKinney P, Katrana DJ. Prevention of injuries to the greater auricular nerve during rhytidectomy. *Plast Reconstr Surg* 1980; 66:675.

30. Aston SJ. Platsyma muscle in rhytidoplasty. *Ann Plast Surg* 1979; 3:529.

31. Cardoso de Castro C. The anatomy of the platysma muscle. *Plast Reconstr Surg* 1980; 66:680.

32. Vistnes LM, Souther SG. The anatomical basis for common cosmetic anterior neck deformities. *Ann Plast Surg* 1979; 2:381.

33. Conner TJ, Bellville JW, Wender JH, et al. Evaluation of intravenous diazepam as a surgical premedicant. *Anesth Analg* 1977; 56:211.

34. Baker DC, Conley J. Avoiding facial nerve injuries in rhytidectomy: anatomical variations and pitfalls. *Plast Reconstr Surg* 1979; 64:781.

35. Ellenbogen R. Pseudo-paralysis of the mandibular branch of the facial nerve after platysmal facelift operation. *Plast Reconstr Surg* 1979; 63:364.

36. Owsley JQ. Aesthetic facial surgery. Philadelphia: Saunders, 1994; 53.

37. Webster RC, Smith RC, Karolow WW, et al. Comparison of SMAS-plication with SMAS-imbrication in facelifting. *Laryngoscope* 1982; 92:901.

38. Ellenbogen R, Karlin JV. Visual criteria for success in restoring the youthful neck. *Plast Reconstr Surg* 1980; 66:826.

39. Singer R. Improvement of the "young" fatty neck. *Plast Reconstr Surg* 1984; 73:582.

40. Ellenbogen R, Karlin JV. Regrowth of platysma following platysma cervical lift. Etiology and methodology of prevention. *Plast Reconstr Surg* 1981; 67:616.

41. Feldman JD. The corset platysmoplasty. *Plast Reconstr Surg* 1990; 85:333.

42. Jost G, Levet Y. Parotid fascia and face lifting: a critical evaluation of the SMAS concept. *Plast Reconstr Surg* 1984; 74:42.

43. Robles JM, Tagliapietra JC, Grandi MA, et al. Refinements in the treatment of the superficial musculoaponeurotic system: the retroauricular flap and the zygomatic folled flap. *Ann Plast Surg* 1985; 14:302.

44. Gleason MC. Brow lifting through a temporal scalp approach. *Plast Reconstr Surg* 1973; 52:141.

45. Gradinger GP. Editorial comments on aesthetic plastic surgery of the chin. In: Kay BL, Gradinger GP, eds. *Symposium on problems and complications in aesthetic plastic surgery of the face.* St. Louis: CV Mosby, 1984; 319.

46. Pitanguy I. Chin problems. In: Kay BL, Gradinger GP, eds. *Symposium on problems and complications in aesthetic plastic surgery of the face.* St. Louis: CV Mosby, 1984; 91.

47. Peterson R. Presented at American Society of Aesthetic Surgery, Las Vegas, 1982.

48. Illouz YG. Body sculpturing by lipoplasty. New York: Churchill Livingstone, 1989.

49. Hetter GP. Facial lipolysis. In: Hetter GP, ed. *Lipoplasty: the theory and practice of blunt suction lipectomy.* Boston: Little, Brown, 1984.

50. Monasterio FO, Olmeda A. Excision of the buccal fat pad to refine the obese midface. In: Kay BL, Gradinger GP, eds. *Symposium on problems and complications in aesthetic plastic surgery of the face.* St. Louis: CV Mosby, 1984; 91.

51. Tessier P: Face lifting and frontal rhytidectomy. In: Ely JF, ed. *Transactions of 7th International Congress of Plastic and Reconstructive Surgery.* Rio de Janiero, Sociedade Brasileira de Cirurgia Plastica, 1980; 393.

52. Psillakis JM, Rumley TO, Camargos A. Subperiosteal approach as an improved concept for correction of the aging face. *Plast Reconstr Surg* 1988; 82:383.

53. Hinderer UT, Urriolagoitia F, Vildosola R. The blepharoperiorbitoplasty: an anatomical basis. *Ann Plast Surg* 1987; 18:437.

54. Ramirez OM. The subperiosteal rhytidectomy: the third generation facelift. *Ann Plast Surg* 1992; 28:318.

55. Krastinov-Lolov D. Mask lift and facial aesthetic sculpting. *Plast Reconstr Surg* 1995; 95:21.

56. Hamra ST. Composite rhytidectomy. *Plast Reconstr Surg* 1992; 90:1.

57. Stuzin JM, Baker TJ, Gordon HL. The extended SMAS flap in the treatment of the nasolabial fold. Presented at the American Society for Aesthetic Plastic Surgery Meeting, Chicago, April 1990.

58. Aiache AE, Ramirez OH. The suborbicularis oculi fat pad: an anatomial and clincial study. *Plast Reconstr Surg* 1995; 95:37.

59. Terino EO. Alloplastic facial contouring by zonal principles of skeletal anatomy. *Clinic Plastic Surg* 1992; 19:487.

60. Binder WJ. A comprehensive approach to aesthetic contouring of the midface in rhytidectomy. *Facial Plast Surg Clinic NA* 1993; 1:231.

61. Herhahn FT. Submental and submandibular adiposities. In: Hetter GP, ed. *Lipoplasty: the theory and practice of blunt suction lipectomy.* Boston: Little, Brown, 1984.

62. Courtiss EH. Suction lipectomy of the neck. *Plast Reconstr Surg* 1985; 76:882.

63. Lewis CM: Lipoplasty of the neck. *Plast Reconstr Surg* 1985; 76:248.

64. Pitman GH. Suction lipectomy of the face and body, precision and refinement. *Instruct Courses Lect* 1988; 1:71.

65. Klein JA. The tumescent technique. Anesthesia and modified liposuction technique. *Dermatol Clin* 1990; 8(3):425.

66. Toledo LS. Syringe liposculpture: a two-year experience. *Aesthetic Plast Reconstr Surg* 1991; 15:321.

67. Gasparotti M. Superfical liposuction: a new application of the technique for aged and flaccid skin. *Aesthetic Plast Surg* 1992; 16:141.

68. Becker H. Subdermal liposuction to enhance skin contraction: a preliminary report. *Ann Plast Surg* 1992; 28(5):479.

69. Gonzalez-Ulloa M, Simonin F, Flores ES. The anatomy of the aging face. In: Hueston JT, ed. *Transections of the 5th International Congress of Plastic and Reconstructive Surgery.* Sidney: Butterworth, 1971; 1059.

70. Lewis CM, Toledo LS. Contour augmentation. In: Gasparotti M, Lewis CM, Toledo LS, eds. *Superficial liposculpture. Manual of technique.* New York: Springer-Verlag, 1993; 80.

71. Wilkinson T. Fat grafting. In: Wilkinson T, ed. *Practical procedures in aesthetic plastic surgery.* New York: Springer-Verlag, 1994; 47.

72. Baker TJ, Gordon HL. Complications of rhytidectomy. *Plast Reconstr Surg* 1967; 40:31.

73. Aston SJ, Pober JM. Basic principles of aesthetic surgery of the face, neck and brow area. In: Georgiade, et al, eds. *Essentials of plastic, maxillofacial, and reconstructive surgery.* Baltimore: Williams & Wilkins, 1987.

74. Baker DC. Complications of cervicofacial rhytidectomy. *Clin Plast Surg* 1983; 10:543.

75. Pitanguy I, Pinto AR, Garcia LC, et al. Ritidoplastia em homens. *Rev Bras Cir* 1973; 63:209.

76. Baker DC, Aston SJ, Guy CL. The male rhytidectomy. *Plast Reconstr Surg* 60:514.

77. Rees TD, Lee YC, Coburn RJ. Expanding hematoma after rhytidectomy. *Plast Reconstr Surg* 1973; 51:149.

78. Barton FE. Rhytidectomy. *Selective Readings in Plastic Surgery* 1983; 2:20.

79. Rees TD, Aston SJ. Complications of rhytidectomy. *Clin Plast Surg* 1978; 5:109.

80. Fodor PB. Platysma SMAS rhytidectomy: a personal modification. *Aesthetic Plast Surg* 1982; 6:173.

81. Rees TD. Facelift. In: Rees TD, Woodsmith D, eds. *Cosmetic facial surgery.* Philadelphia: WB Saunders, 1973; 203.

82. Rees TD, Aston SJ. Clinical evalution of submusculo-aponeurotic dissection and fixation in facelifts. *Plast Reconstr Surg* 1977; 60:851.

83. Aston SJ. Problems and complications in platysma-SMAS cervocofacial rhytidectomy. In: Kaye BL, Gradinger GP, eds. *Symposium on problems and complications in aesthetic plastic surgery of the face.* St. Louis: CV Mosby, 1984; 132.

84. Nelson D, Gingrass RP. Anatomy of the mandibular branches of the facial nerve. *Plast Reconstr Surg* 1979; 64:479.

85. Guerrero-Santos J, Sandoval M, Salazar J. Long-term study of complications of neck lift. *Clin Plast Surg* 1983; 10:563.

86. Guerrero-Santos J. Surgical correction of the fatty fallen neck. *Ann Plast Surg* 1979; 2:389.

87. Ellenbogen R. Transcoronal eyebrow lift with concomitant upper blepharoplsaty. *Plast Reconstr Surg* 1983; 71:490.

88. Pitanguay I. Indications for and treatment of frontal and glabellar wrinkles in 3,404 consecutive cases of rhytidectomy. *Plast Reconstr Surg* 1981; 67:157.

89. Kaye BL. Problems and complications in the forehead lift. In: Kaye BL, Gradinger GP, eds. *Symposium on problems and complications in aesthetic plastic surgery of the face.* St. Louis: CV Mosby, 1984; 77.

90. Kaye BL. The forehead lift: A useful adjuct to face lift and blepharoplasty. *Plast Reconstr Surg* 1977; 60:161.

91. Correia P de C, Zani R. Surgical anatomy of the facial nerve as related to ancillary operations in rhytidoplasty. *Plast Reconstr Surg* 1973; 52:549.

92. Marino H. The surgery of facial expressions. In: Hueston JT, ed. *Transactions of the 5th International Congress of Plastic and Reconstructive Surgery.* Melbourne: Butterworth, 1971.

93. Aston SJ, Pober JM. Aesthetic surgery of the face, neck and brow area. In: Georgiade GS, et al, eds. *Textbook of plastic, maxillofacial and reconstructive surgery.* 2nd ed. Baltimore: Williams & Wilkins, 1992;609.

94. Vinas JC, Caviglia C, Cortinas JL. Forehead rhytidoplasty and brow lifting. *Plast Reconstr Surg* 1976; 57:445.

95. McKinney P, Mossie RD, and Zakowski ML. Criteria for the forehead lift. *Aesthetic Plast Surg,* 1991; 15:141.

96. Knize DM. Transpalpebral approach to the corrugator supercilii and procerus muscles. *Plast Reconstr Surg* 1995; 95:52.

97. Flowers RS, Capaty GG, Flowers SS. The biomechanics of brow and frontalis function: its effect on blepharoplasty. *Clin Plast Surg* 1993; 20:255.

98. Ramirez OM. Endoscopic technique and facial rejuvenation: an overview. Part I. *Aesth Plast Surg* 1994; 18:141–147.

99. Bostwick J III, Nahai F, Eaves FE III. Face and neck lift: In: Bostwick J. *Endoscopic plastic surgery.* St. Louis: Quality Medical Publishing, 1995; 23.

100. Aiache A. Endoscopic facelift. *Aesthetic Plastic Surgery* 1994; 18:275–278.

101. Gasperoni C, Salgarello M. MALL liposuction: the evolution of subdermal superficial liposuction. *Ann Plast Surg* 1994; 18:253.

50

Blepharoplasty, Forehead and Eyebrow Lift

John M. Shamoun, M.D., F.A.C.S., and Richard Ellenbogen, M.D., F.A.C.S., F.I.C.S.

Surgical procedures to improve the appearance of the eyelids date back to the 10th century A.D., when Arabic surgeons removed redundant skin to improve eyesight (1). In 1951 Castanares helped to clarify the etiology of this fullness and developed the foundation for modern cosmetic blepharoplasty based on his accurate description of protruding fat compartments. Cosmetic blepharoplasty has now become the most popular cosmetic procedure in the United States.

The focus of this chapter is the current appraisal of patient selection, concepts, operative techniques, principles of treatment, and theories of management essential to rejuvenation of the periorbital region. Regrettably, some historical landmarks, many good techniques, and the observations of several experienced authors cannot be included here in a single chapter.

AESTHETIC CONSIDERATIONS

Congenital variations and involutional changes in the upper third of the face may need to be corrected in order to achieve adequate facial harmony. Young patients, both male and female, have become aware that malpositions of structures (i.e., eyebrow ptosis or low-set lateral canthi), or malformations of structure (i.e., "puffy" lower eyelids, upper eyelid hooding, excessively thick orbicularis oculi) are inherited and are not merely signs of aging. On the other hand, many older patients notice involutional changes and seek consultation with the desire to look younger.

There is no one absolute aesthetic ideal that makes a person attractive. It is all the features taken together that yield a pleasant result. What is aesthetically pleasing to different racial groups is variable, as well as what is seen as masculine or feminine. More important, even within a given racial group or sex, there are many different structural arrangements that are recognized as beautiful.

Specific structural differences exist between aesthetic ideals for eyelids and eyebrows in males and females. Females frequently have high arched brows, a deep high superior sulcus and a well-defined eyelid crease. Males frequently have straight low-set eyebrows, a minimal sulcus, and a low subtle eyelid crease. Clearly then, different procedures must be employed for men and women.

ASSESSMENT AND PLANNING

Each patient must be evaluated individually. In planning surgery for a young woman who has congenital low-set eyebrows, the sophisticated aesthetic surgeon (as well as the patient) may realize that the brow looks more pleasing in this lower position. The woman with this heavy "cat eye" wants

to look better, not different. Converting her to a wide-eyed, high-browed eye would in most cases be devastating.

Other patients may start with more ideal features, but owing to illness, stress, time, gravity, and chronic sun damage, develop aging changes with progressive downward migration of the eyelid soft tissues. These older patients frequently have eyebrow ptosis, dermatochalasis, blepharoptosis, lateral canthal dystopia, and/or lower eyelid laxity. Each finding may be present to some degree. Often patients have combinations of congenital variations and involutional changes. Knowing how the patient looked during his or her youth enables the surgeon to set realistic goals for the procedure. Reviewing the patient's old photographs will help determine which components of the changes are acute, involutional, or congenital.

It is important to ask the patient what he or she desires, and to demonstrate realistically what can be performed, to avoid a surgically accomplished strange new look and a displeased patient. In addition, it is crucial for the aesthetic surgeon to focus on functional problems as well as appearance. Structural integrity must be created or preserved before redraping skin over a stable foundation.

Upper Lids

NORMAL ANATOMY

The upper eyelid is comprised of three lamellae: the anterior, consisting of skin and orbicularis oculi muscle; the middle, consisting of orbital septum, eyelid retractors, and tarsus; and the posterior, consisting of the conjunctiva. Variations exist in structure of non-Asian and Asian eyelids (Fig. 50–1). The orbicularis oculi muscle serves as a sphincter to close the eyelids, and is divided into pretarsal, preseptal, and orbital portions. The temporal branch of the facial nerve innervates all three sections of the muscle. A rich vascular supply accounts for almost all bleeding during blepharoplasty procedures. Deep to the orbicularis muscle lies the orbital septum, which originates at the arcus marginalis (a thickening of the orbital periosteum). There are generally two fat pads in the upper eyelid, central and medial (Fig. 50–2). Lying lateral, beneath the orbital rim, is the lacrimal gland. It is distinguished from fat by it paler color and firm, rubbery consistency. Posterior to the central fat lies the levator muscle and its aponeurosis, which inserts over the anterior surface of the tarsus. The Müller muscle, innervated by the sympathetic nervous system, arises from the posterior surface of the levator muscle and courses inferiorly to insert on the superior edge of the tarsus.

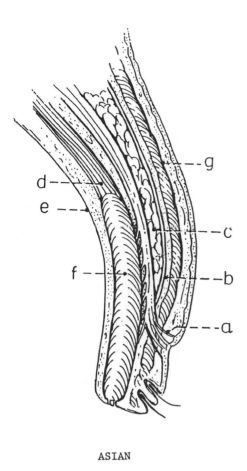

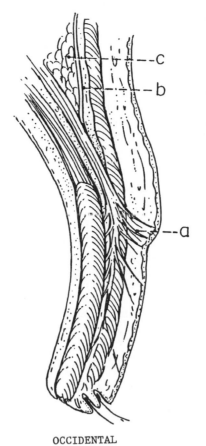

ASIAN   OCCIDENTAL

FIG. 50–1. Comparison of the anatomy of the non-Asian upper eyelid with the Asian upper eyelid: a = fibers of levator aponeurosis passing into orbicularis muscle; b = orbital septum; c = preaponeurotic fat; d = Müller muscle; e = conjunctiva; f = tarsus; g = orbicularis.

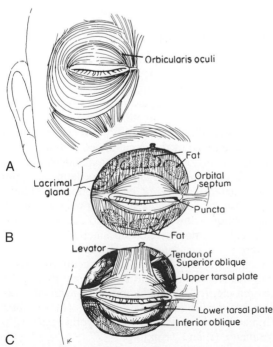

FIG. 50–2. **A,** extent of the orbicularis oculi muscle (eyelid sphincter). **B,** the fat compartments and the relationship of the lacrimal gland. **C,** the orbit, with only the superficial fat removed, reveals the superior oblique and inferior oblique tendons.

The upper eyelid crease represents the superiormost attachment of the levator aponeurosis to the skin and muscle. The upper eyelid crease usually lies 10 to 12 mm above the lid margin in women and 7–8 mm above the lid margin in men.

Each of the four eyelids has a palpebral artery medially (from internal carotid) and lacrimal artery laterally (from external carotid). These vessels lie just anterior to the fat pads and can be swept aside during fat excision.

Anatomic features commonly found in Asians include flat faces, shallow orbits, prominent globes (3), and epicanthal folds, although regional anatomic variation is significant. Anatomic studies in Asian eyelids have demonstrated that the orbital septum fuses with the levator aponeurosis below the superior tarsal border (2–4), which allows the preaponeurotic fat to rest in a lower position. This produces a thicker, or fuller appearing, upper lid; as a result, the Asian eyelid crease is lower and often poorly defined or incomplete. The fuller Asian eyelid also results from four fat pads, which include the subcutaneous fat, pretarsal fat, submuscular or preseptal (ROOF) fat, and preaponeurotic fat (5).

ETIOLOGY

Significant disparity exists in the nomenclature for upper-lid deformities (6). Common and scientific terms include baggy eyelids, ptosis atonia, ptosis lipomatosis, blepharochalasis, dermatochalasis, herniated orbital fat, and temporal hooding.

Baggy upper or lower eyelids result from various factors. Nonsystemic causes include (a) bulging or pseudo herniation of fat, (b) laxity and/or redundancy of skin and muscle secondary to loss of elasticity in the aging process, (c) hypertrophy of the orbicularis oculi muscle, (d) brow ptosis, (e) lacrimal gland ptosis, or (f) any combination of the above. Systemic causes of eyelid pathology include thyroid disease, chronic allergy, and kidney disease. Excessive alcohol, female hormonal cycles, and chronic sinusitis may also be contributory. Most experts believe that heredity is the most influential factor.

PREOPERATIVE PSYCHOLOGIC EVALUATION

A psychologic assessment is performed by taking a careful history of the patient's (a) motivation and expectations for surgery, (b) emotional reaction to the perceived deformity, and (c) overall response to the interview process. Patients present with a variety of complaints. They may have congenital features that they perceive to be unpleasing. They may have heavy eyelids that preclude wearing eye makeup to their satisfaction. Selection of cosmetic blepharoplasty patients must always be balanced between what the patient expects and what realistically can be accomplished (17). It is important for the plastic surgeon to recognize patients who may be prone to dissatisfaction. Danger signals for patient dissatisfaction include unrealistic expectations, extrinsic motivation for the operation, presence of emotional crisis or illness, and a disapproving spouse or lover (17).

It is important for all patients to be given a preview, or simulation, of their appearance after surgery. Patients can be shown how they will look by using a bent applicator stick in the upper lid sulcus (Fig. 50–3). Some individuals will reject surgery when they observe a prospective result that makes them look different but not better.

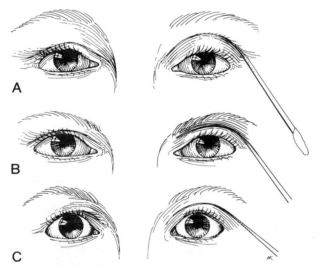

FIG. 50–3. Preoperative upper blepharoplasty evaluation. **A,** bent applicator stick is placed in the sulcus, simulating the result produced by blepharoplasty. A good relationship between brow and sulcus improves the eye. **B,** with a low brow, the eye takes on an angry or intense appearance. **C,** a bulging or exophthalmic eye may appear more bulging, or staring, after upper blepharoplasty. In these cases, the hood is beneficial and should not be removed.

PREOPERATIVE EVALUATION

Before surgery, each patient should have a complete history and physical examination, including diabetes, renal, neurologic, thyroid, autoimmune, and allergic evaluations. The preoperative medical assessment should include bleeding and clotting studies (preferably Wright simplate bleeding time), cardiac evaluation (pressure on the eye may cause bradycardia), and hypertensive analysis. Surgery should be postponed if there is an increased risk of bleeding or uncontrolled hypertension. Asthmatics and heavy snorers frequently cough after anaesthesia, increasing bleeding risk. All drugs that prolong clotting time should be discontinued 2 weeks before and 1 week after surgery. Drugs used to treat common causes of pain (e.g., headache, arthritis, premenstrual cramps) frequently cause bleeding and must be discontinued (Fig. 50–4).

Each patient should have a complete eye exam before surgery. Special attention must be paid to the best corrected visual acuity, tear quality and quantity, and any corneal pathology. Patients with evidence of dysthyroid ophthalmopathy, keratoconjunctivitis sicca, proptosis, amblyopia, retinitis pigmentosa, or VIIth cranial nerve compromise should be identified because of their increased risk for postoperative complication. Patients with a history of glaucoma, blepharochalasis syndrome, retinal surgery, cataract surgery, refractive surgery (RK), and strabismus should also be noted.

The most useful test for the plastic surgeon to measure adequate tear production is the Schirmer test. Although not totally reliable, filter paper placed in the lateral third of the lower lid with dim light and no topical anesthetic will measure basal and reflex rate. After 5 minutes normal wetting is between 15 and 30 mm, hyposecretion between 5 and 10 mm, and dry eye less than 5 mm.

ANATOMIC EVALUATION

Preoperative clinical photography is essential in documenting existing eyelid and periocular anatomy. The photographs are used for preoperative surgical planning, intraoperative decision making, and postoperative documentation. It is extremely important to eliminate distortion in eyelid photographs by controlling head tilt, brow relaxation, the visual focal point, the plane of the camera, and lighting, as well as dynamic muscle action (8). The recommended views include (a) full face, in repose and smiling, to delineate wrinkling; (b) closeup anterior views of eyelids and periorbital structures in repose, smiling, upgaze, and downgaze; (c) closeup lateral and oblique views of eyelids and periorbital structures in repose and smiling; (d) closeup anterior views with eyes totally closed.

Before upper-eyelid surgery the surgeon should note an anatomic evaluation of several components that include (a) skin, (b) muscle, (c) fat, (d) height of supratarsal crease, (e) brow height, (f) orbital rim projection, (g) exophthalmos (19), (h) canthal slant, (i) preexisting eyelid laxity, (j) ptosis, (k) asymmetry, (l) and wrinkling.

As aging takes place, a reduction in collagen and sebaceous secretions contributes to upper-lid skin laxity (9). Redundancy of the orbicularis oculi (the eyelid sphincter) and attenuation of the lateral canthal ligament also contributes to

SOME DRUGS THAT CAUSE BLEEDING PROBLEMS

Two weeks prior to surgery, vitamin E., aspirin, or aspirin containing ibuprofen should be discontinued because they promote bleeding.

FIG. 50–4. Some drugs that cause bleeding problems. Two weeks before surgery, vitamin E, aspirin, or aspirin-containing ibuprofen should be discontinued because they promote bleeding.

Some Products Containing Aspirin or Aspirin like Affects

Aleve	Dislcid	PC-Caps
Alfaxan	Dolobid	Percodan
Anacin	Easprin	Pepto Bismol
Anexsia	Ecotrin	Persantine
Ansaid	Empirin	Propoxyphene
Anti-Inflammatory	Equagesic Tabs.	Robaxisal
Agents	Excedrin	Rowasa
A.S.A.	Feldene	Roxiprin
Ascriptin	Fiorinal	Salflex
Aspergum	Indocin	Salsalate
Axotal	Halfprin	Salsitab
Azdone Tablets	Lortab ASA	Sine-off
B.A.C. Tablets	Marplan	Soma Compound Tabs.
BC Powder	Meprobamate	St. Joseph Products
Bufferin	Midol	Supac
Butazolidin	Mono-Gesic	Synalgos DC Caps.
Cama Arthritis	Norgesic	Talwin Capsules
Pain Reliever	Nsaids	Tolectin Products
Cantharone Plus	Orphengesic	Trilisate
Clinoril	Orudis	Voltaren
Congespirin	Oxycodone	Zorprin
Damason-P	Panasal Tabs.	
Darvon	Parnate	

Products Containing Ibuprofen

Aches-N-Pain	Meclomen	Ponstel
Advil	Medipren	Rufen
Anaprox	Midol 200	Sine-Aid
Co-Advil	Motrin	Toradol
Advil Cold/Sinus	Nalfon	
Haltran	Naprosyn	
Ibu-Tab	Nuprin	

Anticoagulants

Coumadin	Heparin	Periactin
Dicumarol	Panwarfin	

lid laxity (10,11). There are proponents of the theory of herniated excess fat with aging (12), while others postulate bulging of the septum as causative factor.

Orbital fat is the space filler and shock absorber of the orbit. The globe floats upward into the orbit in a supine position, resulting in more fat in the upper lids and less fat in the lower lids. The aesthetic surgeon, when excising fat, should take into account these gravitational changes. Removing excess lower-eyelid fat can contribute to a "hollowed out" upper orbit resulting in a gaunt, cadaverous appearance.

Anatomic Variants of the Upper Eyelid

TRUE DERMATOCHALASIS

Excess skin alone, or true dermatochalasis, is seen in older individuals with involutional changes and deep-set upper eyes, or in those who have had a previous blepharoplasty. Patients with this isolated finding are rare.

BLEPHAROCHALASIS SYNDROME

Blepharochalasis syndrome is a condition of recurrent bouts of nonspecific inflammatory edema over a period of time that produces changes in the eyelid. It usually occurs in young to middle-aged females and may be associated with allergies. The changes usually consist of redundant erythematous skin, atrophy of the nasal fat pad, and possible dehiscence of canthal tendons (13).

EXCESS SKIN, MUSCLE, AND FAT WITH LOW SUPRATARSAL CREASE (Asian-Type Eyelid)

Many women with excess skin, muscle, and fat who have low supratarsal creases are improved by excising excessive skin, muscle, and fat in combination with supratarsal fixation 9 to 11mm above the lid margin. In non-Asian patients, the supratarsal crease frequently blends into the orbitopalpebral furrow when opening the eyes.

Asians can be grouped into two categories as to their preference of crease height: (a) those who wish to look as non-Asian as possible, desiring large eyes and high creases; and (b) those who wish to have a more Eurasian-type crease, which remains low. This latter group, who wish to maintain their ethnicity and simply highlight their eyes, represent the majority. If an Asian upper blepharoplasty is performed with aggressive fat excision, it yields a hollow-eyed, aged look and an unhappy patient. It is important to realize that sunken eyes in most Asian patients results in an aged look. For a more natural, aesthetic double lid, in most Asian patients the surgeon should perform a 5-6-7 mm supratarsal fixation suture with limited fat excision. Many Asians, when shown what a forehead lift will do, prefer this look. Epicanthal fold removal generally is not desired. It may be performed directly or, in may cases, with dorsal nasal augmentation only.

EXCESS SKIN, MUSCLE, AND FAT WITH HIGH SUPRATARSAL CREASE

In this condition, on elevating the overhang of the upper lid, the tarsal crease is seen 8 mm or more above the lashline (Fig. 50–5). In the authors' experience, this is the contour most frequently requiring surgery. These patients often have orbicularis muscle hypertrophy with marked fat deposits. On occasion, more muscle than skin is removed to achieve the nonhooded, deep-set youthful eye. This is a particularly satisfactory operation for women who do not like to wear makeup because it creates a deep, defined shadow.

The postoperative appearance of a deeply contoured, high supratarsal crease is not attempted in males. Men almost universally have lower brows, and a high supratarsal crease may create an angry appearance or a feminine look. A more conservative surgical excision is therefore indicated in males.

LOW OR PROMINENT ORBITAL RIM

In some patients, the orbital rim extends caudad almost to the lashline and must be removed by osteotomy or burring of the bone. Caution in contouring is necessary to avoid entry into the frontal sinus. The procedure can be performed through a transcoronal or blepharoplasty incision when needed. Frontal bossing, medial or lateral, can also be reduced this way.

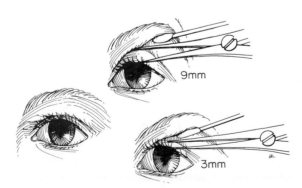

FIG. 50–5. A, the hooded eye can have a low or high supratarsal crease (see Figs. 51–8 through 51–10). **B,** applicator delineates the high crease, the most commonly operated contour, in the author's experience. **C,** the low supratarsal crease.

PROTUBERANT EYES OR MINIMAL EXOPHTHALMOS

The protuberant eye is a unique problem, and upper blepharoplasty sometimes accentuates the problem, producing a staring look. The approach to this condition should be either extremely conservative or refusal of surgery. It is essential that patients with this condition be shown the simulated result with an applicator stick. Removing fat will not decrease the protrusiveness of the globe. Orbital decompression is necessary for this.

PROMINENT OR PROLAPSED LACRIMAL GLAND

When present, this gland is suture fixated to the periosteum, above and behind the superior orbital rim. Excision of the gland is not undertaken because it could lead to dry eye syndrome.

PTOSIS

Patients requesting blepharoplasty who present with incidental mild ptosis must be distinguished from the elderly patient who presents with decreased vision and moderate-to-severe ptosis. The former patient is concerned with aesthetics and the latter with vision. Acquired blepharoptosis can be corrected by (a) conjunctivomüllerectomy, (b) levator advancement, or (c) Fasanella Servat procedure. A conjunctivomüllerectomy is the procedure of choice for the cosmetic patient with only a mild (<2.5 mm) ptosis. Advantages of conjunctivomüllerectomy include the ability to perform correction under general anesthesia and lack of need for overcorrection (unlike the levator advancement technique). In addition, the procedure is forgiving, predictable, and associated with minimal complications. The phenylephrine test is used preoperatively to unmask contralateral ptosis and quantitate muscle resection (14). Levator advancement techniques require patient cooperation, intraoperative decision making, and adequate anesthesia without producing levator akinesia.

True ptosis must be distinguished from pseudoptosis. Pseudoptosis is an optical illusion created when tarsal creases are of different heights. The eyelid with the lower crease appears ptotic. To evaluate, have the patient look up; the coverage of the pupils will be the same unless the pseudoptotic lower eyelid is truly ptotic.

LOW BROW

The height of the brow is one of the most important presurgical evaluations because an individual's brow is inextricably related to facial expression. The brow shape and position sets the gestalt when looking at any face. Even an expert blepharoplasty will not relieve the tired expression produced by a ptotic brow (15) (Fig. 50–6). The brow lift is discussed later in this chapter.

UPPER BLEPHAROPLASTY

Authors' Operative Technique

Anesthesia

After all evaluations (medical, cardiologic, coagulative, psychologic, ophthalmologic, and anatomic) are completed satisfactorily, surgery may be performed in the office, hospital, or outpatient center. Either general sedation, or sedation combined with local anesthesia, may be used. Usually an

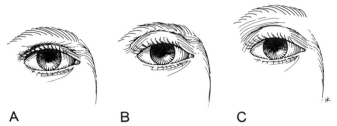

FIG. 50–6. **A,** the brow at the orbital rim with dermatochalasis. **B,** after blepharoplasty, a low brow still gives a tired expression and connotes anger. **C,** when brow is elevated, the appearance of tiredness is improved.

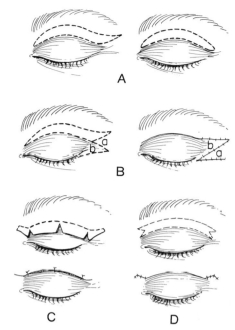

FIG. 50–7. Excisions for upper blepharoplasty. **A,** typical ellipses of excess tissue for upper blepharoplasty. **B,** the Z-plasty of Lewis (51) elevates the lateral canthus. **C,** the excise-as-you-go technique of Silver (33). **D,** the lateral V closure.

adrenalin-containing solution (1:100,000 to 1:200,000) is injected to help delineate tissue planes and promote hemostasis. Hyaluronidase (Wydase) can be used to ensure spreading of the anesthetic.

Patients should be under complete monitoring (using a precordial stethoscope for auditory safety because the anesthetist is away from the head). In addition, medications to control nausea (Reglan capsules and Zofran) and hypertension, and to decrease intraocular tension (intravenous mannitol and acetazolamide, Diamox) should be in the operating room for emergencies. Except for steriod contraindications (recent bleeding ulcers, diabetes, Addison disease), 4 to 12 mg of dexamethasone (Decadron) can be administered intravenously to keep operative and postoperative swelling to a minimum. A small suction and adequate bipolar cautery with backup must be available.

Before the administration of any preoperative medication, the patient is evaluated in a sitting position, fully awake. The individual is instructed to look upward at a 45° angle while the lateral extent of the hood is marked. An assistant elevates the eyebrow until the skin is smooth and no wrinkles are present. For women, a final measurement of 9 mm from the lashes at a midpoint between the canthi is appropriate; for men, or those with lower brows who do not desire a brow lift, 5 to 7 mm is suitable. The medial extent of the hood is marked with a dot placed 4 mm medial and 4 mm cephalad to the medial canthal ligament. A toothless Adson forcep is used to imbricate the skin until the eyes begin to open; this is the most cephalic mark. The marks are connected to outline the excision of skin.

Surgical Techniques

In the operating room and under anesthesia, 2 ml of 1% lidocaine (Xylocaine) with 1:100,000 adrenalin and 1 ml Wydase/10cc local, is injected per lid. The edema is expressed and the skin is incised after waiting a minimum of 10 minutes. In most upper blepharoplasty techniques, either skin, muscle, fat, or a combination of components is removed. Marking of the ellipse varies with other authors (Fig. 50–7). Some merely create a tarsal crease, whereas others elevate the lateral canthus. Some surgeons use a separate technique to fix the supratarsal crease, but others are of the opinion that a fixation is never necessary. The orbital septum is exposed completely to reveal the orbital fat. Entering the septum through small holes over each fat pocket can lead to incomplete removal of excess fat and difficulties

in identifying bleeding, as well as scarring of levator, which limits excursion of the upper lid. Generally, the fat pockets are emptied at a point even with the orbital rim. It may be convenient for surgeons who perform this operation infrequently to draw a grid on the Mayo stand and place the fat in the appropriate box to avoid omission of a fat pad or creating assymetry. Any redundant orbital septum should be trimmed at this time.

If there is lateral hooding, the redundant orbicularis muscle is excised. The lateral orbicularis is then reapproximated using one or two 6-0 absorbable sutures. Care is taken in placing these sutures to avoid bunching and to prevent postoperative "lumpiness." The skin is then reapproximated from lateral to medial using a running 6-0 fast absorbing suture.

No postoperative bandages or blindfolds are needed; they hinder more than they help. Iced saline or iced water compresses on the eyes and sleeping in an elevated position are endorsed by the authors, as are sunglasses during the first weeks after surgery. Patients are then instructed in skin care and fashion makeup. Contact lenses are allowed after 7 days with gentle insertion techniques.

If a brow-lift is performed at the same time, an alternate technique is used to prevent lagophthalmos (Fig. 50–8). An approach other than transcutaneous to upper-lid blepharoplasty is through a coronal incision, as reported by Dingman. This approach may be utilized when a brow-lift is performed and fat alone is to be removed from the upper eyes. Disadvantages include difficulty in removing medial fat and continuity of the forehead dissection with the septum, which results in extra swelling and bruising.

Fat must also be removed from the upper eyelid medial compartment through a transconjunctival approach, as reported by Nahai.

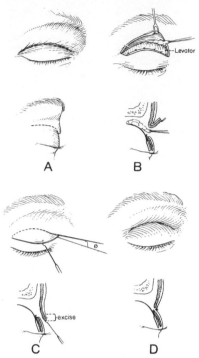

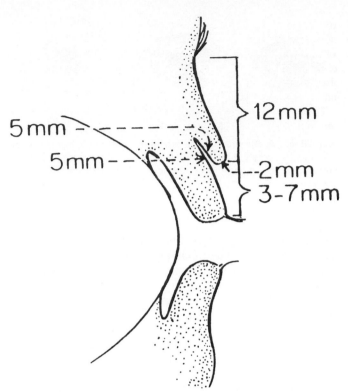

FIG. 50–8. Concurrent blepharoplasty procedure with brow-lift. **A,** marking is made at 9 mm before injection of Xylocaine with adrenalin and Wydase. **B,** an incision is made through the skin and the orbicularis. An adhesion is made between orbicularis and levator with 6-0 white silk and the fat pockets are sculpted. **C,** with eyes closed, excess skin and muscle are excised. Occasionally, merely creating the fixation is sufficient to eliminate dermatochalasis by redraping. **D,** the eye should remain closed or slightly open medially after excision and closure. (From Ellenbogen, R. Transcoronal eyebrow lift with concomitant upper blepharoplasty. *Plast Reconstr Surg* 1983; 71:490).

FIG. 50–9. Twenty-six to thirty millimeters of skin is necessary on the upper lid between brow and lid margin for normal contour, normal invagination, and normal closure. This allows a normal minimum of 1 cm for the invagination process, 12 mm from fold to brow, and 3 to 6 mm of visualized pretarsal skin. One to two millimeters are necessary for the bend. Less skin prevents lid-fold invagination or restricts proper brow positioning (insufficient skin for eye closure). (From Flowers R. *Clin Plast Surg* 1993; 20:2).

AESTHETIC COMPLICATIONS OF UPPER BLEPHAROPLASTY

It is well established that too-aggressive upper-lid excisions are the most common sign of inexperience and of failure after lid blepharoplasty. Aggressive excisions deliver thick, coarse juxtabrow skin down onto thinner skin of the upper lid, where it neither looks good nor functions correctly. An even greater tragedy is the inability to perform a subsequent corrective brow elevation without risking exposure of the cornea.

There is an absolute requirement for upper-lid skin. Flowers reports that a minimum of 27 mm (preferably 30 mm) of skin is necessary on the upper lid for optimal appearance and function (16) (Fig. 50–9). Shorr leaves more upper lid skin in men (24 to 25 mm) than in women (18 to 20 mm) to create a greater fold (17). Emphasis should be on what is left in place, and not on what is removed. A fine scar is a necessity for success. Connecting the thicker, red, vascular preseptal skin to the thin, pale, pretarsal skin leaves a color differential that is noticeable in some cases.

Overaggressive fat excision from all compartments may result in a hollow, gaunt, cadaverous appearance, which becomes more noticable with age.

Cutting through the white levator aponeurosis will show the very reticular capillary pattern of the Müller muscle.

Cautery or severence of the lacrimal gland, superior rectus, superior oblique, or retaining ligaments is theoretically possible. Bleeding complications will be discussed later.

Eyebrow Lift (Forehead Lift)

The primary indication for brow-lift has been eyebrow malposition from aging changes or from congenital variation. However, as many, if not more, eyebrow lifts are performed for other indications, including frown muscle imbalance, forehead rhytids, and abnormal unattractive expression.

In general, a brow-lift is indicated if the medial brow, lateral brow, or both are at or below the supraorbital rim by palpation. Indications have been reduced to a measuring of angles by the authors.

Several surgical approaches (open incisional or closed endoscopic), in several different locations (temporal, coronal, forehead, hairline, upper bleph) as well several different planes (subcutaneous, subgaleal, subperiosteal) have been advocated to address a range of patients anatomic deformities (18–20).

Browpexy has been advocated for isolated mild lateral brow ptosis and as a stabilizer of the brow during upper-lid blepharoplasty (21).

Connell advocates hairline incisions for patients with unusually high foreheads, coronal incisions for patients with low-normal hairlines, two-thirds or lambdoidal incisions for bald patients, and W-incisions or interlocking M-incisions for male-pattern baldness (18). Sokol and Sokol (22), as well as Knize (23), describe performing brow-lifts through blepharoplasty incisions. Almost without exception, a transcoronal incision is used by the authors (24).

The brow-lift performed directly above the brows is condemned for its deep, unrepairable scars.

NORMAL BROW TOPOGRAPHY

The relative position and height of the medial-to-lateral portion of the eyebrow, and its distance from the supraorbital rim, connote specific emotions for our society. High medial-slanting eyebrows denote sadness; low medial-slanting eyebrows denote anger or evil; flat low-set eyebrows denote fatigue; eyebrows with a "normal" arch denote happiness (Fig. 50–10). This is important in terms of preoperative evaluation and surgical planning.

Eyebrow position clearly sets the tone for facial expression. Aside from congenital variation, there is a clear difference between a man's and a woman's eyebrows. Mens' eyebrows are straighter, thicker, and lower-set, with only a subtle arch centrally. Many women will try to achieve an arch if it is lacking. They will also tweeze their eyebrows laterally down to a narrow line, raising the eyebrow away from the upper lid, in hopes of achieving a softer appearance. A lower and thicker eyebrow in most woman encroaches upon their upper lids and conflicts with their makeup's goal of calling attention to the eyes. Many women now utilize tattoo to treat brows that were over-tweezed when they were younger.

Several authors have defined the normal eyebrow topography. These definitions are based on spatial, numerical, or simply visual guidelines and all assist in establishing proper relationships in the upper third of the face (24–26).

Westmore's model for the ideal eyebrow arch is the most useful in evaluating the shape of the eyebrow (Fig. 50–11). The medialmost point lies 1 cm above the supraorbital rim. McKinney describes the ideal brow as lying 1 cm from brow to supraorbital rim, 1.6 cm from brow to crease, and 2.5 cm from brow to midpupil (25,26). Additional visual criteria described by Matarraso include (a) the medial upper-lid fold should not extend more medial than the lashes, (b) the lateral supratarsal skin fold should not go far beyond the lateral orbital rim, (c) the thickened brow skin should not rest on the eyelid skin.

EVALUATION

In evaluating any potential brow-lift patient, a test is performed to determine whether a concomitant blepharoplasty is also indicated (Fig. 50–12).

Another modality to determine if an eyebrow lift will be beneficial is to measure the superciliary angle B to Y to B. (Y being the midpoint between the canthi). If the angle is greater than 90°, an eyebrow lift is indicated. After a eyebrow lift the angle is less than 90° (Fig. 50–13). If both blepharoplasty and brow-lift are indicated, the procedures may be performed concurrently. Alternately, blepharoplasty may be performed as a 1st or 2nd stage procedure (i.e., before or after brow-lift). We believe a more exact upper-lid blepharoplasty can be performed after a brow-lift is performed. An interval of at least 3 months between staged procedures is recommended.

It is very important to identify a low brow before any upper-eyelid surgery. Certain patients may need, not a blepharoplasty, but correction of a ptotic brow. The age or race of the patient should not mislead the surgeon into ruling out a blepharoplasty, a brow-lift, or both. Each patient must be individually evaluated.

During the initial preoperative consultation, the surgeon explains how determination of brow position, frown muscle imbalance, forehead rhytids, lateral brow laxity, and/or unattractive expression can be modified to to bring about an improved periorbital appearance. Concomitantly, the surgeon simulates the aesthetic enhancement in front of a mirror to demonstrate the potential for improvement. Disadvantages must be discussed: possible higher forehead, hair thinning, and numbness.

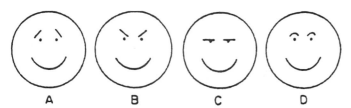

FIG. 50–10. A, Eyebrows that are lower laterally than medially transmit sadness. **B,** eyebrows that are lower medially than laterally transmit anger. **C,** low eyebrows transmit tiredness. **D,** properly aligned eyebrows with medial and lateral approximately at the same height allow the happy face actually to appear happy.

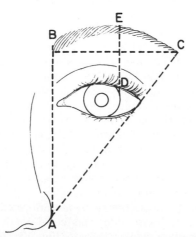

FIG. 50–11. Westmore's model for eyebrow arch. Line A-B from where the ala meets the face, extended cephalad from the medial canthus produces point B, the medialmost extent of the eyebrow. Line A-C to the lateral canthus establishes point C, the lateralmost extension of the brow. B and C are at the same height. Line D-E parallels line A-B at the temporal limbus of the iris to establish point E, the highest point of the eyebrow.

ANATOMY

The four major muscles of the forehead and eyebrow are the occipitofrontalis, orbicularis oculi, corrugator supercillii, and procerus (Fig. 50–14). The occipitofrontalis allows the scalp

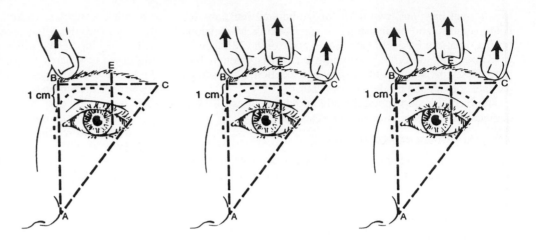

FIG. 50–12. The test for whether concurrent blepharoplasty is indicated. *Left:* Caudalmost hairs of the medial eyebrow are lifted 1 cm over the supraorbital rim by palpation. *Center:* If, when lifting the lateral points of the arches to an equal height C, and lifting E slightly higher, blepharochalasis still exists, then blepharoplasty is indicated. *Right:* If, with this maneuver, the tarsal crease is distinct and without overhang, blepharoplasty is not indicated.

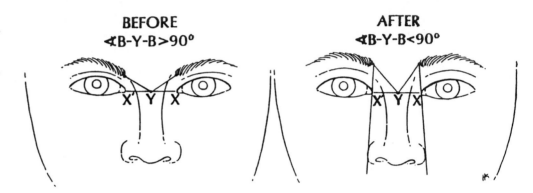

FIG. 50–13. Before B-Y-B angle is measured (Y being the intercanthal point, B being the inferior medial brow point). If the angle is more than 90°, then eyebrow lift is indicated. After B-Y-B, angle will be less than 90°.

to move anteriorly and posteriorly. The orbicularis closes the eyelid. In doing so, it also pulls down the skin of the forehead, temple, and cheek. The corrugator arises from the nasal process of the frontal bone and inserts into the skin of the medial brow. It produces vertical wrinkles of the forehead. The procerus arises from the nasal bone and is continuous with the medial margin of the frontalis. It pulls down the medial end of the eyebrow and produces horizontal wrinkles over the nose. In the forehead region, all muscles are innervated by the temporal branch of the facial nerve, except for the procerus, which is innervated by the buccal branch of the facial nerve.

In the region of the eyebrow, the muscle plane is firmly fixed to the skin of the forehead. The muscle plane is secured to the frontal bone periosteum by a firm attachment on the underside of the brow fat pad. These attachments primarily extend over the medial one-half to two-thirds of the orbit along the supraorbital rim. It is the lack of deep attachments laterally that results in earlier and greater ptosis of this portion of the eyebrow (27).

MARKING FOR A TRANSCORONAL BROW LIFT

With experience in more than 850 patients over an 18-year period, we have determined the constant points on the transcoronal incision, which translate predictably to the lift of points B-E-C on the eyebrow on cephalic traction at surgery (Fig. 50–15). Marking is done preoperatively with the patient seated and awake, and takes about 15 minutes. The cephalic border of the eyebrows are marked B-E-C for

reference (see Fig. 50–15). A point 6 to 7 cm posterior to the frontal hairline at the midline (with nasal root F as reference) is marked G, and the hair is parted symmetrically antihelix to antihelix after being completely saturated with sterile KY Jelly (Johnson and Johnson) to keep the hair in place. No hair is cut off. Point E is extended cephalically parallel to the midline (F-G), from the temporal iris limbus to where it meets the incision (H). (This is within a few millimeters of a constant of 4 cm on all patients.) The distance between the midline, G and H, is the same as between the highest part of the arch of the eyebrow and the midline. The hair is parted and braided and held in place with sterile aluminum foil. Point C is extended cephalically to point I on the incision, 6 cm from point H. The patient is instructed to raise the eyebrows. The transverse line where the frontalis muscle is to be interrupted (J-K) is drawn in the second transverse forehead crease cephalically. Interrupting the frontalis below this line does not allow the patient enough frontalis to raise the eyebrows postoperatively.

The frontalis transection will be performed internally at J-K and is only 5 cm wide. This corresponds to the width between the supratrochlear nerves (Fig. 50–16). The supratrochlear nerves pass directly cephalically (Fig. 50–17). This limited midline transection reduces the postoperative numbness and itching experienced with earlier procedures. When the flap is in traction, it will heal and create an adhesion between the skull and the subcutaneous tissue (Fig. 50–18). We believe this makes the procedure one of the most per-

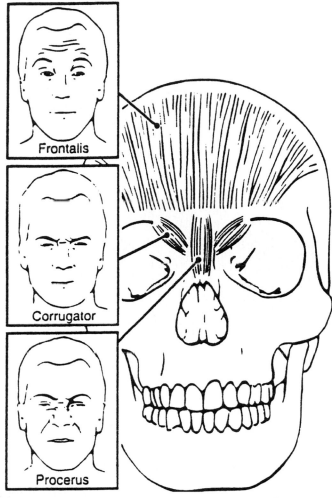

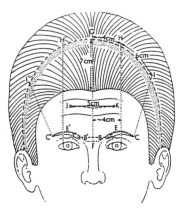

FIG. 50–15. The supratrochlear nerves pass directly cephalically from a nearly constant distance of 2.5 to 2.7 cm from the midline. Therefore, the transection at J-K is 2.5 cm or less.

FIG. 50–14. The frontalis elevates the brows. The corrugators lower and move the brows medially. The procerus lowers the medial brow and wrinkles the nose.

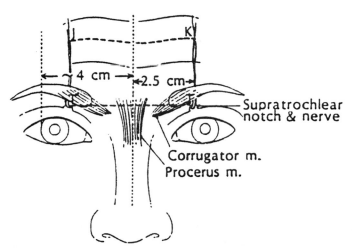

FIG. 50–16. The distance of the supratrochlear nerves from the midline bilaterally is 2.5 to 2.7 cm. The supratrochlear nerves pass directly cephalically; consequently, the transection at J-K will preserve part of that and all of the nerves lateral to it.

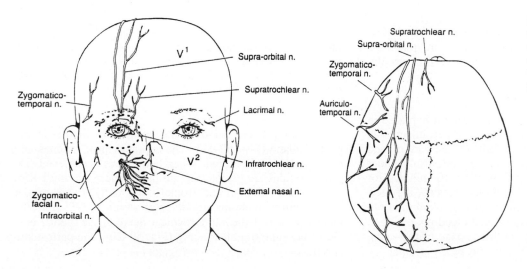

FIG. 50–17. The nerves of the forehead. The supraorbital nerves within the forehead are preserved with the limited J-K transection. This limits annoying numbness and itching.

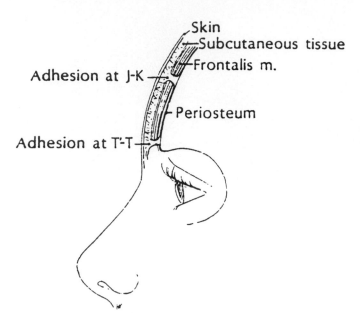

FIG. 50–18. An adhesion is formed between the skin and the skull at the J-K transection postoperatively. This accounts for the permanence of the lift.

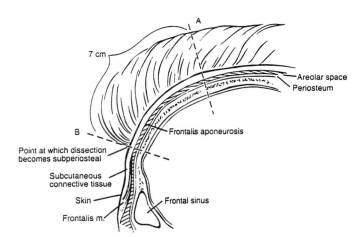

FIG. 50–19. The dissection is subperiosteal. The periosteum is very filmy and is actually areolar tissue until the hairline is met caudally.

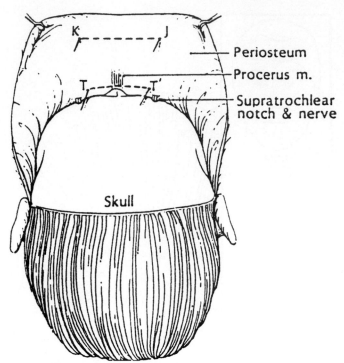

FIG. 50–20. Needles are pushed through and through the flap at K-J and T-T to insure a proper transection.

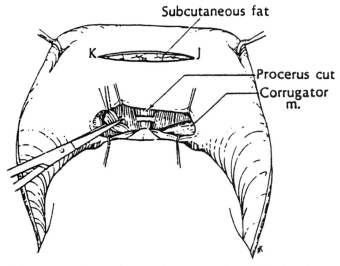

FIG. 50–21. Transection to subcutaneous fat at K-J; after the periosteum at T-T is cut, the periosteum is pulled back to expose the process and corrugators. The procerus is cut across until it retracts and the corrugators are removed.

manent operations. The supratrochlear notches are marked and the T-T' connects them. Between them are the three muscles—procerus, frontalis, and corrugator—that usually have to be corrected.

SURGICAL TECHNIQUES (24, 28)

Under general or sedation anesthesia, the patient is placed in a head-elevated (30°) position. The surgeon then injects 100 to 80 cc of 0.25% Xylocaine, 1:200,000 adrenalin, and Wydase 150 units (Hyaluronidase, Wyeth) uniformly under the proposed dissection area. After waiting 10 minutes for vasoconstriction to take place, the surgeon makes the incision with a no. 15 blade, beveling carefully to avoid injury to the hair bulbs. There is minimal incisional bleeding, owing to the large amount of fluid in the confined space of the scalp. A sterile metal comb removes the hair cut by the scalpel.

Dissection is carried over the orbital rim in the subperiosteal plane (Fig. 50–19). The supratrochlear notches and nasal bones are identified. When hemostasis is achieved, 25-gauge needles are placed through the forehead on line J-K to ensure transection of the frontalis internally at the proper level. A cut is made through the periosteum at T-T' from the medial border of the supratrochlear nerve to the medial border of the supratrochlear nerve (Fig. 50–20). The periosteum is retracted to expose the corrugators (Fig. 50–21).

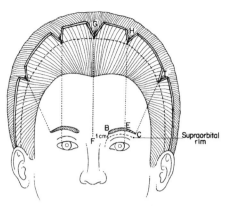

FIG. 50–22. Point G is elevated high enough to create 1 cm between the caudalmost hairs of the medial eyebrow and the supraorbital rim; I is elevated to raise C to the same height as B; H then achieves the highest point of the arch (E).

Great care is taken with removal of the supercillii muscle to preserve the supratrochlear nerves and the vascular pedicle. A transverse cut through the procerus at the intercanthal line eliminates the procerus wrinkle. The periosteum is returned to its original position, but not sutured; this prevents the depression encountered by other techniques when the periosteum and other tissue is removed. Using a D'Assumpçao face-lift marker, the surgeon lifts the flap at point G until the caudal hairs of the medial eyebrow are 1 cm above the caudalmost supraorbital rim in a straight line viewed anteriorly (Fig. 50–22). The flap is incised perpendicularly to its edge and tacked with 3-0 nylon.

Point I is then lifted until points B and C are at the same level and viewed from the foot of the table. The lift at this point is generally less at points H and G, even when these points are of equal height preoperatively. The surgeon measures the distance and performs a lift on the right side to the same degree as the left, checking for symmetry at the foot of the table. Point H is then lifted, so that E is the highest point of the brow bilaterally, and tacked with 3-0 nylon. Excess scalp between the tacking stitches is excised and carefully beveled to preserve hair bulbs.

A few Vicryl 3-0 sutures close the galea; staples complete the closure. The tacking stitches are then removed. The operation rarely takes over 45 minutes. A dressing with light compression is placed over the entire dissected area for 1 day. The patient is allowed to shampoo after 2 days with baby shampoo. Staples are removed in 2 weeks. A shine appears over the forehead that lasts for 4 to 13 weeks. Blepharoplasty is performed immediately following the forehead lift if necessary.

DISCUSSION

Transcoronal forehead lift with frontalis and procerus muscle interruption and corrugator muscle excision has proven to be an acceptable operation for transverse forehead wrinkles, vertical frown wrinkles, and ptosis of the eyebrows and forehead. This operation creates a quantitative measure of how much to lift and avoids the look of perpetual surprise.

Westmore's cosmetic technique for achieving a correct arch in the makeup studio can be applied to all techniques of eyebrow lifts, and specifically to the transcoronal technique.

After careful measurement and evaluation of many patients, a system of marking has been standardized to the points determined on the transcoronal incision that set the heights of the inner and lateral boundaries on the new brow. The problems previously experienced (e.g., numbness, itching, depression between the brows, paralyzed brow, brows too high) have been all but eliminated by these simple modifications of the muscle transection and excision.

The "endoscopic-assisted forehead lift" is currently being used to describe several different operations, including excision of frown muscles; complete forehead lifts comparable to conventional approaches utilizing fixation screws or tie-over bolsters; and a combination of open/closed lift with skin excision at the anterior hairline. Ongoing experience with this technique will determine its potential for further refining aesthetic procedures. Early reports from authors show decrease in hair loss, numbness, and itching. Other authors, after a larger series, show similar hair loss, numbness, and inability to eliminate the deep corrugator lines or maintain the lift.

COMPLICATIONS OF THE BROW LIFT

Untoward sequelae of brow-lift must be distinguished from complications. They may include temporary hair shock (curly when originally straight, or have different texture), headache, transient or permanent numbness, itching, temporary or permanent hair loss, or a change in frontal hairline.

Complications described have included hematoma, infection, flap necrosis, lagophthalmos, forehead lag, corneal abrasion, nerve injury, alteration in expression, reflex sympathetic dystrophy, patient dissatisfaction, surface contour irregularity, widened scar, spot necrosis, alopecia, and oculocardiac reflex.

Lower Lids

NORMAL ANATOMY AND TOPOGRAPHY

The normal youthful lower eyelid is characterized by an almost horizontal rim, so that with few exceptions there is no scleral show. It is suspended by the medial and lateral canthal tendon attachments to the bony orbit.

The horizontal level of the lateral canthus lies 1 to 2 mm superior to the medial canthus in non-Asians (3 mm in Asians), and is less firmly supported than the medial canthus. The slant of the eyelids depends mainly on the quality of the lateral canthal tendon. A lateral downward slant may be either a congenital variant (similar to that seen in Treacher Collins or blepharophimosis syndrome), secondary to trauma, or involutional. There are also ethnic variations (greater lateral upward obliquity) as seen in the Annamite, Chinese, Min-Huong, and Cambodian populations. A subgroup of people have large eyes in which lifelong lateral temporal bowing or scleral show is present on straight gaze. No functional problem exists for them, and many of these eyes are youthful and pleasant in appearance.

The normal lower eyelid courses upward or horizontally from the medial canthus to the punctum, lies tangent to the inferior limbus centrally, and then curves upward again to insert into the lateral orbital rim.

The lower eyelid consists of three lamellae: anterior, middle, and posterior. The anterior lamellae is analogous to the

FIG. 50–23. The lower lid anatomy demonstrates the essential structures and their relationships.

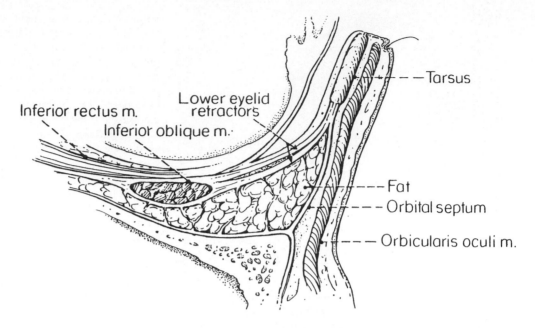

upper eyelid, consisting of thin eyelid skin and orbicularis oculi muscles. Deep to this is the middle lamellae, consisting of the orbital septum and the tarsus. The septum originates at the arcus marginalis of the inferior orbital rim and inserts into the inferior edge of the tarsal plate. In Asian lower eyelids, the orbital septum fuses with the lower eyelid retractors in a slightly higher position, contributing to a fuller eyelid. It is most commonly this middle lamella (septum) that undergoes contracture during lower-lid transcutaneous blepharoplasty, leading to the single most common complication of retraction without ectropion.

The lower eyelid's tarsal plate is only 4 mm high as compared to 10 mm in the upper eyelid. The posterior lamellae consists of the inferior retractors (analogous to the levator Müller muscle complex in the upper eyelid) and the conjunctiva. These lower-lid retractors originate from the inferior oblique muscle anteriorly and the insert on the inferior margin of the tarsus. Between the septum and the lower lid retractors lies three fat pads: medial, central, and lateral (Fig. 50–23).

EVALUATION

Preoperative evaluation must involve an assessment of the tendency for downward migration of the lower eyelid to avoid the telltale sign of lower eyelid malposition with temporal scleral show, ectropion, and loss of the almond-shaped aperture. Lower-eyelid hypotonia is present frequently in the elderly and in middle-aged males. When laxity exists, the surgeon should at least consider one of several tightening or suspension techniques.

Preoperative evaluation should also include (a) bags or dark circles (herniation, periorbital fat, or visible orbital rim), (b) periocular pigmentation, (c) skin laxity, (d) presence of scleral show, (e) muscle hypertrophy, (f) festoons, (g) exophthalmos or protuberant globe, (h) malar hypoplasia or tear trough, (i) asymmetries, (j) canthal obliquity, and (k) dynamic or static wrinkling. As with the upper lids, all of these factors must be evaluated. Preoperative photos, discussed earlier, are helpful as preoperative, intraoperative, and postoperative references.

Anatomic Variants of the Lower Eyelid

BAGS OR DARK CIRCLES (WITHOUT SKIN REDUNDANCY)

Even in the presence of large bags, no skin or muscle should be excised. The convexity of the bulge is converted to a concavity by fat removal (Fig. 50–24). Small herniations in young patients are often hereditary. Such individuals are good candidates for a skin-muscle flap or a transconjunctival approach for fat removal (30,31).

An alternative technique for lid correction, by repairing the orbital septum, has its proponents. This technique for correction of palpebral bags is based on preservation of the bulging fat and correction of the support layer. Mendelson and Camirand state that most cases of aging lower eyelids have as primary pathology a weakness of the orbital septum. Repair of this weakened orbital septum involves suturing the septum-capsulopalpebral fascia to the arcus marginalis, thus preserving fat (32,33).

PERIOCULAR PIGMENTATION

If periocular pigmentation is preexisting, it must be pointed out to the patient. This is checked by asking the patient to tilt the head upward, allowing light to fall perpendicular to the skin. The discoloration that remains is due to pigmentation and not shadow. Hyperpigmentation of the skin cannot be

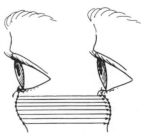

FIG. 50–24. Only fat should be removed in huge lower-lid bags with no skin excess. The convexity is converted to a concavity.

changed by blepharoplasty. However, the removal of "bags" and filling the nasojugal fold will eliminate some of the shadow cast on these areas, thus lightening the discoloration. The use of Kojic acid, hydroquinone steroid creams, Retin A, and glycolic acid combinations have been recommended as bleaching creams with moderate success. Ultra pulse CO_2 laser has been utilized recently and determination of long-term benefits is pending investigation.

SEVERE SKIN LAXITY

Severe skin laxity is frequently seen in smokers, heavy ethanol users, and those exposed to sun; it may also be hereditary. Some authors recommend a separate skin flap for excess skin redundancy (34). Skin excision of the lower lids must be conservative in all procedures. Attempting to eliminate the wrinkles and fine lines of the lower lid by removing a great deal of skin will invariably result in pulling of the lid margin downward, causing scleral show, rounding, or ectropion.

HYPERTROPHIC PRETARSAL ORBICULARIS MUSCLE

This entity, as described by Flowers, is seen in some persons with semiconstant smile, creating a false impression of excess lid skin and hypertrophy of the orbicularis muscle. Sometimes it is unconscious; almost always it is correctable with relaxation, the occasional exception occurring in an Asian patient (8). Loeb has had success in excising this (35).

FESTOONING OR ORBICULARIS LAXITY

Festoons are distinct bulges that are seen caudal to the bulges of herniated fat. They represent sagging of the malar and orbital portions of the orbicularis muscle. In the correction of pure skin-muscle festoons (present when the septum is firm and the orbital fat does not bulge), the orbital septum is left undisturbed and the surgical steps are directed at wide undermining, excision, and lateral cephalad tightening of the slack muscle and skin. True festooning must be differentiated from secondary "cheek pads" (also known as malar mounds, malar bags, pomettes, cheek bags, cheek pouches, or malar pads). These prominences at the malar eminence are formed of fat and connective-tissue fibers, and are associated with peripheral fibers of the orbicularis oculi. They are treated by defatting or liposuction with a small cannula. There is controversy as to whether they are actually retro orbicularis or mainly superficial to the orbicularis.

EXOPHTHALMOS

Only fat is removed in patients with exophthalmos; however, scleral show may still be the outcome. As with the upper lids, the approach is extremely conservative. The correction can sometimes accentuate the exophthalmic look even more. For severe cases with exposure problems, orbital rim implants and lateral or inferior orbital decompression will improve the projection. Symmetry is difficult.

MALAR HYPOPLASIA

Lower eyelid position, structure, function, and appearance depends on the relationship of the ocular globe, lower eyelid, and malar eminence. This relationship is crucial in planning lower-eyelid blepharoplasty (36). A positive relationship (positive vector) is when the most anterior projection of the globe lies behind the lower eyelid margin, which lies behind the anterior projection of the malar eminence. A negative relationship (negative vector) is when the most anterior projection of the globe lies anterior to the lower lid and malar eminence. These negative-vector patients often have scleral show. The hypoplastic malar eminence, with its associated negative support relationship, requires lower-lid and lateral tightening, with repositioning to obtain optimal results (36). Suborbital alloplastic augmentation has also been advocated to achieve optimal results in these difficult patients. Unlike the tear trough deformity (a cosmetic deformity resulting from an inadequate maxillary face), custom rim and prefabricated implants for the correction of inadequate projection have significant functional importance. It is difficult for the eyelid to function properly from an inadequate bony foundation. These rim implants for inadequate rim projection deformities can be custom-made or prefabricated (silicone or polyethylene) and are used in post trauma, Graves ophthalmopathy, and normal variation etiology reconstruction (17).

TEAR TROUGH DEFORMITIES

The nasojugal groove, or inadequate maxillary face, deformity (also referred to as the tear trough deformity) can be of congenital, developmental, or iatrogenic origin. When severe, it gives the eye an unaesthetic or morbid appearance. Flowers documents the groove extending well beyond its usual boundary (8). One of the causes appears to be a fixation of the orbital septum at the level of the inferior-medial portion of the arcus marginalis. In part, the groove is created by the triangular gap between the orbicularis and lateral border of the levator labia alequae nasi muscle. In youth, this gap is filled by fat. With the passage of time, atrophy of the fat occurs and the groove begins to deepen. Hamra has nicely demonstrated how to use fat sliding, orbicularis repositioning, and composite rhytidectomy to obliterate the groove. Loeb describe free fat grafts, as well as sliding fat grafts (37), to permit leveling of the groove. Flowers prefers tear trough implants of varying shapes and sizes to mask this deformity (38). The deformity can be corrected in conjunction with, or independent of, orbital rim augmentation.

LAUGH LINES, WRINKLES, AND CROWS' FEET

Patients must be informed that blepharoplasty alone will not improve fine wrinkles around the eyes. However, the wrinkles are less noticeable when the bags are removed. Eyelid peels are recommended by several authors, usually as a procedure after blepharoplasty for fine wrinkles. An interval of 4 to 6 weeks after surgery is recommended for optimal results. Procedures for crows' feet have been devised by Aston (39), Connell (40), and Camirand (41). All involve undermining the lateral orbicularis skin and transecting the sphincter. They are performed through a forehead lift, face-lift, or blepharoplasty incision.

Recent advances with botulinum neurotoxin have shown excellent temporary benefit in managing lateral canthal crows' feet, lower-eyelid orbicularis muscle folds, and glabellar folds (42). Injections range from 2 to 10 units and are placed directly into the muscles. Injections often need to be repeated every 3 months. There is risk of orbicularis and/or levator paralysis resulting in ectropion or ptosis if large doses are utilized.

FIG. 50–25. A, planes of dissection for lower blepharoplasty. **B,** skin flap between skin and muscle. **C,** skin-muscle flap between muscle and conjunctiva, exposing orbital septum.

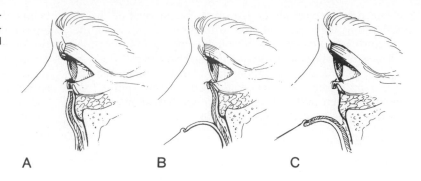

The ultra pulse CO_2 laser has been show by Weinstein and others to give improvement of crows' feet and periorbital rhytides. The results have been limited to the rhytides present in repose (static) and not movement (dynamic).

COLLAGEN

The efficacy and longevity of collagen injections around the eyes are still debatable. Most early reports indicate transitory and unsatisfactory results.

SURGICAL TECHNIQUE

There are four commonly used incisions in lower-eyelid blepharoplasty: The short subciliary incision from the punctum to the canthus (generally used for fat excision only), the extended subciliary incision from the punctum past the lateral canthus (generally used for fat removal, skin and muscle tightening, and canthopexy), and the transconjuctival incision (used for fat removal when no skin or muscle are to be excised) (Fig. 50–25). The fourth commonly used incision is the lateral canthopexy Z-plasty of Lewis (43). The use of stab wounds for fat removal has also been reported. This approach, as well as a transconjuctival approach, has a place in secondary lower-lid blepharoplasties when residual fat has been left behind.

There are basically two dissection planes: (a) the skin flap between the skin and the orbicularis muscle, and (b) the skin-muscle flap between the orbicularis muscle and the lower lid retractors-conjunctiva (Fig. 50–25). It is felt that a skin flap is necessary when redundant, crepey skin is present. When a skin flap is utilized, the removal of fat is achieved by a stab wound in the orbicularis. Conservative skin removal is the rule. It is helpful to place the lower lid slightly above the inferior limbus before excising skin. The skin-muscle flap technique without skin removal is our preference. It is important to leave as much pretarsal orbicularis intact, necessitating only a small amount of skin undermining, before cutting through the orbicularis; this helps preserve tone to the lower lid. This approach also allows muscle excision without skin excision in prominent ridges (44), and permits visualization of the nasojugal fold for fat or sliding, if needed.

We endorse a conservative approach to lower-lid surgery, using the short subciliary incision whenever possible. Some redundancy is preferable to scleral show. We also endorse a low threshold for lid-tightening procedures.

The lower lids are injected with 2 cc 1% Xylocaine, 1:100,000 adrenalin, and 1 cc Wydase. The incision is made with small straight ribbon scissors. A 5-0 silk suture is placed through the tarsal plate and behind the head as a traction suture; it is attached to a hemostat to facilitate dissection as the conjunctiva is held tense. The fat pockets are removed flush to the orbital rim when necessary. Fat is saved and, in the event of overresection, it can be placed as a free graft (44). Some observers believe that the normal youthful lower lid has a fullness below the lashes, and therefore suture orbicularis to the tarsal plate (45) or overlap orbicularis (46) to create fullness. The flap is then laid over the incision and excess tissue is removed.

Ristow advocates using a combination anterior-posterior approach to lower-lid blepharoplasty. This entails the use of a subciliary incision for skin excision and transconjunctival incision for fat removal. Others (and most oculoplastic surgeons) advocate a transconjunctival approach with chemical peel or CO_2 laser. Advantages include an intact orbital septum and orbicularis (middle lamellae) that contributes to immediate lower-eyelid support (17).

Patients with festoons, ptotic cheek fat/orbicularis muscle, thick orbicularis oculi muscles, or hyperpigmentation are not good candidates for transconjunctival blepharoplasty.

Complications of Blepharoplasty

DRY EYE SYNDROME

Postsurgical dry eye (recurrent bouts of irritation of the eyes with burning and itching) may occur. Those more prone to this condition include older patients, those with marginal lacrimal function, and those with exophthalmos. It is important to realize that any patient may experience a postoperative dry eye syndrome. A preoperative Schirmer test may be predictive of this outcome in those who are prone. An absence of lysosome in the tears is diagnostic of keratoconjunctivitis sicca (Sjögren syndrome) (47). Conservative therapy consists of lubricating the cornea and conjunctival surfaces with wetting agents. Medications with high viscosity (e.g., ointments) last longer but blur the vision. Treatment can include topical lubricants (polyvinylpyrrolidone, polyvinyl alcohol, methyl cellulose, or petroleum jelly), eye drops (1 to 2% polyvinylpyrrolidone, mucopolysaccharide), mucolytic agent (acetyl cysteine 10%), nighttime taping, patching, and protective contact lenses (scleral and soft) (7).

SCARRING

This complication is one that is fortunately rare. Black and Asian patients are more prone than whites to development of hypertrophic scars. Scars that extend beyond the orbital rim (thicker skin) have a greater propensity for scarring, thus extensions medially or laterally should be avoided. Hypertrophic scars, or web scars, usually respond to nonsurgical treatment such as pressure, massage, and/or judicious use of steroids.

CYST AND SUTURE TUNNELS

Inclusion cysts, or milia, commonly occur in areas of suture trauma. If they fail to resolve spontaneously they may be treated by unroofing, incision and drainage, or excision. Epithelial tunnels are secondary to leaving sutures in too long. They are treated by marsupialization of the tracts. Subcuticular closure will prevent these tunnels from forming (48).

PIGMENTARY PROBLEMS

After blepharoplasty, a hypopigmented scar may occur; it may be invisible or quite noticeable. When there is a fine reticular pattern of blood vessels in the eyelid skin before surgery, it may appear to the patient that the vessels are more visible after surgery. Actually, the skin is stretched over the vessels because the skin that formerly blended the vessels inconspicuously to brow skin has been removed, thus creating a sharp demarcation postoperatively.

Increased pigmentation is more often seen in the lower eyelids than the upper. It is usually seen in patients who have excessive bruising, hematomas, or slough caused by hemosiderin deposition. Increased telangiectasia may also be seen after subcutaneous dissection.

Dark circles have been attributed to increased pigment, increased vascularity, or shadowing. They are believed to be either congenital, postallergic, posttraumatic, or postinflammatory. Treatments include Retin A, hydroquinone, chemical peels, kojic acid, or cryotherapy. Vascular lesions have responded well to treatment with the candela laser at a wavelength of 585 nm. Experimental treatment of pigmented lesions with the Q-switched Ruby laser at 694 nm has also resulted in improved results (17). The dark circles that may appear in some Asian or dark-skinned patients may persist for 6 months or longer. Sunscreens are recommended, and bleaching agents may be of some benefit.

INFECTIONS

Fortunately, clinically significant infections are rare in the periorbital area because of the clean nature of the operation and excellent vascularity. Chronic blepharitis, although rare, may be aggravated by blepharoplasty. Ophthalmologic consultation is indicated for management. Any preexisting atopy can be aggravated; thus, postoperative cosmetics are restricted for at least 10 days. Orbital cellulitis progressing to blindness has been described after blepharoplasty.

PTOSIS

Ptosis may be produced by injury to the levator muscle during the procedure. More commonly it is transitory, associated with edema, hypotonicity, or supratarsal fixation, and resolves within 6 to 8 weeks. Orbicularis injury, as well as superior or inferior oblique paresis, have been reported.

BLEEDING

Bleeding can occur anywhere in the wound, but most often is associated with the incisions from the cut orbicularis oculi muscle.

Acute periorbital hematomas may occur immediately after injection and are controlled by digital pressure. Localized periorbital hematomas presenting in the postoperative period should be evacuated at the bedside or in the office. Diffuse hematomas are slowly reabsorbed during a 2-week period. The resorption may be assisted by warm compresses. A subscleral hematoma (red eye) usually resolves spontaneously and may benefit from warm compresses. The retrobulbar hematoma is a rare occurrence and has been related to transient and permanent visual disturbances (49). Blood seeps into the orbit and compromises the fine ciliary vessels to the optic nerve. All cases of blindness are associated with an unrecognized hematoma.

The symptoms of retrobulbar hemorrhage consist of mydriasis, chemosis, proptosis, and pain (50). Pain is the predominant symptom. The eye may be woody, firm, and not ballottable. Conjunctival capillaries become injected, and extraocular movements may be limited. Visual loss may or may not occur. Retrobulbar hematomas may result from unusually deep or "blind" injection into the fat compartments or from excessive traction on the fat. Treatment involves opening and exploring the wound, opening the septum widely, and lateral canthotomy with cantholysis, 20% mannitol intravenously (2 mg/kg, the first 12.5 mg given over 3 to 4 minutes), 500 mg acetazolamide intravenously (continue Diamox 250 mg orally every 6 hours for 3 days), inhalatation of 95% oxygen and 5% carbon dioxide, decadron 10 mg, and ophthalmologic consultation (51). Treatment rarely involves orbital exploration with bony decompression. Anterior chamber paracentesis has a limited role and is associated with many complications. If managed appropriately within 10 to 12 hours, visual loss is usually restored within minutes to hours.

To prevent blindness, the surgeon must prevent bleeding. Useful maneuvers include: opening the septum widely, avoiding buttonhole incisions, careful hemostasis, avoiding face-down position postoperatively, and monitoring ocular vital signs.

DIPLOPIA AND ENOPHTHALMOS

Injury to the inferior or superior oblique muscles during fat removal has resulted in visual disturbances consisting of diplopia or double vision. Diplopia can result from deep scarring secondary to overaggressive fat excision in lower-lid blepharoplasty. The inferior rectus muscle may become scarred to the orbital rim, or transected, in transconjunctival approaches. Patients with deeply set eyes and prominent orbital rims are predisposed to a "skeletonized appearance" if excessive fat is removed. Correction of this deformity is both difficult and disappointing.

LAGOPHTHALMOS

Inability to close the eyes completely is not unusual in the postoperative period. This condition may require taping, artificial tears, and possibly Lacri-Lube if corneal abrasion is imminent. It is usually temporary and self-limiting, requiring no treatment.

CLOSED-ANGLE GLAUCOMA

This entity has been reported as a complication of blepharoplasty by Green and Kadri (52). The glaucoma may be precipitated by the operation. This occurrence may be avoided by careful preoperative history, and measurement of intraocular pressure when indicated. Patients who have glaucoma have a history of pain around the eye, ocular irritation, conjunctival infections, headaches, nausea, and vomiting. They may or may not have visual loss, field defects, or blurring (7).

LOSS OF EYELASHES

Eyelash loss is usually produced by infection, cutting the bulbs of the lashes during incision, dissection while injecting with local anesthetics, or cauterization (7). Numb eyelashes in female patients using mascara is frequent and usually self-limiting.

ASYMMETRY

Before surgery, the patient must be evaluated for asymmetry, ptosis, and pseudoptosis (one tarsal crease lower than the other, simulating ptosis). All patients have asymmetry, some more than others. Symmetrical operations on asymmetrical eyelids will magnify the deformity. Iatrogenic asymmetry can result from unequal skin excisions and malposition of incisions or supratarsal creases.

LID CONTOUR IRREGULARITIES

Irregularities are possible from both incomplete and excessive excision of fat. Incomplete excision is treated by repeat surgury to remove the fat. Depressions can be treated by free-fat grafting, fat sliding, or the like (36,37).

POSTOPERATIVE EDEMA AND INDURATION

Edema is caused by interruption of lymphatics in the lateral portions of the eyelids and is seen most commonly after extensive submuscular dissections. Conjunctival edema (chemosis) is usually caused by wide undermining of the orbicularis muscle. Extensive edema may lead to conjunctival prolapse, which can be irritating to the patient. This is managed by warm compresses, diuretics, steroid drops, lid exercises, and eyelid patching during sleep. It may last for several months.

RETRACTION (SCLERAL SHOW)

The most common complication of lower-eyelid blepharoplasty is lower-eyelid retraction with middle lamellar shortening. The middle lamella (orbital septum) becomes scarred and vertically shortened. Patients with laxity of the lower eyelids are predisposed to develop this complication if it is unaddressed at the time of surgery. Treatment is the same as for ectropion and involves lysis of the middle lamellar cicatrix and resuspension with or without an autogenous spacer.

ECTROPION

Ectropion of the lower eyelid may be temporary (secondary to healing and wound edema), and may last several months or be permanent. Early postoperative ectropion is common in the lateral portion of the lower eyelid, and is caused by a combination of edema, wound contraction, muscular hypotonicity from dissection or injection, and possibly by partial denervation of the orbicularis muscle (7).

Temporary ectropion usually subsides in a few weeks. If persistent, it should be treated with taping, exercises, massages, and corneal protection. Causes of permanent ectropion include: excessive skin, muscle, or fat resection; middle lamella (septum) contracture with vertical shortening; scar fixation of lid to orbital floor; gravitational drag of cheek on the lid, paresis of orbicularis muscle; postoperative hematoma; orbicularis contracture; or, it may have no discernable cause (7).

Patients who are prone to develop ectropion demonstrate scleral show and lid hypotonicity preoperatively. They should be managed conservatively with a procedure to increase lower-lid support. These procedures have included muscle plication, suspension, dermocanthal support, tarsal plate resection, or lateral canthal elevation.

A round eye with scleral show, inferior displacement, and lower eyelid retraction (with or without ectropion) predictably occurs in the small but significant percentage of patients with a lax lower eyelid not addressed at the time of blepharoplasty. These patients often require skin grafts and canthal, as well as lower-eyelid, tightening techniques. Some continue to be unhappy and present the plastic surgeon with the most difficult of challenges. The Madame Butterfly procedure with hard-palate graft spacer serves as a superior alternative in dealing with these complex secondary cases (53,54).

EPIPHORA

Epiphora may be produced by hypersecretion of tears or improper processing of tears. Blepharoplasty itself causes a temporary reflex hypersecretion of tears from the lacrimal gland. Corneal irritation or abrasion may also cause a hypersecretion. Improper processing may be produced by hypotonicity of the orbicularis from injection, injury to the lacrimal punctum, ectropion, or lagophthalmos (7).

HOLLOW SUNKEN ORBIT

The overdone upper eyelid is perhaps the most difficult of all problems to correct. It is more commonly encountered in patients with deep-set eyes. Pearl fat grafts have been described as a method of soft-tissue augmentation, with variable and highly unpredictable results. Only careful sculpting of fat with an understanding of gravitational changes can help prevent this deformity from occurring.

References

1. Stephenson KL. The history of blepharoplasty to correct blepharochalasis. *Aesthet Plast Surg* 1977; 1:177.
2. Onizuka T, Iwanami M. Blepharoplasty in Japan. *Aesthet Plast Surg* 1984; 8:97–100.
3. Doxanas MT, Anderson RL. Oriental eyelids. *Arch. Ophthalmol.* 1984; 102:1232–1235.
4. Hisatomi C. Anatomical considerations concerning blepharoplasty in the Oriental patient. *Adv Ophthal Plast Reconstr Surg* 1983; 2:151–165.
5. Uchida J. A surgical procedure for blepharoptosis vera and for pseudoblepharoptosis orientalis. *Br J Plast Surg* 1962; 15:271–276.
6. Sayoc BT. Blepharochalasis in upper eyelids, including its classification. *Am J Ophthal* 1957; 43:970.
7. Klatsky S, Cohen M, eds. *Mastery of plastic and reconstructive surgery.* New York: Kuttke Brown, 1994.
8. Flowers S. Diagnosing photographic distortion: decoding true postoperative contour after eyelid surgery. *Clin Plast Surg* 1993; 20:387–392.
9. Rees TD. *Aesthic plastic surgery.* Vol. 11. Philaelphia: WB Saunders, 1980.
10. Wilkins RB. Evaluation of the blepharoplasty patient. *Ophthalmology (Rochester)* 1978; 85:73.
11. Flowers R. Correction of lower lid laxity by tightening the canthal ligament. Maui, Hawaii, California Plastic Surgery Society, 1984.
12. Putterman AM, Urist MJ. Baggy eyelids: a true hernia. *Ann Ophthal* 1974; 6:290.

13. Wilkins RB, Hunter GJ, McCord CD, et al. Blepharoplasty: cosmetic and functional. In: McCord CD, Tanenbaum M, eds. *Oculoplastic surgery.* New York: Raven Press, 1987; 451. Single stitch, nonincision technique. *Plast Reconstr Surg* 1989; 83:236.

14. Dresner SC. Comprehensive Blepharoplasty Options and Finesse Symposium, Jules Stein Eye Institute UCLA, Feb 17, 18, 1995.

15. Kaye BL. The forehead lift: a useful adjunct to facelift and blepharoplasty. *Plast Reconstr Surg* 1977; 60:161.

16. Flowers S, Caputy G. Flowers S. The biomechanics of brow and frontalis function and its effect on blepharoplasty. *Clin Plast Surg* 1993; 20:2.

17. Shorr N, Bayliss HI, Goldberg RA. Comprehensive cosmetic blepharoplasty. Options and Finesse Symposium, Jules Stein Eye Institute, UCLA, February 1995.

18. Connell BF, Lambros VS, Neuohr HG. The forehead lift: techniques to avoid complications and produce optimal results. *Aesth Plast Surg* 1989; 13:217–238.

19. Papillon J. The subcutaneous browlift. Presented at Pan Pacific Surgical Association, Honolulu, January 1988.

20. Washio H, Giampapa V, Colen H. Foreheadplasty: a selective approach. *Ann Plast Surg* 1982; 8:141.

21. McCord CD, Doxanas MT. Browplasty and browpexy: an adjunct to blepharoplasty. *Plast Reconstr Surg* 1990; 86:248.

22. Loikol AB, Sokol TP. Transblepharoplasty brow suspension. *Plast Reconstr Surg* 1982; 69:940.

23. Knize DM, Transpalpebral approach to the corrugator supercilii and procerus muscles *Plast Reconstr Surg* 1995; 95:52.

24. Ellenbogen R. Transcoronal eyebrow lift with concomitant upper blepharoplasty. *Plast Reconstr Surg* 1983; 71:490.

25. McKenney P, et al. Mathematics of the forehead lift. Presented at the 22nd annual meeting of the American Society of Aesthetic Plastic Surgery, Orlando, April 1989.

26. McKenney P, Mossie RD, Zukowsky ML. Criteria for the forehead lift. *Aesthet Plast Surg* 1991; 15:141.

27. Shorr N, Seiff S. In: Hornblass, ed. *Oculoplastic surgery management of eyebrow ptosis.* New York: Williams & Wilkins, 1989.

28. Ellenbogan R. Transcoronal eyebrow lift: a technique to minimize postoperative complaints. *Plast Surg Techniques* 1995; 1:1.

29. Hinderer UT. Correction of weakness of the lower eyelid and lateral canthus. *Clin Plast Surg* 1993; 20:2.

30. Tomlinson FB, Hovey LM. Transconjunctival lower lid blepharoplasty for removal of fat. *Plast Reconstr Surg* 1975; 56:314.

31. Ristow B. Cohen M, ed. *Mastery of plastic surgery.* New York: Little, Brown, 1994.

32. Mendelson BC. Herniated fat and the orbital septum of the lower lid. *Clin Plast Surg* 1993; 20:2.

33. Camirand A. Plastic surgery of the eyelids: operative techniques. *Plast Reconstr Surg* 1994; Nov.

34. Casson P, Siebert J. Lower lid blepharoplasty with skin flap and muscle split. *Clin Plast Surg* 1988; 15:299.

35. Loeb R. Aesthetic blepharoplasties based on the degree of wrinkling. *Plast Reconstr Surg* 1971; 47:33.

36. Jelks GW, Jelks EB. Preoperative evaluation of the blepharoplasty patient. *Clin Plast Surg* 1993; 20:2.

37. Loeb R. Fat pad sliding and fat grafting for leveling lid depressions. *Clin Plast Surg* 1981; 8:4, 757.

38. Flowers S. Tear trough implants for correction of tear trough deformity. *Clin Plast Surg* 1993; 20:23.

39. Aston SJ. Orbicularis oculi muscle flaps: a technique to reduce crows' feet and lateral canthal skin folds. *Plast Reconstr Surg* 1980; 65:206.

40. Connell BF, Marten TJ. Surgical correction of the crows' feet deformity. *Clin Plast Surg* 1993; 20:2.

41. Camirand A. Treatment of dynamic crows' feet while performing a blepharoplasty. *Aesthet Plast Surg* 1993; 17:17–21.

42. Guyuron B, Huddleston SW. Aesthetic indications for botulinum toxin injection. *Plast Reconstr Surg* 1994; 93:913–918.

43. Lewis JR Jr. The Z-blepharoplasty. *Plast Reconstr Surg* 1969; 44:331.

44. Loeb R. Necessity for partial resection of the orbicularis oculi muscle in blepharoplasties is some young patients. *Plast Reconstr Surg* 1977; 60:176.

45. Sheen JH. Tarsal fixation in lower blepharoplasty. *Plast Reconstr Surg* 1978; 62:24.

46. Bela Fodor P. Lower lid "tarsal fixation" blepharoplasty: a personal technique. *Aesth Plast Surg* 1989; 13:273–277.

47. Graham WP, Mesner KH, Miller SH. Keratoconjunctivitis sicca symptoms appearing after blepharoplasty. *Plast Reconstr Surg* 1976; 57:57.

48. Morgan SC. Orbital cellulitis and blindness following a blepharoplasty. *Plast Reconstr Surg* 1982; 69:823.

49. DeMere M. Blindness and eyelid survey. *Aesthet Plast Surg* 1978; 2:41.

50. Hepler RS, Sugimura GI, Straatsma BR. Discussion of "successful early relief of blindness occurring after blepharoplasty," by Hueston H. *Plast Reconstr Surg* 1976; 57:223.

51. Carraway JH, Miller JR. Treatment and prevention of complications of blepharoplasty. *Perspectives in Plastic Surgery* 1994; 8:1–24.

52. Green MF, Kadri SW. Acute closed angle glaucoma. A complication of blepharoplasty: report of a case. *Br J Plast Reconstr Surg* 1974; 27:25.

53. Shorr N. Madame Butterfly procedure with hard palate graft. *Facial Plastic Surgery* 1994; 10:1.

54. Shorr N, Fallor MK. "Madame Butterfly" procedure: combined with cheek and lateral canthal suspension procedure for post blepharoplasty "round eye" and lower eyelid retraction. *Ophthal Plast Reconstr Surg* 1985; 1:229–235.

51

Facial Contouring: The Next Generation

Edward O. Terino, M.D., F.A.C.S., L.L.D. and Mark Vincent Sofonio, M.D.

Earlier chapters on chin and cheek implants have considered these techniques ancillary, or accessory. But recent technology enables surgeons rapidly to design and manufacture anatomically styled silastic implants that accurately imitate nature's subtle facial contours. The ability to use these implants safely and with minimal morbidity has elevated facial contouring to a primary and essential level.

Three-dimensional "sculpturing" procedures are a new development in facial plastic surgery. These techniques include jowl and neck fat removal, as well as repositioning of the malar fat pad. In addition, subperiosteal and endoscopic lifting techniques to alter facial contour are gaining popularity (1). These recent techniques attempt to create three-dimensional changes in facial structure through soft-tissue manipulations; consequently, they suffer from lack of permanence. In contrast, alloplastic facial augmentation produces permanent and effective three-dimensional alterations in facial contour with low risk and minimal morbidity. Moreover, the advantages of alloplastic techniques versus craniofacial autologous osseous engineering include their ready exchangeability and reversibility. These qualities provide a generous margin of safety and flexibility, so that the variations of surgical judgment and the imprecisions in physician-patient communications—which can produce different end results, sometimes unsatisfactory to the patient—can be corrected if necessary.

The Significance of Facial Contouring

Strong skeletal contours enhance beauty. Redraping and redistributing the soft tissues over a strong facial skeleton enhances restoration and rejuvenation of the face. Augmentation of the midface with implants of permanent volume can alter the atrophic soft-tissue changes that produce a sunken, drawn look. Hereditary midfacial structure can also produce this unattractive appearance and can be similarly corrected. This alloplastic skeletal augmentation is called "surgery of the 4th plane" because it is performed on the basic bony foundation above which lie the other three planes: (a) skin, (b) fat, (c) superficial musculoaponeurotic system (SMAS) (2).

This 4th- plane surgery of the face depends on the unique implantation of volumetric alloplastic implants. Utilization of different shapes and sizes and placement in differing positions alters facial contours in a designated and controlled fashion that produces predictable results. Dividing the facial skeleton into specific zones of anatomy assists the surgeon both in choosing appropriate implants and placing them properly to achieve a desired effect.

This chapter describes the concepts and techniques of using alloplastic implants which we have developed over the last 15 years to augment the malar, midface, and premandible regions. We will also present further considerations on premaxillary augmentation.

Facial Aesthetics and Volume-Mass Relationships

The position, shape, form, and color of accessory aesthetic facial units (e.g., eyes, eyebrows, lips, hair) against a skeletal framework of certain volume-mass promontories are what determines the sociocultural determination that a face is beautiful, attractive, or unattractive. A gross imbalance of these elements is considered "ugly."

The most important facial promontories are (a) the malar, midface prominence, (b) the nasal size and projection, (c) the entire mass of the lower-third facial segment (jawline and mandible segment), and (d) of lesser significance, the supraorbital brow ridges (3) (Fig. 51–1).

The essential principle of facial aesthetics is the appreciation of the fundamental laws governing an aesthetic balance of the volume-mass relationships in the face. These laws are straightforward. Altering any one of the three facial bony promontories directly and inversely affects the aesthetic importance of the others. When one structure is larger and takes up more space, another appears relatively diminished. As nasal significance is reduced, malar and mandibular volume and projection assume more importance. Two or more significant masses further reduce the size significance of the 3rd (or 4th). By accenting the malar, midface complex, the surgeon diminishes the significance of the nose and chin. By enhancing both the mandibular and malar areas, the surgeon effectively reduces the relative magnitude of the nose. Thus, the architectural laws of proportion dictate that the strength of the mass and volume characteristics of each promontory affects the relative balance of one to the other. Simultaneous changes in more than one have even greater significance than altering one alone.

Applications of Balance Principles

Patients with round, full, fleshy facial contours and an abundance of subcutaneous tissues and fat rarely appear beautiful by contemporary standards. Lean-faced individuals with a long facial contour often have inadequate skeletal promontories in the malar and/or mandibular region, as well as deficient midfacial submalar soft tissue. These faces have aes-

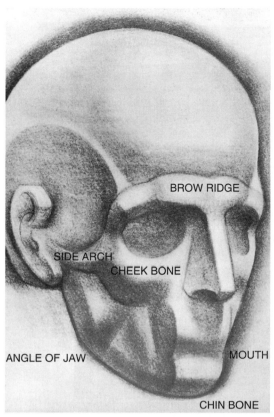

FIG. 51–1. Major facial promontories in artist's rendition of contemporary man.

FIG. 51
malar (z

thetic imbalance (Fig. 51–2). Both of these facial types, and persons with combinations of these deficiencies, can see significant improvement when the volume-mass balance of the skeletal promontories is rearranged by alloplastic onlay techniques.

Extensive experience has conclusively demonstrated to us that the volume of augmentation necessary to produce a significant change in appearance is considerable and requires much larger alloplastic implants in the malar, midface, and premandible region than were previously considered necessary. Additionally, alterations in the size, shape, and positioning of these implants, even to a minor degree, create significant yet subtle nuances of change in the appearance of the human face.

Analysis by Zonal Principles

To facilitate an analysis of facial aesthetics, zonal principles of skeletal anatomy in the malar-midface and premandible regions was developed (4). Zonal analysis enables the surgeon to choose implant size and shape and to determine positioning with certainty.

The malar space is that part of the face which, when augmented appropriately, produces an aesthetic change in cheek and midface contour (Fig. 51–3). To determine how to augment this space, it is useful to think of the malar-midface aesthetic unit in five distinct anatomic zones (Fig. 51–4).

Zone 1 covers the largest surface area and includes the major portion of the malar bone and the first third of the zy-

gomatic arch. Augmentation of zone 1 produces the greatest volumetric filling of the upper cheek and maximizes anterior-posterior projection of the malar eminence (Fig. 51–5).

Zone 2 overlies the middle third of the zygomatic arch. Enhancement of this zone, along with zone 1, increases accentuation of the cheekbone laterally, giving greater width to the upper third of the face. This creates a high-arched appearance that is particularly useful for individuals with a narrow upper face or a long face. It should be noted, however, that when zones 1 and 2 are overaugmented an abnormal, unattractive, knobby protuberance or "skeletal" appearance may result (Fig. 51–6).

Zone 3 is the paranasal area that lies midway between the infraorbital foramen and the nasal pyramid. A vertical line drawn downward from the infraorbital foramen marks the medial extent of the usual dissection for malar augmentation. This line also represents the lateral border of zone 3. When paranasal augmentation occurs in zone 3, it produces medial fullness to the face—often in the upper-medial nasolabial area, which can be unattractive, producing a "chipmunk-cheek" effect. The skin and subcutaneous tissues are thin in that region. Consequently, any implant placed there must be extremely tapered and perfectly positioned. Augmentation of zone 3 may be indicated for reconstructive purposes (e.g. following trauma, or to correct hereditary deficiencies).

Zone 4 overlies the posterior third of the zygomatic arch. Augmentation in this area is never needed and would produce an unnatural appearance. Moreover, dissection there is dangerous because the tissues are adherent to the bone and there is a possibility of injury to the zygomatic and temporal branches of the facial nerve, as well as to the temporomandibular joint (TMJ) capsule itself. Symptoms and deformities have resulted from operations in this area (5).

Zone 5, the submalar zone or "submalar triangle," is bounded posteriorly by the tendinous origins of the masseter muscles and the canine fossa of the maxilla. The superior boundary is the inferior bony margin of the malar eminence, which constitutes the first two-thirds of the zygomatic arch. The medial extent of the submalar space ends at the lateral border of the nasolabial mound and sulcus. Its roof consists of the inferomedial portion of the entire malar space. It contains overlying facial musculature fat and soft tissue of the midface region. The inferior border is a lower limit selected by the surgeon where the natural dissection plane is terminated that separates the masseter from the overlying facial musculature. This lower-limit dissection sulcus is similar to that created in breast augmentation; it determines the inferior aspect of midfacial contour fullness. Dissection and implant placement into this lower sulcus is required to simulate soft-tissue restoration within the midface by alloplastic implants.

Natural aging, as well as hereditary characteristics, cause soft-tissue deficiency deformities in the midface region. These are accentuated by the overhanging prominence of the solid maxillary malar eminence, as well as by the medial, downward sagging of the nasolabial mound. The result is a midface sulcus or depression that defines and underlies a submalar zone. In many individuals, midfacial atrophy creates a tired or haggard appearance, even at ages in the thirties and forties. Augmentation within the submalar zone beneath this soft-tissue sulcus brings back a fuller, rounder, and more youthful contour (Fig. 51–7).

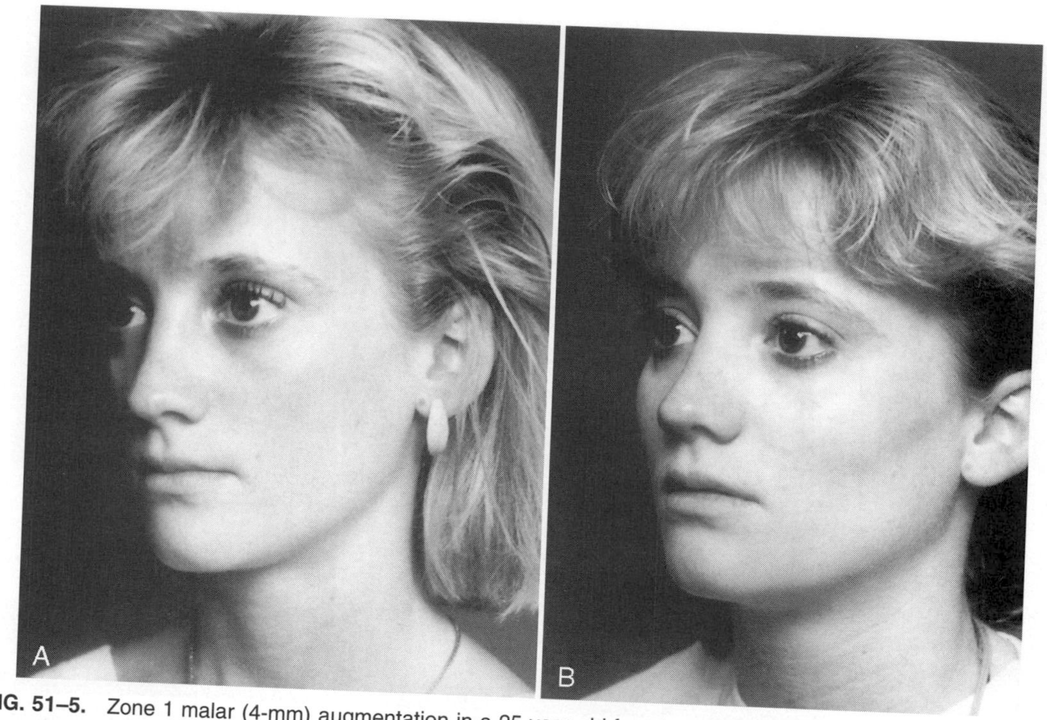

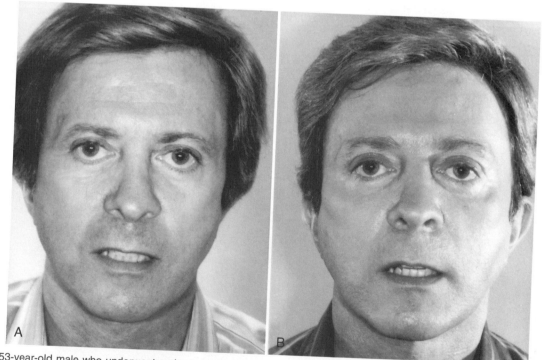

FIG. 51–5.   Zone 1 malar (4-mm) augmentation in a 25-year-old female. Note increase in relative anterior posterior projection of the malar eminence.

FIG. 51–6.   A 53-year-old male who underwent malar augmentation with traditional small, high-profile implants. The patient is left with a skeletal appearance. Contemporary Terino implants are wider and have smaller profiles (cf. Fig. 51–11).

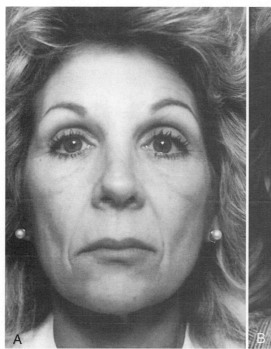 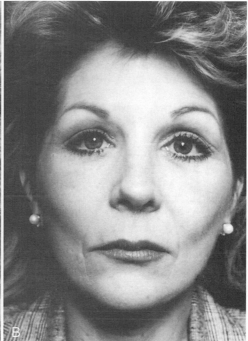

FIG. 51–7. A 52-year-old female with midface submalar triangle soft-tissue deficiency whose youthful appearance was restored by malar and submalar (zone 1 and SM, 4 mm) augmentation. Rhytidectomy was also performed.

The use of a large shell implant in the submalar zone effectively recreates the patient's maxillary architecture (Fig. 51–8). A contoured implant that extends down over the inferior border of the malar bone creates additional vertical length from the lateral canthus down into the midcheek, submalar region. This not only gives the illusion of correcting the midfacial soft-tissue deficiency but also appears to augment the overall size of the patient's own malar bone structure, especially vertically. When the malar shell is positioned slightly higher in zone 1, over the inferior aspect of the malar bone, and extended downward into the submalar zone, a completely united, full, round "apple cheek" contour is created.

Types of Midfacial Deformities

An alternative method of facial analysis was developed by Binder (6). This classification into types of midfacial appearances is essentially correct. Because of its usefulness, it is reprinted here with certain modifications in Table 51–1.

A type 1 pattern consists of patients with insufficient malar and suborbital skeletal development who do possess good midfacial soft-tissue fullness (Fig. 51–9). There is basic deficiency in the zone 1, zone 2, and possibly zone 3 regions. Malar shell implants are chosen to augment the malar-zygomatic promontory and perhaps even the suborbital deficiency.

A type 2 facial pattern consists of midfacial soft-tissue deficiency in the submalar zone 5, in the presence of adequate zone 1 and zone 2 malar development (Fig. 51–10). Correction of this deficiency consists of placing malar shells of various sizes and thickness, 1 to 2 cm inferior to the lower border of the malar bone, over the masseter tendon. In this location they provide anterior projection for a flat face.

Alloplastic augmentation into submalar zone 5 is the most frequently needed procedure for improving facial contour.

When a generous-size shell is placed into the lower aspect of zones 1 and 2, as well as downward into the submalar zone, a round, full, apple-cheek contour results. Augmentation of the submalar space alone restores the soft-tissue deterioration of the aging face to a more youthful fullness. Frequent use of submalar augmentation is mandatory for the surgeon who wishes to maximize alloplastic augmentation contour modalities for the patient's best advantage.

Type 3 deficiency is a more extreme version of type 2 and is rare (Fig. 51–11). It consists of dramatically prominent malar eminences accompanied by severe volumetric deficiency in the submalar aspect of the midfacial unit. This patient often has thin skin and spare soft tissues. An abrupt transition from the strong malar bone to an area of extreme deficiency and hollowness within the submalar region makes the patient appear extremely gaunt, emaciated, and skeletal. Two-dimensional rhytidectomy skin-tightening techniques can only accentuate this unattractive appearance.

Type 4 is rare and is represented in the combination of severe malar-suborbital hypogenesis, as well as deficiency of the midfacial soft-tissue aesthetic unit (Fig. 51–12). This volume deficient midface requires augmentation of both the malar and midface zones (1 and submalar 5). In this situation a large shell or combined implant augments both the malar eminence and the submalar triangle. Occasionally, it is useful to add augmentation of zone 2, the mid aspect of the zygomatic arch, in order to broaden a narrow face.

Type 5 facial deficiency consists of significant suborbital bone deficiency with a visible arcus marginalis attachment that creates a shadowed infraorbital sulcus or valley. This is frequently medial in the zone 3 (tear-trough) region and requires augmentation to correct. This can be either autologous or alloplastic.

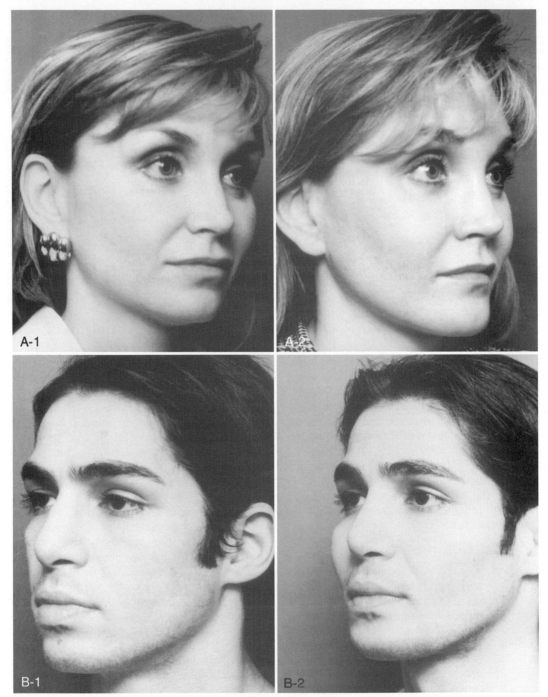

FIG. 51–8. A, 25-year-old female with mild submalar deficiency. Augmentation of SM zone 5 with a 3-mm implant affords the patient a fuller and rounder facial appearance. Vertical-extension chin implant also placed (4 mm). **B,** 25-year-old male who desired strong chin, nasal and malar prominences. Small malar (zones 1 and 2, 4 mm) implants and 5-mm anatomic chin implant improved cheek projection to create aesthetic balance.

Table 51–1
Patterns of Midfacial Deformities Correlated Anatomic Facial Zones and Types of Implants

Deformity Midfacia	Description of Zonal Facial Deficiency	Type of Implant Required	Type of Implant Used
Type I Zones 1 & 2	Primary malar hypoplasia; adequate submalar fullness	Requires projection over the malar eminence (Zones 1, 2)	Malar Implant: Terino "shell type" which can also extend into submalar space for more natural result
Type II Zones SM 5 & Lower Zone 1	Submalar deficiency; Flattened appearance Adequate malar bones	Requires anterior projection. Implant placed over face of maxilla and masseter tendon in submalar space. Provides midfacial fill.	Implant placed in midfacial region (Submalar)
Type III Zone SM5	Extreme malar-zygomatic prominence with abrupt transition to a deep submalar recess, usually thin skin	Requires creation of smooth anatomic transition between malar and submalar regions; (Lower Zone I and SM5)	Large Shell Augmentation Submalar implant (generation II): more refined; U-shaped to fit within submalar space and around inferior border of prominent zygoma within submalar space
Type IV Zones 1, 2 & SM5	"Volume Deficient" Face— A "Combined" Deformity Malar hypoplasia Submalar deficiency	Requires anterior and lateral projection; "volume replacement Implant; for entire midface restructuring	Jumbo "Combined" submalar-malar shell Implant: provides lateral (malar), and anterior (submalar) projection. Fills large midface void
Type V	Infraorbital "Tear Trough" deformity (suborbital rim depression or recess)	Requires site-specific augmentation over entire infraorbital rim	Tear-trough Implant; to fit site-specific suborbital hollowness
Type VI Premaxilla	Premaxilla Peripyriform Deficiency	Peripyriform Augmentation (Premaxilla and Lateral nasal base)	Unique Peripyriform Design (Brink)

Modified from Binder WS. A comprehensive approach for aesthetic contouring of the midface in rhytidectomy. *Facial Plastic Surgery Clinics of North America* 1993; 1:231.

A type 6 face has a retrusive central maxillary appearance. This facial deficiency is a lesser variant of a cleft lip and nose deformity (a Crouzon appearance). A peripyriform premaxillary alloplastic augmentation can successfully improve this deficiency.

A thorough understanding of (a) the zones of facial anatomy, (b) their interrelationships, and (c) the six facial types, gives the surgeon the ability to create a variety of facial contours that accommodate each patient's individual needs or desires. The three critical parameters which the surgeon must control, of course, are (a) appropriate choice of implant shape, (b) size, and (c) precision zonal placement.

Zonal Anatomy of the Lower Third Aesthetic Facial Unit

Recently improved chin augmentation techniques now enable surgeons to augment the entire premandible contour from angle to angle. Anatomic extensions onto a central implant create a lateral widening in the lower third aesthetic facial unit. Traditional implants were placed centrally between the mental foramina and often produced an abnormal, unattractive, round protuberance (7). Traumatic transection of the origins of the mentalis muscle during these procedures can allow downward dislocation of the overlying soft-tissue mound and musculature to produce a "witch's chin," or drooping chin deformity (Fig. 51–13). This is more likely in patients who have an inherited round, globular, and protuberant central soft-tissue chin mound. This central protuberance becomes even more aesthetically undesirable during the process of aging as the patient develops an adjacent lateral "prejowl sulcus" where the central chin mound is separated by the anterior masseteric ligament from the more lateral sagging lower cheek jowl elements (skin, SMAS, and fat). This sulcus is also known as the "marionette groove," or the anterior mandibular sulcus (8).

Aesthetically correct augmentation of the jawline is best achieved when one understands the zonal anatomy of the mandible (Fig. 51–14).

The "premandible space" is that anatomic region of the lower face which when volumetrically augmented creates significant contour alterations in the shape and volume of the lower third of the face and the entire jawline (Fig. 51–15).

The central mentum between the mental nerves can be considered zone 1. Zone 2 extends into the middle of the lateral aspect of the horizontal ramus to the region of the oblique line. With the use of "extended anatomic contour" implants into this zone, the surgeon gains the ability to widen

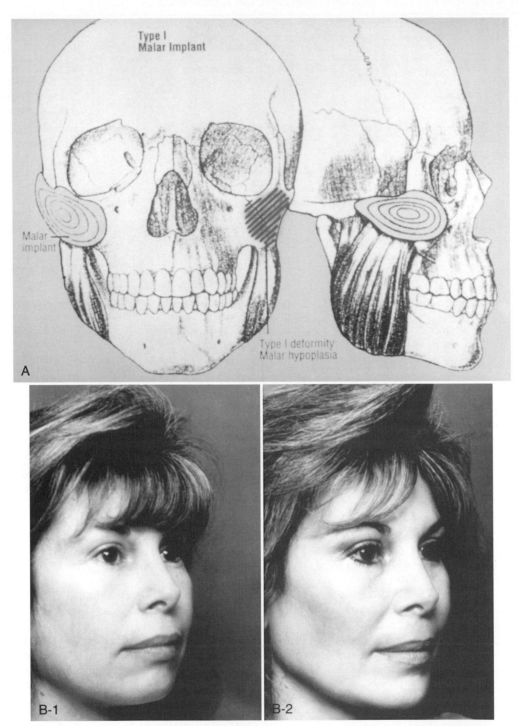

FIG. 51–9.   A, type I facial deficiency of left malar eminence. Correction of this deficiency is accomplished by zones 1 and 2 augmentation. (From Binder WJ. A comprehensive approach for aesthetic contouring of the midface in rhytidectomy. *Facial Plastic Surgery Clinics of North America* 1993; 1:231–255.) **B,** 45-year-old female with type I deficiency. Correction with zones 1 and 2 (4 mm) augmentation. Chin implant also placed.

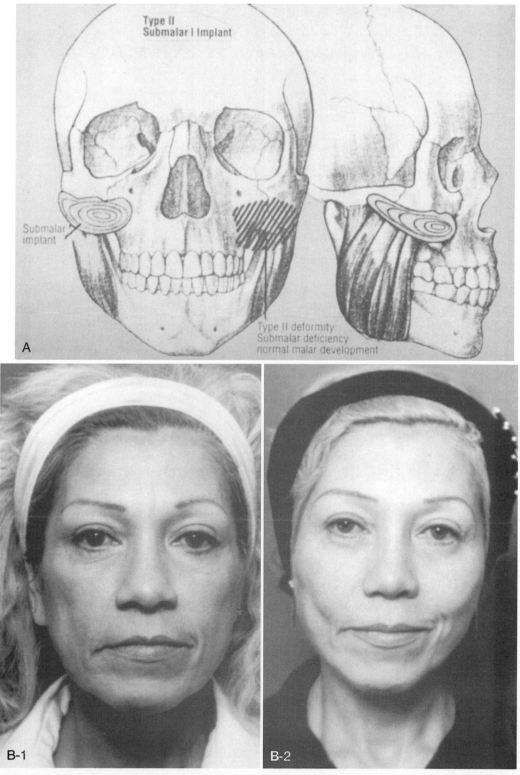

FIG. 51–10.   A, type II submalar deficiency with normal malar eminence (anterior and posterior illustration). Lateral drawing illustrates submalar zone (SM) position of the submalar implant. (From Binder WJ. A comprehensive approach for aesthetic contouring of the mid-face in rhytidectomy. *Facial Plastic Surgery Clinics of North America* 1993; 1:231–255.) **B,** 58-year-old female with type II deficiency corrected by submalar (4 mm) augmentation.

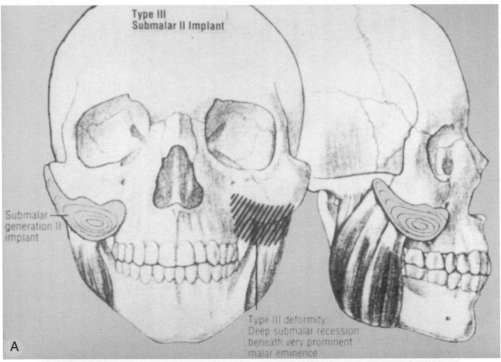

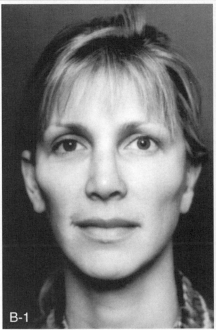
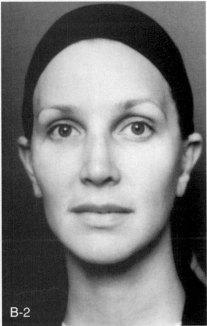

FIG. 51–11. **A,** type III marked submalar deficiency with marked malar prominence. This deformity is rarely encountered naturally, but can be created artificially by improper malar augmentation of zone 1. (From Binder WJ. A comprehensive approach for aesthetic contouring of the midface in rhytidectomy. *Facial Plastic Surgery Clinics of* *North America* 1993; 1:231–255.) **B,** 36-year-old female with a type III deformity from misplaced, overaugmented zone 1 malar implant. Aesthetic balance was achieved by appropriate malar and submalar (zone 1 and SM, 4 mm) midface contouring.

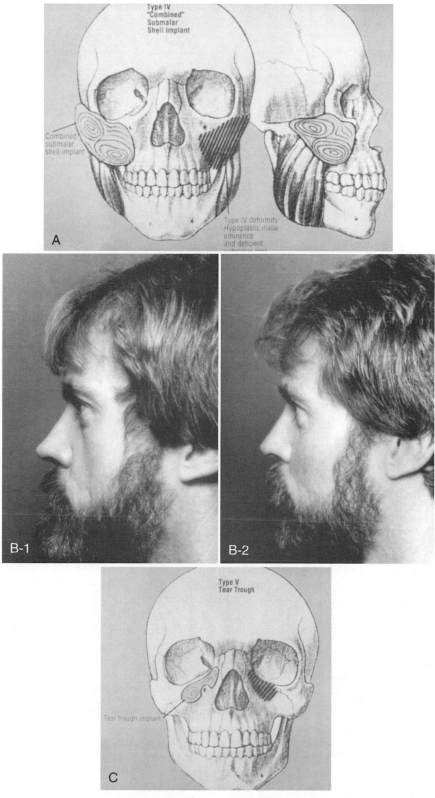

FIG. 51–12. **A,** type IV combined submalar and malar deficiency. (From Binder WJ. A comprehensive approach for aesthetic contouring of the midface in rhytidectomy. *Facial Plastic Surgery Clinics of North America* 1993; 1:231–255.) **B,** 40-year-old male with type IV volume deficiency corrected by combined malar and submalar augmentation, 5-mm implant. **C,** type V tear-trough deficiency.

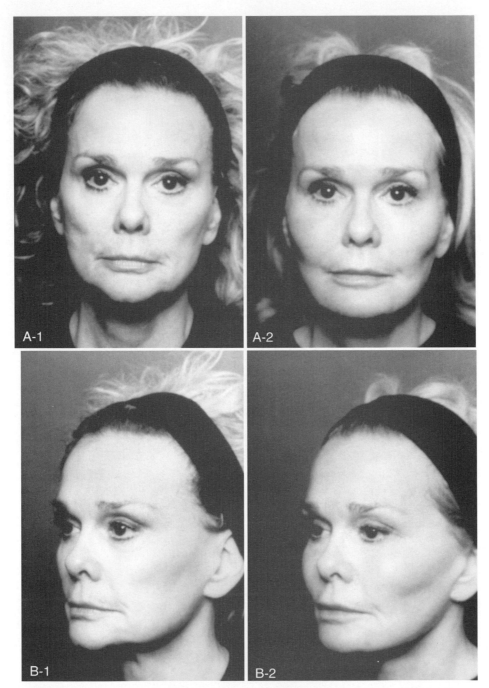

FIG. 51–13. **A,** 50-year-old female with "witch's chin" deformity and midface submalar atrophy. Correction of chin deformity using an extended anatomic chin implant (zone CM, 4 mm and ML, 3 mm) and midfacial deformity correction by submalar zone augmentation (SM, 4 mm). **B,** oblique view of same patient.

FIG. 51–14.   A, facial contouring by zonal anatomy. The four zones of the premandible space: CM, central mentum; ML, midlateral zone; PL, posterolateral zone; SM, submandibular zone. **B,** diagram showing the four zones of the premandible space.

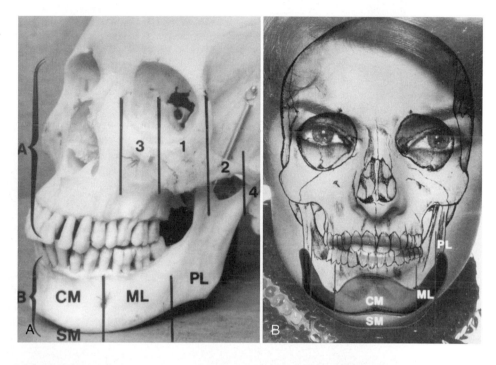

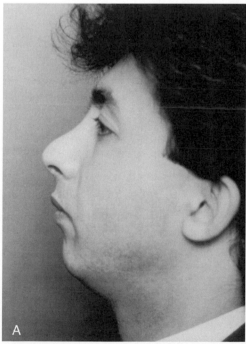
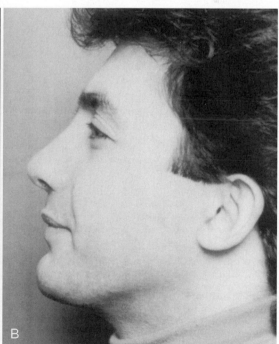

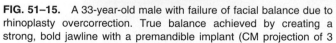

FIG. 51–15. A 33-year-old male with failure of facial balance due to rhinoplasty overcorrection. True balance achieved by creating a strong, bold jawline with a premandible implant (CM projection of 3 mm and ML projection of 10 mm). Secondary augmentation rhinoplasty was also necessary.

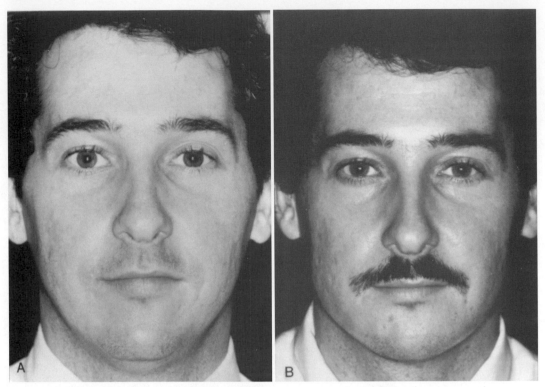

FIG. 51–16. Facial contouring of premandible in a 38-year-old male who desired a strong, more-defined jaw. Extended anatomic contour implant widens middle jaw (CM and ML zones), while PL zone augmentation provides a more sculptured appearance.

the middle aspect of the jawline and the lower third facial segment.

A third zone (posterolateral, PL) overlies the posterior aspect of the horizontal ramus, extending from the oblique line posteriorly and including the angle of the mandible as well as the lower third of the ascending ramus. Augmentation of this posterolateral zone 3 widens the face at the posterior jawline and gives sculptured definition to the mandibular angle (Fig. 51–16).

A fourth premandibular zone exists beneath the inferior border of the mandible. This can be referred to as the submandibular zone (SM). Traditional chin implants have lacked the ability to extend deficient mandibles and faces in a vertical direction. A special design implant, however, is now available that wraps around the inferior bony margin of the mandible; it increases the vertical height of the face from the lower lip to the inferior chin line. This submandibular-zone implant presently has dimensions of 4 mm vertically and 4 mm anteriorly (Fig. 51–17). By augmenting the lateral aspects of both the submandibular (SM) zone and the midlateral zone (ML) simultaneously, it is possible to correct the prejowl sulcus ("marionette groove") (Fig. 51–18).

Qualities of Ideal Facial Implants

An ideal implant should be (a) easy to place, (b) nonpalpable, (c) readily exchangeable, (d) malleable, (e) conformable, (f) acceptable to the body, (g) resistant to infection, and (h) modifiable by the surgeon (Table 51–2). The size and shape of the implants are critical in creating specific and varied facial contours. When an appropriate implant has been selected and the proper techniques used, the potential for mobility and displacement is negligible.

When placed directly on bone (subperiosteal), smooth silicone implants become fixed rapidly and securely by circumferential fibrosis (capsule formation). They can be removed easily and exchanged when necessary or desirable. On the other hand, porous implants permit ingrowth. Examples are Proplast-HA, Porex, and hydroxyapatite, as well as fenestrated implants or implants with Dacron backing (9). Such implants are associated with a consistently predictable, significant rate of infection. Tissue ingrowth makes implants much more difficult to exchange or modify, and can result in excessive trauma, nerve damage, and fibrotic deformity.

Silastic implants survive the onset of inflammation and even gross purulence. If inflammation, cellulitis, or abscess occur, prompt use of antibiotics and (perhaps) drainage techniques can resolve the situation successfully (10). Infected porous implants, however, must always be removed. Despite the excellent salvage potential with silicone implants, surgeons should not be complacent and expect a cure in all cases. Disastrous consequences have been reported from facial implant infections; thus individualized judgment must be exercised.

Successes from using contemporary anatomic facial-implant styles are based on their ability to conform to the facial skeleton in both the malar and premandible regions (Fig. 51–19). These contoured facial implants are larger, which enables them volumetrically to fit the dimensions of the aesthetic facial units. This minimizes migration, misplacement, and contour irregularities.

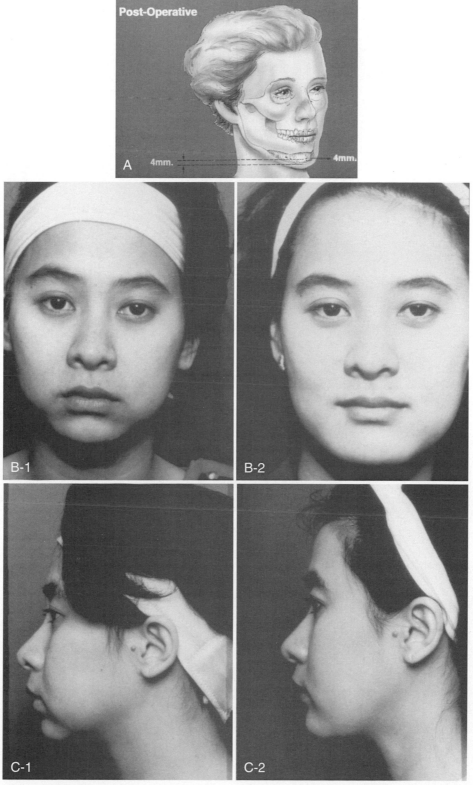

FIG. 51–17. Premandible submandibular augmentation can alter both the anterior projection and vertical length of the chin. **A,** illustration demonstrates positioning of this innovative implant. **B,** 26-year-old female who underwent submandibular augmentation with a vertical extension implant (CM and SM zones, 4-mm implant). Three-millimeter submalar implants were also placed (frontal view). **C,** oblique view.

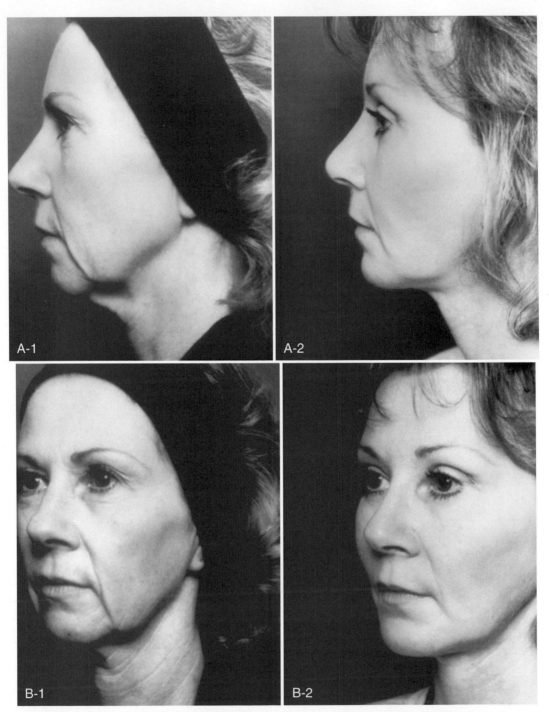

FIG. 51–18.   A 50-year-old female with excessive prejowl sulcus formation. Premandibular augmentation in zones CM (4 mm) and ML (3 mm) augment traditional rhytidectomy well and provide more permanent correction of this deformity. **A,** lateral view. **B,** oblique view.

Ideal facial implants should be malleable and compressible to facilitate insertion through small apertures in the soft-tissue envelope of the face. This minimizes wound dehiscence and extrusion. The necessity of using larger implants makes the above qualities even more important. Often implants of 10 to 20 cm² are needed for proper contouring. Silicone rubber implants fabricated with a medium-grade consistency make it possible to perform these procedures with ease.

Finally, the ability to modify silicone implants easily before or during surgery avoids both intraoperative problems and postoperative contour irregularities. Instead of dissecting into areas where nerve or muscle damage is possible, the surgeon can easily diminish the implant size or alter its configuration without compromising the resulting contour.

Choosing Implants

Even for the most experienced surgeon, it is difficult to contour a face to the patient's satisfaction. Choosing implant size and shape appropriately and positioning them properly still relies on the surgeon's artistic perception and individual judgement. Genetic asymmetries are common, and are only correctable by using implants that differ in size, shape, and

position. Technical precision and standardized implant measurements remain to be perfected. The infinite variations of facial form defy routine analysis for determining aesthetic guidelines.

Nonetheless, certain probabilities exist. Four-millimeter augmentation in the malar-midface zones will almost always

Table 51–2
Comparison of Qualities of Most Commonly Used Facial Implant Materials

Ideal Characteristics	Materials		
			Other
	Silastic		(Hydroxyapatite, MedPore)
Exchangeable		++++	+
Conformable		++++	++
Modifiable		+++	+++
Host acceptable	++++	+++	
Nonpalpable		+++	+
Insertable		++++	+++

++++, most ideal; + least ideal

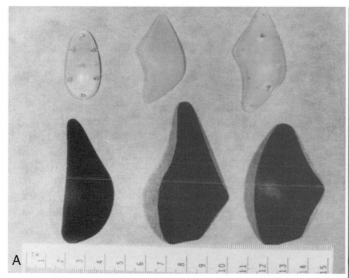

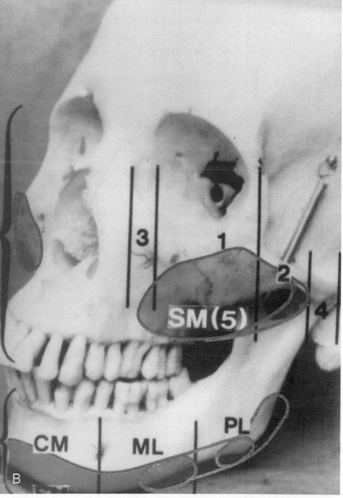

FIG. 51–19. Malar augmentation utilizing larger, broader implants. **A,** historically implants have been smaller (right superior), creating a knobby, unnatural result. Contemporary implants are larger (left inferior) and produce a more aesthetic result. Note that simple intraoperative contouring of implants can easily change the shape of the implant to conform to the patient's bony architecture when necessary. **B,** typical contemporary Terino malar shell design covering zone 1 and submalar zone 5.

be optimum. Occasionally, a 3-mm shell may be needed for a subtle effect, or a 5- to 6-mm implant may be called for to produce a bolder, more dramatic result. In the pre-mandible region, 5 to 7 mm of projection in the central mentum is most suitable for the majority of the patients. Eight to ten millimeters are necessary for severe microgenia. Three to four millimeters of midlateral zone augmentation are provided by the lateral anatomic extensions on the implants. This volume usually is adequate to widen the lower-third facial jawline segment. The posterior angle (PL zone) is usually contoured adequately with an 8-mm lateral extension.

The immediate future of implant technology will involve computerization with three-dimensional imaging and surface laser scanning (11). These modalities will eventually provide more accurate and definitive determinations for alloplastic volumetric augmentation.

Unfortunately, physician and patient dissatisfactions from the results of facial implant augmentation presently constitute the major "complication." As experience with alloplastic facial contouring increases, this disadvantage will diminish dramatically.

Preoperative Evaluation and Planning

For all plastic and reconstructive procedures, preoperative evaluation and planning assures successful results. Elective aesthetic surgery demands accurate communication with patients. It is necessary for the surgeon thoroughly to duplicate the patient's own analysis and perception of the face and their expectations from the surgery.

Aging patients simply want to appear their best. People learn to accept the slow, gradual changes that take place in the soft-tissue contours of their faces. They can, therefore, accept the technical limitations of routine two-dimensional rhytidectomy techniques. They usually perceive and appreciate significant postoperative improvement. Patients 40 years of age or older are not comfortable with the facial image of a 20-year-old. Three-dimensional alloplastic facial contouring techniques can radically change a patient's inherited anatomic configuration when compared to standard SMAS or subperiosteal rhytidectomy techniques alone. After alloplastic facial-contour surgery in the younger age group, especially that done for enhancement, patients may need to accept an entirely different facial image.

Precise implementation of facial form remains difficult. The "zero meridian" concept, cephalometric measurements, CEMAX, MRI, and three-dimensional CT techniques are the major tools of the aesthetic facial surgeon (11). Nonetheless, it is imperative that the surgeon knows exactly what facial image the patient desires (e.g., strong, bold, well-defined features and classic contours, or more subtle appearances).

It is extremely helpful to have patients bring modified photographs of themselves or examples of desired facial contours from fashion magazines and other sources. The object is to have them choose images they feel are similar to themselves, and which they want to create with specific contour characteristics, especially in the skeletal zones to be augmented. This evaluation of a patient's "ideal scene" by the use of visual images has greatly improved our understanding of our patients' expectations.

Personality Assessment of the Cosmetic Surgery Patient

The current exploding demand for aesthetic facial surgery has been accompanied by an equal explosion in the number of patients dissatisfied with their results. It has therefore become critical for the specialty of plastic surgery to examine preoperatively the characteristics of patient's personalities that effect their outlook on the results of their surgery.

For the past 5 years, we have consistently used the Oxford Capacity Analysis (OCA) personality profile assessment to qualify or disqualify patients for surgery. Experience since 1989 in more than 1000 patients has demonstrated an accuracy of approximately 95% in predicting perioperative behavior of severe dissatisfaction; the OCA has also shown that 10% of patients will express some form of threat (12).

Alloplastic Facial Augmentation with Rhytidectomy and Rhinoplasty

Perhaps the most value is achieved by facial contouring when it accompanies traditional two-dimensional tightening procedures for rejuvenation and restoration of the face. Enhancement of the facial skeleton in the jawline, malar, or malar/midfacial aesthetic units creates a definitive and permanent improvement in facial appearance. Techniques involving deep-plane dissections and subperiosteal face lifting depend upon releasing the zygomatic and masseteric ligamentous attachments from the subperiosteal or subSMAS plane.

But even after these advanced techniques are performed, patient dissatisfaction frequently arises from unrealistic expectations of the patient or the surgeon. Desired results achieved by placing aging atrophic, attenuated facial tissues under tension often dissipate rapidly within the first months after surgery; even worse, too much tension can result in an artificially "pulled" face. It seems unreasonable that displaced and atrophied malar fat can be dissected and sutured without a compromise of its blood supply that leads to further atrophy and further loss of volume. It would also seem that subperiosteal elevation and repositioning might deteriorate with time. Alloplastic restoration of midfacial and malar fullness, however, is both permanent and predictable and gives the surgeon a powerful tool for three-dimensional facial change (Fig. 51–20).

Disruption of the zygomatic ligaments and anterior masseteric ligaments during facial contouring helps maintain the repositioned submuscular aponeurotic elements. A volumetric silastic implant can act as an interpositional spacer and prevent reattachment of these ligaments to their original positions (13). All newer aesthetic facial techniques involve more extended dissections, with prolonged edema and induration of tissues. Alloplastic facial implant placement does not increase this morbidity. However, patients must be forewarned that predictable, gradual, and long-term improvement in contour occurs after all contemporary facial procedures and often requires 6 months to 1 year to achieve final appearance.

"Profileplasty" is a term traditionally applied to nose-chin relationships. Because the original central implants were

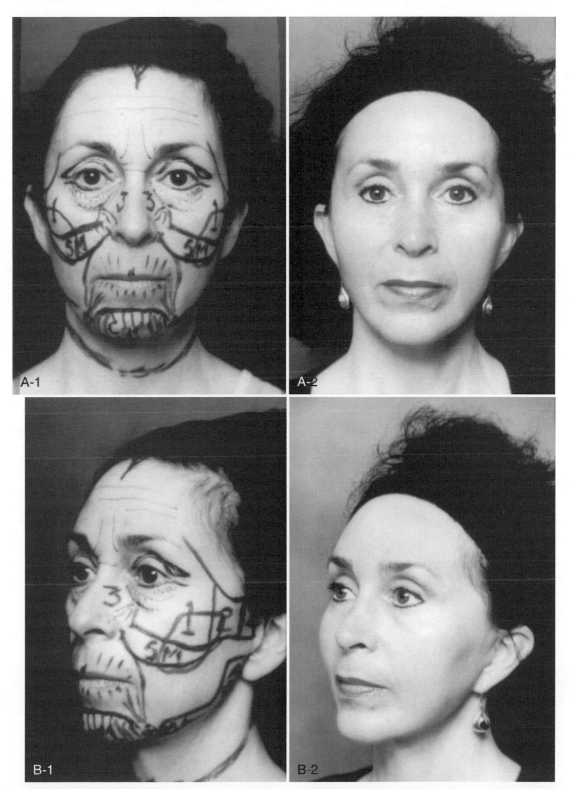

FIG. 51–20. Almost no other aesthetic surgical procedure demands as much precise preoperative communication as facial contouring. We have patients bring in pictures of desired appearances. Detailed preoperative markings and discussion of implant choices with the pa-tient are mandatory. Video imaging is also useful. This is a 40-year-old female following malar and premandible augmentation in addition to rhytidectomy, browlift and perioral dermabrasion. **A,** frontal view. **B,** oblique view.

small, nasal reduction during the early surgical attempts to achieve balance had to be excessive. Newer implants have been designed that can extend across the entire anterior surface of the mandible from angle to angle. They can also extend into the submandibular region to create significant vertical augmentation of the lower-third facial segment. In combination with anatomically designed malar/midface implants, optimum nasal contouring is facilitated, because less reduction in size is necessary.

Sequence of Events for Combined Aesthetic Surgery Techniques

At the present writing, we do not customarily insert malar implants through a coronal approach. We prefer the intraoral route over a subciliary or a preauricular face-lift incision. None of these routes is disadvantageous for surgeons experienced in these operations. When placing these implants, lower-lid and malar midface suspension techniques minimize chances of lower-lid retraction, especially if a subciliary route is utilized. It seems only reasonable that by disrupting the facial ligaments during dissection and interposing implants beneath the SMAS the repositioning will be maintained. This would also be true for the premandible segment when subperiosteal face lifting techniques are used. Placement of premandible implants is done immediately following the neck dissection and platysma plication.

Operative Technique

SUGGESTIONS

1. Stay on bone. When implants are placed directly on bone (subperiosteal), a firm and secure attachment to the skeleton is formed. Capsular contracture has not been seen with anatomic implants, perhaps because of their solid consistency or the inability of a capsule to be constrictive when implants are directly on bone (14).
2. Be gentle in elevating the soft tissues in the malar and premandible regions. Avoid excessive trauma, which can produce mental-nerve symptoms, both transient and prolonged but rarely permanent. Paresis or paralysis of the zygomaticus, the orbicularis oculi, and even the frontalis muscle can occur.
3. Expand the dissection space adequately in either the malar or the premandible regions to accommodate the chosen prostheses comfortably. Elevation of the soft tissues into areas adjacent to bone should be done only gently and with a blunt-edged elevator.
4. Minimize bleeding by using both local and general anesthesia. Maintenance of systolic blood pressure between 90 and 110 mm Hg provides optimum hemostasis when combined with infiltration of a dilute lidocaine 0.1% solution containing adrenalin (1:800,000). Clonidine 0.1 mg is also given orally immediately before surgery to stabilize blood pressure and pulse (Table 51–3).

DETAILS

Once the basic principles of dissection are understood, the remaining technical aspects of facial implantation in the

Table 51–3
Ideal Anesthesia for Alloplastic Facial Contouring

I. General anesthesia
  A. Maintain blood pressure at 90–100 mm Hg systolic.
  B. Clonidine 0.1 mg p.o. preoperatively.

II. Local anesthesia
  A. Lidocaine solution   0.1% - 0.2%
  B. Adrenalin   1:800,000
  C. Generous tissue infiltration into malar and/or premandible space (20–30 cc each)

malar, midface, and premandible regions are straightforward.

The various routes for entering the malar space, including the submalar region, are as follows: (a) intraoral, (b) lower blepharoplasty—subcilial, (c) rhytidectomy, (d) zygomaticotemporal, and (e) transcoronal.

The intraoral route has been the traditional and most frequent approach to maxillary malar and midface augmentation. A 1-cm incision is made through the mucosa in a vertically oblique direction. It is located over the anterior buttress of the maxilla, just above the canine and approximately 2 cm medial to the orifice of the Stensen duct.

A subperiosteal, spatula-shaped elevator with a 1-cm wide blade is thrust directly through the zygomaticus muscle onto bone in a vertical orientation at the inferior base of the maxillary buttress, and in the apex of the gingival-buccal sulcus. The overlying soft tissues are swept obliquely upward over the maxillary eminence by keeping the elevator directly on bone (Fig. 51–21). The elevator should always be kept on the bony margin along the inferior border of the malar eminence and zygomatic arch. Manual palpation of the zonal design previously marked on the malar space is performed, while the underlying elevator separates the tissues from the bone. This maneuver includes palpating the orbital rim and the upper and lower borders of the zygoma as the elevator dissects the subperiosteal space within these areas.

Once bony margins are reached, the space is expanded further by means of a rounded and blunter spatula elevator. Do not use force when dissecting the soft tissues. The infraorbital nerve should not be dissected. By using a careful scraping motion, the periosteum may be lifted inferior to the infraorbital foramen until the nerve and foramen are seen. Frequent irrigation is performed with antibiotic solution (bacitracin 50,000 units/L normal saline).

Once the space is mobilized, the chosen implant is introduced with a long, straight, nonserrated clamp placed transversely across the upper end of the implant and inserted into the posterior zygomatic tunnel. Traction is maintained by two 3-0 Ethibond sutures placed first through the implant tail and then passed transcutaneously posterior to the temple hairline (Fig. 51–22). Positioning can be confirmed by passing a spatula periosteal elevator, both anterior and posterior to the implant. Fiberoptic Aufricht retractors are used to illuminate the

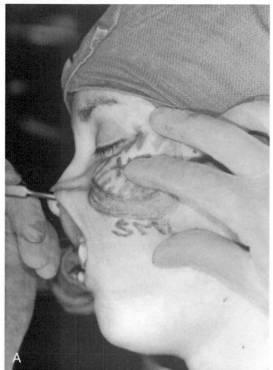

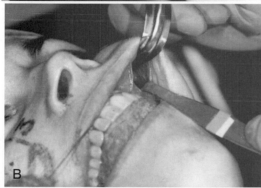

FIG. 51–21.   A, malar shell augmentation by the intraoral route. Soft tissues are elevated over the malar region by staying on the bone with an elevator and controlling the space between the index finger and the thumb. **B,** completed malar pocket.

operative space, reveal the internal anatomy, and confirm the correct position of the implant.

In the submalar zone, the soft tissues are swept off the shiny white fibrous tendon of the masseter muscle in an inferior and outward direction. The submalar space can be opened inferiorly by approximately 1 to 2 cm, depending on the desired cheek shape and the corresponding implant necessary to achieve it.

When adequate anesthesia techniques are used, the intraoral approach permits excellent visualization of the skeletal anatomy and musculature, which in turn facilitates accurate implant placement into zones 1, 2, and 5 (SM).

Closure of the vertical intraoral incision is secure because the muscle pillars of the zygomaticus, which overlie the

maxillary buttress, can be fixed firmly with sutures to provide a sturdy two-layer closure. Traditional transverse incisions through these muscles produce traumatic transection, which results in transient and perhaps even permanent functional damage. This can inhibit normal lip elevation.

Another significant disadvantage of the intraoral approach is that it weakens the inferior aspect of the dissection space, thereby increasing possibilities of rotational asymmetry and slippage of the implant into an undesirable medial inferior position. As noted, augmentation using a subcilial blepharoplasty or rhytidectomy approach is easily performed if desired by the surgeon. Detailed descriptions of these approaches have been discussed elsewhere (2).

PREMANDIBLE AUGMENTATION

To extend a centrally placed implant into the ML and PL zones, dissection is performed along the inferior mandibular border into the "safe zone" posterior to the mental nerve. There is significant constriction and adherence of the tissues to the bone surrounding the mental foramen at the origin of the anterior mandibular ligament. Once these are released, dissection of the tissues from the posterolateral zone occurs easily.

The premandible space can be accessed by either the standard intraoral route or the submental route. The author uses the submental approach exclusively for operations that require additional surgery in the submental and submandibular region, such as liposculpturing and platysma plication and contouring.

In both approaches, the incisions are 2 cm long and transverse. The intraoral incision is through mucosa only. The mentalis muscles are then divided vertically through their midline raphe to avoid transection of the muscle bellies and total detachment from their bony origins. This aperture provides direct access downward onto the bony plane and eliminates the muscle weakening that occurs with customary transection methods (Fig. 51–23).

By elevating the tissues directly from bone (subperiosteal), the muscle attachments are removed from their origins along the inferior margin of the mandible; this does not endanger the mental nerve. The mandibular branch of facial nerve VII does, however, cross just anterior to the midportion of the mandible in the ML. Consequently, it is important not to traumatize the tissues that overlie and constitute the roof of the premandible space in that region. The mental nerve foramina can vary in number and location.

Additional incisions may be made posterior to the mental nerve to place accurately the lateral mandibular bars and implants that extend into the ML and PL zones. A 1-cm vertical mucosal incision made in front of the first molar, followed by direct penetration through the muscle onto the mandibular bone, allows access to and easy dissection of the premandible space beneath. This aperture helps to place the lateral mandibular bars accurately and position the posterior extensions of other implants when augmenting the central mentum and the midlateral zones at the same time.

To position a premandible implant with long extensions, a tunnel or space must be created to be posteriorly longer than the implant. The implant can then be inserted from the cen-

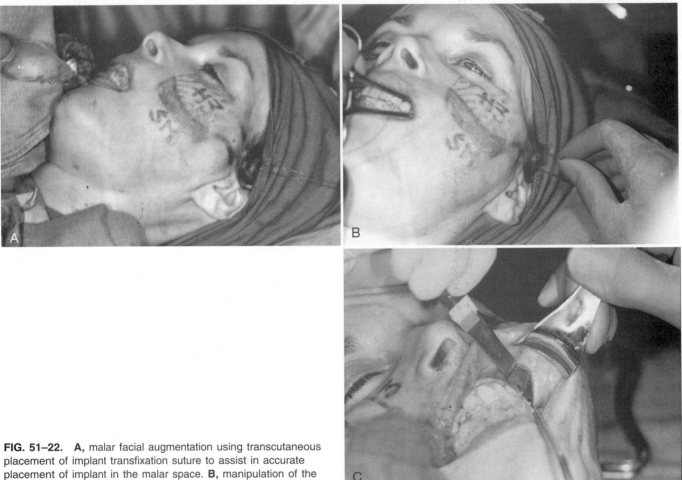

FIG. 51–22. **A,** malar facial augmentation using transcutaneous placement of implant transfixation suture to assist in accurate placement of implant in the malar space. **B,** manipulation of the implant. **C,** implant in final position.

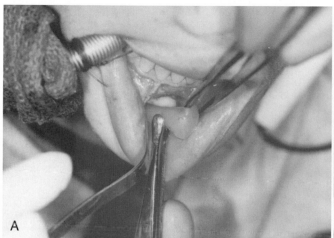

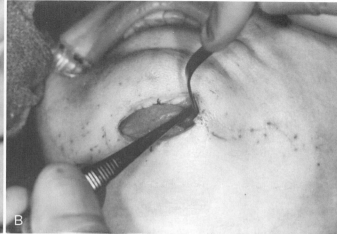

FIG. 51–23. **A,** facial contouring by premandible augmentation showing intraoral insertion of a large extended anatomic implant.

B, facial contouring by premandible augmentation showing submental insertion of a large extended anatomic implant.

Table 51–4
Frequency of Complications with Chin Implants (Author's Experience)

Asymmetries		20%	
Malposition		5%	
Hematoma/seroma/Infection	0.5%		
Mobility		10%	
Extrusion			0.1%
Nerve dysfunction (Temporary)	10%		
Sensory (Permanent)	1.0%		
Motor (Permanent)	0.5%		

Frequency of Complications with Malar Implants

			% of MDs
Asymmetries		10%	
Malposition		5%	
Hematoma/seroma/infections	0.5%		
Extrusion			0.1%
Nerve dysfunction (Temporary)	8%		
Sensory (Permanent)	0.1%		
Motor (Permanent)	0.5%		
Ectropion			
(subcilial route)	0.5%		

tral incision far into one side, folded upon itself, and introduced into the opposite mandibular tunnel.

Posterolateral implants are placed through either an ML or PL incision. The PL incision is transverse and located 1.5 to 2 cm anterior and adjacent to the angle of the mandible.

A curved elevator is used to dissect around the inferior and posterior aspects of the angle and the ascending ramus. In this way, implants designed to fit securely around the angle of the mandible can be positioned accurately. A two-layer closure of muscle and mucosa is optimum for all facial implant incisions.

Complications

Although placement of mid and lower face implants is technically not difficult, a few occasional problems can develop (5). The incidence of complications arising from the experience of the ASPRS membership was investigated in a survey in 1991 (10). Our experience shows the following complications from facial augmentation, in order of importance and frequency:

1. Asymmetries, 10%
2. Malposition, 5%
3. Hematoma, seroma, and infection and removal, 0.5%
4. Infraorbital nerve sensory dysfunction (intraoral route), 0.1%
5. Zygomaticus lip elevation motor dysfunction (intraoral route), 0.5%
6. Lower eyelid ectropion (subcilial route), 0.5% (Table 51–4).

Detailed discussion and treatment of these complications are beyond the scope of this chapter, but have been discussed extensively elsewhere.

Conclusions

Plastic surgeons are now better prepared to fulfill the primary goal of facial cosmetic surgery. By manipulating and combining the various new techniques, they can restore, rejuvenate, or enhance facial form and affect aging changes. The ability to improve facial contour by alloplastic onlay techniques significantly enhances hereditary deficiencies in youth as well as age.

Whereas soft-tissue techniques are essentially two-dimensional, skeletal augmentation represents surgery of the deepest plane and is three-dimensional in nature. The use of implants on this skeletal plane represents volume and mass alteration of facial form. Manipulations of the other three planes (i.e., skin, subcutaneous fat, and SMAS) are attempts to reverse aging qualities of loosening, sagging, and drooping in a two-dimensional fashion.

Skeletal augmentation now represents a final phase for facial plastic surgery. Three-dimensional volume-mass modifications of the 4th plane skeletal framework enable surgeons to dramatically or subtly alter inherited facial images, as well as to compensate for the deterioration, sagging, and diminution of facial tissue mass that comes with age.

Now virtually all aspects of the facial skeleton can be augmented satisfactorily. It can truthfully be said that alloplastic implants may become the "open sesame" of aesthetic surgery, the door through which almost magical facial changes can be made, depending on the imagination and skill of the surgeon.

References

1. Ramirez OM. The subperiosteal rhytidectomy: the third-generation face lift. *Ann Plast Surg* 1992; 28:218.
2. Terino EO. Alloplastic facial contouring: surgery of the fourth plane. *Aesth Plast Surg* 1992; 16:195–212.
3. Tolleth H. Concepts for the plastic surgeon from art and sculpture. Facial aesthetic surgery: art, anatomy, anthropometrics, and imaging. *Clin Plast Surg* 1987; 14(4):585–598.
4. Terino EO. Alloplastic facial contouring by zonal principles of skeletal anatomy. *Clin Plast Surg* 1992; 19:487.
5. Wilkinson TS. Complications in aesthetic malar augmentation. *Plast Reconstr Surg* 1983; 71(5):643.
6. Binder WJ, Schoenrock LD, Terino EO. Augmentation of the malar-submalar/midface. *Facial Plastic Surgery Clinics of North America,* 1994; 2:265.
7. Binder W, Kamer F, Parkes M. Mentoplasty: a clinical analysis of alloplastic implants. *Laryngoscope* 1981; XCI(3):383–391.
8. Wolfe SA. Aesthetic procedures on the chin. In: Regnault P, Daniel RK, eds. *Aesthetic plastic surgery: principles and techniques.* Boston: Little, Brown, 1984.
9. Jobe R. Polymers in craniomaxiliofacial surgery. In: Ousterhout D, ed. *Aesthetic contouring of the craniofacial skeleton.* Boston: Little, Brown, 1991; 165–174.
10. Terino EO. Complications of chin and malar augmentation. In: Peck G, ed. *Complications and problems in aesthetic plastic surgery.* New York: Gower Medical Publishers, 1991.
11. Hoffman W. Three-dimensional evaluation of facial form. In: Ousterhout D, ed. *Aesthetic contouring of the craniofacial ckeleton.* Boston: Little, Brown, 1991; 109–115.
12. Terino EO. The significant economic loss from serving dissatisfied patients. Presented at the annual meeting of the American Society of Aesthetic Plastic Surg, San Francisco, 1995.
13. Binder WJ. Submalar augmentation: a procedure to enhance rhytidectomy. *Ann Plast Surg* 1990; 24:200–212.
14. Parkes ML. Avoiding bone resorption under plastic chin implants. *Arch Otolaryngol* 1973; 98:100.

52

Dermabrasion, Chemical Peel, and Collagen Injection

Michael Breiner, M.D., Samuel Stal, M.D., F.A.C.S., and Melvin Spira, M.D., D.D.S., F.A.C.S.

A primary function of the skin is to serve as a barrier to insult from the environment. The external assault of the sun combined with the normal aging process often leaves our skin with pigmentation and texture irregularities. Many of these conditions are amenable to surgical therapy and adjunctive procedures.

Dermabrasion

Dermabrasion is a surgical procedure that abrades successive layers of skin, permitting a controlled removal of epidermis and upper dermis to a depth sufficient to treat disease, tumor, or deformity. It is primarily employed to treat acne and associated posttraumatic scars, skin rhytids, and traumatic tattoos. The physiologic basis of healing after dermabrasion rests upon the capacity of the skin to regenerate its epidermal cover by epithelialization through skin appendages, primarily the pilosebaceous units.

HISTOPATHOLOGY

Destruction of the upper layer of the skin with dermabrasion is similar to that induced by chemical cauterization, superficial thermal burn, or the removal of a split-thickness skin graft. There is, however, one important difference. Whereas other techniques will leave thicker tissue behind in areas of hyperkeratosis, dermabrasion tends to even things out. Initially following dermabrasion, a coagulum forms on the surface of the wound or overlying gauze dressing. Early mitotic activity that begins in the cells of the pilosebaceous unit immediately underlying the wound surface provide a source of epithelialization during the healing period. Thus, epithelial-cell outgrowth from the shaft of the hair follicles (the roots of which are invariably undisturbed, being located in the depth of the reticular dermis and subjacent subcutaneous tissue) provides a thin layer of epidermis whose development is usually complete 5 to 7 days following abrasion. Concomitant dermal regeneration occurs with fibroblast proliferation and new capillary formation. New collagen formation associated with the edema of wound healing gives the skin an early smooth, erythematous appearance. The gross changes in the appearance of the epidermal surface result from replacement of collagen in the papillary layer of the corium and from increased vascularity. The presence of increased elastic tissue in the dermis after healing, believed by some to account in part for the change in final skin appearance, has not been consistently observed following dermal regeneration (1). After tissue maturation occurs and the edema subsides, the skin is not as smooth as it was in the early postoperative period; this retreat from the early promise of an optimal effect can be disappointing to both surgeon and patient (2).

Repigmentation is an interesting component in the wound healing process. Skin repigmentation originates from the melanoblasts in the basal layer of the epidermis, occurring after epidermal regeneration and dermal regrowth. Regeneration begins in the deeper epithelial elements within the pilosebaceous unit, which contain fewer melanoblasts. The ability to regenerate skin pigment is lessened as the planing or abrading of the skin increases in depth. Development of hyperpigmentation in newly abraded areas exposed to sunlight is recognized clinically but difficult to demonstrate in controlled studies. Baker and coworkers (3,4) postulated that the quantity of melanin granules in the basal epidermal layer is permanently reduced, leading to permanent lightening of skin color and the inability to develop a deep suntan following dermabrasion or chemical peel. The consistency of these color changes often remains variable.

As healing is completed epidermal thickness is regained, although the full thickness of the original dermis is never recovered, the corium remaining thinner than it was before surgical intervention (Fig. 52–1). Thus, the number of times the surgical procedure can be repeated depends not only upon the thickness of the original skin, the number of pilosebaceous units, and the natural skin pigmentation, but also on the depth of the original surgical abrasion or chemical peel. Superficial abrasions can be repeated, but an aggressive initial approach may limit the surgeon to a single procedure if the complications described below are to be avoided. Good judgment in the selection of cases and utilization of appropriate technique is extremely important.

INDICATIONS

Acne-induced scarring is the skin problem most commonly treated by dermabrasion. It is generally recommended that surgery be postponed until the acute infection and eruption of acne has subsided. With the emergence of new drugs, including cis-retinoic acid (Accutane), the natural course of acne has at times been significantly diminished. Dermabrasion can be employed either to level the skin where acne pitting and scarring have occurred or to open residual cysts, sinus tracts, or epithelial tunnels to allow drainage and healing, with a second procedure aimed at reducing scarring and smoothing the skin.

Irregular, uneven scars in which one border is higher or lower than the other can be improved by dermabrasion. Dermabrasion can be especially helpful in traumatic wounds

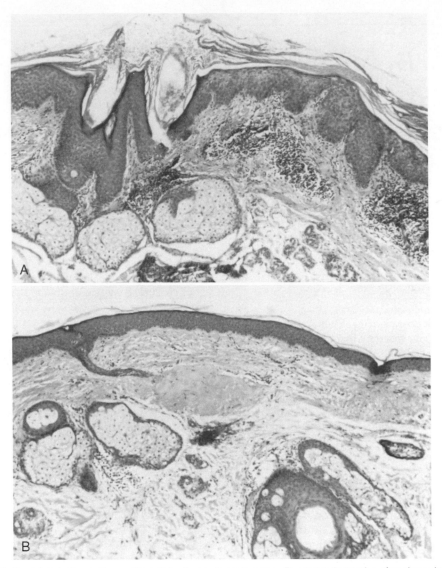

FIG. 52–1. Histologic sections of the skin. **A,** predermabrasion. **B,** status 6 months after dermabrasion.

where there is a "rolling up" of the epidermis and papillary dermal layer that occurs with healing. The surgeon can either lower the raised scar or feather out the depressed scar into the surrounding normal skin.

Rhytids have been treated by dermabrasion sufficient to partially efface fine skin crenulations without violating the deeper dermis. The technique is particularly useful for perioral rhytids. Currently, however, most surgeons have switched to chemical peeling at this site, because the peel is faster and more likely to produce an even effacement. Furthermore, there has been a lot of enthusiasm regarding the role of the ultrapulse CO_2 laser in treating both fine and deep rhytids. Initial results of using this new laser technique has been promising, but the long-term benefits of either dermabrasion or chemical peels have yet to be determined (personal experience).

Traumatic tattoos, as well as some commercial and home-made tattoos, have been treated by dermabrasion with varying degrees of improvement (Fig. 52–2). Although the best time to treat traumatic tattoos is at initial presentation (often, aided by loupe magnification), the dermabrader has been shown to be a useful adjunct in treating traumatic tattoos. However, we believe dermabrasion is unsatisfactory for the treatment of professionally applied tattoos, where various pulse lasers are gaining in popularity. In most professional tattoos, the pigment is embedded so deeply that its removal violates the reticular dermis, or even the subcutaneous tissue; thus, while the pigment can be removed, the residual scarring is often unacceptable. At one time there was much enthusiasm about treating pigmented nevi—especially the giant hairy bathing-trunk nevus—with dermabrasion, but this is no longer recommended therapy. Johnson and others (5, 6) have shown that light dermabrasion done before 3 months of age can remove the nevus cells, which are very superficial, and leave minimal scarring. However, because of conflicting reports in the literature concerning the efficacy of dermabrasion for pigmented nevi and the significant risk of morbidity of such surgery in infants, we find there is little role in dermabrasion for treating such deformities (Johnson, personal communication) (Fig. 52–3).

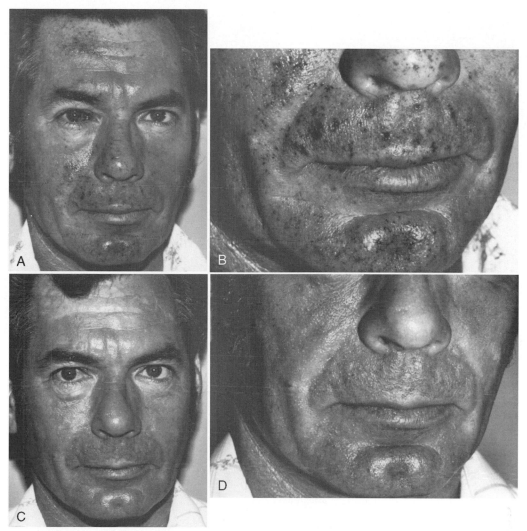

FIG. 52–2. Forty-six-year-old man involved in explosion. **A,** full face photo showing severe tattooing. **B,** closeup of cheek and perioral re- gion. **C,** appearance 6 months postoperatively. **D,** closeup of postop- erative appearance. (Photographs courtesy of D.R. Wiemer, M.D.)

Specific skin tumors, keratoses, sebaceous adenomas, and particularly rhinophymas, can also be effectively treated by dermabrasion (7). Hyperpigmentation has been treated with dermabrasion, although we have found other modalities, in- cluding chemical peel and topical application of hydro- quinone derivatives, to be more advantageous in terms of uniform color, lower expense, and fewer complications.

CONTRAINDICATIONS

Individuals with deep skin pigmentation respond differently to dermabrasion. The problem relates to the usual depth of dermabrasion and the ability of the skin not only to reform the epithelium and dermis but also to repigment from the melanoblasts of the basal layer. Thus, in dark-skinned indi- viduals, there may be a noticeable area of hypopigmentation corresponding to the dermabraded areas. Although this is not a complication but the normal healing process of the derm- abrasion, patients need to be aware of this expected side ef- fect. Burn scars, hypertrophic scars, and keloids do not re- spond well to dermabrasion because they lack the adnexal units from which epidermal healing arises. To a lesser extent,

the same problem exists in radiation dermatitis, primarily be- cause the adnexal pilosebaceous structures have been injured or destroyed. In our opinion, even the more superficial ma- lignancies should not be subjected to dermabrasion as a treat- ment modality, nor should pigmented lesions that are suspi- cious for malignant melanoma. Finally, in patients with bloodborne viral diseases, the risk to operating-room person- nel from aerosolizing tissues must be considered. The patient may be best served by a deep chemical peel.

EQUIPMENT

Motor-driven serrated wheels can be covered by different materials, but diamond fraises are preferred. Straight hand- pieces are generally mounted on a flexible cable or shaft, with rotary power supplied by a high-speed motor or com- pressed air. In the past 2 decades, small dermatones have also been used to remove successive layers of epidermis and der- mis in a process called *dermaplaning*. However, we find that using dermatones makes it more difficult to predict the depth of planing, which can lead to uneven scarring.

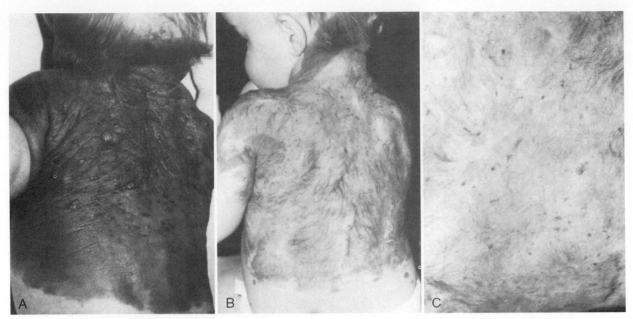

FIG. 52–3. Child with large hairy nevus. **A,** preoperative photograph taken at 4 weeks of age. **B,** child at 13 months after dermaplaning. **C,** closeup showing decrease in pigmentation but still incomplete removal.

SURGICAL TECHNIQUE

The choice to perform the procedure under anesthesia depends on the amount of dermabrasion to be performed as well as the desires of the patient. The area to be dermabraded is first cleansed with a germicidal soap and then degreased with various agents. Whether the procedure is done under intravenous sedation in a hospital, or in an office setting, regional blocks are often helpful to permit adequate anesthesia to areas to be dermabraded (Fig. 52–4).

The deepest scars are stained with methylene blue. Next, two 4 × 4 gauze packs are placed in the patient's mouth, proving sufficient tension for the procedure. The area to be dermabraded is sprayed with a freon spray, which not only puts more tension on the skin but also acts as a local anesthetic. Once these modalities have been accomplished, the dermabrader is kept at right angles to the skin at all times. It is important that all gauzes, gloves, and body parts, especially eyelashes, are kept out of the way of the spinning drums (a spoon placed over the patient's eye is an excellent precaution). In treating deep acne scars, the endpoint of the dermabrasion often is the lowest part of the acne scar; the methylene blue will have gravitated to this lowermost depression and is a helpful depth indicator. It is important to feather out all the areas of dermabrasion, but do not extend more than 1 to 2 cm below the mandible or dermabrade either the upper- or lower-eyelid skin. When dermabrading the forehead and the vermillion area, it is often necessary to feather the process into the hairline as well as into the vermillion border. This is also true for chemical peels. It is important that protective eyewear be used, in addition to regular operating-room protocol, because the spinning motion of the dermabrader will splatter blood and debris.

Once the dermabrasion is complete, small pinpoint bleeding edges are usually controlled easily with pressure and

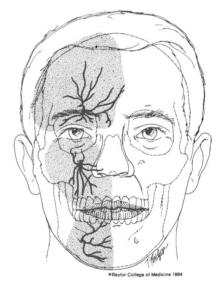

©Baylor College of Medicine 1984

FIG. 52–4. Sites of regional local blocks useful in head and neck area.

epinephrine-solution (1:1000) soaked gauze sponges. The surface is covered with an antibiotic ointment and a nonadherent gauze dressing. The next morning, the patient is allowed to shower and to begin a regimen of gently cleansing the skin with a mild soap at least twice a day. After cleansing, the antibiotic ointment and fine-mesh gauge are reapplied. Generally, antibiotics are not used in the postoperative period. Nonallergenic cosmetics can safely be used 2 to 3 weeks after treatment. A patient undergoing the trilogy of procedures—chemical peel, dermaplaning, and dermabrasion—is seen in Figure 52–5. Another patient, treated by dermabrasion, is seen in Figure 52–6.

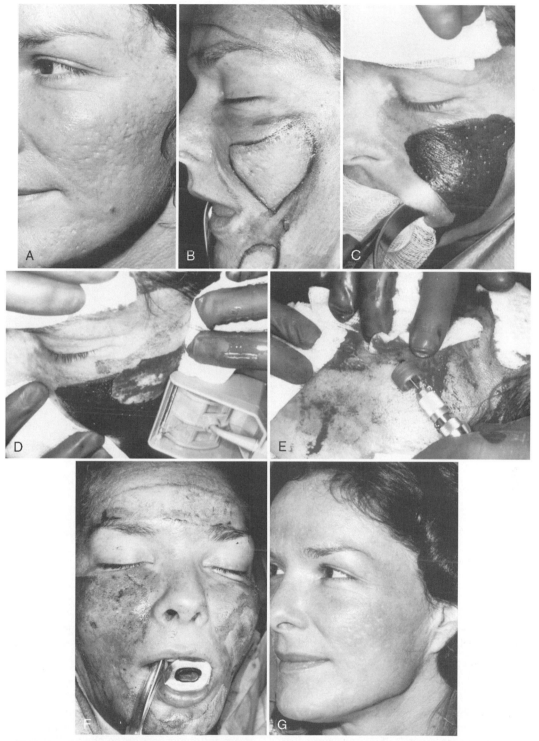

FIG. 52–5. Operative sequence of dermabrasion. **A,** preoperative photograph of 22-year-old white female with nonactive acne scarring, worse in the malar and perimental area. **B,** areas to be dermaplaned are outlined with methylene blue. The adjacent area is first peeled, with the peel carried slightly into the islands marked out for derm-abrasion to ensure a good overlap. **C,** areas previously marked for planing are painted with gentian violet to help in depth excision, and 4 × 4 gauze packs are placed in the patient's mouth for stabilization. **D,** Davol battery-operated dermatome is used to plane the area with countertension. The thickness of skin removed is about 0.015 inch. **E,** final step is dermabrasion to feather out the dermaplaned area. **F,** pa-tient immediately postoperatively. **G,** patient 2 years postoperatively.

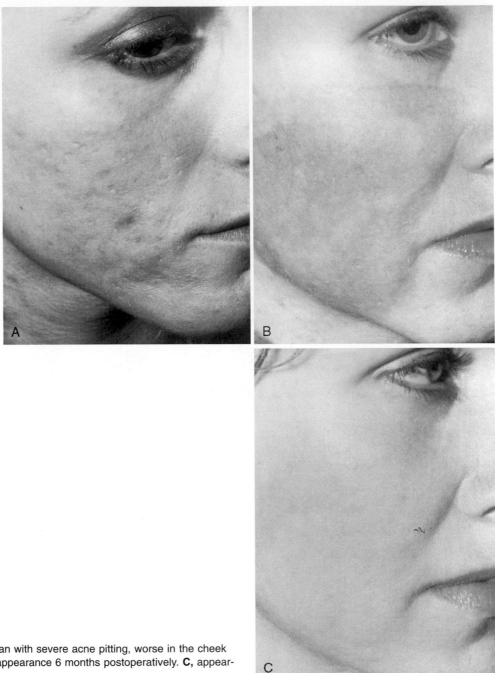

FIG. 52–6. Twenty-one-year-old woman with severe acne pitting, worse in the cheek area. **A,** preoperative appearance. **B,** appearance 6 months postoperatively. **C,** appearance 18 months postoperatively.

RHINOPHYMAS

Rhinophyma is managed by a technique of scalpel excision of the involved tissue followed by dermabrasion to recontour the nose. We prefer to complete one side of the nose first, achieving the desired contour, and then proceed to the other side; this provides a guide as to how much tissue must be removed. Care is taken not to expose the nasal cartilages and to avoid excessive contouring around the alar rims. Because of the propensity for scarring in this area, it is often better to treat the rhinophymas twice, being conservative with the treatment, rather than to trim the nose excessively during the initial procedure.

COMPLICATIONS

Because the cutaneous complications of dermabrasion and chemical face peeling are similar, they are discussed together in the following section on chemical peel.

Chemical Peel

Chemical face peeling, chemosurgery, and chemoexfoliation are terms that are synonyms for the application of an acid or escharotic to the skin. Although this is a very old technique, chemical peeling has become increasingly popular over the past 30 years—primarily for treatment of facial rhytids, abnormal pigmentations, acne scarring, and keratoses. A plethora of chemical agents have been used; we shall discuss phenol, trichloracetic acid (TCA), and the glycolic (alpha hydroxy) acids (8–12). Although there are dramatic differences in the techniques for applying these various acids, the histopathologic features of the chemical peel agents are similar.

PHYSIOHISTOPATHOLOGY

The chemistry and toxicology of phenol has been extensively studied (8,9). Complications are primarily cardiologic, and are manifested by muscular weakness, faintness, weak and irregular pulse, deep respiration, dilated pupils, coma, and possibly even death. Because phenol is selectively cleared by the liver and the kidneys, there is a potential for both hepatic and renal toxicity, especially in patients with damaged livers and reduced creatinine clearance. In contrast, neither TCA nor the glycolic acids have been associated with cardiac, hepatic, or renal toxicity.

Phenol is an acid that causes immediate coagulation of cellular protoplasm. It produces an immediate frost, or whitening, when applied to the skin, which is followed by erythema an hour or so later. The early penetration of phenol, unlike the other acids, exerts a local anesthetic effect, although there is an initial burning sensation. Histologically, the reaction sequence is that of an initial keratocoagulation and epidermal lysis, with a deeper zone of cellular destruction involving only the upper papillary layer of the dermis. A thin crust (superficial eschar) develops, consisting of keratin, necrotic epidermis, and a proteinaceous precipitate interspersed with a cellular exudate. Epidermal regeneration from the pilosebaceous unit begins on the 3rd or 4th day and is usually completed by the 7th to 8th day. Two weeks following application, the epidermal layers appear to be healed, with partial reformation of the rete pegs and an intact but thin stratum corneum; however, dermal reaction is still apparent. Dermal thickening secondary to an inflammatory reaction, with intercellular edema accompanied by perivascular infiltration, is replaced early by a fibroblastic proliferation and deposition of new collagen. Dermal fibrous layers in the papillary dermis persist through the 3rd month as a distinct zone of young collagen with no new elastin noted. With healing of the epidermis, the skin surface is erythematous, then gradually becomes pink, and finally fades over a period of weeks to months (1). Cosmetics containing some green pigment can be used to help mask this erythema. Histologically, there is a diminution in the quantity of melanin granules in the basal layers of the epidermis similar to that seen following dermabrasion (13,14). This phenomenon has not been demonstrated with either TCA or glycolic peels; it is probably responsible for the bleaching of skin following chemical peeling and the inability thereafter to achieve a suntan.

PATIENT SELECTION AND INDICATIONS

The ideal peel patient is middle-aged and fair-skinned, with numerous rhytids and skin pigmentations. Those with darker skin are usually not ideal candidates for phenol peels because of the associated hypopigmentation. However, occasionally darker-skinned individuals may be candidates for the lighter TCA and glycolic peels. Phenol peels need to be approached with some caution in the male patient, whose skin is gener-

ally thicker and who will rarely wear cosmetics to camouflage any difference in skin color between treated and untreated areas. Here again, a TCA or glycolic peel may be more effective.

Spotty hyperpigmentation of pregnancy does lend itself, in select cases, to improvement through chemical peeling. However, in most patients we attempt to induce satisfactory pigmentary improvement using more conservative measures, such as topical application of one of the hydroquinone derivatives (e.g., Solaquin Forte). With sensitive skin, a skin test is recommended when using this particular hydroquinone.

The patient on contraceptive hormonal medications should discontinue medication before chemical peeling to prevent the development of chloasma. We believe that the patient who possesses rhytids and considerable skin redundancy should have a rhytidectomy 3 to 6 months before chemical peeling. When rhytids are present in the perioral, periocular, and forehead areas, peeling can be carried out at the same time as the rhytidectomy at the expense of increased morbidity; an important consideration is that in most patients the chemical peel is an adjunct to the surgery, not a substitute for it. However, the surgeon should use extreme caution before attempting to use any peel agents on skin flaps because of the potential complication of full-thickness skin loss. Other pigmentation changes and/or pigmentary problems (e.g., freckles, lentigos) can be successfully treated with chemical peels. Although chemical peeling has been used for hyperkeratosis and other precancerous lesions in the past, the effectiveness must be compared to other surgical and nonsurgical treatment regimens. Finally, rhytids and pigmentary changes on the dorsum of the hand can be improved with some of the lighter peels, particularly the glycolic acids, and superficial acne scarring can be improved with deep chemical peeling, particularly phenol. However, in our experience, these patients are usually best treated by dermabrasion.

The phenol peel carries one of the highest morbidities in terms of early postoperative patient appearance. Fourteen to twenty-five days must elapse before cosmetics can effectively cover the treated areas and mask the erythema; obviously, this is particularly problematic for the male patient. Because of the amount of morbidity, informed consent is of the greatest importance (as with any chemical peel). Preoperatively, just as in dermabrasion, the patient must be told that larger skin pores, permanently lightened skin, and inability to tan deeply are not complications but sequelae from the phenol peel. The complications for chemical peels are generally the same as for dermabrasion and will be cited below.

PREOPERATIVE PREPARATION

When a full face phenol peel is performed, the surgeon can use personal preference in choosing an analgesic and sedative. Total facial phenol peels are often performed in the hospital, and patients may be admitted overnight for comfort. In general, however, TCA and glycolic acid peels are done in the office and patients are sent home immediately following the peel. It is appropriate to do small areas of phenol peeling (e.g., perioral and touch-up areas) in the office under appropriate light sedation.

A medicated shampoo and face wash are given the night before surgery. The surgical preparation consists of washing the face with soap and water, usually followed by alcohol and ether for degreasing. The purpose of the degreasing is to remove the superficial oils that may interfere with the penetration of the chemical peel. For a phenol chemical peel, we employ the mixture originally described by Litton (8) and subsequently modified by Baker and Gordon: 3 ml of USP phenol 88%, 2 ml sterile water, 3 drops croton oil, and 8 drops Septisol (11). The croton oil is a keratocoagulant that assists in the penetration of the phenol agent and the Septisol acts as an emulsifent. We recommend that the phenol solution be mixed fresh for each application.

PROCEDURE

Although there are similarities among the techniques for using phenol, TCA, and glycolic acid, there are several differences that are highlighted in the appropriate sections. When considering total-face phenol peeling, essentials include appropriate vital-sign monitoring, maintaining an intravenous pathway, and continuous ECG monitoring.

The surgeon's assistant stirs the peel mixture continually to prevent layering, using standard cotton-tipped applicators. The surgeon begins by dipping an applicator into the phenol mixture and expressing the excess liquid by lightly rolling the cotton-tip against the glass container. The cauterant is then applied to the skin by stroking the cotton-tipped applicator in the direction of the lines of least skin tension. The peel is carried directly into the brow and into the hairline in the forehead and temple areas.

In the upper eyelid, the peel is carried down to the superior palpebral furrow or upper border of the tarsal plate; the lower lid is carried to within 1 mm of the free ciliary margin. In peeling the lips, the peel is applied just into the vermillion. Anatomic units are treated one at a time; generally, with phenol peels, we recommend waiting approximately 5 minutes between peeling large anatomical subunits. (Because of the relatively low toxicity associated with TCA and glycolic acids, it is not necessary to pause between peeling anatomical subunits.)

When peeling the entire face, we have found it easiest to peel approximately 1.5 to 2 cm below the lower border of the mandible, feathering out the peeled area with an almost dry cotton-tipped applicator. The dermis of the neck is relatively thin, so we recommend using neither phenol nor TCA on the neck because of the potential for full-thickness skin loss and hypertrophic scarring; similarly, we suggest great caution in using light glycolic acid peels on the neck.

Extreme care is taken to avoid the eyes during the mixing and application of phenol. If the phenol does get into the eyes, flush them immediately with isotonic saline. (Bottled isotonic saline should be included on any chemical peel tray.) If the phenol accidentally gets onto an area of the skin where it is not desired, skin coagulation can be minimized with the rapid application of available alcohol or saline.

One advantage of the phenol peel is that there is an immediate frosting of the skin, which indicates a good take; the physician knows immediately the areas that have been treated with the phenol. In contrast, TCA does not cause an immediate frost, and generally the skin takes about 1 to 3 minutes before turning a whitish color; there is no frosting associated with glycolic acid peels. The frosting reflects immediate denaturing of the superficial epithelium and upper dermis.

Once the total face has been peeled with phenol, many authors recommend waterproof taping the area for deeper pen-

etration. Care is taken not to tape the pretarsal skin of either the upper or lower eyelids. In the submandibular and submental region, the tape is carried to within 1 cm, but not beyond, this peeled area. The tape forms a tight mask, covering the skin and providing an occlusive dressing under which the phenol may exert a macerating, more deeply penetrating effect (Fig. 52–7). An alternative to taping is simpler and probably just as effective: applying a thick layer of either Vaseline, vitamin A and D cream, or Polysporin to the peeled area.

POSTOPERATIVE CARE

The decision to admit a patient postoperatively should be based on the comfort level of the patient, the amount of surface area to which the phenol will be applied, and the general condition of the patient. If the patient is hospitalized for a short period of time, it is generally wise to administer intravenous fluids at least for the first 24 hours; many patients may be reluctant to take fluids by mouth because of facial edema, the presence of tape, and general discomfort. Appropriate analgesics, together with a mild tranquilizer, are usually given, and because most patients experience periocular swelling, "blind precautions" should be ordered for at least the first 24 to 48 hours.

Most phenol peels are now performed in an outpatient setting. It is crucial that the patient be accompanied by a responsible adult who can remain with the patient for at least the first 24 hours. The patient should be encouraged to drink from a straw, which is neater and more comfortable than drinking from a cup or glass. Smoking is prohibited, and talking is discouraged. The patient should be sent home with adequate analgesics and something for sleep. Excessive perioral movement may dislodge the tape, causing an early drying effect of the perioral area and obviating the macerating effect of the tape.

If tape has been applied, it is necessary to remove it within 36 to 48 hours after application. This is a relatively painful procedure and we encourage the use of adequate analgesia. The surgeon removes the tape as gently as possible; gentle sweeping movements under the adhesive with a moistened, cotton-tipped applicator may be helpful. Patients should be forewarned that after removal of the tape they will experience a weeping epidermal surface resembling a second-degree burn. Excess exudate is gently removed with moistened gauze sponges, and ointment may be applied to the entire peeled surface. Thymol iodide may be used as a drying agent.

We emphasize that the postoperative management is critical and the patient must be highly motivated. The patient is encouraged to shower three times daily and to gently wash the face with a bactericidal soap. After showering, the patient reapplies the ointment or thymol iodide powder. By the 7th day, the patient can be started on a corticosteroid cream to hasten the involution of skin edema and erythema. Once the face has reepithelialized completely, a nonallergenic foundation can be applied. The patient is also instructed to avoid sun exposure as much as possible; if it is necessary to be outdoors, a cream or lotion of SPF 15 and a wide-brimmed hat will give some protection.

Pruritus may be a problem during the postoperative period; it can usually be controlled by an antihistamine. Ice packs also may be helpful to relieve the symptoms. Additionally, topical

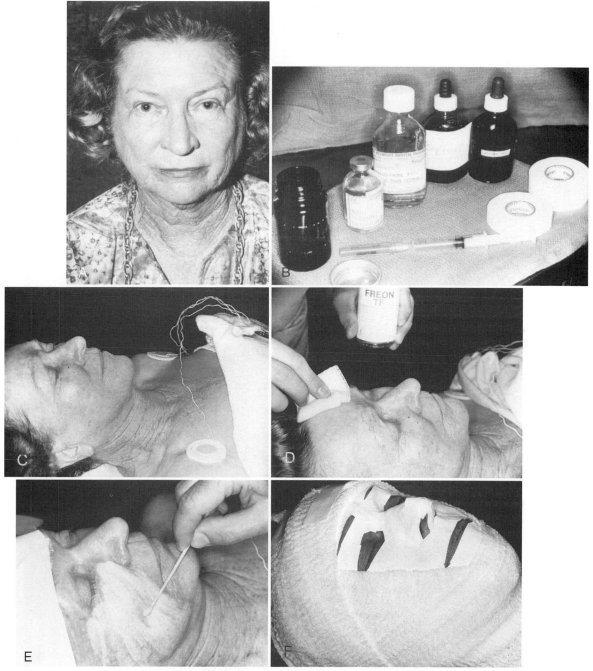

FIG. 52–7. Operative sequence of chemical peel. **A,** preoperative appearance of 60-year-old patient with facial rhytids. **B,** minimal equipment necessary on a Mayo stand. **C,** appropriate monitoring for vital signs includes an electrocardiogram. **D,** skin is cleansed with Freon solution. **E,** cotton-tipped applicator containing solution being applied to the skin by rolling in direction of least skin tension. Anatomic units are treated sequentially. **F,** photograph of taping taken immediately postoperatively, with care taken not to tape the pretarsal area of either the upper or lower lids. A light gauze dressing is applied for a 24-hour period.

antihistamines not only relieve itching but also provide a moist environment. The application of refrigerator-cooled Crisco to relieve pruritus, burning, and eschar discomfort has also been advised.

Any minor trauma to the new epidermis formation can cause bleeding and, ultimately, scarring. It is therefore critical that the patient refrain from any activity that could cause minor trauma—which includes picking at the eschar. We have, on occasion, asked the patient to wear white cotton gloves at night when inadvertent minor trauma to the face has been inflicted during sleep.

Over the past 2 to 3 years, we have been using the tape mask procedure less and less, reserving taping for patients who have deep rhytids. As stated earlier, some authorities feel that liberal application of an ointment can produce the same deep, penetrating results as taping.

The effectiveness of the phenol chemical peel is well documented in the patients seen in Figures 52–8 and 52–9.

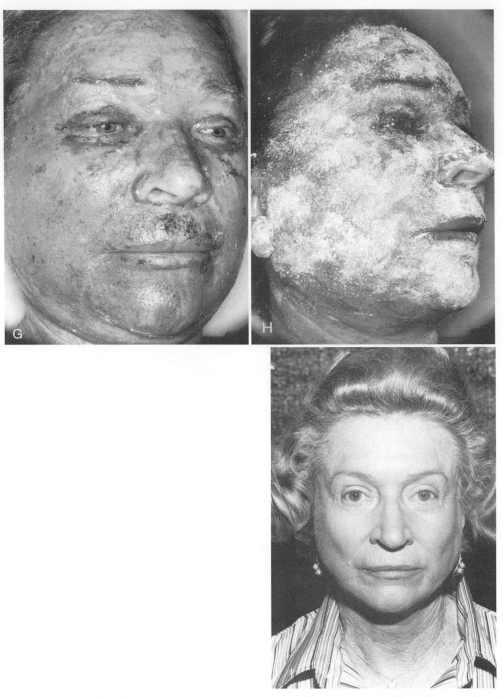

FIG. 52–7.   *continued*   **G,** patient's appearance 48 hours after tape removal. **H,** single application of thymol
iodide is used to initiate drying. **I,** patient 6 months postoperatively.

TRICHLORACETIC ACID (TCA) PEEL

Recently, there has been renewed interest and enthusiasm for
using TCA (12). Trichloracetic acid does not produce as dramatic an effect as phenol, but it is generally better tolerated
by patients because the healing time is much faster. The indications for TCA peel are essentially the same as phenol
with two main exceptions: (a) the TCA peel is not as efficacious in eliminating the deep rhytids, especially those that
are perioral; and (b) the TCA peel is probably better at treating pigmentary changes, especially blepharomelasma.

Trichloracetic acid can either be used by itself or combined
with the pretreatment regimen employing Retin-A (15). Pretreating the patient with Retin-A cream 0.025% nightly for 2
to 3 weeks will create a more profound effect. The concentration may be progressively increased to 0.05% and then to
0.1% before the actual peel. Excessive redness or dryness may
necessitate decreasing the dosage or stopping the drug.

The strength of TCA can be varied anywhere from 10 to
25%, 35 to 50%, and 50 to 75%. As the strength of the TCA
is increased, so are the effects. When using an intermediate

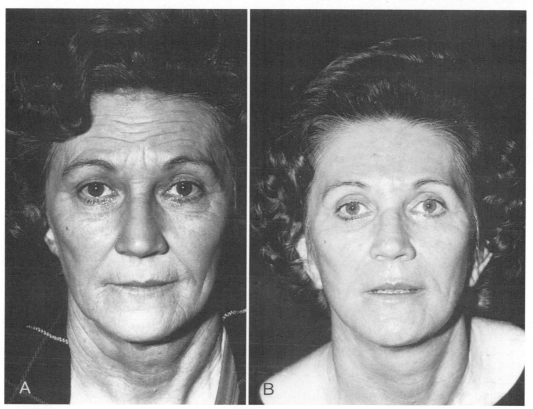

FIG. 52–8.   Fifty-year-old woman with facial rhytids. **A,** appearance before chemical peel. **B,** appearance 2 years after full face peel.

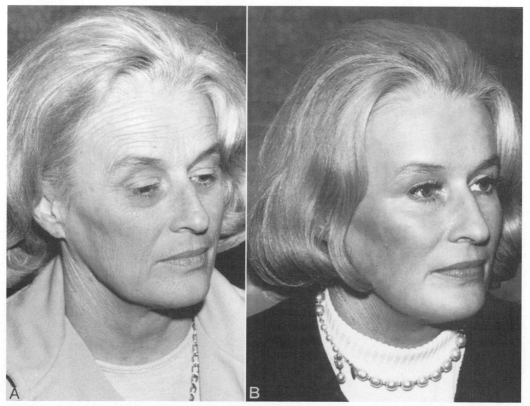

FIG. 52–9.   Fifty-two-year old female with facial rhytids. **A,** appearance before chemical peel. **B,** appearance 2 years after full face peel.

peel (i.e., 35 to 50%), multiple peels may be necessary at 4- to 6-week intervals to achieve the desired results. A 75% concentration TCA peel will have essentially the same histologic changes as a phenol.

Patients tolerate well an intermediate peel of between 35 and 50%. Patients usually experience a 4- to 7-day period of epidermal desquamation (tantamount to a 2° sunburn). After approximately 6 to 7 days, and sometimes sooner, the patient may apply hypoallergenic makeup. Because of the short "down time" compared to phenol peel, TCA peels have been increasingly popular in patients who do not have the luxury of being cloistered for up to 2 weeks. However, it must be emphasized to the patient that they may need successive, intermediate TCA peels to achieve the desired result.

Other advantages of the TCA peel include (a) less edema and postoperative discomfort, (b) no need for local anesthesia, and (c) less systemic toxicity.

The disadvantage of the TCA peel is that the results are not nearly as profound as a phenol peel. One particular disadvantage is that the TCA peel is much more technique-dependent than the phenol peel. When applying TCA, frosting occurs approximately 2 to 4 minutes after application. There have been reports of full-thickness skin loss and subsequent scarring from reapplying the TCA to the same area in expectation of an immediate frost. We recommend that the TCA be applied by applicator swab or by a gauze sponge in aesthetic units.

Another potential problem that is unique to TCA is that it can cause transitory hyperpigmentation (unlike phenol, which can cause profound hypopigmentation). Consequently, in the patient with very fair skin it may be necessary to pretreat with, for example, Solaquin Forte cream for 1 to 2 weeks. In addition, it is critical that, during the healing process and up to 1 year, the patient wear sunblock of at least SPF 15; otherwise, the hyperpigmentary changes may be more profound. Hyperpigmentation is transitory, generally lasting between 1 and 3 months, and can be best treated postoperatively with Solaquin Forte.

GLYCOLIC ACID PEELS

The glycolic (alpha hydroxy) peels are quite different from the standard phenol and TCA peels. The lay term, "fruity acid peels" (they are derived from fruity acids or sugar cane), implies harmlessness, and it must be emphasized to your patients that these agents are still acids and are not innocuous. Histologic effects of glycolic acid peels are not as dramatic as phenol but, with increasing concentrations, these peels will cause discohesion of keratinocytis and epidermal lysis. The indications for glycolic peels are essentially the same as outlined above; however, they are probably best for fine wrinkles, uneven skin tones, and melasma (16).

The peels come in various concentrations including 30, 50, and up to 70%. Of all the chemical peels, the use of glycolic acid is the most technique dependent. After degreasing and cleansing of skin, to provide better penetration with glycolic acid, the surgeon scrapes the superficial layer of epidermis with a no. 10 blade. Once the epidermal planing has been performed, the acid is applied in aesthetic units with either a cotton-tipped applicator or sponge.

The penetration of glycolic acid is time dependent. Generally, the acid is left on the affected area for a period of be-

tween 2 and 6 minutes. The longer the acid is kept on the skin, the deeper is its penetration. When the proper time has elapsed, the acid is neutralized with cold, wet compresses; or, the patient can get up and splash the face with cold water. Unlike phenol and TCA peels, there is no frosting associated with glycolic acid peels. The clinician may notice some erythema and increase in skin turgor, but these are subtle changes and it is more important to time the acid treatments than to rely on clinical examination for its effectiveness.

Glycolic acid peels are well tolerated without the use of any anesthesia. The patient may experience some light flaking of the skin. After the procedure patients may be sent home with weak glycolic-acid solutions that they begin applying 24 hours after the peel. Generally, the patient can use hypoallergenic makeup immediately after the peel. The relatively noncaustic effect of this peel has earned it the nickname of the "lunchtime peel."

To achieve any significant results, the patients will need to be peeled once a week or once every other week for a period of 4 to 6 treatments. The most common side effect is persistent erythema, which can be treated with hydrocortisone cream.

The glycolic acid peels have become popular because of limited down time. However, this must be balanced with the necessity for 4 to 6 repeat peels; and, these peels certainly do not achieve the dramatic results of the other chemical peels. The primary indication for a glycolic acid peel is in younger patients who are just beginning to see signs of small rhytids and pigmentary changes.

COMPLICATIONS

Chemical peel and dermabrasion, while different in a physical sense, are similar in that they both accomplish removal of the epidermis and top layers of the dermis. Consequently, cutaneous complications seen after each of these procedures are similar.

Excessive skin bleaching may result in a demarcation line between treated and untreated skin (Fig. 52–10). The changes in the skin following these procedures include a thinning of the skin, a change in the character of the collagen in the papillary layer of the dermis, and a permanent reduction in the melanin-containing cells of the basement membrane. The deeper the process is carried, be it dermabrasion or chemical

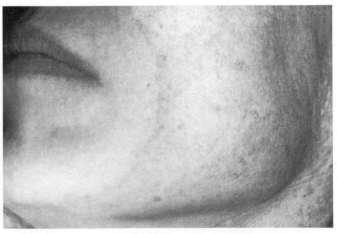

FIG. 52–10. Line of demarcation after isolated perioral peel.

peel, the more effective it is in removing wrinkles, scars, and pigmentation, and the greater the permanent lightening of the skin will be. The problem of color change is often aggravated by a fine zone of hyperpigmentation at the junction of treated and untreated skin. This demarcation line can develop despite extending the peeled area beyond the taped portion, feathering out the peeled area with a lighter concentration of the chemical, or using a lighter dermabrasion. We advise carrying the peel under the jaw line into a shadowy area or repeeling or light dermabrading the demarcation line. The demarcation effect is much more noticeable following sun exposure, especially when no sunscreen has been used to filter out the sun's rays; the neck becomes tan while the face remains light. The use of opaque cosmetics may help.

Splotchy hyperpigmentation is most often seen in darker-skinned patients; often it existed prior to treatment and was, in part, a reason for the peel or dermabrasion. Proper patient selection may help avoid this problem. Although hyperpigmentation problems are much more common with TCA peels, they can occur with phenol peels as well. Hyperpigmentation has not been found as much with glycolic acid peels. To avoid this problem, local areas can be pretreated with Solaquin Forte, which may also be used to improve the problem after the peel.

In the absence of any frank areas of skin loss or skin necrosis, scars and contractures have been noted following perioral peel when the peel has been combined with an extended surgical rhytidectomy and the cheek skin has been undermined to the nasolabial folds.

One to two months after the peel, isolated small scars have been noted along the lower border of the mandible and on both the upper and lower lips adjacent to the vermilion ridge. These are related to localized skin tensions combined with localized areas of deeper skin loss. This complication can usually be avoided by confining the treatment to the epidermis and papillary and upper reticular dermis, particularly in those areas where hypertrophic scar formation or contractures are most common (perioral area, neck). Just as continual motion is probably a factor contributing to the development of hypertrophic scarring over the sternum and anterior chest, repetitive small-muscle action in the perioral area may disturb the healing process sufficiently to induce scarring. Baker and Gordon limited taping to the vermilion ridge itself when doing a perioral peel to reduce vertical wrinkles or rhytids (17). In treating scar contractures where mouth opening is limited, small injections of triamcinolone (Kenalog) hasten maturation of the scar and decrease the contracture. Excision, combined with a small Z-plasty, adequately corrected the problem in another case in which scarring occurred after dermaplaning and dermabrasion for acne scars. Patient compliance, light massage, and "tincture of time" are other factors that can make the treatment of this very difficult problem easier (Fig. 52–11).

Fortunately, full-thickness skin loss is rare. We reported one case that followed a brow lift (18). Using the formula given and the technique described above, this has not occurred in any other case from excessive depth of the peel. In our single case, skin necrosis developed following simultaneous undermining of the peeled area and the application of the chemical. Possibly, edema resulted in an impaired local blood supply that led to the skin necrosis. In our opinion, this complication can be avoided by never treating the same area of skin with simultaneous peeling and undermining; the two procedures should be separated by a minimum of 6 weeks. In treating this complication, epithelialization from the remaining dermal appendages and the peripheral skin should be allowed. The surgeon must refrain from the impulsion to débride these areas. The resultant healed scar will often be more acceptable cosmetically than a skin graft. Surgical revision may be necessary later (Fig. 52–12).

Pinhead-sized, whitish nodules, 1.0 to 1.5 mm in diameter can be quite a nuisance both to the patient and the physician. They represent epidermal cysts that result either from blockage of the pilosebaceous orifice or from mechanical intrusion of a portion of the epidermis into the dermis followed by proliferation of the embedded epithelium. The condition frequently occurs within the first few weeks, and even up to 3 months, after skin treatment. Very small milia may resolve on their own and the process can be accelerated by having the patient gently wash the area with a mildly abrasive soap or buff-buff, providing the peeled area has adequately healed. Large milia may be expressed easily using an 18-gauge needle.

Although bacterial infections are very uncommon after a chemical peel and dermabrasion, herpetic infections may be devastating. It is important to get a good history from your patient before embarking on a chemical peel concerning eruption of cold sores or other perioral and intraoral herpetic infections. If the patient does have a history of herpetic infections, we recommend pretreating these patients with acyclovir (Zovirax 200 mg 5 times per day for 5 days) both before and after the peel. Additionally, if herpetic infections do occur in the peeled or dermabraded area, we advise getting an infectious disease consultation; the dosage of Zovirax may need to be increased. Herpetic infections will manifest themselves as small, clear, whitish nodules occurring in the peeled areas that may either be pruritic or quite painful. If a patient exhibits perioral herpetic activity on the day of the peel, we will delay the peel until the lesions have entirely healed.

CONCLUSION

There is no denying that there are unfortunate side effects, annoying complications, and frankly unfavorable results accompanying dermabrasion, dermaplaning, and chemical peeling; however, these procedures, when properly employed in select patients, can give effective, consistent, and long-lasting results. Generally, the patient who is adequately informed preoperatively of the minor undesirable effects will accept them well. Frank complications can usually be avoided by adhering to proper patient selection, by using the standard technique, by adapting the technique to the skin being treated, and by appropriate postoperative care.

Injectable Collagen

The work with bovine collagen by Knapp and colleagues in 1977 began a new era in the treatment of soft-tissue contour irregularities (19). While injectable collagen is not, by far, a permanent remedy to soft-tissue contour irregularities, it has proved to be a extremely useful adjunct to traditional surgical therapies for soft-tissue defects.

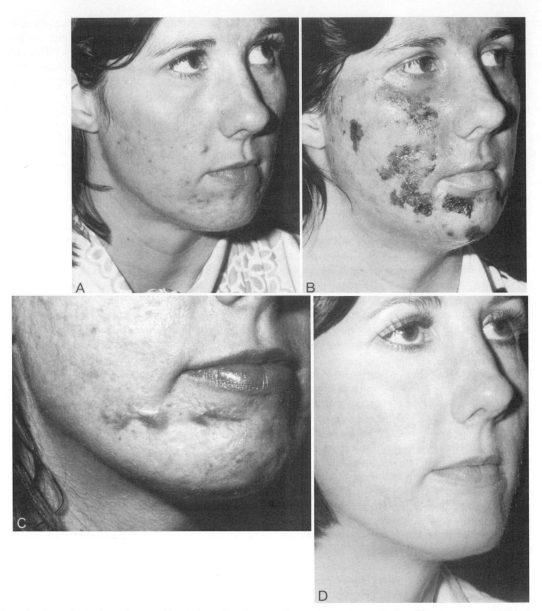

FIG. 52–11. Complication of scarring after combined dermabrasion and peel. **A,** patient preoperatively, with acne scarring, worse in the cheek perioral area. **B,** patient 5 days after dermabrasion. **C,** patient 6 months postoperatively, with severe scar contracture. **D,** patient 18 months postoperatively, after three injections with dilute Kenalog, massage, and partial excision.

MATERIALS

The collagen molecule consists of three polypeptide chains bound together into a triple helix (20). Extensive cross-linkage exists within and between collagen molecules. By removing the end peptide and modifying the triple-helix collagen molecule, the major source of antigenicity is reduced. As reported by Chvapil (21), the characteristics of collagen medical products are closely related to the extent of cross-linkage; the greater the degree of cross-linkage, the slower is the resorption.

The animal studies by Knapp and coworkers (19) with the purified, reconstituted fibrous dispersion isolated from cowhide showed that there was an intense, leukopolymorphic nuclear neutrophilic response at 12 to 72 hours after local injection. This early response subsided within 1 week and was followed by an influx of vascular channels and fibroblasts. In 1 month, neuvascularization was nourishing the fibroblasts. The tissue at the injection site was found to be soft, with good tensile strength, the stabilized implant neither migrating nor becoming encapsulated during the 6-month study.

The injectable collagen commonly used today (Zyderm) is a fibrous dispersion packaged by the Collagen Corporation. Containing physiological saline and 0.3% lidocaine in fluid form that allows injection through a 30-gauge needle, it has been finely filtered and purified by a process that renders it sterile (22). As long as Zyderm is kept at 0° to 5° C, its molecules remain suspended and separated. When the material is brought to 37° C, it undergoes fibrous transformation into a gel and then into an opaque, semisolid mass of orderly, condensed fibrous collagen. The product is dispensed, prepack-

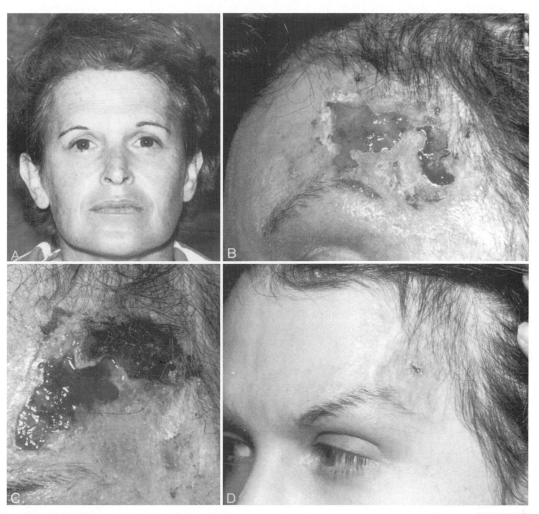

FIG. 52–12. Example of full-thickness skin loss after peel. **A,** preoperative photograph of patient scheduled for full face peel. **B,** status 5 days after peel, with a full-thickness loss of the forehead skin. **C,** appearance 21 days postoperatively with diminution of the open area treated by local wet-to-dry dressing. **D,** appearance 6 months postoperatively, with complete epithelialization.

aged, in 1-ml tuberculin-type syringes and should be refrigerated until use. Within 72 hours of implantation, the saline carrier is resorbed and the suspended collagen fibers come out of dispersion and form a soft, palpable implant. The collagen is this implant constitutes approximately 3.5% of the total injected volume (Zyderm I) and serves as a matrix into which fibroblasts and capillaries grow. The newly vascularized implant becomes incorporated into host tissues (21). Zyderm II, constituting approximately 6.5% of the total injected volume, incorporates an even greater amount. Zyplast (3.5% collagen) is cross-linked by glutaraldehyde treatment during preparation. It is used to correct tissue deficiencies below the skin and is longer lasting than either Zyderm I or II.

PATIENT SELECTION

A complete medical history is obtained from each patient, and a skin test is administered to determine any preexisting sensitivity to the implant. Patients with a personal or family history of autoimmune disorders or collagen vascular diseases were initially excluded from the clinical trials by the manufacturer. Thus, collagen should not be used on individuals with a documented personal history of autoimmune disease.

The test is administered as an interdermal injection in the volar forearm and is monitored for 4 weeks for signs of sensitivity. A positive skin test is defined by the Collagen Corporation as any erythema, induration, tenderness, or swelling at the test site, with or without pruritus, that persists for more than 6 hours or appears more than 24 hours after implantation or onset of a rash, arthralgia, or myalgia. Clinical experience with this material reveals that, immediately upon injection, a wheal and flare appear; these usually subside within 3 days in a negative test and the test site becomes virtually undetectable. A positive test result is usually characterized by a firm, erythematous nodule that appears days or weeks after test implantation. In national clinical trials, unfavorable skin tests occurred in 248 of 9427 patients, an incidence of 3% (23).

The first test does gives a positive reaction in 90% of all patients who will eventually react to the collagen. The other 10% react only after a second dose. Double testing, in our opinion, must be performed when any unusual response or equivocal result occurs. The consistency in appearance of a test site can help predict the efficacy of the collagen. If the test implanted area remains fairly soft and pliable, the patient is a good candidate for treatment. Interestingly, patients who are known to be alcoholic abusers must be warned to abstain from alcohol for 1 month before test-dosing with collagen. Alcohol, and other vasoactive agents, have been implicated in reducing positive test sites (24). Our experience is that, regardless of the concentration of the collagen or the injection technique employed, resorption of the collagen implant has almost always occurred 2 to 6 months postimplant. Consequently, successful therapy with injectable collagen requires initial overcorrection and repetitive injections, and the patient needs to be informed that this is a maintenance therapy. We have not had a single case of permanent overcorrection.

INDICATIONS FOR INJECTIONS

When considering patients for the use of injectable collagen, the overall temporary benefit of the injectable collagen must be compared to the other, more permanent, treatment modalities described earlier in the chapter (e.g., dermabrasion) (Fig. 52–13). Injectable collagen has been used successfully in the treatment of saucer- and crater-type acne depressions. It is important that the areas need to be overcorrected. Icepick acne scars are probably best treated by different modalities (e.g., direct excision).

One of the more popular indications for injectable collagen is the treatment of nasolabial folds. Injectable collagen, although temporary, can give you dramatic improvement in the nasolabial fold. Other facial rhytids, and lateral crows' feet, can also be improved temporarily by injectable collagen (Fig. 52–14).

Depressed scars can also be temporarily improved by injectable collagen. Infiltration of the collagen will balloon out the depressed area, thereby precluding a shallower depression. In contour deformities following procedures such as rhinoplasty and cleft lip, injectable collagen has been found to be extremely useful in correcting small asymmetries (Fig. 52–15).

Generally it is helpful to mark the soft-tissue defect to be corrected with a fine felt-tip pin. If large areas are to be injected, local regional blocks with 1% lidocaine decreases patient discomfort. After prepping the area with alcohol, 30-gauge needles are used to inject the collagen. It is imperative

that the collagen be properly placed in the dermis, with enough material used to illicit a small wheal and tissue blanching.

There are basically three techniques of injection: (a) inserting the needle, creating a tract, and injecting the collagen as the needle is withdrawn; (b) inserting the needle interdermally, fanning it from one area to another, and injecting as it is advanced; and (c) multiply reinserting the needle at a 45° angle to the area being treated (Fig. 52–16).

According to Kaplan and colleagues (24), successful therapy with collagen depends on how much the tissue can be extended and overcorrected. Our experience with Zyderm demonstrates that appreciable improvement is obtained only when a lesion can be corrected from 1.5 to 2 times its initial depth. Overcorrection resolves within 2 to 3 days of injection when absorption of saline occurs. The condensed implant represents only a fraction of the original volume. If the more-concentrated Zyderm II or Zyplast is used, overcorrection is still essential; however, less resorption will occur.

COMPLICATIONS

As stated earlier, incidence of positive test-site responses in national surveys was 3%. Of these, 230 patients had localized reactions, 20 had distal or systemic reactions without test-site involvement, and 34 had responses that were both localized and systemic. Systemic reactions include arthralgia, myalgias, fever, malaise, generalized rash, and edema. Additionally, severe problems of late hypersensitivity at the injection site that resulted in erythema, visible induration, and symptomatic pruritus have been reported (23). The use of antihistamines and topical steroids may help improve these transient symptoms.

CONCLUSION

There is no doubt that many soft-tissue contour irregularities can be temporarily improved by the use of collagen. The benefits of injectable collagen, as discussed, need to outweigh its transient nature, repetitive need for treatment, and expense. It has been our experience that the areas best treated with injectable collagen are laugh lines and nasolabial folds.

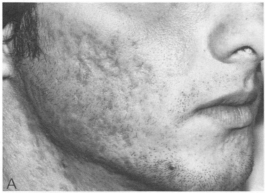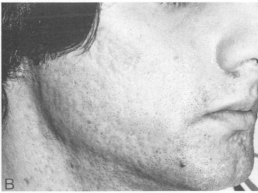

FIG. 52–13. Twenty-five-year old male with severe acne treated with combined dermabrasion and collagen injections. **A,** preoperative appearance. **B,** appearance 3 months after dermabrasion and five treatments with Zyderm I. (Photographs courtesy of D.R. Wiemer, M.D.)

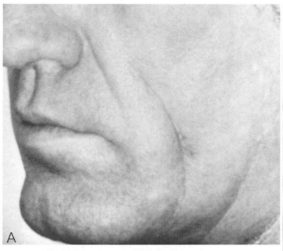

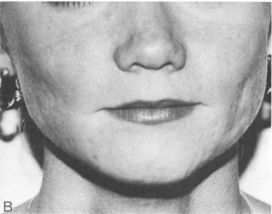

FIG. 52–14. Forty-two-year-old white male with deep nasolabial folds as well as adjacent deep rhytids causing a very stern appearance. **A,** preoperative appearance. **B,** appearance after three treatments with Zyderm I. (Photographs courtesy of R. Kriedel, M.D.)

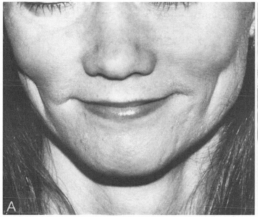

FIG. 52–15. Twenty-year-old female with extremely prominent depression of cheek in dimple area causing an atrophied appearance, especially when smiling. **A,** preoperative appearance. **B,** appearance after three treatments with Zyderm II.

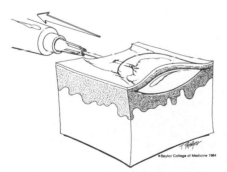

FIG. 52–16. Technique of collagen injection in the upper dermis.

References

1. Spira M, Dahl C, Freeman R, et al. Chemosurgery: a histological study. *Plast Reconstr Surg* 1970; 45:247.
2. Campbell RM. Surgical and chemical planing of the skin. In: Converse JM, ed. *Reconstructive plastic surgery*. 2nd ed. Philadelphia: WB Saunders, 1977; 442.
3. Baker TJ, Gordon HL, Seckinger DL. A second look at chemical face peeling. *Plast Reconstr Surg* 1966; 37:487.
4. Baker TJ, Gordon HL, Mosienko P, et al. Long-term histological study of the skin after chemical face peeling. *Plast Reconstr Surg* 1974; 53:522.
5. Mopper C, Mercannini ES. The inadequacy of dermabrasion in therapy of nevi. *Can Med Assoc J* 1960; 83:1015.
6. Cronin TD. Extensive pigmented nevi in hair-bearing areas: removal of pigmented layer while preserving the hair follicles. *Plast Reconstr Surg* 1953; 11:94.
7. Spira M, Freeman R, Arfai P, et al. Clinical comparison of chemical peeling, dermabrasion, and 5-FU for senile keratoses. *Plast Reconstr Surg* 1970; 46:61.
8. Litton C. Chemical face lifting. *Plast Reconstr Surg* 1973; 51:645.

9. Baker TJ. Chemical face peeling and rhytidectomy. A combined approach for face rejuvenation. *Plast Reconstr Surg* 1962; 29:199.

10. Ayres S III. Superficial chemosurgery. In: Epstein E Jr, ed. *Skin surgery*. 4th ed. Springfield, IL: Charles C Thomas, 1977; 552.

11. Baker TJ, Gordon HL. Chemical peel with phenol. In: Epstein E Jr, ed. *Skin surgery*. 4th ed. Springfield, IL: Charles C Thomas, 1977; 613.

12. Wolford FS, Dalton WE, Hoopes JE. Chemical peel with trichloracetic acid. *Br J Plast Surg* 1972; 25:333.

13. Baker TJ, Gordon HL. Chemical face peeling and dermabrasion. *Surg Clin North Am* 1971; 51:387.

14. Morgan JE, Gilchrest B, Goldwyn RM. Skin pigmentation, current concepts and relevance to plastic surgery. *Plast Reconstr Surg* 1975; 56:617.

15. Hevio O, et al. Tretinoin accelerates healing after trichloracetic acid chemical peel. *Arch Dermatol* 1991; 127:678.

16. Moy LS, Murad H, Moy RL. Glycolic acid peels for the treatment of wrinkles and photoaging. *J Dermatol Surg Oncol* 1993; 19:243.

17. Baker TJ Jr, Gordon HL. Chemical face peeling. In: Goldwyn RM, ed. *The unfavorable result in plastic surgery*. Boston: Little, Brown, 1977; 345.

18. Spira M, Gerow FJ, Hardy SB. Complications of chemical face peeling. *Plast Reconstr Surg* 1974; 54:397.

19. Knapp TR, Luck E, Daniels TR. Behaviour of solubilized collagen as a bioimplant. *J Surg Res* 1977; 23:96.

20. Selmanowitz VJ, Orentreich N. Medical grade fluid silicone: a monographic review. *J Dermatol Surg Oncol* 1977; 3:597.

21. Chvapil M, Kroenthal RL, Van Winkle W. Medical and surgical applications of collagen. *Int Rev Connect Tissue Res* 1973; 6:1.

22. Stegman SJ, Tromovitch TA. Implantation of collagen for depressed scars. *J Dermatol Surg Oncol* 1980; 6:150.

23. Kamer FM, Churukian MM. Clinical use of injectable collagen. *Arch Otolaryngol* 1984; 110:93.

24. Kaplan EN, Falces E, Tolleth H. Clinical utilization of injectable collagen. *Ann Plast Surg* 1983; 10:437.

Suggested Readings

Alt TH. Occluded Baker-Gordon. Chemical peel: review and update. *J Dermatol Surg Oncol* 1989; 15:980.

Brody HJ. Complications of chemical peeling. *J Dermatol Surg Oncol* 1989; 15:1010.

Goldman PM, Freed MI. Aesthetic problems in chemical peeling. *J Dermatol Surg Oncol* 1989; 15:1020.

Knapp TR, Kaplan EN, Daniels JR. Injectable collagen for soft tissue augmentation. *Plast Reconstr Surg* 1977; 60:398.

Stagnone JJ. Superficial peeling. *J Dermatol Surg Oncol* 1989; 15:294.

Stenzel KH, Miyata T, Rubin A. Collagen as a biomaterial. *Ann Rev Biophys Bioeng* 1974; 3:231.

53

Aesthetic Rhinoplasty

Fernando-Ortiz Monasterio, M.D.

The nose, because of its central location, is an important element in facial aesthetics. The size and shape of the nose varies with the race and sex. It is conditioned by the volume and strength of the osteocartilaginous framework and the thickness of the soft-tissue cover. Its appearance is also closely related to the whole face, with which it should have a harmonious relation.

Rhinoplasty is one of the most common aesthetic operations in plastic surgery. It is a complex procedure requiring understanding of the anatomy and how each element contributes to the shape of the nose. The surgeon must have a clear idea of the desired result and how each alteration of the nasal structures will contribute to achieve this goal. Numerous techniques have been described to perform a rhinoplasty. Many of them may produce excellent results in the hands of experienced surgeons and in many instances a specific problem can be solved using two or more different ways depending on the surgeon's personal preference and expertise.

This chapter includes ideas proposed by many authors. This technique has evolved as the result of personal experience, careful observation, and evaluation of long-term results. The operative procedure I describe here can achieve predictable results with a minimum of complications (1–5).

Initial Consultation

The goals of a rhinoplasty are to obtain a pleasing aesthetic result and to have a satisfied patient. These two objectives may not necessarily coincide, and it is important to understand the expectations of the patient before the operation.

Some patients have an objective view of their particular problem and expect results that can be reasonably obtained by the operation. Others may want a change that will not be harmonious with the face or that cannot be achieved by an operation. Sometimes a minimal or nonexisting deformity is magnified, or problems in other areas of the face are related to the nose. Also, some patients expect unrealistic changes in facial beauty or in their quality of life that are beyond the scope of the surgery.

A careful preoperative evaluation of these expectations is important to prevent many unpleasant postoperative problems. When necessary, the patient is seen several times in the office before planning an operation. When faced with anxious, depressed, overdemanding, or unrealistic patients, the surgeon should explain that surgery is not likely to fulfill their expectations and refuse to operate. In my experience, it takes more time to refuse to operate in a cordial way than to propose an operation, but it is worth the effort to build a successful practice.

Examination

It is important to examine the whole face. The patient should be comfortably seated on a rotating stool. To assess symmetry, an imaginary vertical line is traced from the hairline to the chin, dividing the face in two halves. The surgeon observes the position of eye canthus, nasal alae, and buccal commissures, as well as deviation of the nasal pyramid. When the nose is examined in a full face view, the dorsum appears as two parallel or slightly concave lines extending from the brows to the tip of the nose. The width of the alar base should correspond to the intercanthal distance (Fig. 53–1). If the lateral aspect of the ala extends more than 2 mm beyond a vertical line traced from the medial canthus, it suggests that the base is broad and will require a resection of the nostril sill. The domes of the alar cartilages should ideally protrude slightly above the dorsum, producing two prominent points. A third point of prominence must show at the midline at the junction of the middle crus with the medial crus. A superiorly based triangle is then highlighted by the three points.

On the profile view, the face is divided by four imaginary horizontal lines: at the hairline, at the brows, at the base of the columella, and at the chin. An extra line can be traced at the stomiun to analyze the proportions of the lower third of the face. This view, dividing the face in three sections, gives a general impression of vertical facial harmony (Fig. 53–2). Facial convexity and nasal and chin projection in relation to the rest of the face can be appraised on the profile view.

The length of the nose is measured from the nasion to the most prominent point of the tip. The nasion is the lowest point on the frontonasal groove; it should be located at a point between the margin of the upper lid and the upper edge of the tarsal plate with the eye open and looking straight ahead (Fig. 53–3). When the nasion is located at a lower level, it suggests underprojection of the dorsum that may require grafting. When located too high, bone resection at the glabellar area may be necessary. The dorsum should be straight, with the tip protruding about 2 mm further.

Tip projection can be assessed by tracing a horizontal line from the alar cheek junction to the tip. A vertical (perpendicular to the Frankfurt plane) tangential to the upper lip is traced. If more than 60% of the horizontal distance is in front of the vertical line, the tip is overprojected (Fig. 53–4); the opposite suggests underprojection. The angle formed by the

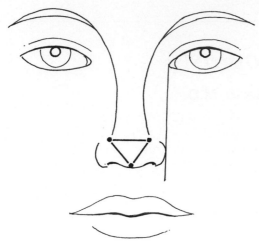

FIG. 53–1.   In the full face view, the nasal pyramid should be limited by two parallel or slightly concave lines extending from the brow to the tip. The domes should protrude at two symmetrical points highlighting the tip. The width of the nasal base should be equal to the intercanthal distance.

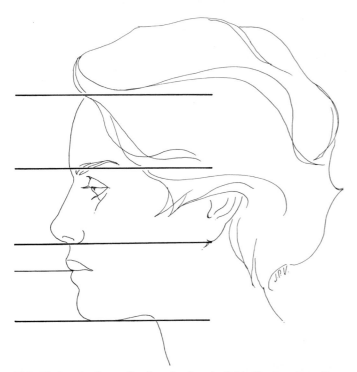

FIG. 53–2.   On the profile view, the face is divided by imaginary lines into three sections. The vertical harmony and the proportions of the nose in relation to the rest of the face, as well as the facial convexity and the prominence of the nose and the chin, can be evaluated.

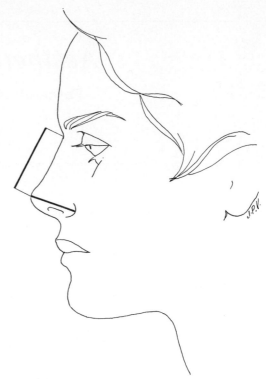

FIG. 53–3.   The length of the nose is measured from the nasion (the lowest point of the frontonasal groove) to the most prominent point of the tip. Tip projection is measured from the alar–cheek junction to the most prominent point of the tip.

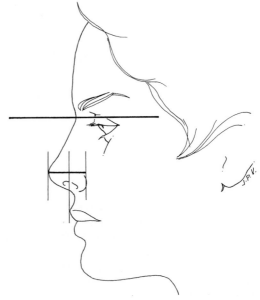

FIG. 53–4.   The nasion should be located at the level between the upper-lid margin and the upper edge of the tarsal plate, with the eyes open in frontal gaze; a nasion located on a lower position suggests the need for a dorsal graft. To assess tip projection, a horizontal line parallel to the Frankfurt plane is traced from the alar–cheek junction to the tip. When this is crossed by a vertical line tangential to the upper lip, it should be divided in two roughly equal segments. When more than 60% of the nose is in front of the vertical line, it suggests overprojection; the opposite suggests an underprojected tip.

columella and the upper lip should be between 95° and 105° for the females and 90° to 95° for the males (5–7).

By palpation, the surgeon determines the vertical length of the nasal bones as well the thickness and elasticity of the cartilaginous framework and the thickness and fixation of the skin to the underlying structures.

The examination is completed with the inspection of the nasal cavities with a frontal light, using a nasal speculum.

At the end of the examination, full face, basal, profile, and three-quarters photos of the patient should be obtained. Using the negatoscope, the surgical plan is traced on the back of the profile photo. The predicted result is discussed with the patient—with or without the photos, depending on medico-legal considerations.

General Technique

ANESTHESIA

With few exceptions, I prefer to perform all complete rhinoplasties under general anesthesia through orotracheal intubation combined with local infiltration. A solution of 0.5% lidocaine and 1:80,000 epinephrine is injected along the incision lines, followed by infiltration in the areas of dissection in the nasal pyramid, the tip, and the columella. Submucosal infiltration is made on both sides of the septum when septoplasty or graft harvesting is contemplated. Nasal packs with 2% lidocaine are inserted intranasally.

For smaller procedures, and under special conditions, a combination of intravenous sedation and local anesthesia may be used. In these cases, a meticulous infiltration at the paranasal area, at the base of the columella, and at the glabellar region must be combined with topical application of 5% cocaine or 2% lidocaine in the nasal cavity.

INCISIONS

The *intra*cartilaginous incision is my choice for most rhinoplasties. The *inter*cartilaginous incision is adequate, but may easily produce a small webbing when it is extended along the caudal edge of the septum. The *infra*cartilaginous incision (rim incision) following the caudal margin of the alar cartilage is convenient for the refinement of a very wide tip or for secondary corrections around that area.

The intracartilaginous incision is located at the middle of the alar cartilage at roughly the same distance from the cephalic and the caudal edges (Fig. 53–5). It extends from the lateral end of the lateral crus to the dome and slightly into the middle crus. When resection of the caudal edge of the septum, septoplasty, or graft harvesting are contemplated, the incision is extended along the caudal edge of the septum to the base of the columella (see Fig. 53–5). This vertical extension is made only on one side, except when caudal septal resection is indicated. The intracartilaginous incision includes only the vestibular skin and the perichondrium (1,13).

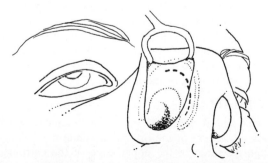

FIG. 53–5. Dotted line showing the location of the intracartilaginous incision. It may be extended inferiorly along the caudal edge of the septum when septal work or graft harvesting are contemplated.

DISSECTION

To preserve function, it is important to maintain the continuity of the mucosal lining by performing the whole operation through an extramucosal approach. With fine sharp-pointed iris scissors, the mucoperichondrial flap is elevated in a cephalad direction to the level of the upper edge of the alar cartilage (Fig. 53–6). At this point, the fine ligament joining the upper and the lower cartilages is cut with a no. 15 blade, extending the subcutaneous dissection over the cartilaginous dorsum (Fig. 53–7). This is then completed with subperiosteal dissection of the bony dorsum with a Joseph periosteal elevator (Fig. 53–8).

Except when the skin is very thick the dissection of the dorsum should be limited, providing only the necessary space to introduce a rasp. Limiting the dissection preserves the circulation and decreases postoperative edema.

To preserve the continuity of the mucosal lining when a large dorsal hump is to be resected, it is necessary to dissect a subpericondrial tunnel along both sides of the anterior edge of the septum (Fig. 53–9). The tunnel is extended laterally

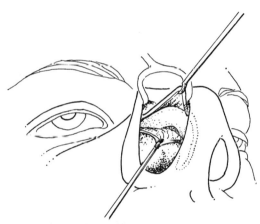

FIG. 53–6. The mucoperichondrial flap is elevated, exposing the cephalic edge of the upper lateral cartilage and the intercartilaginous ligament.

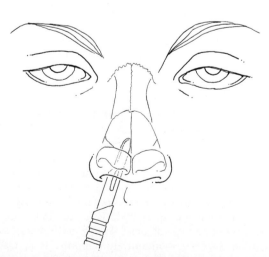

FIG. 53–7. A no. 15 blade is introduced through the intercartilaginous space in order to do a subcutaneous dissection of the lower dorsum.

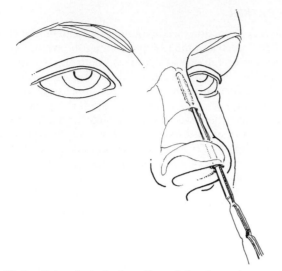

FIG. 53–8. Subperiosteal dissection of the bony hump with a Joseph periosteal elevator.

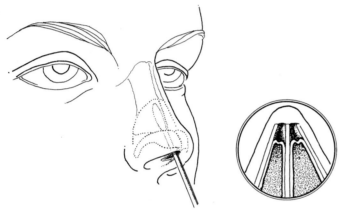

FIG. 53–9. Dissection of the mucosal lining along the cartilaginous dorsum. A tunnel is made on each side of the anterior edge of the septum before removing the hump.

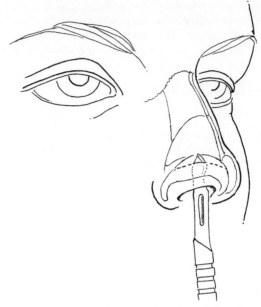

FIG. 53–10. Resection of the cephalic edge of the alar cartilage from the lateral end of the lateral crura to the dome.

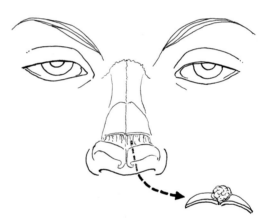

FIG. 53–11. Resection of the two segments of the alar cartilages in one block with the fatty tissue located between the domes.

under the medial portion of the upper lateral cartilages. The dorsal hump can then be removed, while the undermined mucosa remains intact (8).

TIP CONTOURING

In most cases, only a limited resection of the upper edge of the alar cartilage is necessary to refine the tip. The extent of the resection is determined preoperatively, depending on the projection and shape of the cartilages (7,9). A strip of cartilage 4 to 6 mm wide is usually removed from the cephalic edge of the alar cartilage from the lateral end of the lateral crus to the dome, extending slightly into the middle crus when the tip is wide (Fig. 53–10). It is necessary to leave a section at least 4 to 5 millimeters wide of the alar cartilage to maintain tip support. It is also very important to preserve the continuity of the cartilaginous arch to achieve a pleasant contour as well as symmetry of the tip. Transection of the arch will result in visible irreg-

ularities under the skin when the postoperative edema subsides. Transection may also produce collapse of the arch and asymmetries of the nostrils.

Further tip refinement can be achieved by resection of the fatty tissue located between the alar domes (Fig. 53–11). To facilitate the cephalad rotation of the tip, the alar cartilages are then freed from the skin with curved Fomon scissors, dissecting in a retrograde direction. With the previous maneuvers, the tip is refined and rotated superiorly, achieving some tilt-up and shortening of the nose.

PLUNGING TIP

The lower lateral cartilages may have a caudal orientation, resulting in descent of the tip and an acute nasolabial angle. Although resection of the upper edge of the cartilage automatically results in cephalad rotation, it must be remembered that the fibrous attachment of the lateral crura, with the accessory cartilages, extends the structural support of the tip to

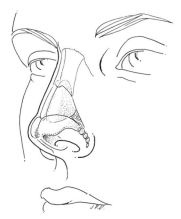

FIG. 53–12. Diagram showing the structural support of the nose. The alar cartilages extend laterally and inferiorly to the base of the nostril through fibrous unions with the accessory cartilages. For mechanical purposes this alar arch works as a unit. The two domes are joined by a loose ligament. Another ligament joins the upper and lower lateral cartilages in the overlapping area. These anatomic details are important for the correction of an overprojected or drooping tip.

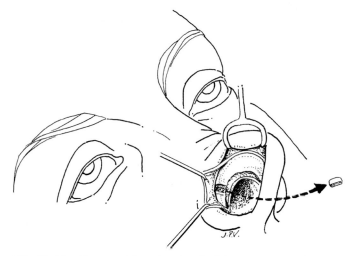

FIG. 53–13. To correct the plunging tip, it is necessary to interrupt the continuity of the arch formed by the upper lateral and its attachments with the accessory cartilages. This eliminates the "memory" of the cartilages, allowing the cephalad rotation of the tip.

the base of the nose, almost completing the circle around the nostril (1,10) (Fig. 53–12). To allow free cephalad rotation of the tip and to prevent relapses, it is necessary to transect the cartilaginous arch laterally to the lateral crura. The shape of the tip is thus preserved, while the "memory" of the cartilage is eliminated.

Caudal descent of the tip may be associated with a short medial crura, requiring freeing of the cartilages from the columellar base and the insertion of the cartilage strut (9,11).

TIP PROJECTION

Overprojection of the tip ("Pinocchio" nose) requires reduction to harmonize with the nasal dorsum. Some surgeons prefer to resect a section of the cartilage at the level of the dome or at the junction of the dome with the medial crura. Others prefer to resect the domes and replace them with an umbrella-shaped cartilage graft. These techniques produce good results in the hands of very experienced surgeons, but asymmetries and irregularities may frequently result.

For the less-experienced surgeon, I suggest a safer technique. Consider the structural support of the tip as two cartilaginous arches joined at the midline. Each arch has two support columns: one is the medial crura and the other is the extension of the lateral crura through its fibrous attachment with the accessory cartilages, which extends to the pyriform area at the base of the nostril (1). It is preferable to resect a section of the arch, lateral to the lateral crura (Fig. 53–13). This decreases the lateral support of the arch. If more reduction is necessary, a resection of the medial crura immediately above the base at the columella decreases the projection of the medial column. By this method, the cartilage arch remains intact at the level of the dome, avoiding postoperative deformities (Fig. 53–14).

Underprojection of the tip may be corrected by medial rotation of the lateral crura, which are sutured to each other at the midline. This is better accomplished through an infracartilage incision and extensive dissection of the alar cartilages,

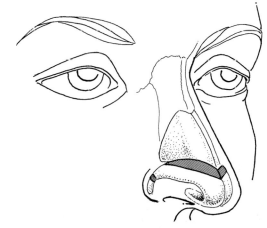

FIG. 53–14. Resection of a segment of the accessory cartilages lateral to the lateral crura to decrease tip projection.

allowing medial rotation and suture at the midline. The exposure provided by the infracartilaginous incisions allows a very accurate joining and suture of domes at the midline to achieve symmetry.

Tip projection can also be increased by the insertion of a cartilage graft at the tip (11–15).

DORSAL RESECTION

Resection of the dorsum should be conservative, in order to preserve the structural support of the nose. Overresection is the most common cause of secondary deformities such as concave dorsum, open roof, collapse of the internal valve, and supratip projection.

The use of a rasp allows progressive resection and the possibility to palpate every few strokes (Fig. 53–15). Minimal pressure is required when a good sharp instrument is used. The cartilaginous dorsum is then resected with a no. 11 blade with the tip amputated (Fig. 53–16).

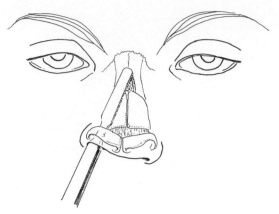

FIG. 53–15.   Resection of the bony hump with a rasp.

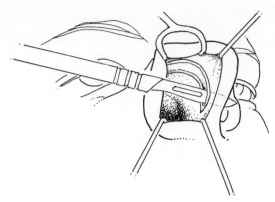

FIG. 53–17.   To resect the caudal edge of the septum (when the columella protrudes inferiorly), the incision is extended along the septal edge.

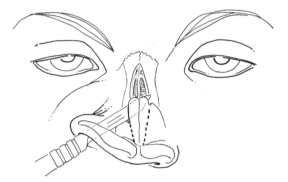

FIG. 53–16.   The cartilaginous hump is resected with a no. 11 blade that has the tip amputated.

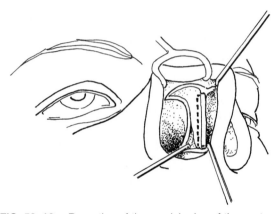

FIG. 53–18.   Resection of the caudal edge of the septum.

SEPTAL SURGERY

Septal corrections, or harvesting cartilage grafts, is done at this stage, before the lateral osteotomies. The intracartilaginous incision is extended on one side along the caudal edge of the septum to the base of the columella (Fig. 53–17). Subperichondrial and subperiosteal dissection is carefully done on both sides of the septum, following the four-tunnel routine. The lower tunnels are dissected first, followed by the superior tunnels, and then the two pockets are joined. This maneuver prevents tearing of the mucosa at the level of maximum convexity or angulation. The curved segments of the septum are removed, taking care to maintain an L-shaped portion for support (Fig. 53–18). The resected pieces may be crushed and replaced between the mucopericondrial layers. Scoring or crushing of convex areas in situ may be necessary to achieve symmetry. Reinforcement of these areas with cartilage struts inserted as splints is often desirable to restore the structural support decreased by crushing or scoring. Resection of the caudal edge of the septum, when necessary, is done at this time.

There is seldom an indication for turbinectomy. Turbinates are always hypertrophic on the concave side of the deviated septum. Total resection of a turbinate results in loss of function. Partial resection and luxation are frequently followed by relapse of the hypertrophy. The procedure *may* be indicated in selected cases and in very narrow noses. Good functional results are achieved if the septal deviation is corrected by widening of the angle formed by the anterior edge of the septum and the medial edge of the upper lateral cartilages with spreader grafts.

The basic rhinoplasty procedure is almost complete at this stage, except for the lateral osteotomies that I prefer to perform at the last step of the procedure.

The mucosal incisions along the caudal edge of the septum and the domes are sutured at this time with fine absorbable material. Complimentary maneuvers such as tip or columella grafting or resection of the sill of the nostrils are done at this time.

NASAL BASE

Ideally, the width of the nasal base should correspond to the intercanthal distance. A vertical line drawn from the medial canthi should be tangenitial to the most prominent lateral point of the ala. If the alar base extends more than 2 mm lateral to the vertical lines, the nasal base is too wide.

Excessive width of the alar base is corrected by the resection of a wedge of tissue from the nostril sill. It is important to maintain the resection at the horizontal segment of the nostril. When the resection is made more lateral, it will produce a distortion of the nostril. Inferiorly, the resection should extend only to the alar–lip junction. Extending the incision into the alar–cheek junctions is not indicated because it results in a visible scar that is impossible to correct. The shape and size of the wedge varies with the particular problem. It can be triangular with the vertix at the nostril–lip junction, in order to correct alar flaring, without altering the diameter of the nostril. When the transverse diameter of the nostril is wide, a block is resected that extends into the nasal cavity. The edges of the wound must be approximated with meticulous care using monofilament nylon sutures. The stitches are removed in 3 days to prevent epithelialization from the numerous sebaceous glands in this area (Fig. 53–19).

The correction of a prominent tip in the narrow nose automatically results in alteration of the long axis of the nostrils. This type of nose, initially considered narrow, may also require a discrete wedge resection of the sill at the end of the procedure in order to achieve a harmonious, refined nose.

OSTEOTOMIES

The resection of the hump produces a flat plateau along the nasal dorsum. This open roof must be obliterated by medial mobilization of the nasal skeleton on both sides. Narrowing of the nasal pyramid is simultaneously accomplished. This maneuver may not be necessary in exceptional cases when dorsal resection was minimal, when the nose is very narrow, or when cartilage or bone grafting of the dorsum is contemplated. Many surgeons prefer to do the lateral osteotomies through an incision on the nasal vestibule at the pyriform area, followed by subperiosteal dissection that forms a tunnel along the line of the osteotomies. This is an excellent approach, requiring considerable expertise to cut the bone at the appropriate level while preserving the integrity of the nasal mucosa. I prefer to use the percutaneous approach. An osteotome, 2 mm wide, is introduced through the skin at a point about 3 mm medial and caudal from the medial canthus of the eye (Fig. 53–20). The site of the osteotomy is located exactly at the junction of the nasal pyramid with the anterior aspect of the maxilla, which is easily found by direct palpation. Several small cuts are made in the bone through the same incision by altering the position of the osteotome. The osteotomy extends from the pyriform aperature inferiorly to the frontonasal suture superiorly. No subperiosteal undermining is done and the nasal mucosa is intact, although an occasional perforation is not significant.

Once the lateral osteotomy is made on both sides, the sides of the nasal pyramid are displaced medially by manual pressure. A pseudogreenstick fracture is actually accomplished. The manual pressure produces a partial disruption of the frontonasal suture, which acts as a hinge for the skeletal rotation (Fig. 53–21).

When the bone resection of the dorsum was minimal, it is necessary to do medial osteotomies before infracturing the nasal bones. These are done at each side of the septum in a cephalad direction. For these, I use a 5-mm osteotome introduced through the intracartilaginous incisions. When the dorsal hump originates very high at the glabella, or in the presence of a very wide nose, it may be necessary to resect a small wedge of bone from each side of the septum to allow

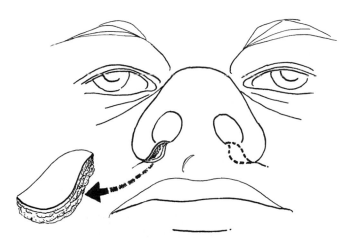

FIG. 53–19. When the alar base is too wide, a wedge is resected from the nostril sill. The edges are sutured with fine monofilament nylon.

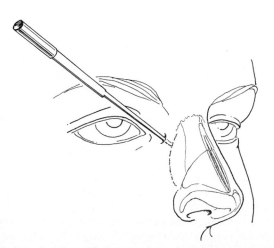

FIG. 53–20. A 2-mm chisel is introduced percutaneously about 3 mm medial and caudal to the medial canthus. The osteotomy is done along the dotted lines through the same skin hole.

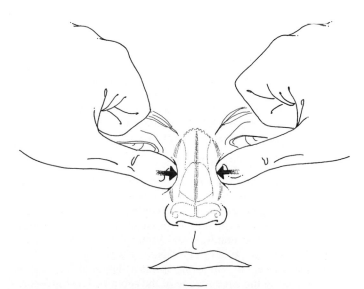

FIG. 53–21. By manual pressure the bones are displaced medially, closing the roof and narrowing the nasal pyramid.

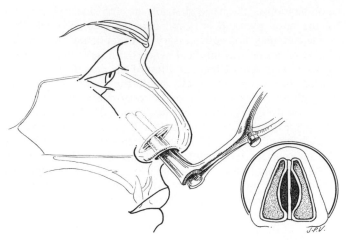

FIG. 53–22.   To obtain a septal graft, the mucopericondrium of the septum is widely dissected on both sides. An incision is made in the cartilage parallel, and about 5 mm posterior to, the caudal septal edge. The graft is harvested with a swivel knife while the mucosal flaps are spread with a nasal speculum.

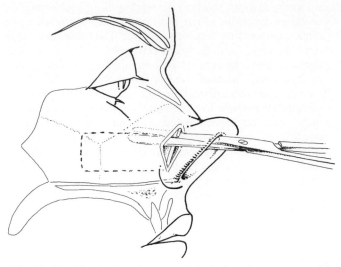

FIG. 53–23.   To obtain a larger graft including the vomer, straight Mayo scissors are used.

the medial displacement of the skeleton. In some cases, when the initial dorsal resection was extended to the nasion, the medial osteotomies may be unnecessary.

The infracture of the skeleton is easily accomplished by manual pressure. If the bone does not move, it is convenient to revise the lateral osteotomies to avoid conminuted fractures. The greenstick fracture produces a perfectly stable pyramid that prevents telescoping of the segments.

Rasping of minor bone irregularities is easily accomplished at this time because of the stable pyramid. Preservation of the mucosal lining and of the soft-tissue attachments externally contribute to the stabilty of the mobilized segments and to maintaining optimal vascular supply. Postoperative edema and ecchymoses are minimal.

The 2 mm stab incision made with the osteotome is not sutured. Scars are always invisible; no secondary correction has ever been necessary in my series.

DRESSING

Intranasal packing with moderate pressure is introduced at this time. The nose is draped with micropore tape and covered with a light, plastic nasal splint. The nasal packs are removed in a few hours (before leaving the hospital). When septal grafts are harvested, I leave the packs for 24 hours. When a septoplasty is performed, the packs are left for 2 to 3 days. The nasal splint is removed in 10 days.

AUGMENTATION TECHNIQUES

Within the concept of augmentation we include those procedures in which cartilage or bone grafts are used to increase or camouflage irregularities or to complement the nasal structural support. The optimal donor area is the septum, followed by ear concha and condrocostal grafts from the chest wall. Parietal or iliac bone is rarely used.

To harvest septal grafts, the intracartilaginous incision is extended along the caudal edge of the septum. The mucoperiosteum is carefully dissected on both sides (Fig. 53–22). A section of cartilage, sometimes including bone, is resected,

preserving always an L-shaped portion of the septum to maintain support. For this, an incision is made on the septum parallel to its caudal edge and a segment of the cartilage is harvested with the swivel knife. Heavy Mayo scissors are used to cut the septum when a larger graft, including Vomer, is necessary (Fig. 53–23). The mucosa is closed with fine interrupted absorbable sutures and the nasal cavities are packed for 24 hours.

For the conchal graft, a retroauricular incision is preferable. A fairly large graft can be obtained that includes the whole concha and preserves the antihelix. The conchal cavity is carefully packed with moist cotton to preserve the shape of the ear.

Chondrocostal grafts are obtained through a submammary incision in females and a lower oblique incision in males. A large section of costal bone and cartilage can be harvested through a small incision with careful subperiosteal and subpericondrial dissection, aided by a bayonet-shaped costotome.

TIP GRAFTS

Cartilage grafts to the tip are indicated to (a) increase the anterior projection; (b) obliterate irregularities, which can be congenital or resulting from previous nasal surgery or trauma; and (c) to improve definition and angularity when the skin is very thick (7,14).

Tip grafts are inserted through a small rim incision near the alar dome. With blunt iris scissors, a fairly large pocket is dissected under the skin from the upper part of the columella to the upper edge of the alar domes (Fig. 53–24). This is the area covered by thick skin that is firmly attached to the nasal SMAS by perpendicular trabeculae extending from the dermis (16). Freeing the dermal fixation allows the skin to drape nicely. To prevent displacement of the graft, one or two nonabsorbable sutures are inserted through the skin, including the graft (Fig. 53–25). These sutures are fixed with tape to the skin and removed in 4 to 5 days. The shape of the graft is determined by the particular problem presented by each

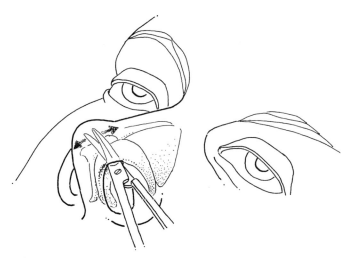

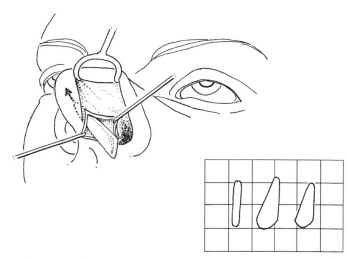

FIG. 53–24. Cartilage graft inserted into the columella through a small mucosal incision near the base. Insert shows different designs for columella strut (scale = 1cm/square).

FIG. 53–26. Small infracartilaginous incision near the dome and dissection of a wide pocket between the dermis and the superficial fascia of the SMAS of the nose.

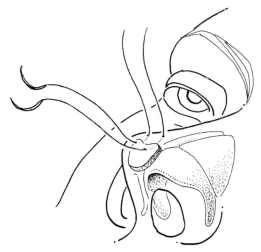

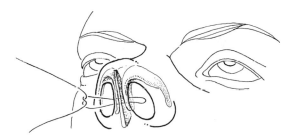

FIG. 53–27. Tip graft is placed in front of the alar domes. Pull-out nylon sutures are used as temporary fixation.

FIG. 53–25. The columellar graft is placed between the two medial crura in a sagittal position.

nose; the basic shield design proposed by Sheen can be used (15,17). When the skin is very thin, it is convenient to crush the cartilage slightly to prevent visible irregularities. When the skin is thick, a stiffer cartilage is convenient to provide better support. Two-layer grafts may also be used when more volume or stronger support is necessary. The ideal material for these grafts is the septal cartilage, but equally good results may be obtained with conchal cartilage. Costal cartilage may also be used when these donor areas are not available or when an exceptionally strong support is required. The tendency of the costal cartilage to curve and buckle after carving must be taken into consideration. It is safe to carve the relatively small tip or columellar grafts from the central core of the costal cartilage (18).

COLUMELLAR GRAFTS

The indications for cartilage grafts of the columella are (a) to increase the structural support of the tip; (b) to elongate the

medial crura once the lower end has been freed from the septum and the connective tissue at the base of the columella; (c) to correct a receding columella and nasal spine; (d) to obliterate the vertix of the nasolabial angle projecting the base of the columella anteriorly. This gives a visual impression of a more open nasolabial angle without cephalad rotation of the tip, which exposes the inside of the nares; (e) to camouflage a very long upper lip, as is frequently seen in older patients; and (f) to camouflage a low alar margin hiding the columella on the lateral view.

Technique

The columella graft may be introduced through the intracartilaginous incision as a complement of a primary rhinoplasty or through a small incision near the base of the columella on one side (Fig. 53–26).

With curved Fomon scissors, the surgeon dissects a pocket between the two medial crura to the base of the columella. The graft is introduced into the pocket and maintained in position with a through-and-through catgut suture (Fig. 53–27).

The shape and size of the graft vary with the particular problem presented by each case. The graft may consist of a strut 3 to 4 mm wide and about 15 to 20 mm long when only structural support is necessary. When columellar projection is required, a triangular piece is carved that is 15 to 20 mm long

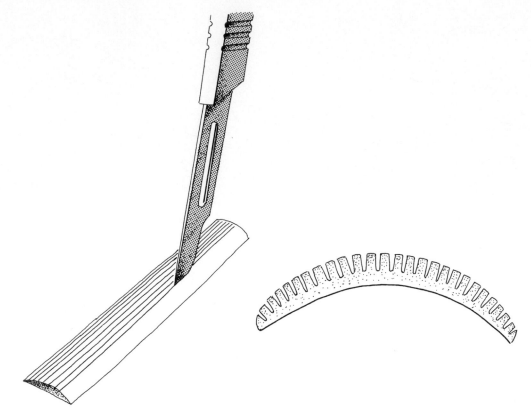

FIG. 53–28. Diagram showing the cartilage graft for the dorsum. Multiple longitudinal partial-thickness cuts release surface tension on one side, producing a convex graft.

and 8 to 12 mm wide at the base. The wide section is located in front of the nasal spine in order to project the columellar base anteriorly and caudally (6,19,20). The graft is introduced in a sagittal position between the two medial crura. It should not extend to the nasal tip, to avoid its protrusion at this area.

DORSAL GRAFTS

The indications for dorsal grafts in primary rhinoplasty are (a) to correct a low nasion, (b) to augment dorsal projection, and (c) to produce an impression of refinement and angularity when the nose is broad and the skin is thick.

In secondary rhinoplasty, the dorsal grafts are indicated to (a) minimize the effects of overreduction, (b) close an open roof, (c) camouflage irregularities, and (d) open a collapsed cartilaginous vault.

Technique

Through the rhinoplasty incision in primary rhinoplasty, or through a small intercartilaginous incision in secondary cases, a pocket is dissected along the dorsum (subperiostially, if possible) to the level of the nasion. The dissection of the pocket is limited to approximately the size of the graft to achieve a snug fit that prevents displacement and eliminates the need for fixation. In secondary rhinoplasty, irregularities of the pyramid should be removed with a rasp to produce a flat bed. A strut, 6 to 8 mm in width and about 4 cm long, is cut from the septal cartilage. Multiple longitudinal partial-thickness cuts are made on one side of the graft to release the

surface tension (18); this automatically produces a curved contour similar to the nasal dorsum (Fig. 53–28).

The graft should be made of one piece from the nasion to the tip to obtain a permanent regular contour. When more volume is required on certain areas, an extra piece of cartilage is added to the undersurface of the graft. Ear conchal cartilage may be used when the septal cartilage is not available. A fairly large piece can be obtained while preserving the antihelical fold and the navicular fossa. Careful crushing is necessary to eliminate the "memory" of the cartilage and produce a straight strut. Good results can be obtained with this graft, but the septal cartilage is used whenever possible (11).

When a major dorsal augmentation is required, a chondrocostal graft is preferable. The rib is split, using a 12-millimeter osteotome, removing only the cortical layer on one side, so the graft is made of one cortex with the cancellous bone. The graft is shaped with a Tessier crusher and cut to the proper size with heavy, straight scissors. The chondrocostal joint and a small segment of cartilage, no longer than 10 mm, may be left to achieve more volume at one end of the new dorsum. The graft is inserted into the dorsal pocket. A very fine K-wire introduced percutaneously may be used for fixation near the radix.

Complications and Bad Results

Complications of rhinoplasty during the early postoperative period are relatively rare. Infection is uncommon because of the rich blood supply, even when bone or cartilage grafts are used, but antibiotics may be indicated in these cases.

Hematoma is also rare because the nasal incisions are not sutured completely, allowing drainage, and because of the compression produced by the splint over the nasal pyramid. Intraseptal hematoma may occur after septal graft harvesting or septoplasty. To prevent this complication of excessive transoperative bleeding, it is convenient to make a stab wound on one side of the septal mucoperiosteum near the nasal spine posteriorly, and to carefully pack the nasal cavities. An undetected intraseptal hematoma may result in cartilage necrosis and loss of nasal support. Careful inspection and cleaning of the nasal cavity allows early diagnosis of a hematoma. In this case, the sutures along the caudal edge of the septum are removed and the hematoma is drained by aspiration and compression.

Nasal bleeding may occur within the 1st week after surgery. It usually comes from the mucosal incisions on the septum and can be controlled by meticulous aspiration of blood clots and repacking. Severe hemorrage uncontrollable by repeated packing is a rarely seen but serious complication. The patient should be examined under general anesthesia in a dark operating room. Using an adequate headlight, a nasal speculum is introduced and the previously infractured nasal bones are separated to allow proper exposure of the bleeding area. A thin, metalic suction tube covered by insulating material (except for the tip) is used, and the bleeding vessel is cauterized through the suction tube.

Unfavorable results may be considered as complications inherent to the procedure or as deficiencies in planning or performing the operation. Overresection is the most common cause of poor aesthetic results and it requires replacement of the missing structures by bone or cartilage grafts at a later date. Undercorrection is a more benign problem with a simpler solution. Skin necrosis and subsequent scarring result from an incorrect plane of dissection or from attempts to thin the soft-tissue cover by defatting. Mucosal scarring and stenosis result from improperly placed intranasal incision and resection of the mucosal lining.

Secondary rhinoplasty, with few exceptions, is a complex procedure requiring careful evaluation of the deformity to determine the participation of each anatomic element. When performing a secondary procedure, the surgeon must have a clear plan for the operation and the patient must be well informed about the possible outcome. Secondary rhinoplasty should never be attempted shortly after the primary operation. For minor correction, a lapse of 6 months may be adequate, but very often a year must pass before the scar tissue is mature and circulation is improved.

Missing pieces of the structural support should be replaced by grafts. Other elements must be repositioned. Scar tissue is resected and mucosa or skin replaced by flaps or grafts.

References

1. Aiache G, Levignac J. *La rhinoplastie esthétique.* Paris: Mason, 1986.
2. Aufricht G. Joseph's rhinoplasty with some modifications. *Surg Clin North Am* 1957; 51:299.
3. Ortiz Monasterio F. Rhinoplasty in the non-caucasian nose. In: Gruber RP, Peck GC, eds. *Rhinoplasty: state of the art.* St. Louis: CV Mosby, 1993.
4. Peck GC. Basic primary rhinoplasty. *Clin Plast Surg* 1988; 15:15.
5. Rees TD, ed. *Aesthetic plastic surgery.* Philadelphia: WB Saunders, 1980.
6. Gunter JP, Rohrich RJ. Augmentation rhinoplasty: dorsal onlay grafting using shaped autogenous septal cartilage. *Plast Reconstr Surg* 1990; 86:39.
7. Peck G. *Rhinoplasty.* Philadelphia: JB Lippincott, 1990.
8. Ortiz Monasterio F. *Rhinoplasty.* Philadelphia: WB Saunders, 1994.
9. Gunter JP. Anatomical observation of the lower lateral cartilages. *Arch Otolaryngol* 1969; 89:599.
10. Zide BM. Nasal anatomy: the muscles and tip sensation. *Aesthetic Plast Surg* 1985; 9:193.
11. Ortiz Monasterio F, Olmedo A, Ortiz Oscoy LO. The use of cartilage grafts in primary aesthetic rhinoplasty. *Plast Reconstr Surg* 1981; 67:592.
12. Ortiz Monasterio F, Olmedo A. Rhinoplasty on the mestizo nose. *Clin Plast Surg* 1977; 4:89.
13. Ortiz MF, Michelena J. The use of augmentation rhinoplasty techniques for the correction of the non-caucasian nose. *Clin Plast Surg* 1988; 15:57.
14. Sheen JH. Achieving more nasal tip projection by the use of a small autogenous vomer or septal cartilage graft. A preliminary report. *Plast Reconstr Surg* 1975; 56:35.
15. Sheen JH. Secondary rhinoplasty. *Plast Reconstr Surg* 1975; 56:137.
16. Letourneau A, Daniel RK. The superficial musculoaponeurotic system of the nose. *Plast Reconstr Surg* 1988; 82:48.
17. Sheen JH. *Aesthetic rhinoplasty.* 2nd ed. St. Louis: CV Mosby, 1987.
18. Gibson T, Davis WB. The distortion of autogenous cartilage grafts: its cause and prevention. *Br J Plast Surg* 1958; 4:257.
19. McKinney P, Stalnecher ML. The hanging ala. *Plast Reconstr Surg* 1984; 73:427.
20. Millard DR. Alar margin sculpturing. *Plast Reconstr Surg* 1967; 40:337.

54

Secondary Rhinoplasty

George C. Peck, M.D., F.A.C.S., and George C. Peck, Jr., M.D.

Although statistics are difficult to obtain, secondary rhinoplasties may occur in 10 to 30% of all rhinoplasties. In many instances, secondary surgery is a result of overreduction, poor judgment, or lack of experience. In some cases, the surgeon is too conservative. It is always better to underresect than overreduce. A secondary rhinoplasty requiring a little more reduction is much easier than a secondary rhinoplasty that requires major reconstruction.

Secondary rhinoplasty is problem-solving rhinoplasty, not cookbook rhinoplasty. Sometimes only subtle changes are necessary. Other times, major reconstruction is required to achieve the desired functional or cosmetic result. Secondary rhinoplasty, like all secondary surgery, is more difficult because of altered anatomy and scar tissue. Successful surgery depends on a combination of perceptive evaluation of the patient to identify the problem(s) with the knowledge and technical skill to solve them. This chapter identifies the most common problems requiring secondary rhinoplasty and our techniques for solving those problems. The problems can be categorized as nasal tip, supratip, middle vault, alar rim, columellar, nasolabial angle, saddle nose, and thick-skin nasal deformities. Open rhinoplasty is a category that has recently been added in response to increased incidence.

Evaluation of the Patient

An accurate diagnosis requires a comprehensive history and physical examination, including an internal and external examination of the nose and septum. The surgeon informs the patient of the diagnosis, the procedure, the risks, and the alternatives. The patient must have realistic expectations of the probable cosmetic result. Delay secondary surgery for at least 1 year after primary rhinoplasty so that all edematous changes resolve and healing is complete.

Nasal Tip Deformities

Inadequate nasal tip projection is the most common problem after rhinoplasty; generally it indicates that the nasal tip fails to project 1 to 2 mm beyond the dorsal line. The etiology of inadequate tip projection is twofold: inadequate projection of the alar domes, or loss of septal support. Inadequate alar dome projection is the result of weak lower lateral cartilages or overzealous resection. The treatment is an onlay graft. A 4 – 9-mm section of convex cartilage from either lower lateral cartilage or conchal cartilage.

Through an infracartilaginous stab incision, the surgeon makes a horizontal pocket over the alar domes. The pocket is the exact size of the graft, preventing graft movement or misalignment. Figures 54–1, 54–2, and 54–3 shows the surgical technique to place an onlay graft.

Another cause of inadequate tip projection is inadequate septal support. On physical examination, the surgeon can push the nasal tip onto the nasal spine when there is inadequate septal support. In profile, the patient may have a drooping nasal tip that is accentuated with smiling. The umbrella graft—a rectangular strut capped by an onlay graft—corrects the drooping tip and inadequate tip projection. The strut is usually from conchal cartilage, or septal cartilage if available. Using an infracartilaginous incision on the side of the columella, the surgeon places the strut in a vertical pocket from the nasal spine to the nasal tip between the medial crura. Figures 54–4 and 54–5 illustrate the correct placement of the strut and the onlay grafts. Figures 54–6 through 54–9 show the results of the umbrella graft.

THE PINOCCHIO TIP

The Pinocchio tip deformity is characterized by excessive nasal tip projection (Fig. 54–10). This deformity is not usually corrected by the standard sculpturing of the lower lateral cartilages because leaving only 2 mm of cephalad lower lateral cartilage may lower tip projection enough to produce acceptable aesthetic lines. In severe cases, the surgeon may need to amputate the alar domes and reconstruct the nasal tip with an umbrella graft. Amputation of the nasal domes is reserved for isolated cases that do not respond to the standard sculpturing techniques (Fig. 54–11).

THE THICK SEBACEOUS NASAL TIP

This nasal tip is a result of hypertrophic sebaceous glands in the nasal tip skin. The nasal tip skin does not conform over the sculptured lower lateral cartilages and remains ill defined despite the usual reduction technique. Selective patients will have a significant improvement with the umbrella graft and external shaving of the nasal tip skin. The technique is similar to the external shaving of a rhinophyma. Complications include hypopigmentation (frequent) and scarring (uncommon).

THE BROAD NASAL TIP DEFORMITY

An abnormally wide lower lateral cartilage dome produces the broad nasal tip deformity. The angle between the medial and lateral crura approaches 90°. Bifidity is usually associated with this problem. Surgical correction requires the lateral rotation technique: complete mobilization of the lateral crus, partial cross cutting of the domes, and excision of the

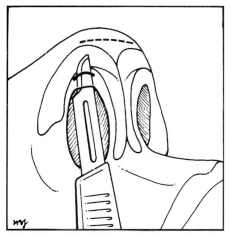

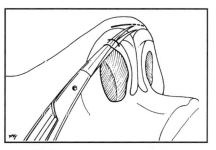

FIG. 54–2. Dissection of the horizontal pocket overlying the alar domes.

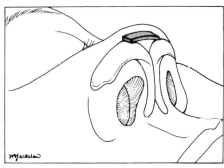

FIG. 54–3. The perfect position for the onlay graft.

FIG. 54–1. The infracartilaginous incision used in placement of an onlay graft.

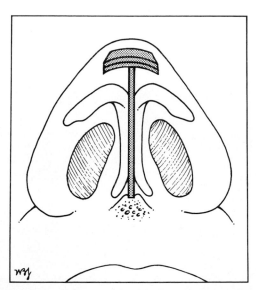

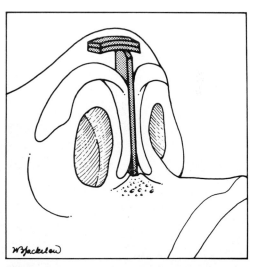

FIG. 54–4. The umbrella graft is composed of a cartilaginous strut between the medial crura from nasal spine to nasal tip and capped with an onlay graft(s).

FIG. 54–5. An oblique view of the umbrella graft.

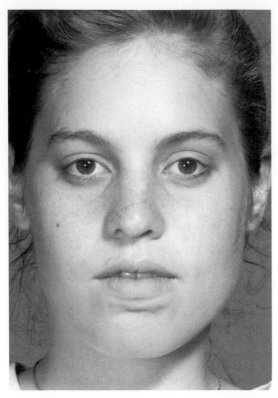

FIG. 54–6. A young woman with a wide bridge and an ill-defined nasal tip presenting for a secondary rhinoplasty.

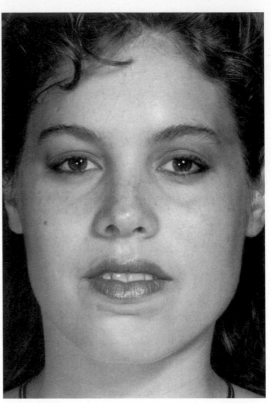

FIG. 54–8. One year after secondary rhinoplasty, the patient has a narrower bridge and a defined nasal tip.

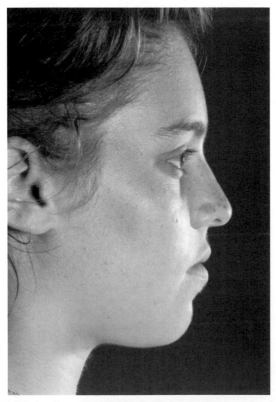

FIG. 54–7. Inadequate nasal tip projection is diagnosed in the lateral view.

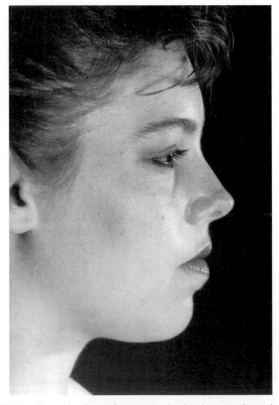

FIG. 54–9. An umbrella graft corrects the inadequate tip projection.

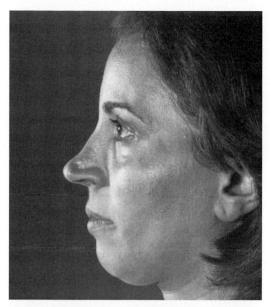

FIG. 54–10. A secondary Pinocchio deformity characterized by excessive nasal tip projection.

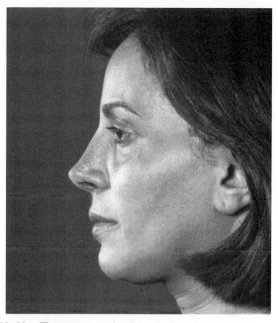

FIG. 54–11. The postoperative lateral view shows the improvement achieved by amputation of the domes and reconstruction of the nasal tip with an onlay graft.

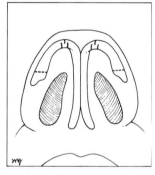

FIG. 54–12. Partial cross-cutting of the domes, and excising 4 to 5 mm of the lateralmost segment of the lower lateral cartilage, corrects the broad nasal tip.

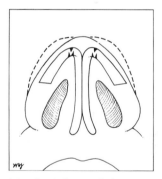

FIG. 54–13. The lateral rotation technique creates a more acute angle at the alar domes, and a narrower tip.

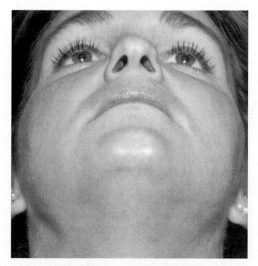

FIG. 54–14. A broad nasal tip.

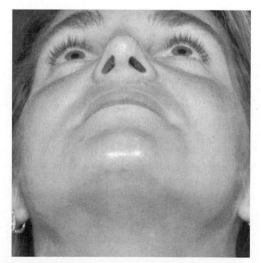

FIG. 54–15. Correction of the broad nasal tip with the lateral rotation technique.

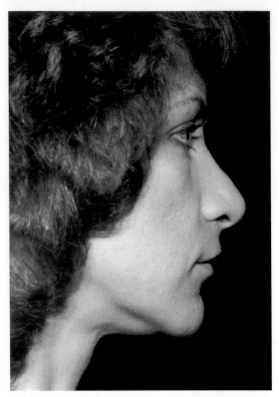

FIG. 54–16. A parrot-beak defomity with a high supratip and inadequate tip projection.

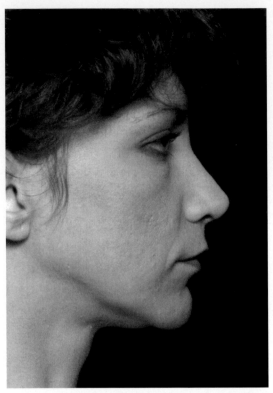

FIG. 54–17. A postoperative lateral view showing resolution of the problem by lowering the supratip septum and reconstruction of the nasal tip with an umbrella graft.

most lateral segment of the lower lateral cartilage. This produces a more acute angle at the dome, narrowing the nasal tip (Figs. 54–12 to 54–15). Suturing the medial crura together or camoflaging the deformity with a cartilage graft corrects the bifid deformity.

SUPRATIP DEFORMITIES

A high supratip septum is the most common cause of supratip fullness after rhinoplasty. Other causes include inadequate resection of the cephalad portion of lower lateral cartilage, scar tissue, and fibrofatty tissue. Surgical correction includes appropriate lowering of the septal cartilage and sculpting of the lower lateral cartilages with the resection of all scar tissue and fibrofatty tissue. A parrot-beak deformity—a high supratip septum with inadequate nasal tip projection—requires reduction of the high supratip septal cartilage and reconstruction of the nasal tip with an umbrella graft (Figs. 54–16, 54–17).

Middle Vault Deformities

Difficulty breathing, and airway obstruction as a result of a pinched middle vault, occur with overresection of the upper lateral cartilages. On physical examination, the patient may have inspiratory collapse of the nasal walls and a severe airway obstruction. Treatment consists of reconstruction of the upper lateral cartilages with triangular cartilage grafts. Spreader grafts can also increase the diameter of the middle vault. Caution must be taken to keep the spreader grafts above the nasal valve; otherwise, further compromise of the

airway occurs and compounds the problem. In our experience, the triangular filler grafts reconstruct normal anatomy and act as batons in a sail supporting the lateral nasal walls (Figs. 54–18 to 54–22).

Alar Rim Deformities

The most common defects of the alar rim are notching, total collapse, pinched tip, alar base deformities, and the veiling of the alar rims. Reconstruction of the alar rims requires convex conchal cartilage grafts that conform to the desired shape of the alar rim. A pocket along the alar rim keeps the cartilage graft in place without sutures (Figs. 54–23 to 54–28).

The modified Weir's technique corrects alar base assymmetry and the flared nostril. Excision of a wedge of nostril described by Millard is the technique of choice for the veiled alar rims.

Columellar Deformities

Defects of the columella are of the retracted or hanging types. Overresection of the caudal septum, vestibular lining, or nasal spine cause the retracted columella. Reconstruction requires cartilage grafts to fill the defect. The surgeon uses a rectangular graft to reconstruct the posterior two-thirds of the columlla and a triangular graft to reconstruct the anterior one-third.

Correction of the hanging columella requires further resection of the excess caudal septum and removal of the appropriate amount of vestibular lining. Failure to take the appropriate amount of vestibular lining is a common cause of recurrence (Figs. 54–29, 54–30).

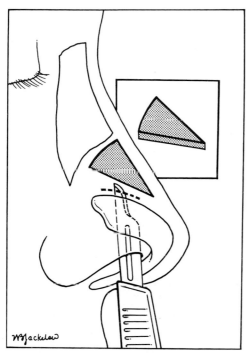

FIG. 54–18. The incision to place triangular filler grafts in the treatment of middle vault deformities.

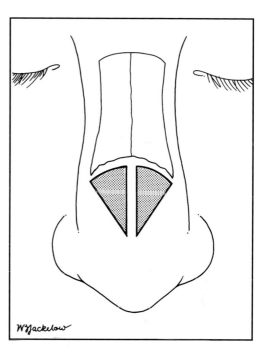

FIG. 54–19. Correct placement of the triangular filler grafts.

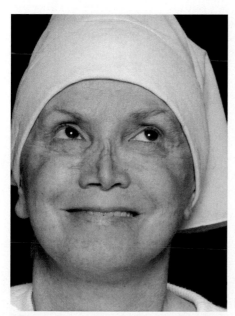

FIG. 54–20. A patient with total collapse of the bony vault, middle vault, and alar rims as a result of overreduction.

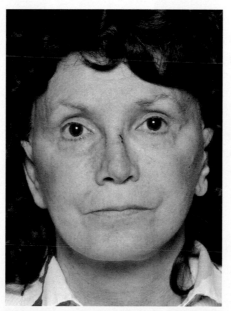

FIG. 54–21. Reconstruction of the bridge, middle vault, and alar rims using cartilage grafts. The middle vault was reconstructed with triangular filler grafts.

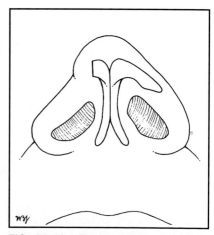

FIG. 54–22. Total collapse of the alar rim, caused by resection of the lateral crura.

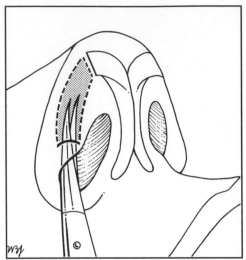

FIG. 54–23. The incision and dissection of the pocket, horizontal to the alar rim.

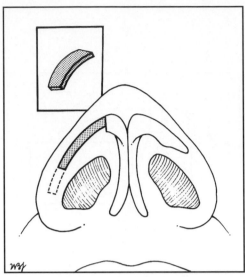

FIG. 54–24. Reconstruction of the right lateral crura with a convex cartilage graft.

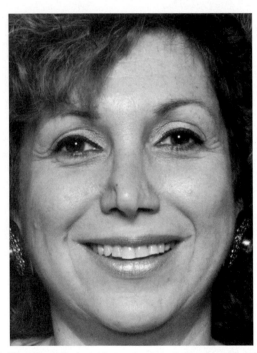

FIG. 54–25. Frontal view of a secondary deformity with collapse of the alar rims.

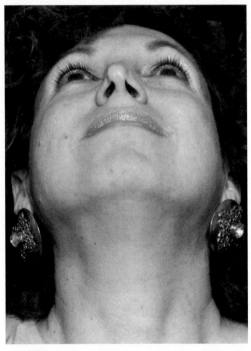

FIG. 54–26. Worm's eye view of the secondary deformity with collapse of the alar rims.

The Overshortened and Turned Up Nose

The overshortened and rotated tip produces a piglike appearance; it is one of the most feared and yet avoidable aesthetic catastrophes. Overreduction of the caudal septum is the most common cause, and retraction of the skin envelope in the postoperative period compounds this disaster.

The ideal nasolabial angle is 90° to 95° in males and 95° to 100° in females. Reconstruction of the overrotated and overshortened nose requires cartilage grafts to the anterior and posterior segments of the columella (Figs. 54–31 to 54–34). However, the patient may need multiple surgeries to expand the contracted skin envelope while maintaining adequate blood supply for cartilage graft survival. Overly aggressive reconstruction leads to blanching of the skin and a compromised blood supply.

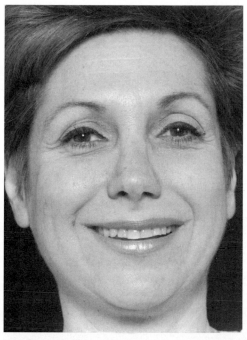

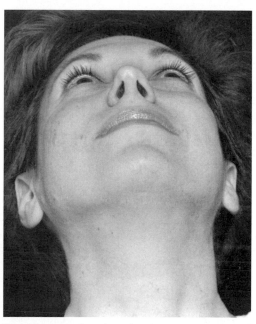

FIG. 54–27. Postoperative view showing reconstruction of the alar rims.

FIG. 54–28. Postoperative view showing reconstruction of the alar rims.

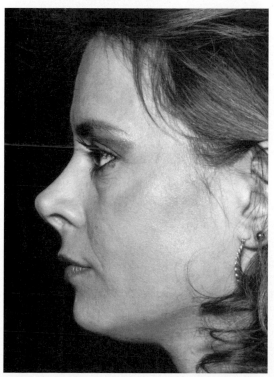

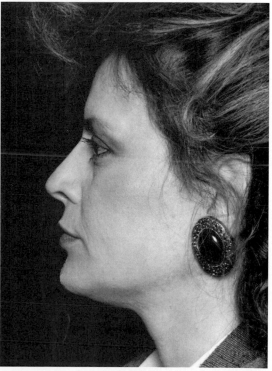

FIG. 54–29. A hanging columella that resulted from excess caudal septal cartilage.

FIG. 54–30. Correction of the hanging columella by shortening the posterior two-thirds of the columella without rotating the nasal tip.

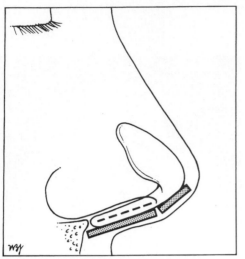

FIG. 54–31. The lateral view of the reconstructed posterior two-thirds of the columella with a rectangular cartilage graft and the anterior one-third of the columella with a triangular cartilage graft.

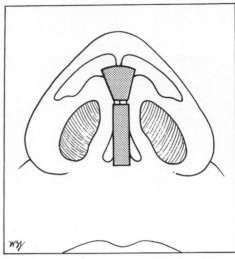

FIG. 54–32. The worm's eye view of the reconstructed posterior two-thirds of the columella with a rectangular cartilage graft and the anterior one-third of the columella with a triangular cartilage graft.

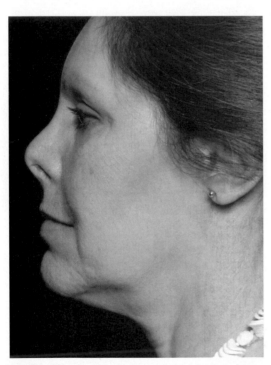

FIG. 54–33. An overrotated and overshortened nose.

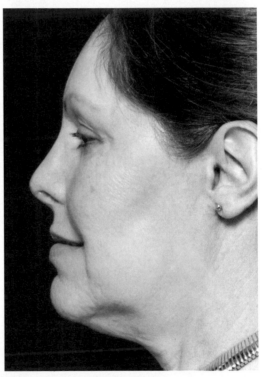

FIG. 54–34. A 1-year postoperative view after reconstruction of the columella.

Saddle Nose Deformity

The most common cause of a saddle nose deformity is trauma. Overreduction of the nasal dorsum and loss of septal support produces a saddle deformity. Moderate saddle deformites respond to septal or conchal dorsal cartilage grafts. A dorsal hull-shaped conchal cartilage graft corrects the deformity while keeping the edges of the graft from showing through the skin. Severe saddle deformities require a bone graft. Our preference is the iliac bone graft, which is easy to shape, and has a very high survival rate and low morbidity (Figs. 54–35 to 54–38).

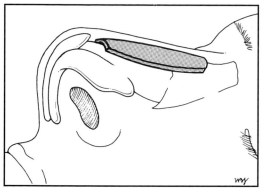

FIG. 54-35. The inverted hull-shaped cartilage graft, used to reconstruct the moderate saddle deformities, extends from the intercanthal line to the supratip.

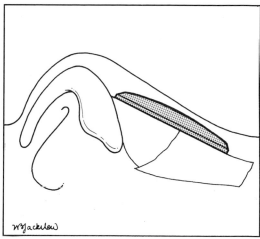

FIG. 54-36. Placement of a dorsal bone graft to correct a saddle deformity.

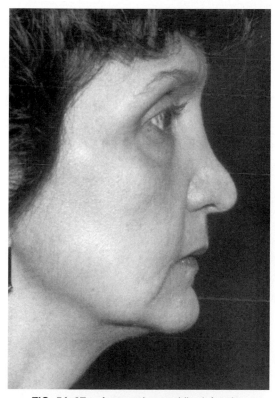

FIG. 54-37. A secondary saddle deformity.

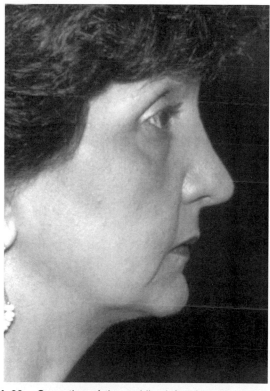

FIG. 54-38. Correction of the saddle deformity with an iliac bone graft.

Open Rhinoplasty Deformities

As a result of the increasing popularity of open rhinoplasty, the open rhinoplasty deformity is becoming very common. The most common problems are the columellar scar and the retracted columella. All complications of the closed rhinoplasty technique are also possible with open rhinoplasty, including inadequate nasal tip projection, the ill-defined nasal tip, the Pinocchio nasal tip, the broad nasal tip, supratip deformities, middle vault deformities, alar rim deformities, columellar deformities, the overshortened nose, and the saddle nose deformity. Aesthetic catastrophes arising from lack of experience, or poor judgement, are reported after open rhinoplasty. One aesthetic catastrophy involved the loss of the nasal tip, which required nasal reconstruction with a forehead flap. This is certainly a significant and avoidable complication. Open rhinoplasty may sometimes be indicated; however, the inexperienced surgeon should proceed with caution and understand that open rhinoplasty is not a panacea.

Conclusion

Secondary rhinoplasty is problem-solving rhinoplasty requiring a range of responses from subtle solutions to more complex reconstructions. This chapter isolates the many types of secondary problems and their treatment. All secondary procedures utilize the closed rhinoplasty approach. Reconstruction involves only autogenous tissue to reestablish the normal anatomy.

Suggested Readings

McCarthy J. Rhinoplasty. In: McCarthy J, ed. *Plastic surgery.* Philadelphia: WB Saunders, 1989.

Peck GC. *Techniques in aesthetic rhinoplasty.* 2nd ed. Philadelphia: JB Lippincott, 1990.

Peck GC, Peck GC Jr. Complications in aesthetic rhinoplasty. In: Peck GC, ed. *Complications in aesthetic surgery.* Philadelphia: Gower, 1994.

Sheen JH. *Aesthetic rhinoplasty.* 2nd ed. St. Louis: CV Mosby, 1987.

55

Aesthetic Surgery of the Ears

Bruce S. Bauer, M.D., F.A.C.S.

Although we generally think of prominent ears when considering aesthetic surgery of the ear, surgeons performing otoplasty need to be familiar not only with procedures for correcting prominence but also with those for correcting constriction of the ear, deformities of the crura (e.g., Stahl ear), cryptotia, and a host of more minor deformities. Although this discussion concentrates on treatment of ear prominence, the overlap of some of the characteristics of prominent ears and the more complex deformities of the constricted ear warrants at least a capsule summary in this chapter.

In any discussion of aesthetic ear surgery, it is necessary to emphasize the incredible variation in ear deformities and the need to analyze each case carefully before beginning correction. No single procedure will be effective in all cases, and a facility with many techniques provides the flexibility necessary to correct all aspects of the deformed ear and obtain symmetry between the two ears, particularly when they are different at the start. Many of the techniques used are minor variations on a similar theme; others take different approaches and still yield comparable results. Surgeons must find the approaches that are most effective in their own hands.

Prominent Ears

HISTORY

In earlier editions of this book, Elliott (1) gave an excellent review of the history of otoplasty. Given that most of today's techniques have arisen as either modifications of earlier procedures or responses to problems inherent in earlier techniques, I have retained much of Elliott's review.

Although Diffenbach (2) reported correction of a posttraumatic prominence of the ear as early as 1845, the earliest elective otoplasty for ear prominence was reported by Ely (3) in 1881. He incised through-and-through the conchal cartilage and allowed the would to heal by secondary intention. The correction was staged with the two sides done in separate operations approximately 6 weeks apart.

In 1910, after the earlier efforts by Morestin (4) and Gersuny (5) with cartilage and skin excisions to change cartilage spring, Luckett (6) identified the failure of scaphal folding to be the cause of ear prominence and described a combination of cartilage excision and suturing to create the antihelical fold. The Luckett procedure was advocated as recently as 1962. Converse and colleagues (7) described a procedure in 1955 that combined posterior abrasion with cartilage incision, and recognized that these procedures would be en-

hanced by excising a rim of excess concha where conchal hypertrophy plays a roll in ear prominence.

The experiments of Gibson and Davis (8) led to a series of procedures, reported in 1963, in which the anterior perichondrial surface was scored to create the necessary shaping of the antihelix, the best recognized being the Stenstrom technique (9). With anterior scoring (in combination with posterior skin excision), Stenstrom was able to create a soft antihelical contour; unfortunately, his technique often resulted in an overcorrection of the ear prominence when it was also used to treat conchal hypertrophy.

During the same year, Mustardé (10) published a mattress-suture technique for folding the scapha that was similar to that published by Owens and Delgado (11) in 1955. Davenport and Bernard (12) improved on the results by using more sutures. Both Elliott (1) and Spira and coworkers (13) adopted this refinement in their subsequent publications (1). Of interest, Mustardé in his later writing denied the benefit of perichondrial scoring. He also continued to treat the associated conchal hypertrophy seen in many cases by converting the excess concha to antihelix (14). Although a review of these cases demonstrated overcorrection, hidden helix, and recurrence, the Mustardé technique grew in popularity, perhaps because of its simplicity, but too often without Davenport's refinements.

Conchal reduction has been performed by anterior and posterior approaches, as well as by rim excisions and base excisions (7,15–17). Others after Gersuny advocated mastoid sutures to correct the conchal prominence; this approach was popularized by Furnas (18). In the description of his technique, Furnas cautioned about visible distortion of the concha and potential deformity of the external auditory meatus. As pointed out by Elliott (19), these distortions were seen only when the Furnas technique was used to reduce the height of the lateral wall in a severe deformity, and I would agree that the suture techniques tend to be better suited for treatment of mild-to-moderate degrees of conchal hypertrophy, but may not as effective as direct excision of cartilage (20).

Elliott also pointed out the benefits of developing a postauricular pocket in combination with conchal mastoid sutures, and stressed the effect this dissection had on correction of the anterolateral rotation of the concha over the fulcrum of postauricular soft tissue. Senechal and Peck (21) arrived at the same conclusion quite independently. Elliott also stressed the fact that most authors ignore rotation of the ear as a contributing factor to prominence, except as it relates to conchal hypertrophy; he believed that the quality and facility of many setbacks could be improved by the simple addition of a postauricular pocket (19).

Treatment of the prominent earlobe was reviewed by Spira and coworkers (13). They favored a dermal-mastoid suture, which Elliott and others, myself included, have used to resolve the occasional residual prominence uncontrolled by helical tail sutures. Goulian and Conway (22) were the first to suggest fixing the tail of the helix lower on the posterior surface of the concha. Resection of the tail of the helix is generally not desirable (16) but, unlike Elliott, I believe that resection of a prominent antitragus, along with reduction of a large lobule, may at times yield a desirable result with a markedly prominent lobule. Review of long-term results will demonstrate that scars from these approaches are barely perceptible.

ANATOMY AND GOALS OF TREATMENT

Although most cases of prominent ear result from an inadequate formation of the antihelical fold, there are many cases in which conchal hypertrophy either contributes to the prominence or is the primary cause (23). In addition, there may be varying degrees of prominence of the antitragus and lobule, and these components may be the most resistant to correction. When choosing otoplasty techniques, there may also be considerable variation in the anatomy of deformity between the two ears on any given individual; as a result, the approach to correction of ear prominence may differ on the two sides in order to produce a symmetrical final result (20).

The final element of prominence that must be taken into account is the influence of the skeletal base upon which the ears rest. Patients presenting with ear prominence secondary to, and accentuated by, cranial deformities (e.g., positional, nonsynostotic plagiocephaly and/or torticollis) may require asymmetrical positioning of the entire ear to obtain a final result of balance and symmetry.

While otoplasty techniques vary from one case to another, the overall goals remain the same. In McDowell's (24) classic paper on correction of prominent ears, he cited as particularly important (a) correction of ear protrusion without severe setback, (b) retention of a visible smooth helix, at least on the upper half of the ear, (c) preservation of a postauricular sulcus, and (d) ear symmetry. Elliott wisely suggested that patient satisfaction was the most important goal, noting that the occasional patient may desire over- or under-correction. He also suggested that an additional goal be the reconstruction of a soft, natural scaphal fold in the proper location.

Finally, reduction of the lobule, scapha, or even the entire ear, may enhance the result in select cases, but these needs are not common (1,19,27).

SURGICAL TECHNIQUES

This chapter will concentrate on reviewing the techniques we have found most effective in correcting (a) the typical prominence that arises from insufficient formation of the antihelical fold and (b) those that are the result of conchal hypertrophy. Additional comments will concern the variation in technique necessary when both elements of prominence require treatment and when overall reduction in ear size is required.

Creating the Antihelical Fold

A review of both plastic surgical and otolaryngological literature (6,9,14,16,18,23–28) demonstrates a multitude of techniques for correction of the antihelical fold. In general, these techniques can be grouped into those involving scoring or abrasion of the cartilage to control the direction and extent of folding and those that rely on suture fixation of the reshaped cartilage (10–15,18). There are also a number of procedures that use a combination of these techniques (1,18,20,28). I generally prefer the combination of techniques.

The cartilage scoring techniques noted above vary, based on whether the cartilage is scored (9) or actually cut through the newly created antihelical fold (6)—and, when scored, whether the scoring is on the anterior or posterior surface of the cartilage (5–9). While, in skilled hands, any technique can be accomplished well, the risk of a sharp antihelical fold is considerably increased by a full-thickness cut in the cartilage (6,27); alternative techniques are available that readily avoid this problem.

My preferred technique is a modification of the procedure described by Stark and Saunders (2,7), in which posterior skin excision is combined with dermabrasion of the posterior cartilage surface to guide the creation of a smooth antihelical fold; permanent sutures are placed to create the desired degree of folding. Sutures are placed from the scapha and helical sulcus to the mastoid fascia in the original description; to this, I add sutures between the scapha and concha, helical sulcus and concha, and concha and mastoid, as needed (20) (Fig. 55–1).

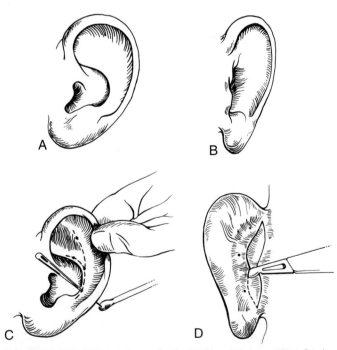

FIG. 55–1. Creation of the antihelical fold using a modified Stark-Saunders technique. **A, B,** preoperative views of ear with deficient antihelical fold. **C,** proposed line of the new antihelical fold is tattooed with methylene blue using a straight needle. **D,** ellipse of skin in dumbbell shape is excised.

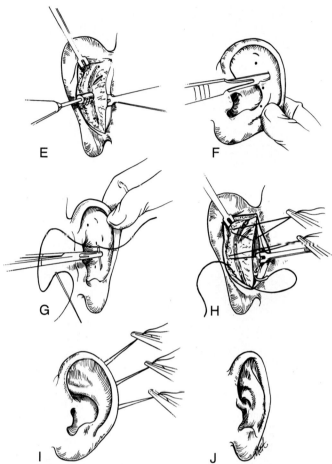

FIG. 55–1. *continued* **E,** after exposing the posterior surface of the cartilage, this surface is dermabraded along the proposed line of antihelical fold: postauricular skin undermined to helix and mastoid area. **F, G,** 1–2 mm stab incisions are made in the skin at the site of suture placement and the nylon sutures are passed from anterior to posterior, catching the anterior perichondrium and cartilage. **H,** sutures placed from scapha and helical sulcus to mastoid, possibly scapha to concha, and helical tail to concha, as needed. **I, J,** once the nylon sutures are tied, creating the antihelical fold and correcting the prominence the skin closure is accomplished with chromic gut.

Conchal Reduction

Although some degree of conchal hypertrophy is not uncommon with ear prominence, in our experience the patients who present with dissatisfaction over the results of a previous otoplasty attest to the fact that conchal hypertrophy is often missed or ignored as an important element of the initial prominence.

The techniques for correction of conchal hypertrophy, once properly identified, include lowering the concha with creation of a the new antihelical fold, conchal setback with conchal mastoid sutures, and conchal reduction. The reduction procedures can be divided into those that excise cartilage alone (14,19,20,23,27), usually through a posterior approach, and those that resect both cartilage and skin through an anterior approach. While minor degrees of conchal prominence

are well handled with creation of the new antihelical fold (20,26) or with conchal mastoid sutures, I believe that most cases with significant degrees of conchal hypertrophy require cartilage excision.

The choice of posterior or anterior approach to the cartilage excision is one of personal preference; either is effective, and the surgeon gains facility with the approach used most frequently. In my opinion, there is considerably more control with an anterior approach similar to that described by Elliott (19,28) than a posterior, and in cases where the resection will be a centimeter or greater in width, the extra skin remaining after a posterior approach may not shrink down sufficiently to avoid leaving a visible fold in the conchal floor. This fold may be more visible that a fine anterior scar, which is rarely visible by 1 year postotoplasty (Fig. 55–2).

Combined Otoplasty Techniques (Fig. 55–1)

A brief review of some key points in my approach to otoplasty will include my own modifications of the technique described initially by Stark and Saunders (25) and explain how this approach is combined with conchal reduction. The versatility of my approach makes it well suited for patients whose prominence arises both from inadequate formation of the antihelix and a moderate degree of conchal hypertrophy.

The procedure begins with a careful reassessment of the deformity and the similarities and differences of the two ears. The proposed site of the antihelix is tattooed with methylene blue, and the postauricular skin excision is carried out to expose the line of the tattoo. Typically, the exci-

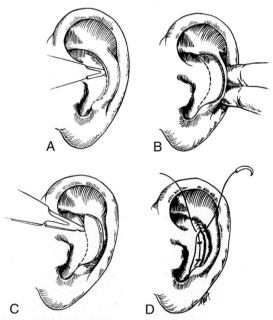

FIG. 55–2. Conchal reduction through an anterior approach similar to that described by Elliott, but typically with both skin and cartilage excision unless minimal cartilage excision is needed. **A,** "rim" incision made along vertical wall of concha, through skin and cartilage. **B,** manual positioning of ear determines the excess cartilage (and skin, if desired). **C,** the excess is excised. **D,** cartilage and skin are then sutured (with clear nylon in the former, chromic gut in the latter).

sion is done in a dumbbell-shaped ellipse, the size dictated by the degree of prominence. Care should be taken to not excise too much of the skin posterior to the lobule in order to avoid later loss of the sulcus.

The antihelical fold is now created by dermabrading the posterior cartilage surface to soften the cartilage over a broad area on either side of the tattoo marks, then further thinning the cartilage along the area of the fold until it bends easily without a sharp fold. Excess thinning can be easily prevented with repeated check of the cartilage flexibility. If the plan is to include reducing the concha, the cartilage (or skin and cartilage) excision should be at least 1 cm below the antihelical fold to prevent a forward springing of the cut edge of the cartilage as the antihelical fold is created.

The cartilage shaping is now guided with a series of permanent sutures. In the majority of cases, three sutures are used, one each between the scapha and mastoid, superior helical sulcus and mastoid, and inferior helical sulcus at the level of, or into, the helical tail and mastoid. If a conchal resection has been performed at the same time, it may be necessary to place additional sutures between the scapha and concha (above the level of excision) and between the helical sulcus and concha at a similar level. Care must be taken to assure that the sutures catch full-thickness cartilage and anterior perichondrium (posterior perichondrium has been abraded). This is most easily accomplished with small (1 to 2 mm) incisions in the anterior skin, as initially described by Stark and Saunders (25). After placement of all sutures, the sutures are tied to create the new antihelical fold and to adjust the overall prominence of the ear. Additional maneuvers may be required to correct a still-prominent lobule (any of the techniques mentioned above being useful at various times). Emphasis should again be placed on avoiding excessive skin excision in an effort to avoid disturbance of the normal sulcus.

Skin closure is generally accomplished using absorbable sutures, both in the conchal and postauricular suture lines. The ear dressing is one of personal preference. Care must be taken to avoid pressure on the ear. While we do not use any drains in our otoplasties, some surgeons use a small suction drain for the first 24 hours after surgery. The dressing is generally left intact for about a week. We then recommend a protective headband at night for an additional 2 weeks.

Results and Complications

We have found the combined approach to otoplasty results in a desirable outcome in the majority of cases (see Figs. 55–3, 55–4). While we have not used anterior scoring of the perichondrium, recurrence of upper pole prominence has not been a problem provided that we have adequately corrected it in the first place. With correct analysis of the deformity and proper application of the various techniques, a sharp antihelical fold, hidden helix, and overcorrection of prominence are readily avoided. However, occasional patients present with a degree of lobule prominence so great that the correction may fall short of ideal; we have found a minor touch-up in the office readily solves the problem. It may help, in patients where there seems to be some potential for this problem to arise, to discuss the possibility ahead of time with the child and parents during a review of possible complications. The

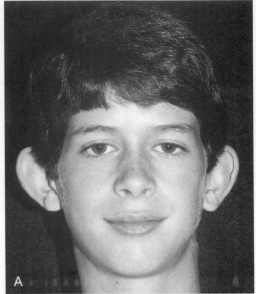

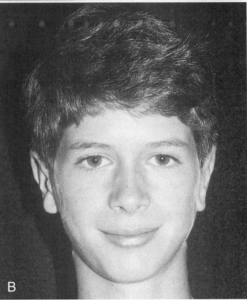

FIG. 55–3. Patient with ear prominence secondary to deficient antihelical fold. **A,** preoperative view of deformity. **B,** postoperative view 1 year following correction.

discussion should include hematoma, infection, chondritis, inadequate correction requiring revision, and possible asymmetries, particularly when the opposing ears start out with considerably different deformities (1,27).

The Constricted Ear

ANATOMY AND CLASSIFICATION

The term "constricted ear" was suggested by Tanzer (29) to describe a group of ear deformities in which the helical rim seemed tight, as if constricted by a purse string. This spectrum of deformities was previously classified separately (and with frequent confusion) as "cup ear" and "lop ear." Tanzer classified constricted ears based on the extent of cartilage and skin deformity. Group I had a minor deformity involving the

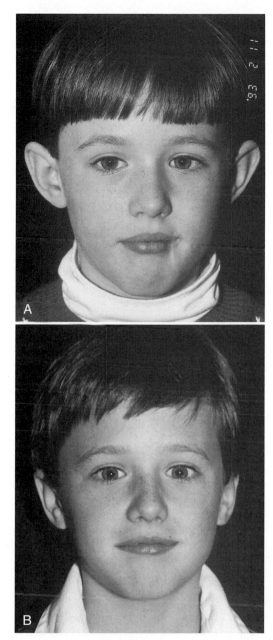

FIG. 55–4. Patient with ear prominence secondary to conchal hypertrophy and deficient superior crus formation. **A,** preoperative view. **B,** postoperative view 1 year following surgery.

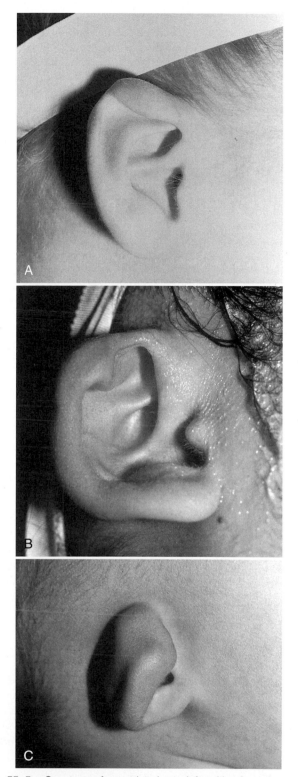

FIG. 55–5. Spectrum of constricted ear deformities from **A,** group I minor lidding, to **B, C,** group IIa,b, with increasing degree of constriction and deficient skin and cartilage, toward a tubular ear similar to an atypical/conchal type microtia.

helix alone, giving a hooded or lidded appearance to the ear. Group II had moderate-to-severe deformities involving the helix and scapha, and was further divided depending on the need for supplemental skin at the margin of the auricle (Group IIb involves deficiency of both cartilage and skin). Group III had extreme cupping, with a tubular form to the ear approaching the appearance of (or in fact being the same as) an atypical or conchal-type microtia (Fig. 55–5). This latter group was often, like the microtic ear, associated with deformities of the external auditory meatus and canal (29).

Cosman (30) described four fundamental elements of ear constriction that varied depending on the severity of the deformity. These were (a) lidding, (b) protrusion, (c) decreased vertical ear size, and (d) low ear position. These aspects correlate well with Tanzer's groupings (29). Lidding or hooding is secondary to helical overhang, arch shortening, and flattening. Protrusion is secondary to shortening of the helical arch, vertical compression of the scapha, and flattening of the antihelical crura. Decreased ear size results from decreased skin envelope, conchal widening, and angulation, and an actual decrease in auricular cartilage size. The low ear position is similar to that seen in other severe auricular malformations and appears to be of similar etiology.

GOALS OF TREATMENT

Since the presentation and spectrum of constricted ears is widely variable, the treatment must be individualized to the specific deformity. There is often some degree of constriction in prominent ears, and the surgeon should have a working knowledge of procedures for treating constriction. Certainly, some of the techniques of cartilage shaping and control of ear prominence are equally applicable to repair of both types of deformity. The moderately severe constricted ear presents one of the greatest challenges to the reconstructive surgeon; in some cases, it is more difficult to correct than the microtic ear.

Techniques vary in their ability to increase the vertical height through cartilage reshaping, alone or in combination with additional cartilage graft of auricular cartilage (contralateral or ipsilateral concha) or costal cartilage (29–32). A review of the literature on treatment of constricted ears reveals one consistent shortfall of the approaches described. While each technique increases the vertical height of the ear, few if any are capable of establishing a *normal* vertical ear dimension. In fact, a careful inspection of the 17 techniques illustrated in the excellent review paper on constricted ears by Cosman (30) demonstrates that only one technique accomplishes this.

In the case of bilateral constriction, obtaining symmetry between the two sides may not be a problem, but when the contralateral ear is of normal size the surgeon must either accept that there will be a discrepancy between the reconstructed and normal side or, as suggested by Brent (33), reduce the size of the normal ear to match the reconstructed side.

OVERVIEW OF TREATMENT TECHNIQUES

Group I

The minor deformities of the helical rim alone can be corrected either by readjusting the rim to gain additional vertical height or by full-thickness excision of the lid. This excision is approached directly through exposure of the lid of extra cartilage and skin excision, placing the final scar just within the helical rim (29–31) (Fig. 55–6).

Group II

In the moderate deformities (Group IIa, Fig. 55–7), the height discrepancy can be corrected either by V–Y advancement, "banner flaps," or augmentation of the cartilage with a contralateral conchal cartilage graft (29–32). The more severe cases (Group IIb, Fig. 55–8) may require splitting the constricted segment and again using an auricular cartilage graft in combination with local skin flap for coverage of the

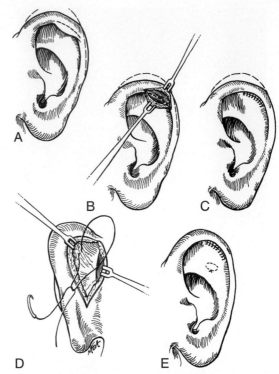

FIG. 55–6. Treatment of group I constriction. **A,** the deformity is shown in relation to the normal vertical dimension (in broken line). **B,** the skin of the helical lid is incised and the cartilage overhang exposed. **C,** the closure can be carried out just within the helical rim. **D,** a posterior skin excision and permanent suture from scapha to mastoid can be used, if needed, to correct associated protrusion of the upper pole in a similar fashion to a standard otoplasty.

anterior skin defect (33). The cartilage deficit may also be corrected with a chondrocutaneous flap from the ipsilateral concha. The cartilage defect in the moderate constriction is best visualized, and therefore corrected, by degloving the ear and getting a direct look at the deformed cartilage (31,32).

Group III

If the constriction is of a tubular variety, with a height difference of as much as 1.5 cm, correction will require addition of both skin and cartilage. These deformities are best treated similar to a conchal-type or atypical microtia, using a costal-cartilage framework splice into the usable portions of the constricted remnant (31,32).

While the figures give a brief overview of several of the more useful techniques for Group I and II constriction, the reader is referred to the cited authors for a review of greater depth.

Nonoperative Treatment of Congenital Deformities

Prominent and constricted ears, along with cryptotia and Stahl ear, have each been treated and corrected (at least partially) by nonoperative splinting techniques. First described by Matsuo and colleagues (34) and then by Brown and coworkers (35), the approach is based on experimental evidence that auricular cartilage is soft and malleable during the

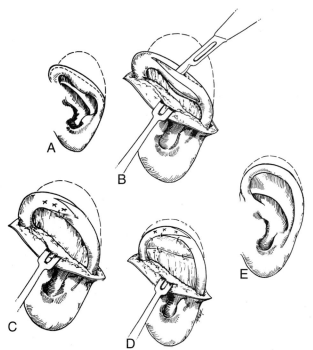

FIG. 55–7. Treatment of group II constriction by the Tanzer "double banner flap." **A, B,** the deformity is visualized by degloving the ear, and anterior and posterior leaves are formed from the helical curl. **C,** the banner flaps are rotated and slid along each other, widening the radius of curve of the helical rim, then sutured together in the expanded form. **D,** support for the marked vertical increase (particularly in group IIb) is obtained with a conchal cartilage graft from the same or opposite ear. **E,** the completed repair still falls short of "normal height" (typically, this is secondary to limitation in skin coverage).

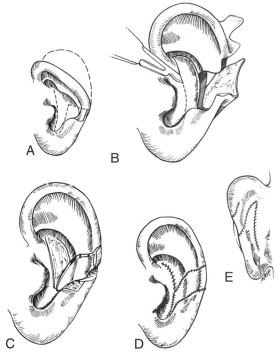

FIG. 55–8. Treatment of group IIb constriction, using an approach similar to Kislov, but supplying the cartilage support and part of the additional skin anteriorly with a chondrocutaneous island flap (rather than conchal graft alone, with need to bring the posterior skin flap further anterior). **A,** the constricted ear is split at the junction between the mid and lower third while a postauricular flap (PA) is developed for partial coverage of the resulting anterior defect. **B, C,** a chondrocutaneous island flap is transposed out of the concha on a fascial pedicle deep to the concha and spliced into the skin cartilage defect in the antihelix and helical rim (excluding the skin of the rim itself, which will wrap from behind using flap PA). **D, E,** the repair is completed when flap PA is transposed to cover the helical rim, following placement of whatever permanent sutures are needed to modulate the degree of correction of ear prominence. Anterior and posterior suture lines are demonstrated, as is the fact that this approach provides the additional skin and cartilage support to gain the full "normal height" of the ear (illustrated by the broken line shown adjacent to the preoperative view of deformity in **A**).

neonatal period while maternal estrogen levels are still high. Once these levels drop (usually after 2 weeks of age) the cartilage becomes more firm and will hold the shape into which it has been molded.

The nonoperative approach has been applied most successfully to prominent ears, constricted ears, and Stahl ear. The main risk is that of skin necrosis arising from pressure of the splint material, but with softer materials now available (the dental compound first described was held in place with Steri-strips), this is rarely a problem. The technique has not been used widely because of the narrow window of opportunity during which the splinting can be applied and the fact that many of the patients are not referred soon enough after birth. Given the opportunity, nonoperative management should be considered and applied in the appropriate cases as part of our armamentarium of treatment techniques for aesthetic correction of the ear.

References

1. Elliott RA. Aesthetic surgery of the ears. In: Georgiade GS, et al, eds. *Plastic, maxillofacial, and reconstructive surgery.* 1st ed. Baltimore: Williams & Wilkins, 1987; 729–736.
2. Rogers BO. Ely's 1881 operation for correction of protruding ears: a medical "first." *Plast Reconstr Surg* 1968; 42:584.
3. Ely ET. An operation for prominent auricles. *Arch Otolaryngol* 1881; 10:97. (Reprinted in *Plast Reconstr Surg* 1968; 42:582.)
4. Moréstin H: De la reposition et du plissement cosmétiques du pavillon de l'orielle. *Rev Orth* 1903; 4:298.
5. Gersuny R. Uber einige kosmetische operationen. *Wien Med Wochenschr* 1903; 53:2253.
6. Luckett WH. A new operation for prominent ears based on the anatomy of the deformity. *Surg Gynecol Obst* 1910; 10:635. (Reprinted in *Plast Reconstr Surg* 1969; 43:83.)
7. Converse JM, Nigro A, Wilson FA, et al. A technique for surgical correction of lop ears. *Plast Reconstr Surg* 1955; 15:411.
8. Gibson T, Davis WB. Distortion of autogenous cartilage grafts: its cause and prevention. *Br J Plast Surg* 1958; 10:257.
9. Stenstrom SJ, Heftner J. The Stenstrom otoplasty. *Clin Plast Surg* 1978; 5:465.
10. Mustardé JC. Correction of prominent ears using simple mattress sutures. *Br J Plast Surg* 1963; 16:170.
11. Owens N, Delgado DD. Management of outstanding ears. *South Med J* 1955; 58:32.
12. Davenport G, Bernard FD. Experience with mattress suture technique in correction of prominent ears. *Plast Reconstr Surg* 1965; 36:91.
13. Spira M, McCrea R, Gerow F, et al. Correction of principle deformities causing prominent ears. *Plast Reconstr Surg* 1969; 44:150.

14. Mustardé JC. The treatment of prominent ears by buried mattress sutures. A 10-year survey. *Plast Reconstr Surg* 1967; 39:382.

15. Ju DM, Li CH, Crikelair GF, et al. Surgical correction of protruding ears. *Plast Reconstr Surg* 1963; 32:283.

16. Webster GV. The tail of the helix as a key to otoplasty. *Plast Reconstr Surg* 1969; 44:455.

17. Courtiss EH, et al. Otoplasty: direct surgical approach. In: Master FW, Lewia JR Jr, eds. *Symposium on aesthetic surgery of nose, ears, and chin.* St. Louis: CV Mosby, 1973.

18. Furnas DW. Correction of prominent ears by conchal-mastoid sutures. *Plast Reconstr Surg* 1968; 42:189.

19. Elliott RA, Hoehn JG. Otoplasty for prominent ears: a complete approach. *Int Microform J Aesthet Plast Surg,* 1972A.

20. Bauer BS. Management and therapy of congenital malformation and traumatic deformities of the pinna. In: Alberti PW, Rubin RJ, eds. *Otologic medicine and surgery.* Vol. 2. New York: Churchill Livingstone, 1988; 1025–1072.

21. Senechal G, Peck A. *Chirurgie du pavillon de l'oreille.* Paris: Arnett, 1970.

22. Goulian D, Conway H. Prevention of persistent deformity of tragus and lobule. *Plast Reconstr Surg* 1960; 26:399.

23. Davis J. Prominent ears. *Clin Plast Surg* 1978; 5:471.

24. McDowell AJ. Goals in otoplasty for protruding ears. *Plast Reconstr Surg* 1968; 41:17.

25. Stark RB, Saunders DE. Natural appearance restored to the unduly prominent ear. *Br J Plast Surg* 1962; 15:385.

26. Elliott RA. Otoplasty: a combined approach. *Clin Plast Surg* 1990; 17:373.

27. Elliott RA. Complications in the treatment of prominent ears. *Clin Plast Surg* 1978; 5:479.

28. Hinderer UT, del Rio JL, Fregenal FJ. Otoplasty for prominent ears. *Aesth Plast Surg* 1987; 11:63.

29. Tanzer RC. The constricted (cup and lop) ear. *Plast Reconstr Surg* 1975; 55:406.

30. Cosman B. The constricted ear. *Clin Plast Surg* 1978; 5:389.

31. Davis J. Repair of severe cup deformities. In: Tanzer RC, Edgerton MT, eds. *Symposium on reconstruction of the auricle.* St. Louis: CV Mosby, 1974; 134.

32. Kislov R. Surgical correction of the cupped ear. *Plast Reconstr Surg* 1971; 48:121.

33. Brent B. Panel: aesthetic otoplasty. *Aesthetic Surgery* 1992; 12:4.

34. Matsuo K, Hirose T, Tomono T, et al. Nonsurgical correction of congenital auricular deformities in the early neonate: a preliminary report. *Plast Reconstr Surg* 1984; 73:38.

35. Brown FE, Colen LB, Addante RR, et al. Correction of congenital auricular deformities by splinting in the neonatal period. *Pediatrics* 1986; 78:406.

56

Hair Restoration Surgery

Thomas J. Hubbard, M.D.

For most people, hair is an important part of self-image. A full head of hair is associated with youth, health, and virility in our society. As aesthetic surgery has become more acceptable to men, an increasing number are considering surgical options to address their hair loss problem. Coincidentally, available surgical options are now numerous. However, the increase in number and sophistication of surgical modalities has still not produced one ideal solution that is applicable to all problems. In fact, what appears to be a straightforward problem is actually as complex as any in plastic surgery. Variables such as color, texture, and density of hair, as well as scalp color and laxity are not just incidental; each has an enormous influence on the final aesthetic result. To add to the complexity, consider that the surgical result will change over the years as alopecia continues to progress. Simply filling bald areas with hair is not sufficient. It is important to avoid creating new problems, such as unnatural hair lines, maldirection of hair growth, a pluggy look, or scars that are difficult to conceal. Excellent results can be obtained with hair restoration surgery, but long-term planning after careful consideration of the many variables is essential. Candidates must be patient, because the multiple stages may require 1 to 3 years and additional procedures may be necessary in the future with progression of the alopecia.

Etiology

Male pattern baldness is clearly related to androgens, but the exact mechanism is not known. Testosterone level in balding individuals does not influence the onset rapidity or pattern of baldness. Androgens stimulate the growth of hair over much of the body but, in those who are genetically susceptible, bring about the loss of hair in certain areas of the scalp. The inheritance of androgenic alopecia continues to be debated. It may be polygenic with variable penetrance and expression (1). Hair loss can begin any time after puberty; the first change is usually bitemporal recession. This occurs in 96% of white males, many of whom are not destined to sustain further hair loss (2). In those males who are, the bitemporal recession progresses, or further hair loss begins in the crown or frontal area. Unfortunately, there is no way to predict the pattern and severity of androgenic alopecia, but generally loss of hair in the second decade portends more severe patterns of loss (3). Norwood (4) has shown that more severe balding can begin later in life and, once balding begins, it is unlikely to stop. Norwood suggests that the incidence of more severe balding is probably higher than earlier studies indicated (5).

Androgenic alopecia also affects women, but it presents later in life. It is manifested by a diffuse thinning over the entire top of the scalp with preservation of the hairline. Some contend androgenic alopecia is just as common in women as in men (3). Much controversy remains over both the etiology and treatment of this condition. Norwood (6) does not recommend endocrine studies for these women patients unless there is evidence of virilization.

Hair Transplantation

Hair transplantation is the backbone of hair replacement surgery. It is the primary or secondary mode in almost all cases. Often it is used alone, employing grafts of various sizes in a carefully planned multistage approach. At other times, grafts accompany scalp reductions or scalp flaps.

In 1959 Orentreich (7) showed donor dominance in which grafts retain their persistent growth characteristic when moved to another site. This redistribution of "permanent" hair is the basis of all hair replacement surgery, reductions and flaps included.

Management of male pattern baldness is primarily a matter of choosing a redistribution technique. Grafting would always be one of the first choices but is not necessarily the simplest or even the least expensive modality. Due to the inelasticity of the scalp, reductions and flaps are usually not simple. Without a quick and easy solution available, the philosophy of management is based on aesthetics.

Hair transplanting in its early years was met with considerable excitement. The effected change in appearance was striking but, with the passage of time, the procedure developed some disappointment and a tainted reputation. Much had to be learned about where and how to recreate a natural hairline and selection of proper candidates. Probably most damaging of all was the unnatural "pluggy" appearance produced by large grafts. In the 1980s, minigrafting and micrografting evolved through the work of Marritt (8), Bradshaw (9), and others. Using different-sized smaller grafts, "corn rowing" (the doll's head appearance) can be almost completely avoided and results dramatically improved.

Some controversy remains as to what exactly constitutes a micrograft, a minigraft, and a standard graft. Knudsed (10) recently proposed that standard grafts are greater than 2.5 mm, minigrafts are less than 2.5 mm, and micrografts contain only 1 to 2 hairs (Fig. 56–1).

The majority of surgeons now employ a variety of grafts according to zones. The frontal hairline, for example, should be comprised exclusively of micrografts for a zone 0.5 to 1

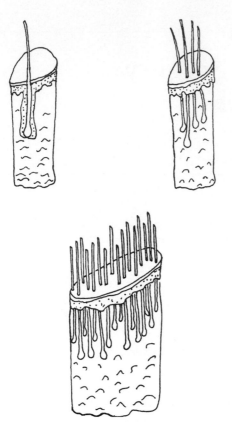

FIG. 56–1. Micrograft, minigraft, and standard graft.

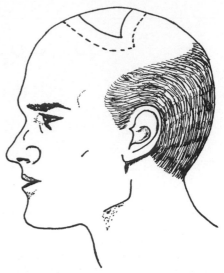

FIG. 56–2. One design of a frontal forelock. Space between fore-lock and rest of hair-bearing scalp is filled or partially filled with mi-crografts. Micrografts are placed within the dashed line and minigrafts within the solid line.

cm in width, followed posteriorly by minigrafts that are ei-ther all one size or increasing sizes by zones (11). Standard grafts, if used at all, are placed further back. Results vary considerably. In a particular candidate, a natural-appearing hairline can be created with large standard grafts. Con-versely, in the patient with coarse black hair and a light scalp, even using micrografts exclusively may not give a 100% nat-ural appearance.

Zones of varying-size grafts should be considered at other border areas as well. In more severe balding, it may become difficult or impossible for grafts to span the distance between the temporal fringes because donor hair in these patients is limited. For these patients, either no surgery or creation of an isolated frontal forelock is planned (12) (Fig. 56–2). This forelock can have considerable density centrally and frontally, but only micrografts and very small minigrafts should be used along the borders. The anterior border of a crown to be left bald should be approached in a similar fash-ion. As grafting proceeds back to this border, grafts should become smaller, progressing to micrografts. If there is patient resistance to leaving bald lateral alleys, these can be man-aged with micrografts.

Planning is essential in hair transplantation. Poor planning can easily lead to unsatisfactory results, which may be impos-sible to correct completely. This may be because of unantici-pated progression of hair loss, exhaustion of grafts, or mis-sized, misplaced, or misdirected grafts or scars. For men in their late teens and early twenties, future hair loss patterns are uncertain. Their emotional pleas for a low hairline and com-plete, high-density coverage of all balding areas may sway the

surgeon toward higher risk plans. Better results are achieved by using small grafts to cover small areas. The smaller the graft size, the more natural is the appearance. With minigrafts covering a limited area, the patient who unexpectedly termi-nates hair restoration surgery at an early stage usually won't be left with any significant deformity. Neighboring hair is gradually lost with further progression of male pattern bald-ness, and the grafts become more exposed or prominent. If they are small and there is little contrast between hair and scalp color, grafts can remain natural in appearance. The size of the area grafted can always be increased later as donor re-serves allow. Moving the hairline down should be considered only after multiple stages when donor reserves are sufficient. Simple grafting of a bald crown alone, or including that with other areas of grafting in early stages, presents considerable risk. There will always be progression of crown baldness and this can result in a halo deformity around the old grafts (Fig. 56–3). The surgeon is then forced into chasing the receding fringe with more grafts—a futile attempt when donor reserves are limited. Furthermore, an already depleted donor area will restrict efforts to reconstruct the frontal area, which may not have been a problem initially but becomes a great concern to the patient 10 years later.

Norwood (13) describes six major factors in patient selec-tion and planning: classification, color, curl, texture (caliber), density, and amount of donor hair. These factors dictate the safe surgical options, with classification the most important. The most popular classification scheme is that of Norwood types I through VII (Fig. 56–4). Savin (14) recently intro-duced a classification scheme with three types of baldness: front of scalp, mid area, and vertex, each graded one through seven. Evaluation is done on hair parted down the middle. Using Norwood's classification, scheme types III, IV, and V are usually good candidates. The candidacy of type VI and VII depend greatly on the other major factors. Unfortunately some types III, IV, and V are destined to join groups of greater baldness severity (Fig. 56–5).

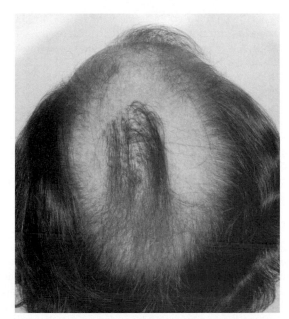

FIG. 56–3. Halo deformity resulting from progression of baldness following inappropriate grafting to vertex. (Photo courtesy of E. Marritt.)

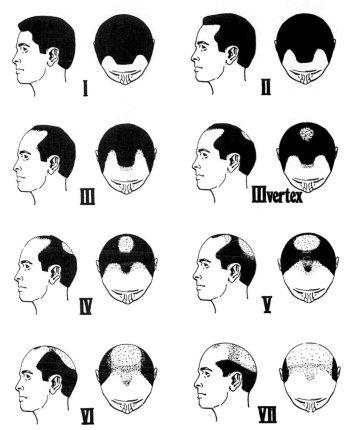

FIG. 56–4. The Norwood classification scheme of male pattern baldness. (From Norwood OT. Male pattern baldness: classification and incidence. *Hair Transplant Forum*, 1993; 3:5.)

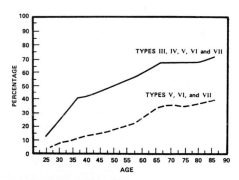

FIG. 56–5. Norwood's graph of balding. The incidence of cosmetically significant male pattern baldness increases with age. The rate of severe baldness is relatively low until later decades. (From Norwood OT. Male pattern baldness: classification and incidence. *Hair Transplant Forum*, 1993; 3:5.)

Hair and scalp color have considerable influence on hair restoration surgery results. When there is little contrast between hair and skin, an optical illusion effects a more dense and natural appearance. Colors, in order of preference, are white, salt-and-pepper, blonde, light brown or red, darker brown, and black (15). Black hair on a light scalp is quite problematic; more and smaller grafts are required to soften the contrasting effect. Scalp coloring agents such as COUVRÉ (Spencer Forrest Laboratories, Westport, CT) and Derm Match (Derm Match, Inc., Potomac, MD) can help. With more severe balding there is limited donor hair, and the surgeon must consider creating a diffuse, thinned appearance with micrografts, an isolated frontal forelock—or question candidacy.

Curliness is favorable because it inherently covers and camouflages any tufted arrangement. Hair transplantation in African Americans have this advantage. In fact, minigrafts may sometimes be substituted for micrografts at the hairline with very curly hair; but, more caution is necessary in harvesting these patients because the bulb may lie obliquely in the dermis and fat (16).

Thick-textured hair has the advantage that its larger volume covers well, but it also creates more striking contrast with the underlying skin, possibly rendering a less natural appearance. Also, it is more difficult to style. Therefore, the surgeon may choose less-coarse hair to graft the hairline by harvesting from the low occipital area or just above the ear. This hair can more easily be combed straight back, and a finer texture is generally more natural at the hairline. However, the inferior occipital hair does tend to thin more rapidly than a more superior donor area (15).

Greater density is surely an advantage in the donor area. In fact, low density in the donor area may rule out candidacy for hair transplantation. But dense hair in the donor area also produces dense grafts. This may hint at a pluggy appearance in those with the dark hair–light scalp combination. For these patients, smaller minigrafts or micrografts should be used. Consideration should be given to using dense grafts as small punch grafts rather than placing them in slits, which can compress the hair even more densely. This is especially true in tight scalps.

With coarse dark hair in a light scalp, a wider zone of micrografts is necessary in front, followed by smaller than usual minigrafts. A natural hairline may still be difficult to accomplish, so the patient should consider eventually combing the hair forward and across rather than straight back. In a patient with limited donor hair, the surgeon may consider densely grafting a zone at the hairline and along the part side, with more sparse grafts elsewhere. By combing back and away from the part, an illusion of more hair can be accomplished. In the patient with more severe balding, if it is consistent with his goals, a diffuse, thinned look through micrografts can be a safe and predictable approach. According to Stough (17), this method requires three to five sessions and employing 400 to 1000 grafts per session. It results in a see-through look, but there is little or no scar around the grafts and they can often be indistinguishable from native hair.

Anesthesia

Patients are initially placed prone on a Pron-Pillo (Robbins Instruments, Inc., Chatham, NJ). Although many surgeons use no sedation, I prefer intravenous sedation with pulse oximeter monitoring. Antibiotics are probably not necessary, but I give all patients Decadron 8 mg to avoid postoperative forehead edema. Postoperative prednisone for several days is also helpful. After intravenous midazolam and ketamine, the donor area is anesthetized with 0.25% lidocaine with 1:400,000 epinephrine. This dilution allows a larger-volume injection for more turgid tissue and precise beveling parallel to the hair follicle. It also facilitates more liberal use of 1% lidocaine with 1:100,000 epinephrine to the recipient area, where maximal hemostasis is extremely important. The recipient (usually frontal) area is injected at the same time (while under influence of the ketamine) and then augmented later after harvest, when the patient is turned supine just before creating the needle hole, slit, or punch recipient sites. For maximal hemostasis, injection should be into the dermis as well as subgaleally. A 0.5% bupivacaine with 1:100,000 epinephrine block is administered at the end of the procedure.

Hairline

The inspection of any natural hairline demonstrates that it is actually not a line at all. The best reproduction is accomplished by treating it as a zone, incorporating a deliberate irregularity and scatter in minigraft placement (17) (Fig. 56–6). A conservative approach to planning would be placing the hairline 9 cm above a horizontal line drawn just above the eye-

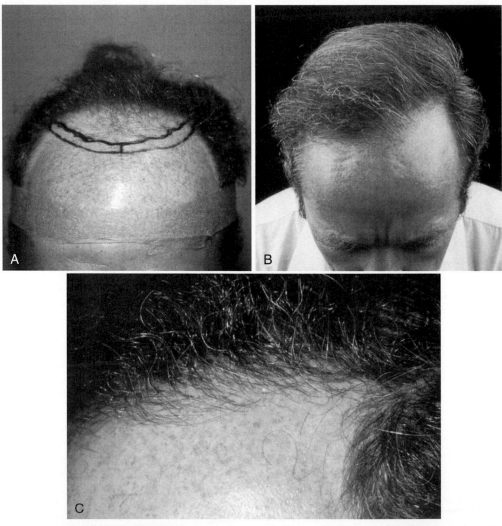

FIG. 56–6. **A,** conservative hairline is drawn, with plans for a feathering zone of 1.5 to 2 cm that consists only of single-hair grafts. Posteriorly, the surgeon will place 1.25-mm minigrafts of up to 4 hairs. **B,** same patient after 5 sessions averaging 400 grafts per session. **C,** closeup of the hairline showing deliberate irregularity of the feathering zone. (Photo courtesy of D. Stough.)

brows (11). Every centimeter the hairline is brought down has enormous ramifications in terms of grafts. Depending on grafting technique, the surgeon may be committing to another 500 to 1000 grafts with each centimeter of advancement. If the temporal fringe is high enough, the anterior hairline can be designed to connect to it. Micrografts are placed in the hairline zone in 16- or 18-gauge needle holes angulated forward about 45°. Of course, surgical plans vary greatly, but a reasonable approach is to plan 100 micrografts placed along the hairline zone along with a variable number of minigrafts behind it at each session. Grafts are placed with a fine jewelers forceps. Grasp the fatty tissue beneath the bulbs and leave the graft slightly protruding. Uebel (18) incises with a Beaver Mini-blade only 2 to 3 mm deep, not transgressing galea. Each graft is placed immediately following recipient slit preparation with not less than 2 to 3 mm between each graft. Other surgeons prefer to incise more deeply, create all the recipient sites first, then place all the grafts. It is not clear yet how tightly grafts can be packed before survival is affected. Surely a density of packing in one session could be reached that would compromise vascularity to the grafts and even risk local scalp necrosis. Rassman (19) feels survival is excellent with even 1 mm or less between slits.

Donor Hair Harvesting

Determining safe donor-area boundaries is a necessary prerequisite to harvesting. Alt (20), and more recently Unger (15), published parameters for mapping safe donor regions. These are useful guides, but nothing is 100% reliable because of the inherent unpredictability of male pattern baldness.

Traditional harvesting was done with multiple punches to the donor area, usually removing usually 4-mm plugs. The ratio of scar to hair is high with this technique and it results in decreased donor density. Harvesting strips with multi-blade knives is preferable, and the previous scar is removed with each session, leaving only one linear scar. Linear narrow scars in the back of the head and/or temporal donor areas are nearly impossible to see and hair density has not been altered. Further, most people can lose 40 to 60% of their donor hair with no significant compromise to the donor area (12). The depth should include approximately 2 mm of subfollicular fat. Harvesting deeper than this leads to unnecessary bleeding and possible damage to the occipital nerves. Two- and three-millimeter spacers between three or four blades are common. It is easier to separate the hairs into micrografts and minigrafts with 2-mm strips. Determining the necessary width and length is a difficult part of harvesting, especially for the inexperienced. Haber (21) has developed a reference table to aid in determining dimension. A necessary first step is determining donor hair density; it is best done under magnification because multiple hairs may exit a single follicular orifice. Knowing donor hair density and planned graft size, reference tables will provide multistrip length of harvest using the triple blade knife with 2-mm spacers. Stough and Pomerantz (22) have also developed reference tables for harvesting.

Harvesting a single ellipse (e.g., 8 – 1.5 cm, or 12 – 1 cm) is preferred by a number of surgeons. These sizes of ellipses are consistent with large graft sessions. After excision, the ellipse is sliced transversely and the resulting short strips cut into grafts of the desired number of hairs. Wide ellipses require undermining and may leave less desirable scars.

Selective donor harvesting allows for considerable artistic flair (15). The densest hair comes from the middle of the occipital area, becoming more sparse superiorly, inferiorly, and anteriorly. Consider grafting the most dense hair in the frontal area several centimeters behind the hairline with less dense hair to the hairline and part side. Likewise high-caliber or coarse hair should be avoided in the hairline and part line areas if possible. Very coarse hair, even employed as one- or two-hair micrografts, does not look as natural as fine hair harvested from the inferior occipital and temporal areas (15).

Ideally, the surgeon should have one or more technicians assisting, depending on session size. Assistants work on a side table, preferably under magnification, cutting the strips into grafts. Early in the procedure, the surgeon tests the first couple of grafts in recipient holes to ensure proper fit.

Graft Placement

There is considerable debate whether minigrafts should be placed in holes taken with small punches or slits made with a blade. Slit grafting is faster, as it eliminates the step of removing bald plugs at recipient sites, but grafts placed in holes yield better results (12). Especially with dark hair and a light scalp, slit grafting compresses the graft, resulting in even more contrast and less natural appearance. With more favorable color and texture settings, though, slits may well be appropriate. Further, they scar less and pose less potential risk to surrounding hair and blood supply.

For the best results, grafts should be placed slightly protruding. The minimal early protrusion flattens and leads to a normal contour. In a rare case when slight protrusion persists, it is easily corrected with light electrodesiccation (23). A depression is addressed with dermabrasion, light electrodesiccation to the surrounding skin, or graft replacement.

After placement of grafts, small crusts form, which gradually fall off in the first 2 weeks. Most of the hair falls out and true growth is noted in the 2nd or 3rd month—longer in later stages or in the setting of scar. The next grafting stage can be in 4 to 8 months (18). The patient won't see a final result until more than a year following the last grafting procedure.

Scalp Reduction

The most common adjunct to hair transplantation is scalp reduction. The idea was introduced synergistically in 1977 by the Blanchard brothers (24) and the Unger brothers (25). Scalp reduction is most useful for the crown and midscalp. In theory, scalp reduction decreases the total surface area of baldness so that more is accomplished with a given number of grafts. Results have improved over time with the addition of preoperative massage, wide undermining, and tissue expanders. The surgeon can employ a variety of incision patterns to customize direction of advancement and better hide scars. However, even with multiple operations, patients with extensive baldness and/or a tight scalp may still be disappointed by final results that include a widened scar and misdirection of hair. Some experienced scalp-reduction surgeons, including Norwood, have greatly decreased or abandoned the procedure altogether (23–25).

The classic midline elliptical scalp reduction is falling out of favor. The midline posterior scar with hair diverging away from it ("slot deformity") is difficult to conceal with styling

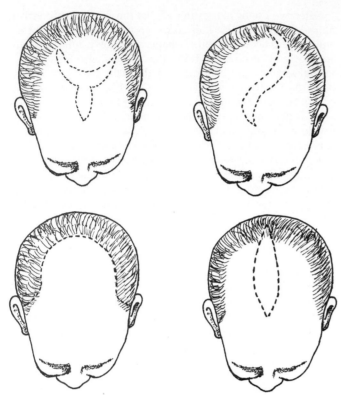

FIG. 56–7. Popular incision patterns for scalp reduction.

and even with grafts. Frechet introduced flaps to redirect local hair and conceal the midline scar, or other reduction patterns, as a response to this created deformity (26); the U-shaped pattern can avoid slot creation. Also, since little bald scalp is undermined, it is theoretically anchored and little or no "stretch-back" occurs. Further, its surgical exposure is the best for more aggressive undermining. Variations of the midline elliptical pattern can avoid a slot deformity. One approach is just to veer off the midline posteriorly in one direction or the other. Other options that help to conceal scar are the S and Y patterns (Fig. 56–7). Unger enumerates advantages and disadvantages of each (25).

Scalp reduction is done in the office, on an outpatient basis, under local anesthesia and intravenous sedation. It is most easily performed with the patient in a prone position, using a Pron-Pillo or bulky pillow under the chin. Undermining is done below the galea and is extensive laterally and over a variable distance posteriorly. The amount to be removed is determined by overlap or use of a D'Assumpçao clamp (Padgett Instruments, Kansas City, MO). Closure is with two layers, a 2-0 absorbable like PDS deep and 4-0 nylon or chromic. Minimal tension on the closure provides for much better quality scars and minimal "stretch-back" (25). The risk of bleeding from galeotomies is not justified by the small increase in skin excision (25). There should be at least 2 months between procedures, with 1 month of massage before each reduction.

A variety of plastic surgery techniques and innovations have been employed in recent years to solve the problem of the galea's resistance to stretch. The most rapid and effective tool is tissue expansion, which was adopted initially for trau-

matic defects of the scalp and then for male pattern baldness (27,28). Individual follicles are abstracted by a factor of 2 to 3 times normal, but this doesn't significantly affect scalp cosmetic appearance (29). One or more expanders is placed through an incision at the balding fringe. Saline injections are done on a weekly basis for 8 to 12 weeks. Discomfort is worse after the earlier injections but usually lasts only a few hours. The expanded scalp is highly vascular and can be applied as simple advancements or rearranged in flaps. Anderson (30) has developed a technique to mobilize expanded scalp as flaps to the hairline, called the bilateral advancement transposition flap. A third flap—a triple advancement transposition flap—may be simultaneously transposed from the expanded occipital area (Fig. 56–8). Random flaps reconstruct the hairline. Total scalp coverage can be obtained with one expansion, but not uncommonly another expansion is necessary.

Anderson prefers to wait 2 to 3 months before placing another expander. He has demonstrated that large areas of scalp can be completely surrounded by incisions and still survive as long as no undermining of the central area is done. Although expansion accomplishes rapid and dramatic results, the patient should be counseled beforehand that some sessions of minigrafting and/or micrografting may be necessary. A hairline created by a flap will always have a scar and present an unnatural transition from forehead to dense scalp. Single-hair grafts to camouflage this may be desirable.

Despite the multiple advantages of scalp expansion, the attendant short period of disfigurement is unacceptable to many patients. An alternative method of scalp reduction called an extension was proposed by Frechet (26). There is no visible deformity of the scalp while the expansion is accomplished. Hooks on both ends of a stretched sheet of silastic engage galea of hair-bearing scalp on both sides of the bald area. (These hooks are available in a variety of sizes through MXM Laboratories, Antibes, France, Fax: (27) 93652536.) While there is usually a delay of several months between scalp reduction stages, Frechet recommends reduction and placement of an extender with only 1 month's delay until the next reduction. He describes the appropriate choice of extender length and amount of stretch on placement to avoid excessive pain (26). Measurements of bald scalp excision at time of extender removal are understated because of compression. Some feel the primary action of the extender is to prevent stretch-back (32), while others have observed that it significantly augments and accelerates scalp reduction (25). Frechet's work with extenders and midline ellipse reduction has been duplicated by an American group with equally impressive results (33).

Much work is being done now in applying extenders to other patterns of reduction such as the "U." With this pattern of reduction, the central flap of bald scalp can be elevated for placement of the extender with no risk to vascularity (Fig. 56–9). Custom extenders (materials from Applied Biomaterial Technologies, Inc., Silverdale, WA) make innovations simple to fabricate in the office. To date there are no significant series with multiple vector extenders. These may play a role in the future by pulling temporal hair medially while advancing occipital hair superiorly. Frechet doubts multidirectional extenders will have much future in scalp reduction, as there is a limit to the amount the central area of bald scalp can be compressed (34).

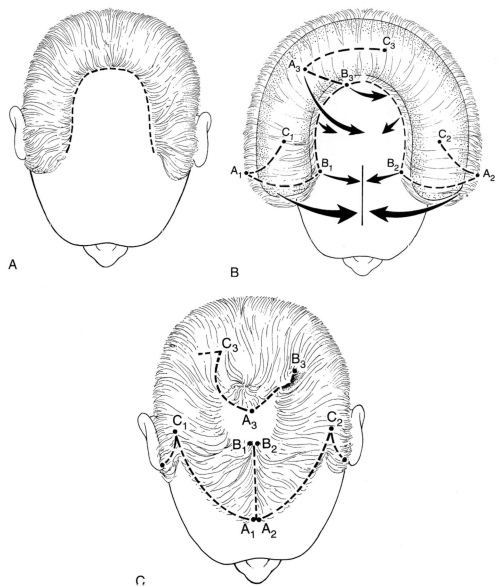

FIG. 56–8. **A,** incision along the fringe for placement of the expander. **B,** expanded hair-bearing area with triple advancement transposition (TAT) flap markings. If the posterior expanded scalp is simply advanced without creation of a random occipital flap, then a bilateral advancement transposition (BAT) procedure is performed. **C,** expected amount of coverage following the TAT procedure. (From Anderson RD. Scalp expansion for the treatment of male pattern baldness. In: Rohrich RJ, ed. *Perspectives in plastic surgery.* St. Louis: Quality Medical Publishing, 1994; 8:78, 79.)

Another adjunct to scalp reduction is use of the Sure-Closure device introduced by Hirshowitz (35). Stough (36) accomplishes 20 to 30% more scalp excision with a 30–60 minute application of the device at the time of reduction. Others, myself included, have found it time consuming and of little benefit.

More and more aggressive scalp reductions have led to a group of procedures that not only stretch the hair-bearing scalp but, by undermining completely past it into elastic neck skin, also shift the hair-bearing unit upward. Although their biomechanics differ significantly, the dramatic results of "hair lifts" rival those of tissue expansion.

Marzolla first introduced this more extensive dissection through the occipitalis insertion, cutting the occipitalis artery, and undermining down to the hairline (37) . With the anterior extent of the incision into the sideburn for more exposure, the scalp could then be advanced both medially and anteriorly. Most other scalp reduction patterns actually pull the temporal hairline posteriorly to some degree. Bradshaw applied a bilateral advancement simultaneously and Brandy added refinements including prior occipital artery ligation that greatly reduced the incidence of local scalp necrosis (38). With occipital artery ligations 4 to 8 weeks before the extensive scalp lift, a delay is accomplished that forces dependence of the occipital scalp on the superficial temporal artery system. Brandy calls his extensive scalp-lift the bilateral occipitoparietal flap (Fig. 56–10). It can be followed by what he describes as the bitemporal flap (38), which can entail similar aggressive undermining, if necessary, to excise

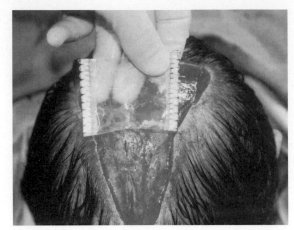

FIG. 56–9.   A homemade extender about to be placed in a reduction with Y pattern.

the remaining bald scalp with a veer to the incision posteriorly. The latter aspect of the design usually avoids a slot formation creating a cowlick arrangement to the vertex hair.

The scalp-lift procedures have their drawbacks, and patients should be chosen carefully. The posterior hairline comes up significantly and baldness behind the ear is increased. There have been disappointed patients who referred to their hair as "a mop on my head" (39). Some will need grafting behind the ears and longer growth of the posterior hair. As the incision needs to be extended, for exposure, toward or well into the sideburn anterior to the superficial temporal artery, the scar may be a problem. With much anterior advancement, the scar may be immediately at the hairline, but with further temporal recession the scar may become exposed. Either way, micrografting may be necessary. Dividing the occipital nerves will lead to an area of anesthesia, which usually is not a problem if the patient is forewarned. Finally, as with any reduction procedure, balding will continue and further procedures may be necessary. Swinehart (40) describes the ideal criteria for scalp-lifting to be a loose scalp, relatively stable hair loss pattern, maximum coronal alopecia width of 12 to 13 cm, and tall posterior and lateral donor areas.

Despite its drawbacks, the scalp-lift procedure in properly selected patients can yield extremely impressive results and very satisfied patients. Variations on the theme can be quite useful. I prefer to limit the anterior extent of the incision and avoid occipital artery ligation. This requires dissection and preservation of the occipital neurovascular bundles at the time of surgery. Much occipital scalp advancement can be accomplished without dissecting all the way to the hairline. This limits elevation of the line and baldness behind the ear. Also, with preservation of the vasculature, I have had no problems simultaneously applying a temporal-to-temporal extender.

Flaps

Dramatic results in the treatment of alopecia have been obtained by various flaps; the most popular, described by Juri (41), is the parietooccipital flap. It is a multiple-stage flap that reconstructs the hairline. There are occasional candidates

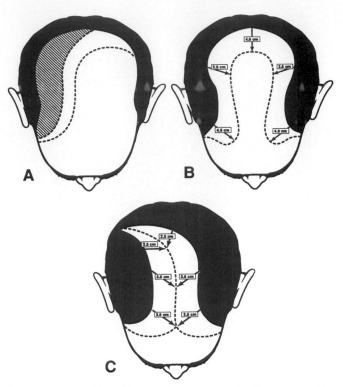

FIG. 56–10.   **A,** Marzola procedure compared with a paramedian scalp reduction. One occipital neurovascular bundle is divided. **B,** bilateral occipoparietal flap. The occipital vessels were divided at a previous stage. **C,** bitemporal flap. (From Brandy DA. Scalp lifting: an 8-year experience with over 1230 cases. *J Dermatol Surg Oncol* 1993; 19:1006.)

for this procedure but, because of a number of disadvantages (42), it is falling out of favor. The hair orientation is the wrong direction. Without tissue expansion, donor area closure is difficult and limits flap width. Tension on closure can leave noticeable scarring. The area harvested may be at considerable risk for hair loss later with progressive alopecia. There are limitations to hairline shape and the scar along the hairline can't be avoided.

Summary

The armamentarium of the aesthetic surgeon addressing male pattern baldness has expanded dramatically in the past 10 years. Coincidentally, there has been recognition of the great complexity of multiple parameters requiring consideration in developing a surgical plan. Not the least of these is the dynamic nature of the balding process, which Marritt describes as ". . . more cunning, unpredictable, relentless, and remorseless than most of us ever could have imagined. . ." (43). With such a challenging problem, more innovative and unique procedures will arise and more medical options will be at our disposal. We can hope that, with further studies and research, there will be more consensus on treatment philosophies and techniques.

References

1. Kuster W, Happle R. The inheritance of common baldness: two B or not two B? *J Am Acad Dermatol* 1984; 11:921.
2. Hamilton JB. Patterned loss of hair in man: types and incidence. *Ann NY Acad Sci* 1951; 53:708.

3. Messenger AG. The control of hair growth and pigmentation. In: Olsen EA, ed. *Disorders of hair growth diagnosis and treatment.* New York: McGraw-Hill, 1994; 39–58.
4. Norwood O. Classification and incidence of male pattern baldness. In: Norwood O, ed. *Hair transplant surgery.* 1st ed. Springfield, IL: Charles C Thomas, 1973.
5. Norwood O. Male pattern baldness classification and incidence. *Hair Transplant Forum* 1993; 3:5.
6. Norwood O. Female androgenic alopecia. *Hair Transplant Forum* 1994; 4:3.
7. Orentreich N. Autografts in alopecias and other selected dermatogical conditions. *Ann NY Acad Sci* 1959; 83:463.
8. Marritt E. Single-hair transplantation for hairline refinement: a practical solution. *J Dermatol Surg Oncol* 1984; 10:962.
9. Bradshaw W. Quarter-grafts: a technique for minigrafts. In: Unger WP, Nordstrom RE, eds. *Hair transplantation.* New York: Marcel Dekker, 1988; 333–350.
10. Knudsed R. Presentation at the 2nd annual meeting of the International Society of Hair Restoration Surgery, Toronto, 1994.
11. Buchwach K. Standard grafts, minigrafts and micrografts. *Facial Plastic Surgery Clinics of North America* 1994; 2:149.
12. Marritt E, Konior RJ. Patient selection candidacy and treatment plan for hair replacement surgery. *Facial Plastic Surgery Clinics of North America* 1994; 2:111.
13. Norwood O. Patient selection, hair transplant design and hairstyle. *J Dermatol Surg Oncol* 1992; 18:386.
14. Savin RC, personal communication.
15. Unger W. The donor site. In: Unger W, ed. *Hair transplantation.* 3rd ed. New York: Marcel Dekker, 1995; 183.
16. Randall J, Schauder C. Current concepts in alopecia correction in the black patient. *Am J Cosm Surg* 1993; 10:3.
17. Stough D. Single-hair grafting for advanced male pattern alopecia. *Cosmetic Dermatology* 1993; 6:11.
18. Uebel CO. The punciform technique with 1000 micro and minigrafts in one stage. *Am J Cosm Surg* 1994; 11:293.
19. Rassman WR. Megasessions: dense packing. *Hair Transplant Forum* 1994; 4:3.
20. Alt T. The donor site. In: Unger WP, Nordstrom RE, eds. *Hair transplantation.* New York: Marcel Dekker, 1988; 145.
21. Haber R. Accurate estimation of graft requirements when utilizing multibladed knives. Presented at the 2nd annual meeting of the International Society of Hair Restoration Surgery, Toronto, 1994.
22. Stough D, Pomerantz M. The donor area. *Facial Plast Surg Clin North America* 1994; 2:139.
23. Unger W. Complications of hair transplantation. In: Unger W, ed. *Hair transplantation.* 3rd ed. New York: Marcel Dekker, 1995; 363–374.
24. Blanchard G, Blanchard B. Obliteration of alopecia by hair-lifting: a new concept and technique. *J Natl Med Assoc* 1977; 69:639.
25. Unger M. Alopecia reductions. In: Unger W, ed. *Hair transplantation.* 3rd ed. New York: Marcel Dekker, 1995; 509–624.
26. Frechet P. Scalp extension. In: Unger W, ed. *Hair transplantation.* 3rd ed. New York, Marcell Dekker, 1995; 625.
27. Argenta LC. Controlled tissue expansion in recontructive surgery. *Br J Plast Surg* 1984; 37:520.
28. Manders EK, Au VK, Wong RK. Scalp expansion for male pattern baldness. *Clin Plast Surg* 1987; 14:469.
29. Argenta LC, Anderson RD. Tissue expansion. In: Unger WP, Nordstrom RE, eds. *Hair transplantation.* 2nd ed. New York: Marcel Dekker, 1988; 519–561.
30. Anderson RD. Scalp expansion for the treatment of male pattern baldness. *Perspectives in Plast Surg* 1994; 8:1.
31. Frechet P. Scalp extension. *J Dermatol Surg Oncol* 1993; 19:616.
32. Brandy DA. The principles of scalp extension. *Am J Cosm Surg* 1994; 11:245.
33. True R, Elliott R. Clinical aspects of scalp extension. Presented at the 2nd annual meeting of the International Society of Hair Restoration Surgery, Toronto, 1994.
34. Frechet P. Personal communication.
35. Hirshowitz B, Lindenbaum E, Har-Shai Y, A skin-stretching device for the harnessing of the viscoelastic properties of skin. *Plast Reconstr Surg* 1993; 92:260.
36. Stough DB. Sure Closure. *Hair Transplant Forum* 1994; 4:3.
37. Alt TH. History of scalp reductions and paramedian method. In: Norwood O, ed. *Hair Transplant Surgery.* 2nd ed. Springfield, IL: Charles C Thomas, 1984: 221–244.
38. Brandy DA. Scalp lifting; an 8-year experience with over 1230 cases. *J Dermatol Surg Oncol* 1993; 19:1005.
39. Manders E. Personal communication.
40. Swinehart JM. Current controversies in hair replacement surgery. *Am J Cosm Surg* 1994; 11:283.
41. Juri J. Use of parieto-occipital flaps in the surgical treatment of baldness. *Plast Reconstr Surg* 1975; 55:456.
42. Anderson RD. Expanded bilateral advancement transposition (BAT) and triple advancement transposition (TAT) flaps for treatment of male pattern baldness. *Am J Cosm Surg* 1994; 11:255.
43. Marritt E, Dzulow L. A redefinition of male pattern baldness and its treatment implications. *J Dermatol Surg Oncol* 1995; 21:123.

57

Body Contouring of the Abdomen, Thighs, Hips, and Buttocks

Richard A. Mladick, M.D., F.A.C.S.

The introduction of lipoplasty (suction removal of fat) stimulated a new awareness of the possibilities for sculpting the figure. However, many contour problems still require a traditional surgical contouring procedure to correct unsightly skin, weak musculoaponeurotic systems, and sagging tissues. This chapter discusses body contouring procedures with and without lipoplasty for the abdomen, hips, thighs, and buttocks. With proper technique, these procedures can provide excellent corrections and a high degree of patient satisfaction.

Etiology

Both heredity and environmental factors play an important role in a person's body shape. Heredity is the primary determinant of our basic body habitus (1). It is heredity that causes the unsightly, diet-resistant fat bulges in many individuals of average weight. In the female, these inherited accumulations usually occur in a gynecoid distribution in the lower abdomen, hips, saddlebags, and inner thighs. In males, accumulations of diet-resistant fat occur in an android distribution in the flanks (love handles), abdomen, and chest. Illouz pointed out that Latin people often have fat hips and thighs (a violin shape); Nordic people have fat around the lower abdomen and hips (a tire or safety-belt shape); Asian people have upper-torso fat (a kimono-type distribution); and black people have fat buttocks (steatopygia) (2). Heredity may also be responsible for weak lower-abdominal muscles, which results in a round, protuberant abdomen. Tall individuals with a marked lordotic posture may have a protruding abdomen. Congenital lipodystrophy is a less-frequently-seen problem of heredity. The lipodystrophy patient is disproportionately large below the waist, often having huge fatty hips and thighs, and sometimes fat legs to the ankles. This may occur with or without a history of high caloric intake.

Environment plays an important role, as in the very obese patient with a lifestyle of little exercise and a high caloric intake. Abdominal surgery, and some neurologic lesions, may result in a bulging abdomen from weakened or denervated muscles and/or hernias. Pregnancy is one of the major causes of stretched abdominal musculoaponeurotic systems and loose skin. The deformity may vary from merely a rounded protruding lower abdomen to one with severe diastasis of the rectus abdominis muscles and extensive striae.

Time, and repeated weight loss and weight gain, have additional deleterious effects on skin tone. This may vary from a hanging abdominal panniculus to severely dimpled cellulite-type skin. No matter what the cause of the contour problem, if the patient is healthy, a body contouring procedure can often achieve improvement.

Anatomy

ABDOMEN

The multilayered abdominal wall has its principle blood supply coming superiorly and inferiorly. The innervation comes from the lateral oblique direction. The skin of the lower abdomen is more movable because it is less firmly attached, covering softer areolar subcutaneous tissue. In the upper abdomen, the skin is less mobile and more firmly attached by many retinacula to the deep fascia. This is the reason lipoplasty more easily removes the lower abdominal fat.

The anterior abdominal musculoaponeurotic system consists of the external obliques, the internal obliques, and the transversus abdominis (which are muscular laterally but converge into aponeuroses medially), and the vertically directed rectus abdominis muscles, which lie within the two layers of the aponeuroses—the anterior and posterior rectus sheath. The sheath of the rectus is strong and criss-crosses in the midline to form the linea alba. Increased abdominal pressure (e.g., during pregnancy) may widen the linea alba, causing a diastasis of the recti. The smaller triangular muscle, the pyramidalis, is superficial to the rectus muscle in the midline lower abdomen. Midway between the umbilicus and the pubis, the posterior rectus sheath ends in a free semicircular margin (a semicircular fold of Douglas). Below the semicircular fold, the transversalis fascia covering the deep surface of the transversalis muscle is very strong.

The main blood supply for the midanterior abdominal wall comes from the superior and inferior epigastric arteries. The superior epigastric artery lies deep in the rectus sheath, and descends to anastomose with the inferior epigastric artery.

The anterior lateral abdominal wall derives its blood supply from the lateral six intercostal and four lumbar arteries and the deep circumflex iliac arteries. These arteries run with the intercostal, iliohypogastric, and ilioinguinal nerves, piercing the lateral rectus sheath and freely anastomosing with the epigastric system. It is helpful for the surgeon to remember the major zones of abdominal blood supply (Fig. 57–1).

The superficial veins of the upper abdomen are the superior epigastric, the intercostals, and the axillary. The lower abdomen drains into the inferior epigastric and superficial circumflex iliac veins. Deep veins run with the deep arteries, and they are so named.

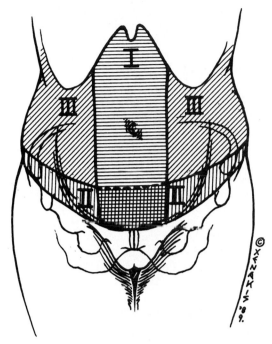

FIG. 57–1. Zones of blood supply to the abdominal wall. Zone I, superior-inferior epigastric system. Zone II, superficial epigastric, superficial external pudendal, and circumflex iliac system. Zone III includes branches from the intercostal and lumbar arteries.

The lymphatics divide into those draining the supraumbilical region, flowing to the thoracic group of axillary nodes, and those draining the inferior umbilical region, flowing to the superficial nodes of the groin.

Nerves to the anterior abdominal skin are derived from the anterior rami of 6th to 12th thoracic nerves and the first lumbar nerve (the iliohypogastric and the ilioinguinal nerves). The lower six thoracic nerves run between the internal oblique and transversus to the lateral border of the rectus, where then they penetrate the subcutaneous tissues. As the rami of the lumbar nerve pass the anterior superior spine, they pierce the internal oblique and run between the internal and external oblique before they become superficial.

The location of the nerves is important because damage to the motor nerves may denervate musculature, producing an abdominal wall bulge or hernia.

THIGHS

In the lateral and medial thighs, there is a definite, deep subcutaneous fat layer that is amenable to suction removal (3). There are no significant structures in the subcutaneous layer except the saphenous vein medially; all other vital structures lie below the deep investing fascia (fascia lata). In the lateral thigh, there is a supratrochanteric gluteal depression which lies between the iliac crest (hip) bulge superiorly and the lateral femoral (saddle bag) bulge inferiorly. In most patients the lateral thigh skin is thick and firmly attached. The medial thigh skin is thinner and more mobile and often hangs loosely. The anterior and posterior thighs have only one layer of subcutaneous fat, making lipoplasty more difficult in these areas (3).

BUTTOCKS

The buttocks are firm and normally convex in the young, with little or no skin hanging over the gluteal crease. The skin is very thick and firmly attached to the underlying subcutaneous fat. The buttock skin frequently has changes of cellulite due to poor tone from damaged elasticity. The thickness of the subcutaneous fat varies in different patients and there is only one layer, unlike the lower abdomen. In older patients, the gluteal muscles lose tone and the retinacular attachments from the skin to the deep fascia stretch. This causes the skin to sag and droop. There are no vital structures in the subcutaneous layer of the buttocks, just smaller cutaneous nerves and vessels.

Treatment Alternatives

The surgeon has three types of procedures for body contouring: lipoplasty, conventional surgery, or a combination of the two. Each of these procedures is indicated for a specific problem. Therefore, the surgeon must identify the problem (or problems) before selecting the correct procedure. Lipoplasty is most successful for patients with definitive accumulations of subcutaneous fat (bulge), reasonably good skin tone, and realistic expectations. When lipoplasty alone can provide the correction it is ideal, because of the small incisions, little morbidity, and quick recovery. For patients with stretched, saggy skin and weak and bulging muscles, conventional surgery is necessary. However, conventional surgery has increased morbidity and scars and a higher incidence of complications. Certain patients require the combination of conventional surgery and lipoplasty; however, in some cases the combination may increase the risk of complications. The liposuction technique has improved over the years, so that surgeons no longer suction only in the deep subcutaneous layer. Gasparotti (4), Toledo (5) and others have emphasized the merit of syringe suctioning in the superficial subcutaneous layer to gain smoother results and obtain increased skin retraction. Gasperoni (6,7) also advocated using much thinner (1.8 to 3 mm) cannulas, along with aggressive suctioning of both the deep and subdermal fat layers, to obtain enough skin retraction to eliminate the need for some dermolipectomies. Whether the actual skin retraction with any form of liposuction is that significant is not yet clear; but it is clear that it will not replace the need for skin excision in patients with significant preoperative skin laxity.

Diagnoses: Evaluating the Problem

ABDOMEN

The surgeon notes the patient's height, weight, and body habitus and examines the patient standing, sitting, and lying down. Morbidly obese patients are usually not candidates for any type of plastic surgery. With the patient standing, the surgeon checks skin elasticity, rebound, and looseness. The pinch test (between thumb and index finger) measures the subcutaneous fat. When there is good skin tone, no overhanging redundant skin, and a pinch test of more than 1 inch, lipoplasty alone may correct the problem. The indications for an abdominoplasty are poor skin tone, excess skin, and weakness of the musculoaponeurotic system. When the standing patient bends forward in a diver's position, the weakened abdominal muscles will bulge, further defining their role in the problem. The patient's voluntary contraction of the abdominal muscles provides further testing of muscle tone and indication of any hernias.

Grasping and pinching together the loose skin with the patient sitting on the side of the examining table identifies the location and extent of skin redundancy. By comparing the results of this examination to those of the same examination in the standing patient, the surgeon determines whether a modified abdominoplasty or a full abdominoplasty is necessary. The full abdominoplasty resection extends from the suprapubic area to above the umbilicus. In these cases, the umbilicus must be relocated to a new opening as the undermined flap moves downward. When there is only a modest redundancy of lower abdominal skin, the smaller elliptical excision of a modified abdominoplasty suffices. In the modified abdominoplasty, the umbilicus is either left untouched or is shifted slightly (1 to 1.5 cm) lower (8). This slight lowering of the umbilicus helps smooth the small supraumbilical folds and epigastric looseness.

The patient then lies on the examining table and raises the head and shoulders to tighten the muscles. This allows the surgeon to again check the musculoaponeurotic system for hernias, weakness, and diastasis of the rectus muscles.

HIPS

Hip rolls are convex, rounded bulges just superior and posterior to the iliac wing. Many patients have a fatty hip bulge that is not harmonious with their lateral profile line. For the proper analysis of this bulge, the surgeon must distinguish the contribution of the subcutaneous fat, loose skin, and wings of the iliac bone. The pinch test determines the amount of subcutaneous fat and the skin elasticity. The pinch test should measure at least 1 inch for lipoplasty to be effective. Lipoplasty alone corrects the hip bulge in most patients. In almost 90% of patients treated for saddlebag bulges, lipoplasty also treats the hip rolls. In abdominoplasty, adjunctive lipoplasty decreases the hip roll fat to minimize the lateral dog-ears. In some patients who have achieved a large weight loss the hip and flank skin is so loose and redundant that a long, horizontal flank excision is necessary. For patients with large, fat hips and loose stretched skin, both lipoplasty and excisional surgery are necessary. In the more severe cases, where a hundred or more pounds have been lost, treatment may require almost circumferential excisions.

THIGHS

Contour abnormalities often exist in the lateral thigh (saddlebag area) and medial or inner thigh, but are infrequently found in the anterior and posterior thighs. The surgeon observes the anterior, posterior, and oblique profile with the patient standing. This careful exam notes the stria, dents, waves, and tightness or looseness of skin. Lipoplasty corrects the discrete saddlebag bulge when the skin tone is acceptable. Lipoplasty alone is also sufficient for other thigh areas if the problem is merely subcutaneous fat and not excessive skin. The pinch test should measure at least 1 inch and ideally there should be good elastic rebound of the skin. In the inner thigh, there is more often some loose, hanging skin complicating a simple lipoplasty correction. Pinching the loose, hanging skin easily measures the amount of redun-

dancy. When skin redundancy is significant, excisional surgery and lipoplasty are combined. If the pinch test measures over an inch anteriorly, posteriorly, laterally, and medially, the thigh problem is circumferential; Therefore, the treatment will need to be circumferential.

BUTTOCKS

The examination notes the overall shape, size, and symmetry of the buttocks and the amount of skin overhanging the gluteal crease. The youthful buttocks have a gentle upward-curving gluteal crease with little or no overhang. The pinch test checks the amount of subcutaneous fat and skin tone. Lipoplasty alone suffices for large buttocks with good skin tone and little or no skin overhang of the gluteal crease. The pinch test should measure a minimum of 1.5 inches on the buttocks for lipoplasty to be successful. For the smaller sagging, loose buttocks, the traditional excision operation (buttock lift) is indicated. For the larger sagging buttocks, a combination of lipoplasty and skin excision is necessary.

Contouring Procedures

Body contouring surgery carries the risk of any major surgical procedure. Therefore it is important first to evaluate the patient's general health. As with all cosmetic procedures, the patient must have an acceptable medical status and realistic expectations. The various procedures for body contouring are discussed here as appliable to patients who are good candidates.

Abdominoplasty

HISTORY

The French surgeons DeMars and Marx (9) first reported the abdominal wall lipectomy in 1890, but it was not until 1899 that Kelly (10) reported this technique in the United States. Since then, many reports have described a variety of techniques (11–24). Much of the literature before 1978 emphasized the shape and location of the skin excision. Since 1978, the emphasis has been on different ways of handling the musculoaponeurotic system, the umbilicus, and adjunctive lipoplasty (8,9,25–32).

TECHNIQUE

Surgical Planning

Preoperatively, the surgeon marks out the anatomic reference points, incisions, and location of the fat and skin removal with the patient standing. These reference points and a line drawn vertically from the xiphoid through the umbilicus to the midpubis helps maintain symmetry and helps locate a new opening for the umbilicus. Marks on the xiphoid, costal margin, and anterior/superior iliac spine are also reference points. Careful palpation is important to locate any hernial protrusions, especially in previous scars. In most cases, there is a correction of the musculoaponeurotic system (rectus sheath) laxity. Plication or imbrication securely tightens the rectus sheath from the pubic area to the umbilicus and often from pubis to xiphoid.

The surgeon plans the incision appropriately for each patient's particular problem, anatomy, and previous scars. For the average patient with excess skin from weight loss or pregnancy, the transverse incision is similar to those described by Regnault, Callia, Grazer, or Pitanguy (9). I favor one similar to Regnault's but slightly higher (Fig. 57–2). When excessive skin looseness requires a large skin resection, the incision extends far laterally to avoid dog-ears. However, if there is a large upper abdominal transverse or oblique scar, extensive undermining from a very low transverse incision may lead to complications. The upper abdominal scar interferes with axial blood supply and may lead to a slough of the lower few centimeters of the flap. There is also an increased risk for lower abdominal flap slough in patients who smoke.

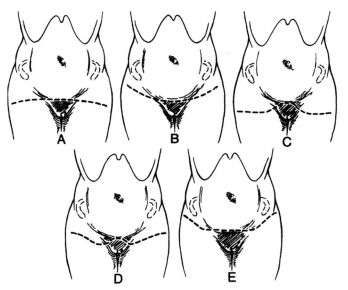

FIG. 57–2. Incisions used for abdominoplasty: **A,** Pitanguy; **B,** Grazer; **C,** Callia; **D,** Regnault; **E,** author's incision, just above pubic hair and angled slightly higher laterally.

For patients with midline scars or a massive weight loss with accompanying excessive skin, the transverse ellipse may be combined with a vertical ellipse, forming a T-incision. The vertical component may be small or large and may extend to the xiphoid, permitting excision of a large amount of skin.

The safest approach for very obese, high-risk patients with a massive panniculus is a simple transverse elliptical excision. This excision around the base of the panniculus avoids undermining of skin flaps (Fig. 57–3). For those patients with extensive girth, Gonzales-Ulloa described the belt lipectomy to permit a more complete resection of the abdomen and flank areas (9,15,33,34).

Surgical Procedure

For all abdominoplasty procedures, the patient is supine with arms abducted on arm boards. A table that flexes in the middle and a pillow under the knees helps position the patient for the closure. Preoperatively applied thromboembolic stockings help prevent phlebitis in high-risk patients. A Foley catheter is helpful for those patients with a history of difficulty voiding.

Performing adjunctive lipoplasty first makes undermining of the skin easier and almost bloodless. A word of caution is warranted, however, about combining major undermining and adjunctive lipoplasty because of an increase in complications (8,31). Even without lipoplasty, the extensive undermining from suprapubic area to the xiphoid and costal margin can decrease circulation to the lower few centimeters of the flap. Adding the trauma of lipoplasty and the tension of the skin closure can cause a slough of the lower few centimeters of the flap. However, adjunctive lipoplasty with a modified abdominoplasty does not increase complications. In these patients there is less undermining; therefore, any area in the abdomen or flanks may be suctioned (8,31) (Fig. 57–4).

FIG. 57–3. Simple wedge resection of large panniculus is a conservative, low-risk procedure for the high-risk patient.

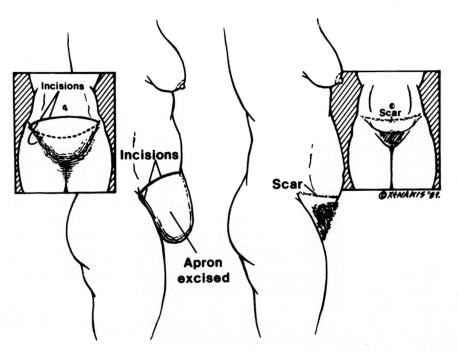

FIG. 57–4. Modified versus major abdominoplasty. **A,** modified abdominoplasty. Undermining extends to just above the umbilicus; smaller elliptical skin flap is resected. Adjunctive lipoplasty is safe and unlimited. Umbilicus is shifted up to 1.5 cm downward by transecting and reinserting its base in the linea alba. **B,** major abdominoplasty. Undermining extends to costal margin and xiphoid. Wide excision is performed to include all skin to umbilicus, which is shifted to new skin opening. Adjunctive lipoplasty is somewhat risky and should be limited because it may increase complications.

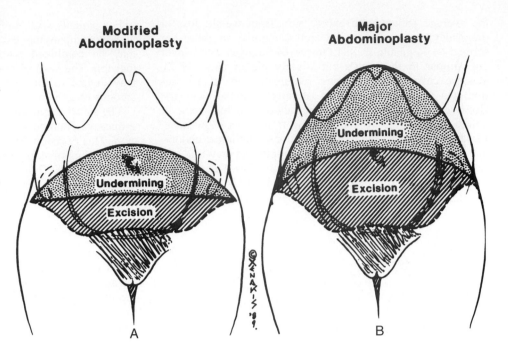

The injection of a large quantity of local anesthetic with epinephrine makes the subcutaneous fat turgid and easy to suction, decreases blood loss, and provides a certain amount of comfort postoperatively. The preinjection of fluids can be done with the tumescent technique, in which a very large quantity of fluid is injected up to 1 to 2 times the amount to be removed (35–39). This fluid is usually made up by adding 1 ampule of epinephrine to 1 liter of saline or Ringer lactate.

In a modified abdominoplasty, the undermining stops at the umbilicus or slightly above (8,31,40). Plication in one or more layers with permanent sutures of the lower abdominal musculature extends from the pubis to the umbilicus or slightly higher. For lowering the umbilicus, the umbilical stalk is transected flush with the linea alba. After tucking in the protruding properitoneal fat, permanent sutures close the opening in the linea alba. One 2-0 absorbable suture reattaches the umbilical stalk 1 to 2 cm inferiorly. After flexing the table, traction pulls the skin flap downward for the elliptical resection. The amount of tissue resected may be more or less than the preoperative markings and depends on the surgeon's intraoperative judgment of the tension.

In a major abdominoplasty, the undermining continues to the xiphoid and costal margin. When the undermining reaches the umbilicus, a diamond-shaped incision outlines the umbilicus, which is freed from the skin flap. Splitting the flap in the midline to the old umbilicus makes the cephalad dissection easier and helps expose the upper abdomen. After completing the undermining, plication of the rectus sheath corrects the diastasis and the bulging muscles. Permanent 2-0 sutures in layers provide a secure plication or imbrication of the aponeurotic system (Fig. 57–5). The advantage of plication is that the rectus sheath and external oblique do not have to be opened and undermined. For imbrication, the anterior sheath and external oblique are elevated and pulled to the midline. Whether imbrication or plication is used, the correction extends from xiphoid to the pubis. In rare cases

with very weak fascia and muscles, the plication or imbrication may be reinforced by oversewing with a nylon mesh. The major contribution of this plication is to flatten the bulging anterior abdomen, but Psillakis believes plication does not narrow the waist (41). To achieve narrowing of the waist, he advocates transposing flaps of the external oblique to the midline (41). An alternative method of narrowing the waist is to plicate the external oblique muscles vertically, horizontally, or obliquely. The plication must not be too tight around the umbilical stalk, to prevent strangulation.

In the major abdominoplasty, the next step is precisely locating the new opening to be cut for the umbilicus. This is done by placing a short, right-angle instrument directly over the retracted umbilicus (Fig. 57–6). With downward traction on the flaps simulating the closure, the protruberance of the vertical end of the retractor indicates the location of the umbilicus. This location should coincide with the preoperative measurements from the costal margin, xiphoid, and anterior iliac spines. Guerrerosantos (42) believes the location of the umbilicus should be 1 cm above a horizontal line drawn between the two iliac crests. The surgeon confirms the accuracy of the new umbilical location before excising the diamond-shaped portion of skin. After fitting the umbilical skin into the new opening, absorbable sutures secure it in a one-layer closure. Baroudi (30) advocates shortening the umbilical stalk by tacking the umbilicus down to the fascia before skin closure. An alternative approach is to catch the deep fascia with the skin-closure sutures as the umbilical skin is sutured in place.

After relocating the umbilicus, multiple absorbable tacking sutures are placed from the subcutaneous tissue to the musculofascial layer to help advance the flap downward, taking tension off the final closure line. These sutures form attachments that change a large "dead space" into smaller compartments, which helps prevent large seromas or hematomas. Two suction drains (one brought out each side) help prevent fluid accumulations under the skin flap. In both the

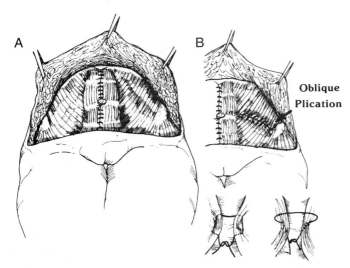

FIG. 57–5. The rectus abdominus fascia and the external oblique fascia are plicated.

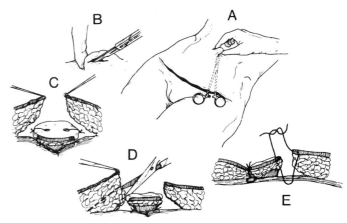

FIG. 57–6. **A,** the location of the umbilicus is established at the level of anterior superior spine. **B,** a horizontal incision at this point delivers the umbilicus. **C, D,** the surrounding flap is defatted and beveled. **E,** the umbilicus and the surrounding flap are sutured to the abdominal fascia for creation of the umbilical dimple.

modified and major abdominoplasties, the technique of skin resection is the same. After completing the tightening of the musculoaponeurotic system and the umbilical work, flexion of the table allows better downward traction on the skin flap. Vertical cuts in the flap help determine the line of resection (Fig. 57–7). The first cut is in the midline and a temporary tacking suture secures the flap. For the lateral flap resection, downward traction slightly toward the midline reduces the lateral dog-ears. The preoperative markings are only a guide as the surgeon adjusts the resection line according to the tension. The resection continues superiorly in the plane between the Camper and Scarpa layers to remove the lower 2.5 to 8 cm of the Scarpa fascia from the underside of the flap. Additional defatting may be done on the underside of the flap around the umbilicus. If liposuction has been done first, then the Scarpa fascia is mostly stringy fibrous remnants with very little fat, which dissects away in almost bloodless fashion. When liposuction has not been done, the Scarpa fascia is thicker and there will be a few more intact small vessels to coagulate.

Final closure consists of multiple tacking sutures from the deep subcutaneous layer to the fascia, a subcuticular layer, and a subcuticular pull-out suture on the skin. After completing the closure, sterile surgical tape strips cover the wound and an elastic wraparound Velcro binder provides moderate pressure to the flap. A recovery bed flexed in the middle like the operating room table helps decrease skin tension. Ice bags may be applied on top of the abdominal binder. As soon as patients have recovered from anesthesia, they are allowed to walk to the bathroom. It may be difficult for patients to stand erect for the first few days and they will tend to bend over when they walk. Assistance is necessary for the early trial periods of walking. If voiding is difficult in the first 8 to 10 hours postoperatively, catheterization is necessary. Those patients with significant blood loss should have a postoperative hemoglobin check. On the first postoperative day, patients take short walks in the room. By the end of the week, walking is easy and the posture is normal. Drains are removed on the 3rd or 4th postoperative day, and sutures be-

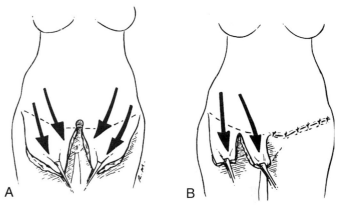

FIG. 57–7. The redundant abdominal apron is resected in stages. Note that traction is medially positioned to minimize the lateral redundancy.

tween 7 and 14 days after surgery. Light activities are acceptable at the end of the week. By the second week, patients may return to almost normal activities (except lifting, pushing, or sports). Compression continues with a binder or a girdle for 4 to 6 weeks. If muscle plication has been extensive, heavy activities and sports are to be avoided until the end of the 6th week.

Alternative Procedures

Less common procedures are the midabdomen abdominoplasty advocated by Stuckey (43) and Baroudi's reverse abdominoplasty (44). The reverse abdominoplasty incision uses the horizontal inferior incision of a reduction mammoplasty to pull the upper abdominal skin upward (Fig. 57–8). The reverse abdominoplasty is ideal for those patients who have excessive redundant skin in the upper abdomen. It is easiest in those patients who need a large reduction mammoplasty that requires a long, continuous horizontal incision. The midabdominoplasty is often the solution for patients with extensive scarring or striae localized to the midabdominal area. The

FIG. 57–8. Reverse abdominoplasty. **A,** lateral view of skin excision to correct loose epigastric skin. **B,** upward traction on undermined epigastric skin to delineate amount of resection. **C,** reduction and reverse abdominoplasty completed.

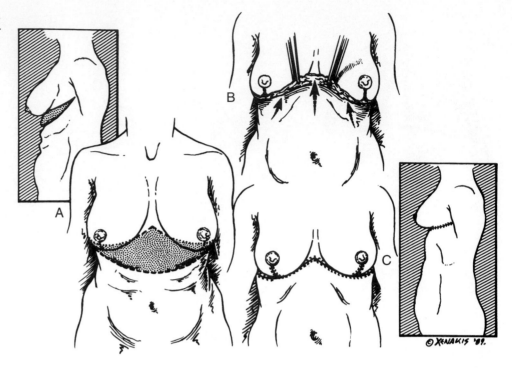

midabdominal ellipse totally removes the stretched, wrinkled, striae-marked skin of the midabdomen, which is otherwise not completely corrected by the standard low transverse incision.

COMPLICATIONS

As with all major surgical procedures, the complications range from minor problems to death. While liposuction of the abdomen has minimal complications, the complication rate for an abdominoplasty is significantly higher. With proper patient selection, careful preoperative preparation and planning, and meticulous surgical technique, the complication rate should be minimal.

Hematomas and seromas are the most common complications. Meticulous hemostasis, drains, and tacking sutures can decrease their occurrence.

Prompt drainage of hematomas may help prevent skin necrosis or infection. The hematoma can be drained by inserting a suction tube through a small stab incision or a slight separation of the incision. After draining a hematoma, it may be necessary to leave a small drain in for 1 to 2 days, and also to continue good compression with a binder or girdle.

Seromas often occur after the first week, and can be persistent. In most cases, aspiration with a needle and syringe is sufficient. It may be necessary to aspirate the seroma five or six times before it resolves. A small collection of serum reabsorbs without treatment over a few weeks. With good sterile technique, there is little chance of infection from aspirations.

Skin sloughs are very rare after modified abdominoplasties but occur more often after major abdominoplasties (8,31). The incidence of skin slough increases in the major abdominoplasty when adjunctive liposuction is also used. The most common area for a skin slough is in the lower midline of the flap. The avascularity of the flap may not be noticeable during the surgical procedure. Any eschar is wiped with alcohol and covered with antibiotic ointment and sterile dressings. The goal is to keep it as an inert scab as long as possible. It is débrided conservatively as the scar separates. This allows the rest of the flap to heal securely. Total débridement of the eschar is necessary when inflammation develops. After débridement, the area is closed secondarily or allowed to heal by secondary epithelialization. An alternative approach for a small slough is early excision as soon as it demarcates and immediate secondary closure.

Fortunately, with expert surgical technique, skin slough is rare. Smokers, older hypertensive patients, diabetics, and those patients with upper abdominal scars are at higher risk for this complication. It is not possible to do anything about the latter three, but in preparation for surgery all smokers should stop using tobacco for at least 10 days before surgery.

A small skin slough at the lower end of the flap will not have a significant effect on the result. Whether by secondary closure or healing by secondary intention, the appearance of the scar will be surprisingly good. Only if there is a major slough will there be a cosmetic problem. These large sloughs require some other type of closure, such as a skin graft. This may significantly compromise the appearance of the abdomen. However, later revision of these major complications can produce very acceptable results.

Dehiscence may result from faulty surgical technique or too much tension on the wound closure. Insufficient deep dermal sutures and inappropriate activities will compromise the repair. The judgment of the surgeon in resecting just enough but not too much of the flap is critical in maintaining proper tension on the closure. A severe coughing spell (often seen in smokers) or straining in the constipated patient are two possible causes of dehiscence. Cough suppressants in smokers and stool softeners for older patients are helpful. By leaning slightly forward the first week, the patient can take tension off the wound. If a dehiscence occurs, a secondary closure with large tension sutures can usually correct the problem.

Administration of prophylactic antibiotics 45 minutes before surgery, irrigation of the wound with an antibiotic solution during surgery, and careful closure and drainage will minimize the infection rate. Patient selection is also important. Open sores or skin eruptions on the abdomen are indications to cancel surgery until a later date. The treatment of an established postoperative infection includes the standard measures of incision and drainage, irrigation, culture and sensitivity, antibiotics, and warm moist compresses.

The major problems with the umbilicus are abnormal shape, abnormal location, scarring, and partial or total necrosis. Recreating the exact-sized, diamond-shaped, neo-opening in the abdominal wall avoids distortion of the umbilicus. A diamond shape has less contraction and a more natural appearance than an oval shape. The position of the umbilicus may be out of the midline to one side or it may be too high or too low. Carefully measuring from known reference points ensures the proper location of the umbilicus. If the umbilicus ends up in an abnormal location, it is possible to move to the normal location but there may be additional scarring.

Umbilical necrosis is extremely rare, but may result from a severely defatted umbilical stalk or one squeezed too tightly by plication of the rectus sheath. When the surgeon plicates around the base of the umbilicus, there should be enough room for the fingertip. An avascular umbilical stalk may become a focus of infection. An established umbilical slough should be débrided and the surrounding skin edges tacked down to fascia to help create a neo-umbilicus. Scarring at the very base of this neo-umbilicus may actually help the result look more natural. The intentional resection of the umbilicus and the reconstruction of a totally new umbilicus (neo-umbilicus) is an excellent option that produces a fine cosmetic result without a preumbilical scar.

Most abdominplasty scars are entirely acceptable and often superb. In cases of marginal necrosis, excessive tension, or simply inherent poor wound healing, however, the scars may end up spread, red, and hypertrophic. Keloid formation is theoretically possible, but is exceptionally rare. In general, keloid formation occurs primarily in blacks, and usually in those patients who have a previous history of keloids.

Excision and revision can correct most hypertrophic or keloidal abdominal scars. On occasion, treatment of recurrent scars may include a short course of superficial radiation therapy after the scar excision. Intralesional cortisone injections are also helpful for the more minor hypertrophic scars. These injections are also especially helpful for small hypertrophic scars that appear around the umbilicus. The excision and revision of small hypertrophic periumbilical scars can be difficult, and there is a significant incidence of recurrence.

Deep thrombophlebitis brings the risk of an embolus breaking off, with severe or even fatal complications. Thrombophlebitis in the calf is more likely in the older patient who does not mobilize early. Thrombophlebitis may actually develop while the patient is on the operating table. The high-risk patient should wear thromboembolic stockings during surgery and for the 1st week postoperatively. However, the prevention of deep-calf thrombosis does rule out an embolus. Pulmonary emboli are most often from the femoral and iliac

veins, and it may not be possible to detect these emboli ahead of time (45). Early mobilization is important to avoid phlebitis and/or pulmonary embolus. Serial compressive pneumatic leg sleeves (sequential or intermittent compression devices) are another way to help promote venous flow. Regimens of preoperative low-dose anticoagulants have no proven degree of success and are not routine for most surgeons (45–47). Both fat emboli and fat emboli syndrome are theoretically possible; however, in the almost 500,000 pure liposuction procedures reported, there have been no proven cases of fat emboli. These complications are extremely rare, even after major abdominoplasties. Prevention of hypovolemia with proper fluid replacement and maintaining an albumin level above 3.5 g/dl are two of the more important measures to prevent fat emboli (48). Intravenous alcohol as a treatment or prevention of fat emboli is contraindicated and dangerous (48).

Virtually all abdominoplasty patients have a significant area of anesthesia or hypesthesia on the lower end of the flap for weeks or months after surgery. In a major abdominoplasty this anesthesia may last up to a year. The surgeon must be careful to avoid the ilioinguinal, iliohypogastric, and lateral femoral cutaneous nerves when placing deep sutures laterally. Hypesthesia and anesthesia may occasionally be long-term, but sensation does return eventually, although not always completely.

Abdominal wall, and even underlying viscus perforation, from liposuction cannulas has occurred in rare cases with disastrous results. The surgeon must be extremely careful when using very small cannulas because they may act like stilletos; this is especially important in patients with previous abdominal surgery. In these patients, the subcutaneous fat may make it difficult to detect a small incisional hernia preoperatively. The surgeon should always be aware of the tip of the cannula and be certain that it is superficial to the deep fascia. If an abdominal wall perforation is suspected during liposuction, the best way to verify this is to directly inspect the fascia for perforation by making a small miniabdominal incision or using endoscopic equipment. When a perforation is suspected postoperatively, the patient must have an immediate general surgical consultation; diagnostic ultrasounds, CAT scans, MRIs, or other tests may be indicated.

Contouring of Hips, Buttocks, and Thighs

Liposuction has markedly decreased the need for conventional body contouring procedures in the hips. However, in those patients with marked skin redundancy and sag, body contouring procedures still play an important role.

HIPS (LOVE HANDLES IN MALES)

Lipoplasty alone corrects most contour problems of the hip area. A skin excision is rarely necessary, except in patients who achieve marked weight loss resulting in extreme skin redundancy. In addition, those patients with a very large abdominal panniculus often need an extension into the hip area to avoid lateral dog-ears. In some cases, the hip excision extends posteriorly onto the back.

In some patients, both lipoplasty and skin incision are necessary to correct hip contour problems (Fig. 57–9). In those cases, the adjunctive lipoplasty should be done before the skin excision. With or without lipoplasty, the hip area is

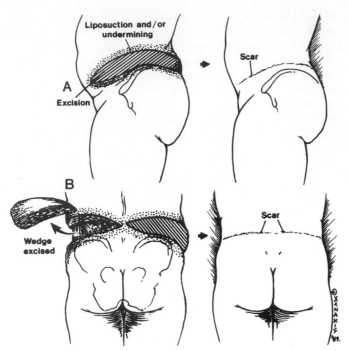

FIG. 57–9. Flank liposuction and excision. **A,** the entire area and periphery is first treated with liposuction and then wedge resection is done in ellipse. **B,** deep sutures close off dead space; scars may actually meet in posterior midline.

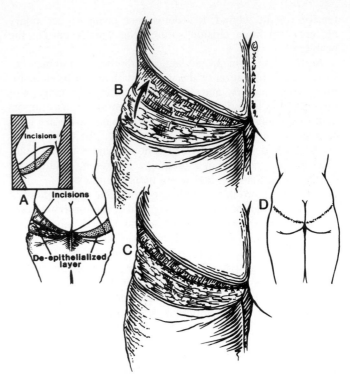

FIG. 57–10. Buttock-thigh plasty. **A,** elliptical incision with dotted area deepithelialized on superior portion of inferior flap. **B, C,** deepithelialized portion is brought upward and tacked to deep fascia under superior flap. **D,** superior flap is pulled downward for closure. Incision shown is for an ellipse through the midbuttock area, used primarily to lift the buttocks. For elevation of the lateral thigh, a lower incision running in the gluteal crease, not laterally on the thigh, is generally used.

treated under general anesthesia. The supine-lateral decubitus position is ideal for these long flank incisions (49). The head and shoulders remain almost supine and the trunk turns at the waist, bringing the hip and flank to excellent exposure. The long transverse elliptical excision may actually meet in the posterior midline with the incision from the opposite hip (8). The surgeon can predetermine the width of the skin excision by pinching and lifting the maximum amount of skin. The measuring and marking of the transverse ellipse is done with the patient standing.

There is little or no undermining of the skin flaps because this is usually more of a wedge resection. During the closure, tacking to the deep fascia obliterates the dead space. Drains are optional because there is little or no room for hematoma. A pressure dressing with a commercial girdle in females or a stretchable abdominal binder in males provides constant compression.

Complications are rare with surgery in the hip area. If the subcuticular closure is inadequate, the scars may indent or even spread. In general, hip contouring is a very safe and forgiving procedure.

THIGHS

Lateral Thigh

Since the introduction of lipoplasty, fewer patients require lateral thigh-lifts. Most of the patients who do require a thigh-life have a history of lipodystrophy and such an extensive bulge that liposuction alone can only partly correct the problem. In these patients, a true redundancy of skin remains in the lateral thigh and a lateral thigh-lift becomes necessary.

The patient stands for the examination and measurements. Lifting and bringing the redundant skin together allows the

surgeon to estimate the excision. In some very fat, bulging thighs it is not possible to predetermine the exact extent of the skin resection until after lipoplasty is done. It is important to be conservative; the resulting closure may spread or actually dehisce if the excision is too wide.

The incision for the lateral thigh-lift usually extends in a semicircular manner from the inferior gluteal crease anteriorly. It continues around the lateral hip superiorly onto the anterior thigh. Medially, the incision extends from the gluteal crease into the perineal crease. The incision will be essentially circumferential if the medial thigh-lift is also being done (50,51). Regnault (52) believes the incision should always be 2 cm above the location of the final scar, because it will drift down with tension. The lateral thigh-lift incision does not always heal as kindly as some of the other body-contouring incisions.

The procedure is done under general or epidural anesthesia in the supine lateral decubitus position. The resection carries through the skin and the subcutaneous tissue down to the investing fascia of the muscle. Undermining is conservative in the lateral thigh-lift, as the skin pulls up easily. Extensive undermining of the distal flap may produce necrosis of the lateral thigh skin. When there is a deep supratrochanteric depression, Regnault and Daniel (52) advocate leaving a deepithelialized island of dermafat in the depression, which is either left flat or plicated double. An alternative approach is to deepithelialize a portion of the inferior flap and tuck it under the undermined superior flap (53) (Fig. 57–10). The deep

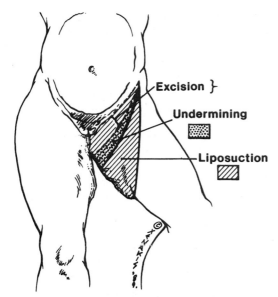

FIG. 57–11. For the patient with fat medial thighs and loose skin, liposuction and resection are combined. The upper ellipse is excised; next, the area below is undermined approximately 2 cm and 40 to 50% of the medial thigh is treated with liposuction.

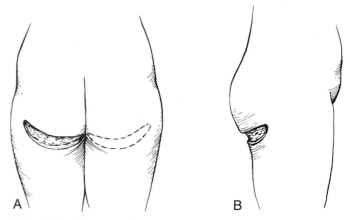

FIG. 57–12. Wedges of buttock tissue can be removed to create a new buttock.

subcutaneous closure with 2-0 absorbable sutures also catches the deep fascia. This deep dermal closure is critical to the strong support necessary for this wound, and is done with interrupted 2-0 absorbable sutures. Suction drains and compression garments are advised.

If lipoplasty is an adjunct, it is done first with a no. 6 cannula (8). Lipoplasty is done both from an incision on the lateral buttocks and an incision in the buttock crease; these two incisions provide cross-tunneling from different directions. In cases of extensive cellulite and/or looseness of the lateral thigh and buttocks, a buttock and lateral thigh-lift can be done with a transverse flank-thigh-buttock incision as outlined by Lockwood. This technique also corrects the supratrochanteric depression, as well as making the buttock more rounded and youthful. Lockwood emphasizes the tight closure of the superficial fascial layer (54–57). Lockwood has also made an important contribution in advocating the use of a circumferential pretunneling maneuver without liposuction all along the thigh to the knee level. This atraumatic undermining with the Lockwood tunneling instrument releases the superficial fascial system from the deep fascia, allowing an easier lift of the skin.

Medial Thigh

The medial thigh is an area that frequently needs a skin excision (traditional thigh-lift) as well as liposuction. This is because the medial thigh skin is not only often redundant and loose but also often accumulates a thick, deep fat layer. This fat causes the two medial areas to bulge and rub together.

An elliptical excision is marked out with the patient standing. The upper incision is placed just above the groin crease, in the perineal crease, and extends posteriorly in the gluteal crease. Guerrerosantos (53) advocates placing the incision above the inguinal crease as it will drift down later. The resection is usually 2 to 4 cm in width and, when the skin is very loose, a vertical V-shaped wedge is added in the midline

to the horizontal ellipse. If lipoplasty is necessary, it is done before the skin incision, using a no. 4 cannula. The entire area is first injected with a dilute xylocaine with epinephrine. Then lipoplasty is done, followed by the skin resection, which includes all the underlying subcutaneous tissue to the investing fascia. Care is taken not to overresect the area. Little or no undermining is necessary (Fig. 57–11).

In closing, the inferior thigh flap advances upward and the deep dermis is sutured to the Colles fascia or other deep investing fascia around the perineum, as advocated by Lockwood (54). This helps support and pull up the skin flap, taking the tension off the skin closure. By suturing the flap to deep fascia (Colles), there is a secure closure without distortion of the vulva (54). A drain is usually unnecessary in this area. The closure is done in two or three layers, and often the final layer on the skin is a subcuticular absorbable suture.

Postoperatively, the patient wears a girdle, which provides firm compression and support. Activities are limited for the first 5 to 7 days. Most of these patients have an excellent result and seem well pleased with the correction.

Buttocks

Liposuction can help the patient with very large, firm, protruding buttocks, but those patients with large, soft, sagging buttocks need a body-contouring procedure. The excision of the redundant loose skin of the buttocks can be done either in the inferior gluteal crease or in the midbuttock area. Either way, the excision lifts the overhanging tissue to a more superior position. Guerrerosantos (53) combines the buttock work into a hip-buttock-thighplasty with almost a circumferential incision (53).

With the patient standing, the buttock skin is grasped in the midgluteal area and pinched to determine the amount of skin resection. Then the same type measurement is done just above the inferior gluteal crease. The surgeon discusses with the patient the two possible approaches. For the crease approach, an elliptical excision with one limb in the inferior gluteal crease and the other horizontally across the lower buttock includes the hanging skin (Fig. 57–12). The alternative approach is to plan an elliptical excision in the midbuttock area. In either location, the incision carries down through the subcutaneous tissue to the underlying gluteal fascia overlying the muscles. Guerrerosantos (53) deepithelializes the distal portion of the inferior flap and undermines the inferior flap enough so it may be pulled upward. The deepithelialized portion slides upward and medially and underneath the superior flap (see Fig. 58–10). It is tacked down to the underlying gluteal fascia for support (53). Guerrerosantos believes this gives more secure healing and eliminates depressions in the gluteal and supratrochanteric area. In some cases, it may be advisable to put some 2-0 absorbable catgut tacking sutures to help plicate the fascia and gluteal muscles to tighten up the buttocks. This deep tightening is easier when the incision is in the midbuttock region.

References

1. Markman B. Anatomy and physiology of adipose tissue. *Clin Plast Surg* 1989; 16:235.
2. Illouz YG. LFDs or "reserve fat." *Body sculpturing by lipoplasty.* New York: Churchill Livingstone, 1989.
3. Illouz YG. The anatomy of subcutaneous fat. *Body sculpturing by lipoplasty.* New York: Churchill Livingstone, 1989.
4. Gasparotti M, Salgarello M. Rationale of subdermal superficial liposuction related to the anatomy of the subcutaneous fat and the superficial fascial system. *Aesth Plast Surg* 1995; 19:13.
5. Toledo LS. Syringe liposculpture: a 2-year experience. *Aesth Plast Surg* 1991; 15:321.
6. Gasperoni C, Salgarello M. Rationale of subdermal superficial liposuction related to the anatomy of the subcutaneous fat and the superficial fascial system. *Aesth Plast Surg* 1995; 19:13.
7. Gasperoni C, and Salgarello M. MALL liposuction: the natural evolution of subdermal superficial liposuction. *Aesth Plast Surg* 1994; 18:253.
8. Mladick RA. Lipoplasty as an adjunctive procedure. In: Jackson IT, ed. *Perspectives in plastic surgery.* St. Louis: Quality Medical Publishing, 1989.
9. Schurter M, Letterman G. Abdominoplasty. In: Gonzalez-Ulloa M, et al, eds. *Aesthetic plastic surgery.* St. Louis: CV Mosby, 1988; 1.
10. Kelly HA. Excision of fat of the abdominal wall-lipectomy. *Surg Gynec Obst* 1910; 10:229.
11. Babcock W. The correction of the obese and relaxed abdominal wall with special reference to the use of buried silver chain. *Am J Obstet* 1916; 74:596.
12. Baker TJ, Gordon HL, Mosienko P. A template (pattern) of abdominal lipectomy. *Aesth Plast Surg* 1977; 2:167.
13. Dufourmentel C, Mouly R. *Chirurigie plastique.* Paris: Flammarion, 1959; 381.
14. Elbaz JS, Flageul G. *Chirurigie plastique de l'abdomen.* Paris: Masson, 1971.
15. Gonzalez-Ulloa M. Circular lipectomy with transposition of the umbilicus and aponeurolytic plastic technique. *Cir Y Cir* 1959; 27:394.
16. Grazer FM. Abdominoplasty. *Plast Reconstr Surg* 1973; 51:617.
17. Pitanguy I. Abdominal lipectomy: an approach to it through an analysis of 300 consecutive cases. *Plast Reconstr Surg* 1967; 40:384.
18. Regnault P. Abdominoplasty by the "W" technique. *Plast Reconstr Surg* 1975; 55:265.
19. Sersons D, Martins LC. Dermolipectomia abdominal: abordage geometrico. *Rev Latino Am Cir Plast* 1972; 16:13.
20. Somalo M. Cruciform ventral dermal lipectomy swallow-shaped incision. *Prensa Méd Argent* 1946; 33:75.
21. Thorek M. Plastic reconstruction of the female breast and abdomen. *Am J Surg* 1939; 43:268.
22. Planas J. The "vest-over-pants" abdominoplasty. *Plast Reconstr Surg* 1978; 61:694.
23. Schwartz AW. A technique for excision of abdominal fat. *Br J Plast Surg* 1974; 27:44.
24. Galtier M. Surgical treatment of the abdominal wall obesity with ptosis. *Mem Acad Chir* 1955; 81:12, 234.
25. Freeman BS, Wiemer DR. Abdominoplasty with special attention to the construction of the umbilicus: technique and complications. *Aesth Plast Surg* 1978; 2:65.
26. Avelar J. Abdominoplasty: systematization of a technique without external umbilical scar. *Aesth Plast Surg* 1978; 2:141.
27. Baroudi R, Keppke EM, Tozzi Neto F. Abdominoplasty. *Plast Reconstr Surg* 1974; 54:161.
28. Baroudi R. Body Sculpturing. *Clin Plast Surg* 1984; 11:419.
29. Psillakis J. Abdominoplasty: some ideas to improve results. *Aesth Plast Surg* 1978; 2:205.
30. Baroudi R. Umbilicaplasty. *Clin Plast Surg* 1975; 2:431.
31. Vogt PA: Abdominal lipoplasty technique. *Clin Plast Surg* 1989; 16:279.
32. Matarraso A. Abdominolipoplasty. *Clin Plast Surg* 1989; 16:289.
33. Gonzalez-Ulloa M. Belt lipectomy. *Br J Plast Surg* 1960; 13:179.
34. Somalo M. Circular dermolipectomy of the trunk. *Semana Med* 1940; 1:1435.
35. Samdal F, Amland PF, Bugge JF. Blood loss during liposuction using the tumescent technique. *Aesth Plast Surg* 1994; 18:157.
36. Samdal F, Amland PF, Bugge JF. Plasma lidocaine levels during suction-assisted lipectomy using large doses of dilute lidocaine with epinephrine. *Plast Reconstr Surg* 1994; 93:1217.
37. Klein JA. The tumescent technique: anesthesia and modified liposuction technique. *Dermatol Clin* 1990; 8:425.
38. Klein JA. Tumescent technique for regional anesthesia permits lidocaine doses of 35 mg/kg for liposuction. *J Dermatol Surg Oncol* 1990; 16:248.
39. Lewis CM, Hepper T. The use of high-dose lidocaine in wetting solutions for lipoplasty. *Ann Plast Surg* 1989; 22:307.
40. Greminger RF. The mini-abdominoplasty. *Plast Reconstr Surg* 1987; 79:356.
41. Psillakis JM. Plastic surgery of the abdomen with improvement in the body contour: physiopathology and treatment of the aponeuroti musculature. *Clin Plast Surg* 1984; 11:465.
42. Guerrerosantos J. Abdominoplasty—some technical details. Gonzalez-Ulloa M, et al, eds. *Aesthetic plastic surgery.* St. Louis: CV Mosby, 1988; 53.
43. Stuckey JG: Midabdomen abdominoplasty. *Plast Reconstr Surg* 1979; 63:333.
44. Baroudi R, Keppke EM, Carvalho CG. Mammary reduction combined with reverse abdominoplasty. *Ann Plast Surg* 1979; 2:368.
45. Hume M. Pulmonary embolism. In: Glenn WWL, et al, eds. *Thoracic and cardiovascular surgery with related pathology.* 3rd ed. New York: Appleton-Century-Crofts, 1975; 552.
46. Francis CW, Marder VJ, Evarts CM, et al. Two-step warfarin. *JAMA* 1983; 249:374.
47. Mitchell JRA. Can we really prevent postoperative pulmonary emboli? *Br Med J* 1979; 1:1523.
48. Moylan J. Current treatment of embolic disease. *Clin Plast Surg* 1989; 16:381.
49. Mladick R. Positioning and incisions. In: Hetter G, ed. *Lipoplasty.* 2nd ed. Boston: Little, Brown, 1991.
50. Baroudi R. Body contour surgery. *Clin Plast Surg* 1989; 16:263.
51. Baroudi R. Torsoplasty. In: Gonzalez-Ulloa M, et al, eds. *Aesthetic plastic surgery.* St. Louis: CV Mosby, 1988; 139.
52. Regnault P, Daniel R. Secondary thigh buttock deformities after classical techniques. *Clin Plast Surg* 1984; 11:405.
53. Guerrerosantos J. Hip-buttock-thighplasty: some technical details. In:Gonzales-Ulloa M, et al, ed. *Aesthetic plastic surgery.* St.Louis: CV Mosby, 1988; 235.
54. Lockwood TE. Fascial anchoring technique in medial thigh lifts. *Plast Reconstr Surg* 1988; 82:299.
55. Lockwood TE. Transverse flank-thigh-buttock lift with superficial suspension. *Plast Reconstr Surg* 1991; 87:1019.
56. Lockwood TE: Lower body lift with superficial fascial system suspension. *Plast Reconstr Surg* 1993; 92:1112.
57. Lockwood TE. Superficial fascial system (SFS) of the trunk and extremities: a new concept. *Plast Reconstr Surg* 1991; 87:1009.

58

Aspirative Lipoplasty

Gregory P. Hetter, M.D., F.A.C.S., and Peter B. Fodor, M.D., F.A.C.S.

Curette Techniques

SCHRUDDE TECHNIQUE

Lipexheresis was the term used by Schrudde (1) to describe his technique of removal: blind undermining with long scissors, followed by the use of a sharp uterine curette. Prolonged drainage, lymphorrhea, hematoma, and skin necrosis prevented this technique from gaining many adherents although, in his hands, the results appeared credible.

FISCHER TECHNIQUE

The first surgeon to apply suction with a sharp mechanically driven curette was Georgio Fischer (2). He used an instrument called a planotome to make a plane in the fat, thus severing the lymph and blood vessels and the retinacula cutis. With suction attached, he then used an electrically driven blade at the tip of the curette to snip off globules of fat. The complications were similar to those of lipexheresis. Fischer's efforts first became known in Europe in 1976. Many problems encountered by other surgeons led to limited acceptance of the machinery (which Fischer manufactured and sold) and the technique.

KESSELRING TECHNIQUE

Ulrich Kesselring (3) devised a large-bore instrument with a sharp, back-cutting blade that was employed after a plane was made with a scissors, much as in the Schrudde technique. Kesselring, however, attached suction to evacuate the fat. He worked deep on the muscle fascia with the blade facing upward to carve fat away toward the surface. Working in the deep fat compartments was an important advance in technique. Kesselring introduced his technique in 1978 and had performed 36 operations with excellent results by 1982. He limited his procedure to young women who had good skin tone and small amounts of excess fat in the lateral thigh. Later Kesselring adopted the basics of the Illouz technique.

TEIMOURIAN TECHNIQUE

Bahman Teimourian (4) used a technique similar to that of Kesselring. He used a scissors for undermining, followed by curetting with a modified fascia lata stripper attached to suction. Later, he used the same types of instruments as Kesselring, as well as others of his own design. Bolder than Kesselring, Teimourian extended his procedure to many areas of the body. He reported a 30% complication rate, which characterized all the curette techniques. Teimourian, however, recog-

nized early the value of separate tunnels. His technique subsequently evolved into a cannula technique.

CANNULA TECHNIQUES

Yves-Gerard Illouz (5) began using a blunt Karman cannula attached to very high vacuum in 1977. He used no undermining, no sharp instruments, and, importantly, spared most of the structures intervening between the muscle fascia and the skin; this was the vital step that had not previously been understood. This maneuver reduced complications and allowed for the dynamic spread of suction lipoplasty, because other surgeons could consistently reproduce his results. Illouz gradually extended this technique to almost every area of the body.

The cannula (Fig. 58–1) is pushed through the deep fat, and the mechanical thrust plus the suction avulses fatty globules. The molecular force of the vaporization of tissue fluids caused by the near-total vacuum forces the fragments up the suction line (Fig. 58–2). A honeycomb pattern results in the fatty tissue, sparing most vessels, nerves, and skin ligaments. When an area is opened for resection of skin after fat extraction, the septa between muscle fascia and skin form sponge-like networks.

Biochemistry and Histology of Fat

Studies, primarily by French (6) and Swedish (7) investigators, have demonstrated that fat cells (adipocytes) possess two chemical receptors for catecholamines: epinephrine and norepinephrine. The beta-1 receptors are lipolytic and secrete lipase, which causes triglycerides (fat) within the adipocyte to split into fatty acids and glycerol. These substances can then pass through the cell membrane into the general circulation, where they are metabolized under normal conditions. It is particularly important to know that fasting or starving, or using tobacco or caffeine, can cause the release of catecholamines that activate beta-1 receptors and thus cause lipolysis.

The alpha-2 receptors conversely block lipolysis, yet they are also stimulated by catecholamines. They are antagonists to the beta-1 receptors. These receptors have been found to be particularly prevalent in areas such as the lateral thigh, lower abdomen, and buttocks, the areas often clinically called diet-resistant. Whereas catecholamines induce lipolysis in areas of metabolically active fat with many beta-1 receptors, such as the upper body, breast, and face, the same hormone blocks lipolysis in areas of so-called reserve fat such as the buttocks, thighs, and lower abdomen where alpha-2 receptors predominate.

FIG. 58–1. Illouz cannula; inset shows lumen.

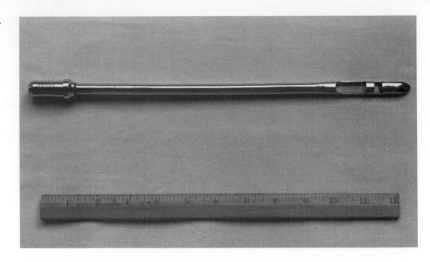

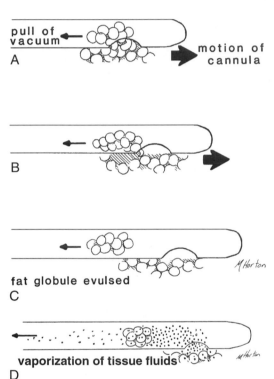

pull of vacuum ←

A

motion of cannula →

B

fat globule evulsed

M Horton

C

vaporization of tissue fluids

M Horton

D

FIG. 58–2. **A,** the vacuum pulls a fat globule into the lumen of the cannula. **B, C,** the movement of the cannula causes evulsion of the fat globule. **D,** the vaporization of the tissue fluids provides the motive force that pushes the fragments toward the collection bottle. (Reproduced with permission from: *Lipoplasty: the theory and practice of blunt suction lipectomy.* Copyright © 1990 by Gregory P. Hetter. Published by Little, Brown, p. 151.)

The *reserve fat,* a term coined by Illouz (8), has been shown to be more receptive to glucose than the more superficial active fat. The reserve fat cells are larger and can hypertrophy faster than those of the active fat. Metabolically the reserve fat areas resist weight loss, particularly during fasting or when catecholamines are stimulated by drugs such as amphetamines or their derivatives, but increase easily in the presence of glucose. This research explains the common clinical syndrome seen in a dieting woman who has lost upper-body fat (face,

shoulders, breasts, and upper abdomen) and in fact appears gaunt, except that her outer thighs appear larger after weeks of fasting. In fact, the number and type of receptors appear to form a genetic basis for these problems; the cause does not appear to be acquired habits or upbringing.

Anatomy

SUBCUTANEOUS ANATOMY

The superficial fascia is an important membrane in some areas of the body, rudimentary in others, and fused with the muscle fascia in most. The fat above the fascia is divided by vertical arches of connective tissue called retinacula cutis. These fibers are anchored to the undersurface of the dermis above and the superficial fascia below (Fig. 58–3). The retinacula cutis are somewhat elastic but have limits to their stretch, hence the dimples (peau d'orange) seen in cellulite during fatty hypertrophy or when large amounts of fluid are injected beneath the skin. The fat fills in the spaces within this complex honeycomb network of fascial extensions. Here beta-1 receptors predominate.

Beneath the superficial fascia lies the deeper laminar fat (reserve fat of Illouz), where the separations are horizontal rather than vertical and alpha-2 receptors predominate. This configuration is macroscopically clear during abdominoplasty when the incisions for the hypogastric dermolipectomy are carried out (Fig. 58–4).

Within the confines between the superficial fascia and the dermis lie the arcades of capillaries, nerves, and lymphatic vessels. Excessive surgical intervention in this layer may lead to destruction of the retinacula cutis, with the probability of surface irregularities and irregular shrinkage, vascular pattern abnormalities, and dysesthesias and hypesthesias. Selective surgical treatment of tethering retinacula cutis can, however, relieve some of the dimples of cellulite. Depending on the area, superficial suction can give further improvement in good hands.

Most of the commonly recognized areas of localized fatty deposits are defined by the superficial fascia's enveloping the deposit and fusing with the muscle fascia at the perimeter of the deposit (Fig. 58–5). This fusion is strong and is readily felt when a blunt cannula is passed along the abdominal wall. Laterally, the cannula meets real resistance at the point of fu-

Cellulite

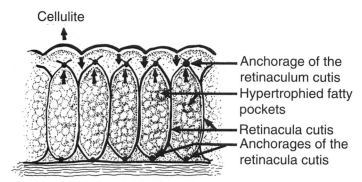

Anchorage of the
retinaculum cutis

Hypertrophied fatty
pockets

Retinacula cutis

Anchorages of the
retinacula cutis

FIG. 58–3. The "cellulite" phenomenon and the Chesterfield sofa. (Reproduced with permission from Illouz YG, de Villers YT: *Body sculpturing by lipoplasty.* English edition. Edinburgh: Churchill, Livingstone, 1988, p. 35.)

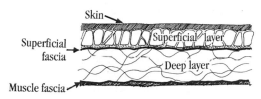

Skin

Superficial layer

Superficial fascia

Deep layer

Muscle fascia

FIG. 58–4. The horizontal architecture of the deep fat compared with the vertical compartmentalization of the superficial fat. (Redrawn after Illouz and reproduced with permission from Hetter G: Blunt suction assisted lipectomy. In: *Mastery of plastic and reconstructive surgery.* Copyright © 1994 by Mimis Cohen. Published by Little, Brown, p. 218.)

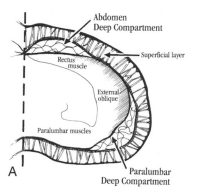

Abdomen
Deep Compartment

Superficial layer

Rectus muscle

External oblique

Paralumbar muscles

A

Paralumbar
Deep Compartment

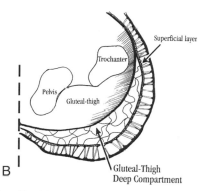

Superficial layer

Trochanter

Pelvis

Gluteal-thigh

B

Gluteal-Thigh
Deep Compartment

FIG. 58–5. Localized fatty deposits in the trunk and thigh showing the layers. Note that, at the perimeter of the localized deposits, the fascia superficialis fuses with the muscle fascia. (Redrawn after Markman.)

sion. When punching through this resistance, the surgeon leaves the subfascial space and enters the subcutaneous space, usually with a divot or dimple as a result.

The most common surgical violation of this fascial fusion is in the lateral thigh, where the superficial fascia fuses with the fascia lata. This is a tough fusion. When the surgeon passes the cannula from the infragluteal crease too far around the curve of the trochanter, a punch through the fascia results in extraction of superficial fat, and surface irregularities result.

SUPERFICIAL FASCIAL SYSTEM

Other areas of well-defined localized deposits encased in their fascial envelopes are the anterior neck, the hypogastrium, the lateral thigh, and the upper posterior arm. Various fascial condensations throughout this system account for the buttock fold (or lack thereof), fatty rolls on the back, and the submammary fold. This whole system is referred to as the superficial fascial system (SFS). Anatomic studies describe both deep and superficial subcutaneous fat compartments. In body regions such as the neck, lower abdomen, and outer thighs, these compartments are separated by a well-defined fascial layer (9). In the epigastrium, hip rolls, and knees, the SFS is less well-defined and is more like a fibrous honeycomb.

Fodor (10) has written that this system of fibrous attachments (SFS) is probably the human derivative of the panniculus carnosium. Many surgeons feel that the vertical fibrous attachments, or retinacula cuti, play an essential role in

postliposuction skin contracture. In conventional blunt suction lipectomy (BSL), suction of the deep fat compartment is the most common.

Superficial suction, or just cannula undermining in the superficial compartment, may help promote postoperative skin contracture. But any errors of technique are highly visible (11).

Fat removal from the superficial layer should be performed as evenly as possible; otherwise grooves and irregularities may result. With considerable experience, the surgeon can skillfully combine both deep and superficial suction. Most suction of the submental region is superficial to the platysma and hence in the superficial layer. Similarly, the epigastric region, breast, calves, and ankles are areas lacking the superficial fascia; hence, the fat is superficial only.

So far there is not a clear consensus on whether all body regions treatable by traditional deep suction do well with superficial suction. It seems that body areas such as the outer thighs, back, and hip rolls, where the dermis is thicker, do better with this technique.

Physics and Equipment

Physics has been forgotten by most surgeons. There are two ways to move the dislodged fat down the cannula or tube. The first is to have an air line to the tip of the cannula or an open wound where air enters the lumen and carries the fat fragments back down the tube towards the vacuum. Such systems work with pressures of one-quarter to one-half atmosphere (190–380 mm Hg at sea level). The other is to produce so nearly an absolute vacuum that tissue fluids "boil."

The molecules from the boiling tissue fluids push the fatty fragments down the cannula towards the vacuum (see Fig. 58–2). At 20° C (68° F) tissue fluids vaporize, or "boil," when the surrounding pressure has been reduced to 17 mm Hg. This is achieved by typical vacuum pumps, but it can also be achieved when a closed syringe plunger is withdrawn and near-vacuum is achieved. This is the basis for syringe-driven suction (SDS). The suction pump is the traditional approach, but good results can be achieved with either method.

Fournier (12) recommended the use of a syringe to replace the aspiration pumps. Many came to believe that this was essential for their superficial technique.

The advantages of the syringe technique are: the elimination of aerosols and noise, a closed "anaerobic" system, the ease of washing and storing harvested fat, and the ease of transporting the equipment to another facility. However, the syringe technique may be more time-consuming and untidy. We favor syringes for the initial infiltration with wetting solutions, small fat removals, touchup procedures, and harvesting fat for the purpose of autologous fat transfer; we favor the pump for removals of size. The skill of the surgeon is far more important than the type of suction source employed.

CANNULAS

The cannula should be blunt, with the lumen sufficiently far back to avoid removal of subdermal fat. The shortest cannula that can be used to reach the area to be defatted allows for the best control by the surgeon. The finer the tunnels, the less the subsequent waves or irregularities. In general, 4- to 6-mm

cannulas are used for major body work. For facial and neck areas, 1.5-, 2.4-, and 3.8-mm single-hole Illouz cannulas are common. Multihole cannulas can extract fat quickly and therefore require close attention while in use.

Cobra cannulas, which have their lumens at the tip, are useful in fibrous areas such as the epigastrium and the calves. Where the operative plane is fairly level, the risk of subdermal removal is less. Three- to five-millimeter cobra cannulas are common. The finish around the lumens should be smooth and burr-free and should have edges that feel dull to the finger.

Focused-energy cannulas have excited interest. Two types have been tried. A laser-tipped unit underwent a multicenter study (13); the result was not to seek F.D.A. approval. Ultrasound focused-energy cannulas have many advocates in Europe (14) and South America. They also have strong detractors because of damage to both fat and skin. They are not F.D.A.-approved in the United States at this time, and are currently under investigation.

BIOHAZARDS

Biohazards have not yet been proven to be associated with the use of suction pumps (15). Vaporization of tissue fluids raises the possibility that bacterial and viral particles may be exhausted into the operating room. It is recommended that a special filter be placed between the collection jar and the pump to reduce this risk. These filters can stop particles larger than 0.3 microns, have a large surface area to allow good air flow, and are reasonably priced. *It is recommended that such filters be used with all machines at all times.* Ideally, the exhaust should be vented to the outside air after the filter is passed. Plastic collection jars and disposable tubing avoid the risks associated with cleaning blood-contaminated jars and tubing.

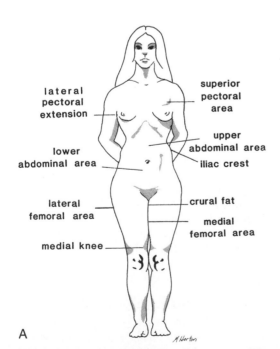

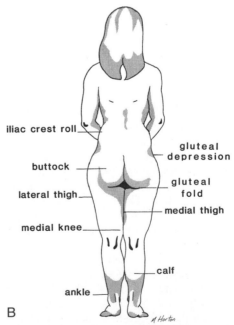

FIG. 58–6. A, female, anterior view. **B,** female, posterior view. (Reproduced with permission from: *Lipoplasty: the theory and practice of blunt suction lipectomy.* Copyright © 1990 by Gregory P. Hetter. Published by Little, Brown, p. 67.)

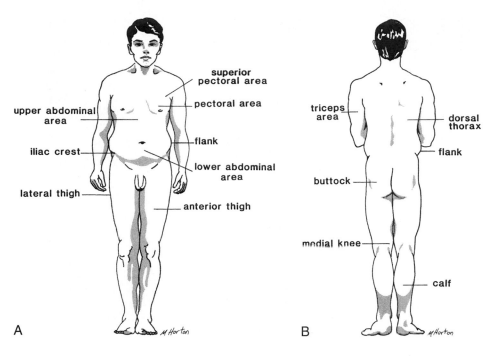

FIG. 58–7. A, male, anterior view. Underlined areas are typical male problem areas. **B,** male, posterior view. (Reproduced with permission from: *Lipoplasty: the theory and practice of blunt suction lipectomy.* Copyright © 1990 by Gregory P. Hetter. Published by Little, Brown, p. 68.)

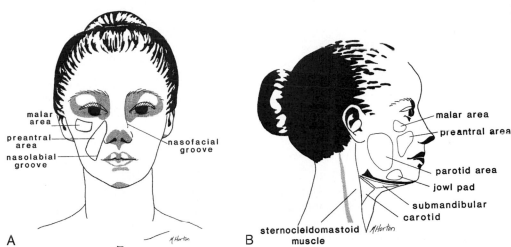

FIG. 58–8. A, anterior view of head and neck. **B,** lateral view of head and neck. (Reproduced with permission from: *Lipoplasty: the theory and practice of blunt suction lipectomy.* Copyright © 1990 by Gregory P. Hetter. Published by Little, Brown, p. 72.)

Evaluation

NOMENCLATURE

Figures 58–6 and 58–7 show the correct names of the areas in which aspirative lipoplasty is performed on the torso and limbs. The nomenclature of the face and neck is depicted in Figure 58–8.

PATIENT EVALUATION

Patient evaluation is the most important step for the surgeon. Wrong choices lead to unsatisfactory results, repeat surgical interventions, accusatory patients, and lawsuits. The patient should be evaluated for body-image disturbances, including bulimia and anorexia nervosa. Patients who exhibit low self-esteem, marked anxiety, fear, paranoia, or unrealis-

tic expectations are not good candidates for aesthetic surgery (16).

The medical evaluation should rule out a history of thromboembolic disease, bleeding disorders, chronic lung disease, brittle cardiovascular system, and acute or chronic systemic diseases. The evaluation should include nutritional practices. Many people follow bizarre diets and are chronically malnourished with low iron stores, low albumin levels, low potassium levels, or all three. Others use steroids or diuretics to influence some aspect of their physiology. Taking vitamins in megadosages is common (recall that vitamin E can influence clotting, for example).

Because the usual technique of blunt-suction lipectomy involves suction pumps that exhaust aerosolized tissue fluids into the operating room, it would be imprudent to operate on

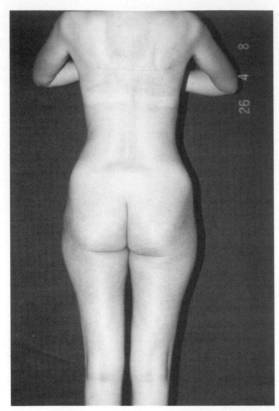

FIG. 58–9. Patient with good skin turgor and highly localized deep fatty excess of lateral thighs (and small crural excess). Note thin limbs. (Reproduced with permission from Hetter G: Blunt suction assisted lipectomy. In: *Mastery of plastic and reconstructive surgery.* Copyright © 1994 by Mimis Cohen. Published by Little, Brown, p. 228.)

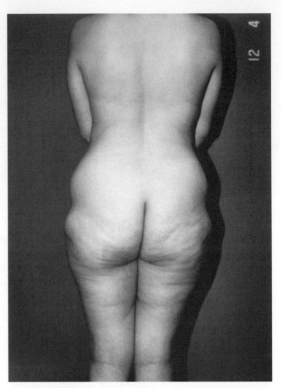

FIG. 58–10. Patient with obvious excesses of iliac crest roll and lateral and medial thighs. Note asymmetry and fat on triceps area of upper arm, indicating modest overweight but reasonable skin tone. (Reproduced with permission from Hetter G: Blunt suction assisted lipectomy. In: *Mastery of plastic and reconstructive surgery.* Copyright © 1994 by Mimis Cohen. Published by Little, Brown, p. 228.)

patients with live virus in their blood and tissue fluids. The testing and exclusion of patients who are positive for hepatitis B surface antigen or core antigen, Hepatitis C antibody, or HIV-III antibody, is necessary.

A sedimentation rate is recommended to detect cryptic infectious processes and connective-tissue diseases. A complete blood count and liver enzyme, sugar, and potassium level are useful to help rule out common problems.

A thorough history is essential. Special importance should be placed on the pulmonary history to rule out restrictive lung disease. The history of bleeding disorders should be elicited. A history of thromboembolic disease, together with smoking, overweight, and use of oral contraceptives, places the patient at high risk for pulmonary embolus following blunt-suction lipectomy.

PHYSICAL EVALUATION

A complete physical examination, including deep tendon reflexes, is useful; An abnormal tendon reflex may be a signal of a spinal disk problem, which could be aggravated when the patient is turned on the operating table. The patient with poor neck posture should be noted and the neck placed similarly on the operating table to prevent cervical root injury. On the basis of the history and physical and laboratory examinations, the surgeon may wish to refer the patient for specialty evaluation.

AESTHETIC EVALUATION

The ideal candidate for body surface lipolysis (BSL) is a young and relatively thin adult, with a highly localized fatty excess and taut skin (Fig. 58–9). The average candidate is 30 to 45 years of age, weighs 10 to 20 pounds over ideal, may have striae from pregnancy or weight fluctuations, and has some degree of skin relaxation (Fig. 58–10). The skin must be evaluated in addition to the fat excess. Usually, BSL will suffice; however, the patient should be informed that subsequent suctionings and an ultimate dermolipectomy may be necessary. Patients in this age group are more difficult to satisfy than younger patients. The less-than-ideal candidate is older than 45 years of age, is more than 20 pounds overweight, or has a history of fluctuating weight with clearly loose skin. Scars, striae, waves, cascading, the beginning of an abdominal apron, buttock ptosis, or a combination of these features is present on examination. Younger patients in this group tend to be critical of their postoperative results, whereas those older than 55 years are more readily satisfied.

Dermolipectomies, combined with BSL, may be needed. The patient should be aware that the extent of the initial suctioning may be limited by loose skin. Secondary suctioning after interim skin contraction may be required, as well as eventual dermolipectomy. The limiting factor of the procedure is the condition of the skin.

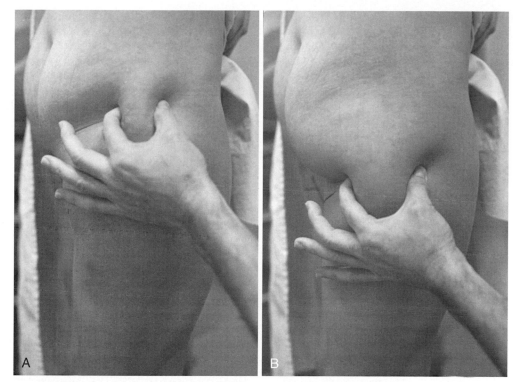

FIG. 58–11. **A,** pinch test above the saddlebag area shows the diet-responsive superficial fatty layer to be about 3 cm. **B,** pinch test at the saddlebag area shows the fat to be 7 to 8 cm. Subtracting the 3 cm of superficial fat leaves the 4- to 5-cm deep layer, or reserve fat of Illouz. This amount would be removed by the procedure. (Reproduced with permission from: *Lipoplasty: the theory and practice of blunt suction lipectomy.* Copyright © 1990 by Gregory P. Hetter. Published by Little, Brown, p. 174.)

It is wise to show the patient by the pinch test where the area of fatty excess is localized and how it differs from surrounding areas. This demonstration is easily understood by patients (Fig. 58–11). The fat of the thigh is palpated above, below, and anterior to the saddlebag and the area of localized excess is determined. If the area of the apparent excess is clearly composed of fat (rather than the trochanter), the area is treatable. Often in men with large "beer bellies," pinching the hypogastrium reveals the same amount of fat there as laterally; there is, in fact, no substantial localized deep fat, and the bulge is from intraabdominal fat that causes the abdominal wall to bulge forward. Suction, of course, leads to disappointing results in such patients. This determination of localized fatty excess demonstrates to the patient two important concepts: (a) not all fat is to be removed, and (b) what remains is more important than what is removed.

The surgeon must be able to pinch at least 1 inch of fat to consider removal on the torso. The pinch test doubles the thickness of the underlying skin-fat complex. Generally, excess lateral thighs measure 3 to 5 inches, abdomens 2 to 6 inches, iliac crests 1 to 4 inches, and knees 1 to 2 inches.

Visual inspection is not enough for an aesthetic evaluation. Evaluation of the skin turgor, elasticity, and strength is also important. Striae are a sign of poor skin elasticity. When pinched skin does not instantly return to the normal position, an operation is contraindicated; there is no potential for retraction. Pointing out areas of waves, dimpling (cellulite), and looseness is vitally important. The posterior photographic view needs to be shown to patients as an important part of their aesthetic education, demonstrating what can and, just as important, what cannot be done about their concerns.

Anesthesia

General anesthesia is the most convenient for large removals. Epidural anesthesia is often used, but it requires somewhat more recovery time. Neuroleptic anesthesia with a clysis of local anesthesia is used by some practitioners.

Anesthesiologists are generally unaware of the degree of the subcutaneous vascular injury produced by BSL and the degree of ongoing serum loss over the following 18 to 24 hours. Experience has shown that removals of less than 1500 ml of fat in healthy young adults rarely are associated with problems. As the volume of fat removed increases above 1500 ml, and as the size of the body surface area damaged increases above 15%, however, the frequency of complications rises, especially in older patients.

PRECAUTIONS

Experience between 1982 and 1989 (17) has shown that whenever the area of injury exceeds 15% of body surface area, the hemodynamic morbidity rises out of proportion to the additional percentage removed. In such situations, autologous blood transfusion increases safety.

A low serum albumin level predisposes to a number of chemical disturbances after any severe injury. A low albumin level may be insufficient to bind the free fatty acids released during lipectomy. This situation in turn sets in motion a neutrophil-mediated injury to the lung tissue, resulting in the condition known as "fat embolus syndrome" (18). The characteristics are pulmonary edema, low PO_2, and failure of gas transfer at the alveolar level. Low tissue perfusion caused by hypovolemia may exacerbate this syndrome, with a lethal outcome. Any patient who has an insufficient quantity of, or an inappropriate type of, intravascular resuscitation after the trauma of extensive suction lipectomy may be at risk.

Almost all lethal complications of suction lipectomy stem from failure to maintain a normal intravascular volume, with resultant poor tissue perfusion. In reviewing lethal outcomes in which the end stage was massive infection, acute respiratory distress syndrome, pulmonary embolus, or myocardial infarction, the authors found that the primary physiologic deficit not initially corrected was hypovolemia.

Fluid resuscitation of the patient undergoing large amounts of fat extraction is extremely important and requires planning. The size of the area of damage, the volume of resection, pretreatment with or without adrenalin, the amount of subcutaneous wetting solution (clysis), and the preoperative hematocrit and albumin are factors.

There is considerable difference in the requirement for intravenous fluid resuscitation, depending on the amounts of wetting solutions injected. Where no wetting solutions are used, large amounts of intravenous fluids, including autologous blood, are necessary with a large removal (Table 58–1).

Utilizing the "superwet" technique, which involves injecting at least an amount of wetting solution equal to the anticipated removal, the amounts of intraoperative and immediate postoperative fluids has been reduced, as has been the need for autologous blood.

No good recommendations for fluid resuscitation can be given for the "tumescent," technique since there is such a huge crystalloid load given by clysis. The need for intravascular fluids may well show up much later, when the patient is no longer monitored. Fluid need is unpredictable and must be based on laboratory findings and vital signs. Patients should be followed closely.

Table 58–1.
Fluid Resuscitation Regimen

Size of Removal	Amount and Type of Perioperative Fluid Replacement
1. <500 ml	2 L crystalloid
2. 500–1000 ml	3 L crystalloid
3. 1000–1500 ml <15% body surface area (if >15%, treat as in 4)	3 L crystalloid plus 1 unit of Hespan prior to ambulatory discharge
4. 1500–2000 ml <15% body surface area (if >15%, treat as in 5)	3 L crystalloid plus 1 unit of autologous blood
5. 2000–2500 ml <15% body surface area (if >15%, treat as in 6)	3 L crystalloid plus 2 units of autologous blood and possible overnight monitoring
6. 2500–3000 ml >15% body surface area	4 L crystalloid and 3 or more units of autologous blood and probable overnight monitoring in a hospital setting

In all cases, there is a reduction of circulating blood volume over the 12 to 36 hours after the operation, as serum and blood leaks into the wounded areas. Therefore, orthostatic tests of standing and lying blood pressure and pulse are often more revealing than hematocrit changes. Patients may require intravascular volume expansion to prevent oliguria, tissue hypoxia, hemoconcentration, and embolic phenomena.

Planned autologous whole-blood transfusions of 1 or 2 units are very useful in large removals and allow a safer and more rapid recuperation.

Patients lose heat because of the large area of the body exposed and because of the vaporization of tissue fluids. To minimize this loss, the body should be covered as much as possible, an endotracheal humidity trap should be used, and intravenous fluids should be warmed. The patient's head may be covered with plastic to retain heat. The operating room can be maintained warmer than usual.

In the recovery period, oxygen should be administered; oxygen consumption may be enormous as the body restores natural temperature by the muscle activity seen clinically as shivering.

Procedures

DETERMINING OPERATIVE TECHNIQUES

The patient should agree to the area to be treated and the incision sites on the day of the operation, so that no misunderstanding can later be claimed. Patients occasionally add or delete an area during this marking. A polaroid photograph of the markings can be taken to document any change that contradicts earlier office notes. The markings are done with a broad, felt-tipped indelible marking pen just before going to the operating room.

Before marking is done, the patient's fatty deposits should be evaluated by both sight and touch with the patient standing. Turning the patient slowly, in side lighting and in light from above, reveals areas of irregularity, high spots, waviness, and depressions. These areas should be marked and pointed out to the patient. Some surgeons use many colors for emphasis.

The areas of claimed fatty excess are also judged by the "pinch test." The areas of excess beyond normal superficial body fat are noted in centimeters. A topographic map of the deformity is marked out. The surgeon decides where maximal extraction should be performed (where plus signs are placed), where crisscrossing should be carried out, and where simple undermining without suction should be done (mesh undermining). Figure 58–12 shows a patient marked to illustrate these concepts.

Depressions and valleys should be noted with minus signs and should be avoided to prevent worsening such areas. When the patient is on the operating table, such an area may no longer appear as a depression because of shifting of the fat. The tactile pinch test probably provides the most information about the thickness and quality of the fat to the surgeon both before and during the procedure. This test should be performed during marking immediately preoperatively. The normal superficial fat (by pinch) varies between 1.5 and 3.0 cm in nonobese people.

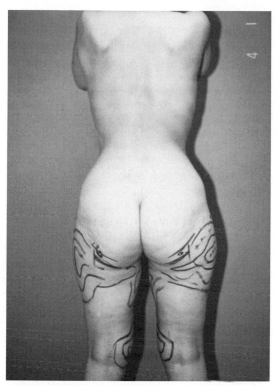

FIG. 58–12. Topographic markings show the contour. *Plus* marks show their greatest excess. *Minus* marks show dimples. Heavy marks show area to extend the gluteal fold. (Reproduced with permission from: *Lipoplasty: the theory and practice of blunt suction lipectomy.* Copyright © 1990 by Gregory P. Hetter. Published by Little, Brown, p. 106.)

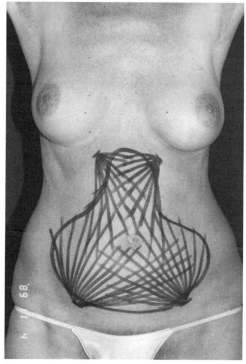

FIG. 58–13. Drawing on a patient illustrating the approach to the epigastrium though two rib margin incisions and to the hypogastrium through two high inguinal incisions, allowing complete crisscrossing of both areas. (Reproduced with permission from: *Lipoplasty: the theory and practice of blunt suction lipectomy.* Copyright © 1990 by Gregory P. Hetter. Published by Little, Brown, p. 158.)

Before the marking is completed, an appraisal of the surrounding subcutaneous thickness should be made by pinching these tissues (see Fig. 58–11). If 2 to 3 cm can be pinched above and below a saddlebag, and the localized fatty deposit is 6 to 7 cm, the goal of the extraction process should be to reduce this excess to the level of the surrounding 2- to 3-cm thickness and not more.

Treatment is carried out in the prone position for thoracodorsal rolls, iliac crest rolls, sacral bulge, buttock, lateral thigh, subgluteal areas, posterior medial thigh, medial knee, and calf, with the chest supported by chest rolls and the arms in a "hands up" position. Great attention must be paid to the placement of the patient on chest rolls: use of a soft mattress, protection of bony prominences, care in turning, and the prevention of brachial plexus injuries. The neck must be placed in the normal postural position to avoid potential pinching of the cervical roots. For the breast, abdomen, flank, anterior thigh, anterior medial thigh, and suprapatellar area, the patient is placed in the supine position.

The lateral decubitus position (19) allows a patient to be turned from side to side and many but not all posterior areas can be adequately reached. This saves time and personnel by avoiding the turning of an anesthetized patient. The supine frog-leg position is useful for medial thighs, knees, and medial calves. Incisions to reach these areas should be as close as possible to the fatty excess. To provide the best control, the surgeon uses as short a cannula as possible to reach the

area involved. To reach the epigastrium, two incisions beneath the breasts is ideal (Fig. 58–13). For dorsal rolls, paraspinal incisions are used. Figure 58–14 shows approaches to the back and posterior extensions of the iliac crest fat, which can only be treated successfully with the patient in the prone position.

The "tumescent" technique, as popularized by the dermatologist Klein in 1988 (20), is the very gradual (up to 3 hours) instillation of wetting solution until the limb is white, there is tissue turgor, and a peau d'orange appearance of the skin. Advocates of this technique have told me they inject under pressure between 3 and 6 ml of wetting solution per ml of estimated aspirate to obtain tissue turgor. Thus, many liters of fluid might be injected, which amounts to a highly variable clysis.

The pressure of the infiltrate is such that it exceeds the capillary pressure and almost no blood is seen during the removal. The subsequent tissue-damage cycle is probably unaltered. The removed aspirate has much more of the instilled wetting solutions in it than with other methods. The volumes removed, as reported by advocates of the technique, are often much larger than with other methods and cannot be compared with volumes removed when smaller amounts of wetting solutions are instilled. A statistically valid "lipocrit" study is needed to compare the true amount of fat removed as a percentage of total aspirate, for these techniques are now in vogue.

We recommend the "superwet" technique. Approximately 1 to 1.5 ml of wetting solution for each ml of anticipated as-

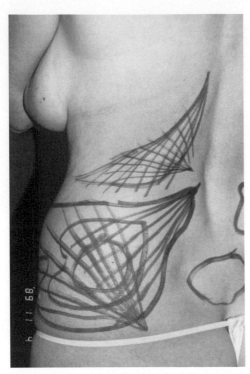

FIG. 58–14. Paraspinal incisions are used to reach the most medial extension of the iliac crest folds and the dorsal rolls. Crisscross lipoplasty may be used through two paraspinal incisions as shown for a dorsal roll. The iliac crest roll is treated through a more lateral upper buttock port and a paraspinal port. (Reproduced with permission from: *Lipoplasty: the theory and practice of blunt suction lipectomy.* Copyright © 1990 by Gregory P. Hetter. Published by Little, Brown, p. 159.)

pirate is injected sequentially throughout the intended areas of removal during the surgery. Injection is performed with fine, multiholed, long blunt cannulas along the deep, intermediate, and superficial plane. We use Ringer lactate or saline containing epinephrine 1:800,000, with or without xylocaine $\frac{1}{8}$%. Some surgeons believe the lidocaine reduces postoperative pain caused by spinal cord memory. Some surgeons instill anesthetic solutions and/or antibiotic solutions as a "wash out" or irrigation at the end of the procedure.

Generally, we believe the "super-wet technique" has the benefits claimed for the "tumescent technique" of low blood loss, lesser need for immediate colloid and crystalloid replacement—without the disadvantages of lengthy anesthesia time, the hazard of delayed fluid uptake by large clysis, the need for drainage sites, the risk of pulmonary edema (21), and the potential for xylocaine toxicity. The maximum xylocaine dose in the PDR today is still 7 mg/kg. Some proponents of the tumescent technique use up to 70 milligrams of xylocaine per kilogram. This danger is amplified by the fact that xylocaine absorption from the subcutaneous fat can peak as late as 16 hours after the injections (as shown by Klein), at which time the patient usually has been discharged from the surgical facility.

Finally, it must be stressed that the amount of wetting solutions (crystalloid) delivered alters the amounts of intravenous fluids required over time. Each surgeon must therefore develop a physiologically correct program to maintain as normal an intravascular volume as possible throughout the procedure and the first few days of postoperative fluid requirements. This requires monitoring of the patient's reclining and standing blood pressure, pulse, and HCT or Hb in the postoperative period. Monitoring of oxygen saturation with oximetry is useful for the early recognition of fat embolism syndrome or pulmonary edema from other causes. Most catastrophic outcomes could have been prevented by proper serial monitoring of the patient's vital signs, including orthostatic hypotension, hematocrit, and oxygen saturation. There is bleeding in the tissues, both acute and delayed, which is not measured by performing a "lipocrit" on the aspirate. Typically, the patient's hemoglobin will fall substantially (1 to 3 grams/L) at 5 days (22). Therefore, a yellow aspirate *does not* mean that the operated area will not eventually lose blood and/or serum into a fourth space.

Pretunneling is simply passing a cannula that is not connected to suction through the incision to the proper plane. The feel of running through superficial fat where there are many retinacula cutis is "gritty," whereas the deep reserve fat produces an easier, smoother passage. Too pointed a cannula does not give this important information. When suction is applied, the cannula has more resistance to movement, which detracts from this tactile information.

By passing the cannula into the proper plane and developing the plane with regular radiating thrusts, a kind of pseudoplane is developed at or just below the superficial fascia (Figs. 58–15, 58–16). When no suction is attached, a puncture into the superficial fat causes no lasting defect, as would happen if suction were attached (Fig. 58–17). Pretunneling is useful in defining the depth, extent, and character (or "feel") of the fat.

For most body areas, start at the side of the bulge and work toward the other in a regular, even manner. Using a single-hole 4-, 5-, or 6-mm Illouz blunt cannula, turn the hole away from the muscle fascia by about 30% in the proceeding direction. Stop after making about 10 passes, or when you can feel that little more fat is forthcoming or the fat becomes bloody. At that point go on to the next tunnel and so on, over the whole area. Where plus signs indicate more fat to remove, make a few more passes. The length of the pass is determined by the topographic map. The edge of the deposit is feathered by thrusts of different length or by using a smaller cannula at the periphery.

When removing the cannula, break suction to avoid overextracting around the entry site. The pinch and roll test is performed regularly throughout the procedure to monitor progress. It should be remembered that what is pinched is two thicknesses of fat.

When about 65 to 70% of the extraction is complete, use a second incision to cross-tunnel at right angles to the first tunnels. The remaining 30 to 35% of the procedure is completed using both directions. The pinch and roll test is performed often to avoid the unpleasant surprise of an overextracted area. Small lumps or islands of fat can be grasped with the control hand and speared with a smaller cannula. In this manner any remaining irregularities are extracted.

What is *not* done is as important as what is done. No side-to-side windshield wiper motion is performed; this motion could injure the SFS and the vessels and nerves. The cannula lumen is not turned toward the surface. Persistently over-

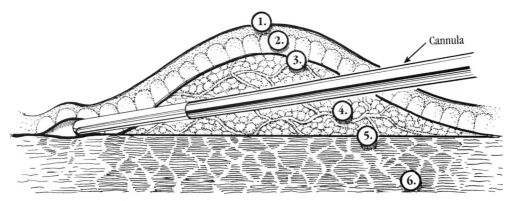

FIG. 58–15. The cannula has punctured the fusion of the superficialis fascia and muscle fascia and has entered the superficial fat. No dimple or divot results from this maneuver if no suction is present. **1.** Skin. **2.** Superficial fat. **3.** Superficial fascia. **4.** Deep fat. **5.** Muscle fascia. **6.** Muscle. (Reproduced with permission from: *Lipoplasty: the theory and practice of blunt suction lipectomy.* Copyright © 1990 by Gregory P. Hetter. Published by Little, Brown, p. 160.)

working a bloody area is not done. Excessive cross tunneling may lead to a cavity and then a pseudobursa. Overthinning beyond the normal thickness of surrounding superficial fat is not recommended.

MESH UNDERMINING

When extraction is complete, the edges of the extracted area are loosened, simply by passing a very blunt Illouz cannula into the surrounding area without suction. This maneuver tends to break up the edge and allow some recontouring of the adjacent tissue. The theory behind such a maneuver is that there are three phases to the improvement seen from BSL: (a) immediate fat cell extraction, (b) subsequent fat cell death, and (c) fibrosis and retraction (23). Mesh undermining is believed to cause some additional fat cell death at the periphery, which allows a more even transition.

The hardest thing to know in all endeavors is when to stop. Several factors influence the decision. When mostly blood and little or no fat appears in the tube, it is time to move on to the next tunnel. Some patients have very fibrous fat and bleed a great deal, so that little fat can be obtained. When the skin becomes wavy, especially in the lateral thighs or abdomen, it is reasonable to stop. Some superficial suction with small cannula may increase skin retraction, but be very careful. A secondary suction may be done 6 months later, after skin retraction has occurred. To go far beyond the ability of the skin to retract risks uneven contraction or ptosing of the skin because of a lax SFS. It is important to compare the extracted area to the surrounding normal areas and the evenness within the extracted area. The areas should be uniform as you pinch and roll. Observe the areas from side to side and from directly above the operating-table level to judge the "skyline" view on both sides for symmetry and contour. Small refinements can be made with a 3- or 4-mm cannula. Fat may be injected by the syringe technique to fill in areas marked with minus signs or overresected. The feel of the passage of the cannula changes as the procedure progresses. The feeling is difficult to describe, but it is grittier, because the passage is through fibrous shrouds drawing into the lumen of the cannula rather than through fatty substance. Overresections are often done because patients have emphasized that they desire a flat stomach or

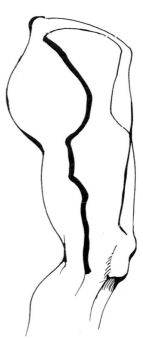

FIG. 58–16. Fusion of the fascia superficialis to the fascia lata. In front of this line, only superficial fat is found in the upper thigh. Violating this fusion results in superficial extraction, with resultant dents anterior to this line. (Reproduced with permission from Hetter G: Blunt suction assisted lipectomy. In: *Mastery of plastic and reconstructive surgery.* Copyright © 1994 by Mimis Cohen. Published by Little, Brown, p. 219.)

straight thighs. The natural curves of the body should be known and respected. If less fat is left over the trochanter than over the surrounding areas, a female patient will appear masculine in the posterior view. The surgeon can always remove more fat later, if necessary. In the areas where irrigation can be undertaken easily (iliac crest, calves and ankles, face and neck), it has proved useful. When blood and fatty fragments are removed, both swelling and bruising are reduced and hemosiderin pigmentation is less likely. Saline solution or saline containing antibiotics is instilled through a syringe, and a folded towel is rolled along the op-

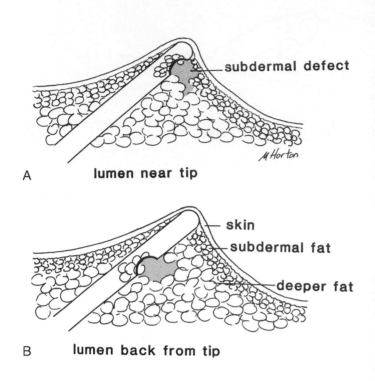

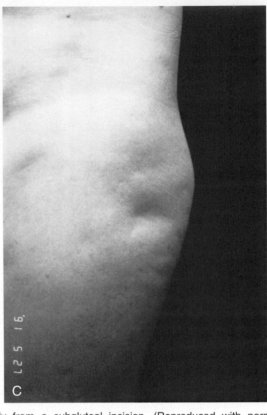

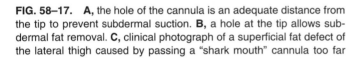

FIG. 58–17. A, the hole of the cannula is an adequate distance from the tip to prevent subdermal suction. **B,** a hole at the tip allows subdermal fat removal. **C,** clinical photograph of a superficial fat defect of the lateral thigh caused by passing a "shark mouth" cannula too far laterally from a subgluteal incision. (Reproduced with permission from: *Lipoplasty: the theory and practice of blunt suction lipectomy.* Copyright © 1990 by Gregory P. Hetter. Published by Little, Brown, p. 234.)

erated area toward the entry sites to express it. It may also be suctioned away if tunnels are in confluence.

ILIAC CREST AND DORSAL ROLLS

The bulk of the iliac crest roll is suctioned laterally with a 5 or 6-mm, single-hole Illouz cannula through a lateral port. Dorsal rolls may be separate from each other and are formed by fibrous elements attaching to deeper structures. Some of these can be extracted accurately only with the patient in the prone position. An incision is made approximately 4 or 5 cm from the midline; a 4-mm cobra cannula is used for these dorsal rolls or iliac crest extensions and for the posterior flank area.

LATERAL THIGHS

Five or six-millimeter Illouz cannulas are used through an infragluteal incision 3 to 5 cm lateral to the ischial tuberosity, and an iliac-crest incision about 10 to 12 cm from the midline.

Suction is applied after thorough pretunneling. The first two-thirds of the removal is made through the infragluteal incision and the final third through both incisions. The most anterior portion of the saddlebag is approached from the iliac-crest incision, because it is a much straighter approach. The results of trying to curve around the trochanter from the infragluteal incision were illustrated in Figure 58–17C. A typical example of lateral thigh and iliac crest reduction is shown in Figure 58–18.

MEDIAL THIGHS

The danger in operating on the medial thigh is overextraction, because the skin is thin and fine (in contradistinction to the lateral thigh). A posterior infragluteal incision can be combined with an anterior inguinal incision if the patient is to be turned. Cannulas in the 3- to 5-mm range usually are best. The frog-leg position allows approach from above and below. An inguinal incision and a mid-thigh incision allow a good crisscross approach (Fig. 58–19). Many times a medial thighplasty must be added when the skin is very flaccid (24).

ANTERIOR AND CIRCUMFERENTIAL THIGHS

The suprapatellar fat often hangs over the patella. This fat may be approached from two parapatellar incisions. A crisscross lipoplasty is carried out with 3- to 4-mm cobra or Illouz cannulas. The inferior anterior thigh is reached from these same incisions, and similar 4- to 5-mm cannulas are used. The whole anterior thigh has only superficial fat. It may be debulked from above and below but great care needs to be exercised to prevent subdermal vascular damage and grooving (25). An anterior thigh suction is shown in Figure 58–20.

KNEES

The approach to the medial knee may be from the medial popliteal fossa. This fat should come out easily with almost

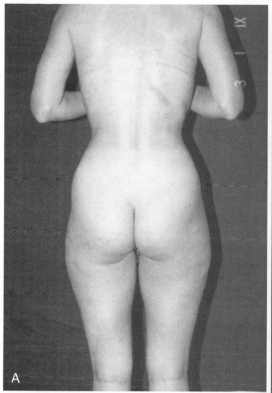
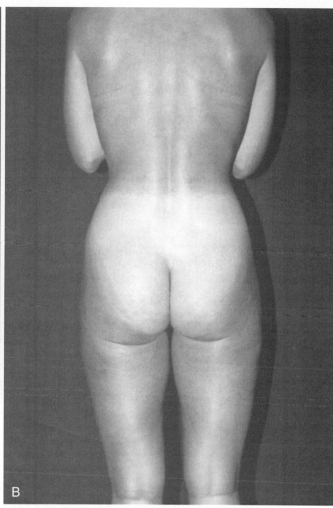

FIG. 58–18. **A,** preoperative posterior view of 31-year-old woman with asymmetric iliac crest excess and large asymmetric lateral thigh deposits. (The excess is greater on the right side.) **B,** postoperative view shows better symmetry and the open S-line from rib cage to midthigh, uninterrupted by bulges or waves. The buttock folds have been defatted to accentuate them. (Reproduced with permission from Hetter G: Blunt suction assisted lipectomy. In: *Mastery of plastic and reconstructive surgery*. Copyright © 1994 by Mimis Cohen. Published by Little, Brown, p. 236.)

no blood, and a 4- or 5-mm Illouz cannulas is a good choice depending on bulk (26). The inferior hook of fat below the level of the joint is more fibrous, and a 4-mm cobra cannula is useful.

ABDOMEN

There are two distinctly different anatomic areas of the abdomen. The epigastric fat is more fibrous, bleeds more, and lacks a discrete superficial fascia starting several centimeters above the umbilicus. Two incisions either beneath the breasts or at the fibrous fat pads overlying the flare of the ribs allows good access (see Fig. 58–13). In some people, these fat pads are quite prominent. Crisscross lipoplasty is carried out with 4- or 5-mm short cobra or Illouz cannulas over the whole epigastrium through these two incisions. The return of mostly blood rather than a full reduction often signals the endpoint of the operation; a reduction of the pinch by half is about the most one can hope to achieve. Pseudobursas can occur here if tissue damage is severe by oversuctioning (27).

The deep *hypogastric* fat is softer, is less bloody (if adequate suprafascial epinephrine is used), and has a well-demarcated superficial fascia. Two incisions just above the inguinal crease allow crisscross tunneling. Pretunneling is performed to delimit the deep compartment. Thereafter, extraction begins laterally, proceeding medially toward the umbilicus. The endpoint is reached when the thickness of the hypogastric pinch test is the same as the surrounding lateral superficial fat (in the hypochondrium). After the surgeon performs the extraction on the other side, crisscrossing from the opposite side is carried out. A variety of cannulas in the 4- to 6-mm range is acceptable. Extraction in the superficial fat, if desirable, is best accomplished with 4-mm cannulas. The periumbilical fat is more resistant to removal and requires extra attention. A typical reduction is shown in Figure 58–21.

MALE FLANKS

The male flanks lack superficial fascia, and the extraction is from the superficial fat. There are many retinacula cutis. The fat is very fibrous. The material extracted is usually bloody. Plenty of epinephrine and a 20-minute wait are useful. A centimeter of undamaged fat beneath the skin ensures a better result. Several entry sites and short 4- and 5-mm cobra can-

FIG. 58–19. Intraoperative photographs shows approach to medial thighs through inguinal port and a small midthigh incision using a relatively short cannula for maximal control. (Reproduced with permission from: *Lipoplasty: the theory and practice of blunt suction lipectomy.* Copyright © 1990 by Gregory P. Hetter. Published by Little, Brown, p. 343.)

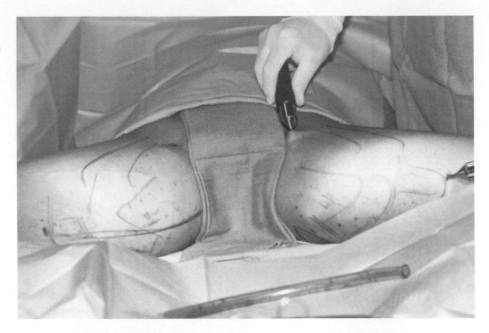

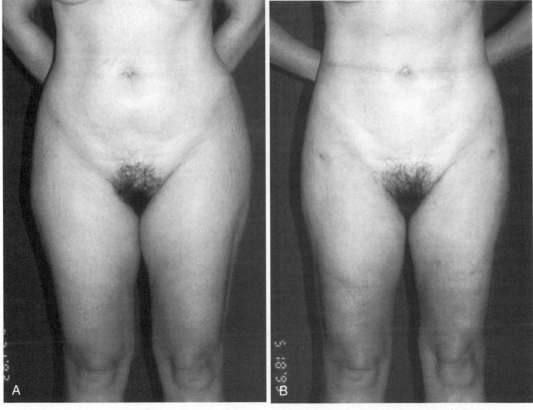

FIG. 58–20. **A,** preoperative anterior view of 36-year-old woman before two suction sessions. **B,** postoperative anterior view, 5 months following second session. First session removed 850 ml from the iliac crest areas, 950 ml from the lateral thighs, 125 ml from the medial thighs, 200 ml from the knees and 775 ml from the abdomen, for a total of 3000 ml of almost pure fat. Second session, 11 months later, removed 1300 ml from the anterior and medial thighs and 150 ml from the left lateral thigh because of asymmetry.

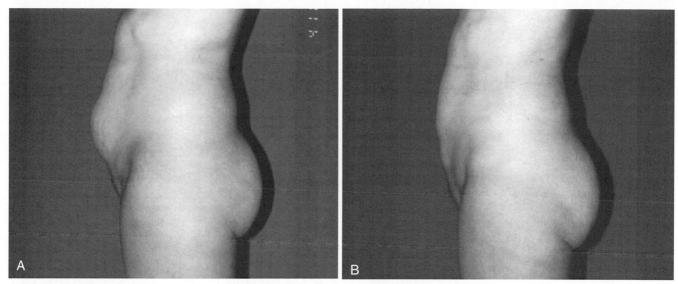

FIG. 58–21. **A,** preoperative lateral view of 32-year-old woman seeking removal of fat from abdomen, hip rolls, and lateral thighs. **B,** post operative lateral view, 3 months following removal of 600 ml from each hip roll, 1000 ml from the abdomen, and 400 ml from each lateral thigh.

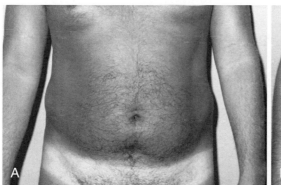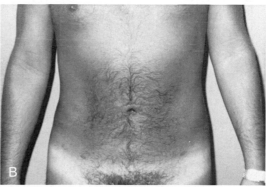

FIG. 58–22. **A,** preoperative view of typical male flanks with confluent hypogastric excess not amenable to remedy through exercise. **B,** postoperative view after suction of flanks and hypogastrium showing more youthful figure. (Reproduced with permission from: *Lipoplasty: the theory and practice of blunt suction lipectomy.* Copyright © 1990 by Gregory P. Hetter. Published by Little, Brown, p. 326.)

nulas are our usual choices. The endpoint is usually bloody extract and a reduction to half the beginning thickness by pinch and roll. A typical result of hypogastric and flank suction in a male patient was shown in Figure 58–22.

BUTTOCKS

There are many pitfalls associated with sculpting the buttock region (28). Poor results are common because of the difference between male and female anatomy, the interrelationship between hip rolls and lateral thigh bulges, and the static and dynamic anatomy. The novice should approach this area with caution. The inferior medial area of the buttock should *not* be suctioned. Serial suctions of up to 12.5 liters have been reported with good results by Ersek (29).

GYNECOMASTIA

Gynecomastia responds well to blunt-suction lipectomy. A periareolar incision is often used but an axillary and/or infra-mammary incisions allow a better access. Illouz or cobra cannulas are useful in 4- to 6-mm sizes. If the tissue is very fibrous, it can be grasped with the control hand like a sausage and speared by the cannula; extraction occurs as the control hand squeezes the tissue around and into the cannula. Criss-crossing is necessary for good results.

The glandular component may easily be underestimated, and gland resection through a periareolar incision may become necessary. Mammograms are helpful in defining fatty-glandular composition (30). Sometimes an areolar reduction is also necessary. Little glandular removal is possible by suction alone, although it is often mentioned.

PECTORAL FAT PAD

Some women complain of fatty excess at the junction of the anterior axillary fold and the tail of the breast in the superficial fat. This fat is easily removed by light suctioning with a 4-mm Illouz, single-hole cannula through a small axillary incision.

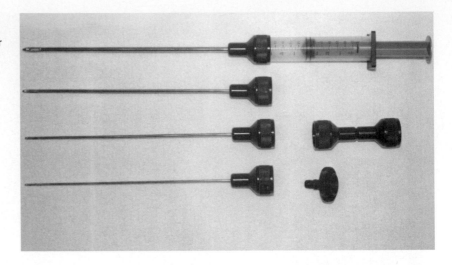

FIG. 58–23. SDS designed by Louis Toledo (JMJ Products), for the extraction, washing, and reinjection of fat. (Reproduced with permission from Hetter G: Blunt suction assisted lipectomy. In: *Mastery of plastic and reconstructive surgery.* Copyright © 1994 by Mimis Cohen. Published by Little, Brown, p. 239.)

CALVES AND ANKLES

Careful preoperative evaluation, marking, and planning are necessary. There is only superficial fat and it is neither uniform from high calf to ankle nor circumferentially. At least six entry sites allow access to all areas: two on either side of the Achilles tendon, two high on the posterior calf, and usually one low and one high anteriorly. Depending on bulk, 4-, 5- or 6-mm cannulas are used. The extraction is essentially circumferential except for the area above the tibia. A 2.5-mm cannula is useful around the ankle. Frequent pinch and roll tests are necessary to control the removal, and an even removal is difficult.

Saline irrigation of the operated area washes out many fatty fragments and blood. These breakdown products cause an increased oncotic pressure, with resultant prolonged edema and pain that adversely affects skin shrinkage and may lead to hemosiderin deposits. Drains can be placed for 24 hours when necessary. Tourniquets may be used, as described by Stallings (31).

FACE AND NECK

The use of suction techniques in fat removal from the face and neck has gained adherents since its introduction by Illouz. In open facelift techniques, it has replaced the scissors in removing neck fat quickly.

"Less is more" is the best rule of thumb when performing facial suction; the nasolabial line, particularly, can be overextracted. Grooving and fixation of dermis to underlying facial muscles are common lasting aesthetic complications that are difficult to treat.

Fat Injection

Fat injection remains a controversial subject (32–34). The authors maintain a skeptical viewpoint but use fat injection for postoperative divots and dimples and for filling the gluteal depression on occasion. It appears useful in nasolabial folds and hemifacial atrophy. Lip enlargement is a controversial area.

The fat is harvested with a syringe-driven system (SDS) (Fig. 58–23). Some surgeons inject it as is, others wash it in Ringer lactate or saline solution and reinject it with the same

harvest system in multiple tunnels. A graduated controlled injection gun is useful for even deposition of the injected adipose graft. Whether the apparent bulk that remains is based on living cells, microcysts, or some other phenomenon has not been determined. The procedure has potential, as shown in Figure 58–24.

It is the only technique available for the filling of iatrogenic divots or grooving. A divot noticed during the operation should be refilled immediately using the SDS. Using fat from the suction bottle is not practical. Touch-ups years later appears to have some benefit. It is not accepted to inject fat for breast augmentation; it can cause confusion in the interpretation of mammograms because of resulting calcifications.

Treatment of Cellulite

The anatomic basis for cellulite was shown in Figure 58–3. The theory behind the treatment is to cut the restraining retinacula cutis to release a dimple. Toledo devised an instrument to cut these retinaculae and claims good results. This operation needs to be approached cautiously.

Postoperative Care

Fluid shifts in BSL of the torso can be large, with massive third-space sequestration. This acute sequestered edema is mobilized, as in a burn patient, after several days. The need for attention to these fluid and hemodynamic shifts is only one reason this procedure should be performed by surgeons adequately trained in the physiology of shock and trauma. Hypovolemia, oliguria, fat embolism syndrome, shock, renal shutdown, pulmonary embolism, and myocardial infarction may follow injudicious ambulatory discharge of patients without adequate blood and fluid replacement. Most surgeons give a cephalosporin intravenously before the start of the operation. Most important, the *barrel of the cannula should never be touched with a gloved hand.* If touched, it should be wiped clean with saline containing antibiotic. Some surgeons irrigate the operated areas with a very dilute solution of aminoglycoside. Various binders and girdles are useful for the abdomen, iliac crest, thighs, buttocks, and knees. The constant mild pressure is believed to reduce edema. Girdles are usually worn for 1 to 2 weeks. Constric-

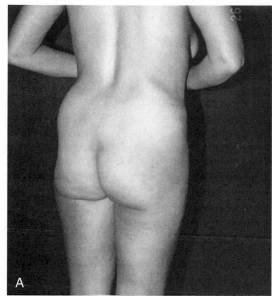
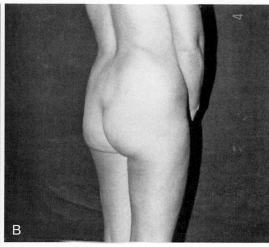

FIG. 58–24. **A,** preoperative view showing very large iliac crest roll and marked gluteal depression. **B,** postoperative view at 15 months showing filling out of gluteal depression by injection of 150 ml of fat per side harvested from the iliac crest with the SDS and injected into multiple tunnels. (Reproduced with permission from Hetter G: Blunt suction assisted lipectomy. In: *Mastery of plastic and reconstructive surgery.* Copyright © 1994 by Mimis Cohen. Published by Little, Brown, p. 240.)

tion around the knee may lead to an embolic phenomenon and should be checked. Surgeons working superficially usually tape.

Additional amounts of protein, iron, zinc, and vitamin C are recommended. Generally patients are asked not to smoke and are encouraged to have a diet rich in seafood, vegetables, and fruits in addition to supplements. Physical therapy modalities, primarily massage and ultrasound, are utilized by Hetter but not by Fodor. Ultimately, the results are probably indistinguishable at 1 year. During the convalescent phase, patients find the experience comforting and it maintains patient compliance and communication. The worried or anxious patient is especially well served by bi- or tri-weekly massage treatments.

GENERAL CONVALESCENCE

Five phases of convalescence of lipoplasty patients have been recognized by Hetter (35): (a) bandage phase (days 1 to 7); (b) fatigue phase (days 7 to 15); (c) disappointment phase (days 16 to 25); (d) relief phase (days 26 to 42); (e) satisfaction phase (after 6 weeks). Appropriate nursing and physician support during these phases mitigates problems. The massage therapist is invaluable during the disappointment phase.

The remodeling of the tissues is relatively complete 3 months after the procedure, except for the ankles, which may take 6 to 9 months for remodeling. Changes continue for as long as a year while collagen contracture and fatty remodeling progress.

TOUCH-UPS

Every patient is told preoperatively that touch-ups may not be discussed until 3 months after the operation. Fat injection and fine cannula recontouring are usually done 4 to 6 months postoperatively, generally with the SDS technique.

SEQUELAE

The following are commonly seen after BSL: (a) mild over or under resection; (b) temporary hypesthesia; (c) mild waviness; (d) occasional minor dent or divot; (e) faint hemosiderin deposits; (f) Transient pain; (g) some asymmetry; (h) transient fatigue. These sequelae usually resolve within 3 months, although some areas take longer to resolve than others. In order of rapidity of healing, the areas are the neck, knees, iliac crests, lateral thighs, abdomen, and calves.

AESTHETICALLY UNFAVORABLE RESULTS

The boundary between expected sequelae and aesthetically unfavorable results is hard to define and may vary from one patient to another, depending mainly on the skin condition before the operation. The following are problems that lead most often to lawsuits claiming malpractice: (a) grooving of the skin; (b) multiple dents and divots; (c) localized overresections (dishing out); (d) generalized overresections, such as flat thighs, flat buttocks, skinny thighs, or no remaining iliac crest roll; (e) generalized washboarding; (f) androgynous appearance; (g) buttock ptosis; (h) skin adhesions to muscle fascia; (i) subdermal damage to the vasculature (reticulate pattern); (j) skin loss.

All of these aesthetic problems can be minimized or prevented by careful work and anatomic knowledge. An example of excessive superficial suction is shown in Figure 58–25.

SEVERE COMPLICATIONS

The most common life-threatening medical complications are as follows: (a) fluid overload with pulmonary edema; (b) pulmonary embolus; (c) fat embolism syndrome, a variant of ARDS; (d) myocardial infarction; (e) renal shutdown; (f) massive infection; (g) viscus perforation, including intestine, spleen, liver, and lung; (h) death from xylocaine toxicity.

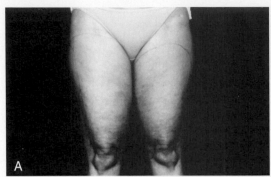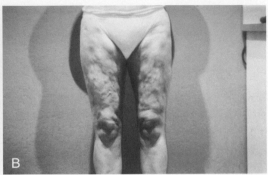

FIG. 58–25. A 43-year-old woman referred for aesthetic complications following superficial suction of the thigh. **A,** preoperative views obtained from referring surgeon. **B,** postoperative views several months later. Note abnormal vascular pattern, shriveled skin envelope discoloration and irregularities.

Pulmonary embolus and myocardial infarction may be random events; however, postoperative hypovolemia caused by inadequate blood and fluid resuscitation may lead to either of these complications as well as renal shutdown. The fluid loss continues in the wound for 12 to 36 hours, and the intravascular volume may reach its nadir 18 to 24 hours postoperatively.

A word about fat embolism syndrome is in order. Restrictive lung disease such as emphysema or acute restriction of lung excursion caused by abdominal or chest operations and dressings (abdominoplasty with fascial plication or subpectoral augmentation) may predispose to this syndrome. A healthy lung making good excursions is the best prevention. Many surgeons send patients home with an incentive spirometer to use postoperatively.

Suction of a large body surface area combined with procedures that limit diaphragmatic or chest excursion increases the risk, as does a low albumin level. Fat embolism syndrome should not be confused with fat embolism, which is common and generally benign. The treatment of these complications is much more difficult than their prevention. Despite all precautions, however, fat embolism syndrome may appear. Excessive fluids may push a patient with poor cardiac reserve into pulmonary edema. The differential diagnosis between the two is difficult.

Infection is best prevented by never touching the cannula shaft with the gloved hand. Many surgeons irrigate with antibiotic containing solutions while others give intravenous antibiotics before starting. Poor tissue perfusion due to hypovolemia or poor oxygenation due to fat embolism syndrome or pulmonary edema increase the chance for organisms carried into the tissues to survive.

Several deaths preceded by seizures following large clysis with xylocaine have been noted many hours following the procedure (36).

LESSER COMPLICATIONS

Other complications, from lesser to greater frequency, are: (a) anemia; (b) seroma; (c) hematoma; (d) incision site infection; (e) sensory nerve damage with persistent dysesthesias or hypesthesias; (f) muscle or muscle fascia damage with persistent pain; (g) pseudobursa formation.

Summary

Lipoplasty procedures have become one of the most commonly performed procedures in plastic surgery. Blunt-suction lipectomy makes possible lipoplastic operative procedures without skin removal. Lipoplasty combined with conventional dermal lipectomies improves the results of these operative procedures by extending the defatting beyond the previous operative field.

References

1. Schrudde J. Lipexeresis in the correction of local adiposity. Abstract. First Congress of the International Society of Aesthetic and Plastic Surgeons, Rio de Janeiro, 1972.
2. Fischer A, Fischer GM. Revised technique for cellulitis fat. Reduction in riding breeches deformity. *Bull Int Acad Cosm Surg* 1977; 12(2):40.
3. Kesselring UK, Meyer R. A suction curette for removal of excessive local deposits of subcutaneous fat. *Plast Reconstr Surg* 1978; 62:2:305–306.
4. Teimourian B, Fisher JB. Suction curettage to remove excess fat for body contouring. *Plast Reconstr Surg* 1981; 68:1:50–58.
5. Illouz YG. Une nouvelle technique pour les lipodystrophies localisees. *Rev Chir Esth Franc* 1980; 6:19.
6. Berlan M, Lafontan M. Alpha-2 receptors. *Quotidien du Med* (suppl. to no. 2855) 1983; 19:35–40.
7. Bjorntorp P. Human adipose tissue: dynamics and regulation. *Adv Metab Dis* 1971; 5:277.
8. Illouz YG. The study of subcutaneous fat. In: Hetter GP, ed. *Lipoplasty: the theory and practice of blunt suction lipectomy.* Boston: Little, Brown, 1990; 77–99.
9. Lockwood TE. Superficial fascial system (SFS) of trunk and extremities: a new concept. *Plast Reconstr Surg* 1991; 87(6):1009–1018.
10. Fodor PB. From the panniculus carnosus (PC) to the superficial fascia system (SFS). *Aesth Plast Surg* 1993; 17(3):179–181.
11. Gasparotti M, Lewis CM, Toledo LS. *Superficial liposculpture and manual of technique.* New York: Springer-Verlag, 1993.
12. Fournier PF: *Liposculpture: ma technique.* Paris: Arnette, 1989.
13. Apfelberg DB, Rosenthal S, Hunstad JP, et al. Progress report on multicenter study of laser-assisted liposuction. *Aesth Plast Surg* 1994; 18(3):259–264.
14. Zocchi M. Clinical aspects of ultrasonic liposculpture. *Perspect Plast Surg* 1993; 7(2):153–174.
15. Cukier J. Circumventing potential problems: suction lipoplasty, biohazardous aerosol, and exhaust mist—the clouded issue. *Plast Reconstr Surg* 1989; 83(3):494–497.
16. Lewis CM. Patient selection: psychological aspects. In: Hetter GP, ed. *Lipoplasty: the theory and practice of blunt suction lipectomy.* Boston: Little, Brown, 1990; 113–117.
17. Hetter GP. Blood and fluid replacement for lipoplasty procedures. *Clin Plast Surg* 1989; 16(2):245–248.

18. Laub DR. Fat embolism and fat embolism syndrome. In: Hetter GP, ed. *Lipoplasty: the theory and practice of blunt suction lipectomy.* Boston: Little, Brown, 1990; 219–222.
19. Mladick RA. Positions, incisions, and pretunneling. In: Hetter GP, ed. *Lipoplasty: the theory and practice of blunt suction lipectomy.* Boston: Little, Brown, 1990; 163–172.
20. Klein JA. The tumescent technique anesthesia and modified liposuction technique. *Derm Clin* 1990; 8(3):425–437.
21. Gilliland M. Tumescent liposuction complicated by pulmonary edema: a case report. (Submitted to *Plast Reconstr Surg.*)
22. Samdal F, Amland PF, Bugge JF. Blood loss during liposuction using the tumescent technique. *Aesth Plast Surg* 1994; 18(2):157–160.
23. Fournier PF. *Liposculpture: the syringe technique.* Paris: Arnette, 1991; 77.
24. Lockwood T. Fascial anchoring technique in medial thigh lifts. *Plast Reconstr Surg* 1988; 82(2):299–304.
25. Mladick RA. Circumferential "intermediate" lipoplasty of the legs. *Aesth Plast Surg* 1994; 18(2):165–174.
26. Fodor PB. Lipoplasty of the knees and anterior thighs. *Clin Plast Surg* 1989; 16(2):361–364.
27. Ersek RA, Schade K. Subcutaneous pseudobursa secondary to suction and surgery. *Plast Reconstr Surg* 1990; 85(3):442–445.
28. Illouz YG, de Villers YT. *Body sculpturing by lipoplasty.* Edinburgh: Churchill Livingston, 1989; 154.
29. Ersek RA, Bell HN IV, Salisbury AV. Serial and superficial suction for steatopygia (Hottentot bustle). *Aesth Plast Surg* 1994; 18(3):279–282.
30. Fodor PB. Management of gynecomastia. *Probl Plast Reconstr Surg* 1992; 2(3):422–435.
31. Stallings JO. Lipoplasty of the calves and ankles. In: Hetter GP, ed. *Lipoplasty: the theory and practice of blunt suction lipectomy.* Boston: Little, Brown, 1990; 354.
32. Illouz YG. Fat injection: a four-year clinical trial. In: Hetter GP, ed. *Lipoplasty: the theory and practice of blunt suction lipectomy.* Boston: Little, Brown, 1990; 239–246.
33. Chajchir A, Benzaquen I, Wexler EM, et al. Fat injection. *Aesth Plast Surg* 1990; 14(2):127–136.
34. Toledo LS. Syringe liposculpture: a two-year experience. *Aesth Plast Surg* 1991; 15(4):321–326.
35. Hetter GP. Convalescence. In: Hetter GP, ed. *Lipoplasty: the theory and practice of blunt suction lipectomy.* Boston: Little, Brown, 1990; 215–217.
36. Gilliland M. Personal communications, 1995.

59

Lipoplasty and a Step Beyond

Ted Lockwood, M.D., F.A.C.S.

Aspirative lipoplasty has become synonymous with body contouring surgery over the past 15 years (1–3). And yet, liposuction deals with only one element of the aesthetic body contour deformity. While excess fat deposits are the major component of body contour problems, skin laxity and skin contour irregularities—cellulite—are a significant problem in many women.

There are two basic methods to deal with body contour deformities: liposuction and excisional lifts. Significant improvements and refinements have occurred in the past few years in both areas of body contour surgery (4–15). However, there continues to be much confusion regarding the indications for liposuction and for excisional lifts. There is no need for such confusion because generally these two techniques are not indicated for the same body contour problem.

Liposuction deals with localized fat deposits and with thick subcutaneous fat layers, and excisional lifts deal with significant laxity of the skin and soft tissues. Often the aesthetic contour deformity in a given patient consists of both excess fat deposits and skin laxity; therefore, it may require a combination of liposuction and lifting techniques for optimal results.

Patient Evaluation

The human body is a three-dimensional figure; body contour surgeons must learn to assess and treat aesthetic contour deformities in a three-dimensional fashion. The body can be divided into circumferential aesthetic units, from the breasts to the pubis for the trunk and from the breasts to the knees for the thighs or thigh/trunk problems. Surgery on one part of the trunk aesthetic unit (e.g., the abdomen) without careful consideration of its effect on the overall aesthetic balance of the circumferential trunk can lead to mediocre results and an imbalance in truncal contours. For example, simply flattening a protuberant abdomen in a patient with a significant hip/back fat deposit may create the illusion of a wider, square or boxy hip profile that is noticeable in clothing. In patients who have aesthetic deformities of both the trunk and thighs, dramatic sculpturing of the trunk aesthetic unit may create the illusion of much larger thighs, leading to an imbalance of the trunk/thigh aesthetic. This concern should be carefully discussed preoperatively; concomitant or staged thigh contouring may be required for an optimal outcome.

Photograpic Documentation

Documenting skin quality photographically is particularly challenging, but essential in body contour surgery. The most common long-term aesthetic complication of liposuction is skin laxity with surface contour irregularities (cellulite), resulting in an acceleration of the aged appearance of the skin. In body lifts requiring long incisions, an accurate documentation of the degree of skin laxity problems and their improvement postoperatively is necessary to justify long incisional scars. There are several photographic tips that we have found helpful. In addition to nude photos, we suggest that the surgeon photograph the patient with the same dark bikini underwear before and after surgery designed to compress the soft, loose fat and skin that was producing "bikini overhang." Use a moderate-to-dark background with overhead lighting and no flash (ASA 400 Ektachrome). Replace fluorescent bulbs with Spectralite bulbs for natural colors. Available-light photography most accurately demonstrates subtleties of skin contour irregularities, while flash techniques "fill the shadows," losing surface detail. Be careful to avoid light-colored backgrounds and bikinis because the backlighting effect produces loss of surface detail.

Liposuction

Liposuction is used for the majority of body contour problems. There are marked variations in the nature and extent of familial fat deposits, so each patient should be carefully studied before the development of a surgical plan. Rather than suctioning just the standard localized fat deposits, such as the abdomen and hips, a sculpturing of the entire aesthetic unit toward the aesthetic ideal should be performed. This may require suctioning of the waist, back, and costal margins as well as etching of the midline epigastric valley. Liposuction usually results in some degree of skin retraction, depending on skin quality and body location. However, in many cases this retraction is short-lived or nonexistent. Long-term studies of liposuction patients commonly reveal progressive skin relaxation, as might be expected with the aging process. Exceptions to this basic principle may be patients under 35 years of age, or favorable body locations in areas over natural musculoskeletal concavities (e.g., the waist, epigastrium).

Superficial liposuction within the superficial fat layer beneath the dermis has given the promise of more significant skin retraction than standard level liposuction (5–7). However, in my experience, superficial liposuction has not produced a major improvement in skin quality on a long-term basis (over 1 year) in most body locations. And, more important, superficial liposuction has resulted in permanent and often dramatic skin/fat contour aesthetic deformities even when used by experienced surgeons (Fig. 59–1). Since many of the contour irregularities produced by superficial liposuc-

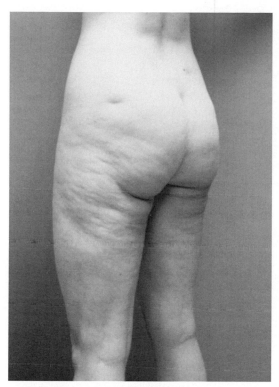

FIG. 59–1. As seen in this 30-year-old woman, superficial liposuction of the lateral thighs may result in contour irregularities that may not be correctable by any treatment. I do not recommend superficial liposuction in the lateral or medial thighs for most patients, with the exception of patients with a thick, immobile superficial fat layer.

fat. The infusion fluid I prefer contains 50 cc ½% xylocaine and 1 cc epinephrine 1:1000 in each 1000 cc of lactated Ringer solution. For the usual body contour patient, I use both superficial and deep liposuction techniques. Figure 59–2 demonstrates the liposuction technique I currently use for most patients with trunk and thigh fat deposits and reasonable skin tone.

Excisional Lifts

Excisional lifts are designed to treat skin quality problems of the aesthetic body contour deformity. Laxity of skin and cellulite will occur in all women with the normal aging process. It would seem likely, therefore, that excisional lifts play an increasingly important role in most practices as our population ages. However, liposuction almost completely dominates the field of body contour surgery today. Why have so many surgeons turned away from excisional lifts, recommending liposuction for most of their patients? I believe the predominant reason for this change in treatment strategy is not a different population base, but rather disappointment with the aesthetic results of classic excisional lifts (16). The argument can be made that, instead of placing long incisions on the body and obtaining mediocre results, we lower our aesthetic goals and use liposuction alone to gain as much improvement as possible without the long incisions. There is a certain logic to this argument, but we are still left with compromised goals and reduced expectations in body contouring patients. Liposuction will remain the mainstay for patients who present primarily with localized fat excess and fat disproportion. However, in many patients, skin laxity and cellulite are the primary elements of the aesthetic deformity.

In the last decade, significant progress has occurred in the understanding of aged aesthetic body deformities, allowing new body-lift designs based on modern surgical principles (9–15). Body lifts are a useful adjunct to liposuction, and should be considered when developing an overall surgical plan for an individual patient. Clear indications for trunk and thigh lifts include skin laxity without significant fat deposits, excessive skin laxity and cellulite, patients in which skin tightening is their primary goal, medial thigh deformities in patients over 35 years old, and buttock ptosis.

Lifts may be used at the time of initial liposuction or may be required to treat skin laxity and contour irregularities that appear after liposuction. Patients should be aware of the limitations of liposuction and that subsequent body lifting may be required to gain optimal body contours. Having this discussion prior to initial liposuction helps the patient understand that skin tone is the primary determinant of the aesthetic success or failure of liposuction, even with the best liposuction technique. Patients who understand this principle rarely have unrealistic expectations about the results of liposuction and are reasonably prepared to consider body lifts in the future, if needed.

The excisional lifts presented in this chapter are based on a careful analysis of youthful aesthetic anatomy as well as both youthful and aged body contour aesthetic deformities. These body lifts have proven to be effective and long-lasting, with low risk of significant complications. Key technical elements of all of these lifts include: incisions placed in current high-cut bikini lines, superficial fascial system (SFS) suspension with permanent sutures, direct undermining through

tion may not be correctable with any degree of predictability, I would urge caution with its use. Superficial liposuction does have a selective role in body contouring procedures, which will be outlined later in this chapter.

Liposuction, in general, has a limited aesthetic life. We should assume that our patients may desire skin quality improvements in addition to body contour improvements as they age. Therefore, any surgical plan should reflect these principles. Just as liposuction of the neck does not eliminate the need for face/neck lifting in the future, liposuction of the body may be only the first step in body contouring for a given individual.

There are well-defined indications for liposuction with which there is general agreement. These include localized fat deposits with minimal skin laxity, thick subcutaneous fat, body areas poorly treated by lifts (upper back, arms, axilla, legs, knees), and excisional scars that would be unacceptable to the patient. In addition, fat deposits overlying natural musculoskeletal concavities such as the lower back, waist, and epigastrium respond well to a combination of superficial and deep liposuction even with moderate skin laxity.

Currently, liposuction should use smaller cannulae (3 to 5 mm), preinjection with dilute epinephrine/local anesthetic solutions, and a combination of deep and superficial liposuction, depending on the body location and the anatomic level of the excess fat deposit (i.e., excess superficial fat or a deep fat deposit). Deep liposuction refers to aspiration deep to the top 1 cm of fat, and superficial liposuction within the top 1 cm but preserving 2 to 3 mm of subdermal

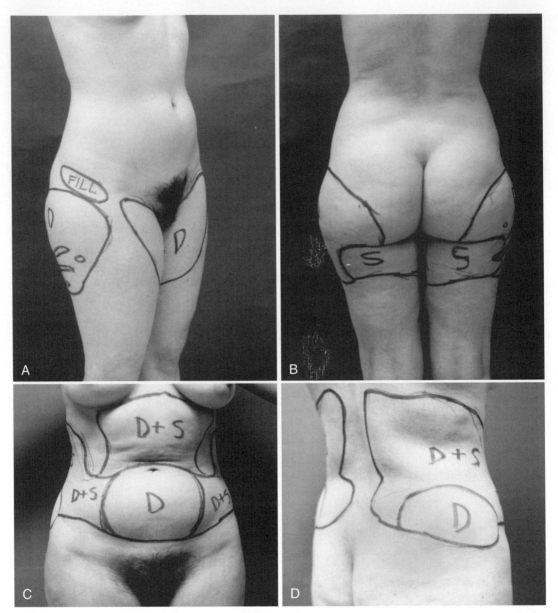

FIG. 59–2.   Current technique for trunk/thigh liposuction in average patients. **A, B,** 37-year-old woman with fat deposits of the medial, lateral, and posterior thighs, along with a few cellulite dimples of the trochanteric area. Deep liposuction is performed for the medial and lateral thigh fat deposits and superficial liposuction for the upper posterior thighs. Subdermal transection of cellulite bands with a picklefork cannula, along with fat injection, may improve isolated dimples. In addition, lipofilling of the lateral gluteal recess can help smooth the lateral contours to a mild degree. **C, D,** 37-year-old woman with circumferential truncal fat deposits. Thorough liposuction in both the deep and superficial planes is performed in the epigastrium, waist, and lower-back areas. For the average patient, deep liposuction alone is used for the hypogastrium and iliac-crest fat deposits.

SFS proximal zones of adherence, and discontinuous cannula undermining.

HIGH-LATERAL-TENSION ABDOMINOPLASTY

Modern abdominoplasty techniques were developed in the 1960s. The advent of liposuction has reduced the need for classical abdominoplasty and allowed more aesthetic sculpturing of the entire trunk. However, the combination of significant truncal liposuction and classical abdominoplasty is not recommended because of increased risk of complications.

Although the surgical principles of classical abdominoplasty have certainly stood the test of time, they are based on two theoretical assumptions that may prove to be inaccurate. The first assumption is that wide direct undermining to costal margins is essential for abdominal flap advancement. In fact, discontinuous undermining allows effective loosening of the abdominal flap while preserving vascular perforators. The second inaccurate assumption is that, with aging and weight fluctuations (including pregnancy), abdominal skin relaxation occurs primarily in the vertical direction from xiphoid to pubis. This is true in the lower abdomen, but a strong SFS

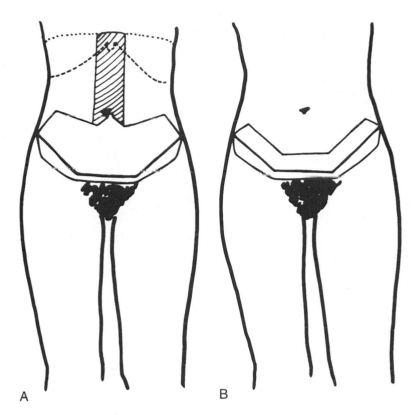

A   B

FIG. 59–3. **A,** high-lateral-tension abdominoplasty design, standard pattern for patients with significant vertical epigastric laxity. In these patients, the umbilicus usually is loosely anchored, lax, and mobile. Direct undermining initially is limited to the paramedian area to allow muscle plication (cross-hatched area). Wider discontinuous undermining and liposuction are performed as needed. Bold line = planned line of closure; solid lines = estimated resection lines. **B,** high-lateral-tension abdominoplasty design, modified pattern, for patients with limited true vertical epigastric excess. In these patients, the umbilicus usually is stable and fixed with a normal to high position. The umbilical stalk is transected to allow muscle plication and is reinserted at or slightly below its original location. Direct and discontinuous undermining and liposuction are performed as needed.

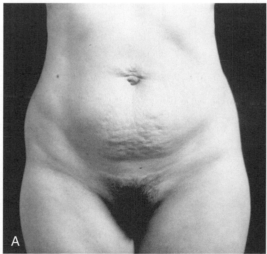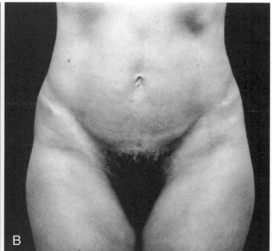

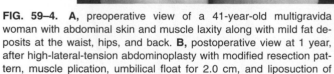

FIG. 59–4. **A,** preoperative view of a 41-year-old multigravida woman with abdominal skin and muscle laxity along with mild fat deposits at the waist, hips, and back. **B,** postoperative view at 1 year, after high-lateral-tension abdominoplasty with modified resection pattern, muscle plication, umbilical float for 2.0 cm, and liposuction of waist, hips, and back. The incision line has faded and is hidden in skimpy bikinis. The abdominal contours have a natural aesthetic balance. (Reprinted with permission from Lockwood T: High-lateral-tension abdominoplasty with superficial fascial system suspension. *Plastic and Reconstructive Surgery,* 1995; 96:603.)

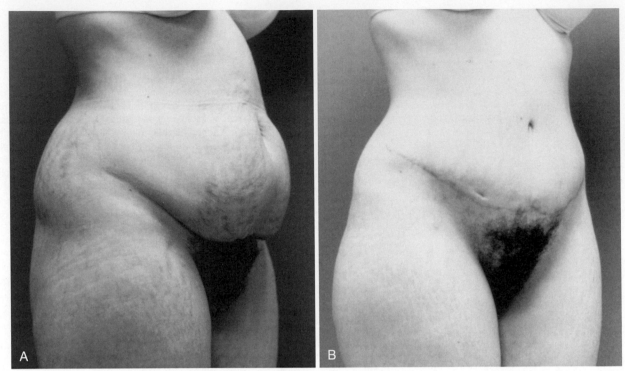

FIG. 59–5. **A,** preoperative view of a 29-year-old woman with familial truncal fat deposits and severe abdominal laxity and striae following three pregnancies. **B,** postoperative view at 10 months after standard abdominal resection, muscle plication, umbilical transposition, and superficial and deep liposuction of the hips and lower back, along with limited liposuction in the epigastrium. (Reprinted with permission from Lockwood T: High-lateral-tension abdominoplasty with superficial fascial system suspension. *Plastic and Reconstructive Surgery,* 1995; 96:603.

adherence to the linea alba in the epigastrium limits vertical descent in most patients. Epigastric laxity frequently results from a progressive horizontal loosening due to relaxation of the tissues along the lateral trunk (12). Experience with the lower body lift procedure has shown that significant lateral truncal skin resection results in epigastric tightening. In these patients, the ideal abdominoplasty pattern would resect as much or more laterally than centrally, leading to more natural abdominal contours.

The high-lateral-tension abdominoplasty, with and without truncal liposuction and other aesthetic procedures, has been performed in over 75 patients (13). The primary indication for surgery is moderate-to-severe laxity of abdominal skin and muscle with or without truncal fat deposits. Complication rates were at or below historical controls and were not increased with significant adjunctive liposuction. Key technical elements of this procedure include: (a) direct undermining limited to the paramedian area, (b) discontinuous undermining to costal margins and flanks as needed (with vertical-spreading scissors or cannula undermining), (c) skin resection pattern with significant lateral resection and highest-tension wound closure placed laterally, (d) superficial fascial system (SFS) repair with permanent sutures (0 or 2-0 Nurolon) along entire incision, and (e) liberal use of adjunctive liposuction in the upper abdomen and in the lateral and posterior trunk (Figs. 59–3, 59–4, and 59–5).

MEDIAL THIGH LIFT

The medial thigh aesthetic deformity frequently presents a challenging problem to the body contouring surgeon. Skin

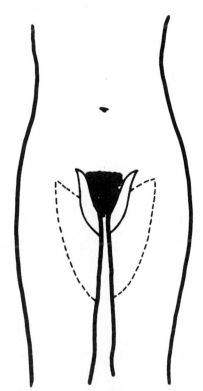

FIG. 59–6. Current medial thigh-lift resection pattern has rotated more anteriorly because most of laxity occurs at the anteromedial thigh area. The entire procedure is now performed in the supine position. Deep liposuction of the medial thigh fat deposit can be safely liposuctioned at the time of the lift (dotted line).

laxity in the medial thigh is frequently the earliest sign of aging in the thighs and is one of the first signs of significant ptosis in the body (2). The skin of the medial thigh is quite thin and inelastic, resulting in early relaxation with age and poor retraction after liposuction. Conservatism is usually recommended in liposuction of the medial thighs. By the 35 years of age in most patients, actual or potential laxity of the medial thigh tissues can lead to disappointing results after liposuction alone. Laxity of the medial thighs may occur at even earlier ages in patients with a history of significant obesity in childhood or early adulthood or in patients with the familial trait of thin, lax skin.

The classic medial thigh-lift has been plagued with persistent problems including inferior migration and widening of scars, lateral traction deformity of the vulva, and early recurrence of ptosis. In an attempt to limit untoward results, the medial thigh-lift was modified to allow anchoring of the inferior skin flap to the tough, inelastic deep layer of the superficial fascia of the perineum (9). Using the Colles fascia as the central anchor for the medial thigh-lift has produced more consistent, long-lasting results, decreasing the risk of problems commonly associated with the classic skin-suspension medial thigh-lift.

Since the fascial anchoring technique for medial thigh lifts was originally described in 1987, numerous technical refinements have been developed to provide enhanced safety, predictability, and aesthetics (15). The surgical principles of the medial thigh-lift have evolved to allow more accurate patient selection, individualized operative planning, and standardized surgical technique. Significant actual or potential laxity of the medial thigh tissues remains the standard indication for medial thigh lifting today. Liposuction of moderate to severe fat deposits of the medial thighs often leads to skin relaxation, especially after 30 years of age. Moderate-to-severe skin laxity will require thigh lifting, along with liposuction of any medial thigh fat deposits. For milder cases of skin laxity, a more limited medial thigh-lift may provide optimal thigh contours and skin tightening with improved aging potential in the region.

The medial thigh-lift design has changed significantly since the original description, due to a better understanding of thigh aesthetic deformities. Since the majority of skin laxity in this area occurs at the juncture of the anterior and medial thighs, the standard surgical resectional pattern has rotated anteriorly, allowing the entire procedure to be performed in the supine position (Fig. 59–6). In contrast to previous descriptions, the incision should not extend into the buttock fold posteriorly. The resectional ellipse can be limited for milder cases of medial thigh laxity or extended to the anterior superior iliac spine for more extensive problems in the anterior thigh and inguinal areas. The actual skin resection has become more conservative over the years, averaging 5 to 7 cm of stretched skin at the anteromedial corner of the thigh. The anchoring of the perineal-thigh crease into the Colles fascia provides an additional 3 to 5 cm of lift. More conservative resection has decreased wound complications from overresection while still providing consistent contour improvements. Superficial undermining over the soft-tissue bundle that extends from the femoral

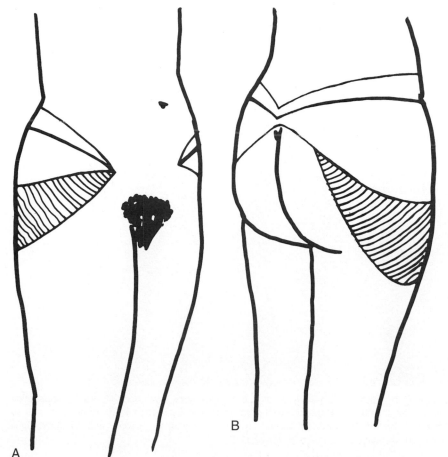

FIG. 59–7. A, preoperative markings for the transverse flank/thigh/buttock lift for the usual patient, anterolateral view. The bold middle line is the planned line of closure, with the estimated amount of skin redundancy above and below that line marked as resection lines. Areas of cross-hatching denote direct undermining through the superficial fascial system (SFS) zone of adherence that begins inferior to the inguinal ligament and extends into the lateral gluteal recess. **B,** preoperative markings, posterolateral view, for either the transverse flank/thigh/buttock lift or the lower body lift (see Fig. 59–8). No undermining is performed near the gluteal vessels to maintain strong thigh flap vascularity. The high-cut bikini pattern separates the major vascular territories of the trunk and thighs; resecting redundant tissue in this region will allow optimal blood flow to both flap edges.

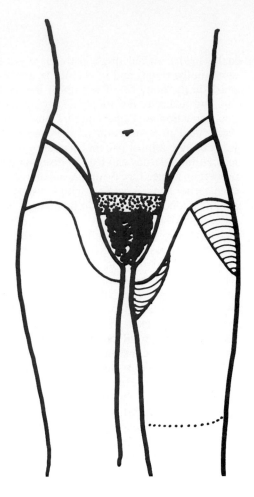

FIG. 59–8. Preoperative markings for the lower body lift, anterior view. The bold line within high-cut bikini outlines is the planned line of closure, with the resection lines on either side. The cross-hatched areas denote direct surgical undermining while discontinous cannula undermining extends to the knee if necessary (see Fig. 59–7B for the posterior view of the lower body lift markings).

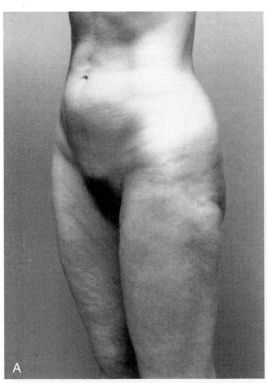
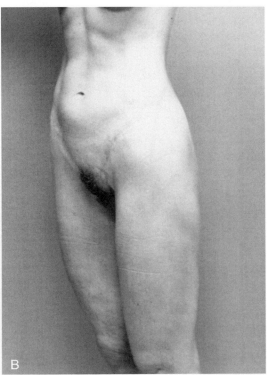

FIG. 59–9. **A,** preoperative view of a 44-year-old woman, 5 years after thigh liposuction with marked laxity of lower trunk and thighs and skin contour irregularities. Redundant skin and fat should be pinched and lifted at the hip level to assist in proper patient selection. **B,** post-operative result at 6 months, after lower body lift without liposuction. (Reprinted with permission from Lockwood T: Lower body lift with superficial fascial system suspension. *Plastic and Reconstructive Surgery* 1993; 92:1112.)

triangle to the mons pubis preserves the external pudendal vessels, reducing the risk of lymphatic complications. Blunt dissection through this soft-tissue bundle at the mons pubis exposes the Scarpa fascia or muscular fascia, either of which can be used for anchoring of the thigh flap.

Permanent anchoring sutures into the Colles fascia are now used for all patients (0 Nurolon). In addition, anchoring sutures must also be placed into the Scarpa fascia anteriorly and into the buttock fold SFS posteriorly. To more securely hold the thigh flap into position, the anchoring suture is placed into the thigh SFS and dermis, instead of dermis alone as initially reported. The actual incisional closure line is forced onto the relaxed vulvar tissues to decrease the risk of scar widening or migration.

TRANSVERSE THIGH/BUTTOCK LIFT

The thigh/buttock lift of Pitanguy was originally designed in 1964 to allow direct excision of trochanteric fat deposits (17). For nearly 30 years, the Pitanguy lift was also used as the standard procedure for laxity and cellulite of the lateral thigh and buttock region. However, Pitanguy's procedure was infrequently performed because of problems including noticeable scars, early recurrence of deformities, unnatural contours, significant wound complications, long operative times, and prolonged postoperative disability.

With the advent of liposuction and a better knowledge of the vascular anatomy of skin and the anatomy of the superficial fascial system (10), a new thigh/buttock lift procedure was designed using a transverse resection of redundant skin and fat of the trunk, with an incisional scar within high-cut bikini lines (11) (Fig. 59–7). Using appropriate direct and discontinuous cannula undermining as well as SFS suspension with permanent sutures (1 Nurolon), the transverse thigh/buttock lift provides numerous advantages for truncal contouring. There is improved skin-flap vascularity, strong yet dynamic fascial support, simultaneous tightening of lax flank and abdominal tissues in addition to lifting the buttock and lateral thighs, and a stable scar that remains hidden in bikini lines.

The transverse thigh/buttock lift can be used alone or in combination with medial thigh lifting, termed the lower body lift (12) (Figs. 59–8, 59–9), or with high-lateral-tension abdominoplasty in 1 or 2 stages (13). Patients presenting with skin laxity and cellulite of the lateral thigh/buttock region frequently have associated laxity problems in the abdomen, flanks, and medial thighs. These patients almost always require excisional treatment of multiple areas of the body to keep the aesthetic harmony intact. Once significant experi-

ence is gained with the transverse thigh/buttock lift, it is often used in combination rather than as an isolated procedure.

MULTIPLE BODY CONTOUR PROBLEMS

To develop a surgical plan in patients with multiple body contour problems, visualize the lower body lift incision on each patient and use that portion of the lower body lift incision that adequately treats the aesthetic deformity for that individual. If there is moderate-to-severe abdominal laxity, an initial abdominoplasty will be required before thigh lifting. Mild-to-moderate abdominal laxity will be improved with either the transverse thigh/buttock lift or the lower body lift.

Conclusion

In conclusion, body contour surgeons will need expertise in both liposuction and lifting techniques to deal with the variety of aesthetic deformities of the trunk and thighs. Often the combination of liposuction and lifts produces superior results compared to those obtained by either technique alone.

References

1. Illouz YG. Body contouring by lipolysis: a 5-year experience in over 3000 cases. *Plast Reconstr Surg* 1983; 72:591.
2. Illouz YG, De Villers Y. *Body sculpturing by lipoplasty.* New York: Churchill-Livingstone, 1989.
3. Hetter, G, ed. *Lipoplasty: the theory and practice of blunt suction lipectomy.* 2nd ed. Boston: Little, Brown, 1990.
4. Fournier P. *Liposculpture: the syringe technique.* Paris: Arnette, 1991.
5. Toledo L. Syringe liposculpture: a two-year experience. *Aesth Plast Surg* 1991; 15:321.
6. Gasperoni C, Salgarello M, et al. Subdermal liposuction. *Aesth Plast Surg* 1990; 14:137.
7. Gasparotti M. Superficial liposuction: a new application for the technique for aged and flaccid skin. *Aesth Plast Surg* 1992; 16:141.
8. Baroudi R, Moraes M. Philosophy, technical principles, selection, and indications in body contouring surgery. *Aesth Plast Surg* 1991; 15:1.
9. Lockwood T. Fascial anchoring in medial thigh lifts. *Plast Reconstr Surg* 1988; 82:299.
10. Lockwood T. Superficial fascial system (SFS) of the trunk and extremities: a new concept. *Plast Reconstr Surg* 1991; 87:1009.
11. Lockwood T. Transverse flank-thigh-buttock lift with superficial fascial suspension. *Plast Reconstr Surg* 1991; 87:1019.
12. Lockwood T. Lower body lift with superficial fascial system suspension. *Plast Reconstr Surg* 1993; 92:1112.
13. Lockwood T. High-lateral-tension abdominoplasty with superficial fascial system suspension. *Plast Reconstr Surg* 1995; 96:603.
14. Lockwood T. Brachioplasty with superficial fascial system suspension. *Plast Reconstr Surg* 1995; 96:912.
15. Lockwood T. Technical refinements in medial thigh lifting. Submitted for publication.
16. Regnault P, Daniel R. Secondary thigh-buttock deformities after classical techniques: prevention and treatment. *Clin Plast Surg* 1984; 11:505.
17. Pitanguy I. Trochanteric lipodystrophy. *Plast Reconstr Surg* 1964; 34:280.

FIVE

Breast and Chest

60

Congenital and Developmental Deformities of the Breast and Breast Asymmetries

James G. Hoehn, M.D., F.A.C.S. and Gregory S. Georgiade, M.D., F.A.C.S.

Most humans demonstrate a natural asymmetry of their body halves (1). Minor differences in individual breast contour, volume, or position on the hemithorax are usually accepted as normal by the patient. However, major variations may present significant physical, social, and psychologic concern (2–4).

The patient seeking correction of breast asymmetry presents a unique challenge to the reconstructive surgeon. The decisions regarding treatment and its timing will reflect an accurate analysis of the problem, a sensitivity to the patient's wishes, and a thorough understanding of the surgical techniques available for reconstruction of the three individual components of the breast—the gland, the skin cover, and the nipple-areolar complex (3).

Classification

Any classification of congenital, developmental, or traumatic breast asymmetries might well be structured around the entities that the reconstructive surgeon must develop: the breast mound, its skin cover, and the nipple-areolar complex. Any definitive classification, such as those proposed by Maliniac (5), Simon and colleagues (4), and Regnault (6), will provide for both etiological causes and defect presentation. What is important to the surgeon is a realization that asymmetry classified by etiology will include congenital, traumatic, inflammatory, and neoplastic conditions, whereas a classification by anatomic presentation would recognize position, number, size, and shape of the breasts and the nipple-areolar complexes. The numerous subcategories developed by combining these groups would be unwieldy. The most useful clinical descriptions would combine the etiological cause as a modifier to the anatomic presentation.

Incidence

Because patients with minor variations do not present for correction, there is no practical way to estimate the true incidence of breast asymmetry. Hueston reported that 10% of his patients requesting breast surgery had done so for a major complaint of asymmetry (7).

Normal Growth and Development

Although the understanding of breast asymmetry remains elusive, there are known genetic and hormonal facts that are relevant to the clinical presentation of this deformity. It is appropriate to review briefly the normal embryology of the breasts and its supporting structures, as well as their subsequent growth and development as a basis for developing

treatment protocols (5,8–10). In addition, various hormonal influences act on the breast gland at each stage of development, and are reviewed.

For purposes of understanding the factors that affect final breast contour, shape, and pendulousness, the breast can be considered to be made up of only two structures, the breast gland and the surrounding skin. The mass, shape, and volume of the glandular component defines the ultimate breast appearance, and the skin only expands to accommodate the underlying gland.

BREAST EMBRYOLOGY

The primordia of the human breast first appear between the limb buds on the ventral surface of the embryo as two ectodermal ridges known as mammary ridges or "milk lines" at about the 5th week of intrauterine life (Fig. 60–1). Projected on the fully developed fetus, these ridges extend from each axilla to the ipsilateral groin. The duration of the mammary ridges on the fetus may vary, but normally a coalescence of cells persist in the cranial one-third of each ridge to become the future breast. These persisting elevations, known as the breast anlagen, will determine the future position of the breast. Additional mammary gland anlagen will persist along this line in lower mammals, but in humans regression is the rule. Persistence of definable breast structures in aberrant locations occurs only in 1 to 5% of persons (back, axilla, abdomen).

At about the 6th gestational week, the ectoderm overlying the breast thickens, and by the 10th week the ectoderm burrows into the mesenchyme, stimulated by the action of maternal and placental hormones to form the mammary bud. Concurrently, the remaining mammary anlagen regress. Soon thereafter, vasculogenesis around the mammary bud begins, and about the 15th week, epidermal sprouts appear that will become the mammary ducts. The developing breast is sensitive to the action of testosterone hormonal inhibition for several weeks at this juncture. The absence of testosterone in the female fetus (or the absence of testosterone receptors, as in the testicular feminization syndrome) allows female breast development to proceed. Conversely, the presence of testosterone in the male fetus apparently induces rapid mesenchymal proliferation that effectively "strangles" the epidermal sprouts and obviates further breast development (11).

Ductal development continues in the 20th to 32nd week under the varying influences of estrogen, insulin, and glucocorticoids. During this time, the breast ducts canalize and lengthen. From the 32nd to 40th week, the relatively straight ducts arborize into the normal lobular-areolar pattern under the influence of progesterone, while estrogen, insulin, and the glucocorticoids assume a permissive role.

The common terminus of the ducts elevates to form the nipple. Although this elevation is commonly seen at birth, it may require future growth to make its presence known. The surrounding areolas, with the progenitors of the specialized lubricating glands of Montgomery, as usually identifiable to the naked eye in the 20-week-old embryo (2).

At birth, the normal breast (anlagen) has the complete adult complement of 15 to 20 lobes of glandular tissue. Each lobe is a separate system of alveolar-lobular cells specialized for milk production and a system of smaller collecting ductules that connect with a major duct exiting ultimately via the nipple. Until puberty, breasts grow in proportion to the body size. Thelarche (the earliest breast growth, which is not in proportion to the body size) usually represents the first sign of puberty (10). In the presence of prolactin or growth hormone, the rising estrogen levels at puberty stimulate the ductal system to elongate and to branch, while vascularity, stroma, and fat deposition all increase until the characteristic ductal spacing of the adult breast has occurred. When balance of the hypophyseal-pituitary-ovarian axis is established and ovulatory cycles begin, the breast comes under the influence of progesterone from the corpus luteum, which stimulates development of the acinar, or milk-secreting, structures. With continued cyclic flux of ovarian hormones, the breasts continue to develop until approximately 30 years of age. Functional maturity (milk production) is dependent on the hormonal changes that occur during pregnancy and is sustained as long as the functional stimulus of breastfeeding continues.

At birth, and for a few weeks afterward, transient breast enlargement occurs in the newborn as a result of the transplacental influence of maternal steroids, but it will usually subside spontaneously with postnatal metabolism of the residual hormones.

In the male, the androgen/estrogen imbalance seldom permits significant breast enlargement. Few well-documented hormonal studies performed in the male patient with gynecomastia are available. However, similar asymmetrical presentations of gynecomastia do occur. The size and configuration of the ultimate breast is thereby determined by the finite number of cells in the developing primordia and the vigor of the cellular response to the hormonal situation (2).

CHEST WALL EMBRYOLOGY

The configuration of the chest wall upon which the breasts are located depends primarily on the development of the ribs and sternum and, to a lesser degree, on the relative position of the vertebral bodies. The ribs arise from the costal processes of the embryonic vertebral masses (Fig. 60–2A) (8). In the thoracic and upper region, these processes become bars of varying length that follow the developing body curvatures and encircle the upper portion of the thoracoabdominal cavity. The majority join the ventral sternal

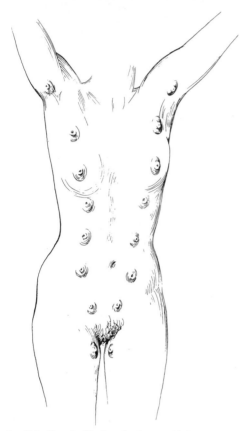

FIG. 60–1. Primitive "milk lines" along which accessory nipples, areolas, or breasts may develop. (From Georgiade NG, Georgiade GS, Riefkohl R. Esthetic breast surgery. In: McCarthy JG, ed. *Plastic surgery.* Philadelphia: WB Saunders, 1990; 3840; modified after Arey [8].)

FIG. 60–2. Development of the anterior ribs and sternum during fetal life. **A,** mesenchymal stage (modified after Peter Kingsley). **B,** cartilaginous stage (at 9 weeks). **C,** ossification centers in a child. (From Arey LB. *Developmental anatomy.* Philadelphia: WB Saunders, 1954; 410).

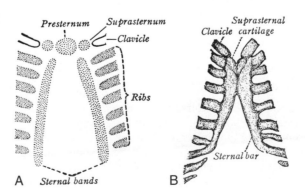
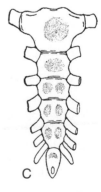

primordia and can be recognized as early as the 6th week of embryonic life. The ribs unite in a craniocaudal direction to complete the thoracic cage (Fig. 60–2B, C). The breast anlagen are supported on this developing and migrating chest wall and thus are subject to any positional errors that may occur.

Errors in Growth and Development

It seems unlikely that circulating hormones could act selectively on breast primordia of equal quantity in similar local environments to effect asymmetry, unless the vascular supply was shown to be significantly asymmetrical. Thus, where the transport systems are symmetrical, hormonal influences should not be a prime factor in the production of breast asymmetry in either sex. However, genetic defects and errors in the embryologic development of the breast and thoracic cage can account for the wide spectrum of asymmetries that are seen in clinical settings.

ABSENCE OF STRUCTURES

The absence of a structure follows a total failure of its anlage (agenesis) or a developmental failure of its anlage (aplasia). When the nipples and areolas are present and equal, an asymmetry of the breast may not be evident until the growth changes of puberty. Absence of the nipples (athelia) and are-

ola always accompanies glandular absence (amazia) to produce a total absence of the breast (amastia), because the nipple-areolar complex is required for the development of the glandular portion of the breast (see discussion above) (Fig. 60–3A). This presentation should be accurately diagnosed in the newborn, because athelia is rarely seen as an isolated defect except in ectodermal dysplasia syndromes (13,14). Despite the absent breast mound, a hypoplastic nipple-areolar complex is almost always found on examination (Fig. 60–3B, C). Unilateral congenital amastia is rare, but Trier found 20 cases in his review of the literature in 1965 (14).

Deformities of the breast have been associated with Poland syndrome, which consists of unilateral breast hypoplasia, deficiency of the pectoralis major and minor muscles, and varying degrees of deformities of the ipsilateral upper extremity, usually syndactyly of the central digits (15–19) (Fig. 60–4). However, many of the reported cases demonstrate minimal deformities of the upper quadrant or upper extremity, which must be present for the diagnosis to be made.

EXCESS STRUCTURES

Ectopic clusters of primordial breast cells retained along the milk line will produce supernumerary nipples (polythelia) and areola in about 5% of patients (13). Curiously, it is more frequently seen in males. The supernumerary nipples are

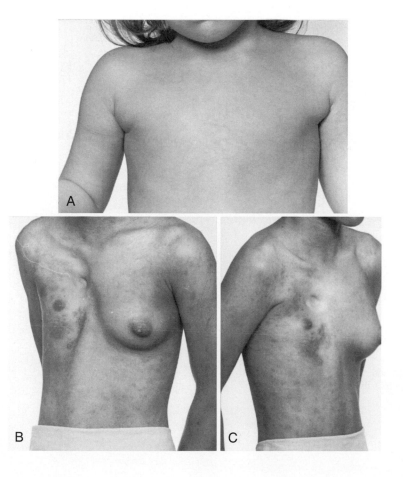

FIG. 60–3. **A,** 2-year-old female patient with nipple-areolas absent. **B, C,** 12-year-old patient with amastia. Note complete absence of breast tissue, with presence of a hypoplastic nipple-areola complex.

FIG. 60–4.   A, 14-year-old girl with breast asymmetry and unilateral breast hypoplasia with diminished development of the pectoralis major and minor muscles. This is a variation of Poland syndrome. **B,** postoperative appearance follows transfer of latissimus dorsi muscular flap and simultaneous augmentation. Note slight increase in size of reconstructed breast in anticipation of future patient growth.

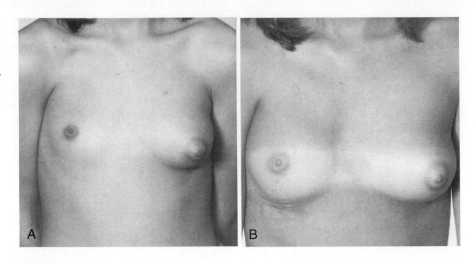

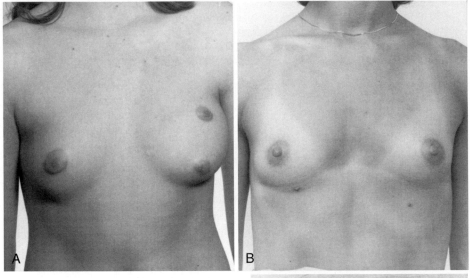

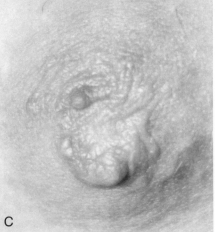

FIG. 60–5.   A, 11-year-old girl with supernumerary nipples and areolas. **B,** 21-year-old female with multiple asymmetric supernumerary nipples. **C,** closeup photo of a bifid nipple.

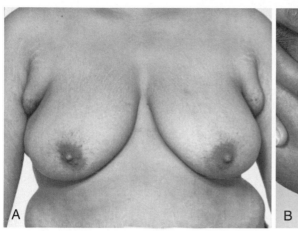
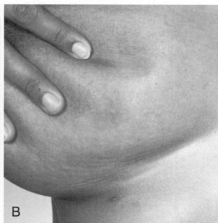

FIG. 60–6. **A,** 26-year-old patient with bilateral axillary ectopic breast tissue. **B,** 26-year-old patient with ectopic mammary tissue in the infra-mammary area. (From Georgiade GS, Lanier VC. Developmental breast abnormalities in children. In: Serafin D, Georgiade NG, eds. *Pediatric plastic surgery.* St. Louis: CV Mosby, 1982; 785.)

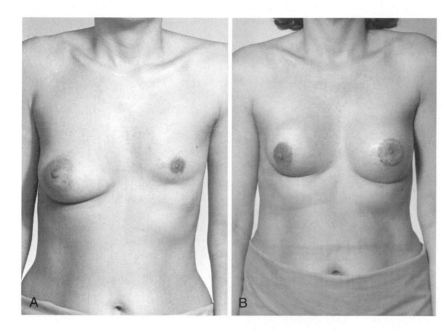

FIG. 60–7. **A,** 33-year-old patient with hypomastia with associated small nipple and areola. **B,** the same patient 3 years after reconstruction, with augmentation and areola sharing procedure.

seen most commonly on the anterior chest and abdomen (Fig. 60–5A, B) but may occur in the axilla or groin as well.

The bifid nipple can be considered an intraareolar form of polythelia, in which both nipples drain functional glandular tissue (10) (Fig. 60–5C).

Retention of extra aggregations of glandular anlage will produce ectopic breast (polymastia). Two percent of patients have ectopic breast tissue, which will occur along the developmental milk line from the axilla to the groin. The most common site is the axilla, followed by the inframammary area (Fig. 60–6). The ectopic breast tissue may include an overlying nipple-areolar complex. Ectopic foci of breast tissue may only become apparent during or after pregnancy and lactation, when hormonally stimulated. Fully developed breasts have also been reported on the back, documenting an embryologic migratory arrest of breast primordia during chest wall development (20,21).

VARIATIONS IN LOCATION

The location of breast structures will depend upon the loci of developing cell aggregations along the mammary ridge and

the developing chest wall. Ectopic nipple, areolar, and glandular tissue usually results in supernumerary structures, but minor variations in the location of two asymmetrical breasts are common.

VARIATIONS IN SIZE

Normally, the sizes of the nipple, areola, and gland show great variation from patient to patient (13). These variations are disturbing when they are asymmetrically present on the same patient. The size of the breast will vary with the individual cellular complement, which is embryologically determined, and the vigor of the response to hormonal stimulation.

The cellular response may be one of increased unit size (hypertrophy) or an increase of cellular numbers (hyperplasia). Similarly, decreased cellular numbers in the primordia (hypoplasia) will produce a small unit (Fig. 60–7). A difference in the number of cells in the primordia would logically set the stage for asymmetry. If cell numbers are finite, and if the hormonal stimulation can be assumed to be equal, then the differences in breast size should depend on the differences in the ability of the cell to respond. The quality of the cell and its ability to respond to hormone stimulation may conceivably be altered by trauma (e.g., surgery, radiation), chronic inflammation, or neoplasm. If the quality of the cells is similar, then the number of cells would account for the majority of congenital asymmetries (2).

Beginning with puberty and continuing through adolescence, some breasts are unusually sensitive to hormonal stimuli. Growth of one or both breasts leading to hypertrophy may occur with apparently normal hormonal function. Massive hypertrophy (virginal hypertrophy) consists histologically of vascular, fibrous, and stromal elements rather than glandular tissue. The causes of massive virginal hypertrophy are not well understood but may relate to progesterone stimulation of the estrogen-primed breast (Fig. 60–8).

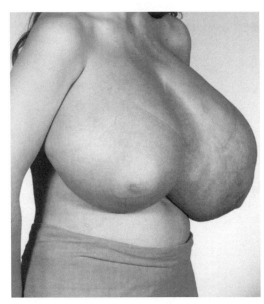

FIG. 60–8. A 13-year-old patient with mammary hypertrophy (gigantism).

VARIATIONS IN SHAPE

The shape of the breast depends primarily upon the arrangement of glandular tissue, the fibrous support structures, and the skin envelope. On the basis of the previous discussions, it might be logical to conclude that quadratic deficiencies are probably related to the pattern of cellular distribution within the anlage (2). Upper-quadrant deficiencies, however, may be related to the effects of gravity.

Aberrations in spatial relationships between the skin, the fibrous support structures, and the gland may produce a breast contour known as the tuberous breast (22,23) (Fig. 60–9). During pubertal development, the circumference of the zone of skin attachment between the breast and the chest wall apparently remains at or near the prepubertal diameter. The skin distal to this attachment expands in the normal fashion to accommodate the developing breast gland. However, complicating this anatomic deformation is laxity of the periareolar fibrous tissue, which allows afascial herniation of some or all of the breast gland, with resulting dilation of the areola. This constellation of deformities may produce a grotesque appearance (Figs. 60–9B and 60–10).

The effects of gravity on the breast mass and the quality and relative size of the skin envelope will influence breast shape in all patients. A significant sagging of the breast (ptosis) may be unilateral, an isolated defect, or it may further complicate another asymmetry. In older females, the relative disproportion of the decreasing glandular mass (atrophy) and its atonic or stretched skin envelope results in ptosis of varying degrees. This disproportion is also seen in the young postpubertal female, especially after childbirth (postpartum atrophy). This deformity may be psychologically distressing enough when bilateral and equal, but is of greater concern when superimposed on asymmetry (Fig. 60–11).

VARIATIONS IN THE NIPPLE-AREOLAR COMPLEX

Size, color, and texture of the nipple, areola, and subjacent Montgomery glands vary widely from patient to patient

FIG. 60–9. A, 25-year-old patient with small, tuberous breasts. **B,** 22-year-old patient with another variant of the tuberous breast.

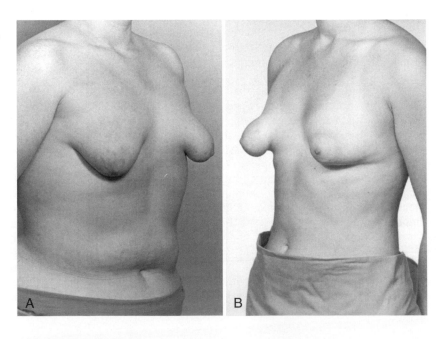

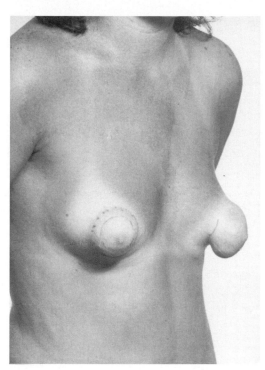

FIG. 60–10. This 15-year-old patient has herniation of the glandular tissue into the base of the nipple area.

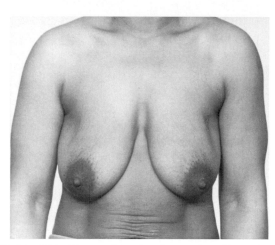

FIG. 60–11. This 30-year-old patient has a class III ptosis and associated asymmetry with markedly decreased breast volume.

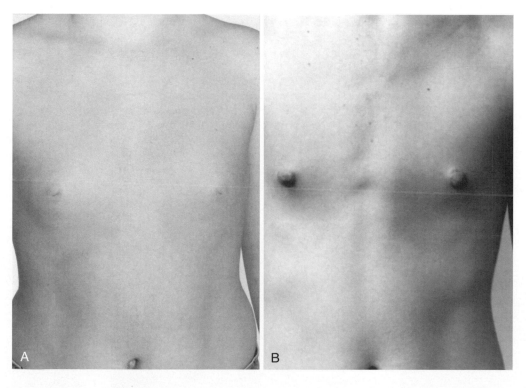

FIG. 60–12. A, 12-year-old male with bilateral inverted nipples. **B,** the same patient 3 years after nipple reconstruction using the Broadbent technique.

(13). In some patients, however, the dermal support of the areola is apparently weak or absent, allowing the breast glandular tissue to "herniate" into the areola guided by its attachment to the nipple (2,24). During the course of development this may distend the areola, and patients have been seen with the majority of their glandular tissue within the areola (see Fig. 60–10).

Excessive projection of the nipple beyond the normal 10 to 12 mm seen in the adult female breast is termed "nipple hypertrophy." It is an unusual occurrence, and many cases are associated with hypomastia. Occasionally, functional nipple hypertrophy is seen following prolonged nursing.

An inverted nipple may be congenital or may be acquired from malignancies, infection, or surgical deformation.

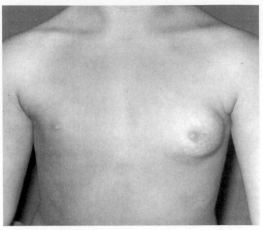

FIG. 60–13. An 11-year-old female with a large angiomatous mass involving the subareolar and left chest area.

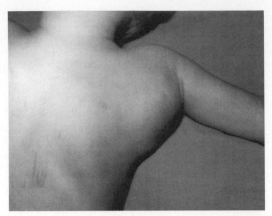

FIG. 60–14. A 7-year-old female patient with a large hemangioma involving the left chest and axilla.

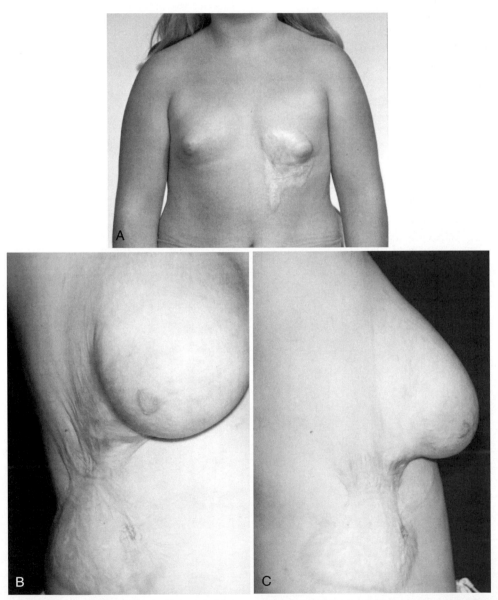

FIG. 60–15. **A,** 11-year-old female with distortion in size and shape of the left breast and nipple-areola area following a 3rd-degree thermal burn that was allowed to heal without skin grafting. **B,** anterior view of right breast of a 20-year-old female with a major burn scar deformity, showing contracture across the lateral inframammary fold and anterior axillary line that produced downward and outward deformity of the nipple-areola complex. **C,** lateral view, demonstrating the skin deficit produced by the burn scar contracture.

Congenital inverted nipples may have as much as a 50% familial tendency, as reported by Skoog (25). The typical congenital inverted nipple consists of three components: (a) fibrous bands and a hypoplastic ductal system that tether the nipple in the inverted position; (b) a lack of smooth muscle fibers, which prevent normal eversion, in the nipple; and (c) fibrous tissue found beneath the inverted nipple that is only half the normal thickness (Fig. 60–12). However, inverted nipples are usually functional in milk production and sexual stimulation.

VARIATIONS IN CHEST WALL STRUCTURE

Asymmetry of the breast may either complicate, or result from, a deformity of the chest wall, the sternum, or the vertebral column (18). Problems can occur in the transport of the breast anlage on the maldeveloped chest wall (as in scoliosis), or there may be unilateral underdevelopment of the bony thorax, its covering muscles, and the ipsilateral breast in almost any combination (e.g., Poland syndrome, mentioned above).

Patients with scoliosis will frequently appear to have asymmetrical breasts; however, the discrepancy is one of position rather than size. The breasts may be of equal size, but they appear unequal because the asymmetrical chest wall positions one breast inferiorly and posteriorly to the other (2).

Acquired Asymmetry

The number, size, shape, and position of the breasts may be altered by trauma, surgery, inflammation, or neoplasm. Failure of patient development can result from a variety of acquired conditions and may be unilateral. Among the more common iatrogenic causes of total breast failure are surgical removal of a tender mass from beneath the areola of a prepubertal childhood female (prepubertal mastitis) or the irradiation of a benign tumor (e.g., a large chest-wall and/or axillary hemangioma) (Figs. 60–13, 60–14). Distortion or incomplete breast development may be seen after significant burns of the anterior chest and breast (Fig. 60–15).

In the young adult, the benign giant fibroadenoma is a tumor capable of producing a gross unilateral enlargement of the breast (Fig. 60–16). In rare instances, a low-grade malignancy, cystosarcoma phylloides, may present in the adolescent patient, also producing unilateral asymmetry. The premalignant and malignant tumors of older patients may also cause gross unilateral distortion, and the associated deformities of simple, modified (Fig. 60–17A), or radical (Fig. 60–17B) mastectomy are well known and well discussed in the literature (26). To review the etiologies and the treatment of these conditions is beyond the scope of this presentation (26–30).

Infection (mastitis) does not occur frequently in the antibiotic era but has produced contour deformities in the past. Cu-

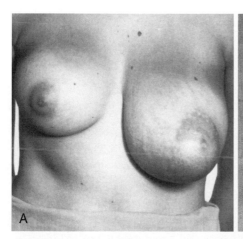 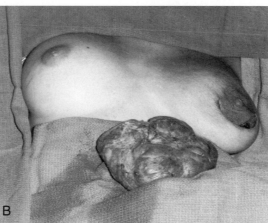

FIG. 60–16. **A,** 17-year-old patient with a large fibroadenoma involving the left breast. **B,** the size of this benign fibroadenoma at the time of excision.

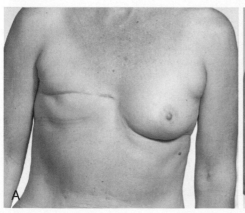 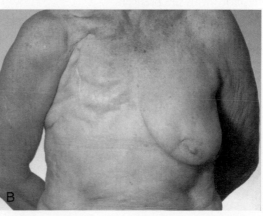

FIG. 60–17. The types of resultant postoperative deformity created by (**A**) modified radical mastectomy, and (**B**) radical mastectomy (Halsated).

taneous infections are seen but rarely penetrate to the glandular tissue in the absence of invasive trauma. Fortunately, infection severe enough to result in an irreversible asymmetry is rare.

Patient Evaluation

The clinical evaluation of the patient with asymmetrical breasts requires a detailed history, psychosocial evaluation, and physical examination. This information is collated for the patient in the postexamination patient conference (3,30).

PREEXAMINATION HISTORY

As with most surgical candidates, a focused history will be supplemented by an inventory of the patient's general condition. This sequence will highlight the patient's presenting complaint. The specific history of breast development and breast pathology will focus the consultative direction. Specific historical events that may explain asymmetrical deformities are explored in greater detail. An adequate history always lends increased safety to any surgical procedure by offering the opportunity to correct systemic or regional medical conditions that might interfere with anesthesia or surgery (2,10).

PSYCHOSOCIAL EVALUATION

The motivation and stability of the patient seeking elective correction of breast asymmetry deserves special evaluation if a successful result is to be achieved. The patient with a gross asymmetry has usually been subjected to great psychosocial pressures from efforts to hide the deformity. The motivation for correction is usually even greater than that seen in patients with symmetrical deformities (2).

Judgement of the psychologic stability or instability is important. It must be weighed against the severity of the deformity, the complexity of the appropriate surgical reconstruction, and the likelihood of obtaining an anatomic improvement that will be pleasing to the patient and acceptable to the surgeon. Early in the era of elective mammaplastic surgery, a psychiatric consultation was frequently mandatory, especially preceding augmentation mammaplasty (31). Today, based on increased personal experience and the published experience of others, the plastic surgeon routinely assumes the responsibility for the psychosocial evaluation (32). Occasionally, more than a single preoperative consultation is required to arrive at a decision, but the experienced surgeon's familiarity with the preoperative emotional stress and the postoperative stability and gratitude expressed by the majority of these patients will usually result in a decision to proceed with corrective surgery. Occasionally, a second opinion may clarify the appropriate course, but only the obviously unstable patient will need formal psychiatric consultation.

PHYSICAL EXAMINATION

The physical examination may confirm or deny suspicions gained from the history. The clothed body posture, noted while taking the history, is now contrasted with the unclothed presentation. Unless a complete physical examination is indicated by the history, the office examination is generally lim-

ited to the upper torso, and the general physical examination is done on the day of surgery.

The examination of each breast should include evaluation of the skin cover, nipple, areola, and gland with the patient standing, first with the arms by the sides in a relaxed attitude and then with the arms elevated over the head. The gland and axillary lymph node fields are also evaluated with the patient in the supine position with the arms both abducted and adducted on the chest wall. This detailed breast examination should uncover the majority of pathologic changes.

Examination of the muscles of the chest wall and the configuration of the bony thoracic cage—including sternum, ribs, vertebral column, and scapulae—is essential and should be carried out anteriorly, posteriorly, and from each side. Variations in the anteroposterior and transverse dimensions of each hemithorax are noted, and the vertical alignment of the thoracic cylinder is observed. Differences in muscle mass and shoulder position may be significant (18). Detection of a small scapula on the same side as a hypoplastic breast may indicate the necessity for further evaluation to exclude other bony congenital abnormalities (2).

Finally, a comparison of the breasts and an evaluation of their relationships to each other, to the chest wall, and to the body as a whole will be needed for definition of symmetry or lack thereof. The relative volume, shape, and position of the breasts and the size, color, and relative location of the nipples and areolas are compared, as are shoulder levels and thoracic contours. Techniques for elevation of breast volume have been described, but their inherent volumetric discrepancies are usually so significant as to preclude their routine use (33–35). Mammography is used only when the neoplasm is suspected in the preoperative patient.

PHOTOGRAPHIC RECORDS

Before the patient re-dresses, a photographic record is made. Nelson and Krause (36) have discussed the standard views, which include an anterior view with the arms slightly abducted (which becomes the reference view); an anterior view with the arms elevated above the head, which allows documentation of the glandular size and contours; and right and left lateral oblique views with the arms at rest and elevated over the head to define the profile of the breast. Special views are added as required to document unusual anatomic presentation. Emphasis should be placed on consistency of composition and reproduction in the sequential photographic record (36).

POSTEXAMINATION CONFERENCE

The consultation is completed with a review of the patient's desires regarding breast size and contour. Then, the surgeon's opinion of the realistic goals of surgical treatment is presented and the goals are compared. The closer the goals of patient and surgeon, the more satisfactory will be the outcome of the surgical correction.

The required surgical scars, and their placement, are emphasized, and if there are limitations to the ultimate cosmetic result because of the nature or severity of the deformity, these limitations are clearly defined. It is important to document these limitations and their discussion in the patient's record. Any surgical procedure that will interfere with the

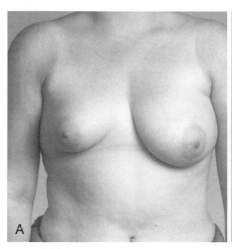 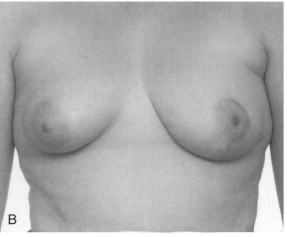

FIG. 60–18. **A,** 22-year-old patient with micromastia of one breast and macromastia of opposite breast. **B,** the same patient 15 months following a reduction mammaplasty and mastopexy.

ductal integrity (e.g., breast reduction or mastopexy, nipple reduction, correction of bifidity, or correction of inversion of the nipples) should be discussed in detail. The probable inability to breastfeed any future children should be explained in detail to the patient and her mother. If breastfeeding is desired, certain surgical procedures should be postponed until after childbearing is completed.

If the clinical history and presentation suggest tumor as the causative factor, an appropriate tumor management protocol must be established until the proper histologic and clinical staging can be established. The experienced surgeon, with adequate pathology laboratory support, can offer immediate reconstruction of the breast.

Finally, the more common potential complications are discussed. When all questions have been answered and the patient seems adequately informed about the proposed therapy, the conditions are properly set for patient cooperation and mutual satisfaction.

Surgical Planning

The individual requirements and desires, the available tissues, and the techniques required for reconstruction are inventoried and recorded during the patient evaluation. Any special or unusual problems deserve special notation, with subsequent study or consultation on the part of the surgeon. Selection of techniques that are both established and familiar to the surgeon will tend to enhance the result and minimize difficulties in execution.

CORRECTION OF GLANDULAR ASYMMETRY

If the history and physical examination indicate that an appropriate breast exists on one side, the other breast can be augmented, reduced, expanded, or repositioned to produce the desired balance in size, contour, and position. When a greater volume is desired in both breasts, balance is achieved by unequal augmentation. The weight and physiologic descent (postsurgical ptosis) should be anticipated preoperatively for either the augmented or the reduced breast. The greater weight of the silicone gel-filled prosthesis will produce breast ptosis faster than saline-filled prosthesis. Some

quadratic defects may benefit from the use of custom prosthesis to achieve better symmetry.

When both breasts are larger than desired, the amount of gland excision can be varied as each side is reduced. More unusual asymmetries will require special, and often unique, planning. Volume match of the breast gland is usually easier to obtain than symmetry of position and shape.

Perhaps the most difficult deformities of glandular inequality to balance aesthetically are micromasty on one side and macromastia on the other (Fig. 60–18). Correction of each of these basic problems is quite different. When they present concurrently, the surgeon is faced with the difficult problem of judging the operative position of the reconstructed breasts. The decreased weight of the reduced breast will slow the rate of physiologic ptosis on that side, while the weight and volume of the prosthesis will gradually stretch the skin envelope and increase the rate of descent of the augmented breast. When an associated ptosis must be corrected along with the augmentation and/or reduction, the result may be more satisfactory, because scars are now bilateral, the quality of the skin envelope is likely to be equal, and the volume of the cover and contents can be more effectively controlled.

The advent of tissue-expansion techniques has provided the reconstructive surgeon with a new method for treating glandular asymmetry. An expansion device with a buried injection reservoir is placed and the volume can be increased and adjusted over a period of time. The tissue expansion device can be replaced by a permanent prosthesis when the desired size and ptosis matches the fully developed opposite breast (Fig. 60–19). Recently, a double-lumen gel/saline expandable prosthesis has been described that is designed to allow removal of only the filling port and connecting tubing (16). Satisfactory results in the treatment of glandular asymmetry, tubular breasts, and Poland syndrome with athelia have been reported (14,16,37). The use of this prosthesis in the adolescent patient, with a treatment protocol of gradual volume expansion over several years to keep pace with the unaffected breast as it enlarges and descends, offers correction at a much younger age. This treatment protocol also allows a potentially reversible correction (device removal) if delayed breast development should occur.

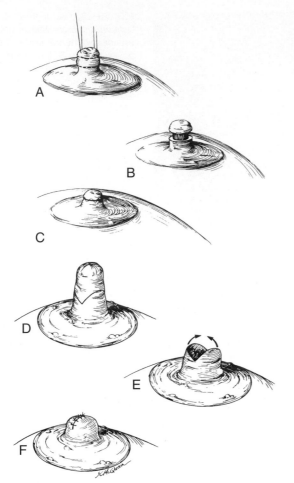

FIG. 60–19. A–C, the preferred technique for nipple reduction. **D–F,** alternate method of a lesser nipple reduction, of particular use in an older patient.

CORRECTION OF NIPPLE-AREOLAR ASYMMETRY

Nipples may vary greatly in their presentation, color, and prominence. Simple reduction of nipple height can be accomplished by several techniques for balance (13,38) (see Fig. 60–19). Correction of nipple inversion is more difficult, as noted by the large number of proposed corrections in the literature (25) (see Fig. 60–12). Most produce inconsistent results at best.

Variations in the size and color of the areolas may be improvable. When the areola is being repositioned for any reason, a simultaneous reduction of its circumference is readily accomplished. Enlargement, on the other hand, is more difficult, and the results are less aesthetic. Physiological areolar enlargement may follow augmentation. Areolar sharing, saving, and tattooing have their advocates (38–43).

Total reconstruction of an absent nipple and areola is somewhat more complex (10). However, Georgiade and others (43) improved the aesthetic results through their work utilizing a large chest flap to construct the nipple and thick areola in the postmastectomy patient. This procedure was later modified by Little and Spear (38). Currently, three techniques seem to offer the most reproducible results for the appropriate indications. Free grafts of oral mucosa reproduce the lighter pink nulliparous areola and free grafts of labia minora or upper, inner thigh provide the darker brown pigmentation for the multiparous nipple and areola. Both of these techniques are frequently augmented or supplanted by tattooing (38,39,42–44). Timing of nipple reconstruction is somewhat procedurally dependent. Most surgeons will delay total nipple/areolar reconstruction until the breast mound has settled, which may be as long as 6 months.

Attention must also be paid to the relative size and position of the nipple-areolar complex and the effects of any herniation present preoperatively. Reconstruction of the areolar hernia, and reduction of the areolar size with reconstruction of the dermal planes beneath the nipple and perhaps subpectoral placement of the prosthesis, are all useful adjuncts in correcting this severe problem.

With most ptosis and reduction procedures, allowance must be made for a postoperative descent of the breast mass toward the lower quadrants. This maybe accompanied by an upward and medial migration of the nipple and areola.

CORRECTION OF CHEST-WALL ASYMMETRY

Reconstruction of chest-wall deformities will depend upon the severity and location of the defect. Minor deformities can be minimized by the addition of breast volume or the rearrangement of the breast mass. More significant deformities may be improved by the use of the custom-made prostheses created from a moulage model (2), or by reconstruction with a choice of several skin or myocutaneous flaps (45,46). The former approach is considered for pectoral muscle deficiency and the latter has been used for correction of pectus excavatum (47). Bony reconstruction of rib-cage and sternal defects is usually not indicated in the absence of cardiopulmonary dysfunction, except in severe cases of pectus carinatum. A muscle flap transfer, or repositioning of the insertion of the latissimus dorsi myocutaneous flap in postmastectomy reconstruction, may add that final touch of symmetry in the selected case (17,48).

CORRECTION OF ACQUIRED ASYMMETRICAL DEFECTS

Many of the factors in surgical planning for the correction of developmental errors will obviously apply to a variety of acquired deformities as well. The cause of the deformity may alter treatment choices.

Posttraumatic deformities are unusual and varied, and their treatment is highly individualized. Contracted burn scars, for example, may limit breast development or distort existing structures and require release of interpositional flaps (Z-plasties) or skin flaps (49). Treatment protocols may also include repositioning of the remaining breast structures and, occasionally, augmentation with or without tissue expansion, as discussed above (26,37,50). In general, the use of myocutaneous flap techniques for breast reconstruction (transabdominal rectus myocutaneous flap) or the latissimus dorsi myocutaneous flap have obviated the use of the breast-sharing techniques (15,26).

CORRECTION OF TUMOFACTIVE ASYMMETRY

Unilateral gigantomastia with glandular hyperplasia may require breast reduction and supplemental hormonal therapy to achieve control of the problem. Regrowth is occasionally seen, and total mastectomy to control glandular growth has been required (40,51). Then, breast reconstruction is appropriate as for any mastectomized patient.

Giant fibroadenomata of the breast displaces the glandular breast and stretches the skin envelope severely. The tumor is readily separated from the cover and gland, but tailoring of the skin brassiere is usually required. The less common cystosarcoma phylloides is considered to be a low-grade malignant disease and is capable of producing gross asymmetry. There is incomplete agreement on its management but resection of the tumor is required. Once the ablation is complete, appropriate reconstruction can be carried out, depending on the clinical and histologic staging (52–54) (Fig. 60–16).

Surgical Regimens

PREOPERATIVE PREPARATION

Augmentation procedures and minor revisions are usually accomplished on an outpatient basis. Patients requiring a reduction mammaplasty or correction of a major chest-wall deformity are usually admitted following surgery for a short hospital stay. Skin hygiene and the removal of axillary hair are done by the patient before entering the hospital.

ANESTHESIA

Most breast procedures, except for reconstruction of the nipple-areolar complex and minor revisions, are performed under general anesthesia for patient comfort. Simple augmentation mammaplasty may be performed under local infiltration anesthesia supplemented by intravenous short-acting sedation under appropriate circumstances.

OPERATIVE SEQUENCE

Neither augmentation, reduction, nor reconstruction should present great technical difficulties for the accomplished surgeon. When bilateral augmentation is required, it may be helpful to operate first on the breast that is nearest to the desired volume. Then, the contralateral breast is either augmented or reduced to match. Insufflation of the dissected cavity, the "air pocket technique," is a useful technique to determine both the size requirements and the contours achieved by the pocket dissection (45).

However, when an augmentation and a reduction are required on the same patient, the reduction is usually done first and the resulting volume matched with augmentation. If there is any question about the limitation of volume by the skin brassiere, it may be better to do the augmentation first.

It is helpful to have a wide range of prosthetic sizes available when treating any type of asymmetry. In addition, the use of an inflatable permanent prosthesis or a tissue-expansion device to correct the specific problem will have been identified and procured in the preoperative evaluation.

Prosthetic placement in either the subglandular or the submuscular dissection plane is left to the choice of the surgeon with the notation that, in contradistinction to the standard augmentation mammaplasty, anatomic variations resulting in a thin or small pectoralis major muscle may significantly restrict the muscle coverage available. The submuscular position is favored by most surgeons to minimize encapsulation of the prosthesis.

POSTOPERATIVE CARE

Some form of mild compression dressing is used after all mammaplasties. Augmented breasts are fitted with a gentle compression brassiere (without wire inserts). Patients having breast reduction or mastopexy procedures are dressed with a bulky anterior compression dressing secured with tape. Suction drains are rarely used for any type of mammaplasty unless indicated by the clinical situation. Antibiotics are continued for 5 days after surgery when used in conjunction with prosthesis placement. Restriction of mild activities is minimal, with patient comfort as a gauge, but vigorous physical activities are avoided for 1 month.

COMPLICATIONS

The shape of the breast is not always ideal after reduction and repositioning procedures, but this is more often an inherent fault of the procedure rather than of the surgeon. Good results have been obtained with a wide variety of techniques, but no one operation may be best for all patients, and the procedure chosen should fit the patient.

Serious postoperative complications (e.g., massive hematoma, infection, tissue slough, loss of a prosthesis) should be rare when the surgery is carefully planned and executed. Meticulous hemostasis is essential in all breast surgery, and the attentive surgeon is ever alert for excessive bleeding, especially where glandular tissue has been divided and fascial planes widely opened. Late serum or serosanguineous collections may be removed under antibiotic coverage, with salvage of the prosthesis in most cases. Early replacement of a lost prosthesis is urgent, especially after subcutaneous placement, when the expanded skin with a subjacent capsule tends to wrinkle.

Malposition of a mammary prosthesis is a preventable complication for which reoperation may be required (Fig. 60–20). Enlargement of the existing pocket is not always successful and, in our experience, formation of a new pocket in the submuscular plane (but in the correct location) is the best approach. Ptosis of the breast over the surface of a prosthesis that is adherent to the chest wall is seen less commonly since the introduction of the patchless prosthesis. Management of skin excesses by mastopexy can improve the ptotic condition, but the patient must be aware of the aesthetic limitations.

It is now well accepted by most surgeons that the placement of a silicone device anywhere in the body generates a fibroblastic response. This response, when seen in the postoperative breast surgery patient, is termed *encapsulation*. Although it can change a soft, natural contour into a firm, unattractive, spherical mass (Fig. 60–21), encapsulation must still be regarded as a natural bodily response to a foreign body, and thus be considered "normal" (54,55). Various therapeutic regimens to control encapsulation, such as prolonged binding of the breast, proved unacceptable to most patients (and were ineffective as well). Steroids, placed intraluminally in the prosthesis and intraoperatively in the dissected pocket, have been used in both primary and secondary augmentation procedures with only mixed success. Most well-controlled studies have indicated that there seems to be little long-term benefit in maintaining freedom from encapsulation, and there have been significant complications reported from such attempts (55).

FIG. 60–20. Breast asymmetry caused by malposition of a breast prosthesis. **A,** left lateral oblique view demonstrating deformity of the left breast caused by superior malposition of the breast prosthesis. **B,** left lateral oblique view demonstrating restoration of the appropriate contour by open capsulotomy and repositioning of the prosthesis in the submuscular position. A mastopexy has been performed on the right breast to correct the Class I ptosis.

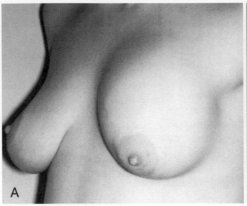 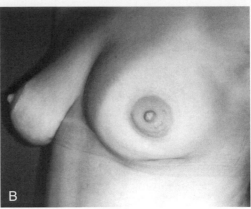

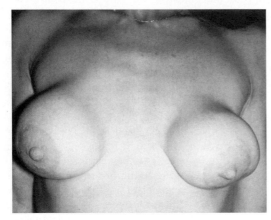

FIG. 60–21. Breast asymmetry secondary to severe fibrous capsular contracture of long duration.

Baker and colleagues (56) described the manual external closed capsulotomy, and this was the primary method of managing mild and moderate breast encapsulation. Some have found this open capsulotomy of benefit for moderate to severe capsular contracture. Relocation of the prosthesis in a newly created pocket below the pectoralis major muscle has produced satisfactory results. However, the controversy surrounding the silicone gel breast implants has emphasized the fragile and finite nature of the shell of the implant. Closed capsulotomy is rarely performed now, and only with the fullest of informed consents.

The surgeon should have an appreciation of the limited life span of silicone gel implants and be prepared to exchange them if the implants rupture. Replacement with another silicone gel implant is still possible with strict compliance to the bureaucratic and legal guidelines. Frequently, however, patients will request saline-filled implants instead. The less-than-satisfactory results with saline-filled breast implants has been noted.

The loss of nipple sensation and erection is predictable with free nipple/areolar transplantation, but may be noted as a complication of any operation on the breast. Temporary loss of sensation is reported occasionally after simple augmentation, but it is usually avoidable if the 4th and 5th intercostal nerves are preserved during the operative dissection (45,57,58). We are at a loss to explain the wide variations of patient response to seemingly similar operative techniques, but the inconsistent anatomy of the neurovascular perforator from beneath the serratus anterior muscle may play a role. If lateral movement of this nerve is required for good access to the dissection pocket, it may be gently mobilized and reset laterally, thus enhancing preservation of nipple erection and sensation. With recognition of this variation, postaugmentation sensation may be more consistent.

Acknowledgment. The authors wish to acknowledge that patients cared for by James A. Edmond, James L. Dolph, Debbie A. Kennedy, and Marc E. Gottlieb are included in the cases presented.

References

1. Gorney M, Harries T. The preoperative and postoperative consideration of natural facial asymmetry. *Plast Reconstr Surg* 1974; 54:187.
2. Elliott RA Jr, Hoehn JG. Asymmetrical breasts. In: Georgiade NG, ed. *Aesthetic breast surgery.* Baltimore: Williams & Wilkins, 1983; 110.
3. Elliott RA Jr, Hoehn JG, Greminger RF. Correction of asymmetrical breasts. *Plast Reconstr Surg* 1975; 56:260.
4. Simon BE, Hoffman S, Kahn S. Treatment of asymmetry of the breasts. *Clin Plast Surg* 1975; 2:375.
5. Maliniac JW. *Breast deformities and their repair.* Baltimore: Waverly Press, 1950; 153. (Reissued by Krieger Publishing Co., Huntington, New York, in 1971.)
6. Regnault P. Ptosis, asymmetry, tubular breast and congenital anomalies. In: Owsley JQ, Peterson R, eds. *Symposium on aesthetic surgery of the breast.* St. Louis: CV Mosby, 1978; 109.
7. Hueston JT. Unilateral agenesis and hypoplasia: difficulties and suggestions. In: Goldwyn RM, ed. *Plastic and reconstructive surgery of the breast.* Boston: Little, Brown, 1976; 361.
8. Arey LB. *Developmental anatomy.* Philadelphia: WB Saunders, 1954; 410, 452.
9. Chatterton RT Jr. Mammary gland: development and secretion. *Obstet Gynecol Ann* 1978; 7:303.
10. Vanik RK, Georgiade GS. Congenital and developmental breast anomalies. In: Georgiade NG, et al., eds. *Essentials of plastic, maxillofacial and reconstructive surgery.* Baltimore: Williams & Wilkins, 1987; 673.
11. Porter JC. Hormonal regulation of breast development and activity. *J Invest Dermatol* 1974; 63:85.
12. Jacobs LS. The role of prolactin in mammogenesis and lactogenesis. *Adv Exp Med Biol* 1977; 80:173.
13. Teimourian B, Adham MN. Congenital anomalies of nipple and areola. In: Georgiade NG, ed. *Aesthetic breast surgery.* Baltimore: Williams & Wilkins, 1983; 347.
14. Trier WC. Complete breast absence. *Plast Reconstr Surg* 1965; 36:430.
15. Amovoso PJ, Augelasts J. Latissimus dorsi myocutaneous flap in Poland syndrome. *Ann Plast Surg* 1981; 6:287.
16. Becker H. Expansion augmentation. *Clin Plast Surg* 1988; 15:587.
17. Hester TR, Bostwick J. Poland syndrome: correction with latissimus muscle transposition. *Plast Reconstr Surg* 1982; 69:226.

18. Pers M. Aplastias of the anterior thoracic wall, the pectoral muscles and the breast. *Scand J Plast Reconstr Surg* 1968; 2:125.
19. Ravitch MM. Poland syndrome—a study of an eponym. *Plast Reconstr Surg* 1977; 59:508.
20. Castano M. Dorsal scapular supernumerary breast in a woman. *Plast Reconstr Surg* 1969; 43:536.
21. Kaye BL. Axillary breasts. *Plast Reconstr Surg* 1974; 53:61.
22. Rees TD, Aston SJ. The tuberous breast. *Clin Plast Surg* 1976; 3:339.
23. Teimourian B, Adham MN. Surgical correction of the tuberous breast. *Ann Plast Surg* 1983; 10:190.
24. Bass CB. Herniated areolar complex. *Ann Plast Surg* 1978; 1:40.
25. Skoog T. An operation for inverted nipples. *Br J Plast Surg* 1952; 5:65.
26. Hartrampf CR Jr, Scheflan M, Black PW. Breast reconstruction following mastectomy with a vascular island rectus abdominus myocutnaeous flap. Presented at the annual meeting of the American Association of Plastic Surgeons, Williamsburg, VA, May 1981.
27. Bostwick J, Scheflan M. The latissimus dorsi musculocutaneous flap: a one-stage reconstruction. *Clin Plast Surg* 1980; 7:71.
28. Gant TD, Vasconez LO. Latissimus dorsi musculocutaneous flap breast reconstruction. In: Gant TD, Vasconez LO, eds. *Postmastectomy reconstruction.* Baltimore: Williams & Wilkins, 1976; 103.
29. Snyderman RK, ed. *Symposium on neoplastic and reconstruction problems of the female breast.* St. Louis: CV Mosby, 1973; 65.
30. McGregor GI, Knowling MA, Este FA. Sarcoma and cystoscarcoma phylloides tumors of the breast: a restrospective review of 58 cases. *Am Jour Surg* 1994; 167:477–480.
31. Corso PF. Plastic surgery of the unilateral hypoplastic breast: a report of eight cases. *Plast Reconstr Surg* 1972; 50:134.
32. Grossman AR. Psychologic and psychosexual aspects of augmentation mammaplasty. *Clin Plast Surg* 1976; 3:167.
33. Gifford S. Emotional attitudes toward cosmetic breast surgery: loss and restitution of the "ideal self." In: Goldwyn RM, ed. *Plastic and reconstructive surgery of the breast.* Boston: Little, Brown, 1976; 103.
34. Bouman FG. Volumetric measurement of the human breast and breast tissue before and during mammaplasty. *Br J Plast Surg* 1970; 23:236.
35. Brody GS. Breast implant size selection and patient satisfaction. *Plast Reconstr Surg* 1981; 68:611.
36. Kirianoff TG. Volume measurements of unequal breasts. *Plast Reconstr Surg* 1974; 54:616.
37. Nelson GD, Krause JL Jr. *Clinical photography in plastic surgery.* Boston: Little, Brown, 1988; 82, 84–85.
38. Argenta LC, Vander Kolk C, Friedman RJ, et al. Refinements in reconstruction of congenital breast deformities. *Plast Reconstr Surg* 1985; 76:73.
39. Little JW, Spear SL. The finishing touches in nipple areola reconstruction. *Perspect Plastic Surg* 1988; 2:1.
40. Georgiade N. *Breast reconstruction following mastectomy.* St. Louis: CV Mosby, 1979.
41. Mayl N, Vasconez L, Jurkiewicz M. Treatment of micromastia in the actively enlarging breast. *Plast Reconstr Surg* 1974; 54:6.
42. Millard DR Jr. Nipple and areola reconstruction by split-skin graft from the normal side. *Plast Reconstr Surg* 1972; 50:350.
43. Wexler RM. Areolar sharing to reconstruct the absent nipple. *Plast Reconstr Surg* 1973; 51:176.
44. Georgiade G, Riefkohl R, Georgiade N. To share or not to share. *Ann Plast Surg* 1985; 14:180.
45. Brent B. Nipple-areolar reconstruction following mastectomy: an alternative to the use of labial and contralateral nipple areolar tissues. *Clin Plast Surg* 1979; 6:95.
46. Hoehn JG, Elliott RA Jr. Use of an air pocket for estimation during augmentation mammaplasty. *Plast Reconstr Surg* 1979; 63:273.
47. Hoffman S. Recurrent deformities following reduction mammaplasty and corection of breast asymmetry. *Plast Reconstr Surg* 1986; 78:55.
48. Masson JK, Payne WS, Gonzalez JB. Pectus excavatum: use of preformed prosthesis for correction in adults. *Plast Reconstr Surg* 1970; 46:399.
49. Pierre M, Jouglard J. Treatment of unilateral congenital hypoplasia or absence of the breast. Presented at the annual meeting of the American Society of Plastic and Reconstructive Surgeons, Houston, TX, October 1974.
50. Neale HW, Smith GL, Gregory RO, et al. Breast reconstruction in the burned adolescent female (an 11-year, 157-patient experience). *Plast Reconstr Surg* 1982; 70:718.
51. Versaci AD, Balkovich ME, Goldstein SA. Breast reconstruction by tissue expansion for congenital and burn deformities. *Ann Plast Surg* 1986; 16:20.
52. Ship AG, Shulman J. Virginal and gravid mammary gigantism: recurrence after reduction mammaplasty. *Br J Plast Surg* 1971; 24:396.
53. Donegan WL. Sarcomas of the breast. In: Spratt JS, Donegan WL, eds. *Cancer of the breast.* Philadelphia: WB Saunders, 1967; 246.
54. Hafner CD, Mezger E, Wylie JH. Cystosacroma phylloides of the breast. *Surg Gynecol Obstet* 1962; 115:29.
55. Mandel MA, DePalma RG, Gogt C, et al. Cystosarcoma phylloides: treatment of subcutaneous mastectomy and immediate prosthetic implantation. *Am J Surg* 1972; 123:718.
56. Baker JL Jr. Augmentation mammaplasty. In: Owsley JQ, Peterson RA, eds. *Symposium on aesthetic surgery of the breast.* St. Louis: CV Mosby, 1978; 256.
57. Baker JL, Bartles RJ, Douglas WM. Closed compression technique for rupturing a contracted capsule around a breast implant. *Plast Reconstr Surg* 1976; 58:137.
58. Craig RDP, Sykes PA. Nipple senstivity following reduction mammaplasty. *Br J Plast Surg* 1970; 23:165.
59. Townsend P. Nipple sensation following breast reduction and free nipple transposition. *Br J Plastic Surg* 1974; 27:308.

61

Augmentation Mammaplasty

H. Hollis Caffee, M.D., F.A.C.S.

Breast augmentation is an aesthetic surgical procedure that until recently was one of the most frequent in the practice of plastic surgery. In general, the operation yields very satisfactory results and the vast majority of patients would have the operation again (1). Recently, the operation has become the source of great controversy that has only minimal basis in science, but was generated by a curious mixture of the media, the tort system, and politics. Despite the fact that the operation yields consistently good results, it does have problems, some of which have known significance and others for which the significance is unknown.

History of Breast Augmentation

The first reported attempts at breast augmentation were paraffin injections in 1904. The results were disastrous, leaving patients with hard masses and draining sinus tracts. In the 1950s and 1960s, some practitioners began injecting liquid silicone. The initial results from these injections were often good, but most patients eventually developed painful nodularity and inflammation that could only be corrected by mastectomy. Incredibly, this practice can still be found today, but is employed only by unscrupulous physicians and—perhaps more often—by lay people. The history of breast augmentation is, essentially, the history of implant development and that history is still evolving.

Surgically placed implants appeared in 1958; the first of these were Ivalon sponges, made from polyvinyl alcohol. Fibrous tissue invaded these sponge implants, causing them to shrink and become hard. Attempts to solve this problem by covering the sponge with various plastic envelopes were still not satisfactory and breast augmentation fell into disrepute (2).

In 1963, Cronin and Gerow (3) reported the use of the silicone gel prosthesis, which remained the standard until recently. The implant industry was not subject to government regulation initially, and even after the FDA was given a mandate to regulate medical devices several years went by before the attention of that agency was directed toward the gel implant. As the time of the hearings approached, a very vocal minority of implant patients directed a campaign alleging a wide variety of diseases that they claimed were a result of silicone exposure. They were joined in this effort by the trial lawyers and "consumer advocate" (4) organizations. Just as the time for a decision was due from the FDA, the commissioner, David Kessler, called for a moratorium on the use of gel implants and later restricted them to tightly controlled protocol studies, effectively ending the use of the device (5).

The saline-filled implant, which had been in use almost as long as the gel-filled implant, became the implant of choice. The regulatory future of the saline-filled implant is still uncertain, and to date no other material has been found to be satisfactory for construction of a breast implant.

Preoperative Considerations

PREOPERATIVE EVALUATION

During the initial patient interview, the patient's motives for seeking breast augmentation should be explored. Those patients who are trying to improve their own self-image are usually appropriate candidates. However, some women will seek breast augmentation at the urging of a male partner, or they may want larger breasts in order to gain the attention of a potential male partner. This group should be considered to be questionable candidates because they may be bitterly disappointed if they do not get the anticipated response. Most women who seek breast augmentation are mature and in stable relationships. Often they are troubled by postpartum atrophy and will sometimes relate that during pregnancy was the only time they were happy with the appearance of their breasts. Younger women who request augmentation are typically those with minimal breast development. They will usually relate a feeling of inadequacy. It is important to recognize that, with few exceptions, the women who request augmentation do not perceive themselves as normal and seeking larger than normal breasts. They consider their condition to be an abnormality that they wish to correct. Most will request enough augmentation to bring them up to a size they consider to be average.

A thorough history should be obtained with emphasis on any preexisting breast disease or family history of breast cancer. The physical examination should be complete, and must include careful palpation for any breast masses or enlarged axillary nodes. Patients with any suspicious finding in the history or physical examination, and probably any patient over the age of 35, should have preoperative mammography. Aesthetic defects in the breasts, other than small size, should be noted because they might indicate a variation in the surgical technique. The ptotic or tuberous breast might not be corrected with just an implant, and the possibility of a combination of mastopexy and augmentation should be discussed with these patients. If the breasts are asymmetrical in size or position, the patient should be made aware of any differences she may not have noticed before. A difference in size can usually be improved with implants of different sizes, but the patient should be told that it is not expected that the breasts be identical.

As with any aesthetic procedure, preoperative photographs are essential. Most patients are unable to remember how small they were once they incorporate their new breast size into their body image. This lapse of memory can occur as early as the first dressing change and it is sometimes useful to be able to remind the patient of her preoperative appearance if problems develop later.

The initial consultation is the appropriate time to discuss the anticipated size change that the patient can expect. It may be useful to question the patient about the size brassiere she wears and the size she would like to wear. However, it is difficult to translate that information into a specific implant volume. This is largely due to the way brassiere sizes are determined. The brassiere manufacturing industry defines brassiere sizes according to a standard method of measurement. Band size is determined by measuring around the chest just below the breasts and then adding either 5 or 6 inches to the resulting measurement, whichever is required to result in an even number. (This is why all brassiere sizes have even numbers.) A measurement around the breasts at the point of maximal projection equal to the band size is defined as a AA cup and should occur only if there is no breast tissue. If the breast measurement is one inch larger than the band size the cup is defined as A and for each additional inch the cup size increases one letter. The volume of implant required to increase the brassiere size by one cup size will be subject to multiple factors and cannot be extrapolated from one patient to the next. Most women are not aware of the measurements from which brassiere sizes are determined and derive their own size by trial and error. Therefore, it may be difficult for them to visualize the anticipated change. One simple method to help the patient and surgeon arrive at an informed decision regarding the choice of implant size is through the use of sizers. The patient can try putting various size implants into a brassiere. If implant sizers are not available, plastic bags filled with water are a satisfactory alternative (6).

PREOPERATIVE MANAGEMENT

Very little preoperative care is required for augmentation patients. All patients should be warned to avoid aspirin in all of its forms because of the associated increased bleeding. Any infection, even if it is minor and at a remote site, is a good reason to postpone the surgery until the problem has resolved. The patients are nearly always normal, healthy women, so hospitalization should not be needed for this operation, even if general anesthesia is planned. Antibiotics have not been found to reduce the risk of infection for this operation (7).

Operative Techniques

Augmentation mammaplasty can be done with either local or general anesthesia. Local anesthesia is often chosen by the patient in order to minimize the cost. In most cases, local anesthesia is completely satisfactory, although the dosage should be closely monitored because the total dose required often approaches the toxic limit. The risk of toxicity can be lessened by using epinephrine in the solution and by injecting the second side after the first side is nearly completed.

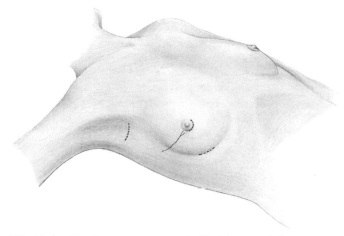

FIG. 61–1. The three common surgical incisions are inframammary, axillary, and intraareolar. Note the position of the 4th intercostal nerve, which provides sensation to the nipple-areola complex.

Lidocaine (0.5%) with 1:200,000 epinephrine is a good combination. The pain of injection can be greatly reduced by buffering the lidocaine with sodium bicarbonate.

All patients should be premedicated with a drug such as diazepam or midazolam to reduce anxiety. Narcotic analgesics are also helpful to reduce the pain associated with the injection of local anesthetics. Some surgeons have found the use of subanesthetic doses of ketamine helpful (8). When using large doses of local anesthetics, and the potent drugs just mentioned, it is imperative that the surgeon be thoroughly familiar with the pharmacology of these drugs and be prepared to manage any adverse reactions. Cardiac monitoring and pulse oxymetry are useful in addition to monitoring of vital signs. Adequate resuscitation equipment and trained personnel must be immediately available.

There are some significant variations in the operative approach. The most commonly used incisions are the inframammary, axillary, and periareolar (Fig. 61–1). The inframammary approach has the advantage of simplicity; the retromammary or submuscular space can be exposed easily with minimal dissection and retraction. The disadvantage is that, of the three choices mentioned, the inframammary incision results in the most conspicuous scar. The axillary incision results in the least visible scar, but provides the least exposure. The periareolar incision usually results in an inconspicuous scar that normally will be out of the public view. The exposure is limited by the diameter of the areola, so there are some patients for whom this approach is not practical. This incision is best made just inside the edge of the areola from the upper medial quadrant to the lower lateral quadrant. After the areola is incised, the dissection may go subcutaneously around the lower border of the gland or directly through the gland. The theoretical objection to cutting through the gland is that ducts are transected and that this might interfere with lactation or introduce contamination. In practice, however, no adverse effects of incising the gland have ever been demonstrated (9,10).

With any of these techniques, attention must be given to the sensory innervation of the nipple-areola complex. The sensory branch to the nipple comes from the fourth inter-

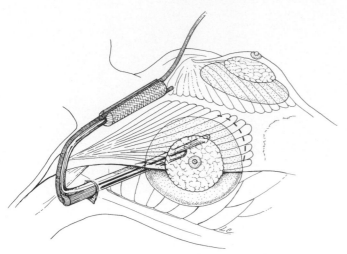

FIG. 61–2. The use of an endoscopic retractor and long cautery instruments makes it possible to create a very precise subpectoral pocket and partially detach the pectoralis origin.

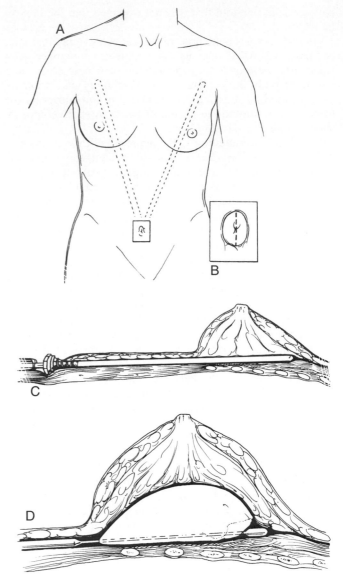

FIG. 61–3. **A,** The insert shows the type and location of the umbilical incision. **B,** the endoscopic approach to the breast. **C,** the position of the endoscope and GSI balloon expander. **D,** the inflated balloon expander is shown overexpanding the submammary pocket. (This is subsequently removed and replaced with the final saline implant to be filled to the desired volume). (Illustration courtesy of G. Georgiade.)

costal nerve and is remarkably constant. It pierces the deep fascia at the lateral border of the pectoralis major and passes through the lateral part of the breast gland to the midlateral position of the areola. Regardless of which incision is used, the nerve is at risk and should be protected (11,12). The other nerve at risk is the intercostal brachial nerve, which can be easily injured with the axillary approach.

The axillary approach has the disadvantage of very limited visibility making precise control of the inframammary line and hemostasis difficult. In the past it was done as a blind procedure using blunt dissection. With the introduction of endoscopic retractors, the axillary approach has renewed appeal (13–16). (Fig. 61–2). The endoscopic approach can be carried out via a 2-cm axillary incision. More recently, a 2-cm inframammary incision and a GSI balloon dissector have been used endoscopically to create the pocket with the insertion of an appropriately sized inflatable implant. The most extreme application of endoscopy to breast augmentation has been the use of an umbilical incision which is being advocated increasingly for selected patients. The use of the umbilical incision and approach for breast augmentation, utilizing endoscopy and the GSI tissue expansion technique with the insertion of an inflatable implant, adds another dimension to the surgeon's options for augmentation mammaplasty (17) (Fig. 61–3).

Other than the location of the incision, the other major variation in operative technique is in the final location of the implant. The original technique was to place the implant behind the breast gland on the anterior surface of the pectoralis fascia. (Fig. 61–4). Subsequently, some surgeons began placing the implant behind the pectoralis muscle (18) (Fig. 61–5). This technique covers only the medial portion of the implant with muscle, so those who place great importance on muscle coverage place the implant under both the pectoralis major and serratus anterior in order to obtain complete muscle coverage. (Fig. 61–6). There is reason to believe there is a lower incidence of scar capsule contracture when the implant is behind the muscle (19). The disadvantages of submuscular technique are the more difficult exposure and dissection and

a tendency for the muscle to flatten the implant, resulting in less projection and too much fullness in the upper breast. The problems with breast shape tend to disappear over the first few months as the muscle adapts to the presence of the implant. A common error in submuscular augmentation is to place the implant too high, where the dissection is easier. It is important to be certain that the pocket is low enough. Creating a low enough pocket used to be a major problem with the transaxillary approach, but endoscopic dissection has been helpful in this regard.

Regardless of whether a retromammary or submuscular position is chosen, it is important to dissect a large enough space to accommodate the implant with room to spare. Hemostasis should be meticulous and the wound should be thor-

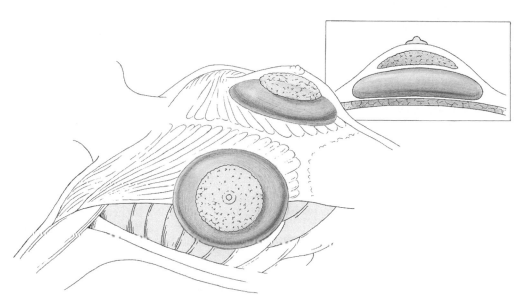

FIG. 61–4. In most cosmetic augmentation mammoplasties, the implant is behind the breast gland on the surface of the pectoralis fascia.

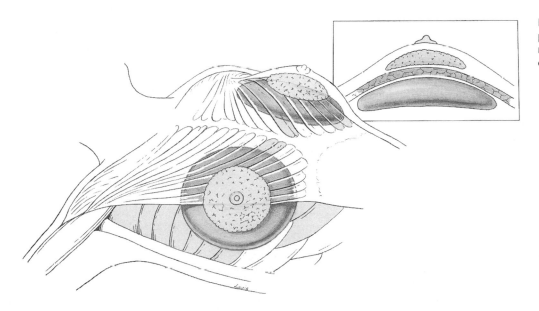

FIG. 61–5. The implant may be placed behind the petoralis major muscle which, however, will cover only part of the implant.

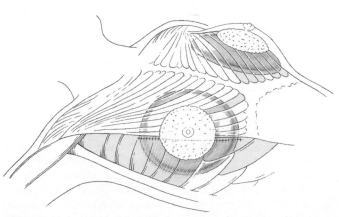

FIG. 61–6. In order to have the implant completely covered with muscle, it is necessary to use both the pectoralis major and the serratus anterior muscles.

oughly irrigated to avoid leaving clots behind. Lighted retractors, headlights and long cautery instruments can be helpful in this task. Drains should not be necessary in this operation. Dressings vary considerably according to the preference of the surgeon. In addition to covering the wound, the dressing can function to support the weight of the implant for patient comfort. Often a soft elastic brassiere with gauze in it is all that is required.

Types of Implants

The only implant currently available for breast augmentation is a silicone rubber (elastomer) bag filled with saline. In the past, the silicone gel–filled implant was chosen more often because of its more natural consistency. However, with sufficient tissue cover, saline-filled and gel-filled implants are indistinguishable.

Implants are available with either a smooth or textured surface. One of the most successful implants in the past was covered with a polyurethane foam, which apparently gave it a considerable advantage in resisting contracture. The purpose of the textured silicones was to achieve this contracture resistance without adding another material. Controlled studies support the use of textured implants, but they have not been universally adopted, since they seem to have a greater propensity to have visible wrinkles, and the greater thickness of the elastomer makes them more likely to be palpable (20).

Saline implants are filled at the operating table by inserting a fill tube through a valve. Some surgeons prefer to fill the implant after it is in the pocket in order to use a smaller incision. Implants come with a labeled volume that can be exceeded by about 10%. Underfilling implants is to be avoided, as it can lead to folds in the implant that may be palpable and will probably lead to a greater risk of leakage through fold flaws. Overfilling the implant helps avoid wrinkles, but the more the implant is filled the firmer it will be.

Implants should be handled with great care to prevent damage or contamination. Implants tend to attract particulate matter such as glove powder, dust from the air, or lint from cloth or paper. They should be kept in the manufacturer's package until just before use and then handled only with well-washed gloves. When closing the wound, care must be taken to avoid puncturing the implant with an instrument or a needle (21,22).

Postoperative Care and Complications

Breast augmentation patients who do not experience complications require minimal postoperative care. A mild analgesic such as codeine is usually sufficient for pain control. Because the operation is nearly always an outpatient procedure, a companion should be instructed to report any significant pain not relieved by analgesics, particularly if it is unilateral.

Complications of breast augmentation are infrequent, but include such problems as implant puncture, hematoma, and infection. Implant puncture will be apparent within hours as the saline leaves the implant and is absorbed. The occasional hematoma will present as pain and swelling, and sometimes ecchymosis. In general, if a hematoma is large enough to be detected, the patient must be returned to the operating room for evacuation of the blood and control of the bleeding point if one can be found. Fortunately, infection is rare, but when it does occur the implant must be removed. A possible exception to this rule is superficial infection that does not involve the implant space. As soon as the infection has resolved and the wound has healed, it is safe to replace the implant, but it may be wise to wait a few weeks for the scar to soften (23).

UNFAVORABLE RESULTS

The two most common adverse effects of augmentation mammaplasty are sensory disturbances and capsular contracture. Sensory disturbances are usually transient, but may be permanent in as many as 15% of patients. Laceration of the 4th intercostal nerve would be expected to produce permanent anesthesia of the nipple, and must be avoided.

By far the most troublesome problem with breast implants has been scar capsular contracture. All implants become encapsulated with scar, which would ordinarily be of no consequence. However, in some patients the scar will contract, resulting in a deformation of the implant and increasing firmness.

The incidence of capsular contracture varies widely with various clinical reports, and it is difficult to determine because of the subjective nature of the diagnosis. The incidence seems to have decreased since the introduction of the textured implants and is probably in the range of 10%.

Implant capsules, like any other scar, contract through action of myofibroblasts. Beyond that, the etiology remains unknown. Any irritant, such as gel leaking from a gel filled implant, or subclinical infection from low levels of bacterial contamination, can probably contribute in some cases, but most of the time there is no readily apparent explanation.

A variety of measures have been suggested to prevent capsular contracture. Textured implants have reduced, but not eliminated, the problem. Antiseptic irrigations may or may not reduce the risk of contracture. Submuscular placement of the implant may reduce contracture or may cover the contracted capsule with more tissue, making it less apparent.

The local use of steroids has been tried with mixed results. Placement of a low-solubility steroid in the wound at the time of closure is probably not effective because it does not persist long enough. Placement of soluble steroid in the saline seems to reduce contracture, but has resulted in some disturbing side effects including thinning of the overlying skin and even implant extrusion. These problems seem to be dose related (24–27).

Another unfavorable result that may present at any time is deflation of a saline implant. Deflation was once a common problem, but with the use of room-temperature vulcanizing elastomers the incidence is quite low, probably under 5% at 10 years. When deflation occurs the only treatment is implant replacement, which fortunately is a relatively simple procedure (28,29).

The unfavorable results just mentioned have aesthetic or convenience consequences. A more troubling effect of breast implants is their tendency to obscure a mammogram. Both gel-filled and saline-filled implants are radioopaque (30). The tendency to obscure a mammogram can be at least partially overcome by using a "displacement" view in which the technician pulls the breast forward and pushes the implant back (31). This maneuver is facilitated by submuscular placement of the implant and is largely prevented by capsular contracture. There is considerable interest in the development of a radiolucent implant to overcome this problem (32).

An adverse outcome that has been increasingly recognized is the so-called silent rupture, a problem with gel implants analogous to deflation of a saline implant. The frequency of this problem seems to be related to the age of the implant (33). It is not clear whether implants weaken with time (or perhaps the older implants were weaker when they were made). The gel tends to be contained by the capsule, although silicone may be found in axillary lymph nodes. The medical consequences of a contained rupture, if any, are uncertain. Implants have been alleged to cause a variety of systemic symptoms, even when they are not ruptured. So far, epidemiological studies have failed to support these allegations (34).

TREATMENT OF ESTABLISHED CAPSULAR CONTRACTURE

Once a contracture occurs, it can only be relieved by capsulotomy. Originally, capsulotomy was done by reopening the wound and then incising the capsule around its base, and sometimes across the dome as well (35). Later, it was discovered that the capsule could be ruptured by closed compression (36). Closed capsulotomy is not entirely without danger, although it does avoid an operation when it is successful. Often the release is incomplete, or the capsule cannot be ruptured at all. The principal danger is implant rupture, which will deflate a saline implant or extrude gel from a gel-filled implant. Extruded gel must be removed because it will form granulomas and may migrate along tissue planes (37,38).

The other problem with capsulotomy by either open incision or closed capsulotomy is recurrence of the contracture. The risk of recurrence has been variously reported to range from 30 to 80%, and seems to increase with repeated capsulotomies. There are probably some patients who can only be relieved of contracture by implant removal without replacement (37,38).

In summary, augmentation mammaplasty is an operation that has been of considerable benefit to the vast majority of women who choose to have it done, even if they do not get a perfect result. The problems associated with the operation are usually easily managed, although in some cases this will require additional surgery. The problem of capsular contracture has been reduced with advances in implant design. The problem of the obscured mammogram may be reduced in the future with newer implant designs now on the horizon.

References

1. Hetter GP. Satisfactions and dissatisfactions of patients with augmentation mammaplasty. *Plast Reconstr Surg* 1979; 64:151.
2. Letterman G, Schurter M. History of augmentation mammaplasty. In: Owsley JQ, Peterson RA, eds. *Symposium on aesthetic surgery of the breast.* St. Louis: CV Mosby, 1978.
3. Cronin T, Gerow F, Augmentation mammaplasty: A new "natural feel" prosthesis. In: Broadbent TR, ed. *Transactions of the Third International Congress of Plastic Surgery.* Amsterdam, Exerpta Medica Foundation, 1963.
4. Redick LP. Sidney Wolfe, David Kessler, and the FDA: medical clearinghouse (letter). *Plast Reconstr Surg,* 1990; 5:932.
5. Coleman EA, Kessler LG, Wun LM, et al. Trends in the surgical treatment of ductal carcinoma in situ of the breast. *Am J Surg* 1992; 164:74.
6. Brody G. Breast implant size selection and patient satisfaction. *Plast Reconstr Surg* 1981; 68:611.
7. LeRoy J, Given KS. Wound infection in breast augmentation: The role of prophylactic perioperative antibiotics. *Anesthetic Plast Surg* 1991; 15:303.
8. Vinnik CA. An intravenous dissociation technique for outpatient plastic surgery: Tranquility in the office surgical facility. *Plast Reconstr Surg.* 1981; 67(6):799.
9. Courtiss EH, Webster RC, White MF Selection of alternatives in augmentation mammaplasty. *Plast Reconstr Surg* 1974; 54:552.
10. Courtiss EH, Goldwyn RN, Anastasi GW. The fate of breast implants with infections around them. *Plast Reconstr Surg* 1979; 63:812.
11. Courtiss E, Goldwyn R. Breast sensation before and after plastic surgery. *Plast Reconstr Surg* 1976; 58:1.
12. Farina MA, Newby BG, Alani HM. Innervation of the nipple-areola complex. *Plast Reconstr Surg* 1980; 66:497.
13. Price CI, Eaves FF III, Nahai F, et al. Endoscopic transaxillary subpectoral breast augmentation. *Plast Reconstr Surg* 1994; 94:612.
14. Ho L. Endoscopic assisted transaxillary augmentation mammaplasty. *Brit J Plast Surg* 1993; 46:332.
15. Troilus C. Total muscle coverage of a breast implant is possible through a transaxillary approach. *Plast Reconstr Surg* 1995; 95:509.
16. Chajchir A. Benzaquen I, Spagnolo N, et al. Endoscopic augmentation mastoplasty. *Aesthetic Plast Surg* 1994; 18:377.
17. Johnson G, Christ J. The endoscopic breast augmentation: the transumbilica insertion of saline-filled breast implants. *Plast Reconstr Surg* 1993; 92:801.
18. Truppman ES, Ellenby JD. A 13-year evaluation of subpectoral augmentation mammaplasty. In: Owsley JQ and Peterson RA, eds. *Symposium on aesthetic surgery of the breast* St. Louis: CV Mosby, 1978.
19. Mahler D, Hauben D. Retromammary versus retropectoral augmentation: a comparative study. *Ann Plast Surg* 1982; 8:370.
20. Burkhardt, BR, Demas CP. The effect of Siltex texturing and povodine-iodine irrigation on capsular contracture around saline inflatable breast implants. *Plast Reconstr Surg* 1994; 93:128.
21. Mladick R. No-touch submuscular saline breast augmentation. *Aesthetic Plast Surg* 1993; 17:183.
22. Lavine D. Saline inflatable prostheses: 14 year experience. *Aesthetic Plast Surg* 1993; 17:325.
23. March JL, Stevens WG, Smith GL, et al. Reinsertability after breast prosthesis pocket infection: an experimental study. *Plast Reconstr Surg* 1982; 69:234.
24. Peterson IID, Burt GB. The role of steroids in prevention of circumferential capsular scarring in augmentation mammaplasty. *Plast Reconstr Surg* 1974; 54:28.
25. Perrin ER. The use of soluble steroids within inflatable breast prostheses. *Plast Reconstr Surg* 1976; 57:163.
26. Carrico TJ, Cohen IK. Capsular contracture and steroid-related complications after augmentation mammaplasty: a preliminary study. *Plast Reconstr Surg* 1979; 64:377.
27. Caffee HH. The effects of intraprosthetic methylprednisolone on implant capsules and surrounding soft tissue. *Ann Plast Surg* 1984; 12:348.
28. Gibney J. Saline breast implant deflaton rate. *Plast Reconstr Surg* 1995; 95:1329.
29. Gylbert L, Asplund O, Jurell G. Capsular contracture after breast reconstruction with silicone-gel and saline-filled implants: a 6-year follow-up. *Plast Reconstr Surg,* 1990; 85:373.
30. Silverstein MJ, Handel N, Gamagami P. The effect of silicone-gel-filled implants on mammography. *Cancer* 1991; 68:1159.
31. Eklund GW, Busby RC, Miller SH, et al. Improved imaging of the augmented breast. *Am J Roentgenol* 1988; 151:469.
32. Young VL, Diehl GJ, Eichling J, et al. The relative radiolucencies of breast implant filler materials. *Plast Reconstr Surg* 1993; 91:1066.
33. Peters W, Keystone E, Smith D. Factors affecting the rupture of silicone-gel breast implants. *Ann Plast Surg* 1994; 32:449.
34. Sanchez-Guerrero J, Colditz GA, Karlson EW, et al. Silicone breast implants and the risk of connective tissue diseases and symptoms. *N Eng J Med* 1995; 332:1666.
35. Freeman BS. Successful treatment of some fibrous envelope contractures around breast implants. *Plast Reconstr Surg* 1972; 50:107.
36. Baker JL, Bartels RJ, Douglas WM. Closed compression technique for rupturing a contracted capsule around a breast implant. *Plast Reconstr Surg* 1976; 58:137.
37. Nelson GAD. Complications from the treatment of fibrous capsular contracture of the breast. *Plast Reconstr Surg* 1981; 66:969.
38. Little G, Baker JL. Results of closed compression capsulotomy for treatment of contracted breast implant capsules. *Plast Reconstr Surg* 1980; 65:30.

62

Management of Complications Following Augmentation Mammaplasty

G. Patrick Maxwell, M.D., F.A.C.S., and Patricia A. Clugston, M.D., F.R.C.S.(C.)

Until recently, augmentation mammaplasty was one of the most commonly performed plastic surgical procedures. Complications, particularly serious ones, are rare; but, minor complications do occur, despite careful patient selection and surgical technique (1,2). It is particularly important to discuss potential complications with all perspective augmentation patients, because litigious attitudes have increased as a result of the FDA moratorium (January 1992) on silicone gel implants, the earlier removal of polyurethane implants from the market, and the recent global settlement package announced by the major implant manufacturers.

This chapter describes the potential complications and their appropriate treatment options. Complications will be categorized as those that occur in the immediate or early postoperative period and those that occur on a delayed basis.

Acute and Early Postoperative Complications

HEMATOMA

Hematomas usually occur in the early postoperative period, but may occur as late as 7 to 14 days postoperatively. Although diffuse oozing from multiple sites can be the cause, more commonly, previously controlled arterial bleeders break loose postoperatively. The incidence in most series is 1 to 3% (3). Percutaneous suction drains do not prevent hematomas; rather, careful hemostasis within the operative pocket before implant insertion is imperative.

Clinically, hematomas present with increasing size of the breast mound associated with increasing pain and firmness. Failure to recognize and treat significant hematomas around breast prosthesis results in delayed ecchymosis that is most noticeable on the lower chest wall. The presence of a hematoma may be associated with an increased risk of periprosthetic infection and/or delayed capsular contracture (3,4).

Hematomas of any significant degree should be drained surgically; this typically requires return to the operating room and a general anesthetic. The implant is removed, all clot is evacuated, and the source of bleeding is identified and controlled with electrocautery. The pocket should be irrigated with an antibiotic solution before reimplantation of the device, and perioperative systemic antibiotics may be indicated. If early adequate evacuation of the hematoma is successful, the final augmentation mammaplasty result should not be affected.

SEROMA

Dissection of a subglandular or subpectoral pocket creates a large, raw surface that oozes blood initially, later becoming serous in nature. Textured devices induce a controlled inflammatory response that may lead to greater serous collection around these prostheses as compared to smooth-walled devices (5,6). This may be an indication for the placement of a suction drain in the periprosthetic space, to minimize serous fluid collection and to increase tissue adherence at the implant-capsule interface. However, many surgeons individualize the use of drains, reserving their use for those cases of revision capsulotomy, capsulectomy, or placement of a temporary or permanent expander for reconstructive purposes.

Seromas typically present with a soft, nontender swelling that results in asymmetry. Since they are self-limiting, with spontaneous resolution occurring over 7 to 14 days, surgical intervention is unnecessary. Patient reassurance is required during this period of observation.

ASYMMETRY

Breast implant asymmetry, noted in the early postoperative period but not believed to be secondary to seroma formation, probably is the result of a technical error in preoperative planning or operative execution that resulted in implant malposition. Occasionally, asymmetry may result from the surgeon's not appreciating a preoperative volume discrepancy between the breasts, or from positional asymmetry of the nipple-areolar complex that has become more apparent following the augmentation procedure.

With textured implants, and particulary anatomically designed devices, these problems can be avoided by meticulous preoperative markings of the planned positioning of the implant base (and of the new inframammary fold, if it requires lowering), careful pocket dissection intraoperatively, and intraoperative assessments of the implant position and adequacy of the pocket by placing the patient upright at 90° (7).

If the implant malposition results from overdissection of the inframammary fold, taping of the fold and wearing an underwire bra on the side that is too low may allow adherence of the dissected flaps, thereby limiting the lower extent of the pocket. This is most beneficial if initiated early. If the implants seem more superiorly located initially, then a circumferential elastic bandage wrap of the superior breast poles may help the implants settle. If true implant malposition occurs, and it is not improved by taping, revision of the implant pocket should be done on a delayed basis (several months) once tissue healing and equilibrium is achieved.

ALTERATIONS IN NIPPLE AREOLAR COMPLEX (NAC) SENSIBILITY

Dissection of a subglandular or subpectoral pocket can result in inadvertant injury to the lateral cutaneous branches of the intercostal nerves, particularly those felt to provide sensation to the NAC (8,9). This can result in hyperesthesia, hypoesthesia, or anaesthesia. It is believed that subglandular dissection places these nerves at increased risk because they are more tethered to the overlying glandular tissue and underlying pectoral fascia, and are thereby prone to traction or direct injury (8,10). In the subpectoral dissection, the nerves are often visualized; if dissection is carried out bluntly and with caution, injury is less common. Most series report an incidence of altered sensibility of approximately 15% (8). The majority of these patients' symptoms improve with time, but they should be informed that this may take several months. A small number of patients will have permanently diminished or absent sensibility postoperatively, as a result of a complete nerve injury. These cases are typically the result of overly aggressive dissection of the lateral pocket with the electrocutting or sharp dissection, and this should generally be avoided.

In those patients with bothersome hyperesthesia of the NAC, a soft barrier dressing will offer some subjective improvement by decreasing the contact from motion of the overlying clothing.

ALTERATION IN ARM SENSATION

Intercostalbrachial nerve injury has been reported following transaxillary augmentation. This is typically transient and improves with time (11).

INFECTION

Infection rarely occurs in the early postoperative period following breast augmentation. The risk is slightly increased by the placement of a foreign body in the human body. Local and systemic antibiotic prophylaxis are commonly used perioperatively despite lack of reproducible evidence to suggest routine utilization (3,13).

Infection can generally occur in two forms. The incidence reported in most series is about 2% (3,13). The most common offending organism in the early postoperative period is *Staphylococcus aureus,* followed by *S. epidermidis* (3). Clinically, the patient complains of discomfort, warmth, swelling, and erythema, most commonly 5 to14 days postoperatively. The less serious form represents a superficial wound infection, or cellulitis. Early, appropriate treatment with oral antibiotics usually results in resolution. Failure to resolve suggests that the antibiotic therapy is inadequate either in specificity, dose, and/or delivery, or that the diagnosis is incorrect and a more serious form, a purulent periprosthetic infection, is present. Signs of this condition are typically more significant, with greater swelling, pain, and tenderness. The erythema is more extensive and the skin often has a shiny appearance with localized edema. This condition requires intravenous antibiotic therapy, implant removal, and drainage of the pocket (13,14). Most authors recommend the implant be removed for a period of 3 months, at which time reimplanta-

tion may be attempted (13). Because of the implications of implant removal following complication of a primary aesthetic procedure, some have reported implant salvage following drainage of the periprosthetic space abscess, soaking of the implant and pocket irrigation with betadine, and a full course of appropriate systemic antibiotics (15). Despite reported success with such cases, this is generally not recommended.

GALACTORRHEA

Galactorrhea is a rare complaint following augmentation mammaplasty. It is hypothesized to result from sensory stimulation of the dorsal root ganglion with retrograde activation of the pituitary/hypothalamic axis, resulting in increased prolactin production (16). These patients are usually on oral contraceptives, in whom estrogen and progesterone are falling, and they present with spontaneous lactation about 7 to 14 days postoperatively. Prolactin suppression with oral bromocriptine is effective treatment (16).

MONDOR DISEASE

Mondor disease is a rare occurrence (<1%). It can be seen following any type of breast surgery, and occasionally occurs spontaneously. It represents a superficial thrombophlebitis of the larger veins that are often present in the subcutaneous tissue overlying the lower breast parenchyma and upper abdominal wall (17). It presents with a thick tender cord extending from the lower breast onto the upper abdominal wall. The occurrence is most common following an inframammary incision. There is no risk of embolic phenomena, and the treatment is conservative, with antiinflammatory medication and intermittent cool packs for symptomatic relief (17).

SUBCUTANEOUS FLEXION CONTRACTURE BANDS

Some authors refer to these subcutaneous cords as Mondor disease; however, we do not believe they represent a superficial thrombophlebitis; we treat them as subcutaneous fibrotic contractures. They present in the early postoperative period, are commonly tender, and are demonstrated by arm abduction. They can occur in the inframammary region following an inframammary fold approach, and in the axilla following transaxillary access. They commonly resolve after 1 to 2 months. We recommend treatment with massage, with the arm in the abducted position.

PNEUMOTHORAX

This is possible, but it is a very rare occurence. Pneumothorax can result from a needle puncture during infiltration of local anaesthetic into the breast tissue, from intercostal nerve blocks, or as a result of errant intraoperative dissection. Depending on the degree of injury to the pleura, this can be manifest intraoperatively or postoperatively when the patient is removed from the ventilator. Hypoxemia and shortness of breath require a careful and thorough physical examination, blood gas determination, and chest radiograph. If a pneumothorax is confirmed and the patient is symptomatic, chest tube placement is indicated. If the patient is asymptomatic and the volume of the pneumothorax is small, conservative therapy with serial x ray may be warranted in some cases.

Delayed Complications

IMPLANT PALPABILITY

Implant palpability is dependent on many factors, including surface morphology, implant fill volume and material, thickness of the overlying soft tissue, and location of the implant relative to the pectoralis muscle (18). This is generally most common in the lower pole of the breast, and tends to be more frequent in saline-filled devices, especially in the case of underfill. *Knuckling* is a type of palpable fold that results from the implant folding on itself, and is typically seen in the setting of capsular contracture.

The immobility of textured devices (textured silicone and polyurethane) results in an increased likelihood that the edge of the implant is palpable; this is especially true if the overlying soft tissues are thin (19).

Currently, with the restricted use of silicone gel prostheses and the lack of any other alternative cohesive gel fills, there is no simple solution to these problems of implant fold irregularities, which are more common with saline-filled devices because of the noncohesive nature of the filler.

IMPLANT DEFLATION

Deflation can occur with saline-filled implants or double-lumen implants. It is much more obvious in the former, where the volume of saline is greater. It can result from valve failure, which is now uncommon, or as a result of fold flaws (20,21). A recent series of long-term follow-up with saline inflatable devices showed a deflation rate of 20% with posterior retention valved devices (Heyer Schulte 1800 series), and 0.56% with anterior diaphragm valves (Heyer Schulte 1600 series) that had been available in the latter years of this series (20). The posterior valve system was subsequently redesigned to a leaf valve system by Mentor Corporation in 1984. The likelihood of fold flaw failures is greater if the implant is underfilled (22).

Deflation most commonly occurs suddenly, and may be associated with a warm flushing feeling. Occasionally, it is a slow process with gradual loss of implant volume. The removal and replacement of the implant is the only appropriate treatment. If this is done soon after deflation, the pocket should be well maintained, and the need for capsulotomy can be avoided unless some degree of capsular contracture was present before the deflation.

Asymmetry

Implant asymmetry can result from technical errors, as discussed earlier, and from the changing soft tissues overlying the implant that result in implant distortion or malposition. The most common cause of asymmetry in the delayed setting is capsular contracture, discussed below. Lateral malpositioning of the implant and loss of the intermammary cleavage can occur over time and is most commonly seen when implants are placed retropectoral with inadequate release of the inferomedial sternal insertion of the pectoralis major muscle (11,18). This is less commonly observed with textured implants, which are more likely to be immobile and remain in place. Treatment of this latter problem requires either further release of the remaining pectoral muscle insertion inferomedially or dissection of a new retroglandular pocket and change of implant location (9,11,18).

An unnaturally constricted lower breast pole can be seen postaugmentation as a result of inadequate release of the original inframammary fold. This may be seen unilaterally or bilaterally when lowering of the fold is desired to achieve optimal dimensional augmentation. In its worse form, this is referred to as a "double bubble" deformity (18–23) (Figure 62–1). The only treatment for this is surgical, with further release of the constricted pocket inferiorly; change of location of the implant to a retroglandular position is often beneficial (12,18,23).

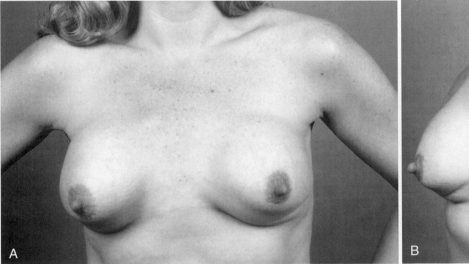
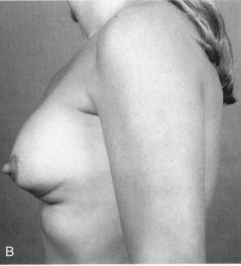

FIG. 62–1. Lateral and AP views of patient with inadequate release of a constricted lower pole following augmentation mammaplasty, demonstrating a "double bubble deformity."

Upper Pole Fullness

Despite some patients' desire for upper pole fullness and increased cleavage, this is not an aesthetically natural result. It typically reflects too superior a location of the implants. This is most commonly seen with round-based, smooth-walled implants when inadequate lowering of the inframammary fold has been carried out. In early reports of transaxillary augmentation done without the aid of the endoscope, in which release of the inferomedial insertion of the pectoralis muscle was not complete, this was an all-too-common sequelae (11). The other situation in which upper pole fullness is problematic occurs when capsular contracture is present and the implant is forced into a more spherical dimension.

The treatment for this deformity is repositioning of the implant and lowering of the inframammary fold (if necessary). The availability of anatomically designed textured implants, careful preoperative planning and surgical execution should allow the surgeon to avoid such deformities. If this deformity is a result of capsular contracture with implant distortion, then open capsulotomy or capsulectomy will also be required.

Upper Pole Rippling

Upper pole rippling is seen in women who otherwise would have an excellent aesthetic result. The causes of this are implant fill material and volume, along with the presence of partial adherence owing to surface texturing, thin overlying soft tissues, excessive relative pocket size, and the absence of capsular contracture. Since the underfill of saline implants contributes to this problem and also to the increased risk of fold flaws, underfilling is strongly discouraged (22).

This has become more common with increased use of textured devices (silicone and polyurethane), particularly the saline-filled prostheses. The rippling or pleating is seen primarily in the superomedial aspect of the breast and is most noticeable when the patient is in the upright position or with forward trunk flexion (Figure 62–2). Treatment of this deformity is in its infancy, but most feel changing the implant to a retropectoral position helps camouflage it. Presently, we are using the endoscope to help visualize this deformity from the capsule-implant interface before surgical correction, in an attempt to understand the pathophysiology.

Silicone Gel Bleed

Gel bleed refers to the passive diffusion of fluid silicones (non cross-linked silicone, polydimethylsiloxane—PDMS) through the silicone elastomer envelope (13,24). The degree to which this happens is dependent on the type of implant and whether it is low-bleed or not. Low-bleed implants, which were developed by altering the silicone elastomer envelope, have generally been on the market since 1985, and are believed to decrease the amount of gel bleed by approximately tenfold (24). Cohesive silicone gel implants have recently become available in Europe and South America. These gels have significantly less small-molecular-weight fluid silicone and thereby are believed to have less potential for diffusion (gel bleed) across the low-bleed silicone elastomer envelope. The presence of a double lumen provides added protection against gel bleed, providing the outer lumen is the saline reservoir. Gel bleed in itself is not felt to be injurious; however, with older implants in which the amount was higher, it could be the source of siliconomas (discussed below).

Implant Rupture

The rupture of the outer silicone elastomer envelope is more common with older style implants that had thin silicone elastomer shells. With silicone gel implants, the silicone gel is most commonly contained within the existing capsule. Occasionally, the capsule does not contain the silicone gel and it extends into the extracapsular tissues. Free extracapsular silicone can be ingested by cells of the reticuloendothelial system and cause a foreign-body reaction, resulting in local siliconomas or invading regional lymph nodes (24,25).

Diagnosis of ruptured gel implants, in which the gel is contained in the capsule, is not always straightforward. Clinical examination is often not conclusive, particularly if there is any degree of capsular contracture present. Most now believe that ultrasound is more accurate than mammography for this purpose, providing the ultrasonongrapher is experienced in this area (25–28). Magnetic resonance imaging (MRI) has been suggested to be a more sensitive and specific diagnostic aid, providing it is equipped with a breast coil, but this is a costly method (28). Others have utilized direct visualization of the implant surface endoscopically to diagnose implant shell disruption (29). (See also Chapter 63.)

Controversy exists regarding the risk of rupture in silicone gel implants, but most now agree that, if the diagnosis is made, the implant should be removed along with any free gel. Some prefer to achieve this by carrying out a capsulectomy, and attempt to leave the disrupted silicone elastomer and silicone gel within the capsulectomy specimen.

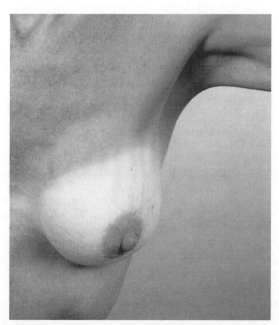

FIG. 62–2. A patient with subglandular textured saline prostheses with visible upper pole rippling.

Siliconomas

Siliconomas result from the immune system's attempt to wall off the foreign material (free silicone gel), which ultimately results in a mass. Clinically, siliconomas cause concern because of the difficulty in distinguishing them from malignant lesions. They can occur locally around the implant, within intraparenchymal nodes or regional lymph nodes (25). This differentiation requires biopsy, with histologic confirmation of those characteristic of siliconomas. These include central refractile silicone particles surrounded by foreign-body giant cells and fibrosis (30).

Carcinogenicity

Concerns regarding carcinogenicity of silicone and, in particular, free silicone gel or fluid silicones, has been fueled by laboratory evidence of fibrosarcomas developing in a high percentage of rats implanted subcutaneously or injected within the intraperitoneal cavity with silicone gel. There is criticism regarding the significance of this evidence as related to humans, because the rodent model is inbred and felt to be very susceptible to "solid-state carcinogenesis" (31). Fibrosarcomas of the breast are rare in humans, and no epidemiologic studies support an increased risk of these tumors in women with implants. Both extant large epidemiologic studies with long term follow-up show a lower incidence of carcinoma than expected compared to the general population (32,33). Some investigators have raised a question regarding later-stage presentation of breast carcinoma in women with breast prosthesis as a result of mammographic interference (discussed below) (34).

Systemic Responses

Anecdotal reports of a link between silicone gel implants and various connective-tissue diseases have resulted in significant changes in the practice of aesthetic breast surgery (35–39). Studies reporting since the moratorium was announced in 1992 have failed to support any causal relationship between any connective-tissue disorders and silicone implants (40–42). Regardless of the scientific literature, several lawsuits have successfully produced awards in favor of the plaintiffs and against the implant manufacturers, and availability of these implants remains significantly restricted in North America. There is a need for further research in this area to determine if fluid silicones (PDMS) incite an immunologic reaction systemically; this would allow the medical community, implant manufacturers, and patients to reach a consensus with regard to these reports and the future of silicone gel prostheses.

With the concern regarding silicone gel implants, many patients have requested explantation followed by reimplantation with saline devices. Other patients have requested explantation alone. This latter group of patients must be informed of the potentially poor aesthetic result that is likely because of the loss of breast volume, relative secondary skin excess, and resultant ptosis that is common postoperatively.

Polyurethane Prostheses Degradation

Polyurethane-covered implants are no longer available for market use in North America. Despite this, many patients who were implanted with these devices in the 1980s may require future surgery or may present with concerns regarding the long-term safety of these devices.

Separation and degradation of the polyurethane cover on these gel-filled implants has been seen clinically since their introduction. Microencapsulation of the polyurethane particles is felt by most to be the reason these implants are associated with a decreased rate of capsular contracture (5,19,43–45). In vivo fragmentation and degradation of polyurethane foam has been shown to occur in the laboratory, resulting in formation of 2,4 toluene diamine (TDA), a known chemical carcinogen in animals (5,19,45). Whether this hydrolysis occurs in humans in vivo is disputed, and if it does, the significance of the amount of TDA formed is questioned. Based on an in vitro experiment to simulate the physiologic situation, the lifetime cancer risk to the patient associated with the amount of TDA formed from complete breakdown of the polyurethane foam present on implants would be less than 1 in 1 million (46).

While the silicone elastomer-containing silicone gel can be easily removed with the polyurethane-impregnated capsule following delamination, it is probably advisable to perform a total capsulectomy. This capsule is generally thicker and more vascular than that found around other devices. Its removal can be accomplished without too much difficulty, unless it is located under very thin soft tissues or in a total submuscular pocket. These latter situations require technical skill and diligence.

Mammographic Interference (Also see Chapter 63)

It is an accepted fact that the presence of breast implants, placed either subpectoral or subglandular, interferes with the mammographic assessment of the breast. The degree to which implants interfere is dependent on several factors, including the position of the implant relative to the pectoral muscle, the amount of native breast parenchyma present, the degree of capsular contracture, and the mammographic technique used (47–54). Retroglandular implant position is felt to interfere to the greatest degree, with reports of 49 to 83% of the breast parenchyma obscured with routine views on compression mammography (47,49,51). This can be improved to 39% if additional views using the displacement technique described by Eklund and coworkers are added. With implants in the retropectoral position, breast parenchyma is better visualized with standard compression mammography, with approximately 28% of the breast parenchyma obscured. The degree of interference is further reduced to 9% if displacement techniques are added (47). It is generally felt that posterior breast tissue is best visualized with standard compression views, and anterior tissues with displacement techniques (47,49). Capsular contracture greatly interferes with the ability to carry out either technique. The additional use of focal compression and magnified images, of areas of concern in the breast and areas of microcalcification seen on preliminary films, is also recommended.

Most people feel plain film mammography to be the screening method of choice for breast carcinoma. But, xeromammography is associated with a four to tenfold increased radiation exposure and the breast cannot be compressed with this technique; therefore, the percentage of breast tissue obscured by implants is greater, and for these reasons xeromammography is no longer recommended for screening, particularly in women with implants (48).

Despite this interference with routine mammographic screening, there have been studies that suggest that the pathologic stage of breast carcinoma in women with breast implants is no worse than in women without implants (52,53). Women with implants should be encouraged to carry out monthly self breast examinations and undergo yearly clinical examination as well as mammographic screening as recommended based on their age and other risk factors.

Soft-Tissue Problems

CAPSULAR CONTRACTURE

Placement of any foreign material within vascularized tissue results in the body's attempting to wall it off, which results in a bursa-like pocket surrounding the implanted material. This is commonly referred to as a capsule. If the capsule surrounding a breast implant remains soft and compliant, then the resultant breast remains soft. If the capsule thickens and contracts concentrically, then the breast feels firm, and a capsular contracture is present. A method for grading the degree of capsular contracture has been proposed by Baker and others and is often referred to in clinical series when reporting the incidence of capsular contracture in breast augmentation (55,56). The incidence of capsular contracture varies greatly, and has been reported as low as 2% in series with polyurethane foam–surfaced devices to as high as 75% with smooth-walled devices (5,57,58). Most recent clinical series of primary augmentation report an incidence of 5 to 25% for Baker III and IV contracture (42,60,61).

The etiology of capsular contracture remains elusive, and is felt by most to represent a multifactorial pathogenesis. Various theories have been proposed but there is no consensus with regards to a specific etiology. Low-grade infection with *S. epidermidis,* undrained hematomas, gel bleed, foreign-body reaction, implant geometry, and an increased myofibroblast activity, have all been postulated as contributing factors (57,59,62–64). Reduction in the incidence of capsular contraction rates has been shown with submuscular placement of implants, saline-filled implants, textured-surfaced (silicone or polyurethane) implants, intraluminal steroid instillation, displacement exercises to maintain a pocket larger than the implant dimensions, and antibiotic pocket irrigations prior to implant placement (57–61,65). Recent clinical reports and laboratory models have supported a significant reduction in the incidence of capsular contracture rates with textured silicone elastomer saline-filled devices, at least in the early postoperative follow-up reported since these devices were made available in the late 1980s (59,60,66).

Treatment of established capsular contracture is primarily surgical. The practice of closed capsulotomy has fallen out of favor in recent years, because the risk of implant rupture is felt to increase with implant age (particularly older, thin-walled implants) and in view of the concerns regarding the effects of extracapsular silicone gel (13,17). Surgical treatment includes open capsulotomy, partial or complete capsulectomy, change of implant position to subpectoral, and the use of saline textured implants (17,18,57,58). The cautious use of intraluminal steroids (20 mg solumedrol per implant) has been advocated by some investigators with a minimal risk of steroid-related soft-tissue atrophy (67–68). The most beneficial treatment appears to be total capsulectomy and replacement of implants with textured saline devices into a newly dissected preferably subpectoral pocket. The role of displacement exercises is not clear with textured devices, as the role of adherence, formation of a double capsule (i.e., a capsule within a capsule), and use of recently available anatomically designed implants makes the beneficial effects uncertain and perhaps contraindicated.

TISSUE THINNING

Tissue thinning is most commonly seen if steroids are injected within the implant lumen and to a lesser degree within the implant pocket. It typically occurs from injudicious use of nonsoluble steroids in attempts to prevent capsular contracture and presents several years after implantation. If appropriate dosages and techniques are used, significant atrophy is extremely rare. It can result in parenchymal, subcutaneous, and skin thinning, and occasionally leads to impending implant extrusion or frank exposure (67,68). Surgical intervention is warranted prior to exposure, at which time relocation of the implant to a retropectoral location may be required. Occasionally, temporary implant removal is required. Parenteral vitamin E may help to counteract the effect of the steroid, as there has been some studies to suggest that the release of steroids from the implant can persist for years (the diffusion half-life of methylprednisolone has been shown to have been approximately 20 months) (69–71).

MUSCULAR DISTORTION OF THE IMPLANT

This occurs with retromuscular placement of implants, primarily if inadequate release of the inferomedial sternal pectoral attachments has been achieved. It results in diagonal compression of the implant, with loss of lower-pole projection during dynamic pectoral contractions (9,12,72). This is justification in female body builders not to undertake retromuscular augmentation. Correction of this problem requires further surgical release of the lower pectoral insertion or, more commonly, change of implant location to a retroglandular position.

CUTANEOUS SCARRING

Occasionally, despite good technique, cutaneous scarring can be a problem postoperatively, and can be seen both in the periareolar and inframammary locations. Axillary scars are generally well tolerated unless the orientation of the scar is placed across the lines of tension and not in the transverse folds. Little more than local measures to speed scar maturation can be offered to patients with problematic scars. Occasionally, scar revision is undertaken in a delayed manner for inframammary incisions that have spread.

References

1. Cronin TD, Greenberg RL. Our experience with the Silastic gel breast prosthesis. *Plast Reconstr Surg* 1970; 46:1.
2. Williams JE. Experience with a large series of Silastic breast implants. *Plast Reconstr Surg* 1972; 49:253.
3. Courtiss EH, Goldwyn RM, Anastasi GW. The fate of breast implants with infections around them. *Plast Reconstr Surg* 1979; 63:812.

4. Williams C, Aston S, Rees TD. The effect of hematoma on the thickness of pseudosheaths around silicone implants. *Plast Reconstr Surg* 1975; 56:194.

5. Hester TR: The polyurethane covered mammary prosthesis: facts and fiction. *Persp Plast Surg* 1988; 2:135.

6. Barone FE, Perry L, Keller T, et al. The biochemical and histopathologic effects of surface texturing with silicone and polyurethane in tissue implantation and expansion. *Plast Reconstr Surg* 1992; 90:77.

7. Maxwell GP. Transaxillary subpectoral augmentation mammaplasty. In: Georgiade NG, Georgiade GS, Riefkohl R, eds. *Aesthetic surgery of the breast.* Philadelphia: WB Saunders, 1990; 75.

8. Courtiss EH, Goldwyn RM. Breast sensation before and after plastic surgery. *Plast Reconstr Surg* 1976; 58:1.

9. Farina MA, Newby BG, Alani HM. Innervation of the nipple-areolar complex. *Plast Reconstr Surg* 1980; 66:497.

10. Spear SL, Matsuba H, Little JW. The medial periareolar approach to submuscular augmentation mammaplasty under local anaesthesia. *Plast Reconstr Surg* 1989; 84:599.

11. Tebbetts JB. Transaxillary subpectoral augmentation mammaplasty: long-term follow-up and refinements. *Plast Reconstr Surg* 1984; 74:636.

12. Tebbetts JB. Transaxillary subpectoral augmentation mammaplasty: a 9-year experience. *Clin Plast Surg* 1988; 15:557.

13. McGrath MH, Burkhardt BR. The safety and efficacy of breast implants for augmentation mammaplasty. *Plast Reconstr Surg* 1984; 74:550.

14. Biggs TM, Cukier J, Worthing LF. Augmentation mammaplasty: a review of 18 years. *Plast Reconstr Surg* 1982; 69:445.

15. Wilkinson TS, Swartz BE, Toranto R. Resolution of late-developing periprosthetic breast infections without prosthesis removal. *Aesthetic Plast Surg* 1985; 9:79.

16. Rothkopf DM, Rosen HM. Lactation as a complication of aesthetic breast surgery successfully treated with bromocriptine. *Br J Plast Surg* 1990; 43:373.

17. Green RA, Dowden RV. Mondor disease in plastic surgery patients. *Ann Plast Surg* 1988; 20:231.

18. Biggs TM, Yarish RS. Augmentation mammaplasty: retropectoral versus retromammary implantation. *Clin Plast Surg* 1988; 15:549.

19. Hester TR, Nahai F, Bostwick J, et al. A 5-year experience with polyurethane-covered mammary prostheses for treatment of capsular contracture, primary augmentation mammaplasty, and breast reconstruction. *Clin Plast Surg* 1988; 15:569.

20. Lavine DM. Saline inflatable prostheses: 14 years' experience. *Aesthet Plast Surg* 1993; 17:325.

21. McKinney P, Tresley G. Long-term comparison of patients with gel and saline mammary implants. *Plast Reconstr Surg* 1983; 72:27.

22. Spear SL. Breast reconstruction with expanders and implants. Presented at Advances in Breast Surgery, Symposium 1, Nashville, TN, May 1994.

23. Maxwell GP. The importance of the inframammary fold in aesthetic and reconstructive surgery. Presented at the annual meeting of the American Society for Aesthetic Plastic Surgery, Los Angeles, 1987.

24. Dunn KW, Hall PN, Khoo CTK. Breast implant materials: sense and safety. *Br J Plast Surg* 1992; 45:315.

25. Leibman AJ. Imaging of complications of augmentation mammaplasty. *Plast Reconstr Surg* 1994; 93:1134.

26. van Wingerden JJ, van Staden MM. Ultrasound mammography in prosthesis-related breast augmentation complications. *Ann Plast Surg* 1989; 22:32.

27. Levine RA, Collins TL. Definitive diagnosis of breast implant rupture by ultrasonography. *Plast Reconstr Surg* 1991; 87:1126.

28. Andersen B, Hawtof D, Alani H, et al. The diagnosis of ruptured breast implants. *Plast Reconstr Surg* 1989; 84:903.

29. Dowden RV, Anain S. Endoscopic implant evaluation and capsulotomy. *Plast Reconstr Surg* 1993; 91:283.

30. Williams CW. Silicone gel granuloma following compressive mammography. *Aesthetic Plast Surg* 1991; 15:49.

31. Oppenheimer BS, et al. Further studies of polymers as carcinogenic agents in animals. *Cancer Res* 1955; 15:333.

32. Deapen DM, Brody GS. Augmentation mammaplasty and breast cancer: a 5-year update of the Los Angeles study. *Plast Reconstr Surg* 1992; 89:660.

33. Berkel H, Birdsell DC, Jenkins H. Breast augmentation: a risk factor for breast cancer? *N Eng J Med* 1992; 326:1649.

34. Schirber S, Thomas WO, Finley JM, et al. Breast cancer after mammary augmentation. *South Med J* 1993; 86:263.

35. Brozena SJ, Fenske NA, Cruse CW, et al. Human adjuvant disease following augmentation mammaplasty. *Arch Dermatol* 1988; 124:1383.

36. Spiera H. Scleroderma after silicone augmentation mammaplasty. *JAMA* 1988; 260:236.

37. Varga J, Schumacher HR, Jimenez SA. Systemic sclerosis after augmentation mammaplasty with silicone implants. *Ann Int Med* 1989; 111:377.

38. Sergott TJ, Limoli JP, Baldwin CM, et al. Human adjuvant disease, possible autoimmune disease after silicone implantation: a review of the literature, case studies, and speculation for the future. *Plast Reconstr Surg* 1986; 78:104.

39. Press RI, Peebles CL, Kumagai Y, et al. Antinuclear autoantibodies in women with silicone breast implants. *Lancet* 1992; 340:1304.

40. Gabriel SE, O'Fallon WM, Kurland LT, et al. Risk of connective-tissue diseases and other disorders after breast implantation. *N Eng J Med* 1994; 330:1697.

41. David P. Augmentation mammaplasty: beauty or the beast. *J Rheum* 1993; 20:927.

42. Brody GS, et al. Consensus statement on the relationship of breast implants to connective-tissue disorders. *Plast Reconstr Surg* 1992; 90:1102.

43. Ersek RA. Rate and incidence of capsular contracture: a comparison of smooth and textured silicone double-lumen breast prostheses. *Plast Reconstr Surg* 1991; 87:879.

44. Melmed EP. Polyurethane implants: a 6-year review of 416 patients. *Plast Reconstr Surg* 1988; 82:285.

45. Pennisi VR. Long-term use of polyurethane breast prostheses: a 14-year experience. *Plast Reconstr Surg* 1990; 86:368.

46. Jacobson ED. Food and Drug Administration: open letter to the American Society of Plastic and Reconstructive Surgeons, April 24, 1991.

47. Eklund GW, Busby RC, Miller SH, et al. Improved imaging of the augmented breast. *Am J Roentgenol* 1988; 151:469.

48. Glicksman CA, Glicksman AS, Courtiss EH. Breast imaging for plastic surgeons. *Plast Reconstr Surg* 1992; 90:1106.

49. Silverstein MJ, Handel N, Gamagami P. The effects of silicone-gel filled implants on mammography. *Cancer* 1991; 68 (suppl):1159.

50. Gumucio CA, Pin P, Young VL, et al. The effect of breast implants on the radiographic detection of microcalcification and soft-tissue masses. *Plast Reconstr Surg* 1989; 84:772.

51. Silverstein MJ, Handel N, Gamagami P, et al. Mammographic measurements before and after augmentation mammaplasty. *Plast Reconstr Surg* 1990; 86:1126.

52. Silverstein MJ, Handel N, Gamagami P. Breast cancer diagnosis and prognosis in women following augmentation with silicone gel–filled prostheses. *Eur J Cancer* 1992; 28:635.

53. Carlson GW, Curley SA, Martin JE, et al. The detection of breast cancer after augmentation mammaplasty. *Plast Reconstr Surg* 1993; 91:837.

54. Hayes H, Vandergrift J, Diner WC. Mammography and breast implants. *Plast Reconstr Surg* 1988; 82:1.

55. Baker JL Jr. Classification of spherical contractures. Presented at the Aesthetic Breast Symposium, Scottsdale, Arizona, 1975.

56. Burkhardt BR, Schnur PL, Tofield JJ, et al. Objective clinical assessment of fibrous capsular contracture. *Plast Reconstr Surg* 1982; 69:794.

57. Burkhardt BR. Capsular contracture: hard breasts, soft data. *Clin Plast Surg* 1988; 15:521.

58. Puckett CL, Croll GH, Reichel CA, et al. A critical look at capsule contracture in subglandular versus subpectoral mammary augmentation. *Aesth Plast Surg* 1987; 11:23.

59. Burkhardt BR, Dempsey PD, Schnur PL, et al. Capsular contracture: a prospective study of the effects of local antibacterial agents. *Plast Reconstr Surg* 1986; 77:919.

60. Hakelius L, Ohlsen L. A clinical comparison of the tendency to capsular contacture between smooth and textured gel-filled silicone mammary implants. *Plast Reconstr Surg* 1992; 90:247.

61. Burkhardt BR, Demas CP. The effect of Siltex texturing and povidone-iodine irrigation on capsular contracture around saline inflatable breast implants. *Plast Reconstr Surg* 1994; 93:123.

62. Rudolph R, Abraham J, Vecchione T, et al. Myofibroblasts and free silicon around breast implants. *Plast Reconstr Surg* 1978; 62, 185.

63. Lossing C, Hansson HA. Peptide growth factors and myofibroblasts in capsules around human breast implants. *Plast Reconstr Surg* 1993; 91:1277.

64. Baker JL Jr, Chandler ML, LeVier RR. Occurrence and activity of myofibroblasts in human capsular tissue surrounding mammary implants. *Plast Reconstr Surg* 1981; 68:905.

65. Gylbert L, Asplund O, Jurell G. Capsular contracture after breast reconstruction with silicone-gel and saline-filled implants: a 6-year follow-up. *Plast Reconstr Surg* 1990; 85:373.

66. Clugston PA, Perry LC, Hammond D, et al. A rat model for capsular contracture: the effects of surface texturing. *Ann Plast Surg* 1994; 33:595.

67. Peterson HD, Burt GB Jr. The role of steroids in prevention of circumferential capsular scarring in augmentation mammaplasty. *Plast Reconstr Surg* 1974; 54:28.

68. Perrin ER. The use of soluble steroids within inflatable breast prostheses. *Plast Reconstr Surg* 1976; 57:163.

69. Ellenberg AH, Braun H. A 3½ year experience with double lumen implants in breast surgery. *Plast Reconstr Surg* 1980; 65:307.

70. Cucin RL, Guthrie RH, Graham M. Rate of diffusion of Solu-medrol across the silastic membranes of breast prostheses: an in vitro study. *Ann Plast Surg* 1982; 9:228.

71. Morykwas MJ, Argenta LC, Oneal RM, et al. The fate of soluble steroids within breast prostheses in humans. *Ann Plast Surg* 1990; 24:427.

72. Maxwell GP, Tornambe R. Management of mammary subpectoral implant distortion. *Clin Plast Surg* 1988; 15:601.

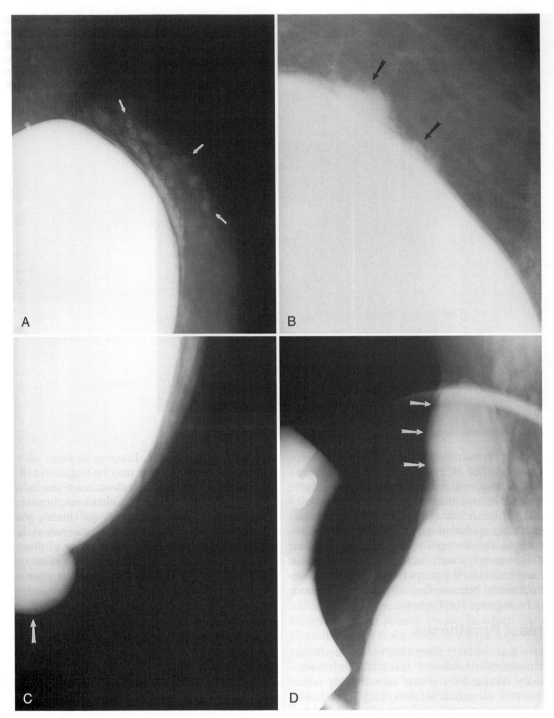

FIG. 63–4. Mammographic findings of implant rupture. **A,** mediolateral oblique mammogram of the left breast demonstrates free silicone globules within the breast parenchyma (arrows). Some have rim calcifications. **B,** craniocaudal mammogram of the left breast shows a small, irregular protrusion of silicone away from the expected smooth contour of the implant (arrows). **C,** coned mediolateral oblique mammogram of the left breast demonstrates a smooth protrusion of the inferior aspect of the left implant (arrow). **D,** mediolateral oblique mammogram of the right breast shows streaming of silicone away from the superior aspect of the implant into the axilla (arrows). Free silicone is also seen in the surrounding area.

also be seen in cases of heavy gel bleed. Silicone can occasionally be seen in mammary ducts following rupture. False positive exams may occur when residual silicone from a previous implant rupture is identified; therefore, comparison with earlier films and knowledge of past surgical history are important to avoid misinterpretation. Findings such as tenting of the implant, capsular calcification, and rounding of the implant are nonspecific and are not indicative of rupture. The absence of mammographic abnormality does not exclude implant rupture; false negative mammograms occur for several

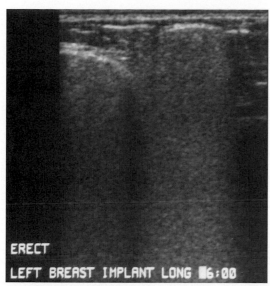

FIG. 63–5. Sonogram of the ruptured implant seen in Figure 64–4C shows two echogenic columns that obscure underlying structures. This is known as the snowstorm sign and corresponds to extracapsular silicone.

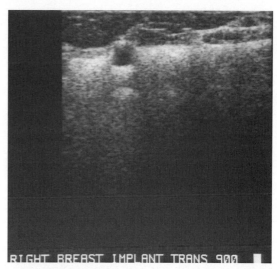

FIG. 63–6. Sonogram demonstrates a hypoechoic nodule with echogenic backwall and echogenic reverberation in the tissue deep to the nodule, consistent with a free silicone globule within the parenchyma.

reasons. Intracapsular rupture, which accounts for a large number of ruptured implants, is not seen on film screen mammograms. Extracapsular rupture, particularly small silicone droplets, may evade detection on craniocaudal and mediolateral oblique views if they are located posteriorly within the breast because they are obscured by the large opaque prosthesis. Additional focal compression views may be useful for evaluating these posterior regions if rupture is suspected clinically. The posterior half of subpectoral implants cannot be imaged using film screen mammography, and posterior portions of subglandular implants are rarely seen, limiting mammographic sensitivity.

In evaluating double lumen implants, mammographic detection of an outer saline lumen implies that both lumens are intact. Absence of detection of the outer lumen signifies deflation of the saline lumen but does not address the issue of integrity of the inner silicone lumen. Deflation of the outer saline lumen is common over the natural history of double lumen implants. Some patients may have a double lumen implant on one side and a single lumen implant on the other; in these cases, knowledge of implant type and surgical history is important for accurate evaluation.

Many patients are having silicone implants replaced with saline implants. Mammography readily detects deflation of saline implants, demonstrating marked wrinkling and collapse of the shell, with decreased or no remaining saline identified.

SONOGRAPHY

In patients with clinically suspected rupture who have mammographic findings that are negative or indeterminate, ultrasound is a useful adjunctive exam. Ultrasound of an intact implant reveals a large anechoic, smoothly margined prosthesis with reverberation echoes seen superficially. Findings that are suspicious for rupture include the "snowstorm" pattern (a column of echodense noise with well-defined anterior

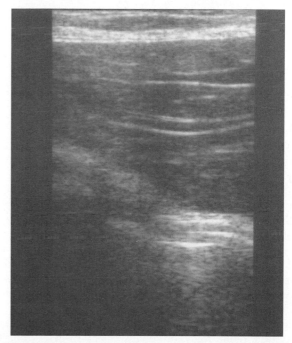

FIG. 63–7. Sonogram of the left prosthesis in a patient suspected to have implant rupture shows numerous parallel white lines within the dark implant. This stepladder sign corresponds to the collapsed shell of the implant.

and poorly defined posterior margins corresponding to free silicone in soft tissues adjacent to the implant) (Fig. 63–5), hypoechoic nodules with echodense backwalls and posterior echogenic reverberation (Fig. 63–6), corresponding to free silicone globules in the parenchyma, and the "stepladder" sign (parallel echogenic lines within the implant) (Fig. 63–7), signifying intracapsular rupture (15–18).

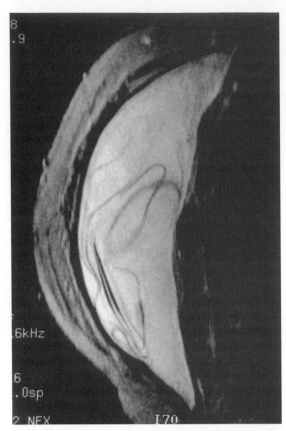

FIG. 63–8.   Sagittal T2-weighted FSE image of the breast shows hyperintense silicone surrounded by a black fibrous capsule. There are curvilinear black lines ("linguine" sign) within the bright silicone, corresponding to the collapsed implant shell.

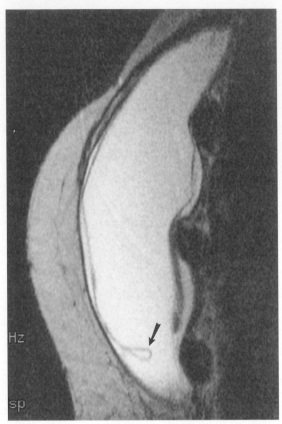

FIG. 63–9.   Sagittal T2-weighted FSE image of the breast shows subtle signs of intracapsular implant rupture and shell collapse. A black line paralleling the fibrous capsule is seen within the bright silicone; this corresponds to the implant shell that has been displaced away from the fibrous capsule by a small amount of silicone that has leaked from the prosthesis. A more focal area of shell displacement is shown by the "teardrop" sign (arrow).

Sonography also has limitations in evaluating implants. In several small series, the snowstorm pattern has been a reliable sign for rupture; however, false positives can occur. Parenchymal cysts may be confused with the hypoechoic nodules with echogenic reverberation if care is not taken to document the presence of the echogenic reverberation. The hypoechoic nodules may also be misleading in patients who have residual silicone left over within breast parenchyma from earlier implant rupture and exchange. While intracapsular rupture can be detected sonographically by the stepladder sign, nonspecific echogenic lines are frequently identified within the implants. These may correspond with intracapsular rupture, radial folds, or collapsed saline shells from double lumen implants, and caution should be taken in diagnosing intracapsular rupture in these patients.

MAGNETIC RESONANCE IMAGING

Magnetic resonance imaging has the highest sensitivity (95%) and specificity (93%) of all imaging modalities in evaluating implant integrity and is the method of choice to detect ruptured implants (14). Dedicated breast coils or other surface coils (shoulder coil, flexicoil) are necessary to achieve high-resolution images of the implants. The patient is placed in the coil in a prone position to limit respiratory motion artifact, and images are obtained in at least two planes to assess the breasts and implants adequately.

Intracapsular rupture is best detected by MRI, demonstrated by low-intensity curvilinear lines (the "linguine sign") (Fig. 63–8) located within the high-intensity silicone (19). These lines represent the ruptured and collapsed silicone shell surrounded by free silicone that is contained within the fibrous capsule. Two other signs of intracapsular rupture are the "teardrop sign," where the shell is focally displaced away from the fibrous capsule in a teardrop configuration and parallel low-intensity lines just inside the fibrous capsule on multiple consecutive images (Fig. 63–9). Some false-positives could occur with the teardrop sign or parallel line sign in cases of heavy gel bleed (20). The signs of intracapsular rupture should not be confused with normal radial folds, which are infoldings of an intact silicone shell. More prominent, complex radial folds are often seen in double lumen implants where the outer saline lumen has deflated but the inner gel lumen is intact; these may be more difficult to differentiate from ruptured implants.

Mammography Following Prosthesis Explantation

Many patients with silicone prostheses are electing to have the implants removed and not replaced, either due to implant complications or because of recent concerns about the safety of silicone implants. The mammographic appearance in these patients ranges from a nearly normal parenchymal pattern to severe distortion. Residual fibrous capsules, free silicone, fat necrosis, and spiculated masses may be identified (22,23). Seromas may develop in residual fibrous capsules in cases where implants were removed through capsulotomy. Mammography of these seromas shows large, irregular, or well-circumscribed masses that could be confused with residual silicone, saline implants, or malignant lesions (24). Knowledge of the spectrum of mammographic findings following implant removal is necessary in order to avoid unnecessary biopsy in these patients.

References

1. Eklund GW, Busby RC, Miller SH, et al. Improved imaging of the augmented breast. *Am J Roentgenol,* 1988; 151:469–473.
2. Snyderman RK, Lizardo JG. Statistical study of malignancies formed before, during or after routine breast plastic operations. *Plast Reconstr Surg* 1960; 25:253.
3. Pitanguy I, Torres ET. Histopathological aspects of mammary gland tissue in cases of plastic surgery of the breast. *Br J Plast Surg* 1964; 17:97.
4. Fajardo LL, Roberts CC, Hunt KR. Mammographic surveillance of breast cancer patients: should the mastectomy site be imaged? *Am J Roentgenol* 1993; 161:953–955.
5. Propeck PA, Scanlan KA. Utility of axillary views in postmastectomy patients. *Radiology* 1993; 187:769–771.
6. Rissanen TJ, Makarainen HP, Mattila SI, et al. Breast cancer recurrence after mastectomy: diagnosis with mammography and US. *Radiology* 1993; 188:463–467.
7. Lee CH, Poplack SP, Stahl RS. Mammographic appearance of the transverse rectus abdominus musculocutaneous (TRAM) Flap. *Breast Dis* 1994; 7:99–107.
8. Mund DF, Wolfson P, Gorczyca DP, et al. Mammographically detected recurrent nonpalpable carcinoma developing in a transverse rectus abdominus myocutaneous flap. A case report. *Cancer* 1994; 74:2804–2807.
9. Mendelson EB. Evaluation of the postoperative breast. *Radiol Clin North America* 1992; 30:107–138.
10. Miller CL, Feig SA, Fox JW. Mammographic changes after reduction mammoplasty. *Am J Roentgenol* 1987; 149:35–38.
11. Fajardo LL, Bessen SC. Epidermal inclusion cyst after reduction mammoplasty. *Radiology* 1993; 186:103–106.
12. Baber CE, Libshitz HI. Bilateral fat necrosis of the breast following reduction mammoplasties. *Am J Roentgenol* 1977; 128:508.
13. Steinbach BG, Hardt NS, Abbitt PL. Mammography: breast implants—types, complications, and adjacent breast pathology (review). *Curr Probl Diagn Radiol* 1993; 22:43–86.
14. Everson LI, Parantainen H, Detlie T, et al. Diagnosis of breast implant rupture: imaging findings and relative efficacies of imaging techniques. *Am J Roentgenol* 1994; 163:57–60.
15. Rosculet KA, Ikeda DM, Forrest ME, et al. Ruptured gel-filled silicone breast implants: sonographic findings in 19 cases. *Am J Roentgenol* 1992; 159:711–716.
16. Ganott MA, Harris KM, Ilkhanipour ZS, et al. Augmentation mammoplasty: normal and abnormal findings with mammography and US. *Radiographics* 1992; 12:281–295.
17. Harris KM, Ganott MA, Shestak KC, et al. Silicone implant rupture: detection with US. *Radiology* 1993; 187:761–768.
18. DeBruhl ND, Gorczyca DP, Ahn CY, et al. Silicone breast implants: US evaluation. *Radiology* 1993; 189:95–98.
19. Gorczyca DP, Sinha S, Ahn CY, et al. Silicone breast implants in vivo: MR imaging. *Radiology* 1992; 185:407–410.
20. Mund DF, Farria DM, Gorczyca DP, et al. MR imaging of the breast in patients with silicone-gel implants: spectrum of findings. *Am J Roentgenol* 1993; 161:773–778.
21. Berg WA, Caskey CI, Hamper UM, et al. Diagnosing breast implant rupture with MR imaging, US, and mammography. *Radiographics* 1993; 13:1323–1336.
22. Hayes MK, Gold RH, Bassett LW. Mammographic findings after the removal of breast implants. *Am J Roentgenol* 1993; 160:487–490.
23. Stewart NR, Monsees BS, Destouet JM, et al. Mammographic appearance following implant removal. *Radiology* 1992; 185:83–85.
24. Soo MS, Kornguth PJ, Georgiade GS, et al. Seromas in residual fibrous capsules after explantation: mammographic and sonographic appearances. *Radiology* 1995; 194:863–866.

64

Hypermastia and Ptosis

Gregory S. Georgiade, M.D., F.A.C.S., and Nicholas G. Georgiade, M.D., F.A.C.S.

Improvements in the state of the art in the reduction of hypertrophied breasts with and without associated ptosis has produced a number of procedures yielding acceptable to excellent results. No one procedure has presently been designed to manage the wide range of mammary hypertrophies (1).

Anatomic Factors

BLOOD SUPPLY TO THE BREASTS

The blood supply to the breast is primarily from three plexuses, the perforating branches of the internal mammary artery through the pectoral muscles supplying the upper and inferior medial aspects of the breast (these are mainly the upper four perforating mammary branches). The upper and lateral portion of the breast is supplied by branches of the lateral thoracic or external mammary artery. The branches of the lateral thoracic artery coalesce with the internal mammary branches, supplying approximately 75% of the blood supply to the nipple-areola area. The lesser blood supply is via the intercostal perforating arteries, which represent the third group of vessels supplying the lateral and infralateral areas of the breast; these collateralize with the external mammary artery branches and posterior aortic perforating arteries (2). This supports the authors' concept of continuity of the dermal blood supply and glandular tissue.

INNERVATION OF THE BREAST

The breast, and particularly the nipple-areolar area, is supplied by the lateral cutaneous intercostal nerves—primarily from the 3rd to the 6th intercostal nerves—which innervate the lateral breast area, and the 4th and 5th intercostal nerves innervating, in particular, the nipple and the areolar area. The internal mammary nerves perforate through the pectoralis musculature and join with the intercostal innervation to the medial inferior aspect of the breast. The superior aspect of the breast is innervated by the 3rd and 4th branches of the cervical plexus.

Hypermastia

A breast of less than 500 grams is amenable to a number of reduction procedures utilizing various types of dermal flaps for transporting the nipple-areola complex to its new location. Early techniques were described by Arie (3) and Pitanguy (4) (Fig. 64–1A) using a superior dermal pedicle and by Strömbeck (5) using a horizontal dermal pedicle. Since then, techniques by Dufourmentel and Mouly (6), by Skoog (7) using a lateral dermal pedicle nipple-areolar flap (Fig.

64–1B) and others (8–16) have utilized various other types of dermal flaps with the nipple-areolar complex transferred on these pedicles. The greater the distance the dermal pedicle is to be transferred superiorly, the greater will be the traction on the dermal pedicle, making nipple transposition more difficult (Fig. 64–1C,D). The massive breast hypertrophy is managed by amputation and free full-thickness nipple-areola grafts (17) (Fig. 64–1E).

LIPOSUCTION OF THE BREAST

Liposuction alone, or as an adjunctive procedure, can be carried out via two small incisions medially and laterally in the premarked new inframammary line or as described by Le Jour (18,19) in the medial inframammary dermal location (Fig. 64–2). The second option is to proceed with deepithelialization of the inferior dermal pedicle and then the medial or lateral liposuction (Fig. 64–3). The third option is to liposuction the usual areas of excess fat accumulation, particularly the medial and lateral areas, just during the final stages of closure following reduction mammaplasty.

REDUCTION UTILIZING DERMAL FLAPS

Superiorly Based Dermal Flap

The use of a superiorly based dermal flap has been described by Weiner and colleagues (8) and Cramer and Chong (9). The nipple-areolar pedicle can be elevated as much as 6 cm without increasing the potential loss of vascularity and nipple sensation (see Fig. 64–1D).

Vertical Bipedicle Dermal Flap

The vertical bipedicle dermal flap of McKissock (10) has been found to be a predictable method of breast reduction with particular value in the removal of up to 1000 g of breast tissue. With associated marked ptosis of the breasts, it is more difficult to accurately position and match the nipple-areola complex of both breasts, and partial necrosis of the areola occurs occasionally. This difficulty has been noted particularly when the superior dermal pedicle is over 6 cm in length and there is any torsion on the dermal pedicle.

Superior Horizontal Dermal Flap

The superior horizontal dermal flap described by Arie (3) and redefined by Pitanguy (4) has produced excellent results (Fig. 64–4). This technique was further changed by Ribeiro (11) by placing an underlying inferior pedicle flap in order to result in a more protrusive conical breast.

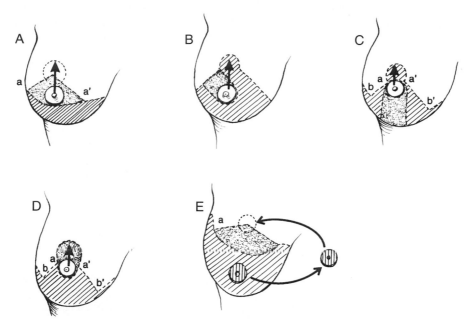

FIG. 64–1. **A,** Arie Pitanguy dermal flap. **B,** lateral Skoog dermal pedicle nipple-areolar flap. **C,** inferior dermal pedicle flap. **D,** superior based dermal flap. **E,** Rubin breast amputation reduction mammaplasty procedure. The nipple-areola from the amputated specimen is transferred as free full-thickness grafts.

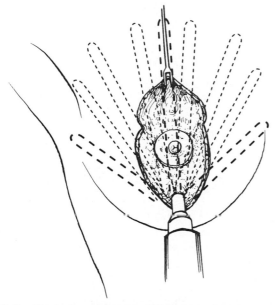

FIG. 64–2. The LeJour technique of liposuction of the hypertrophied breast.

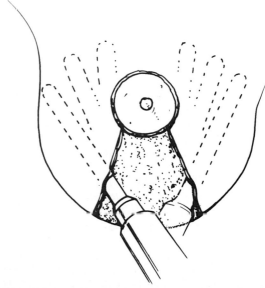

FIG. 64–3. Liposuction medial and lateral to the inferior dermal pedicle before the mammary resection.

Classic Pitanguy Reduction

The width and level of the future breast resection is determined by the inframammary crease E (see Fig. 64–4) and points A, B, and C that are equidistant from the nipple. Points D and E delineate the limits of the future resection and the new inframammary resection. The points are now marked with brilliant green. The epidermis is removed within points ABC in the periareolar area. The breast tissue with skin is then excised as a unit BE:CD. A keel-type excision is carried out in the subareolar area, with the degree of excision depending upon the desired reduction in size of the breast form. The breast is then closed in three layers. With the patient in a semi-upright position, the location of the nipple is determined and placed slightly lower than the optimal site. The nipple sites are determined utilizing a suture from the sternal notch and manubrium and equidistant from the midline. Liposuction of the breasts is carried out medially and laterally for the final tailoring of the breast form. Drains are inserted laterally in each breast. The skin is then closed with interrupted and continuous subcutaneous 5-0 nylon sutures. A figure-eight dressing is applied.

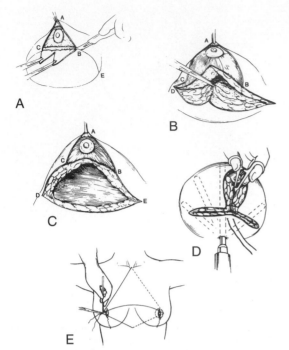

FIG. 64–4. **A,** area of epidermis to be removed is marked (points A, B, C, E). **B,** areas of breast skin resection are shown as CB-DE. **C,** area of excision (D, C, B, E). **D,** areas of liposuction and closure technique. **E,** final check for positioning of the nipple is determined with the patient in the semi-upright position. A suture from the sternal notch and another suture from the mid manubrium determine the nipple position bilaterally.

The limitations of this procedure appear to be the larger breast (exceeding 1000 grams), and the difficulty in elevating the dermal nipple-areolar pedicle in the ptotic breast. This latter problem has been partly resolved by partially incising the inferiomedial and lateral aspects of the dermal areolar flap.

Inferiorly Based Dermal Flap

The inferiorly based dermal flap described by Robbins (12), Courtiss and Goldwyn (13), and Georgiade and colleagues (14) was a natural progression in the state of the art of breast reduction (see Fig. 64–1C). Certain important modifications have been found to be most valuable in attaining the best possible result with inclusion of an inferior dermal pyamidal breast pedicle for simultaneous correction of ptosis (15,16,20–23). We have modified this procedure as discussed below.

Inferiorly Based Dermal Pyramidal Flap

Our modification maintains a broad-based flap of breast tissue, so that sufficient blood supply and tissue remain at the base of the pyramidal flap to support the nipple-areola complex (Fig. 64–5). This technique has the advantage of resulting in a breast that is easily shaped and can be elevated to any desired height. In addition, since there are seldom neurovascular changes to the areola and nipple, and no disruption of underlying breast parenchyma, lactation is still possible (16).

The amount of breast tissue to be removed, and the position of the nipple-areola complex, are usually determined preoperatively with the patient in an upright or standing position (see Fig. 64–5).

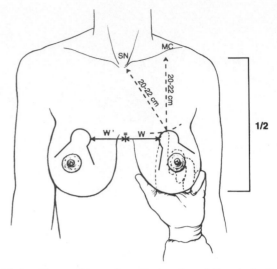

FIG. 64–5. The markings place the location of the nipple, the distance of the new nipple from the midline, and the width of the breast dermal pedicles and future skin flaps.

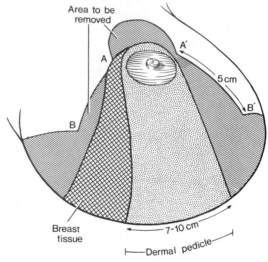

FIG. 64–6. The pyramidal dermal breast flap is outlined. Note the increased width at the base with the increase of ptosis. The dermal pedicle width is variable, depending on the desired eventual breast mound size.

The distance from the clavicular notch to the new areolar site is calculated at approximately 20 cm and slightly above the inframammary line (see Fig. 64–5). The amount of skin excision and breast coning is then determined. The calculated resultant skin flaps should be able to be approximated with only slight tension on the flaps. The distance between the flaps will vary from 8 cm to more than 16 cm for the breast resection of more than 1200 g. The distance from each areola to the midsternal line should be equal ($W_1 = W_2$) and is usually 10 to 12 cm from the midsternal line (see Fig. 64–5). The flap is marked with gentian violet or brilliant green, which is preferred because it is discernible after skin preparation. The skin flaps overlying the resected breast tissue should be maintained at 1.5 cm in thickness (Fig. 64–6). Coning of the breast tissue and liposuction can be carried out

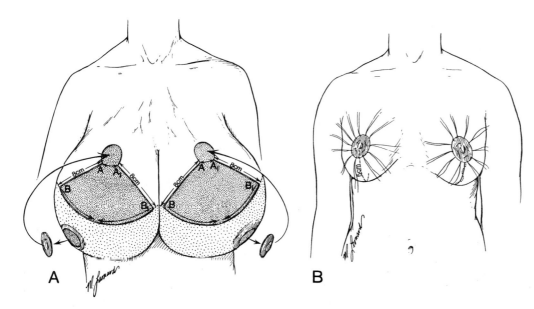

FIG. 64–7. **A,** the width of the breast amputation and dermal pedicle may vary depending on the size of each breast. The nipple-areolas are excised from the breast tissue specimen. **B,** the position of the new nipple areola site is determined with the patient in a semi-upright position and the nipple-areola specimen placed on the dermal base as a free graft.

at this time (see Fig. 64–3). The skin flaps are then adjusted and approximated using 4-0 Dexon or Vicryl sutures; the areola is approximated in its new position utilizing 5-0 Prolene sutures for the circumareolar skin approximation and 4-0 Prolene subcuticular sutures for vertical and horizontal skin approximation. Paper tape is then applied to the appropriate skin edges. *Note:* A suction drain is inserted into each lateral breast flap before the final dermal approximation.

A bulky mechanics waste dressing is applied and an 8-inch stockinette cut on the bias is used to wrap and support the breast, using a figure-eight configuration. The breasts are examined within 24 hours for any sign of hematoma, drains are removed 24 hours postoperatively, and the sutures are removed on the day 12 postoperatively.

GIGANTISM OF THE BREAST

The use of a breast amputation and free nipple grafting technique (17) is reserved for the breast reductions over 2500 grams, when the use of the inferior dermal pedicle technique is not feasible. The reduction of massive breasts will not yield a consistently satisfactory aesthetic result because of the difficulties in symmetrically matching the breasts after reduction and in predicting accurately the vascularity and symmetry of the free nipple-areola grafts after grafting (Fig. 64–7). The technique as described by Rubin (17) appears to yield a satisfactory postoperative aesthetic result.

Breast Ptosis

The breast in the young adult female is located over the pectoral muscle, starting usually at the second intracostal space and extending over a surface inferior to the 6th rib. The nipple is usually slightly lower than the center of the breast, with increased inferior shifting with age below the submammary fold.

The ptotic breast will have excess skin, causing the nipple-areola complex to be located at various positions inferiorly depending on the degree of ptosis. The ptotic breast may have an associated hypertrophy of the breast tissue or, in most types of ptotic breasts, there may be varying amounts of breast tissue and fat atrophy.

The type of ptosis must be considered before any attempt to correct. The two major types of ptosis usually fit into either glandular or true ptosis. Where the entire glandular tissue including the nipple skin and gland is involved, there is considered to be a glandular ptosis. True ptosis appears to be directed to the excess skin above the nipple areolar area (24). (See also Chapter 66.)

MANAGEMENT OF PTOSIS WITHOUT BREAST REDUCTION

Minimal Ptosis

In minimal breast ptosis the nipple is at the level of the inframammary fold. Correction can usually be carried out with a small augmentation using 140- to 160-ml prostheses. Inflatable prostheses can be inserted via an inferior periareolar incision in a subcutaneous or submuscular position. An axillary approach (and, more recently, an endoscopic transumbilical approach) can be used. (See Chapter 61, on augmentation mammaplasty.)

Occasionally, after reevaluation of the position of the nipple, a slight elevation of the areola can be carried out by deepithelialization of a determined amount of superior skin with advancement of the areola into this new position (Fig. 64–8). The redundant infraareolar skin is tailored and excised with an oblique lateral excision or, if practical, the skin may be redraped using a Benelli-type periareolar suturing technique (25) (Fig. 64–9).

Intermediate Ptosis

There is an excess of skin brassiere in intermediate ptosis, with the nipple as much as 3 cm below the submammary fold. If there is adequate breast volume, then the new nipple and areola position is marked once again on the breast at the level of the inframammary fold. Loss of tissue substance, with resultant breast atrophy, necessitates not only augmentation to the atrophic breast mound but also skin draping. The markings for the contemplated new nipple-areola position are made, but the repositioning is not executed until the augmentation has been carried out. The augmentation procedure is performed

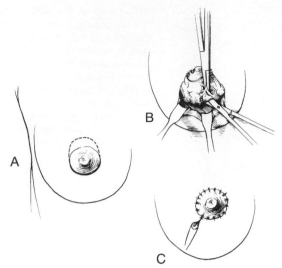

FIG. 64–8. **A,** simple elevation of the nipple-areola attained by superior deepithelialization and superior advancement. **B,** augmentation of the breast via an inferior periareolar approach can be carried out simultaneously. **C,** alternate procedure shows excision of the lateral inferior areola skin when the Benelli-type closure is not feasible.

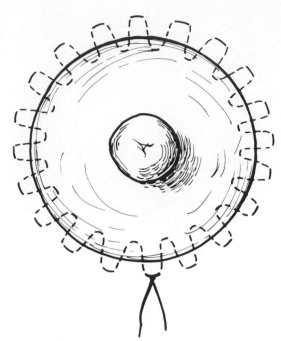

FIG. 64–9. The approximation of the redundant periareolar skin is carried out by utilizing a permanent 3-0 subcuticular suture (Benelli technique).

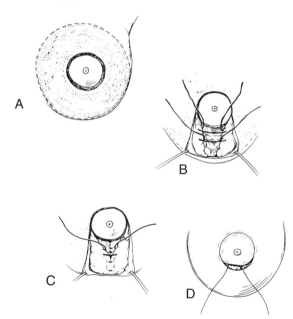

FIG. 64–10. **A,** area of undermined skin flaps. **B,** variable V-type inframammary excision and closure, with invagination and reversal of interrupted permanent sutures. **C,** second layer of invaginated inframammary periareolar sutures. **D,** subcuticular approximation of periareolar skin.

via a circumareolar incision in the lower half of the areola. Through this incision, the breast tissue is separated from its fatty layer inferiorly to the pectoral muscle. An incision is made through the pectoralis musculature. The plane of dissection then goes beneath the pectoral muscle, creating a large pocket. A decision is made as to the appropriate size, and an inflatable mammary implant is then inserted. The pectoral muscle, and then the breast tissue, are approximated over the prosthesis with a number of deep nylon sutures.

The final determination of the new nipple-areola height is then made. The actual final position will vary from the initial contemplated position because of the augmentation mammaplasty that has been carried out. There is usually a decrease in the ptosis following an augmentation procedure. After an adjustment of the initial estimated height of the nipple-areola, the area is deepithelialized and the nipple-areola complex is advanced superiorly to its new position. The infraareolar skin is tailored in an oblique manner to conceal the eventual scar in a more optimal lateral position.

The second option is the use of a Benelli-type periareola skin closure (see Fig. 64–9). *Note:* With this technique there is always a varying degree of redundancy and irregularity of the skin closure that gradually improves in 6 to 9 months; however, some patients may object to this periareolar irregularity. The periareolar irregularity may be improved by releasing the permanent subcuticular suture after 6 months.

Marked Ptosis

The skin brassiere in marked ptosis is excessively elongated, with the nipple positioned more than 3 cm below the inframammary crease and at the most inferior portion of the breast. Management involves skin redraping and repositioning of the nipple. An augmentation may or may not be desirable, depending on the ultimate breast size desired and the amount of concomitant atrophy of the breast tissue. The tech-

nique previously described can be used. If feasible, a rotation invagination technique can be utilized that involves an extensive undermining of the skin, with the areola left attached to the mammary gland (26) (Fig. 64–10). The inferior undermined mammary tissue is then invaginated with the lateral and medial glandular tissue to the mid breast area, with interrupted 3-0 nylon sutures overcorrecting the ptosis (Fig.

64–10B,C). The skin is then reapproximated with a two-layer subcutaneous closure with absorbable sutures (Fig. 64–10D). If the amount of redundant skin is greater than 7cm, markings for an inferior dermal pedicle or superior pedicle flap can be made, as in a reduction mammaplasty, with only minimal breast resection.

References

1. Georgiade NG, Serafin D, Riefkohl R, et al. Is there a reduction mammaplasty for all seasons? *Plast Reconstr Surg* 1979; 63:765.
2. Richboung B. Anatomie appliquée DV sein annal de chirurgie. *Plastique Esthetique* 1992; 37:603.
3. Arie G. Una neuva technica de mastoplastia. *Rev Iber Latino Am Chir Plast* 1957; 3:28.
4. Pitanguy L. Breast hypertrophy. In: *Transactions of the second international congress of plastic surgery.* Edinburg: E & S Livingstone, 1960; 509.
5. Strömbeck JOP. Mammaplasty: report of a new technique based on the two-pedicle procedures. *Br J Plast Surg* 1960; 13:79.
6. DuFourmentel L, Mouly R. Plastic mammaire par la methode oblique. *Ann Chir Plast* 1962; 6:45.
7. Skoog T. A technique of breast reduction. *Acta Chir Scand* 1963; 126:1. (Originally published in: *Plastic surgery.* Stockholm: Almquist and Wifsell, 1927; 345.)
8. Weiner DL, Aiache AE, Silver L, et al. A single dermal pedicle for nipple transposition in subcutaneous mastectomy, reduction mammaplasty or mastopexy. *Plast Reconstr Surg* 1973; 51:115.
9. Cramer LM, Chong JK. Unipedicle cutaneous flap: areola nipple transposition on an end-bearing superiorly based flap. In: Georgiade, NG, ed. *Reconstructive breast surgery.* St. Louis: CV Mosby, 1976; 143.
10. McKissock PK. Reduction mammaplasty with a vertical dermal flap. *Plast Reconstr Surg* 1972; 49:245.
11. Ribeiro L. A new technique for reduction mammaplasty. *Plast Reconstr Surg* 1975; 55:330.
12. Robbins TH. A reduction mammaplasty with the areola-nipple based on an inferior dermal pedicle. *Plast Reconstr Surg* 1977; 59:64.
13. Courtiss EH, Goldwyn RM. Reduction mammaplasty by the inferior pedicle technique. *Plast Reconstr Surg* 1977; 59:500.
14. Georgiade NG, et al. Reduction mammaplasty utilizing an inferior pedicle nipple-areola flap. *Ann Plast Surg* 1979; 3:211.
15. Hinderer UT. Evolution of technique in mammoplasty. Personal choice. *Worldplast* 1995; 1:11.
16. Georgiade G, Riefkohl R, Georgiade N. The inferior dermal-pyramidal type breast reduction: long-term evaluation. *Ann Plast Surg* 1989; 23:203.
17. Rubin LR. The massive hypertrophic breast: surgical treatment. In: Georgiade NG, ed. *Reconstructive breast surgery.* St. Louis: CV Mosby, 1976; 218; and Georgiade NG, Georgiade GS, and Riefkohl R, eds. *Aesthetic surgery of the breast.* Philadelphia: WB Saunders, 1990; 505.
18. LeJour M. Vertical mammaplasty liposuction of the breast. *Plast Reconstr Surg* 1994; 94:1.
19. Courtiss E. Reduction mammaplasty by suction alone. *Plast Reconstr Surg* 1993; 92:1276.
20. Seyfer A. Reduction mammoplasty using the inferior glandular pyramid pedicle. In: Georgiade N, Georgiade GS, Riefkohl R, eds. *Aesthetic surgery of the breast.* Philadelphia: WB Saunders, 1990; 363.
21. Moufarrège R. Plastie mammaire à pedicule dermoglandulaire inferieur. *Ann Chir Plast* 1982; 27:294.
22. Moufarrège R. The total dermoglandular pedicle mammaplasty. In: Georgiade NG, Georgiade GS, Riefkohl R, eds. *Aesthetic surgery of the breast.* Philadelphia: WB Saunders, 1990; 371.
23. Hester TR, Bostwick J, Miller L, et al. Breast reduction utilizing the maximally vascularized central breast pedicle. *Plast Reconstr Surg* 1985; 76:890.
24. Brink R. Management of true ptosis of the breast. *Plastic Reconstr Surg* 1993; 91:657.
25. Benelli L. The Benelli periareolar mammaplasty: the "round block" technique. In: Georgiade NG, Georgiade GS, Riefkohl R, eds. *Aesthetic surgery of the breast.* Philadelphia: WB Saunders, 1990; 747.
26. Erol O, Spira, M. A mastopexy technique for mild to moderate ptosis. *Plast Reconstr Surg* 1980; 65:603.

Suggested Readings

Bostwick J. *Aesthetic and reconstructive breast surgery.* St. Louis: Quality Medical Publishing, 1990.

Breast surgery. *Clinics in Plastic Surgery* 1976; 3:(2).

Georgiade NG, Georgiade GS, Riefkohl R, eds. *Aesthetic surgery of the breast.* Philadelphia: WB Saunders, 1990.

attachment of the breast to the chest wall, it is essentially to limit the separation initially to that which is absolutely required. When the circle sutures are placed, the bunching of tissue should be at the inferior edge of the circle between 5 and 7 o'clock. This is the area that will rest upon the brassiere and give a more rapid smoothing of the folded tissue.

The initial cut is made with cautery just inside the skin edge, as noted above. It is then quite easy to separate the subcutaneous soft tissue from the breast if this area has been infiltrated with the "super wet" technique.

The "super-wet" technique is a modification of local anesthesia. After the preliminary medication orally and intravenously, 30 mg of Ketamine is administered intravenously. After 1 minute, small stab wounds are made in the drawn circle lines and the blunt cannula is introduced. Using the Hunstad pump, 400 to 500 cc of lactated Ringer solution with ⅛% xylocaine and 1:1,000,000 epinephrine are infiltrated into the subcutaneous tissue. Additional infiltration is placed into the axilla and the base of the breast, if liposuction in that area is anticipated. Bleeding is reduced and patient comfort is enhanced. The volume of infusate allows an easy separation of subcutaneous fat from breast parenchyma.

It is essential to leave excess fat on the flaps. Thickness can be adjusted later in the procedure. Leaving a thick cushion not only ensures protection from trauma and a better blood supply, but also gives a smoother contour to the created mound by draping it with a thicker blanket.

Once the chest wall has been identified, further dissection is carried out laterally and medially, as indicated, based on the amount of tissue advancement and/or resection that will be required.

EXCISION, FOLD OR OVERLAP?

Once the inferior half of the breast has been exposed, it is easy to judge the amount of tissue that will be utilized, where it will be positioned, and/or how much will be removed by liposuction or direct midline wedge excision. For *implant replacement* cases, a vertical split is made from the areola to the inframammary fold. The length of these flaps is shortened to 5 to 6 cm in length by lateral excisions. After removing the old prosthesis and the capsule, as indicated, the new prosthesis is placed in its higher position. The left-to-right overfolding is carried out by advancing one wing upward and suturing it into the pectoralis fascia; two fixation sutures set the inferior edge at the position of the new inframammary fold. The opposite side is then folded over this one, giving a "lateral pants-over-vest" reinforcement. This dual reinforcement has proved advantageous in slowing or preventing future inferior ptosis.

For the *mastopexy* patient with sufficient tissue who does not require (or request) a breast prosthesis, the infolding technique of Erol is used. A minimal amount of undermining is required. A single no. 1 Dexon suture can be placed in the midline fascia, roughly at the level of the proposed new areolar position (Fig. 65–1). This suture is used to bring the initial infolded edges together. Additional infolding sutures are placed in several layers, using slower dissolving sutures such as PDS or no. 1 Vicryl. There is no advantage in substituting nondissolving sutures such as braided nylon or mersilene. Infolding is continued until the breast mound has been com-

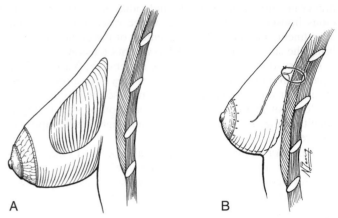

FIG. 65–1. **A,** cross section showing implant in ptotic breast. **B,** the implant has been removed. The suture is shown elevating the inferior ptotic breast pedicle to the proposed new areolar position.

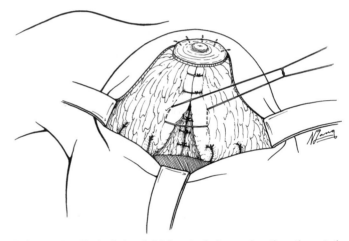

FIG. 65–2. Erol, Spira infolding technique elevating the ptotic breast.

pleted. Then, additional sutures are added to fix the inframammary fold at its new position (Fig. 65–2).

Most mastopexy patients and reduction patients require some tissue removal. A midline wedge is excised as a triangle, from areolar edge to the lower edge of the breast tissue. This procedure may be described as a "subcutaneous Pitanguy wedge excision." Lateral wedges are removed as well, to shorten the nipple to inframammary fold distance as described. For moderate reductions, large reductions, and some mastopexy patients, this wedge of tissue is gauged to narrow the base of the breast, reduce the volume to the desired size, and create a projecting cone when closed in multiple layers (Fig. 65–3).

On completion of these maneuvers, a breast cone at a higher position, firmly anchored to pectoralis fascia, has been obtained.

ELEVATING THE NIPPLE AREOLAR COMPLEX

Although the circumareolar technique has been used with success in patients in whom the new nipple position is 6 cm or more from the edge of the reduced-diameter areola, better results are obtained when a small circle is required. These patients are better suited for circumareolar lift or reduction. In all but those patients who have suffered vascular compromise because of prosthesis failure, it is wise to excise a wedge of tissue above the areola. Inverted 2-0 absorbable sutures (Dexon or Vicryl) are used to fix the areola at its new position. These 3–4 anchoring sutures also bring in the lateral skin edges. Without this maneuver, the nipple is adrift in the middle of the circle and may easily lie at an abnormal position when the circular sutures are completed.

At this point, the surgeon has created a new breast shape of the size and projection required, with the skin held back for visualization and access. Judgement is now made as to whether liposuction should be employed in the posterior portions of the breast to equalize or reduce upper or lateral fullness. Liposuction is most often used to reduce the axillary tail fullness or the fat pad that is often found at the superior

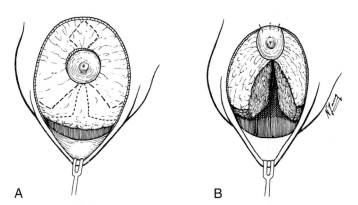

FIG. 65–3. A,B, various possibilities for excision of excess breast tissue. From Wilkinson TS. *Circumareolar Techniques for Breast Surgery.* New York: Springer-Verlag, 1995.

edge of the axilla. A single entry point is used to minimize trauma to the incoming vessels or nerves.

ADVANCING THE CIRCLE TO THE AREOLA

The goal is to advance the skin and subcutaneous tissue to the areola without tension. Direct suturing resulted in the megaareolae that plagued earlier efforts. A dual advancement system is not only effective but also saves operating room time.

The first Benelli suture is of nonabsorbable material. The initial knot is placed 1cm below the areolar edge and the tissue bites are made at intervals 1 cm below the skin edge into the dermis and 0.5 cm below the areolar edge, into the deepithelialized ring. When this circle is complete (Fig. 65–4), the skin edges touch without tension but are not secured.

The second Benelli suture should be absorbable. One of the minor complications is suture extrusion, and this is handled easily if the suture resorbs. This knot is also buried. Suture bites are into the deepithelialized skin a few millimeters below the edge and into the deep deepithelialized area just below the skin edge of the nipple itself. On completion of this circle, the edges should touch and evert (Fig. 65–5).

Small irregularities are corrected by loosely tied 6.0 nylon tacking sutures. When the circle sutures are correctly placed, only one or two tacking sutures should be required. It is prudent to place one in the midline to make sure that the central area, in which the suture knots are buried, will remain sealed.

DRAINAGE

In all cases, it is necessary to drain the fluid that accumulates, both from the super-wet technique and from the operative procedure itself. Generally preferred is a small lateral stab wound and a suction or penrose drain for 24 hours.

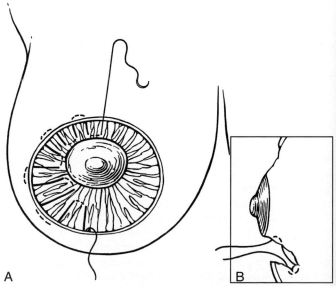

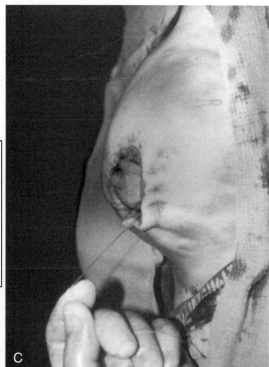

FIG. 65–4. A, initial suture is nonabsorbable and placed 1 cm below the areolar margin. **B,** side view shows the position of the permanent dermal suture, advancing the skin with a continuous suture placed approximately 0.5 cm into the deepithelialized periareolar circle. **C,** appearance of the loose periareolar skin condensed to a workable quantity of redundant skin utilizing the initial suture placement with a pursestring effect.

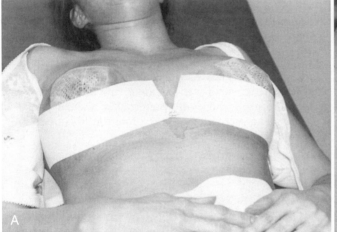

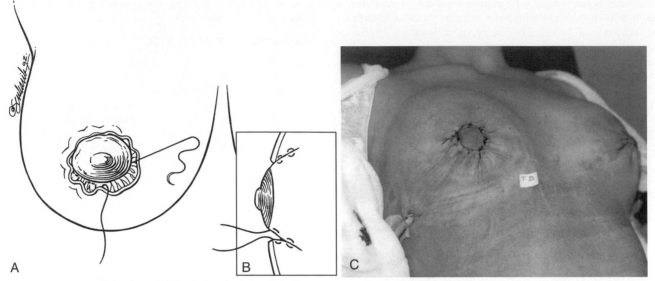

A

B

C

FIG. 65–5. A, the second suture of absorbable material is shown in the deepithelialzed periareolar dermis just below the skin edges, avoiding tension on the areolar; however, the areolar and breast tissue will approximate without tension. **B,** side view of the position of second suture. **C,** appearance of the completed periareolar closure. Some nylon skin sutures may be indicated for closer approximation.

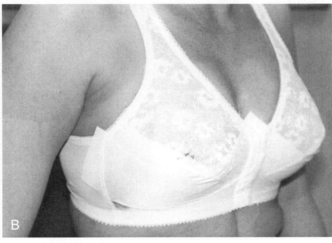

A

B

FIG. 65–6. A, mesh paper tape dressing applied to operative areas for up to 48 hours. **B,** wireless support brassiere is worn within 36 hours following surgery over the supporting underlying tape dressing.

From Wilkinson TS. *Circumareolar Techniques for Breast Surgery.* New York: Springer-Verlag, 1995.

At the end of the procedure, $\frac{1}{2}\%$ marcaine with epinephrine is placed into the deep subcutaneous tissues laterally and medially using a 20-gauge spinal needle. Additional marcaine placed into the subcutaneous pocket provides topical anesthetic before it drains away. Supportive dressings are then applied.

AFTERCARE

Aftercare for the minimal ptosis procedure and minor or major reduction procedures is similar to that employed for T-scar procedures, with a few exceptions. Because there will be fluid exudate from the entire circle, tape reinforcement is delayed for 24 to 48 hours, after which mesh paper tape (3M company) is applied that immobilizes a 4-cm square area, yet allows full drainage through the interstices of the tape (Fig. 65–6). Antiseptic gauze is used initially in the dressings

and later placed over the mesh tape until there is no further fluid escape. At this point, wide support tapes are placed. "Foam" elasticized tape is the current preference. This tape forces the still-lax inferior skin to conform to the secured subcutaneous mound. This tape may be changed as needed and is helpful for the first 7 to 10 days.

As a general rule, patients are placed into a front-hook support bra without wires beginning 24 to 36 hours following surgery (Fig. 65–6B). Because the internal mound is breast tissue, additional external support is required for at least 30 days after surgery. Once the incisions are dry, the mesh tape is gently removed, and 1-inch paper tape is applied around the periphery of the circle primarily as a protection against trauma. This tape is sealed with a waterproof material, collodion, so that the patient may shower with the brassiere in place. After two weeks, the patient is allowed to sit in a warm tub with added bath oils. Hydrotherapy and heat are means of reducing tissue edema. At the end of 30 days, the patients change to a softer, more elastic form of the support bra, which is used for an additional period of several weeks.

Because the lower flap has been completely reflected, it is wise to advise patients to avoid underwire brassieres for at least 6 weeks following surgery. To avoid flattening of the reconstructed cone, the patient must not sleep face downward during this time and should wear a supportive night brassiere for at least that length of time, and perhaps longer.

Complications

Complications of the circumareolar mastopexy, or reduction, are divided into the time frames that preceded many technical innovations. Flattening of the breast mound and expansion of the areola were not completely controlled, even with multilayered sutures and internal cone formation. These complications soured many surgeons on the procedure and led to its virtual abandonment.

With the introduction of newer techniques, the circumareolar procedures are becoming more popular, particularly for younger patients and clothes-conscious middle-aged patients who are physically active.

Long-term ptosis will still occur with any type of breast reduction; it will occur no more or no less with the circumareolar techniques. With additional care in multilayered "basket weave" suturing of the subcutaneous cone, and additional attention to suture repositioning of the inframammary fold, this has been a minor and infrequent complication. Stitch abscesses still occur and, on occasion, may involve the second dissolvable suture. If this occurs, the suture may be simply clipped flush with the skin and tacking sutures from the surface employed to close the gap. Minor revisions are carried out at 6 months.

Scar hypertrophy has surprisingly been uncommon, perhaps because of the tension-free closure as well as the limitation of this procedure to healthy women with good skin tone.

There may be a degree of rippling in the lower half for up to 18 months. In many instances, the smoothing is completed by 3 months, but this is the exception rather than the rule. Postoperative massage with creams and aloe vera–vitamin E oils may be helpful, as are elastic brassieres that exert pressure on the lower half folding. Occasionally, a revision of this area has been required because of unexpected stretch of the areola, irregularity of the scar, or persistent edge folds. Fortunately, these are not common and require only minor surgical touch-ups, with rapid healing owing to the position of the scar revision.

More serious complication of areolar loss has occurred in patients in which deviations from the standard procedure were undertaken. As with other reductions and mastopexies, inspection of nipple areolar color and congestion is required. Should there be color changes, it is a simple matter to clip the circumareolar suture to relax the tension. It can be replaced after a short delay without consequence. Tissue losses may be secondary to delayed hemorrhage.

Circumareolar surgery is definitely a hands-on plastic surgical procedure that is very technique dependent. With increasing familiarity, complications have been reduced to a level consistent with, or lower than, those obtained with standard inferior or superior, or double pedicle, techniques. The advantage is that the scar becomes acceptable rapidly, and one avoids the complications attended upon the T-scar junction or scar migration beyond bathing attire.

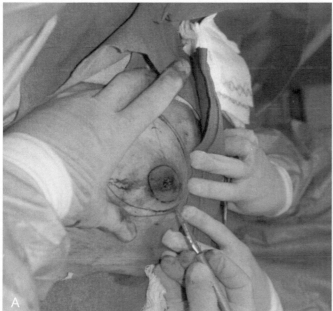 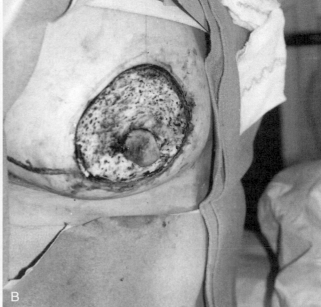

FIG. 65–7. **A,** in this patient with a typical mastopexy/moderate-reduction, the ellipse has been drawn with the upper point measured at 19 cm and the lower point at the ellipse at 9 cm above the inframammary fold. The nipple has been reduced to 3½ cm. **B,** the initial skin incisions are made and the area is completely deepithelialized, leaving the nipple in its original position.

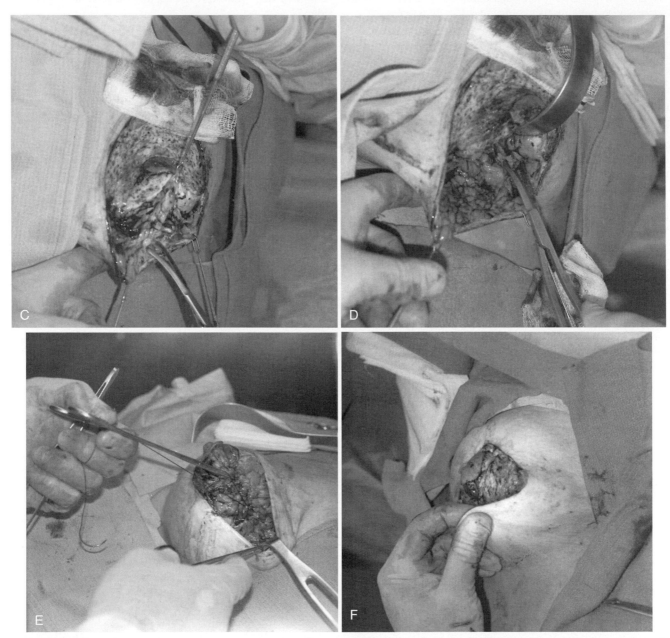

FIG. 65–7. (continued)   **C,** with the breast mass on traction, a
curved flat-bladed dissection scissors is used to separate the subcutaneous tissue from the mass of the gland between 3 and 9 o'clock.
D, with a retractor in place, the inframmmary fold is identified, and
dissection is carried upward for several centimeters so that the new
inframammary fold can be reset at a higher position. **E,** the first anchoring sutures and infolding sutures are placed at this point. **F,** the
areola has been moved to the upper portion of the ellipse, here
viewed from the left side. The triangle has been excised, and anchoring sutures bring the skin in to the edge of the nipple across its
upper border. The second layer of infolding sutures is placed and a
decision has been made regarding the distance to be excised so that
the new nipple will lie approximately 5 cm from the new inframammary fold. The last of these sutures is to insure that the lateral margins of the breasts are fully rotated medially.

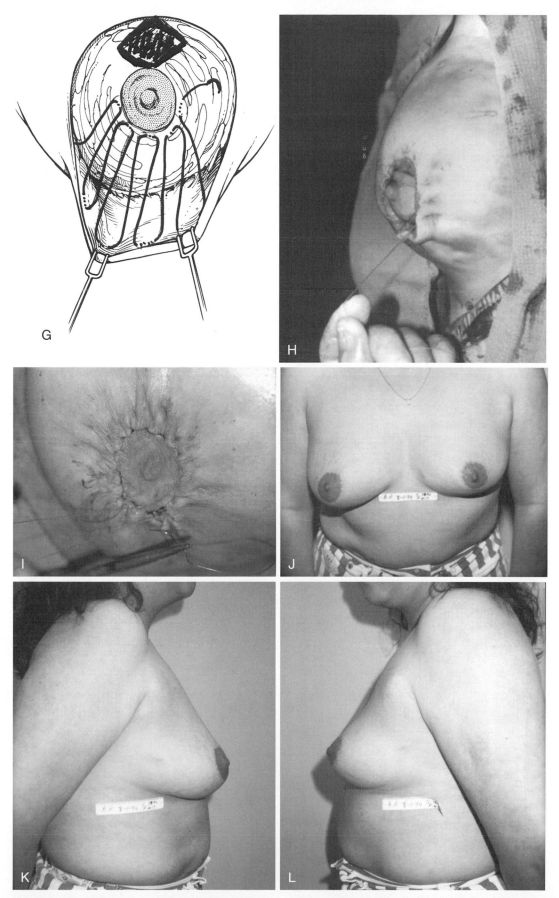

FIG. 65–7. (continued) **G,** placing the first "tissue advancement" nonabsorbable Benelli suture. The diamond excision above the areola will be closed with tacking sutures to elevate the areola before completing the circular suture. **H,** side view of the purse-string effect of the permanent suture placed approximately 0.5 cm into the deep-ithelialized periareolar circle. **I,** the second Benelli absorbable suture close to the areolar skin and breast skin. At this time, a few nylon tacking sutures are usually required to insure the deep position of the circular suture knots and for closure of any areas of separation. **J, K, L,** postoperative appearance 18 months postmastopexy of this same patient. Note minimal periareolar irregularities. **J, K, L,** postoperative appearance 18 months postmastopexy of this same patient. Note minimal periareolar irregularities. Figures A-G and I-L from Wilkinson TS. *Circumareolar Techniques for Breast Surgery.* New York: Springer-Verlag, 1995. Figure H from Wilkinson TS. *Practical Procedures in Aesthetic Plastic Surgery.* New York: Springer-Verlag, 1994.

Summary

A patient who has had a typical mastopexy and moderate reduction mammaplast is shown in Figure 65–7.

References

1. Rossell E, Stark RB. Circumareolar mastopexy. American Society of Plastic and Reconstructive Convention, Hollywood, FL, October 1976.
2. Bartells RJ, Strickland DM, Douglas WM. A new mastopexy operation for mild or moderate breast ptosis. *Plast Reconstr Surg* 1976; 57:687.
3. Erol O, Spira M. Mastopexy technique for mild to moderate ptosis. *Plast Reconstr Surg* 1980; 65:603.
4. Georgiade NG, ed. *Aesthetic breast surgery.* Vol. 7. Baltimore: Williams & Wilkins, 1983; 71–86.
5. Louis JR, ed. *The art of aesthetic surgery.* Vol. 127. Boston: Little, Brown, 1989; 833–836.
6. Proceedings of the International Society, Elsevier Science Publishers, B.V. Plastic Surgery, 1992. Vol. II. In: Hinderer UT, ed. *Principles of circumareolar mastopexy, as applied to breast repair and reconstruction.*
7. Hinderer UT. Primera experiencia con una nueva tecnica de mastoplastica para ptosis ligeres. Presented at the Sixth National Reunion of Spanish Society of Plastic and Reparative Surgery, Bulletin Madrid, 1969.
8. Hinderer UT. Mammary plastic modeling with superficial dermopexy and retromammary dermopexy. *Revista Esp de Cir Plast* 1972; 1:65.
9. Hinderer, UT. Reduction and augmentation mammoplasty: remodeling mammoplasty with superficial and retromammary mastopexy. *Internat Micr J Esth Plastic Surg* 1972; E.
10. Spear SL, Kassan M, Little JW. Guidelines in concentric mastopexy. *Plast Reconstr Surg* 1990; 85:961.
11. Gasperoni C, Salgarello M, Gargani G. Experiences and technical refinements in the "donut" mastopexy with augmentation mammaplasty. *Aesthetic Plast Surg* 1988; 12:11.
12. Dinner MI, Artz JS, Foglietti MA. Application and modification of the circular skin excision and pursestring procedures. *Aesthetic Plast Surg* 1993; 17:301.
13. Benelli L. Technique de plastic mammaire "round block." *Rev de Chir Esth de Langue Francaise* 1988: 13, 50, 7.
14. Benelli L. A new periareolar mammoplasty: "the round block" technique. *Aesthetic Plast Surg* 1990; 14:93.
15. Toledo LS, Matsudo PK. Mammoplasty using liposuction and the periareolar incision. *Aesthetic Plast Surg* 1989; 13:9.

Suggested reading

1. Wilkinson TS, ed. *Practical procedures in aesthetic plastic surgery,* New York: Springer Verlag, 1994.
2. Wilkinson TS, ed. *Circumareolar techniques for breast surgery.* New York: Springer Verlag, 1995.

66

Medical Management of High-Risk Diseases of the Breast

Kenneth Scott McCarty, Jr., M.D., Ph.D., Barry Lembersky, M.D., and Edwin B. Cox, M.D.

Patients can be divided into three broad groups with respect to the risk of breast cancer. The first group includes women who have been diagnosed and treated for breast cancer and who are concerned about the risks of distant metastases and recurrence, as well as second primary lesions (in patients who elected breast conservation) (1). The second group includes patients who have been identified as having some factor associated with an increased risk of breast cancer (e.g., atypical epithelial lesions, family history, genotypic risk) (2,3). The third group—by far the largest, and the one in which most new breast cancers will occur—is made up of those with no currently identifiable factors for increased risk of breast cancer. More than 80% of primary breast cancers are observed in patients with no identifiable increased risk factor (4).

Understanding breast disease and breast cancer risk begins with an appreciation of the physiology of the breast. The breasts undergo dramatic changes during puberty, with menstrual cycling, during pregnancy and lactation, with the climacteric, and with menopause (5,6). Each individual's breasts are affected to some degree by these normal life events. The role of medical management in diseases of the breasts has been extended through increasing awareness of the benefits and risks of hormone replacement therapy (HRT) in the perimenopausal and menopausal period (7). Signs and symptoms of breast conditions that would previously have ceased with the menopause may now continue. However, the use of HRT often has beneficial effects on quality of life and, recent evidence suggests, on duration of life (7). In addition to effects on cardiovascular health, bone integrity, skin quality, and genital functionality, for one-third of women symptoms of hot flashes and their effect on sleep and mood are significant considerations. One of the principal concerns regarding the use of HRT involves the issue of their effects on the breast and on the risk of breast cancer. Understanding how to assess risk of breast cancer is a critical part of the medical management of breast disease and assessing patients for hormonal therapies. Such therapies have significant effects in preserving skin and tissues turgor and texture and are of concern to patients and to plastic surgeons (8).

In addition to considerations of breast cancer risk, patients whose presenting concerns focus on symptoms and signs of diseases of the breast often involve complex medical and endocrinologic considerations that underlie these findings and symptoms (9). These range from the influence of thyroid deficiency on cystic change and mastodynia to the influence of obesity on androstenedione conversion to estrone and the ef-

fect on breast density, and include the effects of commonly prescribed medications such as phenylephrine on breast secretions (10,11).

Benign Breast Conditions

Anxiety regarding breast cancer is the primary reason most women seek evaluation of a perceived abnormality in their breast. This remains true despite the fact that the great majority of breast complaints and conditions will be shown to be due to benign conditions (12). This fact does not reduce the intensity of the anxiety and distress that these conditions may produce. This anxiety is heightened by publicity presenting the incidence of breast cancer in American women in terms of lifetime risk, a concept that is often misunderstood. While the risk for a given individual at a given age before 70 does not rise above a fraction of 1%, the often-cited "lifetime" cumulative risk is calculated to be nearly one woman in nine (13,14). This is a lifetime cumulative risk of breast cancer for a woman who lives beyond 85 years of age. Concern is, however, heightened by the realization that the signs and symptoms of benign breast lesions mimic the signs and symptoms that we recognize and teach our patients suggest the possibility of breast cancer (15).

Attention may be drawn to the signs of a breast disorder by symptoms of pain and tenderness, the observation of a lump or thickening on examination, or the presence of a nipple discharge. These are the observations that bring the patient to the physician and are, as already stated, in the vast majority of encounters, benign, imparting no increased risk of breast cancer (12). They nonetheless require attention and evaluation to exclude malignancy. The observation by the physician or patient of a palpable mass, thickening or distortion of the breast, or the presence of patient-described symptoms makes the interaction a diagnostic rather than a screening event and requires an active management plan to optimize the evaluation and diagnosis of signs and symptoms and to minimize discomfort, morbidity and anxiety (16).

Women in their reproductive years have a nodular texture to their breasts that is maximal in the late luteal phase of the menstrual cycle. The nodules are produced by the lobules and glandular units of the breast interspersed in fatty tissue and fibrous stroma. The lobules are comprised of clusters of terminal ductule and acini that undergo a characteristic pattern of proliferative changes and secretory activity associated with the cyclic variation in hormonal levels experienced with normal menstrual cycles (5,6). In the breast, in distinct contrast to the uterus, the proliferation of the breast epithelium is

incidentally in biopsy specimens obtained in the course of evaluating signs and symptoms caused by other breast lesions, as noted earlier. Epithelial hyperplasia has been correlated with increased cancer risk. Atypical lobular and ductal hyperplasias describe epithelial proliferative changes most closely associated with cancer risk (26). Atypical hyperplasia is found in nearly 4% of otherwise benign breast biopsies (2). Such change carries with it a fourfold increased risk of breast cancer in the patient whose biopsy displays these changes (2). It should be emphasized that a biopsy revealing epithelial hyperplasia in one breast does not predict in which breast a subsequent cancer might occur; cancer may arise with equal frequency in either the ipsilateral breast biopsied or the breast contralateral to the biopsied breast. Alternately stated, cancer arises in either breast with nearly equal frequency regardless of the breast from which the biopsy containing atypical hyperplasia was obtained. Even epithelial hyperplasia without atypia is associated with an increased cancer risk estimated at 1.6 times the expected rate in women without epithelial hyperplasia (2). A biopsy that is benign, but contains areas of atypical hyperplasia, thus serves to identify individuals at significantly higher risk of breast cancer. If, in addition to the presence of atypical hyperplasia, family history is positive for breast cancer in a first-order relative, the relative risk is further increased from fourfold to nearly ninefold (3,26).

Several modalities exist to evaluate breast symptoms. The first measure is a thorough review of relevant history, including family history, personal history of breast disorders, menstrual history, reproductive history, hormonal review of systems with emphasis on ovarian and thyroid function, use of contraceptive or other medications, and breast trauma. The family history should include the age and number of first-order female relatives and the breast cancer history for each. Variations in symptoms, or the size of a palpable nodule, with the menstrual cycle are often important clues suggesting benign disease. Dietary and smoking habits and the consumption of products containing xanthine may influence symptoms of benign breast disease, especially cysts.

Physical examination should address the size, general contour, symmetry, and form of the breast, with the patient examined in recumbent and upright position. The patient should be asked to demonstrate any lesion she has felt and positioned for examination to demonstrate the lesion. Puckering of the skin or retraction of the nipple in some cases may only be observed with the patient's hands raised over the head or placed on her hips with the pectoralis contracted. Palpation should be done with proper positioning of the patient using a small wedge or pillow under the shoulder to allow the breast to flatten by gravity against the chest wall. The general texture of the breast, as well as specific lesions, should be evaluated. Optimally, the physician makes notes of the size, character (solid or fluctuant, resilient or firm, smooth or lobulated, movable or fixed, round or irregular) and location of masses so as to allow an objective evaluation of changes with subsequent examinations.

After the history, physical examination, and additional studies as indicated, a decision must be made as to whether the findings point compellingly away from cancer. In a woman less than 30 years of age, the presence of a smooth, round, discrete, and freely movable mass may be so characteristic of a benign lesion that reasonable treatment options

would include simply observing the patient for one or two menstrual cycles, or recommending a several-month trial of a rigorously xanthine-restricted diet and complete cessation of cigarette and nicotine use. A careful search for medication use that may be stimulating breast secretions is also indicated, and in specific circumstances a trial of danazol or similar agent may be appropriate.

In many situations, the characteristics of the lesion as observed with physical examination and the clinical history do not allow immediate disposition. In this event, the next level of evaluation of a palpable nodule includes needle aspiration and/or ultrasound—procedures of low morbidity and minimal cost that may serve to define the nature of the lesion. If the lesion is cystic in character, needle aspiration may yield fluid and result in the collapse of the palpable mass. If no mass remains after aspiration and the fluid is not sanguinous, the diagnosis of cystic duct dilation is supported and no further studies are needed. If the fluid is bloody, cytologic examination of this fluid may be of some benefit. In the event that there is no fluid obtained and the mass is solid, the physician may acquire diagnostic material by a thin-needle aspiration biopsy using the same apparatus used to attempt to acquire the fluid. Use of the fine-needle aspiration biopsy technique should only be considered if there is a cytopathologist available who is capable of properly interpreting the specimen obtained. If none is available, the patient is better served by the performance of a core-needle biopsy or open biopsy.

Mammography is best considered as a detection method rather than a diagnostic method although the image may provide diagnostic clues with degrees of probability that a lesion is of a particular histology. The mammogram may draw attention to a specific area warranting diagnostic evaluation. This evaluation must eventually involve tissue acquisition if a suspect lesion persists or if the suspicion is high enough on initial examination. Biopsy directed by a needle placed under mammographic guidance permits the more selective biopsy of the abnormal area(s), obviating the need for large, disfiguring biopsies in many cases. Mammography cannot, by itself, exclude the possibility that a given lesion is malignant, nor does it always detect lesions that are present. Mammography may appropriately sway the decision toward performing a biopsy in an otherwise equivocal situation.

Tissue biopsy provides the material to define the nature of a clinically observed lesion. If biopsy were entirely innocuous, its use would probably be justified in all cases of a clinically (mammographic or physical exam) apparent lesion. However, biopsies themselves may result in tissue scarring and the formation of masslike lesions that confuse and confound subsequent diagnostic evaluation; the use of open biopsy should be therefore be selective and carefully reasoned. The use of thin-needle aspiration biopsy has been limited as a result of reports of false-positive rates at one major medical center as high as 1% and false-negative rates of 15 to 20%. Despite these serious considerations, no reasonably suspicious persistent lesion of the breast should be passed by without either histologic or cytologic evaluation. Multiple biopsies may be required to ascertain confidently that malignancy is not present.

Guidelines for biopsy evolve from experience with breast lesions and incorporate subtle aspects of size, texture, mobility, and contour of the lesion, as well as, in some cases, the mammographic and ultrasound findings. In presence of any complexity, referral to a specialist in breast disease is to be preferred over well-meaning but ill-advised decisions by an observer not familiar with the subtleties of breast disease.

Gail and associates (27) developed a relative risk scale for breast cancer that has been advocated by some and used in the breast cancer prevention trial of the National Surgical Breast Program. In this setting, a minimum relative risk to enter the prevention trial is developed for age groups divided in 5-year intervals from 35 to 55 years of age. The estimated number of women in the 35-year-old age group who are considered at high enough risk by the NSABP Breast Cancer Prevention Trial use of the Gail model is 3 women per thousand, while at 50 years of age, the proportion is 93 women per thousand population (28). Few of the patients modeled at high risk actually develop breast cancer. More accurate means of selecting patients at truly high risk need to be developed.

TREATMENT OF BENIGN BREAST CONDITIONS

In considering intervention, it must be kept in mind that many breast lesions are self-limited and are only detected when transient hormonal aberrations or other temporary factors affect their detectability. If a lesion is only palpable premenstrually at the point of maximal progesterone stimulation and regresses after the menstrual period, the nature of the lesion is likely benign and no other measures are needed beyond a clearly articulated plan to reevaluate the lesion after several menstrual cycles.

Lesions that persist, particularly when multiple, may be a reflection of heightened end-organ responsiveness or persistent hormonal (or xanthine) stimulation. Hormone ingestion and absorption, as seen with estrogen-containing creams, have been implicated in exaggerated breast glandular nodularity, as has thyroid dysfunction and obesity. Other exogenous factors, such as caffeine or nicotine, have been associated with the stimulation of cyst formation (29). The approach to the correction of the cystic condition begins with the modification of the hormone use, correction of thyroid dysfunction if present, and (if possible) complete restriction of caffeine and nicotine use or exposure. Vitamin E, administered in conjunction with restriction of nicotine and caffeine consumption, has been helpful in reducing nodularity and mastodynia in many women, even though rigorous proof of its efficacy is lacking. It is important to exclude thyroid dysfunction, or correct it if present. Some have had success with the use of iodide preparations in cystic change and mastodynia, although controlled trials of these agents are needed (30). Undiagnosed palpable or imaged lesions should be diagnosed before considering hormone replacement therapy for menopause, although estrogens and estrogen combinations may be judiciously considered for use after effective treatment of breast cancer (31).

In some cases, exaggerated nodularity and mastodynia may persist despite the measures outlined above. In situations in which mastodynia is a significant problem to the patient, a trial of Danazol may be considered. Danazol is a synthetic androgen, and should be used only with caution and careful monitoring of symptoms and side effects. Timing of the initiation of its use in premenopausal women is important. One difficulty is the frequent return of symptoms when Danazol is discontinued, even after prolonged use (32).

The approach to the patient with atypical hyperplasia on biopsy and a family history of first-order relatives with breast cancer, or demonstration of BRCa1 or similar genes, is particularly difficult. In considering treatment directed at reducing the risk of subsequent breast cancer, attention must be paid equally to the breast in which the atypical hyperplasia biopsy was obtained and to the contralateral breast, because we cannot predict the site or side of future neoplasm based on the site of the biopsy. Bilateral subcutaneous mastectomy is a treatment option considered for high-risk patients at several institutions where the expertise is available to perform this procedure properly. The removal of the majority of the glandular portion of the breast facilitates monitoring of the patient by conventional methods, in experienced hands, and the procedure of bilateral subcutaneous mastectomy is amenable to immediate reconstruction. Tamoxifen as a potential chemopreventive agent is also under trial, although concerns regarding its long-term use have arisen (19).

Benign breast lesions, largely insignificant in themselves, cause much concern in relation to risk of breast cancer. Most such lesions have no significant relationship to cancer, nor do they carry any increased risk of that individual patient developing breast cancer. Conservative management, including reassurance, is usually appropriate and effective once the diagnosis is clear. Persistent benign lesions can often be ameliorated by simple measures such as modification of estrogen/progesterone use (e.g., birth-control pills), correction of thyroid deficiency, caffeine and nicotine restriction, vitamin E administration, or Danazol. Cysts can be aspirated as a diagnostic/therapeutic procedure. Biopsy should be used judiciously. Complex examinations, or patients with high-risk lesions or family history, should be referred to a breast specialist, given the many guises of breast cancer.

CARCINOMA IN SITU

Carcinoma in situ of the breast is divided into two subtypes: lobular and ductal. Lobular carcinoma in situ (LCIS), like atypical hyperplasia, is a microscopic diagnosis and is discovered incidentally in a biopsy specimen obtained in evaluating a mass or mammographic abnormality produced by another breast lesion. LCIS does not produce calcification, mass effects, or other physical changes detectable clinically. Lobular carcinoma in situ has a high incidence of multicentricity and bilaterality; biopsy revealing LCIS in one breast does not predict in which breast subsequent cancer might occur. Invasive breast cancer occurs in 15 to 35% of patients with LCIS treated by biopsy alone. Management of patients with LCIS requires that attention be paid to both breasts (33).

Ductal carcinoma in situ (DCIS) presents most often as a microscopic finding although in contrast to LCIS, DCIS may be associated with calcification on mammography. No mass or palpable abnormality is seen with DCIS as with LCIS. Ductal carcinoma in situ is less likely than LCIS to be multicentric or bilateral relative to LCIS. In patients with DCIS treated by biopsy alone, subsequent invasive breast cancer is observed in 14 to 60%, usually in the ipsilateral breast (34).

Invasive Carcinoma of the Breast

Invasive breast cancer departs from the behavior of the lesions addressed up to this point, bringing with it the potential for metastatic spread, and death. Recognition of the association of invasive breast carcinoma with disease dissemination has led to the use of systemic therapies and local treatments in an attempt to forestall or prevent clinical emergence of metastatic disease.

The adjuvant therapies in common use are chemotherapy, hormonal therapy, and combined chemoendocrine therapy. Each of these modalities is effective in delaying disease recurrence in distinct subgroups of patients, underscoring the fact that each works by a different mechanism. In appropriately selected patients, adjuvant chemotherapy and/or hormonal therapy results in approximately 25% reduction in the risk of relapse and 15% reduction in the risk of death.

However, adjunctive therapies have real costs in terms of time, money, and toxicity, so their usage has to be carefully tailored to each patient's situation in order to optimize the benefit. Empirically proven prognostic factors that may aid in selecting patients for adjuvant systemic therapy include size of the tumor, histologic grade, number of axillary nodes to which tumor has metastasized, age, menopausal status, hormonal receptor content, cell kinetics (mitotic rate, S phase fraction), and growth factor content. The first six are those in nearly universal usage, while the rest remain research tools because of their cost and unavailability, as well as the need for development of validated algorithms incorporating them as prognostic factors.

The presence of metastatic tumor in the ipsilateral axillary lymph nodes is the most powerful prognostic factor in metastatic breast carcinoma. The number of lymph nodes provides a quantitative means of estimating the risk (probability of metastasis in the individual patient compared to all patients with similar-stage disease). Even in those with negative nodes, a substantial risk for subclinical metastatic disease is present. This is true even if the primary tumor is small, although the probability is less. Below 1 cm in diameter, the probability of recurrence is in the range of 5 to 10%—low enough to be offset by the costs and long-term adverse effects that could result from adjuvant therapy. Tumors greater than 1 cm generate a proportionately higher risk of having disseminated, despite netative nodes, and attempts to lower this risk are warranted, even if that means using relatively toxic treatments. The average node-negative primary breast cancer carries a risk of metastatic disease and death of nearly 30% in the 10 years from the time of diagnosis. Considerable attention is being given to the treatment of node-negative breast cancer and clinical trials are in progress to identify the optimum treatments. Slightly over half of all invasive breast cancers have negative lymph nodes at diagnosis and thus account for the majority of breast cancer deaths. Likelihood of dissemination increases with increasing number of nodes found to contain tumor. In the absence of systemic adjuvant therapy, eventual disease recurrence is experienced by 55% of those with one to three nodes involved, about 65% of those with 4 to 7 nodes, about 75% in those with 8 to 12 nodes, and 90% of those with 13 or more nodes. Clearly, these serious risks justify intensive treatment efforts.

Although controversies abound in regard to fine points of adjuvant therapies, several principles are commonly agreed upon. Adjuvant chemotherapy has its highest level of effectiveness in premenopausal women, whereas hormonal adjuvant therapy is most beneficial in postmenopausal women.

The greater effectiveness of hormonal adjuvant therapy in postmenopausal women is at least partly explained by the progressive rise in percentage of estrogen receptor–positivity with increasing age. No entirely satisfactory explanation for the relative ineffectiveness of chemotherapy in older women has been found. In premenopausal women, chemotherapy would nearly universally be prescribed where adjuvant therapy is indicated. In estrogen receptor–positive postmenopausal women, the antiestrogen compound tamoxifen is most often used. In estrogen receptor–negative postmenopausal women, there is less general agreement on optimum therapy, although most clinicians prescribe chemotherapy if the patient is in otherwise good health. Where there is access to treatment on a clinical trial, it would seem best to participate in these studies that are designed to offer the best-known treatment while at the same time adding to our understanding of this disease (1).

References

1. Early Breast Cancer Trialists' Collaborative Group. Systemic treatment of early breast cancer by hormonal, cytotoxic, or immune therapy: 133 randomized trials involving 31,000 recurrences and 24,000 deaths among 75,000 women. *Lancet* 1992; 339:1–15, 71–85.
2. Harris JR, Lippman ME, Veronesi U, et al. Breast cancer. *N Eng J Med* 1992; 327:319–328, 390–398, 473–80.
3. Chen Y, Chen CF, Riley DJ, et al. Aberrant subcellular localization of BRCA1 in breast cancer. *Science* 1995; 270:789–791.
4. Seidman H, Stellman SD, Mushinski MH. A different perspective on breast cancer risk factors: some implications of the nonattributable risk. *CA Cancer J Clin* 1982; 32:301–313.
5. Vogel PM, Georgiade NG, McCarty KS Jr., et al. The correlation of histologic changes in the human breast with menstrual cycle. *Amer J Pathol* 1981; 104:23–34.
6. Anderson TJ, Battersby S, Macintyre CCA. Proliferative and secretory activity in human breast during natural and artificial menstrual cycles. *Amer J Pathol* 1988; 130:193–204.
7. Grady D, Rubin SM, Petitti DB, et al. Hormone therapy to prevent disease and prolong life in postmenopausal women. *Ann Int Med* 1992; 117:1016–1037.
8. Wernick M, Manaster G. Age and the perception of age and attractiveness. *Gerontologist* 1984; 24:408–414.
9. Daniel CW, Silberstein GB. Developmental biology of the mammary gland. In: Nevill MC, Daniel CW, eds. *The mammary gland.* New York: Plenum, 1987; 3–36.
10. Schindler AE, Ebert A, Friedrich E. Conversion of androstenedione to estrone by human fat tissue. *Journal of Clinical Endocrinology and Metabolism* 1972; 35:627–630.
11. Martinez L, Castilla JA, Gil T, et al. Thyroid hormones in fibrocystic disease. *Eur J Endocrinol* 1995; 132:673–676.
12. McDivitt RW, Stevens JA, Lee NC, et al. Benign breast disease histology and the risk for breast cancer. *Cancer* 1992; 69:1408–1414.
13. Boring CC, Squires TS, Tong T. Cancer statistics, 1992. *CA Cancer J Clinicians* 1992; 42:19–38.
14. Cancer Statistics Review 1983–1987. In: Ries LAB, Hankey BF, Edwards BK, eds. National Institute Division of Cancer Prevention and Control Surveillance Program. *NIH Publication N.* 90-2789; 1990.
15. Shingleton WW, McCarty KS Jr. Breast carcinoma: an overview. *Gynecologic Oncology* 1987; 26:271–83.
16. Bonadonna G. Conceptual and practical advances in the management of breast cancer. *J Clin Oncol* 1989; 7:1380–1397.
17. Hutter RVP. Consensus meeting: is "fibrocystic disease" of the breast pre-cancerous? *Arch Pathol and Laboratory Medicine* 1986; 110: 171–173.
18. Greenwald P, Kelloff G, Burch-Whitman C, Kramer BS. Chemoprevention. *CA Cancer J Clin* 1995; 45:31–49.
19. National Cancer Institute. Adjuvant therapy of breast cancer: tamoxifen update, November 28, 1995.
20. Page DL, Dupont WD. Anatomic markers of human pre-malignancy and risk of breast cancer. *Cancer* 1990; 66:1326–1335.

21. Fiorica JV. Fibrocystic changes. *Obstet Gynecol Clin North Am* 1994; 21:445–452.

22. Dupont WD, Page DL, Rogers LW, et al. Influence of exogenous estrogens, proliferative breast disease, and other variables on breast cancer risk. *Cancer* 1989; 63:948–957.

23. McGrath PC. The role of the surgeon in breast disease diagnosis. In: Powell DE, Stelling CB, eds. *The diagnosis and detection of breast disease.* St. Louis: Mosby–Year Book, 1994; 80.

24. Page DL. Cancer risk assessment in benign breast biopsies. *Human Pathol* 1986; 17:871–873.

25. Hijazi YM, Lessard JL, Weiss MA. Use of anti-actin and S-100 protein antibodies in differentiating benign and malignant sclerosing breast lesions. *Surg Pathol* 1989; 2:125–135.

26. Page DL, Dupont WD, Rogers LW, et al. Atypical hyperplastic lesions of the female breast. A long-term follow-up study. *Cancer* 1985; 55:2698–2708.

27. Gail MH, Brinton LA, Byar DP, et al. Projecting individualized probabilities of developing breast cancer for white females who are being examined annually. *Journal of the National Cancer Institute* 1989; 81:1879–1885.

28. Fisher B, Redmond CK, Wickerham DL, et al. National Surgical Adjuvant Breast Project breast cancer prevention trial information handbook, May 1992; 2.16.

29. Minton JP, Abou-Issa H, Reiches N, et al. Clinical and biochemical studies on methylxanthine-related fibrocystic breast disease. *Surgery* 1981; 90:299–304.

30. Ghent WR, Eskin BA, Low DA, et al. Iodine replacement in fibrocystic disease of the breast. *Can J Surg* 1993; 36:453–460.

31. Isaacs CJD, Swain SM. Hormone replacement therapy in women with a history of breast carcinoma. *Hematology Oncology Clinics of North America* 1994; 8:179–195.

32. Andrews WC. Hormonal management of fibrocystic disease of the breast. *J Reprod Med [suppl]* 1990; 35:87–90.

33. Beute BJ, Kalisher L, Hutter RVP. Lobular carcinoma in situ of the breast: clinical, pathologic, and mammographic features. *Amer J Roentgenol* 1991; 157:257–263.

34. Eusebi V, Feudale E, Foschini MP, et al. Long-term follow-up study of in situ carcinoma of the breast. *Seminars in Diagnostic Pathology* 1994; 11:223–235.

67

Surgical Management of High-Risk Diseases of the Breast

Gregory S. Georgiade, M.D., F.A.C.S., and Kenneth S. McCarthy, Jr., M.D., Ph.D.

In the past 10 years there have been notable advances in the identification of subsets of patients with a significantly increased risk of developing breast cancer. This has been through the identification of BRCA1 and BRCA2 genes, as well as other genetic markers associated with breast cancer (1–3). These mutations were initially demonstrable in a relatively small subset of breast cancers (4), but changes related to the gene may play a role in a larger proportion of patients (5).

While means of identifying women at risks up to 80% of developing breast cancer have been emerging (1–5), medical strategies based on the concept of chemoprevention of breast cancer have been undergoing clinical trials (6). The largest of these trials, involving the prophylactic use of tamoxifen (an antiestrogen with some estrogenic effects), was based in large part on the observed reduction in *clinically manifest* second breast cancers, observed in contralateral breasts in randomized controlled clinical trials in which patients received adjuvant tamoxifen for a breast cancer in the opposite breast (7,8). Unfortunately, as treatment has continued beyond 5 years with rerandomization for patients to receive additional years of tamoxifen, the number of *clinically manifest* contralateral breast cancers has increased in the arm of the trial where tamoxifen was continued as compared to those who discontinued tamoxifen (9). The fact that these are clinically manifest cancers is important because of the lead time necessary for a breast cancer to become clinically manifest. This suggests that a strategy is limited that is based on agents that provided apparent benefit through only 5 years of use for a disease which may take 10 or more years to express itself clinically. Thus, just as a popular wave of breast conservation for manifest cancers crests, glandular mastectomies with reconstruction reemerges as a potentially important option for patients with demonstrably increased risks of breast cancer (10). The glandular mastectomy not only removes the majority of tissue at risk for developing overt cancer but it also allows definition of the presence of dysplastic lesions and early, not yet clinically manifest, breast cancers (11).

The procedure of a subcutaneous mastectomy appears to be valuable in selected breast disease patients (11–16). The decision to carry out a subcutaneous mastectomy should be discussed with the patient at length, emphasizing that it is basically not an aesthetic procedure, although every attempt will be undertaken to make the result as aesthetically satisfactory as possible. Other possible problems arising from this procedure, such as possible tissue necrosis, capsular contracture, rupture of the prosthesis, infection, decreased nipple-areolar sensation, and location of the operative scar, should be brought to the patient's attention before surgery. The fact that all of the breast tissue is not removed with this surgical techniques should be discussed.

Surgical Technique

MODERATE BREAST VOLUME

The breast with a volume up to 400 grams usually can be managed using a curved incision 8 cm in length in the infralateral mammary crease line and approximately 5-5.5 cm inferior to the areolar border. The technique of removal of the breast tissue is performed after exposure of the inframammary plane. The dissection and separation of the breast tissue from the pectoralis muscle fascia is carried out until the entire breast tissue has been undermined. After this, the breast resection is undertaken, starting along the medial border of the breast tissue and extending medially and superiorly. Traction on the breast parenchyma, utilizing a pair of Lahey clamps, expedites sharp separation of the breast tissue from the subdermal fat layer. Traction on the breast mound is maintained by the assistant's use of a Deaver retractor. When the dissection approaches the subareolar area, a slight increase in thickness of the breast flap is allowed so that a button of tissue is left to protect the vascularity of the nipple-areola complex. A heavy black suture is now placed on the breast specimen where the nipple ducts have been separated from the specimen. This allows the pathologist to evaluate accurately the histologic appearance of these ducts at this level. (*Note:* We have found that approximately 1% of nipples must be removed as a result of pathologic findings.)

The breast resection is carried laterally, with retraction on the axillary portion of the pectoralis muscle; the tail of the breast is dissected free, and axillary nodes are sampled, if possible. The tail of the specimen is marked with a long white suture for identification and orientation by the pathologist.

Creation of a subserratus, subpectoral pocket is next initiated. An incision over the inferior portion of the 7th rib is made through the serratus fascia and muscle with sharp dissection. A pocket is developed with sharp dissection extending into the subpectoral space. Release of the medial pectoral fibers in the region of the rectus muscle fascia is carried out, extending the subpectoral pocket. Care must be taken to limit the subpectoral axillary portion of the dissection. Overzealous dissection in this area will allow the prosthesis to migrate into the axillary area after insertion (Fig. 67–1).

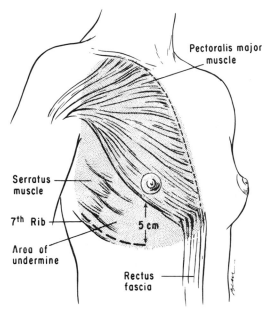

FIG. 67–1. The creation of the subserratus subpectoral pocket. Note extension of the pocket to and under the insertion of the rectus fascia.

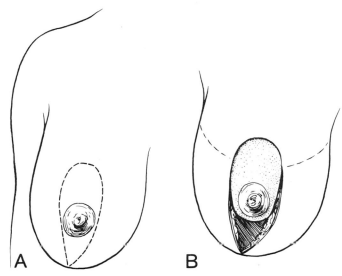

FIG. 67–2. **A,** mastopexy precedure is performed after the subcutaneous mastectomy and the subpectoral prosthesis implantation. The redundant skin is redraped and the nipple-areolar complex is elevated to the desired height with deepithelialization of the superior dermal pedicle. **B,** redundant skin is excised in an inferior oblique manner.

As a rule, in this group of patients the inserted saline prosthesis is approximately the same size as the amount of breast tissue removed. In resections of smaller breasts, the prosthesis is usually slightly larger to allow for better breast contour. Two suction drains are inserted through separate stab wounds into the subpectoral and suprapectoral axillary areas. The muscle layer is closed with interrupted 3-0 nylon sutures that are approximated to the tissue slightly above the region of the incised serratus muscle. This allows for the expanded submuscular pocket layer and permits the prosthesis to be in a slightly lower position than the pectoralis muscle, so that the prosthesis will be directly under the crest of the breast mound. The remaining sutures in the subdermal layer are 4-0 Dexon or Vicryl, followed by a running 4-0 monofilament nylon suture. A compression dressing using mechanics waste is placed in a doughnut fashion over the breast mound, followed by a stockinette cut on the bias in a figure-eight manner, which provides support and compression to the breast during the immediate postoperative course. Examination of the breasts is carried out within 24 hours to rule out the presence of a hematoma or ischemia of the breast tissue.

MODERATE BREAST VOLUME AND PTOSIS

The patient with ptosis and moderate breast volume is managed as described above. However, the nipple-areola complex and skin are advanced superiorly over the pectoral muscle using an Elastoplast tension dressing to elevate and maintain the nipple-areola complex in a more superior position during the healing phase and to minimize the postoperative ptosis (17). This dressing is maintained for 12 to 14 days. The patient with a greater degree of ptosis will need a mastopexy procedure and some skin redraping. This procedure is carried out at the completion of the subcutaneous mastectomy and after insertion of the prosthesis. The patient is placed in an upright position and the desired degree of correction is marked with brilliant green above the present areola. Markings are made in a semicircular manner to conform with the desired new position of the areola. After this, deepithelialization is carried out within the marked area and the areola is advanced and sutured into its new position, utilizing interrupted 5-0 Prolene sutures (Fig. 67–2). The inferior portion of the areola is incised, releasing the areola and allowing it to advance superiorly. The gap that results is closed with resection of a small V-shaped wedge of skin that is approximated, creating a new inferior areola area (18).

LARGE BREAST VOLUME AND PTOSIS

Larger, hypertrophied, ptotic breasts (over 400 grams) will usually require a combination of procedures, including a reduction mammaplasty and mastopexy carried out at the time of the mastectomy (19). Preplanning and premarking of the skin with the patient in upright position is our choice; this allows for the planning of a large, inferior, wide dermal pedicle with retention of a narrower superior dermal pedicle—to maintain, if possible, the vascularity of the nipple-areola complex (Fig. 67–3). If there is any question about the vascularity, then the nipple-areola is removed as a free graft. Following the subcutaneous mastectomy, with insertion of the subpectoral implants and redraping of the breast flaps, the nipple-areolar grafts are applied. The positioning of the nipple-areolar site is determined usually with the patient in a semiupright position on the operating table, and the grafts are attached and fixed over a bolus for 1 week.

STAGED SURGERY

Some surgeons may stage the procedures, inserting the prostheses at a later date. This is a reasonable approach in situations in which there is concern about potential problems with the vascularity of the skin and nipple-areolar complex (20–23).

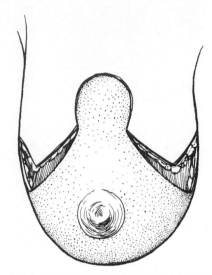

FIG. 67–3. The subcutaneous mastectomy of the larger breast reduction has a wide dermal base to allow the maximum vascularity to the nipple-areolar complex. The dermal pedicle is folded under the approximated medial and lateral breast flaps directly over the pectoral muscle.

Postoperative Management

Postoperative management of the subcutaneous mastectomy includes leaving the drains in place until drainage has decreased completely, over a period of 4 or 5 days or to a maximum of 10 ml. Sutures should be removed on the 7th postoperative day, except in those patients who have undergone a reduction mammaplasty. In this group, the sutures should remain for approximately 12 days. After this, the patient can start on multirotary arm motions, allowing the pectoralis muscle to be stretched for loosening of the tissues. It has been our experience that daily rotary arm motions, both forward and backward, have minimized the effects of contractions occurring with the prosthesis in the submuscular position. Patients can usually return to their normal routine within 12 to 14 days postoperatively and to more strenuous activity shortly after.

References

1. Miki Y, Swensen J, Shattuck-Eidens D, et al. A strong candidate for the breast and ovarian cancer susceptibility gene BRCA1. *Science* 1994; 266:66–71.
2. Wooster R, Neuhasen SL, Mangion J, et al. Localization of a breast cancer susceptibility gene, BRCA2, to chromosome 13Q12-13. *Science* 1994; 265:2088–2090.
3. Easton DF, Bishop DT, Ford D, et al. Breast cancer Linkage Consortium. Genetic linkage analysis in familial breast and ovarian cancer: results from 214 families. *Am J Hum Genet* 1993; 52:678–701.
4. Futreal PA, Liu Q, Shattuck-Eidens D, et al. BRCA1 mutations in primary breast and ovarian carcinomas. *Science* 1994; 266:120–122.
5. Langston AA, Malone KE, Thompson JD, et al. BRCA1 mutations in a population-based sample of young women with breast cancer. *N Engl J Med* 1996; 334:137–142.
6. Greenwald P, Kelloff G, Burch-Whitman C, et al. Chemoprevention. *CA Cancer J Clin* 1995; 45:31–49.
7. Fisher B, Constantino J, Redmond C, et al. A randomized clinical trial evaluating tamoxifen in the treatment of patients with node-negative breast cancer who have estrogen-receptor-positive tumors. *N Engl J Med* 1989; 320:479–484.
8. Scottish Cancer Trials Office (MRC). Adjuvant tamoxifen in the management of operable breast cancer. The Scottish trial. *Lancet* 1987; 2:171–174.
9. National Cancer Institute: Update. Adjuvant therapy of breast cancer, tamoxifen update, November 28, 1995.
10. Collins FS. BRCA1: lots of mutations, lots of dilemmas. *N Engl J Med* 1996: 334:186–188.
11. Georgiade NG, Georgiade GS, McCarty KJ Jr. Subcutaneous mastectomy: an evolution of concept and technique. *Ann Plast Surg* 1982; 8:8–19.
12. Jarrett J, Cutler R, Teal D. Aesthetic refinements in prophylactic subcutaneous mastectomy with submuscular reconstruction. *Plast Reconstr Surg* 1982; 69:624.
13. Woods J, Irons G, Arnold P. The case for submuscular implantation of prosthesis in reconstructive breast surgery. *Ann Plast Surg* 1980; 5:115.
14. Georgiade N. *Reconstructive breast surgery.* St. Louis: CV Mosby, 1976.
15. Shons AR, Press BH. Subcutaneous mastectomy. Indications, technique and applications. *Arch Surg* 1983; 118:844.
16. Ariyan S. Prophylactic mastectomy for precancerous and high-risk lesions of the breast. *Can J Surg* 1985; 28:262.
17. Georgiade N, Hyland W. Technique for subcutaneous mastectomy and immediate reconstruction in the ptotic breast. *Plast Reconstr Surg* 1975; 56:121.
18. Jarrett JR, Cutler R, Teal D. Subcutaneous mastectomy in small, large, or ptotic breasts with immediate submuscular placement of implants. *Plast Reconstr Surg* 1978; 62:702.
19. Spira M. Subcutaneous mastectomy in the large, ptotic breast. *Plast Reconstr Surg* 1977; 59:200.
20. Woods JE, Verheyden CN. Pitfalls and problems with subcutaneous mastectomy. *Mayo Clin Proc* 1980; 55:687.
21. Woods JE. Subcutaneous mastectomy: current state of the art. *Ann Plast Surg* 1983; 11:541.
22. Woods JE. Detailed technique of subcutaneous mastectomy with and without mastopexy. *Ann Plast Surg* 1987; 18:51.
23. Schuster DI, Lavine DM. Nine-year experience with subpectoral breast reconstruction after subcutaneous mastectomy in 98 patients utilizing saline inflatable prostheses. *Ann Plast Surg* 1988; 21:444.

Suggested Readings

Bostwick J III. *Plastic and reconstructive surgery.* St. Louis: Quality Medical Publishing, 1990.
Georgiade N. *Breast reconstruction following mastectomy.* St. Louis: CV Mosby, 1979.
Georgiade N. *Reconstructive breast surgery.* St. Louis: CV Mosby, 1976.

68

Breast Reconstruction after Mastectomy: Overview and Implant Reconstruction

Gregory S. Georgiade, M.D., F.A.C.S., and Michael J. Sundine, M.D.

Overview

It has been estimated that in 1996 approximately 185,000 American women will develop carcinoma of the breast (1). Thus 1 in 8 women will face the psychologic trauma associated with the illness, along with the emotional trauma arising from loss of a breast.

The emotional impact of a mastectomy may be profound. Not only does the patient have to deal with the stress of a potentially life-threatening disease, but she must also adjust to her altered body image and its consequences on her sexual, social, and occupational functioning (2).

A patient newly diagnosed with breast cancer must be followed by a multidisciplinary team who care for patients with breast cancer. Members of this team may include an oncologic surgeon, a medical oncologist, a radiation oncologist, a plastic surgeon, nursing personnel, and a social worker. It should be remembered that patients with breast cancer are heterogeneous (3) and that their treatment must be individualized; this concept is facilitated by the presence of a multidisciplinary team.

As members of the team treating patients with breast cancer, it is important that plastic surgeons understand the rationale for the oncologic procedure to be performed. Based on pioneering work by Veronesi and Fisher, the movement toward breast-conserving therapy has moved rapidly. In an excellent review of the literature, Radford and Wells (4) have defined the important indications and contraindications for breast conservation therapy (Tables 68–1, 68–2).

The goals of breast reconstruction are (a) to create a breast that looks and feels like the resected breast, (b) to allow for undelayed chemotherapy or radiation therapy, or both, (c) to avoid predisposing to local recurrence, (d) to allow immediate or delayed reconstruction, (e) to entail acceptable risks, (f) to avoid predisposing to distant metastases (5).

Patients who are about to undergo mastectomy, or who have had a previous mastectomy, now have more options than at any other time for reconstruction of the breast. The available choices include implant reconstruction alone, tissue expansion followed by the placement of an implant, latissimus dorsi myocutaneous flap with or without an implant, free or pedicled TRAM flaps, free inferior or superior gluteal myocutaneous flaps, free lateral thigh flap, and Rubens flap.

Because of the frustration of both surgeons and patients with inability to create a soft, pendulous breast with a well-defined inframammary fold, surgeons have been increasingly using autogenous tissue for breast reconstruction. Bostwick and Jones (6) have outlined some specific indications for the use of autogenous tissue in breast reconstruction; they include patient preference and mastectomy-site tissue deficiency, arising either from radical mastectomy techniques or from large amounts of skin having been removed at the time of modified radical mastectomy. Also included are patients with recurrent capsular contracture following implant reconstruction, recurrent periprosthetic infection, coverage of high-risk implants, salvage of ruptured silicone implants with granuloma formation, a history of collagen vascular disease, and previous chest-wall irradiation.

The safety of immediate breast reconstruction has been well established (7–14). Immediate breast reconstruction has advantages in terms of aesthetic results, reduced costs, psychologic benefits, and availability to almost all patients. The aesthetic results are improved by cooperation between the oncologic and reconstructive surgeons in reducing the amount of skin removed and preserving natural landmarks (e.g., the inframammary fold). Economically, it is clear that by performing the extirpative procedure and reconstruction during the same hospital admission significant cost savings can be obtained.

Early studies investigating the psychologic impact of breast reconstruction focused on grief theories and assumed that the patient should pass through stages of mourning the loss of her breast. Those patients who sought breast reconstruction were believed to be having difficulty in completing the mourning process (15). Recent studies have shown that the only psychiatric solution to the disfigurement caused by mastectomy is breast reconstruction (16), and other studies have demonstrated that patients who undergo immediate reconstruction have less psychologic stress than those patients who have delayed breast reconstruction (17).

Finally, by performing breast reconstruction at the time of mastectomy, reconstruction is essentially available to all patients instead of that select population who would later be assertive enough to demand it (14).

Patients who are candidates for immediate breast reconstruction are generally those patients who present with early-stage breast disease (i.e., stage I and stage II disease) unless the chest wall is involved, in which case the patient may require chest-wall irradiation. Those patients who present with stage III disease are not candidates for immediate reconstruction, and they may require pre and postoperative chemotherapy in addition to mastectomy and possible irradiation. There are also medical contraindications to immediate reconstruction (18) (Table 68–3).

Table 68–1.
Indications for Breast Conservation Therapy

Tumor size < 5 cm
Well-motivated patient
Resection would not compromise cosmesis
   Acceptable tumor-to-breast size ratio
     Solitary lesion that can be completely excised
   Focal, not diffuse, calcifications

Table 68–2.
Contraindications to Breast Conservation Therapy

Absolute
   Multiple primaries
   Large tumor in small breast
   Gross residual tumor
   Pregnancy
   Collagen vascular disease
   Diffuse microcalcifications
Relative
   Extensive ductal carcinoma in situ
   Young age

Table 68–3.
Medical Contraindications to Immediate Breast Reconstruction

Severe diabetes
Vascular disease
Uncontrolled hypertension
Severe cardiac disease
Obesity
Anticoagulation therapy
Smoking
Collagen vascular disease
Postoperative radiation treatment

There have been many changes in breast reconstruction over the last several years. Among these are the increase in the use of autologous tissue, an increase in immediate breast reconstruction, an increase in the use of free-tissue transfer techniques, and a focus on skin preservation during mastectomy.

In a review of their 13-year experience of 455 postmastectomy reconstructions in 381 patients, Trabulsy and colleagues (19) identified several of the trends noted above. The use of autogenous tissue increased from 13% in the first 5 years of the study period to 37% in the final 4 years. However, the use of the textured silicone saline-filled expander/implant remained the most common method of reconstruction. There was also an increase in immediate reconstruction from 6 to 28% over the same time period. Finally, the use of free-tissue transfer for reconstruction was zero for the first 9 years of the study and increased to 19% in the final 4 years.

The use of skin-sparing techniques, in which the scar at the biopsy site is removed along with the nipple-areolar complex, has allowed plastic surgeons to improve the quality of their results by preserving the inframammary fold and by decreasing the tissue requirements for the reconstruction. Kroll and associates (20) reviewed their experience, in a series of 100 breast reconstructions in 87 patients, of using skin-sparing mastectomy techniques followed by immediate reconstruction. With a minimum follow-up period of 1 year and an average follow-up period of 23 months, a 1.2% local recurrence rate was noted, thus establishing the safety of skin sparing techniques. From an oncologic perspective, it is probably wise to remove the entire nipple-areolar complex at the time of mastectomy and not attempt any "nipple coring" technique to preserve the areola since histologic analysis of the areola has identified the presence of mammary ducts (21).

Historically, there has been some concern that immediate breast reconstruction might seed tumor cells into freshly dissected tissue planes or may mask and impede the detection of a local recurrence. Recurrences in those patients who have undergone implant reconstruction have been found in the skin and subcutaneous tissues and have not been found in the subpectoral space. Slavin and co-workers (22) reviewed a series of 161 patients who had immediate reconstruction using myocutaneous flaps (latissimus dorsi and TRAM) following mastectomy, and they observed a recurrence in 10.6% of the patients. All of the recurrences were found in the skin and subcutaneous tissues adjacent to the mastectomy and flap reconstruction site. They did not observe any concealment of the recurrence of tumor by the use of myocutaneous flaps. Thus it appears that available methods of breast reconstruction do not hinder the detection of local recurrences.

Tissue Expander/Implant Reconstruction

The use of prosthetic materials represented a significant advance for breast reconstruction. Radovan, in 1982, reported the first use of tissue expansion for reconstruction of the breast and ushered in the current method of breast reconstruction (5). Even with the increasing popularity of autogenous tissue reconstruction, the majority of breast reconstruction is still performed using implants (19,23). This technique can produce acceptable results in the majority of patients. Currently, most authors do not place permanent implants at the original operation. Instead, a tissue expander is placed into a submuscular pocket and, after the breast pocket is adequately expanded, the expander is removed and a permanent prosthesis is placed.

Breast reconstruction using a tissue expander followed by an implant offers many advantages that have been nicely summarized by Beasley (24) (Table 68–4). With the use of a tissue expander, the local tissues of the chest are stretched. Thus, the resulting breast mound will have the same skin texture, color, and sensation as the opposite breast; and, by using the patient's mastectomy incision to place the tissue expander, no new scars are introduced (as they are in flap techniques). Also, any donor-site morbidity from a flap procedure is avoided by using tissue expansion. The technique is relatively easy to master and provides for a short operating time and reduced postoperative recovery time.

There are reportedly many disadvantages to implant breast reconstruction (6) (Table 68–5). Often cited are the problems of a poorly defined inframammary fold and lack of natural ptosis; however, in a series of 84 consecutive breast reconstructions using a textured silicone tissue expander, Maxwell and Falcone (25) were able to demonstrate excellent results. Woods and Mangan (23) also found good aesthetic results in

Table 68–4.
Advantages of Implant Reconstruction

Provides donor tissue of similar texture, color, and sensation
Minimal scar formation
Avoidance of problematic donor sites
Decreased operating and recovery time
Technically easy procedure to perform

Table 68–5.
Disadvantages of Implant Reconstruction

Capsular contracture
Lack of natural ptosis
Poorly defined inframammary fold
Implant deflation
Need for multiple procedures
Implant rippling
Poor in irradiated fields
Questionable autoimmune phenomena
Prolonged time for reconstruction
Cost of implants
Need for contralateral breast procedure

reviewing their series of over 300 tissue-expander breast reconstructions. The use of overexpansion and differential expansion with anatomically shaped tissue expanders may help to alleviate some of these problems. Also cited is a significant rate of capsular contracture, which may require revisionary procedures such as capsulotomy, but in the series cited above Maxwell noted that 97% of his breast reconstructions using tissue expanders were moderately to very soft (Baker II).

Other purported disadvantages include: implant failure and deflation, implant rippling, need for multiple procedures, prolonged time for reconstruction, implant cost, poor results in irradiated fields, questionable autoimmune phenomena, and the need for a contralateral breast procedure.

The relationship between silicone breast implants and possible development of connective-tissue disease has received a great deal of attention in the lay media and in the medical literature (29,30). There is mounting scientific evidence that there is no relationship between silicone and the development of connective-tissue disease. In a prospective study by Schusterman and colleagues (26), a series of patients who underwent breast reconstruction using silicone breast implants (308 reconstructions) were compared with a group of patients who underwent autogenous reconstruction (408 reconstructions). In both groups one patient developed an autoimmune disease, and they concluded that the incidence of autoimmune disease was not different between the two groups. Gabriel and associates (27) compared a total of 749 women in Olmstead county, Minnesota, who had received silicone breast implants to 1498 community controls and then reviewed the development of connective-tissue disease. They found no association between the presence of silicone breast implants and the development of connective-tissue diseases (31).

In view of the many possible disadvantages of using tissue expanders for breast reconstruction, it is wise to attempt to optimize results by choosing appropriate candidates for this method of reconstruction. We would agree with Dowden (32) that success in tissue-expander reconstruction is primarily related to patient selection. The patient should have a small- to medium-size breast and should not object to the placement of an implant. It is difficult to obtain satisfactory aesthetic results using a tissue expander to reconstruct a large ptotic breast and these patients are better candidates for a double-pedicle or free TRAM procedure, especially if a procedure on the contralateral breast is not desired. Two groups of patients who tend to have consistently poor results using tissue expanders for breast reconstruction are obese patients and those patients who have had chest-wall irradiation. It is difficult to achieve the definition and size needed in the obese patient (23) and, in addition, these patients have a higher rate of infection/extrusion failures (32). Patients who have had

chest-wall radiation expand poorly and the quality of the result is poor because of the firmness of these irradiated tissues. Those patients who either object to a large operation or who are not medically fit to undergo a large flap reconstruction are good candidates for a tissue-expander reconstruction, as are those patients who object to the scars associated with flap procedures. Finally, many patients may not be candidates for flap procedures because the vascular pedicle has been previously transected during earlier procedures (e.g., subcostal incision from previous cholecystectomy). Slavin and Colen (33) describe the "ideal patient" for tissue expansion breast reconstruction as "a healthy nonsmoker of moderate contralateral breast size with adequate soft-tissue coverage and the absence of previous irradiation who is undergoing reconstruction on a delayed basis." (Table 68–6)

It follows, then, that patients who are obese and have previous chest-wall radiation are not good candidates for tissue expander reconstruction. Also, those patients who have atrophic and tight skin with poor muscle (23) and those with skin flaps of questionable viability (32) are likely to have poor results or implant infection and extrusion. Skin flaps of questionable viability may have led to the high rate of implant loss seen in the series of Slavin and Colen (34). Patients with marginally viable skin flaps or tight skin coverage will require importation of skin through a flap procedure (32,35). Cigarette smoking may be a contraindication to the use of tissue expanders for reconstruction (35,36) (Table 68–7).

The technique of placement of the tissue expander is the same whether the reconstruction is performed on an immediate or delayed basis. An incision is made through the muscle-fascial layer transversely over the 6th–7th interspace in the lateral thoracic region, elevating the serratus muscle as a flap. Sharp dissection is carried out, advancing to the level of the 6th–7th interspace, and is continued beneath the serratus muscle to the pectoralis major muscle (Fig. 68–1). The medial attachments of the pectoral muscle are released and undermined beneath the rectus abdominus fascia, with the undermining carried laterally to the anterior axillary line area. This may be an area of minimal muscle attachment and coverage. In these situations, the pectoralis minor muscle attachments are released and attached to the upper lateral pectoral muscle after the technique of Barwick (personal communication). The desired size of prosthesis or expander may then be inserted. It is our preference at this time to insert a tissue expander for most patients undergoing immediate reconstruction (Figs. 68–2, 68–3).

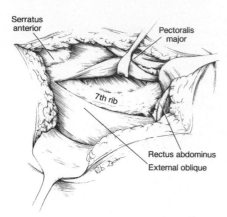

FIG. 68–1. Dissection carried out from the 6th-7th interspace upward beneath the serratus anterior with the pectoralis major muscle, with extension beneath the rectus muscle fascia.

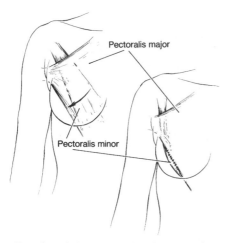

FIG. 68–2. Transfer of the pectoralis minor muscle to the lateral edge of the pectoralis major muscle is carried out in the immediate reconstruction when insufficient tissue remains after modified radical mastectomy.

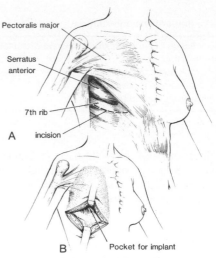

FIG. 68–3. **A,** when the approach is via an inframammary incision, it is carried over the 6th-7th interspace, separating the serratus muscle-fascia layer and dissecting under this muscle layer, extending the dissection under the pectoralis major muscle and above the pectoralis minor muscle. **B,** the pocket with area of undermining extending medially beneath the rectus abdominis fascia.

The muscle pocket is then closed over the tissue expander using interrupted 3-0 Vicryl sutures. The operative wound is closed in two layers with a deep subdermal layer of 4-0 Vicryl. A running 4-0 Prolene subcuticular suture is used to approximate the skin edges, followed by Steri-strips over the suture line. Care is taken not to place so much saline in the tissue expander that undue tension is placed on the skin closure (37).

There have been many recent improvements in breast tissue expander design. The use of a textured design is felt to have multiple advantages, including ease in expansion with lower injection pressures, decreased patient discomfort during the expansion process, less chest-wall compression, and decreased capsule formation (25). This has recently been challenged by May and co-workers (38) in a double-blind study between smooth and textured expander implants. In their series of six patients, four of the six showed decreased intraluminal pressures in the smooth expander from its textured counterpart, and the smooth expander was noted to cause less discomfort during the expansion process than the textured expander. There was no difference between the smooth and textured capsules, but the textured expander did hold its position on the chest wall more effectively. It is also believed that infectious complications may be reduced with the textured expander because of tissue ingrowth and adherence to the expander and its integrated valve. Another fundamental improvement in tissue expander design has been the integrated valve, which requires less tissue dissection and no subcutaneous tunnel dissection, unlike expanders with remote ports; this design also helps avoid the problems of valve rotation with fill-tube kinking (25) (Fig. 68–4).

Other important advances in implant technology include the development of "anatomically shaped" tissue expansion devices. By coupling this design with a textured surface that maintains the proper orientation and position of the implant, the breast pocket is able to be expanded further in the lower pole than in the upper pole, allowing for a more natural appearing reconstructed breast. Hammond and others (39) used a biomechanical model to examine the contour of various breast tissue expanders and found that the anatomic and differential expanders had the most inferiorly located point of maximal projection, but the differential expander also had the greatest upper pole deformity of all of the expanders. The Becker, Gibney, and round expanders were all found to create an essentially round and symmetric profile.

We have used complete submuscular coverage of the tissue expander, as have many other authors (14,23,40). The placement of implants into this location may prevent difficulties with implant infection, exposure, and extrusion. However, there is not agreement on the necessity of complete muscle coverage, and some authors believe that with complete muscle coverage of the expander they are unable to expand the lower pole of the breast effectively. Dowden (32) does not believe that complete muscle coverage of the implant is necessary, and the lower pole of Dowden's tissue expander is covered only by skin and subcutaneous tissue; but, he believes it is important to isolate the skin incision from

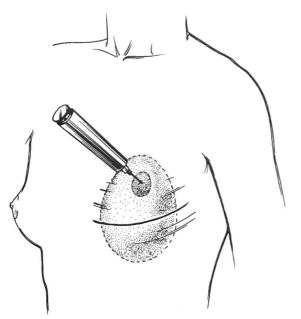

FIG. 68–4. Location of the injection port of an inflatable prosthesis. (From Georgiade GS. Reconstructive and aesthetic breast surgery. In: Sabiston DC, ed. *Textbook of surgery.* 15th ed. Philadephia: WB Saunders, in press.)

Table 68–6.
Indications for Tissue Expander/Implant Reconstruction

Small- to medium-sized breast
Patient not obese and chest wall not irradiated
Patient not opposed to use of an implant
Patient prefers not to undergo an extensive operation
Medical contraindications for a large operation
Patient objects to scars associated with flaps
Not a candidate for autogenous reconstruction because of previous incisions

Table 68–7.
Contraindications to Tissue Expander/Implant Reconstruction

Patients who have undergone chest-wall irradiation
Obese patients
Patients with atrophic and tight skin with poor muscle
Patients with skin flaps of questionable viability

the implant with muscle, especially at the medial and lateral extremes of the incision. A review of 60 consecutive tissue-expander breast reconstructions—in which complete muscle coverage was obtained at one medical center, and the lower and medial aspects of the expander were not covered by muscle at another medical center—demonstrated no difference in complication rates between the two groups (34).

Inflation of the expander usually begins 2 weeks following placement. The patient is then seen at 1- to 2-week intervals and 50 to 100 cc of saline is injected into the tissue expander under sterile conditions. The expansion is usually carried out until approximately 20% overinflation is achieved. This degree of overexpansion is maintained for at least 8 weeks to allow the capsule to mature. At this point the expander may be removed and a permanent prosthesis inserted. Also at this time, any small adjustments in the breast pocket can be made along with nipple-areolar reconstruction and alterations of the contralateral breast.

The pace of the expansion process has recently been challenged by Wickman (41), who randomized a series of patients into a rapid expansion group and a slow expansion group. With the rapid expansion group, the expansion was initiated 1 week postoperatively and the expander was inflated daily, while the slow expansion group began expansion at 2 weeks postoperatively and inflations were carried out weekly. In both groups, the second-stage procedure was performed 3 months after the expansion was completed. Using these methods, there was a significant decrease in the time required to complete the reconstruction. There was a tendency for the rapid expansion group toward firmer breasts than in the slow expansion group, but this did not achieve statistical significance.

The potential complications using tissue expander/implant techniques are numerous; they include hematoma, infection,

flap necrosis, implant deflation, device malfunction, capsular contracture, and implant extrusion and loss. The complication rates have been reported to be as high as a 50% failure rate and up to 18% implant loss rate (32). However, with careful attention to detail and appropriate selection of candidates for this method of reconstruction, the implant loss rate should be able to be kept in the 3 to 4% range.

In terms of the aesthetic results that can be achieved using tissue expansion/implant reconstruction, many authors have achieved a great proportion of good to excellent results (2,23,25,32,35). In an interesting study, Kroll and Baldwin (42) compared the aesthetic results of three different procedures: tissue expansion, latissimus dorsi myocutaneous flaps, and TRAM flaps. In their series, the TRAM flap was the most aesthetically successful technique and tissue expansion had a significantly higher failure rate than the other two techniques. Tissue expansion was also found to be less successful in obese patients.

Management of the opposite breast is usually initiated at the time of the first stage of breast reconstruction if the patient is undergoing delayed reconstruction, or at the time of the second stage of reconstruction if the patient is undergoing immediate reconstruction. There are a number of possibilities that exist, depending on the status of the opposite breast.

A subcutaneous mastectomy can be carried out in highly selected patients if there are severe dysplastic changes in the remaining breast. Such changes are associated with a higher incidence of malignancy in the severely dysplastic breast.

The hypoplastic breast will frequently necessitate augmentation mammaplasty with or without accompanying mastopexy. The increased difficulty of mammography in the augmented breast should be taken into account in patients who have had breast cancer prior to an augmentation mammaplasty on the remaining breast.

The patient with a large, hypertrophied or ptotic breast may require a mastopexy or some form of reduction mammaplasty in order to better balance the final breast forms. This can be carried out during the initial stage of reconstruction, so that any small final revisions may be made without difficulty at a later date, such as at the time of the removal of the tissue expander or nipple reconstruction (37).

References

1. American Cancer Society.
2. Schain WS. Breast reconstruction: update of psychosocial and pragmatic concerns. *Cancer* 1991; 68:1170.
3. Boyd FJ, McKenney SA, Hayes DF, et al. Psychosocial issues in breast reconstruction. *Cancer* 1991; 68:1176.
4. Radford DM, Wells SA. Surgical techniques in breast conservation. *Adv Surg* 1993; 26:1.
5. Hugo NE. Breast reconstruction in the postsilicone era. *Adv Surg* 1993; 27:161.
6. Bostwick J, Jones G. Why I choose autogenous tissue in breast reconstruction. *Cli. Plast Surg* 1994; 21:165.
7. Hueston JT, McKenzie G. Breast reconstruction after radical mastectomy. *Aust N Z J Surg* 1981; 39:367.
8. Georgiade GS, Georgiade NG, et al. Modified radical mastectomy with immediate reconstruction for carcinoma of the breast. *Ann Surg* 1981; 73:565.
9. Georgiade GS, Georgiade NG, et al. Rationale for immediate reconstruction of breast following modified radical mastectomy. *Ann. Plast Surg* 1962; 8:20.
10. Georgiade N, Riefkohl R, Cox E, et al. Long-term clinical outcome of immediate reconstruction after mastectomy. *Plast Reconstruct Surg* 1985; 76:415.
11. Webster DS, Mansel RE, Hughes SE. Immediate reconstruction of the breast after mastectomy: is it safe? *Cancer* 1984; 12:431.
12. Georgiade GS. Immediate reconstruction of the breast following modified radical mastectomy for carcinoma of the breast. *Clin Plast Surg* 1984; 11:383.
13. Frazier TG, Noone RB. An objective analysis of immediate simultaneous reconstruction in the treatment of primary carcinoma of the breast. *Cancer* 1985; 55:102.
14. Noone RB, Frazier TG, Murphy JB, et al. Immediate reconstruction after mastectomy for cancer. *Adv Plast Reconstr Surg* 1987; 4:51.
15. Goldsmith HS, Alday ES. Role of the surgeon and the rehabilitation of the breast cancer patient. *Cancer* 1971; 28:1672.
16. Asken MJ. Psychoemotional aspects of mastectomy: a review of the literature. *Am J Psychiatry* 1975; 132:56.
17. Wellisch DK, Schain WS, Noone RB, et al. Psychosocial correlates of immediate vs. delayed reconstruction of the breast. *Plast Reconstruct Surg* 1985; 76:713.
18. Marcial VA, Nixon DW, Wilson JL, et al. Defining the role of reconstruction. *Cancer* 1991; 68:1178.
19. Trabulsy PP, Anthony JP, Mathes SJ. Changing trends in postmastectomy breast reconstruction: a 13-year experience. *Plast Reconstruct Surg* 1994; 93:1418.
20. Kroll SS, Ames F, Singletary SE, et al. The oncologic risks of skin preservation at mastectomy when combined with immediate reconstruction of the breast. *Surg Gynecol Obstet* 1991; 172:17.
21. Schnitt SJ, Goldwyn RM, Slavin SA. Mammary ducts in the areola: implications for patients undergoing reconstructive surgery of the breast. *Plast Reconstruct Surg* 1993; 92:1290.
22. Slavin SA, Love SM, Goldwyn RM. Recurrent breast cancer following immediate reconstruction with myocutaneous flaps. *Plast Reconstruct Surg* 1994; 93:1191.
23. Woods JE, Mangan MA. Breast reconstruction with tissue expanders: obtaining an optimal result. *Ann Plast Surg* 1992; 28:390.
24. Beasley ME. Discussion: eighty-four consecutive breast reconstuctions using a textured silicone tissue expander. *Plast Reconstruct Surg* 1992; 89:1035.
25. Maxwell GP, Falcone PA. Eighty-four consecutive breast reconstructions using a textured silicone tissue expander. *Plast Reconstruct Surg* 1992; 89:1022.
26. Schusterman MA, Kroll SS, et al. Incidence of autoimune disease in patients after breast reconstruction with silicone gel implants versus autogenous tissue: a preliminary report. *Ann Plast Surg* 1993; 31:1.
27. Gabriel SE, O'Fallon M, et al. Risk of connective-tissue diseases and other disorders after breast implantation. *N Engl J Med* 1994; 330:1697.
28. Sanchez-Guerrero J, Schnur PH, Sergent JS, et al. Silicone breast implants and rheumatic disease: clinical, immunologic, and epidemiologic studies. *Arthritis Rheum* 1994; 37:158.
29. Cook RR, Harrison MC, LeVier RR. The breast implant controversy. *Arthritis Rheum* 1994; 37:153.
30. Bridges AJ, Vasey FB. Silicone breast implants: history, safety, and potential complications. *Arch Intern Med* 1993; 153:2638.
31. Hennekens CH, Lee IM, Cook NR, et al. Self-supported breast implants and connective-tissue diseases in female health professionals. *JAMA* 1996; 275:616.
32. Dowden RV. Selection criteria for successful immediate breast reconstruction. *Plast Reconstruct Surg* 1991; 88:628.
33. Slavin SA, Colen SR. Discussion: analysis of risks and aesthetics in a consecutive series of tissue expansion breast reconstructions. *Plast Reconstruct Surg* 1992; 89:844.
34. Slavin SA, Colen SR. Sixty consecutive breast reconstructions with the inflatable explander: a critical appraisal. *Plast Reconstruct Surg* 1990; 86:910.
35. Cohen BE, Casso D, Whetstone M. Analysis of risks and aesthetics in a consecutive series of tissue expansion breast reconstructions. *Plast Reconstruct Surg* 1992; 89:840.
36. Cohen IK, Turner D. Immediate breast reconstruction with tissue expanders. *Clin Plast Surg* 1987; 14:491.
37. Georgiade GS, Georgiade NG. Breast reconstruction with local tissue. In: Georgiade GS, et al, eds. *Textbook of plastic, maxillofacial, and reconstructive Surgery.* Baltimore: Williams & Wilkins, 1992; 843–845.
38. May JW, Bucky LP, Sohoni S, Ehrlich HP. Smooth vs. textured expander implants: a double-blind study of capsule quality and discomfort in simultaneous bilateral breast reconstruction patients. *Ann Plast Surg* 1994; 32:225.
39. Hammond DC, Perry LC, Maxwell GP, et al. Morphologic analysis of tissue-expander shape using a biomechanical model. *Plast Reconstruct Surg* 1993; 92:255.
40. Little JW, Golembe EV, Fisher JB. The "living bra" in immediate and delayed reconstruction of the breast following mastectomy for malignant and non-malignant disease. *Plast Reconstruct Surg* 1981; 68:392.
41. Wickman M. Comparison between rapid and slow tissue expansion in breast reconstruction. *Plast Reconstruct Surg* 1993; 91:663.
42. Kroll SS, Baldwin B. A comparison of outcomes using three different methods of breast reconstruction. *Plast Reconstruct Surg* 1992; 90:455.

69

Total Autogenous Latissimus Breast Reconstruction

John B. McCraw, M.D., F.A.C.S., Christoph Papp, M.D., and Ann McMellin, M.D.

The standard latissimus breast reconstruction was a dramatic improvement over the subcutaneous and subpectoral implant reconstructions that were the prevailing methods in 1978 (1). The latissimus flap provided muscle coverage of the silicone implant, breast skin replacement, and immediate ptosis, even in the radical mastectomy deformity. Unfortunately, capsule formation around the implant was common and resulted in a round shape, with elevation of the implant over time.

Popularization of the concept of the autogenous flap originated with the TRAM flap, which was described by Hartrampf in 1981 (2). Bohme's description of the buried latissimus myocutaneous flap predated this by 1 year, but it went unnoticed (3). Because some patients were not candidates for the TRAM flap, Papp independently developed the deepithelialized latissimus myocutaneous flap as an alternative volume replacement beginning in 1983 (4). Like the standard latissimus flap, no fat was carried on the surface of the muscle. No implant was needed in obese patients, but a large implant was still required in thin patients. In 1985, McCraw and Papp modified this design by carrying fat on the surface of the latissimus muscle to create the total autogenous latissimus (TAL) breast reconstruction (5).

The total autogenous latissimus breast reconstruction carries the full thickness of back fat with the myocutaneous skin paddle, and carries fat over most of the surface of the latissimus muscle. It is this fat that replaces the lost breast volume, the shape of the upper breast, and the anterior axillary fold. When additional volume is needed, as in a patient who has less than 2 cm of back fat, a small implant is usually adequate to augment the shape of the flap.

The initial design of the total autogenous latissimus flap included a fleur-de-lis, or three-cornered skin paddle, as a way of transferring a large area of skin from the back to the breast. This was soon abandoned because of the unfavorable back scar. A crescent-shaped skin paddle was designed in a favorable skin line to produce a good scar, and the skin paddle was lengthened in order to provide adequate skin replacement. The flap design changed the relationship of flaps and implants, as the autogenous latissimus flap itself restored the shape of the breast, including the anterior axillary fold, while an implant used simply augmented this shape. This is similar to the current use of implants with the TRAM flap, and is contrasted with the standard latissimus reconstruction, in which the implant gives virtually all of the shape (6–7).

Indications

The TAL breast reconstruction is useful for a large variety of deformities, ranging from the quadrantectomy to the irradiated chest.

Quadrantectomy defects are usually less than 50% of the breast volume and can easily be replaced by a partial or complete latissimus flap with fat on the surface of the muscle. Because most of these patients have planned radiation treatments that will cause permanent flap swelling, the TAL reconstruction should be smaller than the breast defect initially.

The *Poland chest wall deformity* is an almost perfect application for this flap because the congenital breast deformity primarily affects the pectoralis muscle and the breast volume. The TAL reconstruction, except in the most severe deformities, with absent latissimus muscles as a part of the deformity, can completely replace the contour of the anterior axillary fold and upper breast, the central breast volume, and the shape of the missing pectoralis major muscle.

Modified radical mastectomy defects typically include an 8 cm – 18 cm deficiency of breast skin that can easily be replaced by the TAL breast reconstruction. In obese patients, the upper fill and anterior axillary fold replacement is frequently better than that achieved by the TRAM flap. When very large skin replacements are needed, a TRAM flap is the better reconstructive choice.

TRAM flap failures can be converted to exceptional results by the addition of the TAL flap. Many times the major area of deficiency with partial TRAM flap loss is in the upper breast and the anterior axillary fold. The TAL flap is an ideal choice for this replacement and usually does not require an implant.

Autogenous conversion of implant reconstructions are becoming more common because of aging implants. This is actually a simple reconstruction, because the primary defect is the breast volume. The TAL reconstruction can usually be done without an implant, or with a very small implant that is used to augment the volume and not for shape. Nipple reconstruction can be incorporated into the TAL reconstruction by designing a fishtail nipple flap on any part of the flap skin.

Alternative autogenous flap sites are essential because any flap can be lost. The TAL breast reconstruction is usually more acceptable than any buttock or thigh flap, and may be chosen by the patient instead of a TRAM flap. As part of our preoperative plan with free TRAM flaps, we routinely discuss the use of the TAL reconstruction in the case of a free-flap failure.

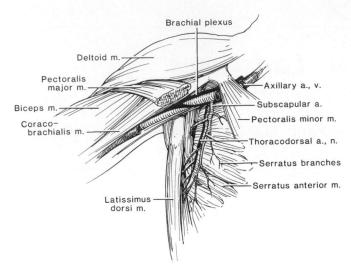

FIG. 69–1. The vascular pedicle is dissected carefully from the serratus and circumflex branches of the thoracodorsal artery.

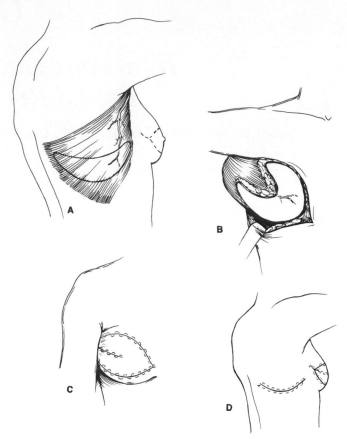

FIG. 69–2. **A,** the latissmus myocutaneous flap outline. **B,** myocutaneous flap being transferred beneath a lateral axillary skin bridge. **C,** transferred flap in its new position. **D,** location of the final incisions.

Completion mastectomies for radiation-lumpectomy are usually associated with locally recurrent breast cancer, which is not metastatic disease. The total mastectomy and skin defect can normally be corrected with the TAL flap, unless there is severe radiation damage that requires massive skin replacement.

Radiation ulcerations require flaps that have robust blood supply that is independent of the bed for flap inset. The vigorous blood supply of the TAL flap is ideal for this application, and the addition of fat on the surface of the latissimus muscle provides additional padding on the surface of the chest.

Flap Design

The TAL flap should be designed preoperatively, marked, and not changed at the time of the operation, when anatomic relationships are altered by the position of the patient on the operating table. There are three essential elements of the flap design, discussed below.

SKIN PADDLE

The skin paddle closure is placed in the proper skin tension lines, parallel to the ribs. The width of the paddle is determined by the ease of closure, and varies between 7 and 10 cm in average-sized patients. The long line of the skin paddle extends from the area below the tip of the scapula to the inframammary fold. This is usually 24 to 30 cm in length. The paddle carries the full thickness of the fat and the volume can be determined precisely (length – width – height) if the tips of the paddle are ignored. A crescent shape with a longer inferior margin of the paddle is always preferred, because this design takes advantage of the laxity of the lower back to facilitate the closure.

LATISSIMUS DORSI MUSCLE

A part, or all, of the latissimus dorsi muscle can be elevated, depending on the volume requirements. If only the anterior half of the muscle is elevated, the skin paddle can be centered over it. The TAL muscle flap can be used for partial

breast defects and raised with an endoscope using very small incisions.

FAT CARRIED BY THE MUSCLE

The latissimus muscle can carry fat over its entire surface, as well as in the area distal to the origin near the iliac crest. It is essential to leave 1 cm of fat with the back skin so that it will not be devascularized by the removal of the muscular perforators. When the patient has 2 cm of fat thickness on the back, 1 cm of fat can be removed with the muscle, which provides a volume of 1 cm multiplied by the surface area of the muscle (20 cm – 20 cm), or 400 grams of fat on the surface of the muscle. When the patient has 3 cm of fat thickness, 800 grams of fat can be carried on the surface of the muscle. Some additional fat near the iliac crest can be left attached to the lower edge of the muscle to provide 100 to 400 grams of fat.

Flap Dissection

Two things make flap dissection difficult: fat covering the surface of the muscle, and the inaccessibility of the thoracodorsal vessels. The fat obscures the usual landmarks on the muscle surface, so that it is necessary to identify the surrounding structures (e.g., the serratus anterior, the external oblique, and the teres major muscles).

The vascular pedicle must be completely dissected away from the serratus and circumflex branches and any fascial attachments to avoid kinking of the pedicle (Fig. 69–1).

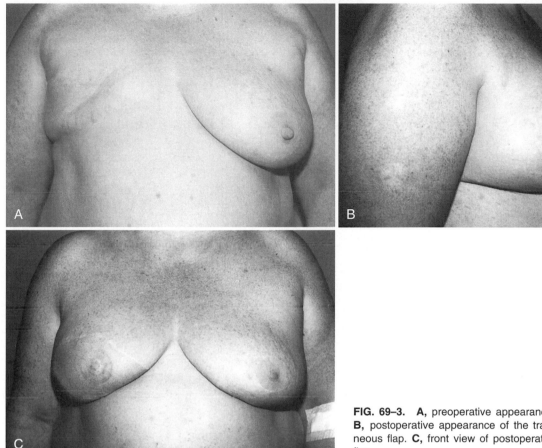

FIG. 69–3. **A,** preoperative appearance of the chest deformity. **B,** postoperative appearance of the transferred latissmus myocutaneous flap. **C,** front view of postoperative latissimus myocutaneous flap.

Flap Shaping

The vascular pedicle is secured anteriorly, and the tendon of the latissimus muscle is attached to the highest point of the anterior axillary fold. The upper fill is recreated first by attaching the anterior margin of the flap to the clavicle and then draping the muscle over the sternum. The inframammary fold is formed next, and the flap is finally folded into a U-shape to make the central cone of the breast. The dog-ear that results from coning the flap can be used as a fishtail bilobed flap for nipple reconstruction (see Fig. 69–1).

Donor Site

Fluorescein is routinely used to assess the viability of the back flaps. The donor site can be expected to form seromas because of the wide area of dissection. It is important to think of "collapsing" the space between the back skin and the chest wall. This is done by adequate suction drainage and immobility of shoulder motion for 1 week. If a seroma develops after the suction drains are removed, it should not be aspirated because this will not remove all of the fluid, and total removal of the fluid collection is essential to the collapse of the cavity. Seromas can virtually always be treated successfully on the first attempt by inserting a small penrose drain if it is placed in the most dependent part of the cavity (Fig. 69–2).

Results

The results of the TAL breast reconstruction are generally above average and can be excellent, depending on the size of the defect. Excellent results are expected in partial defects, Poland deformity, and salvage of failed implant and TRAM reconstructions. Flap loss is less than 2% in the early period. Revisions are usually minor and can be done with local anesthesia. When small saline implants are used to augment the flap shape it is very unusual to have a problem, because these implants range from 100 to 150 cc and only account for about 25% of the breast volume. When it is necessary to use large implants, any changes in the shape of the implant will cause visible changes in the reconstruction (Fig. 69–3).

References

1. Bostwick J III, Vasconez LO, Jurkiewicz MJ. Breast reconstruction after a radical mastectomy. *Plast Reconstr Surg* 1978; 61:682.
2. Hartrampf CR Jr, Scheflan M, Black PW. Breast reconstruction with a transverse abdominal flap. *Plast Reconstr Surg* 1982; 69:216.
3. Bohme PE. Mammarekonstruktion mit dem versecten latissimus dorsisnsellappen. In: Bohme H, ed). *Brustkrebs und brustrekonstruktion.* Stuttgart: Georg Thieme Verlag, 1982.
4. Papp C, Zanon E, McCraw J. Breast volume replacement using the deep-ithelialized latissimus dorsi myocutaneous flap. *Eur J Plast Surg* 1988; 11:120.
5. McCraw JB, Papp C. The fleur-de-lis autogenous latissimus dorsi myocutaneous flap reconstruction. Presented before the annual meeting of the American Association of Plastic Surgeons, Scottsdale, Arizona, May 1989.
6. McCraw J, Papp C. The fleur-de-lis autogenous latissimus breast reconstruction. In: Hartrampf C, ed. *Breast reconstruction with living tissue.* New York: Raven, 1991.
7. McCraw J, Papp C, Edwards A, et al. The autogenous latissimus breast reconstruction. *Clinics in Plastic Surgery* 1994; 21:279.

70

Breast Reconstruction with the Transverse Abdominal Island (TRAM) Flap

Carl R. Hartrampf, Jr., M.D., F.A.C.S., Mark A. Anton, M.D., and Jean Trimble Bried, P.A.

Breast reconstruction with autogenous tissue has a number of distinct advantages over reconstruction with a silicone prosthesis. Breasts reconstructed with natural living tissue have a realistic form, remain soft, and are generally trouble free over a lifetime. The most widely used method of breast reconstruction with autogenous tissue is the transverse abdominal island flap, or TRAM flap, first reported in 1982 (1) and still undergoing refinement today (2,3). The operation is not simple but rather deceptively complex. It requires considerable preparation and experience on the part of the surgeon in order to optimize breast mound aesthetics and to avoid serious complications.

Patient Selection

The TRAM flap reconstructive method is not for every mastectomy patient. Of all the factors influencing the success of this operation, patient selection is the most important.

RELATIVE INDICATIONS

Modified Radical Mastectomy

Patients with this defect who have tight, thin chest-wall skin, have failed previous reconstruction by other methods, have irradiation of the chest wall, or have a large ptotic opposite breast are candidates for the TRAM flap for reconstruction. In addition, many patients who are concerned about the potential dangers of synthetic materials prefer breast reconstruction with autogenous tissue.

Halstead Radical Mastectomy

No procedure can reconstruct the radical mastectomy defect as completely as the TRAM flap. This method will reproduce the anterior axillary fold (the pectoralis major muscle), fill the infraclavicular hollow, and at the same time produce adequate breast volume to match the opposite side. Generally, it takes one-half of the lower abdominal flap to reconstruct the infraclavicular axillary defect and one-half to reconstruct the breast.

Salvage Procedures of the Breast and Chest Wall

The TRAM flap can be especially useful following salvage mastectomy in patients who have experienced failed breast conservation cancer therapy. Marked chest-wall damage and even frank skin ulceration may occur following extensive radiation therapy for breast cancer. These individuals require autogenous tissue reconstruction but have limited options, either because the latissimus dorsi muscle is denervated or because potential recipient vessels for free-flap reconstruction have suffered radiation damage. The TRAM flap can provide the necessary coverage for even the most extensive defect and will introduce badly needed new blood supply to the area.

Subcutaneous Mastectomy Cripple

Those patients who, following subcutaneous mastectomy, have developed severe and often painful capsular contractures following silicone implant reconstruction and who have repeatedly undergone unsuccessful operative attempts to correct this problem with the implant can often be rehabilitated by removing the silicone implant and reconstructing the patient with autogenous tissue.

Congenital and Traumatic Chest-Wall Defects

The TRAM flap also can be useful in patients with Poland syndrome, pectus excavatum, massive sternal resection for neoplasm, and osteomyelitis after coronary bypass surgery.

CONTRAINDICATIONS AND RISK FACTOR ASSESSMENT

This operation necessarily invades tissue planes from the pubis to the upper chest. The tight abdominal closure may compromise pulmonary function. The tissue insult and subsequent stress on the body systems during and following the procedure are considerable. Therefore, candidates should be healthy, have a strong desire for autogenous tissue breast reconstruction, and have realistic expectations of the outcome. Potential physical and emotional constraints to successful results should be carefully assessed, and individuals who fall into a high-risk category should be offered reconstruction with an alternate method.

The absolute contraindications to this operation as an elective breast reconstruction include chronic pulmonary disease, severe cardiovascular disease, uncontrolled hypertension, morbid obesity, and insulin-dependent diabetes. Less obvious risk factors must be carefully noted, because the compounding of these factors in one patient may insidiously increase the chance of a complication beyond the acceptable range. Table 70–1 lists risk factors for complications associated with this operation along with the author's rating estimate (using a scale of 1 to 10) of the severity of that risk. These risk factors can be translated into a patient risk classification that will help in determining who is a candidate for this operation and who is not (Table 70–2). The rating estimates and the patient risk classifications have been arbitrarily assigned

786

Table 70–1.
TRAM Operation Risk Factors and Their Severity[a]

Risk Factor	Score (1–10)
Obesity	
Moderate: ≤25% above ideal body weight	1
Severe: >25% over ideal body weight	5
Small vessel disease	
Light to moderate smoking (0.5–1+ pack/day for 2–10 years)	1
Chronic heavy smoking (10–20 pack years)	2
Chronic heavy smoking (20–30 pack years)	5
Autoimmune disease (scleroderma, Raynaud's, etc.)	**10**
Diabetes mellitus—non–insulin dependent	5
Diabetes mellitus—insulin dependent	**10**
Psychosocial problems	
Unstable emotional state (life crisis)	5
Personality disorder	5
Substance abuse	5
Abdominal scars	
If "planned out" of flap design	0.5
Disruption of vascular perforators; transection of superior epigastric vessels (Chevron incision) abdominoplasty, etc.	**10**
Patient's attitude	
Patient unwilling or unable to invest time required for healing, or objects to abdominal scar	**10**
Surgeon's inexperience	
Less than 10 TRAM flaps	1
Major system disease process	
Chronic lung disease	**10**
Severe cardiovascular disease	**10**

[a]Entries in bold type are contraindications to use of the TRAM flap.

Table 70–2.
Patient Risk Factor Classification for the TRAM Operation

Class I	No risk factors and a score of 0 on the risk rating scale. Patients in this class are most likely to do well with this operation.
Class II	One risk factor or a score of 2 or less. Patients in this category are still good candidates for the TRAM flap, but the surgeon should institute measures to increase safety and to minimize the risk.
Class III	Two risk factors, but a combined score of 5 or less. These patients are marginal candidates for the TRAM flap; complications are likely to occur despite all efforts to prevent their occurrence.
Class IV	Three or more risk factors or a combined score of greater than 5. Patients in this category are NOT candidates for reconstruction with the TRAM flap.

by the author and are not intended to represent a scientifically derived ranking system.

Risks to Smokers

Special attention must be paid to the smoker. Nicotine is detrimental to flap perfusion because it slows blood flow to the flaps and increases platelet adhesiveness (4,5). A patient who is eager to undergo breast reconstruction may not be truthful about efforts to stop smoking. Serum carboxyhemoglobin and urine nicotine will confirm the patient's compliance with the request to stop smoking. A patient should be free of nicotine several months before breast reconstruction and continue free several months afterward.

ASSESSMENT OF ABDOMINAL TISSUE AVAILABLE FOR TRANSFER

Assessment of a patient's eligibility for TRAM flap breast reconstruction requires (a) an estimation of the amount of tissue needed to achieve symmetry with the remaining breast, and (b) an estimation of the available abdominal tissue.

The appropriate breast size is best determined by noting the weight of the mastectomy specimen and the size of the skin ellipse (pathologists should be universally encouraged to weigh all surgical specimens submitted for examination). Al-

though some allowance should be made for specimen shrinkage, the skin ellipse size provides a useful estimate of the chest skin deficit.

After measuring dimensions of 25 TRAM flaps, a comparison of the dimensions of the flap with the weight of the flap was performed using standard linear correlation analysis (5). The result indicated that conversion of the dimensions of the flap to weight is represented by a least-squares line. The coefficient of correlation ($r = .97$) was significant at a 99% confidence level. The following formula, which represents this least-squares line, provides a consistently accurate estimate of total flap weight:

Estimated flap weight (g)
$$= .81 \,[\text{length (cm)} - \text{width (cm)} - \text{thickness (cm)}]$$

Length and width are measured in centimeters at their extreme dimensions (including any bevel of the flap), and thickness is measured in centimeters with nutritionists' calipers at the widest point of the flap outline (with the patient's abdomen relaxed) and divided by two. These simple measurements can be made at the time of initial consultation and can help determine if the patient is a candidate for a TRAM flap and whether a single pedicle (approximately 69% of the total flap weight) or a double pedicle is required.

Pertinent Anatomy

After patient selection, the next most important area to success with the TRAM flap is abdominal wall anatomy. The subtle relationships of the normal, unaltered anatomy are important to appreciate, so that an intact, competent abdomen will result along with a viable, well-sculpted breast.

SKIN AND SUBCUTANEOUS FAT

The skin of the abdomen compares well to the breast in thickness and color, although it is sometimes paler. There is often a characteristic infraumbilical fat deposit in the female that is ideally suited for reconstruction of the breast. It extends from just above the umbilicus to the suprapubic crease (Fig. 70–1). The fat of the abdomen is divided into two layers of Scarpa fascia, and this strong fascia may be used to secure the superior extent of the new breast to the upper limits of the mastectomy defect.

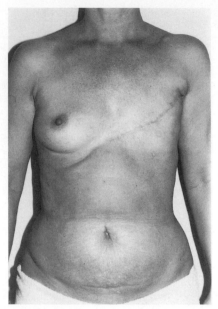

FIG. 70–1. This 53-year-old woman underwent a left modified radical mastectomy for infiltrating ductal carcinoma on January 26, 1983.

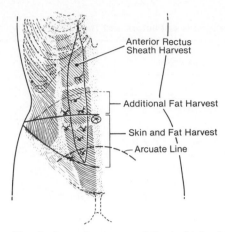

FIG. 70–2. Plan for lower transverse abdominal island flap uses a contralateral vascular pedicle. Note concentration of vascular perforators in periumbilical region and their inclusion in the limited rectus muscle-anterior sheath harvest.

MUSCLE AND FASCIA

The strength of the anterior abdominal wall is mainly provided by five paired muscles and an array of fascial structures. The muscles include the rectus abdominis, external oblique, internal oblique, transversus abdominis, and pyramidalis. These muscles are all attached, directly or indirectly, to three important vertical ligaments: the central linea alba and the linea semilunaris on either side. When the TRAM flap is isolated from surrounding tissues, these ligaments should be preserved in their entirety along with all fascial elements, except for a segment of anterior rectus sheath.

There is no posterior sheath below the arcuate line, which is found about halfway between the umbilicus and the pubis, and therefore most of the rectus muscle and anterior rectus sheath should be left undisturbed in this area to optimize repair of the abdominal wall. This should not be difficult to achieve because the predominant vascular perforators that supply the TRAM flap are found in the periumbilical area (Fig. 70–2). Although the posterior rectus sheath is fairly strong above the arcuate line, it may be attenuated in places, and a sturdy repair of the anterior sheath must always be performed.

The rectus muscle arises from the pubic crest and inserts onto the costal cartilages of the 5th, 6th, and 7th ribs. The muscle is divided into four or five sections by horizontal, tendinous inscriptions. These inscriptions are usually found below the xiphoid process, at the level of the umbilicus, and midway between these two areas. They occasionally occur below the umbilicus. The rectus muscle is firmly adherent to the anterior rectus sheath at the level of these inscriptions, but usually not to the posterior sheath.

NERVES

Intercostal nerves VIII through XII provide sensory supply to the skin of the abdominal wall and motor supply to the anterior abdominal wall musculature. The sensory nerves may be used with microsurgery to provide innervation with the free TRAM flap. The main nerves course between the internal oblique and transversus muscles and enter the posterior aspect of the rectus muscle at the junction of the lateral third and medial two-thirds. Some minor nerve filaments can enter more laterally and supply that aspect of the muscle that is left behind in the operative routine. The iliohypogastric and ilioinguinal sensory nerves run immediately superior and parallel to the inguinal ligament and should be avoided during the abdominal wall dissection and closure.

BLOOD SUPPLY TO ANTERIOR ABDOMINAL WALL

The blood supply to the anterior abdominal wall is provided by the deep superior and inferior epigastric vessels, the superficial inferior epigastric vessels, the superficial circumflex iliac vessels, the VIIIth through the XIIth intercostal vessels, the superficial external pudendal vessels (6–18). The first four are the most pertinent in regard to the TRAM flap procedure.

Deep Superior Epigastric Vessels

The internal thoracic (mammary) vessels run about 1.25 cm from the midline and terminate by dividing into the musculophrenic and deep superior epigastric vessels at the level of the 6th intercostal space. The latter enters the posterior rectus sheath about 1.25 cm from the midline and descends obliquely along the posterior aspect of the costal margin for 1 to 2 cm before turning inferiorly. As they leave the costal margin, these vessels have branches that anastomose with the 8th intercostal (costomarginal) vessels. The deep superior epigastric vessels course on the deep surface of the rectus muscle for a variable distance, but always enter the muscle above the first inscription. They usually enter the central portion of the muscle, but in 12% of cases can originate from the costomarginal artery and enter the muscle laterally (17,18,19). Awareness of these anatomic variations is important when dissecting the muscle pedicle. The pulse of the deep superior epigastric artery is easily palpable above the first inscription, but is often difficult to feel inferior to this point because of progressive branching to reduced-caliber choke vessels and anastomoses with the deep inferior epigastric artery.

Deep Inferior Epigastric Vessels

The deep inferior epigastric vessels arise from the external iliac artery immediately superior to the inguinal ligament, and are usually larger than the superior counterparts. The artery is usually accompanied by two veins. These vessels approach the undersurface of the rectus muscle at the linea semilunaris, 3 to 4 cm below the arcuate line, and ascend posterior to the muscle for a variable distance. At about the level of the arcuate line, the deep inferior epigastric vessels will continue as single vessels (29%) or divide into two (57%) or three (14%) main trunks (20). It is interesting to note that the branching of the deep superior epigastric vessels tends to match that of its inferior counterpart, but left and right sides are often asymmetrical.

Superficial Inferior Epigastric Vessels

The superficial inferior epigastric vessels originate from the femoral vessels just below the inguinal ligament and enter the fat of the anterior abdominal wall at a point about halfway between the pubic tubercle and the anterior superior iliac spine. They course superficial to the Scarpa fascia, and higher up on the abdomen the branches assume a more superficial and medial position. A vein of generous size can usually be found, but in 50% of cases the artery will be nonexistent or too small for microsurgical hookup (personal survey). The superficial inferior epigastric vessels play a significant role in the overall blood supply and venous drainage of the lower abdominal wall because they communicate freely across the midline and also intercommunicate with the deep inferior epigastric vessels.

Superficial Circumflex Iliac Vessels

The superficial circumflex iliac vessels also originate from the femoral vessels just below the inguinal ligament and generally run in the same plane as the superficial inferior epigastric vessels, but lateral to them. The branches of these vessels gradually assume a more superficial and lateral position in the lower abdomen. These vessels are usually large enough for microvascular transfer, and may be considered for microsurgically augmenting a TRAM flap if the lateral tissue is needed.

Lateral Intercostal Vessels

The lateral intercostal vessels are of varying size and number and enter the lateral aspect of the posterior rectus sheath, accompanied by the intercostal nerves. These vessels communicate with the deep epigastric vascular system, but are necessarily divided during isolation of the deep epigastric vascular pedicle.

Perforating Vessels and Vascular Plexi

The perforating vessels that supply the skin and fat of the anterior abdominal wall vary greatly in number, size, and distribution. The superficial superior epigastric vessels originate as perforators from the deep superior epigastric vessels at the most cephalic tendinous inscription. Except for these vessels, most perforators are found anywhere from 1 cm above the umbilicus to the level of the arcuate line (9 cm below) the umbilicus. There is an irregular row of medial and lateral perforators, but the most salient perforator occurs just above and lateral to the umbilicus. Smaller lateral perforators that are found in the lateral 1 to 2 cm of the anterior rectus sheath may be sacrificed, along with the smaller medial ones that occur within 1 cm of the midline, so that as much of the anterior rectus sheath may be preserved as possible. Being able to preserve the important periumbilical perforators with the flap while keeping enough anterior rectus sheath in place to achieve a sturdy closure, is crucial to the success of the TRAM flap operation.

Some of the musculocutaneous perforating vessels extend directly from the deep epigastric system to the subdermal region to form the rich vascular subdermal plexus. Other perforators mainly supply deeper tissues, with some terminal branches that extend to the subdermal plexus and other branches to ramify on the areolar tissue, which is immediately superficial to the external abdominal oblique and anterior rectus sheath fascia (21,22). The TRAM flap needs to be cleanly elevated off the anterior abdominal wall fascia in order to save this prefascial vascular plexus. Both subdermal and prefascial vascular plexi communicate with the superficial epigastric system across the midline (23) and into the lateral reaches of the abdomen.

HEMODYNAMICS

The inferior abdominal tissue is primarily supplied by the deep inferior epigastric vessels (24) and their perforators, but we now know from clinical experience that these vascular areas may be captured by the deep superior epigastric vessels. This phenomenon may be explained in several ways.

There is a direct communication between the deep superior and inferior epigastric systems in every case. Milloy and colleagues (17) demonstrated in cadavers that, in 40% of cases, these anastomoses were large enough to visibly identify. Arteriograms will demonstrate anastomoses between these two systems, even in those that communicate through smaller choke vessels, if the inferior epigastric vessels are first ligated. If these vessels are not initially ligated, the pressure gradients do not allow the communications to be demonstrated. Clinically, it appears that the shift in direction of flow is instantaneous with division of the inferior epigastric system, and that a preliminary "delay" by ligating the inferior epigastric vessels is unnecessary.

Taylor (24) has defined the primary vascular territory of a source artery as an angiosome, and the corresponding venous territory as a venosome. If the primary blood supply to an angiosome is interrupted, it can be secondarily supplied by a source vessel to an adjacent territory. One source vessel can safely perfuse one or two adjacent angiosomes through anastomotic choke vessels (if cutaneous hydrostatic pressure is maintained during surgery and vasospasm is prevented), but attempts to capture any more are unreliable.

The skin around and below the umbilicus is an angiosome and venosome primarily supplied by the deep inferior epigastric system, but when these vessels are ligated, this tissue can be secondarily supplied by the deep superior epigastric system. This system can also supply the next more lateral angiosome, but cannot reliably capture the most lateral territories of the TRAM flap.

Therefore, when a rotational TRAM flap is raised (based on the deep superior epigastric vessels), it depends on complete filling of the deep inferior epigastric artery via choke anastomotic vessels with secondary and tertiary filling of the various skin territories. Even more important, the emptying of the deep inferior epigastric vein into its superior counterpart requires retrograde flow of blood against the venous valves. It appears that this temporary obstruction is overcome when the blood dilates the veins and makes the valves incompetent. However, retrograde flow may not be optimal and this phenomenon may explain why engorgement of the deep inferior epigastric vein and flap occurs more often than desired. The engorgement may be relieved by elevating the flap or temporarily releasing the clamp on the deep inferior epigastric vein.

Perioperative Management

The operative plan is drawn on the patient the day or evening before surgery. The patient maintains a liquid diet for 24 hours before surgery and is given magnesium citrate on the night before surgery and a Fleets enema on the morning of surgery in order to minimize gastrointestinal distention. This mechanical bowel prep is an aid to abdominal wall repair and reduces postoperative ileus.

Intravascular volume is maximized by preoperative intravenous hydration and by replacing blood loss as it occurs intraoperatively with autologous blood. The patient scheduled for a single TRAM flap has two units of blood banked, whereas those patients scheduled for a bipedicled TRAM flap or bilateral reconstruction have three to four units banked.

The patient receives nifedipine 30 mg (long acting) at midnight before surgery. Methylprednisolone (Solu-Medrol) 250 mg is administered at 6 AM on the morning of surgery and once intraoperatively for a total dose of 500 mg. A second dose of nifedipine 30 mg (long acting) is given on the first postoperative evening. Intravenous cefazolin 1 g is given on induction of anesthesia and every 6 hours after that time, and is changed to oral cephalothin postoperatively when the patient is tolerating an oral diet.

The anesthetic routine should maintain normal body temperature and maximize skin blood flow. To accomplish this, the room temperature should be elevated before the patient enters the room. Heated blankets and/or table pads should also be utilized in this effort. Nitrous oxide is not used in order to minimize bowel distention, but paralyzing agents are utilized to minimize the reactivity of the rectus muscle to electrocautery dissection. Patients with an increased risk of deep venous thrombosis are placed on an intravenous heparin protocol or pneumatic compression devices are used.

FLAP AND PEDICLE DESIGN

Before designing the TRAM flap skin island, the surgeon must decide upon the volume and shape of the desired new breast. The weight of the TRAM flap may be estimated, as previously discussed, and if the weight of the mastectomy specimen is known, then it can be determined how much of the lower abdominal tissue will be needed and whether it can be transferred on one or two pedicles.

In single-pedicle reconstructions, it is preferable to use the contralateral rectus muscle pedicle (Fig. 70–3), but the ipsilateral pedicle can also be reliably used if abdominal scars

PEDICLE OPTIONS
Shaded areas of flap possibly unsafe.

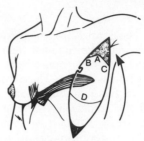
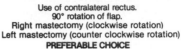
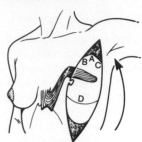

Use of contralateral rectus.
90° rotation of flap.
Right mastectomy (clockwise rotation)
Left mastectomy (counter clockwise rotation)
PREFERABLE CHOICE

Use of ipsilateral rectus.
45°-90° rotation of flap.
GOOD CHOICE

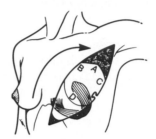
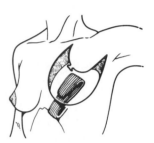

Use of ipsilateral rectus.
135°-145° rotation of flap.
POOR CHOICE

Use of ipsilateral rectus.
0° rotation of flap.
(double fold in pedicle)
UNSAFE CHOICE

FIG. 70–3. Vascular pedicle options for a left modified radical reconstruction. Abdominal scars and other circumstances influence the choice.

(e.g., Kocher incision) present a problem. Whichever pedicle is used, the inferior aspect of the flap should always be swung toward the mastectomy defect, so that it rotates about 90% and the umbilicus points toward the midline. The same type of rotation is used for the double pedicle flap. Other methods and degrees of rotation are available but they have a higher risk of vascular pedicle folding, which causes obstruction to venous return.

If all of the lower abdominal tissue is needed for the reconstruction and one of the superior vascular pedicles had been violated by a previous incision, then a microvascular augmentation of the flap blood supply must be anticipated. The internal mammary vessels can also be used in select cases.

The proposed operative plan is marked with the patient in the standing position (Fig. 70–4). The highest central point of the mastectomy defect is point A and the highest medial and lateral points are points B and C, respectively. The central position of the inframammary line is point D. The superior and inferior extent of the proposed chest skin incision is marked as line EF. Corresponding A' and D' points are marked on the normal breast.

Whether the proposed chest skin incision for insertion of abdominal flap skin completely follows the mastectomy scar or not depends on the judgment of the surgeon. If there is a low, transverse mastectomy scar, the skin between the scar and a point about 1 to 2 cm above the inframammary fold may be elliptically excised with the scar. This can produce a

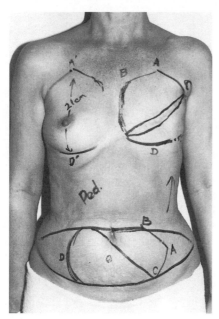

FIG. 70–4. The same patient as shown in Figure 70–1. Plan for procedure is drawn on the skin with a marker that will survive operative prep. Note the limits of the mastectomy **(B, A, C, D)** transferred to the abdominal flap. On the existing breast line, **A'D'** is the approximate flap length necessary to reproduce size and projection of that breast.

natural breast ptosis with the lower breast scar hidden in or near the inframammary fold. With a higher transverse mastectomy scar, the medial extent of the scar may sometimes be ignored and the medial aspect of the chest incision extended down to the inframammary fold. This redesign of the mastectomy scar can accomplish several things: (a) the medial mastectomy scar is not changed, which leaves natural skin color and texture in the "cleavage" area; (b) the horizontal tension across the lower breast skin is released, providing a more natural curve and ptosis to the lower breast; and (c) this orientation allows a longer skin island to be inserted with the TRAM flap without rotating the flap more than 90%.

The standard lower abdominal flap is outlined on the patient (from just above the umbilicus to the pubic crease) and then points A, B, and C are transposed to the flap in the "safe region" on the side of the mastectomy. If reproduction of the opposite breast is desired, the distance over the nipple between points A' and D' on the normal side is measured and then the same distance is marked out from point A to a new point D on the flap. The healthy tissue lateral to point D will be rolled into the lower outer quadrant of the new breast and behind the rest of the flap to increase bulk and projection of the new breast. The skin island to be added to the new breast is then drawn on the flap to make sure that there is sufficient length available with the proposed rotation.

Operative Procedures

A brief review of the single pedicle TRAM flap operation for reconstruction of a modified radical mastectomy defect can be divided into the following steps: (a) chest wall exposure, (b) TRAM flap elevation and vascular pedicle isolation, (c) abdominal wall repair, and (d) shaping of the new breast. The double-pedicle TRAM flap procedure follows the same steps,

but has a number of additional requirements that will be mentioned. For more detailed study of the operative technique, we recommend two videos available through the Plastic Surgery Educational Foundation of the American Society of Plastic and Reconstructive Surgeons (25,26) and the book *Breast Reconstruction with Living Tissue* (27).

CHEST WALL EXPOSURE

The breast envelope is developed by incising the skin along the predetermined skin markings and elevating the chest skin flaps to the limits of the mastectomy defect. Axillary scars are released, to relieve axillary tightness. The inferior skin flap is raised to just above the new inframammary line, but not below point D, because the final level of the inframammary crease will be determined after the abdomen is closed. The goal is to recreate the premastectomy breast envelope, because this, with exact tissue volume and skin replacement, will ultimately determine the shape and size of the new breast.

The subcutaneous tunnel for passage of the TRAM flap is made over the lower sternum, in the midline, and into the epigastric region to establish continuity with the abdominal dissection. It is important to locate the tunnel in the midline because it preserves the natural inframammary adhesion on the mastectomy side. This natural crease serves as a shelf on which the breast flap will rest and can be considered one of the keystones of the breast shaping process.

TRAM FLAP ELEVATION AND VASCULAR PEDICLE ISOLATION

The contralateral vascular pedicle is preferred because it ultimately rests in the tunnel and across the epigastrium in a less compromised position. However, the ipsilateral pedicle can also be safely used when abdominal scarring or other conditions preclude the use of the contralateral pedicle. The transverse abdominal flap (either upper or lower) is always designed to include the periumbilical vascular perforators. The upper skin incision can be made at the upper level of the umbilicus, but additional abdominal fat should be taken with the flap to a level at least 2 cm above the skin incision to protect the large perforators that occur just above the umbilicus. The lower limit of the skin incision is usually in the suprapubic crease. These incisions generally provide a flap 14 to 15 cm in width, which is necessary for adequate breast width replacement. The lateral limit of the flap usually extends beyond the anterior superior iliac spine and can be adjusted up or down to fit the preferred bathing suit of the patient. The length of the flap from the midline (umbilicus) to its most lateral point usually measures 20 cm.

In designing the lower transverse abdominal island flap, it is desirable to keep the abdominal scar as low as possible. However, the first goal of the surgeon is to make a breast that will survive in its entirety and stay soft. Therefore, in some instances the abdominal scar may have to be a bit higher on the abdomen or extend farther in the flanks than the typical abdominoplasty scar, and the patient should be so informed before surgery. The lower limb of the abdominal incision is first incised in a manner that will bevel the abdominal fat away from the flap skin island. The upper limit of the flap is incised from flank to flank and the incision is beveled through the fat at a 45° angle superiorly for 2 to 3 cm. The

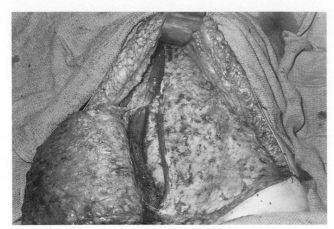

FIG. 70–5. The nonpedicle side of the abdominal flap is elevated across the midline and the right anterior rectus sheath is incised approximately 1 cm from the midline. The rectus muscle is separated from the sheath medially to the arcuate line.

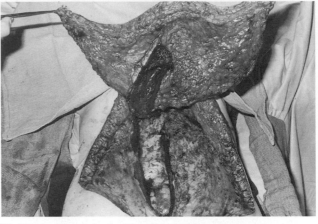

FIG. 70–7. The abdominal flap is isolated on the superior deep epigastric vascular pedicle with a narrow superior segment of rectus muscle.

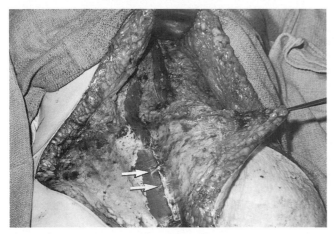

FIG. 70–6. The pedicle side of the flap is elevated to a point approximately 2 cm past the lateral rectus border and the rectus sheath is incised. Note careful preservation of the medial row of large vascular perforators (arrows).

dissection is continued just above the thick abdominal wall fascia onto the lower sternum and costal martins, to connect with the tunnel from the breast pocket.

The exact course of the deep superior epigastric artery is located with a sterile Doppler ultrasound probe and marked with methylene blue. The anterior rectus sheath is opened by two parallel incisions beginning from a common point on top of the sternum at the origin of the rectus muscle and continuing to the upper border of the abdominal flap. The medial rectus sheath incision is placed about 1 cm from the medial rectus border and the lateral incision about 3 cm from the medial incision. This, in effect, isolates a strip of anterior rectus sheath (2 to 3 cm) on the underlying muscle.

The umbilicus is incised circumferentially and kept attached to the linea alba by its stalk with a cuff of surrounding fat to maintain its blood supply. The anterior rectus sheath should be readily visible on the rectus muscle pedicle. This will assure that there is no rotation or torsion of the pedicle. The abdominal flap is first elevated on the side op-

posite the pedicle, extending across the midline to a point approximately 1 cm past the medial rectus border. This dissection is carried out on the surface of the external oblique fascia, thereby taking with the flap the vascular areolar tissue lying just above the fascia (Figs. 70–5, 70–6). The location of the important vascular perforators should be noted as they are encountered on the nonpedicle side so that they can be easily identified and preserved on the pedicle side. The rectus sheath is opened 1 cm lateral to the midline or medial to any significant perforators in that region, and then this incision is connected to the superior, medial rectus sheath incision and extended inferiorly to a point near the arcuate line (halfway between the umbilicus and the pubis). This level is usually not more than 10 cm below the umbilicus.

The flap is elevated on the pedicle side to the lateral row of large vascular perforators that usually occur 2 cm medial to the lateral rectus border (Fig. 70–7). Small vascular perforators that are encountered just at the rectus border or slightly medial to it should be sacrificed. The critical vascular perforators can be visualized by placing gentle traction on the flap and countertraction on the external oblique fascia. Good light and a dry field is important in this phase of the operation. The rectus sheath is opened just lateral to these perforators and the incision is connected with the incision previously made above the flap and with the inferior extent of the medial anterior rectus sheath incision at about the level of the arcuate line. We prefer to leave a strip of rectus muscle medially and laterally in all cases. This maneuver is safe if the surgeon is always aware of the location of the lateral excursion of the superior deep epigastric artery and vein. It is also important to carry out the muscle dissection in a manner that will preserve all vessels running parallel to the fibers of the rectus muscle and to identify the vessels on the posterior sheath before they are divided. If the surgeon is not comfortable with this muscle-sparing maneuver, then the entire width of the muscle can be taken with the vascular pedicle, but the majority of muscle with its overlying sheath should be left undisturbed below the arcuate line. This lower muscle can be preserved by leaving its medial and lateral attachment to the sheath at the transverse tendinous inscription at the level of the umbilicus and by taking a V-shaped segment of muscle to the arcuate line.

The muscle dissection begins laterally by incising the epimysium just lateral to the large perforators and separating the muscle fibers to expose the posterior sheath. The lateral intercostal vessels and nerves are divided between vascular clips or with electrocautery as they are encountered. The deep inferior epigastric artery and vein enter the posterior sheath near the arcuate line, and they are preserved as long as possible (for microvascular hookup if necessary). They are controlled with large vascular clips and divided. Muscle fibers are then separated, a few bundles at a time, up the rectus muscle to expose the posterior sheath and the lateral vessels up to the costal margin. Vessels are not divided until they are identified. The 8th intercostal (costomarginal) vessels are divided as far laterally as possible to avoid kinking or damaging the major vascular pedicle, which courses along the rib margin high in the epigastrium and then enters the substance of the rectus muscle (usually the middle third). It is important to divide the VIIIth intercostal nerve to effect atrophy of the muscle portion of the pedicle in the epigastrium and thereby prevent an unnatural bulge in this region. The muscle fibers above the rib margin are divided laterally to reduce the vascular pedicle to a 2 to 3 cm medial segment of muscle.

When a double-pedicle TRAM flap is elevated, the medial and lateral perforators on both sides are left intact, making it more difficult to incise the medial aspects of the anterior rectus sheaths. This may be accomplished in one of two ways. The rectus muscle may be approached from the lateral anterior rectus sheath opening and elevated off the posterior rectus sheath, and then the medial anterior rectus sheath can be incised from the posterior aspect. Another method entails dissecting the flap off the midline area from an inferior and superior approach, and then incising the medial anterior sheath from the anterior aspect. In the bilateral reconstruction, the flap is divided in the midline and the approach is then the same as with a single pedicle flap.

For the single-flap, double-pedicle breast reconstruction, the ipsilateral vascular pedicle needs to be dissected superiorly a little more than the contralateral pedicle, so that it can reach further up on the chest wall. This maneuver also allows the contralateral pedicle to be positioned more inferiorly in the subcutaneous tunnel than the ipsilateral pedicle, so that they do not cross each other.

Once the musculovascular pedicle with its segment of anterior rectus sheath is freed from the posterior rectus sheath, the entire flap is suspended with a towel clamp and weighed with a calibrated, spring-action weighing device. The least vascularized, lateral portions of the flap may then be excised until the known weight of the mastectomy specimen is approximated. Further tailoring will be done with the flap in the breast pocket. The flap is then passed through the tunnel into the breast pocket, where it is temporarily stapled in place (Fig. 70–8). Great care should be taken to ensure that the rotated rectus muscle pedicle remains flat in the subcutaneous tunnel and does not become folded under the flap. The anterior rectus sheath should be readily visible on the rectus muscle pedicle. This will assure that there is not rotation or torsion of the pedicle.

The flap should be inspected frequently, and if any evidence of venous congestion is present the vascular clips can

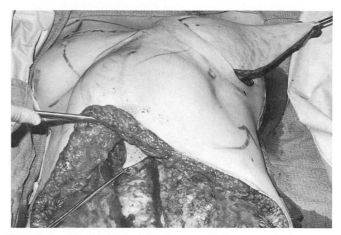

FIG. 70–8. The abdominal flap is rotated 90° counterclockwise and passed into the breast pocket. By using this direction of rotation in this patient the least vascular portion of the flap is placed high, where much of this marginal tissue can be discarded.

be removed from the deep inferior epigastric vessels to decompress the vascular system. The ipsilateral TRAM flap is most difficult to use because the muscle pedicle becomes folded under the flap as it rests in the breast pocket. With this ipsilateral pedicle, the muscle must be swept medially from under the flaps to prevent venous obstruction.

ABDOMINAL WALL REPAIR

When the musculovascular pedicle has been harvested in the manner described, the repair of the abdominal-wall defect can be direct and straightforward, assuring future abdominal wall integrity (28). If the critical supporting structures of the anterior abdominal wall are destroyed during the harvest of the vascular pedicle, then postoperative abdominal wall weakness can be expected or a frank hernia may develop (Figs. 70–9, 70–10).

The anterior rectus sheath is "set up" by first approximating the sheath with skin staples. Occasional 2-0 vicryl sutures are placed in regions where there is tension. A three-layered closure is accomplished with a running double-stranded 0 nylon suture. Healthy bites of anterior rectus sheath and linea semilunaris are taken, and the rectus muscle remnants are incorporated with these sutures. (Fig. 70–11).

The tendon of the internal oblique muscle may not be fused with the external oblique tendon to form the anterior rectus sheath and may retract laterally beneath the fascia of the external oblique muscle. It is imperative to include both of these layers when repairing the anterior rectus sheath. A second continuous suture repair of the anterior rectus sheath is oversewn in the same direction, further tightening and reinforcing the closure. The cephalad closure of the sheath should begin as close to the costal margin as possible without constricting the vascular pedicle (often a 2 to 3 cm space remains). The caudal aspect of the repair should extend down to the pubis in order to minimize any suprapubic bulge.

In our series of 700 patients, a primary repair in the above manner has been possible in 99.2% of single-pedicle reconstructions. Synthetic mesh material has been used in 45.8% of double-pedicle reconstructions and 35.2% of bilateral breast reconstructions. In repairing the abdominal wall after

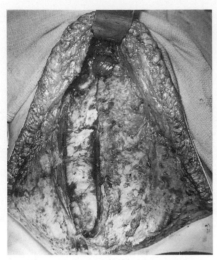

FIG. 70–9.   The abdominal wound as it appears after passage of the flap to the chest. Note the preservation of a full-length lateral strip of rectus muscle with overlying sheath.

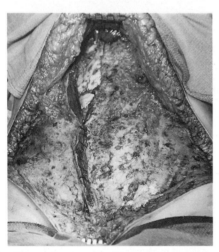

FIG. 70–10.   The rectus muscle with deep layers of medial and lateral sheath has been repaired from the umbilical region to below the arcuate line.

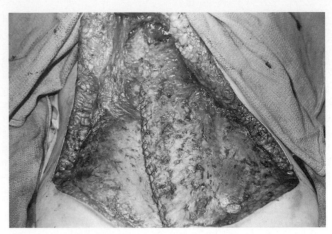

FIG. 70–11.   The anterior rectus sheath has been repaired with a double row of continuous (no. 1) nylon suture.

dermal 4-0 Vicryl suture. The umbilicus is reconstructed by exteriorization, as with an abdominoplasty.

SHAPING OF THE NEW BREAST

The surgeon must be strong and mentally alert for this final step in the operation, for herein lies the essence of the entire procedure. The hard work entailed in bringing a viable flap into the mammary pocket can lead to fatigue, which might cause the surgeon to hasten this essential part of the procedure. It is advisable for the surgeon to take a few minutes break before commencing this step. The experience and artistic ability of the surgeon will be directly reflected in the quality of the final product (29).

The superior portion of the flap should be tapered from the undersurface to give a natural slope to the upper aspect of the breast. While holding this in position, the inferior wing of the flap is gently rolled behind the main body of the flap, in order to maximize the projection of the new breast. The skin edges are then temporarily stapled to the skin of the flap, outlining what will become the skin island. This should approximate the skin ellipse of the mastectomy specimen. Once the contour of the skin island is determined, it is marked, and all skin outside of this area is deepithelialized.

The superior margins of the flap are tacked with several 4-0 Vicryl sutures to the upper limits of the mastectomy defect (Fig. 70–12). Two drains are placed in the breast pocket and brought out through the lateral breast area and contralateral inframammary fold. The flatness and positioning of the vascular pedicle are again checked, as is the gentle rolling under of the inferior wing of the flap. The TRAM flap should be shaped by the breast envelope, much like a normal breast fits into a brassiere.

Once the sculpting of the new breast is completed and the breast has appropriate shape and symmetry in the sitting position, the skin island is sutured to the surrounding skin. This is done with interrupted, deep dermal 4-0 Vicryl sutures, followed by a continuous, superficial dermal 5-0 Vicryl suture. All incisions are covered with sterile paper tape, which remains in place for 2 to 3 weeks (Fig. 70–13).

Nipple reconstruction is best delayed for at least 6 weeks to allow the new breast to become well vascularized. The

bilateral muscle harvest, it is important to perform a simultaneous bilateral repair and then, if the repair is deemed inadequate, sew a Prolene mesh over the primary repair. Synthetic mesh should only be used to reinforce the abdominal wall closure when the surgeon believes it to be inadequate; mesh should not be used as a primary means of closure of the abdominal wall defect (only as an overlay reinforcement, after the best possible muscle-fascia closure has been accomplished). Most women in the mastectomy age range have considerable laxity of the anterior abdominal wall structures and, for that reason, in a single-pedicle reconstruction after the pedicle side has been closed the opposite side of the abdomen is tightened by plicating the anterior rectus sheath with a double layer of 0 nylon.

The abdominal wall area is drained with four Axiom drains; two are brought out through the lateral aspects of the incision and the other two are brought out through separate suprapubic stab incisions. The skin is closed with deep dermal interrupted 3-0 Vicryl sutures and a running, superficial

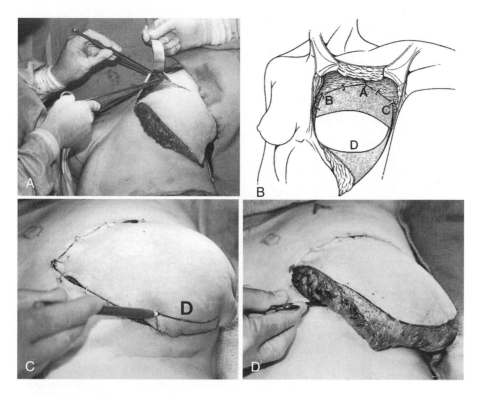

FIG. 70–12. Shaping the new breast. **A, B,** The poorly vascularized portion of the abdominal flap is discarded and the new breast tissue is sutured to the upper limits of the mastectomy defect (points **B, A, C**). **C, D,** The inframammary line of the flap (point **D**) is adjusted to give desired ptosis and projection. Final line at point **D** is incised and the deepithelialized distal flap tissue is rolled in the lower outer quadrant of the new breast.

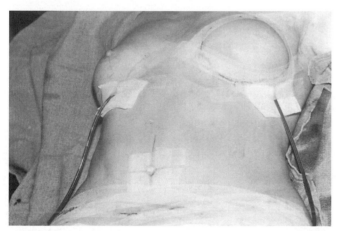

FIG. 70–13. Final skin repair is supported with sterile 1-inch paper adhesive. Without bulky dressings, the new breast is easily monitored for temperature and color changes.

areola color is tattooed into the skin after the nipple reconstruction is well healed (Fig. 70–14).

Postoperative Care

Close clinical monitoring of the flap is essential, and evidence of a hematoma or a persistently cold and mottled flap are indications for immediate reexploration. A warm towel is kept over the breast flap, but no heating elements are used because of a risk of a burn in the insensate new breast. If the flap and patient are doing well, the humidified oxygen and Foley catheter are discontinued on the first postoperative day and ambulation is begun. The diet is advanced slowly and the patient is usually discharged between the 5th and 7th postoperative days.

AESTHETIC MANAGEMENT OF THE CONTRALATERAL BREAST

Breasts are paired organs, and the fundamental goal of reconstruction is to achieve pleasing symmetry with the remaining breast. Aesthetic results in TRAM flap surgery are judged by the final production of breasts that are similar in size, shape, contour, and softness. When the total reconstructive plan includes opposite breast reduction, performing the reduction prior to the reconstruction allows pathologic examination of the reduced breast before committing the entire TRAM flap to a unilateral reconstruction. We choose to perform the reduction either well in advance of the TRAM reconstruction (often on an outpatient basis) or 2 days before the reconstruction, to allow for careful microscopic examination of the specimen. If cancer is found, then a second mastectomy may be performed followed by bilateral reconstruction.

The McKissock pattern for breast reduction with a conservative skin excision produces a more rounded and slightly more ptotic breast than the more usual cone-shaped reduction, and more closely matches an autogenous tissue reconstruction. Although it may seem more difficult to shape the reconstructed breast to match a reduced natural breast, it is often helpful to have an ideal opposite breast as a model.

If the natural breast requires elevation and reshaping (mastopexy), one should consider the same timing considerations applied to breast reduction. The surgical exposure of a large amount of breast tissue is an excellent opportunity to obtain multiple random tissue specimens for pathologic examination. Findings are atypia or malignancy again will indicate the need for an opposite breast mastectomy followed by a bilateral reconstruction.

In some instances, the reconstructed breast has a fuller, more rounded shape than the opposite breast. A subpectoral or submammary implant placed in the remaining breast will

FIG. 70–14.   The patient in Figure 70–1 is shown 10 months after breast reconstruction. The nipple-areola reconstruction was performed 3 months after breast reconstruction.

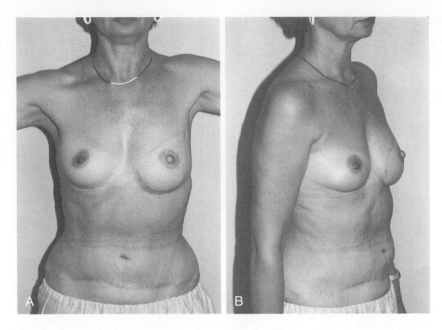

usually achieve a natural symmetry. Of course, any patient contemplating an implant should be adequately informed of the current concerns regarding breast implants and breast cancer detection.

Complications

In our initial series of 500 patients, the cumulative complication rate was approximately 16%. When complications occurred, they were often multiple in a single patient, such as a hematoma leading to infection with resulting fat necrosis or partial flap loss. The complications we experienced included total or partial flap loss, fat necrosis, inadequate abdominal wound healing, pulmonary embolus, deep vein thrombosis, wound infection, and hematoma (Table 70–3).

The two most frequent causes of total or partial flap loss in this series were poor patient selection and the use of the flap beyond its reliable limits. Additional causes included technical error, excessive tension on the vascular pedicle, and venous obstruction arising from hematoma under the pedicle. Our perioperative routine has evolved toward minimizing vasospasm and avoiding technical damage to the vascular system, but as technical advances are made, we become more aware of the critical nature of appropriate candidate selection as the major key to the avoidance of complications.

Areas of fat necrosis occurred more commonly in the first few years of this series and it became clear that the high incidence seen in the early developmental stages of this operation was related to the overdependence on a single pedicle to nourish the abdominal tissue beyond the midline. We now believe that a single pedicle will reliably nourish only 60 to 70% of the total lower abdominal flap in a healthy patient. Cases in which additional tissue volume is needed are managed with a double-pedicle TRAM flap.

Abdominal hernia and abdominal wall weakness are the least likely complications to occur when the operation is properly performed. Conservative rectus muscle harvest and a secure multilayered closure of the anterior rectus sheath are the keys to prevention. Two of the six hernias in this series

Table 70–3.
Complications in 500 Patients

	No. of Patients	%
Deaths	0	0
Flap loss		
100%	2	0.4
>50%	4	0.8
25–50%	7	1.4
<25%	21	4.2
Abdominal hernia	6	1.2
Abdominal laxity	2	0.4
Small rent: upper anterior sheath	2	0.4
Pulmonary embolus	4	0.8
IInfection		
Breast	3	0.6
Abdomen	6	1.2
Hematoma		
Breast	11	2.2
Abdomen	8	1.6
Skin loss (nonflap, requiring graft)	2	0.4
Total	78	15.6

occurred in the first 100 patients. The other four occurred much later during a brief period involving 30 patients when the abdominal closure routine was changed from two layers of nylon suture to one layer of polyglycolic suture followed by one layer of nylon and the application of stainless steel fascial staples. Once the hernia rate was recognized, the traditional two-layer direct closure was reestablished and no hernias have subsequently occurred.

Necrosis of an area of abdominal wall skin between the umbilicus and the transverse abdominal scar occurred in 10 patients, all but one of whom were smokers or ex-smokers. We have minimized this complication by requiring patients to cease smoking for a minimum of 3 months prior to surgery (30), by limited thinning of the upper abdominal skin flap, and by avoiding defatting of the new periumbilical tissue to wound closure in all ex-smokers (31).

Three patients developed deep vein thrombosis and four had pulmonary emboli. Common factors in these cases were excessive operating time, obesity, and past history of deep vein thrombosis. For patients with such a vascular history, or who are between 15 and 20% over their ideal body weight, we have developed a regimen of continuous low-dose heparin (partial thromboplastin time is maintained between 30 and 40 sec) from the night before surgery to just prior to discharge. This dose should not anticoagulate the patient but should maintain normal coagulation factors.

This operation requires extensive tissue exposure of the chest and abdomen. Without meticulous hemostasis, blood collections will occur that will jeopardize the success of the operation. Two constant suction drains are used in the breast (three for bilateral reconstruction) and four in the abdomen. However, even liberal use of drains will not prevent hematoma occurrence if bleeding is not controlled during surgery.

Early in the series, 26% of patients developed persistent abdominal seromas requiring aspiration or drainage. In the last 300 patients, abdominal seroma formation has occurred infrequently, and we attribute this marked decrease to careful hemostasis and external drainage with four small nonirritative silicone tubes. As of September 1995, our series included 729 patients. It is our impression that all of the complications have been reduced. There have been no deaths.

Conclusion

The transverse abdominal island flap operation is a valuable addition to the plastic surgeon's armamentarium for breast and chest wall reconstruction. However, the apparent simplicity of this operation is deceptive and the prudent surgeon will undertake its performance only after adequate study and will then gain experience in a cautious, self-critical manner.

References

1. Hartrampf CR, Scheflan M, Black PW. Breast reconstruction with a transverse abdominal island flap. *Plast Reconstr Surg* 1982; 69:216.
2. Watterson PA, Bostwick J III, Hester TR Jr, et al. TRAM flap anatomy correlated with a 10-year clinical experience with 556 Patients. *PRS* 1995; 95:1185–1995.
3. Jacobsen WM, Meland NB, Woods JE. Autologous breast reconstruction with use of transverse rectus abdominis musculocutaneous flap. Mayo Clinic experience with 147 cases. *Mayo Cln Proc* 1994; 69:635–640.
4. Brown RG, Vasconez LO, Jurkiewicz MJ. Transverse abdominal flaps and the deep epigastric arcade. *Plast Reconstr Surg* 1975; 55:416.
5. Feldman S, Michelow BJ, Hartrampf CR. Method to preoperatively predict the weight of a TRAM flap. *Perspect Plast Surg* 1989; 3(2):91.
6. Fisher J, Bostwick J III, Powell RW. Latissimus dorsi blood supply after thoracodorsal vessel division, the serratus collateral. *Plast Reconstr Surg* 1983; 72:502.
7. Woodburne RT. *Essentials of human anatomy.* 3rd ed. New York: Oxford University Press, 1965; 54.
8. Berrino P, Santi P. Hemodynamic analysis of the TRAM. Applications to the "recharged" TRAM flap. *Clinics in Plastic Surgery* 1994; 21(2):233
9. Georgiade GS, Voci VE, Riefkohl, et al. Potential problems with the transverse rectus abdominis myocutaneous flap in breast reconstruction and how to avoid them. *Br J Plast Surg* 1984; 37:121.
10. Bostwick J III. *Aesthetic and reconstructive breast surgery.* St. Louis: CV Mosby, 1983.
11. Hartrampf CR. *Transverse abdominal island flap technique for breast reconstruction after mastectomy.* Baltimore: University Park Press, 1983.
12. Hartrampf CR. Unilateral transverse abdominal island flap. In: McGibbon BM, ed. *Atlas of breast reconstruction following mastectomy.* Baltimore: University Park Press, 1984.
13. Scheflan M, Dinner MI. The transverse abdominal island flap: Part I. Indications, contraindications, results, and complications. *Ann Plast Surg* 1983; 10:24.
14. Scheflan M, Dinner MI. The transverse abdominal island flap; Part II. Surgical technique. *Ann Plast Surg* 1983; 10:120.
15. McCraw JM, Dibbell DG. Experimental definition of dependent myocutaneous vascular territories. *Plast Reconstr Surg* 1977; 60:212.
16. McCraw JM, Dibbel DG, Carraway J. Clinical definition of independent myocutaneous vascular territories. *Plast Reconstr Surg* 1977; 60:341.
17. Milloy FJ, Anson BJ, McAfee DK. The rectus abdominis muscle and the epigastric arteries. *Surg Gynecol Obstet* 1960; 110:293.
18. Hendricks DL, Wilkens TH, Witt PD. Blood-flow contributions by the superior and inferior epigastric arterial systems in TRAM Flaps, based on laser Doppler flowmetry. *J Reconstr Microsurg* 1994; 10(4):249.
19. Arnold M. The surgical anatomy of the sternal blood supply. *J Thorac Cardiovasc Surg* 1972; 64:596.
20. Moon HK, Taylor GI. The vascular anatomy of the rectus abdominis musculocutaneous flaps based on the deep superior epigastric system. *Plast Reconstr Surg* 1988; 82:815.
21. Pontén B. The fasciocutaneous flap: its use in soft-tissue defects of the lower leg. *Br J Plast Surg* 1981; 34:215.
22. Tolhurst DE, Haeseker B, Zeeman RF. The development of the fasciocutaneous flap and its clinical applications. *Plast Reconstr Surg* 1983; 71:597.
23. Hill HL, Brown RG, Jurkiewicz MJ. The transverse lumbosacral back flap. *Plast Reconstr Surg* 1978; 62:177.
24. Boyd JB, Taylor GI, Corlett RJ. The vascular territories of the superior epigastric and deep inferior epigastric systems. *Plast Reconstr Surg* 1984; 73:1.
25. Hartrampf CR Jr. Breast reconstruction with the transverse abdominal island flap, PSEF Teleplast #8521. Plastic Surgery Educational Foundation, American Society of Plastic and Reconstructive Surgeons.
26. Hartrampf CR Jr, Beegle PH. Unilateral breast reconstruction with a bipedicle TRAM flap. PSEF Teleplast #8923. Plastic Surgery Educational Foundation, American Society of Plastic and Reconstructive Surgeons.
27. Hartrampf CR. *Breast reconstruction with living tissue.* New York: Raven, 1990.
28. Hartrampf CR. Abdominal wall competence and the transverse abdominal island flap operations. *Ann Plast Surg* 1984; 12:139.
29. Elliott LF, Hartrampf CR. Tailoring of the new breast using the transverse abdominal island flap. *Plast Reconstr Surg* 1983; 72:887.
30. Reus WF, Robson MC, Zachary L, et al. Acute effects of tobacco smoking on blood flow in the cutaneous microcirculation. *Br J Plast Surg* 1984; 37:213.
31. Kroll SS. Necrosis of abdominoplasty and other secondary flaps after TRAM flap breast reconstruction. *Plastic Reconstr Surg* 1994; 94:637.

Suggested Readings

Hallock GG. Transverse rectus abdominis musculocutaneous (TRAM) flap from TRAM flap for sequential bilateral breast reconstruction. *Ann Plast Surg* 1995; 34:406.
Marshall DR, Ross DA. A fleur de lys modification of the TRAM flap for breast reconstruction. *B J Plast Surg* 1994; 47:521.
Maxwell GP, Andochick SE. Secondary shaping of the TRAM flap. *Clin Plast Surg* 1994; 21:247.
Mizgala CL, Hartrampf CR, Bennett G. Abdominal function after pedicled TRAM flap surgery. *Clin Plast Surg* 1994; 21:255.
Spear SL, Travaglino-Parda RL, Stefan MM. The stacked transverse rectus abdominis musculocutaneous flap revisited in breast reconstruction. *Ann Plas Surg* 1994; 32:565.
Wilkins EG, August DA, Kuzon WM Jr, et al. Immediate transverse rectus abdominis musculocutaneous flap reconstruction after mastectomy. *J Am Coll Surg* 1995; 180:177.
Williams J Kerwin, Bostwick J III, Bried JT, et al. TRAM flap breast reconstruction after radiation treatment. *Ann of Surg* 1995; 221:756.

71

Microsurgical Breast Reconstruction

Bryan Oslin, M.D., and James C. Grotting, M.D., F.A.C.S.

Although the first postmastectomy breast reconstruction with free-tissue transfer was reported by Fujino (1) in 1976, only recently has the full appreciation of this technique has taken hold. Reconstruction of the breast following mastectomy with tissue expanders and implants offered satisfactory, often excellent, results. However, the difficulty in attaining symmetry with the opposite unoperated breast and the inherent risks of capsular contracture, expander infection or extrusion, and implant rupture prompted many plastic surgeons to consider autogenous tissue as a source for recreating a more natural breast mound. In addition, many patients requesting reconstruction of the breast had undergone radical mastectomy, with subsequent chest-wall irradiation, thus leaving potentially large chest-wall defects to reconstruct. Serafin and colleagues (2) in 1982 reported a series that included 26 patients on whom breast reconstruction was performed using free-tissue transfer. Their indications for free-flap reconstruction at that time included the inability to use the ipsilateral latissimus dorsi musculocutaneous island flap, previous conventional flap failure, and breast restoration with minimal donor-site deformity. Subsequently, Hartrampf's (3) introduction of the transverse rectus abdominis musculocutaneous (TRAM) flap in 1982 established a new standard for correction of the surgically absent breast. With enthusiasm for this autogenous tissue reconstruction, the more complex microsurgical procedures were temporarily disregarded.

The TRAM flap was reliable. Based on its nondominant pedicle, the deep superior epigastric artery, the rectus muscle could supply a large skin territory, more still when both rectus muscle pedicles were harvested. The donor tissue was obtained from an area of abundant fat, and offered a "free" abdominal lipectomy. Moreover, a natural-appearing breast mound was reestablished without the need for an underlying implant, as was often the case with the latissimus dorsi flap. The TRAM flap, however, could not be utilized in patients whose previous abdominal scars violated the muscular pedicle, and was not recommended in markedly obese patients.

As expertise with the TRAM flap increased, there arose new interest in its microsurgical applications (4). In addition to primary microvascular reconstruction, techniques for "supercharging" the TRAM flap were presented—these in an effort to maximize arterial perfusion and minimize flap loss (5). One recurring question was whether the added complexity of the microsurgical reconstruction ensured the same degree of safety as did the conventional technique. This was answered in part by Grotting and colleagues (6) in 1989 in

their review of breast reconstructions comparing conventional pedicled TRAM flaps with microvascular free TRAM flaps. Of 54 patients undergoing immediate breast reconstruction with TRAM flaps following mastectomy, 10 were reconstructed by microvascular free-flap transfer. In their series, they reported no loss of any portion of any free flaps, but approximately 25% loss of one conventional flap. There were no additional complications related to the microsurgical procedure. Other series have confirmed the safety of free flaps for breast reconstruction (8,16).

Rationale for Microvascular Free-Tissue Transfer

Microvascular free-tissue transfer offers several advantages over conventional pedicled transfer of autogenous tissue. These include:

1. Superior vascular reliability
2. No deformity from bulk of transposed pedicle
3. Improvement in donor-site morbidity
4. Ability to gain more stable coverage in radiated fields
5. Choice of donor sites, given body habitus of patient

The dominant vascular supply to the rectus muscle is through the deep inferior epigastric system. Through this vascular bed, a larger TRAM skin paddle can be carried with less risk of ischemia to the peripheral zones of the transverse skin island than can be carried with the conventional superiorly based pedicle flap (7). Thus, one rectus muscle segment will yield enough skin and subcutaneous tissue to reconstruct the breast mound. Because of its more robust vascularity, more aggressive insetting and shaping of the flap can be accomplished than can that of the pedicle flap. Nonetheless, restraint must be exercised in dealing with patients who smoke cigarettes because of the increased risk of partial flap loss and fat necrosis in that population (especially loss of native breast skin flaps (8).

The conventional TRAM flap may produce an epigastric bulge from the fullness of the muscular pedicle that disrupts the contour of the inframammary fold. This bulge might recede with time as the underlying muscle pedicle atrophies, but it often requires secondary procedures to contour. The free TRAM, in contradistinction, requires no pedicle tunneling and allows for a distinct, unviolated inframammary fold.

TRAM donor-site morbidity arises mainly from chronic complications of abdominal-wall hernia or eventration. With the requirements for less rectus muscle, and thus the harvest of smaller rectus fascial segments with free TRAM flaps, the risk of abdominal-wall closure under tension is decreased, even when segments of both muscles are harvested for bilateral procedures; in addition, with more rectus muscle remaining, there is less functional muscle weakness, which has been studied subjectively by Feller (9).

Free flaps in general are preferred for breast reconstruction in which the chest wall has been heavily irradiated and in situations where conventional rotational-flap methods of coverage are deemed unacceptable because of their inclusion in or proximity to the field of radiation. These "salvage" patients, many of whom have undergone extensive chest-wall resection for advanced breast cancer, require stable and reliable soft-tissue coverage—coverage that might not be achieved with pedicled TRAM or latissimus dorsi flaps. The exception to this indication, of course, is when recipient vessels for microvascular anastomosis have been previously damaged or are unavailable.

The patient's body habitus affects the donor-site possibilities. The TRAM flap may not be the best source of tissue for reconstruction for those patients who have a paucity of adipose tissue in the infraumbilical abdomen. Some have prominent "saddle bags" in the lateral thighs or generous gluteal fat deposits, and it is these patients who could benefit from breast reconstruction using either the free lateral thigh flap, based on the tensor fascia lata muscle and its overlying soft tissue, or the gluteal flap, based on the superior or inferior gluteal muscle and its overlying fat and skin. The Ruben fat pad flap, which takes advantage of periiliac adipose tissue, is an additional refinement, as are the deep inferior epigastric artery flap and the superficial inferior epigastric artery flap, which attempt to minimize the donor-site morbidity and abdominal weakness by harvesting no muscle or fascia of the rectus sheath complex (10–12).

Indications for Microvascular Free-Tissue Transfer

It should be emphasized that free flaps for breast reconstruction require a skilled microvascular surgeon. Also necessary is a nursing support staff familiar with the procedure and instrumentation and available for the initial procedure as well as "take-backs" for exploration of a failing free flap. There is no place for a novice microvascular surgeon or one who performs only an occasional free flap.

Indications for free-flap reconstruction of the surgically absent breast include:

1. Large chest-wall defects following radical mastectomy, with or without subsequent radiation therapy, in which no acceptable regional flaps will suffice
2. Previously failed regional flaps
3. Desire to minimize donor-site morbidity, especially in patients with inadequate infraumbilical soft tissue for TRAM flaps
4. Previous operative procedures that violated the conventional TRAM flap pedicle
5. Previous TRAM procedure or aesthetic abdominoplasty
6. Surgeon's preference for microsurgical transfer

The first three indications coincide with those proposed by Serafin in 1982 at a time before introduction of the TRAM flap, when delayed reconstruction was more common and when the initial surgical defects often were more extensive. The remaining indications reflect evolving trends in managing more complex reconstructive needs and in perfecting the aesthetics of breast reconstruction.

As experience with autogenous tissue reconstruction evolved, investigators sought to refine the technique, customizing it for each particular patient. The Ruben flap, lateral transverse (Fig. 71–1) or vertical thigh flap, and the gluteal flaps (Fig. 71–2) exemplify investigators' searches for autogenous tissue outside the boundaries of the TRAM region,

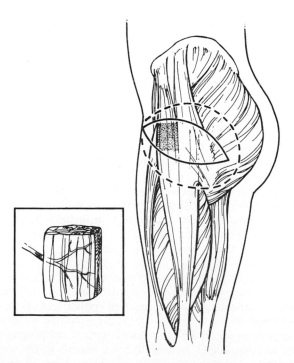

FIG. 71–1. Schematic design of the lateral transverse thigh flap. Based on the tensor fascia lata muscle, the skin can be oriented either horizontally (as pictured) or, as we prefer, vertically.

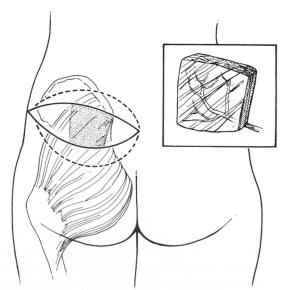

FIG. 71–2. Schematic of the superior gluteal flap based on the superior gluteal artery and vein. By dissecting the pedicle away from the surrounding muscle, a "perforator" flap can be harvested, which has the advantage of a longer pedicle.

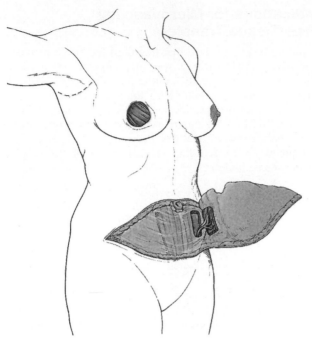

FIG. 71–3. Concept of the skin-sparing mastectomy by using the periareolar approach. In this case, the depicted free TRAM flap is based on the deep inferior epigastric artery and vein.

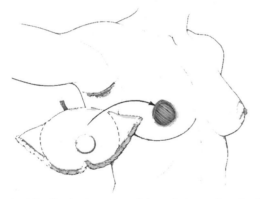

FIG. 71–4. The flap is then passed through the periareolar incision, with the microvascular anastomoses performed through a small separate axillary incision.

especially when the TRAM flap was previously harvested for breast reconstruction or discarded following aesthetic abdominoplasty.

Contraindications to Free Flaps

An intact and untraumatized vascular pedicle is mandatory for a successful free-flap transfer. Patients having undergone previous operative procedures in which the vascular pedicle has been divided will require an alternative source for autogenous tissue for reconstruction. Often, the details of the previous procedure are obscure and careful planning, both preoperatively and intraoperatively, is imperative to prevent mistakes. For example, in planning a free TRAM flap in a woman who had previously undergone a gynecologic procedure through a Pfannenstiel incision, one must assess the in-

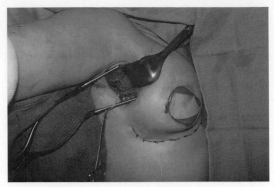

FIG. 71–5. Retractors expose the recipient thoracodorsal vessels for flap revascularization.

tegrity of the deep inferior epigastric artery and vein before division of the upper portion of the rectus muscle, and convert the procedure to a conventional pedicled-TRAM flap if those vessels have been divided. Also, the use of autogenous tissue involving vascular pedicles in an irradiated bed may be hazardous owing to the possibility of radiation vasculitis and fibrosis of the surrounding tissues.

Patients with significant preoperative morbidity, such as severe chronic obstructive pulmonary disease, angina pectoris, insulin-dependent diabetes mellitus, or hepatic or renal dysfunction, present higher perioperative risks from extensive operative dissection, blood loss, electrolyte shifts, and changes in pulmonary mechanics from constricted abdominal girth. Their risk of flap loss also may be greater, either from preexisting vascular disease, from medications that affect vascular tone, or because of altered flap perfusion from low cardiac output or from hypoxemia. Endocrinologic abnormalities, such as pheochromocytoma or other conditions that predispose to intractable blood pressure derangements, should signal the potential for flap compromise, as should intraoperative findings of refractory vasospasm in patients with Raynaud phenomenon.

Timing of Reconstruction

Several reported series have documented no increased risk of breast malignancy or its detection in women having undergone immediate reconstruction following mastectomy (13–15). Because of this information, and the psychologic benefit to women, interest in immediate breast reconstruction continues to increase. Another reason for this trend is the willingness of oncologic surgeons to suggest the option of reconstruction early in the discussion of management.

Benefits of immediate reconstruction include the psychologic boost to the patient who desires an immediate return to "wholeness," the option of employing a skin-sparing technique along with the advantage of the uncontracted breast skin envelope, the already exposed recipient vessels in the axilla, and the avoidance of a second major operation with its attendant anesthetic risk and required convalescent period.

As noted above, interaction with the oncologic surgeon is paramount in achieving the desired goal. If the general surgeon is comfortable technically and oncologically with a skin-sparing mastectomy, the plastic surgeon can utilize the native breast envelope to achieve a more aesthetic result

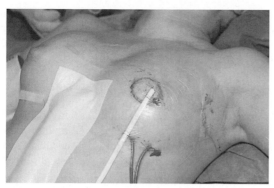

FIG. 71–6. Intraoperative view at the completion of the procedure, showing the TRAM skin island, closed axillary incision, and laser doppler monitoring probe.

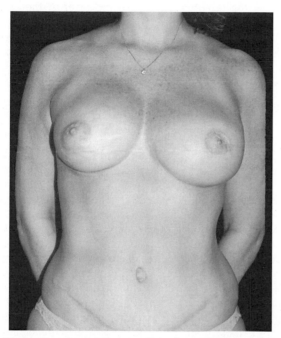

FIG. 71–7. Result of left immediate free TRAM reconstruction through a periareolar incision. Nipple reconstruction and tattooing were performed at 3 months following mound construction.

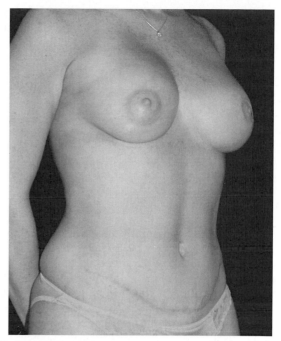

FIG. 71–8. Three-quarter view of the patient in Figure 71–7.

(Figs. 71–3, 71–4, 71–5). A periareolar excision of the breast will allow the resultant "periareolar" scar to be concealed within the tatooed neoareola. The axillary incision, used to expose the axillary nodal contents adequately and to perform the microvascular anastomoses (Fig. 71–6), can be placed such that the reconstructed breast mound appears without scars (Figs. 71–7, 71–8).

One of the primary concerns regarding immediate reconstruction is the effect on initiation of chemotherapy, if needed. Schusterman and colleagues (16) reported on 48 patients receiving conventional TRAM flaps, 21 (44%) of whom required postoperative chemotherapy, with 6 of 21 (29%) delayed because of flap complications. Seven of 20 patients (35%) with free TRAM flaps required postoperative chemotherapy, with 1 of 7 (14%) delayed for flap complications (16).

Our experience at the University of Alabama at Birmingham with 228 patients undergoing immediate breast reconstruction following mastectomy yielded only three patients (1.3%) who experienced delays in initiation of chemotherapy arising from complications of the initial procedure. Each was because of marginal mastectomy flap necrosis; and, all women were given chemotherapy within 3 weeks of the intended initiation date (17).

Preoperative Preparation

Following a thorough discussion of the appropriate options available for breast reconstruction (including expander/implant placement, pedicled flaps, and free flaps), the appropriate informed consent should include not only the benefits of the proposed procedure but also the accepted risks. For free-flap transfer, these risks include the donor-site morbidity of hematoma, seroma, or hernia formation, the risk of infection within the transferred flap or the donor site, the possibility of blood transfusion, the risk of native mastectomy flap ischemia or necrosis, and the risk of free-flap loss, either partial or total. The risk of total flap failure in reported series ranges from 6% (18), to 1.8% (19), to 1.0% (8).

As noted earlier, patients who smoke cigarettes have an increased risk of partial flap necrosis or fat necrosis, in addition to the risk of pneumonia or atelectasis. They should be strongly encouraged to quit for several weeks before surgery and for approximately 6 weeks following the procedure.

Free TRAM Flap: Preparation and Procedure

The patient is admitted to the hospital on the morning of the procedure. Preoperative medications include diazepam 2 or 5 mg by mouth, heparin 5000 units subcutaneously, and cefazolin 1 gram intravenously. Sequential compression hose are placed on both legs. The operating room should be warmed to 70° to 75° F and a forced-air warming blanket placed on the patient to prevent hypothermia. After induction of general anesthesia, a urinary catheter is placed. An arterial catheter is reserved for bilateral procedures and for patients with a significant cardiac history. Avoidance of brachial plexus neuropraxia or pressure-related ischemic phenomena mandates careful patient positioning. The arms are abducted to no greater than 90°, with the forearms in neutral position (thumbs pointing up). The head is turned slightly (less than 20°) to the side opposite the mastectomy. The hips and knees are slightly flexed. The head is supported with a foam ring and the patient's face is padded after confirming the security of the endotracheal tube. The patient is secured to the bed so that she can be positioned sitting for assessment of symmetry during flap insetting. The anesthesiologist monitors the patient from the feet with the use of long circuit tubing, so that the patient's head and shoulder area is accessible for the microscope and the surgical team.

The preoperative preparation must be altered appropriately when harvesting the lateral thigh flap or the gluteal flaps. For harvesting the lateral thigh flap, the patient must be "twisted" slightly on the operating table such that the chest is supine and the appropriate hip is elevated into the correct view for properly visualized dissection. For the gluteal flaps, the patient is placed in the lateral decubitus position, and following the harvest of the flap the position must be changed before vessel anastomosis and flap insetting.

For immediate reconstruction, the dissection of the TRAM free flap can proceed simultaneously with the resection of the breast by the oncologic surgeon. The inframammary fold on the mastectomy side is marked with sutures to aid in preventing dissection below that boundary with disruption of the natural fold. The flap can be designed much like an aesthetic abdominoplasty. The umbilicus is transcribed sharply down to the level of the abdominal fascia, with care taken to preserve adequate tissue around the stalk to avoid ischemia to the umbilicus. The previously marked upper TRAM incision is begun, bevelling away from the flap to include more underlying fatty tissue and possibly more musculocutaneous perforators. The incision is carried laterally and inferiorly following the previously marked lines, down to the level of the abdominal-wall fascia. The superficial inferior epigastric vessels will be crossed, and must be adequately ligated on both sides to prevent inadvertent bleeding. The side opposite the proposed rectus muscle harvest side is elevated at the level of the superior oblique fascia beginning laterally and extending medially on the rectus fascia to the midline. The ipsilateral side is likewise elevated lateral to medial to the lateral aspect of the rectus fascia, at which point care must be taken to dissect slowly to avoid disruption of any lateral perforators piercing the rectus fascia. This part of the dissection is usually done sharply with the knife under loupe magnification. Once the lateral row of perforators is identified, the rectus fascia may be incised longitudinally lateral to this row. The dissection is continued from the inferior aspect of the flap, and the inferiormost perforator is identified, usually at the level of the semicircular line of Douglas. The transverse inferior fascial incision is made at this point. An inferiorly directed incision is made toward the pubis to allow better dissection of the donor vessels. The rectus muscle is reflected

medially for identification, and exposure of the deep inferior epigastric vessels and the 12th intercostal neurovascular bundle, which is ligated and divided. Blunt finger dissection will free the space beneath the rectus muscle and the posterior rectus sheath. Care must be taken, however, to avoid bluntly dissecting beneath the posterior rectus sheath, which is easy to do if the semicircular line is not appreciated. The rectus muscle may then be elevated medially, and the association of the deep inferior epigastric artery (DIEA) and deep inferior epigastric vein (DIEV) with the muscle can be assessed to determine the amount of lateral rectus muscle to spare. An inferior branch from the DIEA and DIEV to the rectus muscle may be divided. At approximately this position the operator must bluntly dissect between the rectus muscle and the DIEA and DIEV pedicle so as to divide the lower rectus muscle transversely. Care must be exercised to avoid injury to the pedicle with this maneuver. Once completed, the dissection of the proximal pedicle to the level of the external iliac vessels may be performed, with a fiberoptic retractor for visualization and gentle retraction on the muscle. A pedicle of 7 to 8 cm is obtained. The DIEA ranges in size from 2 to 3 mm in diameter and the accompanying venae commitantes are usually paired. At this point, the medial rectus muscle is dissected, often sparing a medial strip of muscle.

Before division of the superior margin of rectus muscle, a clear evaluation of the status of the recipient vessels must be ascertained. If the recipient vessels are inadequate, then the flap can be rotated as a superiorly pedicled flap. If the recipient vessels are adequate, the TRAM flap can be explanted and transferred to the recipient site for anastomosis, usually using the thoracodorsal artery and vein, which have been dissected prior to flap vessel division. By anastomosing to the thoracodorsal artery above the branch to the serratus muscle, adequate retrograde filling of the pedicle to the latissimus muscle is maintained to allow for its possible use in the event of a free-flap failure. The technique of the senior author is to anastomose the artery end-to-end under microscopic visualization and to couple the vein ends with an anastomotic coupling device (Precise MAS device, 3M company), most often using the 2.5-mm diameter coupler. Following the microvascular anastomoses, the flap is inset. The abdominal-wall defect may be closed while the microvascular repair is ongoing and, once the patient is positioned upright for flap insetting, the remaining abdominal closure, including insetting of the umbilicus, may be completed (Figs. 71-9, 71-10, 71-11).

Operative Technique for the Lateral Thigh Flap

The skin paddle for the lateral thigh flap, although previously reported as a transverse ellipse, is designed as a vertical ellipse overlying the tensor fascia lata muscle, fascia lata, and subcutaneous fat. This skin paddle orientation allows a better closure in the "vest-over-pants" technique. Raising the flap requires shaping of the subcutaneous fat in the shape of the new breast mound. A cuff of tensor fascia lata muscle, with its pedicle of the lateral femoral circumflex artery and venae commitantes, is included and transferred to the recipient site for vascular anastomosis. The pedicle is long enough to ensure adequate reach to the thoracodorsal vessels. Closure of

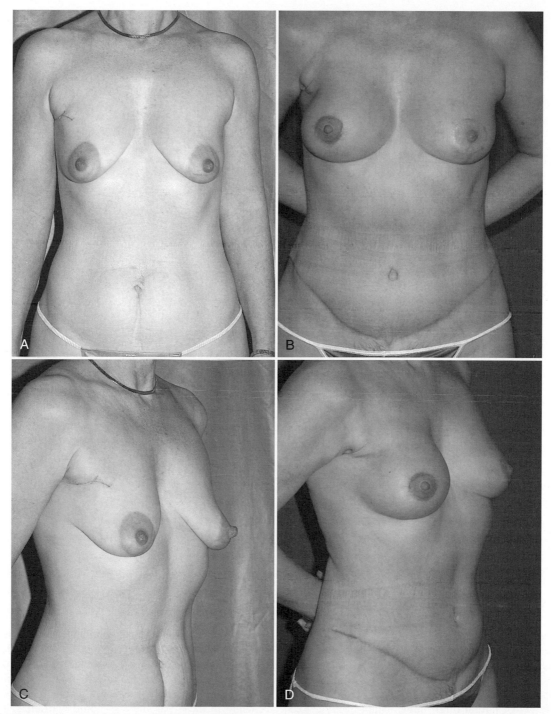

FIG. 71–9. **A,** 47-year-old patient with a small infiltrating ductal carcinoma of tail of right breast (note biopsy scar). **B,** postoperative view following immediate free TRAM reconstruction using the periareolar approach, with microvascular anastomoses performed through the excised biopsy scar incision. Left mastopexy was also performed. **C,** preoperative three-quarter view. **D,** postoperative three-quarter view.

the donor defect requires careful obliteration of dead space, with deepithelialization of one side of the ellipse to fill the defect and allow closure of the skin in a vest-over-pants fashion. Despite the obliteration of dead space, seroma is common and may persist for several weeks to months. The asymmetry of the thighs is noticable, and better symmetry is achieved when both lateral thigh flaps are harvested for bilateral reconstruction of the breasts.

Operative Considerations for the Gluteal Flaps

Both the superior and inferior gluteal flaps offer abundant adipose tissue for breast reconstruction. The resultant scars are maintained within most undergarments and unilateral gluteal harvests cause only small alterations in symmetry.

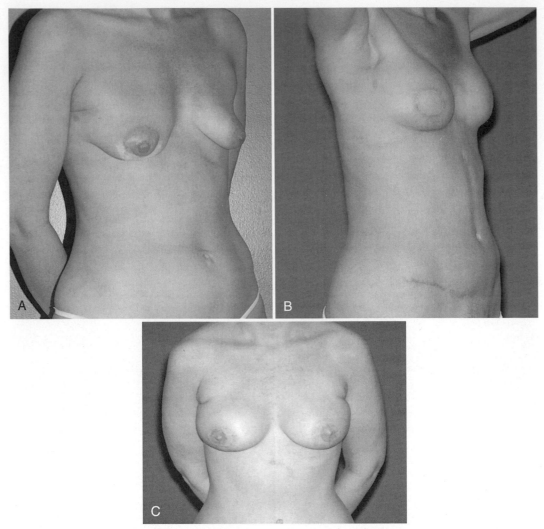

FIG. 71–10. **A,** 44-year-old patient with a left infiltrating ductal carcinoma and right premalignant mastopathy who had a strong family history for breast cancer. **B,** initial result following bilateral mastec- tomy and immediate free TRAM reconstruction. **C,** final result following nipple-areolar reconstruction and tattooing.

The patient is positioned in the lateral decubitus position and draped such that intraoperative turning to the supine position requires no additional prepping. The harvested specimen represents a wedge of skin and adipose tissue and a small cuff of gluteus muscle, either oriented over the superior or inferior gluteal vessels. The pedicle length is shorter than that of the TRAM or lateral thigh flaps, usually only 2 to 3 cm. Although this pedicle can occasionally reach to the axillary vessels (if the thoracodorsal artery and vein are dissected out and elevated towards the midline), the internal mammary vessels are closer. These are exposed by resecting the 3rd costal cartilage, which will yield an artery of 1.5 to 2.0 mm diameter and a vein of 2 to 3 mm diameter.

Postoperative management differs little from that of other free-flap breast reconstructions. The patient is allowed to sit and flex at the hips by the 3rd postoperative day. Closed-suction drains often can be removed before patient discharge.

Postoperative Management

Once the microvascular anastomoses have been completed and the patient has left the operating room, it is imperative that the surgical team be vigilant in assessing the flap. The laser doppler flow probes, which record continuous flow measurements, aid in early detection of vascular insufficiency, but should not supplant more traditional techniques of flap assessment; frequent determinations of flap color, turgor, warmth, and capillary refill also must be made. Any change in these parameters should warrant consideration of reexploration of the anastomoses.

The patient room is maintained warm (75° F, or more). The hydration of the patient is maintained by assuring urine output of >30 mm per hour. Fluid boluses are given for any signs of underresuscitation. An acceptable postoperative hematocrit is 25 to 30%, given that the patient has no significant cardiovascular indication for greater oxygen-carrying capacity. Intravenous rheologic agents or anticoagulants are not routinely administered.

The patient is encouraged to sit in a chair and to ambulate with assistance on the 1st postoperative day, in addition to using an incentive spirometer. Every effort is made to prevent the potential complications of pneumonia and deep venous thrombosis. The sequential-compression hosiery are re-

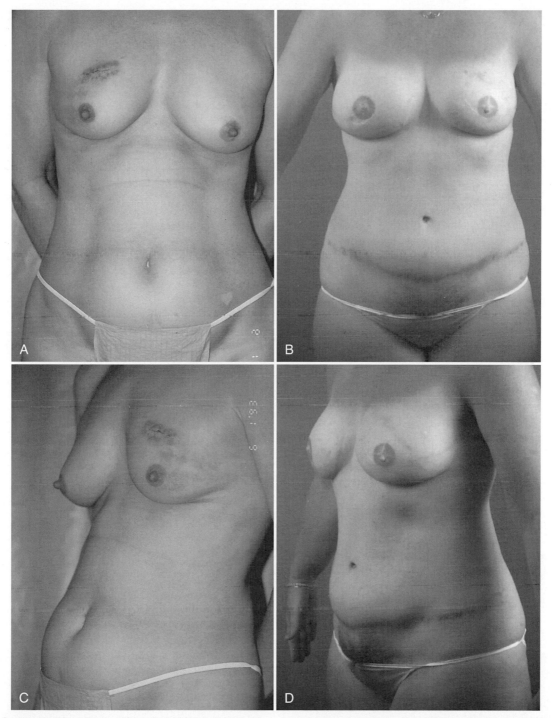

FIG. 71–11.   A, 42-year-old patient with recent biopsy site on left breast revealing ductal carcinoma in situ. She also has a strong family history for breast cancer, compelling her to elect bilateral mastectomies and immediate free TRAM reconstruction. **B,** note how biopsy site location influences the amount of skin removed on left breast, whereas right breast can be reconstructed using the periareolar approach only. **C,** preoperative three-quarter view. **D,** postoperative three-quarter view.

moved by postoperative day 3, when the patient has begun ambulating consistently. No formal physical therapy is indicated to initiate ROM exercises of the shoulder on the operated side. Simple exercises designed to slowly increase shoulder motion are taught, beginning approximately 10 days postoperatively; and, only if the patient has significantly decreased ROM of the shoulder at 3 weeks postoperatively is physical therapy recommended.

Closed-suction drains are removed when the daily output measures less than 30 ml. Usually one or more drains remain at the time of patient discharge, which requires patient teaching for management at home. Activity limitations include no heavy lifting, no strenuous exercise, and no vigorous athletics for 6 to 8 weeks to help prevent abdominal-wall weakness or hernia formation during early wound healing. These restrictions apply to patients undergoing the Ruben fat pad flap as well; lateral thigh flaps and gluteal flaps do not have hernia formation as a potential problem.

Surgical Refinements

Plans can be made for revision of the reconstructed breast with nipple reconstruction and revision of the abdominal donor site at approximately 3 months, or 1 month after completion of chemotherapy (if needed as an adjuvant treatment). The nipple is best reconstructed using a modification of the fishtail flap, which offers adequate projection and leaves the incision within the margins of the neoareola. Nipple sharing offers an alternative method if the contralateral nipple is large. After adequate healing of the reconstructed nipple, usually 6 weeks, the neoareola can be recreated with dermapigmentation. The usual "touch-ups" performed at the time of nipple reconstruction include suction-assisted lipectomy of the flanks, often with excision of the abdominal dog-ears at the lateral abdominal donor sites; also, suction-assisted lipectomy can be used to better contour the reconstructed breast. Care must be taken to suction the flap conservatively because the abdominal fat is very readily aspirated with suction cannulas, and inadvertent over-suctioning can result.

Management of the Failing Free Flap

Subtle changes in the free flap can indicate vascular compromise. A high index of suspicion is needed to ensure that no failing free flap is allowed to necrose. Certainly changes in the arterial or venous doppler signals can herald impending flap failure, as can the gross color changes of venous engorgement or arterial ischemia; however, often the changes are not so evident. Careful comparison with previous exams may suggest progressive alterations in blood flow. Recurrent intraoperative platelet thrombus formation should heighten the surgeon's suspicion that vessel thrombosis may be present.

Prompt return to the operating room for flap exploration is mandatory, given the suspicion of flap failure. At operation, the findings often suggest a technical fault that can be corrected, such as vessel twisting or excessive tension. However, even if the cause is not evident, revision (sometimes with an interposed vein graft) is required. Schusterman and others (8) report in their review of 211 consecutive cases of free TRAM flaps for breast reconstruction a total of seven flap complications of vessel thrombosis, three of which progressed to total flap necrosis. Four were salvaged (57%), yielding a 99% flap success rate.

Complications

The most ominous complication of free-flap breast reconstruction is flap failure. Vessel thrombosis requiring revision is generally successful if repaired early. Partial flap necrosis and fat necrosis are potential problems. Partial flap loss may require revision of the necrotic wound or conservative débridement, with healing by secondary intention. The resultant scar and firmness of fat necrosis may be confused with recurrence of malignancy, but close follow-up by the plastic surgeon, with frequent breast exams, should alleviate that concern, especially when the lesion is appreciated soon after the reconstruction and does not enlarge.

Donor-site complications may also arise following breast reconstruction. The harvest of the TRAM flap, with its attendant violation of the abdominal wall at its most vulnerable region, might result in a fascial hernia. The incidence of abdominal hernia following free TRAM reconstruction is 3 to 6%. Reinforcement with prosthetic mesh, although infrequently needed, will maintain greater abdominal-wall resistance to weakness and thereby reduce the risk of hernia formation. Overall, the risks of free-flap reconstruction do not outweigh the risks from reconstruction using other methods (6, 8).

Conclusion

The trend toward autogenous breast reconstruction, and specifically reconstruction using free-tissue transfer, has proven beneficial to women, and more refinements are likely to follow. The risks of complex reconstruction with the additional complexities of microsurgery have not been shown to increase morbidity or to be detrimental oncologically to the patient.

References

1. Fujino T, Harashina T, Enomoto K. Primary breast reconstruction after a standard radical mastectomy by a free-flap transfer. *Plast Reconstr Surg* 1976; 58:372.
2. Serafin D, Voci VE, Georgiade NG. Microsurgical composite tissue transplantation: indications and technical considerations in breast reconstruction following mastectomy. *Plast Reconstr Surg* 1982; 69:216.
3. Hartrampf C, Scheflan M, Black P. Breast reconstruction with a transverse abdominal island flap. *Plast Reconstr Surg* 1982; 69:216.
4. Holstrom H. The free abdominoplasty flap and its use in breast reconstruction. *Scand J Plast Reconstr Surg* 1979; 13:423.
5. Harashina T, Sone K, Inoue S, et al. Augmentation of the circulation of pedicled transverse rectus abdominis musculocutaneous flaps by microvascular surgery. *Br J Plast Surg* 1987; 40:367.
6. Grotting JC, Urist MM, Maddox WA, et al. Conventional TRAM flap versus free microsurgical TRAM flap for immediate breast reconstruction. *Plast Reconstr Surg* 1989; 83:828.
7. Boyd J, Taylor G, Corlett R. The vascular territories of the superior epigastric and the deep inferior epigastric systems. *Plast Reconstr Surg* 1984; 73:1.
8. Schusterman MA, Kroll SS, Miller MJ, et al. The free transverse rectus abdominis musculocutaneous flap for breast reconstruction: one center's experience with 211 consecutive cases. *Ann Plast Surg* 1994; 32:234.
9. Feller AM. Free TRAM. Results and abdominal wall function. *Clin Plast Surg* 1994; 21(2):223.
10. Hartrampf CR, Noel RT, Drazan L, et al. Ruben's fat pad for breast reconstruction: a periiliac soft-tissue free flap. *Plast Reconstr Surg* 1994; 93:402.
11. Allen RJ, Treece P. Deep inferior epigastric perforator flap for breast reconstruction. *Ann Plast Surg* 1994; 32:32.
12. Grotting JC. The free abdominaplasty flap for immediate breast reconstruction. *Ann Plast Surg* 1991; 27(4):351.
13. Noone RB, Murphy JB, Spear SL, et al. A 6-year experience with immediate reconstruction after mastectomy for cancer. *Plast Reconstr Surg* 1985; 76:258.
14. Georgiade GS, Riefkohl S, Cox E. Long-term clinical outcome of immediate reconstruction after mastectomy. *Plast Reconstr Surg* 1985; 76:415.
15. Webster DJT, Mansel RE, Hughes LE. Immediate reconstruction of the breast after mastectomy: is it safe? *Cancer* 1984; 53:1416.
16. Schusterman MA, Kroll SS, Weldon ME. Immediate breast reconstruction: why the free TRAM over the conventional TRAM flap? *Plast Reconstr Surg* 1992; 90:255.
17. Grotting JC, Urist MM, Passmore AK, et al. Oncologic aspects of autogenous breast reconstruction. *The Breast Journal* 1995; 1(1):36.
18. Arnez ZM, Bajec J, Bardsley AF, et al. Experience with 50 free TRAM flap breast reconstructions. *Plast Reconstr Surg* 1991; 87(3):470.
19. Shaw WW, Ahn CY. Microvascular free flaps in breast reconstruction. *Clin Plast Surg* 1992; 19(4):917.

72

Alternatives in Autologous Free-Flap Breast Reconstruction

William W. Shaw, M.D., F.A.C.S., James Watson, M.D., and Christina Y. Ahn, M.D.

Flap Choices

Although the TRAM flap has become the workhorse for autologous breast reconstruction, not all patients are suitable candidates for this flap (1). Several other autologous free flaps provide useful alternative options, making autologous reconstruction feasable in nearly all patients. These options include the modified deep circumflex iliac artery flap (or Rubens flap), the tensor fascia lata flap (lateral thigh flap), the superior and inferior gluteal flaps, and a number of other flaps. The availability of so many flap choices makes surgical decision making somewhat more complicated. The reconstructive surgeon, therefore, must evaluate each case based on the recipient site requirements, the characteristics of the available donor tissue, the patient's priorities, and the surgeon's own experience. A discussion about flap selection cannot be complete without reference to these issues.

RECIPIENT SITE REQUIREMENTS

Planning for autologous reconstruction always starts with recipient site analysis. Horizontal skin requirements, vertical skin requirements, and three-dimensional volume requirements must be evaluated independently. If the remaining chest wall skin is of poor quality owing to irradiation, scar contractures, or silicone gel infiltration, further skin excision may be needed to achieve a good aesthetic result. Total skin requirements must then include both missing skin and planned excision of poor-quality chest wall skin. Volume requirements may be underestimated as well, due to complete pectoralis muscle absence (radical mastectomy) partial pectoralis deficiencies (Poland syndrome, deep breast cancer resections), muscle atrophy (subpectoral implants), or chest wall depressions (implants, pectus deformity). The size and shape of the contralateral breast must also be considered in flap selection. Finally, ptotic breasts require additional skin in the vertical dimension.

Inadequate skin replacement results in a contracted, flat contour that limits projection and ptosis of the reconstructed breast. Inadequate skin replacement may also compress the flap and compromise blood flow, resulting in flap loss or excessive fat necrosis. Inadequate flap volume may call for supplementation with implants, which fewer and fewer patients are willing to accept (2). For these reasons, adequate skin and volume requirements must be met, or no amount of secondary surgeries will achieve an optimal result. Since these alternative flaps all have less skin surface availability than the unilateral TRAM flap, inadequate skin is more likely to occur unless careful preoperative planning has been done.

PATIENT FACTORS

For autologous tissue breast reconstruction, the TRAM flap should always be considered first. Primary reasons for alternate flap use include inadequate abdominal fat, high-risk abdominal scars, patient preference, and TRAM flap failure. Thin patients with minimal abdominal-wall fat cannot achieve adequate volume with a TRAM flap. A gluteal flap, on the other hand, almost always provides adequate volume (3). Certain abdominal scars are unsafe TRAM donor sites (paramedian scars, abdominoplasty, colostomy, ileostomy) (4). Recent studies have shown that TRAM flaps can be used despite appendectomy, hysterectomy, C-section, and endoscopic cholecystectomy scars (5). Other patients may prefer an alternate donor site for lifestyle, pregnancy plans, or other personal reasons (6). Normal pregnancies and normal deliveries have been reported in TRAM flap patients, however (7). Despite high success rates with TRAM flap reconstruction, failures still occur that require an alternate method for salvage reconstruction. In some patients, only one alternative flap is suitable. In others, many alternatives may achieve a good result. For this reason, the patient should be informed of the pros and cons of the various choices and actively participate in the decision-making process.

FLAP CHARACTERISTICS

The surgeon must have a hands-on familiarity with the special features of each flap: skin surface availability, flap bulk, flap projection (contour), vascular pedicle length, donor vessel diameter, ease of anastomosis, flap reliability, donor-site morbidity, and scar quality (8) (Table 72–1).

TECHNICAL FACTORS

All of these alternative flaps are technically more difficult than the TRAM flap. The most important technical factor is the surgeon's experience. In experienced hands, all of these flaps have been done safely with high success rates. The surgeon must not only be familiar with flap anatomy, but must also have hands-on experience with flap dissection. Attempting a difficult reconstruction method with no clinical experience is likely to give the patient a less-than-optimal result with high morbidity.

Common technical difficulties with alternative flaps include the following:

1. *Skin island design.* Errors in skin island positioning are less forgiving in these alternative flaps, since musculocutaneous perforators are not organized into rows, as they are in the TRAM flap. Precise skin island design and care-

Table 72–1.
Comparison of Flaps for Autologous Breast Reconstruction

	Skin	Bulk	Contour	Donor Appearance	Reliability	Technical Ease
Free TRAM	++++	+++	+++	+++	+++	+++
Pedicled TRAM	+++	++	++	+++	++	+++
Latissimus	+	+	+	++	++++	++++
Gluteus	+++	++++	++++	+++	++	++
DCIA	+++	+++	+++	++	+++	++
TFL	++	++	++	+	+++	++

+ = poor
++ = average
+++ = good
++++ = excellent

ful muscle sparing dissection must be done to preserve vascular supply. Errors in flap sizing are less forgiving, when compared with the TRAM flap. Table flexion helps close large TRAM flap donor sites, whereas flexion maneuvers are not of much benefit in these other flaps. If the skin flap is designed too big, little can be done to help achieve primary closure.

2. *Pedical dissection.* All of these flaps have vascular pedicles in close proximity to important nerves. Unlike the TRAM, where the intercostal nerves entering the rectus sheath are usually transected with impunity, the motor nerves near these vascular pedicles must be spared. Whenever possible, the sensory nerves should be preserved as well. Important nerves at risk for injury include the femoral nerve (TFL flap), the sciatic nerve (inferior gluteal flap), the lateral cutaneous nerve of the thigh, and the cutaneous branch of T12 (DCIA flap). Bleeding during pedicle dissection in the superior gluteal flap may be difficult to control, due to vessel retraction into the greater sciatic foramen.

3. *Donor site closure.* Donor site closure must be done very carefully, or hernias (DCIA flap), seromas (TFL flap), depressions (Gluteal, TFL) or wound dehiscence (too large a skin island) may result. Preoperative patient education about these flap choices must include a discussion about the donor-site scars, contour deformities, sensory deficits, and potential motor nerve injury. Donor-site scars may require revision at the second stage of breast reconstruction.

Recipient Vessels for Alternative Flaps

Because these alternative flaps have unique shapes and short vascular pedicles, the surgeon must also be very familiar with all recipient vessel options (9). Hands-on experience with thoracodorsal *and* internal mammary vessel exposure is mandatory. The surgeon should also be familiar with vascular access to the lateral thoracic, circumflex scapular, and thoracoacromial vessels. Lack of appropriate planning for recipient vessels will result in a malpositioned pedicle or a malpositioned breast mound. Recipient vessel exposure should ideally be finished while flap dissection is still underway, thereby avoiding any delay when the flap is ready for harvest. Vessel exposure is best done with mag-

nification, to avoid injury to the recipient vessels or nearby structures.

Bilateral Breast Reconstruction

In patients with moderate amounts of abdominal tissue, the TRAM flap may be large enough to reconstruct one breast. If used for bilateral reconstruction in the same patient, however, flap volume may be inadequate. For these patients, alternative flaps may give a much better aesthetic result for bilateral breast reconstruction.

Bilateral breast reconstruction has other features that may affect flap choice and operative staging. Bilateral flap harvesting and insetting can be done with minimal patient repositioning in bilateral TRAM, DCIA, and TFL reconstructions. With bilateral gluteal reconstructions, however, the patient must be turned (from side to side or front to back), which lengthens operating-room time and raises concerns about flap vascular compromise. For this reason, bilateral gluteal reconstructions are best staged as two unilateral reconstructions (8).

Preoperative planning is critical in bilateral cases. Intravenous access and patient monitoring should be discussed in advance with the anaesthesiologist, since both arms should be prepped free of lines and monitoring devices. A two-team approach with two surgeons, two scrub nurses, and two circulators help to avoid unreasonably long operating times (8).

Gluteal Flaps

Gluteal free flaps for breast reconstruction were first described by Fujino and associates in 1975 (10). These flaps can be based on the superior or inferior gluteal artery. Although this flap is technically a myocutaneous flap based on a type III muscle, a muscle-sparing harvest can be done so that the majority of the gluteus maximus muscle is preserved. Some authors favor the superiorly based flap; others favor the inferiorly based flap (11,12). The differences are discussed later under flap characteristics.

FLAP ANATOMY AND DISSECTION (Fig. 72–1)

The superior and inferior gluteal arteries are terminal branches of the internal iliac artery that exit the pelvis

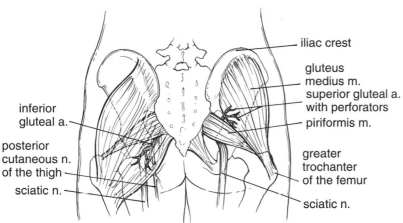

FIG. 72–1. Gluteal flap anatomy.

through the greater sciatic foramen. Above the piriformis muscle, the superior gluteal artery divides into a superficial and deep branch. The superficial branch supplies the upper half of the gluteus maximus and gives rise to cutaneous perforators (13). Below the piriformis muscle, a number of neurovascular structures exit the greater sciatic foramen, including the sciatic nerve, pudendal nerve, inferior gluteal nerve, posterior cutaneous nerve of the thigh, pudendal vessels, and the inferior gluteal vessels. The inferior gluteal nerve (L5,S1,S2) innervates the entire gluteus maximus muscle. The inferior gluteal artery supplies the inferior half of the gluteus maximus muscle and the overlying cutaneous perforators as it descends inferiorly. It terminates as a cutaneous branch that accompanies the posterior femoral cutaneous nerve. This terminal branch forms the basis for the gluteal thigh flap (14). The superior and inferior gluteal arteries are usually accompanied by one vena comitans which drains as separate vessels into the internal iliac vein (15).

FLAP DESIGN AND DISSECTION (Fig. 72–2)

The ipsilateral buttock is chosen as the donor site, allowing for simultaneous recipient and donor sites dissection with the patient in the lateral decubitus position. The gluteal artery flaps are harvested with elliptical skin surfaces and wedge-shaped volumes. The superior gluteal artery flap can be dissected with a horizontal or oblique axis. The oblique skin is-

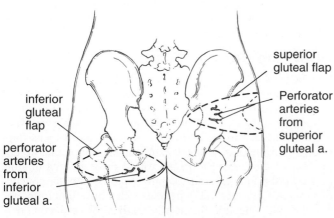

FIG. 72–2. Gluteal flap design.

land axis is centered over a line from the posterior superior iliac spine to the greater trochanter (16). The horizontal skin island is designed directly over the superior gluteal artery perforators, extending laterally off the muscle to include some of the fat overlying the TFL muscle (17).

The inferior gluteal artery flap is usually centered horizontally just above the inferior gluteal crease (18). Inferiorily, the descending terminal branch and the accompanying posterior cutaneous nerve must be ligated and transected, resulting in numbness of the posterior thigh. Care must be taken to avoid injuring the sciatic nerve. The gluteus muscle harvest may leave the sciatic nerve or the stump of the posterior cutaneous nerve of the thigh exposed with minimal soft-tissue cover, causing pain postoperatively. This is a major drawback of the inferior gluteal artery flap.

FLAP CHARACTERISTICS

The gluteal donor site consistently offers adequate flap volume, even in thin patients. The fat tends to be firmer, giving excellent projection to the reconstructed breast. The quantity of skin available is less than that of the TRAM, but comparable to the TFL flap. A superior gluteal flap 13 cm wide by 25–30 cm long can be harvested with primary donor-site closure. The inferior gluteal flap usually yields a smaller skin island and a smaller volume, when compared to the superior gluteal flap.

The major drawback of the superior gluteal flap is the short, vertically oriented vascular pedicle, making both flap harvest and microvascular anastomoses technically difficult. The effective length of the vascular pedicle can be lengthened by intramuscular dissection of the vessels, however. The arterial diameter averages 2.0 mm, although the inferior gluteal artery is somewhat smaller. The accompanying vein may vary from 2 to 5 mm. This vessel diameter discrepancy may make the microvascular anastomoses difficult and limit the recipient vessel choices. Although the thoracodorsal vessels can be used, often the internal mammary vessels must be chosen for adequate flap positioning.

IDEAL PATIENT (Fig. 72–3)

The ideal candidate for a gluteal flap is a thin patient who needs unilateral breast reconstruction and who has high-risk abdominal scars or inadequate volume in TRAM, DCIA, and TFL donor sites. Since the gluteal donor site always has suf-

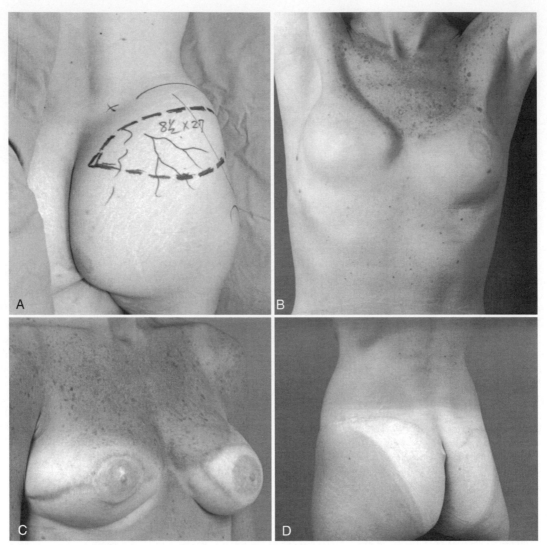

FIG. 72–3.   Bilateral breast reconstruction with staged superior gluteal flaps. **A,** preoperative flap donor site. **B,** preoperative bilateral breast reconstruction. **C,** postoperative bilateral breast reconstruction. **D,** bilateral flap donor site scars.

ficient fat for free-flap harvest, this may be the only flap option for the thin patient. Because this flap is technically difficult to harvest and to inset, other options should be considered first in patients with inadequate fat in other donor sites. Due to patient repositioning problems, it is a better flap for unilateral than bilateral reconstruction. If bilateral gluteal flap reconstruction is chosen, it is best to stage the reconstruction, completing one side at a time.

COMPLICATIONS

Major significant complications of the superior gluteal flap are related largely to surgical technique. Vascular pedicle dissection must be done with precise hemostasis, because of the vertical orientation of the vessel as they exit the greater sciatic foramen. Uncontrolled bleeding rapidly obliterates the bleeding site, like water filling a well, which makes hemostasis very difficult. The microvascular anastomoses can also be very difficult due to a short vascular pedicle (3–5 cm) or vein diameter mismatch. Nevertheless, these problems can be solved

with good technique. Few donor-site complications with the superior gluteal flap have been reported. Significant donor-site morbidity can potentially occur with the inferior gluteal flap, if the sciatic nerve is left exposed by muscle harvest.

Neuromas of the posterior cutaneous nerve of the thigh may result in chronic pain.

DCIA Flap (Rubens Flap)

The DCIA flap was originally described by Taylor and associates (19) as the iliac crest osteocutaneous (or osteomyocutaneous) free flap. Recently, this flap has been modified by Elliot and associates (20) to exclude bone, yet harvest skin and fat. This modification has been named the Rubens flap, referring to the painter Peter Paul Rubens. In his classic depictions of the female form, he would paint an area of fullness over the iliac crest, in keeping with the popular concept of beauty of his day. Many patients today have this (now unpopular) fat collection that is vascularized by cutaneous perforators from the descending branch of the deep circumflex

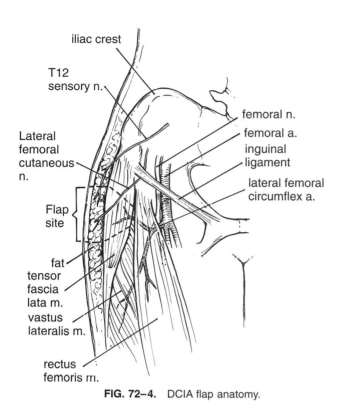

FIG. 72–4. DCIA flap anatomy.

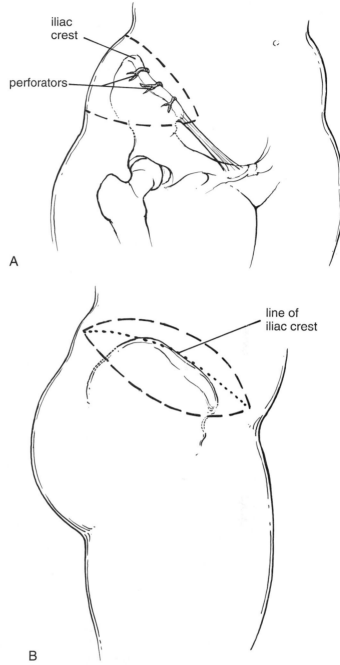

FIG. 72–5. DCIA flap design. **A,** oblique view. **B,** side view.

iliac artery. This iliac crest fullness may be prominent for genetic reasons (pear-shaped body habitus) or arise from previous surgery (abdominoplasty, TRAM flap). In these patients, this is a good alternative for breast reconstruction.

FLAP ANATOMY (Fig. 72–4)

The deep circumflex artery arises from the posterolateral aspect of the external iliac artery and runs laterally, just above and parallel to the inguinal ligament. Just before it reaches the ASIS, the DCIA gives off an ascending branch to the internal oblique muscle, which does not have any significant cutaneous perforators. In this same area, the lateral femoral cutaneous nerve crosses the vascular pedicle and passes under the inguinal ligament as it exits the pelvis to supply the anterior thigh. This pure sensory nerve can be preserved, but it is often injured unintentionally or transected intentionally for exposure purposes. The DCIA continues along the inner surface of the iliac crest, running in a groove where the iliacus muscle and transversalis fascia insert onto bone. Here it gives off cutaneous perforators that exit the external oblique fascia 1 to 3 cm above the iliac crest. One vena comitan usually accompanies the artery, diverging upward as it crosses the external iliac artery and enters the external iliac vein.

FLAP DESIGN AND DISSECTION (Fig. 72–5)

Flap design is based on surface anatomy landmarks of the inguinal ligament, ASIS, and iliac crest. The skin paddle is designed as an ellipse with an axis parallel to the iliac crest. To increase flap fat volume and flap surface area, as much as one-third of the flap can be centered below the iliac crest. This allows for adjacent fat, overlying the TFL and gluteal muscles, to be included with the flap. To protect the vascular pedicle and the cutaneous perforators, the DCIA flap is usually harvested with a cuff of internal oblique transversalis fascia, and periosteum along the inner surface of the iliac crest. This creates the major drawback of the DCIA flap: that of donor-site closure. To repair this defect, transosseous sutures usually need to be placed through the iliac crest to reattach the external oblique, the internal oblique, and the transversalis fascia. This causes a significant amount of donor-site pain during the early postoperative period.

FLAP CHARACTERISTICS

The quantity of skin available with the DCIA flap is less than that of the TRAM, but comparable to the gluteal and TFL flaps. By including fat below the iliac crest, a consistent volume of fat can reliably be obtained in all but the thinnest patients. The vascular pedicle is 5 to 6 cm long (shorter than the free TRAM, comparable to the TFL, and longer than the superior gluteal artery). Vessel diameters average 2.0 mm for the artery and 2.5 mm for the vein. The three-dimensional fat volume projects well in the reconstructed breast.

IDEAL CANDIDATE (Fig. 72–6)

The ideal candidate for a DCIA flap is a gyncecoid (pear-shaped), normal-weight patient who has previously had an abdominoplasty. Patients with other unfavorable abdominal surgical scars that preclude the use of the TRAM are also good candidates. Caution should be taken with patients who have compromised abdominal-wall integrity (e.g., hernia), because this operation also compromises their abdominal-wall strength. DCIA flaps are good options for bilateral breast reconstruction in patients whose abdominal fat would

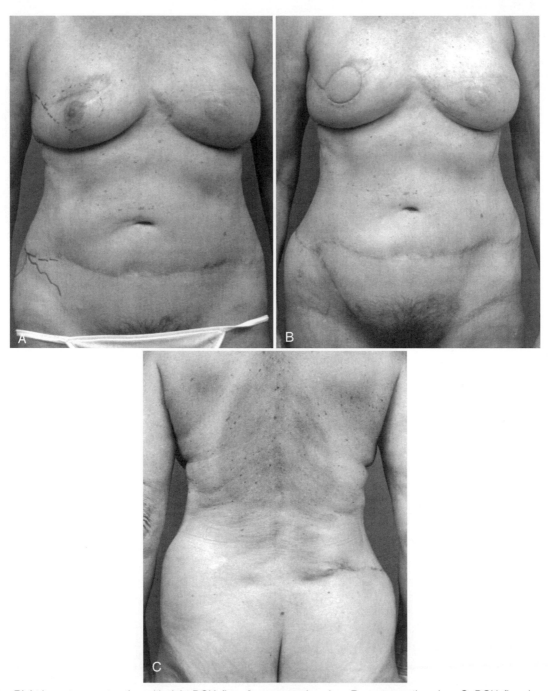

FIG. 72–6. Right breast reconstruction with right DCIA flap. **A,** preoperative view. **B,** postoperative view. **C,** DCIA flap donor site scar.

be inadequate to make two breasts. Bilateral DCIA flap breast reconstruction can also be done with minimal patient repositioning, unlike gluteal flaps.

COMPLICATIONS

DCIA flap complications are related primarily to donor-site closure, pain, and sensory nerve deficits. The DCIA donor wound is one of the few situations in plastic surgery where bone must be apposed to muscle to achieve wound closure. Postoperative donor-site pain is more severe than with other techniques and has been attributed to the transosseous sutures needed to restore abdominal-wall integrity.

Potential sensory nerve deficits can also be of significance. The lateral femoral cutaneous nerve can be preserved, but this may significantly increase the difficulty of flap harvest. Often a second sensory nerve can be found exiting the pelvis lateral to the ASIS; this is a cutaneous sensory branch of T12 that supplies part of the thigh over the proximal TFL muscle and fascia. If either nerve is injured, postoperative paresthesias, numbness, and neuromas may be a problem. All patients should be informed before surgery that some sensory deficit of the thigh will occur.

TFL Flaps

The TFL flap has been described as an alternative breast reconstruction method utilizing one of two basic designs. The lateral transverse thigh flap, as described by Elliot and associates (21), is a TFL flap with a horizontally based skin island that takes advantage of the "saddle bags" that many patients have. A second design is the "oblique" TFL flap, which also captures excess fat, but increases the skin island size that can be taken and still obtain primary closure (22). Both flaps have common anatomy in regards to vascular pedicle, muscle taken, and musculocutaneous perforators that are included.

FLAP ANATOMY (Fig. 72–7)

The TFL muscle itself is a small muscle originating from the anterior iliac crest and inserting into the iliotibial band. It has a type II blood supply from the lateral circumflex femoral artery, which originates from the profunda femoris artery. The lateral circumflex femoral artery passes between the branches of the femoral nerve, behind the sartorius and rectus femoris muscles, and divides into three branches. A descending branch supplies the rectus femoris and vastus lateralis muscle, and a transverse branch supplies the TFL from its deep surface (23). These musculocutaneous perforators are the key to skin paddle design for breast reconstruction. The artery is usually accompanied by two veins measuring 2 to 4 mm in diameter, which empty into the femoral vein (not the profunda femoris vein). Motor innervation of the TFL is the superior gluteal nerve. Sensory innervation of the overlying skin is supplied proximally by the lateral cutaneous branch of T12 and distally by the lateral cutaneous femoral nerve.

FLAP DESIGN AND DISSECTION (Fig. 72–8)

Contralateral or ipsilateral flaps can be used for breast reconstuction, with the patient in the supine position. The transverse skin island (lateral transverse thigh flap) is designed as a horizontal ellipse, with the axis centered over the lateral

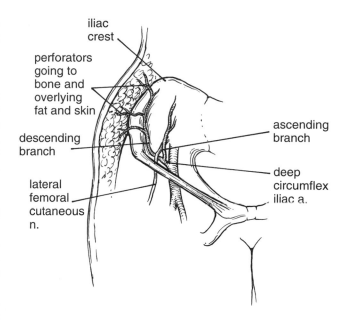

FIG. 72–7. TFL flap anatomy.

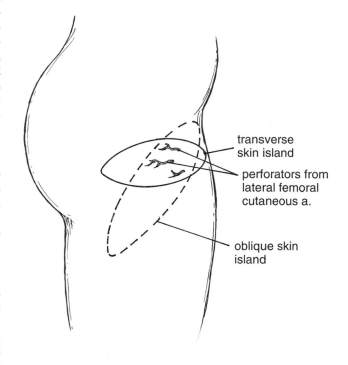

FIG. 72–8. TFL flap design.

femoral circumflex vessels and greater trochanter, extending back to the gluteal crease. The oblique skin-island axis is oriented superomedially and inferolaterally, allowing more skin and fat to be included with the flap without donor-site depression.

Dissection starts with the skin island, beveling out to capture more surrounding fat. A small cuff of TFL muscle, with its accompanying perforators, are taken with the skin island, and the pedicle is then dissected retrograde under the rectus femoris and sartorius muscles. Near the profunda femoris artery, care must taken to avoid injury to the femoral nerve branches.

FLAP CHARACTERISTICS

The TFL flap offers adequate volume in patients with "saddle bags," or collections of fat over the greater trochanter area. The quantity of skin available is limited (7–9 cm in vertical dimension) with the horizontal skin island (lateral thigh flap), but can be as large as 30 cm by 14 cm for the oblique skin island. The vascular pedicle is of adequate length (7–8 cm) and diameter (2–3 mm) to use with nearly all recipient vessels. The major drawback of this flap is donor-site contour irregularities with a scar in a noticeable position. Donor-site depression can be minimized with a muscle-sparing harvest and by limiting the amount of fat harvested. The donor scar may be unacceptable to some patients, and thorough patient education about this scar must be carried out preoperatively.

IDEAL PATIENT (Fig. 72–9)

The ideal candidate for TFL flap breast reconstruction is a patient who is concerned with saddle-bag fat collections, but

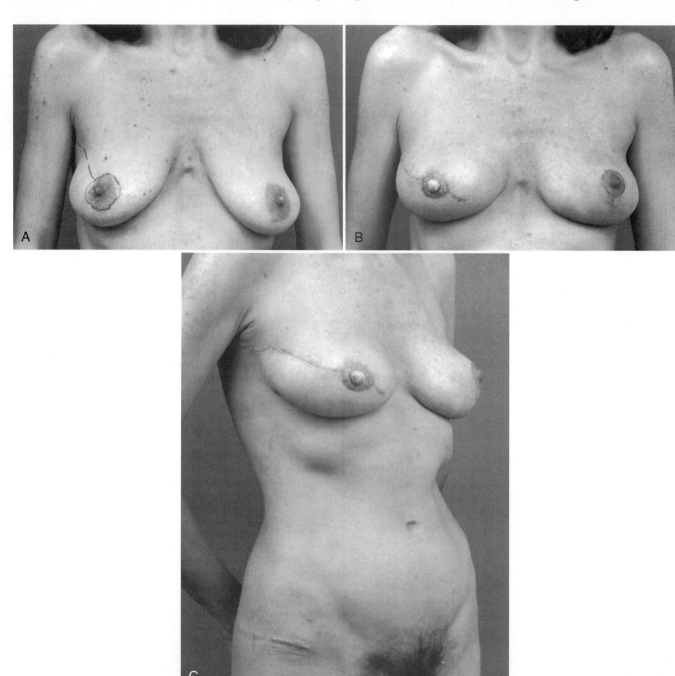

FIG. 72–9. Right breast reconstruction with TFL flap. **A,** preoperative view. **B,** postoperative view. **C,** TFL flap donor site scar.

is unconcerned about having a noticeable thigh scar (after thorough patient education). Unless the patient is willing to accept this scar, other choices should be considered. Because this flap can be harvested with the patient supine (with minimal hip rotation), it is an ideal option for bilateral breast reconstruction, unlike the gluteal flaps.

COMPLICATIONS

The most significant complication unique to the TFL flap is femoral nerve injury. Ambulatory disturbances due to muscle harvest are uncommon, since the TFL is an expendable muscle. Donor-site seroma formation is common, and most authors recommend prolonged closed suction drainage. The most common complaint by patients, however, is the aesthetic aspect of the donor deformity.

Other Free Flaps

Many other alternatives for free-flap breast reconstruction have been reported. Free contralateral latissimus dorsi breast reconstruction has been described by Serafin and colleagues (24). The groin flap, based on the superficial inferior epigastric artery, has been described for breast reconstruction; its small and unreliable vascular pedicle has limited its usefulness, however. LeQuang and associates have described using excess tissue from the opposite breast for reconstruction. The possibility of future breast cancer in the donor breast remains a concern. The bilateral inferior epigastric artery flap (BIEF) has also been advocated by Buncke, but adds the complexity of two vascular pedicles to the breast reconstruction. The gracilis flap has been used by Shaw for breast reconstruction in patients with excess medial thigh fat (22). This flap has limitations in volume and skin island reliability, however.

Recently, Allen and others (25) have described harvesting free flaps with no muscle. These flaps are harvested from the same donor sites, but the intramuscular vessels between the vascular pedicle and the cutaneous perforators are dissected free. This aggressive attempt to minimize donor-site morbidity by harvesting no muscle has been reported with high success rates by those familiar with this technique. The intramuscular dissection required for muscle preservation is a daunting technical challenge and may be associated with a higher risk of flap and vascular pedicle damage, as well as prolonged operating time.

Conclusion

In addition to TRAM flaps, several other free flaps are available for autologous breast reconstruction. In experienced hands, these flaps can be done safely with high success rates (Table 72–2). Because of donor site disadvantages or increased technical difficulty, these flaps are generally considered as secondary alternatives to the TRAM flap. They are an important option in the patient who is unsuitable for a TRAM flap because of a thin abdomen, unfavorable abdominal scars, or other special reasons. In bilateral breast reconstruction these alternatives may be especially useful when the patient's abdominal tissue is inadequate to create two breasts with a good aesthetic result. These alternative autologous tissue options should be made known to patients, regardless of the surgeon's own familiarity. Attempting a new and difficult reconstruction with no prior experience, however, is likely to give the patient a less-than-optimal result with high morbidity. Adequate patient education and surgeon experience should make these options more widely available as viable alternatives for autologous tissue transfer.

Table 72–2.
Flap Success Rates

Flap	Surgeon	Number	Success (%)
Pedicled TRAM	Hartrampf et al. (1)	700	98
Free TRAM	Shusterman et al. (26)	211	99
Superior Gluteal	Shaw	122	98
Inferior Gluteal	Nahai (3)	25	100
DCIA	Elliot	11	N/A
TFL	Elliot et al. (27)	17	94
Perforator	Allen (25)	11	100

References

1. Hartrampf CR. The transverse abdominal island flap for breast reconstruction: a 7-year experience. *Clin Plast Surg* 1988; 15:4.
2. Bostwick J, Jones G. Why I choose autologous tissue in breast reconstruction. *Clin Plast Surg* 1994; 21(2):167.
3. Codner M, Nahai F. The gluteal free flap breast reconstruction. *Clin Plast Surg* 1994; 21(2):289.
4. Ahn C, Shaw W. Unfavorable abdominal scars in TRAM flap harvest. Presented at the 63rd Annual Scientific Meeting of the American Society of Plastic and Reconstructive Surgeons, San Diego, September 1994.
5. Longaker M, Hong R, Colen L, et al. TRAM flap harvest in patients with endoscopic cholecystectomy scars. PSEF Senior Residents Conference, May 1995.
6. Galli A, Adami M, Berrino P, et al. Long-term evaluation of the abdominal wall competence after total and selective harvesting of the rectus abdominis muscle. *Ann Plast Surg* 1992; 28:409.
7. Chen L, Hartrampf CR, Bennett GK. Successful pregnancies following TRAM flap surgery. *Plast Reconstr Surg* 1993; 91(1):69.
8. Shaw WW. Bilateral free flap breast reconstruction. *Clin Plast Surg* 1994; 21(2):299.
9. Shaw WW, Ahn CY. Microvascular free flaps in breast reconstruction. *Clin Plast Surg* 1992; 19(3):917–926.
10. Fujino T, Harashina T, Aoyagi F. Reconstruction for aplasia of the breast and pectoral region by microvascular transfer of a free flap from the buttock. *Plast Reconstr Surg* 1975; 56:178.
11. Shaw WW. Breast reconstruction by superior gluteal microvascular free flaps without silicone implants. *Plast Reconstr Surg* 1983; 72:940.
12. Paletta CE, Bostwick J, Nahai F. The inferior gluteal free flap in breast reconstruction. *Plast Reconstr Surg* 1989; 89:875.
13. Kida MY, Takami Y, Ezoe K. The ramification of the superficial branch of the superior gluteal artery. *Surg Radiol Anat* 1992; 14(4):319–323.
14. Hurwitz DJ, Swartz WM, Mathes SJ. The gluteal thigh flap: a reliable sensate flap for the closure of buttock and perineal wounds. *Plast Reconstr Surg* 1981; 68:521.
15. Serafin D. The gluteus maximus muscle musculocutaneous flap. In: Serafin D, ed. *Atlas of microsurgical composite tissue transplantation*. Philadelphia: WB Saunders, 1996.
16. Strauch B, Yu HL. Gluteus maximus flap. In: Strauch B, Yu HL, eds. *Atlas of microvascular surgery*. New York: Thieme, 1993;102.
17. Shaw WW. Microvascular free flap breast reconstruction. *Clin Plast Surg* 1984; 11(1):333–343.
18. LeQuang C. Two new free flaps developed from aesthetic surgery. II. The inferior gluteal flap. *Aesthet Plast Surg* 1980; 4:159.
19. Taylor GI, Watson N. One-stage repair of compound leg defects with free, revascularized flaps of groin skin and iliac bone. *Plast Reconstr Surg* 1978; 61:494.

20. Hartrampf CR, Noel RT, Drazan L, et al. Rubens' fat pad for breast reconstruction: a perio-iliac soft-tissue free flap. *Plast Reconstr Surg* 1994; 93(2):402–407.

21. Elliot LF, Beegle PH, Hartrampf CR. The lateral transverse thigh free flap: an alternative for autogenous tissue breast reconstruction. *Plast Reconstr Surg* 1990; 85(2):169–178.

22. Shaw WW. Personal correspondence, November 1995.

23. Medot M, Fissette J. The cutaneous territory of the transverse tensor fascia lata flap: further anatomical considerations. *Surg Radiol Anat* 1993; 15(4):255–258.

24. Serafin D, Voci VE, Georgiade NG. Microsurgical composite tissue transplantation: indications and technical consideration in breast reconstruction following mastectomy. *Plast Reconstr Surg* 1982; 70:24.

25. Allen JR, Tucker C Jr. Superior gluteal artery perforator free flap for breast reconstruction. *Plast Reconstr Surg* 1995; 95(7):1207–1212.

26. Schusterman MA, Kroll SS, Miller MJ, et al. The free transverse rectus abdominis musculocutaneous flap for breast reconstruction: one center's experience with 211 consecutive cases. *Ann Plast Surg* 1994; 32(3):234–241.

73

Nipple Areola Reconstruction

Gregory S. Georgiade, M.D., F.A.C.S.

Nipple Areola Location

The location and size of the areola to be constructed is predetermined and marked with a permanent marker with the patient in an upright position. The nipple and areola marking is placed on the reconstructed breast mound at a slightly lower level than the opposite breast mound. The diameter of the new areola is relative in size to the opposite areola and its final location must be at the same distance from the midline as its opposite.

Nipple Reconstruction

NIPPLE SHARING

The nipple sharing technique previously described by Georgiade and colleagues (1) is the simplest and most direct method yielding a protruding nipple with the same color characteristics as the opposite nipple. This technique is particularly desirable when the donor nipple is of sufficient size that will allow it to be reduced in size (approximately 50%). The nipple sharing procedure yields a consistently satisfactory result when the remaining "donor" nipple is large enough in size to be evenly divided. The procedure consists of excising a V-configuration of the donor nipple and transferring this nipple as a free full-thickness graft to the newly prepared bed on the reconstructed breast mound. The new nipple is maintained in this position utilizing 3-0 chromic catgut sutures throughout the entire thickness of the graft and the underlying dermis in a radial fashion, finally attaching the graft to its new bed—which was prepared by depithelialization of the full-thickness skin, leaving a layer of underlying dermis. The donor defect is closed with interrupted 5-0 Vicryl sutures (Fig. 73–1).

LOCAL CHEST FLAP

At the present time, three types of chest flaps have been found to yield satisfactory nipples.

The use of a local full-thickness chest flap, either inferiorly or superiorly based, can be designed and elevated to the desired final position of a new nipple (1) (Fig. 73–2A). The flap is designed to be approximately 35% greater in width and length than the final new nipple. Once the position and size of the areola have been determined on the new breast mound, the flap to be elevated is carefully marked with brilliant green or methylene blue dye. The entire new areola, except for the flap area, is then deepithelialized (Fig. 73–2B). The nipple flap is elevated as a full-thickness flap, including

the underlying subcutaneous tissue (Fig. 73–2B). The newly outlined nipple can be tattooed before elevation; or, tattooing is also easily carried out a few weeks postoperative (2). The quantity of underlying tissue to be incorporated in the flap will vary with the desired size of the new nipple. The elevated nipple flap is surrounded by contiguous thick split-thickness skin flaps resembling bat wings (Fig. 73–2B, C). These split-thickness skin flaps are then wrapped around the newly elevated nipple flap (Fig. 73–2D). The base of the flap is tubed utilizing a 4-0 or 5-0 Vicryl suture at the base of the defect created by elevation of the flap. The defect created by elevation of the flap is covered with a full-thickness groin graft to reconstruct the areola at the same time (Fig. 73–1D, 73–2D). The defect created by elevation of the nipple flap can be closed primarily and then the predetermined areola area is micrpigmented. We have used this technique since 1981 with satisfactory results (1).

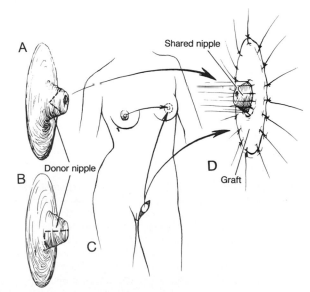

FIG. 73–1. **A, B,** an appropriate-sized opposite nipple segment can be used for reconstruction of a new nipple. **C,** the new areola is reconstructed with a full-thickness skin graft from the inner aspect of the groin (usually lateral to the labia). **D,** the nipple is sutured in place before fixation of the areola graft over a bolus over the nipple-areolar area.

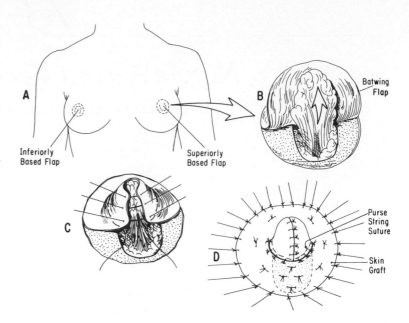

FIG. 73–2. **A,** the nipple flap can be reconstructed using either a superiorly or inferiorly based flap. **B,** the flap is raised including the underlying fat for bulk. Deepithelialization of the new areola area is carried out, creating thick split-thickness surrounding flaps. **C,** the thick split-thickness areola skin flaps are wrapped around the exposed portion of the elevated nipple flap. The excess is trimmed at the nipple base. **D,** the reconstructed nipple. A 4-0 Dexon pursestring suture is placed at the base to maintain the nipple in an elevated and protrusive position. The groin graft is sutured in position with catgut "tacking sutures" and a bolus used to stabilize the graft around the newly created nipple.

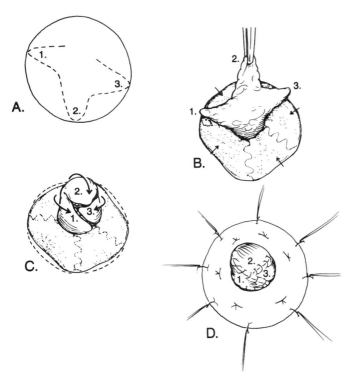

FIG. 73–3. **A,** chest flaps 1 and 3 are marked at different levels on the new planned areola. **B,** flaps 1, 2, and 3 are raised and the sites are closed primarily. The areola is deepithelialized. **C,** flaps 1 and 3 are interpolated around flap 2, which is turned to create the nipple height. Deepithelialization adjustments are made to compensate for primary closure of flap donor areas. **D,** the newly created nipple. A full-thickness groin graft covers the deepithelialized areola area. A bolus is tied over newly created nipple and areolar graft.

The modification of the original "star flap" procedure (2,3) utilizes three flaps based at different positions projecting laterally from the main flap. This modification allows a more precise interpolation of the lateral flaps (5). The tip, 1, of the main flap (Fig. 73–3) is turned over with the interpolated flaps, 1 and 3, beneath the tip of the main flap, (2). A thick groin skin graft is applied to the predetermined deepithelialized area to create the new areola.

The third possibility for a successful nipple reconstruction is a clever use of the midline redundant TRAM flap as described by McCraw (4). This technique is designed to create bilobed flaps of the redundant TRAM flap (Fig. 73–4A). The bilobed flaps, (5), are rotated in opposite directions, creating interpolated flaps and a new nipple with adequate height (Fig. 73–4B-E). Care must be taken preoperatively to accurately plan the location of the nipple areola. The areola is then reconstructed with a suitably pigmented groin graft. (Fig. 73–4D, E).

Areola Reconstruction

Construction of the areola is usually carried out as a free full-thickness skin graft obtained from the inner aspect of the thigh (groin) area. The most posterior portion of the inner thigh crease of the skin will yield a more pigmented areola, which may be more desirable depending on the color tones of the opposite areola (see Fig. 73–1C, D). A tie-on bolus of cotton is used to immobilize the areola graft for 7 days.

The areola can also be created by tattooing without the use of a graft (5–7).

Tattooing

Intradermal tattooing can be carried out either at the time of the initial nipple areolar reconstruction or as an outpatient office procedure post nipple construction.

There is usually some color disparity between the newly constructed nipple areola and the opposite areola. To attain a more acceptable color match, we have been utilizing selective tattoo pigmentation for over 20 years (5,6). Pigment color charts are available, and we use them for attaining the best color match of the pigments. Infrequently, it is necessary to mix the selected basic color with other pigments for the best match. The tattooing can be via a multiple tattoo needle technique or by use of a professional electric vibrating tat-

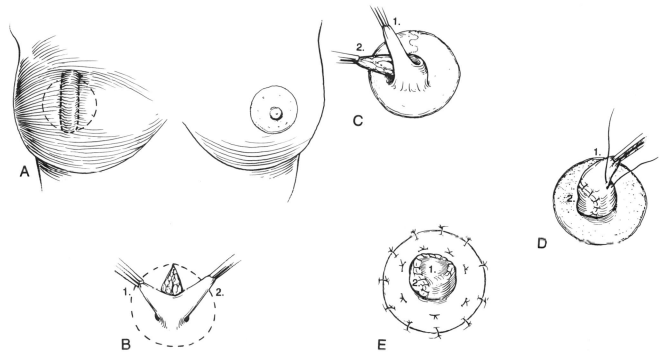

FIG. 73–4.   A, the redundant area of a TRAM flap is marked for the position of a new areola. **B,** flaps 1 and 2 are elevated utilizing the redundant TRAM flap tissue. **C,** Flaps 1 and 2 are now interpolated. **D,** the position of new flaps 1 and 2. The surrounding area of areola is deepithelialized. **E,** the newly reconstructed nipple and full-thickness skin graft.

tooing instrument with multiple needles. One must keep in mind that there is eventually lightening of the original tattooed areas.

References

1. Georgiade N, Riefkohl R, Georgiade GS. To share or not to share. *Ann Plast Surg* 1985; 14:180.
2. Anton M, Hartrampf C. Nipple reconstruction with the star flap. *Perspect Plast Surg* 1991; 5:67.
3. Eskenazi L. A one-stage nipple reconstruction with the "modified star" flap and immediate tattoo: a review of 100 cases. *Plast Reconstr Surg* 1993; 92:671.
4. McCraw J. 1995 construction of nipple via a TRAM flap. Personal communication and illustrations, 1995.
5. Georgiade N. Nipple tattooing. In: Georgiade NG, ed. *Reconstructive breast surgery.* St. Louis: CV Mosby, 1976; 310.
6. Georgiade N. In: Georgiade NG, ed. *Breast reconstruction following mastectomy.* St. Louis: CV Mosby, 1979; 249.
7. Wong RK, Banducel PR, Feldman S, et. al. Reconstruction tattooing eliminates the need for skin grafting in nipple areolar reconstruction. *Plast Reconstr Surg* 1993; 92:547.

74

Gynecomastia

Ronald Riefkohl, M.D., F.A.C.S., George P. Zavitsanos, M.D., and Eugene H. Courtiss, M.D., F.A.C.S.

Gynecomastia is a benign enlargement of the male breast. It is literally translated from its greek origins *gynes* (woman) and *mastos* (breast). Historical writings and artifacts document the presence of gynecomastia as early as 1559 B.C. (1). It has been speculated that historical depictions of Tutankhamen and his father and brothers demonstrate familial gynecomastia (1). Opponents of this theory argue that ancient depictions of breasted male rulers may have been mythologic symbols of their fertile and nurturing qualities (1). During the seventh century A.D., the first surgical treatment of gynecomastia was reported in the writings of Paulus of Aeginata, who lived from 1635 to 1690 A.D. (2). It was not until 1928 that Dufourmentel formally described the intraareolar approach for surgical correction of the gynecomastia (3).

Incidence

The incidence of gynecomastia in the literature varies considerably. Problems arise in the clinical definition and selection bias of studied patient groups. There are three distinct peaks in the age distribution of gynecomastia. Neonatal gynecomastia develops in approximately 60 to 90% of all neonates (4). It is caused by the transplacental migration of estrogens and uniformly resolves. The second peak occurs during puberty (peak 13 to 16 years of age) with an incidence varying between 4 and 69% (4–8). Nydick and colleagues (8) reported an overall incidence of gynecomastia of 38.7% in 1,855 nonobese Boy Scouts 10 to 16 years of age. A peak incidence of 65% was found in boys 14 to 14.5 years of age. In 27% of the cases, gynecomastia persisted for 12 months, and in 7.7% it persisted for 24 months or more (8). The third peak incidence is found in the adult population. Reported incidences, in the literature, vary between 35 and 65%, depending on clinical criteria of gynecomastia and patient selection (1–3). The incidence of bilaterality also varies in the literature. Nydick and colleagues reported on the incidence of 75% bilaterality in pubertal gynecomastia, while other authors report incidences varying from 25% to 50% (1–4).

Clinical Findings

Gynecomastia can be defined as a palpable or visible breast mass that ranges from 1 to 10 cm in diameter, with an average of 4 cm in diameter (5). It can range from a small discoid subareolar mass of breast tissue, often seen in pubertal gynecomastia, to diffuse enlargement of the entire breast. It can be comprised of varying amounts of breast adipose tissue, depending on the etiology and age of presentation. Initial onset can be unilateral and often progresses to bilateral

development. Age of onset varies with clinical etiologies, which may include hormonal changes associated with puberty, endocrine dysfunction, metabolic disorders, drugs, and neoplasms. Patients are often asymptomatic and, in most series, only 10 to 20% of patients experience pain, where as up to 33% may have tenderness (5,16). These symptoms are usually noted in the initial 4 to 6 months of development, particularly in the pubertal patient. By far the most distressing aspect to the patient is the alteration in body image. School-age children particularly are susceptible to the ridicule of peers. Adults may likewise have considerable embarrassment and anxiety regarding gynecoid breasts. The goal in management of gynecomastia should be the restoration of normal male body image. Aesthetic results are of paramount importance in achieving this goal.

Histology

The development of gynecomastia can be divided into three distinct types based on histologic findings. These are described as florid, intermediate, and fibrous types (17). There is generally a progression from the florid type to the fibrous type, depending on the duration of the gynecomastia; this is unrelated to the etiology (18). Gynecomastia of less than 4 months' duration is of the florid type. Fibrous gynecomastia usually develops after 1 year, whereas the intermediate type is typically found between 4 months and 1 year.

In the florid type, there is an increase in the number and length of ducts, proliferation of ductal epithelium, periductal edema, and a highly cellular, fibroblastic stroma with hypervascularity (Fig. 74–1). The florid process may regress or may continue to develop dense fibrosis and hyalinization that are characteristic of the fibrous type.

In the fibrous type, there are dilated ducts with minimal proliferation of epithelium, absence of periductal edema, and a relatively acellular fibrous stroma without adipose tissue (Fig. 74–2). The intermittent type is the overlapping pattern of both the florid and fibrous type; it seldom regresses.

Etiology

The underlying etiology usually involves either the relative or the absolute excess of circulating estrogens, a deficiency of circulating androgens, or a defect in androgens receptors. The key element in the development of gynecomastia centers around an elevated ratio of estrogens to androgens, which can occur through a variety of etiologies (Table 74–1). The clinical etiologies are based on four broad categories: physiologic, pathologic, pharmacologic, and familial. Most pa-

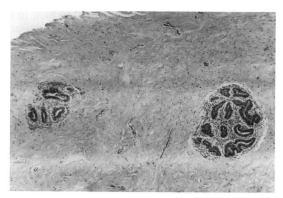

FIG. 74-1.   In the florid type of gynecomastia, there is an increase in the number and length of ducts, proliferation of ductal epithelium, periductal edema, a highly cellular fibroblastic stroma and hypervascularity, and the formation of pseudolobules. (From Georgiade NG, Georgiade GS, Riefkohl R: *Aesthetic surgery of the breast.* Philadephia, WB Saunders, 1990.)

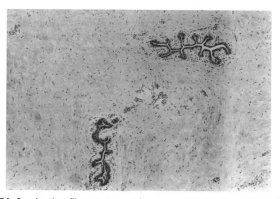

FIG. 74-2.   In the fibrous type of gynecomastia, there are dilated ducts with minimal proliferation of epithelium, absence of periductal edema, and an almost cellular fibrous stroma without adipose tissue. (From Georgiade NG, Georgiade GS, Riefkohl R: *Aesthetic surgery of the breast.* Philadephia, WB Saunders, 1990.)

tients seeking consultation in gynecomastia will be found to have acute or persistent gynecomastia arising from puberty (25%) or idiopathic gynecomastia (25%) (4). A small proportion of patients will have gynecomastia owing to drugs (10 to 20%), cirrhosis malnutrition (8%), primary hypogonadism (8%), testicular tumors (3%), secondary to hypogonadism (2%), hypothyroidism (1.5%), or renal disease (1%) (4).

PHYSIOLOGIC GYNECOMASTIA

The development of neonatal gynecomastia occurs in 60 to 90% of all newborns (4). This is because of the transplacental migration of maternal estrogens, and usually resolves within several weeks (4).

The development of prepubertal gynecomastia is a rare event, with 41 cases described in the literature (19). Unlike pubertal gynecomastia, prepubertal gynecomastia often involves a pathologic etiology and warrants a thorough examination upon initial consultation. Evaluations should include a chromosome analysis and a complete endocrine evaluation including the assay of 11 beta hydroxylase levels (19). Idiopathic prepubertal gynecomastia is rare and usually self-

Table 74-1.
Classification of Gynecomastia by Etiology

Physiologic
  Newborn
  Adolescent
  Aging (involutional)

Pathologic
  Deficient production or action of testosterone
  Klinefelter syndrome
  Androgen resistance
    Testicular feminization
    Reifenstein syndrome
  Defects in testosterone synthesis
  Secondary testicular failure
    Viral orchitis
    Trauma
  Increased substrate for peripheral aromatase
    Adrenal disease
    Liver disease
    Malnutrition
    Hyperthyroidism
  Increase in peripheral aromatase

Drugs

Familial

limited. The severity of gynecomastia will determine the necessity of surgical intervention.

Pubertal gynecomastia is a relatively common finding that occurs in approximately 38% of adolescents. During the transient period from the prepubertal to pubertal phase, there is a thirtyfold increase in the testosterone concentration, whereas the concentration of estrogens increase threefold. The etiology of pubertal gynecomastia is not clear. Some authors speculate that a relative imbalance of estrogen to testosterone may exist in the very early pubertal phase, and that this may be responsible for the initiation of the development of gynecomastia (4). Moore and associates (20) have suggested the possibility of an elevated ratio of estradiol relative to androgens, of adrenal origin, which may be responsible for the initiation of pubertal gynecomastia (20).

Multiple etiologies account for adult-onset gynecomastia, which is relatively common and varies from 35 to 65%, depending on clinical inclusion criteria and physical examination criteria (9–11). Progressive testicular failure, combined with the elevation in lutenizing hormone levels, is a significant factor in the development of gynecomastia associated with aging. Furthermore, there is a simultaneous increase in estrogen-binding globulin, which further decreases the amount of free testosterone (21). Increasing adiposity leads to greater conversion of androgens to estrogens through increased peripheral aromatization in the adipose tissue (4,21,22). These are thought to be the major factors responsible for the gynecomastia associated with aging. Because of the numerous pathologic states that can cause gynecomastia, the diagnosis of physiologic gynecomastia in the adult population remains a diagnosis of exclusion.

PATHOLOGIC GYNECOMASTIA

A wide variety of pathologic states are associated with gynecomastia in the pediatric and adult populations. These in-

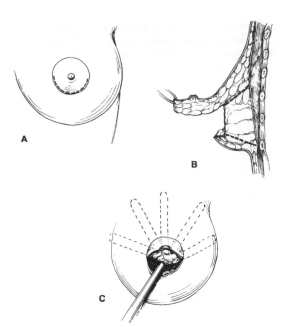

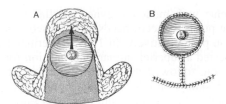

FIG. 74–7. **A,** the nipple-areolar complex may be transposed superiorly on an inferiorly based pedicle, with **(B)** a resulting T-shaped inframammary scar.

FIG. 74–6. **A,** periareolar incision just within the areola. **B,** a sufficient thickness of areolar breast tissue stays with the pedicle to avoid a postoperative depression and "donut" effect of residual breast tissue. The remaining underlying breast tissue is excised tangentially. **C,** the remaining aspects of the breasts are decreased with liposuction in all directions.

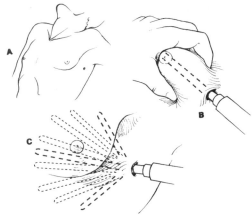

FIG. 74–8. **A, B,** lateral anterior axillary approach to the breast for liposuction. **C,** complete liposuction of the breast is possible with lateral approach.

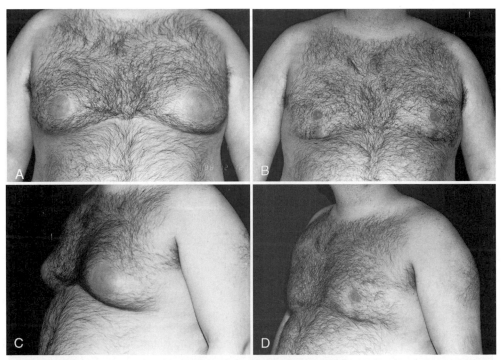

FIG. 74–9. **A,** preoperative frontal view of a 25-year-old male, 5 feet 9 inches tall, and weighing 250 pounds. He complained of large breasts from 12 years of age. **B,** postoperative frontal view 3 years after treatment, showing results of removal of 300 ml of fat by suction, 200 ml of gland per side by resection, and areolar reduction by the VOQ technique of Regnault. **C,** left oblique preoperative view. **D,** left oblique view 3 years postoperatively. (Reproduced with permission from Hetter G: Blunt suction-assisted lipectomy. In: *Mastery of plastic and reconstructive surgery* (pp. 238–239). Copyright 1994 by Mimis Cohen. Boston: Little, Brown.)

Table 74–3.
Complications of Surgical Reduction

Inversion of nipple or areola
Nipple or areola necrosis
Contour deformity
Conspicuous scars
Residual skin redundancy
Inadequate breast excision
Breast asymmetry
Hematoma and fluid collection
Infection

breast. Contouring of the chest wall with direct excision and liposuction will enhance postoperative results. If nipple viability is questionable, then the surgeon can consider free nipple grafting (58).

In summary, skin excision techniques are only warranted in patients with very large gynecomastia, with considerable skin redundancy and laxity, as is often seen in the elderly or massive weight-loss patient (58). With the advent of liposuction in conjunction with direct excision techniques and inframammary fold detruction, there are few clinical circumstances where direct skin excision will be necessary (Figs. 74–8, 74–9). If the surgeon has concerns regarding the adequacy of more conservative techniques, skin excision can always be performed at a later time.

Results and Complications

Usually, patients are enormously satisfied with the postoperative results. These individuals are often ashamed of their transsexual appearance and signs of femininity and are embarrassed to participate in sports or swimming activities. The complication rate is low, and most complications can easily be prevented (Table 74–3). Inversion or folding of the nipple-areolar complex can be prevented by maintaining adequate thickness of tissue on the nipple areolar flap, as well as maintaining adequate tissue on the pectoralis fascia. Nipple-areolar necrosis is unlikely if adequate dermal circulation is present and the tissues are handled gently. Contour and size asymmetries are prevented by carefully marking the extent of the hypertrophied tissue preoperatively and insuring the same thickness of tissue on the nipple-areola and skin flaps on both sides. The advent of liposuction has seemed to decrease the incidence of overresection by allowing a more gradual contouring of the chest wall. In a retrospective review of 38 patients, liposuction in conjunction with excision yielded complications that included seroma (10%), hematoma (5%), underresection (3%), and no cases of overresection (60). Prior to the advent of liposuction, this investigator's early experience with direct excision techniques yielded an overresection rate of 19% and a hematoma rate of 16% (60). The incidence of hematoma and/or seroma can be minimized in the postoperative period with compression garments, particularly with wide areas of liposuction, which will also enhance the aesthetic results. Postoperative suction drains are optional and are used as indicated. Residual skin redundancy is a possibility, particularly with the decreased skin elasticity often seen in the elderly or massive weight-loss patients. Avoidance of this complication involves adequate preoperative planning regarding the necessity of skin excision, as well as

postoperative pressure garments to facilitate a more cephalad repositioning of the nipple to the chest wall.

References

1. Paulshock BZ. Tutankhamen and his brothers: familial gynecomastia in the eighteenth dynasty. *JAMA,* 1980; 244:160–164.
2. Aeginata P. The seven books of Paulus Aeiginata (translated from greek by Francis Adams) London: London Sydenham Society, 1848, Vol. 2, Book 6, Sec. 46.
3. DuFourmentel L. L'incision areolaire dans la chirurgie du sein. *Bull Mim Soc Chir* Paris, 1928; 20:9.
4. Braunstein GD. Gynecomastia. *N Engl J Med* 1993; 328(7):490–495.
5. Nutall FQ. Gynecomastia as a physical finding in normal men. *J Clin Endocrinol Metab* 1979; 48:338–340.
6. Fara GM, Del Corvo G, Bernuzzi S, et al. Epidemic of breast enlargement in an Italian school. *Lancet* 1979; 2:295–297.
7. Harlan WR, Grillo GP, Cornoni-Huntley J, et al. Secondary sex characteristics of boys 12 to 17 years of age: the U.S. Health Examination Survey. *J Pediatr* 1979; 95.293–297.
8. Nydick M, Bustos J, Dale JH, et al. Gynecomastia in adolescent boys. *JAMA* 1961; 178:449–454.
9. Anderson JA, Gram JB. Male breast at autopsy. *Acta Pathol Microbio Immunol Scand,* 1982; 90:633–638.
10. Williams MR. Gynecomastia: its incidence, recognition, and host characterization in 447 autopsy cases. *Am J Med* 1963; 34:103–112.
11. Niewoehner CB, Nuttal FQ. Gynecomastia in a hospitalized male population. *Am J Med* 1984; 77:633–638.
12. Mahoney CP. Adolescent gynecomastia: differential diagnosis and management. *Ped Clin of North Am* 1990; 37(6):1389–1404.
13. Hamer DB. Gynecomastia. *Br J Surg* 1975; 62:326–329.
14. Von Kessel F, Pickrell KF, Huger WG, et al. Surgical treatment of gynecomastia: an analysis of 275 cases. *Ann Surg* 1963; 157:142–151.
15. Wheeler CE, Cawley EP, Gray HT.
16. Knorr D, Bidlingmaier F. Gynecomastia in male adolescents. *Clin Endocrinol Metab* 1975; 4:157–171.
17. Bannayan GA, Hijdu SI. Gynecomastia: clinicopathologic study of 351 cases. *Am J Clin Path* 1972; 57:431–437.
18. Rodriguez-Rigau LJ, Smith KD. Gynecomastia. In: Degroot LJ, ed. *Endocrinology.* 2nd ed. Philadelphia: WB Saunders, 1989; 2207–2209.
19. Haibach H, Rosenhaoltz MF. Prepubertal gynecomastia with lobules and acini: a case report and review of the literature. *Am J Clin Path* 1983; 80:252–255.
20. More DC, Schlaepfer LV, Paunier L, et al. Hormonal changes during puberty. V. Transient pubertal gynecomastia: abnormal androgen-estrogen ratios. *J Clin Endocrinol Metab* 1984; 58:492–499.
21. Stearns EL, MacDonnel JA, Kaufman BJ, et al. Declining testicular function with age: hormonal and clinical correlates. *Am J Med* 1974; 57:761–766.
22. Carlson HE. Gynecomastia. *N Engl J Med* 1980; 303:796–799.
23. Scheike O, Visfeldt J. Male breast cancer: breast carcinoma in association with the Klinefelter syndrome. *Acta Pathol Microbiol Scand* 1973; 81(3):352–358.
24. Jackson VP, Gilmor RL. Male breast carcinoma and gynecomastia: comparison of mammography with sonagraphy. *Radiology* 1983; 149:533–536.
25. Wilson JD. Aiman J, MacDonald PC. The pathogenesis of gynecomastia. *Adv Intern Med* 1980; 25:1–25.
26. Jacobs EC. Effects of starvation of sex hormones in the male. *J Clin Endocrin* 1948; 8:227–232.
27. Ashlar FS, Smoak WM, Gilson AJ, et al. Gynecomastia and mastaplasia in Graves' disease. *Metabolism* 1970; 19:946–951.
28. Smith SR, Cheetri MK, Johanson AJ, et al. The pituitary gonadal axis in men with protein calorie meal nutrition. *J Clin Endocrin Metab* 1975; 41:60–69.
29. Pope HG, Katz DL. Psychiatric and medical effects of anabolic androgenic steroid use: a controlled study of 160 athletes. *Arch Gen Psychiatry* 1994; 51(5):375–382.
30. Aiache AE. Surgical treatment of gynecomastia in the body builder. *Plast Reconstr Surg* 1989; 83(1):61–66.
31. Haagensen CD. Carcinoma of the male breast. In: *Diseases of the breast.* Philadelphia: WB Saunders, 1971; 779–780.
32. Holleb AI, Freeman HP, Farrow JH. Cancer of the male breast. *NY St J Med* 1968; 68:544–553.

33. Male Breast Cancer. In: Fentiman IS, ed. *Detection and treatment of early breast cancer.* Philadelphia: JB Lippincott, 1990; 207–218.

34. Treves N. Gynecomastia: the origins of mammary swelling in the male—an analysis of 406 patients with breast hypertrophy, 525 with testicular tumors, and 13 with adrenal neoplasms. *Cancer* 1958; 11:1083–1102.

35. Kuhn JM, Roca R, Laudat MH, et al. Studies on the treatment of idiapathic gynecomastia with percutaneous dihydrotestosterone.

36. LeRoith D, Sobel R, Glick SM. The effect of clomiphene citrate on pubertal gynecomastia. *Acta Endocrinol* 1980; 95:177–180.

37. Buckle R. Studies on the treatment of gynaecomastia with danazol (Danol). *J Int Med Res (suppl)* 1977; 3:114–117.

38. Buckle R. Danazol in the treatment of gynaecomastia. *Drugs* 1980; 19:356–361.

39. Plano VF. Danazol: review of recent studies. *J Am Osteopath Assoc* 1980; 79:530–534.

40. Jones DJ, Holt SD, Surtes P, et al. A comparison of danazol and placebo in the treatment of adult idiopathic gynecomastia: results of a prospective study in 55 patients. *Ann R Coll Surg Eng* 1990; 72(5):296–298.

41. Parker LN, Gray DR, Lai MK, et al. Treatment of gynecomastia with tamoxifen: a double-blind crossover study. *Metabolism* 1986; 35:705–707.

42. McDermott MT, Hofeldt FD, Kidd GS. Tamoxifen therapy for painful idiopathic gynecomastia. *South Med J* 1990; 83:1283–1285.

43. Gagnon JD, Moss WT, Stevens KR. Pre-estrogen breast irradiation for patients with carcinoma of the prostate: a critical review. *J Urol* 1979; 121:182.

44. Metzger H, Junker A, Voss AC. Irradiation of the breast glands as prophylactic treatment of an estrogen-induced gynecomastia in patients with prostate carcinoma. *Strahlentherapie* 1980; 156, 102–104.

45. Waterfall NB, Glasser MG. A study of the effects of radiation on prevention of gynecomastia due to estrogen therapy. *Clin Oncol* 1979; 5:257–260.

46. Courtiss EH. Reduction mammoplasty by suction alone. *Plast Reconstr Surg* 1193; 92(7):1276–1284.

47. Becker H. The treatment of gynecomastia without sharp excision. *Ann Plast Surg* 1990; 24(4):380–383.

48. Rosenberg GJ. A new cannula for suction removal of parenchymal tissue of gynecomastia. *Plast Reconstr Surg* 1994; 94(3):548–551.

49. Simon BE, Haffman S, Kahn S. Classification and surgical correction of gynecomastia. *Plast Reconstr Surg* 1973; 51:48–52.

50. Webster JP. Mastectomy for gynecomastia through a semicircular intra-areolar incision. *Ann Surg* 1946; 124.

51. Barsky AJ, Kahn S, Simon BE. In: *Principles and practice of plastic surgery.* 2nd ed. New York: McGraw-Hill, 1964; 564–568.

52. Eade GG. The radial incision for gynecomastia excision. *Plast Reconstr Surg* 1974; 54:495–497.

53. Teimourian B, Perlman R. Surgery for gynecomastia. *Aesth Plast Surg* 1983; 7:155–157.

54. Letterman G, Shurter M. Surgical correction of gynecomastia. *Ann Surg* 1969; 35:322–325.

55. Davidson BA. Concentric circle operation for massive gynecomastia to excise the redundant skin. *Plast Reconstr Surg* 1979; 63:350.

56. Cohen IK, Pozez AL, McKeown JE. Gynecomastia. In: Courtiss EH, ed. *Male aesthetic surgery.* 2nd ed. St. Louis: Mosby–Yearbook, 1991; 373–395.

57. Wray RC, Hoopes JE, Davis GM. Correction of extreme gynecomastia. *Br J Plast Surg* 1974; 27:39–42.

58. Courtiss EH, Becker H, Rosenberg GJ, et al. Treatment of gynecomastia. *Aesthetic Surgery* 1994; 4–9.

59. Kornstein AN, Cnelli PB. Inferior pedicle reduction technique for larger forms of gynecomastia. *Aesth Plast Surg* 1992; 16:331–336.

60. Courtiss EH. Gynecomastia: analysis of 159 patients and current recommendations for treatment. *Plast Reconstr Surg* 1987; 79, 740.

75

Mediastinitis

Gregory S. Georgiade, M.D., F.A.C.S., and Robert Rehnke, M.D.

Chest wall defects may be the result of trauma or of mediastinitis following open heart surgery or ablative surgery. Less commonly, thoracic defects may be due to extensive radiation or developmental anomalies.

Management

MAJOR DÉBRIDEMENT

Major débridement involves excision of the margins of soft tissues and débridement of the sternum and any of the involved costocartilages back to normal-appearing ribs. Extensive removal of the infected sternum may result in chest wall instability with ensuing respiratory difficulties (1). Patients with localized infection of the skin and subcutaneous tissue can usually be managed by local excision, débridement and delayed closure with drainage. Complete sternal separation with exposure of the underlying heart and vein grafts in the depths of the wound requires more extensive planning for closure of the defect utilizing a variety of possible muscle transpositions to fill the exposed dead space.

RIB GRAFTS

Autogenous rib grafts are infrequently necessary to stabilize the chest by bridging the sternal defect for future stability. The rib grafts are usually covered by pectoralis major muscle flaps.

PRIMARY CLOSURE

Occasionally, undermining of the chest skin, with medial advancement of these skin flaps and sternal rewiring, will allow delayed primary closure of the chest wound if antibiotic irrigation catheters and chest tube drainage are employed (2). This type of procedure will not be successful in a grossly infected, inadequately débrided environment.

MUSCLE FLAPS

Pectoralis Major Muscle Flaps

Advancement and transposition of one or both pectoralis major muscle flaps is probably one of the most frequently used procedures for reconstruction of the anterior chest wall defects (1–5). It is preferable initially to transfer the nondominant pectoralis major muscle following extensive débridement (5) (Fig. 75–1). If this flap is not sufficient because of the extent of the defect, the opposite pectoralis muscle flap can then be used.

In order to obtain the maximum pectoralis rotation for mediastinal cover, the muscle is dissected free from the overlying skin and the pectoralis major muscle is divided from the humerus in the anterior axillary fold, following separation of the pectoralis major muscle from the underlying chest wall. The attachments to the clavicle are also released. Care must be taken to identify and preserve the thoracoacromial vessels, which enter the pectoralis major muscle along its posterior surface and just lateral to the midclavicular line. The pectoralis muscle flap is then advanced and rotated to cover the mediastinal defect and secured in position by suturing it to the soft tissues on the opposite side of the defect. If necessary, the opposite pectoralis muscle can be used to cover additional areas of the sternal defect (Fig. 75–2).

Pectoralis Major Turnover Flap

The use of the pectoralis major turnover flap (5) is made anatomically feasible because of its dual blood supply. The alternate blood supply to the body of the pectoralis major muscle is based on the internal mammary artery. The branches of the internal mammary artery to the pectoralis major muscle are located lateral to the border of the sternum as they advance into the body of the pectoralis major musculature from the second to the 6th intercostal spaces. The lateral pectoral nerve innervates the medial portion of the pectoralis major muscle. This technique of using the medial portion of the pectoral musculature preserves the anterior axillary fold and the lateral one-third of the pectoralis major musculature and its neurovascular pedicle.

Technically the use of this flap involves the same procedure as previously described in separating the skin from the pectoralis musculature to the lateral clavicular area. The pectoralis major muscle is then separated from the pectoralis minor muscle and underlying chest wall. The pectoralis major muscle is then divided just medial to the entry point of the thoracoacromial blood supply. This provides two-thirds of the pectoralis major muscle for use as a turnover flap. The dissection is then carried medially, elevating the pectoralis major muscle and turning it over into the mediastinal defect (Fig. 75–3). The dissection is carried to within 2 to 3 cm of the sternal border, at which point the branches of the internal mammary artery are identified. This single turnover flap will yield significant muscle bulk. A segmented portion, or all, of the pectoralis major muscle may be used in this fashion (Figs. 75–4, 75–5). The severed lateral portion of the pectoralis major muscle may be sutured to the underlying pectoralis minor muscle.

In patients who have had the internal mammary artery used in a revascularization of the coronary vessels, this type

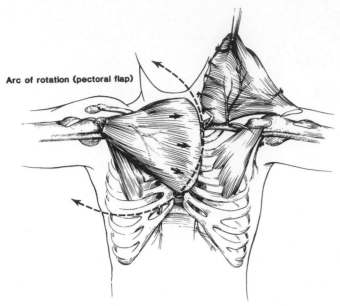

FIG. 75–1. The nondominant pectoralis major muscle with its arc of rotation.

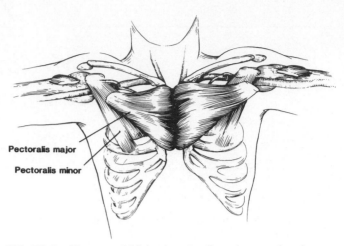

FIG. 75–2. The use of bilateral pectoralis major muscle advancement flaps to fill the midline defect.

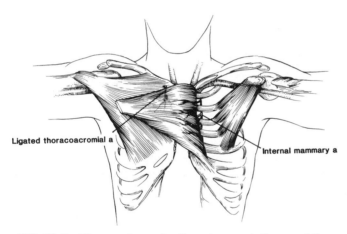

FIG. 75–3. The use of a pectoralis major muscle "turnover" flap.

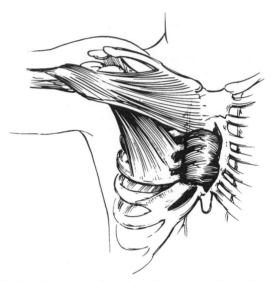

FIG. 75–4. A segmented portion of the pectoralis major muscle used as a "turnover" flap for a smaller defect.

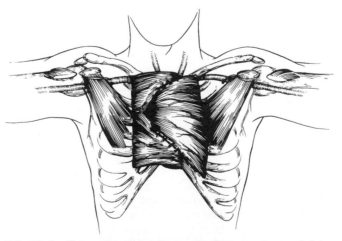

FIG. 75–5. Two entire pectoralis muscle flaps can be used, interdigitated for maximum closure and thickness, to fill the mediastinal defect.

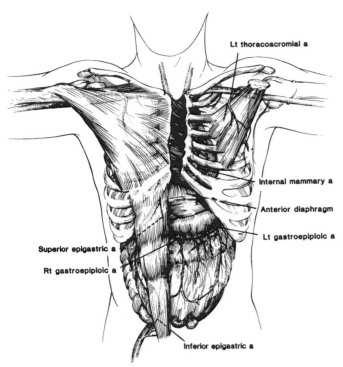

FIG. 75–6. The blood supply of the long flat rectus abdominis muscle, which extends from the pubis to the costochondral area.

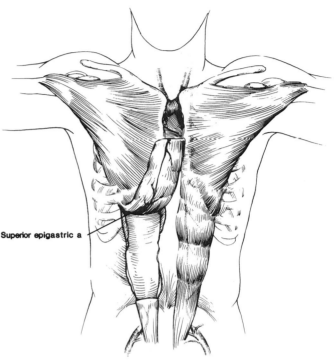

FIG. 75–7. The rectus abdominis muscle is shown being rotated 180° to fill the mediastinal defect.

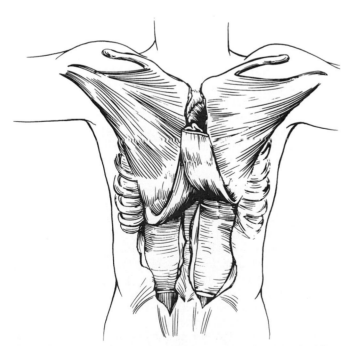

FIG. 75–8. Bilateral rectus abdominis muscles rotated to fill the mediastinal defect.

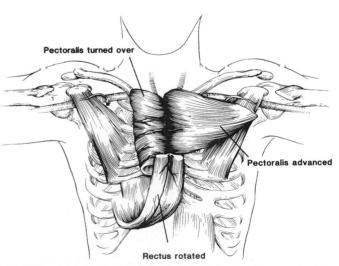

FIG. 75–9. The rectus abdominis muscle being used in combination with a pectoralis major muscle turnover flap and pectoralis major muscle rotation flap.

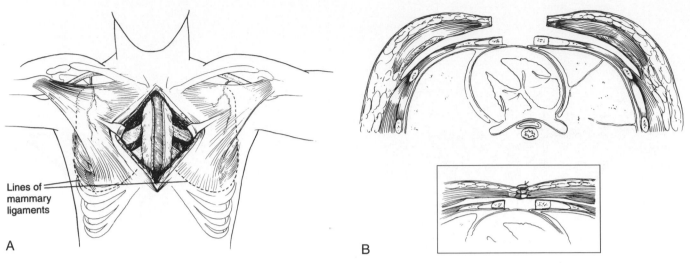

Lines of
mammary
ligaments

A

B

FIG. 75–10. A, the area of dissection is outlined. **B,** the flaps are shown elevated;
insert shows three-layer closure.

of pectoral turnover flap cannot be used reliably on the affected side.

Rectus Abdominis Muscle Flaps

In recent years, the rectus abdominis flap has been used with increasing frequency for coverage of large lower sternal and mediastinal defects (7,8). The paired rectus abdominis muscles are strategically located anatomically. They originate at the pubis and insert in the costochondral areas of the 5th, 6th, and 7th ribs. The superior and inferior epigastric vessels are the only blood supply to these long, flat, anterior abdominal muscles (Fig. 75–6). If the left internal mammary artery has been used in the revascularization of the heart, it is preferable to use the right rectus abdominis muscle.

The contralaeral rectus muscle is usually exposed by a vertical midline incision to just below the level of the umbilicus. The rectus muscle is then undermined and separated slightly below the level of the umbilicus. This muscle is rotated 180°, and can easily fill most inferior mediastinal defects (Fig. 75–7). It is important to use care in dissecting the rectus muscle flap superiorly because the superior epigastric artery and vein are located along the deep surface of the muscle close to the posterior rectus sheath. Care must be taken to identify the location of the superior epigastric vessels as they exit approximately 3 cm lateral to the xiphoid process and behind the 7th costal margin. The muscle is then carefully elevated and transferred counterclockwise for closure of the sternal defect. If necessary, bilateral rectus flaps can be transferred (Fig. 75–8). The rectus abdominis muscle flap can also be utilized to fill a major mediastinal defect in conjunction with pectoralis muscle advancement or turnover flaps (Fig. 75–9).

MYOCUTANEOUS FLAPS

Pectoralis Major Myocutaneous Advancement Flap

An alternative to the pectoralis major muscle advancement or turnover flap is the pectoralis myocutaneous advancement flap. It has been shown to be a quick and simplified approach

to covering sternal wounds, with equivalent efficacy as well as superior functional and aesthetic results (9). This technique is suited for treatment of acute sternal wounds by simultaneous débridement and flap coverage. Since dead space created by débridement is not filled with muscle flaps, but covered with myocutaneous flaps, the mediastinum should be supple, to allow expansion and wound contracture to obliterate the space. A suppurative sternal wound that has been débrided and packed open for several days may yield a stiffened mediastinum with a large dead space that will not close with this technique unless an adjunctive procedure such as an omental flap is used.

Once débridement of the sternum and mediastinum is complete, the procedure is performed in a similar fashion to the pectoralis major advancement flap without the dissection of the plane between the skin and muscle. Electrocautery and blunt dissection is used to separate the pectoralis major and overlying subcutaneous fat and skin from the chest wall. At the medial and inferior aspect of the wound, the dissection continues under the anterior rectus fascia. The dissection must be taken laterally to the anterior axillary line and inferiorly to the 6th intercostal space to divide the mammary ligament, thus allowing mobilization of the flap to the midline without tension (Fig. 75–10). Superiorly, the dissection is performed bluntly in order not to injure the thoracoacromial pedicle. After placement of drains below the flaps and over the mediastinum, the myocutaneous flaps are closed at the midline with large absorbable sutures through the muscle and overlying fascia. The skin is closed in layers. Since the insertion at the humerus is left intact, the functional results and aesthetic outcome is much improved (Fig. 75–11).

SKIN GRAFTING

If the chest skin cannot be closed over the muscle repair, a split-thickness skin graft can be used for adequate coverage of the wound.

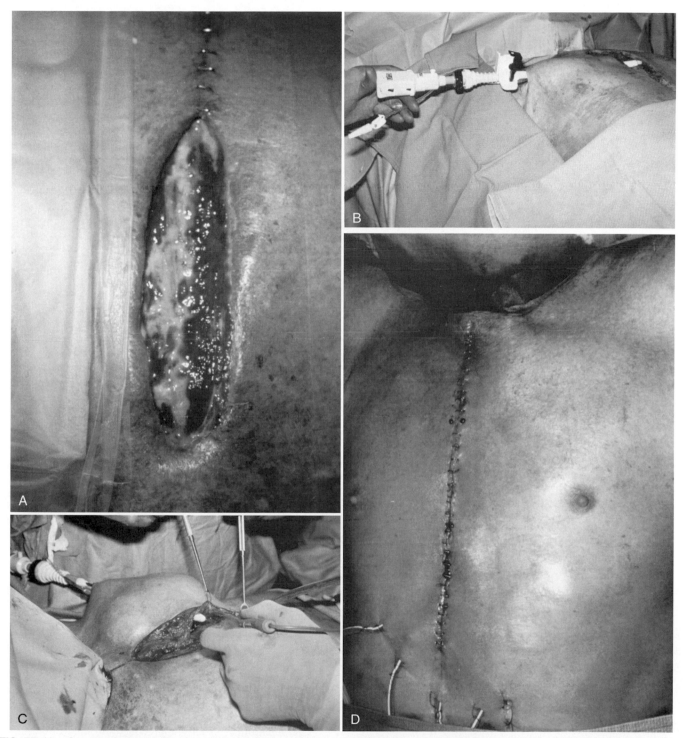

FIG. 75–11. **A,** preoperative appearance of mediastinal wound in a postoperative open-heart patient. **B,** the GSI spacemaker beneath pectoral muscle. **C,** the expander expanded beneath the pectoral muscle with extension to the mediastinal space. **D,** the advanced myocutaneous flaps with closure at the midline (notice the four drains to the subpectoral space).

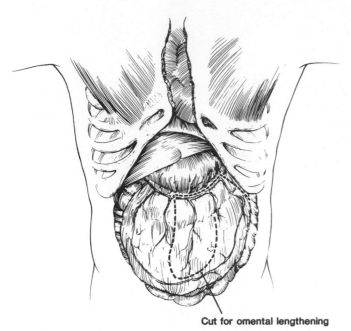

FIG. 75–12. The lines of incision for development of a large omental flap.

Cut for omental lengthening

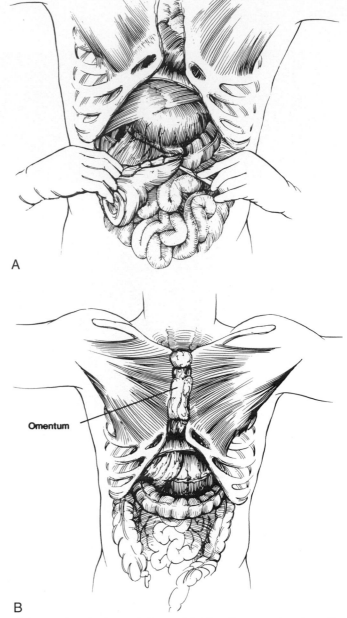

A

B

FIG. 75–13. **A,** the technique of freeing the omentum from the transverse mesocolon and gastric attachments, preserving the integrity of the gastroepiploic vascular arch. **B,** the transfer of the omental flap to the entire length of the mediastinal defect.

Omentum

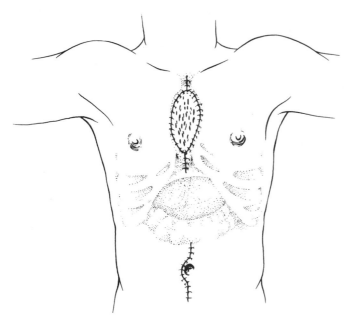

FIG. 75–14. A split-thickness skin graft can be used in covering any residual defect of the skin not approximated. Note the location of the incision and closure used for obtaining the omental flap.

OMENTAL TRANSPOSITION FLAPS

Omental transposition flaps have been found to be particularly useful in filling in the dead space in large mediastinal defects after the use of bilateral internal mammary grafts (10). They can be covered with split-thickness skin grafts or the chest wall skin. A large amount of omental tissue can be obtained based on either the right or left gastroepiploic vessels (Fig. 75–12).

The omentum is usually approached through a midline incision sparing the rectus abdominis muscles, which could be used for later flaps if necessary. The omentum is then freed from left to right, separating the transverse mesocolon attachments, and freed from its gastric attachment, staying close to the seromuscular layer of the stomach but being careful to preserve the integrity of the gastroepiploic vascular arch. The right gastroepiploic artery and vein are usually the vessels of choice (see Fig. 75–12). The omentum is then brought through the diaphragm or abdominal wall (Fig. 75–13). A large mediastinal defect can be filled with a long omental flap transfer. A skin graft can be used to resurface any residual defect (Fig. 75–14).

Summary

There are a wide variety of potential myocutaneous flaps and omental transposition flaps available for closure of mediastinal defects. The choice of the flap to be used for mediastinal coverage should be based on the earlier operative procedure that was employed for revascularization of myocardium. This will define which potential blood supplies to muscles are intact and which have been altered by the procedure. Once this information is available, a planned débridement and closure of choice of the mediastinal defect can be carried out in a timely fashion. Generally speaking, the earlier closure is accomplished, the less morbidity is associated with the patient's mediastinitis, and the better the end result.

References

1. Jurkiewicz MJ, Bostwick J, Hester RT, et al. Infected median sternotomy wound. *Ann Surg* 1980; 191:738.
2. Brant LR, Spencer FC, Trinkle JK. Treatment of median sternotomy infection by mediastinal irrigation with an antibiotic solution. *Arch Surg* 1969; 169:914.
3. Arnold PG, Witzke D, Irons G, et al. Use of omental transposition flaps for soft-tissue reconstruction. *Ann Plast Surg* 1983; 11:508.
4. Nahai F. Pectoralis major muscle turnover flaps for closure of the infected sternotomy wound. *Plast Reconstr Surg* 1982; 70:471.
5. Martin RD. The management of infected median sternotomy wounds. *Ann Plast Surg* 1989; 22:243.
6. Arnold PG, Pairolero PC. Use of pectoralis major muscle flaps to repair defects of anterior chest wall. *Plast Reconstr Surg* 1979; 63:205.
7. Ford TD. Rectus abdominis myocutaneous flap used to close a median sternotomy chest defect. *South Afr med J* 1985; 68:115.
8. Ishii C, Bostwick J, Raine T, et al.. Double-pedicle transverse rectus abdominis myocutaneous flap for unilateral breast and chest wall reconstruction. *Plast Reconstr Surg* 1985; 76:901.
9. Hugo NE, Sultan MR, Ascherman JA, et al. Single-stage management of 74 consecutive sternal wound complications with pectoralis major myocutaneous advancement flaps. *Plast Reconstr Surg* 1994; 93:1433.
10. Herrera HR, Ginsburg ME. The pectoralis major myocutaneous flap and omental transposition for closure of infected median sternotomy wounds. *Plast Reconstr Surg* 1982; 70:485.

Suggested Readings

Seyfer AE, Graeber GM, Wind GG. *Atlas of chest wall reconstruction.* Rockville, MD: Aspen, 1986.

SIX

Genitalia

76

Embryology of Genitalia

**Cary N. Robertson, M.D., F.A.C.S., Carl H. Manstein, M.D., F.A.C.S., and
Mark E. Manstein, M.D., F.A.C.S.**

The embryology of the human sex structures is characterized by two stages of development: an initial stage of gender indifference, and a subsequent stage of male or female differentiation. During the initial stage, a pair of primitive gonads arises from the primordial genital ridge and the genital tract begins its formation. Although rapidly developing, the gonads and the structures that develop along the genital tract remain identical for both males and females until genetically encoded directions alter their course. Until that point, the embryo possesses a sexually bipotential status. Once directed, the gonads begin to form into either testes or ovaries, and the genital tract into corresponding male or female accessory structures. This process of differentiation marks the second stage and occurs during the 8th week in utero (embryo length, 32 mm).

The mechanisms that trigger male and female differentiation are not completely understood. It has been long known that chromosomal sex is established at the moment of fertilization. Only recently has it been appreciated that the actual process of male gonadal differentiation awaits the activation of the histocompatibility Y (H-Y) antigen. Without activation of the H-Y antigen, gonadal development proceeds as female. A current hypothesis is that its release is triggered by an autosomally coded precursor substance that is activated by a Y chromosome. It is clear that the presence of the H-Y antigen is crucial to males of all species. Without it, functional testes would not develop—and without functional testes, the internal and external male genitalia would not form (1,2). The exact locus for testis determination is a region of the short arm of the Y (SRY) chromosome coding for testis determining factor (TDF) (3).

Gender-Indifferent Stage

Once the ovum is fertilized, the initiation of cell division is immediate, and by the 7th or 8th day, the cell mass is a recognizable blastocyst. The cells of the blastocyst continue dividing to produce, by the end of the 2nd week, the so-called embryonic disc, the structure that will develop into the embryo. The embryonic disc consists of an outer layer of ectoderm and an inner layer of endoderm. It rests on the yolk sac within the blastocyst.

At the caudal end of the embryonic disc, a proliferation of ectoderm begins to form a midline groove called the primitive streak. From this groove, between the endoderm and ectoderm, arises a 3rd cell layer, the mesoderm. As the mesodermal cells multiply, they might migrate peripherally, separating the ectodermal and endodermal layers (3) (Fig. 76–1).

Immediately caudal to the primitive streak lies a territory where the ectoderm and endoderm remain adherent without any mesodermal ingrowth. This area is labeled the cloacal membrane, and it will grow and convolute. Further caudal, below the cloacal membrane, is the allantois, which is an outpouching of the posterior wall of the yolk sac that bulges into the connecting body stalk (4).

The most important occurrence in the development of the general body form is the transformation of the flat embryonic disc into a fairly cylindrical embryo attached to the yolk sac by a narrow stalk. With this development comes a rapid growth at both the cephalic and caudal ends and an infolding toward the stalk, especially at these two regions. At the caudal end, this occurs in the following fashion: The germ cells continue to proliferate and migrate, particularly the mesodermal cells; because the cell layers of the cloacal membrane are fused, the mesodermal cells cannot penetrate, merely accumulating around the edges of the membrane and, in so doing, form the cloacal ridge (3).

Growth continues to be quite rapid in the caudal region, which outpaces the slower central portion. This disparity in cell division results in an infolding of the embryo, and the actual tail fold is identifiable by the 21st day. With the "bending" inward, the cloacal membrane and allantois become ventral wall structures, the cloacal membrane now assuming an infraumbilical position. At the caudal end of the embryo, an endoderm-lined tube develops that is termed the "hindgut." It terminates in a cul-de-sac, the cloaca, whose blind ending lies dorsal to the cloacal membrane (see Fig. 76–1).

Cloacal folds continue to grow as the migratory mesoderm is blocked by the fused cloacal membrane. By the end of the 5th week (8 mm) a conical genital tubercle appears in the ventral midline between the cloacal membrane and the allantois. (This tubercle will eventually elongate into the phallus.) At the same time, a wedge of mesenchyme, the urorectal septum, becomes discernable. This septum will descend as it grows, thereby partitioning the cloaca into a urogenital sinus ventrally and a rectum dorsally. When the urorectal septum completes its descent, it fuses with the cloacal membrane to form the perineal body (5) (Figs. 76–2 and 76–3).

Posterolateral anal tubercles also develop toward the end of the 5th week, and the lateral mesoderm proliferates to form urethral and genital folds. A genital ridge arises on the ventromedial aspect of the genital fold and extends longitudinally, protruding into the celom. Concurrently, primitive germ cells begin migrating into this region via the endodermal gut and dorsal mesentery. These germ cells evolve into

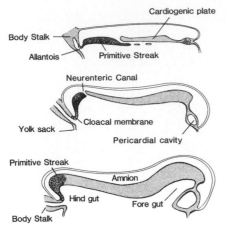

FIG. 76–1. Growth of human embryo: top, approximately 18 days; middle, 24 days; bottom, 28 days.

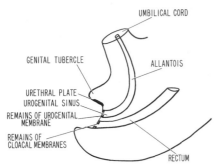

FIG. 76–2. Anatomy of the hindgut by the 6th week shows division of cloaca into rectum and urogenital sinus.

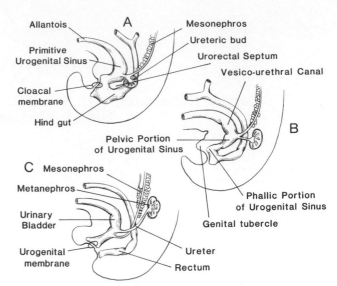

FIG. 76–3. The cloaca is divided into the rectum and the urogenital sinus. **A,** appearance at approximately 5 weeks. **B,** intermediate phase. **C,** appearance at approximately 12 weeks.

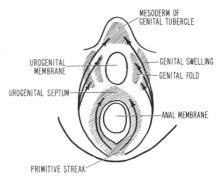

FIG. 76–4. Proliferation of lateral mesoderm creates urethral and genital folds at the end of the 5th week.

the sexually bipotential gonads and the overlying epithelium develops into the sex cords projecting into each gonad. In the male, these sex cords become the seminiferous tubercles (Fig. 76–4).

Closely linked chronologically and spatially to gonadal genesis is the development of the kidney. From the lateral mesoderm on each side arises the urogenital ridge, which undergoes a segmental development; tubules arising first cranially, with differentiation proceeding caudally. The midportion of the renal blastema (mesonephros) becomes organized as the cranial tubules coalesce to create a solid cord (the nephrogenic cord). The cord undergoes canalization to form the mesonephric (Wolffian) duct and, by the 26th day, each duct has a lumen. The mesonephric duct then grows caudally to meet the cloaca, which has already divided into a urogenital sinus or bladder ventrally and a rectum dorsally. As mesonephric ("urinary") pressure increases, the cloacal membrane ruptures, allowing the urogenital sinus to communicate with the exterior. The mesonephric duct then proceeds to degenerate, with its duct persisting in the male as the vas deferens, ejaculatory duct, seminal vesicles, and a portion of the rete testis. The presence of the mesonephric duct, however, is crucial to renal development because the ureteral bud develops from it and grows to meet the developing kidney (metanephros) (6).

The ultimate fate of the urogenital sinus depends on the differentiation of the external genitalia. Convergence of the anterior wall of the urogenital sinus results in the formation of an endodermal urethral plate on the floor of the urethral groove. The urethral groove, laterally flanked by mesoderm, is formed by the elongation of the urogenital sinus. As the urethral plate disintegrates, the urethral groove deepens and an anterior urethra is formed. A premature rupture of the urethral and cloacal membranes leads to exstrophy of the bladder (see Fig. 76–3).

The rectum is an endoderm-lined projection inside the hindgut and cranial to the allantois. It is formed during the folding of the abdominal wall, which grows downward into the cloacal cavity. When the anal membrane ruptures, it serves as the outlet for the rectum.

The paramesonephric (Müllerian) ducts comprise another critical embryologic structure and arise at the level of the 3rd thoracic somite. (The somites are primitive segments of mesoderm that give rise to a specific muscle mass supplied by a spinal nerve.) By the 6th week of development, an area of celomic epithelium at the cephalic end of the mesonephros becomes thickened and invaginates; this creates the bilateral paramesonephric ducts in both sexes (7). The site of infolding becomes the abdominal ostium of the uterine tube in the

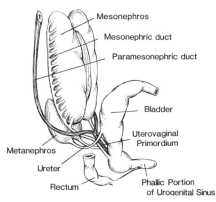

FIG. 76–5. In a 9-week-old fetus, the Müllerian tubercle is created by the uterovaginal primordium bulging into the urogenital sinus.

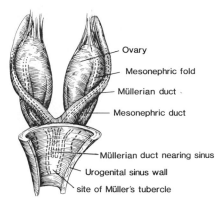

FIG. 76–6. Urogenital ducts at 8 weeks.

female and the scattered indentations form the beginnings of the future fimbriae (Fig. 76–5).

Each paramesonephric duct grows caudally through the mesenchyme. Inasmuch as those ducts course parallel to the mesonephric ducts, the term *paramesonephric* is appropriate. However, the growing caudal tip of the paramesonephric duct lies within the basement membrane of the mesonephric duct, and it is possible that the latter contributes directly to the growth of the former.

As the paramesonephric ducts approach each other caudally, they begin to fuse. (This takes place even as their united tips reach the urogenital sinus.) The external walls merge first; as the cavities come together, the median septum that separates them is resorbed. By 8 weeks, ductal fusion has transpired that creates the genital or uterovaginal canal in the female. Irregularities in the fusion lead to anomalies of the uterus (8) (Fig. 76–6).

Hitherto, the development of the embryo has been identical regardless of sexual chromosomal composition. In this initial sexually indifferent phase of development, the primordia of both sex ducts appear and develop independently of genetic sex or hormonal influence. What follows is the crucial period of gonadal differentiation in which hormonal control of sex duct growth is paramount.

Stage of Sexual Differentiation

Although depicted here as two discrete stages, sexual differentiation is a sequential process that is initiated at conception. In the male, the change from gonad to testes does, however, await activation of the H-Y antigen. A further requirement for male differentiation is that the testes be functional. They must produce hormones. No gonadal hormones are required for the development of the female phenotype, and so if the testes do not function as male endocrine organs the external genitalia become female.

Two secretions from the fetal testes are responsible for the male phenotype. The first is Müllerian-inhibiting substance (MIS). This product of testicular Sertoli cells inhibits the development of Müllerian ducts in the male. Testing for this substance by enzyme link immunoassay (ELISA) techniques may be helpful in difficult intersex cases (9,10).

The second, and far more crucial, factor is the secretion of androgenic steroids, primarily testosterone. The onset of synthesis of these androgenic steroids in the fetal testes oc-

curs just before the onset of male phenotypic differentiation. It is believed that the hormonal synthesis is independent of gonadotropic control and that testosterone itself is responsible for the virilization of the Wölffian duct system into the epididymis, ductus deferens, seminal vesicle, ejaculatory duct, ureter, and pelvis of the kidney. Its metabolite, dihydrotestosterone, induces development of the prostate and male external genitalia. Congenital lack of the reducing enzyme 5 alpha-reductase prevents such metabolite formation and leads to pseudohermaphroditism (10–13).

The onset of endocrine function in fetal gonads takes place early in embryogenesis. Molecular mechanisms by which hormones act during fetal development appear to be the same as those operating in the postnatal state (14).

Sexual Differentiation of the Male

By the 8th week there is an infolded epithelial sheet that has become fenestrated to form primitive sex cords. This sheet continues to proliferate and separate itself from the surface epithelium by the development of the tunica albuginea. The Leydig cells evolve from mesenchyme that is located between the primitive sex cords.

The genital tubercle has meanwhile emerged at a point where cloacal folds join between the cloacal membrane and the allantois. While the genital tubercle is a midline mesodermal mass, it displays a shallow midline depression; this urethral groove extends the length of the tubercle. At the tip of the tubercle an epithelial tag forms from ectoderm. As the genital tubercle elongates, it carries the groove with it, maintaining the tag at its tip. It continues to become the phallus (Fig. 76–7).

The phallus projects in a perpendicular manner to the abdominal wall. With elongation, the urethral groove depends from the opened urogenital ostium far out onto the shaft. By 3 months, the urethral folds begin to close over the urethral groove, and the original urogenital ostium closes. The urethral groove seals together, and the tube of the urethra progresses distally with the urogenital ostium advancing before it. The penile urethra forms on the ventral surface of the genital tubercle. It is this progression of events that explain the anatomic location of the ostium in hypospadias (6). Although most authorities believe that the urethra raises by fusion of the paired urethral folds after rupture of the urogenital membrane, recent investigative work contradicts this (15). Rather,

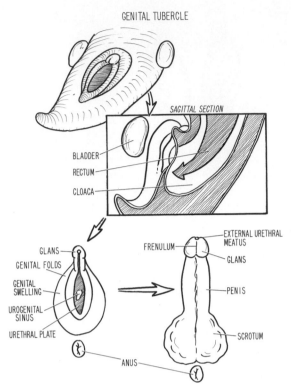

FIG. 76–7. The genital tubercle develops into male genitalia.

studies in pigs propose that the urethral opening, initially situated dorsally, is displaced to the tip of the genital anlage by the rapid ventral growth of the perineum.

Experiments in rats suggest a new concept of urethral development, with subsequent implication in the pathogenesis of hypospadias (16). The malformation may appear when there is an inhibition in the formation of the genitalia. In more proximal hypospadias, the extension of the genitalia is prevented, possibly by chordee, and the penis remains curved. Thus the urethra is relatively too short, and it is the penis rather than the urethra that is the primary dysgenic organ in hypospadias. Perineal hypospadias studies in the rat indicate that there are often marked signs of feminization.

Consolidated mesenchyme in the dorsal portion of the phallus divides in the midline to form the two columns of erectile tissue (corpora cavernosa) and the muscular structures that attach the penis to the bony pelvis. Proximally, the mesenchyme around the urethra becomes the corpus spongiosum. As the glans enlarges, it depends the urethral groove. While the glans begins to close over the groove, the edges do not fuse until later (7).

The urogenital ostium is present as a diamond-shaped opening at the corona. At the end of the 12th week, a roll of skin is appreciable on either side of the urethral opening. A ridge extends to encircle the shaft of the penis, forming the prepuce by growing out to cover the corona. As the prepuce grows, the edges of the meatus reach their final location at the site of the foraminal epithelial tag (7).

Simultaneously, the formation of the scrotum is transpiring. At the 8th week, as the genital tubercle elongates, the labioscrotal swellings appear. These swellings are two cuta-

neous elevations lateral to the testes lateral to the tubercle. The primordial scrotum is sharply separated from the penis by lateral phallic grooves. The labioscrotal swellings fuse in the midline, forming the scrotum. There is a median raphe and septum that acts as a divider, maintaining two separate compartments. One of the hallmarks of the masculinization of the external genitalia is the formation of this raphe rather than the nonunited structures in the female (6).

Sexual Differentiation of the Female

The feminization of the external genitalia is the direct result of absence of, or insensitivity toward, androgens. It is at the 8th week when the embryo, still phenotypically indifferent, possessing paired Wölffian and Müllerian ducts, begins to differentiate. In the normal female fetus, the absence of both androgens and the müllerian regression hormone permits the growth of the Müllerian (paramesonephric) ducts. Devoid of any stimulus, the mesonephric ducts cannot keep pace and become progressively more inconsequential. (Eventually, the Wölffian ducts will persist as more microscopic foci or as minute portions of ductal epithelium buried in vaginal wall, cervix, or broad ligament) (17).

During the 8th week, the paramesonephric ducts coalesce to form the uterovaginal canal. While these ducts are united, they become displaced by the enlarging adrenals and permanent kidneys. The ducts therefore develop two bends that roughly demarcate these regions: (a) a cranial longitudinal portion, the uterine tube; (b) a transverse midportion, the uterine fundus and corpus; and (c) a caudal longitudinal portion that fuses with the other duct to produce a common conduit, the cervic and provisional vagina (4).

The cranial portion of each Müllerian duct maintains its individual existence and becomes a uterine tube, with its patent upper aspect gaining a fringe, or fimbriae, early on. Originally, the future corpus segment of the uterus is seen in the transverse segment of the ducts; after a number of weeks the cranial walls of both these tubes bulge cephalad so that convex dome is added to the original angular junction. This allows the developing uterus to gain significant volume (5).

The cervix emerges from the upper aspects of the lower portion of the ducts, where primary fusion has already transpired. This fused end migrates to the posterior wall of the urogenital sinus and pushes it somewhat caudally, thereby creating the Müllerian tubercle. Between the tubercle and the ducts themselves is a proliferation of cells derived from the urogenital sinus that have been termed the "sinovaginal bulbs." These bulbs undergo rapid hyperplasia and help produce a new longitudinal structure, the vaginal plate. The vaginal plate, in turn, demonstrates active growth caudally, and it follows alongside the urethra down to its separate opening in the vestibule. A central core of the vaginal plate cells then degenerates and sloughs, thus forming the vaginal vault. This canalization is a slow process and is only complete by the 5th month (18).

There is a longstanding controversy as to the exact origin of the cells of the vagina. Presently, five theories are promulgated: (a) mesonephric alone, (b) mesonephric and paramesonephric, (c) paramesonephric only, (d) paramesonephric and urogenital sinus, and (e) urogenital sinus alone. Further

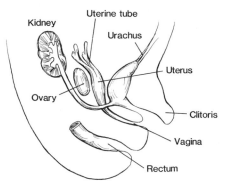

FIG. 76–8. The late developmental stage of female genitalia.

References

1. Bernstein R. The Y chromosome and primary sexual differentiation. *JAMA* 1981; 245:1953.
2. Polani PE, Ainolfi M. The H-Y antigen and its function. *J Immunogenet* 1983; 10:85.
3. Berkovitz GD, et al. The role of the sex-determining region of the Y chromosome (SRY) in the etiology of 46,XX true hermaphroditism. *Hum Genet* 1992; 88:411–416.
4. Arey LB. *Developmental anatomy.* Philadelphia: WB Saunders, 1974; 995–998, 295–341.
5. Jirasek JE. Morphogenesis of the genital system in the human. *Birth Defects* 1977; 13:13.
6. Devine CJ. Embryology of the male external genitalia. *Clin Plast Surg* 1980; 7:141.
7. Bellinger MF. Embryology of the male external genitalia. *Urol Clin North Am* 1981; 8:375.
8. Marshall FF. Vaginal agenesis. *Clin Plast Surg* 1980; 7:175.
9. Josso N, Picard JY, Tran D. Anti-Müllerian hormone. *Birth Defects* 1977; 13:59.
10. Harbison MD, Magid ML, Josso N, et al. Anti-Müllerian hormone in three intersex conditions. *Ann Genet* 1991; 34:226–232.
11. Wilson JD, Griffin JE, George FW. Sexual differentiation: early hormone synthesis and action. *Biol Reprod* 1980; 22:9.
12. Winter JS, Fairman C, Reyes F. Sex steroid production by the human fetus. *Birth Defects* 1977; 13:41.
13. Skandalakis JE, Gray SW, Parrott TS. Sex determination. In: Skandalakis JE, Gray SW, eds. *Embryology for surgeons: the embryological basis for the treatment of congenital anomalies.* 2nd ed. Baltimore: Williams & Wilkins, 1994; 848–876.
14. Jost A, Prepin J, Vigier B. Hormones in the morphogenesis of the genital system. *Birth Defects* 1977; 13:85.
15. van der Putte SCJ. Normal and abnormal development of the anorectum. *J Pediatr Surg* 1986; 21:434.
16. Kluth D, Lambrecht W, Reich P. Pathogenesis of hypospadias: more questions than answers. *J Pediatr Surg* 1988; 23:1095.
17. O'Rahilly R. The development of the vagina in the human. *Birth Defects* 1977; 13:123.
18. Ulfelder H, Robboy SJ. Embryologic development of the human vagina. *Am J Obstet Gynecol* 1976; 126:769.
19. Moore KL: *The developing human.* Philadelphia: WB Saunders, 1977; 220.

investigation is needed, but currently few researchers believe that the mesonephric ducts play a significant role (1).

What is certain is that, unlike the male, the labioscrotal swellings and urethral folds, which are derived from the genital tubercle, do not fuse in a midline raphe. The phallus does not extend outward, perpendicular to the abdominal wall. Rather, the phallus bends caudally and becomes the clitoris (Fig. 76–8). The urethral folds evolve into the labia minora and the labioscrotal swellings into the labia majora. The labioscrotal folds do converge posteriorly to form the posterior labial commissure and anteriorly to form the mons pubis (19).

The hymen emerges at the site of the Müllerian tubercle, initially as a ring-shaped fold between the future vagina and the urogenital sinus. It is formed passively by the invagination of the posterior wall of the sinus, owing to the expansion of the lower end of the vagina. The hymen is composed of vaginal cells and an external layer of sinusal epithelia. Its appearance completes the morphogenesis of the vestibule.

77

Anomalies of the Male Genitalia

Cameron S. Schaeffer. M.D., and Lowell R. King, M.D., F.A.C.S.

Historically, plastic surgeons have played a major role in the care of male patients with surgical genital problems. Although subspecialists in urology are now treating the majority of these patients, the plastic surgeon will be called upon to handle the more complex reconstructive problems. It is, therefore, important for the plastic surgeon to be familiar with the congenital disorders of the male genitalia.

Congenital genital anomalies are frequently associated with other birth defects or are part of a larger syndrome, some of which can be acutely life threatening. The clinician should be alert to other defects, and appropriate studies and consultations should be obtained before surgical correction is undertaken. In most pediatric centers today, the approach to the child with severe genital malformations is often multidisciplinary, involving pediatricians, geneticists, psychologists, endocrinologists, and the reconstructive surgeon.

Embryology

Congenital anomalies of the male genitalia are best understood in the context of normal development (1). Prior to the 9th week of gestation, the fetal genitalia are indeterminate. Under the influence of growth hormone and testosterone from the fetal testes, development proceeds along male lines. This requires the conversion of testosterone to dihydrotestosterone (DHT) by the enzyme 5-alpha reductase. Under the influence of DHT, the genital tubercle elongates to form the phallus, while ventrally, the urethral groove develops from the elongating urogenital sinus. Paired urethral folds coalesce in the midline, beginning proximally and moving distally to form the floor of the urethra (2). This process continues to the glandular corona. Simultaneously, an ectodermal pit at the tip of the glans forms, creating a groove or channel that eventually joins the developing urethra. The lateral wings of the flattened ventral glans roll medially to envelop the distal urethra, giving the glans a conical shape and bringing the dorsal foreskin to the ventrum. Normally, the foreskin completely conceals the underlying glans. The genital swellings fuse posteriorly to form the scrotum, which remains empty until late in gestation when the testes descend. The prominent scrotal and penile raphes testify to the described fusions.

When these processes of ventral fusion and rotation arrest prematurely, hypospadias results. This may vary from mild (incomplete foreskin) to severe (penoscrotal hypospadias). In general, any degree of hypospadias results in a dorsal, hooded foreskin, while deficiency or dysplasia of the distal spongiosal tissue is only seen where the urethra fails to develop. When this occurs, the associated cavernosal tissue is also often deficient, causing ventral chordee or curvature. Isolated chordee does occur and probably represents a disorder of corporal body development, termed *corporal disproportion*. Extremely severe hypospadias closely mimics the female phenotype.

In normal, term neonates, the penis is 35 ± 7 mm in stretched length and 11 ± 2 mm in width (3,4). Accurate measurements can be difficult to make in the squirming patient with a generous prepubic fat pad, and many such patients are mistakenly referred with the diagnosis of microphallus. Released from the maternal hormonal milieu, which causes fetal pituitary suppression, the male neonate experiences a surge of testosterone production that persists for about 4 months. After this period, the penis undergoes very modest growth until the onset of puberty, when the penis can be expected to at least double in size.

Developmental processes are not complete at the time of birth. At birth, the glans is very delicate and easily irritated by urine and feces; the prepuce provides a natural barrier protection. Physiologic adhesions exist between the inner foreskin and glans penis, preventing retraction of the foreskin. In virtually all boys, epithelial ingrowth along each surface causes gradual separation and retractability of the foreskin by 7 years of age. Epithelial debris, visible as white "pearls" beneath the foreskin, may accumulate between the two layers if the normal process of separation does not occur. These sterile keratin deposits should not be confused with smegma, which is the white, cheeselike substance that accumulates under the foreskin with improper hygiene. It is commonly and mistakenly believed that it is difficult to care for the foreskin. It should be washed daily, and it is unnecessary and potentially harmful to fully retract the foreskin before its natural separation from the glans penis.

Congenital Anomalies of the Penis and Foreskin

APHALLIA

Also termed *penile agenesis,* aphallia is an extremely rare anomaly with some fifty reported cases (5,6,7). The scrotum and its contents are usually normal, although cryptorchidism may be present. The urethral meatus is variably found under the pubis, often associated with a small tag of skin. Associated anomalies of the urinary tract are common and should be pursued with ultrasound and voiding cystourethrography prior to sex reassignment.

The aphallic male is probably best reared as a female, and conversion should be accomplished as soon as possible to avoid confusion among the concerned. While penile replacement is technically feasible, the creation of a serviceable phallus typically requires multiple operations, including prostheses for erection that can only be placed after puberty. Such an undertaking should probably be reserved for acquired aphallia when the patient recognizes the loss. For the newborn, congenitally aphallic patient, it is far simpler and more reasonable from a surgical and psychologic standpoint to establish female identity early. This is not a universally held belief. Trengove-Jones argues that with current techniques of phalloplasty the technical difficulties and the psychologic impact of male-to-female gender conversion and the loss of fertility may be avoided (8). That testosterone affects the fetal brain in a fundamental way is well recognized; exactly how those changes mold and contribute to a male's self-perception of gender is unclear and needs further study (9).

MICROPENIS

The term *micropenis,* or "microphallus," usually describes a well-proportioned phallus smaller than two standard deviations below normal (10,11,12). This anomaly occurs when the penis receives inadequate androgen stimulation after 14 weeks of gestation (i.e., after the penis is already formed, or because of a deficiency in penile tissue). Malfunction earlier in gestation results in hypospadias or ambiguous genitalia. In the first trimester, placental HCG is the primary stimulus for fetal Leydig cell secretion of testosterone. Beginning in the 15th week, increased hypothalamic secretion of GnRH induces LH production and thus Leydig cell stimulation. Therefore, inadequate GnRH production or any other failure in this hormonal axis would lead to an arrest in penile growth. Rarely, the testes are lost in the 2nd trimester from a vascular insult. This phenomenon, termed the vanishing testes syndrome, is characterized by a small phallus, a flat, poorly rugated scrotum, and blind-ending gonadal vessels. There may also be a problem with the end organ itself. If the corporal bodies are dysplastic and stringlike, growth will not be induced hormonally.

True micropenis is relatively rare, and most patients referred with this diagnosis are actually misdiagnosed. A generous prepubic fat pad in the chubby infant, a penoscrotal web, or a circumcision complicated by phimosis and concealment are all frequent imitators. Only after careful palpation of the penile shaft to rule out corporal dysplasia, as well as an assessment of penile width and stretched length, can the diagnosis be made. Nomograms should be consulted.

Assessing the phallus's response to exogenous androgen is critical prior to any discussion of gender reassignment. Generally, human chorionic gonadotropin (HCG) is given at a dose of 75 mg/kg intramuscularly biweekly for 3 weeks. If no response is seen, 25 to 50 mg of testosterone enanthate is administered intramuscularly. Response should be assessed in 3 to 4 weeks. Failure to respond suggests end-organ resistance to testosterone, and the likelihood the penis will grow at puberty is slim. The female gender should then be established, and therapy mimics that of penile agenesis except for the phallus. Obviously, the penile urethra must be resected and positioned appropriately on the perineum. If any corporal tissue is removed, care must be taken to avoid disturbing the dorsal neurovascular pedicle to the glans, which should be preserved for sexual function. Wedge resection of the glandular urethra may be a sufficient reduction glanduloplasty, if needed. As with penile agenesis, the surgically corrected microphallic patient should be younger than 18 months of age for psychologic reasons.

When the microphallus does respond to hormonal stimulation, the infant can be safely reared as a male. Usually, the phallus remains small until puberty, so some hormonal assistance may be needed during childhood to bring the patient more closely abreast of his peers. The postpubescent microphallus typically attains an erect length of 8 to 10 cm. Though two standard deviations below normal for adult males, the phallus is serviceable, and no apparent psychologic impact has been consistently described; Shober showed that most such boys grow into well-adjusted men (13).

MACROPHALLUS

Neurofibromatosis will occasionally involve the penile shaft and cause enlargement due to lymphedema, or the lesion may be focal. When the lesion is discreet, excision is the treatment of choice. If lymphedema results in a large and unsightly penis, this condition can be partly corrected by excising all the subcutaneous tissue between the corpora and the skin. This diminishes the girth of the penis, and the skin tends to adhere to the underlying corporal bodies, losing its normal mobility. Other causes of macrophallus include congenital lymphedema, capillary hemangioma, and megalourethra (14).

DIPHALLIA

Diphallia, or penile duplication, is a rare anomaly, with a spectrum between a small accessory penis and true paired duplication (15). Corporal anatomy is variable, with each penis containing one or two corporal bodies. Typically, they are unequal in size and sit side by side. Presumably, this anomaly results from splitting of the genital tubercle. Other genitourinary anomalies (e.g., myelomeningocele, cardiac defects, and anal malformations) are commonly associated with diphallia. Complete evaluation of the urinary tract is mandatory to rule out other anomalies. Treatment is individualized, and should be based on repair and centering of the dominant phallus, with consideration given to urethral anatomy.

PENILE TORSION

Penile torsion is a rotational defect of the penis, usually noted after retraction of the foreskin at circumcision (16). The rotation is usually counterclockwise. Its significance is purely cosmetic, and milder forms can be managed with reassurance alone. Rotations greater than 45° are managed by penile degloving, circumcision, and reconstruction of the subcoronal margin in a fashion that detorses the glans. Severe rotational defects may also require resection of dysgenetic bands or suspensory ligaments at the base of the penis. Care should be taken to avoid the dorsal neurovascular pedicles of the corpora. If the rotation persists, laterally placed, braided nylon sutures between the corporal body and the pubic bone should be corrective (again, avoiding the dorsolateral nerves).

WEBBED PENIS

Webbed penis or "penoscrotal web" are descriptive terms for the congenital anomaly in which the ventral penile and scrotal skin are fused, or there appears to be a paucity of ventral penile skin such that the hair-bearing scrotal tissue reaches the coronal margin (17). The anomaly can vary in severity. It is best seen by stretching the penis cephalad and away from the abdominal wall, often demonstrating a prominent frenulum or true web. Though rare, it is more often seen in association with micropenis and hypospadias (3.5%), when the ventral penile skin is deficient.

The anomaly is first repaired by making a circumferential subcoronal incision and completely degloving the penis, releasing it from its scrotal attachments. This drops the ventral subcoronal margin, which is essentially the anterior aspect of the scrotum, back to the base of penis. The foreskin is unrolled and then brought around to resurface the ventrum of the penis. The penoscrotal angle can be dropped back farther by making two angled incisions at the interface between the rugated scrotal skin and the lateral base of the penis, and closing as a reverse Y-V advancement. If this is performed, postoperative scrotal edema can be anticipated and minimized with catheter drainage and pressure dressings.

CHORDEE WITHOUT HYPOSPADIAS AND HEMIHYPERTROPHY OF THE PENIS

Chordee without hypospadias is a rare condition, often encountered in older children or adolescents who present with downward-curved erections (18,19). As its name implies, the urethra is intact to the tip of the glans; however, this condition can be treated as a mild variant of hypospadias. The foreskin may be incomplete and reside on the dorsum of the penis, and intraoperative ventral inspection may reveal spongiosal dysplasia at the coronal margin. If such dysplasia is present, the urethra is easily entered during circumcision, as the skin is juxtaposed to the underlying urethral lumen. Theoretically, any urethral dysplasia leads to abnormal development of the overlying corporal bodies and ventral chordee. If the spongiosum and urethra in the distal penis are normally formed, then the curvature can be attributed solely to disproportionate formation of the dorsal and ventral aspects of the corporal cylinders themselves, or corporal disproportion.

Irrespective of which variation is encountered, the repair is straightforward. If the patient's primary concern is the asymmetry of the foreskin, the surgeon should resist the temptation to simply excise the hoodlike dorsal foreskin. The patient should first undergo artificial erection to rule out unsuspected chordee, which is corrected first. A careful assessment of the quantity and quality of the ventral shaft skin should also be made, as rotating a portion of the dorsal foreskin to the ventrum may improve the overall cosmetic appearance. If chordee is present, it is corrected by shortening the length of the dorsal corporal bodies in a symmetric fashion. The dorsal neurovascular pedicles are first elevated sharply off the underlying corporal bodies. The point of maximal curvature on artificial erection is then marked with bilateral traction sutures, and a narrow, transverse ellipse of tunica albuginea is excised as described by Nesbit (20). The defect is then closed with 5-0 polyglactin suture. Alternatively, paired, short, symmetric incisions are made in the dorsal aspect of each corporal body at the point of maximal curvature, then closed transversely with interrupted, absorbable suture. If repeat artificial erection demonstrates persistent chordee, the sutures may be removed and longer incisions performed. After the correction is complete, the dorsal neurovascular tissue is replaced, tacking it back into position with fine, interrupted absorbable suture, with care being taken to avoid the dorsolateral nerves. In both maneuvers, the penis is nicely straightened without actually losing length because the ventrum remains undisturbed.

Hemihypertrophy of the penis may be a related condition in which the corporal disproportion is not dorsal versus ventral, but right versus left (21). With penile hemihypertrophy, the penis angulates laterally on erection towards the side with the smaller corporal body. In all but one reported case, the right corporal body has been larger in length and diameter than the left. This congenital condition should not be confused with Peyronie disease, which is an acquired angulation of the penis due to focal scarring of the corporal body. Correction is the same as for chordee, but the excised ellipse or site of incision and plication will be on the lateral aspect of the larger corporal body at the site of maximal curvature. Occasionally, the corpus spongiosum will have to be mobilized to remove a full semicircular ellipse from the side of the corporal body.

Hypospadias and the Principles of Repair

It has been observed that there are things a male should be able to perform both standing and lying down, and that the goal of hypospadias surgery is to permit them. Thus, the correction of hypospadias is both a cosmetic and functional venture. The reconstructive surgeon should settle for nothing less for his patients than a straight penis on erection, a normal caliber urethra, and a meatus at the tip of the glans, as techniques to accomplish these goals have been developed. While a coronal margin meatus permits normal male function, the cosmetic appearance is less than ideal. Furthermore, mild hypospadias is often associated with significant chordee. Artificial erection under anesthesia is mandatory in all hypospadias to rule out chordee, so correcting these milder forms should be accomplished at the same sitting with minimal risk of morbidity.

The modern era of hypospadias repair began over a century ago, and since then hundreds of distinct repairs and modifications have been described, many of which are still in use throughout the world today. Duckett has provided us with a brief overview of the fascinating evolution of surgical technique (22). Obviously, no single operation is universally applicable, so the reconstructive surgeon should be familiar with various repairs that encompass the wide range of anatomic variations seen in this disorder.

Modern hypospadiology is a rewarding and occasionally frustrating pursuit. Much of the success of modern repair is attributed to the earlier age at which the surgery can be performed. After the physiologic testosterone surge in the first 4 months of life, relatively little penile growth occurs until puberty, so the traditional posture of waiting until the child "gets older" is unjustifiable. Berg and co-workers (23) have performed psychiatric evaluations on individuals who underwent hypospadias repair at ages permitting recollection of the deformity and corrective surgery. Overall, these men were functional, yet they faired less well in life than age-matched controls. They had more "neurotic constriction," meaning they used their resources less well, exhibited lower self-esteem and activity, lower capacity for interpersonal relationships, increased hostility, and decreased ego strength. Sexuality and fertility did not seem to be affected (23). Thus, it seems advantageous to complete the repair before the child is old enough to remember the anomaly or the events of the repair (i.e., before 2 years of age). It can usually be accomplished before the onset of separation anxiety, which peaks between 15 and 30 months of age. Modern anesthesia and intraoperative monitoring have made the risks of operating on infants over 60 weeks of gestational age essentially unmeasurable, while improvements in instruments, sutures, urethral catheters, dressings, and optical magnification have negated the "size factor."

Currently, repair is performed in one stage for all degrees of hypospadias severity at 6 to 12 months of age. Should any complications arise, touch-up work can be performed after 6 months of healing and scar remodeling and softening. Any attempt to make corrections before this 6-month healing period, especially closure of urethrocutaneous fistulae, is fraught with additional complications. To promote penile skin vascularity and thickening, and thus postoperative healing, a single dose of parenteral testosterone (25 mg for infants) can be given 4 weeks before surgery. This has the added benefit of modest penile growth. Hormonal stimulation is a critical adjunct in severe hypospadias, or in the setting of a small phallus, to ascertain that the genitalia have normal androgen receptors. Those who fail to respond to parenteral testosterone will not be expected to have normal genital growth at the onset of puberty. Testosterone cream is no longer recommended because of inconsistency of drug delivery via this vehicle, and the risk of absorption in the mother. Chorionic gonadotropin may also be used, but this requires multiple shots. Single-dose parenteral therapy assures delivery, and there is no apparent risk of premature bone maturation. Husmann (24) has cautioned that exogenous androgens may accelerate androgen receptor loss in penile tissue, negatively affecting ultimate penile size. Until further studies are performed, the surgeon should use exogenous hormones selectively (24).

Hypospadias surgery requires a strict adherence to surgical principles and meticulous technique, and the surgeon quickly develops routines that foster consistency, efficiency, and good outcomes. All hypospadias repairs require rote maneuvers, yet the details of the urethroplasty and glanduloplasty must be individualized. Before discussing specific repairs, it is essential to review the routines that lead to success irrespective of method.

Before any elective operation, the patient should be carefully assessed for any illness, especially upper respiratory infections, including otitis media. An unexplained fever should postpone the operation. The patient should also be checked for diaper rash before entering the operating room. Once anesthetized, the lower extremities should be slightly abducted to permit full preparation of the entire scrotum and perineum. The physiologic adhesions between the foreskin and glans should be separated bluntly, and all smegma and keratin pearls removed before preparation. Once draped, a 2-0 silk traction suture is placed in the dorsal midline glans to permit atraumatic manipulation of the penis on the surgical field. A .025 % plain Marcaine penile block can be placed to decrease anesthetic requirements if a caudal anesthetic has not been introduced. Care should be taken to not overdose the Marcaine or use epinephrine, which may lead to vascular compromise

At this point, the type of repair is selected. Generally, this is done on the basis of five criteria: (a) the meatal location; (b) the size of the meatus; (c) the configuration of the glans, especially the depth and width of the urethral groove; (d) the degree or absence of chordee; and (e) the quality and quantity of the ventral skin. Although dozens of repairs are in use today, a small number enjoy wide popularity and can be used for single-stage repair of most presentations of hypospadias. The GAP procedure should be restricted to boys with wide, deep glanular grooves, glanular or coronal hypospadias, and a fixed meatus (25). If the meatus is mobile, that is, if it's ventral lip can be advanced distally, a meatoplasty and glanduloplasty procedure (MAGPI) may be used with a lower risk of fistulization (22). If the meatus is more proximal than the corona and the ventral skin is thick and pliable, a meatal-based flap repair is appropriate (26) (Fig. 77–1). If the glans is conical, the meatal-based flap can be tubularized and tunneled through a cored-out channel in the glans (27,28). For boys with longer defects, or poor quality or scant ventral-shaft skin, the island onlay technique provides reliably vascularized tissue for urethral floor replacement (29) (Fig. 77–2). If the glans is conical, or if the urethral plate must be resected to repair chordee, the vascularized preputial island flap can be tubularized and channeled through a glans tunnel (30,31). Occasionally, the surgeon encounters a patient with a wide urethral plate and a deep glandular groove. Such patients can be safely corrected with tubularization of the plate and glandular groove (32).

Once a repair is selected, the proposed incision lines should be carefully marked with a pen or with brilliant green and a sterile toothpick. The subcoronal incision should leave an adequate cuff of skin so that subsequent closure is not directly to the coronal margin, but to the "mucosal collar" (33). This skin often seems to shrink over the course of the repair, so the incision should be about 8 mm from the coronal margin in the infant. The ventral incision lines are critical both in location and depth. Before cutting across the midline proximal to the meatus, the surgeon must be absolutely certain that a meatal-based flap is not anticipated. Furthermore, the spongiosal tissue here is often hypoplastic or even absent, so it is very easy to enter the urethra. Once the incisions have been made, the penis is completely degloved to the base of the penis. This is done in the avascular plane on top of the Buck fascia. Care must be taken not to enter the Buck fascia, as the dorsolateral nerves, the dorsal vessels, the corpora, and the spongiosum are easily damaged by dissection below this plane. Ventral bands should be sought and released from the surface of the corpus spongiosum. Once the penis is degloved, a Rummel-type tourniquet using a rubber vessiloop rather than umbilical tape can be used to perform artificial erection or to control bleeding. The tourniquet should not be placed over the skin, as this may lead to thrombosis of the preputial vessels, and should it be relaxed occasionally to prevent ischemic damage to the erectile tissue.

5. Johnston WG Jr, Yeatman GW, Weigel JW. Congenital absence of the penis. *J Urol* 1977; 117:508–512.
6. Soderdahl DW, Brosman SA, Goodwin WE. Penile agenesis. *J Urol* 108:496–499.
7. Kessler WO, McLaughlin AP III. Agenesis of the penis: embryology and management. *Urology* 1973; 1:226–229.
8. Trengove-Jones G, Alter G. Total phallic reconstruction. *Dialogues Pediatr Urol* 1995; 18:3.
9. MacLusky NJ, Naftolin F. Sexual differentiation of the central nervous system. *Science* 1981; 211:1294–1303.
10. Lee PA, Mazur T, Danish R, et al. Micropenis I. Criteria, etiologies, and classification. *Johns Hopkins Med J* 1980; 146:156–163.
11. Danish RK, Lee PA, Mazur T, et al. Micropenis II. Hypogonadotropic hypogonadism. *Johns Hopkins Med J* 1980; 146:177–184.
12. Ehrlich RM, ed. Micropenis and penile growth: understanding the underlying factors. *Dialogues Pediatr Urol* 1994; 17:5.
13. Schober JM, Woodhouse CRJ. Micropenis: future social, psychological, and physical considerations. *Dialogues Pediatr Urol* 1994; 17:5.
14. Reid C, Gonzales R. Syndromes associated with micro or macropenis. *Dialogues Pediatr Urol* 1994; 17:5.
15. Elder JS. Congenital anomalies of the genitalia. In: Walsh PC, et al., eds. *Campbell's urology.* 6th ed. Philadelphia: WB Saunders, 1992; 1926.
16. James T. Curiosa pediatrica IV: tortipenis congenitus. *S Afr Med J* 1981; 59 (pt1):19–20.
17. Kenawi MM. Webbed penis. *Br J Urol* 1973; 45:569.
18. Kramer SA, Aydin G, Kelalis PP. Chordee without hypospadias in children. *J Urol* 1982; 128 (pt1):559–561.
19. Cendron J, Melin Y. Congenital curvature of the penis without hypospadias. *Urol Clin North Am* 1981; 8:389–385.
20. Nesbit RM. Congenital curvature of the phallus: report of three cases with description of corrective operation. *J Urol* 1965; 93:230–232.
21. Fitzpatrick TJ. Hemihypertrophy of the human corpus cavernosum. *J Urol* 1976; 115:560–561.
22. Duckett JW. MAGPI (meatoplasty and glanduloplasty). A procedure for subcoronal hypospadias. *Urol Clin North Am* 1981; 8(3):513.
23. Berg R, Svensson J, Astrom G. Social and sexual adjustment of men operated for hypospadias during childhood: a controlled study. *J Urol* AQ 1981; 125:313–317.
24. Husmann DA. Penile growth. *Dialogues Pediatr Urol* 1994; 17:5.
25. Zaontz MR: The GAP (glans approximation procedure) for glanular/coronal hypospadias. *J Urol* 141:359-361, 1989.
26. Mathieu P. Traitement en un temps de l'hypospadias balanique et juxta-balanique. *J Chir* 1932; 39:481.
27. Mustardé JC. One-stage repair. IV. In: Horton CE, ed. *Plastic and reconstructive surgery of the genital area.* Boston: Little, Brown, 1973; 290.
28. Belman AB. The modified Mustardé hypospadias repair. *J Urol* 1982; 127 (pt1):88–90.
29. Elder JS, Duckett JW, Snyder HM. Onlay island flap in the repair of mid and distal penile hypospadias without chordee. *J Urol* 1987; 138:376–379.
30. Asopa HS, Elhence IP, Atri SP, et al. One-stage correction of penile hypospadias using a foreskin tube. A preliminary report. *Int. Surg* 1971; 55:435–440.
31. Duckett JW. Transverse preputial island flap technique for repair of severe hypospadias. *Urol Clin North Am* 1980; 7:423.
32. King LR. Hypospadias: a one-stage repair without skin graft based on a new principle: chordee is sometimes produced by the skin alone. *J Urol* 1970; 103:660–662.
33. Firlit CF. The mucosal collar in hypospadias surgery. *J Urol* 1987; 137:80–83.
34. Gittes RF, McLaughlin AP III. Injection technique to induce penile erection. *Urology* 1974; 4:473–474.
35. Nesbit RM. Congenital curvature of the phallus: report of three cases with description of corrective operation. *J Urol* 1965; 93:230–232.
36. Dessanti A, Rigamonti W, Merulla V, et al. Autologous buccal mucosa graft for hypospadias repair: an initial report. *J Urol* 1992; 147 (pt 2): 1081–1084.
37. Memmelaar J. Use of bladder mucosa in a one-stage repair of hypospadias. *J Urol* 1947; 58:68–73.
38. Dector RM, Roth DR, Gonzales ET Jr. Hypospadias repair by bladder mucosal graft: an initial report. *J Urol* 1988; 140:1256–1258.
39. Snow BW. Use of tunica vaginalis to prevent fistulas in hypospadias surgery. *J Urol* 1986; 136:861–863.
40. Nesbit RM. Plastic procedure for correction of hypospadias. *J Urol* 1941; 45:699–702.
41. Byars LT. Technique for consistently satisfactory repair of hypospadias. *Surg Gynecol Obstet* 1955; 100:184–190.
42. van der Muelen JCH. The correction of hypospadias. In: Whitehead ED, Leiter E, eds. *Current operative urology.* Philadelphia: Harper & Row, 1984; 1243.
43. Orandi A. One-stage urethroplasty. *Br J Urol* 1968; 40:717–719.
44. Johanson B. Reconstruction of the male urethra in strictures. *Acta Chir Scand (suppl)* 1953; 176.
45. King LR. Neonatal circumcision. *Dialogues Pediatr Urol* 1982; 5:5.
46. Maizels M, Zaontz M, Donovan J, et al. Surgical correction of the buried penis: description of a classification system and a technique to correct the disorder. *J Urol* 1986; 136:268–271.
47. Shrom SH, Cromie WJ, Duckett JW. Megalourethra. *Urology* 1981; 17:152–156.
48. Stephens FD. Congenital intrinsic lesions of the anterior urethra. In: *Congenital malformations of the urinary tract.* New York: Praeger, 1983; 128–129.
49. Lancaster PAL. Epidemiology of bladder exstrophy and epispadias: a communication from the international clearinghouse for birth defects monitoring systems. *Teratology* 1987; 36:221–227.
50. Dees JE. Congenital epispadias with incontinence. *J Urol* 1949; 62:513.
51. Arap S, Nahas WC, Giron AM, et al. Incontinent epispadias: surgical treatment of 38 cases. *J Urol* 1988; 140:577.
52. Young HH. An operation for the cure of incontinence associated with exstrophy. *J Urol* 1922; 7:1.
53. Cantwell FV. Operative treatment of epispadias by transplantation of the urethra. *Ann Surg* 1895; 22:689–694.
54. Ransley PG, Duffy PG, Wollin M. Bladder exstrophy closure and epispadias repair. In: Nixon HH, Spitz L, eds. *Operative surgery: paediatric surgery.* 4th ed. Edinburgh: Butterworths, 1988; 620–632.
55. Devine CJ Jr, Horton CE, Scarff JE Jr. Epispadias. *Urol Clin North Am* 1980; 7:465–476.
56. Monfort G, Morisson-Lacombe G, Guys JM, et al. Transverse island flap and double flap procedure in the treatment of congenital epispadias in 32 patients. *J Urol* 1987; 138 (pt 2):1069–1071.
57. Elder JS. Congenital anomalies of the genitalia. In: Walsh PC, et al., eds. *Campbell's urology.* 6th ed. Philadelphia: WB Saunders, 1992; 1927.
58. Lamm DL, Kaplan GW. Accessory and ectopic scrotum. *Urology* 1977; 9:149–153.
59. Alter GJ, Trengove-Jones G, Horton CE Jr:. Hemangioma of the penis and scrotum. *Urology* 1993; 42(2):205–208.
60. Asarch RG, Golitz LE, Sausker WF, et al. Median raphe cysts of the penis. *Arch Dermatol* 1979; 115 (pt2):1084–1086.

78

Congenital Deformities of the Female Genitalia

Gregory A. Dumanian, M.D., and Dennis J. Hurwitz, M.D., F.A.C.S.

Congenital deformity of the female genital tract may be isolated, associated with anomalies of the lower bowel and/or bladder, or part of a complex of anomalies. This myriad of presentations has fascinated physicians for millennia (1).

A common cause of congenital deformities is hormonal imbalance during gestation. Diseases of genetic origin associated with abnormal female development include congenital adrenal hyperplasia, adrenal insensitivity syndrome (testicular feminization), and chromosome aberrations of trisomy D or E. Arrest in development of the cloaca results in severe genitourinary and hindgut deformity; a suspected but still unproven cause is maternal exposure to teratogenic agents. Frequently, as in the case of vaginal agenesis, the etiology is unknown.

In-hospital plastic surgery consultations arise on newborn infants with ambiguous genitalia or with devastating cloacal abnormalities. In the office, adolescents with amenorrhea and newly diagnosed vaginal agenesis present for reconstruction.

Careful physical examination of the newborn uncovers most anomalies. Vaginoscopy establishes the presence and configuration of the vagina and cervix. If abdominal and pelvic radiographs suggest anomalous uterine development or ectopic kidneys, ultrasound exam is indicated. Intravenous pyelography is performed before reconstructive surgery. A lower intestinal workup should be considered.

Computed axial tomography (CT) and laparoscopy are indicated in adolescents with anomalous genitalia, pelvic pain, and masses. Magnetic resonance imaging (MRI) has the advantage of no ionizing radiation in this pregnancy-prone population (2). Examination of nuclear chromatin or, more reliably, a karyotype will establish genetic sex.

Embryology

NORMAL DEVELOPMENT

The development of the female genital tract depends on the complex interplay between fetal genes, intrinsic fetal hormones, and exogenous maternal hormones. Before 10 weeks of gestation, the undifferentiated external genitalia are constituted by (a) a genital tubercle or phallus; (b) the urethral groove, which is limited laterally by the urogenital folds; and (c) the labioscrotal folds (Fig. 78–1). In the female, the genital tubercle develops into the clitoris. The urethral groove re-

mains open to become the vestibule. The urethral folds remain unfused to form the labia minora, while the labioscrotal folds similarly form the labia majora. Exposure to androgen (dihydrotestosterone, or DHT) develops the genital tubercle into the phallus, fuses the urogenital folds to form the penile urethra and causes the labioscrotal folds to form the scrotal raphe. After the twelfth week of gestation, the external genitalia will typically demonstrate either a male or a female appearance.

The undifferentiated paired reproductive ducts are joined to the excretory tract and hindgut in the primitive receptacle called the cloaca. By the sixth week, the urorectal septum separates the intestinal and genitourinary compartments. The latter opens exteriorly shortly thereafter to become the urogenital sinus.

The paired reproductive ducts, now called *Müllerian* ducts, enlarge and fuse into a genital canal. In males, this development is blocked by the production of *Müllerian*-inhibiting substance (MIS), a hormone produced by functional Sertoli cells (3). The proximal portion of the *Müllerian* duct differentiates into the fallopian tubes and uterus. The distal aspect of the *Müllerian* duct lengthens and abuts the urogenital sinus. A lumen between these two structures opens shortly thereafter.

ABNORMAL DEVELOPMENT

The External Genitalia

When uncertainty is present regarding the sex of a child, the child is considered to have "ambiguous genitalia." Microphallus, clitoral enlargement, and partial or total labial fusion are causes of uncertainty. In order to diagnose these infants, a determination is made on physical exam whether the gonads are symmetric in position, either above or below the inguinal ligament. Asymmetry points to true hermaphrodites (a mosaic of XX and XY cells in a single gonad) for infants *without* a Y chromosome on buccal smear. Asymmetric gonad position in combination *with* a Y chromosome on buccal smear implies mixed gonadal dysgenesis. The "streak" gonads in these patients have increased rates of neoplastic transformation and should be removed.

When the ambiguous gonads are symmetric in position and the infant does not have a Y chromosome on buccal smear,

FIG. 78–1. The external genitalia arise at the genital eminence, which is located on the median ventral surface of the body between the umbilicus and tail. The glans portion of the phallus forms the clitoris. The urethal folds elongate and form the labia minora. The genital swellings differentiate into the labia majora. Excessive exposure of these organs to androgen leads to masculization of the genitalia.

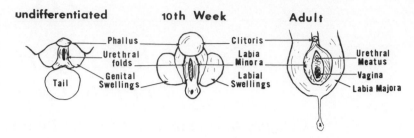

then the child is a female pseudohermaphrodite. The external genitalia in these cases are enlarged due to exposure to supra-normal levels of androgens. The increased androgen level may be due to an inborn metabolism error like that in congenital adrenal hyperplasia. In this syndrome, excess androgens are synthesized by the infant due to an inability to make other related steroids such as cortisol. Enlargement of the clitoris and partial or total fusion of the labia may also be due to exogenous maternal ingestion of androgens with subsequent in-utero exposure of the fetus.

Symmetric gonad position with a Y chromosome on buccal smear implies male pseudohermaphroditism. The cause of this poor response to testosterone may be due to low testosterone production, inability to convert testosterone to DHT, or poorly functional cellular receptors for testosterone. In the classic syndrome of testicular feminization, a familial X-linked disorder, the receptor for testosterone is completely nonfunctional. These children have normal external female genitalia (normal estrogen response), but have no internal female organs (MIS-induced *Müllerian* duct regression).

The Internal Genitalia

The internal female organs, consisting of the majority of the vagina, the cervix, the uterus, and the fallopian tubes, are derived from the *Müllerian* ducts. Abnormalities of these structures can be categorized as a failure of the ducts to form, a failure of the ducts to fuse adequately, or an inadequate dissolution of structures after fusion.

Failure of the *Müllerian* duct–derived structures to form is a fairly common abnormality that occurs once in every 4,000 to 5,000 births, and the cause for this developmental failure is unknown. In the Mayer-Custer-Hauser-Rokitansky syndrome, none of the *Müllerian* derived structures (vagina, cervix, uterus, and fallopian tubes) are present. The vagina is shallow, or presents as a dimple. Combinations of vaginal agenesis with presence of some of the *Müllerian* duct–derived structures also exist. The uterus, when present, is often nonfunctional. A rudimentary uterus may contain enough endometrial tissue to accumulate menstrual blood, causing cyclic lower abdominal pain. In such cases, excision of the rudimentary tissue is required. Vaginal agenesis is associated with other developmental anomalies including ectopic kidneys, uteropelvic obstruction, and lumbar spinal deformity. As has been mentioned, certain familial causes of vaginal agenesis exist (e.g., the testicular feminization syndrome).

Failure of the *Müllerian* ducts to properly fuse can result in duplications of the vagina, cervix, and uterus. Failure of the upper aspect of the ducts to fuse is thought to be the cause of the bicornuate uterus.

Persistence of the urethral membrane of the urogenital sinus is manifest as an imperforate hymen, and this is an example of a failure of dissolution. Newborns with an imperforate hymen may present with hydrometrocolpos, or the distension of the vagina and the uterus with accumulated mucous secretions. An adolescent with an imperforate hymen presents with hematometrocolpos due to the inability to discharge menstrual fluid. Another example of a failure of dissolution is a septate vagina, which may be a cause of dyspareunia. A third example of a failure of dissolution is a transverse annular septum of the vagina, which results from an incomplete perforation of the junction of the urogenital sinus with the *Müllerian* duct. This ring of tissue must be completely excised.

Surgical Reconstruction

For patients with ambiguous genitalia, a thorough physical exam will determine the symmetry of the position of the gonads, and a karyotype will establish the genetic sex. Once genetic and endocrine factors have been determined, a decision regarding the sex of rearing is made. Unless a male identity has already been assumed, genetic females are raised females and male pseudohermaphrodites are sometimes reversed to females. The size of the microphallus is one of the deciding factors in the sex rearing of male pseudohermaphrodites, as some infants are treatable with androgen replacement (4).

CLITOROMEGALY

For female pseudohermaphrodites (excessive androgen exposure), the enlarged size of the clitoris is a source of concern to the family and may interfere with acceptance of the child. Goals regarding clitoral reduction surgery include maintenance of sensitivity of the glans, minimal scars, and near-total excision of erectile tissue. Many techniques have been described that preserve the distal aspect of the glans on its dorsal neurovascular bundle (5). The erectile conjoined corpus cavernosum is excised, while the glans is then sutured to the base of the divided corpora (6). Preservation of too much erectile tissue can be a cause of painful clitoral erections (7). Surgery is typically performed at an early age, often in conjunction with vaginal flap surgery (see below).

Not all cases of clitoral hypertrophy require surgery. Clitoral hypertrophy secondary to maternal ingestion of exogenous androgens or progestational drugs during pregnancy is self-correcting after withdrawal of stimulation.

LABIAL HYPERTROPHY

Hypertrophy of the labia minora is a normal variant. If it is a cause of irritation or embarrassment, the labial excess should be excised.

VAGINAL ATRESIA

Vaginal atresia is defined as the condition in which the small vagina empties into the urethra, rather than externally into the perineum as the vestibule. The distinction between vaginal atresia and vaginal agenesis is important, because local flaps may be used to reconstruct and exteriorize the atretic vagina.

Normally, females have no connection between the urinary and the gynecologic systems. For female pseudohermaphrodites with virilization, the degree of excess androgen exposure can be "measured" by the level of proximity of the connection between the vagina and the urethra. Distal vagino-urethral connections are termed *low vaginal atresia,* while connections proximal to the urethral sphincter are called *high vaginal atresia,* and comprise 5% of the cases. Congenital adrenal hyperplasia due to a 21-hydroxylase enzyme deficiency is a prime cause of vaginal atresia, and the diagnosis is in part made by measurement of an excess of 17-hydroxyprogesterone. Caution in the preoperative preparation of these patients before surgery is mandatory, as they are prone to salt wasting, hypotension, and adrenal insufficiency (3). Also necessary in the preoperative workup of these patients is contrast and endoscopic evaluation of the urinary system, because of the high incidence of associated congenital anomalies. Disastrous injury to a single pelvic kidney in the course of vaginal reconstruction can be averted by preoperative diagnosis of an ectopic kidney.

Low vaginal atresia is corrected with a flap vaginoplasty between the ages of 3 and 6 months (8). A U-shaped flap based posteriorly towards the rectum is raised, and the atretic vagina (which is connected to the urethra) is located. After division of the fistula tract, the vagina is exteriorized by sewing the vaginal cuff to local perineal advancement flaps. Postoperative dilatations of the vagina are frequently required.

High vaginal atresia includes the added surgical dimension of the urinary external sphincter. Division of the fistula tract between the vagina and the urethra puts the patient at risk for urinary incontinence. The atretic vagina is also located further away from the perineum, requiring longer, somewhat precarious local flaps.

The surgical correction for high atresia is delayed until the child is 2 years of age to permit accurate localization of the external urethral sphincter with a nerve stimulator. After insertion of a catheter via the urethra into the atretic vagina, a careful cut-down onto the vagina is performed. The fistula to the urethra is meticulously closed. The vagina is dissected away from both the bladder and the rectum toward the perineum. An added benefit of this mobilization is to cover the urethral fistula closure with viable tissue. The vaginal exteriorization is completed with a posteriorly based U-shaped advancement flap and laterally based transposition flaps (9).

VAGINAL AGENESIS

Progress in the techniques of vaginal reconstruction has paralleled the development of plastic surgery. Surgeons of the early nineteenth century bluntly dissected a space between the rectum and the bladder in order to create a "vaginal cavity," but despite continuous packing they had difficulty maintaining the new opening (1). In order to sidestep the problem of spontaneous closure of the bluntly dissected cavity, Abbé (10) and later McIndoe (11) lined the walls of this cavity with a split-thickness skin graft. The Abbé-McIndoe technique, which uses split-thickness skin grafts with prolonged obturation of the lined cavity has become a standard treatment of vaginal agenesis (12). Patient cooperation in postoperative stenting and dilatation is mandatory. Vaginal reconstruction is done at the time of physical and emotional maturity, and for the highly motivated sexual activity need not be postponed. The complex nature of this disorder in regard to femininity and fertility should prompt a preoperative psychiatric consultation.

The patient's lower bowel is emptied by enema. A split-thickness skin graft of approximately 0.015 inches with a surface area of 24 cm is harvested from the upper lateral thigh or buttock skin. After dressing the donor sites, the patient supine on the operating room table. Laparoscopy may be performed at this time as indicated. A Foley catheter is inserted into the urethra. The bladder is inflated with normal saline and a percutaneous suprapubic catheter is inserted. (The Foley catheter is removed at the completion of the procedure to avoid pressure between it and the vaginal mold, which may injure the posterior urethra.)

The patient's legs are raised into stirrups, and the perineum is shaved. A three-limbed stellate incision is centered over the perineum (Fig. 78–2). The initial sharp dissection is followed by a blunt opening of the easily dissected rectovesical space up to the peritoneal reflection, which lies approximately fifteen cm from the incision. Care must be taken to maintain a uniform width of the tunnel and not to deviate from the midline, which increases the risk of vascular and visceral injury. Hemostasis must be complete.

The skin graft is draped over an appropriately sized vaginal mold. Noncompressible materials such as balsa wood have traditionally been used for the skin graft stent, but recently other materials have been described as easy to use (13,14). The suture line should take a spiral alignment (to help prevent a linear contracture band) and stop before the apex of the mold, where the graft take is most tenuous. The mold may be

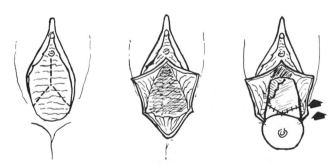

FIG. 78–2. A three-limbed stellate incision is made in the introitus to create three triangular flaps. The vesicorectal space is opened by blunt and sharp dissection. A split-thickness skin graft measuring approximately 1/15,000 inch is draped over the plastic mold, which is covered by adhesive tape and a latex condom to allow suturing of the skin graft. The triangular flaps are interdigitated with the skin graft to avoid circular scar contracture at the introitus. The obturator may be retained with a T-binder or by suturing the labia together over it.

retained by suturing the labia together or fixing the distal end of the mold with an umbilical tape to a T-binder.

The mold is left in place for the first postoperative week while the patient is on bed rest. It is then removed with the patient under sedation. Gentle inspection with the Graves speculum will permit débridement of nontake areas. If graft loss is greater than 2 cm the patient should be regrafted. The mold is returned and left in place for 1 month, to be removed only briefly for cleansing and defecation. After 4 to 6 weeks the original mold may be replaced by a slightly smaller obturator that can be self-retained for 6 months. Brief removal is permissible for coitus, dilating exercises, or hygiene.

The long-term results of this procedure are fair. Fifty consecutive patients who underwent vaginal reconstruction at the Mayo Clinic were followed an average of 6.5 years (15). Only 72% of these patients were coitally active at the time of the survey. In a compilation of 19 separate studies that reported on results of the Abbé-McIndoe procedure in 1,229 patients, 83% were able to have "normal, good or satisfactory sexual relationships (16)."

Potentially to improve results by decreasing the likelihood of vaginal stenosis, Sadove and Horton used full-thickness (as opposed to split-thickness) skin graft vaginoplasties with excellent take (17). They advocated correction in childhood because postoperative stenting is decreased and there is the theoretical potential for vaginal growth with full-thickness grafts.

Skin grafts of the neovagina acquire characteristics of vaginal mucosa, though the cells continue to keratinize (18). Fol-

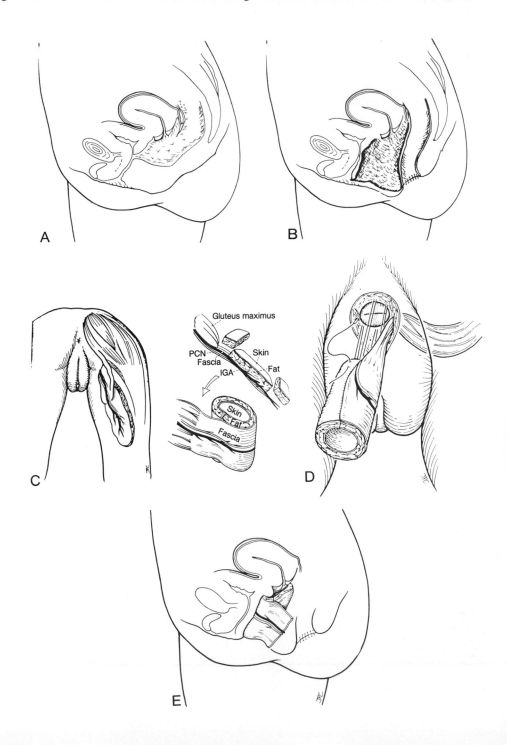

FIG. 78–3. Gluteal thigh flap reconstruction of the vagina in severe persistent cloacal deformity. **A,** the termination of the high imperforate anus in the female forms a common sinus with the vagina and uretha. **B,** the sinus has been excised, the urethra repaired, and the rectal pull-through performed. Skin graft vaginoplasty takes poorly in these wounds primarily because of urine leakage from the repaired urethral fistula. **C,** the gluteal thigh flap is elevated on the inferior gluteal artery (IGA) and posterior cutaneous nerver (PCN) pedicle. After removing the ends of the elliptical flap, the skin is tubed on itself. **D,** the flap is tunneled under the thigh and labia. It is sewn to the proximal cuff of vaginal tissue with a series of polyglycolic acid sutures, which are left long and tied after all are placed. **E,** the tubed flap fills the cavity and creates a vagina.

low-up with Papanicolaou (PAP) smears should be continued indefinitely after reconstruction, because some grafts have degenerated into squamous cell carcinomas (19). Chronic irritation and infection are the possible etiologies for carcinoma that develops an average of 15 years after the reconstruction.

There has been a movement in some centers away from using grafts and toward using vascularized skin in vaginal reconstruction. Abdominal axial flaps have been designed and should be limited to thin patients. Unfortunately, donor site scarring tends to be unsightly (20). Myocutaneous flaps are bulky and may not fit into the narrow rectovesicle space (21). Postextirpative surgery for pelvic carcinoma better utilizes these hearty flaps (22,23). Preliminary tissue expansion of the labia has had limited success, an awkward effort at vaginoplasty (24).

Free-tissue transfer presents the best opportunity to introduce vascularized tissue with a low tendency for contracture into the perineum for reconstruction. The magnitude of the operative procedure must be contrasted to the simplicity of the alternatives (25).

Small and large bowel pedicle grafts were popular for vaginal construction in the early 1900s. Some good results have been reported (26). An added benefit is the ability to perform these reconstructions at an early age because theoretically the vascularized bowel will grow with the patient. Despite advances in operative technique and the use of antibiotics, the procedure remains difficult to perform and may be complicated by prolapse, bowel necrosis, and infection. Invasion of the peritoneal cavity is a distinct disadvantage. Regular douching may be necessary to control vaginal mucous discharge (27).

The nonoperative technique of frequent forceful pressure by glass rods in the region of the rectovesicle septum was developed by Frank in 1938 (28). Few modern surgeons have applied this approach successfully; it should be reserved for the highly motivated patient with a substantial vaginal dimple. Modifications of this tissue-stretching technique by combining it with a vulvoplasty have been described (29). Unsightly scarring, vascular pedicle limitations, skin grafts, and intraabdominal surgery are all avoided with this technique.

IMPERFORATE ANUS AND PERSISTENT CLOACA

Imperforate anus and persistent cloaca are complex malformations with a variety of presentations. Complete examination and diagnosis includes a careful contrast study to unravel the aberrant anatomy. Low rectal lesions have perineal fistulas and rarely involve the genitourinary system. In high lesions there is anorectal atresia, and persistence of the cloaca manifests as a large rectal fistula to the vagina and nearby urethra (Fig. 78–3A). An abdominoperineal-sacral approach preserves as much rectal sphincter as possible for rectal pull-through. Reconstruction of a perineal urethra is also a surgical priority. Usually, insufficient cloacal lining remains for vaginal reconstruction (30). Skin graft vaginoplasty generally results in a poor take in these pelves. Pedicle bowel grafts have been advocated but are unpredictable and complicated by mucosal friability and discharge. Earlier surgeries frequently leave bladder and bowel fistulas. A unilateral tubed gluteal thigh flap was used successfully to solve a difficult problem in a patient at Children's Hospital of Pittsburgh (Fig. 78–3B-E) (31).

Summary

The identification of aberrant or atretic portions of the external female genitalia requires a careful search for accompanying local or systemic deformity. Sex assignments are made early. For patients with clitoromegaly and vaginal atresia, reconstruction of the phallus and labia is performed early in life. Vaginal reconstruction for vaginal agenesis is done at the time of physical and emotional maturity.

References

1. Goldwyn RM: History of attempts to form a vagina. *Plast Reconstr Surg* 1977; 59:319.
2. Barach B, Falces E, Benzian SR: Magnetic resonance imaging for diagnosis in pre-operative planning in agenesis of the distal vagina. *Ann Plast Surg* 1987; 19:192.
3. Donahoe PK, Powell DM, Lee MM: Clinical management of intersex abnormalities, in *Current Problems in Surgery,* Well SA (ed.), Mosby-Year Book, St. Louis MO.
4. Allen TD: Microphallus: Clinical and endocrinological characteristics. *J Urol* 1978; 119:750.
5. Sagehashi, N: Clitoroplasty for clitoromegaly due to andrenogenital syndrome without loss of sensitivity. *Plast Reconstr Surg* 1993; 91:950.
6. Donahoe, PK, Crawford JD: Ambiguous genitalia in the newborn. In KJ Welch et. al. (eds.) *Pediatric Surgery,* Vol 2, 4th ed. Chicago: Year Book Medical Publishers, 1986; p. 1383.
7. Allen LE, Hardy BE, Churchill BM: The surgical management of the enlarged clitoris. *J Urol* 1981; 128:351.
8. Hendren, WH: Reconstructive problems of the vagina and the female urethra. *Clin Plast Surg* 1980; 7:207.
9. Dumanian GA, Donahoe PK: Bilateral rotated buttock flaps for vaginal atresia in severely masculinized females with adrenogenital syndrome. *Plast Reconstr Surg* 1992; 90:488.
10. Abbe R: A new method of creating a vagina in a case of congenital absence. *Med Record NYU* 1898; 54:836.
11. McIndoe A: The treatment of congenital absence and obliterative conditions of the vagina. *Br J Plast Surg* 2:254, 1950.
12. Garcia J, Jones IIW Jr: The split-thickness graft technic for vaginal agenesis. *Obstet Gyncecol* 1989; 49:328.
13. Viegas T, Thomas R, Guido NL: An improvised mould for vaginoplasty. *Br J Plast Surg* 1989; 42:487.
14. Concannon MJ, Croll GH, Puckett CL: An intraoperative stent for McIndoe vaginal construction. *Plast Reconstr Surg* 1993; 91: 367. Also comment, *Plast Reconstr Surg* 1994; 93:1528.
15. Buss JJ, Lee RA: McIndoe procedure for vaginal agenesis: Results and complications. *Mayo Clin Proc* 64:758, 1989.
16. Tolhurst DE, van der Helm TW: The treatment of vaginal atresia. *SGO* 1991; 172:407.
17. Sadove RC, Horton CE: Utilizing full-thickness skin grafts for vaginal reconstruction. *Clin Plast Surg* 1988; 15(3):443.
18. Lelle RJ, Heidenreich W, Schneider J: Cytologic findings after construction of a neovagina using two surgical procedures. *Surg Gynecol Obstet* 1990; 170:21.
19. Baltzer J, Zander J: Primary squamous cell carcinoma of the neovagina. *Gynecol Oncol* 1989; 35:99.
20. Chen Z-J, Chen M-Y, Chen C, Wu N: Vaginal reconstruction with an axial subcutaneous pedicle flap from the inferior abdominal wall: A new method. *Plast Reconstr Surg* 1989; 83:1005.
21. Lilford RJ, Johnson N, Batchelor A: A new operation for the vaginal agenesis: Construction of a neovagina from a rectus abdominus musculocutaneous flap. *Br J Obstet Gynaecol* 1989; 96:1089.
22. Tobin GR, Day TG: Vaginal and pelvic reconstruction with distally based rectus abdominus myocutaneous flaps. *Plast Reconstr Surg* 1988; 81:62.
23. McCraw JB, Massey FM, Shanklin KD, et. al: Vaginal reconstruction with gracilis myocutaneous flaps. *Plast Reconstr Surg* 1976; 58:176.
24. Lilford RJ, Sharpe DT, Thomas DF: Use of tissue expansion techniques to create skin flaps for vaginoplasty: Case Report. *Br J Obstet Gynaecol* 1988; 95:402.
25. Johnson N, Lilford RJ, Batchelor A: The free-flap vaginoplasty; a new surgical procedure for the treatment of vaginal agenesis. *Br J Obstet Gynecol* 1991; 98:184.
26. Hitchcock RJ, Maline PS: Colovaginoplasty in infants and children. *Br J Urol* 1994; 73:196.

27. Turner-Warwick R, Kirby RS: The construction and reconstruction of the vagina with the colocecum. *Surg Gynecol Obstet* 1990; 170:132.

28. Frank RT: Formation of an artificial vagina without operation. *Am J Obstet Gynecol* 35:1053, 1938.

29. O'Brien BMcC, Mellow CG, MacIsaac IA, et al: Treatment of vaginal agenesis with a new vulvovaginoplasty. *Plast Reconstr Surg* 1990; 85:942.

30. Hendren WH: Further experience in reconstructive surgery of the cloacal anomalies. *J Pediatr Surg* 1982; 71: 695.

31. Hurwitz DJ: Reconstruction following radical surgery of the buttocks, perineum and pelvis with the gluteal thigh flap. In Williams B (ed): Transactions of the VIII International Congress of Plastic and Reconstructive Surgery. Washington, DC, Congress of Plastic and Reconstructive Surgery, 1983, p 257.

79

Gender Reassignment Surgery

Milton T. Edgerton, Jr., M.D., F.A.C.S., and Margaretha Willemina Langman, P.S., D.R.A.

Transsexualism is the most complete and profound disorder of gender identity. *Gender identity* is that inner sense of knowing to which sex one belongs. It is one's inner, basic awareness that "I am a male" or "I am a female."

Gender role is the public expression of one's gender identity and can be defined as the sum of the social and cultural activities, including all that one says and does to indicate to others (and to the self) the degree to which one is male or female (1).

Behaviorally, *transsexualism* manifests itself as an individual living in the role of the gender opposite to his or her physical anatomy—either before or after having attained hormonal, surgical, and legal sex reassignment.

The term *transsexualism,* presumably first used by Benjamin (2) in the early 1950s, is now widely recognized. Transsexualism is a true disease, although its etiology continues to be an issue of debate in professional circles; it is a disease in the literal sense of the word "dis-ease"—a lack of ease with the anatomy of the body. Transsexualism is *not* a variation of the norm, but a condition that sits *apart* (L. *dis* = apart) as an abnormal entity differing from *other* normal or pathologic body states.

Cross-gender behavior is described in Greek mythology and is often referred to in classical history (3). Despite these historical references to cross-gender behavior, psychosocial and clinical interest in the phenomenon of transsexualism and its treatment has emerged only in the last two decades. Physicians remain puzzled by the etiology of transsexualism, and controversy continues regarding the treatment of choice. The number of transsexual patients seeking either vaginoplasty or phalloplasty increased dramatically in the 1980s (4).

Why have we seen a dramatic increase in the requests for surgery? A conservative estimate of the number of people suffering from gender dysphoria is 30,000 worldwide (5). In the United States, at least 10,000 people are known to have some form of a gender-identity disorder (5).

Although the cause, or causes, of transsexualism remains elusive, numerous observations and laboratory studies have highlighted the recent increases in human male infertility, the appearance of gender disturbances among nonmating birds, fish, and reptiles, and the appearance of deformed genitalia in alligators and Great Lakes birds who have been exposed to a variety of industrial chemical pollutants. Some of these synthetics may be shown to mimic the actions of estrogens or testosterone when they enter the body. Such influences during gestation, even in tiny doses, have the capacity to alter the brain of a developing fetus so that *gender choice* (the sex of the love object), gender identity, or development of genitalia may be abnormal. Depending on the timing of exposure to such synthetic hormones, from one to three of these midbrain centers may be affected. One possible explanation for the apparent increase in transsexualism may be related to the recent additions of these "synthetic hormones" to our air, water, and soil. At the very least, we need further laboratory studies to test the theories advanced so convincingly in the recent book *Our Stolen Future* (Colburn T, Dumanoski D, and Myers JP. New York: Dutton, 1996).

Research has shown that a substantial amount of sexual education is provided by the media (6). In the entertainment world, cross-gender behavior is openly portrayed. Identification with the apparent success of popular entertainers with cross-gender images reinforces the drive of the young transsexual patient to obtain reassignment surgery.

Society has always been fascinated by ambiguous sexuality and either rejects or endures its manifestations. With more knowledge of, and greater publicity about, transsexualism, more patients publicly admit to their gender dysphoria and their secret longings for cross-gender confirmation. Plastic surgeons have become increasingly successful in devising sophisticated surgical methods of simulating both female and male anatomy. This has further increased the demand by patients for surgical reassignment.

From 1960 to 1970 the ratio of male to female transsexuals requesting surgical reassignment was 4.5:1. However, during the 1980s, the ratio approached 1:1. Patients now apply to gender identity clinics for surgery at a much younger age than a decade ago. Very often these young patients come with the support and encouragement of a parent or close friend. With the evolution of new and improved surgical techniques for genital reconstruction of the transsexual patient, more are electing surgical sex reassignment as the treatment of choice. These changing patterns seem to be a universal experience of gender identity clinics in the United States, as well as abroad.

This trend places an unusual burden on the plastic surgeon and the gender identity team in the treatment selection process. The selection of patients requesting sex reassignment surgery and ancillary procedures to change body configuration is a difficult task, even for clinicians who view such surgery as a legitimate form of treatment and who have had substantial experience with gender disorders. Almost all transsexuals are psychologically complex patients. Each has an absolute conviction that he or she belongs in the opposite

Table 79–1
Obstacles to Formation of University Gender Identity Programs

Lack of physician knowledge of transsexualism
Physician discomfort in relating to gender dysphoria patients
Fear of criticism by uninformed colleagues

Table 79–2
What Urologists, Gynecologists, and Plastic Surgeons Should Do

Work with university gender teams
Avoid solo management of transsexual patients
See patients before and after (long-term) surgery
Offer skills and knowledge of their surgical discipline
By example, encourage residents and students

sex. They believe that through some "mistake of nature" they were born with the anatomically wrong external body. Transsexualism represents the ultimate body disturbance, producing major psychosocial hardships on the patient (e.g., rejection, isolation, social ridicule, alienation, extreme psychic distress). Professional controversy about this disease, as well as personal and moral/ethical biases about the condition, leave many desperate patients without access to reputable professional support (Table 79–1). Because of this, some patients are driven by desperation to request surgery from less ethical, or commercially motivated, practitioners. The resulting inept surgery and inadequate psychological counseling has led to some unsatisfactory results.

How should the medical profession respond? Physicians must be educated to accept the reality of the transsexual syndrome and recognize that it can be treated.

Nontreatment of this disease costs U.S. taxpayers millions of dollars each year in disability, unemployment, and Social Security benefits. The transsexual patient has average intellectual abilities and, in general, *does not suffer from any major mental illness,* but is forced to expend an enormous amount of psychic energy just to deal with the persistent sense of being handicapped. Thus, the transsexual's emotional reservoir becomes depleted and is not available for more productive conversion of energy. The patient may become a parasite on society. The cost to the community of nontreatment accumulates over time, resulting in many transsexuals becoming noncontributing citizens, prone to suicide and secondary mental illness.

Treatment may prevent these undesirable effects, but is necessarily bound to a complete knowledge of diagnostic criteria.

Principles of Diagnosis and Patient Selection

MULTIDISCIPLINARY APPROACH

Careful guidelines for the hormonal and surgical sex reassignment of transsexual patients were made available in 1979 by the Harry Benjamin Foundation, a national interdisciplinary committee on gender dysphoria. However, it was not until 1980, with the publication of the American Psychiatric Association's *Diagnostic and Statistical Manual of Mental Disorders,* 3rd edition (DSM-III) (7), that standard descriptive criteria for the psychiatric diagnosis of transsexualism were released. The responsible and appropriate professional approach to the diagnosis and treatment of transsexualism is multidisciplinary. With such an approach in mind, programs have been established in gender identity clinics in university-based hospitals (Table 79–2). Stringent selection criteria for the treatment of transsexualism will provide diagnostic accuracy, ethical objectivity, and scientific follow-up, along with optimal specialized and cost-effective surgery with minimal patient risk.

DIFFERENTIAL DIAGNOSIS

Diagnostic criteria are defined by the American Psychiatric Association (7) as follows:

1. A sense of discomfort and inappropriateness about one's anatomic sex.
2. A wish to be rid of one's own genitalia and to live as a member of the other sex.
3. The disturbance has been continuous (not limited to periods of stress) for at least 2 years.
4. Absence of physical intersex or genetic abnormality.
5. Absence of any mental disorder, such as schizophrenia.

The psychiatrist's role in the initial stages of the diagnostic process for transsexualism is of the greatest importance. Subgroups of transsexualism include patients whose sexual orientation is reported as asexual, homosexual, or heterosexual. This spectrum of related gender disorders complicates the diagnostic picture. The blurring of diagnostic lines between homosexual and transsexual conditions is very subtle and may confuse those physicians unfamiliar with the manifestations of psychosexual disorders. It is not uncommon that the physician is confronted with a "gender-confused" patient seeking surgical sex reassignment, but who in reality is succumbing to societal pressure to live a heterosexual lifestyle; often these patients are desperately attempting to escape the stigma of homosexuality. If the proper diagnosis is missed and such a patient receives surgical treatment, postoperative crisis may follow. Such an error may lead to suicide or mental incapacity. The true homosexual is rarely dissatisfied with the genitalia, and will feel "mutilated" if castration and penectomy are performed. This is in sharp contrast to the expressions of relief and appreciation consistently reported by the true male transsexual after similar surgery.

Patients who as adults first consult a physician with symptoms characteristic of transsexualism, often give a history of gender identity problems during childhood. This is manifested by extensive, pervasive femininity in a boy or masculinity in a girl (8). Parental and peer interview usually confirm such behavior. A disturbed parent-child or parent-parent relationship is often, but not always, reported by the patient.

Some cases of transvestism, or patients reporting transvestite tendencies for the first time in early adult life, seem to evolve into transsexualism over a period of years. This subgroup of patients needs more long-term study. Caution should be used in offering sex reassignment surgery to these patients.

PATIENT SELECTION

Upon psychiatric referral to our University of Virginia Gender Identity Team, the patient is evaluated by a multidisciplinary team consisting of plastic surgeons, gynecologists, urologists, endocrinologists, psychiatrists, psychologists, and a coordinator.

Even when the diagnostic prerequisites have been fulfilled, certain true transsexual patients might be disallowed surgery. Some of our contraindications to sex reassignment surgery in transsexuals are:

1. Sexual ambiguity: patients who waver in their sexual object choice or sexual role.
2. The very young patient, who cannot give a meaningful informed consent for operation.
3. The emotionally disturbed patient who suffers from bodily delusions, or the overtly paranoid patient.
4. The secretive patient, who cannot establish trust in the team members.
5. The criminal patient (as evidenced from police records).
6. The drifter, or the patient with no close friend or supportive relative.
7. The patient who resists or refuses presurgical psychotherapy.
8. The patient who persists in unrealistic expectations of surgery, or who gives a history of drug addiction.

An occasional homosexual may mimic the history of transsexualism. Such patients may be detected if interviews reveal that they (a) wish surgery primarily to escape the stigma of homosexuality or (b) indicate that they derive erotic pleasure through self-stimulation of their genitalia.

The University of Virginia Gender Identity Clinic uses a special operative consent form for sex reassignment surgery. Every effort is made to help the patient anticipate each new stress before it is encountered. The multidisciplinary team approach is not only efficient and cost effective but it also adds objectivity to the evaluations and reduces the chance of misdiagnosis that might follow examination by a solo physician.

Principles of Treatment

PATIENT PREPARATION FOR SEX REASSIGNMENT SURGERY

It appears evident from experiences of the last 20 years that a substantial fraction of carefully selected transsexual patients benefit from surgical construction of the desired genitalia (9). Expectations for surgical outcome must be reasonable, and psychologic guidance and support play an important role after surgery.

Kohut (10) described the transsexual patient as a person with "marked intrapsychic and interpersonal conflicts, suffering from a disorder of the self." This disorder has its roots in a severely disturbed body image, evident in childhood and culminating in early puberty. Treatment must be viewed as a continuous, collaborative process with patient, psychiatrist, and plastic surgeon actively involved.

Before surgery, the patient is expected to be involved in an active therapeutic program for at least 1 to 2 years. In the therapy period, a number of important issues need to be addressed. These issues include: exploration of the patient's core gender identity; understanding of motivational patterns for surgery; social ramifications of living in the gender of conviction; ways of informing family members of the patients gender dysphoria; implications of losing fertility after surgery; recognition of personal sexual orientation; possible conflicts with religious convictions; legal issues; and impacts of surgery on work opportunities.

During this evaluation process, with the consent of the treating physician, the patient should begin a trial period of cross-living, both socially and at work. *This trial period of actually living in the desired gender is the most important single requirement for patient selection and preparation for surgery.* In addition, hormone treatment can be initiated and the male transsexual may begin electrolysis to remove unwanted facial or body hair. Voice training is helpful for some male transsexuals.

Many patients, especially those who received earlier gender-change surgery, will urge the gender team to bypass psychiatric prerequisites. Such patients are usually quite impatient, lacking the insight, ability, or motivation to become involved in *any* psychiatric relationship. Many have feelings of basic distrust, ingrained over years of frustration in their efforts to get responsible medical treatment. It takes considerable skill and understanding from the psychiatrist and other members of the team to win the confidence of these troubled patients.

Most transsexual patients have a stereotypical view of the female and male roles in a traditional sense. They espouse the idea that external body representation is not aligned with internal image. This myth needs to be clarified in therapy and through trial living.

The role of the psychiatrist is crucial, both in the early stages of treatment and in the transition phase. Psychiatric involvement needs to be intensified during the perioperative and postoperative periods. The psychologic stress of staged surgery and the resulting economic demands have a momentous impact on the patient's emotional equilibrium. This must be anticipated by both patient and medical team.

MALE-TO-FEMALE REASSIGNMENT

Surgical Techniques

It is now possible to create an aesthetically acceptable and functional vagina for the male transsexual patient. Improvements in these surgical techniques have reduced the complications and provided the patients with results that, in some instances, have passed medical examinations as examples of normal female anatomy.

Two surgical approaches for vaginoplasty are generally used, with several alternative methods available for unusual and complex cases.

Penile Flap Method

In the method introduced by the senior author (11), the pliable and moist skin of the male penile shaft is preserved as a pedicled skin and fascial flap (Figs. 79–1, 79–2, and 79–3). The pedicle is shifted posteriorly to the appropriate site for the vaginal introitus, the flap is inverted, and the penile skin becomes the lining for the new vagina (Figs. 79–4 through 79–7). The scrotal tissues may then be used to create the labia and a clitoral hood as a second-stage operation (12) (Fig. 79–8).

This technique has many advantages. The pedicle flap of skin and fascia gives a pliable and noncontracting lining for the vagina (Fig. 79–9), and the patient is not required to use

Surgical Technique

The modern history of phalloplasty and urethroplasty dates back to World War II. Later, the imaginative use of local tubed pedicled tissue led to the development of more sophisticated methods of phalloplasty (9). Earlier reconstructions of the phallus and scrotum required multiple stages over a period of years for completion (14).

At the University of Virginia Medical Center current techniques of female-to-male genitoplasty require three operative stages. In the first stage, the corpus of the phallus is formed. In the second, the urethra is constructed to provide transpenile voiding, while maintaining continence. The third stage is used for ancillary procedures such as scrotal reconstruction with testicular implants, contouring of the glans, vaginal cavity ablation, and the insertion of a special Silastic penile implant (required for additional stiffening by approximately one-half of patients).

Stage 1: Construction of the Phallus

Construction of the phallus can be accomplished by a variety of flap techniques, each having merits and drawbacks (Fig. 79–15). Gillies and Millard (15) and Fumpkin (16) described a random tubed abdominal flap to construct the phallus. Recently, axial pattern skin flaps have proved more dependable. A random-pattern flap that is still used in phalloplasty is the inferiorly based midline abdominal flap. Any skin flap used for phallus reconstruction must be of adequate size. The initial dimensions of the flap are 28 cm × 14 cm. Some flap shrinkage will occur after tubing.

The axial pattern flap that has produced the best results in phalloplasty at the University of Virginia is the groin flap (17). Its arterial supply is axial and is based on the superficial circumflex iliac artery. It is currently the most commonly used flap for phallus reconstruction. This flap is relatively non–hair bearing, allows one-stage elevation and tubing, and the donor scar can be easily hidden. This avoids the scar of the grafted forearm that most males dislike.

Alternatively, an axial-vessel tubed flap may be based on a single superficial inferior epigastric artery. This pattern appears to be less reliable than the groin flap for phallus reconstruction.

After months of testosterone therapy, the skin of the phallus tends to become more hair bearing. Abdominal obesity may limit the reliability of the inferior epigastric axial flap. Removal of the excess fat may cause ischemic necrosis. Previous abdominal or groin scars also reduce the alternatives available for phallus reconstruction.

The gracilis musculocutaneous flap and the "pure" gracilis muscle flap (with skin graft to cover) have been used in phalloplasty (14,18). However, the arterial pedicle is variable in both its location and length, and flaps in patients with heavy legs may prove unduly bulky for penile reconstruction. Considerable atrophy of the skin grafted muscle occurs with time.

Tissue transfer by free flap for construction of the phallus during urethral reconstruction represents an additional alternative in surgical therapy. However, this technique requires specialized equipment, microvascular surgical expertise, and prolonged operating time.

The technique of radial-forearm free flap reconstruction of the phallus is as follows. An Allen test is performed preoperatively to ensure adequate ulnar artery contribution to the vascular arch of the hand. In general, the left forearm is the preferred donor arm when performing the radial forearm flap (when the patient is right-handed). The right groin and vessels of the right leg are utilized for microvascular anastomoses to allow a two-team surgical approach. The course of the radial artery and cephalic vein are mapped preoperatively on the left volar forearm beginning 4 cm proximal to the wrist crease (Fig. 79–16). Making the distal portion of the flap 4 cm proximal to the wrist crease allows the donor scar to be easily concealed by a shirt sleeve. The dimensions of the radial forearm flap should be approximately 12 × 12 cm. The urethral portion of the phallus should be constructed from the ulnar side of the flap, where hair is scarce or absent. Preoperative removal of this hair by electrolysis is usually unnecessary. The portion of the flap that is tubed to from the urethra should be approximately 2 cm in width and 14.5 cm in length. Note that the urethral portion of the flap is made 2.5 cm longer than the proximal portion, which will cover the external surface of the phallus. This is accomplished by designing a 2.0 × 2.5 cm proximal extension onto the flap design. A 1.0-cm strip of skin between the urethral and phallic portions of the flap is then deepithelialized. This denuded

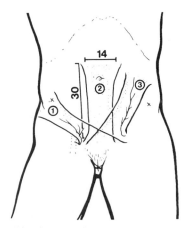

FIG. 79–15. Phalloplasty may be performed using a variety of local axial arterialized or random patterned flaps: (1) the groin flap, based on the superficial circumflex iliac artery; (2) the midline abdominal flap, incorporating the umbilicus, randomly patterned; and (3) the superficial inferior epigastric artery (SIEA) flap.

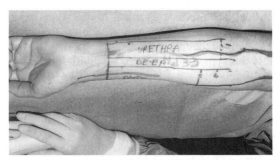

FIG. 79–16. Preoperative markings of the radial forearm free flap for total phalloplasty. Notice that the cutaneous urethral segment is made 2.5 cm longer then the phallic skin segment. The overall dimension of the radial forearm free flap are 12.0 × 14.5 cm.

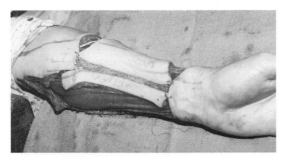

FIG. 79–17. Subfascial plane of dissection of the radial forearm flap.

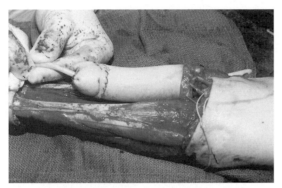

FIG. 79–18. The neophallus is created by forming a tube-within-a-tube. The Surgeon performs a coronoplasty.

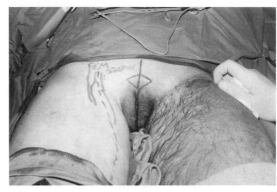

FIG. 79–19. Correct position of the neophallus cephalad to the anterior labial commissure.

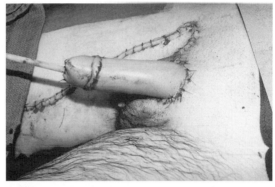

FIG. 79–20. Completed microvascular transfer of neophallus and urethra. Note urethral catheter tip existing through the proximal urethral segment in the superior perineum.

area allows suturing of the urethral tube over a no. 18 French catheter. The radial forearm flap is raised in a subfascial plane, as suggested by Muhlbauer (19) (Fig. 79–17). The median antebrachial cutaneous nerve is included in the flap. This nerve will later be anastomosed to the pudendal nerve at the base of the clitoris. Once the entire flap is raised on its pedicle of radial artery, vein, and nerves, the urethral portion is tubed upon itself over a no. 18 French catheter. The radial portion of the skin flap is then tubed so as to encircle the urethral segment and create a tube-within-a-tube. The distal phallus is closed directly, and a coronoplasty is performed. Up to this point in the operation, the donor vessels are not divided (Fig. 79–18).

The correct position is selected in the midline of the pubic area for placement of the base of the phallus. This midline position should be cephalad to the anterior labial commissure (Fig. 79–19). The prepuce of the clitoris is split vertically and the clitoris is circumscribed to its base. The clitoral frenulum is divided and the clitoris transposed cephalad so that its highly sensitive skin will be incorporated into the base of the new phallus. The right pudendal nerve is then exposed and identified at the base of the clitoris for later microanastomosis to the divided proximal end of the median antebrachial cutaneous nerve that was harvested with the forearm flap. The pubic incision is then curved laterally toward the right groin and extended down the medial aspect of the right thigh. The saphenous vein and common femoral artery are then dissected free of the adjacent fascia. When available, either the medial or lateral superficial circumflex femoral arteries are used as donor vessels. Occasionally, these vessels are too

small or otherwise unsuitable as donor vessels. When this occurs, a reversed segment of the saphenous vein is useful as a vein graft from the common femoral artery to the radial artery of the forearm flap. Venous drainage is readily accomplished by reflecting the saphenous vein superiorly and anastomosing it to the cephalic vein of the free flap. Additional venous anastomoses can be performed from the radial artery venae commitantes to the medial circumflex branches of the saphenous vein.

The pedicle of the completed neophallus has thus been divided and the neophallus transferred to the pubic region. The donor defect in the arm must be skin grafted. Mesh grafts must not be used because they will be aesthetically unacceptable to many patients. Vein grafting of the proximal radial artery to the distal ulnar artery generally is not required.

The nerve anasomosis to the right pudendal nerve is completed first with 8-0 nylon epidural sutures. The artery and veins are then anastomosed in standard microvascular fashion. The proximal urethral segment of the phallus is drawn inferiorly and tunneled through the previously dissected clitoral prepuce. The proximal cutaneous portion of the new urethra is then tunneled through the previously dissected clitoral prepuce. The proximal cutaneous portion of the new urethra is then tunneled through the subcutaneous space of the mons pubis and sutured directly to the superior labia minora remnants. This brings the neourethra into a perineal position and leaves the neophallus in its appropriate position on the mons pubis (Fig. 79–20). At a second stage, the perineal urethra is

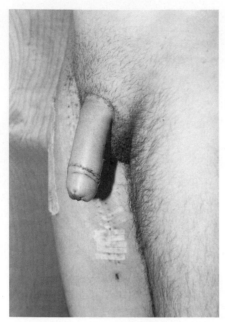

FIG. 79–21.   Early postoperative result of total phallourethroplasty.

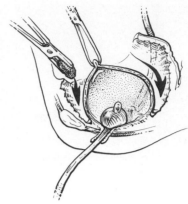

FIG. 79–22.   The bladder-flap method of urethral reconstruction. The urinary bladder is inflated with normal saline. The retropubic and retrovesical areas are dissected. Care is taken not to injure the ureters.

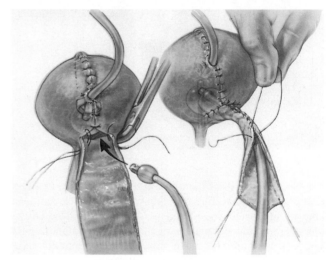

FIG. 79–23.   An anteriorly based flap of full-thickness bladder wall (28 × 4 cm) is created and tubed over a catheter.

joined to the external urethral opening by constructing the intervening segment with labial and vaginal wall flaps, as described by Bouman (20). Large-size adult silicone testicular implants are placed into pockets within each labia majora. These can be placed at the initial operating procedure or during the second stage of perineal urethroplasty (Fig. 79–21).

With improved techniques of phalloplasty, the female transsexual can expect to have a phallus of adequate size for sexual stimulation of a partner. The choice of flap design is individualized and should be based upon surgical judgment that considers such variables as patient obesity, previous abdominal scarring, and the goals of the particular patient. Patients who smoke regularly should be advised that they have four times the wound-healing complication rate of non-smokers.

Stage 2: Urethral Reconstruction

Many methods of penile urethral reconstruction have been tried. These include free split-thickness skin grafts, vein grafts, transplantation of a ureter, and the reverse tubing of skin flaps (21). The senior author has reported building the urethra from a segment of vascularized ileum (9). Ideally, the chosen method of urethral reconstruction should be combined with concurrent phallic reconstruction. This will minimize the number of operative stages. All methods of urethral reconstruction have potential limitations and possible complications. Skin grafts utilized for urethral reconstructions tend to contract and produce urethral strictures or fistulae. Free grafts do not take as well when incorporated into the skin flaps as they do when placed within the vascularized penile tissue (as in hypospadias patients). Such grafts result in a high incidence of postoperative fistuala formation.

Local skin flaps of hair-bearing tissue are sometimes tubed "in reverse" and used for urethral reconstruction. This method has been reported to lead to recurrent stone formation and infundibular folliculitis within the urethra.

When the vaginal remnant of mucosa is used for urethral reconstruction, the results are generally disappointing. Prolonged hormonal therapy usually causes significant thinning and atrophy of the vaginal mucosa, making it a poor and fragile lining for the neouretha.

The most promising technique for total urethral reconstruction at this time appears to be the use of a long, narrow, full-thickness flap of bladder wall (the "bladder flap" technique; Fig. 79–22) to create a musculomucosal urinary conduit from the bladder neck to the tip of the penile glans. It is lined with transitional epithelium (Figs. 79–23 through 79–26). Surgical details of the bladder flap technique currently performed at the University of Virginia Medical Center are reported elsewhere (22). The objection to this operation is the need for a major abdominal operation, but the rich vascularity of the bladder wall makes the flap very safe and the bladder mucosa is the ideal lining for a urethra.

Stage 3: Ancillary Procedures

The third stage of female-to-male genitoplasty is comprised of one or more commonly requested ancillary procedures.

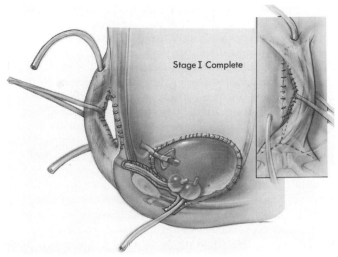

FIG. 79–24. The tubed bladder flap is incorporated into the neophallus as the urethra.

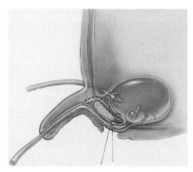

FIG. 79–25. Six weeks later, the cephalic pedicle of the abdominal flap is detached from the abdominal wall. The phallus with its contained urethra is reflected forward and the neoglans contoured. The bladder flap is divided at its base and transposed anterior to the pubic symphysis and anastomosed to the external urethra. *Note:* Urinary continence has been maintained.

These include scrotal reconstruction by use of tissue expanders and testicular implants of silicone gel. Bilateral gracilis musculocutaneous flaps may be used for scrotal reconstruction if the labia are scarred and unsuitable for tissue expansion. The neophallus can be sculpted to improve its aesthetic appearance by a variety of local plastic procedures. These are designed to avoid a phallus that resembles a flap of tissue, and produce a more natural shape about the neck of the glans.

Patients on long-term hormonal supplements frequently experience recurrent episodes of vaginal monilial (yeast) infections. At some point in their care and follow-up, they may require ablation of any residual vaginal pocket. Many patients find this vaginectomy to be very helpful. Care should be taken to avoid injury of the external urinary spincter in removing the lining of the anterior vaginal wall.

Complications

Complete phallourethroplasty requires meticulous attention to detail and careful surgical planning. These procedures should not be attempted by someone not experienced in gen-

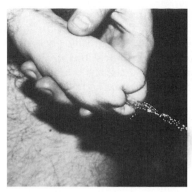

FIG. 79–26. Final result 2 years postoperatively demonstrates satisfactory orthostatic micturition.

ital plastic surgery. Reconstruction of the phallus by any technique carries the risk of tissue necrosis. This complication is more common when the patient is obese or when the surgeon is forced to use random patterned flaps. These flaps must be delayed and moved in stages. Delay of random patterned flaps for phallus reconstruction requires additional time and more procedures. Axial patterned flaps can undergo thrombosis of a critical vessel from either arterial insufficiency or venous thrombosis; either event will lead to partial or total flap necrosis. Venous congestion appears to be a more common problem in the groin or abdominal flaps than arterial insufficiency. In addition, tissue loss may also occur from infection. The viability of the phallic flap can be checked in the operating room by injection of fluorescein intravenuously and examination of the flap with an ultraviolet light.

Urethral reconstruction is more complicated than reconstruction of the body of the phallus, but it adds a pleasing, more functional result for the patient. Fortunately, the bladder wall possesses a vigorous circulation with rich small-vessel intercommunications. This makes its use for long and narrow flaps relatively dependable.

The neophallus generally develops protective sensation over a period of 6 to 12 months. During the interim, the relatively insensate phallus may incur pressure sores. The patient should be made aware of this possibility and warned about wearing constrictive clothing. Improved sensation of the phallus may come in the future from free nerve grafting to the deep pudendal nerves. This method carries a potential hazard. Failure of free nerve grafting may result in additional surgical injury to the pudendal nerve on the side of the operation. This could lead to decreased rather than increased sensation in the reconstructed area. Fortunately, at the present time the desire for erotic sensation in the penis is reasonably well met by retaining an island of normally innervated clitoral tissue. The clitoral tissue can be incorporated into the base of the neophallus to provide erogenous sensation. The labial and periurethral tissues also retain much sensate and erectile tissue.

Scrotal reconstruction can result in extrusion of the implant, infection, tenderness, or perineal fistula. These complications can be avoided by meticulous surgical technique and by tissue-expansion techniques before insertion of the final testicular prostheses.

Although surgical techniques for male genitoplasty are constantly modifed by surgeons working in gender clinics throughout the world, it is already possible for the female transsexual to receive surgical therapy that will satisfy his desire for a phallus of reasonable aesthetic appearance that will allow sexual intercourse and continent orthostatic micurition.

It can be expected that increasing numbers of patients will seek operative help as these surgical procedures continue to improve. Long-term results of patients treated surgically have been encouraging (23). Improved aesthetic and functional results after complete phalloplasty with urethral reconstruction are anticipated for the future. This will lead to an even higher degree of patient benefit and satisfaction.

RESULTS

The senior author's personal series embraces patients treated over an 8-year period (1962 to 1970) at the gender identity clinic at the Johns Hopkins Hospital, and over a 14-year period (1970 to 1984) after this program was transferred to the University of Virginia Medical Center (Table 79–3).

Over 200 male and female transsexuals have been seen and studied during this period of 22 years; 112 received gender reassignment surgery. A multidisciplinary team reviewed all patients both before any recommendations for surgery and postoperatively. Criteria for acceptance for surgery were established and clarified over this period. Almost 25% of the patients were first seen after earlier unsuccessful attempts at surgical reassignment, or after self-mutilation involving castration. The criteria for further reparative surgery were less strict for this group of patients. Continuing patient satisfaction with the surgical approach has led us to believe that we

have been overly conservative in the acceptance of transsexual patients for surgical gender reassignment (Fig. 79–27).

Until some reasonably promising alternative treatment is found for transsexualism, we must recognize that the overwhelming majority (95%) of operated patients give consistent reports of markedly improved self-images and satisfaction (some of our patients are now over 20 years post surgery). The senior author has had *no* patient in his series who regretted the surgical reassignment; this includes those patients who experienced one or more major complications during the reconstruction (Table 79–4).

The postoperative problems encountered by transsexuals are related mostly to wound complications and to economic pressures resulting from high hospital costs that are often not borne by health insurance carriers. We have found transsexual patients to be consistently motivated, cooperative, and deeply appreciative when reasonable surgical results are obtained.

Lundstrom (24) reported on a follow-up of 31 cases of gender dysphoria *not* accepted for sex reassignment; these are compared with a similar group of patients who did receive sex reassignment surgery. Lundstrom found the surgically treated patients to be more content than those treated in other ways.

In reviewing the world literature, Lundstrom found a higher incidence of unsuccessful results (up to 13%) after surgery on male *and* female transsexuals. He postulated that this may be because some reports include operations on effeminate homosexuals or transvestites who might better have been treated with nonoperative methods. The diagnosis of female transsexualism is not so likely to be confused with similar conditions, and fewer bad results can be anticipated.

Older patients (40 years of age or older) may represent examples of true transsexuals whose symptoms are of low intensity (or they may be aging transvestites). Such individuals may be poor candidates for surgical reassignment.

In addition to transsexuals, some "compulsive" transvestites may be proper candidates for sex reassignment. Laub and Fisk (25) have shown that such patients do well after sex-modifying operations, provided they first function successfully over a 1-to 3-year test period in the new sex role. Others (26) believe these atypical subgroups do not adjust as well postoperatively as the core group of transsexuals.

Lundstrom's studies (24) suggest that "*psychosocial* functional capacities of transsexuals appear to be independent of

Table 79–3
Follow-Up Summary

Total number	202
Male transsexual surgery	153
Female transsexual surgery	49
Follow-up (1–21 yr)	
Mean	10.2 yr.
Complication rate	26%
Mortality	0%

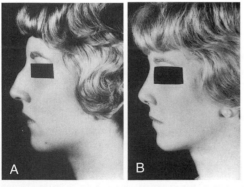

FIG. 79–27. Accessory feminizing operations are often requested by male transsexuals either before or after genital reconstruction. The most common request is for reduction rhinoplasty, as shown in this 22-year-old male transsexual.

Table 79–4
University of Virginia Experience—Male Transsexualism Postoperative Complications (64 of 202 Patients)[a]

Partial failure of skin graft or flap	36
Stenosis in vagina (mild or severe)	21
Rectovaginal fistula	3
Painful erectile tissue (periurethral)	3
Hypertrophic scarring	5
Urethrovaginal fistula	1
Pain in vagina	3
Unsatisfactory appearance of labia	6

[a]Most complications occurred early in the series and are now considered "preventable." Fifteen of the 64 patients required additional operations to correct one or more complications. Fifty-six of the 64 patients reached a point at which they declared themselves "satisfied" with their surgical results.

Table 79–5
Factors Favoring Acceptance of Sex-Reassignment Surgery

Rarity of long-term bad results or regrets of treated patients
Absence of effective nonsurgical treatment methods

sex reassignment and that this consideration is therefore not of fundamental importance in deciding on sex reassignment." He also concluded that patients who do not receive sex reassignment continue to be more dissatisfied with their life situation than those who do (statistically significant at p < .01); we would agree with those conclusions (Table 79–5).

ALTERNATIVE TREATMENT METHODS

Nonsurgical therapy for transsexualism has been tried repeatedly in the past and should be undertaken in the future, if better understanding of this disease were to suggest a new and promising approach.

At present, the efforts to bring harmony into the lives of transsexuals by use of psychoanalysis, psychotherapy, electric shock, hormone therapy, or hypnosis have been very disappointing. Many patients categorically refuse to enter such nonsurgical programs; many others start, but soon drop out of counseling programs as they become discouraged with the lack of relief. Surgeons continue to receive constant pleas for operations from the dropouts of these programs.

Until something more promising is developed, surgical sex reassignment continues to offer more subjective relief for transsexualism than any other known treatment.

Even when surgical gender reassignment is undertaken, patients frequently need supportive therapy. Hormone therapy, electrolysis, grooming and beautification instruction, and group or individual counseling are all of vital importance.

The need for long-term follow-up of each patient cannot be overstressed. Only in this way may future patient selection and treatment methods be improved.

Trends for the Future

Some gender clinics are trying to identify the transsexual during early childhood (8). If this is successful, environmental modification may offer promising treatment. Some animal research would suggest that electrophysiology may yet produce changes in gender identity by selective stimulation of the central nervous system. New psychologic and hormonal methods may develop that will alter gender identity.

Until such a breakthrough occurs, patients with severe and fixed transsexualism deserve the best treatment that medicine can offer. At the present time, this continues to be sex reassignment surgery. These operations at least bring the anatomic and psychologic genders into harmony; they also provide a high degree of subjective relief for the patients.

The public, the insurance carrier, and even the medical profession are all in need of more education on the nature, causes, and treatment of transsexualism.

Results and Initiatives from Other Clinics

Between 1991 and 1996, medical clinics throughout the world have become increasingly active in studying transsexualism and the possible effects of sex reassignment surgery.

Hage and colleagues (27) in Amsterdam have been major contributors and leaders in the European arena. They have recently studied the surgical goals of the female to male transsexual patient. In a review of 200 female-to-male subjects, all but one stressed being able to void in a standing position as a major goal of surgery. In addition, many of these patients had special requests for the reconstruction of genitalia, including a scrotum, aesthetic shaping of a glans, and rigidity in the reconstructed phallus. The demand for these more sophisticated goals has increased as surgical finesse has been developed in many gender clinics.

In Canada, the Clarke Institute and Blanchard's group (28) have investigated the reasons why many transsexuals do not request surgery for the first time until they are in their twenties, or later. Many of these older patients had a history of earlier marriage and, in some instances, the fathering of children. They indicated they would have come to the gender clinic much sooner if they had not been restrained by commitments to wives and children in their attempt, usually futile, to fit into the heterosexual community (28).

Coleman (29) and his team studied a rare subgroup of nine female-to-male transsexual patients who found themselves attracted to homosexual men even after sex reassignment. It is interesting that none of these subjects had received phalloplasty. Following sex reassignment, they reported satisfaction with the surgery as well as with postoperative sexual satisfaction and psychologic adjustment. This group emphasizes that sexual *orientation* is less important than gender *identity* in the decision to offer sex reassignment to a patient with gender dysphoria. Laboratory studies from Germany would indicate that sexual orientation and gender identity are, in fact, determined by two separate centers in the developing midbrain of the fetus.

Hage (30) has reviewed the general medical requirements and consequences of sex reassignment surgery. He continues to stress that diagnosis, counseling, and treatment of gender dysphoria should be restricted to reputable gender teams, including not only surgeons but also behavioral scientists and endocrinologists. He urges such clinics to make it clear to transsexual patients that, in the case of female-to-male sex reassignment, one-stage reconstruction is not feasible, that often many procedures may be required, and that they will be irreversibly infertile after surgery.

Snaith and Hohberger (31) have reviewed the experiences at the University of Leeds. They conclude "gender reassignment for carefully assessed transsexual patients is now an established and accepted practice in many parts of the world." They recommend a book by Morris (1974) for physicians interested in a review of this subject and, for lay persons, a book by Hodgkinson (1987).

Polderman's group (32) in Amsterdam have studied the response of the adrenal glands to long-term administration of testosterone to female-to-male transsexuals. They conclude that "testosterone does increase the response of the adrenal gland to stimulation by ACTH."

Rubin (33) has reviewed the Scandinavian experience with transsexual reassignment surgery. He suggests that current investigations indicate transsexualism may result from mutations in the SRY-gene. He acknowledges that the ideal surgical methods of sex reassignment have probably not yet been developed, but that current surgery does provide social and psychologic rehabilitation. He believes the results in male-to-female transsexuals to be more successful when the operations are carried out in younger patients and an effort is made to preserve the sensation of the glans penis by means of a subcutaneous-tissue neurovascular pedicle. He believes that, when orchiectomy is performed early, the amount of estrogen required will be less.

Sales (34) studied the psychologic problems encountered by the children of transsexual patients who had been born before sex reassignment surgery was readily available and feasible. He stresses that such children usually require psychologic counseling and that, if carried out, the results are likely to be quite helpful.

Snaith and his colleagues (35) carried out a study of 141 Dutch transsexuals. Thirty-six female-to-male and 105 male-to-female transsexuals received sex reassignment surgery. They concluded that "there is absolutely no reason to doubt the therapeutic effect of sex reassignment surgery." These benefits were, in fact, noted even in those who had not completed surgical treatment, as well as in those who had. It was of interest that the female-to-male transsexuals responded just as favorably as the male-to-female group, despite the more complex surgery.

Recently, Huang (36) reviewed 20 years of experience in managing transsexual sex reassignment in Texas. His follow-up included 121 male-to-female transsexuals, ranging from 6 months to 20 years after surgery. The surgical procedures used were varied, and similar to those described in the early portion of this chapter. The subjective responses of the patients indicated satisfaction and confirmed the value of sex reassignment surgery.

Lief and Hubschman (37) conducted a detailed study of orgasm in the postoperative transsexual patient. Fourteen male-to-female and 9 female-to-male patients were studied after sex reassignment surgery. Despite some decline in orgastic capacity in the male-to-female group, they expressed unquestioned satisfaction with sex and with the overall impacts of sex reassignment. The female-to-male group showed an increase in orgastic capacity postoperatively. This was true whether or not phalloplasty had been carried out. Lief concluded that sexual satisfaction was to be expected after patients had their body image surgically changed to confirm their sense of sexual identity.

Tsoi (38) has conducted a follow-up of transsexuals in the Singapore community after sex reassignment surgery. Forty-five male and 36 female transsexuals were followed 1 to 8 years after sex reassignment. Not surprisingly, the male-to-female group had started cross-dressing 4 to 7 years later in life than the female-to-male group. After surgery, 35% had married, and all reported "no problems" in adjusting to their new lives. Overall results were "good" in 44% and "very good" in the remaining 56%. Younger patients seemed to have somewhat better postoperative adjustments. The Asian transsexual patient appears to respond as positively to sex reassignment surgery as those in North America and Europe.

Recent Contributions to the Surgical Technique of Sex Reassignment

Surgeons in many countries, between 1992 and 1996, developed refinements in sex reassignment surgery that add security and finesse to these procedures. Some of these creative ideas are noted below under the heading of the desired anatomic gender.

MALE-TO-FEMALE SEX REASSIGNMENT

Crighton (39), working in Durban, has developed a new technique for dissecting the pocket that will be used to create the new vaginal canal. He lines this canal with a double-layered skin graft that is composed of split-thickness skin superimposed upon a meshed thick dermal graft. The composite graft is used to deepen the vault of the vagina, part of which is lined by peno-scroto-perineal flaps. He finds such grafts do not contract as much as simple split-thickness skin grafts.

He also urges suspension of the vault of the new vagina laterally by threading the testicular cords above the superior pubic rami. In the postoperative period, he finds that use of a vaginal vibrator gives results superior to the wearing of a fitted vaginal mold.

Hage's group in Amsterdam (40) has developed sculpturing techniques in forming the neoclitoris. They use and recommend a free composite graft from the tip of the penile glans to cover a recipient site at the shortened dorsal neurovascular bundle. He reports excellent take of these grafts with few complications and results quite satisfactory to the patient. He believes that use of an alternative neurovascular pedicle flap of the glans tissue is accompanied by an excessive number of vascular complications.

Van Noort and Nicolai (41) have compared construction of the neovagina using only inverted penile skin flaps (11 cases) with vaginal constructions using a combination of penile flaps and scrotal skin flaps (16 cases). Although the cosmetic effect was judged by the surgeon and the patients as superior when only skin inversion flaps were used, the combination of penile and scrotal flaps usually produced a wider and deeper vagina. It should be noted that these penile flaps were all based on an *anterior* pedicle. This consistently results in a vagina of smaller dimensions than when a penile flap is based on a *posterior* pedicle.

Eldh (42) continues to express enthusiasm for preservation of the glans penis in constructing a clitoris in male transsexuals. He dissects the dorsal vessels and nerves of the penis, extending from its base out to the glans. The reduced glans is left as an innervated island flap and repositioned as a clitoris. Nineteen of 20 patients had good healing of the glans and reported sensation in the neoclitoris. He did, however, acknowledge circulatory problems in the flaps of penile skin. This resulted in three patients having unacceptably short vaginas. Since reconstruction of the vagina takes precedent over the clitoris, many surgeons prefer to retain the dorsal vessels of the penis within the penile flap to maximize the vascular security of the new vaginal wall. Nevertheless, good sensation in the clitoris is a desirable goal. Fang and Chen (43), working in Taiwan, compared Rubin's technique of using the corporis spongiosum as the vascular pedicle for the neoclitoris with the use of a dorsal subcutaneous tissue neurovascular pedicle for clitoroplasty. This latter technique proved preferable, in that all of the flaps survived with good preservation of sensation and the absence of any urine leakage. Six of the 9 patients reported sexual satisfaction; he did not comment on the incidence of flap complications in the reconstructed vagina.

Freundt's team (44) in Rotterdam has studied the complication of prolapse of the neovagina in patients whose vaginas were reconstructed using a loop of sigmoid colon. They treated three of these patients with surgical suspension of the vaginal vault. In two cases, they attached it to the Cooper ligament by means of an abdominal approach, and in one the attachment was to the fascia over the sacrum. They concluded that the latter approach was the more dependable.

FEMALE-TO-MALE REASSIGNMENT

Reconstruction of the male genitalia, and indeed of the male chest configuration, offers special challenges for the plastic surgeon.

Hage's team has recommended preconstruction of the penile portion of the urethra in female-to-male transsexuals (45).

The importance to the patient of being able to stand to void following sex reassignment makes the creation of the penile urethra a necessity. This pendulant portion of the neourethra must be connected at its base to a fixed portion of urethra in the perineum. Hage and colleagues describe the use of pedicled abdominal or inguinal skin flaps that were incorporated into the phallus before its transfer to the pubic region in 25 patients, using Snyder's technique (45). Since this technique was successful in all of the patients, they recommend it in any case where the use of a microsurgical free flap technique is not indicated. They point out that the operations are less complex and the complication rate lower than with free flap techniques for construction of the phallus. In a separate publication (46), these same authors compare 31 phalloplasties using the rectus muscle and inferior epigastric artery pedicled skin flaps with use of the radial forearm free flap for phalloplasty. They conclude that, from a cosmetic and functional standpoint, the free flap technique gave better results—in part, because of the protective tactile sensitivity that was obtained in the free flap group. They did, however, note that erogenous sensitivity was not obtained in these flaps and "should not be expected." They confirm the observation of ourselves and others that abdominal skin flaps tend to be excessively thick and not generally desirable for phalloplasty. They also pointed out a high complication rate of urethral fistula formation at the junction between the penile and perineal portions of the reconstructed urethra. At the University of Virginia, we observed the same location for several postoperative fistulae and found it is related to the acute angulation of the urethra at that point. Reconstruction of the urethra can be designed so that a gentle curve is created, thus avoiding the need for later repair of fistulae. If the rectus muscle is used for phalloplasty, it may be covered by split-thickness or full-thickness skin grafts to avoid the heavy bulk of the lower abdominal wall.

Fisch and his team in Germany recommend osseous fixation of penile implants used to stiffen the phallus after phalloplasty (47). We agree with this observation and prefer drilling holes in the pubic bone and passing silastic implant tails through the body canals to make this fixation secure. Although we have generally preferred penile implantation as a secondary procedure, Fisch believes this is better accomplished at the initial stage of phalloplasty.

In a limited number of patients, Hage's group (48) has reported on the construction of a phallus using a lateral upper-arm sensate-free flap in combination with bladder mucosa as a free graft to line the new urethra. Postoperatively, they experienced bladder spasms and meatal stenosis, despite a pleasing cosmetic result. Several secondary operations were required to complete the reconstruction over a 14-month follow-up period, and the donor-site deformity on the arm proved to be significant.

Zia and others (49) have addressed the possible application of human ovarian or testicular cross-sex transplantation in sex reassignment surgery. If such allotransplants can be made functional, they may allow not only a simplified hormone regime after sex reassignment but also, in the distant future, the possible attainment of fertility.

Karim and colleagues (50) have pointed out the importance of near-total resection of the corpus spongiosum and corpora cavernosa in male-to-female transsexual operations. This technical point should be stressed because incomplete resection will commonly result in severe discomfort and pain during sexual activities following surgery. Secondary surgery to remove this painful erectile tissue will usually produce comfort and a satisfied patient.

Fang and Lin (51) have combined several techniques they believe important in phalloplasty. Earlier, they encountered postoperative fistulae in 38 out of 56 urethral reconstructions, but they later found that a prefabricated flap (creating a tube of vaginal mucosa) greatly reduced this fistula. This reconstruction of the perineal or fixed part of the urethra was usually combined with sensate-free forearm flaps to reconstruct the phallus.

Noordanus (52) has described an interesting late salvage of a free flap phalloplasty in a female-to-male transsexual with ischemia that developed 3 weeks after a radial forearm free flap phalloplasty. Seven hours later, in the operating room, venous return was restored by perfusion of the flap and anastomosis with streptokinase. At the University of Virginia, we have noted two similar very late ischemic problems in radial forearm flaps. We believe these resulted from sudden kinking of the venous anastomosis when the effect of gravity on the healed, but now ambulatory, patient caused further sagging of the soft tissues of the phallus. The design and position of the venous anastomosis should be given critical attention at the time of phalloplasty to avoid this late complication.

The gender team in Amsterdam (53) has made an important contribution as to the anatomic features of the anterior vaginal flap that is used for reconstruction of the perineal urethra in the female-to-male transsexual. They illustrate the cleavage plane between the posterior urethral wall and the anterior vaginal wall in developing this flap. They conclude that these two structures may be dissected apart, even in the caudal two-thirds of the urethra. They find the vascular supply to be abundant in the vaginal wall and that the cleavage plane contains longitudinal strands of muscle, fibrous tissue, and elastin.

Hage's group (54) has reviewed the various methods of sculpting the glans following phalloplasty. When abdominal or inguinal skin flaps are used for the phallus, they believe these procedures should be done in secondary procedures to protect the blood supply. They conclude that the technique described by the Norfold group, consisting of coronal ridge and sulcus construction, offers the best result. They have abandoned the earlier technique described by Nunawar.

Sadove and co-workers (55) have advocated a one-stage phalloplasty using a free sensate osteocutaneous fibula flap. While the photographic results appear excellent, only four cases are reported and the follow-up period is short. They believe the donor-site deformity on the leg to be more easily disguised and less troublesome than a forearm flap defect and they point to the advantage of a long vascular pedicle in this flap. Unfortunately, experience with other free bone transplants would indicate that gradual absorption of the bone is its likely fate since, in the postoperative period, this bone graft is not subjected to the preoperative stresses of weight bearing experienced by a fibula. Surgeons should be slow to adopt this technique until this point can be clarified by a much longer follow-up.

Gottlieb and Levine (56) have suggested a new design for the radial forearm free flap phalloplasty. They believe the original design described by Chang and Hwang to be too limited in size and to have a propensity for developing meatal stenosis. They describe four patients with a new design that allows the glans and distal urethra to be formed in continuity with the urethral portion of the forearm flap. In a somewhat similar fashion, Gilbert and his team have described a "cricket bat-transformer" pattern in the phalloplasty they employ.

Several variations have been described in the construction of the scrotum in female-to-male transsexuals. Several authors (57) utilize a V-Y advancement of labial skin flaps to create a bifid scrotum. This technique is accompanied by a modest (5 to 7%) extrusion rate of the testicular implants, but revisions to correct such complications are not difficult. Several authors have noted that tissue expansion prior to the implantation of testicular prostheses has proven unnecessary with scrotal reconstruction.

Hage and Bouman (58) have had some experience with the use of external phallic silicone prostheses for female-to-male transsexuals. Several models have been tried on approximately 120 patients, and the most successful method of fixation involved creation of a bipedicled skin flap in the pubic area, allowing the prothesis to be worn directly fixed to the body. It should be noted that such external prostheses rarely overcome the patient's sense of deformity in the area of reconstruction.

Not only the phallus but also the breast and chest-wall regions deserve attention in sex reassignment of the female-to-male transsexual.

In addition to the authors, Hage and VanKesteren (59) have called attention to the need for more sophisticated chest-wall contouring in the male-to-female transsexual patient. More attention needs to be paid to proper positioning of the nipple-areolar complex and the obliteration of the inframammary crease that is seen even in females with very small breasts. The shaping of the chest to conform to the pectoralis major muscle contours, the obviation of as many chest-wall scars as possible, and the prevention of depressions by removal of breast tissue beneath the areolar complex are all considerations of significant importance.

Surgery for the transsexual patient is still complex and it is undergoing rapid changes, but the existing state of the art makes the outlook enormously more satisfactory for these patients than even a few years ago.

References

1. Edgerton MT Jr, Langman MW, Schmidt JS, et al. Psychological considerations of gender reassignment surgery. *Clin Plast Surg* 1982; 9:355.
2. Benjamin H. *The transsexual phenomenon.* New York: Julian Press, 1966.
3. Green R. Mythological, historical, and cross-cultural aspects of transsexualism. In: Green R, Money J, eds. *Transsexualism and sex reassignment.* Baltimore: Johns Hopkins Press, 1969; 13.
4. Turner UG, Edlich R, Edgerton MT Jr. Male transsexualism: a review of genital surgical reconstruction. *Am J Obstet Gynecol* 1978; 132:119.
5. Lothstein LM. *Female-to-male transsexualism. Historical, clinical and theoretical issues.* Boston: Routledge & Kegan Paul, 1983.
6. Bandura A, Walters RH. *Social learning and personality development.* New York: Holt, Rinehart & Winston, 1963.
7. American Psychiatric Association. Diagnostic and statistical manual of mental disorders, 3rd ed. Washington: author, 1980.
8. Green R. *Sexual identity conflicts in children and adults.* Baltimore: Penguin, 1974.
9. Edgerton MT Jr, Meyer JK. Surgical and psychiatric aspects of transsexualism. In: Horton CE, ed. *Plastic and reconstructive surgery of the genital area.* Boston: Little, Brown, 1973; 117.
10. Kohut H. *The restoration of self.* New York: International Universities Press, 1977.
11. Edgerton MT Jr, Bull J. Surgical construction of the vagina and labia in male transsexuals. *Plast Reconstr Surg* 1970; 46:529.
12. Meyer R, Kesserling UK. One-stage reconstruction of the vagina with penile skin as an island flap in male transsexuals. *Plast Reconstr Surg* 1980; 66:401.
13. McIndoe AH. The treatment of congenital absence and obliterative conditions of the vagina. *Br J Plast Surg* 1950; 2:254.
14. Orticochea M. A new method of total reconstruction of the penis. *Br J Plast Surg* 1972; 25:347.
15. Gillies H, Millard DR. *The principles and art of plastic surgery.* Boston: Little, Brown, 1957.
16. Frumpkin AP. Reconstruction of the male genitalia. *Am Rev Soviet Med* 1944–45; 2:14.
17. Puckett CL, Montie JE. Construction of male genitalia in the transsexual, using a tubed groin flap for the penis and a hydraulic inflation device. *Plast Reconstr Surg* 1978; 61:523.
18. Hester TR, Hill HL, Jurkiewicz MJ. One-stage reconstruction of the penis. *Br J Plast Surg* 1978; 31:279.
19. Muhlbauer W, Herndl E, Stock W. The forearm flap. *Plast Reconstr Surg* 1982; 70:336.
20. Bouman FG. The first step in phalloplasty in female transsexuals. *Plast Reconstr Surg* 1979; 79:662.
21. Arneri V. Reconstruction of the male genitalia. In: Converse JM, ed. *Reconstructive plastic surgery.* Philadelphia: WB Saunders, 1977; 3902.
22. Edgerton MT Jr, Gillenwater JY, Kenney JG, et al. The bladder flap for urethral reconstruction in total phalloplasty. *Plast Reconstr Surg* 1984; 74:259.
23. Foerster DW. Female-to-male transsexual conversion: a 15-year followup. *Plast Reconstr Surg* 1983; 72:237.
24. Lundstrom B. *Gender Dysphoria.* Göteborg, Sweden: Department of Psychiatry and Neurochemistry, St. Jörgen's Hospital, University of Göteborg, 1981.
25. Laub DR, Fisk N. A rehabilitation program for gender dysphoria syndrome by surgical sex change. *Plast Reconstr Surg* 1974; 53:388.
26. Sorensen T, Hertoft P. Sex modifying operations on transsexuals in Denmark in the period 1950–1977. *Acta Psychiatr Scand* 1980; 61:56.
27. Hage JJ, Bout CA, Bloem JJ, et al. Phalloplasty in female-to-male transsexuals: what do our patients ask for? *Ann Plast Surg* 1993; 30(4): 323–326.
28. Blanchard R. A structural equation model for age at clinical presentation in nonhomosexual male gender dysphorics. *Archives of Sexual Behavior* 1994; 23(3):311–320.
29. Coleman E, Bockting WO, Gooren L. Homosexual and bisexual identity in sex-reassigned female-to-male transsexuals. *Archives of Sexual Behavior* 1993; 22(1):37–50.
30. Hage JJ. Medical requirements and consequences of sex reassignment surgery. *Medicine, Science and the Law* 1995; 35(1):17–24.
31. Snaith RP, Hohlberger AD. Transsexualism and gender reassignment. *Br J Psych* 1994; 165(3):418–419.

32. Polderman KH, Gooren LJ, van der Veen EA. Testosterone administration increases adrenal response to adrenocorticotrophin. *Clinical Endocrinology* 1994; 40(5):595–601.
33. Rubin SO. Sex-reassignment surgery male-to-female. Review, own results, and report of a new technique using the glans penis as a pseudoclitoris. *Scand J Urol Nephrol (suppl)* 1993; 154:1–28.
34. Sales J. Children of a transsexual father: a successful intervention. *European Child & Adolescent Psychiatry* 1995; 4(2):136–139.
35. Snaith P, Tarsh MJ, Reid R. Sex reassignment surgery. A study of 141 Dutch transsexuals. *Br J Psych* 1993; 162:681–685.
36. Huang TT. Twenty years of experience in managing gender dysphoric patients: I. Surgical management of male transsexuals. *Plast Reconstr Surg* 1995; 96(4):921–30; discussion 931–934.
37. Lief HI, Hubschman L. Orgasm in the postoperative transsexual. *Arch Sexual Behavior* 1993; 22(2):145–155.
38. Tsoi WF. Follow-up study of transsexuals after sex reassignment surgery. *Singapore Medical Journal* 1993; 34(6):515–517.
39. Crichton D. Gender reassignment surgery for male primary transsexuals. *South African Medical Journal* 1993; 83(5):347–349.
40. Hage JJ, Karim RB, Bloem JJ, et al. Sculpturing the neoclitoris in vaginoplasty for male-to-female transsexuals (review). *Plast Reconstr Surg* 1994; 93(2):358–64; discussion 365.
41. Van Noort DE, Nicolai JP. Comparison of two methods of vagina construction in transsexuals. *Plast Reconstr Surg* 1993; 91(7):1308–1315.
42. Eldh J. Construction of a neovagina with preservation of the glans penis as a clitoris in male transsexuals (see comments). *Plast Reconstr Surg* 1993; 91(5):895–900; discussion 901–903.
43. Fang RH, Chen CF, Ma S. A new method for clitoroplasty in male-to-female sex reassignment surgery [see comments]. *Plast Reconstr Surg* 1992; 89(4):679–82; discussion 683.
44. Freundt I. Toolenaar TA, Jeekel H, et al. Prolapse of the sigmoid neovagina; report of three cases. *Obstet Gynecol* 1994; 83(4):876–879.
45. Hage JJ, Bouman FG, Bloem JJ. Preconstruction of the pars pendlans urethrae for phalloplasty in female-to-male transsexuals. *Plast Reconstr Surg* 1993; 91(7):1303–1307.
46. Hage JJ, Bouman FG, de Graaf FH, et al. Construction of the neophallus in female-to-male transsexuals: the Amsterdam experience. *Journal of Urol* 1993; 149(6):1463–1468.
47. Fisch M, Wammack R, Ahlers J, et al. Osseous fixation of a penile prosthesis after transsexual phalloplasty: a case report. *J Urol* 1993; 149(1):122–125.
48. Hage JJ, de Graaf FH, van den Hoek J, et al. Phallic construction in female-to-male transsexuals using a laterial upper-arm sensate free flap and a bladder mucosa graft. *Ann Plast Surg* 1993; 31(3):275–280.
49. Xia ZJ, Wang C, Hage JJ. The application of human ovaries and testes cross-sex transplantation in sex reassignment surgery of transsexuals. *Plast Reconstr Surg* 1995; 95(1):201–202.
50. Karim RB, Hage JJ, Bouman FG, et al. The importance of near-total resection of the corpus spongiosum and total resection of the corpora cavernosa in the surgery of male-to-female transsexuals. *Ann Plast Surg* 1991; 26(6):554–556; discussion 557.
51. Fang RH, Lin JT, Ma S. Phalloplasty for female transsexuals with sensate free forearm flap [see comments]. *Microsurgery* 1994; 15(5):349–352.
52. Noordanus RP, Hage JJ. Late salvage of a "free flap" phalloplasty: a case report. *Microsurgery* 1993; 14(9):599–600.
53. Hage JJ, Torenbeek R, Bouman FG, et al. The anatomic basis of the anterior vaginal flap used for neourethra construction in male-to-female transsexuals. *Plast Reconstr Surg* 1993; 92(1):102–108; discussion 109.
54. Hage JJ, de Graaf FH, Bouman FG, et al. Sculpturing the glans in phalloplasty. *Plast Reconstr Surg* 1993; 92(1):157–161; discussion 162.
55. Sadove RC, Sengezer M, McRoberts JW, et al. One-stage total penile reconstruction with a free sensate osteocutaneous fibula flap. *Plast Reconstr Surg* 1993; 92(7):1314–1323; discussion 1324–1325.
56. Gottiev LJ, Levine LA. A new design for the radial forearm free-flap phallic construction. *Plast Reconstr Surg* 1993; 93(7):276–283; discussion 284.
57. Hage JJ, Bouman FG, Bloem JJ. Constructing a scrotum in female-to-male transsexuals. *Plast Reconstr Surg* 1993; 91(5):914–921.
58. Hage JJ, Bouman FG. Silicone genital prosthesis for female-to-male transsexuals. *Plast Reconstr Surg* 1992; 90(3):516–519.
59. Hage JJ, van Kesteren PJ. Chest-wall contouring in female-to-male transsexuals: basic considerations and review of the literature. *Plast Reconstr Surg* 1995; 96:386–391.

80

Necrotizing Infection, Lymphedema, and Trauma of the Male Genitalia

Donald R. Laub, Jr., M.D., and Donald R. Laub, Sr., M.D., F.A.C.S.

Surgery of the external genitalia dates back 5,000 years to the description of the care of the circumcised penis in the Eber Papyrus. Mutilation and castration were a form of punishment and degradation visited upon an adulterer, slave, or prisoner of war (1). The history of plastic surgery of the genitalia may have begun with a Roman operation for recreating the prepuce after circumcision. The reconstructive surgeon today may be called upon to help manage a patient with traumatic injury to the genitalia, penoscrotal lymphedema, or the sequelae of necrotizing infections.

Fournier Gangrene

Fournier gangrene is a necrotizing fasciitis of the perineal, perianal, or genital regions that results in gangrene of the overlying skin. It is caused by mixed bacterial flora, usually *Escherichia coli, Klebsiella pneumoniae,* or streptococcus are cultured, but anaerobic organisms should be strongly suspected even if not cultured (2). The microorganisms cause an obliterative endarteritis of the soft tissue that leads to vascular thrombosis and necrosis of the overlying skin. Myonecrosis, however, is generally not present (3). Overall mortality is currently about 21%, although this varies from 7 to 75%, depending on the speed of diagnosis and on premorbid debility (4). In a retrospective study from the Montifiore medical center, it was found that the amount of infected tissue and the degree of surgical débridement did not correspond to survival as well as an overall score of variance from normal values in vital signs and laboratory values (5). Because Fournier gangrene is a necrotizing infection of the fascia, its direction of spread is determined by the fascial planes. Once the infection penetrates the Buck and Colles fascia, it can spread by continuity to the Scarpa fascia and then involve the entire anterior abdominal wall.

Fournier gangrene arises from anorectal or genitourinary sources. The most frequent causes are undiagnosed or undertreated perianal, ischiorectal, or intersphincteric abscesses (6). Diabetes mellitus is the most common comorbid factor, but advanced age, alcoholism, prolonged hospitalization, and malignancy are also frequently mentioned as contributing.

Patients present complaining of pain and swelling. The skin may look normal initially, but will become erythematous and shiny, progressing to ecchymosis, blistering crepitance, and gangrene. Most patient's systemic symptoms are out of proportion to, and may in fact often precede, any visible sign of local infection. Patients will have elevated white-cell counts, fever, and volume depletion. Other nonspecific signs of sepsis, electrolyte disturbances, coagulopathy, anemia, or

thrombocytopenia may be present. Air is present in the soft tissue in 90% of these infections (7), and ultrasound is suggested as a diagnostic modality to differentiate the causes of an "acute scrotum" (8).

The treatment of Fournier gangrene is immediate, wide, radical, surgical débridment. Hyperbaric oxygen treatment has been shown to reduce the need for soft-tissue débridment and reduce mortality (9). The mechanism is direct toxicity of the increased tissue oxygen tension on obligate anaerobic organisms, as well as an increased oxidative activity of neutrophils (10).

Only when serial operative débridment has been completed and the progression of the disease arrested may reconstruction be considered. As Fournier gangrene is a fasciitis and usually does not cause outright myonecrosis, the remaining muscle bed may usually be skin grafted. Flap coverage may be needed for scrotal reconstruction when the testicles and cords are denuded (11), or when a urethral fistula is formed. Kamei and colleagues (12) from Japan describe a gastric and omental flap reconstruction of the urethra.

Lymphedema of Genitals

The lymphatic drainage from the penis and scrotum is to the medial superficial inguinal node. The testes drain directly to the lumbar paraortic nodes via the spermatic vessels, bypassing the inguinal system; therefore, the testes are spared in lymphedema because of obstruction of the inguinal lymphatics.

Lymphedema of the genitals was classified by Bulkley into two broad categories: primary and secondary (13). Primary lymphedema arises from aplasia, hypoplasia, or hyperplasia of the lymphatics, whereas secondary lymphedema is owing to scarring of the lymphatic channels. Primary lymphedema, which is far more uncommon than secondary disease, is subclassified by age of onset: congenital, or Milroy disease; lymphedema praecox; and lymphedema tarda (that developing after puberty). Congenital lymphedema arises from complete aplasia of the lymphatics; it must be differentiated from lymphatic malformations. Lymphatic malformations will manifest as a mass: cystic hygroma or lymphangioma. Hypoplasia of lymphatic channels will usually manifest as lymphedema in puberty, or lymphedema praecox. Hyperplasia of these channels will result in chylous reflux later in life, causing lymphedema tarda (14).

A vericocoele may be mistaken for unilateral—or, on occasion, bilateral—scrotal lymphedema. The diagnosis can be made after examining the patient recumbent; vericoceles will disappear after a time, whereas lympedema will not.

Sequential pneumatic compression devices on the lower legs can give some improvement in lymphedema. The device must be employed at intervals of 2 or 3 days and graduated compression garments used in the interim. In general, the conservative treatment is not advocated in lymphedema; treatment is surgical. There are really two options, lymphoplasty procedures or excisional therapy.

Lymphoplasty procedures use either alloplastic material or transposed autogenous tissue to promote lymphatic drainage. Both techniques work better on less advanced cases, and may have inconsistent results. There are several techniques of autogenous reconstruction. Gillies (15) advocated a procedure using transposed skin to act as a lymphatic bridge for lower-extremity or scrotal edema. McDonald modified this technique in a thigh-to-scrotal anastomosis, which provided improvement in the scrotum, but not the penis (16). The technique of omental transfer has provided some temporary relief, but recurrence generally occurs after the inguinal area scars. There are techniques described for microsurgical lymphovenous shunts (17), but results are uneven, being largely dependent on the skill of the surgeon.

Excisional therapy currently is little changed from the technique of Delpech in 1820, modified by Feins (18); it provides the most consistent relief from lymphedema. The diseased tissue, including subcutaneous tissue and lymphatics, is totally excised down to the Buck fascia on the penis and the spermatic cords and testicles in the scrotum. The reconstruction employs thick (0.018 inch) split-thickness skin grafts for reconstruction of the shaft of the penis. The testicles may be covered with fasciocutaneous flap from the thigh, or the testicle sutured together and skin grafted. The technique is similar to that described below for avulsion injuries.

Trauma

The management of genital injuries should not distract the surgeon from assessing the patient as a whole; life-threatening injuries must be handled first. Basic principles of psychiatry, urology, general surgery, and infectious disease are of critical importance. Psychologic considerations should be an integral part of the treatment program. Patients will be apprehensive about the appearance of the injured genitalia and may suffer dramatic changes in self-image. Psychiatric consultation should be sought in all cases of self-emasculation.

A thorough understanding of penoscrotal anatomy is fundamental to the appropriate diagnosis and management of injury (Figs. 80–1 through 80–4). Salvage and replantation techniques require familiarity with the blood supply, innervation, and relationships of the supporting structures of the penis and testes.

The urethra function must be considered; trauma to the urethra can result in strictures or fistulas. The proximity of the anus may result in wound contamination, thus complicating open-wound management with fulminating, dissecting infections such as Fournier gangrene. If genital injuries extend to the perineum, the anus must be inspected for sphincter function.

The relative mobility of the testes within the scrotal sac and the cremasteric reflex serve as anatomic protective mechanisms against low-velocity trauma (19) (Fig. 80–5).

PENETRATING TRAUMA

Initial evaluation of a penetrating injury requires inspection of the entire perineal area, including a rectal examination. Gross or microscopic hematuria is diagnostic for urethral in-

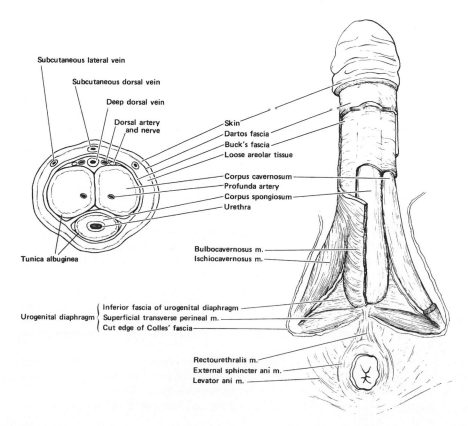

Subcutaneous lateral vein
Subcutaneous dorsal vein
Deep dorsal vein
Dorsal artery and nerve
Skin
Dartos fascia
Buck's fascia
Loose areolar tissue
Corpus cavernosum
Profunda artery
Corpus spongiosum
Urethra
Tunica albuginea
Bulbocavernosus m.
Ischiocavernosus m.
Urogenital diaphragm { Inferior fascia of urogenital diaphragm
Superficial transverse perineal m.
Cut edge of Colles' fascia
Rectourethralis m.
External sphincter ani m.
Levator ani m.

FIG. 80–1. The anatomy of the penile shaft. The urethra is contained within corpus spongiosum, which terminates in the glans penis distally, and the profunda arteries are located within the corpora cavernosa. Each corpus is surrounded by a tunica albuginea. The dorsal arteries and nerves are deep to the Buck fascia. The bulbocavernosus (or bulbospongiosus), ischiocavernosus, and transverse perineal muscles comprise the superficial musculature of the perineum.

FIG. 80–2. The anatomy of the scrotum and its contents. The dartos fascia contains slips of smooth muscle responsible for the characteristic scrotal rugae. Its extension into the perineum is called the Colles fascia and continues into the abdomen as the Scarpa fascia. The external spermatic fascia is derived from the external oblique aponeurosis. The loose areolar tissue between this layer and the dartos is usually the plane of dissection in scrotal avulsion injuries. The cremasteric fascia derives from the internal oblique fascia and the internal spermatic fascia derives from the transversalis fascia. Peritoneal extensions form the tunica vaginalis, a closed sac surrounding the underlying seminiferous tubules. Note that the epididymis lies posterolateral to the testis.

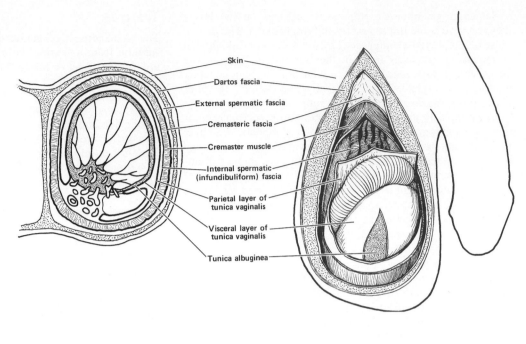

FIG. 80–3. The arterial supply of the penis and scrotum. The internal pudendal artery, a branch of the internal iliac artery, divides into the perineal artery and the profunda and dorsal arteries of the penis. The perineal artery supplies the posterior scrotum and the superficial perineal muscles. The scrotal wall is also supplied by the external spermatic or cremasteric artery in the spermatic cord. The internal spermatic or testicular artery supplies the testis, and the deferential artery supplies the vas deferens.

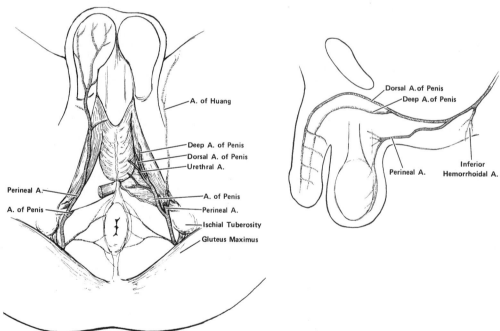

jury, and retrograde urethrography is a useful tool when injury is suspected. Corpus cavernosography may be considered (20), but usually the integrity of the tunica albuginea will be obvious on physical examination. Care must be taken in passing a catheter so that a partial urethral tear is not converted into a complete transsection. If necessary, urinary diversion may be readily established with a suprapubic catheter.

Because contamination is common, operative exploration and débridement are essential in the management of penetrating penile injuries. Perioperative antibiotic coverage for fecal organisms is strongly advocated. Débridement should be conservative, with excision only of clearly nonviable tissue. Surgical aggressiveness will create further hemorrhage within the corpora when hemostasis is already difficult to achieve. Repair of the Buck fascia and the tunica albuginea of the corpora are important in preventing subsequent penile deformity. If the extent of the defect in the Buck fascia or in the corpora does not permit closure without angulation, they should be left open (21). Delayed primary closure of the skin should be considered in severe and highly contaminated injuries.

Urethral lacerations may be repaired primarily with fine chromic suture over a stent or catheter. Attempts at repair where extensive destruction has occurred will result in stricture and fistula formation. In these cases, marsupialization of

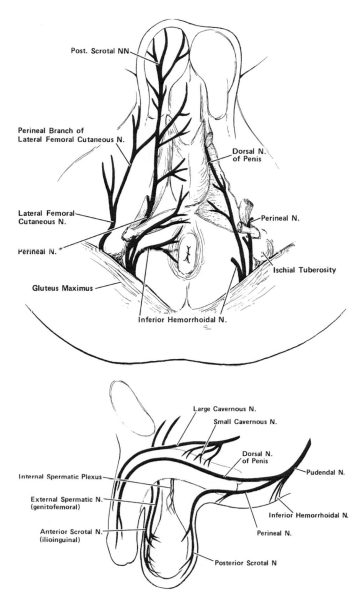

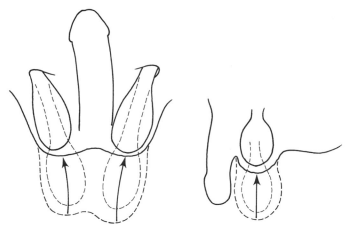

FIG. 80–5. The cremasteric reflex. The cremasteric fascia, innervated by the external spermatic branches of the genitofemoral nerve, may draw the testes up within the scrotum and inguinal canal. This serves as a thermoregulatory and protective mechanism.

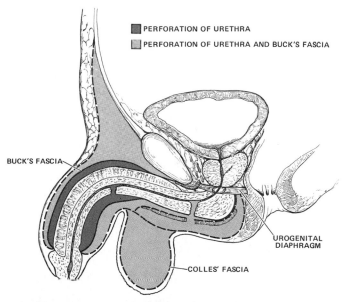

FIG. 80–4. The innervation of the penis and scrotum. The pudendal nerve arises from S2-4 and divides into the inferior hemorrhoidal nerve, the perineal nerve, and the dorsal nerve of the penis. The posterior scrotal wall is innervated by branches arising from the perineal nerve and the lateral femoral cutaneous nerve. The nerve supply of the anterior scrotal wall consists of the external spermatic branches off the genitofemoral nerve and the anterior scrotal branches from the ilioinguinal nerve. The superior, middle, and inferior spermatic nerves within the spermatic cord innervate the scrotal contents.

FIG. 80–6. Urinary extravasation. Urethral penetration with an intact Buck fascia confines extravasation to the area around the corpora. If the Buck fascia is perforated, then extravasation is limited only by the Colles fascia posteriorly, and may dissect underneath the Scarpa fascia anteriorly.

the urethra to the adjacent skin edges with subsequent delayed reconstruction has been recommended (21).

Penetrating injuries of the scrotum also dictate a conservative approach. Testicular salvage may be effected with minimal débridement of necrotic parenchyma and replacement of herniated tubules, closure of the tunica albuginea being accomplished with absorbable suture. If necessary, a dermal-patch graft may be applied. The integrity of the spermatic cord must be assessed. The scrotum should be loosely closed over a Penrose drain. Where extensive scrotal skin loss has

occurred, testicular coverage must be achieved with the residual scrotal skin, grafting, or thigh implantation.

The extent of urinary or hemorrhagic extravasation depends on the location of injury (Fig. 80–6). If the Buck fascia remains intact (as may occur with internal urethral injury or nonpenetrating trauma), extravasation is confined to the space around the corpora. If perforation includes the Buck fascia, urine and blood may extend into the scrotum, perineum, and abdominal wall. The collection is limited posteriorly by the Colles fascia, but may undermine the Scarpa fascia anteriorly and superiorly to the clavicle; if unrecognized, life-threatening infection may ensue. Surgical intervention must include drainage of the extravasated urine with appropriate urinary diversion; antibiotics should be instituted.

Other unusual, but not necessarily uncommon, injuries include penile bites, silicone injections, and injuries of sexual stimulation (e.g., vacuum cleaner lacerations or insertion of foreign objects into the urethra) (22). Risk of infection is of particular concern in bites, where introduction of virulent organisms can lead to cellulitis and gangrene.

BLUNT TRAUMA

Nonpenetrating trauma to the penis and scrotum can create extensive damage. Surgical exploration is indicated to control hemorrhage or repair suspected injury to the testicles, corpora, or urethra.

The approach to the penile shaft may be through a circumferential coronal incision with undermining of the skin proximally to afford complete exposure (23). If the site of injury is well localized, a direct longitudinal incision may be employed. The principles of repair discussed with respect to penetrating injuries apply here as well. The control of hemorrhage and the restoration of the urethra, corpora, and Buck fascia, along with testicular salvage, may be indicated.

Twenty percent of all urethral ruptures are inferior to the urogenital diaphragm; they typically result from straddle injuries (e.g., a bicycle accident or fall on a fence rail). Therapy may be conservative (catheter placement only), or surgical exploration, depending on the extent of the injury.

Penile strangulation may be caused by hair, strings, rings, rubber bands, condoms, catheters, and a multitude of other objects—the result of accident or intention. The nature and motivations of intentional injury have been categorized, ranging from the maintenance of erection to the prevention of enuresis (24). The most frequent presentation is in young children with inadvertent penile encirclement of human hair. Distal swelling of the penis and epithelialization over the hair may allow it to escape detection. This may lead to serious sequelae: urethral transsection, nerve crush injuries, and potential distal necrosis. Treatment consists of removal of the constricting band and repair of the damaged structures.

Avulsions

Avulsions of the penoscrotal skin most frequently occur as a result of machinery accidents, wherein the victim's clothing is forcefully torn away; the skin of the penis is thus separated in the loose areolar plane overlying the Buck fascia (25) (Fig. 80–7). Typically, there is minimal bleeding and little damage to the underlying structures. Scrotal avulsions tend to occur in the areolar tissue beneath the Dartos muscle (see Fig. 80–2).

Penile skin avulsion is best treated with a thick (0.018 inch) split-thickness graft from the thigh or other suitable site. The avulsed skin fares poorly when replaced as a graft, commonly resulting in slough (26). The remaining distal skin should be débrided to the corona to avoid prolonged distal edema arising from disruption of lymphatic drainage. No attempt should be made to stretch residual skin for coverage of the widely denuded shaft. After the recipient bed is adequately prepared, the skin graft should be applied as a single sheet in an interdigitating W-plasty fashion to minimize scar contracture. The bandaging of the penis is difficult; it must secure the graft and provide compression on a mobile struc-

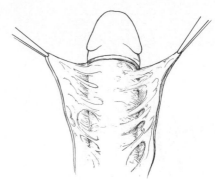

FIG. 80–7. Avulsion of the penile skin. The loose areolar tissue overlying the Buck fascia is typically the plane of dissection in avulsion injuries.

ture. Vaught described an x-ray film stent (27). We utilize a ring-shaped bolus dressing held in place by tie-over silk sutures at the corona and base of the penis. It is left in place for 10 to 14 days.

Other techniques of penile coverage include burial of the denuded shaft within the scrotum and local flap coverage. Results with skin grafting tend to be superior. The treatment of scrotal skin avulsions requires additional judgment because there are several available options. Adequate coverage is critical for preservation of testicular function. Primary closure should be attempted if residual scrotal skin is available. Despite significant initial tension, the scrotum will expand in time. Split-thickness skin grafting of the exposed but undamaged testes has been recommended when insufficient scrotal skin remains (25,26). The testes are sutured to each other for ease of grafting and avoidance of a bifid appearance. This procedure may be technically difficult because of the irregular surface of the recipient bed. Split-thickness skin grafts provide only marginal protection, and graft contracture has been reported to produce testicular distortion and infertility (28). Nevertheless, excellent cosmetic and functional results have been reported.

Burial of the exposed testes in subcutaneous thigh pockets is an appropriate alternative for immediate management. Implantation should be performed immediately under the skin at different levels in the thigh to minimize discomfort on motion. Temperature determinations have demonstrated a comparable environment in the scrotum and the tissue of the superficial thigh. In the deep subcutaneous tissue of the thigh, temperatures are equivalent to intraabdominal recordings, and may be as much as 10° higher. Normal spermatogenesis would be unlikely under these conditions (28). Scrotal reconstruction is performed electively using bilateral thigh flaps (Fig. 80–8). This provides a superior cosmetic result and good sensation.

AMPUTATIONS

Traumatic amputations of the penis are often self-inflicted, a form of focal suicide (29). Success rates of penile replantation are good, even lacking microsurgical techniques, and postreplantation psychiatric prognosis is generally favorable. It is recommended that psychiatric involvement be sought, but the presence of psychiatric disease should not be a contraindication for replantation. In 53 cases of penile self-muti-

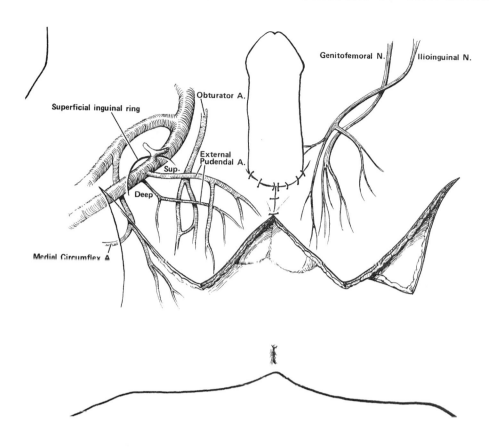

FIG. 80–8. Scrotal reconstruction with bilateral thigh flaps. Medial thigh flaps are raised over the previously buried testes. These flaps have an axial blood supply and are innervated by the genitofemoral and ilioinguinal nerves. The lateral femoral cutaneous nerve of the thigh is "collateral" supply in this area, and its severance in raising the flap is not depicted.

lation, only one postoperative suicide and one repeated attempt at amputation were recorded (30).

Before the development and application of the operating microscope, penile replantation was accomplished with anastomosis of the urethra and corpora. Functional results were generally satisfactory, although skin necrosis typically resulted. The corpora cavernosa are functionally controlled arteriovenous fistulae; replantation by simple reapproximation is possible because of the quantity of arterial blood flowing through the area. Denuding the penis and burying the shaft in the scrotal skin yields consistently good results. Microsurgical replantation of the penis affords the advantages of skin salvage and improved sensation. Cold ischemia times of up to 16 hours have been reported. As with replantation of digits, the replantation should be systematic: exploration for proximal and distal structures is the first step. Any nonviable tissue must be débrided. The penis is stabilized by a urethral stent, and the urethra anastomosed over the stent. The mucosa and the surrounding corpora spongiosum are repaired with absorbable suture. In proximal injuries, the profunda arteries are possible, and should be done next. The tunica albuginea of the corpora cavernosa are repaired with synthetic absorbable suture. Microsurgical repair of the dorsal structures is now possible in the stabilized penis. The paired superficial dorsal arteries, the dorsal vein, and the dorsal nerves are approximated. The Buck fascia and skin are then closed. Urinary drainage with a suprapubic catheter should be maintained for 2 to 3 weeks.

Testicular replantation has met with some limited success because of difficulty distinguishing the distal arteries and veins on exploration.

RECONSTRUCTION OF THE PENIS

Total phalloplasty reconstruction of the penis after traumatic loss, loss from cancer surgery, for microphallus, or for gender dysphoria is a surgical challenge. Microsurgical transfer of distant tissue seems to be essential in order to attain the five ideal goals:

1. A one-stage procedure that can be reproduced
2. Creation of a competent neourethra to allow for voiding while standing
3. The restoration of a phallus that has both tactile and erogenous sensibility
4. Enough bulk to retain a stiffener for use in intercourse
5. A result aesthetically acceptable to the patient

Initial work in the 1940s using abdominal tube pedicle flaps (31), and later work in the 1970s using muscle flaps (32), for reconstructing the penis had problems with flap bulk, insensibility, and extrusion of prosthetic stiffeners. Urinary complications (e.g., fistulae, stenosis) were common. The penis was formed in a one-stage procedure, using the forearm free flap of soft tissue and skin for both urethra and external surface, in 1984 (33). The identification of the deep pudendal nerve of the penis as the conduit of erogenous sensibility has enabled its microsurgical coaptation to the donor nerve in the free transfer (34). As a result of this method, patients have obtained erogenous sensation via normal reflex pathways. Since 1984, other workers have further refined the single-stage radial-forearm flap technique; current results are aesthetic, functional, and have sensibility for protective and erogenous use (35–37). Other microsurgical donor sites employed by various groups include the ulnar forearm (38), lateral upper arm (39,40), and fibular osteocutaneous flaps (41).

Another technique used at our institution utilizes the forearm flap for urethra but not for the external skin covering, thus avoiding the donor-site deformity of a skin graft on the forearm. This flap is combined with the midline lower abdominal flap, both of which are covered with skin graft (42). The resultant flap has two tunnels, one for urinary conduit and one for intermittent use of a prosthetic stiffener. It is our opinion that a split-thickness skin graft produces the best appearance in regard to the surface of the penile shaft.

Summary

The consequences to the patient of penoscrotal injury may be highly leveraged. The reconstructive surgeon is required to draw upon a wide range of knowledge and technique when treating penoscrotal injury. An interdisciplinary effort is clearly of benefit to the patient.

References

1. Rogers BO. History of external genital surgery. In: Horton CE, ed. *Plastic and reconstructive surgery of the genital area.* Boston: Little, Brown, 1973; 3–47.
2. Laucks SS. Fournier's gangrene. *Surg Clin N Am* 1994; 74(6): 1339–1352.
3. Lamb R, Juler G. Fournier's gangrene of the scrotum: a poorly defined syndrome or a misnomer? *Arch Surg* 1983; 118:38.
4. Paty R, Smith AD. Gangrene and Fournier's gangrene. *Urol Clin N Am* 1992; 19(1):149–162.
5. Laor E, Palmer LS, Tolia BM, et al. Outcome prediction in patients with Fournier's gangrene. *J Urol* 1995; 154:89–92.
6. McLaughlin S, Gray J. Delayed recognition of an intersphinteric abscess as the underlying cause of Fournier's scrotal gangrene. *Ann R Coll Surg Engl* 1985; 67:137.
7. Sharfi R. Perineal necrotizing infection. *Curr Surg* 1990; 47:1.
8. Dogra VS, Smeltzer JS. Sonographic diagnosis of Fournier's gangrene. *J Clin Ultrasound* 1994; 22(9):571–572.
9. Riserman J, Zambouni W, Curtis A, et al. Hyperbaric oxygen therapy for necrotizing fasciitis reduces the need for débridments. *Surgery* 1990; 108:847–850.
10. Nachreiner R, Childers BJ, Kizziar, et al. Adjuctive hyperbaric oxygen therapy for necrotizing fasciitis: a ten-year experience. Presented at the meeting of the American Society of Plastic and Reconstructive Surgeon, Montreal, Canada, October 1995.
11. Hallock GG. Scrotal reconstruction using the medial thigh fasaciocutaneous flap. *Ann Plast Surg* 1990; 24:86–90.
12. Kamei Y, Aoyama H, Kauhisa Y, et al. Composite gastric seromuscular and omental pedicle flap for urethral and scrotal reconstruction after Fournier's gangrene. *Ann Plast Surg* 1994; 33:565–568.
13. Bulkley GJ. Scrotal and penile lymphedema. *J Urol* 1962; 87:422–429.
14. Sauer PF, Bueschen , Vasconez LO. Lymphedema of the penis and scrotum. *Clin Plast Surg* 1988; 15(3):507–512.
15. Gillies H, Fraser FR. Treatment of lymphedema by plastic operation. *Br Med J* 1935; 96:96–98.
16. McDonald DF, Huggins C. Surgical treatment of elephantiasis. *J Urol* 1950; 63:187.
17. Huang GK, Hu RQ, Liu ZZ, et al. Microlymphatovenous anastomosis for treating scrotal elephantiasis. *Microsurgery* 1985; 6:36–39.
18. Feins NR. A new surgical technique for lymphedema of the penis and scrotum. *J Pediatr Surg* 1980; 15:787–789.
19. Culp DA. Genital injuries: etiology and initial management. *Urol Clin N Am* 1977; 4:143.
20. Datta NS. Corpus cavernosography in conditions other than Peyronie's disease. *J Urol* 1977; 118:588.
21. Slavtierra O, Rigdon WO, Norris DM, et al. Vietnam experience with 252 urologic war injuries. *J Urol* 1969; 101:615.
22. Citron ND, Wade PJ. Penile injuries from vacuum cleaners. *Br Med J* 1980; 281:26.
23. Culp DA. Penoscrotal trauma. In: Glenn JR, ed. *Urologic surgery.* Philadelphia: JB Lippincott, 1983.
24. Haddad FS. Penile strangulation with human hair. *Urol Int* 1982; 37:375.
25. Gomez RG. Genital skin loss. *Prob Urol* 1994; 8:290–301.
26. Gibson T. Avulsion of penile and scrotal skin. In: Horton CE, ed. *Plastic and reconstructive surgery of the genital area.* Boston: Little, Brown, 1973.
27. Vaught SK, Litvak AS, McRoberts JW. The surgical management of penile lymphedema. *Urol* 1975; 113:204–206.
28. Culp DA, Huffman WC. Temperature determination in the thigh with regard to burying the traumatically exposed testis. *J Urol* 1956; 76:436.
29. Evins SC, Whittle T, Rous SN. Self-emasculation: review of the literature, report of a case, and objectives of management. *J Urol* 1977; 118:775.
30. Henrikson TG, Hahne V. Microsurgical replantation of the amputated penis. *Scan J Urol Nephrol* 1980; 14:111.
31. Gilles HD, Harrison RJ. Congenital absence of the penis with embryologic considerations. *Br J Plast Surg* 1948; 1:8.
32. Persky L, Resnick W, Des Prez J. Penile reconstruction with gracilis pedicle grafts. *J Urol* 1983; 129:603.
33. Kao XS, Kao JH, Ho CL. One-stage reconstruction of the penis with free skin flap. *J Reconstr Microsurg* 1984; 1:199.
34. Gilbert DA, Williams MW, Horton CE. Phallic innervation via the pudendal nerve. *J Urol* 1988; 140:295.
35. Trengrove-Jones G, Colon LB, Horton CE, et al. A new concept in penoscrotal reconstruction: the one-stage free sensory combined penoscrotal reconstruction. Presented at the meeting of the American Society of Reconstructive Microsurgery, Scottsdale, Arizona, 1992.
36. Semple JL, Boyd JB, Farrow GA, et al. The "cricket bat" flap: one-stage free forearm flap phalloplasty. *Plast Reconstr Surg* 1991; 88:514.
37. Gottlieb LJ, Pielet RW, Levine LA. An update on phallic construction. *Adv Plast Reconstr Surg* 1994; 10:267–284.
38. Glasson DW, Lovie MI, Duncan GM. The ulnar forearm free flap in penile reconstruction. *Aust N Z Med J* 1986; 56:477.
39. Shenaq SM, Dinh TA. Total penile and urethral reconstruction with an expanded sensate lateral arm flap. *J Reconstr Microsurg* 1989; 5:245.
40. Young VL, Khouri RK, Le GW, et al. Advances in total phalloplasty and urethroplasty with microvascular free flaps. *Clin Plast Surg* 1992; 19:4.
41. Sandove R, Sengezer M, McRoberts JW, et al. One-stage total penile reconstruction with free fibular osteocoutaneous flap. Presented at the meeting of the American Society of Plastic and Reconstructive Surgeons, Washington, DC, October 1992.
42. Laub DR, Laub DR Jr, Hentz VR. Phalloplasty. In: Marsh JL, ed. *Current therapy in plastic and reconstructive surgery.* Philadelphia: BC Decker, 1989.

81

Penile Scrotal Lymphedema and Scrotal Gangrene

Culley C. Carson III, M.D., F.A.C.S.

The scrotum provides a variety of protective roles in maintaining adequate testicular function for the contained testes. The primary role of the scrotum is to regulate testicular temperature through the function of the Dartos muscle of the scrotum. The Dartos muscle provides mobility of the testes, which is also important for protection from trauma. While scrotal loss has a variety of causes, trauma is the most common, frequently occurring from farming injuries or motor vehicle accidents. Infection, however, is also a common cause of scrotal skin loss and scrotal lymphedema. Because scrotal skin is extremely elastic and has an incredible regenerative capacity, even a small rim of scrotal skin can regenerate or be used to provide complete coverage of both testes, with subsequent enlargement and distension to resume normal scrotal size and function. Because of the extensive blood supply of the scrotum, partial scrotal loss can be compensated for by mobilization of scrotal flaps, with excellent outcome. Following scrotal débridement, therefore, it is essential to retain as much scrotal tissue as possible to assist in later closure.

Penoscrotal Lymphedema (Elephantiasis)

Elephantiasis of the scrotum can be a physically disabling and psychologically distressing condition producing severe difficulty in walking and causing sexual intercourse to be difficult or impossible. While quite common in the tropics, elephantiasis of the penis and scrotum is relatively rare in the United States and the Western Hemisphere. The causes for elephantiasis differ in tropical and nontropical parts of the world. In the Western Hemisphere, simple edema of the scrotal, usually caused by lymphatic obstruction and bacterial infection, represents the most common indication for plastic reconstruction of this enlarged scrotum and penis. Massive elephantiasis caused by filarial infection is more common in the tropics, producing large hydroceles and massive penile and scrotal elephantiasis.

The causes for scrotal and genital elephantiasis were classified by Bulkley (1) into primary, idiopathic, and secondary obstructive forms. The former is usually seen in adolescence as lymphedema praecox. The latter is usually caused by (a) chronic infection by bacteria or filaria, (b) neoplastic lymphatic obstruction; (c) lymphatic obstruction after radiation or surgical lymph node dissection, or (d) chronic edema caused by renal or cardiac failure. Surgical procedures, prostheses, and trauma have also been implicated in scrotal lymphedema (2–4).

MEDICAL MANAGEMENT

The medical management of the underlying cause of scrotal elephantiasis is especially important in initial treatment. Patients with elephantiasis and lymphatic obstruction secondary to malignancy or radiation therapy are especially difficult to treat and, despite surgical excision, may have recurrences of scrotal lymphedema, lower extremity lymphedema, and elephantiasis.

Hidradenitis Suppurativa

Hidradenitis suppurativa is an infection of unknown etiology affecting areas of skin that are rich in apocrine sweat glands. These secondary sex glands occur primarily in the scalp, axillae, breast, umbilicus, groin, and scrotal areas. Simple scrotal infections can usually be medically treated and spontaneous resolution can be expected. Recurrent bacterial infections in these apocrine sweat glands form cystic drainage lesions, from which staphylococcal organisms can usually be cultured. The result of these chronic infections is a progressive brawny edema of the affected areas. Initial medical treatment with long-term culture-specific antibiotics and, occasionally, steroids may limit progression of the disease. Resultant severe elephantiasis of the genitalia is frequently encountered in longstanding hidradenitis suppurativa. Conservative treatment with diuretics, heat, and elevation in addition to antibiotics may be effective with acute swelling and in mild, chronic edema. When the lesions are extensive, however, exteriorization or excision of the entire affected area with direct closure of skin using split-thickness or mesh skin grafts may be required to eliminate these edematous draining areas (4).

Filarial Elephantiasis

Filaria, an endemic parasite in the Mediterranean, Asia, West Indies, and South Pacific produce severe hydrocele formation and scrotal elephantiasis after continued reinfection. A threadlike nematode, *Wuchereria bancrofti,* inhabits the human lymphatics. The parasite is passed through the immediate host mosquito, producing larvae in the human that inhabit the lymphatics. The adult parasites continue to inhabit and obstruct the lymphatics, producing microfilariae that are found frequently in the peripheral blood. Through longstanding infection and continuous inflammation, the lymphatic vessels become fibrotic, thickened and progressively obstructive. The resultant lymphedema produces large hydroceles and scrotal elephantiasis; and, in severe cases, scrotal edema can progress to lymphscrotum (6). The edema fluid in filarial elephantiasis differs from hydrostatic edema in containing protein and having a high cholesterol content. This extreme form of genital lymphedema results in chronic blistering and weeping of lymphatic fluid and is an uncommon result in any forms of elephantiasis other than those caused by filaria. Lymphscrotum usually responds only to surgical reconstruction of the genitalia and excision of the affected area.

Because elephantiasis of the scrotum is the result of filarial infection, usually requiring multiple episodes of inoculation, episodic travel to the tropics by individuals from the Western Hemisphere is unlikely to result in this condition. Patients who have lived in the tropics for long periods and who present with scrotal lymphedema, however, must be suspected of filarial infection, and diagnosis by the detection of *W. bancrofti* microfilariae in the peripheral blood must be undertaken (6). Because *W. bancrofti* is most likely to be found in the peripheral blood during the night, blood samples should be obtained around midnight. These peripheral blood smears must be examined after the lysis of blood red cells and staining of the blood smear with Giemsa or Leishman stain. Microfilariae can also be found in chylous urine and the fluid of hydroceles. Adult worms can be identified in histologic specimens removed at the time of scrotal reconstruction (6). Immunologic identification includes tests of complement fixation and skin tests. These tests, however, are only grouped and species-specific, but they can suggest a filarial etiology for lymphedema.

Differential diagnosis of filarial genital elephantiasis rests on careful history taking and physical examination and may be aided by lymphangiography, which may help distinguish filariasis from nonparasitic forms of lymphatic obstruction (7). Medical management should be initiated in every patient with demonstrated microfilariae. This regimen should include a complete course of antifilarial medication. The standard medication for *W. bancrofti* is diethylcarbamazine (DEC), hetrazan (Banocide), which is effective against both the microfilariae and the adult parasite and may be supplemented with coumarin (8). This drug, which is begun at a low dose, should be increased gradually from 3 to 12 mg/kg per day over a 2-week period (6). Generalized allergic reactions such as urticaria, headache, fever, nausea, and vomiting are common and can be treated with antihistamine medications. Ivermectin is also an effective medication for *W. bancrofti* (6). This agent, which has fewer toxic and allergic side effects than DEC, is less expensive and more convenient in administration. It can be given as a single oral dose of 20 to 25 μg/kg per day. Superimposed infections are common, especially in those patients with lymphscrotum, and treatment should be aimed at eradication of streptococci.

If exposure to the parasites is limited, complete and spontaneous resolution of the disease is common and prognosis is excellent. Frequent reinfection with *W. Bancrofti* often results in genital elephantiasis or chyluria.

Surgical Management

LYMPHATIC DRAINAGE OF THE MALE GENITALIA

Lymphatic channels drain penile and scrotal skin to the medial superficial inguinal lymph node and the groin. Metastases from the malignant disease of the penis and scrotum, therefore, frequently produce palpable adenopathy in the groin. The deep pelvic lymph nodes provide secondary drainage for these organs. The testes themselves are embryonically intraabdominal organs and their lymphatic drainage courses along the spermatic vessels to the area of the renal hilum.

TECHNIQUES

The first reported surgical treatment of scrotal elephantiasis was described by Lanney in 1803 and by Delpech in 1820 (9). Delpech described the excision of a 60-pound scrotal mass with genital reconstruction using abdominal and thigh flaps. Other innovative approaches to restoration of normal genitalia include reports of lymphatic bypass procedures. Orr (10) created a groin-to-scrotum skin bridge with moderate success. Cabanas and Whitmore (11) successfully bypassed lymphatic obstruction in dogs using a modified Touk procedure. More recently, Huang and co-workers (12) have reported successful microlymphaticovenous anastomosis in three patients with satisfactory long-term results. As a practical matter, however, clinical genital elephantiasis is usually of such long duration that lymphatic bypass does not effectively reduce the profound genital abnormalities. Thus, excisional techniques to remove lymphatic scrotal skin are usually the only reliably effective means of restoring genital appearance and function (13).

When scrotal enlargement is moderate and the penile skin is minimally involved, simple primary resection of the brawny, indurated scrotal skin with primary closure will adequately eliminate scrotal enlargement (14–20). This type of excision is best done beginning at the base of the penis and extending an incision along the median raphe of the scrotum to a level approximately 2 cm above the scrotal base. Scrotal contents are then exposed and the testes are examined for the presence of associated hydrocele, common with filarial elephantiasis. While procedures have been used that leave the hydrocele sac intact and inverted after drainage of hydrocele fluid (Lord procedure), the edematous tunica vaginalis frequently will retain an large bulk of tissue, making later scrotal closure difficult. Therefore, the best approach for these associated hydroceles includes delivery of the hydrocele through the midline scrotal incision with blunt separation of adherent subcutaneous tissue. The hydrocele sac is then opened anteriorly and the testis and its adnexa are carefully inspected. All redundant hydrocele sac is then excised close to the testis and epididymis. Hemostasis is best achieved with light cautery along the border of the exposed hydrocele sac but, if necessary, a tightly run locking suture of 30 chromic catgut can be used. It is only necessary to leave an approximately 0.5-cm rim of tissue adjacent to the testis and epididymis. Once the scrotal contents are inspected, the brawny, indurated scrotal skin is resected back to normal-appearing skin, taking care not to damage the spermatic cord and structures. Once this large piece of scrotal skin is removed, the testes are replaced within the remaining scrotal skin and the scrotum is closed in two layers using interrupted, absorbable suture. Perioperative antibiotics are especially important in these cases because an associated skin infection is likely to exist.

Massive elephantiasis of the penis and scrotum that prevents palpation of the testes and underlying cord structures presents a much greater surgical challenge. We have found it best to excise most of the scrotal skin, leaving only a small rim of skin around the edge for creation of a new scrotum. Complete excision of penile skin with split-thickness skin grafting best manages the penile portion of the elephantiasis. If the scrotal contents are not palpable, initial incision should be made at the base of the scrotum to deliver the scrotal contents into the wound before resecting the skin (21). Likewise, an incision over the dorsum of the penis dissected to the level of the Buck fascia exposes the shaft before excision of excess skin.

If adequate peripheral scrotal skin is available, it is best to leave the majority of skin for reconstruction in the posterior portion of the scrotum, allowing a posteriorly based flap of skin in which the testes can reside after closure (Fig. 81–1). This prevents the abnormal appearance of a scrotum produced from purely anteroposterior excision of skin and closure of lateral skin. Similarly, a purely transverse excision creates a large amount of redundant skin at the base of the penis and produces a foreshortened scrotum, which is frequently unacceptable cosmetically (Fig. 81–2).

Management of the penile skin involves complete excision of all skin from the shaft of the penis. It is important to remove the collar of skin just below the corona of the glans (Fig. 81–3). If the skin proximal to the corona is allowed to remain, it will become edematous and cause a "Bishop's collar" deformity. This deformity consists of penile shaft skin to the area of an edematous collar just below the corona penis. Complete excision of all this skin is therefore absolutely nec-

essary before harvesting and placing a split-thickness skin graft. Skin-graft replacement over the shaft of the penis should be obtained from areas of non-hairbearing skin. Mesh skin grafts produce less desirable cosmetic results on the penile shaft but may be acceptable for scrotal reconstruction.

Once harvested, the graft is applied with the suture line on the ventral surface of the penile shaft. This suture line should be interrupted by multiple Z-plasties or zigzags so that penile expansion can take place and scarring and chordee caused by straight-line closure are avoided (Fig. 81–4). In addition, attention must be paid to the penile base to limit "pyramidizing" of the penis and to better define the proximal penile shaft. A further dorsal Z-plasty at the penile base will ensure

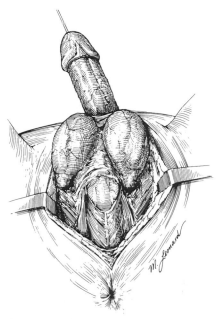

FIG. 81–2. Closure of the scrotum in the midline with dependent straight drainage uses interrupted absorbable sutures.

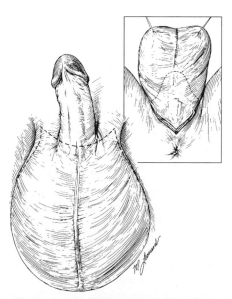

FIG. 81–1. Scrotal elephantiasis is shown with incisions marked. Incision at the base of the penis follows the base of the penis, with wings such that closure can be with entirely healthy skin. *Insert,* Alternative incisions are shown for removal of scrotal skin. The V-shaped incision is used if scrotal skin is entirely abnormal and the lower portion of the scrotal skin cannot be saved. The *dashed line* indicates a scrotal incision, which can be used if the inferior portion of the scrotal skin can be used as a flap to form a cup below the scrotum.

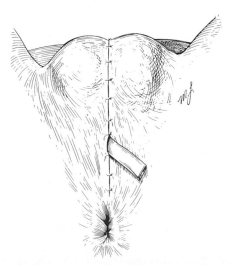

FIG. 81–3. Scrotal skin is removed. The scrotal contents are saved and maintained with their coverings intact. Penile skin is totally débrided to the corona penis.

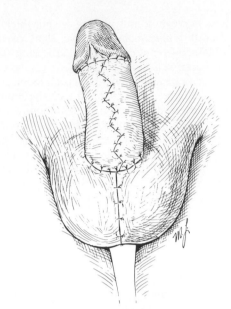

FIG. 81–4.   Scrotal closure with penile skin graft (ventral view). Closure should be performed using a zig-zag or Z-plasty pattern to prevent later scar contracture so that penile expansion during erection can be achieved. Ventral scars allow for an improved cosmetic appearance.

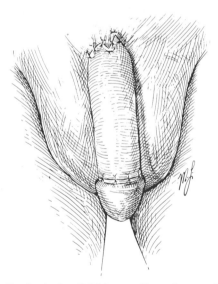

FIG. 81–5.   Penile shaft split-thickness skin graft approximation (dorsal view). The Z-plasty allows for better definition of the penis at the base and prevents contracture of the circular scar. Likewise, improved expansion during erection is allowed.

that base expansion is permitted during erection without a constricting ring of scar tissue (Fig. 81–5). The skin graft should be secured to the deep tissues of the pubic region at the level of the suspensory ligament with several interrupted sutures (Fig. 81–6).

Fournier Gangrene

While not related to elephantiasis of the scrotum, Fournier gangrene is a condition that commonly requires scrotoplasty to reconstruct the male genitalia (22). This rapid-onset scrotal

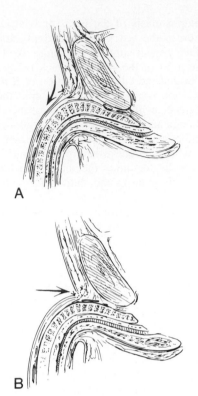

FIG. 81–6.   **A,** Incorrect method: abnormal skin and split-thickness skin graft are sutured directly, decreasing definition of the penis at the penile base. **B,** Correct method; this provides first for suturing of the abdominal skin to underlying tissues, followed by suture of the split-thickness graft to this deep fixed abdominal skin. Definition of the penis at the base is improved using this method.

infection was first described by Fournier in 1884 and, despite a change in its etiology, continues to bear his name (23). The infectious process, which occurs principally in alcoholics and diabetics, is being seen more often in patients immunocompromised following transplantation or in patients with HIV infection (24–27). This infection continues to be most commonly caused by gram-negative rods such as *Escherichia coli* or *Pseudomonas aeruginosa* combined with an anaerobic organism such as bacteroides (28–30). These organisms act synergistically to produce progressive gangrene of the scrotum. Risk factors include diabetes mellitus, alcoholism, genitourinary surgery (especially foreign-body implantation such as in penile prosthesis), immunocompromise, HIV infection, and general debility (24–26,31). Patients usually note the acute onset of scrotal pain, erythema, swelling, and discoloration, progressing rapidly to tissue necrosis without abscess formation. The gangrene is usually limited to the scrotum but may spread beneath the Colles and Scarpa fascia to the abdomen and even as high as the chest wall. Most patients are acutely toxic, with severe fever, chills, nausea, vomiting and even delirium. The mortality rate of these perineal infections continues to be 30% or greater (22). Initial treatment is most important, with prompt, aggressive, surgical débridement. Patients are begun on an aggressive course of triple antibiotic coverage designed for gram-negative rods and anaerobic organisms. Urine is diverted by Foley catheter or superpubic drainage. Débridement is carried out to remove all devitalized

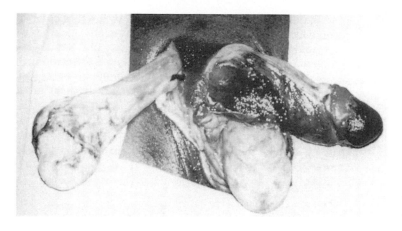

FIG. 81–7. Fournier's gangrene of the penis and scrotum. It was necessary to resect the entire scrotum and penis. The scrotal contents survived.

tissue, leaving multiple drains to limit further disease progression. The scrotal contents and penis are rarely affected by the gangrene and can usually be saved. Occasionally, if primary treatment is delayed, the penis and all scrotal tissue may be lost (Fig. 81–7). In patients with extensive deep-seated gangrene, treatment with hyperbaric oxygen may result in some tissue salvage and limit rapid infection progression (32).

Fortunately, the scrotum, with its capacity to regenerate itself, may spontaneously regenerate once infection is eradicated (29,30). A rim of scrotal tissue must remain to allow this regeneration. If scrotal tissue remains, expectant treatment with whirlpool baths, wet-to-dry dressings, and antibiotics is continued until granulation tissue forms. The scrotum will usually regenerate within 6 to 8 weeks if local treatment is maintained (20). Healing may be hastened by secondary closure, using remaining scrotal skin or a split-thickness skin graft (20,33). A mesh graft, in this situation, may be used to cover the remaining scrotal defect (20,33). These procedures should only be performed after granulation tissue has been established. Meshed skin grafts allow for excellent expanded coverage with reduced risk of graft loss as a result of improved drainage of fluid collections. Because the skin of the anterolateral aspect of the thigh matches the consistency of the scrotum, it is an excellent area for graft harvest. In order to prepare the bed for grafting, granulation tissue is excised because it may be infected. Hemostasis is achieved and the graft applied, covering testes and spermatic cords, and securing the graft in place with staples. Meshed split-thickness skin grafts provide excellent cosmetic results, since their uneven surface re-creates the rugae of the scrotal skin. In order to re-create a normal scrotum, it is essential to create a large enough split-thickness pouch with testicles placed and secured in the most dependent portion of this pouch. Since meshed split-thickness skin grafts can experience significant contractions, scrotal reconstruction in the younger patient may be best performed using nonmeshed grafts. The use of helical skin grafts has been described, with excellent cosmetic results (34). If the entire scrotum is excised, consideration must be given to recreating a scrotum using thigh or abdominal flaps (35). If the testicles are exposed, they can be protected during treatment by implanting them in subcutaneous pockets in the medial thighs. Flaps are outlined and raised from the inner thigh below the level of the penis and based in the medial and superior aspect of the thigh. The two flaps are joined anteriorly and posteriorly, with the testes

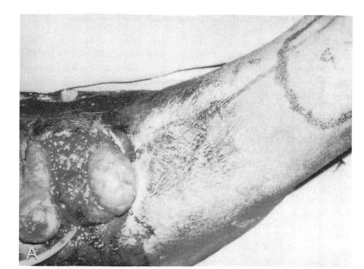

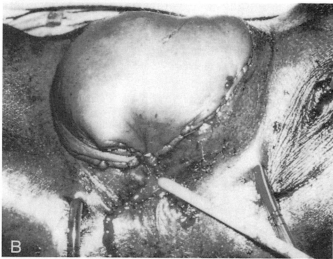

FIG. 81–8. **A,** Gracilis musculocutaneous flap is outlined on thigh. The pedicle enters the muscle approximately 8–10 cm distal to the pubic tubercle. **B,** The flap has been passed through a subcutaneous tunnel and folded on itself to form a scrotum.

within creating a scrotal pouch. The defect left by raising the skin flaps is covered with split-thickness skin grafts. Light compression dressings of fluffs are used postoperatively to eliminate hematoma formation.

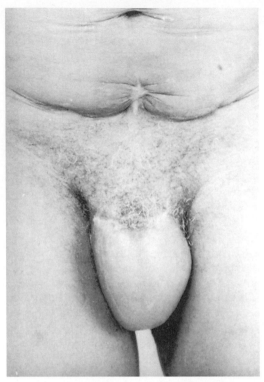

FIG. 81–9. Three months after scrotal reconstruction using gracilis musculocutaneous flaps. The patient declined penile reconstruction.

A single-stage technique for scrotal reconstruction that has proven useful is demonstrated in Figures 81–8 and 81–9. The gracilis musculocutaneous flap is elevated from one thigh. The location of the dominant pedicle of this muscle flap allows the flap to be transposed easily into the perineum. By folding the flap itself, a pouch is created that will easily hold the scrotal contents. The donor site in the thigh can be closed primarily. One theoretical disadvantage of this technique is the thickness of subcutaneous tissue and muscle. If the temperature in the pouch approaches core temperature as a result of its thickness and rich blood supply, an adverse effect on spermatogenesis may occur. The muscle itself will not atrophy to a great extent unless the nerve (which accompanies the dominant pedicle) is severed. If this is done, however, there is an increased risk of damaging the blood supply to the flap.

This major constructive procedure requires prolonged operative time and potential for morbidity. If simpler skin-graft procedures can be performed, they are preferable.

TISSUE EXPANDERS

Tissue expanders have been described for use in scrotal reconstruction where perineal skin is intact (36,37). If perineal skin and underlying skin are preserved following excision of the scrotal skin, tissue expansion may provide an excellent reconstructive procedure. Because Fournier gangrene frequently involves perineal skin, this procedure may be best used for patients with traumatic scrotal avulsion.

Following wound débridement and placement of the testes in thigh or abdominal patches, wound healing is allowed to continue for 4 to 6 weeks. Tissue expanders are then placed in the perineum, with the filling port allowed to

exit through healthy skin in the inguinal or lower abdominal area. These tissue expanders, which frequently have maximum capacities of 200 to 250 ml, are gradually filled to capacity over 6 to 12 weeks. Once capacity has been reached, the testis can be transplanted to the neoscrotum through standard orchiopexy. The cosmetic result obtained from these tissue-expansion techniques is excellent because perineal skin has similar consistency and hair content to that of the normal scrotum. For tissue expanders to work, however, patients must agree to multiple procedures and a prolonged reconstructive course.

References

1. Bulkley GJ. Scrotal and penile lymphedema. *J Urol* 1962; 87:422.
2. Elsahy MI. Syphilitic elephantiasis of the penis and scrotum. *Plast Reconstr Surg* 1976; 57:601.
3. Elsahy MI. Scrotal and penile lymphedema as a complication of testicular prostheses. *J Urol* 1972; 108:595.
4. Dickson RW, Hofsess DW. Non-tropical genital elephantiasis. *J Urol* 1959; 82:131.
5. Rubin RJ, Chinn BT. Perineal hidradenitis suppurativa. *Surg Clin N Am* 1994; 74:1317.
6. Smith JH, Von Lichtenberg F, Lehman JS. Parasitic diseases of the genitourinary system. In: Walsh PC, et al., eds. *Campbell's urology.* Philadelphia: WB Saunders, 1992; 883–927.
7. Janet GH, Taylor GW, Kinmonth JB. Operations for primary lymphedema of the lower limbs: results after 1–9 years. *J Cardiovascular Surgery* (Torino) 1961; 2:27.
8. Casley-Smith JR, Jamal S, Casley-Smith J. Reduction of filaritic lymphedema and elephantiasis by 5,6 benzo-alpha-pyrone (coumarin), and the effects of diethylcarbamazine (DEC). *Ann Trop Med Parasitol* 1993; 87:247.
9. Gibson T. Delpech: his contribution to plastic surgery and the astonishing case of scrotal elephantiasis. *Br J Plast Surg* 1957; 9:4.
10. Orr TG. Elephantiasis nostra of genitalia: report of a case and operative technique. *Surg Clin North Am* 1923; 3:1537.
11. Cabanas RM, Whitmore WF Jr. The use of testicular lymphatics to bypass obstructive lymphatics in the dog. *Invest Urol* 1981; 18:262.
12. Huang GK, Ru-Qi H, Liu Z, et al. Microlymphaticovenous anastomosis for treating scrotal elephantiasis. *Microsurgery* 1985; 6:36.
13. Apesos J, Anigian G. Reconstruction of penile and scrotal lymphedema. *Ann Plast Surg* 1991; 27:570.
14. Boxer RH. Reconstruction of the male external genitalia. *Surg Gynecol Obstet* 1975; 141:939.
15. Dandapat MC, Mohapatro SK, Patro SK. Elephantiasis of the penis and scrotum: a review of 350 cases. *Am J Surg* 1985; 149:686.
16. Das S, Turek D, Amar AD, et al. Surgery of the male genital lymphedema. *J Urol* 1983; 129:1230.
17. Feins NR. A new surgical technique for lymphedema of the penis and scrotum. *J Pediatr Surg* 1980; 15:787.
18. Raghavaiah NV. Reconstruction of scrotal and penile skin in elephantiasis. *J Urol* 1977; 118:128.
19. Altchek ED, Hecht H. A modification of the standard technique for repair of scrotal elephantiasis. *Plast Reconstr Surg* 1977; 60:284.
20. McAninch JW. Management of genital skin loss. *Urol Clin N Am* 1989; 16:387.
21. Hasham AI. Two-stage reconstruction of scrotum for tropical elephantiasis. *J Urol* 109:659.
22. Salvino C, Harford FJ, Dobrine PB. Necrotizing infections of the perineum. *South Med J* 1993; 86:908.
23. Fournier JA. Étude clinique de la gangrene foudroyante de la verge. *Semaine Med* 1884; 4:69.
24. Stephens BJ, Lathrop JC, Rice WT, et al. Fournier's gangrene: historic (1764–1978) vs. contemporary (1979–1988): differences in etiology and clinical importance. *Am Surg* 1993; 59:149.
25. Hughes-Davies LT, Murray P, Spittle M. Fournier's gangrene: a hazard of chemotherapy in AIDS. *Clin Oncol R Coll Radiol* 1991; 3:241.
26. Murphy M, Buckley M, Corr J, et al. Fournier's gangrene of the scrotum in a patient with AIDS. *Genitourin Med* 1991; 67:339.
27. McKay TC, Waters WB. Fournier's gangrene as the presenting sign of an undiagnosed human immunodeficiency virus infection. *Urology* 1994; 152:1552.

28. Jones RB, Hirschmann JV, Brown GS. Fournier's syndrome: necrotizing subcutaneous infection of the male genitalia. *J Urol* 1979; 122:279.

29. Rudolph R, Soloway M, DePalma RG, et al. Fournier's syndrome: synergistic gangrene of the scrotum. *Am J Surg* 1975; 129:591.

30. McAninch JW, Kahn RI, Jeffrey RB, et al. Major traumatic and septic genital injuries. *J Trauma* 1984; 24:291.

31. Walther PJ, Andriani RT, Carson CC, et al. Fournier's gangrene: a complication of penile prosthetic implantation in a renal transplant patient. *J Urol* 1987; 137:279.

32. Hirn M. Hyperbaric oxygen in the treatment of gas gangrene and perineal necrotizing fasciitis. A clinical and experimental study. *Eur J Surg* (*suppl*) 1993; 570:1–36.

33. Vincent MP, Horton CE, Devine CJ. An evaluation of skin grafts for reconstruction of the penis and scrotum. *Clin Plast Surg* 1988; 15:411.

34. Hirshowitz B, Bezald D. Bilateral superomedial flaps for primary reconstruction of scrotum and vulva. *Ann Plast Surg* 1982; 8:390.

35. Coquilhat P, Monod P, Delgove EL, et al. Reconstruction of the penile skin in Fournier's gangrene: the use of a helical skin graft. *Prog Urol* 1992; 2:303.

36. Still EF, Goodman RC. Total reconstruction of a two-compartment scrotum by tissue expansion. *Plast Reconstr Surg* 1990; 85:805.

37. Frohlich G, Stratmeyer R. Reconstruction of the scrotum using a tissue expander. *Urologe A* 1994; 33:159.

SEVEN

Microsurgery

FIG. 82–1.   Six patterns of the vascular supply to the fasciocutaneous plexus. Type A: direct cutaneous vessel; type B: direct septocutaneous vessel; type C: direct cutaneous branch of muscular vessel; type D: perforating cutaneous branch of muscular vessel; type E: septocutaneous perforator; type F: musculocutaneous perforator. (From Nakajima H, Fujino T, Adachi S. A new concept of vascular supply of the skin and classification of skin flaps according to their vascularization. *Ann Plast Surg* 1986; 16:1.)

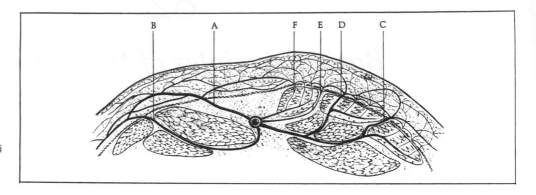

FIG. 82–2.   Patterns of vascular anatomy of muscle. Type I: one vascular pedicle; type II, dominant pedicle(s) plus minor pedicles; type III: two dominant pedicles; type IV: segmental vascular pedicles; type V: dominant pedicle plus secondary segmental pedicles. (From Mathes SJ, Nahai F. Classification system of the vascular anatomy of muscles: experimental and clinical correlation. *Plast Reconstr Surg* 1981; 67:177).

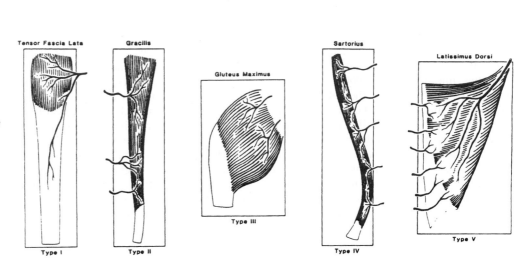

ameter leads to a dramatic decrease in flow. Narrowing related to contraction can usually be overcome by means of mechanical and/or chemical dilation. However, retraction can only be reversed by creating an anastomosis using the same tension as existed before division of the vessel. In free-flap surgery, especially when the recipient vessels are rerouted, this condition is usually not satisfied. Second, the flow through an end-to-end or end-in-end anastomosis depends entirely on the outflow capacity of the vessel. It has been shown that an anastomosis can be a source of microemboli (43) and that the presence of emboli largely depends on the quality of the anastomosis (44). These emboli are able mechanically to block parts of the downstream vascular throughway and are a source of substances such as thromboxane A_2, which is a very potent vasoconstrictor. Both events were found to reduce flow across the anastomosis (45), and may facilitate further platelet aggregation and deposition at the site of the arterial anastomosis, leading to obstruction. The events related to microemboli can also occur in a free flap connected to the main circulation in an end-to-side fashion. However, in an experimental study in which end-to-side anastomoses were used, and in which the downstream flow in some cases was temporarily reduced or even completely stopped, an occluding thrombosis of the actual anastomosis was never found (46). Therefore, preservation of the main circulation along an end-to-side anastomosis may offer an extra safety margin and keep the end-to-side anastomosis open.

END-TO-SIDE TECHNIQUE

No clear consensus exists as to whether part of the wall of the recipient vessel should be excised in preparation for an end-to-side anastomosis and, if it should, in what direction the excision should be performed (parallel or perpendicular to the axis of the native vessel) (46). In coronary bypass surgery, as well as in peripheral bypass surgery, a slit or incision arteriotomy is usually performed parallel to the axis of the recipient vessel (47). In our unit, where we frequently are involved in distal peripheral bypass surgery using microvascular techniques, we often use the same approach, making sure that the minimal length of the anastomosis is 10 mm, but frequently make it 15 to 20 mm. In free-flap surgery, we have adapted the same principles of slit arteriotomy and venotomy and spatulation of the pedicle vessels. However, if the angle of takeoff of the pedicle vessel approaches perpendicularity and the diameter of the anastomosis is shorter than 10 mm, we usually perform an excision of the native vessel wall parallel to the axis of the vessel in order to accommodate the size of the pedicle vessel. However, in an experimental study in which the pedicles of groin or latissimus dorsi free flaps were connected to the femoral artery and vein, Werker found that it was best to excise perpendicular to the vessel axis (46). Whether partial recipient wall excision translates into improved anastomotic patency rates has yet to be determined.

Tools

SUTURES AND SUTURING

A number of tools and techniques have been described to aid in vessel connection. Most investigators advocate the use of a monofilament, nonabsorbable microsuture of varying size, with a curved, round-bodied sharp microneedle. Nevertheless, equally good results in patency have been obtained by using absorbable sutures (48–53). The sutures can be placed in an interrupted, continuous, or combination fashion with equally good patency (54–59). Continuous sutures are only to be avoided in the anastomoses in vessels in children, because they have been found to prevent normal growth and to cause disorientation of the vascular layers and intima hyperplasia (60,61).

Cobbett (62) microsurgically adapted the large-vessel triangulation technique that was initially described by Carrell in 1902 for the creation of an end-to-end anastomosis (34). This technique consists of the placement of three stay sutures 120° apart on the circumference of the anastomosis, and the subsequent addition of as many sutures as necessary between them (Fig. 82–3). The use of this method limits the chance of catching the opposite vessel wall and the subsequent obliter-

ation of the lumen. The technique necessitates the help of an assistant or the use of a double vascular clamp with built-in suture holding frame (63)—the latter only employed when there is enough room to turn the clamp over 180°. To overcome this problem, some authors have advocated the placement of the first suture in the posterior wall, progressing anteriorly on both sides of the first stitch (64,65). Some investigators have advocated the placement of the stay sutures 180° apart, but this method carries a great risk of catching the opposite wall, especially in thin-walled vessels. Additional important aspects of technique are recommended to help insure a successful result: first, to enlarge the surface area of the anastomosis, or to overcome vessel diameter discrepancies, one or both of the vessel ends is cut obliquely or spatulated (Fig. 82–4) (47). Second, to achieve proper eversion of the vessel ends, we advocate the use of horizontal mattress stitches for the stay sutures.

Many of the described techniques apply to the end-to-side anastomosis. Various preferences exist, ranging from performing the anastomosis using simple interrupted stitches to using continuous suturing. Our preference is to create an anastomosis of at least 10 mm and to start with two horizontal mattress stitches at each end of the anastomosis, using 8-0 nylon in most instances. Thereafter, the front and the back wall of the anastomosis are completed using a running 8-0 suture, making sure to evert the vessel walls as much as possible. On the other hand, for the performance of end-to-side anastomoses in an experimental setting without the help of an assistant, one of us has described a modification of the back-wall-first technique, which allows overview of the anastomosis until the last stitch is placed and limits the number of sutures to six (46).

MECHANICAL COUPLERS

In the 1950s, vascular surgeons constructed devices to anastomose larger vessels mechanically (66). These were either staplers or ring-pin systems. The principle basic to all staplers was 180° eversion of the vascular ends over cuffs, and their union by metal staples. Nakayama (67) designed a ring-pin system, which only necessitated 90° eversion of the vessel ends, but this system is designed for larger vessels than are currently encountered in microsurgery. In the performance of microanastomoses, it appeared difficult to achieve 180° eversion of the vessel ends. The anastomotic coupler designed by Daniel (68,69) that relied on this principal was

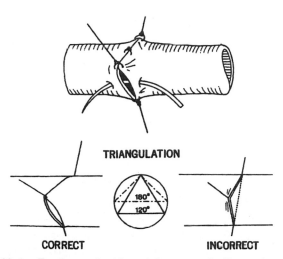

FIG. 82–3. Traction on the triangulation suture facilitates placement of additional sutures, reducing the chances of an accidental anterior-posterior wall suture. (From Daniel RK, Terzis JK. *Reconstructive microsurgery.* 1st ed. Boston: Little, Brown, 1977; 82.)

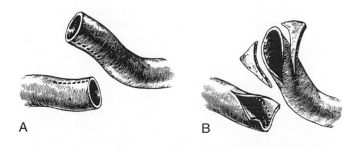

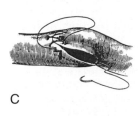

FIG. 82–4. Technique of spatulation for end-to-end anastomosis. **A,** the two ends are slit 180° apart. **B,** the resultant corners and adjacent lateral edges are trimmed conservatively. **C,** anastomosis is begun using two horizontal mattress stitches at each end and completed using two running sutures on each side of the anastomosis. (Modified from Rutherford RB. Basic vascular techniques. In: *Atlas of vascular surgery: basic techniques and exposures.* Philadelphia: WB Saunders, 1993; 40–41.)

never marketed. Ostrup modified and refined Nakayama's ring-pin coupler and developed the UNILINK system, which is currently available in slightly modified form as 3M Precise Anastomotic Coupler (70,71). Basically, each vessel end is passed through one part of the coupler, where it is then everted 90° over pins of the device; subsequently, the two coupler parts are brought together. This results in an optimal intima to intima apposition, without the presence of bonding material inside the vessel lumen. A comparable but less automated system was designed by Liang Siong and subsequently published in Chinese literature (72).

In our hands, application of the 3M system has been limited to the venous microanastomosis, since most often the thickness of the media of an arterial wall does not allow eversion as easily as a venous wall does. Ostrup's group has also reported on the successful application of the UNILINK system for both microvenous and microarterial end-to-side anastomosis in an experimental setting (73,74); however, in a recent publication they stated that clinical end-to-side procedures are rarely possible with the coupler (71). This has been our experience as well.

GLUES

Adhesives are currently being used in many medical specialties to obtain hemostasis, close fistulas, immobilize foreign bodies such as hip prostheses, deliver drugs, and close cutaneous ulcers (75). The two broad types of clinically used adhesives are fibrin glue and the cyanoacrylic glues. Fibrin glue may increase thrombogenicity when applied onto a vessel and is therefore not easily recommended in (micro) vascular surgery. The limitation of cyanoacrylic glues is its potential toxicity (76). The results of experimental application of methyl cyanoacrylate and butyl cyanoacrylate on vessels have been disappointing; they caused thinning of vascular walls, ultimately leading to formation of aneurysms (77–80). Recently a new glue, polyethyleneglycol 400 diacrylate, has been tested in a microvascular setup (80). It remains stable when properly stored, is polymerized by exposure to ultraviolet light, does not augment local vascular thrombogenicity, and is nontoxic to living tissue (82). The glue was found to be able to seal small holes in vessels, but it was not effective enough in early testing to support a sutureless anastomosis. Further study with this glue is indicated.

HYBRID TECHNIQUES

These techniques combine sutures with other methods.

1. *Glues and sutures.* Wrapping a four-suture, end-to-side anastomosis with a spongostan sponge impregnated with fibrogen-thrombin glue was found effective and had several advantages over conventional suturing, including reduction in the number of required anastomotic sutures, ensuring an elastic vascular junction and time savings (83).
2. *Cuff-suture technique.* This technique combines 180° eversion of one vessel end over a cuff and the end-in-end technique, but appears to bear no major advantage when compared to the end-in-end technique (84).
3. *Autogenous cuff technique.* Harris and co-workers (85) have advocated the combining of a limited number of sutures and a autogenous cuff to save time and limit vascular trauma (85).

LASERS

Jain and others, in 1979, were the first to report on vascular anastomosis using a neodymium YAG laser (86). In 1981 the first favorable report using the argon laser appeared (87). From many subsequent reports, it emerged that performance of a microvascular anastomosis using a laser requires less time than conventional techniques and that patency rates were at least equal. Furthermore, clinical results have been good (88–89). However, the reported incidence of pseudoaneurysm formation and rupture at the site of the anastomosis in experimental studies has been high (90–92), and has limited its clinical application. There is an ongoing debate regarding which type of laser has the greatest potential in microvascular surgery. Using the CO_2 laser, the tissue temperature is reported to rise to 80° to 120° C, and adhesion therefore occurs through melting (degeneration) of collagen and coagulation of cells in the media and adventitia (93–97). This coagulum is gradually replaced by fibrous and muscular tissues. To limit tissue damage, the use of low-power CO_2 has been advocated, and it is reported to give fewer problems (98–102). Argon lasers used for vascular anastomoses operate at a temperature of 43° to 48° C, well below the temperature at which collagen degenerates (94). The exact mechanism by which the argon laser fuses tissue has yet to be illuminated, but the widely accepted theory is that protein bonds are degraded thermally, allowing proteins to rebind to adjacent proteins. This results in smooth tissue-tissue connection (103,104). Chikamatsu and colleagues (60) used low-energy conditions in applying the argon laser, and could obtain tissue growth without severe disturbance of the laminar architecture of the vessels and with no aneurysm formation. We conclude that refinements in the technique have decreased the number of complications. However, a standard protocol for laser-assisted vessel anastomosing has yet to be developed.

What Influences the Outcome of a Microvascular Procedure?

The ability to perform the microvascular procedure is of prime importance for the outcome of a microvascular anastomosis. This includes more than the proper placement of sutures or couplers, or the application of any other device to join vessel ends. It necessitates the skill of atraumatic dissection of the blood vessels using sharp instruments and the local removal of overhanging perivascular tissue, without damaging the vessel. Preparation for clinical procedures should take place in the laboratory under supervision of an experienced teacher, and the first exposures to clinical microsurgery should also be carefully guided. It is important that, during the procedure, the microsurgeon attain a comfortable standing or sitting position. Ideally, an assistant should be present who is experienced enough in microvascular surgery to know what is helpful and what is not, and a scrub nurse should be present with interest in the process and dedication to the job. Interest can be encouraged by using a television circuit connected to the microscope. Experience is needed to select the most appropriate site to perform an anastomosis and to recognize damage of the intima. The adequacy of flow through the affected vessels must be demonstrated before the actual anastomosis is performed.

Vasospasm can interfere with the outcome of a microvascular procedure because it becomes more difficult to distinguish the vessel walls during the performance of the anastomosis and because it results in flow reduction once the clamps are released. Spasm can be the result of systemic and local factors. Systemic factors include circulating certain anesthetics, decreased circulating volume, decreased body temperature, catecholamines, nicotine from smoking, and excessive sympathetic stimulation secondary to anxiety and stress. Local factors include vascular trauma, blood or blood products in the operating field, decrease in the ambient temperature, and desiccation. Release of vasospasm by correcting systemic disturbances by the anesthesiologist is mandatory. Local release of spasm is the task of the microsurgeon and can be accomplished either chemically or mechanically. The most widely used topical chemical vasodilators are lidocaine and papaverine. The exact actions of lidocaine are still unrevealed, but it seems to act on both the vascular smooth muscle itself and its nervous innervation without the involvement of any endothelial factors or prostaglandin metabolites (105). An effective dose is 200 mg/ml; as such, the potential for toxicity must be realized. We apply this in a 1-cc tuberculin syringe with a 27-gauge needle in a drop-by-drop fashion. Papaverine at a dose of 30 mg/ml has direct action on vascular smooth muscle, and prevents muscle contraction by inhibiting the oxidative phosphorylation and calcium influx (106). Most microsurgeons apply vessel-dilating forceps intraluminally to stretch the divided vessel ends (21). We prefer to make use of the hydrostatic pressure that can be generated by clamping a vessel on one end and applying gentle bidigital pressure to push the blood towards the clamp. This technique is very effective and results in long-lasting vasodilation. It has not been associated with any increase in thrombotic complications.

During the process of performing an anastomosis, care should be taken to keep the operating field moist with Ringer solution, to prevent desication of the vessel ends and to facilitate suture handling. An occluding thrombus is the fear of every microsurgeon. Perfect technique is probably the single most important factor in preventing this. Apart from this, most experts still recommend the use of a heparinized physiologic solution to wash out the vessel ends (21), even though there is recent experimental evidence that the outcome of a microvascular procedure is not influenced by this irrigation (107). The same group (108), however, showed that intraluminal irrigation with a heparinized solution has benefits in cases where prolonged stasis at the site of a venous anastomosis is induced. In addition to topical measures, some experts advocate the use of systemic treatment with anticoagulants such as dextran, aspirin, low-dose heparin, or a combination of these (21).

Whenever all these demands can be met, microsurgery is an enjoyable event, with a very high success rate.

The Future

It is expected that the time-consuming procedure of microvascular surgery using interrupted sutures will be replaced more and more by the use of running sutures. Furthermore, refinements in laser welding and the development of new glues may take over the role of sutures. The operating microscope itself might also vanish in time. Many microsurgeons prefer to use high-magnification loupes and are able to achieve equally good results (109,110). Furthermore, advances in video technology now enable the surgeon to view a (micro) surgical field on a monitor in three dimensions without the necessity of looking through microscope eyepieces (111). Both techniques allow for more freedom of movement and give comfort in complicated reconstructions where the actual anastomotic site does not lie in a horizontal plane.

References

1. Nylén CO. The microscope in aural surgery, its first use and later development. *Acta Otolaryngol* [*suppl*] (Stockh) 1954; 116:226.
2. Jacobson JH, Suarez EL. Microsurgery in anastomosis of small vessels. *Surg Forum* 1960; 11:243.
3. Holman E, Hahn R. The application of the Z-plasty technique to hollow cylinder anastomoses. *Ann Surg* 1953; 138:344.
4. Shumacker HB, Lowenberg RI. Experimental studies in vascular repair. *Surg* 1948; 24:79.
5. Shumacker HB. The problem of maintaining continuity of aneurysms and arteriovenous fistulas with some notes on the development and clinical application of methods of arterial suture. *Ann Surg* 1948; 127:207.
6. Urschel HC, Roth EJ. Small arterial anastomoses. II. Suture. *Ann Surg* 1961; 153:611.
7. Acland RD. Signs of patency in small vessel anastomosis. *Surg* 1972; 72:744.
8. Buncke HJ, Buncke CM, Schulz WP. Experimental digital amputation and replantation. *Plast Reconstr Surg* 1965; 36:62.
9. Chen ZW, Chen YC, Pao YS. Salvage of the forearm following complete amputation. *Chin Med J* 1963; 82:632.
10. Kleinert HE, Kasdan ML, Romero JL. Small vessel anastomosis for salvage of severely injured upper extremity. *J Bone Joint Surg* [*Am*] 1963; 45:788.
11. Komatsu S, Tamai S. Successful replantation of a completely cut off thumb. *Plast Reconstr Surg* 1968; 42:374.
12. Bakamjian VY. Total reconstruction of the pharynx with a medially based deltopectoral skin flap. *NY J Med* 1968; 68:2771.
13. McGregor IA, Morgan G. Axial and random pattern flaps. *Br J Plast Surg* 1973; 26:202.
14. Daniel RK, Taylor GI. Distant transfer of an island flap by microvascular anastomoses. *Plast Reconstr Surg* 1973; 52:111.
15. Kaplan E, Buncke HJ, Murray D. Distant transfer of cutaneous island flaps in human by microvascular anastomoses. *Plast Reconstr Surg* 1973; 52:301.
16. Harii K, Ohmori K, Ohmori S. Successful clinical transfer of ten free flaps by microvascular anastomoses. *Plast Reconstr Surg* 1974; 53:259.
17. McLean DH, Buncke HJ. Autotransplant of omentum to a large scalp defect with microsurgical revascularization. *Plast Reconstr Surg* 1972; 49:268.
18. O'Brien BMcB, McLeod AM, Hayhurst JW. Successful transfer of a large island flap from the groin to the foot by microvascular anastomoses. *Plast Reconstr Surg* 1973; 52:271.
19. Nakajima H, Fujino T, Adachi S. A new concept of vascular supply of the skin and classification of skin flaps according to their vascularization. *Ann Plast Surg* 1986; 16:1.
20. Mathes SJ, Nahai F. Classification system of the vascular anatomy of muscles: experimental and clinical correlation. *Plast Reconstr Surg* 1981; 67:177.
21. Khouri RK. Avoiding free flap failure. *Clin Plast Surg* 1992; 19:773.
22. Manson PN, Narayan KK, Im MJ, et al. Improved survival in free skin flap transfers in rats. *Surgery* 1986; 99:211.
23. Wright JG, Kerr JC, Valeri CR, et al. Regional hypothermia protects against ischemia-reperfusion injury in isolated canine gracilis muscle. *J Trauma* 1988; 28:1026.
24. Berggren A, Weiland AJ, Dorfman H. The effects of prolonged ischemia time on osteocyte and osteoblast survival in composite bone grafts revascularized by microvascular anastomoses. *Plast Reconstr Surg* 1982; 69:290.
25. Lundborg G. Ischemic nerve injury. *Scand J Plast Surg* (*suppl*) 1970; 6:3.

26. Walkinshaw M, Downey D, Gottlieb JR, et al. Ischemic injury to enteric flaps: an experimental study in the dog. *Plast Reconstr Surg* 1988; 81:939.

27. Jobsis FF, Boyd JB, Barwick WJ. Metabolic consequences of ischemia and hypoxia. In: Serafin D, Buncke HJ Jr, eds. *Microsurgical composite tissue transplantation.* St Louis: CV Mosby, 1979.

28. Cooley DC, Hansen FC, Dellon AL. The effect of temperature on tolerance to ischemia in experimental free flaps. *J Microsurg* 1981; 3:11.

29. Donski PK, Franklin JD, Hurley JV, et al. The effect of cooling on experimental free flap survival. *Br J Plast Surg* 1980; 33:353.

30. Green CJ, Simpkin S. *Basic microsurgical techniques: a laboratory manual.* 2nd ed. Harrow, UK: Northwick Park Institute for Medical Research, in press.

31. Cooley BC. A laboratory manual for microvascular and microtubal surgery. Norwell, MA: Look Inc., 1994. [Look Inc., 80 Washington Street, Norwell, MA 02061.]

32. Acland RD. *Practice manual for microvascular surgery.* 2nd ed. St Louis: CV Mosby, 1989.

33. Lauritzen C. A new and easier way to anastomose microvessels. *Scand J Plast Surg* 1978; 12:291.

34. Carrel A. La technique operatoire des anastomoses vasculaires et la transplantation des visceres. *Med Lyon* 1902; 98:859.

35. Murphy JB. Resection of arteries and veins injured in continuity end-to-end suture: experimental and clinical research. *Medical Record* 1897; 51:73.

36. Bougle J. La suture artenelle. *Arch Med Exp Anat Pathol* 1901; 13:205.

37. Siemionow M. Histopathology of microarterial anastomoses: end-to-end versus end-in-end (sleeve) technique. *J Hand Surg* 1990; 15A:619.

38. Krag C, DeRose HG, Lyczakowski T, et al. Healing of microarterial anastomoses. *Scand J Plast Surg* 1982; 16:267.

39. Wieslander JB, Mecklenburg CV, Aberg M. Endothelialization following end-to-end and end-in-end (sleeve) microarterial anastomoses: a scanning electron microscopy study. *Scand J Plast Surg* 1984; 18:193.

40. Vilkki SK. Microvascular sleeve anastomosis in clinical replantation. *Scand J Plast Surg* 1982; 16:71.

41. Lauritzen C, Fogdestam I, Hamilton R, et al. The sleeve anastomosis in clinical microsurgery. *Scand J Plast Surg* 1979; 13:477.

42. Sumner DS. Essential hemodynamic principles. In: Rutherford RB, ed. *Vascular surgery.* 4th ed. Philadelphia: WB Saunders, 1995.

43. Acland RD, Anderson GL, Siemionow M, et al. Direct in vivo observations of embolic events in the microcirculation distal to a small-vessel anastomosis. *Plast Reconstr Surg* 1989; 84:280.

44. Gu J-M, Acland RD, Anderson GL, et al. Poor surgical technique produces more emboli after arterial anastomosis of an island flap. *Br J Plast Surg* 1991; 44:126.

45. Barker JH, Acland RD, Anderson GL, et al. Microcirculatory disturbances following the passage of emboli in an experimental free-flap model. *Plast Reconstr Surg* 1992; 90:95.

46. Werker PMN, Kon M, Green CJ. Geometrical approach to the end-to-side anastomosis. *Microsurg* 1991; 12:420.

47. Rutherford RB. Basic vascular surgery. In: Rutherford RB, ed. *Basic techniques and exposures.* Philadelphia: WB Saunders, 1993; 40.

48. Mallon WJ, Seaber AV, Urbaniak JR. A comparison of absorbable and nonabsorbable sutures to vascular response in immature arteries. *J Reconstr Microsurg* 1986; 2:87.

49. Cook AF, Azar CA, Dinner MI. The short-term effects of dexon and nylon sutures in experimental microvascular surgery: a quantitative comparison. *J Hand Surg* 1983; 8B:299.

50. Mii Y, Tamai S, Hori Y, et al. Microvascular anastomoses with absorbable and nonabsorbable sutures: a comparative study in rats. *Microsurg* 1980; 2:42.

51. Patel CB, Sykes PJ, Melville-Jones G. A comparison of polyglycolic acid (Dexon) and polyamide (nylon) sutures in experimental microvascular anastomoses. *Int J Microsurg* 1981; 3:285.

52. Thiede A, Lutjohann K, Beck C, et al. Absorbable and nonabsorbable sutures in microsurgery: standardized comparable studies in rats. *Microsurg* 1979; 1:216.

53. Fried MP, Caminear DS, Sloman-Moll ER. The efficacy of absorbable sutures for microvascular anastomoses. *Arch Otolaryng Head Neck Surg* 1990; 116:1051.

54. Guity A, Young PH, Fischer VW. In search of the perfect anastomosis. *Microsurg* 1990; 11:5.

55. Lee BY, Thoden WR, Brancato RF, et al. Comparison of continuous and interrupted suture techniques in microvascular anastomosis. *Surg Gynecol Obstet* 1982; 155:353.

56. Firsching R, Terhaag PD, Muller MW, et al. Continuous and interrupted suture technique in microsurgical end-to-end anastomosis. *Microsurg* 1984; 5:80.

57. Little JR, Salerno TA. Continuous suturing for microvascular anastomosis. *J Neurosurg* 1978; 48:1042.

58. Chen L, Chiu DT. Spiral interrupted suturing technique in microvascular anastomosis: a comparative study. *Microsurg* 1986; 7:72.

59. Eisenhardt HJ, Hennecken H, Klein PJ, et al. Experiences with different techniques of microvascular anastomosis. *Microsurg* 1980; 1:341.

60. Chikamatsu E, Sakurai T, Nishikimi N, et al. Comparison of laser welding, interrupted sutures, and continuous sutures in growing vascular anastomoses. *Lasers Surg Med* 1995; 16:34.

61. Nakashima S, Sugimoto H, Inoue M, et al. Growth of the aortic anastomosis in puppies: comparison of monofilament suture materials, whether absorbable or nonabsorbable, and of suture techniques, whether continuous or interrupted. *J Jpn Surg Soc* 1991; 92:206.

62. Cobbett J. Small vessel anastomosis. A comparison of suture techniques. *Br J Plast Surg* 1967; 20:16.

63. Acland RD. Microvascular anastomosis: a device for holding stay sutures and a new vascular clamp. *Surgery* 1974; 75:185.

64. Harris GD, Finseth F, Buncke HJ. Posterior-wall-first in microvascular anastomotic technique. *Brit J Plast Surg* 1981; 34:47.

65. Acland RD. Practice manual for trainees. Louisville Microsurgery Laboratory. St Louis: CV Mosby, 1975.

66. Androsov PL. New method of surgical treatment of blood vessel lesions. *Arch Surg* 1956; 73:902.

67. Nakayama K, Tamiya T, Yamamoto K, et al. A simple new apparatus for small-vessel anastomosis (free autograft of the sigmoid included). *Surgery* 1962; 52:97.

68. Daniel RK, Olding M. An absorbable anastomotic device for microvascular surgery: experimental studies. *Plast Reconstr Surg* 1984; 74:329.

69. Daniel RK, Olding M. An absorbable anastomotic device for microvascular surgery: clinical applications. *Plast Reconstr Surg* 1984; 74:337.

70. Ostrup LT, Berggren A. The Unilink instrument system for fast and safe microvascular anastomosis. *Ann Plast Surg* 1986; 17:521.

71. Berggren A, Ostrup LT, Ragnarsson R. Clinical experience with the Unilink/3M precise anastomotic device. *Scan J Plast Reconstr Hand Surg* 1993; 27:35.

72. Liang Siong, et al. The using of the 73-2 microvascular anastomotic apparatus in facial-maxillar surgery. *Chin J Stomatol* 1984; 19:190.

73. Ragnarsson R, Berggren A, Ostrup LT, et al. Arterial end-to-side anastomosis with the Unilink system. *Ann Plast Surg* 1989; 22:405.

74. Ragnarsson R, Berggren A, Ostrup LT. Microvenous end-to-side anastomosis: an experimental study comparing the UNILINK system and sutures. *J Reconstr Microsurg* 1989; 5:217.

75. Lerner R, Binur NS. Current status of surgical adhesives. *J Surg Res* 1990; 48:165.

76. Vinters HV, Galil KA, Lundie MJ, et al. The histotoxicity of cyanoacrylates. *Neuroradiology* 1985; 27:279.

77. Green AR, Milling MAP, Green RT. Butylcyanoacrylate adhesives in microvascular surgery: an experimental pilot study. *J Reconstr Microsurg* 1986; 2:103.

78. Weissberg D, Goetz RH. Necrosis of arterial wall following application of methyl 2-cyanoacrylate. *Surg Gynecol Obstet* 1964; 119:1248.

79. Woodward SC, Herrmann JB, Cameron JL, et al. Histotoxicity of cyanoacrylate tissue adhesive in the rat. *Ann Surg* 1965; 162:113.

80. Matsumoto T, Pani KC, Hardaway RM, et al. A method of arterial anastomosis using cyanoacrylate tissue adhesives. *Arch Surg* 1967; 94:388.

81. Dumanian GA, Dacombe W, Hong C, et al. A new photopolymerizable blood vessel glue that seals human vessel anastomoses without augmenting thrombogenicity. *Plast Reconstr Surg* 1995; 95:901.

82. Pathak CP, Sawhney AS, Hubbell JA. Rapid photopolymerization of immunoprotective gels in contact with cells and tissue. *J Am Chem Soc* 1992; 114:8311.

83. Aksik IA, Kikut RP, Apshkalne DL. Extra-intracranial anastomosis performed by means of biological gluing materials: experimental and clinical study. *Microsurg* 1986; 7:2.

84. Deshmukh GR, Yang Y, Tellis VA, et al. A simple cuff-suture technique for microvascular anastomosis. *J Reconstr Microsurg* 1992; 8:491.

85. Harris GD, Finseth F, Buncke HJ. The microvascular anastomotic autogenous cuff. *Brit J Plast Surg* 1981; 34:50.

86. Jain KK, Gorisch W. Repair of small blood vessels with the neodymium-YAG laser: a preliminary report. *Surgery* 1979; 85:684.

87. Gomes OM, Macruz R, Armelin E, et al. Vascular anastomosis by argon laser beam. *Texas Heart Inst J* 1981; 10:145.

88. White RA, White GH, Fujitani RM, et al. Initial human evaluation of argon laser-assisted vascular anastomoses. *J Vasc Surg* 1987; 9:542.

89. Okada M, Simizu K, Ikuta H, et al. An alternative method of vascular anastomosis by laser: experimental and clinical study. *Lasers Surg Med* 1987; 7:240.

90. McCarthy WJ, Cicero JL, Hartz RS, et al. Vascular anastomoses with laser energy. *J Vasc Surg* 1986; 3:32.

91. Quigley MR, Bailes JE, Kwaam HC, et al. Aneurysm formation after low-power carbon dioxide laser-assisted vascular anastomosis. *Neurosurg* 1986; 18:292.

92. McCarthy WJ, Cicero JL, Hartz RS, et al. Patency of laser assisted anastomoses in small vessels: one-year follow-up. *Surgery* 1987; 102:319.

93. Serure A, Whithers EH, Thomsen S, et al. Comparison of carbon dioxide laser-assisted microvascular anastomosis and conventional microvascular sutured anastomosis. *Surg Forum* 1983; 34:634.

94. Kopchok GE, White RA, White GH, et al. CO_2 and argon laser vascular welding: acute histologic and thermodynamic comparison. *Laser Surg Med* 1988; 8:485.

95. Danielsen CC. Precision method to determine denaturation temperature of collagen using ultraviolet difference spectroscopy. *Coll Relat Res* 1982; 2:143.

96. Epstein M, Colly BC. Electron microscopic study of dosimetry for microvascular tissue welding. *Laser Surg Med* 1986; 6:202.

97. Frazier OH, Painvin GA, Morris JR, et al. Laser-assisted microvascular anastomoses: angiographic and anastomopathologic studies on growing microvascular anastomoses—preliminary report. *Surgery* 1985; 97:585.

98. Sartorius CJ, Shapiro SA, Campbell RL, et al. Experimental laser-assisted end-to-side microvascular anastomosis. *Microsurgery* 1986; 7:79.

99. Kiyoshige Y, Tsuchida H, Hamasaki M, et al. CO_2 laser-assisted microvascular anastomosis: biochemical studies and clinical applications. *J Reconstr Microsurg* 1991; 7:227.

100. Nakata S, Campbell CD, Pick R, et al. End-to-side and end-to-end vascular anastomoses with a carbon dioxide laser. *J Thorac Cardiovasc Surg* 1989; 98:57.

101. Guo J, Chao YD. Low-power CO_2 laser-assisted microvascular anastomosis. Experimental study. *Neurosurg* 1988; 22:540.

102. Neblett CR, Morris JR, Thomsen S. Laser-assisted microsurgical anastomosis. *Neurosurg* 1986; 19:914.

103. White RA, Kopchok GE, Donyre C. Argon laser-welded arteriovenous anastomosis. *J Vasc Surg* 1987; 6:447.

104. White RA, Kopchok GE. Laser vessel sealing with the argon laser. *Laser Surg Med* 1987; 7:229.

105. Perlmutter NS, Wilson RA, Edgar SW, et al. Vasodilatory effects of lidocaine on epicardial porcine coronary arteries. *Pharmacology* 1990; 41:280.

106. Hartsock LA, Seaber AV, Urbaniak JR. Inhibition of epinephrine-induced vasospasm with adrenoreceptor blockade in the rat cremaster muscle. *Microsurgery* 1991; 12:55.

107. Rumbolo PM, Cooley BC, Hanel DP, et al. Comparison of the influence of intraluminal irrigation solutions on free flap survival. *Microsurgery* 1992; 13:45.

108. Li X, Cooley BC, Gould JS. The influence of topical heparin on stasis-induced thrombosis of microvascular anastomoses. *Microsurgery* 1992; 13:72.

109. Shenaq SM, Klebuc MJA, Vargo D. Free tissue transfer with the aid of loupe magnification: experience with 251 procedures. *Plast Reconstr Surg* 1995; 95:262.

110. Serletti JM, Deuber MA, Guidera PM, et al. Comparison of the operating microscope and loupes for free microvascular tissue transfer. *Plast Reconstr Surg* 1995; 95:276.

111. Franken RJPM, Gupta SC, Banis JC, et al. Microsurgery without a microscope: laboratory evaluation of a three-dimensional on-screen microsurgery system. *Microsurgery* (in press).

83

Principles of Microneurosurgery

Allen L. Van Beek, M.D., F.A.C.S., and Patricia Bitter, M.D.

We have entered an era when artificial intelligence is becoming a reality, an era when the transmission of information is performed by systems that are actually smaller than the axons required in biologic systems. Even more significant, information can be conducted using these systems infinitely faster and with greater accuracy and sensitivity than in cellular systems. The application relevance of electrical technology to biological systems is immense. The major impediment to its clinical application is the inability to completely understand and control the biologic systems in man.

However, attempting to understand the peripheral nerve, and particularly the injured peripheral nerve, is essential to surgeons if the potentials of new technology are to be incorporated successfully into clinical practice (1–5). Presently, many surgeons still deal with peripheral nerve injuries using techniques described decades in the past (6–9).

Certain refinements in managing nerve injuries have occurred because of improved understanding of microscopic surgery, microsutures, and enhanced visibility. Despite these improvements, the adult sustaining a transsection of a major peripheral nerve never achieves normal function distal to the site of the nerve injury.

Nerve Degeneration and Regeneration

Wallerian degeneration and axonal regeneration are almost simultaneous events. After transsection of a peripheral nerve, the sequence of events that occurs will depend on the diameter of the axon, the thickness of myelin, and the species involved (10–13). After transsection, retrograde degeneration occurs in the proximal stump to at least the 1st or 2nd node of Ranvier. The distal axonal stump, however, undergoes wallerian degeneration from the site of injury to the end organ (Fig. 83–1). After early degeneration in the proximal stump, regeneration begins. Regeneration axon sprouts can be seen within 72 hours egressing from the proximal axon stump. The regeneration axons migrate between the Schwann cell sheath and myelin that is still present. In the distal nerve stump, the myelin tubules are eventually replaced by cords of Schwann cells referred to as Bungner bands. Degeneration quickly results in a decreased diameter of neurotubule surrounding cellular constituents, and regenerating axons are smaller than normal. Therefore, in a whole-nerve preparation, the distal nerve stump diameter decreases in size very early after injury. The decrease in diameter of the distal nerve stump can be as much as 40% within 4 weeks of injury (Fig. 83–2). Since it became recognized that nerves could regenerate, many types of repairs have been advocated. A historical review of nerve repair was recently presented by Snyder and colleagues (8). They pointed out that some of the suture techniques that have been advocated in the past were as useful "as showed on a snake." While the application of microsurgery has helped, history may hold the same indictment for the present techniques of neurorrhaphy.

The first fresh autogenous nerve graft was probably used by Deams in 1896. Bunnell and Boyes (14) and Seddon and others (15) began to use nerve grafts in the 1930s. However, Millesi and colleagues (16) more recently popularized nerve grafting as a reconstructive technique when excessive gaps existed between the proximal and distal stumps of an injured nerve. Nerve grafting techniques were soon followed with the application of the microscope to nerve repairs (17). Visual enhancement of the stumps of nerve allowed better topographical mapping, dissection, and preparation of the nerve stump without injury to other tissues. Minimization of the amount of reactive foreign body in the nerve repair, as well as the volume of foreign body within the nerve repair site, was made possible by improved technology. These refinements have improved the results after peripheral nerve repair. Presently, recent efforts by surgeons managing peripheral nerve injuries are directed at maximizing alignment, enhancing coaption, and decreasing the amount of foreign body and trauma at the injury repair site. Augmentative measures that are being explored include electromagnetic fields generated across the repair site, utilization of tubulization materials to prevent egress of regenerating axons, improving the vascularity of nerve grafts, application of nonsuture repair techniques, and histological mapping of fascicles to enhance alignment (18–27).

Peripheral Nerve Anatomy and Terminology (see also Chapters 10 and 82)

A surgeon who is working with extremity injuries must be aware of the topical linear anatomy of the peripheral nerve. Recognition of this anatomy is essential to avoid confusing the peripheral nerve with tendons, which is a common mistake. The suturing of a peripheral nerve to a tendon stump, while rare, still occurs.

The extrinsic vascularity of the peripheral nerve is readily apparent. Extrinsic blood vessels run between the grooves of fascicles (Fig. 83–3) and similar vessels are not seen on tendons. From the extrinsic vascularity of the nerve, branches supply the internal portions of the nerve (intrinsic vascularity). The generous vascularity within a peripheral nerve can be seen on cross-sectional examination. Axons require a periph-

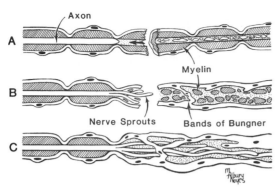

FIG. 83–1. **A,** after nerve transsection, axon degeneration begins. **B,** by 5 to 7 days proximal axon sprouting has occurred. Distally, myelin tubes are fragmenting and Schwann cells are proliferating. **C,** by 21 days, many axons are extending distally and most myelin tubes are replaced by bands of Schwann cells.

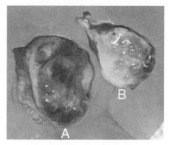

FIG. 83–2. Nerve and fascicle shrinkage occurs in only a few weeks. Specimen A is a proximal slump. Specimen B is a distal stump. Note the change in size present 1 month after injury.

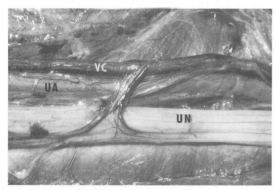

FIG. 83–3. Normal surface anatomy of the nerve. Note the linear vascularity corresponding to interfaces between adjacent fascicles. Also the segmented vascularity is noted: ulnar artery (UA), ulnar nerve (UN), vena comitantes (VC).

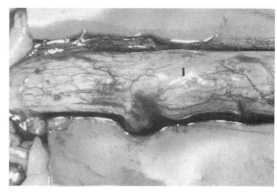

FIG. 83–4. Note the great increase in vascularity in this partially injured (I) nerve 10 days after injury.

eral blood supply to maintain metabolism and membrane potentials, and to maintain a milieu of nutrients. Injury produces a profound increase in vascularity (Fig. 83–4). Restriction of vascularity produces a zone of ischemia and will result in peripheral nerve dysfunction at the site of vascular interruption. Cross-sections of a major peripheral nerve also reveal the nerve's fascicles. Peripheral nerves can usually be divided into fascicular groups, which can be the anatomic basis for some nerve repairs (Fig. 83–5). Surrounding the nerve and each fascicle is the epineurium, which contains sheets of laminated cells that are durable and supportive (the part of the epineurium surrounding the nerve perimeter is the external epineurium). The internal or interfascicular epineurium is located internally, courses between the fascicles, and is continuous with the external epineurium. Supporting connective tissue is thicker in the lower extremity than in the upper extremity, particularly after traumatic insults.

Each fascicle is surrounded by perineurium, a multistriated sheath of cells that seems to be an extension of the pia-arachnoid (Fig. 83–4). It varies in thickness from three to ten cell layers. The perineurium appears to have some semipermeable properties that affect distribution of some pharmacologic agents. Fascicles surrounded by perineurium vary in size from 50 μ to many millimeters. The greater the size of the fascicle the larger the number of axons contained there. In comparison syndromes and after trauma, perifascicular fibrosis may occur. In children, similar anatomic details are present, but on a smaller scale.

Nerve fibers can be myelinated or unmyelinated. Myelinated nerve fibers conduct at a very rapid rate, are larger in

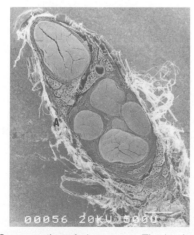

FIG. 83–5. Cross-section of ulnar nerve. The beginning of a nerve branch, vascularity, and surrounding connective tissue **(A)** is depicted. This tissue **(A)** is unacceptable for repair. Two "groups" could be easily created.

diameter, and are more sensitive to stimulation (excitable). Unmyelinated nerve fibers are small in diameter, slow in conduction velocity, and generally associated with basal activity (28,29). Myelinated axons are designed to deal with immediate environmental changes and immediate responses. The actual mechanism of nerve conduction is interrelated with the mitochondria, microtubules, neurofilaments, axoplasmic transport, and metabolism of the axon and its pericaryon. The critical balance between these systems can be altered by changes in vascularity, disease, compression, toxins, radiation, viruses, and autoimmune phenomena. The loss of function in a peripheral nerve is manifested by alterations in the expression of afferent and efferent information, and all the etiologies for this change must be considered. Alteration in nerve function not only produces functional deficits but also a great potential for pain and suffering. While the financial losses associated with peripheral nerve injures are certainly measurable, what is immeasurable is the amount of pain, disruption of life routines, and expenditure of emotional energy that are associated with the frustration caused by peripheral nerve injuries.

CLASSIFICATION OF NERVE INJURIES

A clear classification of nerve injuries is essential and, unfortunately, does not presently exist. However, the classifications of Sunderland and Seddon are probably the most widely recognized (Fig. 83–6). In a Sunderland type I injury, the nerve structure and axon structure are intact but a conduction block exists and, therefore, functional loss is noted. A 1st-degree injury in Sunderland classification is called "neurapraxis" by Seddon. A 2nd-degree injury implies that wallerian degeneration is occurring because of a more severe injury to the axon. However, the epineurium, perineurium, and Schwann cell sheaths remain intact. This is classified as "axonotmesis" in Seddon's classification. An optimistic recovery should be expected because the Schwann cell sheath

is intact. In a 3rd-degree injury, the axon is undergoing wallerian degeneration. The Schwann cell sheath has been disrupted, but the perineurium and epineurium are intact. In a 4th-degree injury, the nerve has a severe stretching injury with wallerian degeneration and a loss of continuity of the Schwann cell's sheath and perineurium; however, strands of epineurium are intact. Attempts at regeneration produce a neuroma in continuity, and some regenerating axons are able to bridge the injury site. In a 5th-degree injury, all nerve structures are transsected. Sunderland 2nd-degree and 3rd-degree injuries are called "neurotmeses" in Seddon's classification. The obvious problem lies in determining what degree of injury is present in closed or stretch injuries when the measurable result in each instance clinically is interruption of function (1,30).

It is unfortunate that injury classifications are not really meaningful clinically because the physician cannot ascertain exactly what structures are intact. Classification systems are further complicated by the different spectrums of injuries encountered. In a clinical setting, the surgeon may see an injury classified as sharp, blunt, multisegmental, avulsion, narrow area of injury, or wide area of injury. However, documentation of the injury mechanism and suspected degree of injury is helpful in estimating the ultimate outcome or explaining why subsequent delayed neurorrhaphy may be required.

Microneurorrhaphy Tools and Materials

As in microvascular surgery, microneurorrhaphy requires special equipment such as jewelers' forceps, microsurgical needle holders, approximating devices, scissors, and other delicate instruments (Figs. 83–7 through 83–9). There are

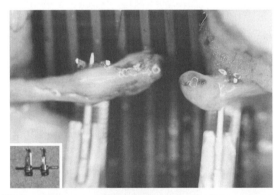

FIG. 83–8. A nerve-approximating clamp (Weck Instruments). The small retaining needle usually holds the nerve's external epineurium.

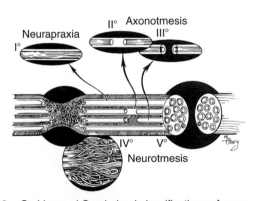

FIG. 83–6. Seddon and Sunderland classifications of nerve injury.

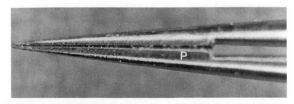

FIG. 83–7. A jewelers' forceps with a typing platform (P) is a very useful tool (Storz Instruments).

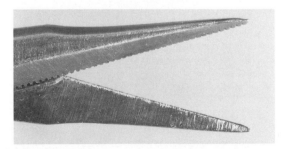

FIG. 83–9. Microsurgical scissors with serrated edges are used to trim fascicles (Storz Instruments).

also unique requirements in microneurorrhaphy that are not encountered when suturing luminal structures. The solid fascicle, with its extruding contents, is often a more difficult problem to solve than suturing an empty lumen. The proper training is essential in this field.

Nerve Repair Sequence

There are many different approaches to nerve repair. Before beginning nerve repair, fractures should be fixed, joints reduced, and tendons repaired. Attempting to perform these maneuvers after repairing structures with microscopic technique will frequently result in either stretching or disrupting of nerves and vascular repairs. Even uncontrolled extremity movements of the patient in the operating room or recovery room can disrupt repairs. Provisions for sequential repair and control of movement is essential. A unique problem occasionally encountered is the flexor carpi ulnaris tendon injury combined with an ulnar nerve and ulnar artery injury. In this instance, accomplishing repair of the flexor carpi ulnaris before microrepair impedes microscopic repair. The solution is to place the tendon stump sutures, but not tie them. After repair of the nerve and artery, it is quite simple to approximate the tendon carefully. This will prevent disruptive movements that could injure the microscopic repair.

Using loupe magnification, the injured nerve is identified and mobilized from its bed for a distance of approximately five times its diameter. This mobilization allows sufficient manipulation of the nerve to allow easier repair. A blue-colored background material is placed behind the nerve to enhance tissues. After dissection of the injured nerve, when nonmicroscopic repairs have been completed, the operating microscope is brought over the field. It is essential to position the operating microscope before beginning the surgical procedures both to save time and to facilitate easier placement. The remaining steps of the microscopic repair are dealt with

individually and sequentially in the discussion that follows.

For trimming and repairing neuromatous stumps, special devices are available. We prefer to utilize an ophthalmic keratome knife with a 30° cutting angle. These blades are extremely sharp, disposable, and usually readily available. The knife may also be used for linear fascicular dissection during neurolysis or when transsection of fascicles or groups of fascicles is required. Trimming the extruding fascicular material is done with a straight microsurgical scissors, and a serrated scissors makes trimming extruding fascicles easier (Fig. 83–10).

When a nerve is transsected, the two stumps retract. The amount of retraction generally varies with the location of the injury. Nerves that are severed at the fulcrum of a joint can either be approximated or distracted depending on the positioning of the joint. We prefer to use a nerve approximating device (31) to control the stumps and hold them in position (Fig. 83–11). Positive stump control permits careful examination, preparation, and suturing of the nerve without struggle. During group fascicular nerve repair, the nerve approximater becomes particularly useful. In addition, because the nerve approximater permits easy nerve rotation, the backside of the nerve is readily accessible. This promotes more accurate alignment and nerve suture. The technique of drawing the nerve together with a stay suture and then using it as a rotating suture is another common method of approximating the nerve.

When repairing extensively injured hands, it often is not possible to use the tourniquet during the nerve repair because of excessive tourniquet time. When the tourniquet is deflated, the stump readily bleeds. Some of this bleeding can be controlled through the use of bipolar cautery. However, when controlling the intrinsic circulation, there is some risk to the adjacent fascicles, even when using a bipolar jewelers' forceps. In that instance, rather than continuing vigorous coagulation in the area, we prefer to use a suction background material (Fig. 83–12). This microsurgical background material has a suction incorporated into it. Continuous suction can be applied in the area of the field to prevent fluid accumulation; this greatly aids visibility on some occasions.

The advent of taper-cut ends on 70- or 100-μ needles makes suture penetration through dense tissue easier. This has enhanced the suturing of nerve. In an effort to minimize trauma, foreign body presence, and suture reaction, it is rec-

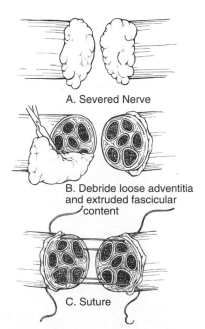

FIG. 83–10. Preparing the nerve stump is a key in nerve repair. Fascicle visibility and definition is one goal. This permits more accurate coaption of the nerve.

A. Severed Nerve

B. Debride loose adventitia and extruded fascicular content

C. Suture

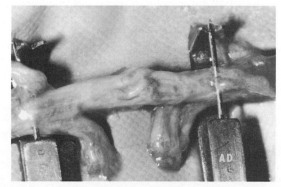

FIG. 83–11. The severed stumps are approximated using a nerve-approximating device (AD) while the groups of fascicles are repaired.

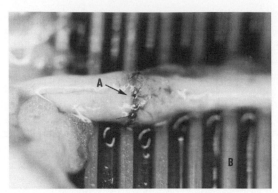

FIG. 83–12.   A, sutured digital nerve. B, a background material with suction incorporated is used to remove excess fluid and enhance visibility.

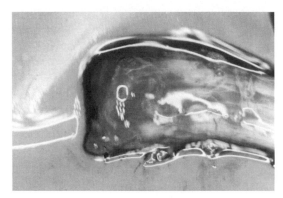

FIG. 83–13.   In the unprepared stump, fascicular anatomy is obscured.

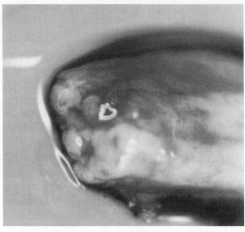

FIG. 83–14.   After initial surgical preparation, fascicular anatomy becomes more apparent. Microscopic visual enhancement is essential to careful stump preparation and examination.

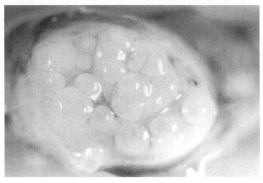

FIG. 83–15.   The appropriate alignment of the nerve's stumps is selected.

ommended that 10-0 and 11-0 sutures be utilized for nerve repairs. Occasionally, a traction stitch of 9-0 nylon can be utilized to coapt some of the external epineurium or adventitia of the nerve trunk.

Stump Preparation

In acute or delayed nerve repair, stump preparation is essential to assure accurate alignment and to minimize fibrosis. In the acute nerve injury, adventitia, epineurial hemorrhage, or extruded fascicular content may blur the stump topography (Fig. 83–13). Careful removal of these tissues under the microscopic (Fig. 83–14) control of hemorrhage is essential before repair. After trimming extruded fascicular content, perineurial collars can usually be identified. The topography of the proximal and distal nerve stumps should be noted and correct alignment determined (Fig. 83–15). If desired, the stimulation techniques of Hakstian (32) or Gaul (33) can be utilized when necessary to aid proper fascicular alignment. During acute repair, the fascicles are usually easy to match when magnified unless there is a segmental loss. In chronic nerve injuries, fascicular fibrosis, edema, swelling, and traumatic distortion affect fascicular topography, and in that instance the stimulation technique would be invaluable. Unfortunately, after 24 to 48 hours fascicular stimulation of the distal nerve becomes impossible because of degeneration in the stump. However, dissection of the distal nerve combined with proximal stimulation may still be of use.

Nerve Repair Techniques

FASCICULAR REPAIRS

An ideal nerve repair provides for the maximal alignment and coapting of fascicles. For this reason, repair of fascicles on an individual basis as a method of nerve repair has been reported. This technique is time consuming and more invasive than standard techniques, but potentially provides a more accurate fascicular alignment than other types of nerve repairs (Fig. 83–16). However, because of the difficulty of this procedure, its invasiveness, and the potential for excessive fibrosis, it is not widely applied in primary nerve injuries. Where single-fascicle repair does become an important technique is in procedures such as toe-to-hand transfer, microneurovascular muscle transfer, and other areas of reconstruction where varied, dissimilar nerve stumps are present. When neurotization is critical and the cross-sectional surface area of the fascicles being coapted is small, accurate alignment of dissimilar fascicles is required if effective regeneration is to be expected.

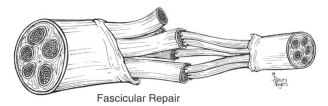

Fascicular Repair

FIG. 83–16. Fascicular repairs are important when dissimilar fascicles are repaired during toe-to-hand, free muscle, and some other elaborate microsurgical reconstructions.

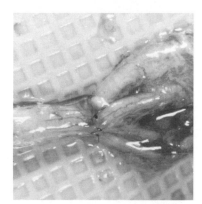

FIG. 83–17. Single-fascicle repair is shown in a free muscle transfer.

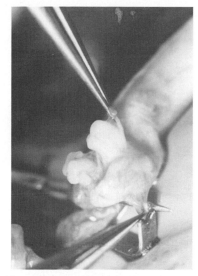

FIG. 83–18. Three groups of fascicles have been separated for repair.

An example of this application is shown in Figure 83–17. A branch of the anterior interosseous nerve containing a single, large fascicle is being connected to the three fascicles of the nerve to the gracilis muscle. In this instance, a single fascicle of the anterior interosseous is larger than the composite three fascicles of the gracilis muscle. Furthermore, if the gracilis muscle has been split based on its fascicular territories to provide independent function, it may be necessary to suture specific fascicles to specific nerve segments; this can only be accomplished by single fascicle repair. This application of single-fascicle repair is the most common and is essential because of the reconstructive goals that are sought. In single-fascicle repairs, the external epineurium, interfascicular epineurium, or perineurium are utilized to approximate the fascicles. Care must be taken to assure that the needle does not pass into the fascicular material during repair, or vital axons will be injured, constricted, or even rendered useless by the suture material.

GROUP FASCICULAR REPAIR

Group fascicular repair is based on the demonstration of Sunderland, and others, that nerves can be dissected in groups of fascicles over long distances. Because large, whole nerves, when sutured using only external epineural technique, may leave poor alignment and gaps within the central part of the nerve, a greater degree of coaption can be achieved by splitting the nerve into its group fascicular components (Fig. 83–18). The most frequent sites of nerve injury at the wrist and forearm—the median and ulnar nerves—lend themselves to this technique. The median nerve at the wrist can be divided into three, or occasionally four, groups. The ulnar is divided into two groups. The composite structure of these groups is well described. The advantage of the repair is that

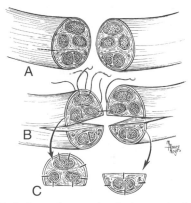

FIG. 83–19. Technique of group fascicular repair. **A,** nerve stumps are divided into groups and mobilized. **B,** groups are accurately coapted using 10-0 nylon suture. **C,** sutures are placed to maximize peripheral fascicle alignment.

it coapts the central nerve and allows for better spatial alignment of the nerve. However, care must be exercised when creating the separation and cleavage in the groups or fascicular crossover damage could occur.

Group fascicular repair should only be performed using the operating microscope to assure that crossovers are not damaged when creating the groups. During group fascicular repair, the nerve is dissected into its component groups for a distance of 5 to 15 mm to allow for easy manipulation of the groups (see Fig. 83–10 and 83–19). The groups thus created are coapted by suturing around the perimeter of each group. Group fascicular repair is reserved for nerves proximal to the palm or forefoot. When using this technique, the nerve approximating clamp is very useful. It holds the nerve in position while the nerve is examined and groups created and then sutured.

EXTERNAL EPINEURAL NERVE REPAIR

In nerves measuring less than 4 to 5 mm in diameter, an external epineurial repair is the most efficacious. This tech-

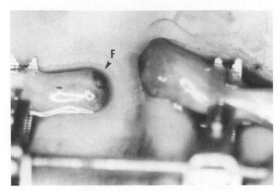

FIG. 83–20. After preparation of stumps, fascicles (F) should be readily visible.

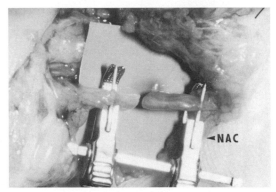

FIG. 83–21. Retracted nerve stumps are secured with a nerve-approximating clamp (NAC). The stumps are then prepared and approximated for suturing. External epineurium and adventitia are pierced.

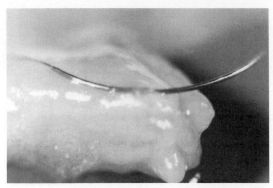

FIG. 83–22. Accurate suture placement is easy using the operating microscope. Loupe magnification is inadequate for reliable repair. The needle should not pierce into the fascicle.

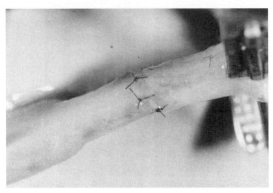

FIG. 83–23. Digital nerve repair.

nique does not imply a lesser degree of alignment or care during the repair. In the external epineurium technique, the operating microscope is still utilized for the repair. In addition, the stumps are examined for the appropriate alignment, preparation, and coaption (Figs. 83–20 and 83–21). It is essential that corresponding fascicles be approximated whenever possible. Clues that can lead to appropriate alignment include vascular anatomy and configuration of transsection site, but most commonly the fascicular topography of the stump is used. The stump topography must be clearly visualized and magnified to allow this to be accurately performed. In our opinion, this can only be done with an operating microscope. Once this has been done, the nerve is coapted by placing sutures through the external epineurium corresponding to each fascicle (Fig. 83–22). For instance, the digital nerve, which contained four to five fascicles, would generally have at least four to five sutures (Fig. 83–23). In some instances, if the nerve is still poorly aligned, additional sutures can be placed, and occasionally two sutures are required to coapt large fascicles.

This is the most common nerve repair. Emphasis is placed on accurate topographic alignment, accurate suture placement to avoid encroachment on the fascicle, and minimizing foreign body presence by using 10-0 nylon. Obviously, in smaller nerves the central component of the nerve is aligned, and in most instances the nerves are exactly coapted because the fascicles will lie on the perimeter. It is only in those nerves in which there are large numbers of central fascicles that the group fascicular technique is indicated.

ADDITIONAL TECHNICAL MANEUVERS

After accurate coaptation of the fascicles of the nerve, the looser adventitial layer of the nerve is usually approximated over the nerve repair site. It can be repaired easily. To coapt this loose adventitial tissue, 10-0 nylon figure-of-eight sutures are used. This probably gives some support to the nerve and provides some additional cushion to the repair site. After repairing the peripheral nerve, careful attention should be given to wound closure. Whenever possible, fat or muscle should cover the nerve. Suturing aponeurosis, muscle, or subcutaneous tissue over nerve repair sites assures at least some protection of the egressing axons of the neuroma from the cutaneous scar. Without this barrier, it is possible for axons egressing from the repair site to become caught in the dermal wound, resulting in recalcitrant sensitivity and pain in the area (neuroma).

TECHNICAL SUMMATION

The technique of microneurorrhaphy is more demanding and time-consuming than the repair of luminal structures. The result of a failed nerve repair remains unseen until months later, when the chronic effects of the failed repair become in-

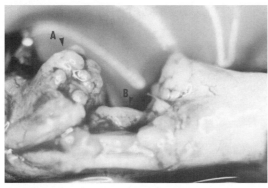

FIG. 83–24. An acute, sharp, partial median nerve transsection with intact fascicles (A) and severed fascicles (B).

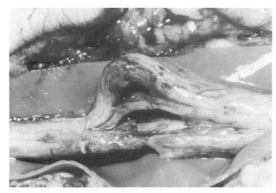

FIG. 83–25. After repair, some tension exists on the repair site and the uninjured nerve forms a redundant loop.

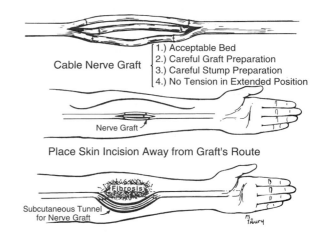

Cable Nerve Graft
1.) Acceptable Bed
2.) Careful Graft Preparation
3.) Careful Stump Preparation
4.) No Tension in Extended Position

Nerve Graft

Place Skin Incision Away from Graft's Route

Fibrosis

Subcutaneous Tunnel for Nerve Graft

Detour Fibrotic Areas

FIG. 83–26. The principles of nerve grafting must be adhered to if the graft is to be successful.

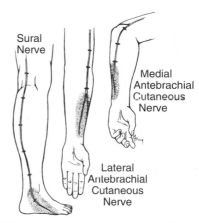

Sural Nerve

Medial Antebrachial Cutaneous Nerve

Lateral Antebrachial Cutaneous Nerve

FIG. 83–27. These nerves are commonly used for donor sites, and the areas of hypesthesia associated with harvesting are stippled. The patient must be informed of this hypesthesia as well as the associated proximal neuroma.

creasingly problematic. If the surgeon cannot do microvascular anastomoses successfully and reliably, it should be left to someone of greater experience or skill. Furthermore, in our opinion, loupes are inadequate magnification for nerve repair.

Partial Nerve Injuries

A partially transsected nerve is not an uncommon entity and often presents technical difficulties (Fig. 83–24). If the injury is old, granulation tissue, edema, and wound reaction fill the gap, and it is easy to underestimate the significance of the injury. In the acute situation, injured fascicles can be readily identified. After nerve mobilization, the injured fascicles can be directly approximated. This will result in some buckling of the intact fascicles (Fig. 83–25). If the gap is long or it is an old injury, tension on the partially injured segments of nerve may prevent direct approximation. In such cases the gap should be spanned by using interpositional cable nerve grafts. Usually grafts are required in partially injured nerves only when the repair has been delayed for several weeks.

Nerve Grafts

Nerve grafting has been advocated, popularized, and carefully studied by Millesi (see Chapter 10). The primary indication for nerve grafting is to span an excessive gap between the proximal and distal stumps of an injured nerve. Excessive mobilization combined with tension at the repair site is particularly detrimental to nerve regeneration. Furthermore,

nerve repairs using excessive mobilization and suture under tension confuse and often delay adequate treatment because some regeneration occurs even across these repair sites. Thus, the hopeful surgeon may delay appropriate treatment even longer, awaiting effective regeneration.

Large-diameter nerves with gaps of over 3 to 5 cm in length invariable require nerve grafts. Nerves with a smaller diameter usually require grafts for gaps over 1 to 1.5 cm.

Nerve grafts are not as good as direct repairs without tension, but they are superior to direct repairs done with tension. Tension can be assessed in the following manner: if two nerve stumps can be approximated with a single suture of 8-0 nylon with the adjacent joints in neutral or slightly advantageous positioning, excessive tension is not present. If the suture breaks or pulls out of the tissue, excessive tension is probably present and consideration of nerve grafting should be made.

NERVE GRAFT RECIPIENT BED (Fig. 83–26)

Nerve grafts are vascularized by the process of inosculation. The time sequence of inosculation is similar to that in skin grafts (5). To enhance inosculation, a very well-vascularized, minimally fibrotic and uninfected bed is desirable. Dense fibrosis from trauma, irradiation, ischemia, or systemic disease provides an undesirable bed. If possible, nerve grafts should detour these areas or an alternative method of treatment should be planned.

Resurfacing techniques using microvascular free-tissue transfers is one modality for providing a suitable graft bed. Simultaneous free-tissue transfer and nerve grafting is not recommended, but silicone rods may be placed through the transferred flap to assure easy passage and circumferential tissue contact when the nerve is repaired 2 to 4 months later.

Vascularized nerve grafts are the newest of nerve graft techniques available to the reconstructive surgeon. This technique is applicable when the recipient bed is densely fibrotic, irradiated, and unlikely to support the process of graft inosculation. When performing a vascularized graft, not only is a nerve graft supplied to span a gap but also the graft is not dependent on inosculation from the bed for circulation; therefore, this type of graft could be used in adverse recipient beds without the risk of graft failure because of fibrosis.

Vascularized nerve graft donor sites are not as forgiving as nonvascularized grafts. The most commonly used vascularized grafts are harvested from the superficial radial, sural, ulnar, and superficial peroneal nerves. The anatomy of these grafts provides vascular perfusion through systems of segmental or linear intrinsic circulation, as described by Breidenbach and others (34–36). The application of these grafts must be limited until additional clinical information is obtained regarding the final result. The donor-site morbidity of these grafts is greater and is combined with greater risk and cost. However, in adverse recipient beds, vascularized nerve grafts seem advantageous (Fig. 83–27).

References

1. Sunderland S. *Nerves and nerve injuries.* Baltimore: Williams & Wilkins, 1968.
2. Landon DN. *The peripheral nerve.* London: Chapman and Hall, 1976.
3. Waxmann SG. *Physiology and pathology of axons.* New York: Raven, 1978.
4. Omer GE, Spinner M. *Management of peripheral nerve problems.* Philadelphia: WB Saunders, 1980.
5. Davis L, Cleveland D. Experimental studies in nerve transplants. *Ann Surg* 1934; 99:271.
6. Sunderland S, Ray LT. The selection and use of autografts for bridging gaps in injured nerves. *Brain* 1947; 70:75.
7. Bjorkesten G. Suture of war injuries to peripheral nerves: clinical studies of results. *Act Chir Scand (suppl)* 1947; 119:1.
8. Snyder GG, Omer GE, Spinner M. *History of nerve repair in management of peripheral nerve problems.* Philadelphia: WB Saunders, 1980.
9. Boyes JH. *Bunnell's surgery of the hand.* Philadelphia: JB Lippincott, 1970.
10. Hubbard JH. The quality of nerve regeneration. *Surg Clin North Am* 1972; 52:1099.
11. Powell HC, Varon S, Lundborg G. Competence of nerve tissue as distal insert promoting nerve regeneration in a silicone chamber. *Brain Res* 1984; 293:201.
12. Van Beek AL, Eder MA, Zook EG. Nerve regeneration: evidence for early sprout formation. *J Hand Surg* 1982; 7:79.
13. Lugennegard H, Berthold CH, Rudmark M, et al. Ultrastructural morphometric studies on regeneration of the lateral sural cutaneous nerve in the white rat after transsection of the sciatic nerve. *Scand J Plast Surg* 1984; 20:27.
14. Bunnell S, Boyes JH. Nerve grafts. *Am J Surg* 1939; 44:64.
15. Seddon HS, Young JZ, Holmes W. The histological condition of a nerve autograft in man. *Br J Surg* 1942; 29:378.
16. Millesi H, Meissl G, Berger A. Further experience with interfascicular grafting of the median, ulnar and radial nerves. *J Bone Joint Surg (Am)* 1976; 58:209.
17. Smith JW. Microsurgery of peripheral nerves. *Plast Reconstr Surg* 1964; 33:317.
18. Rand RN. *Microneurosurgery.* St. Louis: CV Mosby, 1978.
19. Levinthal R, Brown WJ, Rand RW. Comparison of fascicular, interfascicular, and epineural suture techniques in the repair of simple nerve lacerations. *J Neurosurg* 1977; 47:744.
20. Van Beek A, Kleinert HE. Practical microneurorrhaphy. *Orthop Clin* 1977; 8:377.
21. Cham RM, Peimer CA, Hower CS, et al. Absorbable versus nonabsorbable suture for microneurorrhaphy. *J Hand Surg (Am)* 1984; 9:434.
22. Almquist EE, Nachemson A, Auth D, et al. Evaluation of the use of the argon laser in repairing rat and primate nerves. *J Hand Surg (Am)* 1984; 9:792.
23. Hurst LC, Badalamente MA, Blum D. Carbon dioxide laser transsection of rat peripheral nerves. *J Hand Surg (Am)* 1984; 9:428.
24. Taylor GI, Ham FT. The free vascularized nerve graft: a further experimental and clinical application of microvascular techniques. *Plast Reconstr Surg* 1976; 57:413.
25. Terzis J, Faibisoff B, Williams HB. The nerve gap: suture under tension vs graft. *Plast Reconstr Surg* 1975; 56:166.
26. Lundborg G, Rydevik B. Effects of stretching of the tibial nerve of the rabbit: a preliminary study of the intraneural circulation and the barrier function of the perineuerium. *J Bone Joint Surg (Br)* 1973; 55:390.
27. Orgel MG. Experimental studies with clinical application to peripheral nerve injury: a review of the past decade. *Clin Orthop* 1983; 163:98.
28. Dorfman LJ, Cummins KL, Leifer LJ. *Conduction velocity distributions: a population approach to electrophysiology of nerve.* New York: Alan R. Liss, 1981.
29. Sumner AJ. *The physiology of peripheral nerve disease.* Philadelphia: WB Saunders, 1980.
30. Seddon HJ. *Surgical disorders of the peripheral nerves.* Edinburgh: Churchill Livingstone, 1975.
31. Van Beek AL, Zook EG. A nerve approximating device. *Plast Reconstr Surg* 1980; 66:143.
32. Hakstian RW. Funicular orientation by direct stimulation. *J Bone Joint Surg (Am)* 1968; 50:1178.
33. Gaul JS Jr. Electrical fascicle identification as an adjunct to nerve repair. *J Hand Surg* 1983; 8:289.
34. Breidenbach WC. Vascularized nerve grafts. A practical approach. *Orthop Clin North Am* 1988; 19:81.
35. Doi K, Kuwata N, Kawakami F, et al. The free vascularized sural nerve graft. *Microsurgery* 1984; 5:175.
36. Gilbert A. Vascularized sural nerve graft. *Clin Plast Surg* 1984; 11:73.

84

Cutaneous Free Flaps

**Joseph C. Banis, Jr., M.D., F.A.C.S., Paul M.N. Werker, M.D., Ph.D.,
Hussein S. Abul-Hassan, M.D., and John W. Derr, Jr., M.D., F.A.C.S.**

The introduction of free flaps has revolutionized the field of plastic and reconstructive surgery. A continuous flow of research and anatomic dissections concerning cutaneous flaps has led to a widespread increase in the applications and utilization of microsurgically transferred skin flaps. A historical review indicates that cutaneous flaps have been utilized for several centuries. Tagliacozzi (1) performed nasal reconstruction with an arm flap in 1597 and the "Indian" rhinoplasty (2) strongly influenced 19th century European reconstructive surgeons such as Carpue (3), von Graefe (4) and Dieffenbach (5). These flaps, developed and utilized over a period of 500 years, represent isolated events in the slow course of development of this field of surgery. It was not until World War I, and increasingly in the years leading up to World War II, that the principles of flap surgery were conceived.

A wide variety of cutaneous flaps were described and used during this period (3,6–12). The pioneering work of Esser (13), Gillies (8), and McIndoe during and after the First World War included experience with many flaps, large and small, tubed and untubed—all, however, sharing one thing in common; they were random pattern skin flaps and the "delay" procedure was the key to obtaining any significant length of the flap. After the Second World War, many surgeons were involved in the discovery and elucidation of numerous flap territories. These included the forehead, neck, chest, abdomen, and upper back regions (3,7,10–12,14).

Shaw and Payne (15) described the hypogastric flap in 1946. This flap possessed the desirable qualities of both a high length:width ratio and the potential for immediate transfer without a delay procedure. Their short paper "was misunderstood or ignored completely," but "contained the kernel of much later work on axial flaps. The place of the hypogastric flap in the evolution of flap design has to be given to it retrospectively as a result" (16).

This isolated and prescient publication excepted, the mass change in the thinking of flap design started with the description of the deltopectoral flap by Bakamjian in 1965 (17). This flap, which was raised on a single medially based pedicle, flouted all the accepted restrictions of flap surgery and culminated in two other papers searching for an explanation of its viability, when length:width ratios would have suggested necrosis. The first investigation, by Muir and colleagues (18), concluded that the incorporation of an artery in a tubed flap will increase the pressure gradient from one end to the other. In 1970, Milton (19) described his findings concerning skin flaps in pigs, in which flaps were raised with variable lengths but of the same width. In this study, all flaps survived in their entirety. It was clearly demonstrated later that this unexpected finding was the result of the presence of a discrete vessel within the base of each flap (i.e., a so-called axial blood supply to each skin segment) (20). With this new understanding of flap blood supply, McGregor and his colleagues began a search for another donor site similar to the deltopectoral flap. This work resulted in a long, single-pedicled skin flap based on the superficial circumflex iliac system. This flap was named the *groin flap* by McGregor and Jackson in their description of this territory in 1972 (20).

The definition in 1973 of "random" and "axial" skin pattern flaps was a pioneering work of McGregor and Morgan (21) and respects a milestone in our understanding of the anatomy of skin flaps. According to them, a random pattern flap is defined as a flap with a vascular pattern that lacks vascular "bias" in any particular direction and that is subject to relatively strict limitations of length:width ratio. An axial pattern flap may be defined as one constructed around a preexisting, anatomically recognized arteriovenous system. It is independent of length:width ratio.

Axial pattern skin flaps were thus found to be supplied by a system of vessels that run in the subcutaneous fat, parallel to the skin surface. It was soon found that these flaps could be converted into island flaps and transferred as free flaps by isolating the vessels at the points where they emerge and branch off the main circulation. A true example of this sort of flap is the groin flap. The first free groin flap transferred by microsurgical techniques was performed in 1971 by Kaplan (22). The flap, used for intraoral lining, was extruded 2 weeks after surgery. Daniel (23), inspired by the account of Kaplan, performed and reported the first successful microsurgical transfer of a groin flap. Harii (24) performed his first free scalp transfer in 1972 and reported it in a series of cases in 1975 (25). In 1973, O'Brien and Shannugan (26) reported their experience with successful microsurgical transfer of a groin flap. The age of free-tissue transfer was born.

Frustrated by the short length of the superficial circumflex iliac vessels and the bulky nature of the groin flap, Acland (27) studied and described the "lateral groin" or "iliac" flap, which had the advantage of a thinner skin territory and a longer vascular pedicle. At the end of the 1970s, the experimental and clinical work of Taylor (28) demonstrated the advantages of using the deep circumflex iliac system for free groin skin and osteocutaneous flaps.

In the meantime, a further major development in flap surgery came with the understanding that muscles also can be transferred based on their vascular pedicles, as originally described by Ger (29) and Orticochea (30), and that a system of musculocutaneous perforating vessels allows perfusion of the overlying skin territories of many muscles (See Ch. 85). This concept and its widespread applications were described by McCraw and colleagues (31,32) in 1977.

While muscle and musculocutaneous flaps soon filled a major need in reconstructive surgery, and proved to be more reliable than the earlier reported skin free flaps, it became increasingly apparent that these tissues were not appropriate for all defects. The problems with size, bulk, the unchangeable relationship of underlying muscle to subcutaneous tissue and skin, and functional donor deficit (albeit usually minimal) led to a renewed interest in understanding the blood supply of the skin and underlying fascia. Pontén described the concept and use of fasciocutaneous flaps in the repair of soft-tissue defects in the lower leg in 1981 (33). Before that, the existence of fasciocutaneous vessels had been ignored. This is remarkable, since Manchot in 1889 (34) had already described the full vascularity of certain territories of the skin and fascia, and since both Esser (13) in 1917 and Gillies (8) in 1920 suggested that it might be advantageous to include the deep fascia in what are now known as random-pattern skin flaps. Cormack and Lamberty (35) introduced a classification system for fasciocutaneous flaps in 1984, while at the same time Nakajima, (36) developed a classification system that described the complete vascular supply of the skin. These accounts and those by other investigators (35,37,38) paved the way for the acceptance of the concept of fasciocutaneous flaps, and many of the skin flaps described in the 1970s are now recognized.

Many of the currently available fasciocutaneous flaps can be transferred as sensate flaps. Especially in the reconstruction of defects of the mobile tongue, the base of the tongue and the pharynx, application of these flaps might improve functional recovery. Although some groups have substantial early experience in this field (39), long-term results have yet to be published.

Many fasciocutaneous flaps have the potential to be raised together with a segment of bone. The radial forearm flap can carry a piece of radius, the lateral arm flap a piece of humerus, the scapular flap a strip of scapula, and the dorsalis pedis flap the complete second ray or parts of it. On the other hand, in flaps primarily consisting of bone, a skin paddle can be incorporated (see Ch. 86). This is the case in the iliac crest flap and the fibula free flap. One problematic aspect with the use of most of the osteocutaneous flaps is a limited freedom to position the various components of the flap. An exception to this is the free scapular osteocutaneous flap. Various skin paddles and a strip of scapula can be isolated on different branches of the main pedicle. This makes the flap attractive for the reconstruction of complex defects and can compensate for the single major disadvantage of the flap (in most instances of head and neck reconstruction), which is that it necessitates repositioning of the patient during the procedure. The alternative is the combination of several free flaps, wherein for each part of the reconstruction the optimal free flap is selected.

All free flaps that have been discussed thus far have a vascular network consisting of arteries, capillaries, and veins, and are revascularized by connecting the vessels orthotopi-

cally. In 1981 Nakayama (40) introduced an entirely new idea in flap content, when they reported on an experimental study in which flaps with only a subcutaneous venous network produced a reliable take by perfusion of arterial blood. Honda (41) in 1984, and Yoshirmura (42) in 1987 succeeded in clinical application of venous flaps to skin defects of the fingers with exposure of deep structures. These flaps have been described as uni- or bipedicled flaps or as free flaps (43). Fukui (44) reported on a classification system for venous free flaps, which suggests they can be connected to the circulation in one of three ways: venous blood can flow in and out (V–V type), arterial blood can flow in and out (A–A type), or the inflow vein can be connected to an artery and the outflow vein to a vein (A–V type). The results of clinical application of unpedicled venous flaps have not been consistent (45–47). Most clinical reports on application of flaps in the V–V, A–V, and A–A category have shown complete survival in most cases and superficial necrosis in a minority of cases (44,48–54). Chen (54) concluded that venous flaps can be useful for wound coverage of fingers and hand, but that they do not replace cross-finger flaps or other conventional flaps when these simpler flaps are available. One of the major advantages of these flaps as compared to conventional free flaps is that no artery has to be sacrificed. However, guidelines for the use and reliable application of venous flaps have yet to be defined.

This chapter gives a brief description of the most clinically useful and straightforward cutaneous flaps of microsurgical transfer. The three "workhorses" and three lesser used cutaneous flaps are described with particular reference to applicability, pedicle size and length, size of flap territory, potential for sensation, bulk, and potential for composite or multiple flap reconstruction. In addition, a variety of other cutaneous flaps that for a number of reasons do not find their way into our frequent usage are described in a much more limited fashion. The inclusion of a flap into the workhorse or other categories is in no way meant to imply that the lesser or rarely used flaps are not excellent choices for specific circumstances. This accounting (Table 84–1), however is based on the authors' pattern of usage (except where otherwise stated), and may well reflect practice, problems, and referral characteristics peculiar to our own practice and experience. We have mentioned many flaps, but whether they are commonly used is still a matter of the surgeon's preference, recipient site requirements, and (as concerns donor-site acceptability) aesthetic concepts in the community. Additionally, the competent and safe dissection and transfer of any flap is possible only through a thorough knowledge of the flap anatomy. In all cases, a surgeon should become thoroughly

Table 84–1
Cutaneous and Fasciocutaneous Flaps (Anatomical Order)

Workhorses
   Lateral upper arm; radial forearm; scapular
Lesser used
   Dorsalis pedis; groin; scalp
Rarely used
   Lateral thigh; medial thigh; posterior thigh; medial upper arm;
   deltoid; saphenus; sural; transverse cervical; posterior calf;
   deltopectoral; epigastric; venous flaps

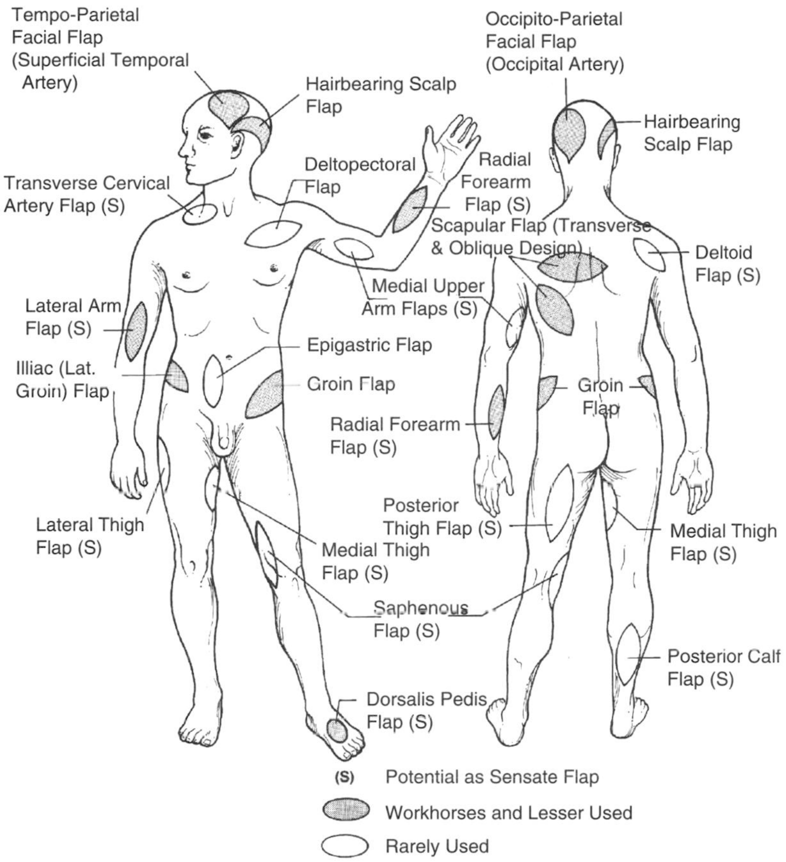

FIG. 84–1. Cutaneous free flap donor site territories.

(Labels on figure:)

Tempo-Parietal Facial Flap (Superficial Temporal Artery)

Occipito-Parietal Facial Flap (Occipital Artery)

Hairbearing Scalp Flap

Hairbearing Scalp Flap

Transverse Cervical Artery Flap (S)

Deltopectoral Flap

Radial Forearm Flap (S)

Scapular Flap (Transverse & Oblique Design)

Deltoid Flap (S)

Medial Upper Arm Flaps (S)

Lateral Arm Flap (S)

Epigastric Flap

Illiac (Lat. Groin) Flap

Groin Flap

Groin Flap

Radial Forearm Flap (S)

Lateral Thigh Flap (S)

Posterior Thigh Flap (S)

Medial Thigh Flap (S)

Medial Thigh Flap (S)

Saphenous Flap (S)

Posterior Calf Flap (S)

Dorsalis Pedis Flap (S)

(S) Potential as Sensate Flap

Workhorses and Lesser Used

Rarely Used

Table 84–2
Advantages and Disadvantages of the Lateral Arm Flap

Advantages
1. Constant vascular anatomy
2. Generally thin, hairless area of skin
3. Potential as sensate flap
4. Potential for use in composite reconstruction with vascularized bone

Disadvantages
1. Occasional small-diameter vessels
2. Donor site visibility on arm may be objectionable to some individuals
3. Donor site must be skin-grafted in larger flaps
4. Potential for radial nerve damage during dissection or donor reconstruction

---

familiar with the flap anatomy in the cadaver lab (or under guidance in the clinical situation) before attempting these dissections in "live" circumstances. The reader is referred to the original articles for further information, particularly for the flaps we classify as lesser used (Fig. 84–1).

Cutaneous Flaps

LATERAL ARM FLAP (Table 84–2)

The first comprehensive clinical study of the lateral upper arm flap was reported by Katsaros (55), although brief reports of the anatomy and the clinical use of the flap were available in 1982 (56). The lateral arm flap is based on the posterior radial collateral vessels. The anatomy of this vascular pedicle is constant, in contrast with the medial arm flap, which has a more variable vascular supply. The territory is of thin-to-medium bulk, is innervated by the lateral brachial cutaneous nerve of the arm, and is often hairless. In addition, vascularized bone (humerus) may be harvested with this flap for composite reconstruction (55).

The flap territory covers the posterolateral aspect of the upper arm between the deltoid insertion and the elbow.

Surgical Anatomy (Fig. 84–2)

Arterial Supply

The vascular pedicle is the posterior radial collateral artery, which is a direct continuation of the deep brachial artery. Extensive dissection and dye injections have clearly delineated a large area of perfusion by this vessel (35,55,57,58). The deep brachial artery arises from the proximal portion of the brachial artery. It accompanies the radial nerve as it winds around the spiral groove of the humerus deep to the triceps muscle. At the midhumeral point (measured from acromion to lateral epicondyle), the artery passes through the lateral intermuscular septum, where it gives off a small, variable anterior radial collateral branch that accompanies the radial nerve as it passes between the brachialis and brachioradialis muscles. The remaining branch, the larger, constant posterior radial collateral artery (PRCA) proceeds distally in the lateral intermuscular septum between the triceps posteriorly and the brachialis and brachioradialis anteriorly. The artery sends numerous branches superficially to the overlying fascia and skin. The ex-

The free neurovascular radial forearm flap in based on the radial artery and one or two of the comitant veins or one or two of the forearm veins (basilic or cephalic vein or one of the interconnecting branches). One or two of the cutaneous nerve branches of the forearm (ulnar, medial, or lateral cutaneous nerves of the forearm) supply sensation to this area and can be incorporated to provide a sensate flap.

Surgical Anatomy (Fig. 84–5)

Arterial Supply

The radial artery is one of the two terminal branches of the brachial artery. Although it is smaller than the ulnar artery, it appears to be the more direct continuation of the brachial

Table 84–3
Advantages and Disadvantages of the Radial Forearm Flap

Advantages
1. A constant anatomy with easy surgical access
2. Thin, pliable skin in relatively large size
3. Great versatility in flap design due to septocutaneous blood supply (Comack & Lamberty, type C)
4. A thin layer of subcutaneous fat that does not usually need secondary defatting procedure and has no tendency to later fat deposition
5. Relatively large nutrient vessels, allowing easy and safe microsurgical anastomosis
6. A long vascular pedicle, which diminishes the need for interpositional vein grafts
7. Adequate drainage with one venous anastomosis from either the superficial or deep venous system
8. Potential incorporation of sensory innervation
9. Possible primary closure in narrow flaps (<3 cm)

Disadvantages
1. If larger flaps are taken, split thickness skin grafts are needed; this may be an offending problem, especially in females
2. The sacrifice of a major vessel of the forearm for only a small piece of skin; this appears not to be a major problem if care is exercised in selecting patients
3. The flap is often hairbearing, which can be a problem in intraoral reconstruction

trunk. It begins at the division of the brachial artery about 1 cm distal to the bend of the elbow and passes along the radial side of the forearm to the wrist, where its pulsation can be readily felt in the interval between the flexor carpi radialis tendon medially and the adjacent lower part of the anterior border of the radius laterally. It then divides and the major dorsal branch winds backward around the lateral side of the carpus, beneath the tendons of the abductor pollicis longus and extensor pollicis brevis and longus muscles to the space between the 1st and 2nd metacarpal bones, where it passes between the two heads of the first dorsal interosseous muscle, finally terminating in the deep palmar arch. In the upper third of the forearm, the brachioradialis is lateral and the pronator teres is medial: in the lower two-thirds (except for the last several centimeters), the brachioradialis is covering the artery and the tendon of the flexor carpi radialis muscle is medial. Juergens and others (65) pointed out that the hand and fingers derive their blood supply mainly from the ulnar artery by means of the deep palmar arch, an important consideration that allows the safe dissection of the radial artery.

Based on observations of the arterial supply of the flap, Song (41) described the forearm flap as somewhat different from the classical axial pattern free flap. The radial artery supplies the flap through numerous branches that pass directly upward in the reflections of the deep fascia in the intermuscular spaces, between the brachioradialis and flexor carpi radialis muscles. Accordingly the intermuscular septum, containing the artery, concomitant veins and septocutaneous vessels must be included in the flap. Mühlbauer and co-workers (60) dissected 20 fresh forearms and described the diameter of the artery at the origin at 2.5 mm and at the wrist as 2 mm. The perfusion study shows that practically all the skin of the flexor aspect of the forearm and a considerable portion of the radiodorsal aspect is supplied by the radial artery.

With regard to this same territory, studies of the forearm angiotomies by Lamberty and Cormack (37) emphasized the importance of the inferior cubital vessel as the vascular supply of the proximal portion of the anterior forearm, which can be raised as a distinct flap, the antecubital flap (66). This vessel originates about 2 to 5 cm (average 4 cm) below the midin-

FIG. 84–5. Surgical anatomy of the radial forearm flap.

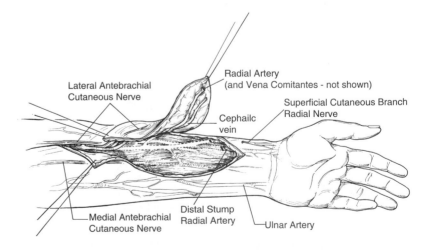

RADIAL FOREARM FLAP

terepicondylar point on the anterior surface of the forearm. This vessel ramifies up to 15 cm in the superficial fascia.

Venous Drainage

Although a major part of the venous drainage of this territory is via the venae comitantes of the radial artery, the flap can be planned to contain both the cephalic vein or the basilic vein, or both. The cephalic vein winds upward from the dorsal venous network, around the radial border of the forearm to its anterior surface, receiving tributaries from both surfaces. Distal to the anterior elbow, it gives off the median cubital vein, which receives communicating branches from the deep veins of the forearm and passes medially to join the basilic vein. The basilic vein originates in the ulnar part of the dorsal venous network of the hand. It ascends for some distance on the posterior surface of the ulnar side of the forearm, but then eventually inclines forward to the anterior surface distal to the elbow.

Neuroanatomy

Lateral Antebrachial Cutaneous Nerve. A terminal branch of the musculocutaneous nerve, this nerve passes deep to the cephalic vein and descends along the radial border of the forearm to the wrist. It supplies the skin over the lateral half of the anterior surface of the forearm and distributes branches that turn around the radial border of the forearm to communicate with the posterior cutaneous nerve of the forearm and terminal branch of the radial nerve.

Medial Antebrachial Cutaneous Nerve. Arising from the medial cord of the brachial plexus (C8-T1), this nerve passes on the medial side of the brachial artery, pierces the deep fascia along with the basilic vein at about the midpoint of the arm, and divides into anterior and posterior branches. The larger anterior branch passes usually anterior to, but occasionally deep to, the median cubital vein. It then descends on the anteromedial aspect of the forearm, distributing filaments to the skin as far distally as the wrist. The posterior branch passes obliquely downward on the medial side of the basilic vein, in front of the medial epicondyle of the humerus, and winds around the back of the forearm, descending on the medial side as far as the wrist. Mühlbauer and others (60) described a diameter of approximately 1.5 to 2.0 mm at the elbow joint for these nerves.

OPERATIVE TECHNIQUE OF FOREARM (RADIAL) FLAP (Figs. 84–6, 84–7)

Flap Design

Mühlbauer and others (60) obtained preoperative angiograms in all their cases. Song (61) based his decision about suitability of hand vascularity on the simple Allen test. The examiner occludes the radial and ulnar arteries at the patient's wrist. The patient then clenches the hand one or more times in order to squeeze the blood out of the hand. After a few seconds, the patient extends the fingers and the blanched color of the hand and fingers is noted. The radial and ulnar arteries are then sequentially released. If the respective arterial tree and arch are intact, a rapid return of color of the palm and fingers is noted. If there is a deficiency in the radial or ulnar artery supply, pallor is maintained for a long period of time after releasing this vessel (65).

The required shape and size of the flap are then mapped on the flexor or radiodorsal surface of the forearm. Soutar and

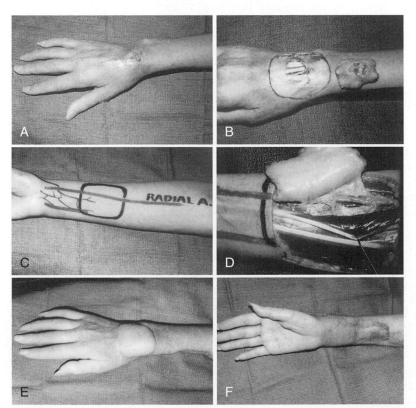

FIG. 84–6. A, B, 54-year-old female sustained a chemotherapy infusion injury to the dorsum of her right hand, shown pre and postexcision, with tendon exposure. **C,** design of a reverse-flow radial forearm flap on the distal forearm is based on the radial artery and superficial veins. **D,** dissected flap under tourniquet ischemia is demonstrated with the areolar vascular communication with the radial artery deep in the muscular cleft. **E, F,** postoperative result of the reconstructed dorsum of the wrist as well as the skin-grafted donor site.

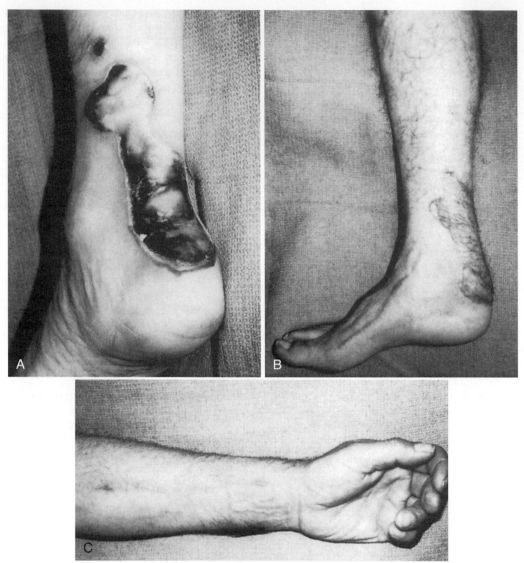

FIG. 84–7. **A,** this 54-year-old male suffered a muffler burn involving his right tendon Achilles. **B,** postoperative result after excision of the wound and radial forearm free flap reconstruction. Note the excellent hair growth and thin but healthy coverage of this territory. **C,** the donor site was closed primarily because a narrow elliptical flap was selected.

colleagues (62) designed the flap on any part of the volar forearm skin. Song (61) stated that the proximal border of the flap can be safely extended beyond the level of the elbow to as far as the lower one-fourth of the upper arm. He explained this large territory of perfusion by the presence of a free anastomosis of the cutaneous vessels between the arm and forearm. In doing this he, in fact, combined the radial forearm flap and the antecubital flap as later described by Lamberty and Cormack (66). It is also possible to design the flap distally based, whereby the skin island is located proximal on the forearm and the distal end of the radial artery and comitant veins are used for revascularization or are left intact in case of a distally based transposition flap (see Fig. 84–6).

Surgical Technique

A pneumatic tourniquet around the upper arm facilitates dissection. Each side of the fascia can be raised along with the fascia until the radial artery is identified. The sequence of eleva-

tion of the pedicle of the flap depends on its position; a distally based flap is best elevated from distal to proximal and a proximally based flap from proximal to distal. The radial artery and venae comitantes are isolated, ligated, and divided first at the site where the elevation starts, after which the flap is raised together with its pedicle. All perforators that leave the vessels on their deep surface have to be divided in this process.

The superficial cutaneous veins can also be used for venous outflow if they are included, and in a proximally based flap the medial and/or lateral antebrachial nerves can be included to create a sensate flap. The superficial branches of the radial nerve should be protected to preserve sensation to the radial aspect of the hand and fingers.

At this stage, the tourniquet is released and the viability of the flap is assessed. One may also test the remaining blood supply of the hand by clamping the radial artery at its origin and at the wrist before dividing it. The flap is transferred once the recipient vessels are prepared. The radial artery may be revascularized at one end or both ends (thus giving this flap the possibility of affording segmental vascular reconstruction if necessary).

Where bone is to be included, the perforators from the radial artery and veins to the flexor pollicis longus (FPL) must be preserved. On the medial side of the intermuscular septum, the radius is exposed by incision of the FPL. On the lateral side of the septum the radius is reached by following the septum until the periosteum is reached. Only the segment of bone between the insertion of the pronator teres and the brachioradialis can be elevated with the flap (61,62). To decrease the likelihood of a radial fracture, no more than one-third of the circumference of the radius should be taken. Furthermore, the bone segment should be cut without sharp angles, rather with gentle curvilinear incisions, thus avoiding "stress risers" in the bone.

Donor Site

After isolation of a narrow flap, the donor site can be closed directly or by advancement of an ulnar artery fasciocutaneous flap (67). A larger donor site must be covered with a skin graft. This can be a split-thickness skin graft taken from the inner thigh. Sometimes part of the donor site can be closed primarily and this usually results in skin redundancy proximal and/or distal to the defect. This skin must be excised and instead of discarding it, it can be employed as full-thickness graft to repair the remaining defect (68). This method is also advantageous because it will restore normal hair growth in the donor site, thereby making the donor site less conspicuous than when using a split-thickness skin graft. No impairment of function because of adhesions or contractures has been reported (60–62,64,65). Some authors have reported a lengthy hospital stay for their patients to assure intensive physiotherapy of the hand postoperatively.

Immediate Reconstruction of Radial Artery. In spite of the fact that the ulnar artery is the major artery of the hand, immediate reconstruction of the radial artery by vein grafts is advised by some, but it is usually not necessary (56,61,62,64).

Reconstruction of the Bone Defect. An upper arm cast should be applied for 4 to 6 weeks, followed by 3 months of protected, progressive load bearing. If there is any doubt about the stability of the remaining radius, the radius should be plated and immediately bonegrafted.

Table 84–4
Advantages and Disadvantages of Scapular Flap

Advantages
1. Provides a huge donor area with unsurpassed potential for a variety of dimensions and designs
2. Can provide multiple flaps on the same CSA pedicle
3. Can provide combinations of skin, bone, and fascia
4. Is a thin, hairless flap
5. Has a constant vascular anatomy with large vessels
6. Provides good intraoperative positioning for two-team procedure for upper extremity and lower extremity defects
7. Donor site is acceptable if closed primarily

Disadvantages
1. Has poor potential as sensate flap
2. Gives an obvious donor site when skin grafted, and when primarily closed the scar may widen

SCAPULAR FLAP (Table 84–4)

The scapular flap was first described by dos Santos (69), who investigated the territory of the skin of the back supplied by the circumflex scapular artery. Her report in the Brazilian literature was initially overlooked but, when discovered, led to many reports validating the clinical usefulness and versatility of this flap (70–74). It is a thin, usually hairless, skin flap from the posterior chest that is perfused by the cutaneous branches of the circumflex scapular artery (CSA). The vascular pattern of this territory makes it possible to raise multiple skin flaps on a single vascular pedicle or to harvest the lateral border of the scapula as an osteocutaneous flap for complex reconstruction. The reconstructive possibilities afforded by this anatomic arrangement are possibly unparalleled by any other donor site currently available (69–72,75).

Surgical Anatomy (Fig. 84–8)

Arterial Supply

The CSA is a large, constant vessel that is the main blood supply to the scapula, the muscles that attach to the scapula, and the overlying skin. The CSA is a main branch of the subscapular artery (SA), with a takeoff from the SA between 2 and 4 cm distal to the origin of the SA from the axillary artery. The CSA runs posteriorly deep to the teres major muscle, giving off muscular branches, and then emerges in the triangular space. This triangle is formed by the teres minor superiorly, the teres major inferiorly, and the long head of the triceps laterally. The CSA courses through the triangular space and within this space sends off muscular and bony branches that supply the lateral border of the scapula through a generous periosteal network of vessels, on both the superficial and the deep surfaces of the bone. These branches are

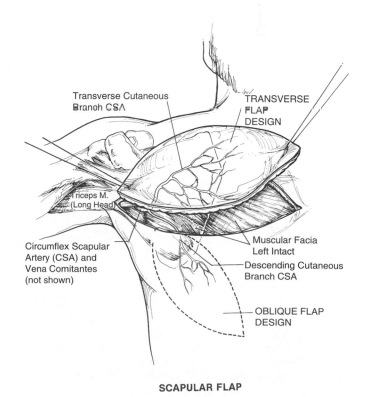

SCAPULAR FLAP

FIG. 84–8. Surgical anatomy of the scapular flap.

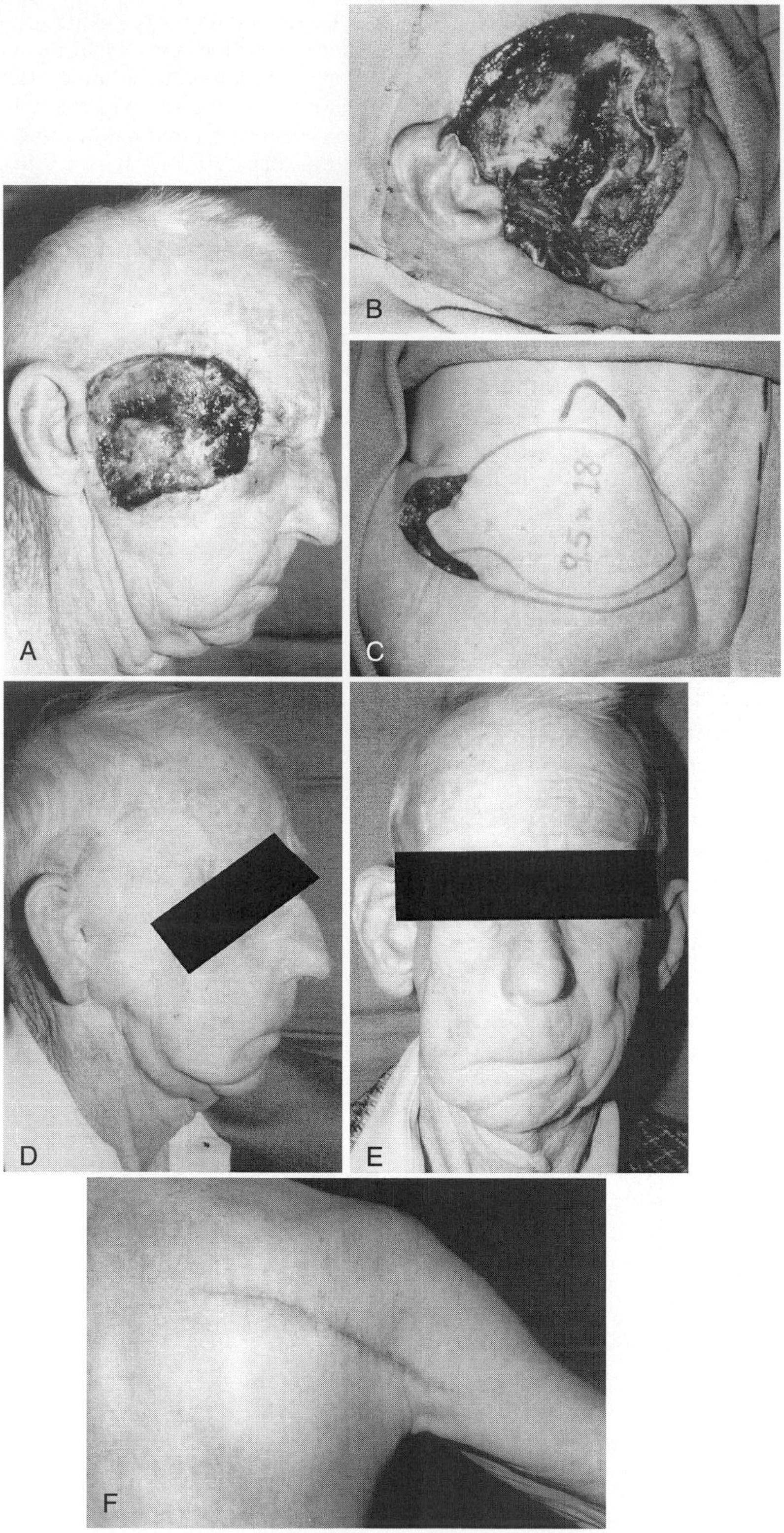

FIG. 84–9. **A,** an 88-year-old male presented with a large right preauricular defect subsequent to multiple previously attempted resections of an apparent squamous carcinoma of the skin. **B,** the extent of additional resection necessary to obtain clear surgical margins, including the lateral orbit, mandible, and resection to the periosterum of temporal bone. **C,** markings and initial stages of elevation of a right scapular free flap (patient's head to left). **D, E,** postoperative appearance is satisfactory with regard to bulk and color of the flap. **F,** postoperative appearance of the donor site, with no functional limitations.

generally about 4 cm from the origin of the CSA from the SA. This point constitutes the division of the CSA into "cutaneous" and "bony" branches. The main cutaneous branch then runs posteriorly around the lateral border of the scapula and divides into two or more major branches. Transverse branches of the CSA travel horizontally, overlying the scapula in a fibroareolar tissue layer, and descending branches travel in this same layer inferiorly toward the tip of the scapula. While these may be only a single vessel, or as many as four terminal cutaneous vessels of the CSA.

While previous authors have emphasized the individual anatomy of each of the cutaneous branches (29,75,76), we do not attempt to differentiate between them because they are all branches of the CSA, and with their extensive vascular interconnections in the fascial tissue layer they can be used singly or in combination to raise one or more individual flaps (all based on the CSA pedicle). The CSA external diameter varies from 1.5 to 4.0 mm, depending upon how proximally the surgeon dissects. Dissection proximally to the SA will result in vessel diameters averaging 4 mm.

Venous Drainage

The flap is drained by the venae comitantes of the CSA, which terminate in the subscapular vein. The external diameter of the venae comitantes ranges form 2.0 to 6.0 mm. The flap can, in all instances, be drained with one of the paired venae comitantes. No superficial veins drain this territory.

Neuroanatomy

The scapular territory is supplied at least in part by the lateral posterior cutaneous branches of the intercostal nerves. Unfortunately, clinical experience suggests little potential for this being used as a sensate flap because of the small size of these nerve branches and the difficulty in dissection. No reports exist of this flap being used as a sensate flap.

Operative Technique (Figs. 84–9, 84–10)

Flap Design

Careful examination of the donor site preoperatively with the patient's cooperation greatly facilitates absolute identification of the triangular space and the CSA. The triangle through which the CSA emerges can be identified by asking the patient to abduct and internally rotate the arm at a 90° position against resistance. With this maneuver, the teres major and triceps muscles contract and the muscle-bounded triangle is easily palpable.

By marking this point, the surgeon has identified the site of emergence of the vascular pedicle, which can then be further confirmed by Doppler ultrasound examination. Additionally, the general region of this space can be identified 2 to 3 cm superior to the posterior axillary fold (which is formed by the teres major muscle). Because the scapular area is so abundantly supplied by vessels in the subcutaneous fascial layer, the flap can be designed in almost any shape desired. The usual shape is an ellipse with a transverse or oblique orientation, one tip overlying the triangular shape.

Surgical Technique

While several methods of elevation are entirely appropriate, we advocate an initial lateral dissection to identify the CSA and partially dissect the pedicle vessels, which can then sim-

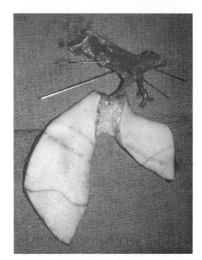

FIG. 84–10. A blood scapular flap has been harvested along with the vascularized lateral border of the scapula for mandibular reconstruction, in combination with internal oral lining and external facial resurfacing using the multiple skin territories available in the scapular region. The outstanding versatility afforded with the use of multiple flaps from this donor territory surpasses that of any other donor territory for this purpose.

plify the remainder of the dissection, as well as ensure the safety of the supplying vessel (by knowing exactly where it is at all times). With a thorough understanding of the flap anatomy, a medial-to-lateral dissection may be easier or faster for some surgeons.

The elevation of the scapular flap begins laterally with a V-shaped incision overlying the triangular space. The incision is deepened to identify the deep fascia. The dissection proceeds medially at this level beneath the deep fascia. No major vessels are cut in this dissection. As the lateral border of the scapula is reached, the inferior border of the teres minor (covered by glistening fascia) and the superior border of the teres major (beefy muscle with minimal fascial covering) are identified. By retracting these two muscles, a loose areolar fatty tissue plane surrounding the pedicle will be identified. By careful dissection in this space, about 7 to 10 cm of pedicle can be obtained up to the subscapular artery. Attention is then directed to raising the main portion of the flap. The muscular fascia covering the supraspinatus and infraspinatus muscles should not be included in the flap. The fascioareolar layer subjacent to the skin must be preserved because it contains the cutaneous branches of the CSA. The plane between these two fascial layers is well defined and easily dissected.

If the lateral border of the scapula is to be harvested as a vascularized bone graft, care should be taken to avoid injury of the nutrient vessels that arise from the CSA (77). The identification of this branch is mandatory in the triangular space; it may be necessary to remove part of the teres major to preserve the vascular supply of the bone.

COMBINING OF SCAPULAR FLAP WITH OTHER FLAPS (69,72,75,78)

Different combinations of the scapular flap with other flaps based on the SA blood supply are possible and may greatly facilitate certain complex reconstructions. These include the latissimus dorsi and serratus anterior flaps, which can supply additional skin, muscle, and bone (rib) if necessary. The technique of raising these combination flaps involves further proximal dissection of the CSA to the point where it forms a common trunk with the thoracodorsal vessels. The SA is used as the pedicle for all of the flaps harvested.

Donor Site

All elliptical flaps up to 13 cm wide can be closed primarily and generally give a reasonable cosmetic result, particularly in males. Larger flaps and multiple flaps must be closed with a combination of primary closure and skin grafting. Whenever possible, it is best to avoid skin grafting on the back because partial failure of graft take is not uncommon. The donor-site scar represents somewhat of a limitation on the use of the flap in women who wear swimsuits or low-backed dresses. Other alternatives for coverage should be explored for individuals to whom these considerations are important.

DORSALIS PEDIS (Table 84–5)

The dorsalis pedis flap was described in 1973 as a potential free flap by O'Brien and Shanmugan (26) and reported in clinical application by McCraw and Furlow in 1975 (79,80). The account of the internal anatomy of the flap reported by Man and Acland (81), along with many surgical reports of raising the flap as a free skin flap, increased the understanding and usage of this skin flap territory (82–86).

It is a thin, sensate, fasciocutaneous flap from the dorsum of the foot. It is based on the dorsalis pedis artery and its venae comitantes. It is possible to include the long and short saphenous veins in this flap. Preservation of the superficial peroneal or deep peroneal nerves in the flap can provide a sensation. The flap may be raised as a skin flap alone. In combination with the second metatarsal bone as an osteocutaneous flap (84), or in combination with 1st and 2nd toe transfers (87).

Surgical Anatomy (Fig. 84–11)

Arterial Supply

The anterior tibial-dorsalis pedis system is the arterial pedicle of the dorsalis pedis flap. At the junction of the middle

and lower third of the lower leg, the anterior tibial artery comes to lie between the tendons of the anterior tibial muscle and the extensor digitorum longus. It is related medially to the tibialis anterior muscle and its tendon and laterally to the extensor digitorum longus tendon. As the anterior tibial artery traverses the lower third of the leg, it comes to lie just lateral to the extensor hallucis longus tendon. As the vessel passes under the extensor retinaculum, it is usually between the tendon of the extensor hallucis longus muscle medially and the tendons of the extensor digitorum longus muscle laterally. It is lying on, and in intimate relation to, the tarsal bones.

The belly of the extensor hallucis brevis muscle covers the proximal part of the artery. More distally, the tendon of the muscle at first lies laterally and then turns medially. The dorsalis pedis artery leaves the dorsum of the foot by passing through the gap between the two heads of the first dorsal interosseous muscle and from that point travels deeply to join the plantar arch. It is in this region that the vascular anatomy is of particular importance. Before the vessel disappears into the sole of the foot, it gives off the first dorsal metatarsal artery (FDMA), a cutaneous branch that travels along the first intermetatarsal space superficial to the first dorsal interosseous muscle. It is this vessel that supplies the bulk of the distal half of the flap territory. At the level of the metatarsophalangeal joints, the vessel bifurcates and sends dorsal branches to the adjacent sides of the 1st and 2nd toes. Immediately proximal to the joint at which the FDMA arises the arcuate artery branches from the dorsalis pedis artery. The arcuate artery gives an identifiable branch that penetrates the proximal end of the first dorsal interosseous muscle (lateral head) and indirectly vascularizes the periosteum of the second metatarsal bone through muscular vessels (84).

The exact nature of the takeoff of the FDMA from the dorsalis pedis artery requires further discussion. This vessel does

Table 84–5
Advantages and Disadvantages of Dorsalis Pedis Flap

Advantages
1. A large terminal artery (2–4 mm) with both deep and superficial venous drainage
2. Incorporation of sensory innervation with a two-point discrimination that can reach 15 mm in its recipient site
3. A neurovascular pedicle of considerable length
4. Extremely thin (thinnest free flap available)
5. Acceptable size for many defects
6. Inconspicuous donor site, especially if skin graft healing occurs without complication; it is possible to achieve primary donor site healing routinely and no significant donor site morbidity

Disadvantages
1. Variable donor site anatomy
2. Sometimes tedious dissection
3. Restricted size
4. Significant donor site delay in healing if poor initial skin graft take occurs
5. Hair bearing

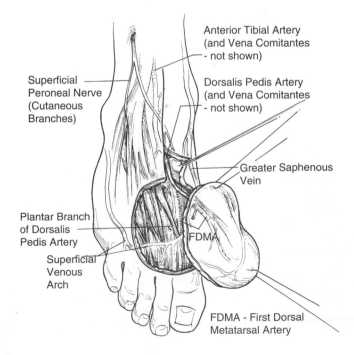

DORSALIS PEDIS FLAP
FIG. 84–11. Surgical anatomy of the dorsalis pedis flap.

not simply branch off the dorsalis pedis artery at right angles; rather, the dorsalis pedis artery usually dives deeply between the two heads of the first dorsal interosseus muscle and the FDMA arises distal to that point. It then travels in recurrent fashion back out of the gap between the two heads of the muscle, and the result is usually a Y-shaped pattern (Fig. 84–12). The surgical significance of this point is that extreme caution must be exercised in raising the flap to avoid (a) dividing the dorsalis pedis artery proximal to the takeoff point of the FDMA, or (b) transecting the FDMA distal to this area, leaving no continuity with the proximal dorsalis pedis pedicle. The FDMA travels fairly superficially after this point and presents few problems in its distal half. However, it may travel considerably deeper along the intermetatarsal space and, therefore, deserves continued caution throughout its entire dissection (81,85,87).

Anatomic variations are not uncommon. In 3 to 5% of cases, the anterior tibial artery is absent or small and the dorsalis pedis artery is supplied by a perforating branch of the peroneal artery (88). Anatomic injection and dissection studies corroborated this anatomic variability in 3 of 23 dissec-

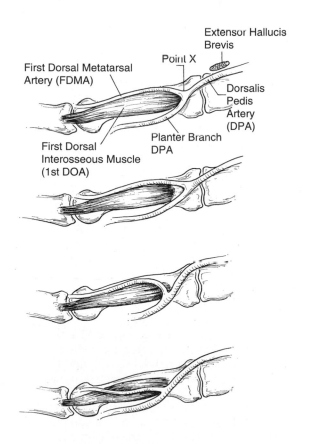

**VARIATIONS IN ORIGIN AND COURSE OF
THE FIRST DORSAL METATARSAL ARTERY**

FIG. 84–12. The variability in the relationship of the first dorsal metatarsal artery (FDMA) to the distal portion of the dorsalis pedis artery (DPA) at the proximal portion of the first web space. Four major variations have been shown, in addition to the situation in which the FDMA appears to arise completely from the plantar arch (not shown). As noted, the FDMA may arise superficially or deeply at an acute or obtuse angle, and travel superficially or deeply through the first dorsal interosseous muscle. Care must be taken, therefore, when dissecting around point X at the proximal portion of the first web space.

tions where the FDMA was absent, with the skin of the distal third area presumably supplied by the subdermal plexus only (81). Additionally, in 18% of cases the dorsalis pedis artery does not directly communicate with the FDMA, making transfer as a free flap impossible (87,89).

Venous Drainage

Two sets of veins of usable size drain the dorsalis pedis flap; these are the superficial dorsal veins of the foot and the venae comitantes of the dorsalis pedis and anterior tibial arteries.

Superficial Veins. The common dorsal digital veins of the toes and perforating veins from the sole of the foot combine to form an irregular arch over the distal part of the dorsum of the foot. The anatomy of this arch is unpredictable but, in many cases, it is drained proximally by lateral and medial veins that become the short and long saphenous veins, respectively. In addition, oblique veins on the dorsum of the foot may unite to form a median superficial vein, which normally joins the long saphenous vein several centimeters above the ankle. This is the most common pattern.

Venae Comitantes. At the level of the ankle joint, the venae comitantes (usually paired) are of a significant caliber, usually from 2 to 5 mm. These veins, although not the primary venous drainage of the skin of the foot, adequately drain this flap territory and are frequently used as pedicle vessels.

Neuroanatomy

The deep branch of the peroneal nerve accompanies the dorsalis pedis artery and supplies sensation to the skin of the first web space. The superficial peroneal nerve branch passes from lateral to medial, above the superficial fascia, and supplies cutaneous sensation to the remaining dorsum of the foot and dorsum of the great toe. The two-point discrimination of the skin of the flap is about 20 to 30 mm (25,85).

Internal Anatomy of the Flap

The original description of this flap included ten fresh amputation specimen dissections to study the fine vascular branches of the anterior tibial dorsalis pedis system. The conclusions from this study were (79):

1. The artery is attached to the flap by a network of fine branches that are essential to the survival of the flap.
2. The major branches are visible for a distance of 3 cm medial and lateral to the parent vessel.
3. The distal branches are most deficient laterally, and are deficient to a lesser extent distomedially. This is a random area of the flap.

A later, detailed study of the fine vascular anatomy included quantification of perforating vessels to the skin and resulted in a better understanding of the blood supply to the flap. In this study, 5.9 perforating vessels were identified in the proximal portion of the flap, 5.7 supplied the midportion, and 6.7 fed the distal one-third of the flap (90).

Operative Technique of the Dorsalis Pedis Flap

Flap Design

The dorsalis pedis flap may extend distally to include the web space of the toes. In its medial and lateral aspects, it includes the long and short saphenous veins, respectively. If small flaps are designed, they should be centralized over the arterial pedicle. A potential flap size of 12 cm by 9 cm has been described in the average adult (91).

The preoperative assessment is of paramount importance. The use of Doppler ultrasound to delineate the anatomy of the dorsalis pedis and FDMA arteries is a satisfactory and efficient technique in our hands. The anterior tibial and dorsalis pedis arteries are followed until the change in signal at the proximal end of the space between the first and second metatarsal bones. Demonstration of continuation of the signal across this point is crucial and indicates continuity of the FDMA (distally) with the dorsalis pedis artery (proximally). Inasmuch as retrograde flow through the plantar system may confuse the findings in the case of an absent or aberrant artery, occlusion of the posterior tibial artery by digital pressure will cause a diminished or absent signal over the FDMA if retrograde flow is present. If no change in signal results from occlusion of the posterior tibial artery, pressure is then applied over the anterior tibial artery. A diminished signal over the first web space with this maneuver confirms the continuity of the FDMA with the dorsalis pedis artery.

Surgical Technique

The use of a tourniquet facilitates dissection. The procedure is tedious, but can usually be done within one tourniquet time (i.e., usually in less than 2 hours). The dissection is started by making a distal incision in the first web space to identify the distal portion of the FDMA. The vessel should not be divided at this point. This indicates the depth of the dissection distally and the size of the vessel expected. The dissection continues by incising the skin down to subcutaneous tissue around the whole flap (Fig. 84–13) The incision is deepened to the level of the deep fascia medially and laterally, taking great care not to injure the paratenon over the extensor muscles.

Medially, the dissection stops at the lateral side of the extensor hallucis longus tendon. The deep fascia is incised to the level of (but not including) the periosteum on the lateral side of the first metatarsal bone and on the cuneiform bones.

On the lateral side of the flap, the paratenon of all extensor tendons is preserved during dissection and all superficial veins are included in the flap. The dorsal veins of the toes are divided as they are encountered. The dissection stops at the medial edge of the second metatarsal bone. The next step is to identify the extensor halucis brevis tendon, which underlies the long extensor of the second toe. This tendon is divided from its muscle bed and may be included in the flap.

Both arterial and venous pedicles are then developed. The extent to which this is necessary depends on the characteristics of the recipient bed. To avoid skin necrosis during isolation of the neurovascular pedicle, a linear incision is made over the course of the artery directly down to the extensor retinaculum but without raising skin flaps. A pedicle of 10 to 15 cm can be easily developed, although the anterior tibial artery above the ankle is rather deeply placed and freeing it of its malleolar and tarsal branches is a tedious procedure.

At this stage, the flap remains completely attached to its vascular pedicle with no division of either the dorsalis pedis artery or FDMA.

The communicating branch of the dorsalis pedis artery after the takeoff of the FDMA is now identified and occluded with a microvascular clamp. Another clamp is applied to the

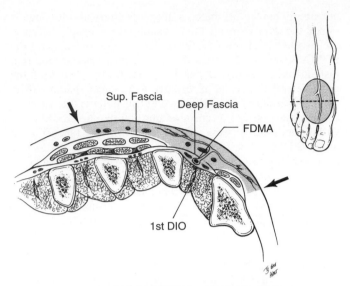

CROSS SECTIONAL ANATOMY OF THE DORSALIS PEDIS FLAP

FIG. 84–13. The plane of dissection of the dorsalis pedis flap, including all the subcutaneous superficial veins and branches of the cutaneous nerves, until one reaches the first web space, where a deeper dissection is carried out down to and frequently within the substance of the first dorsal interosseous (1st DIO) muscle to include the FDMA within the flap. Peritenon is carefully preserved over the extensor tendon to optimize skin graft healing.

distal end of the FDMA and the tourniquet is released. The vascularity of the flap is assessed with inflow only from the dorsalis pedis artery pedicle. If satisfactory bleeding is present, the dissection is completed by ligating the distal FDMA and the plantar communicating branch.

The flap is then freed completely, except for attachment by its arterial and venous pedicles. The flap is detached when the recipient vessels are ready for the anastomosis. Donorsite closure is performed after the anastomosis is complete and the flap is perfused satisfactorily (Fig. 84–14).

Special Notes on Donor-Site Morbidity

McCraw and Furlow (80) reported ten short-term complications in 48 cases of dorsalis pedis flaps. The most commonly expressed reservations concerning this flap refer to the position of the secondary defect, and the difficulty in obtaining primary healing of the skin-grafted donor site (83). It is often considered the exception rather than the rule to get primary healing. Other problems include ridge formation, hypertrophic scars, and lymphedema-like conditions.

A reevaluation of the technique for managing the donor defect of the dorsalis pedis has led to a complete change of donor management. This technique now includes (82):

1. Avoidance of intraoperative donor-site desiccation.
2. The use of sheet or nonexpanded mesh skin graft.
3. The use of minimally compressive bolus dressing (e.g., a Dacron polyester fiberfill bolus dressing only to ensure secure apposition of the skin graft to deeper portions of the defect, particularly the first web space).
4. Avoidance of use of compression bandages on the foot, in order to avoid ischemic necrosis of the skin graft; compression is only used during periods of ambulation to

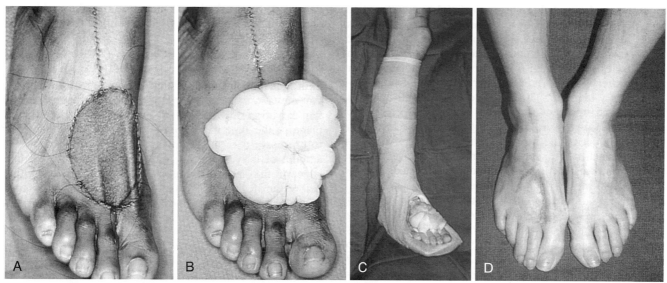

FIG. 84–14. Closure of donor site with split-thickness skin graft. **A,** immediate placement of skin graft following flap elevation prevents desiccation of delicate peritenon and enhances graft take. **B,** tie-over bolus dressing. **C,** graft is protected from motion of underlying tendons with posterior plantar splint. **D,** well-healed donor site following dorsalis pedis skin flap. (From Banis JC. Thin cutaneous flap for intraoral reconstruction: the dorsalis pedis free flap revisited. *Microsurgery* 1988; 9:132.)

Table 84–6
Advantages and Disadvantages of Groin Flap

Advantages
1. Inconspicuous donor site (probably the most inconspicuous free flap donor site currently available with the exception of temporoparietal fascial flap)
2. Large flap
3. Good for pale areas and areas requiring a fair amount of bulk

Disadvantages
1. Bulkiness of the flap, especially in obese patients
2. Small-diameter vessels
3. Short pedicle and anatomical variations of the pedicle vessels

avoid venous hypertension and hematoma collection beneath the graft.

5. Strict elevation of the foot in the early postoperative period. With attention to these basic principles, almost complete primary healing can be achieved with resultant absence of any significant doner site morbidity.

GROIN FLAP (Table 84–6)

The history of the groin free flap has been described already in the introduction. The groin area provides a large skin and subcutaneous tissue territory suitable for free-tissue transfer with minimal donor-site morbidity. This territory is perfused by the superficial circumflex iliac vessels. The donor-site scars are easily concealed by most swimming suits, making this flap more aesthetically acceptable. It does not include any sensory nerves.

Surgical Anatomy (Fig. 84–15)

Arterial Supply

The complexity of the vascular anatomy of the groin is one reason for the dissatisfaction many surgeons feel toward the

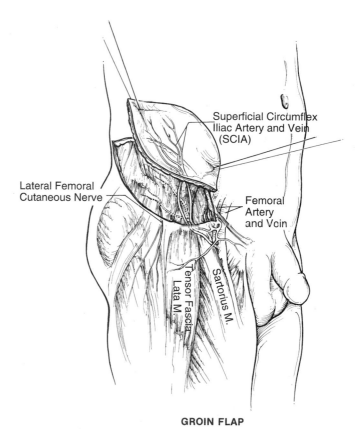

GROIN FLAP
FIG. 84–15. Surgical anatomy of the groin flap.

free groin flap. The vascular anatomy has been investigated extensively both in anatomic and clinical studies (14,23,25,86,92,93). Although the arterial anatomy was thought to be constant in early studies, further cadaver and clinical dissections have demonstrated the reverse to be the

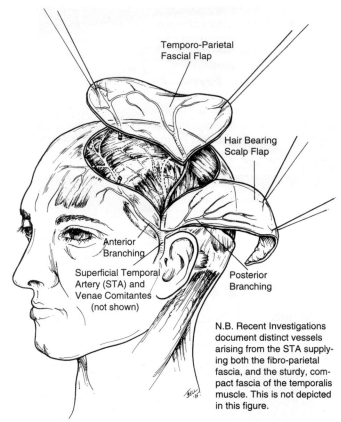

Temporo-Parietal
Fascial Flap

Hair Bearing
Scalp Flap

Anterior
Branching

Superficial Temporal
Artery (STA) and
Venae Comitantes
(not shown)

Posterior
Branching

N.B. Recent Investigations
document distinct vessels
arising from the STA supplying both the fibro-parietal
fascia, and the sturdy, compact fascia of the temporalis
muscle. This is not depicted
in this figure.

FIG. 84–17. Surgical anatomy of the scalp and temporoparietal fascial flap. (*Note:* Recent investigations document distinct vessels arising from the STA and supplying both the fibroparietal fascia and the sturdy, compact fascia of the temporalis muscle. This is not depicted here.)

passes anterior to the tragus. The vein empties into the internal jugular vein. Its diameter is 1.3 to 4.0 mm (82).

Operative Technique (Fig. 84–18)

Flap Design

The pulsation of the STA can be palpated in front of the tragus. A line running cranially drawn from this point extending upward about 5 cm above the zygomatic arch will approximate the course of the STA before division into anterior and posterior branches. A broad variety of flaps may be designed over the temporoparietal area of the scalp.

Flap Elevation

The flap is raised by making an incision along the course of the STA, taking care not to injure the pedicle in the process. The elevation of a hair-bearing skin flap requires elevation of the superficial layer of the temporal fascia with the flap. The plane of dissection will thus be between the superficial and deep temporal fasciae that invest the temporalis muscle. If a fascial flap alone is to be elevated, the plane of dissection is the same on the deep surface, but also must include a delicate dissection of the superficial plane just deep to the level of the hair follicles. Care should be taken to avoid injury to the temporal branch of the facial nerve.

Donor Site

Primary closure of the flap is the rule, especially when raising fascial flaps.

Lesser Used Flaps

DELTOPECTORAL FLAP (17,24,92)

The deltopectoral flap in head and neck surgery has been reported as both a pedicle and a free flap. The free flap is usually based on the second anterior thoracic perforator, which is usually larger than all other perforators. On rare occasions, the 3rd perforator may be larger than the second and can be used for microvascular anastomosis. The artery is about 0.8 to 1.2 mm in diameter and the accompanying vein is 1.2 to 2.5 mm.

The wide use of this flap is limited by the unacceptable scar of the anterior chest, the relatively short vascular pedicle, and the small vessel diameters.

MEDIAL ARM FLAP (56,73,101)

The territory of the inner aspect of the arm is supplied by numerous branches of the brachial artery. The medial arm flap is supplied by the superior ulnar collateral artery, which has proven to be variable and unpredictable. The vessel diameter is about 0.8 to 1.5 mm and the venous drainage is via the venae comitantes. The vessels can be dissected to a length of about 4 to 6 cm. The quality of the skin in this territory is excellent because it is a thin, hairless territory with good color and may be transferred as a sensate flap through the medial antebrachial cutaneous nerve. The flap is overshadowed currently by the constant and more reliable lateral arm flap.

DELTOID FLAP (74,102)

This potentially sensate territory overlies the deltoid muscle and is based on a cutaneous branch of the posterior circumflex humeral artery, which emerges from beneath the deltoid muscle. The vessel diameter is 1.5 to 3 mm and a pedicle length of 4 to 6 cm may be obtained. Sensation is supplied by a cutaneous branch of the axillary nerve. This flap provides thin, pliable, sensate skin that is well suited for the head and neck, foot, and ankle areas. The disadvantages include donor site appearance, flap bulk, and as yet undetermined quality of sensation.

SAPHENOUS FLAP (34,35)

This flap includes the skin on the medial side of the knee, with a perfused territory of at least 29 cm × 11 cm. The vascular supply is the descending genicular artery, a branch of the superficial femoral artery, and its venae comitantes, which can be dissected up to 10 cm above the knee. The flap can be sensate by including the branches of the medial femoral cutaneous nerve or the saphenous nerve. The inconsistency of the vascular pedicle along with the donor site morbidity limits its use as a free flap. As a pedicled flap, it can be used for resurfacing knee injuries.

MEDIAL THIGH FLAP (103)

This flap lies on the medial side of the thigh and is supplied by an unnamed branch of the superficial femoral artery. This cutaneous branch runs in the adductor canal and passes be-

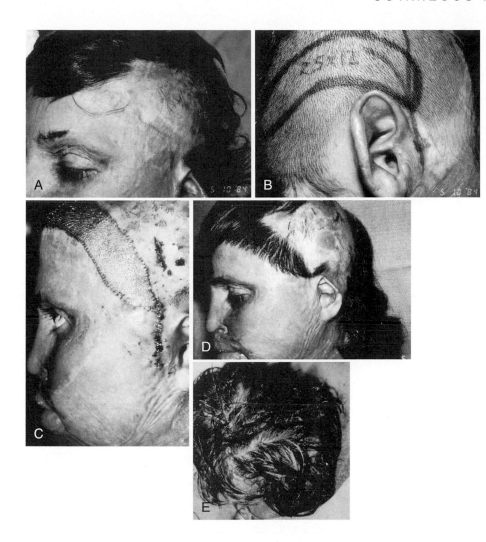

FIG. 84–18. **A,** young male presents with burn scar alopecia of the left scalp region. **B,** design of a right hair-bearing scalp flap based on the superficial temporal artery and vein. **C,** re-creation of the anterior hairline in the early postoperative period. **D,** excellent hair growth 1 month postoperatively. **E,** subsequent tissue expansion of the remaining healthy portion of scalp has resulted in complete scalp reconstruction. (Case courtesy of Dr. Bendy So.)

tween the sartorius and adductor brevis muscles. The artery is constant and varies between 2 and 4 mm in diameter, with a pedicle length averaging 5 cm. The flap may be sensate by including the medial femoral cutaneous nerve. It is important to identify the artery at the apex of the femoral triangle before raising the flap. Donor defects can usually be closed primarily but larger defects must be skin grafted.

LATERAL THIGH FLAP (103)

The lateral side of the thigh is supplied by a cutaneous branch of the 3rd perforating branch of the deep femoral artery and its accompanying vein. The vessel diameter is 3 to 5 mm. The nerve supply is via the lateral femoral cutaneous nerve, which is a branch of the lumbar plexus. In raising the flap, the vascular pedicle can reach 10 cm. The donor defect can be closed primarily or skin grafted depending upon the size of the defect.

GLUTEAL THIGH FLAP (104,105)

The gluteal region extends from the iliac crest to the gluteal crease and overlies the gluteal aponeurosis and gluteus maximus muscle. Subcutaneous fat increases in thickness in the gluteal fold but becomes progressively thinner as one proceeds down the posterior thigh. The entire thigh skin and fat posteriorly overlie the posterior fascia lata, which is a thin but distinct layer of fascia covering the hamstring muscles. The blood supply of this huge area of skin and subcutaneous tissue is the direct cutaneous branch of the inferior gluteal vessels that accompanies the posterior cutaneous nerve of the thigh to the popliteal fossa. This territory has potential as an island pedicle flap but, because of the small size of the cutaneous vessels, has not found wide usage as a free flap. The donor site can be closed primarily if the flap is less than 12 cm in width.

POSTERIOR CALF FLAP (106)

The cutaneous territory of the posterior calf has been investigated as a transpositional fasciocutaneous flap. A free flap can be designed in this territory with a dominant axial vessel that is a direct cutaneous branch of the popliteal artery. Sensation can be provided by including either the medial or posterior cutaneous nerve of the thigh, or the sural nerve. The flap is thin and sensate, and may also be used as a fascial flap.

TRANSVERSE CERVICAL FLAP (107)

The skin of the posterior cervical triangle is nourished by at least one superficial branch of the transverse cervical artery (TCA). Venous drainage is by venae comitants or the external jugular vein. The supraclavicular nerves provide sensation to the flap. The flap is outlined as a transverse ellipse (8 × 15 cm) over the supraclavicular area. The external diameter of the TCA is 1.5 to 2 mm. The donor site can always close directly.

MONITORING FREE CUTANEOUS FLAPS (108)

The critical nature of the problems being treated with free skin flaps, as well as the time necessarily invested in them, dictate that all reasonable measures be used to identify quickly vascular compromise to the transferred tissue. The viability of the flap may be monitored postoperatively by a variety of techniques, each of which currently falls short of fulfilling all the desirable attributes of a monitoring device. Clinical tests of blanch-refill, bleeding, and color require the presence of the operating surgeon, are imprecise and non-quantitative, and are impossible to perform with inaccessible flap locations. The technique for flap monitoring should fulfill these requirements:

1. The method should be reliable, free from mechanical failure, and respond promptly to both arterial or venous obstruction.
2. It should provide a continuous report of the changes in the flap with no limitations.
3. It should be harmless, instantaneous, and easily interpreted even by inexperienced personnel.

Available mechanical-physiological monitoring methods include temperature, photoplethysmography, percutaneous oxygen tension, Doppler ultrasound, laser Doppler (109), radioisotope clearance, and fluorescein injection techniques. The advantages of the noninvasive techniques are obvious because the checks must be made on a repetitive basis. In the current state of the art, no one technique has become the standard and many modalities are in variable stages of clinical trials. The reader is referred to the literature for further elaboration of this complex area.

Acknowledgment

The authors would like to recognize the invaluable assistance of Robin Miller and Lynn Jaggers in the preparation of this chapter.

References

1. Tagliacozzi G. Quoted in: Gnudi MT, Webster JP, eds. *The life and times of Gaspar Tagliacozzi.* New York: Herbert Reichner, 1950.
2. McDowell F. *The source book of plastic surgery.* Baltimore: Williams & Wilkins, 1977; 67.
3. Carpue JC. *An account of two successful operations for restoring a lost nose.* London: Longman, Hurst, Rees, Orme, 1816.
4. von Graefe CF. *Rhinoplastik oder die kunst den verhurst der nase organisch zu erssetzen.* Berlin: Reimer, 1818.
5. Goldwyn RM, Dieffenbach JR. In: McDowell EF, ed. *The source book of plastic surgery.* Baltimore: Williams & Wilkins, 1977; 433.
6. Blair VP. *Surgery and diseases of the mouth and the jaws.* St. Louis: CV Mosby; 1912.
7. DesPrez JD, Kiehn CL. Methods of reconstruction following resection of anterior oral cavity and mandible for malignancy. *Plast Reconstr Surg* 1959; 24:238.
8. Gillies HD. *Plastic surgery of the face.* London: Oxford University Press, 1920.
9. Gillies HD, Millard DR. *Principles and art of plastic surgery.* Boston: Little, Brown, 1957.
10. Owens N. A compound neck pedicle designed for the repair of massive facial defects: formation, development, and applications. *Plast Reconstr Surg* 1955; 15:369.
11. Wookey M. The surgical treatment of carcinoma of the pharynx and upper esophagus. *Surg Gynecol Obstet* 1942; 75:499.
12. Zovickian A. Pharyngeal fistulas: repair and prevention using mastoid-occiput shoulder flaps. *Plast Reconstr Surg* 1957; 19:355.
13. Esser JFS. *Studies in plastic surgery of the face.* Leipzig: FCW Vogel, 1917.
14. McGregor IA. The temporal flap in intraoral cancer: its use in repairing the post-excisional defect. *Br J Plast Surg* 1963; 16:318.
15. Shaw DT, Payne RL. One-stage tubed abdominal flaps. *Surg Gynecol Obstet* 1946; 83:205.
16. McGregor IA. Flap reconstruction in hand surgery: the evolution of presently used methods. *J Hand Surg* 1979; 4:1.
17. Bakamjian VY. A two-stage method for pharyngoesophageal reconstruction with a primary pectoral skin flap. *Plast Reconstr Surg* 1965; 36:173.
18. Muir IFK, Fox RH, Stranc WE, et al. The measurement of blood flow by a photoelectric technique and its applications to the management of tubed skin pedicles. *Br J Plast Surg* 1968; 21:14.
19. Milton SH. Pedicled skin flaps. The fallacy of the length:width ratio. *Br J Plast Surg* 1970; 57:502.
20. McGregor IA, Jackson IT. The groin flap. *Br J Plast Surg* 1972; 25:3.
21. McGregor IA, Morgan G. Axial and random pattern flaps. *Br J Plast Surg* 1973; 26:202.
22. Kaplan E, Buncke H, Murray D. Distant transfer of cutaneous island flaps in humans by microvascular anastomoses. *Plast Reconstr Surg* 1973; 52:301.
23. Daniel RK, Terzis J, Schwarz G. Neurovascular free flaps. *Plast Reconstr Surg* 1975; 56:13.
24. Harii J. *Microvascular tissue transfer: fundamental techniques and clinical applications.* Tokyo: Igaku Shoin, 1983.
25. Harrii K, Ohmori K, Torii S, et al. Free groin skin flaps. *Br J Plast Surg* 1975; 28:225.
26. O'Brien B, Shanmugan M. Experimental transfer of composite free flaps with microvascular anastomoses. *Aust NZ J Surg* 1973; 43:285.
27. Acland RD. The Free iliac flap. A lateral modification of the free groin flap. *Plast Reconstr Surg* 1979; 64:30.
28. Taylor GI, Townsend P, Corlett RE. Superiority of the deep circumflex iliac vessels as the supply for free groin flaps. Clinical work. *Plast Reconstr Surg* 1979; 64:745.
29. Ger R. Surgical management of ulcerative lesions of the legs. *Curr Probl Surg* 1972; 3:25.
30. Orticochea M. Musculocutaneous flap method: immediate and heroic substitute for the method of delay. *Br J Plast Surg* 1972; 25:106.
31. McCraw JB, Dibbell Dg. Experimental definition of independent myocutaneous vascular territories. *Plast Reconstr Surg* 1977; 60:212.
32. McCraw JB, Dibbell DG, Carraway JH. Clinical definition of independent myocutaneous vascular territories. *Plast Reconstr Surg* 1977; 60:341.
33. Pontén B. The fascioucutaneous flap: its use in soft tissue defects of the lower leg. *Br J Plast Surg* 1981; 34:215.
34. Manchot C. *Die hautarterien des menschlichen korpers.* Leipzig: FCW Vogtel, 1889.
35. Cormack GC, Lamberty BG. A classification of fascio-cutaneous flaps according to their patterns of vascularization. *Br J Plast Surg* 1984; 37:80.
36. Nakajima H, Fujino T, Adachi S. A new concept of vascular supply of the skin and classification of skin flaps according to their vascularization. *Ann Plast Surg* 1986; 16:1.
37. Lamberty B, Cormack G. The forearm angiotomes. *Br J Plast Surg* 1982; 35:420.
38. Banis JC Jr, Acland RD. Clinical applications of the scapular skin and osteocutaneous flap. In: Williams HB, ed. *Transactions of the VIII International Congress on Plastic Surgery.* Montreal: IPRS, 1983; 125.
39. Urken ML. The restoration or preservation of sensation in the oral cavity following ablative surgery. *Arch Otolaryngol Head Neck Surg* 1995; 121:607.
40. Nakayama Y, Soeda S, Kasai Y. Flaps nourished by arterial inflow through the venous system; an experimental investigation. *Plast Reconstr Surg* 1981; 67:328.
41. Honda T, Nomura S, Yamauchi S. The possible applications of a composite skin and subcutaneous vein graft in the replantation of digits. *Br J Plast Surg* 1984; 37:607.
42. Yoshimura M, Shimada T, Imura S, et al. The venous skin graft method for repairing skin defects of the fingers. *Plast Reconstr Surg* 1987; 79:243.

43. Thatte MR, Thatte RL. Venous flaps. *Plast Reconstr Surg* 1993; 91:747.
44. Fukui A, Inada Y, Maeda M, et al. Venous flaps—its classification and clinical application. *Microsurgery* 1994; 15:571.
45. Baek SM, Weinberg H, Song Y, et al. Experimental studies on the survival of venous island flaps without arterial inflow. *Plast Reconstr Surg* 1987; 75:88.
46. Thatte RL, Thatte MR. Cephalic venous flaps. *Br J Plast Surg* 1987; 40:16.
47. Thatte RL, Thatte MR. The saphenous venous flap. *Br J Plast Surg* 1989; 42:399.
48. Yoshimura M. A venous skin graft in the treatment of injured fingers. *Jpn J Plast Reconstr Surg* 1984; 27:474.
49. Inoue G, Nakamura R, Maeda N, et al. Arterialised venous flap coverage of a big toe defect resulting from a wrap around flap transfer. *Jpn J Plast Reconstr Surg* 1989; 32:1013.
50. Nakashima S. Experiences with the venous skin grafts. *Jpn J Plast Reconstr Surg* 1989; 32:11.
51. Koshima I, Soeda S, Nakayama Y, et al. An arterialized venous flap using the long saphenous vein. *Br J Plast Surg* 1991; 44:23.
52. Galumbeck MA, Freeman BG. Arterialized venous flaps for the reconstruction soft-tissue defects of the hand. *Plast Reconstr Microsurg* 1994; 94:997.
53. Karacalar A, Ozcan M. Free arterialized venous flaps for the reconstruction soft tissue defects of the hand. *J Reconstr Microsurg* 1994; 10:243.
54. Chen HC, Tang YB, Noordhoff MS. Four types of venous flaps for wound coverage: a clinical appraisal. *J Trauma* 1991; 31:1286.
55. Katsaros J, Schusterman M, Beppu M, et al. The lateral upper arm flap: anatomy and clinical applications. *Ann Plast Surg* 1982; 12:482.
56. Song R. The upper arm free flap. *Clin Plast Surg* 1982; 9:27.
57. Dolman S, Guimerteau JC, Baudet J. The upper arm flap. *J Microsurg* 1979; 1:162.
58. Matloub HS, et al. The lateral arm flap. A neurosensory flap. In: Williams HB, ed. *Transactions of the VIII International Congress of Plastic Surgery.* Montreal: IPRS, 1983; 125.
59. Moffet TR, Madison SA, Derr JW, et al. The extended lateral arm free flap. *Plast Reconstr Surg* 1992; 89:259.
60. Mühlbauer W, Herndl E, Stock W. The forearm flap. *Plast Reconstr Surg* 1982; 70:336.
61. Song R. The forearm flap. *Clin Plast Surg* 1982; 9:21.
62. Soutar D, Scheker L, Tanner N, et al. The radial forearm flap: a versatile method for intraoral reconstruction. *Br J Plast Surg* 1983; 36:1.
63. Soutar D, Tanner NS. The radial forearm flap in the management of soft tissue injuries of the hand. *Br J Plast Surg* 1984; 37:19.
64. Yan Guo Fan, et al. Forearm free skin flap transplantation (in Chinese). *Natl Med J China* 61:139. (Abstracted in *Plast Reconstr Surg* 1982; 69;779.)
65. Juergens JL, Spittell JA, Fairbairn JF. *Peripheral vascular diseases.* Philadelphia: WB Saunders, 1980; 21.
66. Lamberty BGH, Cormack GC. The antecubital fasciocutaneous flap. *Br J Plast Surg* 1983; 36:4.
67. Elliot D, Bardsky F, Batchelor AG, et al. Direct closure of the radial forearm flap donor defect. *Br J Plast Surg* 1988; 41:358.
68. Swartz WM, Banis JC Jr. *Head and neck microsurgery, Ch. 5, Fasciocutaneous and osteocutaneous flaps.* Baltimore: Williams & Wilkins, 1992.
69. dos Santos LF. The vascular anatomy and dissection of the free scapular flap. *Plast Reconstr Surg* 1984; 73:599.
70. Barwick W, Goodkind D, Serafin D. The free scapular flap. *Plast Reconstr Surg* 1982; 69:779.
71. Gilbert A, Teot L. The free scapular flap. *Plast Reconstr Surg* 1982; 69:601.
72. Mayou B, Whitby D, Jones B. The scapular flap. An anatomical and clinical study. *Br J Plast Surg* 1982; 35:8.
73. Kaplan EN, Pearl RM. An arterial medial arm flap. *Ann Plast Surg* 1980; 4:205.
74. Franklin JD, Rees RS, Madden JJ Jr, et al. The posterior circumflex humeral neurovascular free flap. *Plast Surg Forum* 1980; 3:172.
75. Urbaniak JR, Koman LA, Goodner RD, et al. The vascularized cutaneous scapular flap. *Plast Reconstr Surg* 1982; 69:772.
76. Nassif T, Vidal L, Bover J, et al. The parascapular flap: a new cutaneous microsurgical free flap. *Plast Reconstr Surg* 1982; 69:591.
77. Teot L, Bosse JP, Moufarrege J, et al. The scapular crest pedicled bone graft. *Int J Microsurg* 1981; 3:257.
78. Batchelor A, Sully L. A multiple territory free tissue transfer for reconstruction of a large scalp defect. *Br J Reconstr Surg* 1984; 37:76.
79. McCraw JB, Furlow LT Jr. The dorsalis pedis arterialized flap. A clinical study. *Plast Reconstr Surg* 1975; 55:177.
80. McCraw J, Furlow LT Jr. The dorsalis pedis arterial flap. In: Grabb WC, Myers MB, eds. *Skin flaps.* Boston: Little, Brown, 1975; 520.
81. Man D, Acland R. The microarterial anatomy of the dorsalis pedis flap and its clinical applications. *Plast Reconstr Surg* 1980; 65:419.
82. Banis JC Jr, Acland RD, Flynn MB. An evaluation of the dorsalis pedis free flap in immediate reconstruction of anterior oral defects. Proceedings of 50th Annual Convention of the American Society of Plastic and Reconstructive Surgery. *Plast Surg Forum* 1981; IV:83.
83. Franklin J, Withers E, Madden J, et al. Use of the free dorsalis pedis flap in head and neck repairs. *Plast Reconstr Surg* 1980; 63:195.
84. Robinson D. Microsurgical transfer of the dorsalis pedis neurovascular island flap. *Br J Plast Surg* 1976; 29:209.
85. Strauch B, Shafiroff B. The foot, a versatile source of donor tissue. In: Serafin D, Buncke H Jr, eds. *Microsurgical composite tissue transplantation.* St. Louis: CV Mosby, 1979; 345.
86. Taylor GI, Daniel RK. The anatomy of several free flap donor sites. *Plast Reconstr Surg* 1975; 56:243.
87. May J, Chait L, Cohen B, et al. Free neurovascular flap from the first web of the foot in hand reconstruction. *J Hand Surg* 1977; 2:387.
88. Warwick R, Williams PL. *Gray's anatomy.* Philadelphia: WB Saunders, 1973; 1041.
89. Leung P, Wong W. The vessels of the first metatarsal web space. *J Bone Joint Surg [Am]* 1983; 65:235.
90. Hayhurst JW, O'Brien BMcM. Experimental study of microvascular technique, patency rates and related factors. *Br J Plast Surg* 1975; 28:128.
91. Manktelow RT. *Microvascular reconstruction.* Berlin: Springer-Verlag, 1973.
92. Harii K, Ohmori K, Ohmori S. Free deltopectoral skin flaps. *Br J Plast Surg* 1974; 27:231.
93. Ohmori K, Harii K. Free groin flaps; their vascular basis. *Br J Plast Surg* 1975; 28:238.
94. Penteado CV. Venous drainage of the groin flap. *Plast Reconstr Surg* 1983; 71:678.
95. Harashima T, Nakahima T, Yoshimara Y. A free groin flap reconstruction in progressive facial hemiatrophy. *Br J Plast Surg* 1977; 30:14.
96. Buncke HJ, Hoffman WM, Alpert B, et al. Microvascular scalp island transplant between identical twins. *Plast Reconstr Surg* 1982; 60:605.
97. Walton RL, Bunkis J. A free occipital hair-bearing flap for reconstruction of the upper lip. *Br J Plast Surg* 1983; 36:168.
98. Harii K, Ohmori K, Ohmori S. Hair transplantation with free scalp flaps. *Plast Reconstr Surg* 1974; 53:410.
99. Brent B, Byrd HS. Secondary ear reconstructions with cartilage grafts covered by axial, random, and free flaps of temporoparietal fascia. *Plast Reconstr Surg* 1983; 72–141.
100. Abul-Hassin HS, Ulfe E, Acland RD. The superficial and deep temporal fascia: anatomical approach. *Plast Surg Forum* 1984; VII.
101. Newsome HT. Medial arm free flap. *Plast Reconstr Surg* 1981; 67:63.
102. Franklin JD. The deltoid flap: anatomy and clinical applications. In: Buncke H, Furnas D, eds. *Symposium on Clinical Frontiers in Reconstructive Microsurgery,* St. Louis, CV Mosby Co., 1984.
103. Baek S-M. Two new cutaneous free flaps: the media and lateral thigh flaps. *Plast Reconstr Surg* 1983; 71:354.
104. Hurwitz DJ, Swartz WM, Mathes SJ. The gluteal thigh flap: a reliable sensate flap for the closure of buttock and perineal wounds. *Plast Reconstr Surg* 1981; 68:521.
105. Jurkiewicz MJ. Discussion of paper on "the gluteal thigh flap." *Plast Reconstr Surg* 1981; 68:531.
106. Matory W, Walton R, Petry J. Posterior calf fasciocutaneous flap reconstruction of upper and lower extremity defects. *Plastic Surgical Forum VIII,* 1984.
107. Morris R, Fillman D, McCabe J, et al. The transverse cervical neurovascular free flap. *Ann Plast Surg* 1983; 10:90.
108. Jones B. Monitors for the cutaneous microcirculation. *Plast Reconstr Surg* 1984; 73:843.
109. Nilsson G, Tenland T, Oberg P. Evaluation of a laser Doppler flowmeter for measurement of tissue blood flow. *Trans Biomed Eng* 1980; 27:59.

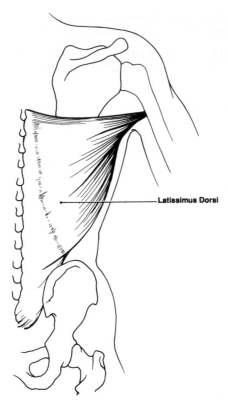

FIG. 85–2. Latissimus dorsi muscle.

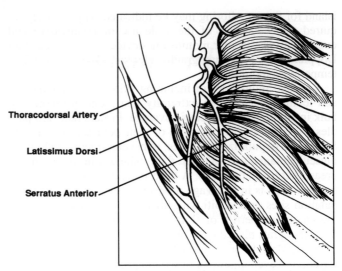

FIG. 85–3. Vascular pedicle to serratus anterior and latissimus dorsi muscle.

• Sensory nerve: The skin overlying the latissimus is supplied by multiple cutaneous branches of the intercostal nerves. Generally, this is not used as a sensate flap.

The Flap

All skin overlying the muscle may be transferred. Random anterior skin over the serratus anterior muscle can be utilized for 3 to 4 cm if skin over the anterior border of the latissimus dorsi is used. Primary closure can be accomplished to a maximum skin island width of about 9 cm. This width will vary with the patient's size and the amount of subcutaneous tissue. When used as a musculocutaneous unit, this flap may be quite thick and therefore unsuitable for certain areas. The latissimus dorsi is the largest transfer available, with a muscle surface area of 25×35 cm^2. The muscle is a workhorse for several areas of reconstruction. It can be used to cover the entire anterior leg, or the entire scalp in incidence of burns, and may be split or combined with the serratus anterior muscle for even greater area.

Functional Loss

The functional loss to the limb girdle with removal of the latissimus dorsi is minimal.

Flap Harvest

It is important to identify the anterior border of the muscle preoperatively by having the patient contract the muscle with the hand supported on the hip in a standing position. Dissection is most easily accomplished beginning from the anterior border. Skin paddles are designed along the long axis of the muscle. If a random position is included over the serratus an-

terior, at least one-half of the total skin island must overlie the latissimus dorsi. Marking of the posterior superior iliac spine and scapular tip is helpful. It is also wise to measure 10 cm from the apex of the axilla and place a mark at the site of the pedicle entrance into the muscle. This allows dissection to proceed rapidly and without fear of pedicle damage until this area is reached.

After preoperative marking, the patient is placed in the lateral decubitus position with an axillary roll. The prepped area should include the arm, posterior trunk to the midline, upper buttock, and lower neck. The prep should also extend forward to the nipple and include the axilla, which should be shaved preoperatively.

If elevation is begun at the anterior border of the muscle, early pedicle identification is possible. If a split latissimus is to be used, the anterior branch of the thoracodorsal artery and its associated motor nerve can quickly be identified at the previously marked point. If only the anterior latissimus muscle or skin-muscle flap is used, it is important to note that a pedicle length of just 7 cm is obtained. Further proximal dissection will denervate and devascularize the remaining posterior muscle, making functional preservation impossible.

If the entire muscle is used, elevation of the skin flaps exposes the muscle origins, which are then released from the lumbosacral fascia and iliac crest. The large secondary perforating pedicles must be carefully identified and ligated to avoid troublesome bleeding. After pedicle identification, division of the serratus branch is completed and the entire flap is reflected toward the axilla. Before releasing the muscle peripherally, marking sutures should be placed along the long axis of the muscle every 5 cm if functional transfer is planned, in order to allow adequate tension adjustment in the recipient site.

Once the flap is reflected toward the axilla and the arm is abducted, the pedicle may easily be seen entering the muscle. Proximal dissection is performed for the previously determined pedicle length and the muscle insertion is divided. The flap is now ready for transfer. Large suction drains should be left beneath the skin flaps and in the axilla to avoid postoperative hematoma or seroma problems.

Special Problems

- Because of patient positioning, this flap frequently cannot be elevated simultaneously with donor-site preparation, particularly if the flap is to be transferred to the upper extremity.
- In obese patients, the musculocutaneous flap may be excessively thick.
- The flap may be too thick for functional transfer to the face, and may be too powerful for functional transfer to the upper extremity (flexors or extensors).
- Despite careful tissue handling, the most distal aspect of the flap may undergo necrosis. This is possibly because of the watershed area between dominant lumbar perforators and thoracodorsal artery axial vessels. Therefore, care should be exercised when the entire latissimus is used.

GRACILIS, TYPE II (DOMINANT PEDICLE AND SEVERAL MINOR PEDICLES (25–27) (FIGS. 85–4 TO 85–6)

Muscle Anatomy

- Origin: the pubic symphysis
- Insertion: medial tibial condyle
- Function: thigh adductor

Vascular Supply

The major pedicle is a terminal branch of the medial femoral circumflex artery, which arises from the profunda femoris artery. One or two minor pedicles enter the distal muscle and arise from the superficial femoral artery.

The dominant pedicle enters the muscle 10 cm below its origin from the pubic tubercle. After leaving the profunda femoris, the vessel lies beneath the adductor longus muscle and above the adductor magnus muscle, giving branches to these before entering the deep medial surface of the gracilis. The artery is approximately 2 mm in diameter and is usually accompanied by one or two veins also measuring 2 mm. The pedicle length is 6 cm.

Innervation

- Motor nerve: The gracilis is innervated by the anterior branch of the obturator nerve. Although the obturator nerve has a variable entrance into the muscle, it is always found above the level of the dominant vascular pedicle. A length of 6 cm may be obtained if proximal dissection is performed between the adductor muscles.
- Sensory nerve: There is no sensory innervation of the gracilis muscle.

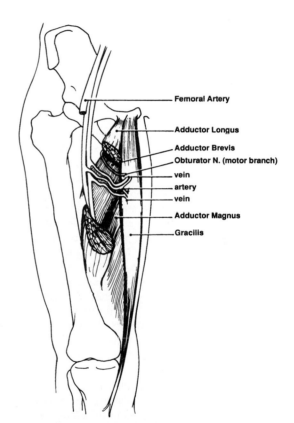

FIG. 85–5. In situ anatomy of dissection of gracilis muscle.

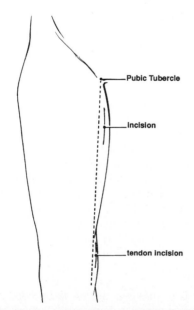

FIG. 85–4. Gracilis flap skin incision. A point is drawn between the pubic tubercle and the adductor tubercle. The incision is made 2 cm posterior to this line and 6 cm cephalad to the tubercle to find the gracilis tendon.

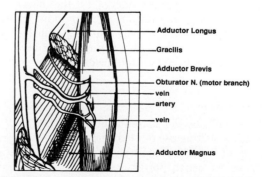

FIG. 85–6. Neurovascular pedicle to gracilis muscle.

The Flap

Usable muscle suitable for transfer may be obtained over an area measuring 6 × 15 cm. If the tendon is included for functional transfer, the long axis can be extended to almost 30 cm.

Although the skin overlying the gracilis muscle is supplied by its musculocutaneous perforators, the distal skin is unreliable when the minor pedicles have been divided. This allows a maximum skin island of 6 × 15 cm (which should be based proximately). For maximum skin use, accurate preoperative marking is especially important in this flap. In obese patients accurate skin design is difficult, and an excessively thick flap may result.

Functional Loss

There is no functional loss with removal of the gracilis. In slender patients there may be a slight contour deformity of the thigh.

Flap Harvest

One of the true advantages of this flap is that simultaneous donor and recipient dissections are frequently possible. Preoperative localization is the key to success in elevation of this muscle. The tendon of the gracilis can be identified by drawing a line from the pubic tubercle to the adductor tubercle. A point 6 cm cephalad to the adductor tubercle and 2 cm posterior to this line will mark the course of the gracilis tendon. The gracilis is sometimes confused with the adductor tendon; the gracilis tendon is usually a round, small tendon just anterior to the semimembranosus.

A small distal incision is then made above the knee and the saphenous vein and muscle belly of the sartorius are seen. These structures are retracted anteriorly, exposing the tendon of the gracilis. To confirm this, look for the tendon of the semimembranosus muscle just posterior to the gracilis. Once the position of the gracilis is assured, traction on the tendon against the overlying skin nicely outlines the cutaneous territory. Remember that the skin overlying the distal portion of the muscle is unreliable when the minor pedicles have been ligated. After incising around the skin island, carefully fix the skin to underlying muscle. The pedicle may now be dissected.

If the adductor longus is retracted anteriorly 10 cm below the pubic tubercle, the gracilis pedicle is immediately seen lying on the adductor magnus muscle. Several muscle branches to the adductors must be divided before complete isolation is achieved. Before division of origin or insertion, sutures are placed at regular intervals if the muscle is to be used as a functional transfer, in order to allow maintenance of the normal length-tension relation when transferred.

Before closure, large suction drains should be left in the bed of the gracilis to avoid troublesome postoperative fluid collections.

Special Problems

- In obese patients, the musculocutaneous flap may be too bulky, necessitating use of a skin graft placed on the muscle.
- When used for functional transfer to the face the gracilis may have too much power; when used in the forearm it may not have enough.

TENSOR FASCIAE LATA, TYPE I (ONE VASCULAR PEDICLE) (28–30)

Muscle Anatomy

- Origin: iliac crest, lateral to sartorius origin
- Insertion: iliotibial tract
- Function: abductor, external rotator of the thigh

Vascular Supply

The single pedicle is the transverse branch of the lateral femoral circumflex artery, which arises from the profunda femoris artery. Running beneath the rectus femoris muscle, this artery gives branches to the vastus lateralis, gluteus minimus, and rectus femoris muscles before terminating in the tensor fascia lata. The pedicle enters the tensor fasciae latae 8–10 cm below the anterior superior iliac spine.

The artery is accompanied by a similarly sized vein that drains into the profunda femoris vein. At their points of origin both vessels are 1.5 to 2.5 mm in diameter. The pedicle length is 6 to 8 cm.

Innervation

- Motor nerve: The tensor fasciae latae is supplied by a branch of the superior gluteal nerve, which enters the muscle just proximal to the vascular pedicle.
- Sensory nerve: There are two major sensory nerves supplying the tensor fasciae latae, making this flap an option for neurosensory coverage. The superior cutaneous territory is supplied by the cutaneous branch of T12, which is located subcutaneously and enters the flap posteriorly and superiorly. The lower portion is innervated by the lateral femoral cutaneous nerve, which enters medially at the level of the vascular pedicle.

The Flap

All of the lateral thigh skin to within 4 cm of the knee may be safely transferred. This would give a maximum flap dimension of 7–9 cm × 22–26 cm. Because of the relative immobility of the lateral thigh, skin flaps wider than 6 cm require skin grafting of the donor site. If the iliac crest is included (making this an osteocutaneous flap), a significant depression superiorly is unavoidable. In general, this flap is thin, especially distally. It has poor motor strength and is usually not used for functional motor transfer.

Functional Loss

Functional loss with removal of the tensor fasciae latae involves decreased sensation in the distribution of the lateral femoral cutaneous nerve. There is also a slight functional deficit in the normal knee. The tensor fascia lata is a secondary restraint (lateral stabilizer). In addition, the iliotibial fascia is sometimes used for knee reconstruction, and harvesting a tensor fasciae latae flap would make this unavailable for future reconstruction.

Flap Harvest

Preoperative flap markings are made by constructing a line from the anterior superior spine to the lateral tibial condyle. The greater trochanter marks the posterior boundary. The distal extent of the flap can be within 4 cm of the knee. The superior border may include the superior iliac crest. The pedicle entrance is marked 10 cm below the anterior superior iliac spine.

It is easiest to elevate this flap from distal to proximal, tacking the cutaneous portion to the fascia on the deep surface. The deep surface of the flap is an excellent plane that allows rapid blunt dissection above the vastus lateralis. When the level of the pedicle is reached, the rectus femoris muscle is retracted medially, allowing dissection toward the profunda vessels. There are numerous small vessels to adjacent muscles that must be carefully ligated. Care must also be taken to identify and preserve the gluteus minimus, which can be inadvertently elevated with the tensor fasciae latae.

If an osteomusculocutaneous flap is planned, preoperative marking will include up to 10 cm of the outer iliac crest and up to 4 cm of skin superior to this bone. Special care must be taken not to disturb the origin of the tensor fasciae latae muscle on the ilium.

If a neurosensory flap is used, the T12 sensory branch or lateral femoral cutaneous nerve can be dissected proximally as needed before vascular pedicle dissection.

For functional transfer, the motor nerve may be dissected proximally between the gluteus medius and maximus. If the flap is intended for restoration of forearm motor function, a useful technique is extension of the tensor fasciae latae fascia distal to the skin island so that facial strips can be used to weave into recipient tendon.

Special Problems

- The majority of this flap has nonadhering fascia on the deep surface, which may cause problems with lack of conformity to the recipient site.
- This muscle has poor motor strength and limited excursion.

RECTUS ABDOMINIS, TYPE III (TWO DOMINANT PEDICLES) (31–33) (FIGS. 85–7 TO 85–9)

Muscle Anatomy

- Origin: pubic crest and symphysis pubis
- Insertion: costal cartilage of 5th, 6th, and 7th ribs
- Function: tensor of abdominal wall and flexor of vertebral column

Vascular Supply

Each of the dominant pedicles supplies just over one-half of a muscle. The lower pedicle is the deep inferior epigastric artery, a branch of the external iliac artery. It arises proximal to the inguinal ligament and travels along the medial border of the internal inguinal ring. From here it penetrates the transversalis fascia and enters the rectus abdominis muscle just below the arcuate line. The artery is usually 2 to 3 mm in diameter and accompanied by one or two similarly sized veins.

The superior pedicle is the superior epigastric artery, a continuation of the internal mammary artery. The superior epigastric artery travels between leaves of the diaphragm and enters the rectus sheath deep to the muscle. It eventually pierces the muscle and travels parallel to the muscle fibers.

There are anastomoses between the leaves of the diaphragm and it enters the rectus sheath deep to the muscle. It eventually pierces the muscle and travels parallel to the muscle fibers.

There are anastomoses between these vessels that are usually sufficient to support the nondominant half, if one of the two pedicles is ligated. Because of the larger size and easier dissection of the inferior epigastric vessel, this is usually used for free transfer. The pedicle length is 5 to 7 cm superiorly and 8 to 10 cm inferiorly.

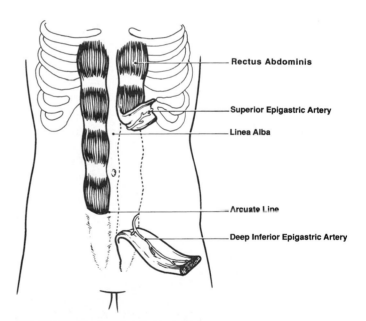

FIG. 85–8. Rectus muscle harvesting.

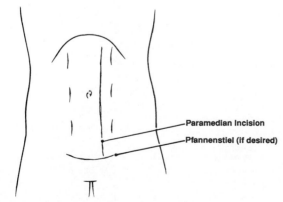

FIG. 85–7. Incision for rectus abdominis flap.

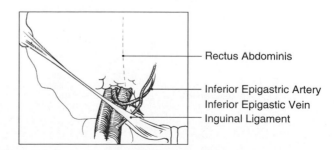

FIG. 85–9. Vascular pedicle to rectus abdominis muscle.

Innervation

- Motor nerve: This muscle has segmental innervation from branches of the 7th through 12th intercostal nerves. These nerves pierce the muscle laterally and are often accompanied by small vessels that must be ligated during flap elevation. Because of the segmental innervation, this flap is unsuitable for functional transfer.
- Sensory nerve: The cutaneous area is supplied by the anterior and lateral cutaneous nerves of T8 to T12. This flap is insensate and is not useful for neurosensory transfer.

The Flap

The rectus abdominis muscle alone can be used for defects of up to 20 cm × 8 cm. The cutaneous area supplied by this muscle is enormous and the flap may be designed vertically, horizontally, or obliquely. It extends reliably from xiphoid to pubis, and from the ipsilateral anterior axillary line to almost the contralateral midclavicular line.

Functional Loss

Use of the superior half of the rectus abdominis does not weaken the abdominal wall, but transfer of the lower rectus does result in variable abdominal-wall weakness and abdominal hernia may occur.

Flap Harvest

If a muscle flap alone is planned, a vertical incision over the muscle allows rapid access. The anterior sheath is opened laterally and the inferior epigastric pedicle is identified at the arcuate line. Sharp dissection is needed in the areas of the four tendinous transcriptions, but the muscle can be bluntly removed from the posterior rectus sheath. Below the arcuate line, care must be taken not to injure the thin transversalis fascia and underlying peritoneum. When sufficient length has been obtained, the superior end of the flap is divided and bleeding confirmed from the muscle edge. The distal attachment is then transected and the muscle allowed to perfuse. The pedicle is then easily dissected across the floor of the inguinal canal back to the external iliac origin.

If a musculocutaneous flap is used, the skin island is incised and tacked to the anterior rectus sheath that is being elevated with the muscle and skin. Closure can usually be accomplished by advancing the external oblique muscle and fascia and suturing it to the remaining rectus fascia along the midline. If the closure is too tight, synthetic mesh should be employed to achieve solid closure.

Special Problems

- This flap provides only soft-tissue coverage and is not suitable for sensory or functional transfer.
- The abdominal-wall defect may lead to significant weakness and, possibly, hernia formation.

SERRATUS ANTERIOR, TYPE III (TWO DOMINANT PEDICLES) (FIGS. 85–3, 85–10 AND 85–11)

Muscle Anatomy

- Insertion: anterior aspect of the first eight to nine ribs
- Insertion: medial border of the scapula
- Function: scapular stabilizer

Vascular Supply

The serratus anterior muscle is supplied by two pedicles, the serratus anterior branch and the lateral thoracic artery. The anterior vascular pedicle can be harvested right below the takeoff of the thoracodorsal artery to the latissimus dorsi. The vascular pedicle as well as the motor nerve separates into fingers of muscles corresponding to the slips of the serratus. This is beneficial, in that the muscle can be split for a facial reanimation. The serratus anterior branch is approximately 1.5–3.0 mm in diameter; the pedicle length is usually 5 × 7 cm.

Innervation

- Motor nerve: The segmental intercostal is T2 to T4.
- Sensory nerve: The sensory innervation is by segmental intercostal nerves 2 to 4 and the nerve to the serratus anterior. If the entire muscle is taken, there may be winging of

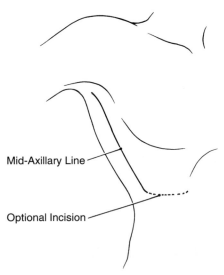

Mid-Axillary Line

Optional Incision

FIG. 85–10. Skin incision for serratus anterior flap.

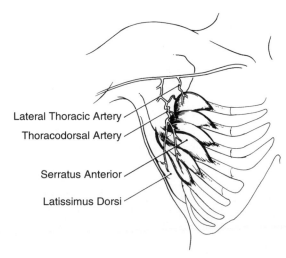

Lateral Thoracic Artery

Thoracodorsal Artery

Serratus Anterior

Latissimus Dorsi

FIG. 85–11. Serratus muscle and in situ anatomy.

the scapula. However, the cephalad and caudad slips can be preserved for function.

The Flap

The size of the serratus anterior flap is 10 cm × 12 cm. A musculocutaneous flap of 5 cm × 15 cm can be elevated.

Functional Loss

No functional loss is experienced with removal of the lower 2 to 3 slips of serratus anterior muscle.

Flap Harvest

A longitudinal incision is made along the anterior axillary line with the patient supine. The subcutaneous tissue is divided, and the serratus is identified right above the ribs.

Muscle is then isolated in the middle slips; usually three slips of the muscle are taken at the level of 6th, 7th, and 8th ribs. Sharp dissection is used to resect the muscle off the chest wall, dividing the posterior muscle anterior to the lateral border of the scapula. The thoracodorsal pedicle is identified, and then the vascular pedicle to the serratus is identified from its takeoff with the branch to the latissimus dorsi. Closure can be done directly. This flap is particularly good for small tissue defects around the foot (e.g., in diabetic or vascular ulcers).

Other Muscles Used for Transfers

PECTORALIS MINOR, TYPE V (11,12)

The pectoralis minor is currently a popular muscle for facial reanimation. While the vascular pedicle is somewhat variable, the branches from the axillary artery and vein are suitable for microsurgical transfer. It is innervated by the medial and lateral pectoral nerves. Elevation is straightforward and functional loss is minimal. The slips of origin on the 3rd, 4th, and 5th ribs may be sutured to the alar base, oral commissure, and upper and lower lips. The coracoid insertion is attached along the zygomatic arch and preauricular fascia.

EXTENSOR DIGITORUM BREVIS, TYPE I

The extensor digitorum brevis is supplied by a branch of the dorsalis pedis artery and vein. It has a single motor nerve that is a branch of the anterior tibial nerve. Because of low muscle amplitude and power, clinical results in facial reanimation have generally been unsatisfactory.

PECTORALIS MAJOR, TYPE V (34)

The pectoralis major is a large, flat muscle that arises from the clavicle, sternum, and 2nd to 6th costal cartilages. It has a large vascular pedicle from the thoracoacromial axis and an effective excursion of 10 cm, making it a potentially effective finger flexor. Because of cosmetic and functional loss, only the sternal head is routinely used for transfer.

References

1. Mathes SJ, Nahai F. *Clinical applications for muscle and musculocutaneous flaps.* St. Louis: CV Mosby, 1982.
2. Shaw WW. Microvascular free flaps: the first decade. *Clin Plast Surg* 1983; 10:3.
3. Jacobson JH, Suarez EL. Microsurgery and anastomosis of small vessels. *Surg Forum* 1960; 11:243.
4. Serafin D, Buncke HJ Jr, eds. *Microvascular composite tissue transplantation.* St. Louis: CV Mosby, 1979.
5. Tamai S, Komatsu S, Sakamoto H, et al. Free muscle transplants in dogs with microsurgical, neurovascular anastomosis. *Plast Reconstr Surg* 1970; 46:219.
6. Ikuta Y, Kubo Tsuge K. Free muscle transplantation by microsurgical technique to treat severe Volkmann's contracture. *Plast Reconstr Surg* 1976; 8:407.
7. Mathes SJ, Nahai F. *Clinical atlas of muscle and musculocutaneous flaps.* St. Louis: CV Mosby, 1979.
8. Mathes SJ, Nahai F, Vasconez LO. Myocutaneous free flap transfer: Anatomical and experimental consideration. *Plast Reconstr Surg* 1978; 62:162.
9. Serafin D, Sabatier RE, Morris RL, et al. Reconstruction of the lower extremity with vascularized composite tissue: improved tissue survival and specific indications. *Plast Reconstr Surg* 1980; 66:230.
10. O'Brien BM, Franklin JD, Morrison WA. Cross-facial nerve grafts and microneurovascular free muscle transfer for long established facial palsy. *Br J Plast Surg* 1980; 33:202.
11. Terzis JK. Pectoralis minor: a unique muscle for correction of facial palsy. *Plast Reconstr Surg* 1989; 83:767.
12. Harrison DH. The pectoralis minor vascularized muscle graft for the treatment of unilateral facial palsy. *Plast Reconstr Surg* 1985; 75:206.
13. Mayou B, Watson JS, Harrison DH, et al. Free microvascular and microneural transfer of the extensor digitorum brevis muscle for the treatment of unilateral facial palsy. *Br J Plast Surg* 1981; 34:362.
14. Tolhurst DE, Bos KE. Free revascularized muscle grafts in facial palsy. *Plast Reconstr Surg* 1982; 69:760.
15. Russell RC, Graham DR, Feller AM, et al. Experimental evaluation of the antibiotic carrying capacity of a muscle flap into a fibrotic cavity. *Plast Reconstr Surg* 1988; 81:162.
16. Ger R. The management of open fracture of the tibia with skin loss. *J Trauma* 1970; 10:112.
17. Byrd HS, Spicer TE, Cierny G III. Management of open tibial fractures. *Plast Reconstr Surg* 1985; 76:719.
18. Gustilo RB, Anderson JT. Prevention of infection in the treatment of 1025 open fractures of long bones. *J Bone Joint Surg [Am]* 1976; 58:453.
19. Hari K. Microvascular free flaps for skin coverage: indications and selection of donor sites. *Clin Plast Surg* 1983; 10:37.
20. Shaw WW. Breast reconstruction by microvascular transfer. In: Brent B, ed. *Artistry of reconstructive surgery.* St. Louis: CV Mosby, 1987; 921.
21. Manktelow RT, McKee NH. Free muscle transplantation to provide active finger flexion. *J Hand Surg* 1978; 3:416.
22. Maxwell GP. Musculocutaneous free flaps. *Clin Plast Surg* 1980; 7:111.
23. Maxwell GP, Manson PN, Hoopes JE. Experiences with 13 latissimus dorsi myocutaneous free flaps. *Plast Reconstr Surg* 1979; 64:1.
24. Tobin GR, Moberg AW, DuBou RH, et al. The split latissimus dorsi myocutaneous flap. *Ann Plast Surg* 1981; 7:272.
25. Harii K, Ohmori K, Sekiguchi J. The free musculocutaneous flap. *Plast Reconstr Surg* 1976; 57:294.
26. Harii K, Ohmori K, Torii S. Free gracilis muscle transplantation with microvascular anastomosis for treatment of facial paralysis. *Plast Reconstr Surg* 1976; 57:133.
27. Heckler F. Gracilis myocutaneous and muscle flaps. *Clin Plast Surg* 1980; 7:27.
28. Hill HL, Nahai F, Vasconez LO. The tensor fascia lata myocutaneous free flap. *Plast Reconstr Surg* 1978; 61:517.
29. Mathes SJ, Buchanan RT. Tensor fascia lata neurosensory musculocutaneous free flap. *Br J Plast Surg* 1979; 32:184.
30. Nahai F, Hill HL, Hester TR. Experiences with the tensor fascia lata flap. *Plast Reconstr Surg* 1979; 63:788.
31. Bunkis J, Walton RL, Matthes SJ. The rectus abdominis free flap for lower extremity reconstruction. *Ann Plast Surg* 1983; 11:373.
32. Bunkis J, Walton RL, Mathes SJ, et al. The versatile rectus abdominis flap. *Plast Surg Forum* 1982; 5:218.
33. Pennington DG, Lai MF, Pelly AD. The rectus abdominis myocutaneous free flap. *Br J Plast Surg* 1980; 33:277.
34. Tobin GR. Pectoralis major segmental anatomy and segmentally split pectoralis major flaps. *Plast Reconstr Surg* 1985; 75:814.

86

Free Vascularized Bone Grafts and Osteocutaneous Flaps

Fu-Chan Wei, M.D., F.A.C.S., and Tarek Abdalla El-Gammal, M.D.

Conventional (nonvascular) bone grafts are entirely dependent on diffusion of nutrients from surrounding tissue bed. For graft incorporation the majority of cells do not survive. The necrotic bone is removed by osteoclasts allowing ingrowth of blood vessels carrying osteoprogenitor cells into the region. This leads to the information of an advancing front of new bone replacing the original bone of the graft, a process called "creeping substitution." A cortical bone graft is thus weakest during the revascularization phase of creeping substitution and is then most likely to fail. Advances in microvascular surgery have made it possible to transfer autogenous bone grafts on vascular pedicles. With the nutrient blood supply preserved, bone cells survive and healing of the graft to the recipient bone occurs by a mechanism similar to fracture healing rather than creeping substitution. Thus, graft incorporation is thus independent of the status of the recipient bed. This is especially significant when the bone defect is situated in a highly scarred or irradiated area that impedes incorporation of conventional autogenous grafts.

History

The first successful clinical vascularized bone transfer was reported by McKee in 1970, who used an anterior segment of rib based on the internal mammary vessels to reconstruct a mandibular defect (1). In 1974, Ostrup and Frederickson experimentally used, a composite graft based on the posterior intercostal vessels in dogs (2). The use of the posterior rib graft was later reported clinically for mandibular reconstruction by Serafin and co-workers (3) and for tibial reconstruction by Buncke et al. in 1975 (4). Taylor and colleagues first reported the use of free contralateral fibula based on the peroneal artery and its venae comitantes for the reconstruction of 12.5 cm tibial defect. Since then, the technique has been used by several authors for the reconstruction of long bone defects of different etiologies. The use of iliac crest osteocutaneous flap, based on the superficial circumflex iliac vessels, was first reported in 1978 by Taylor and Watson for the reconstruction of tibial defects (5). Later reports recommended the use of the deep circumflex iliac artery because of its dominant blood supply to the bone (6).

Current indications for free vascularized bone grafting are broad. Vascularized bone grafting offers significant advantages in bone defects greater than 6 to 8 cm in length resulting from trauma resection of bone tumor or infection requiring extensive sequestrectomy (7–10). In orthopedics, indications include refractory nonunion with failure of conventional techniques, and congenital pseudarthrosis of the

tibia or forearm (11). Future applications may include transfer of a vascularized epiphysis to reconstitute limb growth (12), and transfer of free vascularized allografts (13).

The most popular donor sites for vascularized bone grafts include the fibula, iliac crest, and rib. The vascularized rib graft, because of its curved shape, was initially often used for reconstruction of complex mandibular defects. Because of its size and bone quality, rib grafts have limited use for limb reconstruction. The iliac graft is predominantly cancellous granissor bone which allows it to heal rapidly, and a long vascular pedicle (up to 8 cm). It may be harvested with the overlying skin and muscle as an osteocutaneous flap. The arc of curvature of the iliac crest makes it suitable for reconstruction of mandibular defects, but usually precludes its use for long bone defects. Removal of the iliac crest may lead to an objectionable cosmetic defect, occasionally, an abdominal hernia and possible irritation of the lateral femoral cutaneous nerve of the thigh.

The fibular graft is best suited for reconstruction of long bone defects because of its shape (straight), strength (cortical structure), and length (up to 25 cm). In addition, the fibula can be osteotomized, while preserving its periosteal continuity and blood supply, and folded on itself as a "double-barrel graft" to provide additional strength for bridging femoral or tibial defects (14,15). There is no donor-site morbidity if adequate fibula is left distally to maintain ankle stability.

The vascularized fibula has become an established donor for mandibular reconstruction, since Hidalgo reported his excellent results using this technique in 1989 (16). By making multiple osteotomies, the fibula can be three dimensionally contoured to any desirable shape to reconstruct defects after mandibular resection. The uniform thickness of the fibula and its strong cortical structure are ideal for osteointegration of the dental implants. The distal runoff of its peroneal pedicle can be used as the recipient vessel of a second flap when required (17).

Vascularized Osteoseptocutaneous Fibular Flap

ANATOMY

The nutrient artery of the fibula arises as a branch of the peroneal artery, and enters the fibula at the midshaft. The peroneal artery also supplies several periosteal branches to the fibula. By isolating the peroneal artery at its origin from the posterior tibial trunk, both medullary and periosteal blood supplies are preserved. Chen and Yan described the blood

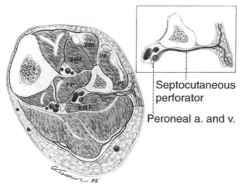

FIG. 86–1. Cross-sectional anatomy of the leg showing the septocutaneous perforator in the posterior crural septum.

supply to the skin on the lateral aspect of the leg which arises from the musculocutaneous branches of the peroneal artery (18). These branches, totaling four or five in number, penetrate the soleus muscle and pass through the deep fascia to supply the overlying skin. Chen and Yan (18) recommended that, in harvesting the fibula as an osteocutaneous flap, these penetrating cutaneous branches be identified along a line approximately 0.3 cm from the posterior border of the fibula, and then the soleus muscle be cut longitudinally 0.5 cm posterior to the points through which the cutaneous branches pass. Wei and co-workers (19) have demonstrated that in cadavers and clinical cases, that some of these cutaneous branches passed entirely in the posterior crural septum (septocutaneous branches), and some of them passed through the flexor hallucis longus, posterior tibia, or soleus muscle before entering the posterior crural septum (musculocutaneous branches) (Fig. 86–1). Wei and others have also demonstrated that one or two sizable septocutaneous branches can provide adequate blood supply to a skin area averaging 24 cm long and 10 cm wide, centered at the posterior fibular margin and the junction of the middle and lower thirds of the fibula. According to their findings, it is unnecessary to preserve an additional border of the soleus muscle through which perforating musculocutaneous branches pass to the skin, as recommended by Chen and Yan (18). This simplifies the technique and saves time.

ADVANTAGE

Inclusion of the skin flap permits not only postoperative monitoring but also simultaneous reconstruction of moderate soft-tissue defects. Donor-site scar is minimal when it is closed primarily. Skin grafting is required if the harvested skin flap is wider than 4 cm. Inclusion of skin attached only by the thin posterior crural septum as a osteoseptocutaneous flap offers distinct advantages over the previous design of the fibula osteocutaneous flap, which was raised with a thick cuff of soleus muscle: (a) the skin can slide freely without being tethered by a bulky muscle cuff, providing greater versatility in wound coverage when the skin defect is not directly located over the bone defect, and (b) the vascular pedicle of the fibula osteoseptocutaneous flap can be easily switched to a new recipient vessel by folding it around the posterior crural septum (19). Although the skin paddle of the fibula osteocutaneous flap has been considered unreliable (16), Wei and

others (17) reported no isolated skin flap loss in 80 extremity reconstructions and 27 composite mandibular reconstructions.

POSTOPERATIVE PLANNING

When raising the fibula as an osteoseptocutaneous flap, a large skin flap extending beyond the junction of the middle and distal third of the leg is more reliable than a small skin flap, because the small flap may miss the perforators. Although the longitudinal axis of the skin flap should coincide with the posterior edge of the fibula, the location of the skin flap need not be centered over the portion of the fibula that is to be used. The skin flap can maintain its vascularity when it is dissected off the bone in the subcutaneous plane. When skin is included for monitoring purpose only, an ellipse of skin about 4 cm wide and 8 to 10 cm long is raised and excess skin is trimmed after the exact location of the perforators is identified.

Sites of fibular osteotomy are determined leaving at least 5 cm of the fibula distally to maintain ankle stability. Even when only a short segment of the bone is needed, it is desirable to remove more bone to facilitate peroneal pedicle dissection. There is no additional functional morbidity from removing a longer segment as long as the ankle mortise is maintained. In children less than 10 years of age, distal tibiofibular synostosis using a transfixation screw is performed to prevent possible proximal migration of the distal fibula with consequent valgus instability.

HARVESTING TECHNIQUE

The procedure is performed under tourniquet with the patient in the supine position and the knee flexed. An elliptical skin incision is made and carried down to the subcutaneous fascia. Care is taken to preserve the lateral sural cutaneous nerve, if any. The skin flap is elevated from the lateral and medial margins towards the posterior crural septum between the soleus and peroneus muscles. The deep fascia is incised along the posterior margin of the peroneal muscles and the anterior margin of the soleus muscle. Inclusion of this part of the deep fascia helps to avoid accidental injuries to the cutaneous branches in the posterior crural septum. Moreover, the superficial peroneal nerve can be preserved. The skin flap is then turned forwards and all sizable vessels seen in the periphery of the posterior crural septum are identified and traced towards their origin. One or two sizable septocutaneous branches can provide adequate blood supply to the skin flap. If no sizable vessels traversing the posterior crural septum are identified, intramuscular dissection of these vessels piercing the soleus muscle is carried out.

After dissection and evaluation of the vessels leading to the skin flap, the flap is turned back to expose the anterolateral aspect of the fibula. Careful attention must be paid not to shear the vessel in the septum. The peroneus longus and brevis are detached from the fibula, leaving only minimal muscle cuffs. The anterior crural septum is incised to allow dissection into the anterior compartment. The periosteum at the planned osteotomy sites is incised and elevated circumferentially. Both ends of the fibula are divided with a Gigli saw. Further dissection is facilitated by traction and rotation of the fibula with bone clamps. Extensor muscles are dissected off the fibula and the anterior tibial neurovascular bundle is iden-

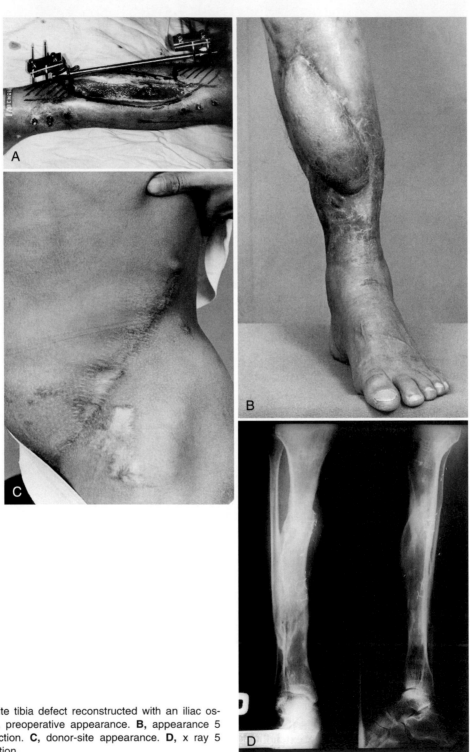

FIG. 86–5.   Composite tibia defect reconstructed with an iliac os-teocutaneous flap. **A,** preoperative appearance. **B,** appearance 5 years after reconstruction. **C,** donor-site appearance. **D,** x ray 5 years after reconstruction.

the cutaneous vessels. The spermatic cord or round ligament is identified and retracted superiorly and medially. The external iliac artery is palpated, and the deep circumflex iliac artery is identified and its origin dissected. The transversalis fascia is divided and the internal oblique and transversus abdominis muscles are separated from the inguinal ligament. The deep circumflex iliac artery is carefully dissected laterally. The internal oblique and transversus abdominis muscles are incised 2 to 3 cm above the iliac crest, raising this width of muscles along the iliac crest. By blunt dissection, the iliacus muscle is separated from the iliac fossa leaving the periosteum intact.

The lower border of the skin flap is incised, and the outer table of the iliac crest is dissected. The attachments of the glutei and tensor fascia lata are dissected from the outer surface of bone leaving the periosteum intact. Osteotomy of the outer and inner tables is performed with an oscillating saw. A straight segment 6-8 cm in length can be obtained. The inguinal ligament and sartorius muscle are incised medial to the anterior superior iliac spine. This leaves the composite flap attached only by the vascular pedicle. After the recipient site is dissected, the pedicle is divided and the flap transferred.

Secure closure of the donor site is essential to prevent hernia formation. The iliacus fascia and muscle are sutured to the transversalis fascia and muscle. The external and internal obliques are sutured to the glutei and fascia lata. The inguinal ligament is attached laterally and the inguinal canal is repaired. During closure, flexion of the hip and knee is helpful in reducing tension on the donor-site closure (Fig. 86–5).

References

1. McKee D. Cited by O'Brien McC. *Microvascular reconstructive surgery.* Edinburgh: Churchill Livingstone, 1977.
2. Ostrup LT, Fredrickson JM. Distant transfer of a free, living bone graft by microvascular anastomosis: an experimental study. *Plast Reconstr Surg* 1974; 54:274.
3. Serafin D, Villareal-Rios A, Georgiade N. A rib containing free flap to reconstruct mandibular defects. *Br J Plast Surg* 1977; 30:263.
4. Bunke H, Furnas DW, Gordon L. Free osteocutaneous flap from a rib to the tibia. *Plast Reconstr Surg* 1977; 59:799.
5. Taylor GI, Miller GDH, Ham FJ. The free vascularized bone graft. *Plast Reconstr Surg* 1975; 55:533.
6. Taylor GI, Watson N. One-stage repair of composite leg defects with free vascularized flaps of groin, skin, and iliac bone. *Plast Reconstr Surg* 1978; 61:494.
7. Taylor GI, Townsend P, Corlett R. Superiority of the deep circumflex iliac vessels as the supply for free groin flaps: clinical work. *Plast Reconstr Surg* 1979; 64:595.
8. Weiland AJ, Moore JR, Daniel RK. Vascularized bone autografts. Experience with 41 cases. *Clin Orthop* 1983; 174:87.
9. Osterman AL, Bora FW. Free vascularized bone grafting for large gap nonunion of long bones. *Orthop Clin North Am* 1984; 15:131.
10. Weiland AJ, Daniel RK, Riley LH Jr. Application of the free vascularized bone graft in the treatment of malignant or aggressive bone tumors. *Johns Hopkins Med J* 1977; 140:85.
11. Chen CW, Yu ZJ, Wang W. A new method of treatment of congenital tibial pseudarthrosis using free vascularized fibular grafts: a preliminary report. *Ann Acad Med Singapore* 1979; 8:465.
12. Nettelblad H, Randolph MA, Weiland AJ. Free microvascular epiphyseal plate transplantation. An experimental study in dogs. *J Bone Joint Surg* 1984; 66A:1421.
13. Shigetomi M, Doi K, Kuwata N, et al. Experimental study on vascularized bone allografts for reconstruction of massive bone defects. *Microsurgery* 1994; 15(9):663.
14. Jupiter JB, Bour CJ, May JW Jr. The reconstruction of defects in the femoral shaft with vascularized transfers of fibular bone. *J Bone Joint Surg* 1987; 69A:365.
15. Wei FC, El-Gammal TA, Lin CH, et al. Free fibula osteoseptocutaneous graft for reconstruction of segmental femoral shaft defects. *J Trauma,* accepted.
16. Hidalgo DA. Fibula free flap: a new method of mandible reconstruction. *Plast Reconstr Surg* 84:71, 1989.
17. Wei FC, Seah CS, Tsai YC, et al. Fibula osteoseptocutaneous flap for reconstruction of composite mandibular defects. *Plast Reconstr Surg* 1994; 93(3):294.
18. Chen ZW, Yan W. The study and clinical application of the osteocutaneous flap of the fibula. *Microsurgery* 1983; 4:11.
19. Wei FC, Chen HC, Chuang CC, et al.. Fibular osteoseptocutaneous flap. Anatomic study and clinical applications. *Plast Reconstr Surg* 1986; 78:191.

EIGHT

Hand

87

Embryology of the Extremities

Ellen Beatty, M.D.

All too often the essential organs of a fetus are formed before the pregnancy is confirmed. This makes protection of an unexpected fetus from known teratogens haphazard at best. The embryonic period includes the first 8 weeks of postovulatory development. After this time, all vital organ systems are present and malformations from external factors such as amniotic bands or contact with the uterine wall are more likely.

Embryology of the Upper Extremities

The earliest detection of an arm bud is in the 3rd week of embryonic development, with the slight elevation of the ectoderm adjacent to the 8th to 10th somites. By the 28th postovulatory day, the arm bud is a definite ridge with scattered thin-walled vessels. In the 4th week, the apical ectodermal ridge has formed with an adjacent marginal vein. At this time, the cervical and brachial plexuses are identifiable and the C4 to T1 nerves have reached the upper end of the limb bud. The 5th week heralds a recognizable hand plate differentiating into a carpal region and distal digital flanges. By the 6th week, major nerves of the arm have advanced to the hand and the chondrification of the humerus has begun. Upon reaching the 7th week and nearing the end of the embryonic stage, the major nerves have reached the hand, and the finger rays have appeared with notches on the plate. The 8th and final week of embryonic development presents a limb with periosteal buds, developing joint cavities, and formation of palmar pads (1). It is obvious that there is much happening during this short span to bring about formation of a structure as intricate as the human upper extremity in 6 weeks from a two cell-layer beginning.

The migration and multiplication of mesodermal cells in the somatopleure to form a ridge along the lateral border of the embryo, known as the Wolff crest, initiates the formation of limb buds (Fig. 87–1). These cells have high RNA content but there is no histochemical difference in any of the cells within this two cell-layered ectoderm for its entire length or as compared to the remainder of the embryo's ectoderm (2). The portion of this crest not related to the limb buds will eventually become absorbed back into the embryo. The mesoderm in the area of the Wolff crest that is destined to produce limb buds then condenses. The ectoderm over the ventral portion of this condensed mesoderm will proliferate and become more adherent to its mesoderm than to the dorsal ectoderm (2). The mesoderm of the bud begins actively increasing, resulting in the caudal growth of the limb. The formation of a thickening in the distal postaxial tip of the bud, known as the apical ectodermal ridge (Fig. 87–2), is be-

lieved to induce the mesoderm to migrate distally under this thickened ventral ectoderm. There is an interdependence between the apical ectodermal ridge and the underlying mesoderm such that without the apical ectodermal ridge further differentiation of distal limb parts ceases. Also, with the "apical ectodermal maintenance factor" from the mesoderm, this ridge flattens and becomes inactive (3). Once the apical ectodermal ridge is formed, the distal limb bud expands to form a hand paddle. At this point the apical ectodermal ridge exists as a rim covering the most distal edge of the hand paddle, and the previously thickened ventral ectoderm in the axillary area has resumed a normal configuration. This apical ectodermal ridge then condenses over the area of digital buds.

Determining regulators of such a complex sequence as limb formation has spurred much interest and experimentation. A large volume of recent work involves the ability of cells in a limb bud to know where they are and what tissue they are destined to be. Several theories have evolved using the gradient of a chemical or a metabolic activity to supply positional information to cells. One phase-shift model proposes "pacemaker" cells that periodically initiate an event, which then propagates through the remainder of the cells by intercellular signaling. Second and 3rd events at different time intervals and propagation speeds provide needed regulation (4). Contrasting this proposal is a widely reported theory defining a positional field of cells, based on a signal from the polarizing zone discovered by Saunders and Gasseling (5), to determine anteroposterior position and a "progress zone" in the distal limb to provide proximodistal position (Fig. 87–3). The polarizing zone originates in the axillary portion of the limb bud (6). This area is proposed to provide a diffusible chemical that will decrease in concentration along the anteroposterior axis and allow induction of limb structures based on the threshold at which each digit or structure will form. This "progress zone" is the mesoderm lying 350 microns beneath the apical ectodermal ridge of the distal bud. Cells of this zone are constantly dividing and only differentiate after leaving this zone. These cells may determine their position in the limb by the number of mitoses or the length of time they spend in the zone; the last cells out being the most distal (5). Much work remains before these interesting theories are proven, but they provide much food for thought on normal and abnormal development.

Cell death in limb formation is an important process that regulates the cessation of function of various tissues at vital times and locations. Developmental defects could be the re-

FIG. 87–7. Serial views of the arteries of the upper extremity show the progression from a median and interosseus system to the dominant ulnar and radial systems in the adult. (After Mazkova, (15))

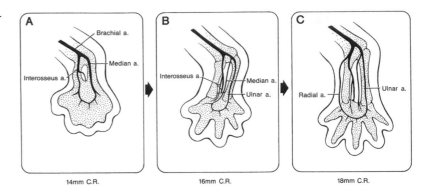

FIG. 87–8. Position changes in the extremities. **A,** initial growth is in a caudal direction with lengthening of the extremity buds. **B,** anterior bends occurs at the knees and elbows during the 6th week. **C,** final rotation of the extremities in the 7th week is in a 90° arc, in opposite directions.

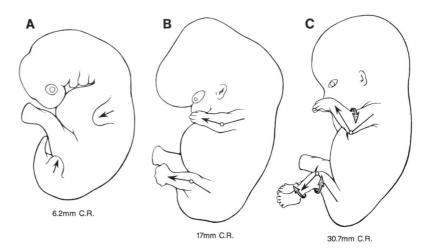

vein will remain functional until the apical ectodermal ridge retains activity only over individual digit formation, at which time individual veins following the general arterial course will have formed (8). The axial artery is seen, in the 12-mm embryo, passing into the distal one-third of the arm to become the capillary network (Fig. 87–7A). In this 5th week of development, at 11 mm, there is a solid median artery on the palmar surface of the muscle blastema of the flexor digitorum profundus and a deeper interosseous artery that joins it to form the brachial artery at the elbow (15) (Fig. 87–7B). In the 15-mm embryo, the ulnar artery can be discerned to the middle of the forearm, where it becomes a capillary network. By 16 mm (now the 6th week), a solid ulnar artery to the palm exists. Not until the embryo is 17–18 mm will the radial artery form, in keeping with postaxial dominance of limb development. The ulnar and radial arteries will continue to enlarge as the median and interosseous arteries decrease in relative size and importance. The interosseous artery will terminate as small arterioles in the carpus (Fig. 87–7C).

Upper-extremity embryogenesis involves four stages of development. The blastema stage will be completed by the 6th postovulatory week. At this point, the next week and a half will be devoted to differentiation of the structures, with basic condensations of cells. The late 7th and the 8th weeks herald formation of the structures and refinements specific to this species. The arrival of the fetal period marks the final-stage, differential growth (16).

Embryology of the Lower Extremities

The development of the lower extremities has a great deal in common with the development of the upper extremities. All of the events from limb bud formation to positional information and structure formation are paralleled, but delayed by as much as several days in lower extremity embryology. Although similar, there are some vital differences in the formation of legs.

The leg's limb bud will form when the embryo is about 4 mm in size, or at about 28 days postgestation (1). This will occur near the 24th to 29th somites. There is an ectodermal thickening on the bud's ventrolateral surface, as in the arm. The apical ectodermal ridge will be present and influencing limb formation throughout the 5th and 6th weeks of embryonic development. At the end of the 4th week of development, spinal segments L1 and L4 will have given off branches toward the bud (1). During the 5th week the foot plate can be recognized, and the tibial nerve will reach the base of this foot plate. At this time, the main trunks of the lumbosacral nerve plexus will be formed. The embryo is between 8 and 11 mm now, and the skeletal condensation had begun. Through the 5th and 6th weeks of development, the femur, tibia, and fibula will begin to chondrify. Some muscles will also be distinguishable at this time (1).

The position of the extremities during development differs (Fig. 87–8). At 5 to 6 weeks of gestational age an embryo's

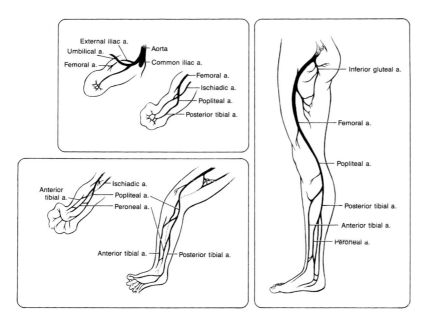

FIG. 87–9. Stages of development of the lower-extremity vessels from the 4-week embryo (upper left) to the adult (right). The gradual involution of early vessels are they are bypassed by flow through later larger vessels leads to the final configuration and many variations. (After Senior, ref. 17.)

limbs point caudally and are also parallel. During the 6th week, both extremities undergo an anterior bend at the elbows and knees. At this time, the palms and soles all face the trunk, but during the following week the extremities undergo a 90° rotation. This rotation occurs in opposite directions, leaving the elbows pointing caudally and the knees pointing cephalad. In the 8th and final week of embryonic development, the lower limbs undergo a further rotation medially. All of these movements leave an embryo with limb surfaces that have dorsal extensors in the upper extremities but dorsal flexors in the lower extremities. This motion also accounts for the curvature of the lower-extremity cutaneous innervation pattern.

Formation of lower-extremity vascular systems is very different (17) (Fig. 87–9). In the lower extremity there is one axial artery, which is a branch of the umbilical artery. This vessel has been identified while the limb bud is still indistinct. In the 5th and 6th weeks, this vessel grows the length of the limb bud and terminates in a plantar plexus and a plexus that perforates the tarsal area (the future dorsalis pedis artery). The 14-mm embryo is noted to have formed a femoral artery anteriorly, which joins the axial artery at the level of the future distal femur. This retained portion of the axial artery will be known as the popliteal artery and is the most permanent section of the initial arterial system. This 14-mm embryo also has developed the future anterior tibial artery and two posterior branches, the peroneal and posterior tibial arteries. The axial artery in the lower leg is now relatively smaller and known as the interosseous artery; by 22 mm of size, this artery will no longer be functional for the length of the lower leg. The origin of the axial artery will become the inferior gluteal artery by the 6th week (18). This complex sequence of vessel formation can be expected to give rise to many anomalies. It is also speculated that deformities such as clubfoot (19), absence of the fibula, and other skeletal dysplasias (20) result when the full sequence of vascular pathway development does not occur. The veins of the lower extremity arise from the initial border vein that follows the apical ectodermal ridge; this vein later forms the greater

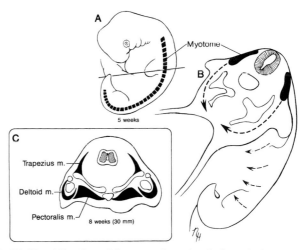

FIG. 87–10. Migration of the mesodermal cells from their paravertebral origin to the lateral and anterior trunk occurs by the 8th week of development.

and lesser saphenous veins and the venous plexus of the dorsal foot (19).

Embryology of the Trunk

Embryology of the trunk begins with the formation of myotomes at the time of notochord development. The cervical, thoracic, and lumbar myotomes will contribute cells to the corresponding areas of the embryo that will later condense into individual muscles. From experimentation, we know that these cells are not regionalized until muscle formation begins in their specific location (18). In the 4th week of development, the thoracic myotomes, rib processes, and spinal nerves are moving into the ventral body wall (Fig. 87–10). In the 5th week, muscles such as the trapezium, latissimus, and serratus anterior are identifiable. The layered abdominal wall is also forming, with the lumbar and sacral areas still trailing. By the 7th week, the body wall muscles can readily be iden-

position on the table, the appearance of the donor site following surgery, and the patient's postoperative needs are also important.

When selecting free tissue transfer, morbidity and efficiency of harvest must be considered. When the donor tissue is a latissimus dorsi free flap, for example, the patient's walking with crutches and moving in bed in the immediate postoperative period is curtailed. Not only is a major blood vessel sacrificed when a contralateral radial artery forearm flap is harvested but also the uninjured hand must be immobilized, decreasing a patient's independence. The supine position is compatible with elevation of the rectus abdominis and groin flaps; however, harvest of a contralateral latissimus dorsi flap requires lateral positioning of the patient.

A patient's gender, culture, and personal preferences affect the type and visibility of defects in appearance of the donor site. The appearance of a rectus abdominis flap harvested through a Pfannenstiel incision is better than that relying on a paramedian incision. The donor sites of both of these are hidden, as compared to the lateral arm flap. In women, the least visible scar for a latissimus dorsi flap, and one easily concealed by underwear, is made by harvest through a carefully designed zigzag incision. Likewise, a design for the groin flap that will be concealed by swimwear is easily made (41).

Skin, nerve, tendon, and bone can be supplied in a single block of tissue. In wounds that require more than one tissue type, the temptation is high to obtain the necessary elements through such a single composite flap. Sites of frequently used composite flaps are the area of the dorsum of the foot, the radial forearm flap, and the lateral arm flap. Composite free tissue can even replace a single metacarpal (23). Taylor and Collett (21) have used the dorsalis pedis artery, extensor tendon, nerve, and second metatarsal to reconstruct a single metacarpal, especially that of the thumb. While this free flap does provide excellent functional results, there may be significant donor-site morbidity. The harvest of several anatomic elements may result in an unsightly defect, an unstable scar, and a functional donor-site deficit; therefore, such composite flaps are not always recommended.

A composite reconstruction for a given defect does not always have to be reconstructed with a composite flap. A composite reconstruction can use nonvascularized corticocancellous bone graft, separately harvested tendon graft, and a flap of vascularized tissue to provide coverage. The result of such a reconstruction can be equal to that of a composite flap with little or no donor-site morbidity.

Larger defects of the dorsum of the hand or first web space can be covered by the versatile ipsilateral lateral arm flap in males. The match of skin color and texture is especially good, and morbidity is restricted to one extremity. Females seem to have difficulty with the donor-site scar created by the lateral arm flap (42), and the groin flap, with its concealed donor site, is preferable here.

Wound Management

DÉBRIDEMENT, THE KEY TO SUCCESS

Once planning is done, the hand is wrapped in a towel, and an Esmarch bandage is applied to the arm to exsanguinate it. Antibiotic is administered before tourniquet inflation and often 4 to 6 hours thereafter. Initially, the tourniquet is kept inflated for a maximum of two uninterrupted hours. A 20-minute break separates each subsequent 1.5-hour session. A bloodless field, made possible by the tourniquet, allows the type of wound excision associated with tumor resection. As proposed by Godina, we term excision of this type "radical débridement," and it constitutes the keystone of the entire procedure.

Débridement is based on the assumption that appropriate soft-tissue coverage can be done. Its goal, like that of tumor surgery, is to remove all compromised or contaminated tissue en bloc. Put concisely, the surgeon's goal is to cut the wound out. Beginning through normal skin (Fig. 88–1), wound excision continues along the entire periphery of the

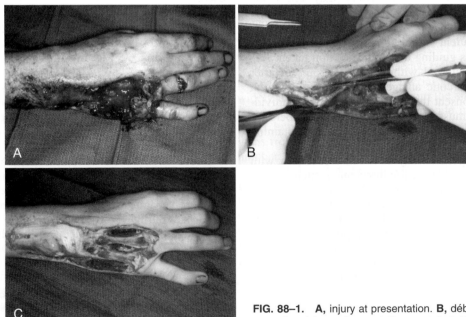

FIG. 88–1. **A,** injury at presentation. **B,** débridement beginning around periphery of wound. **C,** completed débridement.

wound. To preserve uninjured structures, the surgeon identifies a plane of dissection. Bone that provides structural support is cleaned, if necessary by shaving with a grouter. Small fragments of bone that have no soft tissue or substantial articular cartilage attached to them are removed. Tissue of even questionable viability is excised. When only normal-looking tissue is left (Fig. 88–1C), the reconstruction proceeds.

Certain anatomic structures may be excluded from this method of débridement. These include large vessels with normal flow, tendons, and nerves, as long as they seem functional. They are only replaced if, after careful cleansing, they are irregular and friable, because under these circumstances they are unlikely to regain function. This exemption does not apply to muscle, which, if devascularized, must be excised because it will not survive. Radical débridement, however, does respect normal anatomy.

If the dirty wound cannot be made into a clean one, the reconstruction does not proceed. Three elements are required to make this determination: (a) wound excision, as defined above; (b) profuse irrigation of the area, typically with two to three liters of Ringer lactate solution; and (c) the taking of tissue cultures, followed by cleansing with another liter of crystalloid solution. After this, the tourniquet is released so that areas of poor or impaired vascularity will show themselves, significant bleeding points may be seen, and hemostasis secured. The condition of exposed vessels that might need repair by direct anastomosis or by grafting is then determined.

Once the tourniquet has been deflated 20 minutes, the extremity is again exsanguinated and the tourniquet reinflated. The injury is reassessed. Further débridement is done if needed. The wound is again irrigated. Those anatomic structures to be reconstructed are marked and their measurements taken.

If the surgeon at this point doubts that all devitalized elements that could become foci of infection have been removed, reconstruction is postponed, and a pouch with tobramycin beads is applied. Once the time needed for tissue demarcation has passed, usually between 24 and 48 hours, the patient can return to the operating room (depending on the general condition). If all tissues in the wound still appear healthy, débridement is considered complete and reconstruction may begin. We stress that the key to a successful reconstruction is effective wound excision (12,14,24,43).

STARTING THE RECONSTRUCTION

Once débridement is considered complete, a "shopping list" of the anatomic parts needed is made. In the case of wounds requiring only microvascular soft-tissue transfer, the dimensions of the defect and the length of the pedicle is the only information gathered. Lesser wounds may lend themselves to reconstruction with local flap closure or skin grafting. If a complex composite reconstruction will be done during the initial procedure, the amount of missing bone, length of tendon defects, nerve gap, size of the flap, and length of the pedicle are all assessed and measured. The presence of a second team with whom to share the duties of harvesting and reconstruction will enhance the use of surgical time and resources.

Emergency Free Tissue Transfer

Stable bony architecture, adequate débridement, good blood supply adjacent to the recipient site, good recipient vessels, a flap that can at least cover the major structures needing protection and nutrition, skin graft coverage available for structures not at risk, and a patient whose condition will remain stable during surgery are the essential components for emergency free flap coverage. Osteosynthesis, interosseous wires, Kirschner wires, screws, plate-and-screws, or external fixators are methods by which bone fixation may be done. The flap may be applied during the first procedure for healing, and bone grafting done later.

One definition of emergency free flaps is "those that are performed at the end of the primary débridement, within 24 hours of the time of the injury" (43). The senior author has found that patients whose wounds are covered within 24 hours after injury have a better postoperative course, including a lower complication rate, higher flap survival rate, and better functional recovery. To date, emergency free flap coverage for combination injuries has been used in 102 patients with a 95.1% flap survival rate and 6.5% infection rate.

Even free flaps done during the first 3 days after injury do better than those delayed longer and are associated with better survival rates, lower rates of infection, and shorter hospitalization (12). In our unit we have found this also to be the case. Unfortunately, the patient's general condition or that of the injured part does not always allow immediate coverage—or even coverage during the first 3 days. Under these circumstances, staged reconstruction is done. Sundine and Scheker (13) demonstrated that patients with staged reconstructions in dorsal hand defects have a hospital stay, time off work, and number of operations three times greater than patients undergoing one-stage reconstructions.

Staged Reconstruction

When immediate reconstruction is impossible, conservation of health care system resources is achieved if the patient is discharged and taken care of by home health care personnel. Many such patients receive soft-tissue coverage in their first procedure, bone grafting in the second, and tendon grafts or transfers and nerve grafts in the final procedure.

Staged reconstructions require more planning about what is available and what can be spared and are more difficult than those done immediately in one procedure. During dissection through the extensive scar tissue associated with staged reconstructions, blood vessels and nerves are difficult to identify, and even the most experienced surgeon can damage them.

SURGICAL METHODS

One excellent way to describe surgical methods is to present specific cases with increasing demands as to the size of the defect and the elements to be reconstructed. In this section, we will consider all types of defects, from those amenable to skin grafting or local flap closure to those wounds requiring emergency microvascular soft-tissue transfer for coverage of complex defects. Reconstruction for these complex injuries varies from the single flap that provides all necessary components for reconstruction to the fasciocutaneous flap utilized to house elements (including bone, tendon, and nerve) harvested separately from the original flap.

Many wounds not amenable to primary closure can be managed by skin grafting. Certain situations, however, will preclude the use of skin grafts (e.g., exposed bone devoid of periosteum, exposed joint surface, bare tendons stripped of paratenon, or exposed metal used for skeletal fixation). The anatomy of the hand allows closure of small wounds with a myriad of local flaps for resurfacing exposed vital structures. Larger wounds frequently require microvascular free tissue transfer for reconstruction.

Fingertip and Digital Injuries

In fingertip injuries, for loss of digital pulp associated with exposed bone or other vital structures (when digital shortening is not an option), several local sensory flaps can be considered. Small defects in the volar fingertips can be covered with a local advancement flap. Examples of these include the Tranquilli-Leali volar V-Y flap (44) popularized by Atasoy (45), the Kutler double lateral advancement flap (46), and, in the case of more extensive thumb volar tip loss, the Moberg advancement flap (47). Transposition of a neurovascular pedicle island flap from the dorsum of the index finger has also been done successfully for reconstruction of badly injured thumbs (48,49). The Littler palmar heterodigital neurovascular island flap (50) for thumb pulp replacement is less used today. Additionally, Foucher (51) has described the use of homodigital neurovascular island flaps for digital pulp loss. Another flap used for fingertip reconstruction is the thenar flap (52–57), first described by Flatt in 1955. Other illustrations of local flap use in reconstruction of fingertip injuries can also be found in the literature (58–60).

More proximal digital soft-tissue defects can also be resurfaced by a variety of local flaps. Examples of these include neurosensory island flaps (61–63), V-Y advancement flaps (64), cross-finger (65–68), and reversed cross-finger flaps (69,70).

Hueston (71) repaired fingertip injuries and guillotine amputations by directly transposing the volar digital integument distally as a local flap. He preferred this reconstructive method over cross-finger flaps because it (a) is a single-stage procedure, (b) is applicable to multiple adjacent digital injuries, and (c) provides skin coverage of appearance, texture, and sensibility nearer to normal than any cross-finger flap.

Dorsal Hand Defects

For reconstruction of dorsal hand defects, including those requiring coverage of the proximal interphalangeal (PIP) joint, flaps based on the dorsal metacarpal arteries can be used. Small and Brennen (72) reported a series of 20 cases in which a first dorsal metacarpal artery neurovascular island flap for reconstruction of hand defects was employed. Uses included sensory resurfacing of the thumb (six cases) and release of a contracted first web (five cases) in addition to soft-tissue coverage in acute hand defects. Others have described the use of flaps based on the first dorsal metacarpal artery in resurfacing various hand soft-tissue defects (72–74).

Second dorsal metacarpal artery island flaps have also been used by several authors for coverage of local skin defects in the hand (75–77). Possible applications include resurfacing thumb defects and defects on the radial side of the palm and release of first web contractures (i.e., uses similar to those described for the first dorsal metacarpal artery island flap).

Distally based dorsal hand flaps have recently been described by Quaba and Davidson (78) and Maruyama (79). Being reverse flaps, they are not sensate. Many local dorsal hand and web space defects, however, lend themselves to coverage with these reverse dorsal metacarpal flaps.

Palmar Hand Defects

Skin defects are less frequent on the palm than on the dorsal aspect of the hand. Flap coverage is usually necessary for more extensive defects. Several flap techniques are available, depending on the wound requirements.

Moiemen and Elliot (80) discussed a technique of distal palmar soft-tissue advancement into the fingers for proximal defects of their volar aspects, with V-Y closure of the donor defect. Several indications for using this procedure were illustrated in a series of 55 patients.

Earley demonstrated a constant blood supply to the dorsum of the first web skin, allowing its use as an island advancement flap for reconstruction in cases with minor loss of palmar skin or in moderate first web contractures (81).

Use of an island flap supplied by the dorsal branch of the ulnar artery for coverage of the ulnar-sided dorsal and volar wrist as well as proximal hand defects has been described by Becker and Gilbert (82). They originally reported eight cases, one with an island flap, four with pedicled flaps, and three with fascial flaps. A modification of their technique that resulted in improved venous outflow was proposed by Holevich-Madjarova and others (83).

In more extensive defects not reparable by local means, microvascular free tissue transfer of soft-tissue cover is necessary. Some authors have advocated coverage using fasciocutaneous (lateral arm, radial forearm) free flaps for palmar resurfacing (22,25,26). When the palm is the recipient site these flaps may not be entirely satisfactory, however, because the skin cover thus provided is too mobile on the subcutaneous layer. Use of free muscle flaps, specifically the pronator quadratus, followed by skin grafting for coverage of palmar defects has been proposed by Dautel and Merle (84) as an alternative to cutaneous free flap coverage.

Coverage of More Extensive Hand and Upper-Extremity Defects

Every complex extremity wound requiring a distant flap for its reconstruction presents a different defect after wound excision; therefore, no single flap or reconstruction method is suitable for all occasions. When selecting a flap, the surgeon must consider not only the surface-area deficit but also the volume requirements. This concept of volume versus surface area must be clear in the surgeon's mind. When the final defect is a cavity, the flap must fill it. Muscle flaps with their bulkiness can help attain this goal, not only filling the defect but also in contouring to the irregularities found in some wounds. Often, reconstruction of the bony architecture itself eliminates cavities, and soft-tissue reconstruction can proceed with a fascial or fasciocutaneous flap. When extensor tendons are grafted to bridge a defect, a fasciocutaneous flap allowing tendon excursion through its fatty tissue can be used (8).

Microvascular free tissue transfer can also be used to preserve function of elements not directly involved in the trauma. The simplest reconstruction in these cases is a well-

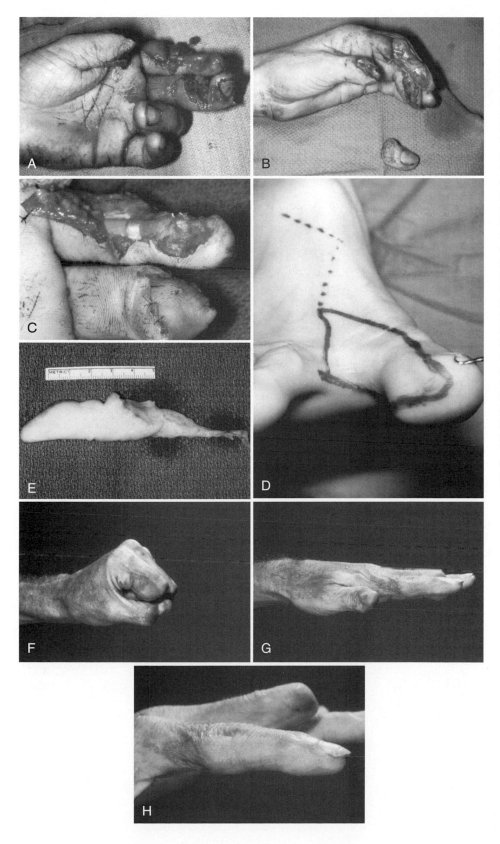

FIG. 88–2.   A, B, a middle-aged laborer who injured his left hand with a circular saw, sustaining amputations of his thumb and middle finger at the distal interphalangeal joint. Additionally, the index finger lost the skin and subcutaneous tissue on its radial aspect, exposing both flexor and extensor tendons; the radial neurovascular bundle was also destroyed. **C,** after wound excision the thumb was replanted and the long finger revised (no distal part was available for replantation). The defect on the index finger extended from the middle of the proximal phalanx to the tip, which was missing most of its pulp. **D, E,** both flexor and extensor tendons required coverage. Sensation on the radial aspect of the index finger is imperative for its function in opposing the thumb during fine manipulation. Glabrous skin is required for the tips of the fingers not only for function but also for appearance. A 2.5 × 8 cm flap from the first web space of the foot was therefore harvested, based on the first dorsal metatarsal artery. This included the lateral aspect of the big toe and its pulp. The deep peroneal nerve was taken with the flap to provide sensation to the radial aspect of the index finger. **F–H,** any other reconstruction would have been less than satisfactory. A therapy program was immediately instituted. The result was recovery of full range of motion for the index finger, with a two-point discrimination of 7 mm.

FIG. 88–3. **A,** a 21-year-old woman had a transmetacarpal amputation of her left hand sustained while operating a punch press. **B,** this crush injury required such wide débridement that, even though the metacarpals ended up shorter than the proximal phalanges, **C,** an extensive skin defect from the carpus to the web spaces remained. The soft-tissue defect not only encompassed the dorsum of the hand but also the first web space and the thumb metacarpal head. The volar forearm had already been incised to harvest the veins necessary to bridge vascular gaps. **D,** her amputation was distal to the superficial palmar arch; both the radial and ulnar arteries had good flow. After the hand was replanted, the extensor tendons and dorsal veins remained exposed. Viable tissue was required both to cover these structures and help ensure survival of the replanted part. Considering the patient's youth and gender as well as the presence of an incision on the volar aspect of the forearm, it was decided to utilize this incision to harvest a distally-based radial artery fascial flap. The flap measured 5 x 16 cm and was raised at the level of the superficial veins, maintaining the viability of the volar skin for direct closure of the donor site defect. Additionally, a bridge of intact skin was preserved at the level of the wrist to minimize scarring between the flexor tendons and the overlying incisions. **E, F,** the flap was passed under the skin bridge at the wrist, turned over, and inset with the subcutaneous fat facing the extensor tendons. **G,** with the original fatty top surface of the fascial flap now facing down, an appropriate paratenonlike plane was provided for optimal tendon gliding, while the smooth fascia, rich in blood supply and ideal for skin grafting, faced up. **H,** in the 13 years since her surgery, she has continued her employment as an assembly line worker, refusing further thumb reconstructive procedures (the flap cover over the metacarpal head has provided enough padding for the stump to work appropriately).

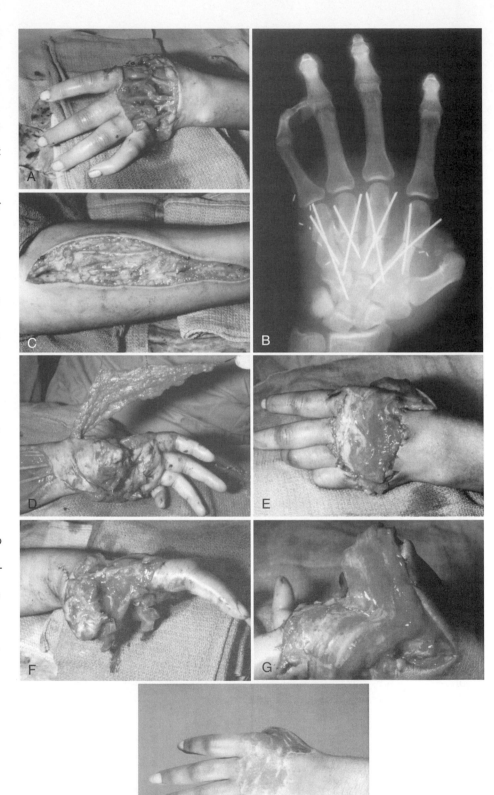

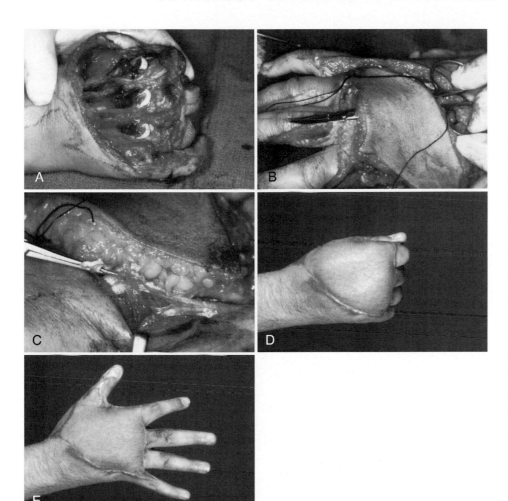

FIG. 88–4. **A,** a 14-year-old boy lost the dorsal skin of his hand and thumb in an MVA. **B,** the metacarpal heads were shaved in an oblique manner and the skeleton of the thumb was lost. It was necessary to provide stability for the thumb with a bone graft and early coverage for the exposed joints so that (a) the cartilage did not suffer permanent damage by desiccation, and (b) the risk of infection would be lessened. The extensor mechanism was damaged within the zone of injury with disruption to the extensor hood and the extrinsic/intrinsic system linkages. Primary tendon grafting was planned to restore extensor mechanism function. A lateral arm flap was used to provide the large area of soft tissue required in this patient, even though it was a bit thick for the dorsum of the hand. The thumb, which had lost skin, tendon, and some bone, was stabilized by means of a segment of bone from the lateral aspect of the humerus. The fascia of the flap was sutured around its margins. Then, tunnels in the direction of each extensor tendon were made using tenotomy scissors (8,39). **C,** the tendon grafts were threaded through the tunnels and connected distally and proximally. **D, E,** shortly after surgery, an extensor outrigger splint was used to initiate early protected motion. Good final function was obtained.

vascularized free flap that allows early mobilization 72 hours after injury (Fig. 88–2). Flaps can cover elements of a replanted part (Fig. 88–3).

Little fat is found between bone and skin in both the wrist and the dorsum of the hand. Thus, soft-tissue loss in those areas often entails the destruction of extensor tendons, and reconstruction must supply tendon grafts as well as vascularized skin. For defects of small size, a relatively small flap with a cuff of fascia that is wider than the overlying skin paddle can be applied to the critical area. A skin graft can then be placed on the fascia of the flap or on the forearm to limit the size of the donor defect.

Composite defects, such as those needing tendon and bone as well as soft-tissue cover, can be reconstructed with a single flap composed of all these structures. This is not recommended, however, in dorsal hand injuries that involve all extensor tendons (8,39) (Fig. 88–4).

Defects of the forearm are treated differently depending on whether the injury is to the proximal, middle, or distal third. A reconstruction is staged when the defect encompasses all the soft tissue of the forearm. The first stage consists of coverage. The groin flap, either as a pedicled or free flap, can be used on the dorsal aspect of the forearm. The free groin flap has the advantage of allowing immediate mobilization of finger joints and elevation of the extremity to reduce swelling.

Primary tendon transfer is done only when the joints to be moved by the transferred tendon are sound. If a fracture necessitates immobilization of the joint that the transferred tendon will act upon, the transfer is definitely not to be done because adhesions will lock the tendon in place. When segmental loss of a tendon causes its muscle to retract, however, a small tendon graft is done primarily to stretch the muscle close to its original anatomic length. In the future, tendon transfer (or perhaps simply tenolysis) is done to restore adequate excursion.

The second stage of reconstruction is the time when tendon transfer is generally done. Likewise, muscle is not transferred to the forearm until the coverage has healed completely and the joints regain motion sufficient to allow the muscle to do its work. Following this two-staged sequence, reconstruction can often achieve good range of motion (Fig. 88–5).

Injuries to the volar forearm, in which are found muscles, tendons, and two major nerves and arteries vital to proper hand function, are treated differently than injuries to the dorsal aspect. When soft tissue is destroyed in this area, revascularization must take place for the hand to survive; only then can attention be directed to reinnervation and motor function. If a substantial amount of tissue is lost (Fig. 88–6A, B), a main goal is to provide muscle (in this case, a latis-

FIG. 88–5. **A,** in an MVA, this patient totally lost the extensor compartment, damaged the wrist joint, and fractured the PIP joints of the long and ring fingers. **B,** after débridement, extensor tendons would need to be replaced if wrist, finger, and thumb function were to be restored. Coverage during the first procedure was done using a groin flap. **C–E,** 6 weeks later, the flap was supple and all joints were mobile, and a second procedure was done involving pronator teres transfer for wrist extension, flexor carpi radialis harvest for finger extension, and palmaris longus for thumb extension. At the patient's request, defatting of the flap was done later.

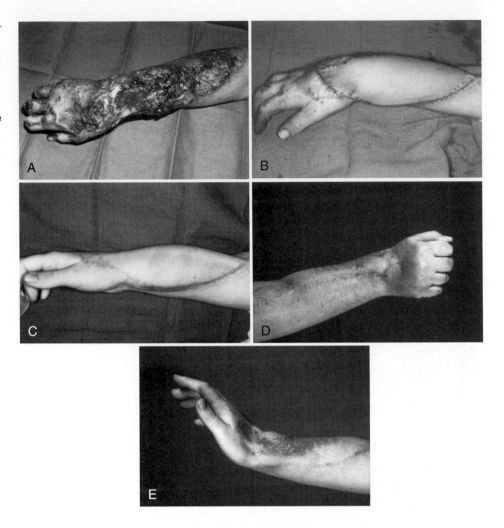

FIG. 88–6. **A, B,** the presenting wound. **C,** in this patient the arm was revascularized by anastomosing a saphenous vein graft end-to-end to connect both ends of the radial and ulnar arteries. Because the nerve staining techniques were not available on an emergency basis, two sural nerve grafts were done as an elective procedure 8 weeks later to repair the gaps in the median and ulnar nerves. **D,** 3 months after injury.

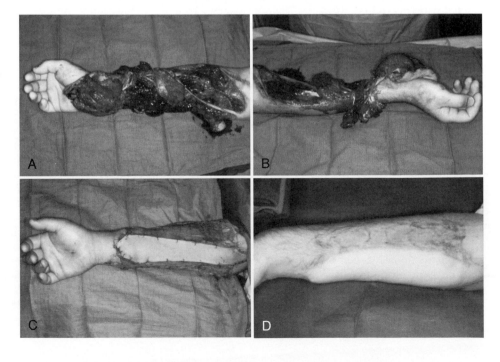

simus dorsi flap) that will bring some function as well as provide coverage (Fig. 88–6C, D). Primary nerve grafting is augmented, if possible, by staining techniques to distinguish motor and sensory fascicles (85).

In the distal forearm, loss of a segment of soft tissue without joint involvement can be treated to some extent by bone shortening without affecting muscle function. If bone is also present, reconstruction addresses bone, tendon, and soft-tissue deficits in that order. Thin or fat individuals are treated differently. A fasciocutaneous flap is the first choice in thin persons, but the panniculus adiposus in fat persons hinders coverage of the defect (Figs. 88–7 and 88–8).

Cutaneous flaps in fat persons are unwieldy. A muscle flap covered by a split-thickness skin graft is more useful and has the added advantage that, if denervated, it loses 25 to 50% of its bulk over time.

Often, injury to the elbow involves a large area of injured skin, lost muscles and tendons, and, occasionally, exposed bones and joints. Especially when a procedure is done to salvage the elbow joint, it will require coverage. Early motion will improve elbow flexion and extension significantly. Thus, coverage with abundant skin, such as that afforded by the scapular flap, is planned for this purpose if the defect is shallow and regular (86–90).

Irregularly shaped defects and those with small cavities needing to be filled are best covered with muscle flaps. The latissimus dorsi muscle flap is the workhorse of this category, but when the patient has injuries necessitating the use of crutches following surgery, a rectus abdominis free flap and skin grafts will both cover the defect and allow adequate range of motion (91) (Fig. 88–9).

Any muscle flap to cover the posterior aspect of the elbow is sutured in place with the elbow fully flexed. Similarly, the elbow is placed in full extension when flaps are applied to its anterior aspect. Because even full-thickness skin grafts contract, preventing full extension, flaps are used to cover antecubital fossa defects, especially if the biceps tendon is being reconstructed at the same time.

In patients with an unreplantable amputation, the length of the proximal stump can sometimes be maintained only through microvascular free tissue transfer. In this situation, a filet flap, which is made of uninjured skin from the amputated part, constitutes one option for coverage of the stump. The patient is spared additional donor site morbidity, and a part is used that would otherwise be discarded.

Postoperative Care

Penrose or silastic drains, several of which are usually inserted under the flap, allow drainage by gravity and so prevent the formation of hematomas. Dry gauze dressing, sufficient to absorb the flap's drainage, is used in preference to circumferential deep dressings. Excess bulk between the fingers can increase edema and venous congestion. The dressing maintains the flap in a position free from tension and eliminates pressure in the area of the vascular pedicle. It is fashioned (a) to prevent the patient from moving the arm behind the back or rolling onto it, and (b) to provide the patient with support and comfort. With the elbow flexed 90° and covered with plaster of Paris, a loose cylinder of foam padding is wrapped around the arm; a window is cut into the padding for observation of the flap.

Kept warm and hemodynamically stable, both patient and flap are monitored carefully, as vessel occlusion can result in a sudden decrease in flap temperature or decrease in laser Doppler readings. Unfortunately, because of heat transfer from the patient's bed, the temperature of even poorly perfused flaps can register in an acceptable range.

Clinical observation, photoplethysmography (PPG), and laser Doppler are used to monitor the patient (92–94). The PPG monitor is first calibrated and a baseline reading taken; then subsequent tracings from the flap are compared to it. Clinical monitoring varies depending on the patient's skin color. In light-skinned patients, both blanching of a portion of a skin flap upon gentle pressure and needle pricks to induce bleeding can help assess the flap's condition. In dark-skinned individuals, for whom the blanching technique is helpful only under special circumstances, flap status is best assessed by needle pricks, PPG, and temperature monitoring. In muscle flaps, stimulating a motor nerve that has been left exposed will cause muscle twitch in a viable flap (Rafael Acosta, M.D., personal communication).

The flap is inspected immediately if its temperature suddenly drops 3° while the patient's body temperature remains unchanged. Tight dressings are promptly released. If the status of the flap does not begin to improve right away, reexploration of the pedicle is done in the operating room. The patients are maintained NPO for 24 hours after the initial procedure, because most problems in this period are related to vascular flow at the site of the anastomoses, such as kinking or hematoma compressing the pedicle. These problems can only be corrected with a quick response to decreased perfusion as shown by continuous monitoring of the flap. After the 3rd day, flap failure is often caused by infection rather than vascular problems.

Flow in the flap and extremity, especially if the injury is extensive or involves crushing, can be assisted by administration of low-molecular-weight dextran (LMD) and low-dose continuous heparin. To a 500-cc bag of LMD we add 5000 units of heparin; an initial bolus of 100 cc is administered, followed by maintenance of a continuous infusion at a rate of 30 cc per hour. The infusion is continued for approximately 5 days; however, it is necessary to watch for hematoma formation under the flap.

DYNAMIC SPLINTING AND PHYSICAL THERAPY

After the drains are removed, usually within 72 hours following surgery, a plaster of Paris splint with an outrigger apparatus is put in place. This allows the commencement of assisted active range of motion exercises. Within 3 weeks, custom-fabricated braces are tailored to a specific range of motion. In patients with no intrinsic muscle function, the splint generally blocks the metacarpophalangeal (MCP) joints in a flexed position but allows distal interphalangeal (DIP) and PIP joint extension. When the intrinsics are intact and the extrinsic extensor tendons have been replaced, MCP joint motion is permitted. Such braces are adjusted as required, depending on the extent of edema and the nature of the repair.

COMPLICATIONS

Complications related to reconstruction in acute hand injuries vary proportionally with the complexity of the procedure. Infection remains a concern despite the excellent and wide

FIG. 88–7.   A, a grain auger fractured both bones of the dominant forearm of a thin man with a segmental injury to the ulna. A radiograph showing extent of injury. **B,** massive soft tissue damage resulted in exposed fractures and wide débridement of muscle bellies, leaving tendons with no proximal attachments. Shown after débridement. **C,** by side-to-side suturing, a common tendon was made to restore motion to the index and middle fingers. While the ring and small fingers were required to share the sublimis, the flexor digitorum profundus was intact. Internal fixation was provided for both forearm bones. **D, E,** a scapular flap was used for skin coverage because a skin graft would have adhered to both muscle and tendon. **F–I,** after recovery, the patient had full ROM. The bulky flap was reduced through defatting and skin shortening. Full pronation, supination, flexion, and extension were present at his final follow-up visit 2 years later.

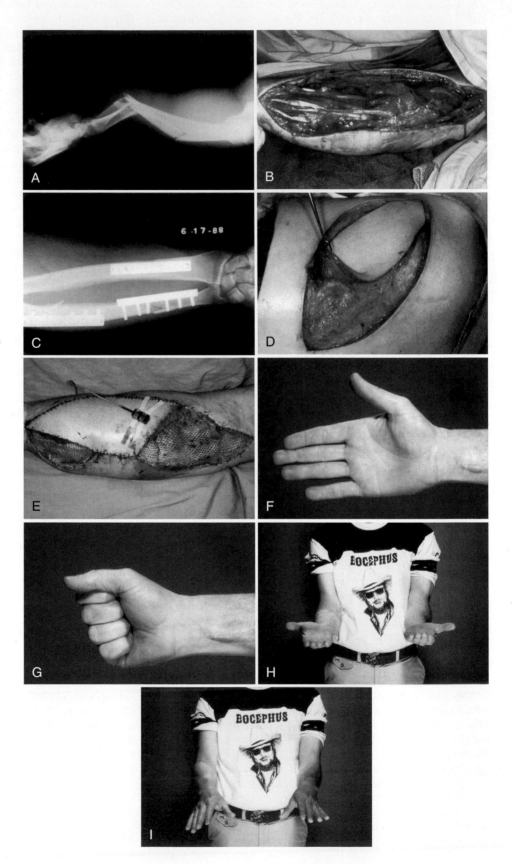

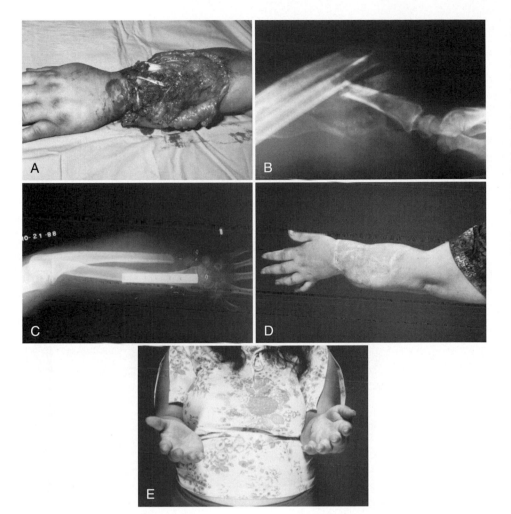

FIG. 88–8. A, B, an MVA caused open fractures of a woman's forearm bones and extensive soft tissue injury. A radiograph and preoperative view of extent of open wound. **C,** her distal radioulnar joint was destroyed. Following complete débridement, the radius and extensor tendons were both shortened. With the establishment of good bony contact, fixation was done with a compression plate. A radiograph shows internal fixation. **D, E,** the fracture site and exposed bone were covered with a latissimus dorsi flap, which in turn had a split-thickness skin graft. While final ROM was only acceptable, her injured hand was able to assist the uninjured hand.

array of antimicrobial pharmaceutical agents available. This risk again underscores the need for complete and thorough wound débridement before initiation of any reconstructive method.

Microvascular free tissue transfer for immediate coverage in acute hand injuries exemplifies the most complex of reconstructive methods. Like any surgical procedure, it entails the risk of various complications, which for purposes of this discussion we are categorizing as early or late. Early complications include the following, the first three of which can cause flap failure: thrombosis at the anastomosis sites; hematoma formation in the same location; infection occurring at either the recipient or donor sites; and failure of split-thickness skin grafts (sometimes used to avoid pressure on the vascular pedicle). Donor-site morbidity, tendon adhesions, joint stiffness, and inadequate return of sensation are examples of late complications.

Superficial infection and skin graft loss were the most common complications occurring in the senior author's series of free flaps done within 24-hours of injury (43). Deep infection caused flap failure in patients who had severe crush injuries and incomplete wound excision of the type described above. This makes it clear that emergency free flaps are not beneficial for all patients. In a limb subjected to a severe crush injury, for instance, amputation may be the only way to

débride the wound adequately. However, if the treating surgeon doubts the viability of tissue in or adjacent to the wound, or if the patient refuses amputation as an option, staged débridement can buy time. As long as the patient's life is not at risk, this may provide both patient and surgeon time to accept what may be an inevitable outcome.

Thrombosis of the vascular pedicle following emergency free flap reconstruction is generally related to poor planning and problems with microsurgical technique. Tension or redundancy in a pedicle, for instance, are both associated with formation of thrombi.

Hematoma accumulation under the flap, a common sequela of inadequate hemostasis and subsequent increased drainage, not only endangers flap viability, as mentioned above, but also increases the risk of infection. While anticoagulation drugs can have great benefit, their advantages must be balanced against the problems that can be caused by hematoma formation.

COMPARISON OF OUTCOMES

While functional outcomes have always been important to health care providers, outcomes regarding cost to the patient and the health care system must also be considered. Time spent with the patient by a variety of providers, and the resources and facilities required for treatment, are factors in

FIG. 88–9. A–C, in this patient, who also had fracture of the ring finger, middle phalanx, and an elbow fracture with bone loss, fractures of the tibia and fibula resulting from an MVA required the use of crutches. Radiographs and view of open wound show extent of injury. **D,** a plate and screw were used for fixation. **E, F,** the ipsilateral rectus abdominis flap that was chosen (91) was anastomosed end-to-side to the brachial artery and to the basilic vein and covered by a full-thickness skin graft that allowed 110° of elbow flexion. The final ROM 2 years after injury.

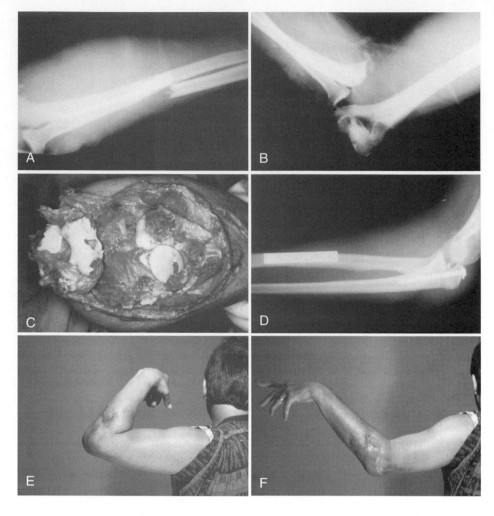

such a determination. Recently, a study by Sundine and Scheker (13) compared various outcome factors of patients having single-stage emergency free flap procedures with those having multistage reconstructions. Regarding return to work, 85% of patients with single-stage reconstruction resumed employment, while only 33% of patients with multistage reconstructions did so. Maximum range of motion was achieved within 6 months by single-stage reconstruction patients, whereas this took 2 years for patients who had multistage reconstruction. The total number of surgical interventions required by these two groups of patients was dramatically different: Patients with emergency free flaps had two, while patients undergoing staged reconstruction had seven.

Conclusion

Treatment of the severely injured arm or hand is founded upon a careful consideration of all injured structures, complete débridement, multifactorial planning of the reconstruction, good surgical technique, and comprehensive, consistent postoperative care and rehabilitation. Each of these elements must be pursued with great diligence for the patient to have a good result. Emergency free tissue transfer is but part of a total reconstructive plan that addresses all damaged and missing structures. One of its primary aims in complex reconstructions is to provide a well-vascularized bed to optimize healing and ultimately restore function to important anatomic elements. The extra effort and energy expended during the first surgery will be time well spent toward the principal goal—rapid return of the patient to independence and a healthy, active life.

References

1. MacGregor IA, Morgan G. Axial and random pattern flaps. *Br J Plast Surg* 1973; 26:202.
2. Haller J. Guy de Chauliac and his chirurgica magna. *Surg* 1964; 55:337.
3. Nicaise E. *La grande chiruragie de Guy de Chauliac.* Paris: Alcan, 1890.
4. Breidenbach WC III. Emergency free tissue transfer for reconstruction of acute upper extremity wounds. *Clin Plast Surg* 1989; 16(3):505.
5. Kleinert HE, Kasdan ML, Romero JL. Small blood vessel anastomosis for salvage of severely injured upper extremity. *J Bone Joint Surg* 1963; 45A:788.
6. Komatsu S, Tamai S. Successful replantation of a completely cut off thumb. *Plast Reconstr Surg* 1968; 42:374.
7. MacGregor IA, Jackson IT. The groin flap. *Br J Plast Surg* 1972; 25:3.
8. Scheker LR, Langley SJ, Martin DL, et al. Primary extensor tendon reconstruction in dorsal hand defects requiring free flaps. *J Hand Surg* 1993; 18B:568.
9. Byrd H, Cierney G III, Tebbetts J. Management of open tibial fractures with association soft tissue loss: external pin fixation with early flap coverage. *Plast Reconstr Surg* 1981; 68:73.

10. Byrd H, Spicer TE, Cierney G III. Management of open tibial fractures. *Plast Reconstr Surg* 1985; 76:719.

11. Cierney G III, Byrd H, Jones R. Primary versus delayed soft tissue coverage for severe open tibial fractures. *Clin Ortho* 1983; 178:54.

12. Godina M. Early microsurgical reconstruction of complex trauma of the extremities. *Plast Reconstr Surg* 1986; 78:285.

13. Sundine M, Scheker LR. A comparison of immediate and staged reconstruction of the dorsum of the hand. Presented at the 25th Anniversary Meeting of the American Association for Hand Surgery, Marco Island, Florida, January 1995. *J Hand Surg* 1996; 21B:216. Accepted for publication in *Br J Hand Surg,* 1995.

14. Foucher G, Citron N. The role of microvascular surgery in acute hand injuries. In: Soutar D, ed. *Microvascular surgery and free tissue transfer.* London: Edward Arnold, 1993; 54.

15. Robbins SL, Cotran RS, Kumar V. Inflammation and repair. In: Robbins SL, Cotran RS, Kumar V, eds. *Pathologic basis of disease.* 3rd ed. Philadelphia: WB Saunders, 1984; 40.

16. Belliappa PP, Scheker LR. Functional anatomy of the hand. *Emerg Med Clin N Am* 1993; 11(3):557.

17. Tubiana R. *The hand.* Vol. 1. Philadelphia: WB Saunders, 1981.

18. Zancolli E. *Structural and dynamic basis of hand surgery.* 2nd ed. Philadelphia: JB Lippincott, 1979.

19. Zancolli EA, Cozzi EP. *Atlas of surgical anatomy of the hand.* New York: Churchill Livingstone, 1992.

20. Tsai TM, Wang WZ. Vascularized joint transfers: indications and results. *Hand Clinics* 1992; 8(3):525.

21. Taylor GI, Collett RJ. Microvascular free transfer of a dorsalis pedis skin flap with extensor tendons. In: Strauch B, Vasconez LO, Hall-Findlay EJ, eds. *Grabb's encyclopedia of flaps.* Vol. II, Upper extremities. Boston: Little, Brown, 1990.

22. Katsaros J, Schusterman M, Beppu M et al. The lateral upper arm flap. Anatomy and clinical applications. *Ann Plast Surg* 1984; 12:489.

23. Scheker LR, Kleinert HE, Hanel DP. Lateral arm composite tissue transfer to ipsilateral hand defects. *J Hand Surg* 1987; 12A:665.

24. Scheker LR. Soft-tissue defects of the upper limb. In: Soutar DS, ed. *Microvascular surgery and free tissue transfer.* London: Edward Arnold, 1993; 63.

25. Muhlbourner W, Herndle E, Stock W. The forearm flap. *Plast Reconstr Surg* 1982; 70:336.

26. Song R, Gao Y, Song Y, et al. The forearm flap. *Clinics Plast Surg* 1982; 9:21.

27. Soutar DS, Scheker LR, McGregor IA, et al. The radial forearm flap. A versatile method for intraoral reconstruction. *Br J Plast Surg* 1983; 36:1.

28. Ohmori K, Harii K. Free dorsalis pedis sensory flap to the hand with microneurovascular anastomoses. *Plast Reconstr Surg* 1976; 58:546.

29. McCraw JB. On the transfer of a free dorsalis pedis sensory flap to the hand. *Plast Reconstr Surg* 1977; 59:738.

30. Man D, Acland RD. The microarterial anatomy of the dorsalis pedis flap and its clinical applications. *Plast Reconstr Surg* 1980; 65:419.

31. Robinson DW. Microsurgical transfer of the dorsalis pedis neurovascular island flap. *Br J Plast Surg* 1976; 29:209.

32. Robinson DW. Dorsalis pedis flaps. In: Serafin D, Buncke H Jr, eds. *Microsurgical composite tissue transplantation.* St Louis: CV Mosby, 1978; 257.

33. Morrison WA, MacLeod AM, Gilbert A. Neurovascular free flaps from the foot for innervation of the hand. *J Hand Surg* 1978; 3:235.

34. Gordon L, Buncke HJ, Alpert BS, et al. Free vascularized osteocutaneous transplants from the groin for delayed primary closure in the management of loss of soft tissue in the hand and wrist. Report of two cases. *J Bone Joint Surg* 1985; 67(A):958.

35. Shah KG, Garrett JC, Buncke HJ. Free groin flap transfer to the upper extremity. *Hand* 1979; 11:315.

36. Harii K, Ohmori K, Torii S, et al. Free groin skin flaps. *Br J Plast Surg* 1975; 28:225.

37. Acland RD. The free iliac flap. A lateral modification of the free groin flap. *Plast Reconstr Surg* 1979; 64:30.

38. Baudet J, LeMaire JM, Guimberteau JC. Ten free groin flaps. *Plast Reconstr Surg* 1976; 57:577.

39. Swartz WM. Immediate reconstruction of the wrist and dorsum of hand with a free osteocutaneous groin flap. *J Hand Surg* 1984; 9(A):18.

40. Scheker LR. Salvage of a mutilated hand. In: Cohen MN, ed. *Mastery of plastic and reconstructive surgery.* Boston: Little, Brown, 1994; 1658.

41. Toth BA, Elliot LF. Aesthetic refinements in reconstructive microsurgery. *Ann Plast Surg* 1989; 22:117.

42. Graham B, Adkins P, Scheker LR. Complications and morbidity of the donor and recipient sites in 123 lateral arm emergency flaps. *J Hand Surg* 1992; 17(B):189.

43. Tranquilli-Leali E. Ricostruzione dell' apice della falange ungeali mediante autoplastica volare. *Infort Traum Lavoro* 1935; 1:186.

44. Atasoy E, Ioakimidis E, Kasdan ML, et al. Reconstruction of the amputated finger tip with a triangular volar flap. *J Bone Joint Surg* 1970; 52A:921.

45. Lister G, Scheker L. Emergency free flaps to the upper extremity. *J Hand Surg* 1988; 13A:22.

46. Kutler W. A new method for finger tip amputation. *JAMA* 1947; 133:29.

47. Moberg E. Aspects of sensation and reconstructive surgery of the upper extremity. *J Bone Joint Surg* 1964; 46A:817.

48. Foucher G, Braun JB. A new island flap transfer from the dorsum of the index to the thumb. *Plast Reconstr Surg* 1979; 63(3):344.

49. Shi SM, Lu YP. Island skin flap with neurovascular pedicle from the dorsum of the index finger for reconstruction of the thumb. *Microsurg* 1994; 15:145.

50. Littler JW. Neurovascular pedicle transfer of tissue in reconstructive surgery of the hand. *J Bone Joint Surg* 1956; 38A:917.

51. Foucher G, Smith D, Pempinello C, et al. Homodigital neurovascular island flaps for digital pulp loss. *J Hand Surg* 1989; 14B(2):204.

52. Flatt AE. Minor hand injuries. *J Bone Joint Surg* 1955; 37B:117.

53. Flatt AE. The thenar flap. *J Bone Joint Surg* 1957; 39B:80.

54. Barton NJ. A modified thenar flap. *The Hand* 1975, 7(2):150.

55. Smith RJ, Albin R. Thenar "H-flap" for finger tip injuries. *J Trauma* 1976.

56. Melone CP, Beasley RW, Carstens JH Jr. The thenar flap—an analysis of its use in 150 cases. *J Hand Surg* 1982; 7(3):291.

57. Dellon AL. The proximal inset thenar flap for fingertip reconstruction. *Plast Reconstr Surg* 1983; 72(5):698.

58. Russell RC, Van Beek AL, Wavak P, et al. Alternative hand flaps for amputations and digital defects. *J Hand Surg* 1981; 6(4):399.

59. Grad JB, Beasley RW. Fingertip reconstruction. *Hand Clin* 1985; 1(4):667.

60. Foucher G, Boulas HJ, Da Silva JB. The use of flaps in the treatment of fingertip injuries. *World J Surg* 1991; 15:458.

61. Bertelli JA, Khoury Z. Neurocutaneous island flaps in the hand: anatomical basis and preliminary results. *Br J Plast Surg* 1992; 45:586.

62. Niranjan NS, Armstrong JR. A homodigital reverse pedicle island flap in soft tissue reconstruction of the finger and the thumb. *J Hand Surg* 1994; 19B:135.

63. Evans DM, Martin DL. Step-advancement island flap for fingertip reconstruction. *Br J Plast Surg* 1988; 41(2):105.

64. Yii NW, Elliot D. Dorsal V-Y advancement flaps in digital reconstruction. *J Hand Surg* 1994; 19B(1):91.

65. Johnson RE, Iverson RE. Cross-finger pedicle flaps in the hand. *J Bone Joint Surg* 1971; 53A(5):913.

66. Kleinert HE, McCalister CG, MacDonald CJ, et al A critical evaluation of cross-finger flaps. *J Trauma* 1974; 14(9):756.

67. Kappel DA, Burech JG. The cross-finger flap: an established reconstructive procedure. *Hand Clin* 1985; 1(4):677.

68. Gault DT, Quaba AA. The role of cross-finger flaps in the primary management of untidy flexor tendon injuries. *J Hand Surg* 1988; 13B(1):62.

69. Atasoy E. The reversed cross-finger subcutaneous flap. *J Hand Surg* 1982; 7(5):481.

70. Martin DL, Kaplan IB, Kleinert JM. Use of a reverse cross-finger flap as a vascularized vein graft carrier in ring avulsion injuries. *J Hand Surg* 1990; 15A(1):155.

71. Hueston J. Local flap repair of fingertip injuries. *Plast Reconstr Surg* 1966; 37:349.

72. Small JO, Brennen MD. The first dorsal metacarpal artery neurovascular island flap. *J Hand Surg* 1989; 13B(2):136.

73. Sherif MM. First dorsal metacarpal artery flap in hand reconstruction. I. Anatomical study. *J Hand Surg* 1994; 19A:26.

74. Sherif MM. First dorsal metacarpal artery flap in hand reconstruction. II. Clinical application. *J Hand Surg* 1994; 19A:32.

75. Earley MJ. The second dorsal metacarpal artery neurovascular island flap. *J Hand Surg* 1989; 14B:434.

76. Small JO, Brennen MD. The second dorsal metacarpal artery neurovascular island flap. *Br J Plast Surg* 1990; 43:17.

77. Hao J, Xing-yan L, Bao-feng G, et al. The second dorsal metacarpal flap with vascular pedicle composed of the second dorsal metacarpal artery and the dorsal carpal branch of radial artery. *Plast Reconstr Surg* 1993; 92(3):501.

78. Maruyama Y. The reverse dorsal metacarpal flap. *Br J Plast Surg* 1990; 43:24.

79. Quaba AA, Davidson PM. The distally-based dorsal hand flap. *Br J Plast Surg* 1990; 43:28.

80. Moiemen N, Elliot D. Palmar V-Y reconstruction of proximal defects of the volar aspect of the digits. *Br J Plast Surg* 1994; 47:35.

81. Earley MJ. The first web flap. *J Hand Surg* 1989; 14B:65.

82. Becker C, Gilbert A. Der ulnaris-lappen. *Handchir Mikrochir Plast Chir* 1988; 20:180.

83. Holevich-Madjarova B, Paneva-Holevich E, Topkarov V. Island flap supplied by the dorsal branch of the ulnar artery. *Plast Reconstr Surg* 1991; 87:562.

84. Dautel G, Merle M. Pronator quadratus free muscle flap for treatment of palmar defects. *J Hand Surg* 1993; 18B:576.

85. Kanaya F, Ogden L, Breidenbach WC, et al. Sensory and motor fiber differentiation with Karnofsky staining. *J Hand Surg* 1991; 16(A):851.

86. Santos LF. The scapular flap: a new microsurgical free flap. *Revista Brasiliera de Cirurgia* 1980; 70:133.

87. Barwick WJ, Goodkind DJ, Serafin D. The free scapular flap. *Plast Reconstr Surg* 1982; 69:779.

88. Gilbert A, Teot L. The free scapular flap. *Plast Reconstr Surg* 1982; 69:601.

89. Hamilton SGL, Morrison WA. The scapular free flap. *Br J Plast Surg* 1982; 35:2.

90. Mayou BJ, Whitby D, Jones BM. The scapular flap—an anatomical clinical study. *Br J Plast Surg* 1982; 35:8.

91. Pennington DC, Lai MF, Pelly AD. The rectus abdominis myocutaneous free flap. *Br J Plast Surg* 1980; 33:277.

92. Buncke HJ, Lineweaver WC, Valauri FA, et al. Monitoring in microsurgery. In: *Transplantation replantation.* Philadelphia/London: Lea and Febiger, 1991; 715.

93. Scheker LR, Slattery PG, Firrell JC, et al. The value of the photoplethysmograph in monitoring skin closure in microsurgery. *J Reconstr Microsurg* 1985; 2(1):1.

94. Girling M. Monitoring in microvascular surgery. In: Soutar D, ed. *Microvascular surgery and free tissue transfer.* London: Edward Arnold, 1993; 26.

89

Replantation of Amputated Parts

Jay A. Goldberg, M.D., Harry J. Buncke, M.D., F.A.C.S., and Greg M. Buncke, M.D., F.A.C.S.

Whereas microvascular surgery has become an integral part of the plastic surgery training regimen, replantation and revascularization of amputated parts has become a ubiquitous procedure in plastic surgery practice. Although currently performed in both the university and community settings, the majority of these procedures should be performed in microsurgery centers. The technical expertise, specialized equipment, staffing, and logistical requirements all demand a concerted team effort that will result in the necessary clinical success and fiscal responsibility required in the 21st century.

Malt and McKhann (1) performed the first replantation on record, reporting 2 cases of arm replantations after train accidents, the first of which was performed in 1962. Research on the reanastomosis of small vessels had started in the late 1950s and early 1960s with the work of Jacobson and Suarez (2), Seidenberg (3), and Buncke and Schulz (4–6). Clinical reports of reanastomosis of small vessels soon followed, by Kleinert and Kasdan (7,8) in North America and by Chien and co-workers (9) and Komatsu and Tamai (10) in Asia. Acland's (11) seminal work on the refinement and standardization of microsurgical instruments, needles, and suture led to the routinely high success rates that we expect today.

The other factor that has resulted in high success rates has been the establishment of microsurgery centers. Only a center can provide the necessary team concept, which includes a qualified surgical team, experienced operating room personnel, dedicated operating room time, appropriate operative microscopes and instrumentation, adept perioperative nursing care, and an experienced hand therapy unit.

The surgery team typically consists of attending surgeons and surgeons in training. The length and tedious nature of replantation procedures necessitates more than one surgical team to maintain at least some "fresh" surgeons. Whether in the university or community setting, a microvascular laboratory is a necessary complement to provide the residents and fellows adequate training on animals both before and in addition to the clinical experience. On occasion, a single surgeon can run a busy microsurgery practice that consists of both elective microsurgery and a heavy replantation component. In order to accomplish this feat successfully, the surgeon must use surgical assistants, physician assistants, and nurse practitioners in lieu of residents and fellows. The surgery team should perform replantation procedures as a consistent portion of their clinical practice. In order to continue to perform these procedures in the present health care climate, surgeons will have to demonstrate that replantation can be performed with a high degree of certainty in a cost-effective manner.

Dedicated operating room time is essential to the expeditious treatment of amputations and devascularizations. Anesthesia personnel should be familiar with adjuvant nerve blocks, either axillary or interscalene, to block sympathetic tone to the involved extremity. Operating room personnel should be well versed in microvascular surgery protocols, surgical techniques, and instrumentation (12). The nurses should know to set up a table at which the amputated part is inspected before deciding the feasibility of replantation. There it is débrided and its structures are tagged. The operative microscope should be tested and readied before inspection of the amputated part. The circulating staff should be familiar with intravenous medications that the anesthesia team will use, and prepare intraoperative irrigation fluids. The operative microscope ideally should have a 200–250 millimeter lens, and an assistant viewing head with an independently controlled zoom, focus, and X-Y control. Television monitors and video equipment allow the whole team to follow the microvascular procedure, promoting teaching and a sense of involvement. Proper care and selection of the surgical instruments to prevent magnetization and/or injury is imperative to a smooth-running procedure.

Perioperative nursing care is important for initial triage, patient preparation for the operation, maximization of the patient's perioperative physiologic status, and monitoring of the replanted part. Functional results are as dependent upon the postoperative rehabilitation as the operative technique. Therefore, close surgeon/therapist interaction significantly improves the results of surgery.

Indications

With high technical success rates a given, indications for replantation now must reflect functional considerations. Although initially most patients think saving a body part is worth all cost and effort, they will not later express appreciation for a cold, painful, stiff appendage. We, as clinicians rather than as technicians, must opt for replantation only if a part has expected function. Furthermore, present cost constraints in the health care system will no doubt make us perform cost/benefit analyses of these technically demanding and expensive procedures.

Absolute indications for replantation in the upper extremity include the amputations of a thumb, multiple digits, and in children (13,14). The thumb should be replanted at any level. Whereas the thumb functions as a post for pinch as well as in grasp, length is important. Even if the nerves or tendons are avulsed from the distal part, subsequent reconstructive procedures are available to provide function. Neu-

conditions such as diabetes or heart disease should be addressed by the anesthesiology team.

Heparin, 2500–5000 units, is administered to the patient. Some surgeons prefer to continue intravenous anticoagulants after surgery; then, a dextran/heparin drip is begun with the completion of the vascular anastomoses. Heparin 10,000 units is added to a 500-ml bag of dextran 40 (low molecular weight). After an initiation of 50 ml over the 1st hour, the solution is adjusted to 25 ml per hour. If vasospasm is encountered, sublingual Nifedipine is very helpful. Antibiotics should be repeated in the operating room at a double dose owing to the large fluid volume changes (i.e., cephalosporin, typically given every 8 hours, should be given every 4 hours). For routine digits, addition of an aminoglycoside and penicillin should be administered in farm injuries.

Bone fixation is completed first. With replantations proximal to the midforearm, in which muscle critical ischemia time is a consideration, a temporary shunt should be used to provide vascular inflow while preparing the bones for fixation (32). Any method with which the surgeon feels comfortable that provides stable fixation is acceptable. As previously mentioned, the fixation should not impede immediate post-operative motion exercises. K-wire fixation is fast, and continues to be the most popular method. However, cross K-wires tend to give the least stability, can unintentionally distract the bones, and sometimes impinge mobile tendons and skin. The pin caps also tend to interfere with the adjacent fingers, if used proximal to the mid-middle phalanx level. Therefore, the cross K-wire technique should be avoided outside of distal replantations. Methods of internal fixation include plates and screws (33), lag screws, and interosseous wiring (34). Steinman pins and Rush rods are used in more proximal extremity replantations. The periosteal stripping necessary for plate placement has not borne out fears of excessive vascular disruption and subsequent bony nonunion usually alluded to in the literature. A smaller H-plate provides adequate stability, ease of placement, and minimal periosteal stripping. In multiple digital replantation, Camacho and Wood (35) demonstrated that a structure-by-structure method achieved better survival and a shorter duration of surgery. Therefore, bony fixation should be completed in all digits prior to soft-tissue repair.

Occasionally, the amputation will occur through a joint without injuring the articular surfaces. The strategy for reconstruction should depend upon the joint location. Because distal interphalangeal joint motion after replantation or simple tendon repair is not functionally significant, the joint should be readily sacrificed to ease vessel and nerve repair. The proximal interphalangeal joint should be salvaged, if possible. The dorsal and volar structures should be repaired. The central tendon should be reinserted into the middle phalanx to prevent boutonniére deformity. Conversely, the volar plate should be distally advanced by incising the proximal check-rein ligaments to prevent the tendency towards flexor contracture. This maneuver is similar to volar-plate arthroplasty after proximal interphalangeal joint fracture-dislocations that include middle phalanx volar lip fractures. One of the authors (JAG) does not repair the collateral ligaments, as early patients in which collateral ligament repairs were completed tended toward joint flexor contracture. Furthermore, Diao and Eaton (36) demonstrated that total collateral ligament excision in the presence of a good soft-tissue envelope did not lead to lateral instability. If the proximal interphalangeal joint is not salvageable, then other modes of reconstruction are warranted. Fusion should be considered for the index and long fingers, the fingers associated with pinch. Arthroplasty is considered for the ring and small fingers, the fingers associated with grasp. Immediate or staged vascularized joint transfer can be considered in young patients, or in those patients with high demand tasks who refuse fusion (37,38). Wrist or ankle joint destruction should be initially stabilized, and later arthrodesis performed in the event of predictable painful and limited motion. Elbow or knee destruction is reconstructed after initial stabilization. Even though total elbow arthroplasty has not been perfected, it is still more functional than arthrodesis. Unfortunately, total knee replacement in the event of significant ligamentous disruption still does not provide a stable knee. However, long-term brace usage does present a smaller energy expenditure than an above-the-knee prosthesis.

Tendon and pulley reconstruction is next completed. Although there are multiple techniques for tendon repair (39–44), the surgeon should incorporate both a core and epitenon suture to allow early postoperative rehabilitation. Finger amputations in zone II present a more difficult decision, whether to repair both sublimis and profundus tendons or to sacrifice one in order to maximize function in the other. Some authors (45,46) suggest sacrifice of the sublimis if both tendons are injured, while sacrificing the profundus if the sublimis is uninjured. If aggressive postoperative rehabilitation in the presence of stable internal fixation is instituted, then the results after repair of both tendons in replantation should come close to those after simple tendon injuries. In the forearm, tendon and muscle repair is completed according to the injury level. In the distal forearm, tendon repair is similar to that in the hand. However, more proximal injuries will involve the muscle-tendon junction, or muscle alone. Tendon should be weaved into the most appropriate muscle as defined by anatomy. Unfortunately, many proximal forearm amputations include crush and avulsion aspects which confuse normal anatomy. Furthermore, associated nerve injury or avulsion may make the remaining muscle nonfunctional. Only experience can guide whether repair of tendons to the remaining muscle will be a futile experience. If the latter is unlikely, then early tendon transfer or innervated muscle transplantation can be useful. Extensor tendons are repaired after the flexor tendon, arteries, and nerves are completed. These repairs are performed in the usual fashion, with simple, horizontal mattress or figure-of-eight suture techniques.

The vascular anastomoses are then performed, arterial and venous, respectively. The dominant artery, whether ulnar in the index and long fingers, or radial in the ring and small fingers, should be repaired first. If this vessel proves adequate flow, then the second vessel is not necessarily repaired. The only situations where both vessels should be repaired is if one digital artery may be sacrificed later to create a local flap. For example, a patient with an amputation through the proximal interphalangeal joint may lead to a replantation with a fused joint. As described by Foucher (38), the distal interphalangeal joint can later be transposed to the proximal interphalangeal joint site to provide a permanent functional reconstruction.

The artery is dissected both proximally and distally for at least a centimeter. Small branches can usually be sacrificed with impunity. The vessel is sharply cut with straight microscissors till normal-appearing intima is demonstrated. If the intima is separated from the rest of the wall, then the surgeon must assume that significant intimal injury will preclude adequate proximal inflow. The tourniquet is deflated to ensure proximal inflow, as demonstrated by pulsatile jet flow. If inflow is inadequate, do not assume that it is vasospasm. Intimal injury more proximal to the site is more likely the cause. Therefore, the vessel should be trimmed back to the level of good flow. Adventitia is excised for several millimeters to prevent interference of the adventitia with the sutures, or entrance into the vessel lumen. The vessel should then be gently dilated with the microdilators. Irrigant fluid is usually injected both proximally and distally. Numerous irrigant fluids have been developed, without specific evidence for the superiority of one or another (47). The typical solution includes a crystalloid, an anticoagulant, and a topical vasodilator. One of the centers (JAG) now uses a combination of Ringer lactate 500 ml, lidocaine 4% 50 ml, and urokinase 100,000 units (48), whereas the Buncke clinic uses a heparin and saline solution. Some surgeons intubate the distal limb to flush the amputated part, while others prefer to irrigate only the vessel ends.

Before placing vessel clamps, the patient is heparinized. The proximal vessel is then clamped with a single microvascular clamp. Choose the smallest clamp available that securely fits the vessel in order to place the least compression on the vessel wall. A colored plastic background material is then placed on the tissue bed under the vessels. An approximating clamp, also the smallest appropriate size, is placed on both limbs. The cross-bar should be on the side opposite the main surgeon. If the vessel ends do not easily coapt, then there is too much tension, and either more dissection or a vein graft is necessary. Vessel redundancy may also lead to postoperative compression and thrombosis. Vein grafts for digital vessels are either harvested from the dorsal surface of other uninjured digits, the volar distal forearm, or the dorsal foot (49). In proximal amputations, arterial autografts from the subscapular arterial tree or omentum may provide better substitutes than vein grafts (50). As in macrovascular surgery, the vein grafts should be reversed to avoid flow obstruction. The vein should also undergo adventitia excision to maximize vein dilatation and blood flow. Alternatively, vessel transposition from adjacent uninjured fingers can prevent the necessity for vein grafting (51) (Fig. 89–2). The anastomotic suture technique can either be performed as the triangulation method (52) or by an open technique (53). These techniques, described elsewhere in this book, are usually chosen based on personal preference rather than any intrinsic superiority. Once the arterial repair is completed, the hand is turned over to perform the venous repair in similar fashion. When feasible, two or three veins are repaired for every artery repaired.

Nerve repair is completed after the arterial and before the venous repair. In replantations proximal to the wrist, where volar veins are abundant, this principle is more loosely applied. Epineural repair is performed in the finger and hand, while group fascicular repair should be performed in the wrist and proximal extremity. Crushing and avulsion injuries may prevent a precise determination of the extent of injury adjacent to the gross transection site. Therefore, primary resection and grafting or secondary reconstruction may be necessary. The principles of nerve repair are more completely detailed elsewhere in this book. (Briefly, crush and high-velocity explosive injuries should be secondarily repaired after 3 weeks to allow a better determination of the extent of nerve damage.) Resection of the damaged nerve, with subsequent nerve graft repair, likely will improve results. However, initial tacking of the nerve ends in a lengthened and stretched position at the first surgery sometimes allows resection and delayed primary repair. Furthermore, one author (JAG) routinely wraps the nerve in the microvascular surgery background sheeting in those cases destined for secondary reconstruction. This allows easy identification of the nerve ends in the scar matrix, and provides a pseudosynovial sheath to allow better nerve gliding for rehabilitation.

Wound closure is crucial to any surgical procedure (Fig. 89–3). In prolonged cases with skin loss, additional swelling

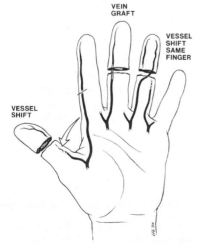

FIG. 89–2. Vessel shift or vein grafting is used to avoid radical bone shortening.

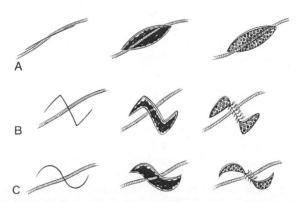

FIG. 89–3. **A,** A poorly planned incision with swelling necessitates placement of skin graft over vein graft. **B and C,** A well-placed zig-zag **(B)** or sigmoid **(C)** incision provides full-thickness coverage of vein graft with lack of tension in spite of swelling.

may prevent wound closure. More proximal replantations also necessitate forearm and hand muscle compartment fasciotomies as well as distal nerve release. Therefore, additional incisions to expose vital structures should be planned so as not to overlie those vital structures (54). Although split or full-thickness skin grafts can be used to cover exposed vessels or vein grafts, they are less desirable than vascularized tissue. Other exposed structures, such as bone, tendon, and nerve, will necessitate either local rotation or free flaps to assure wound closure and early rehabilitation (55). Proximal injuries may present questionably viable muscle and adjacent soft tissues. Second look procedures at 24 to 48 hours offer an opportunity to further débride nonviable tissue, irrigate the wound thoroughly to dilute bacterial inocula, and then obtain wound closure. Muscle can be covered by skin grafts, while other vital structures may need flap coverage. Large loss of muscle and tendon units may necessitate secondary reconstruction via tendon transfer, muscle transfer or innervated muscle transplantation (56).

Postoperative Considerations

A designated and established hand unit with well-trained nursing personnel is the optimal setting for patient care after surgery. If this is unavailable, then an intensive-care unit is necessary for at least the first 24 hours. The patient is kept warm, well-hydrated, and medicated for pain. The replanted extremity is elevated above heart level, and is examined frequently for capillary refill. The replanted part can be monitored by temperature probe, with temperatures greater than 30° C desirable for viability. Intravenous fluids are maintained at a level to produce at least 50 ml of urine per hour. Underlying medical conditions modify the volume and type of fluid administrations. The Foley indwelling bladder catheter is continued while the hydration status is monitored. A PCA intravenous analgesia drip improves pain relief and probably decreases the sympathetic tone caused by pain and anxiety. Both basal and bolus infusion settings optimize pain relief.

Intravenous antibiotics are continued for 24 hours, when oral antibiotics are instituted for a total of 3 days. Antibiotics may be continued in cases of extensive heavily contaminated open wounds, and should be based upon preoperative wound cultures. Mild tranquilizers with a vasodilatory effect, such as chlorpromazine, can be administered with sips of water. A daily baby aspirin is started. Additional medications, such as pentoxifylline, can be started to decrease thrombogenicity of blood. The dextran 40/heparin drip is continued at 25 ml for 3 days. In routine cases, the drip is halved on day 3 at midnight, and discontinued on day 4 at 6 A.M. The patient is discharged that same day. Anticoagulant therapy is modified under certain conditions. Thus, patients with tenuous vascular reconstructions may be fully anticoagulated, or maintained on anticoagulants for a longer time period. On the contrary, it is wise not to anticoagulate patients with large muscle surface injuries to prevent excessive bleeding.

The patient is kept NPO for the first 24 hours. Most vascular complications that are due to technical errors will occur within those 24 hours. The replanted part is monitored both by visual inspection and by objective monitors. A variety of monitors have been developed and utilized with good results (57–59). We prefer temperature and flourescein monitoring

along with clinical evaluation, for their ease and reproducibility. Successful replantation essentially results in a sympathectomized part. Therefore, the clinical appearance consists of a bright pink blush with capillary refill of approximately 1 second and a turgid finger pulp. Crushing injuries or extended ischemia will modify the perfusion quality in the early period after surgery. Slow improvement of perfusion over time is typical in those cases. Clinical changes consistent with vascular compromise include altered capillary refill and tissue turgidity. Venous congestion is the most common cause of vascular compromise after replantation surgery. If vein repair is impossible, leech therapy for 3 to 5 days provides venous decongestion until angiogenesis across the replantation interface is able to drain venous effluent adequately. Both venous or arterial compromise necessitate reexploration and vessel revision. Thrombosed anastomoses should be excised and repaired, either primarily or with new grafts. To reiterate, a trained nursing staff in a hand unit as part of a plastic or orthopedic ward is central to adequate postoperative care.

Rehabilitation after extremity replantation is initiated in the first 3 to 5 days before the patient is discharged. Vessel wall endothelial cell layer covers the sutures and anastomosis within 5 days, and decreases the tendency for subsequent thrombosis. The patient can start "wiggling" the fingers as soon as he or she is alert. A hand therapist examines and starts therapy as soon as the initial bulky splint is changed, on day 4 or 5. The full therapy program is well described elsewhere (60). Briefly, therapy initially consists of joint mobilization and tendon gliding through the tenodesis effect of wrist extension and flexion. In addition, passive holds in the intrinsic plus and intrinsic minus postures cause tendon motion while not overstressing the repair site. Therapy is advanced as tolerated to include active ROM exercises. The patient alternates between the intrinsic plus and intrinsic minus postures to maximize differential tendon gliding. The patient is placed in a dorsal dynamic splint to adequately balance the normally stronger flexor muscle-tendon units with the extensor forces. A protective splint is also supplied to the patient. Additional splinting for contracted joints is added at approximately 3 weeks after surgery. The patient is also followed for return of sensation. As rudimentary sensation appears, sensory reeducation is initiated to both desensitize and maximize functional sensibility (61).

The patient is continually reinforced with the idea that the replantation process is a long and arduous trail, usually lasting at least a year. Further surgery for healing, motion, or sensory function may be necessary. The process continues for 1 to 2 years for extremity replantations proximal to the wrist, and 3 to 5 years for the proximal arm and lower extremity. The team concept, and especially the hand therapist role, is repeatedly emphasized in order to ensure patient compliance with the therapy program and thus to optimize functional restoration.

References

1. Malt RA, McKhann CF. Replantation of severed arms. JAMA 1964; 189:716.
2. Jacobson JH, Suarez EL. Microsurgery in anastomosis of small vessels. *Surg Forum* 1960; 11:243.
3. Seidenberg B, Hurwitt ES, Carton CA. The technique of anastomising small arteries. *Surg Gynecol Obstet* 1958; 106:743.

4. Buncke HJ, Schulz WP. Experimental digital amputation and replantation. *Plast Reconstr Surg* 1965; 36:62.
5. Buncke HJ, Schulz WP. Total ear replantation in the rabbit utilizing microminiature vascular anastomosis. *Br J Plast Surg* 1966; 19:15.
6. Buncke HJ, Buucke CM, Schulz WP. Immediate Nicoladoni procedure in the Rhesus monkey or hallux to hand transplantation utilising microminiature vascular anastomes. *Br J Plast Surg* 1966; 19:332.
7. Kleinert HE, Kasdan ML, Romero JL. Small blood vessel anastomosis for salvage of severely injured upper extremity. *J Bone Joint Surg* 1963; 45A:788.
8. Kleinert HE, Kasdan ML. Anastomosis of edigital vessels. *J Ky Med Assoc* 1966; 63:106.
9. Chien CW, Ch'en YC, Pao YS, et al. Further experience in the restoration of amputated limbs. *Chinese Med J* 1965; 3:225.
10. Komatsu S, Tamai S. Successful replantation of a completely cut-off thumb. *Case Report Plast Reconstr Surg* 1968; 42:374.
11. Acland R. New instruments for microvascular surgery. Br J Surg 1972; 59:181.
12. Nunley JA. Microscopes and microinstruments. Hand Clinics 1985; 1:197.
13. Kleinert HE, Juhala CA, Tsai TM, et al. Digital replantation-selection, technique and results. *Orthop Clin North Am* 1977; 8:309.
14. Zhong-Wei C, Meyer VE, Kleinert HE, et al. Present indications and contraindications for replantation as reflected by long-term functional results. *Orthop Clin North Am* 1981; 12:849.
15. Roszlein R, Simmen BR. Fingertip amputations in children. *Handchir Mikrochir Plas Chir* 1991; 23:312.
16. Wei FC, Epstein MD, Chen HC, et al. Microsurgical reconstruction of distal digits following mutilating hand injuries: results in 121 patients. *Br J Plast Surg* 1993; 46:181.
17. Foucher G, Norris RW. Distal and very distal digital replantations. *Br J Plast Surg* 1992; 45:199.
18. Iglesias M, Serrano A. Replantation of amputated segments after prolonged ischemia. *Plast Reconstr Surg* 1990; 85:425.
19. Russell RC, O'Brien B, Morrison WA, et al. The late functional results of upper limb revascularization and replantation. *J Hand Surgery (AM)* 1984; 9A:623.
20. Axelrod TS, Buchler U. Severe complex injuries to the upper extremity: Revascularization and replantation. *J Hand Surg* 1991; 16A:574.
21. van Adrichem LN, Hovius SE, van Strik R, et al. The acute effect of cigarette smoking on the microcirculation of a replanted digit. J Hand Surg (AM) 1992; 17:230.
22. Schmidt DM, McClinton MA; Microvascular anastomoses in replanted fingers: Do they stay open? *Microsurg* 1990; 11:251.
23. Gelberman RH, Urbaniak JR, Bright DS, et al. Digital sensibility following replantation. *J Hand Surg (AM)* 1978; 3:313.
24. Nunley J, Gabel, GT. Tibial nerve grafting for restoration of plantar sensation. Foot & Ankle 1993; 14:489.
25. James NJ. Survival of a large replanted segment of upper lip and nose. Case report. *Plast Reconstr Surg* 1976; 58:623.
26. Tamai S, Nakamura Y, Motomiya Y. Microsurgical replantation of a completely amputated penis and scrotum: case report. *Plast Reconstr Surg* 1977; 60:287.
27. Pennington DG, Lai MF, Pelly AD. Successful replantation of a completely avulsed ear by microvascular anastomosis. *Plast Reconstr Surg* 1980; 65:820.
28. Jeng SF, Wei FCM, Noordhoff MS. Replantation of amputated facial issues with microvascular anastomosis. *Microsurgery* 1994; 15:327.
29. Partington MT, Lineaweaver WC, O'Hara M. Unrecognized injuries in patients referred for emergency microsurgery. *J Trauma* 1993; 34(2):238.
30. Furnas HJ, Lineaweaver W, Buncke HJ. Blood loss associated with anticoagulation in patients with replanted digits. *J Hand Surg* 1992; 17A:226.
31. Sapega AA, Heppenstall RB, Sokolow DP, et al. The bioenergetics of preservation of limbs before replantation. The rationale for intermediate hypothermia. *J Bone Joint Surg* 1988; 70-A:1500.
32. Nunley JA, Koman LA, Urbaniak JR. Arterial shunting as an adjunct to major limb revascularization. *Ann Surg* 1981; 193(3):271.
33. Lister G. Intraosseous wiring of the digital skeleton. *J Hand Surg (AM)* 1978; 3:427.
34. Melvi HD, Meyer V, Segmuller G. Stabilization of bone in replantation surgery of the upper limb. *Clin Orthop* 1978; 133:179.
35. Camacho FJ, Wood MB. Polydigit replantation. *Hand Clinics* 1992; 8:409.
36. Diao E, Eaton RG. Total collateral ligament excision for contractures of the proximal interphalangeal joint. *J Hand Surg (AM)* 1993; 18A:395.
37. Tsai TM, Wang WZ. Vascularized Joint Transfers: Indications and Results. *Hand Clinics* 1992; 8:525.
38. Foucher G, Lenoble E, Smith D. Free and island vascularized joint transfer for proximal interphalangeal reconstruction: A series of 27 cases. *J Hand Surg (AM)* 1994; 19A:8.
39. Kessler I. The "grasping" technique for tendon repair. *Hand* 1973; 5:253.
40. Robertson GA, al-Quattan MM. A biomechanical analysis of a new interlock suture technique for flexor tendon repair. *J Hand Surg* (BR) 1992; 17B:92.
41. Lee H. Double loop locking suture: A technique of tendon repair for early active mobilization. Part I. *J Hand Surg (AM)* 1990, 15A:943.
42. Savage R, Risitano G. Flexor tendon repair using a "six strand" method of repair and early active mobilization. *J Hand Surg (BR)* 1989; 14B:296.
43. Silfverskiold KL, May EJ. Flexor tendon repair in zone II with a new suture technique and an early mobilization program combining passive and active flexion. *J Hand Surg (AM)* 1994; 19A:53.
44. Strickland JW. Flexor tendon repair-Indiana method. *The Indiana Hand Center Newsletter* 1993; 19A:53.
45. Buncke HJ, Alpert BS, Giebink RJ. Digital replantation. *Surg Clin North Am* 1981; 61:383.
46. May J, Toth BA, Gardner M, et al. Digital replantation distal to the proximal interphalangeal joint. *J Hand Surg (AM)* 1982; 7:161.
47. Geter RK, Winters RR, Puckett CL. Resolution of experimental microvascular spasm and improvement in anastomotic patency by direct topical agent application. *Plast Reconstr Surg* 1986; 77:105.
48. Senderoff DM, Zhang WX, Israeli D, et al. The additive beneficial effect of UW solution and Urokinase on experimental microvascular free-flap survival. *J Reconstr Microsurg* 1994; 9:197.
49. Alpert BS, Buncke HJ, Brownstein M. Replacement of damaged arteries and veins with vein grafts when replanting crushed, amputated fingers. *Plast Reconstr Surg* 1978; 61:17.
50. Godina M. Arterial autografts in microvascular surgery. *Plast Reconstr Surg* 1986; 78:293.
51. Doi K. Replantation of an avulsed thumb with application of a neurovascular pedicle. *Hand* 1976; 8:258.
52. Acland RD. Microvascular anastomosis: A device for holding stay sutures and a new vascular clamp. *Surgery* 1974; 75:185.
53. Harris GD, Finseth F, Buncke HJ. Posterior-wall-first microvascular anastomotic technique. *Br J Plast Surg* 1981; 34:47.
54. Nissenbaum M. A surgical approach for replantation of complete digital amputations. *J Hand Surg (AM)* 1980; 5:58.
55. Lister G, Scheker L. Emergency free flaps to the upper extremity. *J Hand Surg (AM)* 1988; 13A:22.
56. Schecker LR. Salvage of a mutilated hand. In: Cohen M, ed. *Mastery of Plastic and Reconstructive Surgery*. Boston: Little Brown, 1994; 1658.
57. Reagen DS, Grundberg AB, George MJ. Clinical evaluation and temperature monitoring in predicting viability in replantations. *J Reconstr Microsurg* 1994; 10:1.
58. Lowdon IM, Toby EB, Ecker J, et al. Laser doppler monitoring of replants using a small prism probe. *Microsurgery* 1989; 10:175.
59. Graham BH, Gordon L, Alpert BS, et al. Serial quantitative skin surface fluorescence-a new method for postoperative monitoring of vascular perfusion in revascularized digits. *J Hand Surg (AM)* 1985; 10A:226.
60. Chan SW, Jaglowski JM, Kaplan R. Rehabilitation of Hand Injuries. In: Cohen M, ed. *Mastery of Plastic and Reconstructive Surgery*. Boston: Little Brown, 1994; 1745.
61. Dellon AL. Sensory recovery in replanted digits and transplanted toes: A review. *J Reconstr Microsurg* 1986; 2:123.

90

Congenital Hand Deformity

Paul Smith, M.D., F.R.C.S., and Hamish Laing, M.D., M.B.B.S., F.R.C.S.
(Illustrated by David Gault, M.D., F.R.C.S.)

The presence of deformity in a newborn child creates a mixture of emotions in the parents that includes disbelief, anger, guilt, and anxiety about the future. Early consultation with an informed clinician can be reassuring; it is followed by a detailed discussion in the outpatient clinic, when a program of reconstruction can be outlined.

It is essential to gain the confidence of the parents at this stage if a number of complex procedures will be required in the future. Many parents have unrealistic expectations of surgery, and realistic goals must be carefully explained. If multiple congenital anomalies are present, the close cooperation of pediatric colleagues is important.

Appearance and Function

Young children are oblivious to their hand deformities, but later they become aware of parental and peer reactions. If the deformity remains uncorrected the stresses may be considerable especially, at school entry. Thus, the surgeon should not only be concerned with functional disability but also be sensitive to the child's concern about appearance.

The degree of disability suffered varies greatly from a minor deformity such as digital disproportion or disarray, where precision pinch may be all that is missing, to severe bilateral deformity where prehension becomes bimanual. At this level, activities of independent daily living (ADLs) may not be possible, with dramatic consequences on the child's developing personality.

Thus, there is a ladder of functional ability, which surgery can help a child ascend. If judicious surgery is likely to improve functional independence then it should be undertaken, but this may be a difficult decision. Inappropriate surgery may worsen deformity and impair growth and sensibility.

General Principles

The aims of treatment in congenital hand deformities are:

- Restoration of grasp and precision pinch—the basic functions of a normal hand
- Unrestricted growth
- Acceptable appearance

If these goals are already met, then surgery is not indicated. However, annual review to monitor change in function with growth is important.

In children, orthotic, prosthetic, or surgical treatment may be required to achieve these aims. Splinting has a role in correcting deformity by maintaining a corrected position and preventing postoperative scar contracture. While early splinting is most effective, it may be difficult to achieve in small children. Conversely, passive stretching (e.g., in radial clubhand) is easier when the child is small, prior to surgical stabilization.

In some deformities (e.g., complete agenesis at the wrist and phocomelia), prosthetic devices are the only treatment option. These have improved considerably in appearance and function; nonetheless, children often fail to use their unilateral upper extremity prostheses (1).

Careful observation of a child's hand function at play permits accurate assessment of the deformity and planning of surgical correction, which may involve many procedures ranging from bone grafting and flap cover to microsurgical tissue transfer. Emphasis on subsequent growth is essential, and epiphyseal plates must be protected. Sensation is normal in the congenitally deformed hand and great care is required not to damage nerves during surgery. Unsuspected anatomic relationships are common; motor units for planned tendon transfers may be of poor quality and vascular anomalies are frequent.

The timing of surgery is important. The ability to undertake coordinated, purposeful movement in the hand is dependent upon maturation of the peripheral nervous system. Primitive grasp is present at birth; key grip and precision pinch develop later. A persistently abnormal prehensile pattern adversely influences cortical mapping of the affected areas of the hand. In addition, babies below the age of 1 year have not yet developed the fear of hospitals seen in the "terrible two's" (2). Thus, surgical reconstruction should ideally be carried out in the first year of life to provide the infant with everything possible for normal growth and development (3).

Early surgery requires great care because the hand itself is very small. The hand rapidly increases in size during the first 4 years, and so complex procedures such as microvascular transfers using small recipient vessels are best deferred until this time. Arteriography is not essential before such procedures because exploration at the time of surgery will define the vascular anatomy. Another indication for delay is when cooperation is required for complicated postoperative rehabilitation, such as following tendon grafting.

Rarely, surgery must be carried out urgently in the neonatal period in cases of ring constriction syndrome with severe distal lymphoedema. The division of complex syndactyly between digits of different length is undertaken especially early.

At whatever age, the relationship between surgeon, child, and parents is precious. Painful dressing changes should be avoided and are best carried out under general anaesthesia.

Prevalence

The prevalence of all congenital upper-limb malformation is reported to vary between 1 in every 626 births (4) and 1 in every 463 births (5). Syndactyly, polydactyly, and campto-dactyly are the most common deformities. Syndactyly is twice as frequent in males (9.6 per 10,000) as in females (4.9 per 10,000) (6). The prevalence of individual anomalies varies between populations. Temtamy and McKusick (7) found polydactyly in 35 per 10,000 births among African-Americans in Baltimore.

Genetics

While most upper limb deformities are random, about 5% show a familial tendency. Cleft hand, symphalangism, brachydactyly, and camptodactyly often show autosomal dominant inheritance (8). Recessive abnormalities such as acrocephalosyndactyly tend to be more severe. It is important to recognize syndromic hand deformities so that other systems may be examined for anomalies. There have been significant advances in analytical techniques in cytogenetics that allow greater identification of mutations responsible for some hand deformities. All such children should be offered specialist genetic counseling and investigation.

Postnatal Development of Hand Function

Soon after birth, the hands begin to play an important role in the exploration of the environment. Early movements are un-coordinated. At this stage, the hand has two basic abilities: grasp, as in the grip reflex; and use of the flat hand, seen in feeding infants who rest their hands on the maternal breast. As the child matures, patterns of coordinated use develop. By the first birthday, the child is able to oppose the thumb and pick up objects. They can also position the hand and grip firmly.

Postnatal peripheral and central changes in the nervous system lead to an improvement in strength and dexterity. The brain is a sophisticated computer capable of self-programming. Sensory and visual stimulation lead to central software development: an ability that is age related. Peripheral physical changes (myelination) represent hardware alterations, which are most rapid during the first 2 years. Software programming, however, continues throughout life as the individual strives to acquire new skills.

Classification

Classifications of congenital limb deformities are inevitably constrained by our understanding of the developmental processes. These are never perfect and some patients will not fit any particular group (9). The current classification system was proposed by the American Society for Surgery of the Hand and adopted by the International Federation of Societies for Surgery of the Hand. It is based upon the presumed embryologic failure leading to the clinical deformity (10):

1. Failure of the formation of parts (arrest of development)
2. Failure of differentiation or separation of parts
3. Duplications
4. Overgrowth (gigantism)
5. Undergrowth (hypoplasia)
6. Congenital constriction band syndrome
7. Generalized skeletal abnormalities

Failure of the Formation of Parts (Group 1)

In this group there may be a transverse or longitudinal arrest of development.

TRANSVERSE ABSENCE

Transverse deficiencies are the cause of congenital amputation and may occur at any level, although common sites are below the elbow and at the carpus. Surgical reconstruction is not possible, and provision of a prosthesis offers the best form of rehabilitation. This should be introduced at an early age to encourage familiarity, although more complex (and heavy) prostheses must wait until the child is older.

LONGITUDINAL ABSENCE

Isolated absence of the humerus produces a short limb, and while the forearm and hand may be normal there is usually associated shortening of the radius or ulna. Phocomelia ("seal flipper") was more common after maternal thalidomide ingestion during pregnancy.

More distally, defects of the ulnar, central, or radial components of the limb can occur. Central defects produce a cleft hand. In the mildest cases, only the 3rd ray is absent. Absence of the 2nd, 3rd and 4th rays may produce a so-called lobster claw hand (although this offensive term is best replaced by "clefting deformity"). Failure of development of the pre or postaxial segments of the limb may result in a radial clubhand or its ulnar equivalent. In the most severe forms, radial or ulnar failure may be combined with central deficiency.

RADIAL CLUBHAND

Radial clubhand describes radial deviation of the wrist. The frequency of radial ray deficiencies is 1:55,000 births. They are more often unilateral than bilateral, are found on the right side more than the left, and occur in males more than in females (11). In recent years, the most common causative agent has been thalidomide, which recent evidence suggests may have consequences for the children of affected parents.

Other important systems that develop at the same time as the radius may also be affected. Cardiovascular, gastrointestinal, and genitourinary anomalies are associated with radial clubhand—for example, the VATERR association (*v*ertebral anomalies, *a*nal atresia, *t*racheoesophageal fistula, and *r*enal and *r*adial abnormalities). A cardiac septal defect may be associated with radial deficiency (Holt Oram syndrome). Thrombocytopenia may be associated with absence of the radius (the TAR syndrome); this should be considered in children with radial clubhand and a normal thumb. Radial clubhand encompasses a range of deformities from minor to severe. In the most extreme cases, there is thumb hypoplasia or total absence of the thumb, first metacarpal, scaphoid, trapezium, and radius.

The deformity is not confined to the preaxial (radial) border of the limb. The ulna never achieves normal size and is often short and curved; the index and middle fingers are

FIG. 90–1. Radial dysplasia of varying severity, from slight radial shortening and thumb hypoplasia through to complete radial agenesis with marked angulation of the wrist. The "fibrous anlage" is rarely seen; instead, there is marked thickening of the deep fascia.

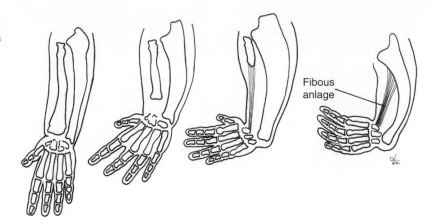

Fibous anlage

often stiff. While it is described that the remnants of the preaxial bones and muscles may be condensed into a fibrous band (anlage) between the proximal forearm and the carpus, it is rarely seen. Instead, the deep fascia of the forearm is diffusely thickened and tight, and there is shortening of skin and muscle-tendon units, which must be released. The radial vessels and nerve are usually deficient (Fig. 90–1).

Elbow movement is often limited by the bony structure of the joint and poor development of biceps and brachialis muscles. This stiffness is pronounced during the first 2 years but may improve with time, so that many children achieve 90° of flexion. Early stiffness is thus not an absolute contraindication to surgical realignment of the wrist; indeed, centralization may encourage increased range of movement at the elbow.

Grasp *should* be improved by centralizing the wrist, since this increases the power of the digital flexors, but in general there is little functional improvement of grasp. Although realignment contributes to improved hand posture, there may be some conflict between the possibility of functional impairment and the desire to improve appearance. Cosmesis, however, is of such importance that many adult patients with established deformity request wrist realignment.

Many children with radial clubhand achieve a surprising degree of function (12). When the deformity is bilateral, however, the combination of a short limb, stiff elbow, and poor hand function makes independent self-care difficult. Because the thumb is often absent or hypoplastic, precision pinch is impaired. Affected children use dorsal prehension and are incapable of fine manipulative tasks; thus, pollicization is often indicated.

Treatment

The deformity is usually mobile, and should be passively corrected by stretching. This is carried out by the parents before each feed and should be continued until surgery. While splinting is desirable to maintain position, it can be very difficult to achieve in small children. If passive stretching achieves a neutral position, the correction may be maintained with tendon transfers. In such cases, some flexion-extension range is maintained at the wrist.

Wrist Centralization

If passive correction to neutral is not possible, it may be necessary to consider soft-tissue release on the radial side. In

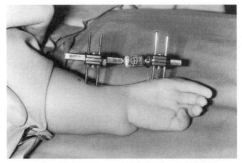

FIG. 90–2. The hand may be centralized on the ulna by distracting the soft tissues with an external fixator (Pennig, Orthofix). The caregivers sequentially distract the device daily. It is then removed and the position held with a K wire for 3 months before tendon transfers are performed.

such cases, there may be evidence of bowing of the ulna on radiographs. Early surgical release is indicated, because growth may increase the tautness of the soft tissues and enhance the curvature.

In the past, excision of some carpal bones was required to reposition the hand adequately. The position was achieved by removing enough of the center of the carpus—usually the lunate and capitate—to wedge the lower ulna in the resulting notch. Such centralization without stabilizing tendon transfers inevitably leads to recurrent deformity. Alternative approaches include incorporating the use of additional tendon transfers, or "radialization," as advocated by Buck-Gramcko (13).

Other options include use of a distracting external fixator (Pennig, Othofix) across the carpus (Fig. 90–2), with release of the skin and tight soft tissues, if needed. The parents are taught to distract the wrist daily until centralization is achieved. The fixator is then removed and the position maintained by a longitudinal K wire for 3 months.

Tendon transfers are also undertaken to stabilize the relocated carpus on the distal end of the ulna. The flexor carpi radialis, extensor carpi radialis longus and brevis, and brachioradialis may be inseparable, and are transferred as a mass dorsally to insert into the extensor carpi ulnaris tendon and become dorsiflexors and ulnar deviators. The forearm and hand are then splinted. Ulnar osteotomy and lengthening can help to compensate for the short forearm (14). Recent advances have allowed the Ilizarov method to be used for this with promising results. If there is significant ulnar curvature, this is best corrected by osteotomy, which can be combined with lengthening if the Ilizarov frame is used.

Pollicization

When the position of the hand has been corrected by wrist realignment and tendon transfers, consideration can be given to thumb function. In most cases the thumb is absent, and in others it is too hypoplastic to be functional. An existing digit can be made into a thumb; the index finger, despite its frequent stiffness, is most commonly used for this purpose. Pollicization is described further in the section on thumb hypoplasia.

The timing of these procedures is important. Wrist centralization may be delayed in an attempt to preserve forearm length. It is now believed, however, that little is lost by early surgery. The wrist is centralized as soon as passive correction has achieved its maximum effect. If pollicization were to be performed before centralization, the tendon balance would be altered by the subsequent wrist procedure; therefore, pollicization is usually performed about 6 months after centralization.

ULNAR CLUBHAND (DISTAL ULNAR DEFICIENCY)

Absence of the ulnar side of the forearm is less common than radial clubhand. A broad spectrum of maldevelopment can occur, from slight hypoplasia of the ulnar digits to total absence of the ulna. Unlike radial deficiencies, the ulnar clubhand is often stable at the wrist, but severe elbow flexion contractures may be seen.

Where the hand deviates ulnarward, corrective splinting of the wrist should be started in the first 6 months. A fibrous condensation replacing the absent ulna may require resection to allow adequate correction. In some cases in which the proximal ulna is present, it can be advantageous to fuse it to the distal portion of the radius to create a "one-bone forearm."

Limb lengthening using Ilizarov distraction may be helpful in cases of significant forearm shortening and can be combined with angulation osteotomy to correct the curvature of the radius.

CLEFT HAND AND CENTRAL DEFECTS

This group includes a range of deformity arising from longitudinal failure of development of the distal central portion of the upper limb. An incidence of 0.4:10,000 births has been reported (5). Cleft hands have the central ray alone missing, with the metacarpal absent or present in a disrupted state. Such anomalies are familial, with dominant inheritance, and are often bilateral with simultaneous involvement of the feet (Fig. 90–3). These were once known as "typical" cleft hands. In severe defects, syndactyly of the border digits is likely. Syndactyly is more frequent between the ring and little fingers than between the thumb and index finger, but when the latter occurs there may be a significant adduction contracture of the thumb that will require early release.

"Atypical" cleft hands are now classified as a variant of symbrachydactyly. Here, the three central rays are missing. The thumb and little finger are present, although they may be hypoplastic. This deformity is usually unilateral, without an associated foot deformity, and often there is no family history.

Functionally, however, they resemble cleft hands and pose similar reconstructive problems. Hands with central defects may function well, but their appearance leads many patients to seek advice about surgery.

Treatment

The first priority is to correct any associated syndactyly of the border digits. This is particularly important if the thumb–index finger web is affected. In the cleft hand, an ingenious method of correcting the cleft devized by Snow and Littler is to deepen the first web space by transposing the index finger ray to the base of the third metacarpal (15) (Fig. 90–4).

The digital neurovascular bundles and the dorsal veins must be carefully preserved. An osteotomy at the base of the index metacarpal allows the ray to be transferred to the third metacarpal. The deep transverse metacarpal ligament is reconstructed and the skin flaps closed without tension.

If the thumb is hypoplastic, a rotation osteotomy or tendon transfers may be necessary to improve function. The cleft may be contracted and require deepening with a Z-plasty to improve function.

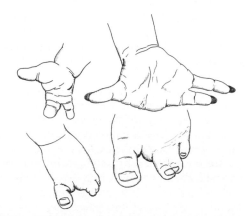

FIG. 90–3. A cleft hand and cleft foot in a mother and her child.

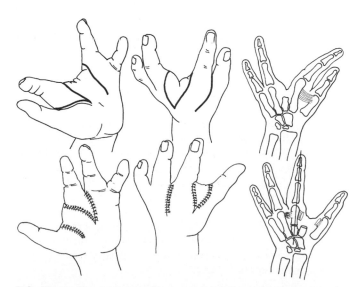

FIG. 90–4. The technique for transposing the index finger into the cleft of the hand described by Snow and Littler. The skin from the cleft deepens the first web space. The second metacarpal is divided and the finger repositioned on the base of the third metacarpal. Once in place, the transverse metacarpal ligament is reconstructed.

SEVERE SUPPRESSION DEFORMITIES

When a distal central defect is associated with a partial or complete radial or ulnar deficiency, the child may be left with a one-digit, (monodactylic) hand. Often such defects are bilateral, and the child lacks the ability to grip with either hand. This can be restored by creating an opposition post against which the remaining digit is able to pinch using skin flaps and bone grafts. Neurovascular free flaps may provide sensation at key points on the opposition post. Toe-to-hand transfer using microsurgical techniques can also restore pinch; however, the toe is transferred to a site where there is tendon and muscle hypoplasia, so function is often poor. Reinnervation of the transferred tissue requires the sacrifice of a cutaneous nerve at the recipient site. If poorly innervated, there will be limited sensory feedback. Such transfers, despite their limitations, do create a fingerlike opposition post in a single stage. The active digit may need repositioning with a rotation osteotomy, tendon graft, or joint fusion to pinch against the new post.

Failure of Separation or Differentiation of Parts (Group 2)

Failure of differentiation of the soft tissues may lead to isolated absence of a muscle or to more complex deformities such as arthrogryposis. In the latter, there is no differentiation between muscle, ligament, and skin, with each merging gradually into the other to produce multiple symmetrical soft-tissue contractures.

There may be fusion of structures, as is seen in syndactyly or synostosis. Synostosis can involve the elbow, radius and ulna, carpal bones, or metacarpals. It rarely requires surgical treatment, although when pronation and supination are severely limited surgical release may be helpful.

SYNDACTYLY

Syndactyly is a common congenital hand deformity with a prevalence of 7 per 10,000 live births in England and Wales (16). Males are affected twice as frequently as females. Between 10 and 40% of the cases are familial, being inherited as a dominant gene with variable penetrance (16). Familial cases are usually bilateral.

Syndactyly is commonly associated with other hand deformities, such as cleft hand and symbrachydactyly, and is associated with some generalized congenital deformities. The 3rd, 4th, 2nd, and 1st interdigital webs are affected in decreasing order of frequency. In *complete* syndactyly, the involved digits are united throughout their length. Within this group, the degree of nail bed fusion influences the quality of the final result. In *incomplete* syndactyly, the common web extends a variable length along the fingers, but not as far as the distal interphalangeal joint.

The deformity may be simple or complex. In *simple* syndactyly, only soft tissue webbing is present, whereas in *complex* syndactyly there is bony fusion between adjacent digits. This may involve all the adjacent phalanges or occur only at the fingertips (acrosyndactyly).

Timing of Surgery

Surgical release is carried out early in simple complete syndactyly to allow growth of affected digits without further angulation. This is especially true for the 1st and 4th webs, where digits of unequal length are tethered. While division of incomplete syndactyly is not mandatory, for aesthetic reasons most parents opt for repair in childhood.

Complex syndactyly may require a series of staged procedures, and in such cases it is also beneficial to commence surgery at an early age. Great care is essential, however, to avoid damage to the delicate digital vessels.

There is rapid growth of the hand prior to 4 years of age, and careful planning of the incisions and skin cover is essential if surgical revisions are to be avoided.

Treatment

The aims of surgical correction of syndactyly are:

1. Creation of a commissure using a flap
2. Separation of the involved digits using a volar and dorsal zig-zag approach
3. Provision of adequate skin cover using full-thickness grafts

The new commissure is best reconstructed using one or more flaps. Many designs have been described to prevent subsequent web creep. At The Great Ormond Street Hospital for Children, we prefer to use two triangular flaps, one dorsal and one volar, which avoids the linear scar across the web that may result from rectangular flaps. Closure of the remaining digit without resort to grafts is rarely possible or sensible, because it inevitably involves compromise in the quality of the result.

After separation of the digits, the marginal scars surrounding the raw surface should be oblique. Volar and dorsal interdigitating flaps are essential to prevent linear scar contractures, which can produce lateral deviation of the digits and advance the new commissure distally (web creep). It is usually possible to achieve skin cover with flaps distal to the proximal interphalangeal joint, but proximal to this skin grafts are required, because the surgeon is trying to cover three surfaces (both digits and commissure) with only two skin surfaces (dorsal and volar).

Adequate skin cover usually requires the use of full-thickness grafts, which contract less than split-thickness grafts. When these are harvested from the groin, it is important to stay lateral to the femoral artery to prevent hair growth in the grafts. If adequate grafts are used, then there is no need to distribute the skin flaps preferentially to one of the two digits, but to do so greatly simplifies the procedure.

In complex syndactyly, where bare bone is exposed in the interdigital cleft, this should be covered with a flap of subcutaneous fat before grafting. Where this is not possible, grafts can be made to take on exposed cancellous bone (Fig. 90–5).

When attempting to provide a commissure of normal depth, it is occasionally necessary to divide the digital artery to one side of the cleft distal to the common digital bifurcation. For this reason, adjacent web spaces should not be released simultaneously. The common digital nerve is split in a proximal direction in such circumstances, and the deep transverse metacarpal ligament may require division. When the nail is conjoined, division results in a defect along the adjacent eponychial borders. Two small transverse flaps from the pulp are useful to reconstruct this defect (Fig. 90–6). Careful hemostasis is essential before suturing of the flaps and appli-

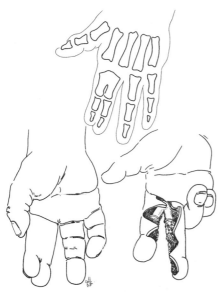

FIG. 90–5. In this case of complex syndactyly, interdigitating zig-zag flaps were used. The bony fusion required division and the two flexor tendons shared a common sheath.

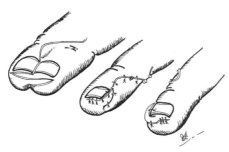

FIG. 90–6. In syndactyly with a common nail, appearance is greatly improved by reconstruction of the lateral nail folds using two transverse pulp flaps.

cation of the full-thickness grafts. A well-padded dressing is applied, and changed under general anaesthesia until the grafts are stable. If further grafting is required, it can be undertaken immediately.

Tissue expansion of the dorsal skin of the interdigital cleft has been attempted in an effort to avoid the need for skin grafting. Our experience has been disappointing, with an unacceptable complication rate and worse outcome than conventional treatment (17). We therefore no longer use tissue expanders for syndactyly correction.

When the wounds have healed, the patient is fitted with a compression glove, and a small overrider pulls the garment down into the web. This encourages the scars to soften.

Causes of Failure

The most catastrophic complication possible is circulatory deficit leading to loss of a digit. To safeguard against this, both sides of the same digit should never be operated on at any one time and the tips of all digits should be inspected after the application of the dressing. If blood flow is compromised, the dressing should be released and if there is no response it is prudent to cut the sutures securing the tightest of the skin flaps.

Infection does occur, and is best treated by frequent and regular dressing changes. A common complication is that of contracture in a longitudinal scar. This may be due to poorly planned incisions or inadequate skin grafting. As the digit grows, such a contracture becomes more obvious. Skin tightness is best corrected by division and insertion of additional skin grafts. Distal creep of the web may necessitate surgical revision. Web creep may result from poor wound healing with fusion of adjacent raw areas, or from design faults when placing the initial incision.

Special Problems

APERT'S SYNDROME

In Apert's syndrome there is complex acrosyndactyly, with all fingers sharing a common nail (Fig. 90–7). In addition, the digits are usually short and deformed and have stiff interphalangeal joints. Movement at the metacarpophalangeal joint is usually preserved. The severity may be classified into three groups according to the degree of thumb involvement.

We now aim to separate the thumb, index, and little fingers from the central mass in one stage using full-thickness grafts. These digits never flex normally, but the patients greatly appreciate the change in appearance of their hands. The first web space must be adequate to allow full use of the thumb. The thumbs of children with Apert's syndrome often deviate radially because of the presence of a delta phalanx, which may be improved by a closing wedge osteotomy at the time of the first procedure. At a later date, the central mass (middle and ring fingers) may be separated if the bony skeleton allows.

EPIDERMOLYSIS BULLOSA DYSTROPHICA

Dystrophic epidermolysis bullosa is a rare, congenital, fragile skin condition in which the hands develop a mittenlike deformity with digital fusion as a result of trauma. The condition has an estimated incidence of 1:300,000 live births (18). Skin blisters form with minimal trauma (the Nikolski sign) and the web spaces are gradually lost from progressive epidermal scarring, which slowly creeps distally until the digits are encased in an epidermal cocoon. At this stage, digital prehension is totally lost. Recent research suggests that the fibroblasts in these children generate over twice the normal contactile force.

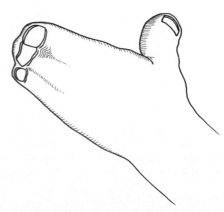

FIG. 90–7. A typical "spoon-shaped" hand in Apert's syndrome. The degree of thumb involvement determines the type of deformity.

A large series of these patients have been treated at The Great Ormond Street Hospital for Children, London. Surgery to the hands is carried out under general anesthesia, and it is possible to use a well-padded tourniquet but skin handling precautions are mandatory. It is essential that the anesthesiologist be familiar with the special problems these children pose. Intravenous lines are difficult to secure, and mouth opening is often limited.

Once inside the epidermal cocoon, it is possible to enter a plane between fused dermal elements of adjacent digits. Flexion contractures of the fingers and the adduction contracture of the thumb are only released when the dermis is incised. It is remarkable that, following prolonged immobilization in a flexed position, the interphalangeal joints in this condition extend as well as they do. The underlying neurovascular bundles are readily seen and preserved. The skin defects are filled with split-thickness grafts harvested from unblistered areas. The skin is harvested with a handheld knife using liberal lubrication, but skin stretching with boards is not permitted. The donor site heals readily and the graft take in the hands is usually excellent. It should be noted that a β-hemolytic streptococcus is often found in the skin blisters of these children.

Dressings with vaseline gauze and wool are applied with meticulous care and are first changed at 2 weeks. Once complete healing is achieved, splints are made to prevent recurrence of the deformity (19). Unfortunately, despite meticulous care of the skin by these children and their caregivers, recurrence of the hand deformity is commonplace, requiring further operations.

SYMPHALANGISM

Symphalangism is the failure of interphalangeal joint differentiation. The capsule and ligaments may be poorly developed; cartilage bars may lie across the joint, and sometimes total bony ankylosis is present. The proximal joints are commonly affected: the distal interphalangeal joints may be spared. Flexion creases are absent opposite the affected joints. Radiographs may show some semblance of a joint space because of the presence of a solid cartilage block. The amount of joint motion varies, but classically it is very limited.

Attempts to improve the range of motion (ROM) of the stiffened joints are rarely successful and may render them unstable. Most patients adapt well to the deformity. Usually the involved digits are short, and there may be an associated syndactyly (symbrachydactyly). In these cases, early release of the conjoined digits is undertaken to diminish any restricting influence on their growth potential.

SYMBRACHYDACTYLY

Children with this deformity have short fingers with rudimentary nails present at the finger tips. This distinguishes it from constriction band syndrome. The bony elements of the digits have failed to develop fully. Four subgroups have been described by Blauth and Gekeler (20). In Poland's syndrome, symbrachydactyly is associated with failure of development of the sternocostal portion of the pectoralis major.

Treatment

Care should be taken when separating syndactyly in the short-finger type because there is often a distal bifurcation of the neurovascular bundles within the digital cleft. Deepening of the first web space may require a local transposition flap. In some patients, the thumb lies in the same plane as the fingers, and an osteotomy of the first metacarpal is required.

In the cleft hand type, function may be improved by deepening the cleft and removing nonfunctioning finger nubbins. However, some boneless digital stumps can be stabilized with a toe phalanx bone graft.

Contractures Resulting from Failure of Differentiation

A number of contractures may result from failure of differentiation, including clasped thumb, camptodactyly, arthrogryposis multiplex congenita, and clinodactyly.

CONGENITAL TRIGGERING

While triggering of the fingers may be seen, congenital trigger thumb is much more common. The parents of children with congenital trigger thumb notice that the child does not extend the thumb. The interphalangeal joint is held in marked flexion and attempted passive extension produces pain. The tendon sheath is thickened at the level of the metacarpophalangeal joint, with an associated nodule in the flexor pollicis longus tendon. One-third of cases spontaneously resolve within 1 year, and so surgery should be deferred until the second year of life. Provided the deformity is corrected by 3 years of age, persistent deformity does not occur. Surgery comprises release of the thickened sheath, but trimming of the tendon nodule is not advised. Because of the potential for damage to other structures, this should not be delegated to an inexperienced surgeon. The excursion of the interphalangeal joint should be seen to be full before closing the wound.

CONGENITAL CLASPED THUMB

While all neonates clutch the thumb, the normal child ceases to clasp the thumb under the fingers by the 3rd or 4th month of life. The congenital clasped thumb is twice as common in males as in females, and is often bilateral. The condition presents with an adducted thumb that is flexed at the metacarpophalangeal joint. There are a variety of causes, including an absence or hypoplasia of extensor pollicis brevis. Sometimes it is associated with abnormalities of the extensor pollicis longus, and on rare occasions there are flexion contractures present.

The various subgroups of congenital clasped thumb have been classified by Weckesser and colleagues (21) into four groups:

- *Group I* has a deficient extensor mechanism, and there is no contracture
- *Group II* has deficient extension, and a flexion contracture is also present
- *Group III* is characterized by hypoplasia of the muscles and tendons and may be a variant of the hypoplastic thumb
- *Group IV* is the association of a deficient extensor mechanism with preaxial polydactyly

Treatment is related to the cause of the deformity. When the extensor tendons are weak, but full extension is possible (group I), prolonged splintage may protect the hypoplastic tendons from the powerful flexor forces. Ideally, splintage should commence before the age of 6 months.

Flexion contractures that remain passively uncorrectable require surgical release. If a Z-plasty is not sufficient, a dorsal rotation flap and skin grafting may be required. Sometimes the flexor pollicis longus requires lengthening (at the wrist) and the transverse head of the adductor may need to be released. Associated tendon hypoplasia or absence requires a tendon transfer. Local tendons (e.g., the extensor indicis proprius) may also be affected, and are thus not suitable for transfer. In such cases, the palmaris longus, brachioradialis, extensor carpi radialis longus, or flexor digitorum superficialis may be used to power thumb extension.

Some flexion deformities prove resistant to all forms of surgical treatment except fusion of the metacarpophalangeal joint in a position of function. Children with arthrogryphosis, cerebral palsy, or Freeman-Sheldon syndrome may present in this way.

CAMPTODACTYLY

This flexion deformity usually affects the little finger, although other fingers may be involved, and it is often bilateral. While most cases are sporadic, some are inherited in an autosomal dominant pattern. There is considerable debate about the etiology and about which are primary and secondary events (22), but examination and surgical exploration reveal a range of abnormalities:

- Shortage of skin and the retinaculum cutis
- Lateral bands that may be adherent to the sides of the proximal phalanx
- An abnormally inserted lumbrical
- A short sublimis tendon that may have an abnormal origin
- Attenuation of the central slip of the extensor tendon
- Deformity of the neck of the proximal phalanx

Clinically, there are two distinct groups: those with a *static* deformity and those in whom it is *progressive*. The static group should be managed conservatively; some find splintage can be useful. Regular review is important because there may be worsening with hand growth during the first 4 years of age and at puberty.

Surgery is reserved for children with rapidly progressive deformity, and should address all the abnormalities listed above. It is not surprising that the results are often disappointing.

CLINODACTYLY

Clinodactyly is congenital lateral deviation of a digit from its normal longitudinal alignment. Any digit may be involved. The usual deformity is a radial deviation of the little finger at the distal interphalangeal joint, but clinodactyly can also occur at the proximal interphalangeal joint. Abnormal development of the middle phalanx is commonly responsible for malalignment of the interphalangeal joint surfaces. This is often a dominant trait, and it may occur bilaterally. An incidence of 9.9:1000 live births has been reported (23). Marked clinodactyly is associated with mental retardation, and it is common in children with Down syndrome. It rarely requires treatment, unless it is so severe as to interfere with function. In fingers of normal length, a closing wedge osteotomy is in-

dicated. In short fingers, an opening wedge osteotomy and bone graft may be undertaken. Any associated soft-tissue contracture will also require release.

The deformity may be due to a delta phalanx in which the proximal epiphysis is C-shaped, extending along the length of the bone and continuous with the distal epiphysis. This has also been described as a longitudinally bracketed diaphysis. Resection of the isthmus of the continuous C-shaped epiphysis and replacing it with a fat graft has given promising results (24). Until this technique is confirmed, osteotomy remains the mainstay of treatment.

An opening wedge osteotomy is often limited by skin shortening and requires a bone graft. A closing wedge osteotomy loses length in the digit. A "reverse" wedge with an angulation of half the required correction, taken from one side of the delta phalanx and inserted into the other, avoids this but is very demanding to perform in a small digit. A dome-shaped osteotomy allows correction while retaining length. All may require revision after subsequent growth is complete.

If the delta phalanx is supernumerary, it should be removed and the collateral ligament reconstructed. This is often the case in a triphalangeal thumb. All surgery for clinodactyly is difficult and the results are unpredictable. It is therefore best to avoid surgery in minor cases and to delay surgery, if the deformity is pronounced, until about 6 or 7 years of age.

Duplications (Group 3)

Duplication is one of the commonest malformations in the hand. All digits in the hand may be duplicated, the most common being the little finger. In the African-American population, prevalence is as high as 1:300 live births. A true prevalence of ulnar polydactyly is difficult to establish because those that look like skin tags are often ligated soon after birth.

Duplication is less common in the European population, with the thumb being more frequently affected. There are three degrees of polydactyly:

- *Type I:* an extra soft tissue mass not attached to the skeleton
- *Type II:* an extra digit, or part thereof, containing normal components articulating with a metacarpal or phalanx
- *Type III:* an extra digit with normal components articulating with an extra metacarpal

Treatment depends on the type of duplication. Only in type I is simple amputation adequate. In other cases, surgery may involve ligament reconstruction or an osteotomy to reorientate the joint surface of a shared joint. There is always hypoplasia of both component parts, and the digit that remains following surgery will often be smaller than normal. When abnormal Y-shaped tendons or neurovascular bundles are present they need careful splitting.

RADIAL POLYDACTYLY (DUPLICATE THUMBS)

The prevalence of radial polydactyly is 0.08 per 1000 live births (7). Duplication may occur at any level, either arising from a common joint or a bifid phalanx or metacarpal. Wassel (25) classified these deformities into seven sub-groups (Fig. 90–8):

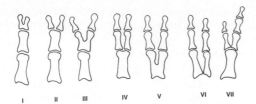

FIG. 90–8.   Classification of bifid thumbs according to the underlying bony configuration as described by Wassel.

Type	Description	Frequency
Type I	Bifid distal phalanx	2%
Type II	Two distal phalanges arising from the interphalangeal joint	15%
Type III	Bifid proximal phalanx	6%
Type IV	Bifid thumb arising at the metacarpophalangeal joint	43%
Type V	Bifid metacarpal	10%
Type VI	Bifid thumbs arising at the carpometacarpal joint	4%
Type VII	Bifid thumb with triphalangia	20%

Although the two elements of a duplicate thumb are often symmetrical, the bony elements of an accessory thumb may be different in size and configuration. Sometimes, the same skin and subcutaneous envelope surrounds all skeletal elements such that the complex looks like a single digit.

When the intrinsic muscles divide to insert into separate compartments of the thumb, the abductor and opponens insert into the radial duplicate and need to be relocated if this digit is discarded. Sometimes, instead of being on the radial side of the hand, the accessory thumb lies in the first web area.

Where the accessory digit is displaced from the main skeletal axis of the thumb, simple excision is the appropriate treatment, but this is rarely the case. If one of the thumb components is significantly smaller, its removal is justified. In the distal duplications of types I and II, where there is a common interphalangeal joint and the two components are of equal size, the Bilhaut Cloquet technique is appropriate (26). Nail deformities are invariable, but the central split in the new nail can be avoided if a complete nail is taken from one of the thumbs.

In type IV duplication, the radial digit is sacrificed if the two are of equal size and function. This preserves normal sensation on the important ulnar side of the thumb, and maintains stability in pinch, because the ulnar collateral ligament of the metacarpophalangeal joint remains undisturbed. Reinsertion of the thenar muscles is required, and the intact ligament of the deleted digit is used to reconstruct the radial collateral ligament. If the metacarpal head is wedge shaped, then an osteotomy to realign the articular surface is necessary. The long flexors and extensors may insert eccentrically to the distal phalanx and thus contribute to malalignment of the digit. If the lateral fibers of the tendon are released and turned over toward the center of the phalanx, a normal tendon pull may be created.

It is important to point out to the parents that the remaining thumb is always hypoplastic; otherwise, they may regard this as a consequence of surgery.

Radial polydactyly may be associated with a triphalangeal thumb. Retention of the biphalangeal component is a desirable but difficult decision if this is hypoplastic. When two triphalangeal thumbs are present, the radial one is usually excised. Removal of an extra phalanx runs the risk of instability, and formal fusion is preferable unless the extra phalanx is trapezoidal or delta shaped.

CENTRAL POLYDACTYLY

Duplication of the index, middle, and ring fingers is most often associated with a complex form of syndactyly, but can occur in isolation. The hypoplastic digit may be hidden. The ring finger is most commonly duplicated, and the index finger least commonly. This is often inherited as an autosomal dominant trait (27).

The nerves and vessels in the vicinity of the extra digit usually take an anomalous course. Because the accessory digit displaces the normal phalanges from their longitudinal axis, early removal is recommended. The remaining digits are often stiff, despite a relatively normal appearance. Abnormal transverse metacarpals may be seen in this condition.

LITTLE-FINGER POLYDACTYLY

Type I duplication of the little finger is inherited as a dominant trait. It is common in blacks and is easy to treat by direct excision. When there are bony connections, adequate tissue from the accessory digit should be retained to reconstruct ligaments. It is useful to conserve a slight excess of skin before closure, so that in the final trimming a Z-plasty can be incorporated.

Overgrowth or Gigantism (Group 4)

MACRODACTYLY

Macrodactyly is a congenital, localized, pathologic enlargement of skeletal and soft tissues, giving a disproportionately large digit (Fig. 90–9). Involvement may be limited to the digits, or extend to the hand and forearm. It is noted at birth or shortly thereafter. All structures of the digit are enlarged, and the condition should not be confused with tumors and special tissue malformations (e.g., vascular malformations). True macrodactyly involves the bones, whereas tissue edema associated with the ring constriction syndrome is a pseudomacrodactyly. True macrodactyly is rare and usually occurs

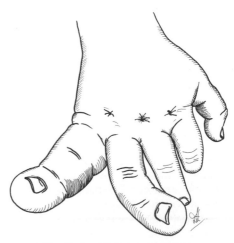

FIG. 90–9.   Digital macrodactyly.

as an isolated deformity. Some cases are associated with syndactyly. The majority of cases are unilateral, and the index finger is frequently affected. When multiple digits are affected (70% of cases), the involved digits are adjacent. The condition is more common in males. Isolated macrodactyly is not familial; a somatic mutation is thought responsible. Syndromic macrodactyly does show a familial tendency. Enlarged digits are found in neurofibromatosis, congenital partial gigantism, Ollier disease, Maffucci syndrome. Klippell Trenaunay syndrome, and congenital lymphedema.

There are two clinical types of macrodactyly: *static,* in which the digital involvement remains in the proportions established at birth; and *progressive,* in which there is an aggressive enlargement of the involved digits, changing the proportions noted at birth. With growth of the digits, lateral curvature may be noticed. The progressive growth of these digits tends to stop when the epiphyses close. Such fingers are not only unsightly but also stiff and difficult to camouflage.

The nerves supplying the digit are frequently enlarged, and Kelikian used the term *nerve territory orientated macrodactyly* (NTOM) to describe the most common form of macrodactyly. Marked soft-tissue hypertrophy on the palmar surface causes the distal interphalangeal joint to assume a hyperextended position, obstructing flexion of the finger. With age, osteophytes appear, giving the fingers a knobby appearance. Calcified deposits in tendons often occur.

Reducing the size of these digits is difficult. For the most grotesque flail, stiff, and anesthetic digits, amputation is indicated. To halt growth when the digit reaches the estimated normal adult size, epiphyseal arrest is achieved by ablating the epiphyseal plate. While this prevents longitudinal growth, circumferential growth may continue.

For patients whose digit is already beyond adult size, reduction osteotomies may be indicated. Excess tissue is later removed from one-half of the finger at a time. Subcutaneous fat and some skin are removed at each stage. Because this interrupts the cutaneous blood supply, wound healing is often poor. Removal of bone from the phalanges with a high-speed burr also helps to decrease the bulk of the digit. Whatever surgical procedures are undertaken, ROM is invariably compromised. Although the size can be reduced, the final result is likely to be a relatively stiff, abnormal looking finger.

Undergrowth or Hypoplasia (Group 5)

The most common type of hypoplasia seen in the hand affects the thumb. When only the fingers are involved, surgical treatment is rarely required. Short metacarpals may be associated with specific syndromes (e.g., Turner syndrome, XO). Short phalanges (brachydactyly) most commonly affect the border digits. Short digits are often seen in association with syndactyly.

THUMB HYPOPLASIA

A spectrum of deformity ranging from a minimally short thumb to an absent thumb has been classified by Blauth (28). Short thumbs are a common feature of many syndromes (e.g., Apert, Carpenter, and Rubinstein Taybi). Web space correction is sometimes all that is required to improve function. The surgical treatment is governed by the degree of hypoplasia:

- *Grade I:* the thumb is slightly small, but all the normal components are present. Surgery is not required and function is not impaired.
- *Grade II:* the thumb is slightly small, but in addition there is hypoplasia of the thenar muscles. This leads to an adduction contracture of the first web space. The ulnar collateral ligament of the metacarpophalangeal joint is lax, and there may be insertional anomalies of the extrinsic muscles. Release of the first web space, opponensplasty, reinsertion of the extrinsic tendons, and ligamentous reconstruction of the metacarpophalangeal joint may be required.
- *Grade III:* the thenar muscles are absent and the extrinsic tendons are abnormal or absent. There is associated skeletal hypoplasia and limited movement at the carpometacarpal joint. Manske has described two sub-groups:
  - *Grade IIIA,* where the metacarpal shaft is of reasonable size
  - *Grade IIIB,* where the majority of the metacarpal is absent
  In grade IIIA there have been promising results using free metarsal and joint transfers. In grade IIIB pollicization of the index finger is preferable.
- *Grade IV:* the floating thumb (pouce flotant) is attached to the hand by skin only and has no function. Pollicization should be carried out within the first year of life.
- *Grade V:* total aplasia of the thumb. Here too pollicization is the appropriate treatment.

Techniques

Release of the Web

Widening and deepening of the contracted first web space in grade II hypoplasia requires the release of skin and any underlying tight, deep fascia. A Z-plasty or four-flap Z-plasty may considerably improve the contracture but, when the space is markedly shortened, a transposition flap from the dorsum of the index finger may be required (Fig. 90–10). The donor defect is covered with a full-thickness skin graft. In cases in which hypoplasia is combined with duplication, the skin from the filleted discard may help to deepen the web (29).

Opponensplasty

Restoration of opposition requires the transfer of an active muscle unit. The superficialis tendon of the ring finger (30) or the abductor digiti minimi (31) can be used. The superficialis tendon of the ring finger has the better range of excursion. The tendon is exposed through an incision at the level of the proximal digital crease. It is retrieved distal to the flexor retinaculum and rerouted to be looped through the proximal phalanx and distal metacarpal, thus reconstructing the lax ulnar collateral ligament.

The entire abductor digiti minimi may also be mobilized to power opposition. The tendon is passed through a tunnel and sutured to the hypoplastic abductor pollicis brevis. This gives some bulk to the thenar eminence, but a separate reconstruction of the ulnar collateral ligament is required.

Stabilization of the Metacarpophalangeal Joint

When the ulnar collateral ligament is lax, it may be reinforced with a free tendon graft. In the very young, the thick

FIG. 90–10. A Z-plasty combined with a dorsal rotation flap to correct an adduction contracture of the first web space. The donor site is reconstructed with a skin graft.

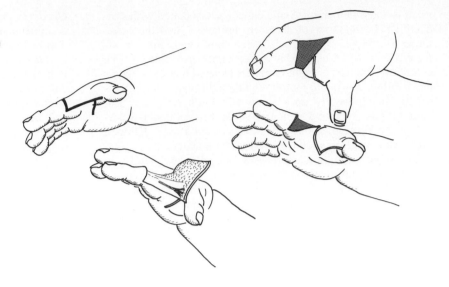

periosteum may hold stitches. If holes in the bones are required to secure the reconstructed ligament, great care should be taken not to damage the growing epiphyses. Stability of the thumb is especially difficult when its muscles are underdeveloped. In some cases, arthrodesis may be required, but once again care is necessary to preserve the epiphyseal plate at the base of the proximal phalanx.

Tendon Adjustment

When the normal skin creases of the thumb are absent or poorly developed, or when there is deviation of the distal interphalangeal joint, anomalies of the extrinsic tendons may be present. In some cases, where the thenar muscles are absent, the flexor pollicis longus may run a very superficial course, connecting with the extensor pollicis longus and brevis tendons and inserting into the lateral digital sheet to exert an abductor force on the distal phalanx. Useful flexion and extension may not be possible, and this complex may exert a powerful abductor force on poorly stabilized joints of the thumb. The anomalous flexor extensor connection (pollex abductus) needs division. The power of the existing flexor may be improved by reinsertion of the tendon.

Pollicization

The creation of a new thumb from an existing digit is the procedure of choice in advanced hypoplasia and aplasia of the thumb. Although the index finger is often stiff in children with radial clubhand, pollicization is also used to reconstruct precision pinch in these children.

Procedure for Pollicization

Preservation of Neurovascular Structures

Arteriography is not required routinely, but may be of value when there is specific concern about the vascular supply, for example in some severe deformities associated with longitudinal hypoplasia of the forearm.

Skin Incisions

At the base of the index finger an incision is fashioned to form a long V on the dorsal aspect extending to a point overlying the shaft of the metacarpal. It is carried through skin

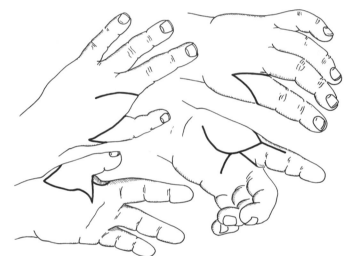

FIG. 90–11. Skin incisions for pollicization of the index finger.

only to preserve vessels and nerves. A short V is used on the volar surface (Fig. 90–11).

Both neurovascular bundles are kept intact if present, however one vessel is usually dominant. On the ulnar side of the digit, the nerve is dissected from the common digital nerve toward the base of the palm. The arterial branch to the radial side of the middle finger is ligated to mobilize the ulnar digital vessel of the index. On the dorsal aspect, two veins should be preserved.

Skeletal Adjustment

The transverse metacarpal ligament is divided and the metacarpal shaft is exposed to allow excision. The ideal position and length of the new thumb is determined preoperatively by the ROM and the length of the other digits. The intrinsic muscles are stripped off the shaft, their distal tendons divided and the shaft of the bone removed, leaving the metacarpal head. The digit is then rotated about its long axis and dropped down into its new position. A rotation of up to 160° is often required to achieve pulp-to-pulp pinch, and it must be remembered that this position frequently regresses when the muscles are reattached and the skin sutured. A lesser degree of rotation may give poor results.

The head of the metacarpal is preserved and the metacarpophalangeal joint becomes the new carpometacarpal joint. To prevent hyperextension of the thumb, the head of the metacarpal is rotated to tighten the volar plate before a K wire is fed up through the joint and proximal phalanx. The distal interphalangeal joint should not be immobilized because adjustment of the tendon transfers will be compromised. Once the position is confirmed, the wire is driven down into the carpus to secure the digit (Fig. 90–12).

Tendon Transfers

The tendon of the first dorsal interosseous is moved one joint distally and attached to the radial side of the base of the middle phalanx to function as a short abductor. The palmar interosseous tendon is sutured to the ulnar side of the middle phalanx to act as an adductor. The extensor tendons are divided and shortened. The two flexor tendons do not need to be shortened in young children, because they readjust their length over the ensuing 6 months. Flexion adequate for thumb function can be expected. In older children, shortening to an appropriate length speeds recovery.

Postoperative Management

A well-padded dressing is applied so that the tips of the digits can be inspected. In older children, a plaster cast is useful. Absorbable sutures are used. The dressing and K wire are removed at 4 weeks. Taping the remaining digits together or wearing a mitten will encourage prehensile use of the new thumb.

Judicious hand therapy can speed up rehabilitation; otherwise, it takes up to 6 months for the final functional result to be seen.

Complications

The most devastating problem is necrosis, which occurs as a result of tight dressings, hematomas, or vessel thrombosis, although this is exceedingly rare. The thin skin flaps are transposed through large distances, and may show marginal necrosis. This usually heals without significant scarring.

Joint imbalance can occur if the metacarpal head is not rotated to prevent hyperextension of the thumb. Tendon imbalance may compromise the function of the new thumb. If the nerve supply to the dorsal interosseous muscle is damaged, a superficialis tendon opponensplasty (32) can correct the deformity.

HYPOPLASTIC DIGITS

Short and underdeveloped digits are associated with many types of congenital hand deformity. Rudimentary digits are often little more than skin tubes with a deficiency of underlying bone and tendon. While surgical treatment is not always warranted, the digits can be augmented by free phalangeal transfer from the toe and subsequent distraction lengthening (33,34). A toe phalanx is usually harvested from the second toe through an incision on the dorsum, splitting skin and the extensor mechanism (Fig. 90–13). The phalanx is harvested with its periosteum. Sewing the flexor and extensor tendons together to prevent shrinkage in the donor toe is counterproductive and should not be undertaken. The free phalangeal transfer is fixed in position with a single K wire, if there is suitable adjacent bone, and sutured to the flexor and extensor tendons. These transfers give good length and create a new functioning joint.

Distraction lengthening may be applied to a phalanx or a metacarpal. Transverse K wires are inserted and the bone is sectioned subperiosteally between them. Using distraction apparatus fitted to the wires, up to 1 mm of distraction per day can be achieved. The eventual defect between the bone ends is filled with a bone graft at a second operation. It is important not to stretch the digit more than the local circulation

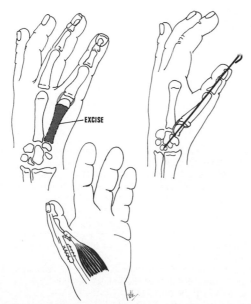

FIG. 90–12. The index digit is shortened and moved into its new position. The volar plate is tightened by rotating the head of the metacarpal and a longitudinal K wire is inserted. The exensor tendon is shortened and the intrinsic muscles are used to create adductors and abductors of the new thumb.

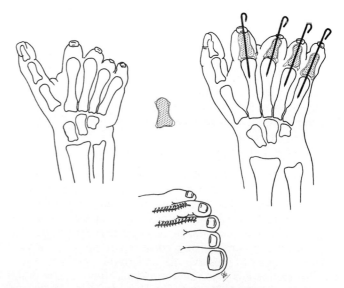

FIG. 90–13. Free phalangeal transfers for brachydactyly. The phalanges are harvested with periosteum and growth plate and placed into a subcutaneous pocket.

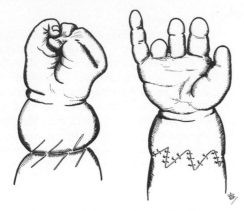

FIG. 90–14. Ring constriction syndrome. The fingers were fused at their tips before separation. The constriction band at the wrist has been excised and closed with multiple Z-plasties.

will permit. In selected cases, free toe-to-hand transfer may be appropriate.

Congenital Constriction Band Syndrome (Group 6)

Ring constrictions occur in about 1:15,000 live births (35). They consist of annular grooves running around a limb or digit. The creases may be only part-circumferential, often on the dorsum. In some of the deepest grooves, granulation tissue may be present. Neurovascular compromise distal to the groove may lead to edema, poor capillary refill, and decreased sensation. Autoamputation may have affected adjacent digits at the same level as the ring constriction (Fig. 90–14).

Digits may be joined at the level of such autoamputations. In these cases, they fuse distally, and tiny sinuses exist that resemble web remnants. When the fingers are separated, there are skin defects at the contact points. Ring constriction is associated with clubfeet, cleft lip and palate, and cranial defects. The etiology of this condition is uncertain. It has been assumed that bands of amnion have wrapped around the limbs; however, Streeter (36) claimed that focal necrosis of fetal germinal tissue was responsible.

The condition has been classified into four degrees of severity:

1. Simple ring constriction
2. Ring constriction with distal deformity
3. Ring constriction associated with fusion of the distal parts (acrosyndactyly)
4. Autoamputation

For simple ring constriction, staged excision of the ring and Z-plasty closure gives good results. Unless the groove is particularly deep, the surgery is not urgent. When there is functional impairment of venous or lymphatic drainage, surgery should be undertaken early to prevent progressive lymphedema. When excising constriction rings, great care should be taken to preserve the underlying nerves and vessels. Where there is associated acrosyndactyly, release of the tips of the involved digits should be performed by the time the child is 1 year of age. Tiny bulbous distal fragments are of little use other than as a source of full-thickness skin grafts.

In type 4 ring constriction, toe-to-hand transfers may be appropriate.

Summary

The surgery of congenital hand deformities is complex and requires a balance so that optimizing function does not impair growth. Early comprehensive surgery is advised so that redistributed or augmented tissues will be incorporated into developing patterns of behavior. Because repeated operations are often required, it is important to maintain the confidence of the patient and parents throughout the treatment program by creating realistic expectations for the outcome of each stage.

References

1. Ahstrom JP, Thomson HG, Lindsay WK, Williams HB. Panel discussion, congenital hand deformity. In: Kernahan DA, Thomson HG, eds. *Symposium on pediatric plastic surgery.* St Louis: CV Mosby Company, 1982; 21:438.
2. Richman N, Lansdown R. *Problems of preschool children.* New York: John Wiley & Sons, 1988.
3. Eaton RG. Hand problems in children—a timetable for management. *Pediatr Clin North Am* 1967; 14:643.
4. Conway H, Bowe J. Congenital deformities of the hands. *Plast Reconstr Surg* 1956; 18:286.
5. Rogala EJ, Wynn-Davies R, Littlejohn A, Gormley J. Congenital limb anomalies, Frequency and etiological factors. *J Med Genet* 1974; 11:221.
6. Office of Population Census and Surveys: Congenital malformation statistics—notifications England and Wales. HMSO Series MB3 (3). London: Her Majesty's Stationery Office, 1989.
7. Temtamy S, McKusick V. Polydactyly. *Birth Defects* 1978; 14:364.
8. Wynn-Davies R, Kuczynski K, Lamb DW, Smith RJ. Congenital abnormalities of the hand. In: Lamb DW, Kuczynski K, eds. *The Practice of Hand Surgery.* Oxford: Blackwell Scientific Publications, 1981; 289.
9. Lösch GM, Buck-Gramcko D, Cihak R, Schrader M, Seichert V. An attempt to classify the malformations of the hand based on morphogenetic criteria. *Chir Plast* 1984; 8:1.
10. Swanson AB, Barsky AJ, Entin MA. Classification of limb malformation on the basis of embryology failures. *Surg Clin North Am* 1968; 48:1169.
11. Kelikian H. *Congenital Deformities of the Hand and Forearm.* Philadelphia: WB Saunders Company, 1974.
12. Lamb DW. Radial club hand. *J Bone Joint Surg (Am)* 1977; 59:1.
13. Buck-Gramcko D. Radialization as a new treatment for radial club hand. *J Hand Surg (Am)* 1985; 10:964–968.
14. Dick HM, Petzoldt RL, Bowers WR, Rennie WR. Lengthening of the ulna in radial agenesis—a preliminary report. *J Hand Surg* 1977; 2:175.
15. Snow JW, Littler JW. Surgical treatment of cleft hand. In: *Transactions of the Fourth Congress of the International Society.* Excerpta Medica Foundation, 1967; 888.
16. Flatt AE. *The Care of Congenital Hand Anomalies.* St Louis: CV Mosby, 1977.
17. Ashmead D, Smith PJ. Tissue expansion for Apert's syndactyly. *J Hand Surg (Br)* 1995; 20B:3:327.
18. Davidson BCC. Epidermolysis bullosa. *J Med Genet* 1965; 2:233.
19. Mullett FL, Smith PJ. Hand splintage following surgery for dystrophic epidermolysis bullosa. *Br J Plast Surg* 1993; 46:192.
20. Blauth W, Gekeler J. Symbrachydaktylen (Beitrag zur Morphologie, Klassifikation und Therapie). *Handchirurgie* 1973; 5:121.
21. Weckesser EC, Reed JR, Heiple KG. Congenital clasped thumb (congenital flexion adduction deformity of the thumb). *J Bone Joint Surg (Am)* 1968; 50A:1417.
22. Smith RJ, Kaplan EB. Camptodactyly and similar atraumatic flexion deformities of the PIP joints of the fingers. A study of 31 cases. *J Bone Joint Surg (Am)* 1968; 50A:1187.
23. Marden PM, Smith DW, McDonald MJ. Congenital anomalies in the newborn infant including minor variations. A study of 4412 babies by surface examination for anomalies and buccal smear for sex chromatin. *J Pediatr* 1964; 64:357.
24. Vickers D. Clinodactyly of the little finger: a simple operative technique for reversal of the growth abnormality. *J Hand Surg (Br)* 1987; 12:335.

25. Wassel HD. The results of surgery for polydactyly of the thumb. *Clin Orthop* 1969; 64:175.
26. Bilhaut M. Guérison d'un pouce bifide par un nouveau procédé opératoire. *Congr Fr Chir* 1890; 4:576.
27. Temtamy S, McKusick VA. Synopsis of hand malformations with particular emphasis on genetic factors. *Birth defects* 1969; 3:125.
28. Blauth W. Der Hypoplastiche Daumen. *Arch Orthop Unfallchir* 1967; 62:225.
29. Lister GD. Upper extremity. In: Mustarde JC, Jackson IT, eds. *Plastic Surgery in Infancy and Childhood.* Edinburgh: Churchill Livingstone, 1988; 581.
30. Herrick RT, Lister GD. Control of first web space contracture. Including a review of the literature and a tabulation of opponensplasty techniques. *Hand* 1977; 9:253.

31. Huber E. Hilfsoperation bei median uslahmung. *Dtsch Arch Klin Med* 1921; 136:271.
32. Buck-Gramcko D. Pollicization. In: Serafin D, Georgiade NG, eds. *Pediatric Plastic Surgery.* St Louis: CV Mosby Company, 1984; 2:1005.
33. Matev IB. Thumb reconstruction in children through metacarpal lengthening. *Plast Reconstr Surg* 1979; 64:665.
34. Carroll RE, Green DP. Reconstruction of hypoplastic digits using toe phalanges. *J Bone Joint Surg (Am)* 1975; 57A:727.
35. Patterson TJS. Congenital ring-constrictions. *Br J Plast Surg* 1961; 14:1.
36. Streeter G. Focal deficiencies in fetal tissues and their relation to intrauterine amputation. Carnegie Institute of Washington Publ 44, *Contrib Embryol* 1930; 22:1.

skin incision for harvesting the pedicle overlies the neurovascular bundle in a straight line. It is extended into the palm to allow visualization and mobilization of the neurovascular bundle for 8 to 10 centimeters. The flap is elevated at the level of the flexor sheath, taking all subcutaneous tissue. The recipient site is prepared by removal of a block of skin and underlying tissue of the same dimensions as the flap. A palmar incision is then extended from the recipient site to the proximal extent of the donor incision for burying the pedicle. Alternatively, the flap may be tunneled beneath intact skin to the recipient area, although this carries a higher risk of pedicle torsion (34). The flap is placed in its final position and the incisions closed without tension. The donor defect has typically been covered with a full-thickness skin graft. However, it has been our experience that with the use of subperiosteal mobilization of the remaining tissue, primary closure is usually possible (Fig. 91–13) and obviates some of the adverse sequelae related to an insensate skin graft (35).

The neurovascular island flap is almost always useful for restoring at least protective sensation to an otherwise anesthetic digital surface. However, results vary widely in terms of the critical capability of the transferred sensation. Some authors report two-point discrimination capability in the normal range, while others have reported only protective sensation (33,36). Surely technical precision in elevating the flap plays some role, but other factors such as lack of cortical reeducation or wound healing problems may decrease the quality of the result. Along with the sensory loss that occurs to the donor, there is a significant incidence of pain and/or paresthesias in the donor or recipient digits. These problems therefore demand very careful patient selection to optimize the outcome.

Other Techniques

Continuing advances in microsurgery have allowed other options in the treatment of fingertip amputations. The technical difficulty of very distal replantation along with questionable benefit makes such treatment a "long run for a short slide." However, some authors have shown that an acceptable survival rate (though usually lower than in more proximal replantation) can be achieved with artery only or arteriovenous anastomosis (37–39). Discriminating sensation has been reported by some to be excellent, as well as providing a very satisfactory aesthetic result (40). When successful, such a distal replant offers the potential for excellent function and a better cosmetic result than other methods of reconstruction. Delayed free-tissue transfer from the toes also yields functional results, while restoring physical appearance to nearly normal (8,42,43).

When flap coverage is needed but options within the hand have been exhausted, we have generally used either the groin flap or the radial forearm flap as the workhorse choices. The prolonged period of immobilization and necessity for a second surgical procedure tend to argue against the groin flap, but in some cases it is still the best choice. Excessive bulk may be a problem with either of these alternatives, but this can be avoided by taking a fascia-only radial forearm flap with a skin graft to provide a less bulky and more serviceable fingertip in a one-stage procedure.

References

1. Zook EG, Guy RJ, Russell RC. A study of nail bed injuries: causes, treatment, and prognosis. *J Hand Surg* 1984; 9A:247.
2. Zook EG, Van Beek AL, Russell RC, et al. Anatomy and physiology of the perionychium: a review of the literature and anatomic study. *J Hand Surg* 1980; 5:528.
3. Zook EG. Anatomy and physiology of the perionychium. *Hand Clin* 1990; 6:1.
4. Glicenstein J, Dardour JC. The pulp: anatomy and physiology. In: Tubiana R, ed. *The hand.* Vol. 1 (116–120). Philadelphia: WB Saunders, 1985.
5. Shepard GH. Management of acute nailbed avulsions. *Hand Clin* 1990; 6:39.
6. Shepard GH. Treatment of nail bed avulsions with split-thickness nail bed grafts. *J Hand Surg* 1983; 8:49.
7. Saito H, Suzuki Y, Fujino K, et al. Free nail bed graft for treatment of nail bed injuries of the hand. *J Hand Surg* 1983; 8:171.
8. Allen MJ. Conservative management of finger tip injuries in adults. *Hand* 1980; 12:257.
9. Bossley CJ. Conservative treatment of digit amputations. *NZ Med J* 1975; 82:379.
10. Chow SP, Ho E. Open treatment of fingertip injuries in adults. *J Hand Surg* 1982; 7:470.
11. Holm A, Zachariae L. Fingertip lesions: an evaluation of conservative treatment versus free skin grafting. *Acta Orthoped Scand* 1974; 45:382.
12. Louis DS, Palmer AK, Burney RE. Open treatment of digital tip injuries. *JAMA* 1980; 244:697.
13. Atasoy E, Godfrey A, Kalisman M. The "antenna" procedure for the "hook-nail" deformity. *J Hand Surg* 1983; 8:55.
14. Porter RW. Functional assessment of transplanted skin in volar defects of the digits: a comparison between free grafts and flaps. *J Bone Joint Surg* 1968; 50A:955.
15. Schenck RR, Cheema TA. Hypothenar skin grafts for fingertip reconstruction. *J Hand Surg* 1984; 9A:750.
16. Kutler W. A new method for finger tip amputation. *JAMA* 1947; 133:29.
17. Shepard GH. The use of lateral V–Y advancement flaps for fingertip reconstruction. *J Hand Surg* 1983; 8:254.
18. Atasoy E, Ioakimidis E, Kasdan ML, et al. Reconstruction of the amputated finger tip with a triangular volar flap. *J Bone Joint Surg* 1970; 52A:921.
19. Moberg E. Aspects of sensation in reconstructive surgery of the upper extremity. *J Bone Joint Surg* 1964; 46A:817.
20. Kiem HA, Grantham SA. Volar-flap advancement for thumb and finger tip injuries. *Clin Ortho* 1969; 66:109.
21. O'Brien B. Neurovascular island pedicle flaps for terminal amputations and digital scars. *Br J Plast Surg* 1968; 21:258.
22. Stevenson TR. Fingertip and nailbed injuries. *Ortho Clin North Am* 1992; 23:149.
23. Gurdin M, Pangman WJ. The repair of surface defects of fingers by transdigital flaps. *Plast Reconstr Surg* 1950; 5:368.
24. Cronin TD. The cross finger flap: a new method of repair. *Am Surg* 1951; 17:419.
25. Hoskins HD. The versatile cross-finger pedicle flap. *J Bone Joint Surg* 1960; 24A:261.
26. Nishikawa H, Smith PJ. The recovery of sensation and function after cross-finger flaps for fingertip injury. *J Hand Surg* 1991; 17B:102.
27. Johnson RK, Iverson RE. Cross-finger pedicle flaps in the hand. *J Bone Joint Surg* 1971; 53A:913.
28. Kleinert HE, McAlister CG, MacDonald CJ, et al. A critical evaluation of cross finger flaps. *J Trauma* 1974; 14:756.
29. Barton NJ. A modified thenar flap. *Hand* 1975; 7:150.
30. Russell RC, Van Beek AL, Wavak P. Alternative hand flaps for amputations and digital defects. *J Hand Surg* 1981; 6:399.
31. Smith RJ, Albin R. Thenar "H-flap" for fingertip injuries. *J Trauma* 1976; 16:778.
32. Melone CP Jr., Beasley RW, Corstens JH Jr. The thenar flap: an analysis of its use in 150 cases. *J Hand Surg* 1982; 71:291.
33. Littler JW. Neurovascular skin island transfer in reconstructive hand surgery. In: Wallace AB, ed. *Transactions of the International Society of Plastic surgeons, Second Congress,* 175–178. London: E & S Livingstone Ltd, 1960.
34. Tubiana R. Island flaps. In: Tubiana R, ed. *The hand.* Vol. II (299–312). Philadelphia: WB Saunders, 1985.

35. Puckett CL, Howard B, Concannon MJ. Primary closure of the donor site for the Littler neurovascular island flap transfer. *Plast Reconstr Surg,* 1996; 97:1062.
36. Murray JF, Ord JVR, Gavelin GE. The neurovascular island pedicle flap. *J Bone Joint Surg* 1967; 49A:1285.
37. Foucher G, Norris RW. Distal and ver distal digital replantations. *Br J Plast Surg* 1992; 45:199.
38. Koshima I, Soeda S, Moriguchi T, et al. The use of arteriovenous anastomosis for replantation of the distal phalanx of the fingers. *Plast Reconstr Surg* 1992; 89:710.
39. Yamano Y. Replantation of fingertips. *J Hand Surg* 1993; 18B:157.
40. Chen CT, Wei FC, Chen HC, et al. Distal phalanx replantation. *Microsurg* 1994; 15:77.
41. Daniel RK, Taylor GI. Distant transfer of an island flap by microvascular anastomoses. *Plast Reconstr Surg* 1973; 52:111.
42. Foucher G, Merle M, Maneaud M, et al. Microsurgical free partial toe transfer in hand reconstruction: a report of 12 cases. *Plast Reconstr Surg* 1980; 65:616.
43. Morrison WA, O'Brien BM, MacLeod AM. Thumb reconstruction with a free neurovascular wraparound flap from the big toe. *J Hand Surg* 1980; 5:575.

92

Tendon Injuries of the Hand

Donald M. Ditmars, Jr., M.D., F.A.C.S., Morton L. Kasdan, M.D., F.A.C.S., and Nan Boyer, O.T.R., C.H.T.

Restoration of function after injury is the goal of hand surgeons. Movements of the fingers are a primary part of hand function and are the result of synchronized contractions of flexor and extensor muscles extrinsic to the hand and intrinsic hand muscle groups. Injuries to the extensor tendons, although common because of their thin protective cover, respond well to good wound care, approximation, and splinting because of the small amplitude of tendon motion (1). Wounds heal all layers with the same scar. This resulting scar attaches all cut tissues to each other and must selectively remodel over time for the hand to regain function. Adhesion of the overlying skin to the extensor tendon repair causes dimpling without much interference in function. In contrast, the flexor tendon sheath, through which the repaired flexor tendons must glide for a longer distance, provides a firm base for scar attachment. This makes mandatory the precise repairs of lacerated flexor tendons with skilled, coordinated postoperative management. A severed tendon can be a source of prolonged disability for the patient and should be approached with a carefully formulated plan, usually involving the services of a skilled hand therapist.

Emergency physicians and trauma surgeons must be able to recognize tendon injuries and refer them to surgeons skilled in hand surgery who have the competence to perform the repairs, treat unusual problems or unexpected complications, and coordinate the various phases of hand therapy. The result of tendon repairs in the hand depends on knowledge of anatomy, history of the injury, accurate examination, utilization of appropriate repair processes, and patient involvement. This chapter defines the functional anatomy, diagnosis, techniques of repair, and rehabilitation of hand tendon injuries.

Flexor Tendons

ANATOMY

Tendons from muscles originating in the forearm are considered extrinsic, whereas those with muscles entirely in the hand are considered intrinsic. The extrinsic flexor tendons begin in the distal third of the forearm. The deep group, the profundi, originate from a common muscle. As a result, blocked flexion of one profundus limits the flexion of the rest—the "quadriga" effect (2). Innervation of the two ulnar heads is from the ulnar nerve, and that of the two radial heads is from the median nerve. Each superficialis tendon is attached to a separate muscle belly, allowing it to act independently. All four of the superficialis tendons are innervated by the median nerve (3). Both groups of four tendons and the

flexor pollicis longus pass through the carpal tunnel with the median nerve, the superficialis tendons lying volar to the profundi. This relationship continues until the level of the proximal phalanges, where the superficialis tendons split to form the Camper chiasm (3), through which the profundus tendons pass on their way to insert into the distal phalanges. The two slips of the superficialis partially decussate at the proximal interphalangeal joint and insert on the middle phalanx (Figs. 92–1 and 92–4). Thus, the superficialis tendons flex the metacarpophalangeal and proximal interphalangeal joints, providing independent action for each finger, and the profundus tendons flex the distal interphalangeal joints.

The lumbricals (usually four) are intrinsic muscles originating from the radial sides of the profundus tendons in the midpalm just distal to the transverse carpal ligament with the fingers extended (4). The lumbricals are drawn into the carpal tunnel with finger flexion (5). These worm-shaped muscles turn into tendons in well-protected, deep tunnels that angle dorsally across the metacarpophalangeal joints volar to the axis of rotation at an angle of approximately 30° to join the lateral bands in the proximal phalanges. They and the interosseous muscles provide independent flexion of the metacarpophalangeal and extension of the interphalangeal joints (2).

The ulnar bursa of the palm is the sheath enveloping the flexors of the index, long, ring, and little fingers. It ends in blind diverticula about halfway along the metacarpals of the index, long, and ring fingers and is prolonged distally to join with the digital synovial sheath of the little finger (6). The index, long, and ring extrinsic flexor tendons exit the ulnar synovial bursa 2.5 cm proximal to the digital flexor sheaths, which begin at the level of the metacarpal necks, extending to the distal phalanges (Fig. 92–2). These sheaths are lined with synovium, sealed at both ends except in the little finger (6). The radial bursa surrounds the flexor pollicis longus until its insertion on the distal phalanx (6,7) (see Fig. 92–2). This bursal configuration is the anatomic basis for the classic "horseshoe abscess" noted in the older literature (9).

The mechanically efficient proximity of the flexor tendons to the bones and joints is maintained by the flexor tendon sheath, with condensations of fibrous tissue at strategic locations called pulleys. Five thick, distinct annular pulleys, three thin, cruciate-synovial bands, and a palmar aponeurotic band prevent bowing of the tendons on flexion of the fingers (10) (see Fig. 92–1). Three pulleys serve the same function for the thumb (Fig. 92–3). The 2nd and 4th annular pulleys in the fingers are the most important to maintain satisfactory flexion, and should be reconstructed if destroyed (11,12).

NUTRITION AND HEALING

The mesotendon is the source of nutrients for the flexor tendon proximal to the synovial sheath. Two sources have been definitely identified within the sheath: vascular and synovial fluid perfusion.

The segmental blood supply of the tendons is from: vessels through muscular branches in the forearm; vessels in the surrounding connective tissue via the paratendon, mesotendon, and vincula; vessels from the bone; and, minimally, vessels from the periosteum near the tendon insertion (13). The length of segmental supply from the musculotendinous junction is 2 cm and that from the vincula is 1 to 2 cm (14) (Fig. 92–4). These arteries enter the dorsal aspect of the tendon and must be preserved by minimizing mobilization during preparation for repair. Dissected segments of tendon longer than 2 cm function as free tendon grafts (14). Sutures are preferentially placed nearer the volar surface to least interfere with the intratendinous circulation so as to promote healing with minimal scar. This may be most important in the midproximal phalangeal segment, where the longitudinal intrinsic vessels meet the vincular system (15).

In the past 3 decades, many studies have been done of synovial nutrition of the flexor tendons within the synovial sheath (16). Tracer studies using hydrogen tritiated proline, sulfur-35, and other metabolic markers demonstrated that, for nutrition, diffusion was more effective than perfusion. Indeed, when the tendon was isolated from vascular connections, diffusion could provide the total nutritional requirement to all segments. Tendons without blood supply exhibited "local intrinsic cellular fibroplasia" within a synovial pouch of a rabbit (17). When the sutured segment of a flexor tendon was isolated with a semipermeable membrane, this evidence of healing occurred without surface macrophages. These latter cells were of an origin extrinsic to the tendon and contributed to the restoration of the tendon surface. Because the longitudinal, intrinsic tendon vasculature is easily occluded by sutures, synovial nutrition may be required in all intrathecal repairs. These studies are evidence

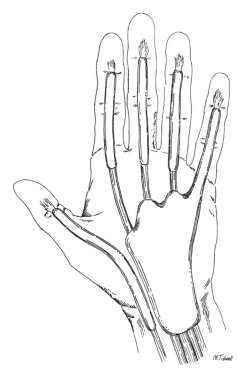

FIG. 92–2. Radial and ulnar bursae. Note that the middle three fingers have discontinuous bursae and only the little-finger bursa is continuous with the ulnar bursa.

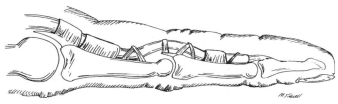

FIG. 92–1. The flexor tendons pass through a series of pulleys to insert on the distal phalanges.

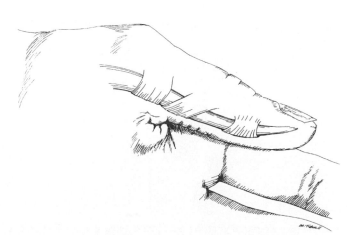

FIG. 92–3. The pulleys of the thumb.

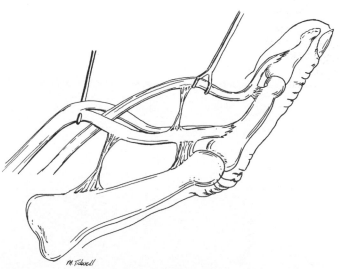

FIG. 92–4. Schematic diagram of the blood supply to the flexor tendons in the hand, through the vincula.

that sheath repair is indicated when primary tendon repairs or secondary tendon grafts are performed (18).

Tendons heal utilizing the usual wound healing processes found in other tissues, with a blending of inflammatory, fibroblastic, and remodeling phases. Tendon healing is very responsive to the initial phase, which can be accentuated and prolonged by contamination and tissue damage, resulting in delayed total healing time and increased scarring (19). Fibroblasts are demonstrated in clean wounds at 2 days, with collagen production commencing at the 4th or 5th day. The total collagen content is stabilized by the 4th to 6th week; however, achievement of final strength requires remodeling of the collagen fibers in response to stress. Peacock's principle of "One wound, one scar" indicates that the tendon and its surrounding tissues heal with one matted scar (1). The challenge to the hand surgeon is to encourage strong, longitudinal tendon healing while minimizing the surrounding scar to allow the gliding of the tendon that is required for function. A method for selectively controlling this process does not exist, but it is recognized that adherence to certain treatment principles will have a beneficial effect on wound healing (20,21):

1. The smaller the mass of collagen in the wound, the more satisfactory is the remodeling process. Atraumatic surgical technique is consequently important to minimize tissue injury, thus lessening the inflammatory phase and the resulting scar.
2. A hematoma must be avoided, because the presence of clotted blood causes greater scar deposition.
3. Young persons frequently have better results in spite of a tendency to form hypertrophic cutaneous scars around tendons, which will adversely affect the final range of motion. Plans for postoperative therapy will have to be formulated accordingly.
4. Postoperative therapy balances the stresses at the repair site to promote remodeling by encouraging polarization of collagen fibers without rupture of the repair. The observation of the relationship of stress to healing forms the basis for carefully timed programs of mobilization following tendon repair.

DIAGNOSIS

At times, making an accurate diagnosis of a divided flexor tendon can be difficult. A skin laceration is not always a reliable indication of damage to the underlying anatomy. For example, if trauma occurs when the finger is flexed, the end of the cut tendon is actually situated more distally than the surface wound (Fig. 92–5). Partial tendon lacerations and avulsions may also pose diagnostic problems (22). In any event, if the general condition of the patient permits, any question of possible tendon laceration should be resolved by surgical exploration.

TECHNIQUE OF REPAIR

Adherence to basic principles of meticulous surgical technique is of paramount importance for satisfactory results. Repairs must be performed in an unhurried fashion. They should be done in the operating room, where adequate assistance, proper lighting, and special instruments are at hand, rather than in the emergency room's busy atmosphere. The surgeon usually uses two- or four-power loupe magnification to enhance the same nontraumatic technique originally described by Bunnell over 70 years ago (23).

Using regional block or general anesthesia, surgery is performed in a bloodless field produced by a pneumatic tourniquet. The calibration of this instrument is checked for accuracy before its use. The cuff is inflated to approximately 100 mm Hg above the patient's systolic pressure. The exact safe tourniquet duration varies in the literature (24). We use 2 hours as a limit. If longer tourniquet time is needed, the cuff is deflated, and after 20 minutes it is reinflated.

The wound is liberally cleansed, irrigated, and débrided. The lacerated tendon is treated gently. It is handled only with gloved fingers and secured with a suture. Metal instruments are seldom used, except to grasp the frayed ends destined to be trimmed away before repair (Fig. 92–6). If necessary, a specially designed instrument or a rubber catheter is threaded through the pulleys to retrieve the portion of the tendon that retracted proximally into the palm, wrist, or forearm. After the tendon is brought into the wound, the proximal stump is held in place by transversely impaling it with a straight nee-

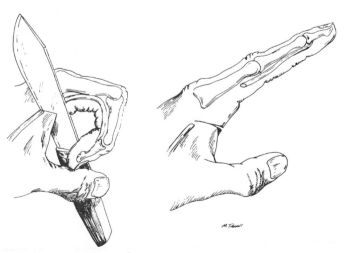

FIG. 92–5. Flexor tendon laceration with the finger flexed produces a cut end more distal than the skin laceration.

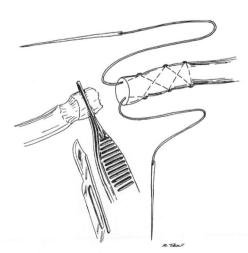

FIG. 92–6. Preparation of the cut tendon. Note that the instrument only grasps the portion to be removed.

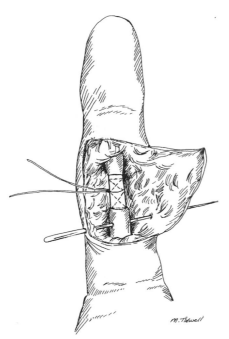

FIG. 92–7. The proximal tendon end may be held in place with a transfixion needle to prevent its retraction.

dle, permitting the repair to be performed without tension (25) (Fig. 92–7). A core, grasping suture is inserted for strength followed by a delicate epitenon circumferential suture for surface accuracy. Nonreactive suture material is used to approximate the tendon ends and postoperative mobilization is carefully supervised. By observing these principles, the surgeon will find fewer adhesions may form.

INCISIONS

The classical elective approach to the flexor tendons in the digits is the midlateral incision originally described by Bunnell (23). This incision offers several advantages. Its location on the lateral aspect of the finger leaves no scars on the volar skin that could result in tenderness or a flexion contracture. The nerve and blood supply of the volar skin is uninterrupted because the neurovascular bundle is raised with the volar flap. Furthermore, if more proximal structures require exposure, the incision can be extended into the palm in a curvilinear fashion, avoiding an unbroken, longitudinal scar.

The midlateral incision has a significant disadvantage. It is an indirect approach to the flexor tendons, necessitating extensive dissection and risking possible injury to the collateral ligaments, lateral bands, and retinacular ligaments. Damage to these structures can lead to joint stiffness or flexion contracture.

The zigzag incision was developed by Bruner in 1967 to avoid such problems (26). This incision is used when it is necessary to extend the wound in order to provide an unobstructed view of damaged structures. It is also employed for elective exposure of the flexor tendons. The incision is planned so that it does not cross flexion creases in the fingers, thereby avoiding potential scar contractures. The angles of the chevron-shaped flaps are greater than 90°, assuring adequate vascularity of the volar skin. If additional exposure is required, the incision is continued proximally, its line break-

ing at the flexion creases in the palm and wrist. Transverse limbs of the incision can be placed in flexion creases as a Z-plasty.

SUTURE MATERIAL AND METHODS

The ideal suture causes minimal tissue reaction, and is of small caliber, pliable, strong, and easy to handle. Once tied, it should hold a knot securely, showing little tendency to unravel (27). Many sutures are available that meet the needs of the hand surgeon. Nylon, polyester, and polypropylene are available in monofilament or multifilamentous strands; these produce little tissue reaction and are suitable for tendon repair (28). One of the earliest materials used in tendon surgery was stainless steel, which was advocated by Bunnell, who placed pull-out sutures at the time of repair and then removed them 3 or 4 weeks later.

Tensile strength is greater in stainless steel than in nylon or polyester; however, manipulation and knotting does diminish its strength. Tensile strength is not of maximum importance. If proper technique is used, there is no tension on the repair, and the integrity of the tendon need not rely on suture strength. Therefore, even though a polyester or nylon suture is not as strong as stainless steel, it is easier to handle and is, for many surgeons, the preferred material (29).

A secure repair results from a core suture technique that utilizes loops of suture to obtain lateral purchase on the tendon. Longitudinal pull is converted to oblique and transverse forces, which hold the tendon together in the early phases of healing when softening occurrs (30). Simple sutures tend to pull through the longitudinal tendon fibers.

The classical criss-cross, described by Bunnell in 1918, was the standard method until the last decade. Most hand surgeons prefer a variation of the Kessler technique (a modification of the Bunnell technique), or the Tsuge technique, which are considered less compromising to the intrinsic blood supply of the tendon (31,32). The 4-0 suture is placed to include 1 cm of tendon on either side of the laceration and tightened just enough to approximate the cut ends (29). The repair is completed with a superficial running suture of 5-0, 6-0, or 7-0 monofilament to invaginate protruding fibers and eliminate raw surfaces, thereby enhancing the smoothness of the repair (Fig. 92–8).

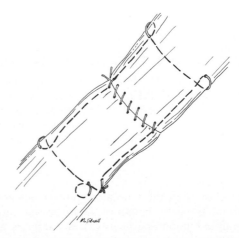

FIG. 92–8. Kessler tendon suture. The running circumferential suture should be 6-0 or 7-0 monofilament.

TIMING OF REPAIR

There are several advantages of primary tendon repair:

1. The original length of the tendon often can be retained.
2. There is a shorter period of disability necessitated by wound healing and late grafting.
3. There is often less joint stiffness.
4. When necessary, secondary tenolysis yields better results when primary tendon repair has already been performed (33).

Skin closure at the time of injury with deferred tendon repair is called "delayed primary repair." This term is arbitrary; "primary" and "delayed primary" are often used interchangeably. Tendon repair can be done up to 14 days after injury without adversely affecting the ultimate result (34–36).

Failure of the primary repair severely compromises the patient's ultimate recovery (22). Equal and sometimes even better results can be obtained with delayed primary repair when the situation merits its use. If the wound or the patient's general condition does not permit primary repair, the skin may be closed and tendon repair delayed. The hand is dressed and elevated, and appropriate antibiotics and tetanus prophylaxis are administered. Repair is performed when the condition of the patient and injured tissue are satisfactory.

Several conditions contraindicate primary repair. Repair can be delayed if:

1. The wound contains crushed, potentially nonviable tissue.
2. The pulley system has been destroyed.
3. The patient is uncooperative.
4. The wound is severely contaminated and cannot be adequately decontaminated by irrigation, débridement, and administration of systemic antibiotics. The "6-hour golden period" is an obsolete concept, and exceeding the 6-hour time limit past wounding does not contraindicate closure (37).
5. The surgeon is inexperienced or fatigued.
6. The general condition of the patient prohibits surgery.

At times, it is not possible to repair the tendon within 2 weeks (e.g., in cases of heavy wound contamination). In such cases, it is necessary to wait from 2 to 4 weeks, until the wound has healed and tissues have softened. A secondary repair is then attempted, often with difficulty because of tendon retraction and scarring. It is reasonable to repair the tendon as soon after injury as possible (21).

PROGNOSIS RELATED TO FLEXOR TENDON ZONES

The hand is divided into clinically significant zones on the basis of the anatomy of the tendons and their sheaths. These were originally described by Verdan (38), and later modified by Kleinert and colleagues (39). Prognosis of wound healing is related to the zone in which the injury occurs (Fig. 92–9).

Zone 5

Zone 5 extends from the musculotendinous junction in the forearm to the proximal border of the transverse carpal ligament. Multiple tendon and neurovascular injuries are common here. Primary repair is preferred, and it is generally successful in this region.

Zone 4

Zone 4 lies beneath the carpal tunnel, in the region between the proximal and distal borders of the transverse carpal ligament. Unless tissue is severely damaged, both superficialis and profundus tendons are repaired. The transverse carpal ligament should be divided to visualize the injury and prevent postoperative carpal-tunnel syndrome. Frequently, the hand surgeon must perform a partial flexor tenosynovectomy if the synovium is edematous and hemorrhagic (33).

Zone 3

Zone 3 extends from the distal border of the transverse carpal ligament to the beginning of the flexor tendon sheath. Repair of both superficialis and profundus tendons in this region usually has a favorable result.

Zone 2

Zone 2 extends from the distal palmar crease to the flexion crease of the proximal interphalangeal joint. Here the superficialis and profundus tendons are in close proximity within their shared fibrous sheath. Bunnell termed this region "no man's land," believing that the results of primary repair in this area were so poor that no one should try it. Ignoring his own advice, Bunnell himself proceeded with repair in this zone, but recommended against it in his teachings, perhaps reflecting his concern that much damage might be done if such cases were undertaken by unqualified surgeons. Bunnell's suggested treatment was skin closure and subsequent reconstruction with a tendon graft (27,40).

Improved techniques now permit successful primary repair of both superficialis and profundus tendons within zone 2. Successful primary repair results in better function and less disability. Because space in the sheath is limited, a window is cut so that the tendons are clearly visible. Some surgeons ex-

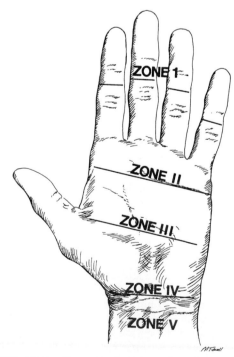

FIG. 92–9. Flexor tendon injury zones (see text).

cise a portion of the sheath around the repair site, whereas others close the sheath (27).

Zone 1

Zone 1 is distal to the insertion of the flexor digitorum superficialis. There are several methods described for tendon repairs in this region. If the laceration is within 1.5 cm of the superficialis insertion, Kleinert and others (41) recommended advancement and attachment of the profundus ends into the substance of the distal phalanx. Other options for repair include primary repair, tendon graft, arthrodesis, and tenodesis of the distal interphalangeal joint.

There is only one long flexor tendon to the thumb, the flexor pollicis longus, which runs in its tendon sheath. If this tendon is cut within its sheath, an intact vinculum usually makes retrieval of the proximal portion easy. Without vincular support, the proximal end may retract into the palm or wrist, necessitating the use of tendon retrieval devices and additional incisions.

PARTIAL LACERATIONS

Some authors suggest repair of the partially cut flexor tendon, whereas others favor refraining from surgical intervention (42,43). Advocates of repair suggest that suturing a partial laceration prevents rupture in the postinjury period and avoids potential "triggering," as well as problems arising from adhesions. If less than one-third of the tendon is involved, we use a small-caliber, continuous suture in the epitenon. If more of the tendon is cut, then we place a supporting stitch.

In one study, the author demonstrated that wound healing progresses just as well without repair if the tendon laceration is minimal (43). It is appropriate to close the wound and start a controlled mobilization program similar to that following a complete flexor tendon repair. This form of treatment is said to enhance gliding and make tendon rupture less likely.

AVULSIONS

Avulsion of the flexor digitorum profundus can result when the finger is forcibly extended during maximum contracture of the profundus muscle. This injury is commonly seen in football players, occurring when a tackler grabs the uniform of an opposing runner. The ring finger is involved in approximately 75% of cases, although avulsions have been reported in all digits. Diagnosis of this injury can be difficult because the radiographs are usually negative and the patient usually can flex the proximal interphalangeal joint. The patient often dismisses the injury as a "sprain."

Three main types of avulsions of the profundus tendon insertions were classified by Leddy, according to the vascular damage, in order to help determine recommendations for timing the repair (44):

1. The tendon retracts into the palm.
2. The tendon retracts to the level of the proximal interphalangeal joint.
3. A bony fragment is connected to the avulsed profundus stump.

In the first type, both vinculae are ruptured and repair is indicated within the first 7 to 10 days. The vinculum longum

remains intact in type 2, allowing up to 3 months for repair. Because both vincula remain intact in type 3, the decision for surgery is not based upon vascularity.

Simultaneous distal phalangeal fractures and dislocations should be repaired at the same time as the tendon advancement. The longer immobilization required may result in limited distal interphalangeal joint motion (45).

POSTOPERATIVE SPLINTING AND MOBILIZATION

Children are remarkable in that their hands can be splinted for 3 weeks or longer with expectations of good motion. An adult finger splinted for several weeks will develop joint stiffness, which, added to adhesions between a repaired tendon and surrounding tissues, will result in interphalangeal joint immobility. This poses an especially serious problem in zone 2, where the tendons are enclosed within the fibrous sheath. The recognition that both tendon gliding and joint motion are required in the immediate rehabilitation period has resulted in controlled-motion protocols (46–48). Indiscriminate mobilization can disrupt the repair. Early, controlled motion maintains joint mobility while reducing or attenuating tendon adhesions. The patient facing repair of a flexor tendon injury must be prepared for a postoperative rehabilitation period that can last up to 3 months before resumption of unrestricted activities. Alternatives to tendon repair should be considered for the patient who demonstrates an inability to responsibly participate in the postoperative treatment program.

The controlled mobilization program is begun 1 to 3 days postoperatively (49). The wrist is splinted in 20° of flexion, with the involved metacarpophalangeal joint(s) in 40° to 60° of flexion. The interphalangeal joints are passively flexed with a fishing line that has been attached by a loop to a dressmaker's hook glued to the finger nail. The line is threaded through a safety pin in the palm dressing or strap and secured proximally to a spring or flexible rubber band (Fig. 92–10). This dynamic traction device passively flexes all finger joints. The patient is instructed to actively extend the finger within the splint against the line tension, which protects the tendon repair by synergistic relaxation of the flexor muscles. Excess tension on the repair is avoided by the blocked extension of the wrist and metacarpophalangeal joints. The line tension can be adjusted by moving the proximal attachment of the spring or band on the proximal splint strap to allow the finger to be actively extended within the limitations of the splint. The patient is instructed to perform this exercise 10 times every waking hour (50).

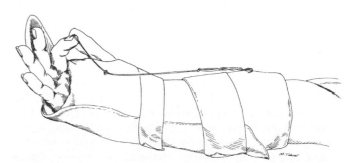

FIG. 92–10. Method of dynamic splinting for flexor tendon injuries (see text).

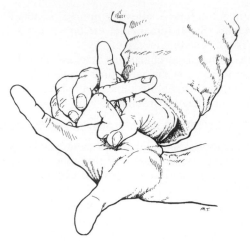

FIG. 92–11.   Immediate postoperative joint mobilization. The interphalangeal joints are completely passively flexed to the distal palmar crease daily by the surgeon/therapist.

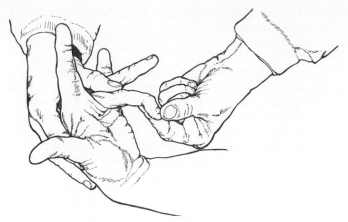

FIG. 92–12.   Postoperative proximal interphalangeal joint mobilization. All joints are flexed except the one being extended. The distal interphalangeal joint is passively flexed while passively extending the proximal interphalangeal joint, with the wrist and metacarpophalangeal joints flexed to minimize flexor tendon pull.

A daily supervised, protected ROM program is begun by the surgeon or therapist soon after surgery. The finger position within the dynamic splint achieves neither full extension nor flexion. Full passive flexion is initiated immediately by the patient after instruction (Fig. 92–11). Passive extension is performed at least 3 times a week by the surgeon/therapist, with protection of the repair. All joints are passively flexed except the one being extended (Figs. 92–12, 92–13). Daily supervision is continued for 2 weeks or longer, until the patient can extend the finger completely.

At 3 weeks, the splint is altered to further extend the metacarpophalangeal joints with the wrist neutral, thus allowing more excursion against the rubberband resistance. At 4 weeks, the dorsal splint can be removed, leaving the line/rubberband attached to a wristlet. Wrist exercises are encouraged. During the 5th week, the rubberband is discontinued; the patient actively flexes without resistance. For the following 2 weeks, active interphalangeal joint flexion, with blocking of proximal and middle phalanges in the line of tendon pull to enhance gliding, is monitored weekly. Any swelling or stiffness will require resumption of daily therapy sessions for further protected ROM exercises, including scar and edema control with massage and pressure. Progressive resistive exercises are instructed weekly during the 3rd month. A residual interphalangeal joint flexion contracture may require a custom dynamic traction splint. This splint has an added benefit of precisely controlling the resistance for the active exercises.

Extensor Tendons

ANATOMY

The extensor tendons are particularly vulnerable to trauma because of their superficial location in a clenched fist. The thin mobile subcutaneous tissue offers little protection. Lacerations of the extensors are common over joints that are easily exposed to contamination. The multiple tendinous interconnections are in a delicate balance of function that is related to the position of the finger (Fig. 92–14). These same interconnections prevent the retraction of the proximal cut

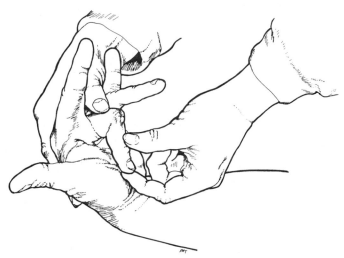

FIG. 92–13.   Postoperative distal interphalangeal joint mobilization. The proximal interphalangeal joint is passively flexed to relieve the tension on the flexor tendon repair, while the distal interphalangeal joint is being passively extended.

tendon ends, making extensive dissection unnecessary. They also make static splinting an integral part of the treatment of extensor tendon injuries. From the metacarpophalangeal joint distally, splinting alone may be the primary treatment because the tendon ends can be held in approximation by joint hyperextension (51–54).

The extensor system is composed of extrinsic and intrinsic muscles. The extrinsic muscles originate proximal to the wrist, their tendons passing over the dorsal aspect to insert into the hand and fingers. At the wrist, they are held in position by a transverse retinacular band that prevents dorsal bowing on wrist extension. The tendons are held in horizontal position under the extensor retinaculum by vertical bands that form the six dorsal compartments through which all extrinsic extensor tendons pass (Fig. 92–15):

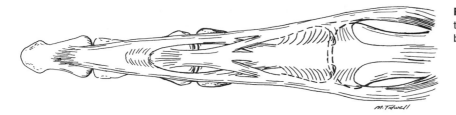

FIG. 92–14. Anatomy of an extensor tendon. Note the complex interrelationship of central slip, lateral bands, and intrinsics.

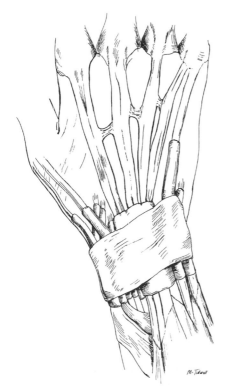

FIG. 92–15. Anatomy of the extensor tendons on the dorsum of the hand. Note the extensor retinaculum and the six dorsal compartments. The tendons on the dorsum of the hand are interconnected (juncturae tendineum).

1. First: abductor pollicis longus and extensor pollicis brevis
2. Second: extensor carpi radialis longus and brevis
3. Third: extensor pollicis longus
4. Fourth: extensor indicis proprius and extensor digitorum communis
5. Fifth: extensor digiti minimi
6. Sixth: extensor carpi ulnaris

Multiplicity of the first-compartment tendons and tunnels is frequent. The number and position of the extensor tendons are more variable on the ulnar side of the hand (55).

On the dorsal surface of the hand, at the level of the distal third of the metacarpals, the extensor communis tendons are interconnected by juncturae tendineum (Fig. 92–15). The extensor communis tendon to the little finger lies adjacent to the one to the ring finger, splitting from it just proximal to the metacarpal head. At this point it resembles a junctura, and indeed is absent in over 50% of hands. The proprius tendons to the index and little fingers are both ulnar to their respective communis tendons as they traverse the dorsum of the hand. The extensor digiti minimi often has more than one tendon,

the most radial slip commonly being mistaken for the extensor communis to the little finger. The extensor tendons are centralized on the metacarpal heads by fibers of the sagittal bands.

In the midproximal phalangeal level, the lateral bands split from the communis tendon (with the proprius tendons of the index or little fingers), which continues as the central tendon distally to insert into the dorsal lip of the base of the middle phalanx at the proximal interphalangeal joint. The lateral bands, as they cross the proximal interphalangeal joint, are joined by the tendons of the lumbrical and interosseous muscles. In full proximal interphalangeal joint flexion, the lateral bands spread apart enough so that they are at the joint axis, thus exerting no extension force in this position. The central tendon is responsible for the first 50% of proximal interphalangeal joint extension, with the lateral bands assuming progressively more effect as extension continues (56,57). In full extension, the lateral bands are taut on the dorsum of the proximal interphalangeal joint; the central tendon is totally lax in this position. The lateral bands join distally to form the tendon slip that inserts into the dorsal flare of the base of the distal phalanx, thus acting to extend the distal interphalangeal joint. The proximal/volar origin and the distal/dorsal insertion of the Landsmeer oblique retinacular ligament, which parallels the course of the lateral bands distal to the proximal interphalangeal joint, are farther apart in proximal interphalangeal extension. This ligament therefore indirectly acts as an extensor of the distal interphalangeal joint as the proximal interphalangeal joint is extended. Part of the transverse retinacular ligament tethers the lateral bands, limiting their volar excursion.

Two extrinsic extensors extend the thumb. The extensor pollicis brevis inserts into the proximal phalanx to extend the metacarpophalangeal joint. The extensor pollicis longus inserts distally to extend both joints. The 3rd dorsal wrist compartment is a sheath that limits bowing of the extensor pollicis longus and maintains the tendon in a position ulnar to the radial styloid, allowing the thumb to be elevated above the palmar plane. A sagittal band extending approximately 1.5 cm proximal to the metacarpophalangeal joint maintains the ulnar relationship of the extensor pollicis longus to the extensor pollicis brevis. The abductor pollicis longus inserts into the base of the first metacarpal, acting to widen the first web space in the palmar plane.

PRINCIPLES OF WOUND MANAGEMENT

Blunt trauma that leaves the skin intact can cause avulsion injuries or ruptures, especially over joints. Initial function after major tendon damage can be normal because of intact interconnecting retinacular tissue in the extensor apparatus. Later, as the weaker tissues stretch, extension will deteriorate progressively and deformities will insidiously appear (58).

Interconnections between the extensor components at and distal to the metacarpophalangeal joint prevent significant proximal retraction of a lacerated tendon end. Static splinting in extension may be the primary mode of treatment from the sagittal bands distally (53). In most extensor lacerations, a horizontal mattress or figure-of-eight suture is adequate, since splinting of the wrist and involved fingers relieves tension on the repair. If the dorsal wrist retinaculum is incised for exposure of lacerated tendons, a band should be left intact to prevent dorsal tendon bowing. The incised dorsal retinaculum can be made into a square flap and sutured under the repaired tendons to minimize deep adhesions. A laceration of the extensor pollicis longus within the firm sheath of the third dorsal compartment requires the same accuracy of repair as a flexor tendon within zone 2. It may be necessary to open restricting retinacula to prevent adhesions.

Lacerations of the forearm muscles or musculotendinous junctions should be repaired with a 3-0 or 4-0 relatively nonreactive suture. A synthetic absorbable suture is satisfactory in this region. A fasciotomy should be performed if there is notable subfascial edema. Lacerations of the dorsal sensory branch of the radial nerve should be repaired. Even with repair, damage of this nerve can lead to a reflex sympathetic dystrophy that can severely limit the function of an otherwise reconstructed hand.

Lacerations within the first dorsal compartment require releases of all involved tunnels to minimize the chance of posttraumatic de Quervain syndrome. The anterior radial aspect of the ligament should be saved to prevent subluxation of the tendons with wrist flexion.

Lacerated tendons over the dorsum of the metacarpals can retract under the skin. Initial full, active extension is not a guarantee that there is no tendon laceration arising from intact junctura and sagittal bands. These lacerations require careful exploration, precise repair, and postoperative splinting of the wrist and involved fingers in extension.

Wounds at the metacarpophalangeal joint usually occur with the hand in the clenched-fist position. Penetrating wounds easily enter the joint, damaging the articular cartilage. The joint capsule can be identified and repaired as a separate layer. Human bite injuries are initially managed with débridement, antibiotics, delayed wound closure, and frequent followup visits, because they can develop potent infections with joint destruction. Cultures are obtained and intravenous antibiotics are given at the first sign of infection. It is important to obtain radiographs to rule out the presence of foreign bodies such as teeth (59).

Closed rupture of the sagittal band support of the extensor tendon allows the tendon to slip off the metacarpal head with metacarpal joint flexion, usually ulnarly. Acutely, this is associated with pain, swelling, and snapping of the tendon on flexion. The long finger is most often affected. If recognized within 10 days, repair by splinting of the affected metacarpophalangeal joint in extension for 5 to 6 weeks is usually definitive (60). Splint failures and established subluxations require repair.

Boutonnière Deformity

The dorsum of the proximal interphalangeal joint is the site of injuries to the central tendon, which can result in the boutonnière deformity. Open lacerations and closed ruptures or avulsions from the dorsal lip at the base of the middle phalanx allow the lateral bands to slip volarward. A disrupted central tendon cannot initiate proximal interphalangeal joint extension; thus, attempts at extension by direct force volar to the joint axis, via the volarly displaced lateral bands, can result in flexion of the proximal interphalangeal joint with hyperextension of the distal interphalangeal joint. The head of the proximal phalanx will progressively buttonhole through the extensor mechanism (Fig. 92–16).

The above alteration of anatomy is the basis for the "boutonnière test," which can indicate the extent of injury over the proximal interphalangeal joint. The first possibility is that the finger can be actively extended from the flexed position. In this case, enough retinacular tissue is intact to transfer force around the lacerated central tendon to keep it approximated. Simple skin closure and splinting the finger in extension is required. The second possibility is that the proximal interphalangeal joint cannot be extended from the fully flexed position, but can be held in extension after passive positioning. This demonstrates injury to the central tendon, medial interosseous bands, and adjacent supporting retinaculum with intact lateral bands. Tendon repair is indicated, with postoperative splinting in extension for 5 to 6 weeks. Finally, the lack of ability to actively extend the finger or hold it in extension indicates that the central tendon and at least one lateral band have been severed. In this case, interosseous cross-joint pinning of the proximal interphalangeal joint in extension is required to prevent an ulcer at an external splint's dorsal pressure point, which would be located directly on the tendon repair.

Some authors advocate immediate operative intervention for closed injuries (51), whereas others suggest splinting in

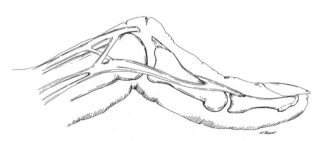

FIG. 92–16. Boutonnière deformity. When the central slip is lacerated, the lateral bands migrate volarly becoming, in effect, flexors of the proximal interphalangeal joint.

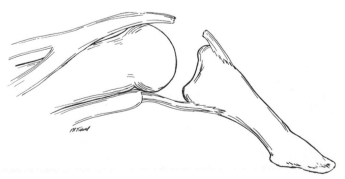

FIG. 92–17. Mallet finger. A small portion of tendon remains attached to the distal phalanx.

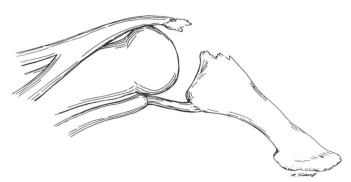

FIG. 92–18. Mallet finger secondary to a fracture of the distal phalanx.

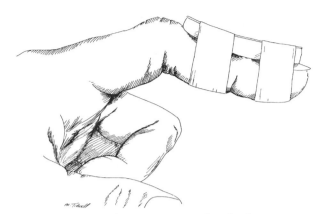

FIG. 92–19. Closed treatment of mallet finger.

extension (61). The boutonnière test will help in the decision. Dynamic splinting to ease the proximal interphalangeal joint into extension may be worthwhile in established boutonnière deformities weeks or months after injury (62). In some cases, this may result in a definitive correction. In others, the contracted retinacular tissues may be stretched enough to allow an anatomic repair. In either case, the postoperative care extends over 6 to 9 months; thus, accurate treatment of the initial injury is much preferred.

Mallet Finger

A mallet finger, or baseball finger, can result from a closed or open tendon injury over the distal interphalangeal joint (Fig. 92–17). A small fragment of the dorsal lip of the distal phalanx may be avulsed (Fig. 92–18). Open repair may be required if a lateral radiograph with the distal phalanx splinted in extension demonstrates volar subluxation of the distal phalanx, indicating significant lateral joint ligament damage. In these cases, the subluxation is reduced and fixed with a fine K wire and the tendon/bone fragment reapproximated with a pullout suture.

Most mallet deformities can be treated by splinting the distal interphalangeal joint in 0° of extension or in slight hyperextension, being careful to broaden the dorsal pressure over the middle phalanx to avoid necrosis (Fig. 92–19). Six to 8 weeks of splinting followed by 2 weeks of night splinting is usually required. Passive stretching of the healed, but stiff, joint is avoided because it can result in recurrence of the deformity. A recurvatum of the proximal interphalangeal joint, or swan neck deformity, can develop in a longstanding mallet finger because the lateral bands are permitted to migrate proximally (53).

Conclusion

The treatment of open and closed injuries of the tendons of the hand requires accurate and timely diagnoses to execute a treatment plan. A thorough understanding of the interactions, variations, and multiplicity of the extensor tendons and the intrinsic mechanism is necessary to achieve the expected good results after injuries.

Even though the principles of surgical repair are well established and techniques are improving, the results following flexor tendon surgery are not perfect, and some controversies still exist: Should continuity of both tendons be restored in "no man's land"? Should the sheath be sutured or excised? Should an incompletely severed tendon be repaired or allowed to heal without surgical intervention? Should early motion be instituted, and how often should it be done? Alternatives to tendon repair should be considered for an unreliable, irresponsible, nonmotivated patient who cannot or will not cooperate with a postoperative treatment program because this behavior is associated with a bad result.

The search for improvements in tendon surgery has stimulated basic science and clinical investigations for over half a century and will continue to pose questions in the future.

References

1. Peacock EE, Hartrampf CR. Collective review: The repair of flexor tendons in the hand. *Int Abstr Surg* 1961; 113:411.
2. Verdan CE. Syndrome of the quadriga. *Surg Clin North Am* 1960; 40:425.
3. Idler RS. Anatomy and biomechanics of the digital flexor tendons. *Hand Clin* 1985; 1:3.
4. Ditmars D. Patterns of carpal tunnel syndrome. *Hand Clin* 1993; 9:241.
5. Cobb TK, An K-N, Cooney WP. Effect of lumbrical muscle incursion within the carpal tunnel on carpal tunnel pressure: A cadaveric study. *J Hand Surg* 1995; 20A:186.
6. Doyle JR, Blythe W. The finger flexor tendon sheath and pulleys: Anatomy and reconstruction. In: American Academy of Orthopaedic Surgery: *Symposium on Tendon Surgery in the Hand.* St Louis: CV Mosby Co, 1975; p 81.
7. Doyle JR, Blythe W. Anatomy of the flexor tendon sheath and pulleys of the thumb. *J Hand Surg* 1977; 2:149.
8. Clemente CD. *Gray's Anatomy of the Human Body,* ed 30. Philadelphia: Lea & Febiger, 1985; p 543.
9. Lampe EW. Surgical anatomy of the hand. *Clin Symp* 1988; 40:1.
10. Doyle JR. Anatomy of the finger flexor tendon sheath and pulley system. *J Hand Surg (Am)* 1988; 13:473.
11. Lister GD. Reconstruction of pulleys employing retinaculum. *J Hand Surg* 1979; 4:461.
12. Manske PR, Lesker PA. Palmar aponeurosis pulley. *J Hand Surg* 1983; 8:259.
13. Peacock EE. A study of the circulation in normal tendons and healing grafts. *Ann Surg* 1959; 149:415.
14. Smith JW. Blood supply of tendons. *Am J Surg* 1965; 109:272.
15. Strickland JW. Flexor tendon injuries, Part 1: Anatomy, physiology, biomechanics, healing, and adhesion formation around a repaired tendon. *Orthop Rev* 1986; XV:632.
16. Manske PR, Lesker PA. Flexor tendon nutrition. *Hand Clin* 1985; 1:13.
17. Lundborg G, Hansson HA, Rank F, Rydevik B. Superficial repair of severed flexor tendons in synovial environment. *J Hand Surg* 1980; 5:451.
18. Lister G. Indications and techniques for repair of the flexor tendon sheath. *Hand Clin* 1985; 1:85.
19. Taras JS, Gray RM, Culp RW. Complications of flexor tendon injuries. *Hand Clin* 1994; 10:93.
20. Ketchum LD. Primary tendon healing: A review. *J Hand Surg* 1977; 2:428.

21. Beasley RW. *Hand Injuries.* Philadelphia: WB Saunders, 1981.

22. Leddy JP, Packer JW. Avulsion of the profundus insertion in athletes. *J Hand Surg* 1977; 2:66.

23. Bunnell S. Repair of tendons in the fingers and description of two new instruments. *Surg Gynecol Obstet* 1918; 26:103.

24. Green DP. General principles. In: Green DP, ed. *Operative Hand Surgery,* ed 2. New York: Churchill Livingstone, 1988; vol 1, p 8.

25. Nicoladone C. Ein Vorschag zur Sechennaht. *Wein Med Wochenschr* 1880; 30:1413.

26. Bruner JM. The zigzag volar digital incision for flexor tendon surgery. *Plast Reconstr Surg* 1967; 40:571.

27. Leddy JP. Flexor tendons: Acute injuries. In: Green DP, ed. *Operative Hand Surgery.* New York: Churchill Livingstone, 1982; vol 2, p 1347.

28. Srugi S, Adamson JA. Comparative study of tendon suture material in dogs. *Plast Reconstr Surg* 1972; 50:31.

29. Kleinert HD, Smith DJ. Primary and secondary repairs of flexor and extensor tendon injuries. In: Flynn JE, ed. *Hand Surgery,* ed 3. Baltimore: Williams and Wilkins, 1982; p 220.

30. Urbaniak JR, Cahill JD, Mortenson RA. Tendon suturing methods: Analysis of tensile strengths. In: American Academy of Orthopaedic Surgery: *Symposium on Tendon Surgery in the Hand.* St Louis: CV Mosby, 1975; p 70.

31. Lister GD, Kleinert HE, Kutz JE, et al. Primary flexor tendon repair followed by immediate controlled mobilization. *J Hand Surg* 1977; 2:441.

32. Tsuge K, Ikuta Y, Matsuishi Y. Intra-tendinous tendon suture in the hand—a new technique. *Hand* 1975; 7:250

33. Strickland JW. Flexor tendon injuries: Flexor tendon repair, *Orthop Rev* 1986; XV:701.

34. Arons MS. Purposeful delay of the primary repair of cut flexor tendons in "some man's land" in children. *Plast Reconstr Surg* 1974; 53:638.

35. Carter SJ, Merheimer WL. Deferred primary tendon repair: Results in 27 cases. *Ann Surg* 1966; 164:913.

36. Masden E. Delayed primary suture of flexor tendons cut in the digital sheath. *J Bone Joint Surg (Br)* 1970; 52:264.

37. Horner RL. Flexor tendon injuries. In: Boswick JA, ed. *Current Concepts in Hand Surgery.* Philadelphia: Lea & Febiger, 1983; p 74.

38. Verdan C. Primary repair of flexor tendons. *J Bone Joint Surg (Am)* 1960; 42:647.

39. Kleinert HE, Kutz JE, Atasoy E, et al. Primary repair of flexor tendons. *Orthop Clin North Am* 1973; 4:865.

40. Bunnell S. *Surgery of the Hand,* ed 3. Philadelphia: JB Lippincott, 1956.

41. Kleinert HE, Forshew FC, Cohen MJ. Repair of Zone 1 flexor tendon injuries. In: American Academy of Orthopaedic Surgery: *Symposium on Tendon Surgery in the Hand.* St Louis: CV Mosby, 1975; p 115.

42. Elias LS, Tountas CP, et al. Partial flexor tendon laceration: A cause of trigger finger. *Orthopedics* 1982; 5:441.

43. Wray RC, Holtmann B, Weeks PM. Clinical treatment of partial tendon lacerations without suturing and with early motion. *Plast Reconstr Surg* 1977; 59:231.

44. Leddy JP. Avulsions of the flexor digitorum profundus. *Hand Clin* 1985; 1(1):77.

45. Ehlert KJ, Gould JS, Black KP. A simultaneous distal phalanx avulsion fracture with profundus tendon avulsion: A case report and review of the literature. *Clin Orthop* 1992; 283:265.

46. Chow JA, Thomas LJ, Dovelle S, et al. A combined regimen of controlled motion following flexor tendon repair in "no man's land". *Plast Reconstr Surg* 1987; 79:447.

47. Saldana MJ, Chow JA, Gerbino P, et al. Further experience in rehabilitation of zone II flexor tendon repair with dynamic traction splinting. *Plast Reconstr Surg* 1991; 87:543.

48. Van Strien G. Postoperative management of flexor tendon injuries. In: Hunter JM, Schneider LH, Mackin EF, and Callahan AD, eds. *Rehabilitation of the Hand, Surgery and Therapy.* Ed 3. St Louis: CV Mosby, 1990; p 400.

49. Duran RJ, Houser RG. Controlled passive motion following flexor tendon repair in zone 2 and 3. In: American Academy of Orthopaedic Surgery: *Symposium on Tendon Surgery in the Hand.* St Louis: CV Mosby, 1975; p 105.

50. Gelberman RH, Nunley JA II, Osterman AL, et al. Influences of the protected passive mobilization interval on flexor tendon healing. *Clin Orthop* 1991; 264:189.

51. Doyle JR. Extensor tendons, acute injuries. In: Green DP, ed. *Operative Hand Surgery.* New York: Churchill Livingstone, 1982; vol 2, p 1441.

52. Tubiana R. Surgical repair of the extensor apparatus of the fingers. *Surg Clin North Am* 1968; 48:1015.

53. Kilgore ES, Graham WP. *The Hand, Surgical and Nonsurgical Management.* Philadelphia: Lea & Febiger, 1977; p 184.

54. Kaplan EB. Anatomy, injuries, and treatment of the extensor apparatus of the hand and the digits. *Clin Orthop* 1959; 13:24.

55. Von Schroeder HP, Botte MJ. Anatomy of the extensor tendons of the fingers: variations and multiplicity. *J Hand Surg* 1995; 20A:27.

56. Micks JE, Reswick JB. Confirmation of differential loading of lateral and central fibers of the extensor tendon. *J Hand Surg* 1981; 6:462.

57. Schultz RJ, Furlong J, Storace A. Detailed anatomy of the extensor mechanism at the proximal aspect of the finger. *J Hand Surg* 1981; 6:493.

58. Kasdan ML, Romm S. Tendon injuries of the hand. Georgiade NG, et al., eds. *Essentials of Plastic, Maxillofacial, and Reconstructive Surgery.* Baltimore: Williams & Wilkins, 1978.

59. Mann RJ, Hoffield TA, Farmer CB. Human bites of the hand, twenty years experience. *J Hand Surg* 1977; 2:97.

60. Araki S, Ohtani T, Tanaka T. Acute dislocation of the extensor digitorum communis tendon at the metacarpophalangeal joint. *J Bone Joint Surg (Am)* 1987; 69:616.

61. Souter WA. The problem of boutonniere deformity. *Clin Orthop* 1974; 104:116.

62. King T. Injuries of the dorsal extensor mechanism of the fingers. *Med J Aust* 1970; 2:213.

63. Kaplan EB. Mallet or baseball finger. *Surgery* 1940; 7:784.

93

Peripheral Nerve Injuries

A. Lee Dellon, M.D., F.A.C.S.

The dysfunction caused by peripheral nerve injury reflects both the unique function of the injured nerve and the mechanism of injury. Diagnosis of peripheral nerve injury, therefore, is based upon knowledge of peripheral nerve anatomy, the ability to evaluate motor function and sensibility, and an understanding of the mechanism of injury. Because most injuries are capable of producing gradations of damage to the nerve's constituent fiber population, this chapter discusses diagnosis and treatment in the context of mechanisms of injury. This chapter presupposes that proper attention will be paid to associated injuries of soft tissue, tendon, and blood vessels in the extremity.

Motor function is evaluated first by manually testing the individual muscle or group of muscles innervated by the peripheral nerve in question. Functional neuromuscular integrity is present if the patient can maintain the position of the part against the examiner's resistance when the part has been placed as if the given muscle were functioning (e.g., the thumb must be maintained in palmar abduction against the examiner's attempt to displace it to test the recurrent (motor) branch of the median nerve). Techniques for manually testing individual muscles (1) and the muscle to be tested for specific peripheral nerves (2) are well described (Table 93–1). Once integrity of neuromuscular function is determined, degree of function may be quantified by manual muscle grading or measuring grip or pinch strength directly. For these assessments of motor function an aware, cooperative patient is necessary, and integrity of bones and joints is assumed. Electrodiagnostic testing may be required for the problem case.

Evaluation of functional sensation should be based upon the neurophysiology of the peripheral nervous system, and this has been reviewed recently (3,4). Sensibility is evaluated first qualitatively with the examiner's moving finger or a tuning fork. This tests for the perception of touch stimuli in the autonomous zone of the peripheral nerve in question. If perception of moving touch or vibration is present, perception of pain and temperature is assumed, inasmuch as dissociation of touch from pain or temperature is present only with lesions in the central nervous system (CNS) (e.g., syringomyelia). Once integrity of the fiber/receptor system is determined, degree of function may be quantified: for example, by recording threshold values—using Semmes-Weinstein monofilaments for cutaneous pressure threshold, or vibrometer (5) for cutaneous vibratory threshold—and innervation density, using static or moving two-point discrimination with a Disk-Criminator [PO Box 16392, Baltimore, MD 21210] (6) (Table 93–2). Electrodiagnostic testing may be required for the problem case.

The classical approach to teaching and writing about nerve injury begins with the classification described by Sir Herbert Seddon (7) in 1942: neurapraxia, axonotmesis, and neurotmesis. This classification is meaningful in terms of understanding the pathogenesis of neural degeneration and the time course of neural regeneration, as well as the degree of recovery after sustaining pure nerve lesions. Unfortunately, many nerve lesions do not fit into these categories. In order to include the complexity of nerve injury, Sir Sydney Sunderland (8) extended the classification to five classes. Sunderland's class 1 lesion corresponds to neurapraxia, may show myelin changes histologically, and has complete recovery in hours to 3 months. A class 2 lesion corresponds to axonotmesis and also has complete recovery, but is generally slower to recover than neurapraxia. Class 3 lesions still maintain intact perineurium, but have axon and endoneural damage. Recovery is still usually complete. Classes 4 and 5 arc nerve-sectioning lesions and do not recover spontaneously. Class 4 is a neuroma-in-continuity with total disruption of the entire nerve and intact epineurium but nerve continuity maintained only by scar. Class 5 is a complete nerve transection corresponding to neurotmesis. There should perhaps be a class "6" wherein the neuroma-in-continuity is partial and some fascicles remain intact. This is a situation frequently seen. This chapter deals with the description, diagnosis, and treatment of nerve injuries as they relate to the mechanism of injury, because it is in this setting that the physician meets the patient.

Nontraumatic Injury

Nontraumatic injury must be considered in each case of peripheral nerve dysfunction because its presence may greatly affect treatment and treatment outcome. This group contains peripheral neuropathies related to systemic diseases (diabetes, alcoholism, thyroid problems, uremia, collagen vascular disease, or arthritis); inherited (Charcot-Marie-Tooth) or acquired (multiple sclerosis, myasthenia) neurologic conditions; infection (Guillain-Barré, leprosy); and exposure to environmental toxins (lead, mercury) (9). The presence of these nontraumatic conditions may predispose the patient to peripheral nerve dysfunction (e.g., rheumatoid arthritis and median nerve compression in the carpal tunnel), and may also delay recovery after treatment of the nerve dysfunction (e.g., alcoholism and nerve regeneration). This group of nontraumatic mechanisms generally involves some form of ionic block, abnormal axoplasmic transport, or abnormal myelination that causes a metabolic dysfunction while the peripheral

Table 93–1
Muscle Function Related to Specific Peripheral Nerve: Localization of Injury Site

Lack of	Suggests Injury to	At
1. Thumb extension, or MP finger extension or ulnar wrist extension	Radial nerve	Proximal forearm, at superficial head of supinator
if also		
Extensor carpi radialis brevis or brachioradialis	Radial nerve	Antecubital fossa, proximal to posterior interosseous nerve
if also		
Triceps	Radial nerve	Proximal humerus
2. First dorsal interosseous	Ulnar nerve	Palm
if also		
Abductor digiti minimi	Ulnar nerve	Guyon's canal
if also		
Flexor profundus to little finger	Ulnar nerve	Proximal forearm
if also		
Ulnar wrist flexor	Ulnar nerve	Cubital tunnel
3. Abductor pollicis brevis	Median nerve	Carpal tunnel
if also		
Flexor sublimis	Median nerve	Midforearm
if also		
Flexor pollicis longus, index profundus, or pronator quadratus	Median nerve	Proximal forearm (anterior interosseous nerve)
if also		
Pronator teres, flexor carpi radialis	Median nerve	Antecubital fossa

Table 93–2
Peripheral Sensibility Correlations[a]

Sensation	Clinical Test	Cutaneous Receptor	Nerve Fiber Property
Constant touch	Finger pressure	Merkel cell–neurite complex	Slowly adapting
Pressure	von Fry Hair (Semmes-Weinstein monofilament)		
Tactile gnosis	Static two-point discrimination		
Moving touch	Finger stroking	Meissner corpuscle	Quickly adapting
Flutter	30-cps tuning fork, vibrometer		
Tactile gnosis	Moving two-point discrimination		
Moving touch	Finger stroking	Pacinian corpuscle	Quickly adapting
Vibration	256-cps tuning fork, vibrometer		
Tactile gnosis	Moving two-point discrimination		

[a]From Dellon AL. *Evaluation of Sensibility and Re-education of Sensation in the Hand.* Baltimore: Williams & Wilkins, 1981.

nerve and its constituent nerve fiber population remain structurally intact.

The diagnosis of nerve dysfunction unrelated to trauma generally requires recognition of the fact that the patient's complaints cannot be explained by dysfunction of a single peripheral nerve (i.e., there is polyneuropathy rather than a mononeuritis). If the complaint involves statements such as "the entire hand" or "the entire foot" goes to sleep or feels cold, or it "doesn't feel right from the elbow (or knee) down," a "stocking-and-glove" type of distribution is being described that may best be explained by a systemic or more central type of problem. There can be multiple peripheral nerve entrapments, such as median at the wrist, radial sensory in the forearm, and ulnar at the elbow, that can give a similar presentation of symptoms, but this is rare, with less than a dozen such patients having been seen in my practice. Such patients are seen usually in a setting of extensive upper-extremity use involving flexion at the wrist and elbow associated with supination/pronation movements (e.g., assembly line workers). Superimposed peripheral nerve compression upon diabetic neuropathy is common and manifests itself not only as multiple nerve dysfunction in the same extremity, mimicking a stocking-and-glove pattern, but also as bilateral carpal/cubital tunnel syndromes and upper- plus lower-extremity combinations, the most frequent being combined carpal and tarsal tunnel syndromes (10–12).

Diagnosis requires an awareness by the examining physician that these conditions, combinations, and superimpositions do occur. The physical examination must include gentle percussion over each peripheral nerve at the site of its likely local entrapment point. Presence of a positive Tinel sign at one of these sites is evidence of local entrapment. Vibratory testing with a tuning fork is accurate, sensitive, and easy to do (13). Documentation of loss of two-point discrimination or muscle atrophy in the peripheral distribution of a particular nerve signals the degree of dysfunction of the nerve (11). In cases of suspected multiple peripheral nerve entrapment or local entrapment superimposed on metabolic neuropathy, electrodiagnostic testing is recommended. Such testing will demonstrate a diffuse slowing of nerve conduction along the entire course of one or more peripheral nerves, with a further incremental slowing across the localized segment of compression. Referral to a neurologist to evaluate the specific type of neuronal dysfunction, to evaluate possible CNS etiologies, and to counsel the patient prognostically is appropriate.

Treatment is directed first at the underlying medical problem. Management is primarily by the patient's internist, neurologist, rheumatologist, or family physician. Surgical intervention is required only for superimposed nerve compression unrelieved by 6 months of medical management and splinting (see section on Nerve Compression).

Nerve Division

Acute injury to the peripheral nerve by means of an object striking it can result in complete or partial division of the nerve (Table 93–3).

In the emergency-room setting, fingers may be examined with a tuning fork without removing bandages, without threatening children, and without causing further excitement to the intoxicated patient (10). Testing with a needle is discouraged because it inflicts further pain, does not help establish doctor-patient rapport, and will engender distrust in the children. In children, evaluation of sensibility in the emergency situation is frequently unreliable, if not impossible, and, if in doubt, diagnosis of a potential nerve injury must be made by surgical exploration of the wound in the operating room with the adjunct of a pneumatic tourniquet.

Complete division of the median, ulnar, or radial nerves should not be a diagnostic problem in the awake, cooperative patient. Division of a nerve in the palm or a digital nerve in the finger, however, can be difficult to diagnose because of overlap in the fingertip pulp from the other digital nerve or in the thumb from the radial sensory nerve. In these overlap situations, the tuning fork is an extremely helpful diagnostic aid (10). Rather than the fingertip, the autonomous zone of the digital nerve over the volar lateral aspect of the distal interphalangeal joint is tested. After the vibrating prong end of the tuning fork is touched to the finger, the patient is asked "Do

Table 93–3
Sensory Area to Test for Unambiguous Diagnosis of Peripheral Nerve Injury

Injured Nerve	Test Area
Digital	Lateral-volar area of distal interphalangeal joint
Median	Index finger pulp
Ulnar, distal ⅓ forearm	Little finger pulp
Ulnar, proximal to mid-forearm	Entire little finger
Dorsal branch, ulnar	Dorsal ulnar aspect of hand
Radial	Dorsal metacarpophalangeal or index or thumb (rarely, no autonomous zone)
Posterior interosseous	None, innervates dorsal wrist capsule
Lateral antebrachial	None, extensive overlap with radial
Medial antebrachial	Medial posterior area, proximal forearm
Musculocutaneous	Radial volar forearm, proximally
Deep peroneal	Web space, big and second toe
Superficial peroneal	Dorsum of foot, proximally
Common peroneal	Entire dorsum of foot
Sural	Lateral aspect of proximal foot
Medial plantar	Big or second toe pulp
Lateral plantar	Little toe pulp
Saphenous	Medial aspect, distal leg
Lateral femoral	Anterolateral thigh, proximally
Femoral	Anterior thigh, distally
Posterior tibial	Pulp of all toes
Calcaneal	Heel

you feel this?" The other side of the finger is tested and the question repeated. Each side is then touched again, asking "Do these feel different?" With a single injury in the palm (partial injury to a common volar digital nerve) or in the finger, the vibratory stimulus will be perceived from both sides of the finger via the intact digital nerve. The stimulus applied to the side with the intact nerve will be perceived as "louder" or "more intense" because the stimulus from the injured side is "dampened" by the greater volume of tissue through which it must travel before it is perceived by the receptors on the noninjured side.

Treatment of the divided nerve is covered in detail in Chapters 10 and 83. My approach is primary repair of all divided nerves, when other factors permit. Surgical débridement plus prophylactic antibiotic coverage (begun intravenously with a cephalosporin at the time of admission to the emergency room) have extended the previously taught "6-hour golden rule." As is described in the following section, nerves divided by crushing or traction injury are probably better treated by secondary débridement when the full longitudinal extent of the scarring can be assessed. Often a nerve graft will be required.

Although the results of nerve repair probably have been improved through the use of microneurosurgery and through the emphasis on grouped fascicular repair and fascicular alignment where appropriate, nevertheless, the functional results of current nerve repair leave much to be desired. It is quite possible that many of the poor results of primary repair are less an indictment of the repair than an indication of failure to select a delayed repair with nerve grafting, thereby leaving at the repair site proximal and distal areas of neural damage that could not be identified acutely. Such a primary repair is destined for a poor result.

Results of treatment of the nerve injured by division can be improved by a program of rehabilitation. Whatever technique is chosen surgically, the operation gives the patient a potential for recovery. Left without rehabilitation, the patient, unless highly motivated, will not recover to fullest potential. Rehabilitation programs have been refined over the last decade and carefully detailed (3,13–16). Once protective splinting is discontinued, at about 4 to 6 weeks after nerve repair or grafting, a graded program to recover full range of motion (ROM) of joints is instituted to regain strength in the remaining innervated muscle groups. The noninnervated muscle groups are splinted, usually to prevent stretch injury to the denervated muscles, although the efficacy of these observations, initially made in patients recovering from polio, has not been proven in patients with posttraumatic paralysis. Similarly, if the nerve repair or graft site is sufficiently proximal to the muscles to be reinnervated so that more than 9 months may be anticipated for reinnervation, electrical stimulation of the muscles may be instituted to prevent muscle atrophy. Again, the efficacy of this approach has not been accepted universally, and patient compliance with the transcutaneous stimuli is usually poor once muscle strengthening is instituted. Although long-neglected, sensory rehabilitation has been emphasized increasingly over the last 12 years. Results previously seen in less than 1% of adults 5 years after nerve repair at the wrist may now be obtained in at least 50% of adults 2 years after nerve repair (3). Sensory reeducation techniques are simple, with a high degree of patient compliance (3,13).

Acutely Increased Compartmental Pressure

Nerve dysfunction arising from acutely increased pressure within a compartment encompasses many causes, including crush, burn, hemorrhage, and fracture (17). The common mechanism among these causes is increased tissue pressure produced by a decrease in the arterial-venous pressure gradient, such that tissue perfusion and oxygen delivery to the tissues is decreased. All tissue within the compartment is at risk of decreased perfusion, subsequent ischemia, and eventual necrosis. Because normal endoneural tissue pressure is higher than other tissue pressure, the endoneural environment is possibly more at risk of ischemia than are other soft tissues.

Regardless of the etiology of the increase in compartmental pressure, the progression of dysfunction is now generally agreed to begin with the sensory component of the nerve going through the compartment (3,17–19). Of the possible modalities of sensation to become altered, touch is altered first. Ischemia and mechanical compression cause dysfunction first of the large, myelinated, group A beta fibers mediating touch perception. Because pain and temperature perception are mediated through the smaller diameter group A delta and C fibers, perception of painful stimuli (testing with a 25-gauge needle) is the last to become altered. (The reverse order is noted for sensory loss induced by local anesthetics.) Because vibration is a touch sensation mediated by the group A beta fibers (see Table 93–2), the tuning fork is the recommended diagnostic tool for detecting increasing compartment pressure in the conscious patient.

Direct crushing injuries like those caused by a clothes roller-dryer, printing or metal press, or rolling mill, usually apply heavy pressures over a varying degree of time (until the machine can be turned off or reversed). Direct crushing injuries like those caused by a closing door, a falling piece of metal or stone, or a sudden blow to a forearm in self-defense, deliver a force that is often of high intensity at the time of impact, but for only a short duration. All forms of crush injury offer four potential mechanisms for nerve dysfunction: (a) direct damage to the nerve; (b) increasing compartmental pressure through bleeding or subsequent edema, with indirect damage to nerve as a result of ischemia; (c) disruption of nerve-fiber continuity, either partial or complete; and (d) late damage to the nerve resulting from progressive fibrosis, inducing chronic nerve compression. Crush injuries damage a nerve over a broader area than a laceration, but not as extensively as a traction or stretch injury. In the acute situation, the chief concern is to relieve the increased compartmental pressure, and not necessarily to treat nerve injury arising from direct disruption of the nerve itself. If this requires an operative decompression, then, depending on how extensive the crush injury has been—and once the bone injury has been stabilized, the blood supply reestablished, and clearly nonviable tissues débrided—the nerves involved may be examined more closely. At this time, if loss of continuity of the nerve is noted, treatment may proceed as for partial or complete nerve division. However, more nerve must be resected (débrided) before repair because of the more widespread nature of the injury. More often than with a simple laceration, delayed repair with nerve grafting will be required. Results of nerve repair for crush injury are generally less satisfactory than for laceration, usually because of failure to resect all injured tissue at the time of repair. Inasmuch as the judgment of how nerve has been damaged by the crush is extremely difficult to make accurately in the acute situation, secondary repair, usually by nerve grafting, is recommended in this situation.

Burns sufficient to cause nerve dysfunction by increased compartmental pressure may be deep 2nd-degree, but are usually 3rd-degree and circumferential. The burn itself does not damage the nerve. Burn injury to a nerve also may occur directly, as in a so-called 4th-degree burn in which the depth of burn goes beyond the skin—or, more usually, with an electrical injury ("burn"). Current experience suggests nerves traversed by electricity in an electrical burn are best left in situ and treated expectantly. If no regeneration has occured after 3 months, these should be managed as neuromas-in-continuity. With a 3rd-degree burn, the increased vascular permeability results in a large increase in extravascular fluid in the compartment. In intubated patients (e.g., those with associated pulmonary injury), rising intracompartmental pressure is easily overlooked because there will be no patient complaints of symptoms of acute nerve compression. Even in the awake burn patient, symptoms of acute nerve compression may never be noticed because of the overall pain and discomfort of the burn itself. As the fluid resuscitation proceeds, the extravascular fluid is constrained by the unyielding burn eschar. Treatment will require escharotomy, and, for the electrical injury, an additional fasciotomy. In these situations, release of the carpal tunnel and the Guyon canal is recommended.

Hemorrhage as a cause of increased compartmental pressure may result from arterial or venous cannulation, usually in a patient on anticoagulants. It has also been noted to occur spontaneously in patients with other hematologic problems, such as leukemia; or, as a complication of diagnostic radiologic procedures such as angiography or cardiac catheterization; or, after fracture, as in an anterior compartment syndrome in the leg after closed tibia/fibula fractures.

The tuning fork presents these patients with a touch stimulus with which they are not familiar. The stimulus is thus perceived as different from the discomfort of the injury. As described above for the digital nerve laceration, the test is done simply by touching the vibrating pronged end of a tuning fork to the index fingertip (to test for increased pressure in the carpal tunnel or in the forearm). The patient is asked "Do you feel anything?" If the response is no, there is significantly increased compartment pressure and surgical intervention is recommended. If the answer is yes, the test is then repeated, comparing the test area with the contralateral area. The patient is asked "Do these feel the same?" If the answer is yes, the pressure is less than 40 mm Hg in a normotensive patient. Nonsurgical therapy is instituted, and the patient is monitored at hourly intervals. If the answer is no, and the perception is that vibration is "less loud" or "farther away" in the test area than 40 to 50 mm Hg in the normotensive patient, surgical intervention or a period of intensive nonsurgical management with frequent monitoring is recommended (13,17,20–22). Nonsurgical management consists of placing the extremity at heart level, institution of medical therapy as required (e.g., reversal of anticoagulation), and correction of malaligned bone segments. Surgical intervention requires release of all involved anatomic compartments.

In the unconscious patient, or until confidence in the tuning fork is gained, the well-documented invasive techniques of direct measurement of intracompartmental pressures are recommended as the guide to surgical intervention (17,21,22).

Traction Injury

Traction on a nerve can produce the full spectrum of degrees of injury. The most common causes of traction today are motor vehicle accidents, particulary those involving motorcycles, in which, depending on the direction of pull on the upper extremity, severe injury to all or portions of the brachial plexus may occur. Similar injury can occur during a fall down steps, when the hand remains grasping the railing as the body falls. Such sudden stretching induces a "palsy," which may recover over a period of up to 3 months if reversible damage has been done, or may result in permanent loss of function if there has been extensive disruption of axons with secondary intraneural fibrosis. Examples of the lesser degree of traction injury are more commonly seen with dislocations; these include ulnar nerve injury at the elbow or common peroneal nerve injury at the knee. Examples of the more severe degree of injury are complete losses of the brachial plexus, with avulsion of the roots from the spinal cord, or with high-velocity missile injuries (23).

Diagnosis of traction injury requires an awareness by the first examining physician that a nerve injury may be associated with other injuries present. Once the area innervated by the nerves in jeopardy is examined, it is usually clear whether the major peripheral nerve in the region is functioning. If the injury has resulted in an open wound that will be explored for vascular or bony injuries, or for débridement of soft-tissue damage, the nerve also should be explored to determine if it is grossly intact. If the wound is closed, surgical exploration should not be carried out solely for the purpose of evaluation of the nerve. With a closed wound, diagnosis will be based on repeated physical examinations and electrodiagnostic studies. Serial electromyography will demonstrate whether the muscle is denervated and beginning to undergo progressive reinnervation (nascent or polyphasic potentials) or remains denervated (spontaneous spike potentials at rest and denervation potentials). Use of the tuning fork is valuable after recovery of the sensory component of nerve function. Perception of both 30 cps and 256 cps recovers at about the same time, within 1 to 12 weeks, if a neurapraxic-type lesion has occurred. Perception of 30 cps recovers sooner than that of 256 cps if more complete nerve disruption has occurred and the nerve is showing evidence of actual regeneration (3,13).

Treatment of traction injuries varies, depending upon the extent of the injury. In general, the extremity is splinted to protect the paralyzed muscles, and physical therapy is initiated to prevent or minimize joint stiffness. This is continued until it is clear that recovery is occurring spontaneously or until surgical exploration is indicated. For injuries with significant force (high-velocity missiles or fracture), if no nerve recovery is noted by 6 months, the nerve should be explored. The most critical treatment consideration at surgery is that traction injuries cause extensive longitudinal damage, resulting in scarring over significantly longer distances than might be expected. Nerve is resected proximally and distally until the cross-sectional area of the nerve trunk is soft, a good fascicular pattern is evident, and no dense white interfascicular or intrafascicular scar is left. This is ascertained by examining the nerve ends under high-power magnification using the microscope. With the exception of the rare case in which the radial nerve can be transposed through a humerous being plated or bone-grafted, or the ulnar nerve can be transposed anteriorly, severe traction injuries of this magnitude require nerve grafting.

Treatment of brachial plexus injuries is evolving, with the development of techniques that offer some hope for restoring elbow flexion and extension, and possibly wrist flexion with protective sensation in the thumb and index finger. When spinal roots have been avulsed, these techniques involve neurotization of the particular plexus segment from intercostal nerves extended with nerve grafts. When spinal roots have not been avulsed, direct nerve grafting within the plexus is possible. The donor nerve is usually the sural nerve, but the ipsilateral radial sensory nerve and the ulnar nerve may be used also (23). The ulnar nerve can be placed as a vascularized nerve graft into heavily scarred beds if there is concern that the beds is not vascularized sufficiently to nourish the multiple fascicular grafts required (24). Treatment of birth palsy remains the most controversial of brachial plexus traction injuries. Recently, a study of 300 congenital palsies has demonstrated that in no case were all five roots avulsed. Thus, there is potential for nerve reconstruction with one of these techniques in every case of congenital palsy (25). A recent monograph provides an excellent contemporary review (26).

Chronic Compression

Chronic compression of a nerve implies an injury whose mechanism combines ischemia and/or mechanical pressure, which may result from a single episode but which usually results from multiple or repetitive insults to the nerve.

A common example of the isolated-event type is a fall in which the elbow is struck, with immediate swelling but without fracture or dislocation. The hematoma and swelling eventually disappear, but 6 to 8 months later there is the insidious onset of ulnar nerve dysfunction. The patient commonly will have seen several physicians, often including a psychiatrist. Electrodiagnostic studies will be normal, and the patient will have seemingly vague complaints of trouble writing, clumsiness, weakness, dropping things, loss of use of the hand, and occasional numbness in the hand. Here, physical examination is critical. Perception of vibration in the little finger is abnormal and may be hypersensitive. The patient also has slightly diminished perception of moving touch over the dorsal ulnar half of the hand, slightly decreased pinch and grip strength, and, most important, a sensitive ulnar nerve in the postcondylar groove. Important negatives on physical examination are: (a) absent tenderness over the anterior scalene muscles, and (b) a negative Roos sign (symptoms not induced after 30 to 45 seconds of opening and closing the fingers with the arm abducted at the shoulder and flexed at the elbow). These negatives effectively rule out thoracic outlet compression of the lower trunks of the brachial plexus, which can stimulate this clinical presentation. Other possible diagnostic considerations are cervical disc disease and gigantomastia (with bra-strap compression of the brachial plexus). These patients have an early cubital tunnel syndrome (formerly called tardy ulnar palsy to distinguish it from posttraumatic ulnar neuritis seen after elbow fractures and presenting with obvious hypesthesia on the ulnar side of the hand and intrinsic wasting).

An increasingly common example of the repetitive type of "trauma" is the cubital tunnel syndrome, described clearly only in 1958–59. This is being seen more often today as occupations require more and more work done with the elbow kept in flexion. Thus, cubital tunnel syndrome patients may present with insidious onset and a history of a past single traumatic event, but also with a more clear-cut history of numbness in the little finger associated with weakness. Questioning reveals that the patient works with the elbow flexed. Examples of such occupations include computer programmer, executive (right arm rests on desk with elbow flexed when writing or using telephone extensively), and meat cutter (left arm constantly flexed holding meat portion while right hand does the cutting). An interesting variant of the "shoulder-hand" syndrome (usually implying stiffness and aching in the shoulder secondary to unusual positioning of the extremity after hand injury) is the cubital tunnel syndrome seen in patients keeping the postraumatic, chronically painful hand held close to the body for protection. The gradual weakness of grip and numbness in the little finger may go unnoticed for years in this situation and is often attributed to simple disuse of the hand.

Chronic nerve compression suggests low levels of increased pressure for a period sufficiently long to produce nerve dysfunction, in contrast to acute compression, in which intracompartmental pressures are greater than 40 to 50 mm Hg. If such pressures are unrelieved for as little as 2 to 4 hours, a loss of conducted action potential and subsequent wallerian degeneration results. Chronic nerve compression pathophysiologically is initiated by altered axoplasmic flow and subsequent progression of paranodal to segmental demyelination (27). Recent experimental models of chronic nerve compression in the rat sciatic nerve (28) and primate median nerve (29) have documented: (a) progressive connective tissue proliferation from extraneural epineural fibrosis, perineural fibrosis, and endoneural fibrosis; (b) loss of myelin of large myelinated fibers before smaller myelinated fibers; (c) uneven distribution of "large fiber dropout" in the overall nerve, with fibers at the periphery of a given fascicle being more susceptible than central fibers, and more-peripheral fascicles being more susceptible than more-central fascicles; and (d) that the end stages of chronic compression also produce distal axonal (wallerian) degeneration and subsequent regeneration. These observations form the basis for interpreting the Tinel sign in chronic nerve compression (30), for understanding the efficacy of intraneural neurolysis (31), and for understanding a two-stage process of recovery after treatment: (a) initial, often "immediate," relief of numbness and tingling or pain after correction of neural ischemia, and (b) delayed recovery of muscle strength, reversal of muscle atrophy, and recovery of two-point discrimination over a time course more consistent with axonal regeneration and remyelination.

The most common site of chronic nerve entrapment is the median nerve at the wrist. The second most frequent, in my experience, is the ulnar nerve at the elbow. The most common site in the lower extremity, although described only as recently as 1962, is the posterior tibial nerve at the ankle—the tarsal tunnel syndrome. With awareness of its existence, the chronic site of nerve injury is probably responsible for much of the "coldness" complained about in feet, as well as the "burning pain." It is probably present to a degree in many people with previous ankle fractures, and chronic venous obstruction with recurrent ankle edema. As is discussed below, it may be responsible for a significant degree of the sensory impairment in diabetic neuropathy. The diagnosis, most commonly in the presence of normal electrodiagnostic studies, is made clinically by abnormal vibratory perception over the toes and a positive Tinel sign over the posterior tibial nerve as it goes beneath the lancinate ligament (flexor retinaculum), and often over the medial and lateral plantar nerves as they go beneath the fascia of origin of the intrinsic muscles. The heel may or may not be involved, depending upon the anatomic site of origin of the calcaneal nerves (14,32).

The next most common site in the lower extremity is the common peroneal as it enters the peroneus muscle fascia over the fibular head. Because the nerve here is both relatively fixed and superficial, it is susceptible to frequent bruising and malpositioning during operations (e.g., total hip replacements). In the trunk, the lateral femoral cutaneous nerve is injured chronically where it exits the pelvis, variously in relation to the iliacus fascia, anterior superior iliac spine, and sartorius muscle. The brachial plexus can be injured repetitively through muscle spasm (myofascial syndrome); job activities (working on an assembly line with hands above shoulders); a variant of the hyperabduction syndrome in which the plexus is impinged on by the pectoralis minor, as seen in ceiling painters or auto mechanics working supine beneath vehicles; weight of breasts transmitted via bra strap; and congenital causes such as cervical rib and bands from the first rib across the plexus. With thoracic outlet nerve compression, in addition to complaints in the hand, there are almost always complaints related to the inner upper arm, shoulder, neck, and chest, and possibly to occipital headaches. The physical examination will not include a positive Tinel at the wrist or elbow, but will include reproduction of symptoms when the arms are extended over the head (positive Roos' sign), and usually tenderness to palpation of the brachial plexus beneath the anterior scalene muscles (14,33).

Returning to some rarer areas of entrapment in the upper extremity, the ulnar nerve can be injured crossing the wrist in the Guyon canal. In this case, grip strength is normal and dorsal ulnar sensation is normal, with variation in intrinsic function and little-finger sensitivity, depending on where in the canal the nerve has been injured. Probably not as rare as the literature would make it seem is compression of the superficial sensory branch of the radial nerve in the forearm. This entrapment was described in German by Wartenberg in 1932 (34), and has now been well described in English (35,36). If the radial sensory nerve is compressed, and this occurs in association with carpal and cubital tunnel syndrome, a stocking-and-glove picture of hypesthesia results, with great potential for a missed diagnosis. One reason this syndrome is little discussed is that patients rarely are aware of altered sensibility on the radial dorsal aspect of their hand, unless it is painful. The diagnosis is made simply by finding abnormal moving touch perception or moving two-point discrimination and a positive Tinel sign over the radial sensory nerve. The Tinel sign will vary in location, depending on where the radial sensory nerve exits from beneath the tight fascia, binding it between the brachioradialis and the extensor carpi radialis longus tendons. This entrapment is commonly misdiagnosed as de Quervain tenosynovitis (37).

Surgical treatment of chronic nerve entrapment is common. The reported results, however, are less than acceptable, in my opinion. From Phalen's first reports (38) of large series of carpal tunnel releases, the impression most people have is that results of carpal tunnel surgery are excellent. In fact, recent series show only 70% excellent results (14). Recent series for ulnar nerve decompression at the elbow have been reviewed extensively (14,39). Regardless of technique, less than 70% of patients achieve excellent sensory results for a severe degree of entrapment, with only about one-third of patients recovering if muscle atrophy was present. Treatment remains without a scientific basis because models for chronic nerve compression have not been available. Most surgical reports of even large series do not stage patients according to degree of disease severity based on careful preoperative testing. Even the few reports on ulnar nerve surgery in which attempts at staging have been made fail to include sensory abnormalities in the staging system. The only report (31) in the English language that addressed the use of intraneural neurolysis as an adjunct to improve results in these cases remains to be substantiated by others. Most surgeons are concerned that extensive intraneural dissection will produce more scarring and result in significant complications, such as causalgia or reflex sympathetic dystrophy. Our research model has demonstrated in the primate model that internal neurolysis can be done safely in the chronically compressed median nerve by a surgeon appropriately trained in microsurgical techniques (40) and, in the rat model, that internal neuroloysis gives significantly better results than simple decompression (41). Guidelines for staging nerve compression and basing treatment upon such guidelines are now available (14).

Note: This treatment scheme should apply to any nerve, regardless of location (upper or lower extremity, proximal or distal), inasmuch as the pathophysiology of chronic nerve entrapments applies to all peripheral nerves.

EARLY CASES

In early cases, patients have symptoms causing them to seek treatment, but may have no physical findings except abnormal vibratory perception (often hypersensitive) and a weakly positive Tinel sign. Medical treatment of underlying inflammatory or endocrine disorder, edema, or vitamin deficiency (B_6) should be begun. Physical therapy is used to relieve any associated muscle spasm, with splinting to relieve nerve compression (e.g., wrist in neutral or elbow extended). Surgery is not recommended, even in the presence of abnormal nerve conduction.

MODERATE CASES

Moderate cases are those in which patients have symptoms causing them to seek attention despite 6 months of "conservative treatment," with physical findings consistent with muscle weakness and diminished perception of vibratory stimulus. If no further nonsurgical measures can be added, and if a period off work or an altered work environment has already been tried, or if the patient refuses further splinting, then surgical treatment, even in the absence of positive electrodiagnostic studies, is recommended. The surgical procedure is total release of the source of nerve compression. (Further technical details of surgical releases are not within the scope of this chapter but are well described (1).)

SEVERE CASES

Severe cases are those in which the patient now has persistent sensory discomfort (the discomfort is not intermittent, does not "come and go") and/or physical examination reveals either abnormal two-point discrimination (>4 mm moving, or >6 mm static) or muscle wasting of any degree. Even if the patient presents this way and has not had previous nonsurgical treatment, and even if electrodiagnostic studies are normal, surgery is recommended. The surgical procedure includes total release of the nerve plus internal neurolysis (because this degree of severity implies presence of significant intraneural fibrosis) (14).

Impeded Neural Regeneration (Neuroma)

If the cell body of a peripheral nerve remains alive after the transection of one of its limbs, neural regeneration at the amputation site is the expected consequence of an effort to restore neural continuity. The range of potential consequences in the scheme goes from an unassisted "spontaneous repair," if the transection is sharp and the ends are not displaced, to a complete block of the proximal end from uniting in any way with the distal end. For mechanisms of injury discussed previously that may result in partial disruption of a peripheral nerve, or after a poor repair, the regenerated neural tissue is partially diverted into surrounding tissues rather than being directed correctly distally. This is a "neuroma-in-continuity." For mechanisms of injury discussed previously that may result in complete division of the nerve, the result of neural regeneration blocked completely is an "end-bulb neuroma." The classical neuroma is a combination of neural regenerating units or clusters, randomly scattered, without fascicular organization and with a mass of collagen.

Because attempted neural regeneration is the inevitable biologic consequence of transecting a peripheral nerve, earlier attempts to "prevent neuroma formation" were not likely to succeed. These attempts involved applying all manner of chemical and physical modalities to transected nerve ends. Mechanical attempts to cap the nerve seem to have been successful only to the extent that the regenerating axon sprouts were prevented from escaping the cap and entering the surrounding tissue. Some neuronotrophic factor (e.g., from denervated skin to transected sensory nerve) may encourage such persistent attempts at distal regeneration (42). Physiologic attempts to prevent neuroma formation, however, appear more promising (i.e., encouraging a perineural environment for the transected end, either by encasing the transected end in its own epineurium or by rerouting the transected end into a vein). Just as tension causes fibrosis elsewhere, a transected nerve left adjacent to an area of movement will be placed under tension, with the subsequent induction of increased collagen in the neuroma itself and adherence of the neuroma to adjacent moving structures. The physiologic approach should be to "control," not "prevent," neuroma formation. Combining these concepts, the approach of implanting a transected nerve end into a muscle, away from joint movements and away from the stimulus of denervated skin, has been investigated in a primate model (42–44). The results of these studies suggest that neural regeneration can be manipulated by altering its microenvironment such that a classical neuroma does not form.

The reason a neuroma is painful is at present unknown. Extensive observations have been documented that neuromas in rodents and primates have spontaneous group A delta as well as C fiber activity, and ephaptic transmission (45). This suggests that, in addition to the local factors, such as the neuroma being superficial and in an area of frequent contact and movement, factors intrinsic to the neuroma may be important in the etiology of neuromatous pain. These observations suggest that treatment of a neuroma clinically may require resection of the formed or "mature" neuroma as well as alteration of its microenvironment.

Diagnosis of pain caused by a neuroma requires three criteria: (a) a well-defined spot where palpation causes pain that radiates into the distribution of the nerve, (b) demonstration of altered sensibility in the area of the nerve distribution distal to the neuroma, and (c) confirmation that the neuroma is contributing to the pain or is its sole source by diagnostic block of the nerve with local anesthetic. Potential for confusion exists in this diagnostic approach unless one is aware of critical areas of nerve overlap; these criteria lead to the diagnosis of neuromatous pain but may not identify the correct nerve. The most common area for this confusion is the dorsal-radial aspect of the hand, where the sensory branch of the radial nerve and the lateral antebrachial cutaneous nerve overlap in 75% of hands (46). Criterion (c) is essential in this area, because a block of both these nerves may be required to achieve pain relief, thereby indicating that the neuroma may be receiving contributions from each of these nerves or that more than one neuroma is present.

Treatment of the neuroma-in-continuity is determined by the amount of function remaining in the injured nerve. This can be determined preoperatively by the clinical assessment of motor and sensory function, as discussed earlier in this chapter, and intraoperatively by nerve conduction studies (47,48). If useful function is present clinically, the preoperative pain symptoms must be treated intraoperatively by identifying (by microintraneural dissection) the injured from the noninjured fascicles. Final selection of the fascicles to be excised and grafted is based on the height, if any, of the compound action potential in the fascicle in question compared with the other fascicles in the nerve. If, after the microintraneural dissection (which is, in fact, an intraneural neurolysis), all fascicles have satisfactory conduction, then treatment is completed for the nerve itself. However, if these fascicles, with or without grafting, are placed back into a scarred bed where they can become adherent to adjacent tendons or overlying denervated skin, then recurrent pain and treatment failure may be anticipated. In these circumstances, interposing a muscle flap between the nerve and these adjacent structures provides a vascularized interface that promotes healing and is a successful salvage procedure or adjunct to the neurolysis/grafting procedure (49,50).

Nerve injection injuries may be considered a special form of neuroma-in-continuity. Depending on whether the agent injected is placed extra- or intrafascicularly, on the particular physical/chemical properties of the injected material, and on the concentration of the agent, intraneural scar of varying degree results from the injury. Diagnosis of a nerve injection injury is established by the history of pain at the injection site associated with severe pain radiating in the distribution of the injected nerve. Treatment should not be immediate surgical exploration. Frequent follow-up examinations are essential to decide appropriate treatment. Initial pain and transient sensory/motor loss should diminish over a 3-month interval. Electrodiagnostic studies are indicated. If recovery is poor, then exploration, neurolysis, or nerve grafting is indicated (51).

Treatment of the painful end bulb or classical neuroma is based upon the following principles, with the specific treatment varying topographically. Ideally, the frustrated proximal axons should be reunited with their original endings, which assumes that the distal site still exists (amputation of the part has not occurred), that a distal nerve segment exists to receive the graft, that donor-site morbidity for the nerve graft is acceptable, and that the path for the nerve graft is both well vascularized and free of scar and tension. If the criterion of scar/tension freedom cannot be met, then, even if the graft is successful in restoring sensibility to the distal area (i.e., the graft is a technical success), pain will still be present because of tension-induced neuroma formation at the proximal and distal graft junctures. This, for example, is the cause of failure of nerve grafts to relieve a painful neuroma of the radial sensory nerve at the wrist, where the radial-ulnar excursion of the nerve is impeded by the graft-neuroma-bed scar distally and the tethered nerve proximally, where it exits from beneath tight forearm fascia and brachioradialis tendon (52).

Nerve grafting as a treatment for painful neuromas is most successful at the level of the common volar digital nerves and proper digital nerves. In these areas, sufficient length of graft can be placed into a bed with good gliding, and proximal and distal graft junctures can be placed away from joint surfaces over near-neutral lines of tension. For painful neuromas at or about the level of the wrist (in particular, for the radial sensory nerve, lateral antebrachial cutaneous nerve, dorsal cutaneous branch of the ulnar nerve, and palmar cutaneous branch of the medial nerve), resection of the neuroma and implantation of the proximal nerve stump into a large muscle belly, away from the musculotendinous region, and into a muscle with small excursion has been found highly effective in relieving pain (53). The brachioradialis muscle has been found to be the ideal recipient muscle. The outcropping thumb muscles, because of their large excursion, have been found unsuitable. The pronator quadratus also is not a suitable site for implantation because, during pronation/supination, the nerve end is subjected to twisting motions and compression beneath the radius and ulna. The placement of neuromas of digital nerves into the muscles of the hand (e.g., the lumbricales), probably fails because of the small cross-sectional area of these muscles, which allow sprouts from the neuroma to escape into surrounding tissue, and because of the relatively large excursion of these muscles, which results either in the nerve's pulling out of the muscle or tension-induced fibrosis about the nerve end. In the areas where the neuroma may be excised and the proximal end of the nerve allowed to lie in a deep subcutaneous plane away from joint movement and denervated skin, such as the upper arm, this "proximal resection" treatment of the neuroma may be sufficient without muscle implantation (43,44,53).

COMPUTER-ASSISTED SENSORIMOTOR TESTING

Quantitative sensory testing has been advocated by the neurologists to measure peripheral nerve function since the early

1980s, because traditional electrodiagnostic testing is painful, expensive, and all too often, for the plastic surgeon's patients, returns with a "normal" interpretation when the patient has clinical symptoms and signs of nerve compression. Quantitative sensory testing can measure the perception of temperature, vibration, or touch. While the tuning fork and the Disk-Criminator have been the mainstays of my office examination technique over the years, in 1992 we first reported the use of computer-assisted measurement of the cutaneous touch threshold. This device causes no pain, is fun for the patient, and is inexpensive for health care insurers, in contrast to nerve conduction studies and electromyography. The Pressure-Specified Sensory Device component measures one- and two-point moving and static-touch thresholds. The motor component, the Digit-Grip, is electromechanic, not hydraulic, and has just + 1% error, in contrast to the curved-handled, hydraulic devices. These computer-assisted devices are IBM compatible, approved by the FDA, and traceable to the National Institute of Standards and Technology. Over the past 4 years, this equipment has been demonstrated to be valid, reliable, more sensitive than electrodiagnostic testing for carpal, cubital, and tarsal tunnel syndrome; able to distinguish diabetic populations at risk for foot ulcerations; serve for screening and surveillance of cumulative trauma disorders in industry; and be able to identify a malinger (54–57). Examples of the computer printouts with these devices are given in Figure 93–1.

PRESSURE SENSORY ONE / TWO POINT DEVICE

LOCATION	1 PT STATIC GM/SQmm	2 PT STATIC GM/SQmm	MM	1 PT MOVING GM/SQmm	2 PT MOVING GM/SQmm	MM
LEFT						
INDEX	0.5	1.0	5.0			
LITTLE	0.8	1.1	5.1			
DORSRADLHND	1.4	6.2	17.0			
RIGHT						
INDEX	2.8	3.9	4.1			
LITTLE	1.5	1.8	6.3			
DORSRADLHND	1.0	12.9	13.1			

A

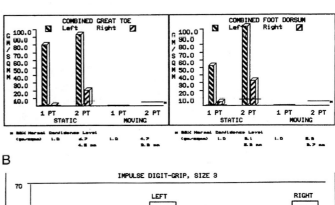

B

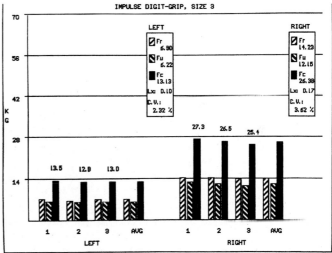

D

FIG. 93–1. Examples of computer printouts with the Pressure-Specified Sensory Device (A,B,C) and the Digit-Grip (D). **A,** the full printout is given, which lists the cutaneous pressure thresholds for one-point static and two-point static touch. In the text is given the distance at which one point is distinguished from two. In the text and on the graph, the cutaneous pressure thresholds are given in grams per square millimeter (units of pressure). During a screening exam, the moving one-point and two-point discrimination thresholds are not done. The horizontal lines are the 99% confidence limits for the pressure thresholds. The right index finger thresholds are elevated, as are the two-point discrimination values, while those for the left index finger and both little fingers are normal. This patient has a carpal tunnel syndrome in the right hand. **B,** for the lower extremity, the patient has elevated thresholds for both the posterior tibial nerve's medial plantar nerve (big toe) and for the peroneal nerve (foot dorsum). This patient had a right tibial and fibular fracture, and now, 6 months later, has findings consistent with tarsal tunnel syndrome and common peroneal nerve compression at the fibular head. In both these patients, the electrodiagnostic findings were normal. **C,** bilateral symmetrical abnormal pressure thresholds for median, ulnar, and radial sensory nerves. This pattern is consistent with a peripheral neuropathy, such as diabetes. **D,** the grip strength measurements of a patient with a left cubital tunnel syndrome are given. The total force in kilograms for the left hand is 13 versus 26 for this right hand-dominant woman, and is therefore weak. The orderly sequence of radial force being greater than ulnar force for each grasp, the coefficient of variation less than 15.0% for each hand and the difference in variation of less than 5% between the hands indicates that this patient has given a maximum effort, and is not malingering.

References

1. Kendall HO, Kendall FP. *Muscles: testing and function.* 4th ed. Baltimore: Williams & Wilkins, 1983.
2. Lister G. *The hand: diagnosis and indications.* 2nd ed. Edinburgh: Churchill Livingstone, 1984.
3. Dellon AL. *Evaluation of sensibility and reeducation of sensation in the hand.* Baltimore: Williams & Wilkins, 1981.
4. Dellon AL, Kallman CH. Evaluation of functional sensation in the hand. *J Hand Surg* 1983; 8:865.
5. Dellon AL. The vibrometer. *Plast Reconstr Surg* 1983; 71:427.
6. Dellon AL. The moving two-point discrimination test: Clinical evaluation of the quickly adapting fiber/receptor system. *J Hand Surg* 1978; 3:474.
7. Seddon JH. A classification of nerve injuries. *Br Med J* 1942; 2:237.
8. Sunderland S. *Nerves and nerve injury,* 2nd ed. London: Churchill Livingstone, 1978.
9. Dykes PJ, Thomas PK, Lambert EH, et al. *Peripheral neuropathy,* 2nd ed. Philadelphia: WB Saunders, 1984.
10. Dellon AL. Improved sensorimotor function in diabetic upper and lower extremities by internal neurolysis (abstr). *Diabetes 36 (suppl):* 1987; 197A.
11. Dellon AL. Optimism in diabetic neuropathy. *Ann Plast Surg* 1988; 20:103.
12. Dellon AL, Mackinnon SE, Seiler WA IV. Susceptibility of the diabetic nerve to chronic compression. *Ann Plast Surg* 1988; 20:117.
13. Dellon AL. Clinical use of vibratory stimuli to evaluate peripheral nerve injury and compression neuropathy. *Plast Reconstr Surg* 1980; 65:466.
14. Mackinnon SE, Dellon AL. *Surgery of the peripheral nerve.* New York: Thieme, 1988.
15. Wynn Parry CB. *Rehabilitation of the hand.* 4th ed. London: Butterworths, 1981.
16. Hunter JM, Schneider LH, Macklin EJ, et al. *Rehabilitation of the Hand.* 2nd ed. St Louis: CV Mosby, 1984.
17. Matsen FA III. *Compartmental syndromes.* New York: Grune & Stratton, 1980.
18. Dellon AL, Schneider R, Burke R. Effect of acute compartmental pressure changes on response to vibratory stimuli in primates. *Plast Reconstr Surg* 1983; 72:208.
19. Szabo RM, Gelberman RH, Williamson RV, et al. Vibratory sensory testing in acute peripheral nerve compression. *J Hand Surg* [*Am*] 1984; 9:104.
20. Effect of increased systemic blood pressure on the tissue pressure threshold of peripheral nerve. *J Orthop Res* 1984; 1:172.
21. Whitesides TE Jr, Haney TC, Morimoto K, et al. Tissue pressure measurements as a determinant for the need of fasciotomy. *Clin Orthop* 1975; 113:43.
22. Mubarak SJ, Owen CA, Hargens AR, et al. Acute compartment syndromes; diagnosis and treatment with the aid of the Wick catheter. *J Bone Joint Surg* [*Am*] 1978; 60:1091.
23. Millesi H. Brachial plexus injuries: management and results. *Clin Plast Surg* 1984; 11:115.
24. Breidenbach W, Terzis JK. Anatomy of free vascularized nerve grafts. *Clin Plast Surg* 1984; 11:65.
25. Gilbert A. Etiology and pathology of obstetrical brachial palsy: a review of 100 operated cases. Presented at a meeting of the American Society of Surgery of the Hand, February 1984.
26. Terzis JK. *Microreconstruction of nerve injuries.* Philadelphia: WB Saunders, 1987.
27. Ochoa J. Nerve fiber pathology in acute and chronic compression. In: Omer GE, Spinner M, eds. *Management of peripheral nerve problems.* Philadelphia: WB Saunders, 1980.
28. Mackinnon SE, Dellon AL, Hudson AR, et al. Chronic nerve compression—an experimental model in the rat. *Ann Plast Surg* 1984; 13:112.
29. Mackinnon SE, Dellon AL, Hudson AR, et al. A primate model for chronic nerve compression. *J Reconstr Microsurg* 1985; 1:185.
30. Dellon AL. Tinel or not Tinel. *J Hand Surg* [*Br*] 1984; 9:216.
31. Curtis RM, Eversmann WW Jr. Internal neurolysis as an adjunct to the treatment of carpal tunnel syndrome. *J Bone Joint Surg* [*Am*] 1973; 55:733.
32. Dellon AL, Mackinnon SE. Tibial nerve branching in the tarsal tunnel. *Arch Neurol* 1984; 41:645.
33. Dellon AL, Hendler N, Hopkins J, et al. Team management of patients with diffuse upper extremity complaints. *Md State Med J* 1986; 35:849.
34. Wartenberg R. Cheiralgia paresthetica (isolierte neuritis des ramus superficialis nervi radialis). *Z Gesamte Neurol Psychiatr* 1932; 141:145.
35. Dellon AL, Mackinnon SE. Radial sensory nerve entrapment in the forearm. *J Hand Surg* [*Am*] 1986; 11:199.
36. Mackinnon SE, Dellon AL, Hudson AR, et al. Histopathology of compression of the superficial radial nerve in forearm. *J Hand Surg* [*Am*] 1986; 11:206.
37. Saplys R, Mackinnon SE, Dellon AL. The relationship between nerve entrapment versus neuroma complications and the misdiagnosis of de Quervain's disease. *Contemp Orthop* 1987; 15:51.
38. Phalen GS. The carpal-tunnel syndrome. *J Bone Joint Surg* [*Am*] 1966; 48:211.
39. Dellon AL. Review of treatment results for ulnar nerve compression at the elbow. *J Hand Surg* [*Am*] 1989; 14:688.
40. Mackinnon SE, Dellon AL. Evaluation of microsurgical internal neurolysis in a primate median nerve model of chronic nerve compression. *J Hand Surg* [*Am*] 1988; 13:345.
41. Mackinnon SE, O'Brien JP, Dellon AL, et al. An assessment of the effects of different treatment strategies, including internal neurolysis on a chronically compressed rat sciatic nerve. *Plast Reconstr Surg* 1988; 81:251.
42. Seckel BR. Discussion of "Treatment and prevention of amputation neuromas in hand surgery." *Plast Reconstr Surg* 1984; 73:397.
43. Dellon AL, Mackinnon SE, Pestronk A. Implantation of sensory nerve into muscle: preliminary clinical and experimental observations on neuroma formation. *Ann Plast Surg* 1984; 12:30.
44. Mackinnon SE, Dellon AL, Hudson AR, et al. Alteration of neuroma formation by manipulation of its microenvironment. *Plast Reconstr Surg* 1985; 76:345.
45. Myers RA, Raja SN, Campbell JN, et al. Neural activity originating from a neuroma in a baboon. *Brain Res* 1985; 325:255.
46. Mackinnon SE, Dellon AL. The overlap pattern of the lateral antebrachial cutaneous nerve and the superficial branch of the radial nerve. *J Hand Surg* [*Am*] 1985; 10:522.
47. Kline DG, Nulsen FE. The neuroma-in-continuity: its preoperative and operative management. *Surg Clin North Am* 1972; 52:1189.
48. Terzis JK, Dykes RW, Hakstian RW. Electrophysiological recordings in peripheral nerve surgery: a review. *J Hand Surg* 1976; 1:52.
49. Reisman N, Dellon AL. The abductor digiti minimi muscle flap. A salvage technique for palmar wrist pain. *Plast Reconstr Surg* 1983; 72:859.
50. Dellon AL, Mackinnon SE. The pronator quadratus muscle flap. *J Hand Surg* [*Am*] 1984; 9:423.
51. Hudson AR. Nerve injection injuries. *Clin Plast Surg* 1984; 11:27.
52. Dellon AL, Mackinnon SE. Susceptibility of the superficial sensory branch of the radial nerve to form painful neuromas. *J Hand Surg* [*Br*] 1984; 9:42.
53. Dellon AL, Mackinnon SE. Treatment of the painful neuroma by neuroma resection and muscle implantation. *Plast Reconstr Surg* 1986; 77:427.
54. Dellon ES, Keller K, Moratz V, et al. The relationship between skin hardness, pressure perception and two-point discrimination in the fingertip. *J Hand Surg* 1995; 20B:44.
55. Tassler PL, Dellon AL. Correlation of measurements of pressure perception using the Pressure-Specified Sensory Device with electrodiagnostic testing. *J Occup Med* 1995; 37:862.
56. Tassler PL, Dellon AL, Sheffler N. Cutaneous pressure thresholds in ulcerated and non-ulcerated diabetic feet, measured with the Pressure-Specified Sensory Device. *J Amer Pod Med Assn* 1995; 85:679.
57. Mitterhauser M, Muse V, Dellon AL, et al. Detection of submaximal effort with computer-assisted grip strength measurements. *J Occup Med* (submitted) 1996.

94

Surgery for Rheumatoid Arthritis in the Hand and Wrist

J.K. Stanley, M. Ch. Orth. F.R.C.S.E., F.R.C.S., and A.J. Beard, F.R.A.C.S.

Rheumatoid arthritis is a whole-body, lifetime, progressive, and incurable disease that by its very nature affects all facets of a person's life and activities. The disease involves all parts of the musculoskeletal system and mesenchymal tissues. The ubiquitous nature of this disease requires careful management planning appropriate to each individual. Thus, consideration must be given to the state of the cervical spine, temporomandibular joints (TMJs), shoulders, and lower limbs; for example, heavy weightbearing on the meticulously reconstructed hand should be avoided by addressing problems in the feet, knees, and hips in advance of any surgery to the hands and wrists.

The cervical spine should be assessed to identify any instability and exclude radicular symptoms and weakness arising from any atlantoaxial pannus that might give rise to compression of the cord or rheumatoid disease–causing irritation or damage to the cervical nerve roots as they exit the intervertebral foramina. Particular care must always be taken to protect the cervical spine during induction of anaesthesia and transferring of the patient from bed to gurney or table. Meticulous positioning of the patient on the operative table protects the osteoporotic bones, stiff joints, thin skin, and prominent pressure points. The use of a rubber bandage exsanguination tourniquet should be avoided to prevent extensive degloving injury to the arm and forearm.

Recurrent aggressive synovitis is the most significant destructive process seen in rheumatoid disease. The synovial tissue proliferates and fimbrillates, increasing many thousands of times in width. The paucity and quality of the synovial fluid, the acid lysozymes, the almost neoplastic aggression of the pannus as it invades from the periphery of the joint, and the fluctuating intraarticular pressure serve to damage the joint progressively. As this occurs, the swelling and distension of the joint causes pressure on the surrounding structures. Pressure on nerves produces compression neuropathies. Pressure on joint capsules and ligaments results in stretching of these structures and associated joint instability.

Extraarticular structures are not exempt from the effects of the disease. The synovial tissue invades tendons directly, weakening them and disrupting their blood supply. The periarticular regions where the synovitis thickens under the collateral ligaments and capsular attachments are particularly prone to the development of erosions and geodes (Fig. 94–1).

Recurrent synovitis is accompanied by attempts at healing, which result in scar formation. Thus, the joints may be stiff from scarring of the soft tissues and destruction of the joint surfaces, or unstable as a result of the capsule, ligament, and tendon damage. Pain results from inflammation, stretching of soft tissues, abrasion of joint surfaces, neurologic damage, and joint subluxations. Muscle weakness and poor tendon excursion further exaggerate the intrinsic joint stiffness and add to the overall effects of the disease.

There are a number of aspects of an accurate and useful evaluation of the patient and in some degree they must be considered in every patient although some will assume more importance in some patients than in others. They are: functional, anatomic, medical, radiologic, psychologic, social, and financial.

Functional Assessment

The rational approach to surgical assessment is to identify functional loss and its anatomic etiology, and then to choose among the surgical procedures in the armamentarium of the individual surgeon. The causes that can be identified in mechanical terms can include pain, deformity, stiffness, and instability; it is these effects of the disease that give rise to the loss of function.

This assessment requires multidisciplinary input. Rheumatologists must consider the complex of medical problems and concentrate on the general rather than the specific. Their approach is medical and includes medication, both systemic and local, and additional and alternate treatments such as orthosis and prosthetics. Surgeons tend to consider the surgically correctable problem and think in terms of pathologic anatomy and the surgical possibilities.

Hand therapists have considerable experience in determining the effects of a particular functional deficit upon the individual's daily activities. The results of surgery are seen by the therapist more frequently than the surgeon and patients often express concerns to the therapist felt too mundane to mention to the surgeon. The therapists are essential in both the assessment of the problem and in formulating the therapy regime before surgery (e.g., joint protection advice, adaptations to the home) and in the rehabilitation phase of the surgical program. The early involvement of the rheumatologist, surgeon, therapist, and patient encourages a positive rapport and establishes well-defined and realistic goals of treatment.

ANATOMIC

An understanding of functional and surgical anatomy is essential. Functional anatomy comprises the anatomic basis of the hand and upper limb in use, and appreciation of the interrelationships of the anatomic units necessary for each defined function is essential; for example, turning a key in a

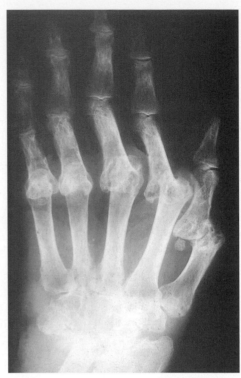

FIG. 94–1. Characteristic radiographic picture of a patient with long-standing rheumatoid arthritis. There is volar subluxation and translation of the wrist, with volar subluxation and ulnar deviation of the MCP joints and dislocation of the MCP joint of the thumb.

lock requires not only appositional grip between index finger and thumb (to hold the key) but also a functional proximal and distal radioulnar joint (to allow adequate supination and pronation to turn the key). The problem is difficulty in turning a key, the obvious pathology is instability of the metacarpophalangeal joint (MCPJ) of the thumb, the treatment is arthrodesis of the MCPJ, the result is a stable thumb—but the patient still will not be able to turn the key if there are problems at the distal radioulnar joint (DRUJ).

The effect of a proposed surgical procedure upon the functional anatomy must also be appreciated; for example, wrist arthrodesis in removing wrist motion will highlight any deficiency in the shoulder as positioning of the hand in space falls to the shoulder rather than the elbow. One of the occasional unwanted side effects of wrist arthrodesis is to precipitate the need for a shoulder arthroplasty.

MEDICAL

The presence of vasculitis (Fig. 94–2) indicates a significant level of the disease and should warn the surgeon of the possibility of wound healing problems.

RADIOLOGIC

The radiographs simply inform the surgeon of three facts about a joint: the residual bone stock, the quality of any remaining joint surface, and the degree of subluxation/dislocation. These facts only serve to highlight to the surgeon those procedures that are technically difficult or impossible, given the state of the joint. Massive bone loss at the wrist (Fig. 94–3) precludes simple synovectomy, radiolunate fusion, in-

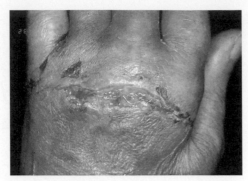

FIG. 94–2. Wound dehiscence occurs more commonly in patients with an active vasculitis, which is seen as splinter hemorrhages or painful rheumatoid nodules.

terpositional arthroplasty, tendon transfer, and total joint arthroplasty. The only reasonable remaining option is arthrodesis.

PSYCHOLOGIC

The attitude of the patient is an important area of assessment. The totally passive patient is difficult to motivate if intensive mobilization is part of the postoperative management. Equally, a clinically depressed patient will not fare well. The formal psychologic assessment of patients is not often performed, but it behoves the prudent surgeon to have some insight into the state of mind of the patient from whom is required significant cooperation.

SOCIAL

The social situation of the patient has a direct effect upon the way in which a problem is tackled; for example, if the patient lives alone significant postoperative help may be required if discharged home early in the rehabilitation phase. The presence of a helpful spouse or partner may be a positive, but overconcern may lead to passive behavior by the patient with a poorer surgical result.

FINANCIAL

Poverty, or the threat to employment by prolonged periods away from work, will determine how patients respond to the suggestion of a surgical procedure, and careful consideration is necessary as to the timing of surgery in these circumstances. Having assessed the overall problem, it is then necessary to examine the problem in a more dispassionate and detached manner, from a purely surgical perspective (Table 94–1).

Any surgical intervention must be clearly defined and have a specific purpose. This may be pain relief, improved range of motion (ROM), correction of deformity, stabilization, prevention of deterioration, or improved cosmesis. In the management of rheumatoid disease there must be a definite functional gain envisaged with each surgical procedure, and it is possible to say that the overriding principle of upper limb rheumatoid surgery is the restoration and preservation of function. In determining which are the best procedures for the patient, the surgeon needs to know the long-term results of the procedures. This requires an understanding of which procedures are possible, which are effective, and finally which are appropriate in the case being considered.

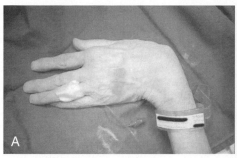

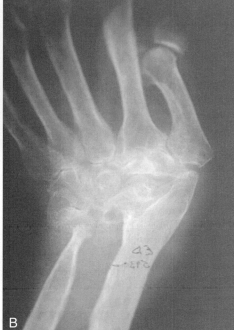

FIG. 94–3. **A,** the clinical picture, and **B,** the radiographic appearance of a wrist with considerable bone destruction and instability. Functional loss is significant.

Table 94–1
Principles of Surgery in Rheumatoid Arthritis

1. There must be with each procedure, a defined, desirable and necessary functional gain and the aim of all procedures must be to restore, maintain, or improve function.
2. There must be an assessment and treatment program tailored to the individual patient.
3. Single-stage surgery is preferable to staged procedures.
4. Realise that rheumatoid disease is a medical, not a surgical, condition and disease progress is inevitable.
5. The solution of one problem is always followed by the presentation of another; thus, a longterm view and strategic plan for a patient is essential.
6. Never operate out of sympathy alone; always have a clear purpose.
7. Test or trial surgery in order to ascertain whether the patient is a "good patient" or not, wastes a valuable opportunity, increases the risk of "surgical fatigue," and therefore should not be considered.
8. The aims of the procedure, which include improvement in motion, stability, deformity, cosmesis, or pain, must be borne in mind and postoperative assessment must take account of the purpose of the surgery.
9. Surgical fatigue may be a major influence upon the patient's mind when discussing further surgical procedures.

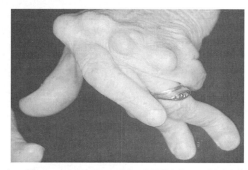

FIG. 94–4. Gross destruction of the MCP joints with instability, stiffness, and pain would be regarded as the end point of this disease.

The surgeon also needs to determine the order of the procedures. Full and complete normal hand function can only infrequently be restored in the patient with rheumatoid polyarthritis; thus, it is necessary to define precisely the aim of any surgical intervention and ensure that the patient and the surgeon understand the realistic outcome, which may well only be a limited one.

Procedures that require multiple stages should be avoided, and most surgical interventions should have a clear func-

tional gain; the luxury of two-stage procedures can only rarely be afforded. A patient with widespread disease, for example, may well require up to 5 or 6 (or more) major joint replacements and other surgery *before* the hands and wrists are considered (Fig. 94–4).

Multiple surgery and completion of a number of procedures under one anaesthetic is attractive, in that this approach reduces the overall rehabilitation period. Ideal combinations include thumb surgery, metacarpophalangeal joint replacement, and wrist procedures. Combinations that have conflicting postoperative regimes (e.g., metacarpophalangeal and interphalangeal joint replacements) are avoided where possible.

The aim of the operation must never be lost sight of; for example, if a joint is unstable, then stability is the aim and some ROM may be sacrificed to achieve it. Alternately, the problem may be stiffness, and in this case ROM remains the purpose of the surgical procedure; therefore it is essential that ROM is not used as a measure of success in the former and compared to the latter. There are two quite different indications and purposes.

Surgical Assessment (see Table 94–1)

The order of priority in management of the rheumatoid hand and wrist is determined in part by the vulnerability of the tissues to damage and the recovery potential of those tissues, and in part to the effect of dysfunction of a part and the effects upon other structures. The summary of the surgical priority is seen in Table 94–2. Although the general rule is "proximal to distal," the particular needs of the patient will override any list, which is only a guide.

Specific Surgical Problems

NERVE

Nerve compression in rheumatoid disease is common and the effects of prolonged compression lead to a poor recovery, particularly in the older patient, if release is not performed early. Hence, nerve decompression surgery takes the first position in the hierarchy of surgical problems. Median nerve compression at the wrist (Fig. 94–5), occurs more commonly in rheumatoid patients than in the general population and incidence of up to 70% (1,2,3,4) is reported. The symptoms of median nerve compression are often precipitated by flexor tendons synovitis within the carpal tunnel. During decompression of the median nerve in the carpal tunnel, the flexor tendons should be inspected and any proliferative synovitis excised. This synovitis may extend to a point which lies 10 cm proximal to the wrist crease and all of this synovitis should be removed. Scarring of the epineurium of the median nerve may result in a poor result from carpal tunnel surgery, and an epineurotomy may be required. Extensive surgery within the carpal tunnel always necessitates a very active postoperative regime to maintain individual ROM of the tendons and in particular the differential motion of the tendons and the nerve.

Table 94–2
Surgical Priorities

Nerve
Flexor tendons
Wrist
Thumb
Metacarpophalangeal (MCP) joints
Extensor tendons
Proximal interphalangeal (IP) joints
Distal interphalangeal (IP) joints

Other compressive neuropathies encountered in rheumatoid disease involve the anterior interosseous branch of the median nerve, the ulnar nerve (which can be compressed at the elbow or the wrist) and the posterior interosseous branch of the radial nerve at the level of the supinator muscle. Compression of the nerve at this level results in the paresis of the extensor digitorum communis, extensor indicis proprius, and extensor digitorum minimus, demonstrated clinically as the inability to extend the fingers. This may mimic multiple extensor tendon ruptures (5) (Fig. 94–6).

Nerves can also be compromised in rheumatoid disease by vasculopathy. These are divided into distal sensory neuropathy and combined sensorimotor neuropathy and are reported in 1 to 18% of rheumatoid patients (6,7). The distal sensory neuropathy is the more common type and has the better prognosis. It presents as a patchy glove and stocking hyperaesthesia. The combined sensorimotor neuropathy is a more severe neuropathy caused by vasculitis of the epineurial arteries, producing nerve ischemia, axonal degeneration, and neuromal demyelination. It may present acutely as a mononeuritis multiple or a polyneuropathy. These patients usually have a high titre of rheumatoid factor. Treatment is medical, with high doses of steroids aimed at the immune complex–mediated necrotising vaculitis. Morbidity rates up to 63% have been reported (8). Surgery is contraindicated in these patients.

FLEXOR TENDONS

The earliest sign of rheumatoid involvement in the flexor tendons may be triggering of the tendons of the fingers or thumb. This is often the first presentation of rheumatoid arthritis. The triggering frequently responds to local injections of steroids. If this fails, surgical decompression is necessary (Fig. 94–7).

Triggering of the thumb may present as a painful nodule on the flexor aspect at the base of the thumb, or as a fixed flexion deformity of the thumb, or as a painful click as the interphalangeal joint (IPJ) is flexed or extended. The tendon sheath of the thumb starts just proximal to the flexor crease at the base of the thumb. A tender nodule is often palpable and is the result of synovitis and invasion of the tendon.

Triggering of the fingers may occur at either the neck of the flexor sheath or at the decussation of the superficialis tendon. If the nodule is large enough, it will be trapped in the flexor sheath, thus preventing active flexion and mimicking a tendon rupture (9).

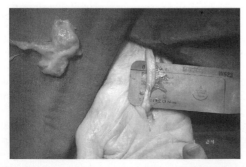

FIG. 94–5. Prolonged compression of the median nerve gives rise to irreversible changes, added to here by steroid injection into the nerve.

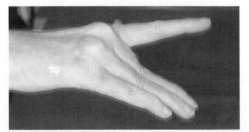

FIG. 94–6. Rupture of the extensor tendons usually commences from the ulnar side with the silent rupture of extensor digitorum minimus, followed by the obvious rupture of common extensors in sequence.

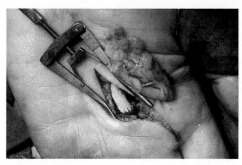

FIG. 94–7. Rheumatoid synovitis involving the tendon at the level of the fibrous flexor sheath in the palm gives rise to significant impairment of flexor tendon function.

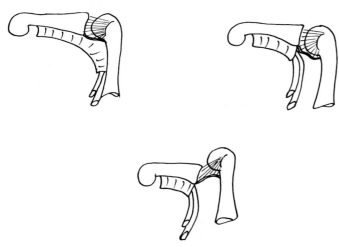

FIG. 94–8. Wide excision of the A1 pulley changes the mechanics of pull of the extensor tendons and predisposes toward volar subluxation of the MCP joint.

Wide division of the length of the A1 pulley encourages the more direct pull of the flexor tendons upon the proximal phalanx; therefore, there is an increased volar subluxation force applied to the MCPJ (10) (Fig. 94–8). This approach also deals inadequately with the synovitis invading the tendon. Improved results come from the performance of a tenosynovectomy by sharp dissection, opening the sheath between the A1 and A2 pulleys by a trapdoor flap, and ensuring any intratendinous nodules are excised, including those that lie hidden on the deep surface of the superficialis tendon (9).

Extensive synovitis may involve the flexor tendons at the wrist, palm, or finger, and if this has not responded to adequate medication and therapy for a period of 3 months then tenosynovectomy must be considered. Synovectomy is performed by excision from proximal to distal using sharp dissection. The incision may have to extend from 10 cm proximal to the wrist crease, crossing it at an angle, extending the incision as for a carpal tunnel decompression. A transverse incision in the palm at the proximal level of the fibrous flexor sheaths allows excellent exposure of the palm, and individual Bruner incisions in the finger are necessary for full exposure. The median nerve and its branches should be identified and preserved. Any adhesions between the superficialis and profundus tendons should be freed. The results of synovectomy of the tendons in the forearm and palm are reported as being

very beneficial. Digital synovectomy is technically more difficult but the results can be worthwhile (11–13), although less likely to give as good a result as wrist and palm surgery.

Longstanding multiple flexor tendon ruptures are a disaster for the patient, and for the surgeon this is a situation almost impossible to treat effectively. This problem severely compromises the function of the hand and makes the surgical restoration of that function very difficult. Prolonged tenosynovitis may threaten flexor tendon rupture, making early detection and intervention essential. More common than rupture is flexor tendon involvement, presenting as a problem with tendon gliding that results in loss of active flexion compared to passive flexion. This is due to adhesion formation between the superficial and deep tendon and between the superficial tendon and the proximal phalanx. This tenodesis effect may also present as weakness and/or loss of dexterity. These adhesions form during the resolution of the acute synovitis and often present months and sometimes years later. Treatment must be directed towards a tenolysis and a synovectomy, rather than just a synovectomy. The problems of flexor tendon dysfunction are often masked by joint stiffness or muscle weakness, which further complicates the assessment and rehabilitation of these patients.

Tendon rupture can result from direct invasion of the tendon by synovial tissue, which also disrupts the blood supply, rendering a section avascular. Rupture can also be caused by abrasion of the tendon over a spur of bone, produced by rheumatoid erosion of the bone or by osteophyte formation as a consequence of osteoarthritis complicating a burnt out rheumatoid joint. Play of the tendon over such a spur abrades the tendon, eventually rupturing it; however, this may not be the end of the matter because once the first tendon fails it allows adjacent tendons to come into contact with the spur in sequence.

The flexor pollicis longus tendon is most prone to rupture by this mechanism, but the profundus tendon to the index finger is also affected on occasion. A spur of bone caused by erosion of the scaphoid or trapezium has been shown to protrude through the floor of the carpal tunnel (14). The ulnar finger flexor tendons are at risk for abrasion in the region of the hook of the hamate (15) or the pisotriquetral joint. The extensor tendons may be abraded and rupture in a similar fashion by the distal radioulnar joint (16).

The risk of tendon rupture is increased by injection of steroids, which weakens the tendons significantly (17).

Pain with resisted flexion of the interphalangeal joint of the thumb suggests threatened rupture of the flexor pollicis longus. Inability actively to flex the IPJ indicates a possible complete rupture. The spur in the floor of the carpal tunnel is exposed through a longitudinal incision in the palm between the thenar and hypothenar muscles, taking particular care to avoid damage to the palmar cutaneous branch of the median nerve. The flexor retinaculum is divided under direct vision and the median nerve gently retracted radially and the flexor tendons ulnarward. The spur may be seen but is better felt as it arises from the scaphoid or trapezium and should be removed with bone rongeurs (Fig. 94–9). The capsular defect is repaired and the tendons are inspected. If the tendon is moderately abraded but in continuity, then reinforcing with a core suture and débriding the loose fibers may suffice. If the tendon is significantly abraded, then excision of the damaged portion and end-to-end tenorrhaphy may be required.

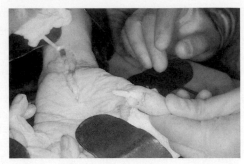

FIG. 94–9. Flexor pollicis longus rupture occurs at the level of the scaphotrapezial-trapezoidal joint, but the tendon stump can "die back" for a distance of 2 or 3 cm.

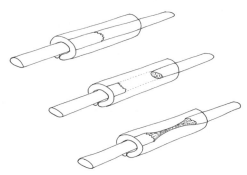

FIG. 94–10. The results of one-stage tendon grafting may not be impressive with regard to ROM of the IP joints, but provides excellent power in pinch, which is an important aspect of hand function.

When complete rupture is present, the proximal end will have recoiled and retracted significantly into the forearm, particularly if any significant delay in diagnosis has been occasioned. If the two ends are not apposable, then end-to-end tendon repair is not possible and a one-stage tendon graft utilizing palmaris longus or a second toe extensor as the donor tendon will be required (Fig. 94–10). Alternately the less functional procedure of arthrodesis of the IPJ of the thumb may be chosen. This will prevent hyperextension and restore pinch; however, IPJ flexion is important for picking up fine objects and the lack of motion at this joint combined with the weakness of thumb flexion due to the lack of flexor pollicis longus very significantly weakens the power of pinch.

The flexor tendons to the fingers can rupture in the carpal tunnel, the palm, or the flexor sheaths. The profundus tendons in the carpal tunnel lie in their own separate synovial sheath and may rupture without significant involvement of the superficialis tendons. This is demonstrable clinically as absence of distal IPJ flexion, but may be mimicked by synovial thickening in the tendon sheath or distal IPJ destruction. When the flexor digitorum profundus is ruptured distal to the origin of the lumbrical, then the lumbrical acts to extend the distal interphalangeal joint, which results in extension at the distal interphalangeal joint as the metacarpophalangeal and interphalangeal joints are flexed. This gives rise to paradoxical extension of the interphalangeal joints when the patient attempts to flex the fingers (the so-called quadrega syndrome).

When the site of rupture cannot be found, despite tracing the tendon from the carpal tunnel through the palm and along

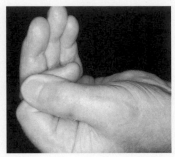

FIG. 94–11. Rupture of flexor tendons may occur silently, often during a period of florrid synovitis. The tendon fails, probably because of prolonged ischemia, but the intact synovial sheath allows healing to occur. The tendons appear to be intact but lengthened, with poor power and excursion. This results in significant functional impairment.

the flexor sheaths, then rupture in continuity should be suspected (18) (Fig. 94–11). This is presumed to be an ischemic rupture of the tendon within the sheath, which provides a mold for the formation of a fibrous repair that occurs with the proximal end in a retracted position and results in an elongated tendon that is functionally severely impaired. It is therefore imperative to ensure a full passive ROM before making this diagnosis. Treatment consists of shortening the tendon and performing an anastomosis by weaving the divided tendon through itself. Success depends upon three factors: (a) the length of time since the rupture and the resultant contracture of the muscle belly, (b) the excursion of the motor unit, and (c) the status of the joints of the thumb.

Repair of ruptured flexor tendons in any situation can be technically difficult, but in this situation rupture is accompanied by significant fibrillation and ischemia and direct repair is usually not possible and tendon transfer or grafting is almost always required. The results of grafting are frequently disappointing in the index finger, and less than perfection is possible in the thumb; hence, the sense of urgency and high priority placed upon the early consideration for treatment that impending ruptures receive and the need for immediate surgery for any ruptures that do occur.

WRIST

The wrist presents as the first evidence of rheumatoid disease in only 2.5% of patients, but eventually there is involvement of the wrist joint in 95% of patients with this disease (19). Rheumatoid involvement of the wrist may sometimes result in a wrist that continues to move despite significant destruction, eventually forming a ball-in-socket type of secondary degenerative arthrosis; in the juvenile and young adult, the carpus may spontaneously ankylose.

Usually, however, the majority of patients continue to deteriorate as more ligamentous and bone loss accrues. The classic deformity of the wrist in rheumatoid disease is a combination of volar subluxation, radial deviation, ulnar translocation, and supination of the carpus in association with carpal collapse, distal radioulnar joint destruction, and progressive loss of bone stock from the distal radius (Fig. 94–12). This deformity results from the synovitis destroying the retraining structures, including the volar and dorsal carpal ligaments and capsule. Early involvement also occurs in the distal radioulnar joint, where stretching of the triangular fi-

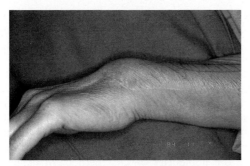

FIG. 94–12. The characteristic volar subluxation and supination of the hand.

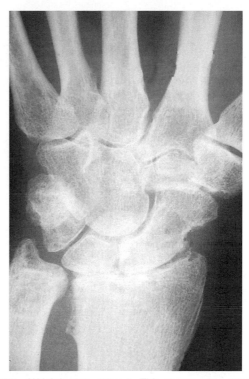

FIG. 94–14. Wrightington, stage 1. This shows early erosions with soft-tissue swelling and normal anatomy; it is suitable for conservative management.

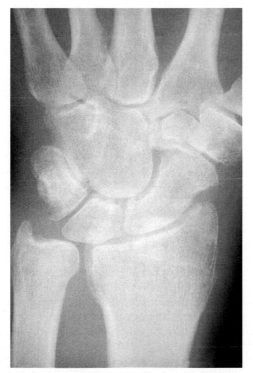

FIG. 94–13. A radiograph demonstrating translocation and translation with good preservation of joints, indicating that a reconstructive program is likely to succeed.

brocartilage complex and its attachments allows the extensor carpi ulnaris tendon to sublux ulnarward and volarly to become a wrist flexor, losing its important stabilizing role over the distal ulna, which dislocates dorsally. Later, the intercarpal joints and radio carpal joints are also destroyed (19) (Fig. 94–13).

The Wrightington classification of the wrist radiographs proposes the surgical options that are appropriate for the four stages of damage (20). The first, or therapeutic, stage (Fig. 94–14) is the ideal stage for synovectomy, rebalancing, and stabilization of the soft tissues. The second, or reconstructive, stage (Fig. 94–15), identifies those patients who would best benefit from limited wrist arthrodesis. The third stage (Fig. 94–16), with loss of all joint surfaces, invites the surgeon to consider arthroplasty or arthrodesis, and the fourth, irretrievable, stage with its significant loss of bone stock (Fig. 94–17) requires arthrodesis of the wrist.

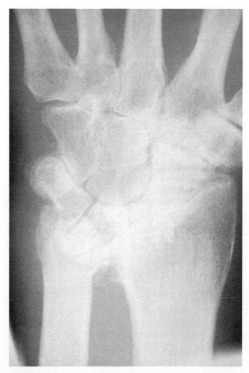

FIG. 94–15. Wrightington, stage 2. The translation and translocation is not associated with significant joint damage at this stage; therefore, a wide range of reconstructive surgery could be performed.

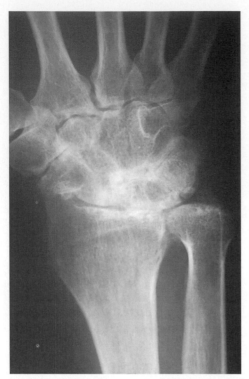

FIG. 94–16. Wrightington, stage 3. Loss of joint surface in the midcarpal joint and the radiocarpal joint; but, preservation of the bone stock indicates that this is the salvage stage of the devolution of wrist disease in rheumatoid. The choices for surgery are fewer in this group.

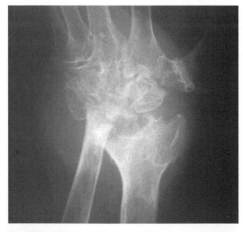

FIG. 94–17. Wrightington, stage 4. The massive bone loss precludes almost all surgery except arthrodesis. This would be regarded as the irreversible stage.

Therapeutic

STAGE 1

Early treatment includes intraarticular steroid injection, splintage, disease modifying drugs, and synovectomy of the extensor tendons and carpus with reconstruction of the distal radioulnar joint and exteriorization of the extensor tendons. The double breasting of the capsule and extensor retinaculum creates a dorsal stabilization. Synovectomy has been criti-

cized as a preventive procedure and is less commonly performed in some areas than in others, perhaps because of local referral patterns, but this procedure still enjoys reasonable popularity in European circles (21).

Arthroscopic synovectomy is being developed that may avoid the major nature, the significant discomfort, the long period of rehabilitation, and the risk of postoperative stiffness associated with open synovectomy (22), but arthroscopic synovectomy is a technically difficult technique requiring sufficient time and a particular expertise that is likely to restrict the popularity of this method. In open synovectomy, the wrist is approached through a dorsal longitudinal incision and the fourth extensor compartment is opened on the radial side, creating an ulnar-based flap of extensor retinaculum. The extensor tendons are carefully débrided using sharp dissection and reconstructed as required.

For radiocarpal and intercarpal disease, a volar approach for synovectomy has also been described (23); however, this runs the risk of further damaging the important volar carpal ligaments, the very structures that the procedure is attempting to protect. This approach is also technically more challenging.

STAGE 2

When there is early, localized involvement of the radiocarpal or intercarpal joints, then interpositional arthroplasty (24) or limited carpal fusions may be considered. These allow the maintenance of some movement at the wrist, while relieving the symptoms and preventing further deterioration. Radiolunate fusion, as described by Chamay (25), has proven very successful (Fig. 94–18) in stabilizing the wrist while maintaining a total arc of motion of up to 70° (26) of flexion and extension and allowing sufficient radioulnar deviation. Before considering this operation, there is an absolute requirement for a functioning, pain-free midcarpal joint; to this end, the capitate head can be replaced in combination with radiolunate fusion or even radioscapholunate arthrodesis (26).

A transverse excision of the distal ulna, as described by Darrach (27,28) (Fig. 94–19) has stood the test of time. This technique results in disturbance of the triangular fibrocartilage complex and ulnar sling mechanism and, it has been suggested, may contribute toward further ulnar translocation of the carpus.

This is a disputed claim, and the senior author's experience is that only when there is gross instability with radial deviation of the wrist prior to surgery is this a significant risk. It may also result in a painful instability of the distal ulnar stump in some patients, in addition to impaction against the distal radius, ulnar sensory neuromas, and rupture of extensor tendons (18,29–31). All of these have been reported as complications of this surgery.

A matched ulna resection (27) is recommended by some if there is destruction of the distal radioulnar joint and painful or limited supination and pronation (Fig. 94–20).

Sauve and Kapandji (32) (Fig. 94–21), proposed arthrodesis of the distal radioulnar joint and creating a pseudarthrosis by excising a more proximal portion of the ulnar (32). This is a useful procedure in those wrists that have developed translocation; the presence of the ulnar head allows the extensor carpi ulnaris tendon to stabilize the carpus in relation to the ulnar head and to stabilize the pseudarthrosis; however, this procedure may be complicated by painful im-

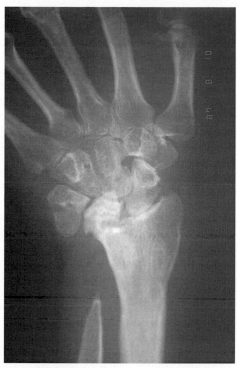

FIG. 94–18. Radiolunate fusion stabilizes the wrist, prevents translocation, translation, and volar subluxation, and preserves function for a considerable time, but requires good midcarpal joint function.

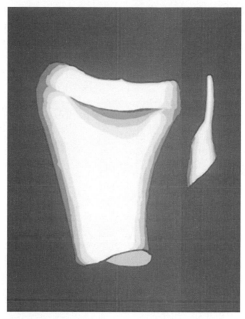

FIG. 94–20. More recently, to preserve distal ulnar stability, the matched ulna procedure has been proposed (shown here in diagrammatic form).

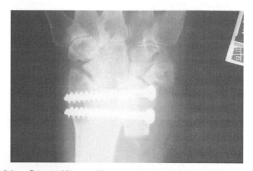

FIG. 94–21. Sauve Kapandji arthrodesis of the distal radioulnar joint with a proximal excision of a segment of ulna.

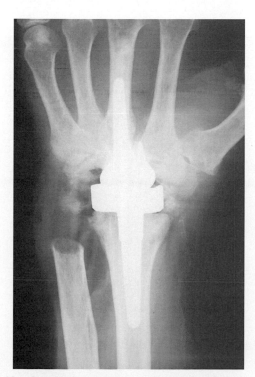

FIG. 94–19. Simple excision of the distal ulna is a popular and successful procedure in rheumatoid disease.

paction of the distal part of the proximal ulnar against the radius, with instability at this point (31).

Swanson's silastic cap (33) (Fig. 94–22) retained length but destroyed the important attachments to the distal ulna. It suffered from dislocation of the prosthesis and excessive motion of the distal ulnar and is now abandoned (18). Bower's interpositional arthroplasty maintains the ulnar styloid but does not sufficiently decompress the distal radioulnar joint in the rheumatoid patient, and requires the presence of an intact and competent triangular fibrocartilaginous complex (34).

STAGE 3

When significant destruction of the carpus has occurred, then arthroplasty or arthodesis need to be considered. Arthroplasty has the benefit of maintaining a useful functional range of movement. This is particularly important in patients requiring preservation of sophisticated grasp, but with limited power. Alternately, arthrodesis is a single, reliable procedure with a guaranteed result requiring a shorter period of immobilization and quicker rehabilitation and return to function (23).

Wrist arthroplasty was pioneered by Thermistocles Gluck in 1890 (35), and much has happened since. The prostheses are still evolving, but good medium term results are reported, with up to 80% good or excellent results maintained after at least 5 years (36–38). The operation is technically demanding and the results reflect the experience of the surgeon and the activity levels of the patient. Good long-term survival occurs more reliably in low-demand patients with quiescent disease than in high-demand individuals.

The Swanson silastic hinge was initially reported as providing sustained pain relief and was used widely (Fig. 94–23). Long-term studies have identified between 20 and 52% prosthetic failure (37,38). Concern about small-particle granulomatous reaction occurring in response to silicone rubber wear particles in other sites has increased awareness of this problem at the wrist level, and cystic changes suggestive of this problem have also been reported variably from 5 to 70% of cases. Sustained pain relief is being maintained between 50 and 80% after 5 years (37,40). The early results have been published for the total-joint arthroplasties such as the biaxial (41) and the trispherical prostheses (38), and it would seem from these studies that concern remains regarding the problems of fixation and loosening of the carpal component, which may need further development.

Total wrist arthrodesis may occur spontaneously, particularly in the juvenile rheumatoid, but in a position that is functionally unacceptable (usually marked flexion) and requires a corrective osteotomy. The osteotomy significantly changes the balance of the hand—in particular, the excursion of the flexor and extensor tendons, such as they are—with significant changes to the function of the hand and upper limb such that it causes significant concern to the patient. Therefore, an individualized and lengthy rehabilitation program must be coupled with careful counseling of the patient, partner, and relatives, before this seemingly innocuous and simple surgery is performed. Arthrodesis can be successfully achieved using an intramedullary pin (42–44). A longitudinal dorsal approach, as for synovectomy but with removal of all the cartilage and synovium, is used. A stout pin is introduced percutaneouly,

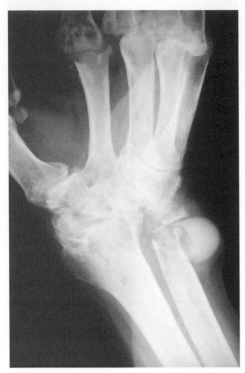

FIG. 94–22. Soft silicone rubber implants, both at the wrist joint and the ulnar head, do not withstand significant deforming forces, and this is particularly true of the ulnar cap, which is shown fractured.

FIG. 94–23. A, Swanson implant in situ with titanium grommets, which were introduced to protect the implant. **B,** a 6-year follow-up of a Swanson silastic implant without grommets. It shows some settling of the implant to 7 mm. This settling is associated with some reduction in ROM but does not impare the overall functional result.

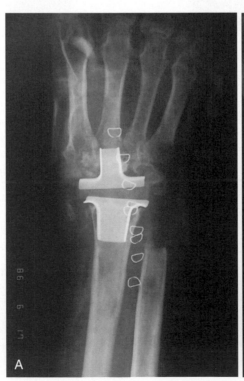
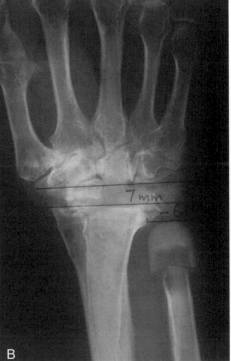

distally through the extensor tendon and the head of the 3rd metacarpal, across the carpus and into the radius. The carpus is held in a reduced position as the pin is advanced. Occasionally, a second pin advanced through the index metacarpal or the second intermetacarpal space, an oblique wire, or staple, may be necessary to control rotation (Fig. 94–24).

The ideal position of wrist fusion needs to be determined individually. Often the neutral (straight) position is functional and cosmetically acceptable. The dorsiflexed position described by Seddon (45) in the polio patient is not desirable in the rheumatoid patient because of the difficulty in attending to perineal hygiene. When bilateral arthrodesis is to be considered, in particular, and in the unilateral cas, a "trial of fusion" is worthwhile, in that the wearing of splints for 6 weeks with removal for skin hygiene only gives a more realistic impression to the patient, therapist, and surgeon of the limitations and secondary effects of wrist fusion. One of the more obvious examples of a secondary, unwanted effect has been discussed above in relation to the shoulder difficulties that may be encountered. It is our experience after 200 arthrodeses that the neutral flexion/extension position for the wrist allows adequate functional access to the perineum for personal hygiene, but that the dominant wrist should as far as is practical retain some motion for the sophisticated manipulative activities, and the nondominant wrist be fused to allow a power grasp for fixing/holding/carrying. Therefore, an arthroplasty or limited intercarpal arthrodesis should be preferred for the dominant hand.

Wrist arthrodesis may also be achieved by the use of a sliding radial bone graft (46). A strut is raised from the dorsum of the radius advanced across the carpus and secured with a screw into the base of the 3rd metacarpal and two screws into the distal radius. Solid union in all cases has been claimed using both techniques (43,44,46).

THUMB

Rheumatoid involvement of the thumb causes a variety of deformities, depending upon which joints are the most significantly affected. These have been classified into five types by Nalebuff (47) (Table 94–3).

Type I

The MCP joint is primarily affected, resulting in flexion of the joint and hyperextension of the interphalangeal (IP) joint. This resembles the boutonnière deformity (Fig. 94–25).

Type II

This occurs when there is subluxation of the carpometacarpal joint and disease of the MCP joint, resulting in flexion of the joint and hyperextension of the IP joint. This type is seen less commonly than types I or III. Treatment involves replacement of the trapezium and MCP joint arthrodesis or sesamoid arthrodesis.

Type III

Type III is a swan neck deformity that results from carpometacarpal disease with subluxation and adduction of the metacarpal and secondary hyperextension of the MCP joint (Fig. 94–26). The treatment regime is similar to type II.

Type IV

Type IV is the gamekeeper's thumb type, which is caused by stretching of the ulnar collateral ligament, resulting in an abduction deformity of the MCP joint (Fig. 94–27). Treatment

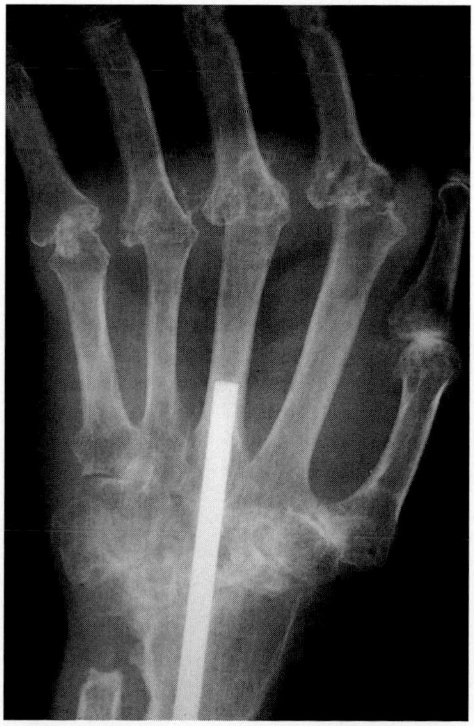

FIG. 94–24. The intramedullary pin is countersunk; it is a simple method of wrist arthrodesis.

Table 94–3
Classification of Thumb Deformity

I	MP disease and flexion of MP and hyperextension of IP boutonnière
II	MP flexion and IP hyperextension and CMC subluxation (rare)
III	CMC disease and subluxation and adduction of MC and secondary MP hyperextension (swan neck)
IV	MP abduction and UCL instability (gamekeepers' thumb)

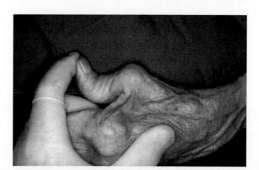

FIG. 94–25. The boutonnière deformity of the thumb may result from failure of the extensor hood at the MCP joint, or rupture of the flexor pollicis longus tendon.

consists of reconstructing the ligament or arthrodesing the MCP joint.

Type V

Type V results from stretching of the volar plate of the MCP joint, resulting in hyperextension of that joint and secondary flexion contracture of the interphalangeal joint. The treatment options are arthrodesis of the metacarpophalangeal joint or sesamoid arthrodesis.

Essentially, it is permissible to fuse two of the three joints and, providing the third joint is stable and mobile, a functional thumb will be maintained. When the carpometacarpal joint is involved, then trapezium arthroplasty or excision arthroplasty with a stabilization procedure is recommended. Disease of the MCP or IP joint is best treated with arthrodesis, except where all three joints are involved, in which case the carpometacarpal and IP joints are arthrodesed and the MCP joint is replaced using a silicone elastomer flexible-hinge finger joint implant (48). If the MCP joint has already been, fused then IP joint replacement is advised, provided the collateral ligaments are sound. However, the final combination depends upon the stability and bone stock of the joints in each individual. Trapezium replacement aims to remove the painful abrading joint surfaces and stabilize the base of the thumb.

It is important to have a stable MCP joint or the thumb metacarpal will adduct, hyperextending the MCP joint and subluxing the base of the metacarpal and the prosthesis if present. An unstable MCP joint may be treated with a sesamoid arthrodesis (49), which will maintain useful flexion, or the joint must be formally arthrodesed.

Arthrodesis of the MCP joint of the thumb can be performed using a number of techniques. A reliable method involves two V-shaped cuts with the apex pointing proximally, as described by Omer (50). The procedure is performed through a dorsal approach. A V is cut into the metacarpal head with the apex proximal. It is sloped slightly volarward. A matching V is cut at the base of the proximal phalanx; using the initial V as a guide (Fig. 94–28) and holding the thumb in the desired position, the cut surfaces are apposed and held with a single lag screw or crossed Kirschner wires. The technique has a high union rate and allows ideal alignment to be achieved easily.

MCP JOINT OF THE

The classic deformity resulting from rheumatoid involvement of the MCP joint is ulnar drift, combined with volar subluxation. The former is composed of ulnar deviation and ulnar translocation, and the latter of both flexion and pronation (Fig. 94–29). This deformity develops as a result of the

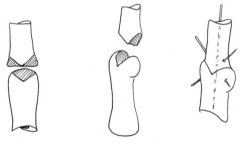

FIG. 94–28. Fusion of the thumb may be performed in many different ways. Our preferred method is the reverse Chevron technique, introduced by Omer, which is simple, stable, and effective.

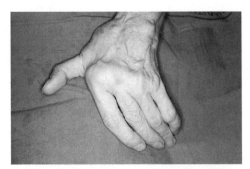

FIG. 94–26. Disturbance of the base of the thumb at the carpometacarpal joint results in the swan neck deformity of the thumb.

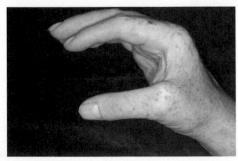

FIG. 94–27. Rupture of the ulnar collateral ligament of the thumb gives rise to instability at this level.

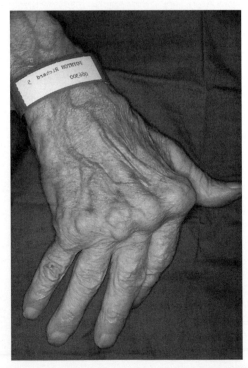

FIG. 94–29. Volar subluxation and ulnar drift of the MCP joints of the hand, which is a common finding in rheumatoid disease.

recurrent or persistent synovial thickening and effusion which, in stretching the capsule and collateral ligaments, allows any imbalance of forces to be unopposed and leads to the collapse of the joint. The direction of collapse is determined by the ulnar pull of the extensor and flexor tendons, which results from the ulnar translocation and radial deviation of the carpus at the radiocarpal joint. This ulnar force is increased by pressure from the thumb during normal pinch, the force of gravity acting on the hand at rest, the anatomic shape of the metacarpal head, the ulnar insertion of the lumbrical, or the ulnar deviation present in the normal hand (51). A common associated deformity is radial deviation of the wrist, which creates the "Z" collapse deformity in compensation for the inappropriate position of the fingers by bringing the finger tips more in line with the long axis of the forearm. The "chicken and egg" argument of which came first still continues with regard to the ulnar deviated fingers/radially deviated wrist and has not been resolved. The truth is that persistence of the radially deviated wrist seems to predispose of a recurrence of ulnar drift of the fingers. Therefore, it is necessary to ensure that the wrist deformity is passively correctable prior to MCP joint surgery, in which event the deformity will tend to correct after surgery without further treatment. A fixed deformity certainly requires some remedial surgery to the wrist.

Surgical intervention at the MCP joint level is aimed at relieving pain, maintaining and restoring function, preventing further deterioration, and improving the appearance of the hand. Any surgery to treat MCP joint disease will require meticulous attention to the soft tissue, and rebalancing aspects of the procedure and the need for an insertion of an implant are related to the quality of the residual articular surface. A Brewerton view of the MCP joint (an anteroposterior view, the wrist extended, the MCP joint flexed to 45°, the tube offset by 15°) (Fig. 94–30), highlights the subcollateral erosions and bone loss effectively and helps predict those joints that will require replacement.

The precise aims of the surgery must be borne in mind when predicting the outcome, for example, pain relief is a good measure of outcome if pain is the major initial problem requiring treatment. It is possible to relieve pain with an arthrodesis, but the functional penalty in the majority of patients is too great.

Soft-tissue reconstruction and synovectomy before significant articular damage has occurred can rebalance the fingers and delay deterioration (46). The surgical procedure is similar to that for a joint replacement, but without the bony

surgery. When subluxation of the joint has occurred, there is usually loss of the dorsal lip of the base of the proximal phalanx and flattening of the volar surface of the metacarpal head. In these circumstances, although the surface of the metacarpal head may seem to be in good condition from the dorsal aspect of the joint, the face of the head is flattened and eroded and simple synovectomy is insufficient to restore joint function. Total joint replacement should be performed in these circumstances.

Metacarpophalangeal joint replacement using Swanson's flexible-hinge spacer has been shown consistently and reliably to produce good long-term results (52–55), principally in terms of pain relief and patient satisfaction, correcting deformity and improving stability while maintaining a functional ROM of up to 56° (56). The joints are approached through either a single transverse or multiple longitudinal incisions. A transverse incision is cosmetically superior but makes the soft-tissue dissection more difficult (57). Postoperative support in an extension outrigger for 6 weeks allows early mobilization of the joints while protecting the extensor mechanism (Fig. 94–31).

EXTENSOR TENDONS

Synovitis of the extensor tendons is very common in rheumatoid arthritis. Synovectomy is advisable when medical treatment fails to control the disease. Exteriorization by placing the extensor retinaculum deep to the tendons further protects the tendons from abrasion and synovitis (58) (Fig. 94–32). Surgery to the extensor tendons is ideally combined with surgery for the wrist. The active therapy program after extensor tendon surgery tends to differ from that of metacarpophalangeal joint surgery; therefore, if there is a decision to replace the MCP joints, any deficit created by loss of active extension is made up by dynamic outriggers, and when there is a good joint range the extensor tendons are repaired. The joint motion is then sufficient to take the extensor repairs through a functional excursion.

Extensor pollicis longus is frequently abraded in the region of the Lister tubercle on the dorsum of the radius (59). Extension of the IP joint of the thumb may still be possible despite complete rupture of the extensor pollicis longus because of the action of the intrinsic muscles. Extensor pollicis longus is necessary for hyperextension and retropulsion of the thumb (i.e., the ability to lift the thumb with the palm of the hand flat on the table).

End-to-end tendon repair is sometimes possible within 3 weeks in acute tendon ruptures. Tendon grafting through a

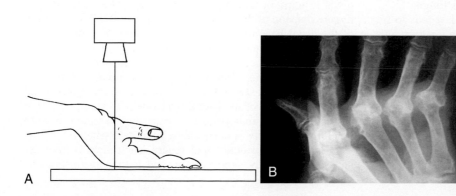

FIG. 94–30. A, diagram of the position of Brewerton's view. **B,** an x ray that shows the subcollateral spaces and the true nature of the damage to the MCP joints.

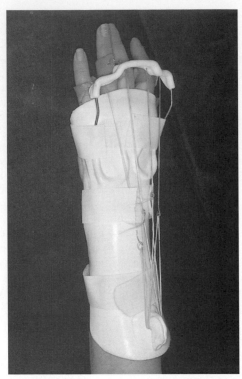

FIG. 94–31. Thermoplastic outrigger splint, which should be individualized for each patient.

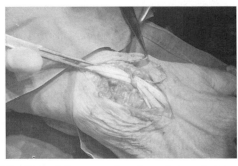

FIG. 94–32. Part of the procedure for extensor tenosynovectomy should include exteriorization of the tendons, but careful centralizing of the tendons is crucial if late deformity is to be avoided.

bed of rheumatoid tissue is compromised by adhesion formation. Tendon transfer is usually the best option, ideally using extensor indicis proprius; alternative motors would be the extensor carpi radialis longus or abductor pollicis longus.

Rupture of the extensor digitorum communis needs to be differentiated from dislocation of the extensor tendons into the intermetacarpal "valleys," volar subluxation of the MCP joints, or posterior interosseous nerve palsy. Early silent rupture of the extensor digiti minimi can be suspected if the patient cannot extend the little finger independently while making a fist with the remaining fingers. This may be the earliest sign of sequential rupture. Significant erosion of the distal radioulnar joint indicates marked instability and also warns of tendon rupture. Six weeks of extensor lively splintage will allow a tenodesis to occur, which leads to an acceptable re-

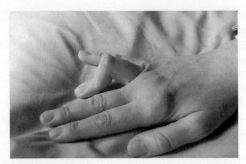

FIG. 94–33. The classical boutonnière deformity is seen here in the ring finger.

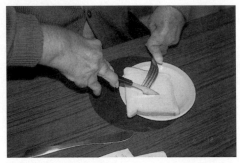

FIG. 94–34. Various deformities of the proximal IP joints can occur. The arthritis mutilans or opera glass hand is seen here.

sult in 50 to 60% of patients in our study with a single tendon rupture; but the mechanism for rupture remains, and some elective remedial procedure for the distal ulna will be necessary.

A single ruptured extensor can be treated by suturing it to an adjacent tendon (buddied), or the extensor indicis proprius can be used to motor the extensors to the ring and little fingers. When there are more than two ruptured tendons, then other motors are required, often with an interposition graft. The results of these complex procedures struggle to justify the effort. Possible additional motors include the flexor superficialis tendon to the ring finger through the interosseous membrane or the extensor carpi radialis longus, palmaris longus, or brachioradialis.

PROXIMAL IP JOINT

Involvement of the proximal interphalangeal joint results in either the boutonnière deformity (Fig. 94–33) with flexion of the proximal IP joint and a secondary hyperextension of the distal IP joint, or the swan neck deformity (Fig. 94–34) with hyperextension of the proximal IP joint and flexion deformity of the distal IP joint. The treatment of these two deformities is based upon a clear understanding that a reconstructive program will require consideration of both cause and effect.

In the boutonnière deformity, there is rupture or attenuation of the central slip of the extensor tendon mechanism and volar subluxation of the lateral bands, which become a flexor force at the proximal IP joint. These are classified as mild when the deformity is correctable, moderate when the deformity cannot be corrected, and severe when there is joint destruction (9). Early synovectomy and tendon reconstruction can prevent or reduce both swan neck and boutonnière deformities (50). However, a structured approach to the problems is essential in order to prevent disappointment.

Treatment involves producing mobile joints through hand therapy, splints, and serial plasters, synovectomy of the proximal IP joint, then reconstruction of the central tendon and repositioning of the lateral bands dorsally. This, in the more established cases, results in a worsening of the hyperextension deformity at the distal IP joint because of the increased tension in the conjoined lateral bands that prevent active motion. The division of the extensor mechanism over the middle phalanx (the Dolphin procedure) (60) will allow active flexion with only a mild mallet finger deformity. An alternate method described by Mateu (61) divides the lateral bands distally, leaving one longer than the other. The longer proximal end is then sutured to the longer distal stump, while the shorter proximal end is used to reconstruct the central slip. This procedure requires a quality of tissue most often seen with the trauma case whereas in the rheumatoid patient such quality is hard to find. The only saving grace of this deformity is that, as the hand and fingers generally are working in flexion, function is often preserved to a remarkable degree. Unfortunately, the long-term results of soft-tissue reconstruction for boutonnière deformity are widely variable and arthrodesis is not infrequently required (62).

Swan neck deformity may result from a number of causes, which result in disturbance of the movement of the proximal interphalangeal joint (Table 94–4). They are classified into four groups depending upon the amount of movement possible and the condition of the joint (47,63) (Table 94–5).

In type I, full flexion of the proximal IP joint is maintained. In this group the initial problem may be hypermobility, attenuation, failure of the volar plate, defunctioning of the flexor digitorum superficialis tendon (which acts as a restraint against proximal IP joint hyperextension), or disease at the distal IP joint that develops a flexion deformity of the mallet type arising from a rupture or attenuation of the extensor attachment to the distal phalanx. This latter circumstance increases the tension within the central slip, creating a hyperextension force across the proximal joint of the finger. Compensatory hyperextension of the proximal phalangeal joint occurs.

When the primary pathology is at the distal IP joint, treatment includes reconstruction of the extensor mechanism attachment to the distal phalanx or distal IP joint arthrodesis.

In type II swan neck deformities, the amount of proximal IP joint flexion depends upon the position of MCP joint. Movement is restricted when the MCP joint is extended and ulnar deviation corrected, and the flexion range is increased when the MCP joint is flexed or ulnar-deviated. This suggests that tightness in the intrinsic system is the major factor. Treatment for type II swan neck deformity is an intrinsic release to correct the cause and then another method to correct the residual deformity.

Type III swan neck deformity is associated with loss of flexion in all positions of metacarpal flexion, but with preservation of the articular cartilage. This results from contracture of the extensor mechanism, collateral ligaments and skin. Attempts to correct this type with manipulation and temporary wiring are occasionally successful and the principle of "cause first, effect second" is often needed in this group. To that end, flexor synovectomy and tenolysis, combined with release of dorsal skin by a curved oblique incision and freeing of the lateral bands from the central slip (Fig. 94–35), may be required. Even release of the accessory collateral ligaments and lengthening of the central slip may be necessary.

In type IV there is, added to the above, destruction of the proximal IP joint, resulting in a fixed contracture of the joint. Treatment involves either arthrodesis or arthroplasty. Arthrodesis is recommended for the index finger and arthroplasty for the ring and little fingers. The middle finger depends upon the individual's requirements.

Arthroplasty of the proximal IP joint in rheumatoid patients provides overall good results (64), with 66% achieving an arc of motion greater than 40°. However, fracture of the prosthesis was demonstrated in 20%, and 21% of fingers with swan neck deformity prior to replacement show recurrence of the deformity. Our experience is that, with time, there is a gradual and progressive loss of ROM over a number of years because of slight sinking of the implant and the development of osteophytes around the implant.

Table 94–4
Cause of Swan Neck Deformity

Mallet finger deformity—attenuation or rupture of the insertion of the extensor mechanism.
PIP joint volar plate stretching or rupture
Interossei and lumbrical tightness
Rupture of flexor digitorum superficialis
Stretching of the flexor digitorum profundus distal to the origin of the lumbrical
Volar subluxation of the MP joint
Volar subluxation of the wrist

Table 94–5
Classification of Swan Neck Deformity

1. PIP flexion maintained in all positions of MP
2. PIP flexion restricted in MP extension and radial deviation
3. PIP unable to flex, joint surface not involved
4. PIP unable to flex, joint disrupted

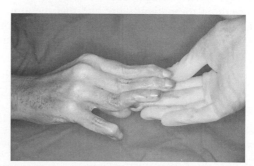

FIG. 94–35. Characteristic swan neck deformities of the proximal IP joints.

Table 94–6
Compatible Surgical Procedures

Extensor tendon and wrist surgery
Carpal tunnel release and flexor synovectomy
Wrist arthrodesis/arthroplasty and MCP replacement
Finger MCP arthroplasty and thumb MCP arthrodesis
Thumb CMC joint arthroplasty and MCP joint arthrodesis, finger MCP
arthroplasty, wrist arthrodesis

Table 94–7
Procedures That Require Conflicting Rehabilitation

MCP and PIP joint arthroplasty
MCP joint and extensor tendon surgery
Flexor and extensor tendon surgery

DISTAL IP JOINT

Synovectomy of the distal IP joint is described, though rarely used (65). The joint is approached through either a Y- or H-incision to protect the germinal matrix of the nail. The insertion of the extensor mechanism is elevated and preserved and the joint is exposed and débrided. When significant destruction of the joint has occurred, fusion is the mainstay of treatment, though arthroplasty is permissable in very special circumstances with reasonable long-term benefit for the stiff finger requiring some motion at one level.

Many different methods have been described to produce a sound fusion of the distal IP joint, including the use of the Herbert bone screw (66), which has the advantage of producing rigid internal fixation without the need for later removal. Other forms of immobilization, including longitudinal and transverse K wires, have reliably effected a sound arthrodesis.

Conclusion

Surgery for rheumatoid arthritis in the hand and wrist requires careful planning on an individual basis, considering all aspects of the disease as well as the patient's requirements. The list of surgical priorities guides the treatment program, which is aimed at preventing irreversible destruction (Tables 94–6, 94–7). The basic principles guide the surgeon in decision making, remembering that the disease process will continue throughout the patient's life and that the aim is to improve the quality of life by relieving pain and restoring and preserving function in order to maintain as independent an existence as possible.

References

1. Chang DJ, Paget SA. Neurologic complications of rheumatoid arthritis. *Rheumatic Disease Clinics of North America* 1993; 19:955.
2. Barnes CG, Curry HLF. Carpal tunnel syndrome in rheumatoid arthritis. A clinical and electrodiagnostic survey. *Ann Rheum Dis* 1967; 26:226.
3. Stanley JK. Conservative surgery in the management of rheumatoid disease of the hand and wrist. *J Hand Surg* 1992; 17B:339.
4. Chamberlain MA, Carbett M. Carpal tunnel syndrome in early rheumatoid arthritis. *Ann Rheum Dis* 1970; 49:149.
5. Marmor L, Lawrence JF, Dubois EL. Posterior interosseous nerve palsy due to rheumatoid arthritis. *J Bone Joint Surg* 1967; 49A:381.
6. Conn DL, Dyck PJ. Angiopathic neuropathy in connective tissue diseases. In: Dyck PJ, et al., eds. *Peripheral neuropathy.* 2nd ed. Philadelphia: WB Saunders, 1984; 2027.
7. Fleming A, Dodman S, Crown JM, et al. Extraarticular features in early rheumatoid disease. *Br Med J* 1976; 1:1241.
8. Conn DL, McDuffie FC. Neuropathy: the pathogenesis of rheumatoid neuropathy. In: Eberl R, Rosenthal M, eds. *Organic manifestations and complications in rheumatoid arthritis.* New York: FK Schattauer Verlag, 1976; 295.
9. Stanley JK. Surgical management of the rheumatoid wrist and hand. In: Beddow FH, ed. *Surgical management of rheumatoid arthritis.* London: Butterworth, 1988; 83.
10. de Jager LT, Jaffe R, Learmonth ID, et al. The A1 pulley in rheumatoid flexor tenosynovectomy. *J Hand Surg* 1994; 19B:202.
11. Flatt AE. *The care of the rheumatoid hand.* 3rd ed. St. Louis: CV Mosby, 1974; 107.
12. Wheen DJ, Tonkin MA, Green J, et al. Long-term results following digital flexor tenosynovectomy in rheumatoid arthritis. *J Hand Surg* 1995; 20A:790.
13. Wyn Parry CB, Stanley JK. Synovectomy of the hand. *Br J Rheum* 1993; 32; 1089.
14. Mannerfelt L, Lund ON. Attrition ruptures of flexor tendons in rheumatoid arthritis caused by bony spurs in the carpal tunnel. *J Bone Joint Surg* 1969; 51B:270.
15. Fowler SB. The hand in rheumatoid arthritis. *Ann Surg* 1963; 29:403.
16. Vaughan-Jackson, OJ. Rupture of extensor tendons by attrition at the inferior radio-ulnar joint. *J Bone Joint Surg* 1948; 30B:528.
17. Möberg E. Tendon grafting and tendon suture in rheumatoid arthritis. *Ann J Surg* 1965; 109:375.
18. Watson HK, Ryu J, Burgess RC. Matched distal ulnar resection. *J Hand Surg* 1986; 11A:812.
19. Hindley CJ, Stanley JK. The rheumatoid wrist: patterns of disease progression. A study of 50 wrists. *J Hand Surg* 1991; 16B:275.
20. Hodgson SP, Stanley JK, Muirhead A. The Wrightington classification of rheumatoid wrist x-rays: a guide to surgical management. *J Hand Surg* 1989; 14B:451.
21. Tilmann K. Recent advances in the surgical treatment of rheumatoid arthritis. *Clin Orthop Rel Res* 1990; 258:62.
22. Adolfsson L, Nylander G. Arthroscopic synovectomy of the rheumatoid wrist. *J Hand Surg* 1993; 18B:92.
23. Clayton ML, Ferlic DC. In: Baumgartner H, et al., eds. *Rheumatoid Arthritis.* New York: Thieme, 1995; 230.
24. Jackson IT, Simpson RG. Interpositional arthroplasty of the wrist in rheumatoid arthritis. *Hand* 1979; 11:169.
25. Chamay A, Della Santa D, Vilaseca A. L'arthrodèse radio lunaire, facteur de stabilité du poignet rheumatoide. *Ann Chir Main* 1983; 2:5.
26. Stanley JK, Boot DA. Radio-lunate arthrodesis. *J Hand Surg* 1989; 14B:283.
27. Darrach W. Anterior dislocation of the head of the ulna. *Ann Surg* 1912; 56:802.
28. Darrach W, Dwight K. Derangement of the interior radio-ulnar articulation. Proceedings of the New York Academy of Medicine. *Medical Record* 1915; 87:708.
29. Gainor BJ, Schaberg J. The rheumatoid wrist after resection of the distal ulnar. *J Hand Surg* 1985; 10A; 837.
30. Van Gemert AML, Spauwen PHM. Radiological evaluation of the long-term effects of resection of the distal ulna in rheumatoid arthritis. *J Hand Surg* 1994; 19B:330.
31. Vincent KA, Szabo RM, Agee JM. The Sauve-Kapandji procedure for reconstruction of the rheumatoid distal radio ulnar joint. *J Hand Surg* 1993; 18A:978.
32. Sauve L, Kapandji IA. Novelle technique de traitement chirugical des luxations recidivantes isolées de l'extremite inferieure du cubitus. *J Chir* 1936; 4:589.
33. Swanson AB. Implant arthroplasty for disabilities of the distal radio ulnar joint. *Orthop Clin North Am* 1973; 4:373.
34. Bowers WH. Distal radioulnar arthroplasty: the hemiresection interposition technique. *J Hand Surg* 1985; 10A; 169.
35. Ritt MJPF, Stuart PR, Naggar L, et al. The early history of arthroplasty of the wrist. *J Hand Surg* 1994; 19B:778.
36. Swanson AB, Swanson GD, Maupin KB. Flexible implant arthroplasty of the radiocarpal joint: surgical technique and long-term study. *Clin Orthop Rel Res* 1984; 187:94.

37. Stanley JK, Tolat AR. Long-term results of Swanson silastic arthroplasty in the rheumatoid wrist. *J Hand Surg* 1993; 18B:381.
38. Figgie MP, Ranawat CS, Juglis AE, et al. Trispherical total wrist arthroplasty in rheumatoid arthritis. *J Hand Surg* 1990; 15A:217.
39. Jolly SL, Ferlic DC, Clayton ML, et al. Swanson silicone arthroplasty of the wrist in rheumatoid arthritis: a long-term follow-up. *J Hand Surg* 1992; 17A:142.
40. Fatti JF, Palmer AK, Greenley S, et al. Long-term results of Swanson interpositional wrist arthroplasty. Part II. *J Hand Surg* 1991; 16A:432.
41. Rattig ME, Beckenbaugh RD. Revision total wrist arthroplasty. *J Hand Surg* 1993; 18A:798.
42. Mannerfelt L, Malmstein M. Arthrodesis of the wrist in rheumatoid arthritis. *Scand J Plast Reconstr Surg* 1971; 5:124.
43. Clayton, ML. Surgical treatment of the wrist in rheumatoid arthritis. *J Bone Joint Surg* 1965; 47A:741.
44. Stanley JK, Hullin MG. Wrist arthrodesis as part of composite surgery of the hand. *J Hand Surg* 1986; 11B(2):243.
45. Seddon HJ. Reconstructive surgery of the upper extremity. Report of the Second International Poliomyelitis Congress (1951). Philadelphia: JB Lippincott, 1952; 226.
46. Stanley D, Getty CJM. Wrist arthrodesis in rheumatoid arthritis. *J Hand Surg* 1993; 18B:377.
47. Feldon P, Millander LH, Nalebuff EA. Rheumatoid arthritis in the hand and wrist. In: Green DP, ed. *Operative hand surgery*. 3rd ed. New York: Churchill Livingstone, 1993; 1587–1690.
48. Ruff SJ, Sonnalrend DH, Tonkin MA, et al. A place for surgery in arthritic diseases. *Med J Aust* 1990; 152:426.
49. Tonkin MA, Beard AJ, Kemp SJ, et al. Sesamoid arthrodesis for hyperextension of the thumb metacarpophalangeal joint. *J Hand Surg* 1995; 20A:334.
50. Millander LH, Nalebuff EA. Preventative surgery—tenosynovectomy and synovectomy. *Orthop Clin North Am* 1975; 6:765.
51. Flatt AE. Some pathomechanics of ulna drift. *Plast Reconstr Surg* 1966; 37:295.
52. Swanson AB. Silicone rubber implants for replacement of arthritic or destroyed joints in the hand. *Surg Clin North Am* 1968; 48:1113.
53. Swanson AB. Implant arthroplasty in the hand and upper extremity and its future. *Surg Clin North Am* 1981; 61:369.
54. Wilson YG, Sykes PJ, Niranjan NS. Long-term follow-up of Swanson's silastic arthroplasty of the metacarpophalangeal joints in rheumatoid arthritis. *J Hand Surg* 1993; 18B:81.
55. Beckenhaugh RD. Implant arthroplasty in the rheumatoid hand and wrist: current state of the art in the United States. *J Hand Surg* 1983; 8:675.
56. Blair WF, Shurr DG, Duckwetter JA. Metacarpophalangeal joint implant arthroplasty with a silastic spacer. *J Bone Joint Surg* 1984; 66A:365.
57. Straub LR. The rheumatoid hand. *Clin Orthop* 1959; 15:127.
58. Clayton ML. The carpal ulnae syndrome. Update. In: Strickland JW, Steichen JB, eds. *Difficut problems in hand surgery*. St Louis: CV Mosby, 1982; 199.
59. Norris SH. Surgery for the rheumatoid wrist and hand. *Ann Rheum Dis* 1990; 49:863.
60. Dolphin JA. Extensor tenotomy for chronic boutonnière deformity of the finger. *J Bone Joint Surg* 1965; 47A:161.
61. Mateu I. Transposition of the lateral slips of the aponeurosis in treatment of longstanding boutonnière deformity of the fingers. *Br J Plast Surg* 1964; 17:281.
62. Kiefhaber TR, Strickland JW. Soft tissue reconstruction for rheumatoid swan neck and boutonnière deformities: long-term results. *J Hand Surg* 1993; 18A:984.
63. Nalebuff EA, Millender LH. Surgical treatment of the swan-neck deformity in rheumatoid arthritis. *Orthop Clin North Am* 1975; 6:733.
64. Swanson AB, Maupin BK, Gajjar NV, et al. Flexible implant arthroplasty in the proximal interphalangeal joint of the hand. *J Hand Surg* 1985; 10A:796.
65. Flatt AE. *The care of the rheumatoid hand*. St Louis: CV Mosby, 1974; 169.
66. Faithfull DK, Herbert TJ. Small joint fusions of the hand using the Herbert bone screw. *J Hand Surg* 1984; 9B:167.

95

Dupuytren's Disease

Robert M. McFarlane, M.D., M. Sc., F.R.C.S. (C.), F.A.C.S.

Although this disease was described and treated by others before, Dupuytren (1,2) was the first to discuss the etiology, describe the anatomy of the diseased fascia, and suggest an appropriate method of treatment. Therefore, the disease rightfully bears his name. The Dupuytren contracture is a disease of fascia, affecting primarily the palmar aponeurosis and its digital prolongations. The pathologic change in the fascia results in flexion contractures, most frequently seen at the metacarpophalangeal joint (MPJ) but also at the proximal interphalangeal joint (PIPJ), and occasionally at the distal interphalangeal joint (DIPJ). Similar pathologic changes in the fascia are occasionally seen in the same patient on the dorsum of the finger (knuckle pads), on the dorsum of the penis (Peyronie disease), and in the plantar fascia (plantar fibromatosis). Because the pathologic process is not confined to the fascia of the palm, it is appropriate to consider this as a disease process rather than simply a local contracture.

Origin, Etiology, and Associated Diseases

Dupuytren's disease (DD) is thought to have originated with the Celtic peoples who occupied all of Europe, including the British Isles, from 1500 B.C. until the Roman conquest of 50 B.C. The disease is extremely common in Europe, and further evidence of a Celtic origin is strongly suggested by an even higher prevalence of the disease in those areas in which the Celtic culture has persisted: parts of Scotland, Ireland, Wales, and Brittany. In 1963, Ling (3) reported the prevalence of a family history in patients seen in a hospital clinic of 24%. When Ling examined their close relatives in the community the prevalence rose to 74%. He concluded that DD was related to a single dominant gene of variable penetrance. There have been no genetic studies since 1963. With the evolution of molecular genetics, it would be appropriate to re-examine this issue to determine if a gene, or genetic mutants, are responsible for DD. This could lead to the identification of susceptible individuals, the prevention of the onset of the disease and possibly appropriate treatment.

The severity of Dupuytren's disease varies considerably. Whether this is because of a variable genetic penetrance or other factors is unknown. Hueston made the astute clinical observation that certain factors determine the severity of disease, which he called the diathesis factors (4). These factors are the age at onset, the family history, the presence of knuckle pads and/or plantar fibromatosis, and the presence of disease on the radial side of the hand. If all of these factors are present in an individual, the disease is bound to be aggressive, difficult to treat, and likely to recur. The most important factors are the early onset of disease (i.e., before 40 years of age) and the presence of knuckle pads or plantar fibromatosis. Either of these factors alone is usually associated with an increased severity. Family history is of prognostic value only if it is positive, because many people do not know the status of their close relatives. As Hueston has emphasized, these features are important in planning treatment, and the surgeon should always examine the dorsum of the digits as well as the feet when the patient is first seen.

In other ethnic strains, both prevalence and severity vary. Egawa in Japan (5) recorded the prevalence in nursing homes over many years and found that it was similar to European studies, but the severity of the disease was less. Very few Japanese with DD develop sufficient finger contracture to require surgical treatment. Only anecdotal reports are available from other countries, but they indicate that the disease is present in the Chinese and other Asians (6), black Africans (7), Asian Indians (8), and Native Americans (personal observation).

Several conditions have been related to DD: gout, pulmonary tuberculosis, neural and vascular thoracic outlet compression, and, more recently, AIDS. However, only three diseases have a statistically significant relationship. Chronic alcoholism has been thought to be related through liver disease, but recent studies suggest that it is more likely due to the volume of alcohol intake than to liver disease (9). The prevalence of DD in epileptics is three times that of the general population.

Opinions differ between a genetic relationship and medication. The most recent studies would favour prolonged barbiturate medication as the causal agent (10). With the introduction of new drugs, it will be interesting to see if the prevalence decreases. It would appear that DD in chronic alcoholism and epilepsy is, at least in part, drug induced.

Dupuytren's disease is extremely common in types I and II diabetics. The prevalence increases with the duration of the disease, rather than with medication (11). This suggests an association with small-vessel disease. Frequently, the disease in diabetics is mild, represented only by the presence of nodules in the palm. Often, the patient presents with trigger finger or carpal tunnel syndrome and is unaware of the presence of nodules. Another feature of diabetes is the so-called limited joint mobility first described by Rosenbloom (12). This is seen in the juvenile diabetic. They are unable to fully extend the interphalangeal joints, but retain full digital flexion.

This is not DD, although these patients can develop DD in later life just as other diabetic patients do.

Pathology

Enzinger and Weiss classify fibromatosis as superficial (Dupuytren type) and deep (13). Thus, the superficial type includes palmar and plantar fibromatosis, knuckle pads, and Peyronie disease. The deep types are the desmoid tumors. Histologically, the types are similar. The predominant cell is the fibroblast, contained in small and large nonencapsulated nodules. Clinically, the two types are different. The DD type is slow growing, forming relatively small nodules that are contained within certain fascial components, whereas the deep type is aggressive, invasive, and forms large tumorlike masses. Presumably the cells of each type, although morphologically similar, are under different control (e.g., growth factors responding to genetic signals).

Millesi believes that the initial lesion of DD is a change in the fibre bundle within the fascia, with disruption of elastic fibres. He has demonstrated fragmentation of elastin and observed absence of elastic tissue as the disease progresses (14). Proliferation of fibroblasts form the pathognomonic nodule. The origin of these cells is unclear. They appear to arise from a perivascular location, from pericytes, endothelial cells, or existing fibroblasts (15,16,17). The very early nodule is composed of active fibroblasts, collagen, and new blood vessels. As the nodule enlarges and contracture occurs, many of the cells have the morphologic appearance of myofibroblasts. As described by Gabbiani (17) and later by Schultz and Tomosak (18), the myofibroblasts contain contractile elements and have cell-to-cell as well as cell-to-stroma connections that strongly suggest the mechanism of joint contracture in DD. The contractile process continues over many years, with the appearance of new lesions and the regression of others. Although the cellular activity in DD is similar to wound healing, the essential difference is that there is continuing cellular activity in DD (19). Nevertheless, in elderly patients the cellular activity and the presence of myofibroblasts diminish so that much of the tissue is tendonlike in appearance, and the few cells remaining are inactive fibroblasts or fibrocytes.

Pathologic Anatomy

The diseased fascia does not develop haphazardly, but within normal fascial structures (20). A clear understanding of the course and relationships of the involved fascia allows the surgeon to perform a complete excision of the diseased tissue without damage to digital nerve or artery, and with more assurance that joint flexion has been corrected and recurrent contractures are less likely.

Only certain components of the fascia of the palm and digits becomes diseased, as illustrated in Figures 95–1 through 95–5. The only cause of MPJ contracture is a pretendinous cord. The natatory ligament is usually involved and prevents side-to-side separation of adjacent fingers, often to the point of causing skin maceration in the web space. Some degree of thumb web contracture is common; it is caused, alone or in combination, by a pretendinous cord to the thumb, the termination of the transverse fibres of the palmar aponeurosis, and the natatory ligament.

PIPJ contracture is caused by a central lateral or spiral cord, either alone or in combination. Also, longitudinally oriented fascia deep to the neurovascular bundle often develops into a retrovascular cord, which also contracts the PIPJ and continues distally to contract the DIPJ.

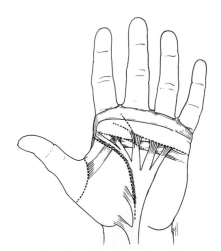

FIG. 95–2. The components of the palmar fascia that become diseased are the pretendinous bands of the palmar aponeurosis, which cause MPJ contracture, the natatory ligament, which draws the adjacent fingers together, and the part of the transverse fibers of the palmar aponeurosis from the index finger to the MPJ crease of the thumb that contributes to thumb web contracture. The pretendinous band to the thumb is usually deficient, as illustrated, but if present can cause MPJ contracture of the thumb. The pretendinous band to the index finger usually terminates in the skin on the radial border of the hand, or is absent, so that MPJ contracture of the index finger is uncommon. The natatory ligament sweeps across the distal palm and terminates at the base of the MPJ crease of the thumb. Thus, three fascial components terminate at this site, and alone or in combination, cause MPJ and thumb web contracture.

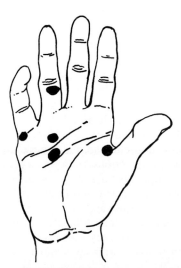

FIG. 95–1. The first clinical sign of DD is a nodule in the palm, which is usually located just proximal or just distal to the distal crease of the palm, in line with the ring and/or small finger. Usually appearing later in the course of the disease are nodules at the ulnar border of the palm, just distal to the distal crease (at the insertion of the abductor digiti minimi tendon), at the MPJ area of the thumb on the ulnar side, and just proximal to the middle crease of the finger.

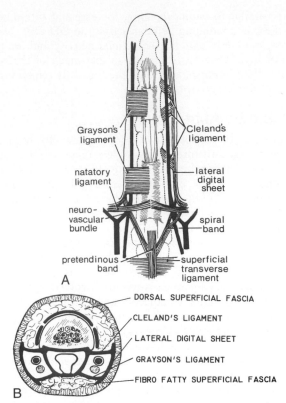

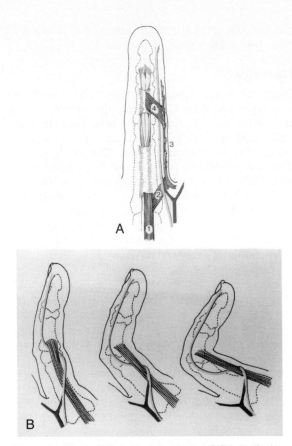

FIG. 95–3. The normal fascial components of the finger. **A,** all components except the transverse fibres of the palmar aponeurosis and the Cleland ligaments can become diseased. **B,** in cross-section, the location of the neurovascular bundle is shown in relation to the flexor tendon sheath and the Cleland and Grayson ligaments. The volar superficial fascia becomes the central cord. The dorsal superficial fascia is the source of knuckle pads.

FIG. 95–5. As the spiral cord contracts the PIPJ, it displaces the neurovascular bundle toward the midline of the finger. **A,** the components of the spiral cord are (1) the pretendinous band, (2) the spiral band, (3) the lateral digital sheet, and (4) the Grayson ligament. **B,** as these components shorten and straighten the neurovascular bundle is drawn to the midline. With increasing PIPJ contracture, the point of maximum displacement of the neurovascular bundle becomes more proximal and superficial, so that it could be cut by the initial skin incision.

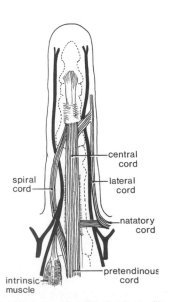

FIG. 95–4. When the normal fascial structures illustrated in Figure 95–3 become diseased and shortened, they form central, lateral, and spiral cords, each of which contracts the PIPJ. The spiral cord arises from the termination of the pretendinous cord (Fig. 95–3) or from an intrinsic tendon, most commonly the abductor digiti minimi.

Treatment

At this time, excision of the diseased fascia is the only definitive method of treatment. Physical methods, such as splinting or stretching, ultrasound or x ray to the involved area, are ineffective if not harmful. Messina (21) has shown that skeletal traction will straighten even a severely contracted finger, but if the fascia is not removed, the contracture recurs. Topical applications and injections of various agents have proven ineffective, although for many years Ketchum (personal communication) has injected steroid into palmar and plantar nodules and knuckle pads, and believes that the progress of the disease is delayed. Because much sophisticated research in cancer and other serious diseases is in progress today, it is likely that methods of controlling cellular activity will eventually apply to DD.

Frequently a person is seen because of concern about a lump in the palm. It may be tender on gripping, or they may believe it could be cancerous. Almost always, an explanation of the nature of the disease satisfies their concern. If not, a steroid injection could be offered to soften the nodule and lessen the pain. Ketchum usually gives two or three injections. My objection to this method of treatment is that the pain almost always disappears as the person becomes accustomed to the nodule, injections are painful, and there is a risk of dermal atrophy with repeated injections. Occasionally a single nodule is very large and interferes with grip. If it is excised, the pretendinous band from which it originated as well as adjacent bands should be removed. The local excision of a nodule is likely to result in a lump of scar and Dupuytren tissue that is larger than the original nodule. On occasion, the palmar skin is firmly adherent to the underlying diseased fascia and drawn into deep folds and pits, which are difficult to cleanse. It is reasonable to remove the fascia while the skin is still salvageable.

The main indication for operation is joint contracture. One should consider contracture at the MPJ and PIPJ differently. Any degree of contracture at the MPJ is readily corrected by incision or excision of the involved pretendinous cord, regardless of the duration of contracture. Usually, the patient is inconvenienced by about 30° of MPJ contracture because the involved finger gets in the way in everyday activities like shaking hands, washing the face, or putting the hand into a pocket or purse. Because the contracture can be corrected readily, the operation can be scheduled at the convenience of the patient.

In contrast, any degree of PIPJ contracture, especially of the small finger, is difficult to correct completely. I have favored operation as soon as joint contracture occurs, in order to remove the disease before the soft tissues about the PIPJ become foreshortened and prevent extension for reasons other than the diseased fascia. However, analysis of this problem (22) reveals that PIPJ contracture of less than 30° is not always corrected by operation and some patients are made worse, especially in the small finger. The extension forces at the PIPJ may be unable to overcome the flexion force of the postoperative scar contracture. Thus, PIPJ contracture is a dilemma for the surgeon. With early operation, the contracture might not be corrected, or might even be worse. With longstanding contracture, it is unlikely that the joint can be fully extended by simply excising the diseased fascia. Most patients with 60° to 90° of contracture should be advised that they are not likely to gain full extension, but will have a residual contracture of some 20° to 40°. This amount of residual contracture is acceptable to most patients. For the younger patient, a capsular release at the PIPJ should be considered at the time of fascial excision (23). With prolonged splinting and therapy, this step is usually successful, although it is not advised in the older patient because full flexion might not be regained. The patient seeks treatment to regain extension of the digit, but the surgeons' goal is not only to regain extension but also to retain full flexion.

Types of Procedures

A variety of procedures have been described to treat DD, depending upon the surgeon's concept of the disease. If it is considered to be a reaction to internal or external forces, then simple incision or partial excision of the fascia is performed. If the surgeon believes that it is akin to a neoplasm, then the fascia is excised. A great variety of incisions have been described; however, the list can be condensed into either a longitudinal or a transverse exposure of the underlying fascia.

Finally, there are different methods of skin closure. The wound can be sutured, skin grafted, or left open.

Thus, there are three considerations to make in planning the treatment of an individual patient: how much fascia to remove, how to expose the fascia, and how to close the wound. With these three options, the surgeon can design a procedure that suits the individual patient. In fact, there is a procedure available for every patient, regardless of age, infirmity, or severity of the disease.

FASCIOTOMY

Fasciotomy is the procedure that was described by Dupuytren, in which the contracting cord is simply incised. It is appealing because it can be performed under local anesthesia with minimal morbidity. Fasciotomy usually corrects MPJ contracture but is less successful in the correction of PIPJ contracture. At the PIPJ, there is a tendency for the contracture to recur, simply because all of the diseased fascia was not incised. The operation is reserved for those patients who cannot tolerate a more extensive procedure because of age or illness and in whom a longterm result is not essential.

An open operation is preferred to subcutaneous fasciotomy. In the palm, there is little danger of cutting a neurovascular bundle at the time of fasciotomy because the bundle is deep to the contracting cord, but a complete fasciotomy can be assured if it is performed under direct vision. In the finger, the fascia often surrounds the neurovascular bundle, so an open operation is much preferred. Having incised the fascia and extended the joint, a skin defect will be created. If a transverse incision has been made, an elliptical defect may require closure by a full-thickness skin graft. However, if a longitudinal incision is made along the contracting cord and converted to a Z-plasty, the flaps of the Z will transpose as the joint is straightened and effectively close the wound without the need for a skin graft.

FASCIECTOMY

With fasciectomy, the fascia is excised on the assumption that the disease process can only be controlled by excision rather than incision of the fascia. Goyrand (24), in 1833, shortly after Dupuytren's publication, suggested that fasciectomy was preferable to fasciotomy. The controversy today centers around how much fascia should be excised. Is it enough simply to break the continuity of the contracting cord by a short excision, or should all of the fascia be excised en bloc, as in a cancer operation? The majority opinion would favor a compromise between these two extremes. Four types of fasciectomy are described.

Local Fasciectomy

Gonzales (25) popularized the excision of a short segment of fascia through a transverse incision, which was then converted into an oval or diamond-shaped defect and covered by a full-thickness skin graft. His results have been satisfactory, although he later reported a tendency for PIPJ recurrence upon long-term follow-up. More recently, Moermans (26) has described a procedure that he attributes to Vilain, in which 1-cm fragments of fascia are excised through multiple curved incisions. He considers his results superior to those of other procedures.

FIG. 95–6.   The recommended incisions. **A,** T-shaped incision exposes all three fascial cords that contribute to MPJ and web space contracture of the thumb. The wound is closed with Z-plasties as required. When a single finger is involved, a midline longitudinal incision is used that extends from the midpalm to just beyond the distal crease of the finger. The Z-plasties are not planned until after resection of the diseased fascia. They are located near flexion creases but in areas where the blood supply to the skin is best. A Z-plasty is not needed at the distal crease of the finger. **B,** when two or more fingers are involved, a transverse incision in or near the distal crease of the palm is used. It usually extends to the ulnar border of the palm, but not often as far radially as illustrated. The finger incisions extend distally as described in **A.** They can join the transverse incision if exposure of the neurovascular bundle and fascia is difficult in the distal palm.

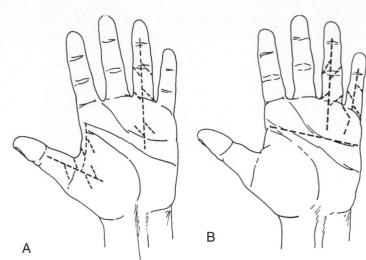

Regional Fasciectomy

In this procedure, the diseased fascia is excised completely, leaving behind the normal-appearing adjacent fascia. This is the most common operation performed today. It is applicable to palmar disease, where the extent of disease is usually well defined, but is less suitable for an operation in the finger, where it is difficult to differentiate between normal and diseased fascia. In fact, more dissection is required in the finger to determine the extent of disease, and normal fascia must be removed in the process. It should also be noted that it is not possible to differentiate normal from diseased fascia by gross appearance, as shown by Brickley-Parsons and colleagues (27); biochemical changes are found in normal-appearing fascia.

Extensive Fasciectomy

The term *extensive* indicates that not only the disease but also the normal fascia is excised. In the palm, this means that the central portion of the palmar aponeurosis is excised. In the finger, an attempt is made to remove all of the disease and potentially diseased cords (i.e., the central, lateral, spiral, and retrovascular cords, as well as the natatory cord in the web space). This operation is performed in order to prevent recurrence of the disease and, if properly done, recurrence is unlikely. However, the extensive dissection is a considerable insult to the hand and the likelihood of complications is increased.

Dermofasciectomy

The term *dermofasciectomy* was introduced by Hueston (28) to describe a procedure in which the skin over the diseased fascia is excised as well as the fascia. Hueston believed that Dupuytren disease originates in the subdermal tissue (superficial to the palmar aponeurosis), and therefore it is necessary to remove the skin in order to eradicate the disease. He would perform a dermofasciectomy primarily for a patient with extensive and aggressive disease because of the potential for recurrence as well as recurrent contracture. Recurrent disease causing MPJ contracture is very uncommon, so that dermofasciectomy is not often performed in the palm. However, recurrent contracture at the proximal interphalangeal joint is not uncommon and dermofasciectomy is the proce-

dure of choice. Hueston advocated the use of a full-thickness rather than split-thickness skin graft.

Author's Method of Treatment (29)

A regional fasciectomy is performed in the palm and an extensive fasciectomy in the finger. The reason for performing a regional fasciectomy in the palm is that there is only one cause of contracture at the MPJ, which is a pretendinous cord. If this cord is removed, MPJ contracture will be corrected and will not recur. I usually remove adjacent pretendinous cords, whether they are thickened or not, as a prophylactic measure against MPJ contracture of the adjacent fingers.

An extensive fasciectomy is advised in the finger, for two reasons: (a) to assure that all of the diseased fascia has been removed and maximum correction at the PIPJ has been achieved, and (b) to remove not only the disease but also the potentially diseased fascia and thus prevent recurrence. Recurrent PIPJ contracture is common and is due to the failure to remove all of the diseased cords that cause PIPJ contracture.

Disease in the thumb and thumb web is usually treated at the time of contracture elsewhere in the hand. The fascia is exposed through a T-shaped incision, so that the three sources of diseased fascia that were shown in Figure 95–2 can be removed.

TYPES OF INCISIONS

If a single finger is involved, a midline longitudinal incision extending from the distal crease of the finger to the mid-palm is preferred (Fig. 95–6A). This incision provides good exposure to perform a regional fasciectomy in the palm and an extensive fasciectomy in the finger. The incision extends to the distal crease of the finger or beyond, to provide exposure over the middle phalanx where the cords that cause PIPJ contracture attach. Also, the lateral and retrovascular cords often attach to the base of the distal phalanx and this tissue can be removed to prevent or correct DIPJ contracture. A straight incision is used instead of a zig-zag incision, because it is easier to design in the severely contracted finger and is much safer in terms of skin viability. It is not always possible to design a zig-zag incision that insures the viability of the skin flaps because the surgeon cannot assess the adherence of the diseased fascia to the skin. It is much safer to perform a dissection through the exposure provided by a midline longitudinal incision and then, at the time of wound closure, design Z-plasties in the areas where the skin has a good blood supply. Gently curved or lazy-S incisions are inappropriate, because they tend to straighten with scar contracture and can, in themselves, be a cause of postoperative joint contracture.

If two or more fingers are involved, the palmar disease is exposed through a transverse incision at or near the distal crease of the palm (Fig. 95–6B). Through this incision it is possible to remove the diseased fascia as well as adjacent (uninvolved) fascia. It is difficult to remove the fascia at the level of the web space, but this can be overcome by further exposure through the finger incision. The fingers are opened through a midline, longitudinal incision. Usually it is not necessary to join the longitudinal incision to the transverse palmar incision, but if the dissection in the distal palm is difficult, especially if it is difficult to visualize one or another neurovascular bundle, then the finger incision can be extended proximally to join the transverse palmar incision.

TECHNICAL CONSIDERATIONS

The use of a tourniquet in all hand operations presents a potential hazard, which is somewhat greater in elderly patients with DD, and in alcoholic and diabetic patients that may have a component of peripheral neuropathy. I prefer a pressure of 250 mm Hg. The tourniquet is released after 90 minutes in those patients in whom the operation will extend beyond 2 hours; it can be reinflated in 20 minutes. Regional is preferred to general anesthesia, as there is evidence that the prevalence of reflex sympathetic dystrophy is less with regional anesthesia (30).

During the past 10 years I have operated upon more patients under local infiltration anesthesia using 0.5% xylocaine containing 1:300,000 epinephrine without a tourniquet (31). I am convinced that the absence of a tourniquet combined with the use of infiltration anesthesia reduces morbidity. I began this technique in elderly patients in whom a regional fasciectomy was performed in the palm for MPJ contracture, and have extended it to some patients with both MPJ and PIPJ contracture of one digit. The infiltration of an anesthetic solution containing 1:300,000 epinephrine produces adequate hemostasis but does not cause spasm in the digital arteries. It is possible to confirm this observation because the arteries are exposed during the excision of disease fascia in the digit. Bleeding is controlled as the operation progresses using a bipolar coagulator. This is certainly a departure from accepted practice and should not be performed by an inexperienced surgeon. I believe the reason an anesthetic solution containing epinephrine is safe is that the present day solutions are purer than in the past. If the surgeon injects this solution with a 30-gauge needle, a small amount of solution can be injected slowly. The value of this procedure is that the patient is not disturbed by a more elaborate anesthetic and most patients do not require other medication. At the completion of the operation there is no concern about a hematoma because the bleeding has been controlled throughout the procedure. A Band-Aid type of dressing is applied and the patient is asked to flex and extend the fingers. This is the initial step in postoperative therapy.

The depth of the skin incision required to reach the diseased fascia is important. In the proximal palm, the incision will extend through skin and a variable thickness of fibrofatty superficial fascia before the diseased palmar aponeurosis is encountered. There is no need to include this fibrofatty tissue in the excision, and having left it attached to the skin means that this skin will have an abundant blood supply. As the incision reaches the distal crease of the palm, the fascia attaches to the dermis and remains close to the dermis to the level of the PIPJ. There is a plane between the fascia and the dermis that can be developed by sharp dissection aided by loupe magnification. This leaves the skin with a precarious blood supply depending upon the extent of the fascial involvement. At the level of the PIPJ crease and distally, the fascia is located deeper as it attaches to the flexor tendon sheath over the middle phalanx. However, the lateral digital sheet will be adherent to the skin as far as the distal interphalangeal joint. At the time of excision of the fascia in the finger, the fascia will be found to be adherent to the flexor tendon sheath over the middle phalanx, but separated from the flexor tendon sheath by a layer of areolar tissue over the proximal phalanx. In the palm, the diseased fascia is superficial to the transverse fibres of the palmar aponeurosis, whereas the neurovascular structures are deep to these transverse fibres. The transverse fibres can be left in situ, but often it is technically easier to remove them than to attempt to separate them from the diseased longitudinal fibres of the pretendinous cords.

The bipolar coagulator is a great asset in hand surgery. It can be used liberally because it causes minimal tissue damage. Using it in combination with loupe magnification allows the many small vessels to be coagulated as the dissection progresses, so that at the end of the procedure bleeding is minimal.

It is important to identify the natatory ligaments as the exposure of the diseased fascia progresses from the palm into the finger. If the adjacent fingers are widely separated, the natatory ligament is under tension and easy to identify. It is superficial to the neurovascular structures, but care must be taken to identify the nerve and vessel passing to adjacent fingers before the fascia is removed.

The neurovascular bundles are usually exposed throughout their course in the finger. It is easiest to expose the bundles distally and proceed proximally. If the surgeon identifies the transverse fibres of the Grayson ligaments, which are superficial to the neurovascular bundles, it is easy to identify the neurovascular bundle distally and proceed proximally into the palm. However, if the neurovascular bundle is displaced towards the midline by a spiral cord, the bundle will disappear into a mass of diseased fascia at the level of the PIPJ. With careful blunt dissection, a passage will be found through this fascia. Upon division of the fascia, the course of the neurovascular bundle will be displayed. Then all of the diseased fascia between, on either side, and deep to the bundles can be excised without damage to the vessels or nerves.

WOUND CLOSURE

A midline longitudinal incision should be interrupted by Z-plasties, preferably two in the finger and one in the palm. Ideally, the Z-plasties are placed at the distal crease of the palm and the proximal and middle creases of the finger. However, they are moved proximally or distally to be placed where the circulation of the skin is best. If the flaps of the Z-plasty are of questionable viability, they can be treated as a free graft by applying a bolus dressing over them.

A transverse incision is very useful in removing widespread disease in the palmar aponeurosis. However, if the incision is closed a hematoma is very likely to develop. This can be prevented by leaving the palm incision open, as recommended by McCash (32). Depending upon the width of the wound, it will heal in 3 to 6 weeks. In addition to avoiding a hematoma, the open palm technique is accompanied by much less pain and swelling in the hand. Patients often regain full finger flexion before the wound is healed.

Our analysis of the results of the open palm technique reveal that PIPJ contracture often persists because of scar contracture. Therefore, if the palm is left open and PIPJ contractures have been corrected, it is recommended that the finger wounds be closed by full-thickness skin grafts. This is especially true when the small finger is involved (22).

Postoperative Management (33)

Ideally, the patient should be seen by a therapist specializing in rehabilitation of the hand, but this is not always possible or practical. The principle of postoperative management is to maintain or increase finger joint extension, but at the same time regain full finger flexion.

Following correction of MPJ contracture, splinting of the involved finger is not necessary if the patient is able to maintain full extension during the period of wound healing. However, following correction of PIPJ contracture, regardless of its severity, splinting is advised. The regime carried out by our therapists is to apply a dorsal forearm-based splint that holds the MPJ and PIPJ in full or at least maximum extension. The splint is more comfortable and more efficient if the wrist is flexed to about 30°. The splint is applied within 3 or 4 days of the operation and is worn all of the time for 3 to 4 weeks. During this time, the patient is instructed to remove the splint frequently for flexion exercises. Thereafter, the patient removes the splint for increasing periods of time during the day until it is only worn during the night. Following the correction of severe PIPJ contracture, it is usually necessary for the patient to wear the splint at night for at least 3 months in order to overcome scar contracture and the inability of the extensor mechanism to maintain extension (34).

Complications

HEMATOMA, SKIN SLOUGH, AND INFECTION

This triad of complications usually occurs in sequence. Hematoma is more likely to occur in the palm than in the finger and should be evacuated before there is loss of viability of the skin or the onset of infection. Small areas of skin loss, such as at the tip of a triangular flap or at the edge of an incision, are allowed to separate spontaneously. Larger areas of skin loss should be excised early and skin grafted. Infection without hematoma or skin loss is unlikely, although it can occur in the presence of intertrigo in the web space if there is severe natatory cord contracture. The webspace should be cleared of intertrigo before operation.

NERVE AND ARTERY LACERATION

The neurovascular bundle is most often damaged in the distal palm when there is severe MPJ contracture. The dissection in this area is very difficult in the presence of MPJ contracture but can be made less difficult by incising the pretendinous cord in order to gain more extension at the MPJ. If the nerve is divided, it is very likely that the artery has been divided as well. Ideally, both artery and nerve should be repaired. Cold intolerance is common in patients with DD and is likely to be aggravated by nerve and/or artery division.

LOSS OF FLEXION

Regardless of the severity of contracture, most patients have full flexion of the digits preoperatively. Loss of flexion postoperatively is disabling and is best managed by prevention with appropriate postoperative therapy. In the postoperative period the patient is expected to maintain extension but regain flexion. The patient cannot be expected to solve this problem alone; the expert help of a therapist is essential.

REFLEX SYMPATHETIC DYSTROPHY

Sympathetic dystrophy occurs in about 5% of patients following an operation for DD (22). It is important to follow the patient closely for signs of undue pain, persistent swelling, and limitation of flexion of the fingers. Often, these signs are not apparent for 3 to 4 weeks after surgery. The best preventive measure is careful observation by an experienced therapist. The basis of prevention (as well as treatment) is appropriate therapy, but a series of sympathetic blocks is indicated if signs of sympathetic overactivity persist.

References

1. Dupuytren G. Permanent retraction of the fingers produced by an affliction of the palmar fascia (English transl). *Lancet* 1933–34; 2:225.
2. Elliott D. The early history of the contracture of the palmar fascia. Parts 1 and 2. *J Hand Surg (Br)* 1988; 13:246, 371. Part 3. *J Hand Surg (Br)* 1989; 14:25.
3. Ling RSM. The genetic factor in Dupuytren's disease. *J Bone Joint Surg (Br)* 1963; 45:709.
4. Hueston JT. State of the art: the management of recurrent Dupuytren's disease. *European Medical Bibliography* 1991; 1:4, 7.
5. Egawa T, Senrui H, Horiki A, et al. Epidemiology of the oriental patient. In: McFarlane RM, McGrouther DA, Flint MH, eds. *Dupuytren's disease.* Edinburgh: Churchill Livingstone, 1990.
6. Liu Y, Chen W. Dupuytren's disease among Chinese in Taiwan. *J Hand Surg* 1991; 16A:779.
7. Mennen U. Dupuytren's contracture in the Negro. *J Hand Surg* 1986; 11B:61.
8. Srivastava S, Nancarron JD, Cort DF. Dupuytren's disease in patients from the Indian sub-continent. *J Hand Surg* 1989; 14B:32.
9. Bradlow A, Mowat AG. Dupuytren's contracture and alcohol. *Ann Rheum Dis* 1986; 45:304.
10. Critchley EMR, Vakil SDM, Hayward HW, et al. Dupuytren's disease in epilepsy: result of prolonged administration of anti-convulsants. *J Neurol Neurosurg Psychiatry* 1976; 39:498.
11. Noble J, Heathcote JG, Cohen H. Diabetes mellitus in the etiology of Dupuytren disease. *J Bone Joint Surg (Br)* 1984; 66:322.
12. Rosenbloom AL, Silverstein JH, Lezotte DC, et al. Limited joint mobility in childhood diabetes mellitus indicates risk for minor microvascular disease. *New Eng J Hand* 1981; 305:191.
13. Enzinger FM, Weiss SW. *Soft tissue tumors.* St. Louis: CV Mosby, 1983.
14. Millesi H. Abstracts of the Third Congress of The International Federation of Societies for Surgery of the Hand, Tokyo, 1986.

15. Kischer CW, Speer DP. Microvascular changes in Dupuytren's contracture. *J Hand Surg (Am)* 1984; 9:58.
16. Shum DT, McFarlane RM. Histogenesis of Dupuytren's disease: an immunohistochemical study of 30 cases. *J Hand Surg* 1988; 13A:61.
17. Gabbiani G, Manjo G. Dupuytren's contraction: fibroblast contraction? An ultrastructure study. *Am J Pathol* 1972; 66:131.
18. Schultz RJ, Tomasek JJ. Cellular structure and interconnections. In: McFarlane RM, McGrouther DA, Flint MH, eds. *Dupuytren's disease.* Edinburgh: Churchill Livingstone, 1990.
19. Delbruck A, Schroder H. Metabolism and proliferation of cultured fibroblasts from specimens of human palmar fascia and Dupuytren's contracture. *J Clin Chem and Clin Biochem* 1983; 21:11.
20. McFarlane RM. Patterns of the diseased fascia in the fingers in Dupuytren's contracture. *Plast Reconstr Surg* 1974; 54:31.
21. Messina A. La T.E.C. nel morbo di Dupuytren grave. *Riv di Chirugie Della Mano* 1989; 26:253.
22. McFarlane RM, Botz JS. The results of treatment. In: McFarlane RM, McGrouther DA, Flint MH, eds. *Dupuytren's disease.* Edinburgh: Churchill Livingstone, 1990.
23. Rives K, Gelberman R, Smith B, et al. Severe contractures of the proximal interphalangeal joint in Dupuytren's disease: results of a prospective trial of operative correction and dynamic extension splinting. *J Hand Surg* 1992; 17A:1153.
24. Goyrand G. Nouvelles recherches sur la retraction permanente des doigts. *Mem Acad Med* 1833; 3:489.
25. Gonzales RI. Dupuytren's contracture of the fingers: a simplified approach to the surgical treatment. *Calif Med* 1971; 115:25.
26. Moermans JP. Segmental aponeurectomy for Dupuytren's disease. *J Hand Surg* 1991; 16B:243.
27. Brickley-Parsons D, Glimcher MJ, Smith RS, et al. Biochemical changes in the collogen of the palmar fascia in patients with Dupuytren's disease. *J Bone Joint Surg* 1981; 63A:787.
28. Hueston JT. Dupuytren's contracture. In: Flynn JE, ed. *Hand surgery.* Baltimore: Williams & Wilkins, 1982; 797.
29. McFarlane RM. Dupuytren's contracture. In: Green DP, ed. *Operative hand surgery.* New York: Churchill Livingstone, 1993.
30. McFarlane RM, McGrouther DA. Postoperative complications. In: McFarlane RM, McGrouther DA, Flint MH, eds. *Dupuytren's disease.* Edinburgh: Churchill Livingstone, 1990.
31. McFarlane RM. State of the art:. The primary treatment of Dupuytren's disease. *European Medical Bibliography* 1994; 4:4.
32. McCash CR. The open palm technique in Dupuytren's contracture. *Brit J Plast Surg* 1964; 17:271.
33. McFarlane RM, McDermid J. Dupuytren's disease. In: Hunter JM, Mackin EJ, Callahan AD, eds. *Rehabilitation of the hand.* St. Louis: CV Mosby, 1995.
34. Smith P, Breed C. Central slip attenuation in Dupuytren's contracture: a cause of persistent flexion of the proximal interphalangeal joint. *J Hand Surg* 1994; 19A:840.

Suggested Reading

Barsky HK. *Guillaume Dupuytren: a surgeon in his place and time.* New York: Vantage Press, 1984.
Hueston JT, Tubiana R. *Dupuytren's disease.* Edinburgh, New York: Churchill Livingstone, 1985.
McFarlane RM, McGrouther DA, Flint MH. *Dupuytren's disease.* Edinburgh, New York: Churchill Livingstone, 1990.
Berger A, Delbruck A, Brenner P, et al. *Dupuytren's disease.* Berlin, New York: Springer-Verlag, 1994.

96

Tumors of the Hand

David T. Netscher, M.D., F.A.C.S., David H. Hildreth, M.D., and Harold E. Kleinert, M.D., F.A.C.S.

Hand tumors arise from any tissue—skin, subcutaneous tissue, tendons, nerve, blood vessels, and bone. Epidermal inclusion cysts and glomus tumors occur more frequently in the hand than in any other part of the body. Benign tumors account for 95% of hand masses if skin cancers are excluded (1). Ganglions represent 60 to 70% of hand tumors, followed in frequency by inclusion cysts, warts, (verruca vulgaris), giant cell tumors of tendon sheaths, foreign body granulomas, lipomas and hemangiomas.

Malignant tumors occur rarely in the hand. Squamous cell carcinoma is the most frequent primary malignancy of the hand (2,3). The dorsum of the hand, together with head and neck regions, have most actinic exposure and hence greatest propensity for squamous carcinoma. The hand accounts for 11% of all squamous cell carcinomas. By contrast with the face, basal cell carcinoma is very rare in the upper extremity (4). Melanoma comprises 1 to 3% of all malignancies and is increasing in frequency at an alarming rate (5). Upper-extremity melanomas account for 12.6% of melanomas in males and 19.1% in females (6).

Soft-tissue sarcomas comprise only 1% of all malignancies of the body, excluding skin tumors (7). Thirteen percent of these sarcomas occur in the upper extremity. Some of the less common subtypes tend to have a predilection for the hand. Epithelioid, synovial, and clear cell sarcomas are relatively rare at other sites, but tend to be more common in the hand (8,9). Most hand sarcomas occur in young patients. Within this spectrum of tumors are those of intermediate malignancy—giant cell tumor and desmoid. Histologic pattern may belie behavior. Juvenile aponeurotic fibroma and nodular fasciitis may appear histologically more aggressive than desmoid, yet are self-limiting. Desmoid behaves malevolently, but may not have malignant histologic appearance (10).

Primary bone tumors of the hand are generally benign. Most common are enchondromas and osteochondromas, except in terminal phalanges where inclusion cysts are the most common (11). Giant cell tumors of bone are relatively rare in the hand compared with other sites in the upper extremity. Of 1,046 benign and malignant primary bone tumors, only 5.8% occurred in the hand and, of the malignant lesions, 1.2% affected the hand (12). Malignant bony metastases to other parts of the body are relatively common, but bones of the hand are rarely affected.

History and physical examination play an integral part in patient evaluation. Rapid growth may indicate an inflammatory process or malignancy, while a history of trauma frequently precedes inclusion cysts, foreign body granuloma, or a traumatic aneurysm. Associated pain may be due to inflammation, osteoid osteoma (classically relieved by aspirin), glomus tumor, intraosseous ganglion, or dorsal wrist ganglion impinging on the posterior interosseous nerve (13). Clinical examination may identify a cystic lesion which could either be a ganglion or inclusion cyst. Ganglions on extensor tendons move with tendon excursion. Many lesions are pigmented, such as vascular tumors, nevi, and melanomas. Nail grooving may be a precursor to mucous cyst emergence. Certain lesions (epidermoid cysts and juvenile aponeurotic fibroma) do not involve the skin surface, but are always adherent to it.

There are many masqueraders. Dorsal wrist ganglion must be differentiated from carpometacarpal bossing (it sometimes causes pain on radial wrist extension and is clearly seen on oblique hand x rays), the anomalous extensor manus brevis muscle (which, unlike ganglion, becomes more prominent on wrist and finger extension) (14), and extensor tenosynovitis. Keratoacanthoma must frequently be distinguished from squamous cell carcinoma by biopsy (15). An ulcer with a red, overgrown granulating base may be a pyogenic granuloma or, more rarely, amelanotic melanoma (16). Subungual melanoma may be indistinguishable from chronic ungual infection or subungual hematoma. Transverse score marks made on the nail proximal and distal to the subungual lesion will distinguish hematoma from melanoma. In the latter, the marks will move relative to the lesion after a 2-week observation period. Bony lesions of hyperparathyroidism may resemble bone tumors.

Examination includes regional axillary and supratrochlear lymph node evaluation. In the presence of malignancy, nodes may be enlarged from secondary infection of malignant ulcers or from tumor metastases. Skin cancers follow a predominately lymphatic course of metastases, as do certain soft-tissue sarcomas—epithelioid sarcoma, synovial sarcoma, clear cell sarcoma, malignant fibrous histiocytoma, and rhabdomyosarcoma.

Special investigations always include hand radiologic evaluations. These may detect lesions arising primarily in bone, or secondary effects produced on bone by adjacent soft-tissue swellings. Subungual glomus tumors may produce bone excavation. Dorsal wrist ganglions occasionally are associated with underlying scapho-lunate dissociation and may be blamed for carpal instability following their excision (17). One-third of volar wrist ganglions are associated with carpal arthritis (18), as contrasted with dorsal wrist ganglions, which are seldom associated with arthritic conditions. Mucous cysts nearly always occur with osteoarthritic changes in the distal interphalangeal joint. Lipoma projects as fat (air density) on radiographs, but other soft-tissue tumors are not radiographically distinguishable unless they produce calcification such as liposarcoma, synovial sarcoma, hemangioma, and juvenile aponeurotic fibroma. Primary bone tumors such as chondromas may also have a classic calcified appearance.

If a soft-tissue lesion is thought to be benign, excision without further workup is appropriate. If primary malignancy of bone or soft tissue is entertained, other studies must be done before biopsy. Computed axial tomography (CT) may help delineate tumor boundaries. Desmoid has identical radiographic density to muscle and is better demonstrated by magnetic resonance imaging (MRI) (19). Radionuclide bone scanning may be used to determine if there is bone involvement by contiguous soft-tissue sarcomas (20). The clarity of CT scan images for hand lesions may be adversely affected by the large amount of bony tissue. Thus, MRI tends to be more useful for hand tumors than CT.

Definitive management of suspected malignancies requires histologic diagnosis (21). Small skin lesions suspected of being carcinoma may be treated by excisional biopsy. Larger skin lesions require incisional biopsy, removing a wedge of both normal and abnormal tissue. Prognosis in melanoma patients at 10 years is not significantly different between patients treated initially with incisional biopsy, minimal margin excisional biopsy, or primary wide excisional surgery (22).

Incisional biopsy is used for tissue diagnosis of bone and soft-tissue tumors because excision violates multiple tissue planes. Needle biopsies generally do not provide sufficient tumor for histologic assessment, but may be appropriate for bone and soft-tissue tumors located deep, where the act of open biopsy will violate several tissue planes (9). The biopsy incision must be placed longitudinally and is performed in such a way that the entire scar and biopsy tract can be excised at the time of definitive surgery (21). The extremity is not exsanguinated with a rubber bandage before tourniquet inflation because malignant cells may be disseminated proximally. Careful hemostasis is obtained and drains are not used. If a bone tumor has soft-tissue extension, it is generally not necessary to obtain an osseous sample, and the soft-tissue sampling may be quite adequate (9). Definitive treatment of such bone and soft-tissue malignancies may be delayed until special tests have been performed on the biopsied tissue; these may include electron microscopy, special stains, and studies for markers.

Cystic Lesions

GANGLIONS

In order of frequency, ganglions occur at the dorsal wrist (60 to 70%), volar wrist (18 to 20%), flexor tendon sheath (10 to 12%), and distal interphalangeal joint (mucous cyst). Less common sites are intraosseous wrist ganglions in association with carpometacarpal boss, extensor tendon, and proximal interphalangeal joint. Occasionally, large distal interphalangeal cysts present volarly and have the appearance of a felon, but without pain.

The usual presenting symptom is a mass. Occasionally, there is associated pain, especially with increased activity.

An intraosseous ganglion presents as aching pain without a mass. Ganglions generally occur between the 2nd and 4th decades of life, though they are not rare in children (23).

Many ganglions resolve spontaneously. Thus, one should delay before planning operative intervention. This applies especially to the so-called occult dorsal ganglion, which may be an unexplained cause of wrist pain and is best initially treated conservatively with symptomatic wrist immobilization, and occasionally by steroid injection (24).

Dorsal Wrist Ganglion (Fig. 96–1)

The dorsal wrist ganglion arises in the scapho-lunate ligament by a tortuous duct to present as a lobulated mass superficial to the capsule (25–28,32–34). As with any other hand operation, surgery is performed in an operating suite with tourniquet control, good regional anesthesia, and loupe magnification. Through a transverse skin incision, the ganglion is mobilized through the extensor retinaculum to the underlying joint capsule. A portion of the capsule through which the ganglion arises is excised. Postoperative wrist immobilization in partial flexion continues for two weeks.

Volar Wrist Ganglion

Volar wrist ganglion is often adjacent to the radial artery (29). Preoperative patency of radial and ulnar arteries is checked by the Allen test. Surgery involves tracing the pedicle of the ganglion to the volar joint capsule and excision of the small portion of involved capsule (Fig. 96–2). In the presence of associated degenerative arthritis, synovectomy and débridement of involved carpal joints is also done. Application of a volar splint with wrist extension completes the operation.

Volar Flexor Sheath Ganglion

Volar flexor sheath ganglion presents as a firm, tender mass near the palmar MP flexion crease and usually arises between A_1 and A_2 pulleys. It is distinguished from a tendon nodule by lack of mobility with finger flexion and absence of triggering. Surgery can often be avoided by rupturing the ganglion with a 20-gauge needle after first obtaining local anesthesia with a 30-gauge needle (31). If surgery is required, the ganglion is traced to its origin from tendon sheath and a small portion of the sheath is excised with the ganglion (Fig. 96–3, Fig. 96–4). Early postoperative motion is encouraged.

The Mucous Cyst

The mucous cyst usually occurs between the 5th and 7th decade (32). Exposure is generally performed through a

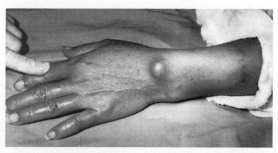

FIG. 96–1. Dorsal wrist ganglion. (Courtesy of JE Kutz, M.D.)

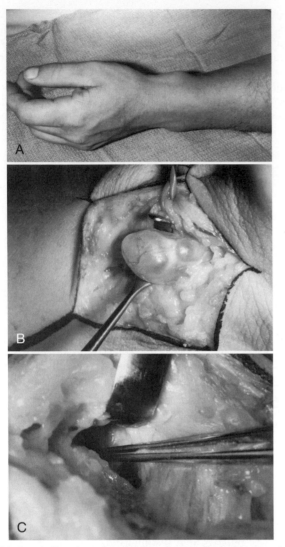

FIG. 96–2. **A, B,** volar wrist ganglion. **C,** ganglion neck extends into wrist joint.

FIG. 96–3. **A, B,** intratendinous extensor ganglion moves distal and proximal to overlying skin mark with finger flexion and extension. **C, D,** ganglion is excised from within the tendon through a longitudinal tendon splitting approach.

curved incision (Fig. 96–5). Skin may need to be excised if it cannot be separated from the underlying cyst. Nail matrix is protected directly under the cyst. The neck of the cyst is traced to the distal interphalangeal joint along the edge of the extensor tendon. Synovectomy and joint débridement of osteophytes lessen possibility of recurrence. Mallet deformity is corrected by tightening the stretched extensor tendon with sutures. The skin defect is then closed as necessary by flap rotation. Transarticular longitudinal Kirschner wire protects the joint in neutral position, and a dorsally applied aluminum splint provides further finger protection (32).

EPIDERMAL INCLUSION (EPIDERMOID, KERATINOUS) CYSTS

These cysts usually occur in the palm and fingertips, and are common in persons whose hands are subjected to repeated minor trauma (laborers and painters) (Fig. 96–6). Unlike ganglions, they are always attached to overlying skin. Occasionally, an inclusion cyst is seen in bone following history of an open bony injury (Fig. 96–7).

These cysts should be excised, because continued growth interferes with nearby structures (33). The entire epithelial sack must be removed or recurrence may occur.

SEBACEOUS CYSTS

These cysts arise from skin appendages and are attached to overlying skin. A dark punctum may be identified. They are very rare in the hand.

Noncystic Skin Tumors

BENIGN SKIN TUMORS

These arise from the epidermal layer, fibrous dermis, or skin appendages.

Verruca Vulgaris (Wart)

This wart is caused by the papovavirus and is transmissible by direct contact or by auto-inoculation. Histologically, there

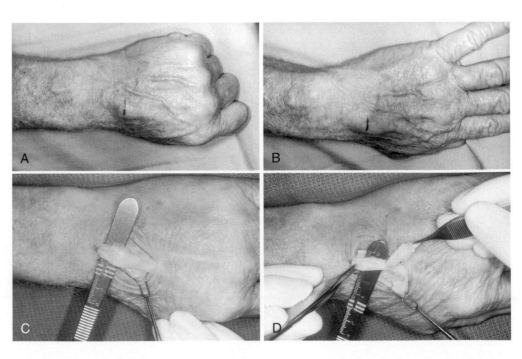

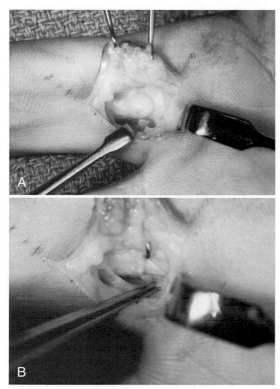

FIG. 96–4. **A,** a 26-year-old presented with painful swelling of the volar ulnar side of the right index finger at the distal palmar crease. Operative finding is ganglion of the flexor tendon sheath. **B,** appearance after ganglion excision.

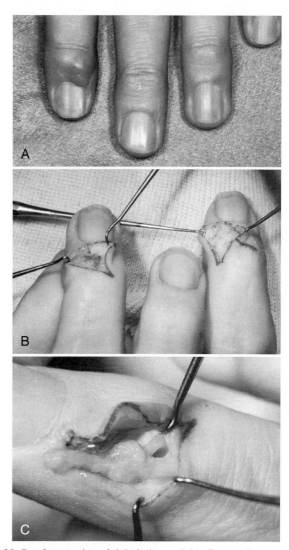

FIG. 96–5. **A,** grooving of right index and ring fingernails as a result of so-called mucous cyst. **B,** appearance at surgery. **C,** neck of cyst extends into distal interphalangeal joint.

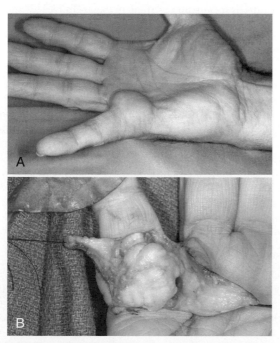

FIG. 96–6. **A,** patient presented with painless swelling at base of little finger. **B,** excision of epidermal inclusion cyst.

are hyperkeratosis, acanthosis, and parakeratosis. Various treatment modalities are appropriate, including application of topical irritants or excision (34). If the wart is shaved to the level of surrounding epidermis and inspected with magnification loupes, a discrete edge is seen. The entire wart can then be sharply curetted from surrounding normal epidermis. Since the basal epidermal layer is not invaded, reepithelialization rapidly occurs. Subungual warts can be treated similarly, after removal of sufficient overlying nail plate to gain access to the wart.

Seborrheic Keratoses

Seborrheic keratoses are common on the dorsum of the hand in the elderly. These superficial scaly plaques are totally removed by shave excision and sutures are unnecessary. Rapid reepithelialization occurs.

Cutaneous Horns

Cutaneous horns require surgical removal. Ten percent have an underlying squamous cell carcinoma (35) (Fig. 96–8).

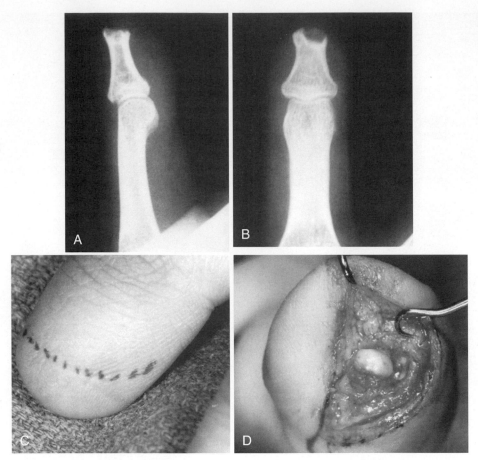

FIG. 96–7. **A,** a previous traumatic amputation of little finger at the distal phalanx. **B,** subsequently, inclusion cyst developed in bone of distal phalanx. **C,** surgical excision of bony inclusion cyst.

that results is often worse than if the lesion is initially excised (36).

Tumors of Epidermal Appendages

Tumors of epidermal appendages occur relatively rarely on the hand as compared to the face and scalp. Pilomatricoma (calcifying epithelioma of Malherbe) is a firm, subcutaneous nodule underlying normal skin (37). It is more frequently seen on the arm than on the hand. Local excision is sufficient treatment (38). Eccrine poroma is a common solitary tumor of the palm. Clinically, it must be distinguished from pyogenic granuloma, amelanotic melanoma, and Kaposi sarcoma (37). It occurs most frequently in middle age. Eccrine spiradenoma occurs between adolescence and middle age. Paroxysmal pain may lead to its being mistaken for glomus tumor or neuroma (37). Excision is definitive.

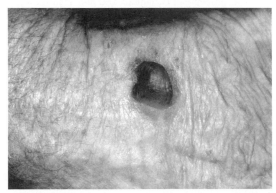

FIG. 96–8. Cutaneous horn on dorsum of hand.

Keratoacanthoma

Keratoacanthoma occurs on exposed body parts such as the face and backs of the hands. They typically occur after 40 years of age, growing rapidly over about 3 weeks into a nodule with central umbilicated keratotic plug. Most authors recommend surgical excision (Fig. 96–9). Although spontaneous resolution may occur within 6 months, the scar

Pigmented Nevi

Pigmented nevi are clusters of melanocytes derived from faulty migration of primitive neural crest cells. Junctional nevi are composed of clusters of melanocytes at the epidermal-dermal border. These are dark, flat lesions. Intradermal nevi are raised and have their nevus cells within the dermis, while compound nevi are also raised but have cells in both

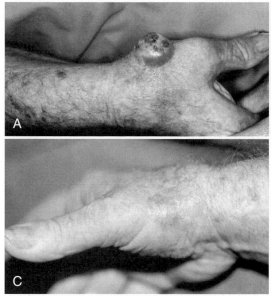

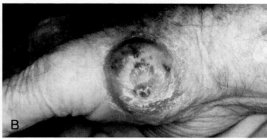

FIG. 96–9. A, B, keratoacanthoma on dorsum of thumb. **C,** healed area after excision.

the junctional area and the dermis. Whenever malignancy is suspected, nevi should be excised. Shave excision is generally condemned. Incomplete nevus excision may leave a margin of cells that later proliferates, giving rise to recurrent nevus (pseudomelanoma). Cellular atypia may lead to confusion with melanoma. Simple reexcision is adequate and informs the pathologist of the previous excision.

Blue Nevi

Blue nevi occur in the mid and deep dermis. Cells are dendritic and associated with macrophages that have phagocytosed the pigment. Spitz nevus was described as "melanoma in childhood," but actually is not a melanoma precursor. The cells are spindle-shaped and the clinical lesion is red-brown and raised. Halo nevus is also not associated with increased risk of malignancy. A halo results from a lymphocytic response caused by an immunologic reaction to nevus cells. The nevus is generally destroyed within 1 to 2 years.

About 1% of newborns have congenital nevi. Most congenital nevi are small, and the nevus cells penetrate the deep dermis and around pilosebaceous structures (39). Giant pigmented nevi can involve the dorsal hand. Staged resection or excision and grafting are then recommended. Predicted malignant transformation is 5 to 8% (40).

Dermatofibroma

Dermatofibroma arises from fibrous dermal tissue and is a firm erythematous plaque sometimes having central umbilication. It is often adherent to overlying epidermis. Surgery is required primarily for diagnosis.

MALIGNANT SKIN TUMORS

Basal Cell Carcinoma

Basal cell carcinoma is rare on the hand and usually located on the dorsum (Fig. 96–10). It is usually an ulcer with raised, pearly edges. Treatment consists of excision with a margin of

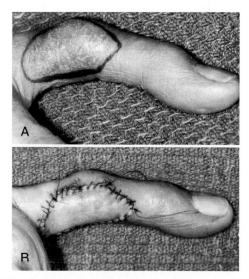

FIG. 96–10. A, this scaly lesion proved to be basal cell carcinoma. **B,** excision followed by full-thickness skin graft.

normal adjacent tissue. Nail bed lesions can be mistaken for paronychial infection, and amputation at distal interphalangeal joint may be required (3).

Squamous Cell Carcinoma

Squamous cell carcinoma may arise de novo or from actinic keratoses. Arsenical keratoses may develop secondary to inorganic arsenic compounds; they have a predilection for palms and soles, unlike the actinic keratoses that occur on the sun-exposed hand dorsum. Radiation dermatitis and prolonged contact with chemicals (especially paraffins and hydrocarbons) may lead ultimately to squamous cell carcinoma.

Bowen's disease is an intraepidermal squamous cell carcinoma (carcinoma in situ) (41). It is a brown verrucous, plaquelike lesion with crusting (Fig. 96–11). Treatment is surgical excision with a margin of normal tissue (42). When

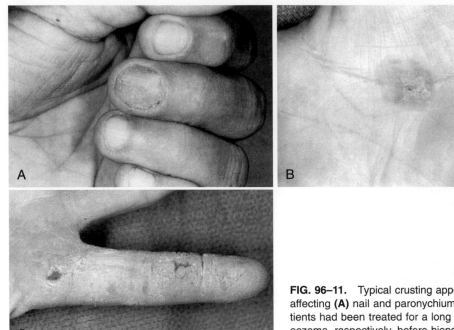

FIG. 96–11. Typical crusting appearance of three patients with Bowen's disease affecting **(A)** nail and paronychium, **(B)** palm, **(C)** index finger. Each of these patients had been treated for a long time for chronic paronychium, dermatitis, and eczema, respectively, before biopsy was done that identified the histologic features of Bowen disease.

nail matrix is involved, amputation at the distal interphalangeal joint is done (43).

Five year mortality of 10% has been reported for squamous carcinoma of the hand, with local recurrence rate of 22% and lymph-node metastatic rate of 28% (44). For lesions under 2.5 cm in diameter, wide excision with 2 to 3 cm clear margins is recommended (Fig. 96–12). However, for larger lesions, because of the high rate of local recurrence, more radical excision is required, which may include ray or segmental amputation. Mohs micrographic surgery and three-dimensional histologic reconstruction with the pathologist at the time of radical resection helps insure complete excision.

Routine prophylactic lymphadenectomy, is not beneficial (45). Lymph-node metastases occur frequently with recurrent hand tumors (67%) (44). Lymphadenectomy is advised for recurrent tumors, even though lymph nodes may not be clinically palpable. Radiation therapy is added to lymphadenectomy if there is extracapsular nodule spread or if nodes are greater than 3 cm in diameter (46).

Squamous cell carcinoma involving nail matrix and paronychium requires distal phalangeal amputation (47).

Malignant degeneration may occur in cicatricial tissue and chronic ulcers (Marjolin ulcer) and, in particular, occurs in burn scars. Marjolin ulcers are said to account for up to 24% of extremity skin carcinomas, and up to 28% of Marjolin ulcers occur in the upper extremity (48,49). Prognosis tends to be poor and relates especially to presence of lymph node metastases (49).

Malignant Melanomas (Fig. 96–13)

Malignant melanomas may arise either in preexisting nevi or de novo (50). There is an association with melanoma and dysplastic nevi. The incidence of dysplastic nevi in the American white population is 5%. They occur in 50% of melanoma patients. Wholesale removal of dysplastic nevi is not justified. If the patient with dysplastic nevi has other family members with dysplastic nevi and melanoma, the melanoma risk is much higher, sometimes approaching 100%. Body photography is commonly used for follow-up for patients with dysplastic nevi, and any suspicious lesions are biopsied. Ophthalmic examination is also recommended because 21% of patients with dysplastic nevi have ocular nevi.

Four histologic melanoma subtypes are recognized:

1. *Superficial spreading melanoma* (75%) occurs in younger patients and has a predilection for sun-exposed areas. There is a prolonged radial growth phase before vertical growth, in the form of nodules, develops.
2. *Nodular melanoma* (10 to 15%) grows rapidly to invade deeper levels.
3. *Lentigo maligna melanoma* (6%) occurs especially in patients over 60 years of age. The Hutchinson melanotic freckle (lentigo maligna) is the precursor. It has a variegated color with a radial growth phase lasting up to 20 years before it becomes invasive. It occurs more frequently on sun-exposed parts.
4. *Acral lentiginous melanoma* occurs most commonly in blacks. It has a predilection for palms, soles, nail beds, and mucous membranes, and has a distinct histologic appearance (51).

Melanoma of the hand is either of subcutaneous or subungual type; there is an almost equal distribution of cases between the two types (52). Frequently there is a delay in treatment, particularly with subungual melanomas, from the time of appearance to the time of diagnosis. Suspicious lesions should be biopsied. Generally excisional biopsy is done after field infiltration of local anesthetic. Frozen section diagnosis of melanoma has many pitfalls

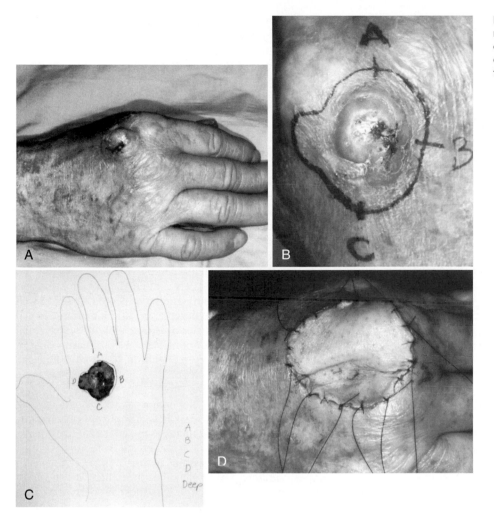

FIG. 96–12. **A,** squamous cell carcinoma. **B, C,** orientation for interpretation of surgical margins on frozen section. **D,** defect after surgical excision, covered by full-thickness skin graft.

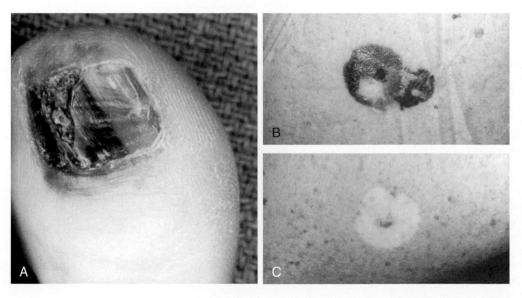

FIG. 96–13. **A,** subungual melanoma showing pigment infiltration at apex of digit and also into eponychial fold. **B,** classic appearance of melanoma with spreading infiltration and central nodularity. **C,** melanoma with surrounding halo of hypopigmentation.

(53). Frozen sections are also 0.1 to 0.4 mm thicker than the permanent sections and thus are unreliable indicators of tumor thickness. Definitive surgical treatment awaits permanent paraffin-section results.

Any subungual pigmented lesion should be biopsied. Under tourniquet control and with loupe magnification, the nail plate is atraumatically removed and a longitudinal elliptical full-thickness excision of the lesion is performed. Depending on lesion size, an incisional biopsy may need to be performed. Careful nail bed repair is done following biopsy by advancement of adjacent tissues and using fine absorbable sutures. The nail plate is then reapplied as a splint.

Benign melanocytic hyperplasia (without evidence of atypia) is completely treated by this excisional biopsy. If there is any evidence of melanocytic atypia, absolute confirmation of complete excision is required. In the absence of a clear margin or recurrence of such a lesion, total nail bed excision and reconstruction with a full-thickness graft is required. Melanoma in situ is similarly treated.

Tumor thickness is the most important prognostic variable (54). The incidence of recurrent metastasis for lesions less than 0.76 mm is 0%, for 0.76 to 1.5 mm is 25%, for 1.5–3.99 mm is 51%, and greater than 4 mm is 62%. Ulcerating lesions also have a poorer prognosis. Once regional lymph nodes are affected (stage II), tumor thickness is no longer of prognostic significance. The margin of excision of cutaneous melanomas has long been debated. But the following are now generally accepted (5, 55): 0.5 to 1 cm margin of skin for in situ melanoma, 1 to 2 cm margin for thin melanomas (less than 0.76 mm), 3 cm margin for intermediate thickness (0.76 to 4.0 mm). Prognosis for patients with subungual melanoma has been regarded as poor (30% 5-year survival). Surgical resection must be individualized. For these lesions, amputation is performed through the joint just proximal to the lesion. If it is felt that a clear margin cannot be achieved because of proximal tumor encroachment toward the joint, then more resection may be required, sometimes even necessitating a formal ray amputation (52). These subungual lesions occur most commonly at the thumb. Following tumor resection, web space deepening by Z-plasty is performed; it will increase functional length for the thumb.

Acral lentiginous melanomas of the palm and sole are often mistaken for warts, and this delays diagnosis. They have been associated with poor 5-year survival of only 30%. However, improved 5-year survival rates at 75% have been reported if these tumors are treated aggressively by wide local excision, regional lymphadenectomy, and hyperthermic isolated limb perfusion with melphalan (56).

The role of elective lymph-node dissection in absence of clinical metastases is controversial. For patients with intermediate-thickness melanomas, and clinically negative nodes, sentinel lymph node mapping may have a role (57, 58). Preoperatively, the lymphatic drainage pattern is identified by radionuclide imaging. Isosulfan blue dye is injected intradermally at the site of the primary melanoma. Axillary lymph-node dissection is performed. A biopsy is performed on the stained "sentinel node" and, based on the presence or absence of metastasis, a determination for further lymphadenectomy is made. This ra-

tionale is based on the fact that malignant melanoma appears to metastasize sequentially within regional lymphatics to the first sentinel lymph node and rarely bypasses this node before metastasizing further. Occult metastases to the regional lymph nodes are very rare (less than 1%) when the sentinel node shows no pathologic evidence of metastatic disease.

5. *Malignant sweat gland tumors* are uncommon, but may masquerade as some of the more common tumors. They are usually slow growing, with episodic bursts of rapid growth. They are frequently painless, red, nodular lesions occurring in the palm of an elderly patient. Malignant eccrine sweat gland tumors may metastasize to both regional lymph nodes, as well as systemically. Local recurrence is common (59,60). Treatment must include wide local excision and therapeutic lymph-node dissection for clinically positive nodes (60). They are unresponsive to radiation therapy or chemotherapy.

6. *Merkel cell carcinoma* is also called "neuroendocrine carcinoma." It is a rare and aggressive neoplasm seen in elderly patients on sun-exposed areas of the extremities and head and neck. It begins as a dermal, slow-growing violaceous nodule that does not ulcerate, but infiltrates deeply. Treatment requires early recognition, wide excision, and lymph-node dissection for adenopathy or vascular invasion. Consideration is given to radiotherapy and chemotherapy because the tumor may respond to both modalities. Systemic disease is nearly always preceded by the appearance of nodal metastases and is uniformly fatal. Some consider elective (prophylactic) regional lymph node dissection to be justified (61).

7. Kaposi sarcoma enters into the differential diagnosis of hand skin lesions, although it is most properly classified as a malignant vascular tumor (Fig. 96–14). It is more

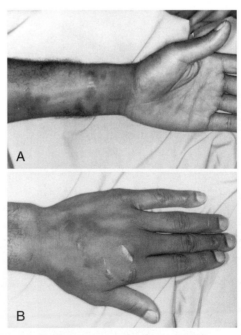

FIG. 96–14. A, B, violaceous skin lesions of AIDS—related to Kaposi sarcoma.

common in lower extremities, but does occur in the hand (62). AIDS-related Kaposi sarcoma must be considered when a patient presents with bluish-red skin plaques. Diagnosis is confirmed by biopsy. Histologically, there are dilation of blood vessels with deposited hemosiderin, dermal lymphocytic proliferation, endothelial proliferation, and sarcomatous tumor with mitoses (62,63). The tumor is radiosensitive. Although good palliation is often achieved with irradiation, residual disease usually remains.

Solid Connective Tissue Tumors

BENIGN SOLID SOFT-TISSUE TUMORS

They are painless, enlarge progressively, and interfere with function only when large enough to obstruct joint motion or distort contours of palmar grasping surfaces. They should be removed for histologic differentiation from the more rare malignant soft-tissue tumors. Most occur in mature adults (except juvenile aponeurotic fibroma).

Giant Cell Tumor

Giant cell tumor of tendon sheath and xanthoma of the tendon sheath are both misnomers. Jaffe (64) has called it localized pigmented villonodular tenovagosynovitis (PVNS). After ganglion, giant cell tumor is the next most common mass occurring in the hand (Fig. 96–15).

Their gross appearance is almost diagnostic with areas of gray, yellow, orange, and brown. Color is affected by the degree of hemosiderin pigmentation, stroma collagenization, and prominence of histiocytes. It usually presents in a digit (most commonly index or little finger) as a painless, slow-growing mass. Any synovial site may be affected—tendon sheath, palmar plate, capsular ligament, and joints (Fig. 96–16). Joint involvement occurs in 20% of cases (65). Two-thirds occur on the volar surface. Dorsal sites include joints and tendon attachments to bone. Fixation occurs to underlying structures, but not to skin. Some have pain and numbness referable to adjacent nerve compression. Range of motion (ROM) is seldom affected; flexor tendon triggering may occur. Untreated, they follow in the path of least resistance and may surround nerves and tendons. They may cause pressure resorption of bone, but bone or cartilage invasion does not occur.

These lesions recur locally (10%) and may also occur at multiple sites (66, 67). Malignant change and metastasis are almost unknown (Fig. 96–17). A more diffuse type of lesion is identified in which there is a more rapid proliferation and less controlled biologic behavior. This should be considered in counseling patients about the possibility of recurrence (68).

Surgical magnification with loupes lessens the likelihood of recurrence. Treatment requires total excision so that every last minute amount of discolored tissue is removed. Care is taken not to probe the lesion directly or to puncture its surface. The lesion is teased out from every nook and cranny involved. "Satellite lesions" must be sought and removed. Partial excision of tendon sheath or joint capsule may be required. Yellow staining of synovium is a clue to joint involvement. If any question remains regarding the adequacy of surgical excision, the collateral ligament of the joint is incised and the joint swung open for adequate inspection under magnification. Synovectomy and bipolar cauterizing of synovial pockets, particularly under the volar plate and collateral attachments, are required if there is joint involvement.

Xanthoma Tuberosum

Xanthoma tuberosum occurs in patients with familial hypercholesterolemia. Lipid deposits infiltrate fibrous tissues, especially tendons. The infiltration is more generalized than the localized deposits of giant cell tumor.

Lipomas

Lipomas are relatively uncommon in the hand. They are more common in women. They may grow to large propor-

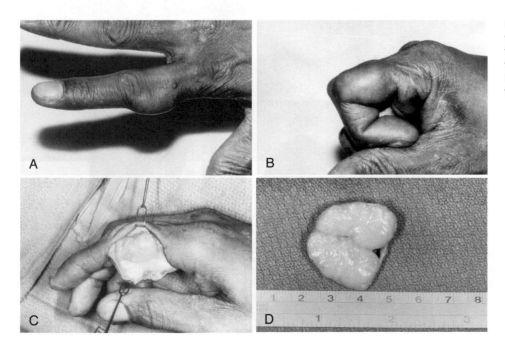

FIG. 96–15. A, B, patient presented with painless swelling on the volar surface of the middle phalanx of the index finger without functional impairment. C, D, excision of yellow-colored giant cell tumor.

MALIGNANT SOLID SOFT-TISSUE TUMORS

Several staging systems have been proposed. All systems basically agree that prognosis, and hence surgical management, are determined by: tissue type, histologic grade, anatomic site, and regional or systemic metastases. The Musculoskeletal Tumor Society (MSTS) spearheaded by Enneking proposed a staging system that was believed to be clinically practical (70):

Stage I: Low-grade without metastases
        A: Intracompartmental
        B: Extracompartmental
Stage II: High-grade without metastases
        A: Intracompartmental
        B: Extracompartmental
Stage III: Regional or distant metastases

Definition of compartments is difficult in the hand and often an impractical consideration. Anatomic boundaries from the wrist proximally to the web spaces distally are poorly defined.

Current American Joint Committee on Cancer (AJCC) staging recommendations (71) base tumor grade on degree of cellularity, pleomorphism, mitotic activity, and necrosis. There are four histologic grades of malignancy. AJCC recommends TNM staging based on tumor size (T1 less than 5cm; T2 greater than 5cm), absence (N0) or presence (N1) of nodal metastases; and absence (M0) or presence (M1) of distant metastases:

Stage I: $G_1N_0M_0$
        A: T_1
        B: T_2
Stage II: $G_2N_0M_0$
        A: T_1
        B: T_2
Stage III: $G_{3-4}N_0M_0$
        A: T_1
        B: T_2
Stage IV: any G, any T
        A: N_1M_0
        B: any N, M_1

Just as with tumor size and anatomic location, biologic behavior is important for surgical planning (Fig. 96–20). For example, a low-grade malignancy of the first web space seen on MRI not to involve neurovascular or musculotendinous structures of index or thumb may be treated by wide excision and preservation of function. Certain tumors are considered high-grade irrespective of their cellular differentiation: rhabdomyosarcoma, angiosarcoma, synovial sarcoma (72). Radiotherapy, chemotherapy and regional node dissection all of have a role (73,74). Rhabdomyosarcoma in particular is sensitive to chemotherapy, yielding very good survival rates when combined with a wide excision (75). Incidence of lymph-node metastasis is low for fibrosarcoma, liposarcoma, leiomyosarcoma, and neurofibrosarcoma, but is high for rhabdomyosarcoma (15%), synovial sarcoma (14%), epithe-

lioid sarcoma (20%), angiosarcoma (11%), and malignant fibrous histiocytoma (10%) (76).

Tumors that involve the distal phalanx are best treated by digital amputation, while those of middle and proximal phalanges are treated by ray amputation with transposition, as indicated. Lesions affecting the metacarpal area frequently involve adjacent metacarpals and so segmental, radial, or ulnar hand amputations may be required. Soft-tissue cover must not be performed with remote tube pedicle flaps since this risks malignant implantation at distant sites.

Desmoid Tumors

Desmoid tumors are rare. They are classified as low-grade fibrosarcomas because of their locally aggressive behavior, despite the benign nature of their microscopic appearance and absence of metastases. Frequency of local recurrence is probably due to difficulty in recognizing clear tumor margins and also to multifocal origin (77). Multiple local recurrences are the rule, and sometimes amputation must be done to prevent further spread (78,79).

Epithelioid Sarcoma

Epithelioid sarcoma is the most common soft-tissue sarcoma of the hand (80). It has an innocuous initial clinical presentation in the superficial subcutaneous tissue as a painless raised nodule. The nodule may ulcerate, leading to mistaken diagnosis of infected wart or foreign body granuloma. When the tumor originates deeper in the hand, it may mimic nodular fasciitis or tenosynovitis. It spreads along tendon sheaths, in subcutaneous lymphatics, or along fascial planes. Vascular invasion indicates very poor prognosis and, when it occurs, amputation is recommended. Regional lymphadenectomy is done if lymph-node metastases are suspected. Recurrent tumors require forearm amputation (81). A combination of surgical excision and high-dose irradiation to primary tumor may yield a more favorable outcome than in the past (82).

Synovial Sarcoma

Synovial sarcoma implies an origin from synovial lining of joints, but less than 10% of cases are intraarticular. They arise in the paraarticular soft tissues, tendons, tendon sheath, and adjacent-to-joint capsules. They present as small, fixed lesions that enlarge slowly and are painful in over 50% of cases. Necrosis and cyst formation are common, leading to mistaken diagnosis of ganglion. Their microscopic hallmark is a biphasic composition, consisting of epithelioid and spindle cells. Calcifications occur frequently. Treatment is by wide local excision, chemotherapy, and regional node dissection (83–85).

Malignant Fibrous Histiocytoma

Malignant fibrous histiocytoma is a rare tumor, but is more common than previously thought, because it was variously grouped with liposarcoma, fibrosarcoma, and rhabdomyosarcoma. It is believed to arise from a histiocytic stem cell. Treatment is radical local excision. Adjuvant therapy and amputation should be considered when it involves skeletal muscle because the metastatic rate is over 40%. In other locations, the prognosis is good, provided local control can be achieved.

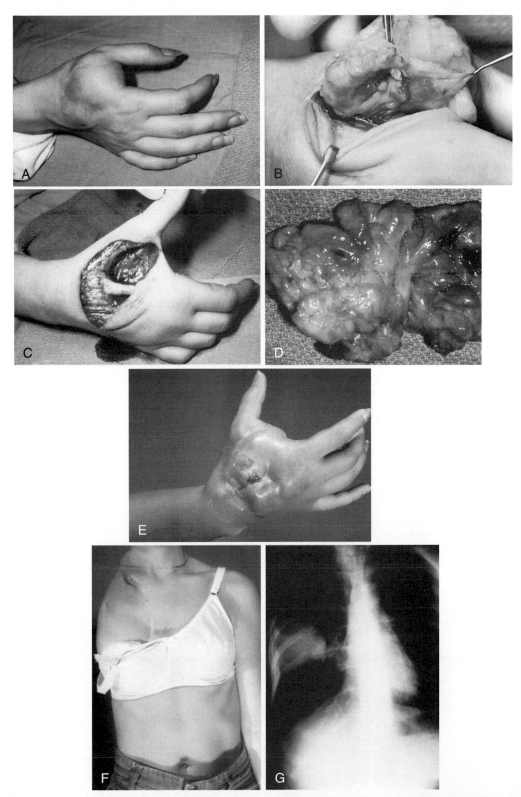

FIG. 96–20. A-D, 17-year-old female presented with swelling on dorsum of hand over the second metacarpal. Biopsy revealed fibrosarcoma. She refused amputation and local wide tumor resection was performed. **E, F,** 3 years later she presented with local recurrence and an axillary mass. Forequarter amputation was performed. **G,** 1 year later she presented with pulmonary metastasis and succumbed to metastatic disease. (Courtesy of J Kutz, M.D.)

Clear Cell Sarcoma

Clear cell sarcoma (malignant melanoma of soft tissue) is an uncommon neoplasm, occurring more frequently in the lower extremity. The prognosis is poor despite radical surgical excision, lymphadenectomy, and adjuvant therapy. At least 50% of patients die of metastases.

Other Sarcomas

Other sarcomas are rare and include fibrosarcoma, rhabdomyosarcoma, and dermatofibrosarcoma protuberans. Fibrosarcoma was considered the most common soft-tissue sarcoma of the body, but now that the classification has become more comprehensive, many cases have been recategorized, so that it is now a rare tumor.

Tumors of Peripheral Nerves

BENIGN TUMORS OF NEURAL ORIGIN

Nerve tumors comprise only 1% of hand tumors (86). They are usually slow growing and minimally symptomatic. Tumors that present with rapid growth along the course of a nerve, associated with pain or neurologic deficits, should raise a concern about malignancy. True tumors of peripheral nerve must be shown to be of neuroectodermal origin, and immunohistochemistry has recently proved useful in identifying such cells by means of antigenic markers (87,88). Recently, chromosomal abnormalities have been identified with genetic defects in the 22 chromosome and 17 chromosome in certain types of von Recklinghausen disease. Nerve tumors in association with von Recklinghausen disease shows similar genetic defects (89,90). Operative evaluation of peripheral nerve tumors is aided by ultrasonography, CT scanning, and MR imaging (91–93). Recently it has been shown that 67 Ga-citrate scintigraphy may be accurate in detecting malignant degeneration of neurofibromas in von Recklinghausen disease (94).

Neurofibroma

Neurofibroma is a tumor composed of Schwann cells, perineurial cells, and fibroblasts. It is the most common benign tumor of nerve. It may occur alone or in association with von Recklinghausen disease. There are three forms: localized, diffuse, and plexiform. Diffuse pattern is also known as molluscum fibrosum and is associated with type I von Recklinghausen disease (95). The lesions are plaquelike swellings of the skin and are thought to result from a diffuse growth pattern within the nerve endings of the skin. The plexiform neurofibroma is pathognomonic for von Recklinghausen disease and is often multicentric over an extended course, creating irregular nerve thickening (Fig. 96–21). Plexiform neurofibromas associated with von Recklinghausen disease have a high potential for malignant degeneration (95). If malignancy is suspected, multiple longitudinally oriented incisional biopsies should be performed. Suspicion of malignancy arises from an onset of pain, neurologic deficit, or large size of the mass.

If it is determined that a neurofibroma should be surgically removed, the lesion will be found to be more centrally located than a Schwannoma, and the fascicles are often intimately involved with the lesion. Isolated tumors involving cutaneous nerves may be surgically excised. If a lesion involves a more significant nerve, then microdissection of the lesion from the nerve should be done, sparing as many normal fascicles as possible. However, frequently primary nerve repair or grafting is required.

Schwannoma

Schwannoma is the second most common benign tumor of nerve and 20% are associated with median, ulnar, or radial nerves (96) (Fig. 96–22). These are usually solitary lesions and occasionally may be associated with von Recklinghausen disease. This lesion is eccentrically located in the nerve and well encapsulated. Since nerve fascicles do not enter the le-

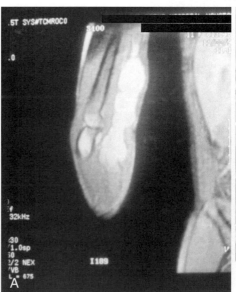

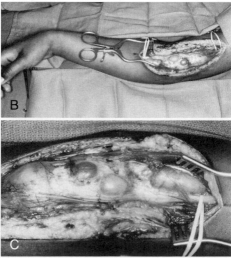

FIG. 96–21. A, classic lobulated MRI appearance of plexiform neurofibroma. **B, C,** lobulated neurofibroma is centrally located in the median nerve and nerve fibers pass through and around the tumor.

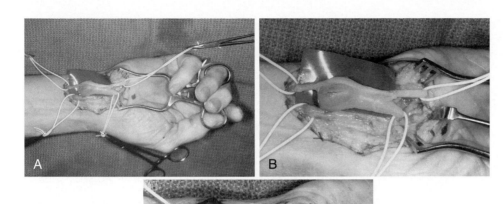

FIG. 96–22.   A, B, Schwannoma of ulnar nerve at wrist is eccentrically located in the nerve. **C,** the tumor is easily shelled out.

sion, it can be removed from the nerve. Microsurgical techniques should be used. Recurrence is rare and malignant degeneration is very uncommon.

Granular Cell Tumor

Granular cell tumor was previously called "granular cell myoblastoma" (97). It has been shown by immunohistochemical staining to be of Schwann cell neural origin. Twenty-five percent of cases may be multiple, and about 20% occur in the upper extremity. It is usually a small (< 3 cm) nontender subcutaneous mass and may or may not be found in association with a nerve. Management is by excisional biopsy, particularly if not directly involving a peripheral nerve.

Neurothckcoma

Neurothekeoma is probably of Schwann cell origin and was previously referred to as a "nerve sheath myoma." It is a slow-growing, asymptomatic, dermal mass, usually less than 1 cm in diameter. Histologically, concentric whirls may be identified as in a pacinian corpuscle, hence giving it a previously used alternate name of pacinian neurofibroma. This dermal lesion is usually easily excised with primary skin closure.

INTRANEURAL TUMORS OF NONNEURAL ORIGIN

Numerous nonneural tumors have been reported in peripheral nerves: lipomas, lipofibromatous hamartomas, and hemangiomas (98). They may present as masses or with motor and neurologic symptoms. Lipomas can be removed completely without neurologic deficit by means of epineurotomy. Treatment of intraneural hemangiomas may involve microsurgical removal.

Lipofibromatous hamartoma is not a true tumor, but a proliferation of fat and fibrous tissue in the nerve (99). This is a very rare condition and most frequently involves the median nerve. Young adults presenting with carpal tunnel syndrome

should be suspected of having this diagnosis. Gross appearance of the nerve is characteristic, with the nerve appearing fusiformly expanded by a fibrofatty infiltrate. The nerve has a lengthened, undulating appearance. When this condition presents as carpal tunnel syndrome, it is best simply to decompress the carpal canal (100). Progressive neurologic deterioration usually occurs. If biopsy is required, it should be taken from the dorsoulnar portion of the nerve to avoid the motor fibers. The tumor can be very difficult to remove and risks injury to the nerve. For recalcitrant symptomatic lesions, nerve resection and grafting may be required.

MALIGNANT SCHWANNOMA

Malignant schwannoma is the most common malignant nerve tumor; it was formerly called "neurofibrosarcoma." The origin for this tumor has been determined to be the Schwann cell. It is clearly a tumor of neural ectodermal origin and, therefore, should not be called a sarcoma (reserved for tumors of mesodermal origin). The majority are found in patients with von Recklinghausen disease. They usually involve deep, large nerves, and almost 20% occur in the upper extremity (101). Surgical management involves en bloc resection, if possible, or amputation. The tumors typically metastasize by a hematogenous route and the lung is the most common site for metastases. Adjuvant radiotherapy and chemotherapy should be considered.

Bone Tumors

BENIGN BONE TUMORS

Benign radiolucent lesions (enchondroma, bone cysts, fibrous dysplasia) are generally treated by curettage and cancellous bone grafting. If pathologic fracture occurs, allow the fracture to heal before performing definitive curettage. Percutaneous intraosseous injection of methylprednisolone (102) has been successfully used for treatment of solitary

FIG. 96–23. **A,** radiographic appearance of a 10-year-old male who presented with a 2-year history of a mass on the left ring finger. **B,** appearance at surgery. Biopsy-proven enchondroma was adequately excised and packed with iliac crest cancellous bone graft. **C,** radiograph 5 years later revealed recurrence. **D,** surgical appearance of recurrent lesion. **E,** defect after curettage. **F,** defect packed with bone graft from distal radius.

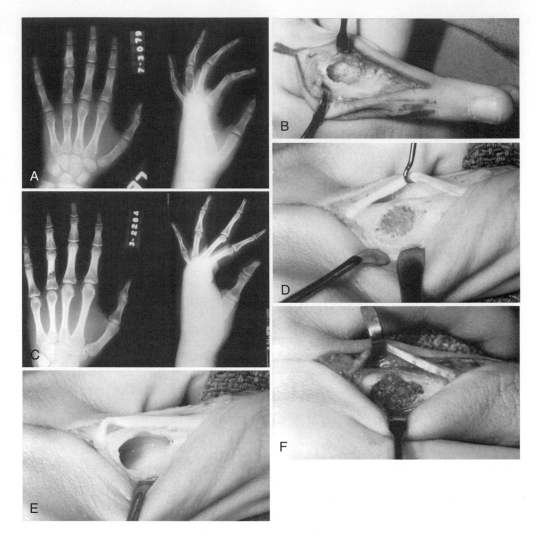

(unicameral) bone cysts. Cyst fluid is aspirated and sent for analysis, and methylprednisolone 50 mg is inserted under radiographic control. If this treatment fails, curettage and bone grafting are done. Giant cell–bearing lesions of bone have high recurrence rate (giant cell tumor 66%, giant cell reparative granuloma 39%, aneurysmal bone cyst 33%) if treated in this manner (103). They are treated more aggressively than bone cysts.

Enchondroma

Enchondroma, the most common primary hand bone tumor, occurs chiefly in the 3rd and 4th decades (Fig. 96–23). It occurs most commonly in the phalanges, usually in the proximal phalanx, and next most frequently in the middle phalanx and metacarpal shaft; least frequent site is the distal phalanx (104). Clinically, it usually presents as pain in the finger, secondary to pathologic fracture. Occasionally, it is discovered incidentally on x ray. Radiographic appearance is that of an eccentrically placed lesion in the metaphyseal or diaphyseal area with varying calcific stippling. Enchondroma may be treated by curettage alone, filling of the residual defect with bone graft being necessary only if structural integrity of the bone has been compromised by the tumor (105). Treatment is

recommended even for a symptomatic incidental and chondromas, in order to confirm the diagnosis and because of the potential for pathologic fracture. Tumor recurrence is infrequent, but can be treated with repeat curettage.

Malignant transformation seldom occurs with isolated enchondromas. However, sarcomatous transformation (usually chondrosarcomas) may be as high as 50% for Ollier multiple enchondromatosis (106) and for Maffucci syndrome (107). Neither of these two conditions is inherited. In both conditions the enchondromas occur throughout the body, with the hand being affected in about 80% of cases. The patients present with growth deformity or pain at the site of pathologic fractures. Once the diagnosis of one of these conditions has been made, whole-body radiographs are required to document the extent of the enchondromas (108). Maffucci syndrome differs from Ollier disease in that it is also associated with multiple soft-tissue hemangiomas and lymphangiomas (107).

Osteochondromas

Osteochondromas (exostoses) are rare hand tumors, although the most common benign tumor of the body (109). In young patients, angular deformities, inhibition of longitudinal

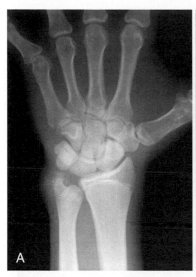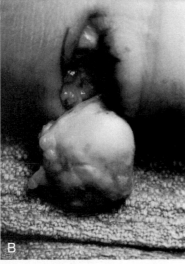

FIG. 96–24. **A,** 15-year-old male presented with a history of the left wrist being stepped on in football practice 8 months before being seen. He complained of "extra bone" in the wrist. The radiograph was interpreted as osteochondroma or calcified hematoma of the ulnar head. **B,** complete surgical excision. Pathologic examination revealed a benign osteochondroma.

growth, and mechanical blockage of joint motion may occur. The patients usually present with a palpable mass and no other significant symptoms (Fig. 96–24). Osteochondroma consists of a bony prominence at the level of the metaphysis covered by a cartilaginous cap over which a bursa commonly develops. Scattered calcification within the cartilaginous cap may be present radiographically, but extensive calcifications should arise the suspicion of malignancy. Surgical treatment of osteochondroma is indicated if the tumor produces pain or disability, has radiographic features suspicious of malignancy, or is cosmetically unacceptable. Malignant transformation to chondrosarcoma for solitary tumors is very rare. If required, corrective surgery is generally completed after epiphyseal closure. Excision must be done with care to include perichondrium and overlying bursa (110).

Multiple hereditary osteochondromatosis is transmitted in autosomal dominant fashion (111). Humerus, forearm, wrist, and phalanges are commonly affected in the syndrome. Patients usually present in the 1st decade of life. Surgery is reserved for correcting deformities, improving limb function and resecting malignancies. Chondrosarcomatous transformation is estimated between 1 and 20% (112).

Unicameral Bone Cysts

Unicameral bone cysts are usually seen in the metaphysis of bones of younger patients. In the metacarpal, they are usually located in the distal third.

Osteoid Osteoma

Osteoid osteoma is an unusual hand tumor with very characteristic presentation (113). It may occur in phalanges, metacarpals, and carpal bones, and presents in the 2nd and 3rd decades of life with a history of aching pain that is greatest at night. Pain is classically relieved by aspirin.

Radiologically, the lesion is seen as an area of cortical sclerosis surrounding a radiolucent area of nidus. It has been reported that 25% of osteoid osteomas are not demonstrable on plain radiographs (114). This often results in a delay in diagnosis. In addition to plain radiographs, bone scans and tomography may be helpful in establishing the diagnosis. Com-

puted tomagraphic scans may also be helpful in lesion localization. In contrast, MR imaging has been found to be confusing in evaluation of osteoid osteomas.

Treatment involves surgical excision. Failure to remove the entire nidus (confirmed by specimen radiography) results in recurrence of tumor and symptoms. It has been reported that after about 8 years following onset, osteoid osteomas may "burn out" (115). This is valuable in management of surgically inaccessible lesions and in the evaluation of asymptomatic osteoid osteomas. If the location of the nidus makes excision difficult without removal of a large block of bone, localization with a CT-guided needle or by radioisotope labeling has proved helpful (116). Some have even refined the technique to nidus removal with a biopsy needle placed under CT guidance (117).

Chondroblastoma

Chondroblastoma is a benign tumor derived from cartilage germ cells. It is a rare bone tumor. It has a predilection for boys in their mid-teens. Characteristic radiographic findings are an eccentric epiphyseal radiolucency, with a smooth sclerotic border adjacent to an open epiphyseal plate. Patients usually present with pain associated with limited motion of the affected joint and soft-tissue swelling.

Chondromixoidfibroma

Chondromixoidfibroma is a rare benign cartilaginous bone tumor. It develops in close association with epiphyseal growth plates.

Giant Cell–Bearing Lesions of Bone

The three lesions in this group have considerable overlap in radiographic appearance, making distinction among them sometimes difficult (103). Aneurysmal bone cysts occur at a young age (2nd and 3rd decades). In the classic case, x ray findings are pathognomonic—an expanded cortex with a lacy pattern inside the lesion. These, unlike giant cell tumor and the reparative granuloma, which are more frequently located in the epiphyseal region, are epiphyseal or diaphyseal lesions. Biopsies should not be performed on the aneurysmal

FIG. 96–25. **A,** aneurysmal bone cyst of the little finger proximal phalanx. **B,** appearance at surgery. **C,** curettage of lesion. (Courtesy of TW Wolff, M.D.)

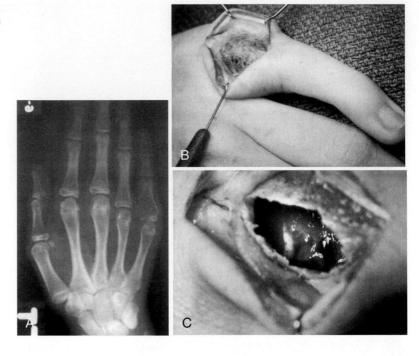

bone cyst because it may be difficult to obtain hemostasis (118). Histologically, there are fibrous septa and cystic blood spaces without endothelial lining (Fig. 96–25). Septa contain numerous giant cells. Treatment consists of curettage and bone grafting, but ray resection may be required for large lesions that manifest local invasion.

Giant cell reparative granulomas are typically found in the hands and feet. They frequently affect the epiphysis and extend to involve articular cartilage.

Giant cell tumor of bone is rare in patients under 20 years of age. Only 2% of all giant cell tumors of bone occur in the hand. The most common site is the distal radius. They behave more aggressively in the hand than at other sites, and 12% become malignant (119). Giant cell tumor is distinguished from enchondroma radiographically by a peculiar "soap bubble" appearance in which numerous trabeculae run through the tumor and divide it into small translucent areas. Later in the disease, these trabeculae disappear.

Some consider histologic grading of giant cell tumors to be helpful (119). Curettage is recommended for grade I, and en bloc resection for grades II and III (110). Others feel that curettage is rarely recommended because it frequently results in recurrence, and that histologic grade and recurrence rate do not correlate. En bloc excision or ray amputation are indicated if the tumor is large, has broken through cortex, or has recurred (119,120) (Fig. 96–26). Recommended treatment for distal radius giant cell tumor is curettage and bone grafting if the lesion is of low grade, occupies less than 50% of distal radius, and has not broken through cortex. If the lesion is of high grade, occupies more than 50% of distal radius, and has broken through cortex, en bloc resection and replacement with vascularized bone graft are done (110). These tumors should not be irradiated for as high as 20% incidence of late sarcomatous change is reported (121,122).

MALIGNANT BONE TUMORS

The AJCC staging system is similar to that for solid soft-tissue sarcomas. Surgery is the mainstay of bone sarcoma treatment. Adjuvant chemotherapy using adriamycin and high-dose methotrexate has produced promising results in controlling microscopic tumor metastases (123–125). Skin coverage must be carefully planned following surgical excision, but major reconstruction may be deferred until final laboratory specimen examination confirms acceptable tumor margins.

Osteogenic Sarcoma

Osteogenic sarcoma is very rare in the hand, presenting as a progressively painful mass in a young patient (1st and 2nd decades). Radiography typically reveals an expansile sclerotic destructive bony lesion. Combination of destruction and proliferation of new bone are usually present. Benign-looking giant cells may on occasion cause confusion with giant cell tumors of bone. It may also mimic metastatic carcinoma to bone.

Chondrosarcoma

Chondrosarcoma is extremely rare in the hand, and usually presents in patients over 40 years. The most frequent site in the hand is the proximal phalanx (126). Radiographs show radiolucent areas with cortical destruction. Small calcified densities are usually present. Prognosis is good with appropriate surgical treatment. Chemotherapy is not helpful.

Ewing Sarcoma

Ewing sarcoma occurs in young patients (1st decade) and may present as an inflammatory process with erythema, swelling, and pain. Radiographically, it is seen as a destructive lytic lesion (127). Resection or amputation is required.

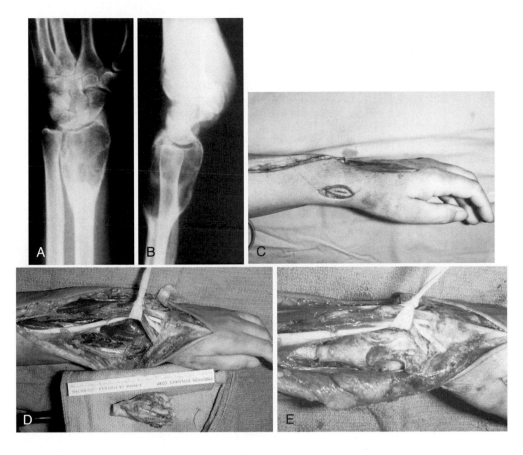

FIG. 96–26. **A, B,** giant cell tumor of the distal radius. **C,** surgical excision planned to include scar of previous biopsy site. **D,** resected tumor. **E,** in this case, reconstruction was performed by distal ulnar transposition and arthrodesis to lunate and scaphoid.

The tumor is radiosensitive, and adjuvant chemotherapy is recommended (128).

Bone Tumors of the Hemopoietic System

Malignant lymphomas of bone are lymphomas that occur primarily as bone tumors (40% of all lymphomas). The upper extremities are involved in 16% of cases. If careful clinical examination reveals other sites of lymphomatous involvement, then the bone lesion should be considered secondary (129). Myeloma is a very common malignant tumor of bone. There is expansion of bone at the site of the lesion. More commonly, classical multiple myeloma appears as numerous round osteolytic lesions with a characteristic "punched out" area (130). For localized lesions, surgical wide excision is recommended, with or without radiation. For disseminated illness, chemotherapy is combined with radiation.

The most common metastatic tumors to the hand skeleton are from lung, breast, and kidney. The hand is involved with metastases only 0.1% of the time, although, considering the entire body, metastatic adenocarcinoma is the most common malignant tumor involving bone. The distal phalanx is the most common site affected by metastatic disease in the hand. Biopsy may identify the primary site. At times, the destructive bony lesion needs to be differentiated from osteomyelitis. Metastatic disease in the hand is a very poor prognostic sign. Most patients are dead from the primary disease within 1 year of diagnosis (131,132).

Vascular Tumors

Hemangiomas are the most frequently encountered congenital anomaly, but many involute. Blood-vessel tumors are not commonly encountered in adulthood. When they do occur, they are frequently noted on the hands. They account for 7% of all hand tumors (133).

HEMANGIOMAS AND VASCULAR MALFORMATIONS

They are not true neoplasms but are sequestra of fetal tissue (hamartomas). They are capable of causing lethal complications and may produce devastating deformity. There are several classifications and the literature is very confusing. The classification most useful diagnostically and therapeutically is that proposed by Upton and Mulliken (134). Hemangioma refers to those lesions that have a rapid growth phase in the 1st year of life and histologically show endothelial mitotic activity and increased mast cell counts. In contrast, vascular malformations show normal endothelial growth characteristics, normal mast cell counts, grow commensurately with the child, and do not undergo spontaneous involution. They may expand with trauma, endocrine modulation (pregnancy and menarche), and in response to certain medications. Vascular malformations contain one or a combination of vascular elements—capillary, venous, arterial, or lymphatic—and are often accompanied by bone and soft-tissue hypertrophy. Malformations are also subclassified according to flow dynamics.

FIG. 96–27. **A,** grossly deforming arteriovenous malformation. **B,** radiograph reveals multiple calcific areas. **C, D,** debulking surgery was performed. **E, F,** postoperative range of motion.

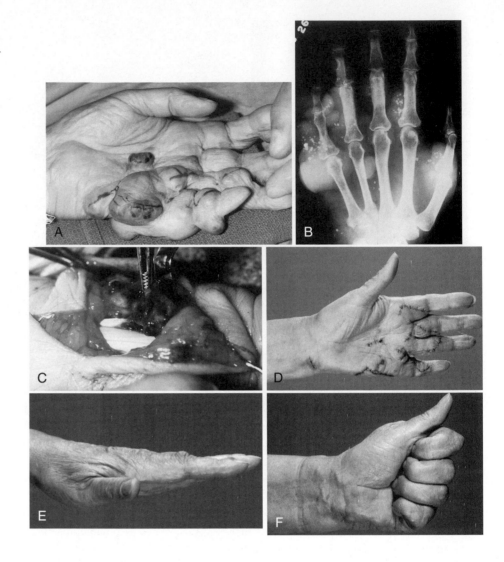

Capillary, venous, and lymphatic elements predominate in low-flow lesions. Arteries and arteriovenous fistulae predominate in high-flow lesions, and they may grow to large proportions that are difficult to treat surgically because the hemodynamic characteristics can open up more proximal arteriovenous connections following excision.

Forty percent of hemangiomas are present at birth. Most of the remainder develop within the 1st year. Females outnumber males in a 5:1 ratio. They may be located in the superficial dermis, in the hypodermis or in both layers. This results in two different clinical appearances, and gave rise to the confusing terms "capillary" and "cavernous" hemangiomas; hemangiomas present uniform histology and the terms "capillary" and "cavernous" should be reserved for vascular malformations. The classical presentation is the superficial strawberry hemangioma. Not all hemangiomas involute, but most (72%) do by 7 years of age. Generally, all lesions that have a good result, show some involution by 4 years. Therapeutic intervention is seldom required. With hand lesions, urgent therapy may be needed if there is significant ulceration and bleeding, widespread hemangiomatosis with high-output cardiac failure, or bleeding because of sequestration of platelets (Kasabach-Merritt syndrome). Systemic (135) or intralesional steroids (136,137) may be effective. Surgery is required only for contour restoration to excise any residual fibrofatty tissue that remains after involution. In contrast to hemangiomas, 90% of vascular malformations are present at birth and there is equal male:female ratio. The typical capillary malformation is the port wine stain. Laser therapy may be helpful in removing the blemish in adults. Venous malformations may result in massive enlargement. Klippel-Trenaunay syndrome is a mixture of venous and lymphatic anomalies with overlying port wine stain plus skeletal overgrowth. Localized malformations over the dorsum of a digit or hand may be easily excised, but massive lesions are best treated by compression. Debulking procedures may be necessary. Arterial high-flow malformations are treacherous (Figs. 96–27, 96–28). There may be massive limb hypertrophy, distal skin may have ulcerations due to "steal" phenomenon, and there may be an associated thrill or bruit. Treatment is initially conservative, with compression. Occasionally, if a digital ray is affected, the entire lesion can be excised. Debulking surgery should not be undertaken without prior angiography. Selective embolization is a last-choice procedure in the upper

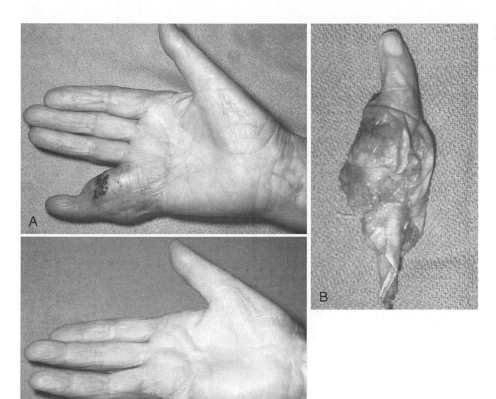

FIG. 96–28. **A,** arteriovenous malformation of the 5th ray. **B, C,** ray resection was performed. The patient has had no further recurrence.

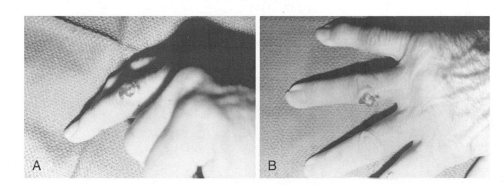

FIG. 96–29. Pyogenic granuloma occurred following minor trauma and was readily treated by simple excision and wound suture closure.

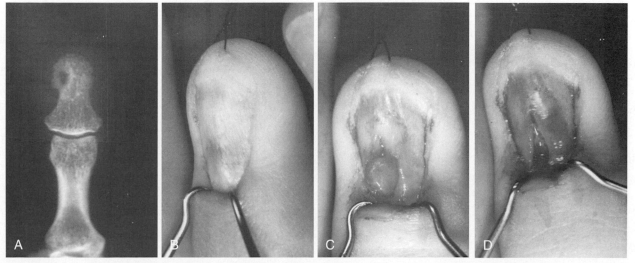

FIG. 96–30. **A,** radiographic appearance of glomus tumor. **B,** appearance after nail removed. **C, D,** magnification is used to aid complete removal.

extremity because of the risk of distal ischemia. Digital tourniquets may prevent embolization into the fingers during the procedure. Vascular malformations, unlike hemangiomas, are not responsive to steroid therapy.

POSTTRAUMATIC VASCULAR LESIONS

Penetrating injury may damage an adjacent vein and artery. Traumatic fistulas form rapidly and surgery must be undertaken early before multiple feeding vessels are "recruited." The natural course is progressive enlargement. Treatment involves fistula excision with separate artery and vein repair. False aneurysms follow an injury that penetrates one wall of a vessel. A pulsatile mass may be felt, and there may be distal digital ischemia secondary to embolic showers. True aneurysms have uniform dilation of vessel wall and may follow a single episode or multiple repetitive episodes of blunt trauma. The most common location is the ulnar artery just distal to the pisohamate ligament. Atherosclerotic aneurysms are rare in the upper extremity. Aneurysms are best treated by resection and vessel repair (138).

PYOGENIC GRANULOMA

It may occur spontaneously or in a region of previous wound puncture. Some consider it to be a variant of hemangioma. Small lesions are treated by cauterization with silver nitrate. Lesions larger than 5 mm, or recurrent lesions after cauterization, are excised surgically. Dissection must continue into subcutaneous tissue to remove the tumor origin (Fig. 96–29).

TRUE VASCULAR NEOPLASMS

Glomus Tumor

Glomus tumor was first described by Masson in 1924 as a tumor of neuromyoarterial apparatus (139). Ten years later, the anatomy was described by Popoff (140). Patients present with a triad of pain, tenderness, and cold sensitivity. Pain is stabbing, and triggered by external pressure or cold. Examination using the head of a pin or closed jewelers' forceps will reveal a single very tender spot. Subungual location is the most frequent site (Fig. 96–30). Examination may show nail ridging. This is a pressure phenomenon, and radiographs may show indentation of the distal phalanx. The tumor is more common in adults and multiple tumors in one fingertip have been reported (141). The next most common site is the volar distal pulp. It may rarely present as an intraosseous lesion at the wrist (142, 143).

Cure rate is 100% if the tumor is completely removed. If the lesion is subungual, the nail is removed and nail matrix incised longitudinally. The lesion can then be bluntly dissected from the nail matrix, which is repaired with 7-0 absorbable sutures.

Malignant Vascular Tumors

Malignant vascular tumors are rare, accounting for fewer than 1% of vascular tumors of the hand. They tend to occur in young men, and require the same surgical approach as other soft-tissue malignancies.

Summary

Benign soft-tissue lesions are by far the most frequent tumors of the hand. Preoperative evaluation of malignant soft-tissue tumors and bone tumors includes bone scan, CT, and MRI. Malignant tumors with propensity for lung metastases should have pulmonary tomograms.

Malignant soft-tissue and bone tumors are generally treated by radical compartmental resection with adequate tumor-free margin. More extensive tumors where adequate margins cannot be obtained require amputation. Reconstruction is easier to perform and psychologically less damaging to the patient at the time of radical resection, unless precluded by a question of tumor margins or poor condition of the patient. Microvascular osteocutaneous and myocutaneous flaps have significantly aided reconstruction after radical tumor surgery.

References

1. Bogumill GP, Sullivan DJ, Baker GI. Tumors of the hand. *Clin Orthop* 1975; 108:214.
2. Lawrence EA, Dickey JW, Vellios F. Malignant tumors of soft tissues of the extremities. *Arch Surg* 1953; 67:392.
3. Butler ED, Hamil JP, Seipel RS, et al. Tumors of the hand. *Am J Surg* 1960; 100:293.
4. Shanoff LB, Spira M, Hardy SB. Basal cell carcinoma: a statistical approach to rational treatment. *Plast Reconstr Surg* 1967; 39:619.
5. Balch CM. Cutaneous melanoma: a review of clinical management. *Texas Medicine* 1987; 83:70.
6. Balch CM, Karakousis C, Mettlin C, et al. Management of cutaneous melanoma in the United States. *Surg Gynecol Obstet* 1984; 158:311.
7. Lawrence W, Donegan WL, Natarajan N, et al. Adult soft tissue sarcomas. *Ann Surg* 1987; 205:349.
8. Rosenberg AE, Schiller AL. Soft tissue Sarcomas of the hand. *Hand Clinics* 1987; 3:247.
9. Mankin HJ. Principles of diagnosis and management of tumors of the hand. *Hand Clinics* 1987; 3:185.
10. Hajdu SI. *Pathology of soft tissue tumors.* Philadelphia: Lea and Febiger, 1979.
11. Smith RJ. Tumors of the hand. *J Hand Surg* 1977; 2:251.
12. Netherlands Committee on Bone Tumors. *Radiological atlas of bone tumors.* Vol 1. Baltimore: Williams & Wilkins, 1966.
13. Dellon AL, Seif SS. Anatomic dissections relating the posterior interosseous nerve to the carpus, and the etiology of dorsal wrist ganglion pain. *J Hand Surg* 1978; 3:326.
14. Reef TC, Brestin SG. The extensor digitorum brevis manus and its clinical significance. *J Bone Joint Surg* 1975; 57A:704.
15. Kern WH, McCray MK. The histopathologic dfferentiation of keratoacanthoma and squamous cell carcinoma of the skin. *J Cutan Pathol* 1980; 7:318.
16. Lister G. *The hand: diagnosis and indications.* Edinburgh: Churchill Livingstone, 1984; 290.
17. Crawford GP, Taleisnik J. Rotatory subluxation of the scaphoid after excision of dorsal carpal ganglion and wrist manipulation. A case report. *J Hand Surg* 1983; 8:921.
18. Croft JD, Jacox RF. Rheumatoid "ganglion" as an unusual presenting sign of rheumatoid arthritis. *JAMA* 1968; 203:144.
19. Bland KI, McCoy DM, Kinard RE, et al. Application of magnetic resonance imaging and computerized tomography as an adjunct to the surgical management of soft tissue sarcomas. *Ann Surg* 1987; 205:473.
20. Enneking WF, Chew FS, Springfield DS, et al. The role of radionuclide bone-scanning in determining the resectability of soft-tissue sarcomas. *J Bone Joint Surg* 1981; 63A:249.
21. Mankin HJ, Lange TA, Spanier S. The hazards of biopsy in patients with malignant primary bone and soft-tissue tumors. *J Bone Joint Surg* 1982; 64A:1121.
22. Griffiths RW, Brigg JC. Biopsy procedures, primary wide excisional surgery and long-term prognosis in primary clinical stage I invasive cutaneous malignant melanoma. *Ann R Coll Surg Engl* 67:75.
23. MacCollum MS. Dorsal wrist ganglions in children. *J Hand Surg* 1977; 2:325.
24. Sanders WE. The occult dorsal carpal ganglion. *J Hand Surg* 1985; 10B:257.
25. Angelides AC, Wallace PF. The dorsal ganglion of the wrist: Its pathogenesis, gross and microscopic anatomy, and surgical treatment. *J Hand Surg* 1976; 1:228.

26. Psaila JV, Mansel RE. The surface ultrastructure of ganglia. *J Bone Joint Surg* 1978; 60B:228.
27. Johnson WC, Graham JH, Helwig EB. Cutaneous myxoid cyst. A clinicopathological and histochemical study. *JAMA* 1965; 191:15.
28. Andren L, Eiken O. Arthrographic studies of wrist ganglions. *J Bone Joint Surg* 1971; 53A:299.
29. Lister GD, Smith RR. Protection of the radial artery in resection of adherent ganglions of the wrist. *Plast Reconstr Surg* 1978; 61:127.
30. Matthews P. Ganglia of flexor tendon sheaths in the hand. *J Bone Joint Surg* 1973; 55B:612.
31. Holm PCA, Pandey SD. Treatment of ganglia of the hand and wrist with aspiration and injection of hydrocortisone. *Hand* 1973; 5:6.
32. Kleinert HE, Kutz JE, Fishman JH, et al. Etiology and treatment of the so-called mucous cyst of the finger. *J Bone Joint Surg* 1972; 54A:1455.
33. Carroll RE. Epidermoid (epithelial) cyst of the hand and skeleton. *Am J Surg* 1953; 85:327.
34. McConahy JG. Common warts. immunity as a result of therapy. *Cutis* 1976; 17:301.
35. Bart RS, Andrade R, Kopf AW. Cutaneous horns: a clinical and histopathologic study. *Acta Dermatol Venereol (Stockholm)* 1968; 48:507.
36. Kopf AW. Keratoacanthoma: clinical aspects. In: Andrade R, et al., eds. *Cancer of the skin*. Philadelphia: WB Saunders, 1976.
37. Zarem HA. Tumors of the epidermal appendages. *Clin Plast Surg* 1987; 14:233.
38. Shenaq S. Benign skin and soft-tissue tumors of the hand. *Clin Plast Surg* 1987; 14:403.
39. Mark FH, Mihm MD, Litelpo MG, et al. Congenital melanocytic nevi of the small and garment type. *Hum Pathol* 1973; 4:396.
40. Quaba AA, Wallace AF. The incidence of malignant melanoma (0 to 15 years of age) arising in "large" congenital nevocellular nevi. *Plast Reconstr Surg* 1986; 78:174.
41. Bowen JT. Pre-cancerous dermatoses. *J Cutan Dis* 1915; 33:787.
42. Paletta FX. Squamous cell carcinoma of the skin. *Clin Plast Surg* 1980; 7:313.
43. Dieteman DF. Bowen's disease of the nail bed. *Arch Dermatol* 1973; 108:577.
44. Schiavon M, Mazzoleni F, Chiarelli A, et al. Squamous cell carcinoma of the hand: fifty-five case reports. *J Hand Surg* 1988; 13A:401.
45. Johnson RE, Ackerman LV. Epidermoid carcinoma of the hand. *Cancer* 1950; 3:657.
46. Ames FC, Hickey RC. Metastasis from squamous cell skin cancer of the extremities. *South Med J* 1982; 75:920.
47. Carroll RE. Squamous cell carcinomas of the nail bed. *J Hand Surg* 1976; 1:92.
48. Ames FC, Hickey RC. Squamous cell carcinoma of the skin of the extremities. *Int Adv Surg Oncol* 1980; 3:179.
49. Novick M, Gard DA, Hardy SB, et al. Burn scar carcinoma: a review and analysis of 46 cases. *J Trauma* 1977; 17:809.
50. Consensus Conference. Precursors to malignant melanoma. *JAMA* 1984; 251:1864.
51. Scrivner D, Oxenhandler RW, Lopez M, et al. Plantar lentiginous melanoma: a clinicopathologic study. *Cancer* 1987; 60:2502.
52. Glat PM, Shapiro RL, Roses DF, et al. Management considerations for melanonychia striata and melanoma of the hand. *Hand Clinics* 1995; 11:183.
53. Shafir R, Hiss J, Tsur H, et al. Pitfalls in frozen section diagnosis of malignant melanoma. *Cancer* 1983; 51:1168.
54. Balch CM, Murad TM, Soong SJ. Tumor thickness as a guide to surgical management of clinical stage I melanoma patients. *Cancer* 1979; 43:883.
55. Veronesi U, Cascinelli N. Narrow excision (1-cm margin): a safe procedure for thin cutaneous melanoma. *Arch Surg* 1991; 126:438.
56. Fletcher JR, White CR Jr, Fletcher WS. Improved survival rates of patients with acral lentiginous melanoma treated with hyperthermic isolation perfusion, wide excision and regional lymphadenectomy. *Am J Surg* 1986; 151:593.
57. Balch CM. The role of elective lymph node dissection in melanoma: Rationale, results, and controversies. *J Clin Oncol* 1988; 6:163.
58. Morton DL, Wond JH, et al. Technical details of intraoperative lymphatic mapping in early stage melanoma. *Arch Surg* 1992; 127:392.
59. Cooper PH. Carcinomas of sweat glands. *Pathol Ann* 1987; 22:83.
60. El-Domeiri AA, Brasfield RD, Huvos AG, et al. Sweat gland carcinoma: a clinico-pathologic study of 83 patients. *Ann Surg* 1971; 173:270.
61. Yiengprukaswan A, Coit DG, Thaler H, et al. Merkel cell carcinoma: prognosis and management. *Arch Surg* 1991; 126:1514.
62. Keith JE, Wilgis EFS. Kaposi's sarcoma in the hand of an AIDS patient. *J Hand Surg* 1986; 11A:410.
63. Muggia FM, Lonberg M. Kaposi's sarcoma and AIDS. *Med Clin North Am* 1986; 70:139.
64. Jaffe HL, Lichtenstein HL, Elsutro CJ. Pigmented villonodular synovitis, bursitis and tenosynovitis. *Arch Pathol* 1941; 31:731.
65. Moore JR, Weiland A, Curtis RM. Localized modular tenosynovitis: experience with 115 cases. *J Hand Surg* 1984; 9A:412.
66. Froimson AI. Benign solid tumors. *Hand Clin* 1987; 3:213.
67. Jones FE, Soule EM, Coventry MB. Fibrous xanthoma of synovium (giant-cell tumor of tendon sheath, pigmented nodular synovitis): a study of 118 cases. *J Bone Joint Surg* 1969; 51A:76.
68. Abdul-Karim FW, El Naggar AK, Joyce MJ, et al. Tenosynovial giant cell tumor: a clinicopathologic and flow cytometric DNA analysis. *Human Path* 1992; 23:729.
69. Leffert RD. Lipomas of the upper extremity. *J Bone Joint Surg* 1972; 54A:1262.
70. Enneking WF, Spanier SS, Goodman MA. The surgical staging of musculoskeletal sarcoma. *J Bone Joint Surg* 1980; 62A:1027.
71. Beahrs OH, Henson DE, Hutter RV, et al. *American Joint Committee on Cancer: manual for staging of cancer*. 3rd ed. Philadelphia: JB Lippincott, 1988.
72. Russell WO, Cohen J, Enzinger F, et al. A clinical and pathological staging system for soft tissue sarcomas. *Cancer* 1977; 40:1562.
73. Rosenberg SA, Tepper J, Glatstein E, et al. The treatment of soft-tissue sarcomas of the extremities. Prospective randomized evaluations of limb-sparing surgery plus radiation therapy compared with amputation. *Ann Surg* 1982; 196:305.
74. Lehti PM, Moseley HS, Janoff K, et al. Improved survival for soft tissue sarcoma of the extremities by regional hyperthermic perfusion local excision and radiation therapy. *Surg Gynecol Obstet* 1986; 162:149.
75. Maurer HM, Beltangady M, Gehan EA, et al. The intergroup rhabdomyosarcoma study. Vol. 1. *Cancer* 1988; 61:209.
76. Suit HD, Mankin HJ, Schiller AL, et al. Staging systems for sarcoma of soft tissue and sarcoma of bone. *Cancer Treatment Symposia* 1985; 3:29.
77. McFarland GB. Soft tissue tumors. In: Green DP, ed. *Operative hand surgery*. 2nd ed. New York: Churchill Livingstone, 1988; 2301.
78. Schenkar DL, Kleinert HE. Desmoplastic fibroma of the hand. Case report. *Plast Reconstr Surg* 1977; 59:128.
79. Lee BS. Desmoid tumor of the hand. Case report and literature review. *J Hand Surg* 1983; 8:95.
80. Campanacci M, Bertoni F, Laus M. Soft tissue sarcoma of the hand. *Ital J Orthotraumatol* 1981; 7:313.
81. Peimer CA, Smith RJ, Sirota RL, et al. Epithelioid sarcoma of the hand and wrist. Patterns of extension. *J Hand Surg* 1977; 2:275.
82. Chase DR, Enzinger FM. Epithelioid sarcoma: diagnosis, prognostic indicators, and treatment. *Am J Surg Pathol* 1985; 9:241.
83. Cadman NL, Soule EH, Kelly PJ. Synovial sarcoma. An analysis of 134 tumors. *Cancer* 1965; 18:613.
84. Hajdu SI, Shiu MH, Former JG. Tenosynovial sarcoma. A clinicopathologic study of 136 cases. *Cancer* 1977; 39:1201.
85. Wright PH, Sim FH, Soule EH, et al. Synovial sarcoma. *J Bone Joint Surg* 1982; 64A:112.
86. Strickland JW, Steichen JB. Nerve tumors of the hand and forearm. *J Hand Surg* 1977; 2:285.
87. Ariza A, Bilboa JM, Rosai J. Immunohistochemical detection of epithelial membrane antigen in normal perineurial cells and perineurinoma. *Am J Surg Pathol* 1988; 12:678.
88. Gray MH, Rosenberg AE, Dickersin GR, et al. Glial fibrillary acidic protein and keratin expression by benign and malignant nerve sheath tumors. *Human Pathol* 1989; 20:1089.
89. Couturier J, Delattre O, Kujas M, et al. Assessment of chromosome 22 anomalies in neurinomas by combined karyotype and RFLP analysis. *Cancer Genet Cytogent* 1990; 45:55.
90. Krone W, Hogemann I. Cell culture studies on neurofibromatosis (von Recklinghausen): monosomy 22 and other chromosomal anomalies in cultures from peripheral neurofibromatosis. *Human Genet* 1986; 74:453.

91. Chui MC, Bird BL, Rogers J. Extracranial and extraspinal nerve sheath tumors: computed tomographic evaluation. *Neuroradiology* 1988; 30:47.

92. Fornage BD. Sonography of peripheral nerves of the extremities. review. *Radiologia Medica* 1993; 85(5 suppl 1):162.

93. Silver M, Patel MR, Vigorito V. Preoperative diagnosis of a forearm peripheral schwannoma. *Ortho Review* 1993; 22:714.

94. Jurgens H, Bier V, Harms D, et al. Malignant peripheral neuroectodermal tumors: a retrospective analysis of 42 cases. *Cancer* 1988; 61:349.

95. Enzinger FM, Weiss SW. *Soft tissue tumors.* 2nd ed. St. Louis: CV Mosby, 1988; 724–815.

96. Rinaldi E. Neurilemomas and neurofibromas of the upper limb. *J Hand Surg* 1983; 8:590.

97. Apisarnthanarax P. Granular cell tumor. *J Am Acad Dermatol* 1981; 5:171.

98. Louis DS. Peripheral nerve tumors in the upper extremity. *Hand Clinics* 1987; 3:311.

99. Paletta FX, Senay LC. Lipofibromatous hamartoma of median nerve and ulnar nerve: surgical treatment. *Plast Reconstr Surg* 1981; 68:915.

100. Amadio PC, Reiman HM, Dobyns JH. Lipofibromatous hamartoma of nerve. *J Hand Surg* 1988; 13:67.

101. Nambisan RN, Rao V, Moore R, et al. Malignant soft tissue tumors of nerve sheath origin. *J Surg Oncol* 1984; 25:268.

102. Scaglietti O, Marchetti PG, Bartolozzi P. The effects of methylprednisolone acetate in the treatment of bone cysts. Results of three years' follow-up. *J Bone Joint Surg* 1979; 61B:200.

103. Dahlin DC. Giant-cell-bearing lesions of bone of the hands. *Hand Clinics* 1987; 3:291.

104. Alawneh I, Giovanini A, Willmen HR, et al. Enchondroma of the hand. *Int Surg* 1977; 62:218.

105. Hasselgren G, Forssblad P, Tornvall A. Bone grafting unnecessary in the treatment of enchondromas in the hand. *J Hand Surg* 1991; 16A:139.

106. Giudici MA, Moser RP, Kransdorf MJ. Cartilaginous bone tumors. *Radiol Clin North Am* 1993; 31:237.

107. Kaplan RP, Wang JT, Amron DM, et al. Maffucci's syndrome: two case reports with a literature review. *J Am Acad Derm* 1993; 29:894.

108. Little C. Ollier's disease: an interdisciplinary approach. *Orthopaedic Nursing* 1994; 13:50.

109. Dahlin DC, Unni KK. *Bone tumors.* 4th ed. Springfield, IL: Charles C Thomas, 1986.

110. Dick HM. Bone tumors. In: Green DP, ed. *Operative hand surgery.* 2nd ed. New York: Churchill Livingstone, 1988; 2347.

111. Jaffe HL. Hereditary multiple exostosis. *Arch Pathol* 1943; 36:335.

112. Schmale GA, Conrad EU, Raskind WH. The natural history of hereditary multiple exostoses. *J Bone Joint Surg* 1994; 76A:986.

113. Doyle LK, Ruby LK, Nalebuff EG, et al. Osteoid osteoma of the hand. *J Hand Surg* 1985; 10A:408.

114. Swee RG, McLeod RA, Beabout JW. Osteoid osteoma: detection, diagnosis and localization. *Radiology* 1979; 130:117.

115. Simm RJ. The natural history of osteoid osteoma. *Aust NZ J Surg* 1975; 45:412.

116. Steinberg GG, Coumas JM, Breen T. Preoperative localization of osteoid osteoma: a new technique that uses CT. *AJR* 1990; 155:883.

117. Voto SJ, Cook AJ, Weiner DS, et al. Treatment of osteoid osteoma by computed tomography guided excision in the pediatric patient. *J Pediatr Orthop* 1990; 10:510.

118. Fuhs SE, Herndon JH. Aneurysmal bone cyst involving the hand: a review and report of two cases. *J Hand Surg* 1979; 4:152.

119. Averill RN, Smith RJ, Campbell CJ. Giant cell tumors of the bones of the hand. *J Hand Surg* 5:39.

120. Patel MR, Desai SS, Gordan SL, et al. Management of skeletal giant cell tumors of the phalanges of the hand. *J Hand Surg* 1987; 12A:70.

121. Harwood AR, Fornaiser BL, Rider WD. Supervoltage irradiation in the management of giant cell tumor of the bone. *Radiology* 1977; 125:223.

122. Shaw JA, Mosher JF. Giant cell tumor in the hand presenting as an expansile diaphyseal lesion. Case report. *J Bone Joint Surg* 1983; 65A:692.

123. Jaffe N, Frei E, Traggis D, et al. Adjuvant methotrexate and citrovorum factor treatment of osteogenic sarcoma. *N Engl J Med* 1974; 291:994.

124. Rosen G, Murphy ML, Huvos AG, et al. Chemotherapy, en bloc resection and prosthetic bone replacement in the treatment of osteogenic sarcoma. *Cancer* 1976; 37:1.

125. Rosen G, Caparros B, Huvos AG, et al. Preoperative chemotherapy for osteogenic sarcoma: selection of postoperative adjuvant chemotherapy based on the response of the primary tumor to preoperative chemotherapy. *Cancer* 1982; 49:1221.

126. Dahlin DC, Salvador A. Chondrosarcomas of bones of the hands and feet. A study of 30 cases. *Cancer* 1975; 34:255.

127. Dryer RF, Buckwalter JA, Flatt AE, et al. Ewing's sarcoma of the hand. *J Hand Surg* 1979; 4:372.

128. Rosen G, Caparros B, Nirenberg A, et al. Ewing's sarcoma: ten-year experience with adjuvant chemotherapy. *Cancer* 1981; 47:2204.

129. Pritchard DF, Krishnan U. Small round cell tumors. In: Bogumill GP, Fleegler EJ, eds. *Tumors of the hand and upper limb.* Edinburgh: Churchill Livingstone, 1993; 392.

130. Schajowicz F, ed. *Tumors and tumorlike lesions of bone and joints.* New York, Springer-Verlag, 1981.

131. Hicks MC, Kalmon EH, Glasser SM. Metastatic malignancy to phalanges. *South Med J* 1964; 57:85.

132. Kerin R. Metastatic tumors of the hand. *J Bone Joint Surg* 1983; 65A:1331.

133. Palmieri TJ. Vascular tumors of the hand and forearm. *Hand Clinics* 1987; 3:225.

134. Upton J, Mulliken JB, Murray JE. Classification and rationale for management of vascular anomalies in the upper extremity. *J Hand Surg* 1985; 10A:970.

135. Zarem HA, Edgerton MT. Induced resolution of cavernous hemangiomas following prednisolone therapy. *Plast Reconstr Surg* 1967; 39:76.

136. Mazzola RF. Treatment of hemangiomas in children by intralesional injections of steroids. *Chir Plast (Berlin)* 1978; 4:161.

137. Sloan GM, Reinisch JF, Nichter LS, et al. Intralesional corticosteroid therapy for infantile hemangiomas. *Plast Reconstr Surg* 1989; 83:459.

138. Wilgis EFS. *Vascular injuries and diseases of the upper limb.* Boston: Little, Brown, 1983.

139. Masson P. Le glomus neuromuo—artierel des regions tachtiles et ses tumeurs. *Lyon Chirurgical* 1924; 21:257.

140. Popoff NW. The digital vascular system with reference to the state of glomus in inflammation, arteriosclerotic gangrene, diabetic gangrene, thrombo-angitis obliterans and supernumerary digits in man. *Arch Pathol* 1934; 18:294.

141. Shugart RR, Soule EH, Johnson EW. Glomus tumor. *Surg Gynecol Obstet* 1963; 117:334.

142. Chi-Wing C. Intraosseous glomus tumor. Case report. *J Hand Surg* 1981; 6:368.

143. Joseph FR, Posner MA. Glomus tumors of the wrist. *J Hand Surg* 1983; 8:918.

97

Basic Principles of Reconstruction of the Thumb

Hung-chi Chen, M.D., F.A.C.S.

Transfer of the banner toe to the thumb occurred in 1900, when Nicoladoni first performed a two-staged toe-to-thumb transfer. In 1966, Buncke successfully carried out single-staged transfer of large and second toes to the thumb in the Rhesus monkey using microsurgical techniques (1). Clincally, Yang (2) transferred the second toe to the thumb in 1966, and Cobbett (3) transferred the great toe to the thumb in 1968, followed by Buncke in 1973.

Toe-to-Thumb Transfer

INDICATIONS

The thumb accounts for at least 40% of hand function. Among the digits of the hand it is the most worthwhile to reconstruct. Before planning surgery, the factors to be considered in toe-to-thumb transfer include: (a) age, (b) occupation, (c) function of the opposite hand and the fingers of the injured hand, (d) level of amputation of the thumb, (e) dominance of the injured hand, and (f) patient's and family's understanding of the procedure after a detailed explanation.

GOALS

The conventional methods for thumb reconstruction have been described by Strickland (4). In comparison with conventional methods, microsurgical toe-to-thumb transfer has the following advantages: (a) it provides pain sensation and mobility, (b) it has glabrous skin with stability in pinch and grip, (c) there is favorable cosmesis, (d) it has growth potential in pediatric patients. A well-reconstructed thumb should also be free of cold intolerance, with minimal morbidity at the donor site. The goals of toe-to-thumb transfer are listed in Table 97–1.

CHOICE OF TOES

The choice of donor toe is dependent on the level of thumb amputation. There are several options for each level of amputation (Figs. 97–1 and 97–2). When there are several options at the same level of amputation, the final choice is influenced by the following factors: (a) the surgeon's experience, (b) the functional requirements of the particular patient, (c) ethnic customs. In Asia and in Europe, people are reluctant to lose the big toe. For example, the second toe is often preferred to the big toe in Asia, because if the big toe is removed from the foot, the patient cannot wear a thong sandal.

Preoperative Preparation

PEDICLED GROIN FLAP

A skin graft is better tolerated at the hand than the foot. A pedicled groin flap can provide good skin coverage, so that the tendons, nerves, vessels, and bone would not be exposed during toe-to-thumb transfer. This flap also provides enough soft tissue for the reconstruction of the first web space. The surgeon should avoid large skin flaps from the dorsum of foot (i.e., the dorsalis pedis flap) while harvesting the toe to minimize donor-site morbidity. Inadequate skin coverage is a major cause of complications in toe transfer, which include tension in wound closure and possible compromise of circulation. Options other than the pedicled groin flap are free flaps (e.g., free groin flap, lateral arm flap, gracilis flap), depending on the requirement of the individual wound.

ELIMINATE INFECTION AND EDEMA

It is essential to eliminate infection and edema before toe-to-thumb transfer. The wound should be closed before toe transfer to minimize possible complications and to assure good tendon function. The patient should also be treated by a hand therapist before toe transfer until the stiffness of all adjacent fingers is minimal. Stiffness of the hand is contraindicated for toe transfer. During physiotherapy, patients may gain knowledge and reassurance about toe transfer from observing other patients who have already had the procedure. This will be helpful in the postoperative period.

CREATE PLASTIC MODELS

We have found it useful to create plastic models before toe-to-thumb transfer (see Fig. 97–2). The model (moulage) is adjusted and changed over the preoperative period. This modeling will help to determine the optimal length and position of the thumb to be reconstructed. Based on the model, the thenar muscles can be trained, if they are still present.

EVALUATE THE VASCULAR SYSTEM

The doppler is noninvasive and can be used for all cases. In clinical assessment, the following items should be checked:

1. Any previous injury to the toes or foot, such as a history of foot fracture, the presence of indurated scar or abnormal pigmentation, or a long history of wearing clogs (Fig. 97–3). X-rays of the foot should be taken if necessary.
2. Induration along the course of the greater saphenous vein, which may have thrombosis. Some patients have throm-

Table 97–1
Goals in Toe-to-Thumb Transfer

Individual Function	Essential Tactics
Sensation	As many nerves should be repaired as possible (on dorsal and volar sides).
Range of Motion	Do toe-to-thumb transfer when the wound has healed (closed). This is essential to prevent vascular problems as well as tendon adhesions.
Power of Pinch and Grip	Good fixation of bone to achieve stability. Good therapy with vocational rehabilitation.
Free of Complications	
1. Infection	Wound healing before toe-to-thumb transfer; sufficient skin for wound closure; good hemostasis to avoid hematoma.
2. Tendon adhesion or disruption	Same as 1.
3. Bone malunion or nonunion	Good bone fixation; careful in therapy.
4. Atrophy of the transferred toe	Avoid long ischemic time or vascular problem.
5. Donor-site morbidity	Careful dissection of the foot; no skin graft at the foot; no tension in wound closure; no hematoma; donor foot splinted after operation.
Patient satisfaction	Good appearance of the reconstructed thumb; good range of movement.
Shortest time before going back to work	Good therapy; desensitization when there is pain.

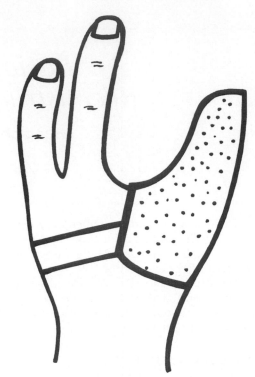

FIG. 97–2. Prosthesis before toe-to-thumb transfer. This helps the surgeon to decide the required length and position of the toe to be reconstructed.

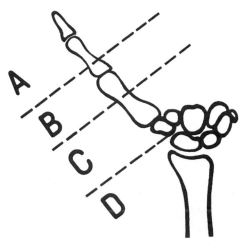

FIG. 97–1. Level of thumb amputation versus choice of toe for thumb reconstruction. See Table 97–5 for description.

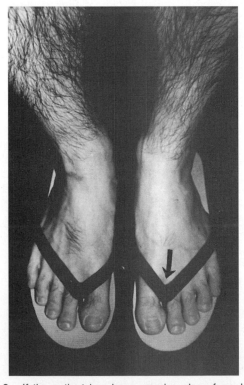

FIG. 97–3. If the patient has been wearing clogs for a long time, and there is induration in the first web space, care should be taken to check for possible injury to the "vital" segment of the vascular pedicle.

bosis of the veins at the dorsum of foot. In these situations, the transferred toes should use the concomitant veins instead of the superficial veins for venous drainage. Angiography is indicated when there is suspicion of vascular injuries, either in the donor site or the recipient site.

3. Measurement of the relative size of the normal thumb, donor-foot big toe, and donor-foot second toe. This is important before toe-to-thumb transfer (Fig. 97–4).

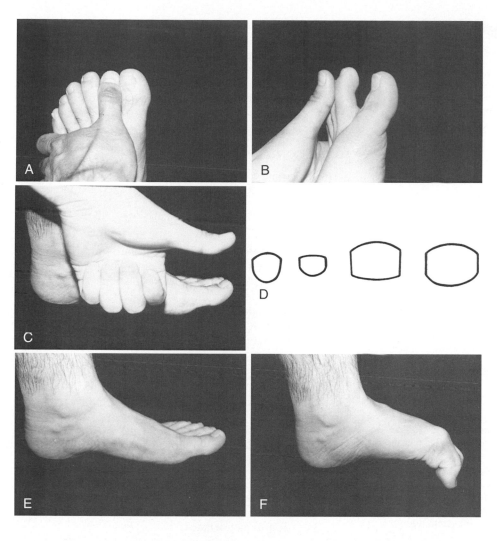

FIG. 97–4. A, AP view. Check the relative size of the big toe and second toe of the donor foot, as well as the thumb of the normal hand. **B,** lateral view. For this patient, the better choice is the second toe. **C,** for another patient, the big toe is the better choice. **D,** the nail is also different in (right to left) the big toe, thumb, second toe, and finger. The nail should be taken into consideration in toe-to-thumb transfer. **E,** the range of motion of the donor toe should be checked in physical examination. In some patients with congenital anomalies, the IP joints of the toes may be stiff. Some other patients (although rare) may have previous injury to the toes. Ask the patient to dorsiflex the toes. **F,** then ask the patient to assume plantar flexion. This is a simple test, but is often neglected. The range of toe movement is recorded before operation.

Anatomy of the Donor Site

The vascular anatomy of the toes had been well documented by Gilbert in 1976 (5) and May in 1977 (6). There are other minor variations, but the determining factor is the position of the first dorsal metatarsal artery in relation to the interosseous muscle and intermetatarsal ligament (7). One constant is the distal communicating branch, which always exists between the first dorsal metatarsal artery and the first plantar metatarsal artery (Fig. 97–5).

The dissection of the toe is made according to the structures required. The reconstructed thumb should have adequate length, with enough web space to provide functional opposition. It must also have good sensibility.

Overcoming Pitfalls in Toe-to-Thumb Transfer

VEIN GRAFTS

Vein grafts can be used more liberally, instead of struggling to obtain enough length of a deep-seated artery of the toe. The latter may cause damage to the donor foot, or even injury to the pedicle artery of the toe. The dominant artery (dorsal or plantar system) is identified by initial dissection in the first web space and then dissection is carried out proxi-

mally. Shortages of arterial length are bridged with vein grafts. This avoids unnecessary damage to the artery, which may not be detected by an inexperienced surgeon. Damage to the artery may be caused by inadvertent use of forceps to pinch the artery, by traction, or even by desiccation; this may lead to thrombosis. While this is not a problem of an experienced surgeon, for a new microsurgeon this is the most common cause of reexploration and failure in toe transfers. Reexploration can be avoided if every step of the dissection is done with direct visualization under loupes. It is clear that struggling in dissection of artery (especially in type III plantar metatarsal artery) should be supplanted with proper use of vein grafts in toe-to-thumb transfer.

NERVE TRANSFER

When there is avulsion of digital nerves that cannot be identified, a nerve transfer can be performed, selecting the appropriate digital nerve from the ulnar side of the long and ring fingers, or from sensory nerve branches of the superficial radial nerve on the dorsum of hand.

METATARSAL HEAD

The metatarsal head of the big toe should be preserved to avoid donor-foot morbidity.

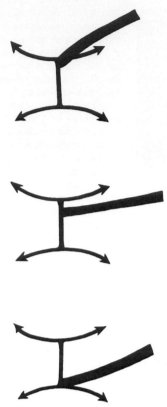

FIG. 97–5. The anatomy of the arteries supplying the big and second toes has a lot of variations. However, it is always safe to dissect distally to proximally, starting from the first metatarsal web. The four arrows indicate the arteries going to the big and second toes. The first dorsal metatarsal artery can be deep or superficial to the interosseous muscle. If dissection is begun from this "arterial framework" at the first web space, it would be easier to decide the major artery supplying the donor toe (dorsal or plantar system artery).

THROMBOSIS

The greater saphenous vein may have thrombosis resulting from an earlier intravenous infusion. This is checked by watching the venous outflow from the cut end of the greater saphenous vein when the artery has not been cut.

VASOSPASM

Vasospasm may be a problem in toe transfer. Toe transfers are different from other free tissue transfers in many ways. Notable is the tendency of vasospasm in the small recipient arteries in the palm (proper palmar digital artery, common palmar digital artery, and digital artery). The strategies for minimizing vasospasm are: (a) at the recipient site use larger recipient arteries, such as the radial artery in the snuffbox; (b) on the donor site, be meticulous in dissection of the vessels. The branches of the artery should be tied, not too close to the main trunk of the artery nor too far away from it, as shown in Figure 97–6. The former will cause narrowing of the lumen, and the latter will leave a blind end that is prone to thrombosis. The untied branch will cause hematoma and spasm. Any trauma during dissection may cause problems in the circulation, so it is important always to use loupe magnification during the dissection. Also, use microsurgical instru-

ments to handle the artery during dissection of the pedicle. Avoid cauterization near the artery, which may induce thrombosis in the artery or spasm of the arterial wall. Good hemostasis is important. Place suction drains away from the pedicle. The pedicle should be well covered, without tension, before wound closure. The entire procedure of toe dissection must be efficient to prevent swelling of the vascular intima. Avoid exposure to cold following surgery.

BONE CONTACTS

Provide broad contact of bone surfaces. A bone peg (Fig. 97–7) or stepwise cut of the bone will increase the contact surface to ensure bone union.

HEMOSTASIS

In comparison with other free flaps, the transferred toe has much less contact with the surface of the recipient site to rely on for neovascularization and inosculation. Therefore, the transferred toe depends on a good feeder artery with long-term patency to prevent atrophy. As with digital replantation, the measurement of temperature is a reliable monitor after toe transfer, but it is not a reliable monitor for other free flaps.

ORDER OF PROCEDURE

If there is only one team, always dissect the recipient site first, so that there will be more time for the dissected tissue to develop spontaneous hemostasis. Time is an important factor in stopping bleeding. In terms of hemostasis, the following order is suggested:

(1) Recipient Site
    Careful hemostasis during dissection
        Tourniquet deflated
        Gentle compression
        Check major bleeders
        Gentle compression with saline swab, and wait for toe harvesting
        Toe transfer
        Check bleeders once more
        Place drains
        Wound closure without tension
(2) Donor Site
    Careful dissection of the toe
        Tourniquet deflated for hemostasis, check bleeders from the toe before transfer
        Place drains
        Wound closure, followed by splinting of foot

Operative Procedures

WRAP-AROUND FLAP (Fig. 97–8)

The wrap-around flap was first described by Morrison in 1980 (8,9). The skin and tissue raised from the big toe provides good sensibility, cosmesis, and strength. When bone graft is required, it can be taken from the iliac crest. The length of the thumb is maintained, but the metatarsophalangeal joint (MP) is not reconstructed. The bone graft might be absorbed in some patients, especially when it is long. In our series, there was no fracture of the bone graft.

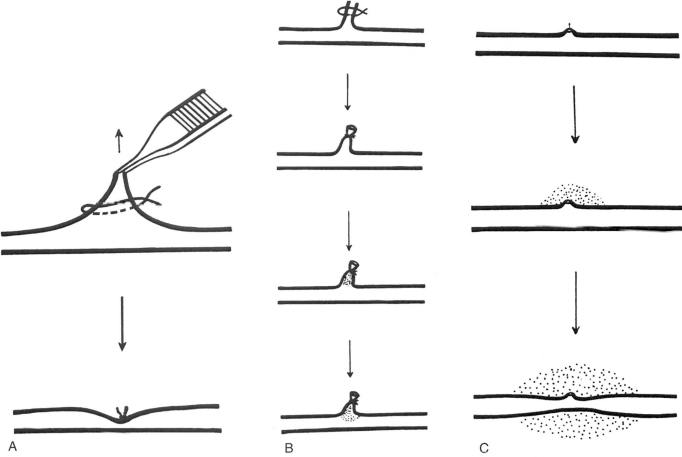

FIG. 97-6. A, when the arterial branch is ligated too close to the artery, it may result in a stricture. **B,** when the arterial branch is ligated too far away from the artery, a blind pouch will be formed. It may develop thrombosis and spread into the lumen, causing problems. **C,** when the arterial branch is not ligated at all, thrombus may develop in the lumen close to the perforation hole. Also, the hematoma outside the artery may cause spasm and compression.

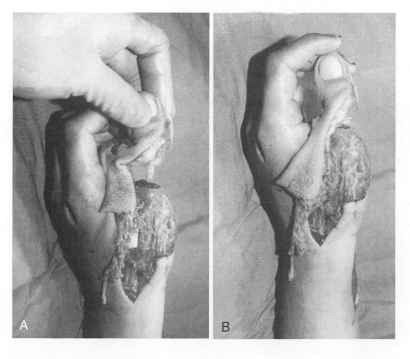

FIG. 97-7. A, a bone peg is useful in toe-to-thumb transfer. It increases the contact surface between the two bones, and therefore increases the stability as well as ensuring bone union. **B,** the bone peg keeps the toe straight. Moreover, the transferred toe can be rotated before a K-wire is inserted if the direction needs to be changed.

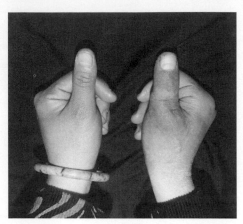

FIG. 97–8.   A wrap-around flap gives a good cosmetic result. Note the exact symmetry of the two thumbs. Patients are happy to show their hands to friends, and are glad to go back to work.

On the donor site, a cross-toe flap can be raised from the second toe to resurface the plantar defect of the big-toe donor site; this helps to decrease donor-site morbidity.

Sometimes there is transfer of pulp tissue without the nail (10–12), and there are other types of partial big-toe transfer (13).

The pulp tissue can be raised from the lateral aspect of the big toe. It can be harvested with the tissue of metatarsal web for simultaneous reconstruction of the thenar web, depending on the tissue requirement of the individual patient (Fig. 97–9).

A variable amount of skeleton can be raised from the big toe. For example, a part of the distal phalanx and even part of the interphalangeal joint (IP) can be harvested (Fig. 97–10). In an effort to reduce the bone and joint, longitudinal osteotomy must be done.

FIG. 97–9.   **A,** the patient had an oblique amputation through the pulp tissue of the right thumb. **B,** for pulp tissue reconstruction, the flap is raised from the lateral aspect of the right big toe. **C,** the pedicle artery is the first dorsal metatarsal artery. **D,** the reconstructed pulp tissue had good sensibility, with 2PD of 8 mm at 1 year follow-up.

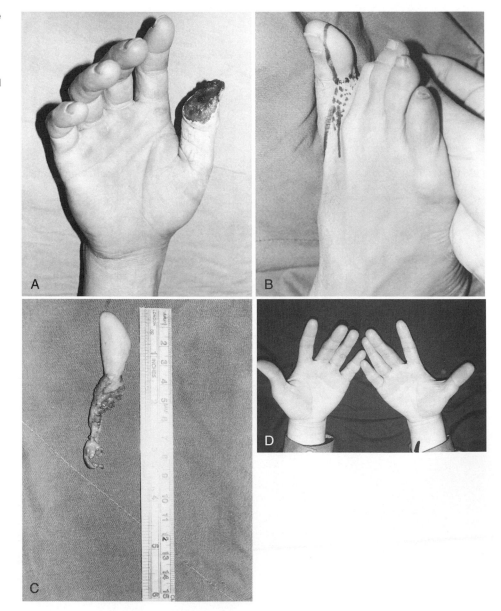

GREAT TOE TRANSFER (3) (Fig. 97–11)

When the entire big toe is transferred, the MP joint is usually not included in the transfer. The entire great toe is less frequently used now, unless the size of the big toe is close to that of the normal thumb. When the size match is good, the functional result is good, allowing more power in the grip.

SECOND TOE TRANSFER (14) (Fig. 97–12)

Transfer of the second toe is indicated in the following situations:

- When the level of thumb amputation is at the proximal metacarpal.
- In the more distal amputation, when the patient does not want to sacrifice a big toe for thumb reconstruction.
- In amputation at the B level, as was shown in Figure 97–1, when the big toe is much larger than the normal thumb.

In our series, the second toe has the following disadvantages in comparison with other methods:

- It provides less stable pinch, because of the smaller area of pulp tissue.
- It provides less gripping power because of its thinner skeleton.
- Its MP joint tends to be in hyperextension, but its IP joint tends to be in hyperflexion. Angled osteotomy at the second metatarsal bone can partially correct the hyperextension at the MP joint, but IP joint hyperflexion is difficult to change. The segment of the second metatarsal bone should be short when angled osteotomy is carried out. The MP joint capsule should be resutured to increase the MP flexion and decrease MP hyperextension. The extensor tendon should be repaired in greater tension. If possible, the intrinsics should be repaired to decrease the IP hyperflexion and to increase IP extension. A comparison is listed in Table 97–2.

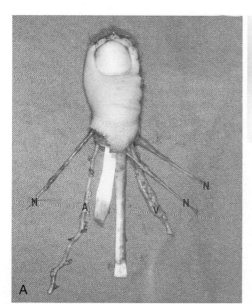

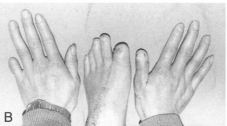

FIG. 97–10. **A,** partial big toe transfer with trimmed IP joint. **B,** appearance is also good, but some patients developed deviation at the IP joint a few years later. It can be fused if there is pain.

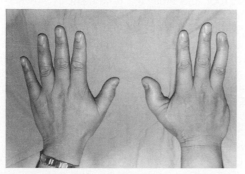

FIG. 97–11.   Transfer of the whole big toe has the advantage of IP movement with good stability. However, it is not so appealing cosmetically.

Table 97–2
Comparison Among Four Common Types of Toe-to-Thumb Transfer

	Big toe	Second toe	Wrap-around	Twisted toe
Hand appearance			+	+
Stability	+	+	+	+
IP joint movement	+	+		+
Sensibility	+	+	+	+
Pinch	+		+	
Grip	+		+	
Donor-site appearance		+	+	+

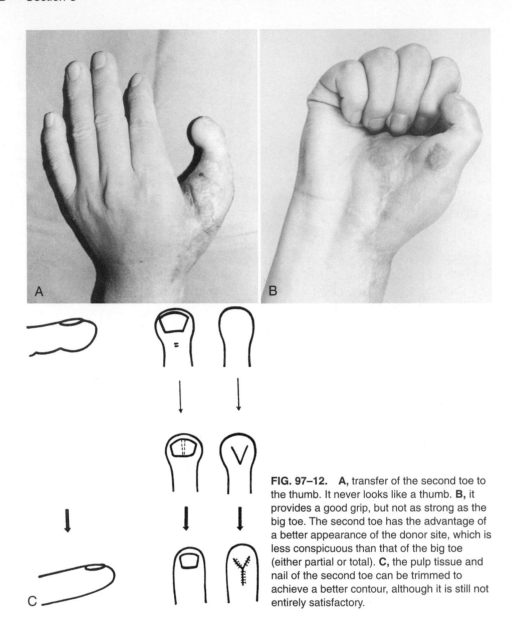

FIG. 97–12. **A,** transfer of the second toe to the thumb. It never looks like a thumb. **B,** it provides a good grip, but not as strong as the big toe. The second toe has the advantage of a better appearance of the donor site, which is less conspicuous than that of the big toe (either partial or total). **C,** the pulp tissue and nail of the second toe can be trimmed to achieve a better contour, although it is still not entirely satisfactory.

- Cosmetically, the second toe is less satisfactory than other choices. The plantar-side soft tissue of the second toe should be reduced primarily before toe transfer; this helps to achieve a better contour. In addition, the soft tissue at the distal phalanx of the second toe can be trimmed. It must be said that a second toe will never look like a thumb.

COMPOUND DIGIT TRANSFER (TWISTED TOE TECHNIQUE) (Fig. 97–13)

This is a combination of the previous methods. It was first described by Foucher (15). The nail, skin, and soft tissue, as well as a piece of bone, are raised from the big toe, while the major bone, joint, and tendon (with or without skin) are raised from the second toe. This will provide stability, with good sensation and satisfactory cosmetic result. It can be used in children, because the compound digit continues to

grow longitudinally. The donor-site morbidity is less than for total great toe transfer (15,16).

On the foot, the great toe donor site is covered with the skin from the second toe, with or without split skin graft. However, this method is more difficult.

The good result is owed primarily to harvesting the IP joint of the second toe. It is not so large as the IP joint of the big toe. Usually, the ipsilateral foot is used as the donor site so that the ulnar side of the pulp tissue is not incised and will have good sensibility.

VILKKI'S PROCEDURE

This procedure was described by Vilkki (17) in 1985. The second toe is transferred to the forearm bone stump when the injury is at, or proximal to, the level of the radiocarpal joint. The transferred toe can pinch the ulnar stump.

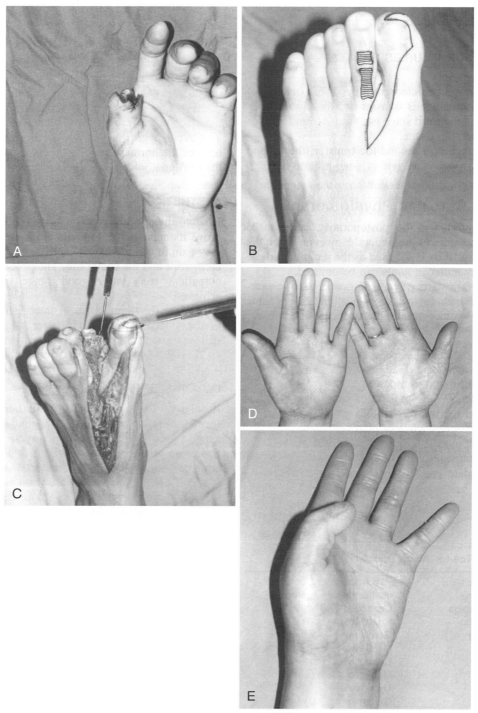

FIG. 97–13. **A,** the thumb had amputation at the proximal phalanx in a crush injury. **B,** a twisted toe transfer is planned. **C,** the skin, nail and soft tissue, as well as a piece of the distal phalanx and tendon, are raised from the second toe. **D,** it has the advantage of good appearance and the capacity of IP joint movement. **E,** the active range of motion at the IP joint is 40°.

Table 97–5
Choice of Toes vs. Level of Thumb Amputation

Level A
1. Partial big toe transfer
   (a) Pulp-tissue transfer
   (b) Wrap-around flap, and other types of its modification
2. Twisted toe transfer

Level B
1. Big toe
2. Second toe
3. Twisted toe transfer

Level C
1. Second toe
2. Combined groin flap, bone graft and twisted toe

Level D
1. Vilkki procedure using the second toe

Therefore, in children it is worthwhile to reconstruct the thumb skeleton with preserved epiphysis.

References

1. Buncke HJ, Sheh KG. The digital transfer. In: Serafin D, Buncke HJ, eds. *Microsurgical composite tissue transfers.* St. Louis: CV Mosby, 1979.
2. Yang D, Gu Y. Thumb reconstruction utilizing second toe transplantation by microvascular anastomoses. A report of 78 cases. *Chin Med J* 1979; 92:295.
3. Cobbett JR. Free digital transfer. Report of a case of transfer of a great toe to replace an amputated thumb. *J Bone Joint Surg* 1969; 51B:677.
4. Strickland JW. Thumb reconstruction. In: Green DP, ed. *Operative hand surgery.* New York: Churchill Livingstone, 1988; 2175–2263.
5. Gilbert A. Composite tissue transfers from the foot. Anatomical basis and surgical technique. In: Daniller A, Strauch B, eds. *Symposium on microsurgery.* St. Louis: CV Mosby, 1976.
6. May JW Jr, Chait LA, Cohen BE, et al. Free neurovascular flap from the first web of the foot in hand reconstruction. *J Hand Surg* 1977; 2:387.
7. Leung PC. The vessels of the first metatarsal web space. *J Bone Joint Surg* 1983; 65A:235.
8. Morrison WA, O'Brien BM, MacLeod AM. Thumb reconstruction with a free neurovascular wrap-around flap from the big toe. *J Hand Surg (Am)* 1980; 5:575.
9. Urbaniak JR. Wrap-around procedure for thumb reconstruction. *Hand Clin* 1985; 1:259.
10. Morrison WA, O'Brien BM, Hamilton RB. Neurovascular free foot flaps in reconstruction of the mutilated hand. *Clin Plast Surg* 1978; 5:265.
11. Morrison WA, O'Brien BM, MacLeod AM, et al. Neurovascular free flaps from the foot for innervation of the hand. *J Hand Surg (Am)* 1978; 3:235.
12. Leung PC, Ma FY. Digital reconstruction using the toe flap. Report of 10 cases. *J Hand Surg (Am)* 1982; 7:366.
13. Wei FC, Chen HC, Chuang CC, et al. Thumb reconstruction with trimmed toe transfer technique. *Plast Reconstr Surg* 1988; 82:506.
14. Leung PC. Thumb reconstruction using second toe transfer. *Hand Clin* 1985; 1:285.
15. Foucher G, Van Genechten F, Morrison WA. Composite tissue transfer to the hand from the foot. In: Jackson IT, Sommerlad BC, eds. *Recent advances in plastic surgery.* Edinburgh: Churchill Livingstone, 1985.
16. Tsai TM, Aziz W. Toe-to-thumb transfer: a new technique. *Plast Reconstr Surg* 1991; 88:149.
17. Vilkki SK. Toe to antebrachial stump transplantation: functional results for new grip reconstruction. In: Brunelli G, ed. *Textbook of microsurgery.* Vol 1. Brescia, Italy: Masson, 1988.
18. Chen HC, Lin CH, Wei FC, et. al. Transposed replantation of fingers at forearm bones in severe segmental injuries across the hand and wrist. *Plast Reconstr Surg* 1994; 94:951.
19. Gilbert A. Toe transfers for congenital hand defects. *J Hand Surg (Am)* 1982; 7:118.
20. Buncke HJ, Harris GD. Toe to hand transplantation in children. In: Serafin D, Georgiade NG, eds. *Pediatric plastic surgery.* St. Louis: CV Mosby, 1984.

98

Hand Infections

Kevin Yakuboff, M.D.

Hand infections in the pre-antibiotic era were associated with significant morbity and even mortality. Acute lymphangitis had a 28% mortality rate, while neglected human bite infections had an associated mortality of 10% (1). Kanavel's (2) detailed anatomic descriptions of the potential spaces of the hand form the basis of understanding how infections develop and spread in the hand and upper extremity (2). Through these studies, proper surgical approaches were developed for drainage of the flexor synovial sheaths, thenar and midpalmar spaces, and fascial planes of the hand. Today, the surgical principles established in Kanavel's time are no less significant in the treatment of established hand infections. Antibiotics alone are curative in only a small number of hand infections because compartmentalization of the hand contains the infection in areas poorly accessible to antibiotics (3). Early and adequate decompression of pus under pressure is necessary to avoid soft-tissue loss in critical anatomic areas. Despite the availability of a powerful antibiotic armamentarium, basic surgical principles remain the primary treatment of established hand infections. These basic principles include adequate surgical drainage through properly placed incisions to avoid damage to adjuvant structures and late scar contracture, appropriate débridement of necrotic tissue, judicious splinting and early mobilization to minimize joint stiffness, and the appropriate use of antibiotics as an important adjunct in preventing the dissemination of established infection.

At high risk for developing severe complications from hand infections are patients who are immunosuppressed, have diabetes, have sustained human or animal bites, or are drug abusers. These patients should receive early and aggressive treatment to avoid long-term complications such as joint stiffness, osteomyelitis, amputation, and even death.

Hand infections in diabetics run a more prolonged and complicated course. Delays in diagnosis and treatment contribute to a higher incidence of stiff digits and amputation (20 to 50%) (4,5). In addition, a higher number of mixed bacterial infections with gram-negative bacilli are encountered in diabetics. All of these facts underscore the need for early, aggressive management.

Felons and Paronychia

Kanavel noted that the distal phalanx is a closed sac, separated from the rest of the digits. This closed pulp space is divided into a latticework by multiple connective tissue septae. The interstices of this latticework are filled with fat and eccrine sweat glands. The dorsum of this pulp space is rigid, being bound by the bony distal phalanx and the nail complex. Any increase in pressure in this unyielding compartment can adversely affect the blood supply to the soft tissue and bone of the distal phalanx.

Felons and paronychia account for approximately one-third of all hand infections seen today (6). Felons are palmar closed-space infections of the distal pulp of the digit. They are characterized by severe pain, redness, and swelling of the digital pulp (Fig. 98–1). A history of minor penetrating trauma is usually present with minor cuts, splinters, or glass slivers being seen as predisposing events. *Staphylococcus aureus* is identified most frequently as the causative agent. Early in these infections there is a phase of cellulitis that can be aborted by soaks and antibiotics. However, once abscess formations have occurred in the closed pulp space, adequate surgical drainage is required to avoid vascular compromise to bone and soft tissue of the distal phalanx. This complication is frequently seen in neglected or endstage felons (Figs. 98–2, 98–3).

Many incisions have been recommended for pulp space drainage. Kanavel recommended a high incision laterally over the distal phalanx that extends over the front of the distal pad (hockey-stick incision). The alligator-mouth incision separating the pulp from the distal phalanx should be avoided because of circulatory compromise, chronic tip instability, and pain. More recently, a palmar, longitudinal incision through the center of the pulp that does not cross the distal interphalangeal (DIP) flexion crease has been recommended (7). This approach provides adequate access to the deep pulp space and heals with a relatively painless scar. Packing of the abscess cavity is necessary to promote adequate drainage and premature closing of the wound. Regardless of incision type, a felon should be drained in the area of maximal tenderness. Untreated felons can result in skin necrosis, osteomyelitis of the distal phalanx, and suppurative flexor tenonsynovitis if infection breaks through into the flexor tendon space.

Herpetic Whitlow (Herpes simplex) has frequently been confused with pulp-space infection of the digits. It is a superficial cutaneous infection that does not involve the deeper tissues of the finger tip. Swelling and erythema of the fingertip make its differentiation from early bacterial felon or paronychia difficult. Herpetic Whitlow typically develops as a painful vesiculopustular eruption over the fingertip (Fig. 98–4). These infections have a high incidence in medical and dental personnel who are in contact with oral secretions and in children following a primary oral herpetic infection (8). The presence of painful coalescing clear vesicals with appro-

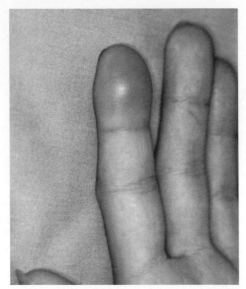

FIG. 98–1.   A typical felon demonstrating swelling and redness of distal pulp.

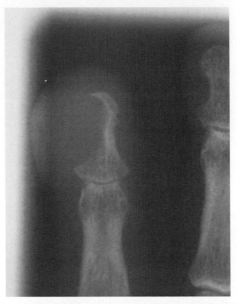

FIG. 98–3.   The same felon showing changes in the distal phalanx.

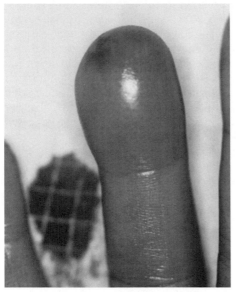

FIG. 98–2.   A neglected felon demonstrating skin necrosis.

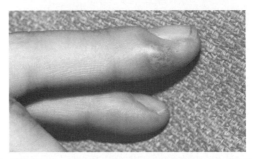

FIG. 98–4.   Coalescing vesicles seen in herpetic Whitlow.

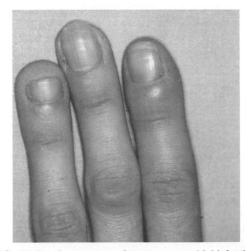

FIG. 98–5.   Appearance of acute paronychial infection.

priate history should make the diagnosis. Herpetic Whitlow is a self-limited process that resolves in 3 to 4 weeks. Nonoperative therapy is indicated. A deep incision in the pulp is to be avoided. Vesicle unroofing and the use of acyclovir have been recommended by some to alleviate painful symptoms (9,10).

Acute and Chronic Paronychia

Infection in and around the nail fold is known as a paronychia (Fig. 98–5). Any break in the seal between the nail fold and nail plate will serve as a portal of entry for infection. Hangnails, manicures, and nail biting are often predisposing events. *Staphylococcus aureus* is the common causative organism. Adequate treatment of a single paronychia involves drainage of the abscess through the nail fold. In more advanced infections, pus can accumulate beneath the nail, lift-

ing off the underlying matrix. In these situations, removal of the nail is necessary for proper drainage. Pus can also spread underneath the nail sulcus to the opposite side, resulting in a "runaround" abscess.

Chronic paronychia is a different disease process with an indolent course marked by exacerbations and remissions, often seen in people whose hands are constantly in a moist environment. Chronic inflammation of the eponychial fold is seen. Often there is separation of the fold from the underlying nail, with intermittent drainage. Fungal and gram-negative microorganisms have been implicated in these chronic infections. In fact, *Candida albicans* has been cultured in 95% of the cases (6). The primary cause of this chronic problem is a combination of proximal nail fold obstruction and fungal infection. Medical treatment of this condition is largely unsuccessful. Eponychial marsupialization, as reported by Eaton, yields the best results (11). In this technique, a crescent-shaped piece of tissue is excised just proximal to the nail fold. Marsupialization combined with topical antifungal agents (Mycolog) provide the highest cure rates.

Tenosynovitis

Pyogenic infection of the tenosynovium involves the flexor tendon sheaths along with the radial and ulnar bursae at the wrist. The anatomic configuration of these sheaths make these closed-space infections. In the fingers, the flexor sheaths begin at the midpalmar crease and end distally just proximal to the distal interphalangeal joint (DIPJ). The flexor sheath of the small finger continues proximally into the ulnar bursa, while the thumb flexor sheath extends proximally into the radial bursa. Both the ulnar and radial bursae extend just proximal to the transverse carpal ligament and connect with the Parona space, a potential space between the flexor pollicis longus and the pronator quadratus muscle. Neglected pyogenic infections of the small or thumb flexor sheaths will predictably spread proximally to the wrist by virtue of their anatomic connections.

Tendon-sheath infections are most often the result of penetrating trauma. Violation of the flexor sheath is likely to occur at joint flexion creases. Tendon sheaths are separated from the skin by only a small amount of subcutaneous tissues at these sites. Neglected pulp-space infections (felons) can rupture into the distal flexor sheath, resulting in tenosynovitis (Fig. 98–6). *Staphylococcus aureus* is the most common causative microorganism. The ring, long, and index fingers are the most frequently involved digits (3). Kanavel's four cardinal signs remain important diagnostic aids:

1. Excessive tenderness over the course of the sheath, limited to the sheath.
2. Symmetrical enlargement (fusiform) of the whole finger.
3. Excruciating pain on passive extensor of the finger, most marked at the proximal sheath.
4. Flexed posture of the involved digit (2).

In early infections, not all four signs will be present. Pain on passive extension (entire sheath) is the most reliable finding in establishing a diagnosis. Early infection (lacking all four signs) may be treated with parenteral antibiotics, but failure to respond to 24 hours of the treatment should result in surgical decompression. Established pyogenic tenosynovitis is a true surgical emergency requiring prompt surgical drainage of the involved tendon sheath (Fig. 98–7). Delays in treatment will result in tendon necrosis and even skin loss in severe cases. Two basic surgical approaches have been described for drainage of the infected tendon sheath: open drainage procedures and closed tendon sheath irrigation. The open technique involves surgical decompression of the entire tendon sheath through combined midaxial and palmar incisions (12). The wounds are left open to drain and heal secondarily. Rehabilitation is prolonged, and permanent finger stiffness is seen in a significant number of patients. This technique is most useful when resection of necrotic tendon is necessary in advanced cases. Closed tendon-sheath irrigation, as first described by Carter and co-workers (13) and reported by Neviaser (14), is most commonly used for treatment of established pyogenic tenosynovitis. The technique involves a proximal palmar incision opening the sheath proximal to

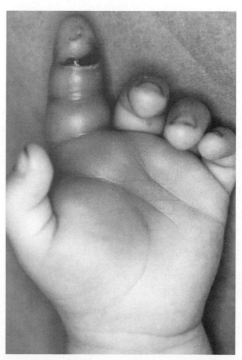

FIG. 98–7. Index finger flexor tenosynovitis. Note pressure necrosis of distal phalanx skin.

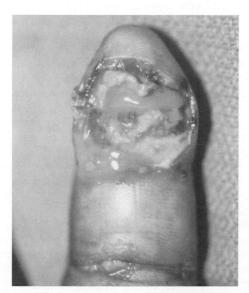

FIG. 98–6. Flexor tenosynovitis resulting from a neglected felon.

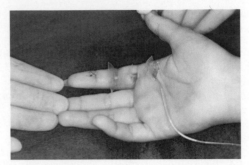

FIG. 98–8. Modified "open" irrigation treatment for pyogenic flexor tenosynovitis. Soft Silastic drains have been introduced behind flexor tendons to promote drainage.

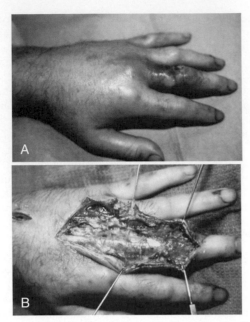

FIG. 98–9. **A, B,** a neglected human bite involving the dorsal subaponeurotic space.

the A1 pulley. A distal midaxial incision at the distal edge of the A4 pulley is made for egress of irrigation solution. A long irrigating catheter (16 to 18 gauge) is placed in the proximal sheath, with a drain left in the distal incision. All incisions are closed, and tendon-sheath irrigation is performed for 48 to 72 hours. Isotonic saline or antibiotic irrigation can be used, and irrigation can be a continuous drip or an intermittent flush every 2 hours. To alleviate the pain associated with saline irrigation, 2 to 3 ml of Marcaine can be injected into the catheter. A modification of this technique involves the use of transverse incisions made in the distal palmar crease and all digital flexion creases (Fig. 98–8). All annular pulleys are preserved and the sheath is opened through incision in the cruciate pulleys. A catheter is inserted proximally in the tendon sheath and silastic drains are used to ensure adequate drainage and egress of irrigant. Irrigation is continued for 48 to 72 hours postoperatively, followed by gentle active and passive range of motion (ROM) after removal of catheter and drains. These incisions ensure adequate drainage, heal quickly, and do not interfere with early rehabilitation plans.

Atypical mycobacterial infections account for a small number of tenosynovitis cases. These are chronic tenosynovial infections most frequently caused by mycobacterium or *Kansasii* and *Marinarum*. These infections are the result of puncture wounds received around aquatic environments. The clinical presentation differs from that of acute pyogenic infections. Chronic swelling involving the affected flexor sheath is the most common finding. There is no disabling pain or loss of function, as seen with acute bacterial infections. The most reliable methods of diagnosis are acid-fast stains and cultures of synovial tissue. The best treatment results are obtained with a combination of extensive tenosynovectomy and postoperative use of antituberculous drugs for 6 to 24 months.

Deep Space Infections

There are four defined, deep spaces in the hand that are clinically significant in hand infections:

1. Dorsal subaponeurotic space
2. Subfascial palmar space
3. Thenar space
4. Midpalmar space

The first two spaces named are the most superficial of the deep spaces of the hand. The dorsal subaponeurotic space is beneath the extensor tendons on the dorsum of the hand. The subfascial palmar space communicates with the dorsal subcutaneous space through the web spaces between the digits. Infections in this subfascial space spread dorsally and are commonly referred to as collar-button abscesses. Palmar spread of infection is limited by the relationship of palmar fascia to skin. Infections in the subpalmar fascia (collar-button) result in a severe amount of dorsal swelling with an abducted finger due to pus-filled web spaces. Drainage is approached through the palmar with unroofing of the palmar fascia.

The dorsal subaponeurotic space usually becomes secondarily infected as the result of penetrating trauma. This deep-space infection is seen frequently with intravenous drug abusers and neglected human bites (Fig. 98–9). A severely swollen dorsum of the hand coupled with appropriate clinical history should prompt surgical exploration. Linear incisions centered in the 2nd and 4th metacarpals will provide adequate access to the space while preserving adequate soft tissue coverage of extensor tendons. Occasionally, direct incision over a pointing abscess is necessary, but it risks exposure and desiccation of extensor tendons.

The thenar and the midpalmar spaces are the deepest of the four potential spaces in the hand. These two spaces can be associated with significant infections, and spontaneous drainage in these areas rarely occurs. Surgical decompression is necessary for a satisfactory result.

The thenar space follows the direction of the adductor pollicis muscle. The dorsal boundary of this space is the adductor muscle, with the volar boundary being the adductor fascia. The space is contiguous with the flexor tendons of the index finger. Radially, the thenar space is confined by the

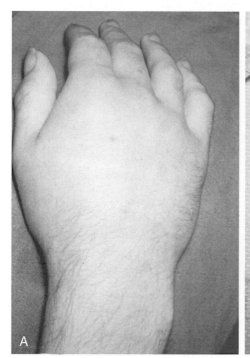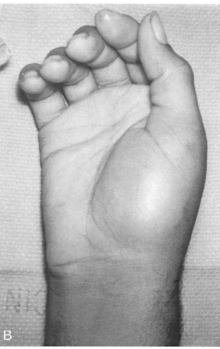

FIG. 98–10. A, B, an undrained thenar space infection with severe dorsal edema and abducted thumb position.

confluence of the adductor muscle, its fascia, and their insertion on the proximal phalanx of the thumb. Ulnarly, the space is separated from the midpalmar space by the oblique septum extending from the palmar fascia to the 3rd metacarpal. Clinically, a thenar space infection presents with marked swelling around the bone of the thenar eminence and into the first web space (Fig. 98–10). The thumb is usually held inward on abducted position; thumb extension and opposition results in severe pain. Established thenar space abscesses will track dorsally through the first web space over the adductor and first dorsal interonneous muscles. Surgical decompression is best approached through a dorsal incision in the first web space, made perpendicular and extending to the web (15). After identifying neurovascular structure, the adductor fascia is unroofed, opening the abscess cavity. Additional palmar incisions are often used to gain the drainage of the area.

The midpalmar space is defined dorsally by the intrinsic muscles and volarly by the flexor tendon. The radial border of this space extends to the oblique septum at the 3rd metacarpal and the ulnar border to the hypothenar musculature.

Midpalmar space infections are less common than thenar space infections and almost always due to direct, penetrating trauma. Clinically, midpalmar space infections result in loss of palmar concavity. Dorsal swelling is also seen. Surgical decompression is best accomplished through wide palmar incisions, with resection of palmar fascia ensuring adequate drainage of the abscess cavity.

Human Bite Infections

Infections secondary to human bites are a frequently encountered clinical problem. Because they are often undertreated and misdiagnosed, the morbidity associated with these infections is severe (Fig. 98–11). Although the hand may become infected through nail biting, finger sucking, or full-thickness bites, the most serious form of human bite infection is the clenched fist injury. This injury commonly occurs during a fight when the patient's clenched fist strikes the tooth of another person. The resulting wound over the head of a metacarpal often results in immediate inoculation of the subcutaneous tissue, subtendinous space, and metacarpal phalangeal joint with saliva (Fig. 98–12). These wounds appear insignificant, and treatment is usually not sought for hours or days after the initial injury. Untreated injuries can result in pyarthrosis of the involved joint a subcutaneous/subfascial spread of infection (Fig. 98–13). Human saliva may contain as many as 100 million microorganisms per milliliter, with over 42 species of bacteria identified in the human mouth (4,16). Human bite infections are polymicrobial. The most commonly cultured organisms are *Staphylococcus aureus* and streptococcus (16–18). *Eikenella corrodens,* a gram-negative facultative anaerobe, has been cultured in 29% of cases (19). The presence of this organism has been associated with more severe human bite infections.

Delay in onset of treatment is directly proportional to unfavorable outcome. In general, human bites treated within 24 hours of injury rarely have serious complications (20). Delay in treatment past 24 hours results in significant morbidity. In optimal emergency-department settings, wounds are débrided, irrigated, and packed open. If joint penetration is established, further exploration and débridement is done in the operating room. More severe infections are taken directly to the operating room. In our patient population, all patients are admitted for 24 to 72 hours. Intravenous antibiotics are administered for *Eikenella corrodens* and gram-positive coverage. This usually is a combination of aqueous Pen G and a 1st- or 2nd-generation cephalosporin. At 24 hours, the wound is reexamined, after which regular wound care and hand therapy

FIG. 98–11. **A, B,** a neglected human bite (clenched fist injury) resulting in destruction of the metacarpal phalangeal joint.

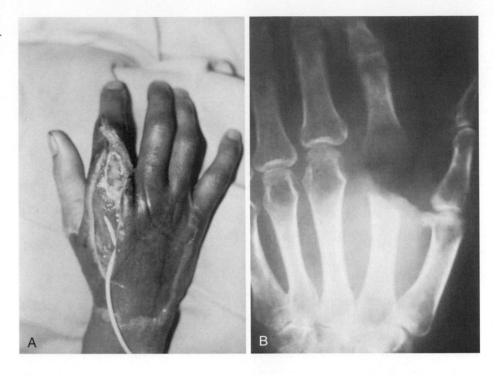

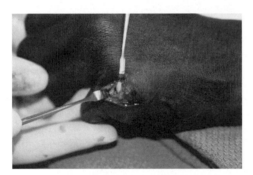

FIG. 98–12. A typical clenched fist injury demonstrating joint space penetration.

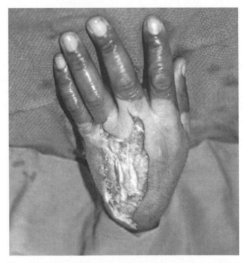

FIG. 98–13. Clenched fist infection, with proximal involvement of subcutaneous and subtendinous spaces.

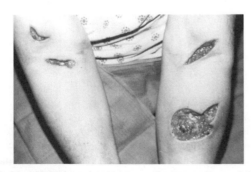

FIG. 98–14. Multiple subcutaneous abscesses in an intravenous drug abuser.

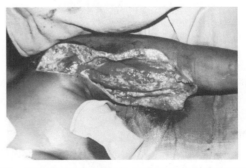

FIG. 98–15. Necrotizing fasciitis in an intravenous drug user that required wide débridement of skin and subcutaneous tissue. *S. aureus* and *E. coli* were cultured from the wound.

begin. Usually, after 48 to 72 hours, treatment is continued on an outpatient basis.

Other Infections

Domestic animal bites are a frequent cause of hand infections. Dog bites are most frequently seen, with more than half involving children. Basic principles of débridement and irrigation apply. Deep puncture wounds are left open, but fresh lacerations can be loosely closed after adequate treatment. Established infections are débrided and packed open. Multiple pathogens, including *Streptococcus viridans, Staphylococcus aureus, Pasteurella multocida,* and bacteroides species are frequently seen. Adequate antibiotic coverage is obtained with penicillin or ampicillin. Cat bites account for only 5% of all animal bites seen, but these injuries can be particularly virulent. These bites result in deep puncture wounds that are difficult to clean adequately. *Pasteurella multocida,* the most frequent pathogen identified, is often inoculated deep into tissues. Excision of these puncture wounds, along with copious irrigation and ampicillin antibiotic coverage, is the recommended treatment regimen (21).

Infection Secondary to Intravenous Drug Abuse

Upper-extremity infections that result from drug abuse continue to be a frequently encountered problem in urban medical centers. The most common sites of involvement are the dorsum of the hand, radial-dorsal area of the wrist, palmar aspect of the forearm, and the dorsum of the fingers at the PIP joint level (22). These patients can present with a wide spectrum of clinical problems including cellulitis, subcutaneous abscesses, flexor tenosynovitis, septic joints, and osteomyelitis (Fig. 98–14). The microorganism involved in these infections comes from a variety of sources including skin, saliva, and bowel. Necrotizing fasciitis is also seen in this patient population. It is a fulminant, life-threatening infection that frequently appears initially as a low-grade cellulitis. This rapidly progresses to necrotizing subcutaneous fasciitis, with skin necrosis and, occasionally, myonecrosis. Meleney (23) originally described this process as a hemolytic streptococcal gangrene, but a mixed flora is present in the majority of cases. Broad-spectrum antibiotics and radical débridement are necessary (Fig. 98–15). Despite this, mortality rates close to 10% are reported (24).

Postoperative Care

Attention to wound care and early initiation on hand therapy are important factors in achieving good functional results in treating hand infection. In general, with significant hand infections, wounds are débrided, irrigated, and packed open. Packing is usually removed 24 hours postoperatively. After packing removal, regular cleansing of the wound is initiated, along with gentle, active ROM under the supervision of a hand therapist. Wound cleansing is best done with mild antibacterial soap and soft scrub brushes. The use of splints may be helpful in enhancing joint motions. Early involvement by a hand therapist is critical in achieving a good functional result.

References

1. McGrath MH. Infection of the hand. In: McCarthy JG, May JW, Littler JW, eds. *The hand. Plastic surgery.* Vol. 8. Philadelphia: WB Saunders, 1990; 5529.
2. Kanavel AB. *Infections of the hand. A guide to the surgical treatment of acute and chronic suppurative processes in the fingers, hand and forearm.* Philadelphia: Lea and Febiger, 1933.
3. Neviaser RJ. Infections. In: Green DP, ed. *Operative hand surgery.* New York: Churchill Livingstone, 1982.
4. Mann RJ, Peacock JM. Hand infections in patients with diabetes mellitus. *J Trauma* 1977; 17:376.
5. Stern PJ, Staneck JL, et al. Established hand infections: a controlled prospective study. *J Hand Surg* 1983; 8:553.
6. Conales FL, Newmyer WL, and Kilgore ES. Treatment of felons and paronychias. *Hand clinics* 1989; 5(4):515.
7. Kilgore E, Brown L, Newmyer W, et al. Treatment of felons. *Am J Surg* 1975; 130:195.
8. Feder HM, Long SS. Herpetic Whitlow: Epidemiology, clinical characteristics, diagnosis, and treatment. *Am J Dis Child* 1983; 137:861.
9. Polayes I, Arons M. The treatment of herpetic Whitlow: a new surgical concept. *Plast Reconstr Surg* 1980; 65:815.
10. Gill MJ, Bryant HE. Oral acyclovic therapy of recurrent herpes simplex injection of the hand. *Antimicrobial Agents & Chemotherapy* 1991; 35(2):382.
11. Keyser J, Eaton RG. Surgical cure of chronic paronychia by eponychial marsupialization. *Plast Reconstr Surg* 1976; 58:66.
12. Frieland AE, Burkhalter WE, Mann RJ. Functional treatment of acute suppurative digital tenosynovitis. *Orthop Trans* 1981; 5:113.
13. Carter SJ, Burman SO, Mersheimer WL. Treatment of digital tenosynovitis by irrigation with peroxide and oxytetracycline. *Ann Surg* 1966; 163:645.
14. Neviaser RJ. Tenosynovitis. *Hand clinics* 1989; 5(4):525.
15. Burkhalter WE. Deep space infections. *Hand clinics* 1989; 5(4):553.
16. Shields C, Patzakis MJ, Meyers MH, et al. Hand infections secondary to human bites. *J Trauma* 1975; 15:235.
17. Dreyfuss UY, Singer M. Human bites of the hand: a study of 106 patients. *J Hand Surg* 1988; 13A:953.
18. Farmer CB, Mann RJ. Human bite infections of the hand. *South Med J* 1966; 59:515.
19. Ragan GM, Putnam JL, Cahill SL. *Eikenella corrodens* in human mouth flora. *J Hand Surg* 1988; 13A:953.
20. McConnell CM, Neale HW. Two-year review of hand infections at a municipal hospital. *Am Surg* 1979; 45:643.
21. Snyder CC. Animal bite wounds. *Hand clinics* 1989; 5(4):629.
22. Reyer FA. Infections secondary to intravenous drug abuse. *Hand clinics* 1989; 5(4):629.
23. Feingold DS. Gangrenous and crepitant cellulitis. *J Am Acad Dermatol* 1982; 6:289.
24. Schecter W, Meyer A, Schecter G, et al. Necrotizing fasciitis of the upper extremity. *J Hand Surg* 1982; 7:15.

99

Fractures and Dislocations of the Hand

John S. Taras, M.D., Richard D. Goldner, M.D., and J. Leonard Goldner, M.D., D.Sc (Hon)

The treatment of hand fractures and dislocations is determined by the circumstances of the injury. While skeletal injuries of the hand can be treated by common principles, many injury patterns have unique factors that must be considered to obtain an optimal outcome (1).

Once the injury occurs, the options for treatment depend upon the extent and severity of the skeletal and soft-tissue injuries. In addition, the patient's age, general health, hand dominance, occupations, avocations, ability to cooperate, and availability for follow-up affect the final choice of treatment.

Diagnosis and Treatment

CLINICAL EXAMINATION OF THE HAND

The injured hand should be examined, before administration of any anesthetic agents, to determine any vascular impairment, tendon, or nerve damage. A sterile bactericidal dressing should be applied over open wounds and a history obtained. Of particular concern are details about the contaminating factors in open injuries (2,3). The type of contaminant should be noted and appropriate antibiotic prophylaxis initiated.

PHYSICAL FINDINGS

The resting position of the hand is observed and deformities noted. Angulation of one or more digits will provide a clue to the mechanism of injury associated with single or multiple fractures or joint dislocations. Alignment of the digits in extension and flexion should be observed for rotational malalignment (4) (Fig. 99–1). Beyond identifying the injury to the skeletal system, a thorough examination of the hand should be performed and recorded. Specifically, the vascular status (5), sensibility, motor function, joint movement, tendon integrity, and wound status should be evaluated in all injuries.

X-RAY EXAMINATION

All injuries with the potential to have caused injury to the skeletal system of the hand should undergo x-ray examination. While most skeletal injuries are apparent on routine posteroanterior and lateral views, special studies may be necessary to identify particular types of injuries. Oblique views are of particular value for carpometacarpal fractures and dislocations. Stress views are used to identify ligamentous instability of the metacarpophalangeal joint (MPJ) of the thumb. Brewerton views may be needed to identify certain fractures of the metacarpal head.

COMPARTMENT SYNDROME

With crush injuries, the surgeon should be suspicious of compartment syndrome. Signs of pain with passive stretch associated with paresthesias in the digit could be secondary to nerve compression or due to the pain from the fractures; however, compartment syndrome should be considered when these symptoms are present. In assessing a crushed, swollen hand, compartment pressure determination is appropriate. If the compartment pressure is above 40 mm Hg in a normotensive individual, then compartment release is advocated. Fasciotomy of the intrinsic muscles of the hand may be accomplished through two dorsal longitudinal incisions between the 2nd and 3rd, and the 4th and 5th, metacarpals. Release of the thenar and hypothenar compartments is achieved through longitudinal incisions over the border of the respective compartments.

ANESTHESIA

In general, closed fractures requiring manipulation for reduction can be managed with local anesthesia. Injuries of the digits can be anesthetized through injection of either 1 or 2% lidocaine or 0.5% bupivacaine without epinephrine at the level of the metacarpal neck. Injection into the digit should be avoided, as this can lead to vascular embarrassment of the digit. Metacarpal injuries can be anesthetized using a wrist block or hematoma block at the site of the injury.

TREATMENT OF NONDISPLACED FRACTURES

Nondisplaced fractures are generally stable and require only buddy taping or simple splinting for 3 weeks (Fig. 99–2). Foam-padded aluminum (with much of the foam removed) or cotton-padded plaster splints should be applied while maintaining the MPJ in flexion and the interphalangeal joint (IPJ) in extension. X-rays should be taken weekly to ensure that no displacement of the fracture occurs.

TREATMENT OF DISPLACED FRACTURES

For displaced fractures, an attempt should be made at closed reduction after appropriate anesthesia has been obtained. After reduction and application of a splint to maintain the reduction, an x-ray is taken to assess the reduced position. If the position is acceptable, splinting is continued for 3 to 4 weeks, with weekly x-rays used to assess any loss of reduction. If, despite reduction attempts, the position of the fracture remains unacceptable, operative fixation of the fracture

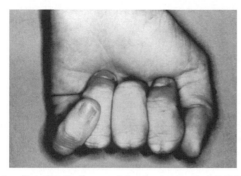

FIG. 99–1. Rotational alignment is checked with full fisting. Overlapping of the digits is observed in this patient with rotational malalignment. Rotational malalignment must be completely corrected to prevent functional impairment.

is indicated. Options for operative fixation of hand fractures include Kirschner wires (K-wires), intraosseous wires, screws and plates, and external fixation.

K-wires have the advantage of versatility and percutaneous placement. They can be removed easily, if percutaneous, or buried just beneath the skin. Their disadvantage is that, when placed percutaneously, they may fix tendons and skin, thereby limiting early mobilization of the adjacent joints. K-wires are biomechanically weaker than other methods of fixation and therefore may limit early mobilization (6). Size 0.032-inch and 0.045-inch diameter K-wires are best suited to fixation of most hand fractures. Recently introduced resorbable K-wires are biomechanically weaker than traditional stainless steel wires, but are useful when an implant needs to be buried in an area where subsequent removal of a permanent implant would prove difficult.

Intraosseous wires require open placement and can be technically challenging. When used, two intraosseous wires should be placed at 90° to each other, or in conjunction with a K-wire

FIG. 99–2. **A,** nondisplaced fracture of the proximal phalanx. **B, C,** it is best treated by buddy-taping, or **(D)** splinting foam-padded aluminum or molded plastic.

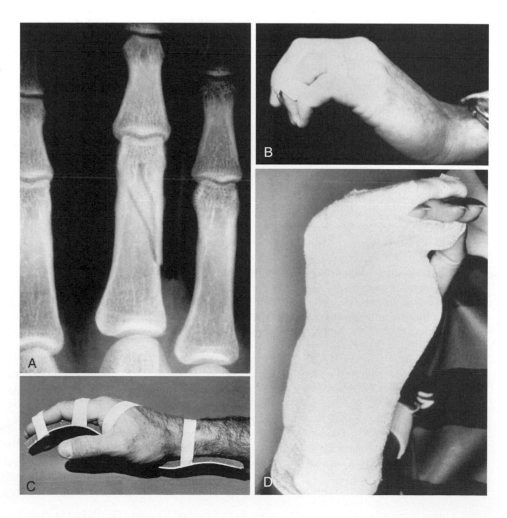

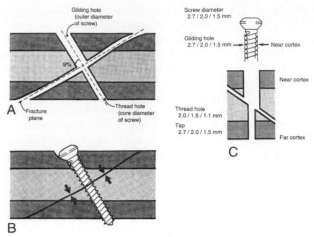

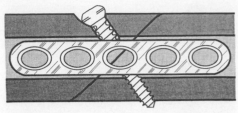

FIG. 99–4. Neutralization plate. After placement of a lag screw through the main fragments, a plate can be applied to obtain further stability. When this plate is used with eccentric drilling of the screws (i.e., without compression) it is termed a neutralization plate. This plate should be applied with at least two screws in each main fracture fragment.

FIG. 99–3. Lag screw. **A,** after the fracture is reduced and held with a clamp, the thread hole is drilled perpendicular to the fracture line, using the drill bit corresponding to the outer diameter of the screw. **B,** after the far cortex is tapped to cut the thread for the screw, the screw is seated so that compression of the fracture site is obtained. **C,** the correct drill and tap sizes for placement of lag screws in the hand.

to create the most stable construct (7–10). We generally prefer creating a more stable fixation construct using screws or plates when open reduction and fixation are required.

Screws and plates provide the most rigid internal fixation in the hand; thus, whenever possible, we use the most stable construct of screws and/or plates when open reduction is required (11,12). Screw fixation alone is appropriate for oblique, spiral, and intracondylar fractures (13). Plates are used for transverse and comminuted fractures. By achieving a stable fixation construct, the digits can be mobilized early after fixation, thus limiting tendon adhesions and joint stiffness. In the phalanges, 1.5-mm and 2.0-mm screws and plates are used, and in the metacarpals 2.0-mm and 2.7-mm implants are most appropriate. It must be kept in mind that fixation techniques with screws and plates are technically demanding, and there is little room for error, especially with implants such as the condylar blade plate.

Incisions should be planned to minimize dissection to avoid unnecessary scarring. In the digits, midlateral incisions are used to avoid disturbing the tendon system (14). The metacarpals are approached through longitudinal dorsal incisions between the metacarpals avoiding the extensor tendons.

At least two screws are needed to completely stabilize a fracture. Oblique and spiral fractures should be greater than twice the diameter of the fractured bone in order for screws to be used alone without fragmentation of the fracture ends. To obtain optimal compression, screws are oriented midway between the plane of the fracture and the longitudinal axis of the bone. When possible, screws should be applied to compress the fracture by overdrilling the proximal cortex to produce a gliding hole, so that the screw threads purchase the distal cortex (Fig. 99–3). The length of the screw used should be adequate to allow one thread of the screw to protrude from the opposite cortex to ensure adequate purchase. Care should be taken to ensure the tips of the screws are not impinging upon the tendons, limiting excursion or causing ten-

don attrition. Intraoperative fluoroscopy is particularly useful in assessing proper implant size and fracture alignment.

Plates are used for transverse and comminuted fractures and come in a variety of shapes and lengths designed for use in the hand. In any application, the plate used should be selected to provide fixation at two sites in each of the main fracture fragments. Straight plates are used for midshaft fractures, and T- or L-shaped plates (or minicondylar plates) are used for fixation of fractures of the neck or base. If fracture is oblique and a plate is used for fixation, then a compression screw can be used across the fracture and a neutralization plate applied (Fig. 99–4).

In certain fractures, it is inappropriate to utilize internal fixation; thus, external fixation is warranted. For open fractures requiring continued wound care because of extensive contamination, external fixation is advisable. Similarly, a pilon fracture, a fracture of the base of the middle phalanx, or a comminuted fracture of the base of the thumb metacarpal can be treated using external fixation (15–17).

TREATMENT OF OPEN WOUNDS

At the time of the initial wound débridement, all tight fascial compartments should be opened, open joints irrigated, and circulation reestablished. Meticulous excision of devitalized tissue and thorough irrigation are essential to prevent infection (2). Treating open wounds openly until it is appropriate to close them by direct suturing or additional soft-tissue coverage, or allowing secondary healing, will eliminate many complications (18). We routinely provide antibiotic prophylaxis for open fractures; a first-generation cephalosporin is given for simple wounds, with penicillin added to bite wounds and aminoglycosides added to farm injuries and severely contaminated wounds.

A simple longitudinal K-wire can be used for temporary fracture stabilization until the wounds have been managed to a point that will allow internal fixation. Likewise, segmental bone loss can be reconstructed after placement of a spacer such as poymethylmethacrylate or silicone. After adequate soft-tissue healing, the spacer is removed and a bone graft inserted.

CLOSED VS. OPEN TREATMENT OF COMPLEX HAND FRACTURES

Certain unstable fractures, if treated closed for a prolonged time, may result in stiffness, particularly in the proximal interphalangeal (PIP) joint, malunion, shortening, and nonunion.

Fractures of the shaft carry a larger risk of complications than do fractures of the base of the proximal phalanx, but both require special attention (19–22).

Eighty percent of extraarticular proximal phalangeal shaft fractures have an acceptable functional result when treated closed. An extensor splint with the wrist dorsiflexed 30°, the MCP joints flexed 70° to 95°, and the IP joints free for active flexion and extension is an acceptable method of management, provided the patient is seen at least 3 times a week during the first 2 weeks so that necessary adjustments are made, and the course of treatment is changed if the alignment and length are not satisfactory (23,24).

Fracture: Dislocation of the Digits by Anatomic Region

DISTAL PHALANX AND DIP JOINT

Distal Phalanx Fracture

With a closed fracture of the distal phalanx, the fingernail is usually elevated from a subungual hematoma expanding within the space between the nailplate and the nailbed, and can be decompressed through a hole made in the center of the nail plate distal to the germinal matrix. Closed fractures of the distal phalanx are treated by splinting with foam-padded aluminum taped in place, a Stack splint, or custom-fabricated thermoplastic material.

Most open fractures of the distal phalanx are contaminated and are treated open. When wounds require care beyond simple closure, a small K-wire can be used to stabilize the fracture fragments; then the soft-tissue injury is treated appropriately (25–27).

Mallet Finger

An extensor tendon tear at the insertion to the distal phalanx, or mallet finger, is managed by a contoured, foam-padded dorsal aluminum splint taped in place over the distal joint in neutral position. Constant splinting is required for 6 to 8 weeks, and the compliant patient is allowed to change the splint every few days without flexing the digit (28). Protective splinting is necessary for as long as 4 months in certain instances. The splint is not discarded until the patient is able voluntarily to hold the distal phalanx against resistance in a neutral position.

When the extensor digitorum communis is avulsed with a segment of bone from the dorsal lip of the distal phalanx, the injury is termed a *mallet fracture* (Fig. 99–5). The fragment may be small, medium, or large, and may include up to 50% of the articular surface. The small and medium fragments are managed with splinting similar to that of a mallet finger. If the fracture fragment encompasses 50% of the articular surface and it has been rotated and displaced dorsally, or the entire phalanx with the palmar articular surface is dislocated palmarward, open internal fixation can be considered. This may be accomplished with a fixation pin or a 30-gauge stainless-steel wire used as a tension band (26,29). Wehbe and Schneider's (26) review suggested that nonoperative treatment of mallet finger was safe and reliable, regardless of fragment size or subluxation.

When a mallet finger or fracture presents late, a period of splinting is again appropriate, but it should be continued for

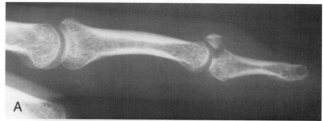
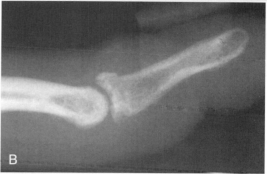

FIG. 99–5. Intraarticular displaced fracture of the proximal end of the distal phalanx. **A,** a bony mallet finger with a dorsal fragment of 40% of the articular surface moderately displaced. Palmar subluxation of the phalanx has not occurred. Anatomic reduction is not essential for satisfactory function. **B,** the degree of extension possible after closed treatment. The distal phalanx was immobilized with a dorsal splint in neutral position. Hyperextension causes ischemia of the edematous dorsal skin and occasionally palmar subluxation of the phalanx. Fifty-five degree flexion was possible. Hyperextension was present.

8 to 12 weeks. When splinting is unsuccessful and function is impaired, or significant pain is present, then a repair of the extensor tendon or arthrodesis can be considered.

Avulsion Fragment from the Flexor Surface of the Distal Phalanx

A bone fragment may be pulled off the distal phalanx when the flexor digitorum profundus is forcibly separated from its insertion as the digit is hyperextended. When this is the case, a palpable mass within the finger or palm is found with the absence of flexion of the distal joint. Lateral radiographs will show a bone fragment if it is attached to the tendon (Fig. 99–6A).

Surgical treatment is necessary to reattach the flexor tendon and the accompanying bone fragment to the distal phalanx (Fig. 99–6B). If the bone fragment is of substantial size, with a portion of the articular surface, then it is fixed to the body of the distal phalanx. If the fragment is small, it can be excised and the flexor tendon reattached to the distal phalanx fracture surface. A polypropylene suture is anchored to the end of the tendon, and the suture is brought through the soft tissue on either side of the phalanx adjacent to the nail plate. The sutures are then tied over the dorsum of the nail. Two interrupted absorbable sutures are placed through the tendon and the fragment and are passed into the adjacent soft tissue. A dorsal plaster splint is applied from the fingertips to the proximal forearm with the wrist in 30° of flexion. The repair is protected for 6 weeks, but passive flexion and dorsally blocked active extension are initiated within 24 hours after repair.

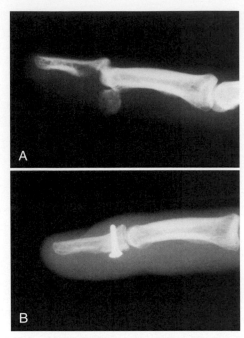

FIG. 99–6. **A,** avulsion of the base of the distal phalanx requires reduction. **B,** in this case, where a large fragment was avulsed, fixation was accomplished with a single 1.5-mm screw.

Collateral Ligament Avulsion from the DIP Joint

An injury will rarely cause radial or ulnar deviation of the distal phalanx without avulsion of the extensor mechanism but with avulsion of the collateral ligament. This injury is usually treated by closed manipulation and a circular cast that covers the entire finger. The cast is preferable to a splint for maintaining the reduction for 3 weeks and allowing the collateral ligament injury to heal. Splinting is then used on the opposite site of the collateral ligament for an additional 6 weeks.

Middle and Proximal Phalanx Fractures

Displacement of the phalangeal fragments depends on the forces that have caused the original fracture and the contractions of the extrinsic muscles, including the extensor digitorum communis, the flexor digitorum profundus, and the flexor digitorum superficialis. In addition, the intrinsic muscle attachments affect the position of the fragments by contraction of the lateral band as they pass over the proximal phalanx, across the PIP joint, and attaches into the distal phalanx. The imbalance between the intrinsics, the extrinsics, and the forces causing the fracture affects the final position. Once the fracture is reduced, the abnormal forces are neutralized (21,30). Phalangeal fractures that present with minimal or no displacement are treated with buddy-taping or splint immobilization. Displaced fractures that can be reduced can generally be managed with splint immobilization, but should be followed by weekly x-rays to ensure maintenance of proper reduction. Fractures that cannot be reduced by closed means require open reduction. The reduction criteria for middle and proximal phalangeal fractures are: less than 10° of lateral deviation, less than 20° angulation in the plane of motion, no rotational deformity, joint gap less than 2 mm, and joint step-off less than 1 mm.

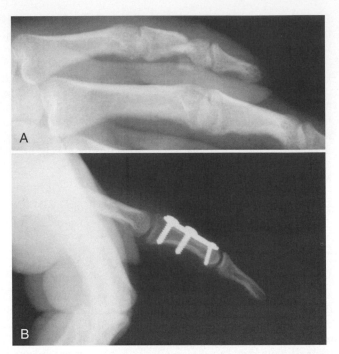

FIG. 99–7. Comminuted displaced fracture of the diaphysis of the middle phalanx of the little finger. **A,** bone defects with displacement of the cortical fragments. Joint surfaces are not involved. This much comminution implies severe soft-tissue injury. **B,** dorsal plate fixation provided stability and allowed early motion; however, the extensive soft-tissue damage, the bulk of the plate that interfered with gliding, and the persistent fibrosis in spite of early motion, resulted in a satisfactory radiograph but about 50% limitation of motion at the PIP and DIP joints.

The surgical approach to the proximal and middle phalanges can be made through either dorsolateral or midlateral incisions (14). The extensor hood is exposed and mobilized dorsally to visualize the fracture. Preservation of the peritenon and the periosteum is important to decrease adhesion formation. The shaft can be approached through the interval between the lateral band and the extensor tendon.

Shaft Fractures of the Proximal and Middle Phalanges

These fractures are usually managed by closed manipulation and extensor splinting, but if significant shortening or angulation occurs and the rotation does not respond to manipulation because of unequal muscle pull or soft-tissue interposition, then open reduction and internal fixation are necessary for anatomic reduction. Fixation may be obtained with pins, tension band wiring, 1.5-mm or 2.0-mm miniscrews—or, in certain severe deformities, a miniplate (31–35) (Figs. 99–7, 99–8).

Mobilization of long, ring, and little finger fractures usually requires that these three digits be taped together after the splinting has been continuous. Since the ulnar three digits flex and extend simultaneously, malrotation is prevented and motion is improved by simultaneous action of the ulnar three digits.

Intercondylar Fracture of the Distal End of the Middle and Proximal Phalanges

If the alignment is in a neutral position, flexion of the middle phalanx over a palmar aluminum splint attached to a plaster

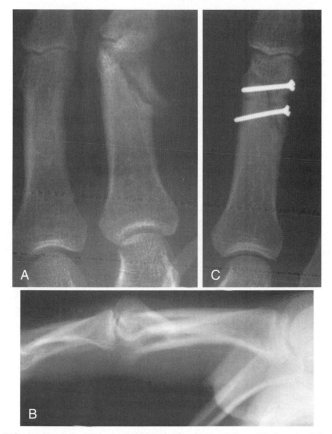

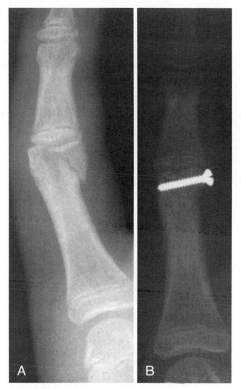

FIG. 99–8. Unstable juxtaarticular fracture of the distal end of the proximal phalanx. **A,** the fracture does not enter the joint. The condyle is displaced and malrotated. **B,** lateral view shows dorsal displacement and malrotation. **C,** lag screw fixation compressed the fragments and allowed early motion. A C wire, if used, requires longer immobilization and provides less rigid fixation.

FIG. 99–9. Intraarticular unicondylar displaced fracture of the distal end of the proximal phalanx. The open physis of the middle phalanx was not involved. **A,** this unicondylar fragment is 60% of the articular surface. **B,** postoperative radiograph showing fixation with full-threaded screw. Early protected motion was initiated, and results were satisfactory.

gauntlet that incorporates the lower forearm and the hand may be sufficient to maintain alignment. Rotation is corrected by observing the fingernail to see that it is directed towards the radial aspect of the palm. Splinting is continuous for 3 weeks, after which time flexion and extension are initiated. The digit is protected for an additional 2 weeks with a removable splint (6,25,27,36).

Intercondylar fractures of the distal end of the middle and proximal phalanges are often displaced. If condyles are spread but the collateral ligaments are intact, a closed reduction by traction followed by percutaneous fixation-pin stabilization may be sufficient (37). If one or both condyles are rotated; however, open reduction from either a medial and lateral incision or a dorsal incision is necessary to realign the fragments and stabilize the condyles to the diaphysis. Open reduction and internal fixation of the condyles may be necessary if the condyles cannot be aligned or if malrotation of one or both condyles persists (Fig. 99–9). Displaced unicondylar fractures can be treated by open reduction and internal fixation with 2.0-mm screws; or, alternately, open reduction and fixation of the condyles can be achieved with 0.032-inch transfixion pins for T- or Y-shaped condylar fractures. Open reduction and internal fixation is best accomplished with a miniplate. A mincondylar plate system is available in 1.5-mm and 2.0-mm sizes (21,28,33). The condylar blade forms an angle of 90°

with the side plate, and the blade length is approximately 14 mm. Proper application of this device requires preoperative planning and previous experience with internal fixation implants (32,35) (Fig. 99–10).

After open reduction, protective splinting is maintained for at least 3 weeks, but during that time daily movement without the splint is initiated. Early motion is helpful to reestablish articular cartilage congruity and to avoid adhesions (19,20,32,33).

PIP JOINT

Dorsal Dislocation of the PIP Joint

Dislocations of the PIP joint are classified by the location of the middle phalanx in relation to the proximal phalanx (palmar, dorsal, lateral).

Dorsal dislocation of the middle phalanx with avulsion of the volar plate from the middle phalanx is a common injury. The lateral radiograph demonstrates displacement and often a small volar fragment from the proximal end of the middle phalanx. To reduce the dislocation, the digit is pulled longitudinally and in slight extension for about 1 minute. As traction is exerted, flexion is continued to about 70°, while gentle but firm compression is applied over the dorsum of the middle phalanx. After reduction, the stability is tested with

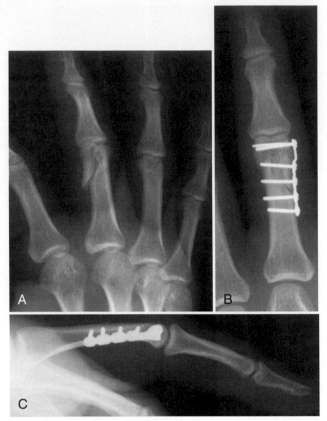

FIG. 99–10. Displaced intraarticular condylar fracture of the distal end of the proximal phalanx. **A,** postinjury, pretreatment displaced intraarticular condylar fracture of the distal end of the proximal phalanx. **B,** fixation with condylar plate applied on the lateral aspect of the phalanx to avoid fibrosis of the extensor mechanism (anteroposterior view). **C,** lateral view showing congruity of the PIP joint and realignment of the natural contour of the phalanx.

attention to the collateral ligaments. If the joint is completely stable, the involved digit is taped to the adjacent one for several weeks to allow assisted motion and to protect the joint from hyperextending. For dislocations that are unstable after reduction, a splint is applied with the PIP joint flexed 20° to 30° for 2 to 3 weeks before joint motion is started. Irreducible PIP joint dislocation may result from interposition of a collateral ligament, lateral band, or volar plate, and open reduction is required.

Dorsal Fracture: Dislocation of the PIP Joint

A dorsal dislocation of the middle phalanx, with a displaced fracture of its volar portion involving greater than 40% of the articular surface, is usually unstable. If the fracture is reduced and stable, it can be treated with a splint that blocks extension but allows flexion (Fig. 99–11). The PIP joint is blocked at 15° short of the point of instability (approximately 40°). The joint is then extended an additional 10° each week for 3 to 4 weeks. An alternative technique involves placing a pin percutaneously into the distal articular surface of the proximal phalanx with the PIP joint flexed (Fig. 99–12). If reduction is not maintained and alignment of the joint cannot be reestablished, then operative treatment is indicated. If the base of the middle phalanx is severely comminuted, the options are to surgically remove the bone fragments and to advance the volar capsule into the defect or to apply a distraction-mobilization device that will allow early motion (32,38,39).

Palmar Dislocation of the PIP Joint

Palmar dislocation of the middle phalanx may disrupt the central slip and dorsal capsule along with the palmar plate and one collateral ligament (40). This may result in flexion deformity of the PIP joint and hyperextension of the DIP joint (boutonniere deformity). The central extensor mecha-

FIG. 99–11. Intraarticular compression fracture of the proximal end of the middle phalanx (PIP joint) and distal phalanx lateral ligament fragment. **A,** fracture dislocation of the PIP joint with 5-mm fragment from the articular surface. Collateral ligament and fragment avulsion of 1 mm of distal phalanx. **B,** comminuted fragments managed in a dorsal splint. Early flexion motion was initiated after 10 days when extensor splint was used. Flexion and extension were limited moderately but overall function was satisfactory.

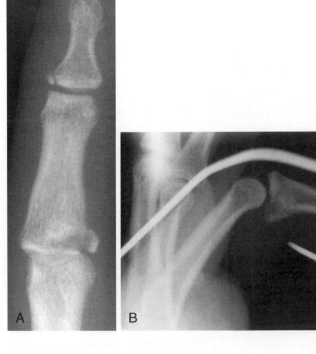

nism is disrupted and the lateral bands, which are normally dorsal to the axis of rotation of the PIP joint, are slipped palmar to that axis. Thus, the lateral bands, which normally extend the PIP joint, now flex the PIP joint and hyperextend the DIP joint. If PIP active extension is absent after reduction, the central attachment of the extensor tendon from the base of the middle phalanx has been disrupted. The PIP joint is immobilized in extension for 4 to 6 weeks, but the DIP joint is allowed to flex. Dorsal avulsion fractures of the middle phalanx having greater than 2 mm of displacement should be reduced and fixed.

Lateral Dislocation of the PIP Joint

Lateral PIP joint dislocation results from a lateral shear stress with collateral ligament disruption, often including a small

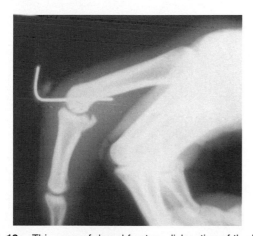

FIG. 99–12. This case of dorsal fracture dislocation of the PIP joint, which could not be successfully managed by splinting, was treated with an extension blocking pin that allows active flexion while preventing recurrent dorsal dislocation.

chip off the base of the middle phalanx. The radial collateral ligament is injured more frequently than the ulnar collateral ligament. Associated avulsion of the palmar plate and extensor mechanism at the base of the middle phalanx is noted. This is diagnosed clinically by stress testing and radiographically by assessing joint asymmetry. If stable, the joint is protected for several weeks. Large displaced avulsion fractures with articular cartilage attached to the fragment and with the fragment displaced and rotated may require open reduction and fixation with figure-of-eight suture or 0.032-inch pins (30,41,42).

METACARPOPHALANGEAL JOINT

Avulsion Fracture from Proximal Phalanx

An avulsion fracture from the proximal phalanx results from unequal rotary traction forces on the collateral ligament. A chip may occur either from the phalanx or the metacarpal head. If the displacement is 1 mm or less, the fracture is treated in a plaster splint with the digit in 20° of flexion at the MCP joint and neutral rotation. If the fragment involves greater than 20% of the articular surface, and is displaced greater than 2 mm, then surgical correction is indicated (29,30,43–45) (Fig. 99–13).

Dorsal MCP Joint Dislocation

The palmar plate and the collateral ligaments are the major supports of the MCP joint. They are relatively weak, and there are no extensions of the palmar plate that are analogous to the ligament prolongations at the PIP joint (checkrein ligaments) (25,30,46). In the "complex" dorsal MCP dorsal dislocation, the palmar plate pulls off the metacarpal and becomes interposed between the proximal phalanx and the metacarpal head, making closed reduction impossible. The metacarpal head is prominent on the palmar surface. The

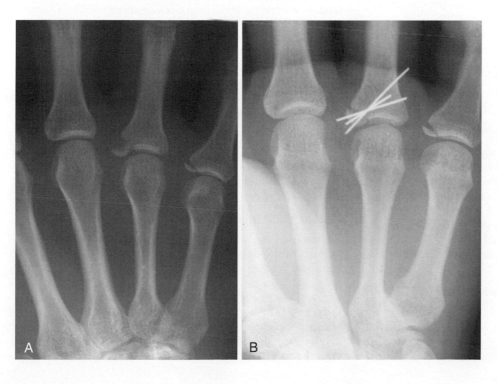

FIG. 99–13. Intraarticular avulsion of a fragment from the proximal end of the proximal phalanx. **A,** the collateral ligament was attached to the displaced intraarticular fragment that was malrotated at the base of the ring finger. The little finger fragment from the same position was displaced 2 mm. **B,** multiple C-wires were inserted under direct vision. Screw fixation of this kind of fragment may cause a stellate fracture of the fragment. The little-finger fragment was treated by closed splinting and early motion.

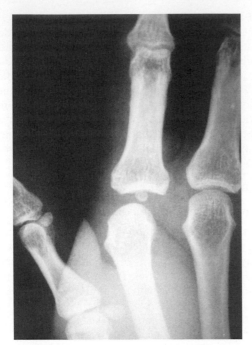

FIG. 99–14. The presence of a sesamoid within the joint on x ray is pathognomonic of an irreducible dislocation.

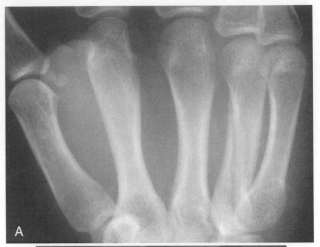

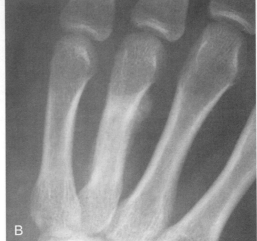

FIG. 99–15. Spiral oblique metacarpal shaft fracture. **A,** long oblique diaphyseal fracture with minimal shortening, mild malrotation, and minimal angulation. The 4th metacarpal is mobile. **B,** the malrotation was corrected under local block anesthesia, the hand was immobilized in a dorsal plaster splint, and abundant callus formed quickly. Motion was initiated on the 2nd day after injury. Final shortening was 2 to 3 mm, and function was excellent.

index finger dislocation is accompanied by a tight lumbrical on the radial side, and the flexor tendons are displaced to the ulnar aspect of the joint, acting like a Chinese finger trap mechanism. As extension or longitudinal traction is applied to the digit, the flexor tendons tighten, and the interposed palmar fibrous plate remains entrapped. This "complex" MCP joint dorsal dislocation is characterized by a palmar prominence of the metacarpal head that compresses the skin, a puckering of the adjacent skin as a result of relative relaxation of that skin, and a prominent dislocated phalanx on the dorsum (46).

A palmar sesamoid, usually contained within the palmar plate of the MCP joint, may become entrapped within the joint. The prereduction radiograph may show the sesamoid within the displaced volar plate. This would be pathognomonic of an irreducible dislocation (Fig. 99–14). The surgeon must recognize that forcible prolonged traction will damage the neurovascular structures and the soft tissues that are subjected to compression while traction is applied (46,47).

We prefer to use a longitudinal dorsal incision for surgical correction of complete MCP joint dislocations (48). The extensor hood is split next to the extensor tendon, and the capsule is divided. The interposed palmar plate is identified and reduced by tucking it back in place with a small elevator. The torn collateral ligaments are identified, and the phalanx is reduced with gentle traction and digital pressure (25,27,46,47,49). Reduction is usually stable, and early motion with extension block splinting can be initiated.

Incomplete (Simple) Dorsal Dislocation of the MCP Joint of the Index Ray

This uncomplicated incomplete dislocation of the MCP joint results from a hyperextension injury that stretches or partially tears the palmar plate from its attachment to the metacarpal neck. The postinjury radiograph will not show the sesamoid as entrapped, and the phalanx will be incompletely displaced dorsally. This injury is managed by slight extension, longitudinal traction, upward displacement of the metacarpal head, and flexion of the digit. Immobilization for 3 weeks using a dorsal flexion splint that allows active flexion during this time usually results in a stable mobile joint (25,27,46).

Palmar MCP Joint Dislocation

Palmar MCP dislocation is rare. Closed reduction may be impossible if the dorsal capsule is avulsed from the metacarpal neck and is interposed between the metacarpal head and the proximal phalanx. Attempted reduction by injecting local anesthetic into the joint may expand the capsule and allow reduction. Alternatively, a dorsal incision through the extensor mechanism is necessary to remove the dorsal capsule by splitting it longitudinally. The phalanx can then be realigned with the metacarpal.

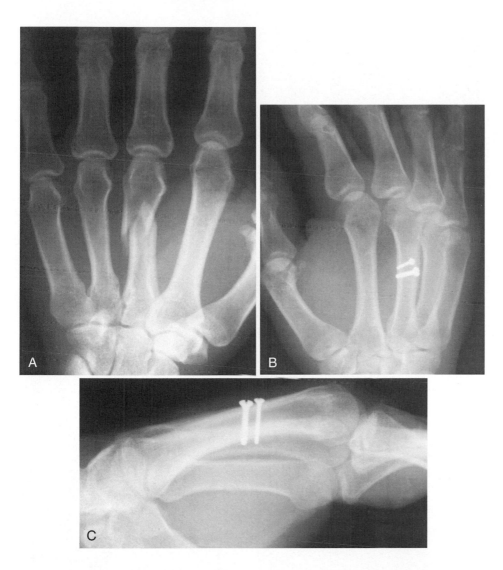

FIG. 99–16. Oblique angulated displaced fracture of the 3rd metacarpal diaphysis. **A,** there is 3 mm of shortening, moderate malrotation, and instability in an otherwise stable metacarpal. **B,** fixation by two threaded screws stabilizes the spiral oblique fracture. A postoperative plaster splint was used for 3 weeks, but early motion was initiated. **C,** lateral view shows the screws fixing both cortices, and the physiologic bowing is restored.

METACARPAL FRACTURES

Biomechanics of the Hand

The 1st, 4th, and 5th metacarpals are mobile and tolerate more residual dorsal angulation than do the stable 2nd and 3rd metacarpals. Shortening and angulation of the 2nd and 3rd metacarpals causes greater functional impairment than of the mobile metacarpals (25,50).

The interossei are attached to the metacarpal shafts, causing dorsal angulation of a metacarpal shaft fracture. Unstable fractures of the 2nd or 3rd metacarpals cause hyperextension at the MCP joint, whereas an unstable fracture of the 1st, 4th, or 5th metacarpal affects both the carpometacarpal (CMC) and MCP joints (but to a lesser degree than those fractures involving the static metacarpals). An anatomic reduction of the fractured shafts of the 2nd or 3rd metacarpals is desirable, whereas a modest degree of dorsal angulation may persist without affecting function after shaft fractures of the 1st, 4th, and 5th metacarpals.

General Concepts of Treatment of Metacarpal Fractures

Metacarpal fractures may be seen at the head involving the articular surface, at the neck with angulation and rotation, through the shaft with angulation and rotation, and at the base with intraarticular fracture and dislocation.

Closed metacarpal neck or shaft fractures with moderate angulation are treated by manipulation under regional anesthesia and stabilization with an extensor splint, with the MCP joints flexed 70° or a palmar splint that molds the metacarpal head upward. The wrist is held in 30° of dorsiflexion to relax the extensor muscles.

Minimally displaced fractures of the metacarpal shaft may be treated by functional bracing (51) or application of a gauntlet cast, an aluminum splint on the digit, and traction of the finger in a splint with the MCP joint flexed 70° and the digit held with clear tape (Fig. 99–15). Options for treatment include intramedullary flexible pin fixation or miniscrew fixation (Fig. 99–16). In addition, unstable metacarpal fractures may be managed with tension band wiring techniques or with miniplate fixation (Fig. 99–17).

Black and colleagues (52) compared several methods of internal fixation techniques for the treatment of metacarpal fractures. For metacarpal fixation, they conclude that dorsal plates with or without lag screws provide significantly more stability than do wire techniques, and the plate approaches that stability provided by normal metacarpal bones (20,25,27,33).

FIG. 99–17. Oblique unstable fracture of the index metacarpal. **A,** this oblique, displaced, malrotated, unstable fracture associated with significant soft-tissue injury was managed by internal fixation. **B,** a plate and lag screws were used to obtain stability before vascular reconstruction and other surgical procedures on this hand. The plate is contoured on the tension side of the fracture to maintain physiologic dorsal bowing.

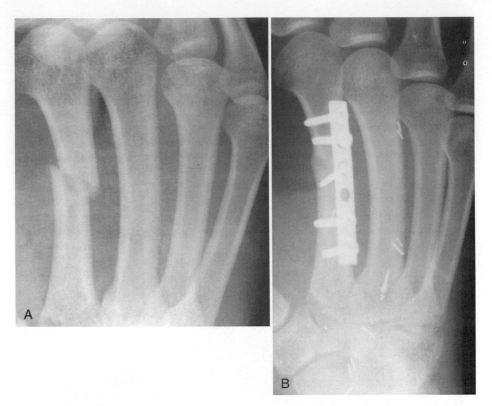

FIG. 99–18. This police officer had a human tooth injury that was not initially recognized as entering the joint. In the absence of proper débridement and antibiotic prophylaxis, a destructive joint sepsis ensued.

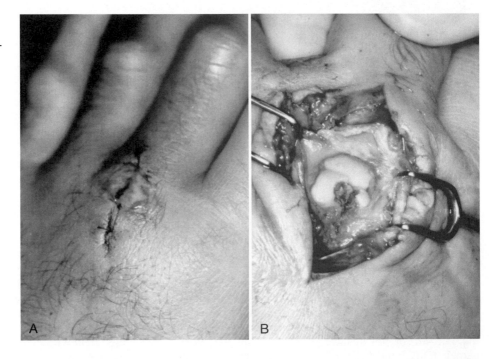

Intraarticular Metacarpal Fracture

Intraarticular metacarpal fractures are usually associated with soft-tissue trauma and, if open, are potentially infected. If a human bite is involved, the area should be excised thoroughly and irrigated, cephalosporin and penicillin given, and the fracture treated by external splints and, if necessary, fixation delayed (Fig. 99–18).

The Brewerton radiographic projection is made with the MCP joint flexed 65°, the dorsum of the hand next to the plate, and the tube angled 15° ulnar-to-radial. This visualizes the metacarpal head and any fractures that might affect it.

If small chondral fragments occur, these are removed. If a large osteochondral fragment is present, open reduction with fixation is performed (53). If the wound is initially open and potentially contaminated, and the decision to use internal fixation is made, the wound is treated open for 3 to 5 days before fixation.

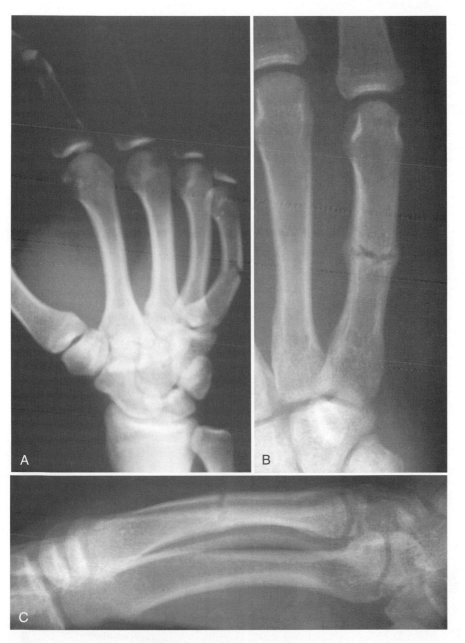

FIG. 99–19. Midshaft angulated fracture of the 5th metacarpal. **A,** the fracture is angulated dorsally. The metacarpal head is directed into the palm; this much angulation in a mobile metacarpal is not acceptable. **B,** after manipulation and splinting, callus formed quickly and satisfactory alignment was maintained. **C,** lateral view shows anatomic position and physiologic dorsal bowing.

A large osteochondral fragment with a collateral ligament attached to the fragment will require open reduction and internal fixation. Transverse fractures at the junction between the articular surface and the diaphysis may undergo aseptic necrosis. These large fragments have been managed by fixation pins passed from the neck directly into the fragment, similar to fixation of a fractured neck of the femur. The extensor mechanism is split from the dorsum, so that the joint surfaces are visible with anatomic reduction obtained and early motion initiated.

Severely comminuted fractures limited to the metacarpal head distal to the collateral ligament are treated with early protected motion. Comminuted intraarticular fractures with severe destruction of the cartilage of the head of the metacarpal are managed by arthroplasty, using a silicone or silicone-Dacron prosthesis, or collagen interposition. In young or middle-aged patients, other options include: an osteochondral allograft of the metacarpal head and part of the

shaft, transfer of a vascularized or nonvascularized autograft of metatarsal head to the metacarpal, an iliac graft with periosteal covering or perichondrium from the rib that may remodel as a metacarpal head, or arthrodesis of the MCP joint.

Metacarpal Neck Fracture

The most common metacarpal neck injury involves the 5th metacarpal and is caused by a direct blow with the clenched fist. This is called a "boxer's fracture." The head of the metacarpal is displaced palmarward, the shaft moves dorsally, and the tip of the little finger rotates toward the radial side of the palm. Soft-tissue swelling occurs on the dorsum, and the alignment of the fragments, except for rotation, is difficult to discern from external examination. A radiograph will show the degree of angulation on the oblique and lateral projections. A dorsal angulation of 40° is acceptable in the 5th metacarpal (13,54), and 30° in the 4th metacarpal, but only 15° dorsal angulation is acceptable in the index and long metacarpals. A fracture of the 5th metacarpal with 15° or less angulation is treated by a short dorsal splint holding the wrist at 30° of elevation and the MCP joint at maximum flexion, which may be only 45° because of edema. The extension splint extends to the PIP joints of the ring and little fingers, and these digits are allowed motion immediately. Immobilization is for 3 to 4 weeks (Fig. 99–19).

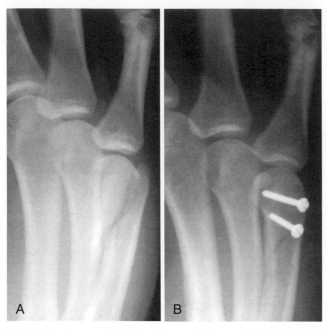

FIG. 99–20. Long spiral oblique fracture of the 5th metacarpal adjacent to the joint. **A,** the long oblique fracture does not involve the articular cartilage. Four mm of shortening occurred, and the fracture was unstable. **B,** internal fixation provided anatomic reduction and allowed early protected motion.

FIG. 99–21. Displaced comminuted midshaft third metacarpal fracture. **A,** moderate angulation occurred, shortening was present, and instability existed. **B,** after traction was applied to the digit, fixation was obtained with percutaneous C-wires that penetrated the index metacarpal before entering the long metacarpal. Adequate length and physiologic rotation were obtained. The pins are inserted after the intrinsic muscles are displaced palmarward. The 3rd metacarpal is about 4 mm more dorsal than the 2nd, and that relationship is maintained if possible.

If the fracture is angled greater than 15°, local anesthesia is used and a reduction is attempted. The distal fragment is disimpacted by traction and manipulation, palmar pressure is applied to the head of the metacarpal through the proximal phalanx, and dorsal pressure is applied to the apex. A dorsal splint that holds the MCP joints of the ulnar three digits in maximum flexion is used, and the PIP joints are free to move. X rays are checked weekly to monitor fracture position, and the splint is replaced if it loosens after swelling subsides with the hand immobilized for 4 weeks.

Excessive flexion of the distal fragment can lead to hyperextension of the MCP joint and discomfort of the metacarpal head, which is prominent in the palm. If the angulation is greater than 40° and there is concern about maintaining the reduction closed, either an intramedullary K-wire is inserted from proximal-to-distal or a percutaneous K-wire is inserted from the ulnar aspect of the metacarpal, avoiding the extensor mechanism. This fixation pin is passed into the 4th metacarpal shaft and remains in place approximately 14 days.

A pretreatment clinical test to determine if closed reduction and cast immobilization are adequate, or whether open reduction might be necessary, was described by Rowland and Green (27). Wrist block anesthesia is used, and when pain is relieved the patient is asked to extend the digits to neutral position. If the little finger shows a position of 45° flexion at the PIP joint and hyperextension at the MCP joint, the metacarpal head should be elevated as close to neutral as possible. Closed manipulation is attempted. The test is repeated and, if improvement occurs, immobilization without pin fixation is considered. If reduction is not possible, percutaneous or intramedullary pinning is considered (36).

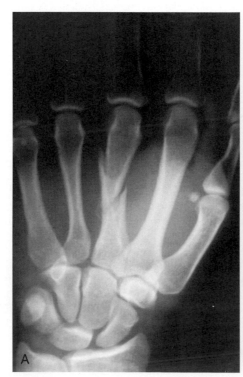
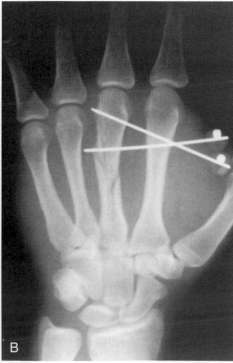

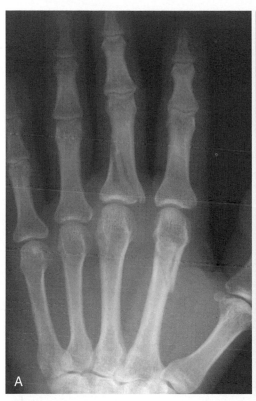
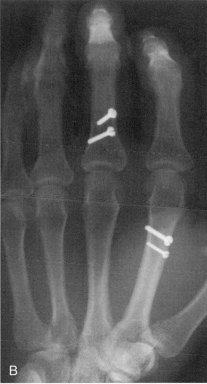

FIG. 99–22. Long oblique fracture of the proximal half of the proximal phalanx of the long finger, with oblique fracture of the distal end of the index metacarpal. **A,** the long finger fracture is malrotated with minimal displacement, and the index metacarpal is in satisfactory alignment. **B,** internal fixation with screws was elected to maintain the existing position and to initiate early motion. The functional end result was excellent.

Transverse and Short Oblique Metacarpal Shaft Fractures

Transverse shaft fractures are usually caused by a direct blow, and result in dorsal angulation secondary to interosseous muscle contractions. The midmetacarpal shaft fracture demonstrates more bowing than the proximal fracture. The intermetacarpal ligaments prevent shortening of 2nd and 3rd metacarpal fracture but have less effect on 4th and 5th metacarpal injuries.

A fracture that is minimally displaced without malrotation is treated by a molded short-arm cast or a hand-based functional brace with padded pressure on the metacarpal, forcing the head upward and the fracture site palmarward (51,55) (Fig. 99–19). Malrotation is determined by testing the position of the fingertip when the MCP joint is in maximum flexion.

Malrotation of the metacarpal shaft, or dorsal angulation greater than 10° in the 2nd and 3rd metacarpals should be manipulated and improved. If this is not possible, open reduction and internal fixation should be considered (Fig. 99–20). Shortening of the 2nd and 3rd metacarpals greater than 3 mm, or a combination of shortening malrotation and angulation, may require open reduction with interfragmentary screws (see Fig. 99–16). Alternatively, the fractured metacarpal can be pinned to the adjacent metacarpal (33) (Fig. 99–21).

Multiple metacarpal fractures may be managed by percutaneous pin fixation after reduction and maintenance of the MCP joints at maximal flexion. Interfragmentary screw fixation for long oblique fractures (Fig. 99–22) or plate fixation for transverse fractures (Fig. 99–23) allows early mobilization in the multiply traumatized hand. The surgeon must remember that the metacarpals are not in a horizontal plane when viewing the metacarpal shafts from the ulnar side. Severely displaced metacarpal shaft fractures that are transverse may require open reduction and rigid miniplate fixation (3,56).

Comminuted Metacarpal Shaft Fractures or Loss of Metacarpal Substance

A comminuted fracture without loss of substance or shortening may be managed closed with a gauntlet cast and an aluminum splint to maintain slight traction, proper rotation, and physiological dorsal bowing (Fig. 99–24). External fixation of closed or open fractures will provide early stabilization, allow easy wound management, and maintain length even with extensive comminution or segmental bone loss, so that bone grafting may be performed as skin coverage is provided. This external fixation technique permits simultaneous soft-tissue and fracture management. Also, while the external fixator is in place for 6 to 8 weeks, bone may form spontaneously to partially fill the gap (15,19,33,36).

CARPOMETACARPAL JOINTS

Fracture: Dislocation of CMC Joints 2 Through 4

Dislocation of the CMC joints, excluding the thumb, is frequently missed in the patient who has had severe hand trauma. The proximal transverse metacarpal arch is flattened, and excessive palmar and dorsal edema occur. Without appropriate radiograph projections, the displacement of the metacarpals may be missed. The metacarpals are usually displaced dorsally, and such injuries most frequently involve the mobile 4th and 5th CMC joints. The radiographic alteration is usually visible on the oblique view of the hand in both supination and pronation (19).

FIG. 99–23. Multiple metacarpal shaft fractures with displacement. **A,** extraarticular oblique fracture of the neck of the second metacarpal with malalignment. Also, there is an oblique fracture of the 3rd metacarpal with moderate displacement and a transverse metacarpal shaft fracture of the 4th metacarpal. **B,** radiograph showing postreduction fixation with 0.026-inch pin for the 2nd metacarpal. This pin migrated moderately and was removed at 3 months. A five-hole plate stabilized the 3rd metacarpal, and a five-hole plate with four screws was used for stabilizing the 4th metacarpal. The extent of the injury is reflected in the internal fixation of both the radius and ulna.

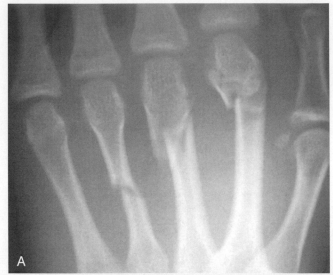

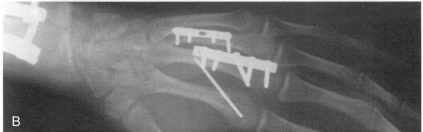

FIG. 99–24. Comminuted 4th metacarpal fracture in satisfactory position. **A,** although comminution has occurred, there is minimal shortening and satisfactory position of the metacarpal. **B,** external splinting was used for this fracture. Position was maintained, and the end result was excellent.

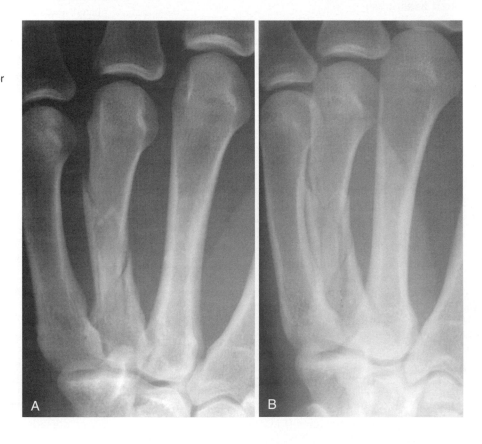

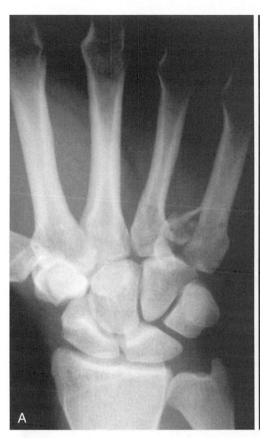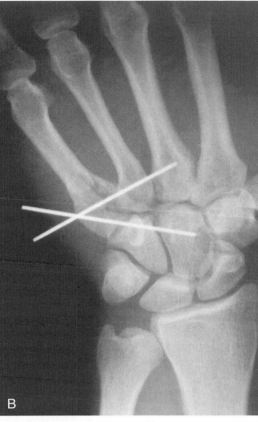

FIG. 99–25. A comminuted, displaced intraarticular fracture at the base of the 5th metacarpal. **A,** the shaft of the metacarpal is displaced to the ulnar side. The articular surface is damaged, and the fragment is about 40% of that surface. **B,** traction and manipulation resulted in satisfactory position. Percutaneous pins were used to maintain the reduction. An image intensifier was helpful.

Reduction of these fracture dislocations is usually accomplished by longitudinal traction and simultaneous digital pressure on the base of the metacarpals, with upward displacement of the distal end of the metacarpal. To maintain reduction, percutaneous fixation pins are used. Placement of transverse pins from one metacarpal to the other is not advisable because this flattens the palm and interferes with anatomic realignment. Supportive splints are changed and readjusted as edema subsides. The pins are maintained for 4 weeks, and the hand is kept in the protective position by removable splints for an additional four weeks.

Fracture: Dislocation of the 5th CMC Joint

Fracture dislocation of the 5th CMC joint may be overlooked because of dorsal edema and a straight lateral radiograph (57). Examination will show severe pain in response to digital pressure over the involved joint. The radiograph should be taken with the forearm in 30° of pronation (oblique pronation). This projection will usually show the dorsal displacement of the 5th metacarpal by the extensor carpi ulnaris muscle. Reduction is obtained by longitudinal traction on the hand, dorsiflexion of the wrist, direct pressure against the base of the fifth metacarpal, and moderate abduction of the little finger with rotary supination maneuver. A percutaneous pin is inserted between the little and ring metacarpals (Fig. 99–25). The pin should be directed from palmar to dorsal to avoid the motor branch of the ulnar nerve. A hand forearm cast is applied for stabilization, and the pin remains in place for 4 weeks.

Thumb Fractures and Dislocations

Fractures at the thumb proximal phalanx and metacarpal are usually caused by a fall on the hand, a twisting mechanism that affects the projected thumb, or a direct blow of the fist against a firm object. Extraarticular thumb proximal phalanx fractures often can be managed with external immobilization, but intraarticular fractures require reestablishing joint congruity and internal fixation (Fig. 99–26).

Extraarticular Fractures of the Thumb

Extraarticular fractures of the thumb usually involve the metaphyseal-diaphyseal junction. The distal metacarpal is extended and abducted, and a counterforce is applied directly over the fracture site as longitudinal traction is applied simultaneously for reduction. Closed manipulation is usually sufficient to correct malposition. The reduction is maintained in a thumb-hand-forearm cast. If the fracture is unstable or if the patient is noncompliant, a 0.045-inch percutaneous fixation pin is used along with the cast.

Intraarticular Fractures of the Base of the First Metacarpal

The Bennett fracture is an intraarticular fracture dislocation of the first metacarpal trapezium joint, with a fragment of the metacarpal held by the intermetacarpal ligament (Fig. 99–27). The remaining metacarpal is displaced laterally by the abductor pollicis longus and simultaneous contraction of the adductor pollicis that pulls the distal metacarpal towards the palm and accentuates lateral displacement of the proxi-

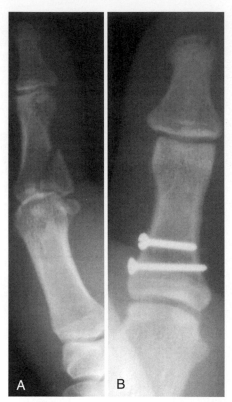

FIG. 99–26. Intra-articular fracture of the proximal end of the proximal phalanx of the thumb. **A,** the large displaced intraarticular fragment is unstable. There is a 3-mm gap, malrotation, and minimal lateral displacement of this 50% fragment. **B,** after fixation with two full-threaded screws, the alignment is anatomic. Early motion was initiated.

mal segment. This deformity is usually managed after obtaining regional anesthesia. Longitudinal traction is applied to the thumb, direct pressure is placed on the base of the first metacarpal, and the first metacarpal head is abducted and extended until a congruous joint results. The mechanism of manipulation is abduction, extension, pronation, and opposition in line with the 1st or 2nd metacarpal. The tip of the thumb is in a horizontal line with the hook of the hamate. The surgeon then inserts a 0.045-inch percutaneous fixation pin 10 mm distal to the articular surface of the first metacarpal and directed toward the base of the second metacarpal (see Fig. 99–27). This fixation is reinforced with a plaster splint or cast that extends to the DIP joint of the thumb, holds the palm and hand in 30° of dorsiflexion, and extends proximally to the forearm.

The Rolando fracture is a comminuted intraarticular lesion of the proximal end of the metacarpal with fragment displacement. The options for treatment of this lesion are (51,55): (a) a transfixion pin through the proximal end of the proximal phalanx with a traction bow and a cast. This mechanism avoids pin fixation of the comminuted area and allows a few degrees of motion once the edema has subsided; (b) percutaneous transfixion with a 0.062-inch pin between the 1st and 2nd metacarpals that will maintain satisfactory position while healing is occurring. The pin should remain in place for approximately 4 weeks; and (c) open reduction,

which may be advisable if the palmar and dorsal fragments are large, malrotated, and displaced, and do not realign with longitudinal traction and palmar abduction. Internal fixation with 2.0-mm screws or fixation pins is possible, after which external plaster splints or casts are used to maintain the position.

THUMB MCP JOINT INJURIES

Ulnar Collateral Ligament Avulsion

Ulnar collateral ligament avulsion (gamekeeper's thumb) is the most common injury involving the thumb MCP joint. The ligament, often with a bone fragment attached, is typically avulsed from the proximal phalanx but can be avulsed from the metacarpal attachment, or the ligament may rupture in its central portion. Additionally, unrecognized injuries occurring with gamekeeper's or "skier's" thumb include tears of the palmar plate or the dorsal capsule. This combination of in-

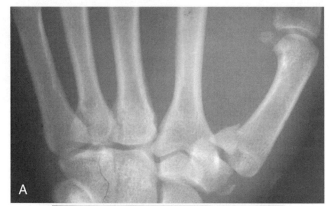

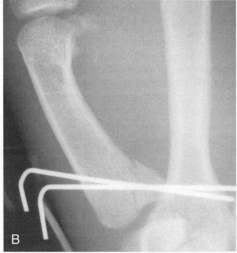

FIG. 99–27. An intraarticular fracture of the base of the first metacarpal (Bennett fracture). **A,** the intraarticular triangular fragment is attached to the intermetacarpal ligament. The abductor pollicis longus displaced the fist metacarpal, and the contraction of the adductor muscle aggravated the deformity. **B,** traction was applied, and closed percutaneous fixation with 0.062-in pins provided satisfactory fixation after the pins were inserted into the 2nd metacarpal. The pins are not required to cross the fracture fragment if reduction is obtained and the pins stabilize the 1st metacarpal to the 2nd.

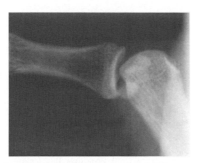

FIG. 99–28. Acute tear of the ulnar collateral ligament, dorsal capsule, and palmar capsule. This stress radiograph demonstrates the severe displacement of the proximal phalanx of the thumb toward the radial side associated with the soft-tissue tear on the ulnar side. With this severe deformity and displacement of the ulnar collateral ligament, open surgery is usually necessary. With lesser tears, closed treatment is satisfactory.

juries results in displacement of the thumb proximal phalanx in a radial palmar direction. Metacarpophalangeal flexion with stress to the radial side is tested and the right and left sides are compared. A stress radiograph is taken, with a fulcrum placed between the right and left metacarpal heads and the phalanges taped together. A deviation of the phalanx of less than 30° indicates a probable incomplete tear. Plaster immobilization, with the digit molded toward the ulnar and dorsal directions of the metacarpal head, is recommended for 4 weeks. Splinting and partial protection are necessary for an additional 6 weeks (19,33,43,47).

If deviation of the MCP joint to the radial side is greater than 30°, a complete ulnar collateral ligament avulsion is suspected, along with a dorsal capsular tear (Fig. 99–28). If the radiograph shows a displaced intraarticular fracture involving more than 20% of the articular surface, open reduction is indicated. If there is an avulsion fracture with displacement of the fragment greater than 5 mm, then open reattachment is indicated (6,22). If the combined information from the history, clinical examination, and stress radiographs under local anesthesia indicates that the ligament is displaced outside the adductor aponeurosis (Stener lesion), open repair is indicated.

PEDIATRIC PHYSEAL PLATE INJURIES

The weakest portion of the immature skeleton is the physeal plate. Most pediatric fractures, therefore, occur through the physeal plate. Fortunately, most pediatric hand fractures do not require reduction (59). If the germinal layer is not traumatized, growth disturbance does not occur. If the germinal layer is affected, there may be a localized disturbance of growth resulting in partial arrest or complete cessation of growth throughout part or all of the physeal plate (60).

If the fracture extends through the junction of the metaphysis and the diaphysis outside the physeal plate, growth will not be disturbed and healing through cancellous bone will occur rapidly. However, malposition of the fragments at this site may result in a deformity that can be improved with remodeling.

If the fracture extends into the joint and through the articular cartilage and involves both the physis and the articular surface, open reduction is usually necessary to realign the cartilage fragments anatomically and to diminish the changes

of growth disturbance and traumatic arthrosis. Intraepiphyseal injuries may involve the secondary centers of ossification and the articular cartilage. These are not visible on radiographs. If the force has been severe and the deformity is obvious, open operation may be necessary to replace these fragments.

Hand Therapy Following Fractures

Depending on their type and location, certain hand fractures may be treated by external immobilization followed by an exercise program. Others are best treated by closed reduction and pinning, or by open reduction and internal fixation. In all hand fractures, however, treating the bony injury is only part of the challenge. Apart from fracture reduction that restores intraarticular congruity and maintains normal length and rotation of the digit, the joints must be appropriately positioned when treating fractures in casts or splints. Immobilization in the "intrinsic plus" position, elevation of the hand to decrease edema, and movement of the uninjured digits are important. Active protected motion of the fractured digit should be initiated as soon as safe, to aid in preventing contractures (61). Internal fixation with miniscrews and plates must be stable, so that active protected motion can be initiated to minimize adhesions and stiffness and to decrease edema.

Although many patients with hand fractures can regain motion and strength in a home exercise program, certain individuals require a vigorous, supervised program consisting of dynamic splinting, edema control, active exercises, and (occasionally) use of a continuous passive motion machine to achieve the best result. Anatomic bony alignment on the radiograph does not always indicate good hand function.

References

 1. Davis TRC, Stothard J. Why all finger fractures should be referred to a hand surgery service: a prospective study of primary management. *J Hand Surg* 1990; 15B:299.
 2. Gustilo RB, ed. *Management of open fractures and their complications. Saunders' monographs in clinical orthopaedics.* Vol 4. Philadelphia: WB Saunders, 1982.
 3. McLain RF, Steyers C, Stoddard M. Infections in open fractures of the hand. *J Hand Surg* 1991; 16A:108.
 4. Royle SG. Rotational deformity following metacarpal fracture. *J Hand Surg* 1990; 15B:124.
 5. Nunley JA, Goldner RD, Urbaniak JR. Skeletal fixation in digital replantation. *Clin Orthop* 1987; 214:66.
 6. Namba RS, Kabo JM, Meals RA. Bio-mechanical effects of point configuration in Kirschner wire fixation. *Clin Orthop Rel Res* 1987; 214:19.
 7. Lister G. Intraosseous wiring of the digital skeletal. *J Hand Surg* 1978; 3:427.
 8. Zimmerman NB, Weiland AJ. Ninety-ninety intraosseous wiring for internal fixation of the digital skeleton. *Orthopaedics* 1989; 12:99.
 9. Hung LK, So WS, Leung PC. Combined intramedullary Kirschner wire and intra-osseous wire loop for fixation of finger fractures. *J Hand Surg* 1989; 14B:171.
10. Green TL, Noellert RC, Belsole RJ, et al. Composite wiring of metacarpal and phalangeal fractures. *J Hand Surg* 1989; 14A:665.
11. Nunley JA, Kloen P. Biomechanical and functional testing of plate fixation devices for proximal phalangeal fractures. *J Hand Surg* 1991; 16A:991.
12. Mann RJ, Black D, Constine R, et al. A quantitative comparison of metacarpal fracture stability with five different methods of internal fixation. *J Hand Surg* 1985; 10A:1024.
13. Ford DJ, El-Hadidi S, Lunn PG, et al. Fractures of the phalanges: results of internal fixation using 1.5-mm and 2-mm A.O. screws. *J Hand Surg* 1987; 12B:28.
14. Field LD, Freeland AE, Jabaley ME. Mid-axial approach to the proximal phalanx for fracture fixation. *Contemp Orthop* 1992; 25:133.

15. Freeland AE. External fixation for skeletal stabilization of severe open fractures of the hand. *Clin Orthop* 1987; 214:93.

16. Parsons SW, Fitzgerald JAW, Shearer JR. External fixation of unstable metacarpal and phalangeal fractures. *J Hand Surg* 1992; 17B:151.

17. Shehadi SI. External fixation of metacarpal and phalangeal fractures. *J Hand Surg* 1991; 16A:544.

18. Suprock MD, Hood JM, Lubahn JD. Role of antibiotics in open fractures of the finger. *J Hand Surg* 1990; 15A:761.

19. Green TL, Noellert RC, Belsole RJ. Treatment of unstable metacarpal and phalangeal fractures with tension band wiring techniques. *Clin Orthop* 1987; 214:78.

20. Hall RF Jr. Treatment of metacarpal and phalangeal fractures in noncompliant patients. *Clin Orthop* 1987; 214:31.

21. Jones WW. Biomechanics of small bone fixation. *Clin Orthop* 1987; 214:11.

22. Reyes FA, Latta LL. Conservative management of difficult phalangeal fractures. *Clin Orthop* 1987; 214:23.

23. Maitra A, Burdett-Smith P. The conservative management of proximal phalangeal fractures of the hand in an accidental and emergency department. *J Hand Surg* 1992; 17B:332.

24. Chow SP, Pun WK, et al. A prospective study of 245 open digital fractures of the hand. *J Hand Surg* 1991; 16B:137.

25. Goldner RD, Goldner JL. Fractures and dislocations of the hand. In: Sabiston DC, ed. *Textbook of surgery.* Philadelphia: WB Saunders, 1986; 1454.

26. Wehbe MA, Schneider LH. Mallet fractures. *J Bone Joint Surg (Am)* 1984; 66:658.

27. Green DP, Rowland SA. Fractures and dislocations in the hand. In: Rockwood CA, Green DP, eds. *Fractures in adults.* 2nd ed. Philadelphia: JB Lippincott, 1984.

28. Stern PJ, Wieser MJ, Reilly DG. Complications of plate fixation in the hand skeleton. *Clin Orthop* 1987; 214:59.

29. Jupiter JB, Sheppard JE. Tension wire fixation of avulsion fractures in the hand. *Clin Orthop* 1987; 214:113.

30. McCue FC, Honner R, Johnson MC Jr, et al. Athletic injuries of the proximal interphalangeal joint requiring surgical treatment. *J Bone Joint Surg (Am)* 1970; 52:937.

31. Vanik RK, Weber RC, Matloub HS, et al. The comparative strengths of internal fixation techniques. *J Hand Surg (Am)* 1984; 9:216.

32. Agee JM. Unstable fracture dislocations of the proximal interphalangeal joint: treatment with the force couple splint. *Clin Orthop* 1987; 214:101.

33. Hastings H. Unstable metacarpal and phalangeal fracture treatment with screws and plates. *Clin Orthop* 1987; 214:37.

34. Brennwald J. Bone healing in the hand. *Clin Orthop* 1987; 214:7.

35. Büchler U, Fischer T. Use of a minicondylar plate for metacarpal and phalangeal periarticular injuries. *Clin Orthop* 1987; 214:53.

36. Green DP, Anderson JR. Closed reductions and percutaneous pin fixation of fractured phalanges. *J Bone Joint Surg (Am)* 1973; 55:1651.

37. O'Rourke SK, Gaur S, Barton NJ. Long-term outcome of articular fractures of the phalanges: an 11-year follow-up. *J Hand Surg (Br)* 1989; 14:183.

38. Eaton RG, Malerich MM. Volar plate arthroplasty for the proximal interphalangeal joint: a 10-year review. *J Hand Surg* 1980; 5:260.

39. Stern PJ, Roman RJ, Kiefhaber TR, et al. Pilon fractures of the proximal interphalangeal joint. *J Hand Surg* 1991; 16A:844.

40. Vicar AJ. Proximal interphalangeal joint dislocations without fractures. *Hand Clin* 1988; 4:5.

41. McElfresh EC, Dobyns JH, O'Brien ET. Management of fracture dislocation of the proximal interphalangeal joints by extension-block splinting. *J Bone Joint Surg (Am)* 1972; 54:1705.

42. Stener B. Displacement of the ruptured collateral ligament of the metacarpophalangeal joint of the thumb. *J Bone Joint Surg (Br)* 1962; 44:869.

43. Coonrad RW, Goldner JL. A study of the pathological findings and treatment in soft-tissue injury of the thumb metacarpophalangeal joint. *J Bone Joint Surg (Am)* 1968; 50:439.

44. Hastings H II, Carroll C IV. Treatment of closed articular fractures of the metacarpophalangeal and proximal interphalangeal joints. *Hand Clinics* 1988; 4:503.

45. Rayhack JM, Bottke CA. Intraosseous compression wiring of displaced articular condylar fractures. *J Hand Surg* 1990; 15A:370.

46. Kaplan EB. Dorsal dislocation of the metacarpophalangeal joint of the index finger. *J Bone Joint Surg (Am)* 1957; 39:1081.

47. Kaplan EB. The pathology and treatment of radial subluxation of the thumb with ulnar displacement of the head of the first metacarpal. *J Bone Joint Surg (Am)* 1961; 43:541.

48. Bohart PG, Gelberman RH, Vandell RF, et al. Complex dislocations of metacarpophalangeal joint, operative reduction by Farabeuf's dorsal incision. *Clin Orthop Rel Res* 1982; 164:208.

49. Neviaser RJ, Wilson JN, Lievano A. Rupture of the ulnar collateral ligament of the thumb (gamekeeper's thumb): correction by dynamic repair. *J Bone Joint Surg (Am)* 1971; 53:1357.

50. O'Brien ET. Fractures of the metacarpals and phalanges. In: Green DP, ed. *Operative hand surgery.* New York: Churchill Livingstone, 1982; 583.

51. Viegas SF, Tencer A, Woodard P, et al. Functional bracing of fractures of the second through fifth metacarpals. *J Hand Surg* 1987; 12:139.

52. Black D, Mann RJ, Constine R, et al. Comparison of internal fixation techniques in metacarpal fractures. *J Hand Surg (Am)* 1985; 10:466.

53. McElfresh EC, Dobyns JH. Intra-articular metacarpal head fractures. *J Hand Surg* 1983; 8:383.

54. Lowdon IMR. Fractures of the neck of the little metacarpal. *Injury* 1986; 17:189.

55. Konradsen L, Nielsen PT, Albrecht-Beste E. Functional treatment of metacarpal fractures: 100 randomized cases with or without fixation. *Acta Orthop Scand* 1990; 61:531.

56. Dabezies EJ, Schutte JP. Fixation of metacarpal and phalangeal fractures with miniature plates and screws. *J Hand Surg* 1986; 11A:283.

57. Viegas SF, Heare TC, Calhoun JH. Complex fracture dislocation of a fifth metacarpophalangeal joint: case report and literature review. *J Trauma* 1989; 29:521.

58. Foster RJ, Hastings H. Treatment of Bennett, Rolando, and vertical intra-articular trapezial fractures. *Clin Orthop* 1987; 214:121.

59. Worlock PH, Stower MJ. The incidence and pattern of hand fractures in children. *J Hand Surg* 1986; 11B:198.

60. Light TR, Ogen JA. Metacarpal epiphyseal fractures. *J Hand Surg* 1987; 12A:460.

61. Wilson RL, Carter MS. Joint injuries of the hand: preservation of proximal interphalangeal joint function. In: Hunter JM, Schneider LH, Mackin EJ, eds. *Rehabilitation of the hand: surgery and therapy.* 3rd ed. St. Louis: CV Mosby, 1990; 284.

NINE

Trunk and Lower Extremity

100

Pressure Sores

David L. Feldman, M.D.

Perhaps more than any other byproduct of modern medicine's ability to prolong human life, pressure sores have become a pariah of patient care. These wounds have been variously termed decubitus ulcers, decubiti, bedsores, and pressure ulcers, but they are most easily defined as ". . . lesion[s] caused by unrelieved pressure resulting in damage of underlying tissue" (1). Although the word *decubitus* derives from the Latin *decumbere* ("to lie down"), this term does not accurately reflect a significant number of pressure sores that are not the results of being in a recumbent position. Similarly, many pressure sores occur in patients not confined to a bed. For these reasons, the terms *pressure sore* or "pressure ulcer" are preferred.

The plastic surgeon may only be called to see the patient with a large pressure sore who needs "flap surgery to close the wound." However, when faced with operating on what is often an elderly, poorly nourished, incontinent, debilitated patient with multiple serious medical problems, surgery seems ill-fated and, in many cases, dangerous. As with any other contemplated procedure, the surgeon must understand the etiology, natural history, and nonsurgical alternatives before resorting to surgery.

The National Pressure Ulcer Advisory Panel (NPUAP) estimated the average per-case cost of pressure ulcer treatment in acute-care facilities to be between $2,000 and $30,000 (2). Others have reported costs to be in the range of $4,000 to $40,000 per pressure sore (3,4), and even as high as $78,000 per pressure-sore admission (5). Alterescu (6) examined the costs associated with the treatment of pressure sores in an acute-care facility that was part of an HMO, and found the cost of treatment for a patient with one or more pressure ulcers to average about $1,300 (6). Preliminary data from a large academic institution showed charges for three consecutive years averaged $26,000 per patient with a primary diagnosis of pressure sore. Of the $2.6 million in charges generated by those patients over that 3-year period, only $1 million had been recovered by the institution at the end of that 3-year period (7).

More impressive are overall health care dollars spent: $500 million per year on pressure relief products alone (8). Loss of productivity and physical and emotional stress has been estimated at $6.5 billion per year (8). Miller and Delozier estimated that the total national cost of pressure ulcer treatment exceeds $1.335 billion (9). In its *Treatment of Pressure Ulcer Clinical Guidelines* (1), the panel reports that if their guidelines reduce the cost of pressure sore treatment by their estimate of 3%, a savings of $40 million would be realized. In the United Kingdom, it has been estimated that the cost of pressure sore treatment by the National Health Service is £150,000,000 ($2 to $3 million) per year (10).

Epidemiology

The 19th century saw pressure sores in young persons with chronic illnesses like tuberculosis, renal disease, and osteomyelitis (11). The majority of patients with pressure sores today are either paralyzed, elderly, or hospitalized (12). The prevalence of pressure sores in acute-care facilities has been reported to range from 3.5 to 29.5% (1). In a 1993 survey of 177 hospitals, Meehan (13) found a prevalence rate of 11.1%, higher than the 9.2% rate the same author found in a similar 1989 survey (14). Allman reported an incidence of 7.7% over a 3-week period in bedridden and chairbound patients during hospital stays (15).

Certain groups of patients have higher rates (e.g., those admitted with femoral fractures, 66% incidence (16), and critical care patients, 33% incidence and 41% prevalence (1). The incidence in paraplegics has been reported to be 21.6%, and that in quadriplegics 23.1% (12). Ischial sores in these patients have been found to occur at a rate of 25 to 85% over a lifetime (17). A prevalence of 20 to 30% within the first 5 years after injury has been reported among patients followed in spinal-cord injury centers in the United States (18). Allman and colleagues (19) followed 286 hospital patients confined to a bed or chair in a prospective inception cohort study (19). He found that nonblanchable erythema, lymphopenia, immobility, dry skin, and decreased body weight were independent risk factors for the development of a stage II pressure sore; the 3-week cumulative incidence with one, two, three or more of these factors was 11.4%, 39.6%, and 67.9%, respectively (19).

Pressure sores occur over bony prominences, and so are most commonly seen at the sacrum (36 to 60%), heel (30%), ischium (6%), and trochanters (6%) (13,20). Other less common areas include the elbow, scapula, occiput, shoulder, and knee. Studies that include a large number of paralyzed patients are more likely to have higher numbers of ischial sores owing to the long hours these patients often spend sitting in a wheelchair.

The largest number of stage IV ulcers are found at the trochanter (18%) and ischium (15%), while stage I and II ulcers make up most of the sacral (82%) and heel ulcers (80%) (13).

Etiology

The formation of a pressure sore is a result of increased tissue tolerance, as mediated by certain intrinsic and extrinsic fac-

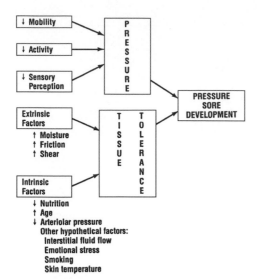

FIG. 100–1. A conceptual schema for the study of the etiology of pressure sores that accounts for the relative contribution of the duration and intensity of pressure and the tissue tolerance for pressure. (Reprinted from *Rehabilitation Nursing,* 12(1), 9, with permission of the Association of Rehabilitation Nurses, 5700 Old Orchard Road, 1st Floor, Skokie, IL 60077-1057. Copyright 1987 Association of Rehabilitation Nurses.)

tors, in the face of applied pressure of a defined duration and intensity (21) (Fig. 100–1). In a 1930 study by Landis (22), it was reported that capillaries close at applied pressures greater than 32 mm Hg. This critical figure, however, may be modified such that in certain patients (e.g., the elderly) lower pressures may result in tissue damage, while in other patients (e.g., the young) higher pressures are required (23). This may explain why long periods of applied pressure do not result in pressure sore formation in certain patients. Kosiak, in his classic studies using dogs (24), showed that ischemic ulcers could be produced with high pressures over a short time, or with low pressures over a long time. He suggested that, with regards to the formation of these wounds, there exists an inverse relationship between pressure and time that follows a parabolic curve. Perhaps more important, he also found that temporary relief of pressure "every few minutes" is essential to prevent irreversible tissue death (24). While many theories have been proposed regarding the mechanism by which tissue necrosis results from pressure, most agree that ischemia and hypoxia are primary factors in the development of necrosis (25). In an attempt to determine the predilection of pressure sores for bony prominences, investigators have proposed two possible theories. Newson and colleagues (26) found that all tissues could tolerate similar pressures, but that those overlying bone experienced higher pressures than soft tissue alone, resulting in higher ulcer rates. Seiler and Stahelin (27) showed that those tissues overlying bony prominences showed a more rapid fall in oxygen tension under increasing pressure relative to other soft tissue. Because the epidermis is able to withstand prolonged absence of oxygen relative to deeper tissues, skin necrosis clinically is the "tip of the iceberg" (25). Deeper tissue (e.g., muscle) is more sensitive to ischemia; however, most of the weight-bearing surfaces of the body have little in the way of muscle padding (28).

Factors that can increase the intensity and duration of pressure include decreased mobility, decreased activity, and decreased sensory perception (21) (see Fig. 100–1).

Moisture, friction, and shear are considered external factors that increase tissue tolerance and predispose to pressure sore formation. Moisture, due mostly to incontinence, perspiration, and wound drainage, can lead to skin rashes and infections that make the skin more susceptible to breakdown (21). Dinsdale showed in a pig model that when friction was applied, lower applied pressures were required to produce an ulcer (29). Shear forces move the skin and superficial fascia relative to the fixed underlying deep fascia and bone, thus disrupting the local blood supply (30).

Intrinsic factors are those that adversely affect the architecture of the supporting structure of the skin and include malnutrition, aging, and decreased blood pressure (21). However, Meijer and colleagues (31), in studying the blood-flow recovery response after pressure application, found no difference between young and old patients not at risk for pressure sore development. These two groups of patients had a mean blood-flow recovery time (as measured using a pressure-temperature-time method) ten times faster than that of older patients who were at risk for pressure sores (31). While diabetes, alcohol abuse, cancer, anemia, and peripheral vascular disease may be associated with pressure sores, the significance of their role lies in the association of these conditions with increasing intrinsic factors, not necessarily with the disease process itself.

Prevention

Prevention of pressure sores lies in the recognition of a potential problem through the identification of patients who are at high risk. If these patients can be recognized early, so that risk factors can be reduced, pressure sores can potentially be prevented. Numerous authors have developed risk assessment tools designed to identify those patients at high risk for pressure sores (32–34). These instruments are mostly subjective assessments made at an initial nursing evaluation and then again periodically during a period of patient hospitalization.

Support surfaces that ideally reduce pressure to below 32 mm Hg can be categorized into either dynamic or static devices. Static devices include elbow pads, gel pads, sheepskin booties, wheelchair cushions, and mattress overlays. Seat cushions can be foam, viscoelastic foam, gel, or fluid flotation types of devices (25). Types of bed overlays include eggcrates, water mattresses, and static or alternating air mattresses. Little in the way of objective criteria from randomized controlled trials exists to assist the clinician in determining an appropriate static device to use in a specific patient. For those patients who are able to participate in their own care, patient education and pressure awareness are probably more important for prevention than the specific static overlay or cushion used.

Dynamic devices include some of the more antiquated bed frames (e.g., Stryker, Foster, CircOlectric, and tilt tables) and the newer beds that support the entire body (eg. low-air-loss, air-fluidized beds). Recently, combinations of low- and high-air loss beds, as well as beds with built in irrigation systems, have become available.

An air-fluidized bed consists of a woven polyester sheet under which high-flow warm air is pumped through a bed of ceramic beads (35). Because the overlying sheet is porous, the "high air loss" can cause a significant drying effect on skin. Allman, in a 1987 randomized trial (36), compared an air-fluidized bed with an alternating air mattress covered by a foam pad and found the former to be more effective in treating pressure sores (36). In a study on healthy volunteers using TcPO2 measurements, Feldman and co-workers (37) found an air-fluidized bed maintained tissue oxygenation on the weighted sacrum and trochanter significantly higher than a standard mattress with or without eggcrate, a low-air-loss bed, and a computer-controlled air mattress bed. Other studies of air-fluidized beds have found these devices effective for prevention and treatment of pressure sores, but they have been uncontrolled (38–40). Other benefits of these beds include a bacteriocidal effect from the desiccation of microorganisms (41,42). While air-fluidized beds are acknowledged by many as the optimal way of supporting a patient and thus preventing and treating pressure-related skin injury, from a practical standpoint their design makes it difficult to move patients in and out of the bed. They are also expensive (costing in the range of $30,000 to $128,000 to purchase, and $55 to $130 per day to rent) (43), air flow from the device can increase insensible water loss (44), and confusion and disorientation can occur due to the sensation of floating (35).

Low-air-loss beds employ computer-controlled inflation of multiple, transversely oriented, cushions, with or without pulsed air. Two recent studies have found low-air-loss beds effective both in preventing and treating pressure sores. Ferrell and colleagues (45) found low-air-loss beds to be more effective than foam mattresses in treating pressure sores in a nursing home population. Inman and others (46) found low-air-loss beds to be a cost-effective method of preventing pressure sores in a critical care setting.

Electrical stimulation has been found to improve the survival of skin flaps in pigs (47) and has also been shown to accelerate the healing rate of stage IV pressure sores in humans (48,49). Increased blood flow to the gluteus maximus muscles and a change in their contour was noted upon electrical stimulation of these muscles (35,50).

Patient Evaluation and Medical Management

Patient's with pressure sores may present to the clinician in a variety of ways, ranging from redness of the skin overlying a bony prominence, to a fulminant necrotizing soft-tissue infection (51). Most patients will have some degree of tissue necrosis, but rarely a true infection. Upon initial presentation, these patients should undergo a workup similar to any patient with an open wound, beginning with a good history and physical examination. Laboratory testing may be limited to a complete blood count, chemistries, and some objective assessment of nutritional status such as serum albumin or transferrin levels. Radiographic studies may be useful in determining the presence of osteomyelitis.

Staging of pressure sores is a useful way of standardizing patient evaluation and subsequent treatment. It also provides a method of communication regarding the severity of a pressure sore amongst the health care team. The Clinical Practice Guidelines of the Agency for Health Care Policy and Research review the four stages of pressure sores (Table 100–1). These

Table 100–1
Clinical Stages of Pressure Sores*

Stage I:	Nonblanchable erythema of intact skin; the heralding lesion of skin ulceration.
Stage II:	Partial thickness skin loss involving epidermis, dermis, or both. The ulcer is superficial and presents clinically as an abrasion, blister, or shallow crater.
Stage III:	Full thickness skin loss involving damage or necrosis of subcutaneous tissue that may extend down to, but not through, underlying fascia. The ulcer presents clinically as a deep crater with or without undermining of adjacent tissue.
Stage IV:	Full thickness skin loss with extensive destruction, tissue necrosis, or damage to muscle, bone, or supporting structures.

When an eschar is present, accurate staging is not possible until the eschar has been removed.

*Adapted from Treatment of Pressure Ulcers Guideline Panel. Treatment of Pressure Ulcers. Clinical Practice Guideline, No. 15. Agency for Health Care Policy and Research, Publication 95-0652. Rockville, MD: Agency for Health Care Policy and Research, Public Health Service, U.S. Dept of Health and Human Services, December 1994.

recommended stages are consistent with those of the National Pressure Ulcer Advisory Panel (2), and are derived from those initially proposed by Shea (52) and the Wound Ostomy and Continence Nurses Society (53).

As in any patient with a large open wound, certain systemic issues must be addressed to aid in wound healing. Associated medical conditions, such as diabetes and cancer, and concomitant infections of the respiratory and/or urinary tracts, must be adequately addressed. Malnutrition is common in many of these patients, as identified by decreased plasma protein levels (54) and low cholesterol and zinc levels (55). Refractory chronic anemia may require red-blood-cell transfusion to improve tissue anoxia (20). In the patient incontinent of stool with a pressure sore in proximity to the stool stream, a temporary (or permanent) colostomy should be considered.

In the nonsurgical management of these patients, four areas relative to the wound itself must also be considered: infection control, dead tissue débridement, pressure avoidance, and dressing use. The bacteriology of pressure sores remains an often-confusing issue. Swab cultures of any open wound will undoubtedly yield multiple organisms but whether a true infection exists (or simply wound colonization) is a more important question. At least two studies have confirmed that anaerobes are more commonly found in nonhealing or worsening pressure sores, and that *Pseudomonas aeruginosa* and Providencia species are more prevalent in progressively worsening sores (56,57). Organisms such as staphylococcus were found in higher concentrations in healing sores (56). From a practical point of view, unless there is evidence of systemic infection (e.g., high white-blood-cell count, fever) with no other obvious source, systemic antibiotic therapy is unnecessary. Local antiinfectives such as acetic acid may be useful when wound cultures grow those bacteria associated with nonhealing or worsening sores. Topical metronidazole gel has also been used to eliminate anaerobic bacteria and their associated odor (58). Bacteremia is uncommon (0.02% of hospitalized patients), but, when present, mortality rate is 50% (20).

Determining the presence or absence of osteomyelitis in a pressure sore can be difficult, its incidence having been reported to be 10 to 65% of pressure sores (59). Initial plain films of the affected area can be difficult to interpret because of heterotopic ossification, demineralization, and air in the soft tissue (60). Bone cultures may also be inaccurate, as there is colonization in virtually all soft-tissue and fibrotic material that is adherent to underlying bone (61). Lewis and colleagues (60) in a prospective review of 61 pressure sores in spinal-cord-injured patients found that a workup consisting of WBC count, ESR, and plain x-ray was 89% sensitive and 88% specific for determining the presence of osteomyelitis; a needle bone biopsy was 73% sensitive and 96% specific. Deloach and co-workers (62) in a prospective review of 14 patients with pressure sores found three-phase radionuclide scanning to be 71% sensitive and 75% specific when correlated with definitive bone biopsy (62). The presence of osteomyelitis may impact on the choice of surgical reconstruction (fasciocutaneous flap versus muscle flap), and the length of postoperative antibiotic therapy. Care should be taken, however, in deciding the amount of bone resection. Ostectomy should be performed only until healthy, bleeding bone is obtained. While in theory inadequately treated osteomyelitis could result in failure of flap reconstruction, pressure sore recurrence usually is a result of hematoma or poor care (63).

Traditional surgical débridement is performed either at the bedside or in the operating room with a scalpel and/or scissors. Blood loss and pain may prevent the removal of all necrotic material in one sitting, requiring multiple bedside or operating-room sessions over a few days or weeks.

Enzymatic débridement can be effected with a variety of chemical agents whose general mode of action is the denaturing of protein. Collagenase, trypsin, fibrinolysin, and Sutilan are but a few of the commonly used débriding agents. These compounds are applied to the wound on at least a daily basis and covered with some type of dressing. Treatment is usually continued for a period of weeks, depending on the amount of necrotic material present in the initial ulcer. Other chemical agents such as povidone-iodine or normal saline, when used in a wet-to-dry dressing, can help mechanically débride a pressure sore. Similarly, whirlpool therapy in large tanks or baths may assist in mechanical wound débridement.

Because of the repetitive blood loss resulting from frequent surgical débridements, and the expense and length of time necessary to débride a wound chemically, laser débridement has become an increasingly used method of débriding pressure ulcers. Using a carbon-dioxide laser with a wavelength of 10,600 microns, débridements can be performed with minimal blood loss, minimal contamination, and the ability to sterilize the ulcer bed (especially useful when laser débridement is immediately followed by flap closure) (64–66). In a recent 2-year review of 150 pressure sore cases treated with the CO_2 laser, it was found to allow earlier rehabilitation of patients, reduce the burden of their care by other health care personnel, and minimize hospital stay and medical costs (67).

Currently used dressings for pressure sores can be best categorized into five groups: traditional, totally occlusive, semiocclusive, alginates, and growth factors. Topical antibiotic solutions such as povidone-iodine, hydrogen peroxide, acetic acid, and sodium hypochlorite (Dakin) make up the bulk of the traditional types of wound care for pressure sores. Gauze dressings can be soaked with these solutions, placed in the wound, and changed every 4, 6, or 8 hours. Their bacteriocidal effect is thought to be responsible for their benefit in aiding in the healing of wounds. Unfortunately, recent evidence suggests that many of these compounds are not only bacteriocidal, but tissue toxic as well (68,69). Some authors have attempted to dilute these solutions to find a concentration that is bacteriocidal but not tissue toxic (70). While povidone-iodine at 1:1000 and Dakin solution at 1:100 were fully bacteriocidal but not toxic to fibroblasts, no such concentration existed for hydrogen peroxide and acetic acid (70). Normal saline, also considered a traditional dressing, is perhaps the most commonly used, and considered by many the most physiologic. While not toxic to the wound (and also not bacteriocidal), normal saline dressings are usually used in a wet-to-dry or wet-to-wet fashion. Relative to some of the newer dressings to be discussed, normal saline dressings are labor-intensive because of the frequency of dressings changes required, and as a result they can be more expensive to use (71).

Hydrocolloid dressings are totally occlusive and are composed of a hydrophobic polymer that is bound to hydroactive particles. The particles in the dressing combine with the wound exudate to form a gel that has been found to promote wound healing. The resultant interaction between the wound and dressing provides a moist environment promoting epithelial-cell migration, prevention of desiccation, and avoidance of wound injury during dressing changes, which need be done only every 3 to 5 days (72). Others have demonstrated that the local wound hypoxia found under these dressings encourages angiogenesis and capillary growth (73). While these dressings are quite useful for superficial stage I or II pressure sores (74), they should not be used in wounds that are grossly contaminated, where their occlusive nature can promote the growth of anaerobic microorganisms (75).

Semiocclusive dressings are very commonly used, not only for pressure sores but also for skin graft donor sites, intravenous sites, and other superficial skin injuries. These dressings are composed of a thin sheet of polyurethane which is synthetic adhesive and moisture-vapor permeable (SAM). Similar to totally occlusive dressings, they promote a moist environment for wound healing and are useful in the treatment of superficial, relatively clean pressure sores. When using these dressings, the caregiver must be careful to note that the pores that allow the transmission of oxygen vapor may close after 2 to 3 days of use, thus converting them from a partially occlusive to a totally occlusive dressing (75).

Calcium alginates were recently introduced in the United States in an attempt to solve the problem of the highly exudative wound. Derived from naturally occurring polysaccharides found in seaweed, the alginate dressings have been found to be highly absorbent, to minimize bacterial contamination, and to avoid disturbance of granulation tissue formation because of their biodegradability (76,77). These dressings come in a rope form, which makes them highly suitable for packing deep pressure sores (e.g., ischial), which can then be covered with a SAM-type dressing and changed every 2 to 3 days. Anecdotal experience with these dressings has been favorable, in our institution and elsewhere, but scientific documentation of their benefits is still lacking (35).

Preliminary studies using recombinant basic fibroblast growth factor, and recombinant human platelet–derived growth factor in the treatment of chronic pressure sores has been beneficial (78,79). Clinical use of these agents is still limited; further studies to evaluate their efficacy are still needed.

With the use of an appropriate dressing regimen, pressure relief, and adequate nutrition, most stage I and II pressure sores will heal within a few weeks. Stage III and IV sores may take longer (3 to 6 months), even with the most diligent wound care, pressure relief, and attention to overall medical condition.

Surgical Treatment

Regardless of the type of reconstruction chosen, if the patient continues to bear weight on that area, recurrent breakdown is likely to develop. Two recent outcome studies from The Johns Hopkins Hospital and the University of Maryland Hospital reviewed the effect of surgical therapy on recurrence (80,81). In the first review, 40 consecutive patients with 68 pressure sores were studied and categorized on the basis of the presence or absence of paraplegia and its etiology (80). Although 80% of the sores were healed at the time of discharge, 61% recurred in a mean of 9.3 months (80). While no recurrences were found in the patient group with paraplegia from a nontraumatic etiology, a 69% patient recurrence (40% pressure sore recurrence) was found in the nonparaplegics, and an 80% recurrence (both patient and pressure sore) was found in the traumatic paraplegics (80). The more recent study reviewed 30 patients and found that within an average time of 19.2 months, 91% of the paraplegic patients had a recurrence of a pressure sore at the same or a different site (81). In the eight nonparaplegic patients, half had surgical treatment with no recurrence, and the other half were considered too ill to undergo surgery.

Basic concepts for the surgical treatment of pressure sores include preparation of the patient both systemically and at the wound site (23). The patient should be prepared for pressure sore surgery much as for any other large surgical procedure: adequate nutrition, absence of concomitant infection, optimization of any other medical conditions. Fecal incontinence is often avoided with a temporary or permanent colostomy, but may be managed with bowel preparation and postoperative medication–induced constipation (82). In paralyzed patients, pharmacologic treatment or surgical ablation may prevent postoperative tension-producing episodes of muscle spasm. Locally, the wound should be granulating, free from purulence, and any bacteria colonizing the wound should be identified so that appropriate prophylactic antibiotic therapy can be instituted. Any potential fistulae between the pressure sore and surrounding orifices (e.g., vagina, rectum) should also be fully evaluated before surgery. A comprehensive discussion with the patient and family must include a commitment to position restrictions for 3 to 4 weeks and awareness of the dangers of continuous pressure, not only at the site of the current pressure sore but also at other potential sites.

Principles of pressure sore surgery were first reviewed by Conway and Griffith in 1956 (83). Complete excision of the sore, surrounding scar, and underlying bursa is first performed. Underlying bone is removed until healthy bleeding bone remains, and resultant dead space is filled with large pedicled flaps, either fasciocutaneous or myocutaneous. Additional points made by Conway and Griffith (83), which remain important even today, include large flap design with an attempt to keep suture lines away from direct pressure areas, and an attempt to avoid violation of adjacent flap territories, which may be needed for future use.

The approach to pressure sore repair is similar to that of any open wound presented to a reconstructive surgeon. In some cases, where there is sufficient soft-tissue laxity, and especially in those patients who are temporarily bedridden, excision and primary closure may be possible. Skin grafts provide poor cover for areas that will ultimately bear weight. Local flaps are the mainstay of pressure sore treatment and may be fasciocutaneous or myocutaneous. Although muscle is not normally found under most weight-bearing surfaces of the body, it has been noted to be advantageous for pressure sore reconstruction because of its ability to bring well-vascularized tissue in sufficient amounts to fill large spaces adequately and thus provide bulk, padding, and durability (23). In addition, muscle flaps have been found to be quite useful in the treatment of osteomyelitis (84,85). Yamamoto and colleagues (86) reported on the superiority of fasciocutaneous flaps in the reconstruction of sacral pressure sores. The authors felt that these flaps have an anatomic structure that resists physical stimulation or external pressure and preserves the ability to use myocutaneous flaps in the future (86). Innervated flaps, either pedicled or free (Fig. 100–10) have been described that restore sensation to a previously denervated area in the hopes of preventing recurrence (87–90).

Tissue-expansion techniques have also been applied to the treatment of pressure sores, despite the conventional concern with using these devices in the presence of an open wound. In one study, expanders were placed under tensor fascia lata flaps and lumbosacral fasciocutaneous flaps in 6 patients (10 flaps), with healing of all sores at 4- to 6-month follow-up (91). The authors found the technique assisted in donor-site closure, and rendered the distal portion of the flaps heartier by virtue of increased vascularity (91). Esposito and colleagues (92) placed expanders under random fasciocutaneous flaps surrounding sacral, ischial, and trochanteric pressure sores in 11 patients. All patients healed at 3- to 25-month follow-up, and the authors concluded that expanders were useful in these patients, as it allowed advancement of sensitive skin useful for pressure awareness and thus future sore prevention (92).

Surgical Techniques

An exhaustive review of all the different techniques available for the surgical closure of pressure sores is beyond the scope of this chapter. Following is a review of the common procedures employed to close sacral, ischial, and trochanteric sores follows as well as a brief discussion of other less common areas where pressure sores are found.

SACRUM

Surgical treatment of a sacral pressure sore requires adequate soft-tissue débridement and excision of any bony ir-

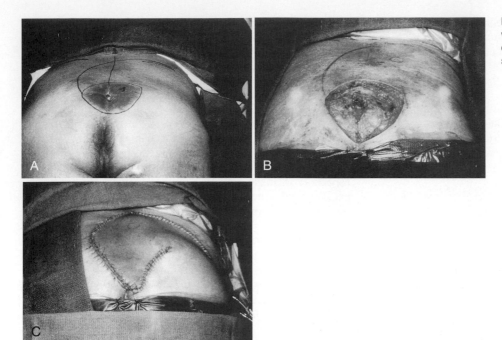

FIG. 100–2. **A,** sacral pressure sore, with proposed flap outlined. **B,** after débridement. **C,** after elevation and insetting of flap.

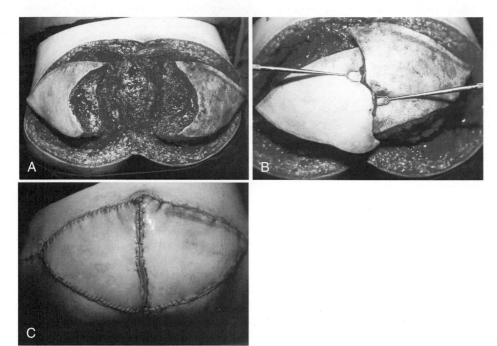

FIG. 100–3. **A,** sacral pressure sore after débridement and dissection of bilateral gluteus maximus myocutaneous flaps. **B,** advancement of flaps. **C,** insetting of flaps.

regularities. Fasciocutaneous flaps used in this area included random rotation/advancement flaps (Fig. 100–1), and transverse lumbosacral back flaps (93). Advocates of fasciocutaneous flaps feel that these flaps avoid loss of function associated with muscle flaps, that muscle does not belong under weight-bearing surfaces such as the sacrum, that sacral pressure sores are mostly skin (thus eliminating the need for large amounts of soft-tissue filler), and that readvancement and tissue-expansion techniques add significant flexibility to the use of these flaps (86,93). Most fasciocutaneous flaps also avoid placing suture lines in pressure areas.

The gluteus maximus is the muscle most commonly used for muscle-flap sacral pressure sore reconstruction (94–96). Unilateral or bilateral gluteus maximus myocutaneous flaps are advanced medially in a V–Y fashion to cover the open wound (Fig. 100–2). The gluteus muscle can also be used with an island of skin (97), and in a way that preserves functional use of the muscle (98).

In our institution, we prefer an attempt at primary closure if enough skin laxity exists. For most sacral sores, especially in nonparalyzed patients, a random rotation/advancement flap based on gluteal or lumbar perforating vessels, with or

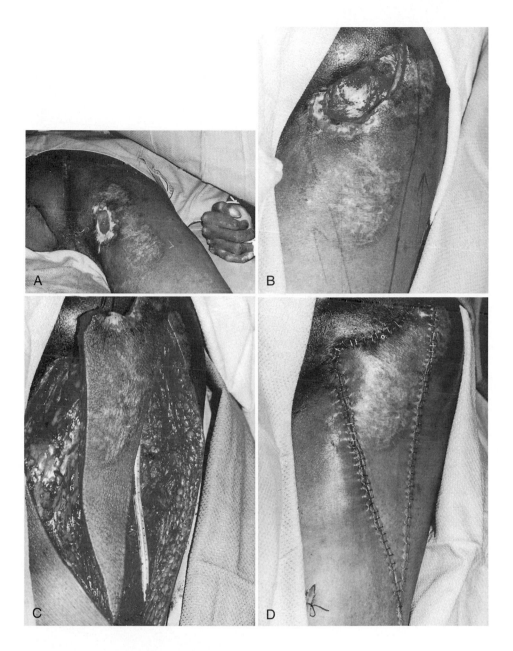

FIG. 100–4. A, right ischial pressure sore in quadriplegic (note left leg hip disarticulation). **B,** after débridement, with proposed flap outlined. **C,** V–Y hamstring advancement flap before insetting. **D,** after insetting of flap.

without a skin graft in the donor area, fills the defect adequately. In paralyzed patients and those with large, deep defects, unilateral or bilateral V–Y gluteus myocutaneous advancement flaps are the option of choice.

ISCHIUM

In the treatment of ischial pressure sores, careful consideration should be given to the ischial ramus. Although ischiectomy has been advocated in the past (99,100), this maneuver will merely transfer pressure to the opposite ischia, making that area more prone to pressure sore formation. Similarly, total bilateral ischiectomy will transfer pressure to the perineum. Possible communication with nearby structures (e.g., rectum, vagina) must be assessed and an adequate soft-tissue débridement, including bursectomy, should be performed.

As with the sacrum, both fasciocutaneous and muscle flaps have been described for treatment of ischial pressure sores. Primary closure may be possible in select patients with ischial tissue laxity. For the paralyzed population V–Y advancement of the hamstring muscles as a myocutaneous unit has proven highly effective (Fig. 100–3). This flap will provide adequate soft-tissue filling of the defect, and allow placement of the suture line above the area of weight bearing (101). As an added benefit, this flap has the ability to be readvanced in recurrent cases (102). Other muscle flaps available include the inferior gluteus maximus (turnover or sliding), gracilis, and rectus abdominis (103–106).

Transposition of the hamstring myocutaneous flap is not recommended in ambulatory patients for whom the posterior thigh "gluteal thigh" flap is the treatment of choice (Figs. 100–4, 100–5). This flap is an axial-pattern fasciocutaneous

FIG. 100–5. **A,** bilateral ischial ulcers. **B,** bilateral posterior gluteal thigh flaps.

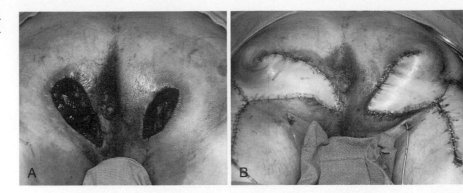

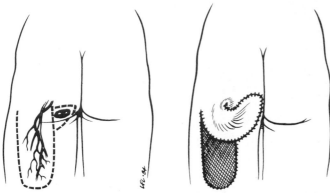

FIG. 100–6. The gluteal thigh flap is an axial flap based on the descending branch of the inferior gluteal artery and also includes the posterior cutaneous nerve. It can be used for coverage of either the trochanteric or ischial areas. When designed as a peninsula fasciocutaneous flap, its transfer will require a relatively large cone of rotation. Depending on the level of cord injury, it has potential as a sensory flap in selected paraplegics.

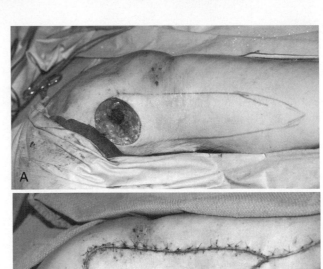

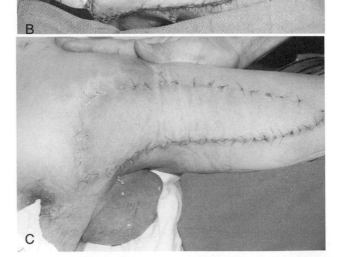

flap based on a subfascial descending branch of the inferior gluteal artery (107). The donor site may be closed primarily, and obligatory inclusion of the posterior cutaneous nerve enables the flap to be sensate. The robust blood supply of this flap has made it useful for coverage of some trochanteric and sacral wounds as well as difficult wounds of the buttock and perineal region (107,108). Tensor fascia lata flaps have also been useful for ischial pressure sores. The flap may be sensate based on the lateral femoral cutaneous nerve, and in some cases the same flap can provide coverage of both an ischial and trochanteric sore (109).

GREATER TROCHANTER

Because of the greater tension of lateral hip tissue, direct closure of trochanteric sores is usually not possible. The tensor fascia lata flap is most often the flap of choice for coverage (Fig. 100–6), its classic use being posterior transposition (109). Siddiqui and colleagues (110) described retroposition of the TFL as a reliable procedure that could be rerotated in recurrent cases (110). The TFL has also been used as a V–Y advancement (Fig. 100–7) and in combination with the gluteus medius (111). Other techniques described for coverage of trochanteric sores include a distally based gluteus maximus flap (112), vastus lateralis myocutaneous flap (113), and gluteal thigh flap (107).

FIG. 100–7. **A,** greater trochanter pressure sore. **B,** V–Y advancement of tensor fasciae latae myocutaneous flap. **C,** early postoperative result.

Perineal defects are often seen in patients who have had earlier treatment of ischial sores. Alternatives to rerotation of previously used flaps are an inferiorly based rectus abdominis myocutaneous flap (114), or a gracilis flap with or without the overlying skin paddle (Fig. 100–8). Heel defects are often best allowed to granulate, and are then skin grafted; however, local flap coverage may be needed, especially on

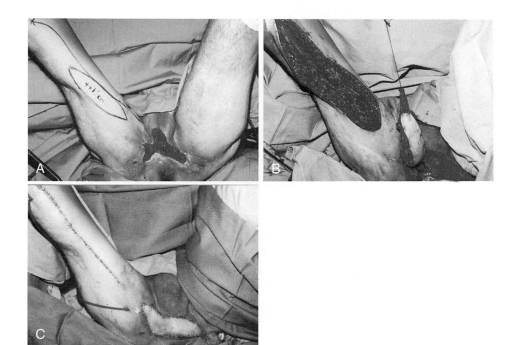

FIG. 100–8. **A,** perineal pressure sore with gracilis myocutaneous flap outlined on right thigh. Note healed incisions from earlier pressure sore surgery. **B,** gracilias flap elevated and tunneled into perineal wound. **C,** after insetting of flap and primary closure of donor site.

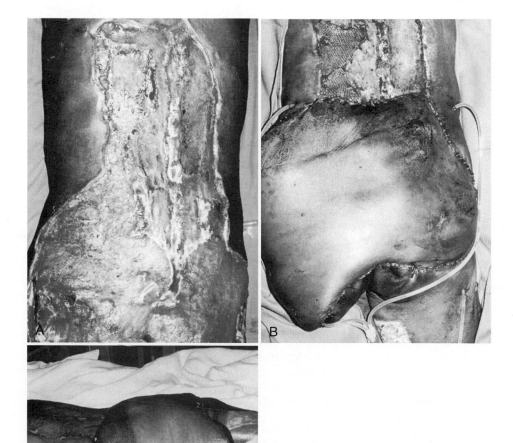

FIG. 100–9. **A,** large open wound of back and buttocks after necrotizing fasciitis of sacral pressure sore in diabetic. Both hip joints are exposed. Partial wound coverage superiorly had earlier been performed with split-thickness skin grafts. **B,** immediately after left total-thigh flap and additional split-thickness skin grafting. Patient had a previous left below-knee amputation. **C,** approximately 6 weeks postoperative showing healed wound.

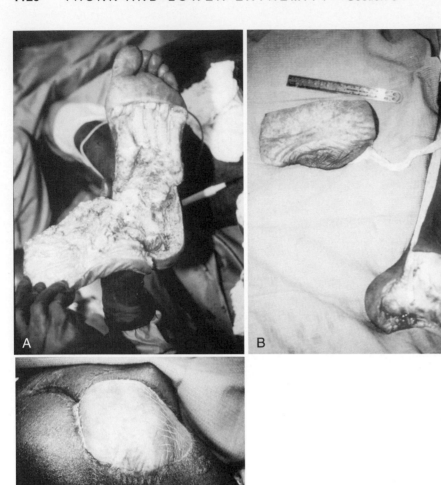

FIG. 100–10.   **A,** dissection of left free foot fillet flap for coverage of a sacral pressure sore. **B,** flap isolated on posterior tibial neurovascular pedicle. **C,** approximately 6 weeks postoperative showing healed flap in sacral area.

the weight-bearing heel. Fasciocutaneous flaps or local muscle flaps (e.g., the flexor hallucis brevis or abductor hallucis muscle) can be used. Occipital wounds can usually be managed with local scalp rotation and advancement flaps. A posteromedial arm flap has been described for coverage of elbow sores (115).

Postoperative Care and Complications

Postoperative care of the pressure sore patient is characterized by attention to pressure relief and wound care. Although it has become almost standard practice for patients to be placed on an air-fluidized bed after pressure sore surgery, a recent prospective randomized trial found a dry-floatation mattress to be as effective as an air-fluidized bed in this setting (116). Fecal incontinence may be managed with pharmacologically induced constipation in those patients who do not have a colostomy (82). Use of clear-film (SAM) dressings over the incisions may help protect them from soilage and still allow for their inspection on a frequent basis. Closed suction drains are maintained until producing less than 10 to 15 cc per day. Patients should remain in the hospital for at least 1 week and may then be discharged if appropriate pressure relief and continued wound care is available as an outpatient.

In the first few weeks after pressure sore surgery, problems with hematomas, recurrent infection, and wound dehiscence can be seen. Many of these problems can be avoided by strict attention to technical details and adhering to general principles of flap design and elevation. Long-term complications have been discussed; almost always, they are secondary to nonavoidance of pressure.

Complex wounds can be found in patients with recurrent pressure sores who have had multiple procedures in the past. In this situation, radical procedures may be indicated to close especially large wounds that may be contributing to protein depletion and systemic deterioration. The total thigh flap, initially described by Georgiade in 1956 (117), entails removal of the femur (including hip disarticulation), amputation of the distal leg, and rotation of the remaining thigh soft tissue for coverage (Fig. 100–9). In a 2-year follow-up of 15 patients treated with total thigh flaps, 10 patients had successful long-term defect closure that did not require further hospitalization (6). Two flap failures were noted from excessive sitting, and two from chronic draining deep-pelvic osteomyelitis. Successful use of a lower-leg fillet free flap for coverage of multiple large, lower back and ischial sores has also been reported (118).

Malignant degeneration in a chronic pressure sore may be considered a form of Marjolin ulcer, initially described in burn scars (119). The incidence of pressure sore carcinoma has been reported to be 0.5% (120), with presentation noted at an average time of 22 years after the development of a sore that remains unhealed (121). While these tumors are usually well-differentiated squamous cell carcinomas, they behave very aggressively, with a high metastatic rate (61%) and a high mortality rate (122). Treatment includes radical surgical resection (including hemicorporectomy in certain cases) and possible elective lymph-node dissection (120). The role of adjuvant chemotherapy and radiation has not been adequately studied.

In an attempt to address the problem of sensory loss as a contributing factor to the etiology of pressure sores, sensate flaps, both pedicled and free, have been used to reinnervate pressure sore–prone areas. In the paraplegic patient, foot fillet flaps may be used based on the posterior tibial neurovascular bundle with nerve anastomoses to an intercostal nerve above the level of sensory denervation (Fig. 100–10). Sensory retraining is necessary, so that the patient will be able to move in response to painful stimuli coming from the newly resurfaced and reinnervated area.

References

1. Treatment of Pressure Ulcers Guideline Panel. *Treatment of pressure ulcers.* Clinical practice guideline, no. 15. Agency for Health Care Policy and Research, Publication 95-0652. Rockville: Agency for Health Care Policy and Research, Public Health Service, U.S. Dept of Health and Human Services, December 1994.
2. National Pressure Ulcer Advisory Panel. Pressure ulcers: prevalence, cost, and risk assessment. Consensus Development Conference statement. *Decubitus* 1989; 2:24.
3. Hibbs P. The economics of pressure ulcer prevention. *Decubitus* 1989; 2:32.
4. Frantz RA. Pressure ulcer costs in long-term care. *Decubitus* 1989; 2:59.
5. Capen DA, Nelson RW, Zigler J, et al. Stage total thigh rotation flap for coverage of chronic recurrent pressure sores. *Contemp Orthop* 1988; 16:23.
6. Alerescu V. The financial costs of inpatient pressure ulcers to an acute care facility. *Decubitus* 1989; 2:14.
7. Feldman DL. Unpublished data.
8. Rodeheaver G, Baharestani MM, Brabec ME, et al. Wound healing and wound management: focus on débridement. *Adv Wound Care* 1994; 7:22.
9. Miller H, Delozier J. Cost implications of the pressure ulcer treatment guideline. Columbia, MD: Center for Health Policy Studies, 1994. Contract No. 282-91-0070. Sponsored by the Agency for Health Care Policy and Research.
10. Phillips TJ. Chronic cutaneous ulcers: etiology and epidemiology. *J Invest Dermatol* 1994; 102:38S.
11. Shaw TC. On so-called bed sores in the insane. *St. Bartholomew Hosp Rep* 1872; 8:130.
12. Barbenel JC, Jordon MM, Nicol SM. Incidence of pressure sores in the greater Glasgow Health Board area. *Lancet* 1977; 2:548.
13. Meehan M. National pressure ulcer prevalence survey. *Adv Wound Care* 1994; 7:27.
14. Meehan M. Multi-site pressure ulcer prevalence survey. *Decubitus* 1989; 3:14.
15. Allman RM, Laprade CA, Noel LB, et al. Pressure sores among hospitalized patients. *Ann Intern Med* 1986; 105:337.
16. Versluysen MJ. Pressure sores in elderly patients: the epidemiology related to hip operations. *J Bone Joint Surg (Br)* 1985; 67:10.
17. El-Torai I, Chung B. The management of pressure sores. *J Dermatol Surg Oncol* 1977; 3:507.
18. Young JS, Burns PE, Bowen AM, et al., eds. *Spinal cord injury statistics: experience of the regional spinal cord injury systems.* Phoenix: National Spinal Cord Injury Data Research Center 1982; 95.
19. Allman RM, Goode PA, Patrick MM, et al. Pressure ulcer risk factors among hospitalized patients with activity limitation. *JAMA* 1995; 273:865.
20. Leigh IH, Bennett G. Pressure ulcers: prevalence, etiology, and treatment modalities. *Am J Surg* 1994; 167:25S.
21. Braden B, Bergstrom N. A conceptual schema for the study of the etiology of pressure sores. *Rehab Nurs* 1987; 12:8.
22. Landis DM. Studies of capillary blood pressure in human skin. *Heart* 1930; 15:209.
23. Granick MS, Eisner AN, Solomon MP. Surgical management of decubitus ulcers. *Clin Dermatol* 1994; 12:71.
24. Kosiak M. Etiology and pathology of ischemic ulcers. *Arch Phys Med Rehabil* 1959; 40:62.
25. Crenshaw RP, Vistnes LM. A decade of pressure sore research: 1977–1987. *J Rehabil Res Dev* 1989; 26:63.
26. Newson TP, Pearcy MJ, Rolfe P. Skin surface PO_2 measurement and the effect of externally applied pressure. *Arch Phys Med Rehabil* 1981; 62:390.
27. Seiler WO, Stahelin HB. Skin oxygen tension as a function of imposed skin pressure: implication for decubitus ulcer formation. *J Am Geriatr Soc* 1979; 27:298.
28. Daniel RK, Faibisoff B. Muscle coverage of pressure points: the role of myocutaneous flaps. *Ann Plast Surg* 1982; 8:446.
29. Dinsdale SM. Decubitus ulcer: role of pressure and friction in causation. *Arch Phys Med Rehabil* 1974; 55:147.
30. Reichel SM. Shearing forces as a factor in decubitus ulcers in paraplegics. *JAMA* 1958; 15:762.
31. Meijer JH, Schut GL, Ribbe MW, et al. Method for the measurement of susceptibility to decubitus ulcer formation. *Med Biol Eng Comput* 1989; 27:502.
32. Gosnell DJ. Client risk for pressure sores. In: Waltz CF, Strickland OL, eds. *Measurement of nursing outcomes. Vol. 1. Measuring client outcomes.* New York: Springer, 1988; 185.
33. Bergstrom N, Braden BJ, Laguzza A, et al. The braden scale for predicting pressure sore risk. *Nurs Res* 1987; 36:205.
34. Norton D, McLaren R, Exton-Smith AN. *An investigation of geriatric nursing problems in hospital.* London: Churchill Livingstone, 1962; 194.
35. Yarkony GM. Pressure ulcers: a review. *Arch Phys Med Rehabil* 1994; 75:908.
36. Allman RA, Walker JM, Hart MK, et al. Air-fluidized beds or conventional beds for pressure sores. *Ann Int Med* 1987; 107:641.
37. Feldman DL, Sepka RS, Klitzman B. Tissue oxygenation and blood flow on specialized and conventional hospital beds. *Ann Plast Surg* 1993; 30:441.
38. Greer DM, Morris EJ, Walsh NE, et al. Cost-effectiveness and efficacy of air-fluidized therapy in the treatment of pressure ulcers. *J Enterostomal Therapy* 1988; 15:247.
39. Parish LC, Witkowski JA. Clinitron therapy and the decubitus ulcer. *Int J Dermatol* 1980; 19:517.
40. Bennett RG, Bellantoni MF, Ouslander JG. Air-fluidized bed treatment of nursing home patients with pressure sores. *J Am Geriatr Soc* 1989; 37:235.
41. Sharbaugh RJ, Hargest TS. Bactericidal effect of the air-fluidized bed. *Am Surg* 1971; 37:583.
42. Sharbaugh RJ, Hargest TS, Wright FA. Further studies on the bactericidal effect of the air-fluidized bed. *Am Surg* 1973; 39:253.
43. Freedman B, Gilbert J, Kaltsounakis LA. Air-support treatment: a case study in the ethics of allocating an expensive treatment. *J Clin Ethics* 1990; 1:298.
44. Treatment of pressure ulcers. In: Abramowicz M, ed. *The medical letter on drugs and therapeutics.* New Rochelle: The Medical Letter, Inc., 1990; 17.
45. Ferrell BA, Osterweil D, Christenson P. A randomized trial of low-airloss beds for treatment of pressure ulcers. *JAMA* 1993; 269:494.
46. Inman KJ, Sibbald WJ, Rutledge FS, et al. Clinical utility and cost-effectiveness of an air suspension bed in the prevention of pressure ulcers. *JAMA* 1993; 269:1139.
47. Im MJ, Lee WPA, Hoopes JE. Effect of electrical stimulation on survival of skin flaps in pigs. *Phys Ther* 1990; 70:37.
48. Kloth LC, Feedar JA. Acceleration of wound healing with high voltage, monophasic, pulsed current. *Phys Ther* 1988; 68:503.
49. Griffin JW, Tooms RE, Mendius RA, et al. Efficacy of high voltage pulsed current for healing of pressure ulcers in patients with spinal cord injury. *Phys Ther* 1994; 71:433.
50. Yarkony GM, Roth EJ, Cybulski GR, et al. Neuromuscular stimulation in spinal cord injury II: prevention of secondary complications. *Arch Phys Med Rehabil* 1992; 73:195.

51. Shibuya H, Terashi H, Kurata S, et al. Gas gangrene following sacral pressure sores. *J Derm* 1994; 21:518.

52. Shea JD. Pressure sores: classification and management. *Clin Orthop* 1975; 112:89.

53. International Association of Enterostomal Therapy. Dermal wounds: pressure sores. Philosophy of the IAET. *J Enterostomal Ther* 1988; 15:4.

54. Mullholland JH, Tui C, Wright AM, et al. Protein metabolism and bedsores. *Ann Surg* 1943; 118:1015.

55. Breslow RA, Hallfrisch J, Goldberg AP. Malnutrition in tube-fed nursing home patients with pressure sores. *J Parenter Enteral Nutr* 1991; 15:663.

56. Seiler WO, Stahelin HB. Recent findings on decubitus ulcer pathology: implications for care. *Geriatrics* 1986; 41:47.

57. Daltrey DC, Rhodes B, Chattwood JG. Investigation into the microbial flora of healing and non-healing decubitus ulcers. *J Clin Pathol* 1981; 34:701.

58. Witkowski JA, Parish LC. Topical metronidazole gel. The bacteriology of decubitus ulcers. *Int J Dermatol* 1991; 30:660.

59. Deloach ED, DeBenedetto RJ, Womble L, et al. The treatment of osteomyelitis underlying pressure ulcers. *Decubitus* 1993; 5:32.

60. Lewis VL, Bailey H, Pulawski G, et al. The diagnosis of osteomyelitis in patients with pressure sores. *Plast Reconstr Surg* 1988; 81:229.

61. Darouiche RO, Landon GC, Klima M, et al. Osteomyelitis associated with pressure sores. *Arch Intern Med* 1994; 154:753.

62. Deloach ED, Check WE, Long R. Diagnosing osteomyelitis underlying pressure sores. *Contemp Orthoped* 1993; 27:240.

63. Thornhill-Joynes M, Gonzales F, Stewardt CA, et al. Osteomyelitis associated with pressure ulcers. *Arch Phys Med Rehabil* 1986; 67:314.

64. Juri H, Palma JA. CO_2 laser in decubitus ulcer: a comparative study. *Lasers Surg Med* 1987; 7:296.

65. Slutzki S. Use of the carbon dioxide laser for large excisions with minimal blood loss. *Plast Reconstr Surg* 1977; 60:250.

66. Zaccaria A, Gudicello F, Dudick S, et al. Treatment of stage IV pressure sores using the carbon dioxide laser. *Contemp Surg (Res)* 1993; 1:7.

67. Lutchman G, Jonnalagadda S, Wang S, et al. Use of CO_2 laser as débriding tool in decubitus ulcer and necrotic wounds. *Am Soc Laser Med Surg* 1991; abstract.

68. Kozol RA, Gillies C, Elgebaly SA. Effects of sodium hypochlorite (Dakin solution) on cells of the wound module. *Arch Surg* 1988; 123:420.

69. Rodeheaver G, Bellamy W, Kody M, et al. Bactericidal activity and toxicity of iodine-containing solutions in wounds. *Arch Surg* 1982; 117:181.

70. Lineaweaver W, McMorris S, Soucy D, et al. Cellular and bacterial toxicities of topical antimicrobials. *Plast Reconstr Surg* 1985; 75:394.

71. Xakellis GC, Chrischilles EA. Hydrocolloid vs. saline gauze dressings in treating pressure ulcers: a cost-effectiveness analysis. *Arch Phys Med Rehabil* 1992; 73:463.

72. Wheeland RG. The newer surgical dressings and wound healing. *Dermatol Clinics* 1987; 5:393.

73. Knighton DR, Silver IA, Hunt TK. Regulation of wound-healing angiogenesis effect of oxygen gradients and inspired oxygen concentration. *Surgery* 1981; 90:262.

74. Gorse GH, Messner RL. Improved pressure sore healing with hydrocolloid dressings. *Arch Dermatol* 1987; 123:766.

75. Marshall DA, Mertz PM, Eaglestein WH. Occlusive dressings. *Arch Surg* 1990; 125:1136.

76. Fowler E, Papen JC. Evaluation of an alginate dressing for pressure ulcers. *Decubitus* 1991; 4:47.

77. Gilchrist T, Martin AM. Wound treatment with Sorbsan—an alginate fibre dressing. *Biomaterials* 1983; 4:317.

78. Robson MC, Phillips LG, Lawrence WT, et al. The safety and effect of topically applied recombinant basic fibroblast growth factor on the healing of chronic pressure sores. *Ann Surg* 1992; 216:401.

79. Robson MC, Phillips LG, Thomason A. Recombinant human platelet-derived growth factor-BB for the treatment of chronic pressure ulcers. *Ann Plast Surg* 1992; 29:193.

80. Disa JJ, Carlton JM, Goldberg NH. Efficacy of operative cure in pressure sore patients. *Plast Reconstr Surg* 1992; 89:272.

81. Evans GRD, Dufresne CR, Manson PN. Surgical correction of pressure ulcers in an urban center: is it efficacious? *Adv Wound Care* 1994; 7:40.

82. Stal S, Serure A, Donovan W, et al. The perioperative management of the patient with pressure sores. *Ann Plast Surg* 1983; 11:347.

83. Conway H, Griffith BH. Plastic surgery for closure of decubitus ulcers in patients with paraplegia: based on experience with 1000 cases. *Am J Surg* 1956; 91:946.

84. Bruck JC, Buttemeyer R, Grabosch A, et al. More arguments in favor of myocutaneous flaps for the treatment of pelvic pressure sores. *Ann Plast Surg* 1991; 26:85.

85. Mathes SJ. The muscle flap for management of osteomyelitis. *N Engl J Med* 1982; 306:294.

86. Yamamoto Y, Ohura T, Shintomi Y, et al. Superiority of the fasciocutaneous flap in reconstruction of sacral pressure sores. *Ann Plast Surg* 1993; 30:116.

87. Spear SI, Kroll SS, Little JW III. Bilateral upper-quadrant (intercostal) flaps: the value of protective sensation in preventing pressure sore recurrence. *Plast Reconstr Surg* 1987; 80:734.

88. Daniel RK, Terzis JK, Cunningham DM. Sensory skin flaps for coverage of pressure sores in paraplegic patients: a preliminary report. *Plast Reconstr Surg* 1976; 58:317.

89. Dibbell DG. Use of a long island flap to bring sensation to the sacral area in young paraplegics. *Plast Reconstr Surg* 1974; 54:220.

90. Hill HL, Nahai F, Vasconez LO. The tensor fascia lata myocutaneous free flap. *Plast Reconstr Surg* 1978; 61:517.

91. Kostakoglu N, Kecik A, Ozyilmaz F, et al. Expansion of fascial flaps: histopathologic changes and clinical benefits. *Plast Reconstr Surg* 1993; 91:72.

92. Esposito G, DiCaprio G, Ziccardi P, et al. Tissue expansion in the treatment of pressure ulcers. *Plast Reconstr Surg* 1991; 87:501.

93. Hill HL, Brown RG, Jurkiewicz MJ. The transverse lumbosacral back flap. *Plast Reconstr Surg* 1978; 62:177.

94. Scheflan M, Nahai F, Bostwick J. Gluteus maximus island musculocutaneous flap for closure of sacral and ischial ulcers. *Plast Reconstr Surg* 1981; 68:533.

95. Parry SW, Mathes SJ. Bilateral gluteus maximus myocutaneous advancement flaps: sacral coverage for ambulatory patients. *Ann Plast Surg* 1982; 8:443.

96. Fisher J, Arnold PG, Waldorf J, et al. The gluteus maximus musculocutaneous V–Y advancement flap for large sacral defects. *Ann Plast Surg* 1983; 11:517.

97. Stevenson TR, Pollock RA, Rohrich RJ, et al. The gluteus maximus musculocutaneous island flap: refinements in design and application. *Plast Reconstr Surg* 1987; 79:761.

98. Ramirez OM, Hurwitz DJ, Futrell JW. The expansive gluteus maximus flap. *Plast Reconstr Surg* 1984; 74:757.

99. Blocksma R, Kostrubala JG, Greeley PW. The surgical repair of decubitus ulcers in paraplegics: further observations. *Plast Reconstr Surg* 1949; 4:123.

100. Arregui J, Cannon B, Murray JE, et al. Long-term evaluation of ischiectomy in the treatment of pressure ulcers. *Plast Reconstr Surg* 1965; 36:583.

101. Hurteau JE, Bostwick J, Nahai F, et al. V–Y advancement of hamstring musculocutaneous flap for coverage of ischial pressure sores. *Plast Reconstr Surg* 1981; 68:539.

102. Kroll SS, Hamilton S. Multiple and repetitive uses of the extended hamstring V–Y myocutaneous flap. *Plast Reconstr Surg* 1989; 84:296.

103. Ger R, Levine SA. The management of decubitus ulcers by muscle transposition-an eight-year review. *Plast Reconstr Surg* 1976; 58:419.

104. Minami RT, Mills R, Paroe R. Gluteus maximus myocutaneous flaps for repair of pressure sores. *Plast Reconstr Surg* 1977; 60:242.

105. Wingate GB, Friedland JA. Repair of ischial pressure ulcers with gracilis myocutaneous island flaps. *Plast Reconstr Surg* 1978; 62:245.

106. Mixter RC, Wood WA, Dibbell DG Sr. Retroperitoneal transposition of rectus abdominis myocutaneous flaps to the perineum and back. *Plast Reconstr Surg* 1990; 85:437.

107. Paletta C, Bartell T, Shehadi S. Applications of the posterior thigh flap. *Ann Plast Surg* 1993; 30:41.

108. Hurwitz DJ, Swartz WM, Mathes SJ. The gluteal thigh flap: a reliable, sensate flap for the closure of buttock and perineal wounds. *Plast Reconstr Surg* 1981; 68:521.

109. Nahai F, Silverton JS, Hill HL, et al. The tensor fascia lata musculocutaneous flap. *Ann Plast Surg* 1978; 1:372.

110. Siddiqui A, Wiedrich T, Lewis VL. Tensor fascia lata V–Y retroposition myocutaneous flap: clinical experience. *Ann Plast Surg* 1993; 31:313.

111. Little JW, Lyons JR. The gluteus medius-tensor fasciae latae flap. *Plast Reconstr Surg* 1983; 71:366.

112. Becker H. The distally-based gluteus maximus muscle flap. *Plast Reconstr Surg* 1979; 63:653.
113. Drimmer MA, Krasna MJ. The vastus lateralis myocutaneous flap. *Plast Reconstr Surg* 1987; 79:560.
114. Pena MM, Drew GS, Smith SJ, et al. The inferiorly based rectus abdominis myocutaneous flap for reconstruction of recurrent pressure sores. *Plast Reconstr Surg* 1992; 89:90.
115. Timmons MJ, Nishikawa H. The posteromedial arm flap for posterior elbow defects. *J Hand Surg* 1994; 19B:303.
116. Economides NG, Skoutakis VA, Carter CA, et al. Evaluation of the effectiveness of two support surfaces following myocutaneous flap surgery. *Adv Wound Care* 1995; 8:49.
117. Georgiade N, Pickrell K, Maguire C. Total thigh flaps for extensive decubitus ulcers. *Plast Reconstr Surg* 1956; 17:220.
118. Chen H, Weng C, Norrdhoff MS. Coverage of multiple extensive pressure sores with a single filleted lower leg myocutaneous free flap. *Plast Reconstr Surg* 1986; 78:396.
119. Berkwits L, Yarkony GM, Lewis V. Marjolin's ulcer complicating a pressure ulcer: case report and literature review. *Arch Phys Med Rehabil* 1986; 67:831.
120. Grotting JC, Bunkis J, Vasconez LO. Pressure sore carcinoma. *Ann Plast Surg* 1987; 18:527.
121. Mustoe T, Upton J, Marcellin V, et al. Carcinoma in chronic pressure sores: a fulminant disease process. *Plast Reconstr Surg* 1986; 77:116.

101

Lymphedema of the Extremities

William C. Pederson, M.D., F.A.C.S.

Lymphedema is a medical malady that has afflicted mankind through the ages. Lymphatic channels were observed as early as the 3rd and 4th centuries BC by Heophilos and Aristotle (1). One of the earliest descriptions of the swelling caused by "elephantiasis" is found in Plutarch's writings from the 1st century. Professor M. Raymond of the Faculty of Medicine in Montpellier, France, published an entire monograph on the subject in 1767 (2) (Fig. 101–1). Despite this long appreciation of the lymphatic system and lymphedema, many of today's surgeons have an understanding of this system and its problems not much more advanced than these earlier physicians. With a proper understanding of the pathophysiology and appropriate management, however, much can be done to improve this condition.

Classification

Lymphedema can be defined as the accumulation of interstitial fluid secondary to stasis of lymph that arises from an abnormality or obstruction of the lymphatic channels. The classification of lymphedema has been based on its etiology as either *primary* or *secondary*. The primary lymphedemas are those with an idiopathic etiology, although their onset is often noted after minor limb trauma or infection. The secondary lymphedemas are those seen after mechanical blockage of an otherwise normal lymphatic system, whether from disease or surgery.

Lymphedema presenting at birth was first described in 1890 by Nonne (3), who called it "elephantiasis congenita," but the eponym of this disease dates from Milroy's description in 1892 (4). Milroy disease is thought to be a sex-linked dominant trait and is an unusual form of lymphedema, seen in only 2% of cases of primary lymphedema. Lymphedema arising after puberty but before age 35 is called *lymphedema praecox* (5). This is the most common form of primary lymphedema, and patients with this type of lymphedema are usually female and most commonly present in the 2nd or 3rd decades of life. Patients with lymphedema developing after the age of 35 are said to have *lymphedema tarda,* which has also been called Meige disease. In my opinion, all patients developing lymphedema after childhood represent a spectrum of the same problem, and this classification of these patients does not address the pathophysiology of the disease. These patients all have lymphatic systems that are inadequate to continue functioning in the face of challenges from local infection, with resultant fibrosis of lymphatics and the nodal system.

Browse (6) has proposed a functional classification of lymphedema based on pathophysiology and, while this has not been widely applied, the system has value because it is based on etiology rather than some arbitrary age of onset. In his scheme, lymphedema can be separated into three types: (a) obliterative, where the lymphatic vessels have been progressively destroyed by recurrent infection; (b) obstructive, in which the proximal lymphatics and/or nodal systems are blocked from developmental abnormalities or surgery; (c) lymphatic valvular incompetence, in which the lymphatic valves are inherently incompetent, which leads to dilation and hyperplasia. This classification system may be helpful in determining therapy, as will be addressed below.

Physiology/Pathophysiology

The lymphatic system acts to carry interstitial fluid and protein away from the tissues, but it is especially important in the transport of large particulate substances and proteins, as these are generally nonabsorbable by the bloodstream. The lymphatics are freely permeable and allow passage of molecules in either direction, but normal intralymphatic pressures are in the subatmospheric range (0 to −16 mm H_2O), which favors the flow of fluids into the lymphatics. The lymphatics have valves and the fluid is pumped proximally by both extrinsic (skeletal muscle) and intrinsic (smooth muscle) action. The lymphatic valves are bi-leaflet, like venous valves, but can only withstand a back pressure of around 50 mm Hg.

The primary lymphatics consist of a dermal network and contain no valves. These primary lymphatics drain into the secondary system, which lies in the subdermal area that contains valves and parallels the superficial venous system. These secondary lymphatics drain into a deeper layer above the fascia that contains more valves and some smooth muscle in the wall. An intramuscular layer of lymphatics also exists that parallels the deep arterial system. This system serves to drain the muscular compartments, joints, and synovium, and seems to function independently of the superficial system. These two systems are probably connected at or near the lymph nodes, but the existence of this separate deep system may partly explain why lymphedema is primarily a problem of the skin and subcutaneous tissues.

Clinically, the primary lymphatic drainage system in the upper extremity can be found beginning distally around the radial wrist, running with the cephalic vein. These large (in the 0.5–1.0 mm range) lymphatic channels parallel the cephalic vein to the antecubital fossa, where they cross over to the area of the epitrochlear node(s) and continue up the inner upper arm following the basilic vein to the axillary nodes. The primary lymphatic channels in the leg begin on

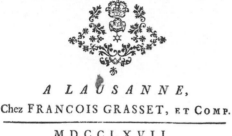

HISTOIRE

DE

L'ELEPHANTIASIS,

contenant auffi

L'ORIGINE DU SCORBUT, DU FEU

ST. ANTOINE, DE LA VEROLE, &c.

avec un Précis

DE L'HISTOIRE PHYSIQUE DES TEMS.

PAR Mᴿ. RAYMOND,

Doĉteur en Médecine de la Faculté de MONTPELLIER,
aggrégé au Collège des Médecins de MARSEILLE, &
Membre de l'ACADEMIE DES BELLES LETTRES
de cette même Ville, &c. &c.

A LAUSANNE,

Chez FRANCOIS GRASSET, ET COMP.

MDCCLXVII.

FIG. 101–1. Frontispiece from Raymond's 1767 monograph on Elephantiasis. (Courtesy of the P.I. Nixon Medical History Library and
Archives, The University of Texas Health Science Center at San Antonio, San Antonio, Texas.)

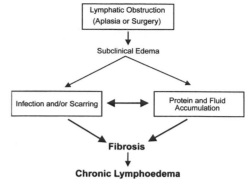

FIG. 101–2. Development of lymphedema after lymphatic obstruction, which proceeds depending on the further compromise of remaining lymphatics.

the dorsum of the foot and can generally be found running
parallel to the saphenous venous system up to the femoral
nodes. Certainly other channels in the limbs exist, but for
lymphatic exploration leading to surgical intervention these
are the best areas. While major connections between the lymphatic system and venous system exist via the thoracic duct,
other smaller lymphatico-venous connections have been
demonstrated in animals and are thought to exist in humans
as well.

When the rate of lymph formation in the tissues exceeds
the rate of lymph return, lymphedema results. This causes a
pooling of proteins and fats in the interstitial spaces, which
leads to an increase in oncotic pressure. The increase in the
protein load causes the osmotic deposition of more fluid and
leads to more edema. The increased protein content of the
edema fluid also leads to fibroblast proliferation with subsequent collagen deposition, resulting in "brawny" edema (Fig.
101–2). This fluid provides an excellent culture media for
bacteria and can encourage recurrent bouts of cellulitis. The
limb with lymphatic obstruction is probably also an im-
munologically isolated site, (7) which promotes infection and
may play a role in the later development of malignancies in
the affected area (8).

PRIMARY LYMPHEDEMAS

The underlying pathophysiology of the primary lymphedemas has been outlined well by Kinmonth, who made a lifelong study of patients with lymphedema (9). In a lymphan-
giographic study of 562 patients with primary lymphedema
of the lower limb, he found that 90% of patients had hypoplasia of the lymphatics and the remaining 10% had hyperplasia. The patients with hypoplasia were found to have
involvement of the distal lymphatics and/or proximal pelvic
nodal basin. The patients with distal hypoplasia have fewer
lymphatic channels than normal and they were usually
smaller than normal. Those with proximal involvement had
small, atrophic pelvic nodes. Pelvic nodal hypoplasia was associated with either normal or hypoplastic limb lymphatic
channels, either condition causing a functional blockage of
lymphatic drainage.

Those patients with hyperplasia were found to have lymphatics larger than normal, with incompetent valves and tortuous channels. Three percent of patients (30% of this group)
had megalymphatics, with huge lymphatic varicosities that
had absent or incompetent valves. Patients with hyperplasia
would fit in the third group of Browse's classification system
(lymphatic valvular incompetence).

Kinmonth (10) noted a relatively high incidence of other,
nonlymphatic, congenital malformations in his patients with
primary lymphedema. In 952 patients with primary lymphedema, he noted 179 other malformations in 166 patients,
for a total rate of 17.4%. These included vascular deformities, gonad dysgenesis, congenital heart disease, and various
other problems. While these malformations are not particularly unusual, one should be aware of the potential for their
presence in patients with primary lymphedema. Lymphedema is also associated with certain syndromes, such as
"yellow nail" syndrome, in which patients have nail abnormalities, lymphedema, pleural effusion and/or pneumonia,
and protein-losing enteropathy (10). Lymphedema is also a
part of the Klippel-Trenaunay syndrome, which is manifested
with multiple hemangiomas and lymphangiomas and resultant overgrowth of the extremity (Fig. 101–3).

While these patients may not present with edema early in
life, over time they develop further obliteration of their lymphatic systems that leads to increasing edema. Studies of the
lymphatics with fluorescent microangiography and pressure
measurements have shown increasing lymphatic hypertension in patients with lymphatic blockage (11). This leads to
valvular incompetence and increasing aplasia and ectasia of
the remaining lymphatics. Recurrent attacks of cellulitis have

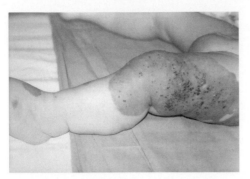

FIG. 101–3. Patient with Klippel-Trenaunay syndrome. Note lymphedematous swelling of leg coupled with hemangioma of thigh. Patient also has overgrowth of left leg and foot.

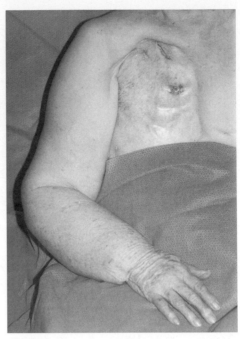

FIG. 101–4. Patient 20 years after Halsted mastectomy and irradiation for breast cancer. Lymphedema developed about 2 years after surgery. Managed successfully with conservative treatment (elevation and compression garment.)

been reported in about 27% of patients in primary lymphedema (12), and this is certainly a contributing factor to the worsening of edema. Kinmouth and colleagues (13) have also documented the phenomenon of lymphatic "die back" of remaining vessels in patients with primary lymphedema, which is the progressive obliteration of distal lymphatics with the passage of time. This process has also been noted in patients with secondary lymphedema, who seem to have sclerosis of the remaining lymphatics over time (14).

SECONDARY LYMPHEDEMAS

Series of secondary lymphedemas reflect the location and referral pattern of their authors, with filariasis being the most common cause worldwide. In the United States, the most common cause is probably the combination of surgery and irradiation for tumors. Lymphedema has been reported secondary to radical mastectomy (15), burn scar excision (16), groin dissection (17), and pelvic surgery (18). Less radical surgery has led to a decrease in the overall incidence of lymphedematous limbs, but the addition of pre- or post-operative irradiation leads to further sclerosis of remaining lymphatics with a resultant increase in edema.

The problem of arm lymphedema after radical mastectomy has been recognized since the development of this operation for breast cancer by W.S. Halsted. Halsted felt that lymphedema after radical mastectomy was not due to the operation itself but rather arose from subsequent infection. This was in part due to the fact that Reichert, working in Halsted's laboratory, was unable to create lymphedema in dog legs even after excision of all soft tissues in the leg (19). This was probably due to the fact that the lymphatic system, particularly in dogs, has a tremendous capacity to regenerate. Clinically, patients who have undergone nodal excision or irradiation rarely develop lymphedema immediately. Those who do go on to have clinical lymphedema usually do not have symptoms for at least 1 year (Fig. 101–4). I believe that this group of patients has some compromise of their lymphatic system to begin with, a feeling echoed by Miller (20). It is interesting to note that patients undergoing replantation of a limb rarely suffer from lymphedema postoperatively. Studies of patients after major limb replantation with lymphatic colloid scintigraphy have demonstrated that only about 50% have objective evidence of lymphatic blockage, although none of these patients had clinically significant lymphedema (21).

Current studies indicate an incidence of postmastectomy lymphedema (based on objective volume measurements) in the range of 7 to 63%. (15,22–24) It should be noted that arm circumference measurements have been found to correlate poorly with actual volume measurements. (22,24) While the performance of axillary clearance vs. node sampling has not shown to increase the incidence of subsequent lymphedema (24), several other factors are important. A study of 136 patients from Scandinavia who underwent mastectomy revealed that several factors were important in the pathogenesis of lymphedema as measured by volume displacement. In this group, a history of one or more infections led to a lympedema rate of 89%. Radiotherapy to the axilla in these patients resulted in a 60% rate of edema, while local irradiation, obesity, and surgery on the side of hand dominance gave rates of lymphedema in the 40% range (23). Patients without these factors had objective lymphedema rates in the 20–30% range. Certainly, as Halsted noted, infection plays a prominent role in the development of lymphedema after surgery, and cases have been reported with the sudden onset of edema 30 years after mastectomy owing to inflammatory processes (24).

Several studies have suggested that lymphatic blockage is not the only factor important in the development of lymphedema after nodal dissection in the axilla. One study has found increased Starling pressures in operated arms, indicating increased capillary filtration in these limbs (26). Others have noted increased arterial inflow (perhaps due to a sympathectomy effect) (27), and venous outflow obstruction (28) in patients after treatment for breast cancer. These factors certainly may play a role in the development of lymphedema, but further work needs to be done as to the therapeutic significance of these findings.

Rates of secondary lymphedema after nodal extirpation in the lower extremity roughly mirror those in the arm. Following groin dissection for treatment of malignant melanoma, lymphedema was found below the knee in about 40% of patients (17). All of the patients in this group were noted to have localized lymphedema of the anterior thigh, however. In patients undergoing pelvic nodal dissection and irradiation for cervical cancer, one study noted that 41% of patients had a >5% increase in volume of at least one leg (18). Twenty-two percent of these patients had clinically symptomatic edema, with 7% having severe swelling of one or both lower limbs.

Lymphedema following severe trauma to the lower extremity has not been well described. Patients who have undergone reconstruction of the limb with severe injury often develop swelling of the ankle and foot at a later time. Generally, these are patients who have had musculoskeletal trauma requiring multiple operations, usually including free flap transfer for soft-tissue injury. Whether the primary etiology of the swelling is venous or lymphatic obstruction is often difficult to ascertain by physical examination, but these patients have clinical symptoms exactly like those with lymphedema. The management of this problem is often difficult, and some patients opt for amputation to alleviate problems with swelling, drainage, and recurrent cellulitis (Fig. 101–5).

Lymphedema of the extremities carries other risks as well as those related to the morbidity from swelling. These complications are probably related to the relative immune incompetence of the lymphedematous limb. Recurrent cellulitis is common, as noted above (7). The development of lymphan-

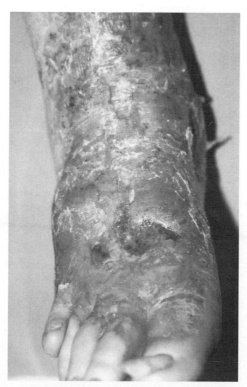

FIG. 101–5. Foot of patient with lymphedema and recurrent infection after severe fracture of distal tibia. Patient developed recurrent infection after minor breakdown of dorsal foot skin.

giosarcoma is a rare but lethal complication of lymphedema (29). This entity was first described in 1948, and is called Stewart-Treves syndrome after these authors (30). It has been reported to have an incidence of 0.45% in women who live 5 years after radical mastectomy (31). Only about 225 cases had been reported as of 1985, and these reports emphasized the necessity of radical surgery (forequarter amputation) for potential cure (32–34). Kaposi's sarcoma has also been reported in the lymphedematous arm, and this further supports the theory that these extremities suffer from a local immune incompetence (8). The question remains as to whether treatment of lymphedema actually decreases the risk of these complications.

Diagnosis and Workup

The etiology of limb edema is often difficult to ascertain, and the workup should exclude other causes of edema whenever possible. Doppler venous studies and/or venography should be used to rule out venous obstructive disease, because 10 to 20% of patients with edema after axillary or inguinal dissection will have combined lymphatic and venous obstruction (35). Evaluation of the lymphatic system in the patient with lymphedema should be undertaken with care, however. While lymphangiography is the "gold standard" for evaluation of the lymphatic system, its use in patients with lymphedema is to be avoided. Lymphangiogram performed in a patient with normal lymphatics results in rapid disappearance of the dye from the lymphatic channels; however studies in patients with lymphatic obstruction show stasis of the dye in the already compromised lymphatics. This causes irritation of the endothelial lining of the lymphatic, with potential worsening of the lymphedema. In a volumetric study of 53 patients undergoing lymphangiography, O'Brien's group found that 32% of patients had an increase in edema following lymphangiography, with 13% having a permanent worsening of their swelling (36). Later surgical exploration of the lymphatics in the patients who had undergone lymphangiogram demonstrated significant scarring and atrophy of lymphatics, even in patients who had no change in their limb after the dye study. Histologic examination of these lymphatic vessels confirmed thickening of the wall and luminal obliteration. For this reason, dye studies should be avoided in patients with lymphedema.

If one is unsure of the level of blockage, the lymphatics can be safely studied with the technique of technetium-99m sulfur colloid scintigraphy (37). While not giving the anatomic detail of dye studies, scintigraphy will delineate lymphatic channels and the adequacy of drainage. This technique can also be used postoperatively to evaluate the results of excisional or microlymphatic surgery.

The use of computed tomographic (CT) imaging of patients to aid in the diagnosis of lymphedema has been proposed (38). A honeycomb appearance of the subcutaneous tissue was noted in 83% of patients with lymphedema in one study, which was not seen in patients with edema from venous stasis. Magnetic resonance imaging (MRI) has also been utilized for the study of these patients. MRI studies reveal muscular edema in patients with venous problems, as compared to subcutaneous swelling (without muscular edema) in those with lymphatic obstruction (39). MRI also reveals a fibrotic honeycomb pattern of the subcutaneous tissue in some patients with lymphedema. While these studies may have some application in very difficult cases or those patients with tumor (or recurrent tumor), their use in most cases is probably not justified for reasons of cost.

Evaluation of treatment methods is also important in documenting the effectiveness of therapy. Measurements of limb circumference are notoriously unreliable, and the best technique is to measure limb volume by water displacement (40) . Measurements are generally recorded in percent difference compared to the normal limb, with 5% usually accepted as the normal limb volume differential.

Treatment

Treatment of lymphedema falls into two general categories, conservative and surgical. Conservative therapy aims at reducing the volume of the limb and avoiding infection, while surgical therapy aims primarily at volume reduction in the limb that has reached a state in which conservative therapy fails to control symptoms. A rational approach to therapy should be applied to every patient when first seen, and surgery reserved for those who fail conservative measures. It should be emphasized to the patient that this is generally a progressive disease that will not spontaneously "go away." Treatment is essentially lifelong, and the support of a knowledgeable physician is essential for the patient's well being and therapeutic success.

CONSERVATIVE THERAPY

A trial of conservative therapy should be attempted in every patient after initial onset of edema. Some would suggest that most patients should be treated conservatively, regardless of the severity of their disease (41). In 1959, Britton (42) outlined five phases of conservative therapy in patients with postmastectomy edema, and these are largely applicable today. Phase I consists of patient education and prevention of infection in the limb. Britton points out the importance of avoiding even the most trivial injury to prevent cellulitis. Phase II consists of the use of antibiotics to control infection, whether it is clinically evident or not. Phase III involves the fitting of an intermittent pneumatic compression device to compress fluid up the limb. He emphasizes the importance of avoiding compression in an extremity with active infection. Phase IV is the fitting of an elastic garment after a plateau in the decrease of edema has been reached with compression. Phase V is the institution of postural exercises to improve posture with respect to the weight of the limb. While the timing of the various phases of treatment in this scheme may need to be modified, it is a good outline of the conservative approach.

The prevention and treatment of infection is an important mainstay of conservative therapy. Infection is almost impossible to avoid completely in these patients, but it is important to try. With proper care of the limb, most patients develop infections only rarely, but there are occasional patients in whom infection poses a recurring problem. These patients may benefit from prophylactic anti-strep antibiotics, but my experience with this approach has been generally poor. Recurrent infections requiring hospitalization and intravenous antibiotics, particularly in the leg, may warrant consideration for amputation.

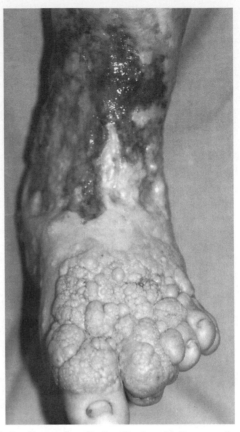

FIG. 101–6. Foot of patient with lymphedema and verrucous changes in toes. Note also skin breakdown around ankle from recurrent infection.

While cellulitis is the most common infective complication, the lower extremity presents other problems as well. Patients with severe lower-extremity edema may develop verrucous changes in the feet and around the toes (Fig. 101–6). This can lead to intertriginous bacterial and fungal infection, with secondary ulceration seen on occasion. While the exact etiology of these warty growths is not known, some feel that they are a result of (rather than a cause of) recurrent infection in the toes (43). The problem of verrucous change and ulceration can be very difficult to treat in the lymphedematous leg, and has been reported to lead to the development of squamous cell carcinoma in longstanding cases (44). While some propose shaving this tissue down to the dermal level and resurfacing the toes with split-thickness skin grafts, I believe this will not eliminate the problem. Distal transmetatarsal amputation offers a reasonable alternative in most patients and affords good control of this problem.

A number of drugs have been proposed for the treatment of lymphedema, but none are in wide usage. Diuretics have been proposed, and may promote an initial decrease in the edema. They are of little use long-term, however, unless the patient is actually fluid overloaded. The benzopyrones have also been utilized in the treatment of lymphedema, as they act to remove protein macrophages from the high-protein edema fluid (45,46). The agent utilized, 5,6,-benzo-α-pyrone, is also know as coumarin (which is not an anticoagulant). Coumarin has been found effective in reducing lymphedema in a dog model (47) and recent studies have shown promise in the treatment of lymphedema after filariasis (48), and in postmastectomy lymphedema (49). The action of this drug is slow, but short-term studies show reasonable tolerance and efficacy. Further studies need to be done, but this drug may become important in conservative treatment. It should be noted that this drug is not presently available for clinical use in the United States.

Conservative approaches in reducing the volume of the lymphedematous extremity are based on mechanical techniques to force fluid out of the limb. This can be simply accomplished by elevating the limb at night, with intermittent periods of elevation during the day. Many patients have made special arrangements at work to allow them to elevate their leg (in patients whose job requires sitting), or to sit and elevate the leg for a certain amount of time each day (in patients who must stand at work). While this approach is useful in patients with mild to moderate edema, it often is of little benefit in those with severe or longstanding edema.

Further diminution in volume can be accomplished by massage or mechanical devices to compress the limb. Massage has been proven effective for the reduction of fluid in the limb (50), and results may be improved when isometric exercises are combined with massage therapy (51). Pneumatic compression devices have been utilized in the treatment of lymphedema for many years (42). Most studies document a significant decrease in edema in the treated extremity, in the range of 15 to 50% (40,52,53). Hands and feet have the most significant improvement based on objective measurements. While a number of devices are available, pumps providing sequential compression (from distal to proximal) seem to make the most sense (53). The use of these devices is usually combined with a compression garment to be worn after the limb volume is down. The primary advantages of this therapy are that it is relatively inexpensive and easy to use.

The problem with these devices, however, is that they require routine daily use to be effective in the long term. The papers cited above described treatment periods of from 4 to 8 hours a day, which theoretically can be done while the patient sleeps. In my experience, however, few patients will continue this regimen very long. Despite the severity of their edema, most patients in my practice find this type of therapy impractical.

Another mainstay of treatment is the use of an elastic compression garment around the limb. This treatment is most useful if the garment is placed after massage or compression therapy, when the limb is in its least swollen state (54). An appropriately fitted compression garment can help to control edema when combined with a program of physical therapy or pumping (40,52,53,55). One study has suggested that a "significant result" can be achieved by use of an elastic garment alone (56).

It is important that the garment fit properly, or it can lead to a worsening of the edema by acting as a tourniquet at the joints or where elastic bands hold the garment in place. The optimal garment is one custom-fitted for the individual. The patient is best measured with the limb in a minimally swollen state, which can be done either after a period of compression therapy or in the morning before the edema has increased from dependency. The best time to measure the patient may be during hospitalization, when elevation and/or pumping of the limb can be assured. Once the patient has a well-fitting garment, it should be put on first thing in the morning. Even brief periods of dependency can markedly increase edema of the foot and ankle. In the case of leg lymphedema, advise the patient to put on the stocking before the foot first hits the floor in the morning. This approach has the advantages of being inexpensive and easy, with minimal interference with daily activities. The disadvantage of compression garments is that they are hot in the summer, and may not be worn for this reason. Patients who are actively using their garments wear them out rather quickly, and should be prescribed several at a time. The patient who presents for followup in the office with a "like new" compression garment each visit (without asking for replacements) is not wearing it, except for the physician's benefit.

Other conservative therapies have been proposed, but are not widely accepted. Electrical stimulation of lymphatic flow has been tried, but was found not to be significantly better than wearing an elastic garment alone (56). Treatment in a dry heat chamber has been tried in China, with one study reporting a 68% decrease in edema in a group of 1045 patients (57). The limb is heated to the range of 100° C for a course of about five treatments, followed by the use of a compression garment. These authors report regeneration of lymphatics based on pre- and post-treatment lymphscintigraphy. Microwave radiation (instead of heat) has also been used, with similar success (58). The results of this type of treatment are intriguing, but further studies need to be completed before it is widely accepted.

SURGICAL THERAPY

The indications for surgical treatment of lymphedema generally follow logically in patients who have failed conservative therapy. Patients who have decreased range of motion (ROM) due to swelling in the upper extremity or those who have problems related to the weight of the limb should be considered for surgical treatment. Some patients present who have problems with the fitting of clothes, despite conservative therapy, and these likewise may be surgical candidates. Patients with recurrent infection and/or chronic drainage from the limb may be surgical candidates, but one must bear in mind that no proof exists that surgical treatment will completely remedy these problems long term. Some authors believe that fewer than 10% of all patients with lymphedema will require surgical treatment (35).

Surgical treatment can be divided into two categories: excisional procedures and physiologic procedures. Excisional techniques aim to decrease girth of the limb by removing some or all of the involved subcutaneous tissues. Physiologic procedures, on the other hand, aim to decrease edema by restoring lymph flow across the area of blockage either via bypass procedures or reliance on lymphatic outflow via tissue with normal lymphatic drainage. The history of the development of procedures for lymphedema gives the reader a feel for the difficulty in handling this problem (Table 101–1).

PHYSIOLOGIC TECHNIQUES

The first attempt at surgical management of lymphedema was by Lis Franc in 1841, who proposed placing stab wounds and needle holes in the extremity to allow the fluid

Table 101–1   Operations for Lymphedema Broken Down Chronologically Into Physiologic and Excisional Procedures

Physiologic	
Lis Franc (1841)	Needle holes & stab wounds
Cornochan (1852)	Ligation of iliac artery
Handley (1908)	Silk thread "wicks"
Kondoleon (1912)	Excised strip of deep fascia
Gillies and Fraser (1935)	Cutaneous flap for drainage
Thompson (1962)	Buried dermal flap
Nielubowicz & Olszewski (1966)	Lymph-node venous shunt
Goldsmith (1966)	Omental flap bridge
Pugnaire (1968)	Mesenteric flap bridge
Politowski (1969) Gilbert & O'Brien (1976)	Lymphaticovenous anastomosis
Kinmonth (1978)	Enteromesenteric bridge
Baumeister (1981)	Lymphatico-lymphatic grafting
Excisional	
Charles (1912)	Excise + FTSG
Sistrunk (1918)	Excision of skin & fascia
Thompson (1962)	Subcutaneous excision/flap
Miller (1973)	Staged subcutaneous excision

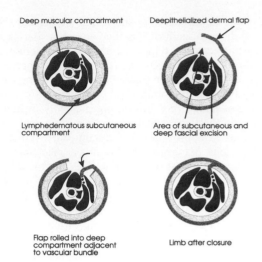

FIG. 101–7. Schematic of Thompson's buried dermal flap procedure for treatment of lymphedema. Note that large segment of subcutaneous tissue is excised.

to drain (1). This technique met with little success, as did the suggestion of Cornochan in 1852 of ligating the iliac artery for control of lymphedema (59). In 1908 Samson Handley proposed the technique of "lymphangioplasty," where silk sutures were placed across the level of lymphatic blockage to act as a wick for fluid egress (60). This technique has been tried with a number of other substances, including nylon, fascia, and various small tubes (61–64). The problem is that the improvement only lasts a few months, and more recent studies have demonstrated the development of scar around the implant (not surprising), which probably blocks further flow of fluid. Likewise, this type of treatment suffers from a high rate of extrusion of the implanted material as the result of infection (65,66). We will see that the problem of scar formation continues to plague attempts at reestablishment of lymphatic flow.

In 1912 Kondoleon proposed the excision of a strip of deep fascia to allow drainage of lymph from the superficial compartment to the deep compartments (which presumably had intact lymphatic drainage) (67). While this operation was supposed to be a physiologic one, Sistrunk from the Mayo Clinic modified the operation in 1918 to include excision of more skin and subcutaneous tissue (up to one-half the circumference of the enveloping fascia) (68). While Sistrunk felt that the decrease in swelling was due to an improvement in lymphatic drainage, his modification of the Kondoleon procedure was the forerunner of most of the excisional techniques described below.

The idea of allowing "normal" tissue to drain a lymphedematous limb prompted Gillies in 1935 to use a pedicled random abdominal flap placed on the leg for lymphatic drainage (69). While he had rather spectacular early success, most other authors have not been as enthusiastic about this technique. The problem lies in the fact that random flaps usually do not have intact major lymphatic channels, which would preclude a reasonable result with this approach. Axial pattern flaps, however, should be expected to contain at least a few lymphatic channels, and they have also been utilized in attempts to reestablish lymphatic flow. In 1981 a fasciocutaneous flap based on the thoracodorsal fascia was reported for treatment of postreplantation lymphedema in the upper arm (70). Although the patient had improvement after this procedure, this flap was performed only 2 months postreplant and one would expect that this edema would have improved with time (21). A latissimus dorsi myocutaneous flap has also been utilized as a "wick" for arm lymphedema after mastectomy, with the pedicled muscle and skin paddle placed into the lymphedematous arm. The reported results of this procedure have been variable (71), with recent case reports showing good results in patients with severe edema (72). The obvious disadvantage of this flap is that it utilizes a muscle which may be needed for breast and/or chest wall reconstruction later. The use of myocutaneous or fascial flaps for the management of lymphedema deserves more attention, but at present they have limited application.

In 1959 Thompson first utilized the buried dermal flap technique for treatment of lymphedema of the lower extremity (73). His rationale was to allow drainage of lymphatic fluid from the subcutaneous compartment via an attached strip of dermis placed into the deep compartment. This was done via a random, deepithelialized flap which was buried in between the muscles ". . . into direct contact with the main vessels of the limb and their accompanying deep lymph trunks" (74) (Fig. 101–7). He noted "good" or "satisfactory" results in the majority of patients treated with this technique in a 10-year survey (74), and found that radioactive iodine clearance from the lymphedematous area was improved in four-fifths of patients studied (75). Other studies have failed to confirm this physiologic improvement in lymphatic drainage, however, and Sawhney suggested that the reduction in limb volume is primarily due to the amount of tissue removed (and is in fact proportional to it) (76).

The first attempt at directly reestablishing lymphatic flow from the lymphedematous limb was made by Nielubowicz and Olszewski in 1966 with the lymph-node venous shunt procedure (77). In their patients with lower extremity lymphedema, anastomosis of cut inguinal nodes to the femoral or saphenous vein produced improvement in the edema. The problem with this procedure is that improvement is not usually longstanding, as the cut face of the node eventually undergoes fibrosis with recurrence of the swelling (78). Goldsmith in 1967 (79) first reported the idea of using a bridge of omentum placed into the lymphedematous limb to allow reconstitution of lymphatic drainage. In a long-term followup paper, he found that only 38% of patients with lower-extremity lymphedema and only 56% of patients with upper-extremity edema had "good" results (80). The problem with this procedure is that the limb lymphatics fail to interconnect spontaneously with the omental lymphatics, despite its rich supply of lymphatic channels (81,82). Use of a piece of small bowel, denuded of its mucosa and placed over the inguinal lymph nodes as a pedicled flap for drainage, was first reported by Pugnaire in 1968 (83). Hurst and Kinmonth later showed that such an enteromesenteric bridge would form lymphatic connections from the limb and allow lymphatic drainage in pigs (84). These authors have reported good results in patients with proximal obstructive disease (whether primary or secondary), and believe it may be the procedure of choice in some patients (85,86). Owing to the potential for intraabdominal morbidity (due to the necessity for small-bowel resection and anastomosis), this approach has not become widely accepted (1).

Early experimental attempts at direct anastomosis between lymphatic vessels and veins were discouraging, with poor patency rates reflecting poor results (87,88). Politowski reported the first attempts at lymphaticovenous shunting in patients in 1969, with 50% showing some decrease in circumference in the limb (89). Improvement in the technique of anastomosis led to improved results, with O'Brien (among others) reporting reasonable results with this technique (90,91). Large series of patients followed for extended periods show that this technique does have some value, however certain points must be emphasized. Patients with longstanding edema (>10–12 years) may have no remaining lymphatics for anastomosis, and should be considered for some other type of therapy. The procedure generally has better results in the upper extremity than the lower, probably because of a less dependent position of the arm, which allows for better drainage via the anastomoses. The methylene blue test, described by Gong, may be helpful in difficult patient selection (92). In this test, methylene blue is injected subdermally in the affected limb; if the blue dye appears in the patient's urine by 1 hour after dye injection, the patient probably has some functioning lymphatic channels (which implies that microanastomoses can be performed).

This technique for identification of the lymphatics is generally done with Patent Blue dye (also know as patent blue V or alphazurine 2G), which is unavailable in the United States.

The dye is of low molecular weight and is not taken up by proteins, which makes it readily diffusible into lymphatic channels (93). When injected intradermally, it stains the lymphatics so that they are identifiable at the time of surgical exploration. I have tried methylene blue and brilliant green for the same purpose, but these dyes provide little staining of the lymphatics in my experience. A mixture containing F.D.A. Blue #1 is utilized in the United States by some radiologists performing lymphangiograms to facilitate cannulation of the lymphatics; this is presumably the same dye and is not officially approved in the United States. Patent blue has been noted to cause allergic reactions in some patients, and an intradermal wheal skin test should be performed prior to actual injection to evaluate for sensitivity.

Finally, critical review of recent reports reveals that many patients had treatment with both microsurgery and resectional surgery (14), which obscures the value of microlymphatic surgery alone (94). Most authors currently believe that this type of surgery can relieve lymphedema, but the question remains as to the longevity of the result (95). The backpressure of the venous system, particularly in the leg, may be high enough to prevent flow of lymphatic fluid across the anastomosis. While it is technically possible to anastomose lymphatics to tiny veins, whether flow will be maintained in the long run is still open to question.

The final and most direct physiologic approach to lymphatic blockage is the use of autologous lymphatic grafts to bridge obstructed segments (96). Baumeister has done much research in this area, beginning with experimental lymphatic grafting in animals (97), and later in applications in patients with lymphedema (98). In a group of 11 patients followed for at least 3 years, his group found a reduction in limb volume of up to 80% (99). These patients were also shown to have a gradual improvement in their lymphedema over the period of the study. This technique deserves further study as it may prove to offer the best physiologic solution for lymphedema.

EXCISIONAL TECHNIQUES

Direct excision of lymphedematous tissues for the treatment of lymphedema secondary to filariasis was first proposed by Havelock Charles of the Indian Medical Services in Calcutta in 1912 (100). In the Charles technique, all lymphedematous tissues superficial to the muscle compartments are excised, and the muscles are resurfaced with skin grafts taken from the excised tissue. This procedure is well-suited to patients with elephantiasis and has the advantage (as proposed by Charles) of avoiding a second wound from skin graft donor site(s). There is generally little recurrence of the edema in the grafted areas, but there can be problems with take of the skin grafts (particularly if full-thickness grafts are utilized). The recurrence of cellulitis seems to be lessened by this procedure, although breakdown of the skin grafts can lead to infection. Long-term followup of patients undergoing the Charles procedure show that the skin graft holds up well but that split-grafted areas of the foot may be prone to some hyperkeratotic changes (101). There can be some increase in the edema of the foot if all of the underlying edematous tissues on the dorsum are not excised (Fig. 101–8). I find that patients may have worsening of the condition of the toes after the Charles procedure in the lower extremity, and will therefore sometimes perform a distal transmetatarsal amputa-

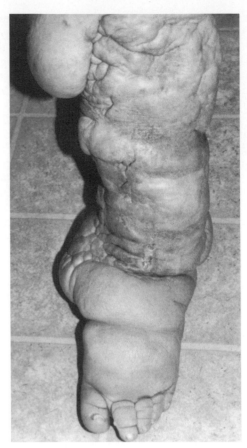

FIG. 101–8. Leg of patient 10 years after Charles' procedure for lymphedema of left leg. Note increased swelling of foot and proximal thigh, as well as verrucous change in grafted calf. Patient was very obese as well.

tion at the time of excision if the toes are very swollen to begin with (Fig. 101–9).

Full-thickness excision is also applicable to the patient with severe involvement of the penis and scrotum. Soft-tissue excision to the deep fascia and coverage with split-thickness skin grafts offers an excellent treatment of penile lymphedema (102).

The Charles procedure is certainly not a cosmetic one in terms of limb appearance, but most patients readily accept this tradeoff if the limb is more functional. Overall the Charles procedure is an excellent option for treatment of patients with severe edema, especially if they suffer from marked skin thickening as is seen in elephantiasis.

The Sistrunk and Thompson procedures, which were described above, were the forerunners of more current partial excisional procedures (68,75). While purported to be physiologic, these two techniques probably provide the majority of their benefit on the basis of the tissue excised, rather than an actual improvement in lymphatic drainage. Homans noted early on that the quality of the result of the Sistrunk operation was directly proportional to the amount of tissue excised (103).

Staged excision of both subcutaneous tissue and skin from the lymphedematous limb is the procedure most commonly practiced today. It is a descendant of the above-mentioned

procedures, but derives its benefit from volume reduction of the limb rather than an improvement in lymphatic flow. The primary proponent of this technique is Miller, who has proven this technique in terms of its safety and efficacy (104–106). This technique involves excision of skin and subcutaneous tissue down to the level of the fascia on both the medial and lateral aspects of the limb. The inner and outer excisions are staged several months apart to avoid complications. In studies of patients having staged subcutaneous excision, Miller has found that up to a 50% reduction in limb volume can be achieved, and many patients have fewer bouts of cellulitis after this treatment (105,106). Most patients continue to have some edema, and thus are placed in well-fitting compression garments in the postoperative period. The complications of this procedure are few, but distal swelling and numbness around the areas of excision are relatively common in my experience. While some authors have expressed concern about the potential for loss of the skin flaps with this operation (107), Miller reported that this occurs infrequently (and will usually heal without further surgery), which has been my experience as well. The foot remains problematic in this regard, particularly in children, as skin loss and/or hypertrophic scarring are common after local excision (108). If properly done, this procedure offers a reasonable compromise for many patients with lymphedema. While it does not totally cure the edema, complications are few and patients generally satisfied with the result.

Liposuction has been recently proposed as a treatment for lymphedema, with somewhat mixed results. One report states that a group of patients had an improvement in limb volume after this procedure, but personal review of this group of patients indicated that treatment with liposuction actually increased the limb volume (109). Another report found an average 6.8% reduction in limb circumference with an 8% reduction in limb volume after liposuction (110), both of which are only marginally significant. This report also noted that the best results were in patients who underwent combined liposuction and resection, which brings the benefit of the added liposuction into question. While reported complications were few, I have seen skin necrosis on the distal extremity after this procedure. It is my opinion that liposuction currently has little place in the treatment of lymphedema, although further work as to the indications and technique may prove its value.

CURRENT APPROACH

Patients with lymphedema are often told that nothing can be done to improve their status, or are left in a state of pseudotreatment with poorly fitting garments and little hope. With a rational approach and an understanding of what can be done, these patients' situations can be improved (Fig. 101–10). It must be emphasized that the problem is not totally curable, however, and treatment is lifelong. As noted above, I believe that all patients should be treated conservatively initially. The problem is that by the time of referral many patients have had marginal conservative treatment and their condition has worsened to the point that surgery may be necessary for adequate improvement. When I am seeing them early, I treat patients primarily with a custom-fitted elastic garment and emphasize the necessity for periods of rest and elevation. I limit the use of pneumatic compression

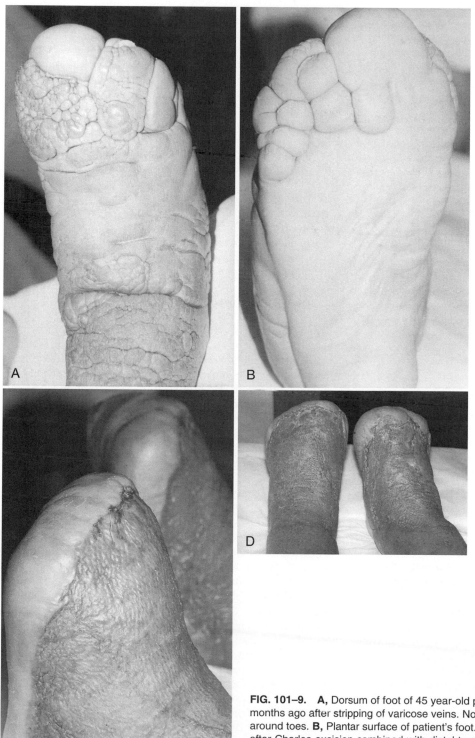

FIG. 101–9.   A, Dorsum of foot of 45 year-old patient who developed lymphedema 22 months ago after stripping of varicose veins. Note severe swelling and verrucous changes around toes. **B,** Plantar surface of patient's foot. **C,** Lateral view of both feet four months after Charles excision combined with distal transmetatarsal amputation of toes. Plantar flap was brought over distal metatarsals and remainder was covered with meshed split-thickness skin grafts. **D,** Dorsal view of feet.

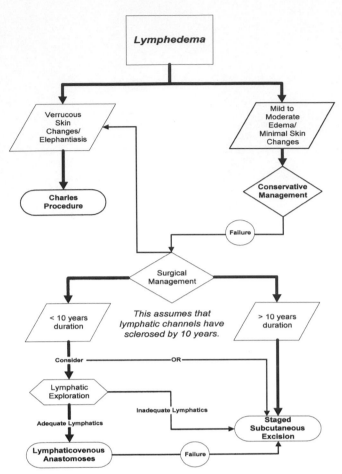

FIG. 101–10. Flowchart for management of lymphedema of the extremities.

devices to those patients who are older (and usually unemployed), who may be poor candidates for later surgery. As noted above, most patients in my experience cannot cope with the regimen necessary to treat their edema effectively with a pneumatic device. I do not routinely give prophylactic antibiotics to my patients, but episodes of cellulitis must be closely watched for by the patient and antibiotics started early if they occur. Patients with recurrent bouts of cellulitis may require continuous low-dose oral anti-strep treatment, but this may not totally alleviate this problem.

The most common patient seen in my practice is one who has been on a conservative regimen for several years and has ongoing problems with limb weight, the fitting of clothes, or recurrent infection. These patients generally are seeking surgical treatment to decrease the size and/or weight of the limb. This group of patients is worked up with evaluation of edema by circumference or volume measurements, status of venous outflow (usually by Doppler exam) to rule out venous stasis, and general medical exam. The option of microsurgical lymphaticovenous anastomosis is discussed with patients with lymphedema of the upper extremity of less than 10 years standing, and in some young female patients with leg edema. While I am not entirely convinced that this procedure is applicable to the lower extremity, cosmetic concerns in younger patients (secondary to scarring from excision), taken with the minimal morbidity

of this procedure, make me continue to offer it to selected patients. Most patients are treated surgically with staged subcutaneous excision; this technique may be performed in those patients undergoing microsurgery as well.

All patients must be free from cellulitis at the time of operative intervention. Many patients with marked skin thickening and verrucous changes may have chronic odor and drainage from the limb. These patients are begun on daily scrubs of the limb with surgical soap and/or vinegar several days before surgery to reduce surface bacteria. All patients undergoing surgery are admitted the night before (assuming the insurance company will allow it) for elevation and/or pneumatic compression of the limb. Surgery on the lymphedematous limb is much easier if the limb is well decompressed at the time of operation, particularly in the case of staged excision. All patients are treated preoperatively and for 5 days postoperatively with systemic antiobiotics.

All surgery on the distal extremity is performed with a proximal sterile tourniquet. The use of an Esmarch (or Martin) bandage for exsanguination may actually decrease the limb volume further if carefully applied before inflation of the tourniquet. I generally perform excision, when needed, on the medial aspect of the limb at the first stage. With this approach, if scarring is severe (which is unusual) the outer excision can be delayed or deferred entirely based on the patient's wishes (Fig. 101–11). I do not attempt to perform an actual subcutaneous excision, but rather remove a block of tissue from the skin surface to the deep fascia. A large segment can be easily removed if the limb has be adequately decompressed before surgery. With this approach, wound healing problems are minimal. I also avoid crossing the elbow or knee at the first stage, and will remove this tissue at the second stage with a Z- or W-plasty type of incision. Suction drains are placed in the depth of all wounds, but these are removed by 3 days postop to avoid retrograde infection (even though they may continue to drain some lymphatic fluid). The second stage can be performed in 6 to 12 weeks on the lateral aspect of the limb following the same protocol.

If lymphatic exploration for potential microanastomsis is performed, some type of dye should be utilized to help identify the lymphatics in the subcutaneous tissues. Patent blue is the gold standard, as noted above, but methylene blue will give some minimal staining of the lymphatic channels. The chosen dye should be injected into the webspaces of the digits before prepping of the limb for surgery. In some cases, the lymphatics will be outlined on the skin after a period of 15 to 10 minutes, particularly with the use of patent blue (Fig. 101–12). In the arm, an incision is made over the cephalic vein at the wrist and along the medial proximal forearm at or near the antecubital fossa. In the leg, incisions are made over the saphenous vein at the ankle, knee, and upper thigh. Appropriate lymphatics and small veins are chosen and anastomoses performed with standard technique using 11-0 nylon. If no patent lymphatics are noted at exploration, subcutaneous excision alone is usually performed. If microanastomoses can be successfully done, dramatic improvement in the edema is usually noted by the first day postop (Fig. 101–13).

Postoperatively, the limb is wrapped in a dressing consisting of a layer of soft foam (about 1 inch thick) held in place with an elastic roller bandage. The inner layer of foam keeps the elastic bandage from bunching up and forming an area of

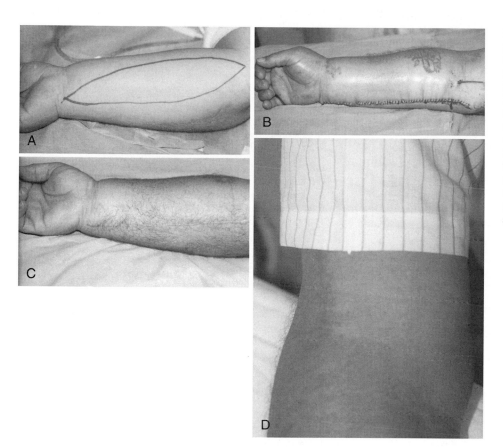

FIG. 101–11. **A,** Arm of patient 10 years after axillary dissection for treatment of malignant melanoma of upper arm. Markings on forearm prior to medial portion of staged subcutaneous excision. **B,** Arm immediately postoperative from medial excision. **C,** Arm six months after completion of medial and lateral staged subcutaneous excisions. **D,** Upper arm after completion of excision. Patient had to have extra fabric sewn into shirt sleeve prior to surgery for fit, now with normal sleeve. It should be noted that patient continues to wear mild compression garment during the day.

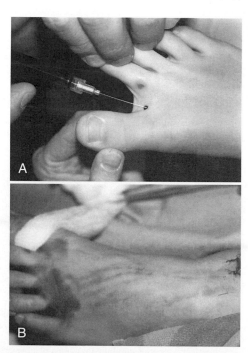

FIG. 101–12. **A,** Injection of Patent Blue into webspace for identification of lymphatics prior to microlymphaticovenous anastomoses. **B,** View of patient 20 minutes after injection of multiple webspaces. Note highlighting of dorsal foot lymphatics from staining after Patent Blue injection.

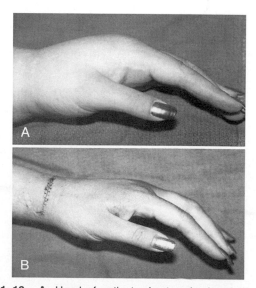

FIG. 101–13. **A,** Hand of patient prior to microlymphaticovenous anastomosis for forearm lymphedema. **B,** View of hand three days postop after performance of four microlymphaticovenous anastomoses at the wrist. Note dramatic improvement in lymphedema of hand. Patient had some recurrence of edema by six months postop, however.

circumferential compression (in effect, it is a tourniquet). On the day of discharge or before, the limb is measured for a custom-made compression garment. The patient is usually discharged with an elastic wrap, and instructed to keep the limb elevated for the period of wound healing (about 3 weeks). When the custom-fitted garment is available, it is to be worn daily as long as the patient is up. The result from microlymphatic anastomosis can be sustained for a prolonged period if the patient is diligent in wearing of the garment. Recurrence of edema may be noted as early as several months, however, and in this case staged subcutaneous excision may be necessary to achieve a reasonable result.

Bibliography

1. Savage RC. The surgical management of lymphedema. *Surg Gynecol Obstet* 1984; 159:501–508.
2. Raymond M. Histoire de L'elephantiasis. Marseille: Francois Grasset, 1767.
3. Nonne MH. Elephantiasis congenita. *Deut Med Wschr* 1890; 16:1124.
4. Milroy WF. An undescribed variety of hereditary oedema. *N Y Med J* 1892; 56; 505
5. Lewis JM, Wald ER. Lymphedema praecox. *J Pediatr* 1984; 104:641–648.
6. Browse NL, Stewart G. Lymphoedema: pathophysiology and classification. *J Cardiovasc Surg* 1985; 26:91–106.
7. Simon MS, Cody RL. Cellulitis after axillary lymph node dissection for carcinoma of the breast [see comments]. *Am J Med* 1992; 93:543–548.
8. Merimsky O, Chaitchik S. Kaposi's sarcoma on a lymphedematous arm following radical mastectomy. *Tumori* 1992; 78:407–408.
9. Kinmonth JB. The Lymphatics: surgery, lymphography and diseases of the chyle and lymph systems. 2nd ed. London: Edward Arnold, 1982.
10. Venencie PY, Dicken CH. Yellow nail syndrome: report of five cases. *J Am Acad Dermatol* 1984; 10:187–192.
11. Bollinger A. Microlymphatics of human skin. *Int J Microcirc Clin Exp* 1993; 12:1–15.
12. Wolfe JHN. The prognosis and possible cause of severe primary lymphoedema. *Ann R Coll Surg Eng* 1984; 6C:251–257.
13. Fyfe NCM, Wolfe JHN, Kinmonth JB. "Die back" in primary lymphoedema. *Lymphology* 1982; 15:66–69.
14. O'Brien BM, Mellow CG, Khazanchi RK, et al. Long-term results after microlymphatico-venous anastomoses for the treatment of obstructive lymphedema. *Plast Reconstr Surg* 1990; 85:562–572.
15. Markowski J, Wilcox JP, Helm PA. Lymphedema incidence after specific postmastectomy therapy. *Arch Phys Med* 1981; 62:449–452.
16. Balakrishnan C, Webber JD, Prasad JK. Lymphoedema of lower extremities following depridement of extensive full skin thickness burns. *Burns* 1994; 20:365–366.
17. Karakousis CP, Driscoll DL. Groin dissection in malignant melanoma. *Br J Surg* 1994; 81:1771–1774.
18. Werngren-Elgstrom M, Lidman D. Lymphoedema of the lower extremities after surgery and radiotherapy for cancer of the cervix. *Scand J Plast Reconstr Surg Hand Surg* 1994; 28:289–293.
19. Halsted WS. The swelling of the arm after operations for cancer of the breast—*Elephantiasis Chirurgica*—its cause and prevention. In: Halsted WS, ed. *Surgical papers by William Stewart Halsted, 1852–1922.* Baltimore: The Johns Hopkins Press, 1924; 90–100.
20. Miller TA. Discussion of "Microlymphaticovenous anastomosis in the treatment of lower limb obstructive lymphedema: analysis of 91 cases." *Plast Reconstr Surg* 1985; 76:680–681.
21. Smith AR, van Alphen WA, van der Pompe WB. Lymphatic drainage in patients after replantation of extremities. *Plast Reconstr Surg* 1987; 79:163–168.
22. Hoe AL, Iven D, Royle GT, et al. Incidence of arm swelling following axillary clearance for breast cancer. *Br J Surg* 1992; 79:261–262.
23. Segerstrom K, Bjerle P, Graffman S, et al. Factors that influence the incidence of brachial oedema after treatment of breast cancer. *Scand J Plast Reconstr Surg Hand Surg* 1992; 26:223–227.
24. Kissin MW, Querci della Rovere G, Easton D, et al. Risk of lymphoedema following the treatment of breast cancer. *Br J Surg* 1986; 73:580–584.
25. Brennan MJ, Weitz J. Lymphedema 30 years after radical mastectomy. *Am J Phys Med Rehabil* 1992; 71:12–14.
26. Bates DO, Levick JR, Mortimer PS. Starling pressures in the human arm and their alteration in postmastectomy oedema. *J Physiol* (Lond) 1994; 477:355–363.
27. Svensson WE, Mortimer PS, Tohno E, et al. Increased arterial inflow demonstrated by Doppler ultrasound in arm swelling following breast cancer treatment. *Eur J Cancer* 1994; 30A:661–664.
28. Svensson WE, Mortimer PS, Tohno E, et al. Colour Doppler demonstrates venous flow abnormalities in breast cancer patients with chronic arm swelling. *Eur J Cancer* 1994; 30A:657–660.
29. Borel Rinkes IHM, de Jongste AB. Lymphangiosarcoma in chronic lymphedema. *Acta Chir Scand* 1986; 152:227–230.
30. Stewart FW, Treves N. Lymphangiosarcoma in postmastectomy lymphedema. *Cancer* 1948; 1:64–81.
31. Schirger A. Postoperative lymphedema: etiology and diagnostic factors. *Med Clin North Am* 1962; 46:1045–1050.
32. Martin MB, Kon ND, Kawamoto EH, et al. Postmastectomy angiosarcoma. *Am Surgeon* 1984; 50:541–545.
33. Kaufmann T, Chu F, Kaufman R. Post-mastectomy lymphangiosarcoma (Stewart-Treves syndrome): report of two long-term survivals. *Br J Radiol* 1991; 64:857–860.
34. Sordillo PP, Chapman R, Hajdu SI, et al. Lymphangiosarcoma. *Cancer* 1981; 48:1674–1679.
35. Gloviczki P. Treatment of secondary lymphedema. In: Ernst CB, Stanley JC, eds. *Current therapy in vascular surgery.* 2nd ed. Philadelphia: Decker, 1991; 1030–1036.
36. O'Brien BM, Das SK, Franklin JD, et al. Effect of lymphangiography on lymphedema. *Plast Reconstr Surg* 1981; 68:922–926.
37. Sacks GA, Sandler MP, Born ML, et al. Lymphoscintigraphy as an adjunctive procedure in the perioperative assessment of patients undergoing microlymphaticovenous anastomoses. *Clinical Nucl Med* 1983; 8:309–311.
38. Hadjis NS, Carr DH, Banks L, et al. The role of CT in the diagnosis of primary lymphedema of the lower limb. *AJR* 1985; 144:361–364.
39. Haaverstad R, Nilsen G, Myhre HO, et al. The use of MRI in the investigation of leg oedema. *Eur J Vasc Surg* 1992; 6:124–129.
40. Raines JK, O'Donnell TF, Kalisher L, et al. Selection of patients with lymphedema for compression therapy. *Am J Surg* 1977; 133:430–437.
41. Wolfe JHN. Progress in the treatment of primary lymphoedema is not surgical. *Acta Chir Scand Suppl* 1990; 555:245–248.
42. Britton RC. Management of peripheral edema, including lymphedema of the arm after radical mastectomy. *Cleveland Clin Quarterly* 1959; 26:53–61.
43. Lewis SR. Colloquium: lymphedema of the extremity. *Ann Plast Surg* 1978; 1:191–192.
44. Epstein JI, Mendelsohn G. Squamous carcinoma of the foot arising in association with long-standing verrucous hyperplasia in a patient with congenital lymphedema. *Cancer* 1984; 54:943–947.
45. Piller NB. Lymphedema, macrophages, and benzopyrones. *Lymphology* 1980; 13:109.
46. Casley-Smith JR. The pathophysiology of lymphedema and the action of benzo-pyrones in reducing it. *Lymphology* 1988; 21:190–194.
47. Knight KR, Khanzanchi RK, Pederson WC, et al. Coumarin and 7-hydroxycoumarin treatment of canine obstructive lymphoedema. *Clin Science* 1989; 77:69.
48. Casley-Smith JR, Wang CT, Zi-hai C. Treatment of filarial lymphoedema and elephantiasis with 5,6-benzo-α-pyrone (coumarin). *BMJ* 1993; 307:1037–1041.
49. Casley-Smith JR, Morgan RG, Piller NB. Treatment of lymphedema of the arms and legs with 5,6-benzo-α-pyrone. *N Engl J Med* 1993; 329:1158–1163.
50. Kurz W, Kurz R, Litmanovitch YI, et al. Effect of manual lymphdrainage massage on blood components and urinary neurohormones in chronic lymphedema. *Angiology* 1981; 32:119–127.
51. Swedborg I. Effectiveness of combined methods of physiotherapy for post-mastectomy lymphoedema. *Scand J Rehabil Med* 1980; 12:77–85.
52. Brennan MJ. Lymphedema following the surgical treatment of breast cancer: a review of pathophysiology and treatment. *J Pain Symptom Manage* 1992; 7:110–116.
53. Richmand DM, O'Donnell TF, Zelikovski A. Sequential pneumatic compression for lymphedema: a controlled trial. *Arch Surg* 1985; 120:1116–1119.

54. Schumacker HB Jr. Management of moderate lymphedema. *Arch Surg* 1981; 116:1097–1098.

55. Campisi C. A rational approach to the management of lymphedema. *Lymphology* 1991; 24:48–53.

56. Bertelli G, Venturini M, Forno G, et al. Conservative treatment of post-mastectomy lymphedema: a controlled, randomized trial [see comments]. *Ann Oncol* 1991; 2:575–578.

57. Zhang TS, Huang WY, Han LY, et al. Heat and bandage treatment for chronic lymphedema of extremities. Report of 1,045 patients. *Chin Med J* 1984; 97:567–577.

58. Zhang DS, Han LY, Gan JL, et al. Microwave: an alternative to electric heating in the treatment of chronic lymphedema of extremities. *Chin Med J* 1986; 99:866–870.

59. Kerstein MD, Licalzi L. Microvascular procedures in the management of lymphedema. *Vasc Surg* 1977; 11:188.

60. Handley WS. Lymphangioplasty: a new method for the relief of the brawny arm of breast cancer and for similar conditions of lymphatic edema. *Lancet* 1908; 1:783–785.

61. Lexer E. Erworbene elephantiasis. *Munchen Med Wochenschr* 1919, 66:1274.

62. Ransohoff JL. Surgical treatment of lymphedema. *Arch Surg* 1945; 50:269.

63. Zieman SA. Re-establishing lymph drainage for lymphedema of the extremities. *J Internat Coll Surgeons* 1951; 15:328.

64. Hogeman K. Artificial subcutaneous channels in draining lymphedema. *Acta Chir Scand* 1955; 110:154.

65. Thompson N. The surgical treatment of chronic lymphedema of the extremities. *Surg Clin N Am* 1967; 47:445.

66. Silver D, Puckett CL. Lymphangioplasty; a ten-year evaluation. *Surgery* 1976; 80:748.

67. Kondoleon E. Die chirurgische behandlung der elefantiastischen oedeme durch eine neue methode der lymphableitung. *Munchen Med Wochenschr* 1912; 59:2726–2729.

68. Sistrunk WE. Further experiences with the Kondoleon operation for elephantiasis. *JAMA* 1918; 71:800–806.

69. Gillies H, Frazer FR. The treatment of lymphedema by plastic operation; a preliminary report. *Br Med J* 1935; 1:96.

70. Freeman BG, Berger A. Treatment of traumatic secondary lymphedema of the upper extremity. *Ann Plast Surg* 1981; 7:411.

71. Medgyesi SA. Successful operation for lymphedema using a myocutaneous flap as a "wick". *Br J Plast Surg* 1983; 36:64–66.

72. Kambayashi J-I, Ohshiro T, Mori T. Appraisal of myocutaneous flapping for treatment of postmastectomy lymphedema: case report. *Acta Chir Scand* 1990; 156:175–177.

73. Thompson N. Surgical treatment of chronic lymphedema of the lower limb. With preliminary report of new operation. *Br Med J* 1962; 58:1566.

74. Thompson N. Buried dermal flap operation for chronic lymphedema of the extremities: ten-year survey of results in 79 cases. *Plast Reconstr Surg* 1970; 45:541–548.

75. Thompson N. Late results of surgical treatment of 50 cases of chronic lymphoedema of extremities using buried dermis flaps. A clinical and radioisotopic evaluation. In: Anonymous transactions of the Fourth International Congress of Plastic and Reconstructive Surgery, Rome 1967. Amsterdam: Excerpta Medica Foundation 1967; 1163–1167.

76. Sawhney CP. Evaluation of Thompson's buried dermal flap operation for lymphoedema of the limbs: A clinical and radioisotopic study. *Br J Plast Surg* 1974; 27:278–283.

77. Nielubowicz J, Olszewski W. Surgical lymphatico–venous shunts. *Br J Surg* 1968; 55:440–442.

78. Calnan JS, Reis ND, Rivero OR, et al. The natural history of lymph node-to-vein anastomoses. *Br J Plast Surg* 1967; 20:134.

79. Goldsmith H, De Los Santos R, Beattie EJJ. The relief of chronic lymphedema by omental transposition. *Ann Surg* 1967; 166:573.

80. Goldsmith HS. Long-term evaluation of omental transposition for chronic lymphedema. *Ann Surg* 1974; 180:847–849.

81. Danese CA, Papioanou AN, Morales LE, et al. Surgical approaches to lymphatic blocks. *Surgery* 1968; 64:821.

82. O'Brien BM, Hickey MJ, Hurley JV, et al. Microsurgical transfer of the greater omentum in the treatment of canine obstructive lymphoedema. *Br J Plast Surg* 1990; 43:440.

83. Pugnaire MD. Linfangioplasia mesenterica en el tratamiento de los elefantiasis de los membros inferiones. *Angiologia* 1968; 20:146.

84. Hurst PA, Kinmonth JB, Rutt DL. A gut and mesentery pedicle for bridging lymphatic obstruction. Experimental studies. *J Cardiovasc Surg* 1978; 19:589–596.

85. Kinmonth JB, Hurst PA, Edwards JM, et al. Relief of lymph obstruction by use of a bridge of mesentery and ileum. *Br J Surg* 1978; 65:829–833.

86. Hurst PAE, Stewart G, Kinmonth JB, et al. Long-term results of the enteromesenteric bridge operation in the treatment of primary lymphoedema. *Br J Surg* 1985; 72:272–274.

87. Laine JB, Howard JM. Experimental lymphatico-venous anastomosis. *Surg Forum* 1963; 14:111.

88. Rivero OR, Calnan JS, Reis ND, et al. Experimental peripheral lymphovenous communications. *Br J Plast Surg* 1967; 20:124.

89. Politowski M, Bartkowski S, Dynowski J. Treatment of lymphedema of the limbs by lymphatic-venous fistula. *Surgery* 1969; 66:639.

90. Gilbert A, O'Brien B, McVorrath JW, et al. Lymphaticovenous anastomoses for obstructive lymphedema. *Br J Plast Surg* 1976; 29:355.

91. O'Brien BM, Sykes P, Threlfall GN, et al. Microlymphaticovenous anastomoses for obstructive lymphedema. *Plast Reconstr Surg* 1977; 60:197.

92. Gong-Kang H, Ru-Qi H, Zong-Zhao L, et al. Microlymphaticovenous anastomosis in the treatment of lower limb obstructive lymphedema: Analysis of 91 cases. *Plast Reconstr Surg* 1985; 76:671–677.

93. Kinmonth JB. Methods of lymphography. In: Kinmonth JB, ed. *The lymphatics: surgery, lymphography and diseases of the chyle and lymph systems.* 2nd ed. London: Edward Arnold, 1982; 1–17.

94. Puckett CL. Microlymphatic surgery for lymphedema. *Clin Plast Surg* 1983; 10:133–138.

95. Puckett CL. Discussion of "Microlymphaticovenous anastomosis in the treatment of lower limb obstructive lymphedema: analysis of 91 cases". *Plast Reconstr Surg* 1985; 76:678–679.

96. Shafiroff BB, Nightingale G, Baxter TJ, et al. Lymphaticolymphatic anastomosis. *Ann Plas Surg* 1979; 3:199–210.

97. Baumeister RG, Seifert J, Wiebecke B. Homologous and autologous experimental lymph vessel transplantation: initial experience. *Int J Microsurg* 1981; 3:19.

98. Baumeister RG, Seifert J, Wiebecke B, et al. Experimental basis and first application of clinical lymph vessel transplantation of secondary lymphedema. *World J Surg* 1981; 5:401.

99. Baumeister RG, Siuda S. Treatment of lymphedemas by microsurgical lymphatic grafting: what is proved? *Plast Reconstr Surg* 1990; 85:64–74.

100. Charles RH. Elephantisis scroti. In: Lantham A, English TC, eds. *A system of treatment.* London: Churchill, 1912; 504–513.

101. Dellon AL, Hoopes JE. The Charles procedure for primary lymphedema: long-term clinical results. *Plast Reconstr Surg* 1977; 60:589–595.

102. Dandapat MC, Mohaptro SK, Patro SK. Elephantiasis of the penis and scrotum. *Am J Surg* 1985; 149:686–690.

103. Homans J. The treatment of elephantiasis of the legs: a preliminary report. *N Engl J Med* 1936; 215:1099.

104. Miller T, Harper J, Longmire WPJ. The management of lymphedema by staged subcutaneous excision. *Surg Gynecol Obstet* 1973; 136:586.

105. Miller TA. A surgical approach to lymphedema. *Am J Surg* 1977; 134:191–195.

106. Miller TA. Surgical approach to lymphedema of the arm after mastectomy. *Am J Surg* 1984; 148:152–156.

107. Edgerton MT. Colloquium: lymphedema of the extremity. *Ann Plast Surg* 1978; 1:188–189.

108. Fonkalsrud EW. Surgical management of congential lymphedema in infants and children. *Arch Surg* 1979; 114:1133–1136.

109. O'Brien BM, Khanzanchi RK, Kumar PAV, et al. Liposuction in the treatment of lymphoedema: a preliminary report. *Br J Plast Surg* 1989; 42:530.

110. Sando WC, Nahai F. Suction lipectomy in the management of limb lymphedema. *Clin Plast Surg* 1989; 16:369–373.

102

Principles of Soft-Tissue Reconstruction of the Lower Extremity

Randolph Sherman, M.D., F.A.C.S., and Jeffrey Scott Isenberg, M.D., M.P.H.

Bipedal ambulation, an activity often taken for granted, is the result of complex and delicately balanced myoneural units powering a lightweight yet strong endoskeleton, otherwise known as the lower extremity. Preserving and reconstructing the lower limb and ensuring functional weightbearing and locomotion has persistently challenged surgeons. For centuries amputation remained the only means of dealing with the massively traumatized or infected lower extremity. While not preserving form, modern prosthetics and a properly performed amputation can provide quite satisfactory ambulation and weightbearing. It is against these results that efforts of lower extremity reconstruction with autologous tissue transplantation must be evaluated.

Preoperative Assessment

Prerequisite in any attempts at limb salvage with autologous tissue is evaluation by a multidisciplinary team composed of the traumatologist, orthopedic surgeon, reconstructive plastic surgeon, and, in selected cases, the vascular surgeon. An insensate weightbearing surface, secondary to loss of the posterior tibial nerve, is considered an absolute contraindication for reconstruction, though a number of relative ones exist (1). In particular, devascularization of the limb, concurrent diaphyseal and major joint fractures, and massive burn injuries with open long-bone fractures should temper the reconstructive surgeons attempt at heroic limb salvage.

Treatment Algorithms

Axiomatic to the reconstructive process is a detailed history and physical examination. Assessment of other injured limbs must include appreciation of the neurovascular elements, soft-tissue envelope, and osseous tissues, with particular attention given the plantar surface of the foot. Underlying medical conditions should be addressed. Radiographic survey generally requires only multiple-view plain x-rays. Angiography plays a limited role in the reconstructive process, and must be utilized selectively. A significant amount of understanding of the wounded extremity is obtained in the operating room, where osseous fixation and wound débridement is conducted (2–4).

A number of studies support early bony stabilization and wound closure (5–11). Advantages include a decrease in the number of anesthesias, time for healing and weightbearing, hospitalization, and complications. It has been our experience that successful reconstruction of the lower limb is possible at any time if the level of débridement is sufficient and creates a clean surgical wound. Multiple débridements at 48–72 hour intervals may be necessary to achieve a surgically clean wound prior to coverage. Antibiotics are considered adjunctive treatment in the management of these complex wounds and should be tailored to wound cultures.

Wound Reconstruction by Region

There are general guidelines for reconstruction of complex wounds of the lower limb. However, in any specific case, the needs of a particular wound may require a combination of regional flaps and/or free-tissue transplantation (12–14).

HIP AND PROXIMAL FEMUR

The proximal femur and hip are invested with a dense layer of muscle units and in most cases do not require microvascular tissue transplantation for wound reconstruction. Furthermore, several robust regional flaps exist that can satisfy most wounds. Chief among these is the inferior-based rectus abdominis muscle or myocutaneous flap. Supplied by its dominant pedicle, the deep inferior epigastric artery, this flap can easily reach any wound of the pelvic girdle or proximal femur. When both dead space fill and cutaneous coverage are needed, a skin paddle can be included. Alternately, when massive wound dead space is encountered, the skin paddle can be deepithelialized and used to assist in filling the dead space (15). Morbidity is minimal in using one rectus abdominis unit if care is taken in reconstituting the anterior abdominal-wall fascia. For small wounds, the tensor fascia lata and gracilis muscle or myocutaneous flaps are often satisfactory. Care in orientation and raising the gracilis myocutaneous flap is required to insure viability of the overlying skin paddle.

DISTAL FEMUR

Options for reconstruction of significant soft-tissue wounds of the distal femur are not as plentiful as those for more proximal wounds, with microvascular tissue transplantation assuming a greater role. Taking advantage of the rectus muscle to transport a generous skin paddle in a reliable and predictable manner, the surgeon can utilize the extended rectus abdominis myocutaneous flap for the most distal femur wounds. Several technical points warrant discussion. First, the skin island is orientated obliquely, curving superiorly and laterally towards the anterior axillary line. Second, to achieve full mobilization, muscular attachments to the pubis must be taken down and the vascular pedicle carefully repositioned, often with partial division of the inguinal ligament needed to prevent kinking. Regionally, a gastrocnemius muscle flap can cover the distal femur, with fascial scoring increasing the length and surface area of the flap isolated on the sural artery and venae comitantes.

KNEE

The gastrocnemius muscle or myocutaneous flap serve well for wounds of this region (16,17). The medial, lateral, or both heads of the muscle may be utilized, though care must be taken to protect the peroneal nerve when mobilizing the lateral head. The myocutaneous flap may include a skin paddle extending distally to a level 5 cm above the medial malleolus (6). This allows more tissue for coverage, but can create a rather unsightly donor defect and for this reason is not very popular. When the gastrocnemius muscles are not suitable, microvascular tissue transplantation is required.

PROXIMAL TIBIA

Here also the bipenate gastrocnemius muscle is the primary source of vascularized soft tissue for reconstruction (18). Exposure has been described via a so-called stocking-seam incision, the flap beneath residual skin bridges. If direct damage to the muscle or its arterial pedicle, the sural artery, is found, microvascular tissue transplantation will be necessary (Fig. 102–1).

MIDDLE TIBIA

Though the cutaneous extension of the gastrocnemius myocutaneous flap can be used for middle-third wounds, the soleus muscle flap is probably more useful because it has the ability to better fill dead space, and with minimal donor-site morbidity. Attention should be given to separating the muscle's distal attachments from the undersurface of the tendoachilles. This is best done sharply with a scalpel to prevent undue trauma to the muscle's distal portion. Several other muscle flaps (including the extensor digitorum longus and tibialis anterior) and fasciocutaneous flaps have been reported for repair of

middle-third wounds. As a group, these flaps can satisfy only the most modest of wounds and are inadequate in any case where a significant dead space is present. Frequently, wounds from the midtibia distal are best satisfied by microvascular tissue transplantation (Fig. 102–2).

DISTAL TIBIA

Soft-tissue reconstruction in this area is viewed by many as the most challenging of all lower-extremity areas. This is because of the lack of significant regional muscle flaps. In fact, it is this lack of regional muscle flaps that greatly simplifies the decision-making process when reconstructing wounds of distal tibia. The vast majority of these wounds are best satisfied by microvascular tissue transplantation (Fig. 102–3). Local flaps such as the peroneus brevis muscle flaps and the soleus muscle, which extends to the level of the malleoli, will only resurface small wounds. A distally based soleus muscle flap has been described, but in our experience this is a very unreliable rotational flap. In cases of low-velocity injury, where only a modest skin defect exists, there is the occasional opportunity to utilize either proximally or distally based fasciocutaneous flaps, incorporating perforators from the posterior or anterior tibial systems or the peroneal vessels. However, any wound of high-velocity etiology, with a significant three-dimensional configuration and expansive zone of injury, will require free-tissue transplantation.

MICROVASCULAR TISSUE TRANSPLANTATION

Over the last two decades, as experience and technical skill in microvascular tissue transplantation has increased, applications of these techniques to lower-extremity reconstruction have also increased, to the point where it is the first choice for coverage. Indications include high-velocity injuries, most middle- and distal-third tibial wounds, radiation wounds, osteomyelitis, and recurrent nonunions. Though over 60 differ-

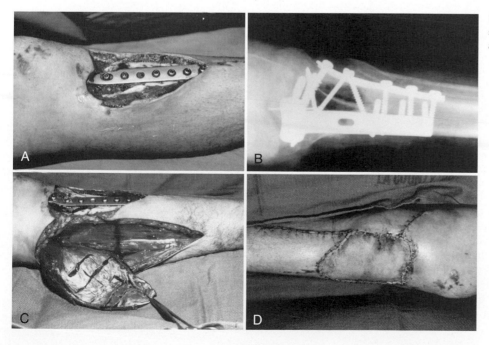

FIG. 102–1. Proximal tibial wound reconstructed with a gastrocnemius muscle flap and partial-thickness skin graft. (STSG).

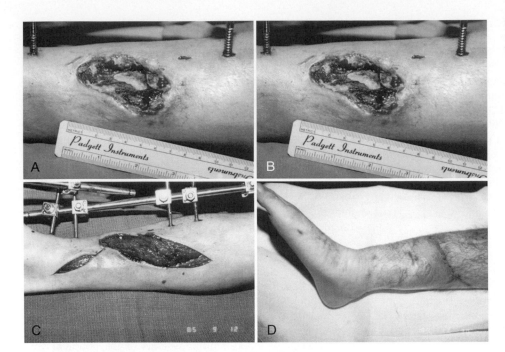

FIG. 102–2. Middle-third tibial defect repaired with a soleus rotational muscle flap and STSG.

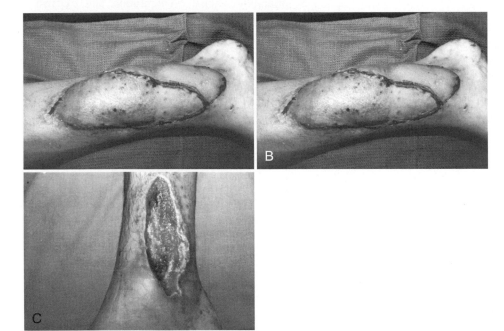

FIG. 102–3. Distal-third tibial wound reconstructed with a microvascular rectus abdominous transplant and STSG.

ent microvascular flaps have been described, in practice the majority of lower-extremity wounds are satisfied by a handful of reliable transfers. In our practice, over three-quarters of wounds are reconstructible with the rectus abdominis muscle transplant, the rest being satisfied by the latissimus dorsi, serratus anterior, and/or gracilis muscle flaps (19–22). These muscle flaps have in common several characteristics that suit their application to lower-extremity reconstruction. Muscle will mold readily to the irregular geometry of complex lower wounds. They are highly vascular, and especially appropriate in the relatively ischemic environment of the traumatic, in-

fected, or irradiated lower-limb wound (23–25). They improve in contour with time (unlike fasciocutaneous transplants to the lower limb, which become edematous in positions of dependency), and when resurfaced with nonmeshed partial-thickness skin grafts, provide very acceptable cosmetic reconstructions. They are easily mobilized, allowing a dual team approach, and all have modest donor-site morbidity. Finally, all travel with relatively long, large vascular pedicles. Successful microvascular tissue transplantation for lower-limb reconstruction requires adherence to the same principles as reconstruction with regional flaps, namely, adequate wound débridement with removal of all scar, necrotic tissue, and avascular bone, rigid bony fixation of unstable osseous elements (generally via external constructs), and microanastamosis of the flap pedicle to suitable recipient vessels.

FOOT AND ANKLE

Reconstruction in this area is made more complex because the reconstruction often must bear weight and yet still conform to the overall shape of the foot to allow shoe fit. More specifically, wounds of the ankle and dorsum should be reconstructed in a fashion that minimizes bulk. Conversely, the plantar surface of the foot requires a certain amount of bulk and durability in its reconstruction. Various local flaps (either fasciocutaneous or muscle) have been reported in this area. All suffer from the same disadvantages, that they required creating another wound in an already wounded foot and they can reconstruct only the smallest of wounds. Once again, it has been our experience that, for all but the most minor of wounds in this region, microvascular tissue transplantation is required. On the dorsal surface, thin flaps, such as the temporoparietal or radial forearm fasciocutaneous flap in adults, or latissimus dorsi muscle with a partial-thickness skin graft in children, are preferred. On the plantar surface muscle flaps with partial-thickness skin grafts provide longlasting coverage and minimize shear. Initially, fasciocutaneous transplantation to this region appears aesthetically superior. With time, however, the flaps gain bulk and become edematous, almost always requiring revision. In contrast, muscle transplants, while initially appearing more bulky, atrophy and improve in contour with time. While the presence of deep pressure sensation in the plantar surface is a requirement for successful reconstruction, transplantation of neurotized flaps for sensory restoration has yet to be clinically substantiated as an addition to return of ambulation.

Special Circumstances

AVULSION-DEGLOVING INJURIES

While at first appearing to the inexperienced eye as straightforward in reconstruction, the degloving injury (whether open or closed) is a significant reconstructive problem. The degloved skin and/or soft tissue envelope, although demonstrating some clinical evidence of viability, is usually crushed and ischemic beyond salvage. Attempts at replacing these soft-tissue elements, particularly if closure is under any tension, result in total necrosis of the avulsed tissue elements. A critical appraisal and liberal débridement are necessary first steps in treating the degloving injury (26).

SEGMENTAL COMPOSITE OSSEOUS DEFECTS

Concurrent soft-tissue and segmental bone defect are frequently encountered where there is to be simultaneous soft-tissue and osseous reconstruction. Presently, two techniques are available for concurrent osseous reconstruction: microvascular fibula transplantation and distraction osteogenesis (Ilizarov technique). Historically, microvascular fibula transplantation gained popularity as the primary means of dealing with osseous defects greater than 6 cm. Though successful in reconstructing large osseous defects, the technique relies on transplant hypertrophy, has an extended postoperative healing phase, and a not insignificant rate of transplant stress fracture. Distraction osteogenesis, a technique recently popularized by Ilizarov, can also facilitate concurrent reconstruction of massive segmental osseous deficits of the lower limb. Unlike microvascular fibula transplantation, this technique is the province of the orthopedic surgeon. Though beneficial, some impact in developing soft-tissue reconstructive options for a given wound may be imposed by the device and require adaptability on the part of the plastic surgeon.

Conclusions

Soft-tissue reconstruction of the lower extremity is predicated upon certain fundamental wound management axioms, including wide débridement of all nonviable tissue and creation of a surgically clean wound, adequate osseous fixation, and obliteration of dead space with well-vascularized soft tissue. Proper patient selection, a sound multidisciplinary approach, and advanced techniques in soft-tissue reconstruction help to ensure an optimal outcome.

References

1. Hansen ST. The Type IIIC tibial fracture: salvage or amputation. *J Bone Joint Surg* 1987; 69(A):79.
2. Behrens F. General theory and principles of external fixation. *Clin Orthop* 1989; 241:15.
3. Burgess AR, Poka A, Brumback RJ, et al. Management of open grade III tibial fractures. *Orthop Clin North Am* 1987; 18:85.
4. Gustilo RB, Anderson JT. Prevention of infection in the treatment of 1025 open fractures of long bones. *J Bone Surg* 1976; 58(A):453.
5. Byrd HS, Cierny G, Tebbets JB. The management of open tibial fractures with associated soft-tissue loss: external pin fixation with early flap coverage. *Plast Reconstr Surg* 1981; 68:73.
6. Byrd HS, Spicer RE, Cierny G III. The management of open tibial fractures. *Plast Reconstr Surg* 1985; 76:719.
7. Caudle RJ, Stern PJ. Severe open fractures of the tibia. *J Bone Joint Surg* 1987; 69(A):801.
8. Ger R. The management of open fractures of the tibia with skin loss. *J Trauma* 1970; 10:112.
9. Godina M. Early microsurgical reconstruction of complex trauma of the extremities. *Plast Reconstr Surg* 1986; 78:285.
10. Stark WJ. The use of pedicled muscle flaps in the surgical treatment of chronic osteomyelitis resulting from compound fractures. *J Bone Joint Surg* 1946; 28:343.
11. Yaremchuk MJ, Brumback RJ, Manson PN, et al. Acute and definitive management of traumatic osteocutaneous defects of the lower extremity. *Plast Reconstr Surg* 1987; 80:1.
12. Mathes SJ, Nahai F. *Clinical applications for muscle and musculocutaneous flaps.* St. Louis: CV Mosby, 1982.
13. McCraw JB. Selection of alternative local flaps in the leg and foot. *Clin Plast Surg* 1979; 6:227.
14. McCraw JB, Arnold PG. *McCraw and Arnold's atlas of muscle and musculocutaneous flaps.* Norfolk, VA: Hampton Press, 1986.
15. Gottlieb ME, Chandrasekhar B, Terz JJ, et al. Clinical application of the extended deep inferior epigastric flap. *Plast Reconstr Surg* 1986; 78:782.
16. Feldman JJ, Cohen BE, May JW. The medial gastrocnemius myocutaneous flap. *Plast Reconstr Surg* 1978; 61:531.
17. Ger R. Muscle transposition for treatment and prevention of chronic posttraumatic osteomyelitis of the tibia. *J Bone Joint Surg* 1977; 59(A):784.
18. Vasconez LO, Bostwick J III, McCraw J. Coverage of exposed bone by muscle transportation and skin grafting. *Plast Reconstr Surg* 1974; 53:526.
19. Bunkis J, Walton RL, Mathes SJ. The rectus abdominis free flap for lower extremity reconstruction. *Ann Plast Surg* 1983; 11:373.
20. Gordon L, Buncke HJ, Alpert BS. Free latissimus dorsi muscle flap with split-thickness skin graft cover: a report of 16 cases. *Plast Reconstr Surg* 1982; 70:173.

21. Meland NB, Fisher J, Irons GB, et al. Experience with 80 rectus abdominis free tissue transfers. *Plast Reconstr Surg* 1989; 83:481.

22. Swartz WM, Jones NF. Soft-tissue coverage of the lower extremity. *Curr Probl Surg* 1985; 22:4.

23. Chang N, Mathes SJ. Comparison of the effect of bacterial inoculation in musculocutaneous and random pattern flaps. *Plast Reconstr Surg* 1982; 70:1.

24. Mathes SJ, Alpert BS, Chang N. Use of the muscle flap in chronic osteomyelitis: experimental and clinical correlation. *Plast Reconstr Surg* 1982; 69:815.

25. Weiland AJ, Moore JR, Daniel RK. The efficacy of free tissue transfer in osteomyelitis. *J Bone Joint Surg* 1984; 66(A):181.

26. Hidalgo DA: Lower extremity avulsion injuries. *Clin Plast Surg* 1986; 13:701.

103

Foot Ulceration in the Diabetic and Vascular Disease Patient

Larry B. Colen, M.D., F.A.C.S., and Tad Heinz, M.D.

The management of the pedal complications of diabetes mellitus is a significant health care problem. Two hundred fifty thousand hospital admissions and approximately 40,000 major amputations are performed yearly for this condition. These challenging patients are at risk for potential loss of the involved extremity as well as for future loss of the contralateral limb. The pathogenesis of many diabetic foot wounds is best characterized as peripheral neuropathy complicated by infrapopliteal peripheral vascular disease. Chronic plantar ulceration is often the mode of patient presentation, although cellulitis and plantar abscess occur in a significant number. Generalized atherosclerosis, osteomyelitis, and Charcot changes may further complicate the management of these patients.

The hypothesis that maintaining an intact skin envelope will decrease the incidence of life/limb-threatening infections seems appropriate. Patients presenting with chronic ulceration are treated with culture-specific antibiotics, surgical débridement, and appropriate wound closure techniques. During the same hospitalization, relevant orthopedic, vascular, and podiatric problems are addressed. The utilization of sophisticated limb salvage techniques, which combine reconstructive approaches and peripheral vascular surgery, has afforded major amputation rates of less than 3%. Multidisciplinary follow-up must be strict to achieve this goal. Patient education concerning foot care is of paramount importance. Feet should be checked daily, using a mirror if necessary, and the skin must be kept clean, dry, and pliable. Callosities must be minimized by use of a pumice stone or by conservative podiatric care. Custom-molded orthotics may be required after loss of foot arches or reconstructive surgery.

The trend in diabetic foot wound management has shifted over the years from primary below-knee amputation to function-preserving surgery using a multidisciplinary approach. Though indications for primary amputation exist (e.g., sepsis, major tissue loss, and nonreconstructible vascular disease), the goal in the management of these patients is to preserve bipedal ambulation. The reasons for this are straightforward and to be discussed below.

In many of the older patients with comorbid factors such as heart disease and prior stroke, the energy expenditure of ambulation with a below-knee, or above-knee, prosthesis may be prohibitive. For example, oxygen consumption of an amputee walking with an above-knee prosthesis is 2.3 times that of an age and disease-matched control (1). Unrestrained above-knee prosthesis walking requires 63% of maximum aerobic capacity at 45% of the control patient's gait velocity.

These results are from the more favorable 30 to 66% of vascular amputees successfully rehabilitated to prosthesis walking (30% for above-knee, 66% for below-knee amputees). Even Symes amputees require 33% more oxygen consumption per unit distance at two-thirds of the control patient's gait velocity. The large number of amputees not successfully rehabilitated comprise those who fail rehabilitation as well as those who are not fitted for prostheses for reasons of dementia, stroke, or debilitation. Crutch walking without a prosthesis requires even higher energy expenditure and universally results in tachycardia. The end result of these energy-inefficient prostheses may be a bed- or wheelchair-bound patient.

Kucan and Robson (2) have stressed the importance of limb-preserving treatment for diabetic patients faced with major amputation because of their risk of contralateral major amputation (30 to 40% within 3 years of their initial presentation). This fact has not changed significantly since the 1960s, despite a decrease in operative mortality from 10 to 1.5%. Forty-nine percent of diabetic patients with a foot infection developed a serious infection in the contralateral foot within 18 months. Ambulation with bilateral prostheses is even less likely than a unilateral prosthesis; only 30% of those with mixed amputations achieved satisfactory rehabilitation (1).

Pathophysiology

The pathophysiology of foot ulceration in the diabetic patient may be divided into four distinct aspects: peripheral neuropathy, peripheral vascular disease, hemorheologic abnormalities, and immune system impairment.

NEUROPATHY

Peripheral neuropathy involving sensory, motor, and autonomic pathways is the fundamental cause of foot disease in the diabetic patient. Considerable effort has been expended over the past decade to better understand the nature of this devastating problem (3). The etiology of diabetic peripheral neuropathy is complex and may be different from patient to patient. Autoimmune mechanisms, as well as microvascular mechanisms, have recently been implicated in the segmental demyelination that is seen on nerve biopsy. The resultant neural edema and slowed axoplasmic flow significantly contribute to the neural dysfunction we have termed "diabetic peripheral neuropathy."

In addition, there exists considerable evidence for peripheral nerve compression, contributing to the underlying metabolic dysfunction in these patients. This "double crush" phenomenon implies that each insult is additive and that they jointly give rise to the observed neuropathy. The compression exacerbates the effect of axonal swelling in a fixed space such as a bony foramen, a muscular band, or a bony or ligamentous tunnel (e.g., tarsal, cubital, carpal) (4–7). Intrinsic muscle weakness of the foot secondary to motor neuropathy contributes to a derangement of the normal toe flexor/extensor balance. This leads to pes cavus deformity, digital extensor subluxation, and subsequent plantar metatarsal head prominence. Loss of the normal transverse and longitudinal pedal arches follow. These Charcot deformities contribute to skin breakdown and ulcer formation. In addition, there is evidence that pressure alone results in increased bacterial localization and replication (8). Denervation alone has also been shown to lead to increased bacterial multiplication relative to the normally innervated limb (9).

The inability to feel pressure or pain as a consequence of sensory neuropathy, in conjunction with abnormal pressure distribution, initiates a deleterious cycle. Autonomic neuropathy results in anhidrosis and hyperkeratosis, leading to callous formation over insensate pressure areas; these may hemorrhage or fissure, and infection ensues. Significant inflow disease, hyperglycemia, compromised immunomodulation, and poor vision secondary to retinopathy contribute to this phenomenon.

VASCULAR DISEASE

Previously, microvascular disease and small-vessel endothelial proliferation were considered the cause for ulcerations found in the diabetic foot (10). The notion that ischemic ulcers occur in the presence of normal pedal pulses continues to be propagated. Upon close inspection, however, these ideas have not been borne out. Subsequent anatomic studies by Strandness (11) and Conrad (12) upon amputated limbs have not supported Goldenberg's original work (13). Diabetics and nondiabetics were found to have equal degrees of intimal hyperplasia. Arteriolar reactivity to papaverine and arteriolar resistance are the same in both groups of patients when treated before undergoing femoral-popliteal bypass graft (14). Transcutaneous PO_2 ($TcPO_2$) measurements in diabetics and nondiabetics with peripheral vascular disease show no significant differences (15). However, other studies have shown that neuropathic diabetics have increased $TcPO_2$ compared to controls and nonneuropathic patients. These same neuropathic diabetics have a much reduced ability to elevate $TcPO_2$ when the skin is warmed to 44° C (16,17). Lack of blood supply is not the primary cause of open wounds in the diabetic foot. The presence of a thickened basement membrane has been confirmed in diabetic capillaries in muscle but not in skin (18). In addition, evaluation of larger arteries reveals a propensity among diabetics towards proximal tibial and peroneal arteriosclerotic occlusive disease (19). As such, these patients may have an ischemic foot below strong popliteal pulsations and yet have nearly "normal" pedal vessels. This pedal sparing occurs more often, in fact, in diabetics than nondiabetics. A good understanding of these predilections is clearly important in order to avoid major amputation in the diabetic patient who presents with this common scenario; for example, femoral-pedal bypass grafting may be performed instead.

HEMORHEOLOGY

Diabetics exhibit alterations in blood flow secondary to serum viscosity elevation and decreased RBC deformability (5). Platelet aggregation, erythrocyte aggregation, and increased fibrinogen levels also play a role in abnormalities of blood flow. Altered viscosity is further exacerbated by serum protein shifts from increased vessel permeability, which allows for the leakage of albumin, and the elevation of several globulins (20,21). It has been linked to the presence of microangiopathy and is most pronounced at low shear rates. Increases in serum viscosity cause greater erythrocyte and platelet aggregation, culminating in rouleaux and platelet aggregates. Platelet aggregation is related to increases in von Willebrand factor levels as well as decreased PGI2 release, fibrinolysis and lipoprotein lipase activity (22). Insulin has been found to quickly reverse some of these viscosity shifts, indicating that they do not all arise from permanent erythrocyte membrane protein glycosylation (23).

Reduced red cell deformability, in contrast with plasma protein changes, is present even in childhood diabetes. Its main manifestation is increased resistance to changes in erythrocyte curvature, which impacts on perfusion of microcirculatory beds. Erythrocyte deformability has been shown to be dependent on adenosine triphosphate (ATP) metabolism (24). Increasing ATP levels thus improves the deformability of rigid, hyperosmolar erythrocytes (25,26). Pentoxyfylline, a methylxanthine derivative, increases erythrocyte ATP levels and offers a clinically promising mode of therapy (17, 27–30). We use pentoxyfylline in all patients being treated for diabetic foot problems.

The energy required to disrupt erythrocyte aggregates and deform rigid erythrocyte membranes has the indirect effect of altering local vessel pressures and shear stress. This leads to greater albumin leak, the synthesis of collagenlike materials, and subsequent stiffening. Pure erythrocyte membrane changes, alone, result in elevated large vessel resistance to flow. This predisposes to large-vessel atherosclerosis.

Possible therapeutic interventions at the hemorheologic level include pentoxyfylline, fish oils (omega-3 fatty acids), aspirin, smoking cessation, and tight glucose control. Fish oils contain eicosapentanoic acid (20C:5) and have been shown to act as a competitive substrate for cyclooxygenase in the prostaglandin cascade. The net effect is to lessen the vasoconstrictive and proaggregatory influence of thromboxane (31). It also lowers the production of platelet-derived growth factor–like protein from endothelial cells, thereby reducing endothelial proliferation (32). Aspirin, in low doses, works through the irreversible inhibition of platelet cyclooxygenase to decrease platelet aggregation. Smoking cessation decreases the vasoconstrictive effect of nicotine and may improve perfusion on marginal areas of flaps and grafts. As discussed above, tight glucose control in diabetics can quickly reverse some of the changes seen in erythrocyte deformability and aggregation.

IMMUNODEFICIENCY

Platelets, polymorphonuclear leukocytes (PMN), and red blood cells are already affected by the diabetic state. The changes in immune system function seen with diabetes stem mainly from polymorphonuclear cell dysfunction, although monocytes and lymphocytes respond abnormally as well.

Chemotaxis, phagocytosis, and bactericidal activity are altered in diabetes. Some of these changes are related to the hyperglycemia of diabetes and are reversible with normalization of serum glucose levels, while others are not. For example, diabetic PMNs showed slowed migration, which was reversible by cell washing and unaffected by the blood glucose level (33). The ingestion of opsonized particles complexed with lipopolysaccharide is equivalent in normal and normoglycemic diabetics but significantly impaired by hyperglycemia in these diabetics. Opsonization itself is adversely altered among diabetics (34). Finally, compared to controls, staphylococcal killing is reduced in diabetic PMNs regardless of blood glucose level.

Cell-mediated immunity is also abnormal. The secondary T-cell response is slowed and monocyte phagocytosis is reduced. This may partly explain the susceptibility of diabetes to fungal infections (35).

Management

The practical approach to the treatment of the diabetic foot wound may be divided into two components: meticulous preoperative evaluation and well-executed medical and surgical management. Preoperative examination and testing should be directed toward diagnosis and optimization of associated medical conditions, evaluation of neurologic and osseous abnormalities including gait disturbances, complete study of the vascular status of the involved foot, and a thorough understanding of the status of the contralateral extremity. Proper management must include the use of broad-sprectrum antibiotics, bedrest with limb evaluation, bone biopsy (if clinically indicated), surgical débridement, liberal use of top-

ical antimicrobials, deep-vein thrombosis prophylaxis, and appropriate vascular surgical intervention before soft-tissue and bone reconstruction. Hyperbaric oxygen therapy has also been shown to be effective in the healing of ischemic lower-extremity ulcers (36–38); however, its role in the management of diabetic ulceration remains controversial. Smoking cessation must be encouraged.

Preoperative Evaluation

The evaluation of the diabetic patient with a foot or leg wound should focus on five major areas: systemic disease, infection, neurologic status, endocrine control, and vascular conditions. Many of these patients have concurrent coronary, cerebrovascular, pulmonary, and renal disease. These need to be conscientiously evaluated and risk assessed, and the patient's medical status must be optimized. Preoperative involvement of anesthesia, cardiology, pulmonary, and renal services may be of great value in managing these complicated patients. Perioperative cardiac monitoring is necessary in many cases.

Deep infection in the foot or leg must be ruled out by inspection and needle aspiration of the plantar space if there is any question (Fig. 103–1). Plain bone radiographs may show evidence of chronic osteomyelitis at the base of an ulcer, but bone culture is often required for definitive proof (Fig. 103–2). This may be done at the time of débridement or when reconstruction is performed. Swab cultures and bone scans are of little value because each is nonspecific. Magnetic resonance imaging (MRI) does show better specificity, compared to bone scan, for identification of pedal osteomyelitis (39), but bears further investigation. Since many of these infections contain more than five organisms, broad-spectrum antibiotics should be used initially and modified as culture reports return.

Careful neurologic examination of the foot and leg allows better discrimination of the degree of neuropathy of the various peripheral nerve territories. If the affected limb is ischemic, bypass grafting or angioplasty may improve symptoms of what may be ischemic rather than "diabetic" neuropathy. Tarsal tunnel syndrome, when a localized Tinel sign is present over the posterior tibial nerve, may be identified. A straightforward nerve decompression may be carried out and is recommended for any neuropathic diabetic patients with localizing electrodiagnostic evidence and/or a

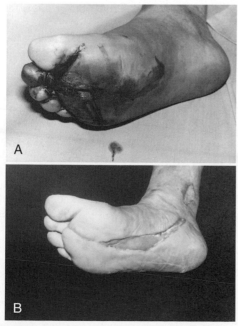

FIG. 103–1. **A**, necrosis and purulent drainage from plantar abscess. **B**, skin graft to nonweightbearing area of foot.

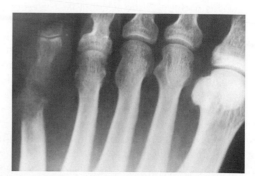

FIG. 103–2.   Joint destruction owing to osteomyelitis of metatarsalphalangeal joint. Note mottling of bone and absence of joint space.

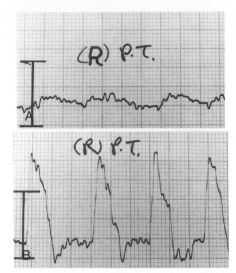

FIG. 103–3. **A,** dampened pressure tracing indicating reduced blood flow. **B,** triphasic Doppler waveform indicating good vascular flow.

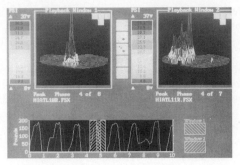

FIG. 103–4. Force pulse diagrams indicating compression points of the foot during gait.

physical exam consistent with nerve compression. Intact innervation of the first web space may allow for the use of neurovascular toe island flaps (40,41). If Charcot neuroarthropathy is evident, treatment must include fusions or tendon transfers. Some degree of neuroarthropathy is present in almost all patients with chronic diabetic foot wounds. Finally, lack of heel sensation must be recognized as a relative contraindication to Syme amputation.

Poor glucose control, as evidenced by high serum hemoglobin A1c levels, must be corrected to improve the rheologic immune dysfunction described earlier. This may be rapidly accomplished by the monitored administration of insulin, preferably by continuous intravenous infusion and intravenous fluid therapy. Endocrine consultation may be necessary for the "brittle" patient. Since infection may cause hyperglycemia, drainage is mandatory.

Vascular evaluation is of paramount importance (42–45). It begins with inspection for the atrophic changes of chronic ischemia and the discoloration and venous changes associated with venous insufficiency. Palpation for pedal pulses will give a "qualitative" assessment of perfusion, but the measurement by Doppler of ankle-brachial indices Doppler waveforms is much more informative (42,43). Ankle-brachial indices above 0.7 are acceptable for reconstruction without correction of inflow, but these values are often artificially elevated because of arterial noncompressibility from medial calcification. Toe pressures greater than 30 to 50 mm Hg are more indicative of healing, and their measurement should be a routine part of the vascular studies. Triphasic and biphasic waveforms are acceptable at the ankle, but lesser-quality signals mandate augmentation of inflow for successful soft-tissue and bone reconstruction (Fig. 103–3).

Duplex scanning, combining real-time B-mode ultrasound imaging with pulsed Doppler capability, may be used to identify areas of adequate vessel diameter or of stenosis in native arteries or bypass grafts of the leg and thigh. This permits preoperative selection of possible targets for free tissue transfer as well as the mapping of flaps based on per-

forators of the leg (26). Color flow analysis, using the Doppler principle and changes in red-cell velocity, allows functional assessment of potentially critical flow-limiting lesions. Duplex scanning is likewise helpful in the preoperative evaluation of the lower extremity venous system. Venous valve competency, as well as vein patency and size, can be analyzed in this fashion. Transcutaneous PO_2 values at one-half of the chest wall control are also helpful indicators of likely pedal healing of flaps, grafts, or other reconstructive procedures.

Angiography, at present, remains the gold standard of anatomic evaluation before arterial bypass grafting or reconstruction of the ischemic limb. Newer digital subtraction techniques decrease the dye load required for a high-quality study in these compromised patients. Isotonic dye should be utilized exclusively in this population, and careful attention must be paid to preangiogram hydration and poststudy renal function. Consultation with the radiologist should stress the need for detailed views of the distal leg and foot, since special techniques (e.g., preinjection reperfusion hyperemia, nitroglycerin infusion) may be required. In special circumstances (i.e., when poor renal function or angiographic dye allergy exist), MR angiography will offer fine anatomic detail equivalent to traditional angiographic techniques. Therapeutic intervention by the radiologists (percutaneous transluminal angioplasty) may be appropriate for such conditions as limited iliac or superficial femoral artery stenoses, but cannot be expected to have the same longevity as bypass grafting. Angioplasty's shorter-lived patency rate may be adequate, however, for healing of soft-tissue reconstructions, especially in the predominantly neuropathic rather than ischemic foot.

Finally, an understanding of gait abnormalities will help construct a complete operative approach to both wound closure and prevention of ulcer recurrence. F-scan gait analysis gives valuable information regarding tendon imbalances and bony prominences that require operative correction (Fig. 103–4).

Principles of Wound Closure

As with any difficult wound, basic principles must be adhered to for therapeutic success. There must be no gross infection, the wound must be in bacteriologic balance, and the foot must be deemed to have adequate perfusion, systemic problems optimized, elevated blood sugars normalized, and foci of osteomyelitis, if present, identified and treated. The closure is tailored to the location and character of the wound.

For example, a second-toe infection from ill-fitting shoes is far different from the large heel wound with calcaneal exposure.

Forefoot, midfoot, and hindfoot areas may subdivide into weightbearing vs. nonweightbearing categories. Additional distinctions are made between superficial and deep wounds, with exposure of tendon, joint, or bone in the latter. The array of surgical options, from primary closure to skin graft, local flap, free flap, or midfoot amputations, must be within the armamentarium of the reconstructive surgeon in order to achieve the goal of bipedal ambulation. Limited toe or ray amputations, or more extensive transmetetarsal or Lisfranc procedures, rather than a complex microvascular reconstruction, may provide the best functional result in many patients with forefoot wounds. In spite of the increasing number and reliability of flaps, both free and pedicled, used in recent years, patient characteristics often influence the choice for closure.

Most of the local flaps for foot reconstruction are dependent upon antegrade posterior tibial artery flow into its medial and lateral plantar branches. The sural artery island flap (46) and the lateral calcaneal artery flap (47) are exceptions based upon the peroneal artery, usually the best preserved of all tibial vessels among diabetic patients (19). Much work had been done on fasciocutaneous flaps of the lower extremity (46,48–50) but their usefulness in this compromised population is yet unclear. Our experience has been limited but such flaps seem most appropriate for smaller wounds.

When wounds are large or local flaps not applicable, free flaps are preferred. A recent review (51) of combined lower-extremity bypass with free-tissue transfer identifies several groups that may benefit. These include those with peripheral vascular disease and plantar ulceration, diabetic neuropathy and ulceration, open midfoot amputations, the rare patient thought appropriate for a nutrient flap, and, possibly, the patient with heavily calcified tibial arteries and distal tissue loss. Duplex scanning and angiography may be used to identify suitable donor areas of native vessels, although, if a long-leg bypass is performed for limb revascularization, suturing the free flap into the bypass vein itself is usually preferred. As a result of this, technically difficult microanastomosis and possible disruption of arterial plaque is avoided. In rare patients, free flaps may provide enough additional runoff to allow a distal revascularization to remain patent. This must be discussed with the vascular surgery team. Bypass grafting may be made directly to a free flap on the foot as a nutrient flap when the arterial system is unreconstructible, but the risk of healing complications and progressive tissue loss around the flap is substantial (22,51). When such reconstructions succeed, long-term improvements in pedal vascularization have been demonstrated angiographically. In general, free-tissue transfers should only be made to adequately vascularized feet. Other contraindications are severe coronary artery disease, severe infections, poor patient motivation, and poor patient understanding of the long-term care necessary for limb preservation (25).

Soft-Tissue Reconstruction

Following control of systemic sepsis, as well as that of the involved extremity, a systematic approach to soft-tissue reconstruction follows. A thorough understanding of the vascular supply to the foot, in conjunction with knowledge of the regional flaps available for wound closure, will assist in obtaining a healed wound. It is most helpful in this regard to approach the plantar foot as having three distinct regions, with the type of closure dependent upon wound location.

FOREFOOT

Chronic ulceration of a single digit with evidence of bone involvement is best treated with single-toe amputation. If no underlying bone infection is suspected, toe-sparing procedures (local flaps, skin graphs) may be utilized; however, all tendon and joint abnormalities that produced the ulceration will need to be corrected in order to prevent ulcer reoccurrence. Toe ulceration is most often exacerbated by peripheral vascular disease, and proper attention to this factor must be given.

Metatarsal head ulceration is the most frequent presenting sequela of Charcot arthropathy. When adequate inflow is present, these wounds are best closed by creative use of toe fillet flaps. An extension of this method, for wounds greater than 2 to 3 cm, is the use of single or mutiple uninvolved adjacent toes for wound closure. The remaining toes are left for possible later use. With this approach, better length and an intact transverse metatarsal arch are preserved. Ray deletions or metatarsal joint resections may be required for evidence of metatarsal osteomyelitis.

Other local flap options for plantar ulcerations are neurovascular toe island (40,41) and plantar V–Y flaps (5,45). (Figs. 103–5, 103–6). The toe island is elevated on its digital neurovascular bundle from the lateral aspect of the great toe and may be dissected proximally for eventual transposition to the mid and forefoot. Two- to three-centimeter defects can be closed in this manner. The donor site is closed primarily or by skin graft. V–Y flaps comprise skin, fat, and fascia, and can be raised singly or in pairs to close up to 4-cm wounds.

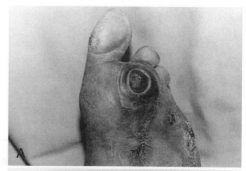
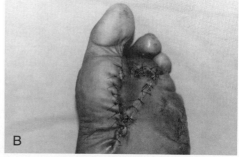

FIG. 103–5. **A,** plantar ulcer over second metatarsal head. **B,** V–Y advancement over metatarsal immediately postoperatively.

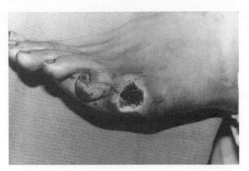

FIG. 103–6.   Fifth toe filleted to cover ulcer.

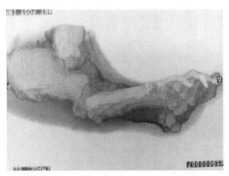

FIG. 103–7.   Tarso-metatarsal collapse due to Charcot arthropathy.

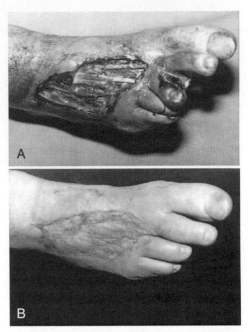

FIG. 103–8.   Dorsal wound. Ray deletion and wound treatment as first stage. **B,** granulation of wound allowed use of STSG.

This is an excellent choice for larger metatarsal head ulcerations. Perfusion is based on the numerous perforating vessels present on the plantar surface of the foot. Elevation involves the release of the plantar fascia circumferentially as well as the vertical slips from the metatarsal bones.

Recurrent ulceration following transmetatarsal amputation may be treated with more-proximal midfoot amputations rather than below-knee amputations. Surgeons should be well versed in the Lisfranc (tarsal-metatarsal junction) amputation as well as the Chopart (intertarsal junction) amputation, both of which allow bipedal, weightbearing ambulation without prostheses (53).

MIDFOOT

Neuropathic disturbances in motor and sensory function play a large role in the etiology of midfoot ulcerations. A spectrum of deformation of the pedal arches from intrinsic muscle denervation can culminate in the Charcot neuroarthropathy found in 2.5% of diabetic patients, most commonly at the tarsometatarsal, metatarsophalangeal, or intertarsal joints (Fig. 103–7). Midfoot closure options include skin grafts, local flaps, and free-tissue transfer. Tarsal tunnel release should be considered as an adjunctive procedure at this time (54). The skin graft (split-thickness skin graft) may succeed in the nonweightbearing portion of this area, but the wound must be in bacteriologic balance and without tendon, joint, or bone exposure (Fig. 103–8). Loss of the longitudinal arch of the foot secondary to neuropathy may eliminate the skin grafts as an option in this area. Toe island and V–Y flaps may be used for closure after judicious bone débridement and contouring is carried out (54). The toe island will need to be more extensively elevated proximally on its plantar or dorsal

circulation in order to reach the midfoot. Transmetatarsal amputation is an acceptable choice for severe wounds at this level. The creative use of plantar or dorsal flaps will allow maximum preservation of length. Transcutaneous PO_2 measurements and toe pressures greater than 30 mm Hg aid in assessment and prediction of uneventful wound healing. Of critical importance for long-term success is the prosthetist's ability and commitment to appropriate orthotics.

Free-tissue transfers of skin or muscle, depending on the requirements, are usually required for midfoot wounds greater than 5 to 6 cm in size (42,44,55,56) (Fig. 103–9). Free-tissue transfer techniques may also allow for closure and salvage of guillotine-type midfoot amputations resulting from infection. When an organized approach to wounds of this area is strictly adhered to, the need for below-knee amputation should be less than 5%, as opposed to greater than 80% reported in patients with coexistent peripheral vascular disease (54).

Midfoot amputations will frequently result in equinovarus deformity, which will predispose the foot to further breakdown. This is a result of the imbalance that occurs among the tibialis anterior, tibialis posterior, and peroneus tendons following the destruction of their points of insertion by the amputation. Correction of foot angulation by tendon lengthening (i.e., tendon Achilles), tibialis anterior anchorage, or transfer, limited fusion or bracing should be considered.

HINDFOOT

Special characteristics of the hindfoot must be recognized when reconstruction is undertaken. Even more than the mid and forefoot, the glabrous skin (with its fibrous septae over a thick heel fat pad) resists impacts and shear forces. The weightbearing demands of the heel must be met. As this is

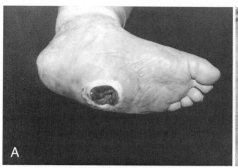
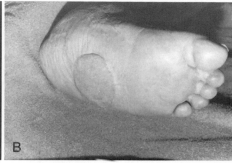

FIG. 103–9.   **A,** midfoot size of defect after débridement requires free flap. **B,** free serratus flap and skin graft for resurfacing of midfoot ulcer.

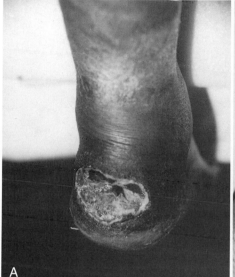
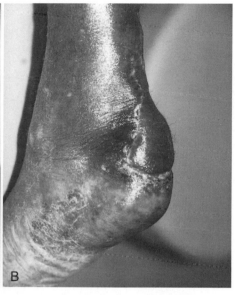

FIG. 103–10.   **A,** heel ulcer amenable to local flap (sural flap). **B,** sural flap, early postoperative (skin and subcutaneous flap).

often difficult to replicate, recurrent breakdown is not uncommon. The Achilles tendon area has a thin, pliable covering over a very mobile structure. The posterior hindfoot is nonweightbearing. Coverage of wounds in this area requires the use of relatively thin, pliable tissue that will adequately cover the Achilles tendon while not restricting ankle motion. Needless to say, flap choices differ greatly depending upon wound location.

Wounds less than 5 to 6 cm in diameter may be closed with a variety of flap options. Most require adequate antegrade blood flow in the posterior tibial artery and may not be suitable for use in patients who have undergone revascularization to the distal anterior tibial or peroneal vessels. Similarly, patients with inflow to the foot supplied only by the anterior tibial/dorsalis pedis axis will have, at best, retrograde flow in the plantar arteries. When the peroneal artery is patent, local flap options for 2- to 4-cm wounds based on this vessel include sural artery island (46) (Fig. 103–10) and lateral calcaneal artery flaps (47). The former is distally based with a pivot point 5 cm superior to the lateral malleolus, and can cover wounds in the posterior hindfoot but not the plantar hindfoot. The loss of sural innervation is minimal.

The latter flap covers posterior and plantar heel wounds up to 2.5 cm in size with potentially sensate pliable cover. Other local alternatives are a suprafascial rotation of the heel pad for small-to-moderate defects of the heel weightbearing area (57,58) (Fig. 103–11). Variations on the medial plantar arterial territory of the posterior tibial artery, such as instep rotation (49) or medial plantar artery flaps (58), may also be used; these require skin grafting of the donor site and thus may be unsuitable for patients with instep weightbearing. V–Y flaps can be used with success in this area for 2-cm defects.

Intrinsic muscle flaps can be used for small-to-moderate defects of the hindfoot. The flexor digitorum brevis is the largest of these and is useful for heel coverage. The plantar fascia is retained with the muscle in order to retain satisfactory bulk. It is usually removed from its origin and insertion and is elevated on its medial and/or lateral plantar vessels (59). The abductor hallucis muscle can cover small wounds in the heel and medial malleolar area, and the abductor digiti minimi muscle can cover lateral mid and hindfoot defects 2 to 3 cm in size.

Patients with wounds over 6 cm in size, or those without posterior tibial artery flow, will usually require free-tissue transfer. Bypass grafts and free flaps may be performed simultaneously or in staged fashion. The posterior tibial artery target is preferable from a microsurgical perspective because the requirement flap pedicle length may often be less than 3 to 5 centimeters. Cutaneous free flaps (e.g., radial forearm, lateral arm, scapular, and parascapular) are advocated for smaller defects because they are from the trunk and upper extremity (with lower incidence of atherosclerotic changes).

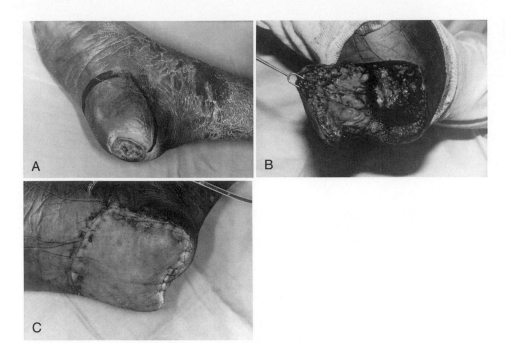

FIG. 103–11.   A, local rotational flap to be used. **B,** flap elevation. **C,** insetting and closure of heel flap.

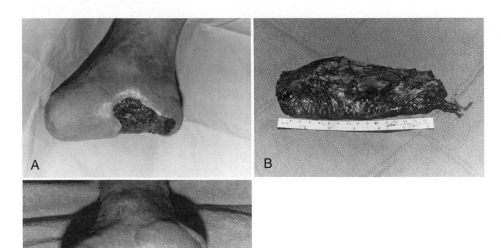

FIG. 103–12.   A, calcineal osteomyelitis requires muscle flap. **B,** rectus abdominis muscle selected for plantar resurfacing. **C,** final result with muscle and STSG after 6 months. Note good contour.

These flaps are thin and pliable and donor-site morbidity is low. In addition, neural coaptation may be performed to the radial forearm and lateral arm flaps, although its value in the neuropathic diabetic is unclear.

When larger or deeper defects necessitate a muscle flap, the serratus anterior, with its long vascular pedicle, may be anastomosed in end-to-side fashion to the posterior tibial or dorsalis pedis arteries more proximally, or to a distal bypass graft. Muscle is preferable in calcaneal or malleolar osteomyelitis because it conforms well to irregular surfaces, has well-proven bacteriocidal activity, and often has adherence to débrided bone, reducing the shear forces that occur during ambulation when skin flaps are used (Fig. 103–12). In most instances, STSG take on a healthy muscle flap is not a problem, but observation of poor skin graft take on free muscle flaps by some authors (56) has prompted a shift toward the use of cutaneous free flaps by these authors.

The subtalar Syme amputation can be performed for certain wounds at this level if adequate heel pad tissue is present. The patient can ambulate limited distances without a prosthesis, which may be a significant advantage for many patients. The tough heel pad is preserved and healing is usually adequate in the well-perfused foot. An experienced prosthetist is needed for proper fitting of a braced appliance.

Adjunctive Procedures

Attention to tendon imbalance, compression neuropathy, and abnormalities of the bony architecture in the diabetic foot has been often disregarded by plastic surgeons. Closure of the soft-tissue defect without recognition of or improvement in the "hard tissues" is short-sighted and doomed to failure. Weightbearing, as discussed earlier, is often abnormal and must be analyzed by gait analysis and treated to avoid recurrent ulceration. Excessive forefoot "loading" from loss of the longitudinal and transverse arches in the neuropathic foot (claw toes), as well as from contracture of the Achilles tendon, results in metatarsal head ulceration that will eventually lead to osteomyelitis. Similarly, disruption of the Lisfranc joint secondary to a "tight" Achilles tendon will lead to midfoot collapse and recalcitrant midfoot ulceration. A sound understanding of these biomechanical abnormalities will contribute to a rational approach to their treatment.

TENDON MANAGEMENT

Both forefoot and midfoot wounds are secondary to excessive loading of these regions during weightbearing. When carefully examined, many patients harboring such wounds will be found to have significant contracture of the Achilles tendon, causing equinous deformity. In its most severe state, barely any weight is borne on the heel pad during gait. Lengthening of the Achilles tendon should be a routine part of the surgical treatment of wounds in these regions. Midfoot collapse at the tarsometatarsal joints (Lisfranc joint) is a predictable sequelae of Achilles contracture. If normal ankle motion during ambulation is restricted because of Achilles tightness, then the Lisfranc joint begins to function "like the ankle" and excessive motion, with ultimate joint failure, results.

Following closure of soft-tissue defects in the forefoot and midfoot, attention should be directed towards lengthening the Achilles tendon. If the Achilles contracture is of long-standing duration, a posterior ankle joint capsulotomy may need to be performed as well in order to completely restore full range of motion (ROM) to the ankle joint. This is best performed immediately following tendon release, with the goal of achieving at least 10° of dorsiflexion.

BONE MANAGEMENT

When forefoot ulceration involves the first metatarsal head region, excision of the medial and lateral seasmoid bones is usually indicated because these structures are usually responsible for the persistence of ulceration in this area. This is best accomplished through the débrided wound on the plantar surface of the foot after retraction of the flexor hallucis longus tendon. Fifth metatarsal head ulceration should be managed with metatarsal head excision at the time of wound closure. Proper management of metatarsal heads II through IV remains controversial (60). Complete excision of a metatarsal head (II, III, or IV) will often result in a "transfer lesion" in an adjacent metatarsal territory. Either resection of the plantar "flare" of the metatarsal head or osteotomy through the neck of the metatarsal angled distally to the plantar surface is our preferred method of treatment. Bone resection may be performed through the plantar approach, whereas osteotomy is accomplished with a linear dorsal incision. If osteotomy is chosen, no formal fixation is currently recommended.

During the closure of midfoot ulceration, resection of bony prominences is necessary. Charcot reconstruction with re-creation of a longitudinal arch and stabilization of the Lisfranc joint is best performed "electively" once all wounds have solidly healed. We currently advocate generous osteotomy through the Lisfranc joint, re-creation of normal anatomic relationships between the metatarsal bases and the tarsal bone, and rigid fixation of the medial column of the foot with an intramedullary screw that traverses the length of the first metatarsal and passes through the medial cuneiform and into the navicular bone. Temporary K-wire fixation of the lateral midfoot completes the procedure. Iliac bone grafts are used when clinically indicated.

TARSAL TUNNEL RELEASE

During the past 5 years, several authors have discussed the potential benefits of tarsal tunnel release in the symptomatic diabetic with neuropathy. As previously discussed, diabetic patients have an increased likelihood of developing compression neuropathy because their underlying "diabetic peripheral neuropathy" renders their nerves more susceptible to compressive forces than nondiabetic nerves. If identified, tarsal tunnel syndrome may be diagnosed and treated with tarsal tunnel decompression at the time of reconstructive surgery for soft-tissue defects. Improvement in plantar sensibility and a decrease in neuropathic pain have been reported in some series (61,62). Whether this significantly contributes to a decrease in ulcer recurrence has not been confirmed.

Diagnosis is best made by eliciting a Tinel sign over the tarsal tunnel located just posterior and distal to the medial malleolus. Nerve conduction studies, if positive, are diagnostic; however, these studies are often equivocal because of the underlying axonal dysfunction related to diabetes mellitus. The use of 30-Hz and 256-Hz vibration perception may further clarify the diagnosis.

A curvilinear incision is made over the tarsal tunnel, beginning at the level of the malleolus and coursing distally towards the instep. Careful incision through the flexor retinaculum (laciniate ligament) will permit visualization of the posterior tibial artery and its associated veins. Just deep to these structures lies the posterior tibial nerve. The nerve divides into three branches; the medial calcaneal nerve (which may exit through the ligament and can be inadvertently damaged if not looked for), the medial plantar nerve, and the lateral plantar nerve. The latter two structures must be followed into their respective tunnels beneath the origin of the abductor hallucis muscle for a thorough release to be accomplished. There is often ligamentous tissue on the deep surface of the abductor hallucis muscle that compresses the medial and lateral plantar branches of the posterior tibial nerve. All structures must be fully released. If there is evidence of intraneural fibrosis, consideration should be given for further neurolysis, though this has been necessary in fewer than 10% of our cases.

The Future

Significant improvement in limb salvage rates have been realized during the past decade; however, much work needs to be done to bring the care of these difficult patients into line with the current changes in our health care delivery system. Though it may appear "obvious" that limb salvage is cost-effective to our society when compared with primary amputation in the subgroup of patients, careful outcome studies will need to be designed in order to better justify the complex surgical approaches outlined in this chapter.

Continued research on the etiology of diabetic neuropathy, as well as atherosclerosis, will provide the necessary foundation upon which preventive management may be successfully instituted. It is becoming clearer that diabetic neuropathy may be a different disease in different diabetic subjects. Autoimmune neuropathy, compressive neuropathy, ischemic neuropathy, and physiologic abnormalities of myo-inositol and sorbitol pathways all play varying roles in the clinical picture we call "diabetic peripheral neuropathy." Exciting results are being realized with innovative, multifaceted approaches to this devastating complication of diabetes mellitus.

Improved understanding of the microvascular and hemorheologic abnormalities continues to be investigated. By interfering with the formation of advanced glycosylation end products (the nonenzymatic glycosylation of proteins such as collagen), aminoguanidine prevents much of the microvascular dysfunction normally seen in untreated diabetic animals. Current clinical trials are underway, looking at the effects of aminoguanidine on the progression of retinopathy in diabetic patients. Though reconstruction of the neuropathic and the ischemic lower extremity remains a demanding challenge for plastic, vascular, orthopedic, and podiatric surgeons, the real challenge lies with our basic science and clinical laboratories.

References

1. Waters R, Perry J, Antonelli D, et al. Energy cost of walking of amputees: the influence of the level of amputation. *JBJS* 1986; 8A(1):42.
2. Kucan J, Robson M. Diabetic foot infections: fate of the contralateral foot. *Plast Reconstr Surg* 1986; 77:439.
3. Cameron N, Leonard M, Roos I. The effects of sorbinil on peripheral nerve conduction velocity, polyol concentrations, and morphology in streptotocin-diabetic rat. *Diabetologica* 1986; 29:168.
4. Dellon A. A cause for optimism in diabetic neuropathy. *Ann Plast Surg* 1988; 20:103.
5. Morain W, Dellon A, Mackinnon S, et al. Current concepts in plastic surgery for the diabetic. *Adv Plast Reconstr Surg* 1987; 4:1.
6. Sammarco G, Chalk D, Feibel J. Tarsal tunnel syndrome and additional nerve lesions in the same limb. *Foot Ankle* 1993; 14(2):71.
7. Upton A, McComas A. The double crush in nerve entrapment syndromes. *Lancet* 1973; 2:359.
8. Groth K. Clinical observations and experimental studies on the pathogenesis of decubitus ulcers. *Acta Chir Scand* (*suppl*) 1942; 87(76):207.
9. Robson M. Difficult wounds: pressure ulcerations and leg ulcers. *Clin Plast Surg* 1979; 6:537.
10. Tooke J. Microcirculation and diabetes. *Br Med Bull* 1989; 45(1):206.
11. Strandness D, Priest R, Gibbons G. Combined clinical and pathological study of diabetic and nondiabetic peripheral arterial disease. *Diabetes* 1964; 13:366.
12. Conrad M. Large and small artery occlusion in diabetics and nondiabetics with severe vascular disease. *Circulation* 1967; 36:83.
13. Goldenberg S, Alex M, Joshi R, et al. Nonatheromatous peripheral vascular disease of the lower extremity. *Diabetes* 1959; 8:261.
14. Bower H, Kaiser G, Willman V. Blood flow in the diabetic leg. *Circulation* 1971; 43:391.
15. Wyss C, Matsen F, Simmons C, et al. Transcutaneous oxygen tension measurements on limbs of diabetic and nondiabetic patients with peripheral vascular disease. *Surgery* 1984; 95:339.
16. Gaylorde P, Fonseca V, Llewellyn G, et al. Transcutaneous oxygen tension in legs and feet of diabetic patients. *Diabetes* 1988; 37:714.
17. Ehrly A. The effect of pentoxyfylline on the deformability of erythrocytes and on the muscular oxygen pressure in patients with chronic arterial disease. *J Med* 1979; 10:331.
18. LoGerfo F, Coffman J. Vascular and microvascular disease of the foot in diabetes. *NEJM* 1984; 311:1615.
19. Haimovici H. Patterns of ateriosclerotic lesions of the lower extremity. *Arch Surg* 1967; 95:918.
20. Rand P, Lacombe E. Hemodilution and blood viscosity. *J Clin Invest* 1964; 43:2214.
21. Macmillan D. The effect of diabetes on blood flow properties. *Diabetes* (*suppl 2*) 1983; 32:56.
22. Colwell J, Lopes-Virella M. A review of the development of large vessel disease in diabetes mellitus. *Am J Med* 1985; 85(5A):113.
23. Vague P, Juhan I. Red cell deformability, platelet aggregation and insulin action. *Diabetes* (*suppl 2*) 1983; 32:88.
24. Weed R, Labelle P, Meirill E. Metabolic dependence of red cell deformability. *J Clin Invest* 1969; 48:795.
25. Nakao M, Nakao T, Yamoro S. Adenosine triphosphate and maintenance of shape of red cells. *Nature* 1960; 187:945.
26. Miller J, Potparic Z, Colen L, et al. The accuracy of duplex ultrasonography in the planning of skin flaps in the lower extremity. *Plast Reconstr Surg* 1995; 95(7):1221.
27. Armstrong M, Kunar D, Cummings C. Effect of pentoxyfylline on myocutaneous flap viability in pigs. *Otolaryn Hd Neck Surg* 1993; 109(4):668.
28. Porter J, Cutter B, Lee B. Pentoxyfylline efficacy in the treatment of intermittent claudication: multicenter controlled, double-blind trial with objective assessment of chronic occlusive arterial disease patients. *Am Heart J* 1982; 104:66.
29. Roeren T, LeVeen R, Nugent L. Photoplethysmographic documentation of improved microcirculation after pentoxyfylline therapy. *Angiology* 1988; 39:929.
30. Schwartz R, Logan N, Johnson P. Pentoxyfylline increases extremity blood flow in diabetic atherosclerotic patients. *Arch Surg* 1989; 124:434. Cronenwett, in press.
31. Singer P, Berger I, Luck K, et al. Long-term effect of mackeral diet on blood pressure, serum lipids and thromboxane formation in patients with mild essential hypertension. *Atherosclerosis* 1986; 62:259.
32. Fox P, DiCorleto PE. Fish oils inhibit endothelial cell production of platelet-derived growth factor-like protein. *Science* 1988; 241:453.
33. Kjersen H, Hilsted J, Madsbad S, et al. Polymorphonuclear leukocyte dysfunction during short-term metabolic changes from normo- to hypoglycemia in Type I (insulin-dependent) diabetic patients. *Infection* 1988; 16; 4:215.
34. Richardson R. Immunity in diabetes: influence of diabetes on the development of anti-bacterial properties in the blood. *J Clin Invest* 1943; 12:1143.
35. Kahn CR, Weir GC, eds. *Joslin diabetes.* 12th ed. Malvern, PA: Lea & Febiger, 1985; 739.
36. Cianci P. Adjunctive HBO therapy in the treatment of the diabetic foot. *Wounds* 1992; 4:158.
37. Hammarlund C, Sundberg T, Hunt T. Hyperbaric oxygen reduced size of chronic leg ulcers: a randomized double-blind study. *Plast Reconstr Surg* 1994; 93(4):829.
38. Kindwall E, Gottlieb L, Larson D. Hyperbaric oxygen therapy in plastic surgery: a review article. *Plast Reconstr Surg* 1991; 88(5):989.
39. Yuh W, Corson J, Baraniewski H, et al. Osteomyelitis of the foot in diabetic patients. *Am J Radiol* 1989; 152:795.
40. Buncke H, Colen L. An island flap from the first web space of the foot to cover plantar ulcers. *Br J Plast Surg* 1980; 33:242.
41. Colen L, Buncke H. Neurovascular island flaps from the plantar vessels and nerves for foot reconstruction. *Ann Plast Surg* 1984; 12:237.
42. Colen L. Limb salvage in the patient with severe peripheral vascular disease: the role of microsurgical free tissue transfer. *Plast Reconstr Surg* 1987; 79:389.
43. Colen L, Mussen A. Preoperative assessment of the peripheral vascular disease patient for free tissue transfer. *J Reconstr Microsurg* 1987; 4:1.
44. Cronenwett J, McDaniel M, Zwolak R, et al. Limb salvage despite extensive tissue loss: free tissue transfer combined with distal revascularization. *Arch Surg* 1989; 124(5):609.
45. Searles J, Colen L. Foot reconstruction in diabetes and peripheral vascular insufficiency. *Clin Plast Surg* 1991; 18(3):467.
46. Masquelet A, Romana M, Wolf G. Skin island flaps supplied by the vascular axis of the sensitive superficial nerves: anatomic study and clinical experience in the leg. *Plast Reconstr Surg* 1992; 89(6):1115.

47. Grabb W, Argenta L. The lateral calcaneal artery skin flap (the lateral calcaneal artery, lesser saphenous vein and sural nerve skin flap). *Plast Reconstr Surg* 1981; 68:723.

48. Healy C, Tiernan E, Lamberty B, et al. Rotation fasciocutaneous flap repair of lower limb defects. *Plast Reconstr Surg* 1995; 95(2):243.

49. Morrison W, Crabb D, O'Brien B, et al. The instep of the foot as a fasciocutaneous island and as a free flap for heel defects. *Plast Reconstr Surg* 1983; 72(1):56.

50. Pontén B. The fasciocutaneous flap: its use in soft tissue defects of the lower leg. *Br J Plast Surg* 1981; 34:215.

51. Colen L, Rubinstein C, Cronenwett J. Lower limb reconstruction with combined distal vascular bypass: surgery and microsurgical free tissue transfer. In: Cronenwett J, *Recent advances in the management of ischemic extremities.* Cronenwett, in press.

52. Karp N, Kasabian A, Siebert J, et al. Microvascular free-flap salvage of the diabetic foot: a 5-year experience. *Plast Reconstr Surg* 1994; 94(6):834.

53. Roach J, Macfarlane D. Pioneer amputators for a new age. *Contemp Surg* 1989; 35:44.

54. Wieman T, Griffiths GD, Polk HC Jr. Management of diabetic midfoot ulcers. *Ann Surg* 1992; 215:627.

55. Lai C, Lin S, Yang C, et al. Limb salvage of infected diabetic foot ulcers with microsurgical free tissue transfer. *Ann Plast Surg* 1991; 26:212.

56. Oishi S, Levin S, Pederson W. Microsurgical management of extremity wounds in diabetics with peripheral vascular disease. *Plast Reconstr Surg* 1993; 92(3):485.

57. Hidalgo D, Shaw W. Anatomic basis of plantar flap design. *Plast Reconstr Surg* 1986; 78:627.

58. Shanahan R, Gingrass R. The medial plantar sensory flap for coverage of heel defects. *Plast Reconstr Surg* 1979; 64:295.

59. Hartrampf C, Scheflan M, Bostwick J. The flexor digitorum brevis muscle island pedicle flap: a new dimension in heel reconstruction. *Plast Reconstr Surg* 1980; 66:264.

60. Patel P, Wiemann J. Effect of metatarsal head resection for diabetic foot ulcers on the dynamic plantar pressure distribution. *Am J Surg* 1994; 167:297.

61. Weiman T, Patel V. Treatment of hyperesthetic neuropathic pain in diabetics: decompression of the tarsal tunnel. *Ann Surg* 1995; 221(6):660.

62. Dellon L. Treatment of symptomatic diabetic neuropathy by surgical decompression of multiple peripheral nerves. *Plast Reconstr Surg* 1992; 89(4):690.

104

Principles of Fasciocutaneous Flaps

Alain Masquelet, M.D., and M. Claudia Romaño, M.D.

There has been extraordinary development over the last 20 years in reconstructive surgery using flaps, particularly by plastic and orthopedic surgeons. The use of these reconstructive techniques has increased the reconstructive armamentarium available to the surgeon.

The rules and principles of the surgery related to fasciocutaneous flaps are different from other tissue transfers (e.g., muscle and bone). The principal reason is that the fasciocutaneous flap is based on the blood supply to the skin, which is usually a smaller vessel and more delicate than the pedicle of large muscles or bone.

The anatomy of muscles and their vascular pedicles have been well described; they can be used as free-tissue transfers. The blood supply of cutaneous flaps is not as well defined; however, the skin and its underlying structures, such as subcutaneous tissue and deep fascia, can be used as a flap with well-identified vascular pedicles. Other territories of skin can be used as pedicles or free flaps if the identified blood supply will allow such transfers.

Surgery using cutaneous flaps is based on two major concepts:

1. The vascular axis supplying a skin territory that can be elevated with reliability from the specific tissue or angiosomes.
2. The idea of the pedicle, which can be used for the technique of island flap.

The idea of axial territory is traditionally attributed to McGregor and Jackson in 1972 (1), and the concept of pedicle flap to Littler in 1953 (2). The first true axial-pattern cutaneous flap was performed by Wood in 1862 (3) to cover an important defect of the hand after the release of a scar. Wood used what he called a groin flap and was guided in the choice of the skin territory by the need to include a vascular axis. The procedure described by Wood predates that described by Shaw and Payne (4) in 1946, and also corresponds to the axial-pattern flap introduced by McGregor and Morgan in 1973 (5).

The concept of island flap was first elaborated by Esser (6), a Dutch surgeon, during World War I. Esser showed that the skin of the hinge of a flap is in no way necessary to keep the flap of tissue alive. Although he applied these procedures only in facial operations, he set the stage for the possibility to extend the concept of the island flap for treating wounds of the lower limbs. The anatomy of the blood supply to the skin was described in the works of Manchot in 1889 (7) and Salmon in 1936 (8).

The connection between the flap concepts and anatomy was difficult to achieve. The emergence of microsurgery (Krizek in 1965 (9), Harii in 1972 (10), Daniel and Taylor in 1973 (11)), with the performance of free-tissue transfers based on specific named vascular pedicles and a skin territory, was important for the proliferative description of flaps that has occurred since that time. The year 1973 is a milestone in the history of reconstructive surgery because it symbolized the fusion of the concept of the axial-pattern flap, the reality of the vascular pedicle, and the technical advance of microsurgery.

Three major advances took place in the early 1980s, which constitute the basis of newly described flaps:

1. The Chinese surgeon Yang Kuo Fan (12) demonstrated that a skin flap could be elevated on an artery that was not, in fact, the vascular axis of the flap. This clinical advance allowed the application of the work of Salmon on *les artères de la peau*.
2. Pontén (13) showed empirically in 1981 the role of the deep fascia in the survival of a peninsular flap taken from the leg with a length:breadth ratio of 4:1.
3. Chinese authors (14) in 1982 proposed distal-based pedicled flaps, which seemed physiologically impossible because they defied Harvey's law for the venous return. This prodigious possibility now allows the solving of the difficult problems of distal defects and can be applied everywhere vascular anastomotic circles exist.

Anatomy

IDENTIFYING BLOOD SUPPLY TO THE SKIN (Fig. 104–1)

Blood supply to the skin is an absolute prerequisite for executing principles of the skin flaps. We have to consider separately the vascular anatomy of the skin and the vascular basis of the flaps to establish reliable flaps that can be transferred without compromising the flap or the limb.

VASCULAR ANATOMY OF THE SKIN

Salmon's studies (8) are valid. He distinguished between direct and indirect arteries. The latter issue from the muscle and cannot provide a pedicle skin flap unless the underlying muscle is included. For a discussion of musculocutaneous flaps, see Chapter 85. Direct arteries are of primary interest because they travel directly to the skin. They originate from a main vascular axis, pass through the fascia, and perfuse the skin. According to their size, length, and direction, they can

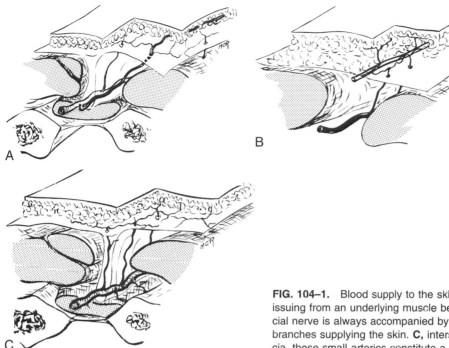

FIG. 104–1. Blood supply to the skin. **A,** a long course artery and a small arteriole issuing from an underlying muscle belly. **B,** neurocutaneous axial network. A superficial nerve is always accompanied by an axial arterial network, which gives many branches supplying the skin. **C,** interstitial arteries. Just after perforating the deep fascia, these small arteries constitute a suprafascial anastomotic plexus.

be classified in two groups: the long course arteries and the interstitial arteries.

Long course arteries are of limited number in the body. They are of a significant size (between 1 and 2 mm at their origin from a main vessel) and they course between deep structures, perforate the fascia, and distribute in the subcutaneous tissue in which their course can be well identified on injected specimens.

Neurocutaneous arteries that accompany the superficial sensory nerves are examples of long course arteries, since they constitute a true vascular axis that provides blood supply not only to the nerves but also (and chiefly) to the skin.

The second group, interstitial arteries, are smaller than the long course arteries. They issue from a deep main vascular axis, course between deep structures either in a very thin membrane (so-called meso) or in a true fibrous septum inserted on a bone, perforate the fascia, and connect via anastomoses to the immediate suprafascial plane. These anastomoses lie on the deep fascia and constitute a vascular network that provides the blood supply to the superior lying skin. This explains why it is mandatory to include the fascia of a flap that is supplied by interstitial arteries.

VASCULAR ANATOMY OF THE FLAPS

Vascular anatomy of the skin flaps can be explained based on the vascularization of the skin. The long course arteries are the basis of flaps with axial vascularisation. The paradigmatic example is the groin flap, described as the first axial-pattern flap. From a surgical point of view, it is very important to understand that it is not necessary to include the deep fascia because the vascular axis courses in the subcutaneous tissue.

The neurocutaneous arteries, well described by Salmon, are the bases of neurocutaneous flaps supplied by the arteries that accompany the superficial nerves. It is important to understand that the term *neurocutaneous* denotes the type of

vascularisation and does not concern the sensibility of the flap. Neurocutaneous flaps are harvested from the leg (saphenous nerve, superficial peroneal nerve, sural nerve) where the sacrifice of a superficial nerve is not harmful (Fig. 104–2).

The interstitial arteries are the basis of flaps that include the main vascular axis from which the small, direct arteries issue. When the main axis is limited to the flap by a loose connective tissue, the flap can be called a mesoflap. The Chinese flap (12) (radial forearm flap) is a good example of a flap based on a meso. In other locations, the linkage between the flap and the axis is fibrous tissue, which is called septum. The posterior interosseus flap (15) is typically a septocutaneous flap, because the posterior interosseus artery is included in a fibrous tunnel that is inserted on the ulna. The lateral arm flap (16) regularly used as a free flap for reconstruction of the hand is also a septocutaneous flap.

It is very important to understand that, for neurocutaneous flap, mesoflap, and septocutaneous flap, the deep fascia should be included because it provides the protection for the suprafascial anastomotic network that allows the harvest of large flaps. It is possible to raise flaps without the fascia but the size of the flap will be limited. For example, the fascia of the forearm can be spared in case of a very small Chinese flap. However, the plane of dissection between the subcutaneous tissue and the fascia is not easy to find; moreover, it is hemorrhagic, thus it is better systematically to include the deep fascia. Thus, we believe that the term *fasciocutaneous* means only that the fascia is included in the flap and does not refer to the vascularization of the flap.

SKIN TERRITORIES, VASCULAR SUPPLY, AND FLAP DESIGN

It would be a mistake to consider that skin territories are juxtaposed and supplied by a single type of vascularization. As a matter of fact, at the level of the limbs some priviliged sites

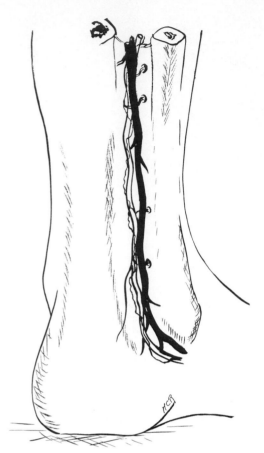

FIG. 104–2. Sural nerve with its blood supply. Several perforators are seen along the course of the nerve. A distally based island sural neurocutaneous flap is based on the lower perforator issued from the peroneal artery (4 to 5 cm proximal to the tip of the lateral malleolus).

are supplied by the three types of vascularisation described above. One of the best examples is the skin of the medial aspect of the leg, which is supplied by interstitial arteries from the tibialis posterior artery, the long course artery of the saphenous nerve, and indirect small arteries emerging from the medial head of the gastrocnemius.

Thus, the same skin territory could be raised as three different kind of flaps, namely:

1. Axial-pattern flap on the neurocutaneous artery (cutaneous branch of descending genicular artery).
2. Flap with meso, including the tibialis posterior artery.
3. Musculocutaneous flap, by raising the medial head of gastrocnemius.

One single source of blood supply is sufficient to nourish the flap by filling the multiple anastomoses between the three systems that constitute the suprafascial network.

One of the major problems in surgical practice is to define the limits of a skin flap. In fact, the territory of a flap is a very ambiguous concept that can be broken down into three parts:

1. First, the anatomic territory can be assessed by dissecting, as far as possible, the vascular axis in injected specimens. This evaluation is static and is valid only for the axial-pattern territory.

2. Second, the physiologic territory corresponds to the territory that is effectively filled by an artery under physiologic conditions in balance with the pressure of the blood flow coming from the other arteries.
3. Third, at least the surgical territory, which is the real territory of the flap, is a potential territory that is achieved when the suppression of the peripheral pressure permits the filling of suprafascial and the subcutaneous network and allows the extension of the anatomic and the physiologic territories.

This very important concept has two consequences:

1. The size of a skin flap is larger than the size that can be based on the identification of the course of the vascular axis.
2. Very large flaps can be based on very small secondary arteries. One example is provided by the posterior flap of the forearm. All the skin of the dorsal aspect of the forearm can survive only on the posterior interosseus artery, the caliber of which is 0.2 or 0.3 mm at the level of the wrist.

CLASSIFICATION OF SKIN FLAPS (17)

Using the above considerations, we can classify the flaps with three criteria:

1. The vascular anatomy of the flap
   Axial pattern flap
   Meso flap or septocutaneous flap
   Neurocutaneus flap
2. The utilization of the flap
   Proximally or distally island pedicled flaps
   Peninsular flaps with a proximal or a distal hinge (Fig. 104–3)
   Free vascularized flaps
   Some flaps, like the radial forearm flap, are very versatile and can be designed for all types of utilization. Other flaps, like groin flaps, are generally used as proximally based peninsular as a pedicled flap. Generally speaking, an axial-pattern flap (with a dead-end vascular axis) cannot be reversed.
3. The component tissues of the flap
   The fascial flap, which includes the deep fascia and a thin layer of subcutaneous tissue to protect the well-vascularized suprafascial network.
   The vascularized fat flap, which is composed of subcutaneous tissue raised between the subdermal and the suprafascial level. This type of flap should be axial pattern.
   The cutaneous flap, including skin and subcutaneous tissue. The plane of dissection passes superficial to the fascia (groin flap and scapular flap).
   The fasciocutaneous flap, elevated en bloc with the skin, the subcutaneous tissue and the deep fascia.

The points to consider regarding the distally based pedicled flap (either as a peninsular or as an island) when it is supplied by a reverse arterial flow, are:

1. The pivot point of the pedicle or the hinge of the peninsular flap should include a part of a vascular anastomotic circle. The first reverse arterial flow flap described was the forearm flap. Reverse flow was indeed insured by the

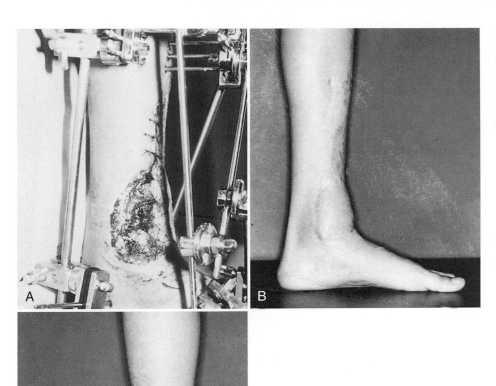

FIG. 104–3. Distally based peninsular supramalleolar flap. **A,** soft-tissue defect of the medial aspect of the lower quarter of the leg. **B, C,** long-term result after coverage by a supramalleolar flap designed on the lateral aspect of the lower leg. This flap is supplied by the perforating branch of the peroneal artery.

anastomosis between radial and ulnar arteries. The extremities of the limbs (fingers and toes) and all the joints are provided with arterial anastomoses that allow the elevation of such flaps.

2. The venous return was considered a mystery for a long time and several explanations were provided; now it has been established that the venous drainage is reversed in the veins and the key of a good venous drainage is to raise the vascular pedicle en bloc as far as the normal venous flow. This key procedure is equivalent to a sympathectomy, which leads to the incompetence of the valves and impedes the flattening of the comitantes veins.

Principles of Elevation

INDICATIONS FOR FASCIOCUTANEOUS FLAPS

Indications for fasciocutaneous flaps are determined by their characteristics. The advantages of fasciocutaneous flaps are well known. They provide a very supple coverage, with a deep gliding surface insured by the fascia. Their disadvantage is the limited blood supply carried to the recipient site; the deep aspect of the fascia is poorly vascularized. For these reasons, a fasciocutaneous flap is preferentially indicated to resurface mobile skin areas and stressed zones and to provide an adequate coverage for tendon units. In contradistinction, a fasciocutaneous flap is not indicated when the defect is a very large cavity, or in case of bone exposure if the bone is infected.

Fasciocutaneous arterialised flaps still find their best indications in the upper extremity since, most of the time, the aim of the treatment is to restore the function of the hand, which requires very supple tissues. This important concept is well supported by the fact that, in the upper extremity, very few muscles can be sacrificed without significant functional loss. On the contrary, numerous fasciocutaneous flaps are available in the upper extremity.

The weightbearing areas of the foot can be readily restored using a fasciocutaneous flap. If the problem is limited to the skin (i.e., unstable or retractile scar), the defect should be treated by skin replacement employing a fasciocutaneous flap when a skin graft is not suitable.

Fasciocutaneous flaps are indicated for treatment of tissue defects when there is no infection of the surrounding tissues.

Soft-tissue defects of the hand are an exception, as in emergencies, when the need for a good functional recovery requires a fasciocutaneous or a fascial flap. We do not advocate the coverage of compound fractures of the leg by fasciocutaneous flaps. The viability of the local and regional skin flaps is not always reliable and bone coverage is better insured by muscle flaps in the leg.

Principles of Fasciocutaneous Flap Surgery

PREOPERATIVE PLANNING

Preoperative planning is fundamental. The procedure, recovery period, and problems must be discussed with the patient. Assessment of the defect is performed and features are noted: size, depth, presence of infection, underlying structures, and condition of neighboring tissues. Several operations are possible. The choice among local flap, island flap, microvascular transfers, or cross-leg flap is based on multiple factors. Age, sex, and occupation are important. Heavy smoking is a contraindication for microsurgical transfer. In diabetics and patients with vascular disease, the distally based pedicle flaps of the lower limb have a high rate of failure. In our opinion, two consultations are needed to determine the choice of the procedure and to be sure that the patient is well informed about the technique used, with details of the donor site, the duration of operation, and the immediate and long-term postoperative care.

Preoperative workup includes an arteriogram, if the patient has been operated on several times previously. We believe that the arteriogram is mandatory for the lower limb to assess the quality of the main axis, the quality of distal anastomosis, and any vascular anomalies. Sometimes, the arteriogram shows the axial artery of the flap when it comes from a secondary axis. Doppler studies can be used to locate the precise emergence of cutaneous perforators (e.g., for the flaps raised from the thigh).

Operative Procedure

The recipient site is prepared first. Flap dissection must be performed according to the definitive shape of the defect. Borders should be excised until the skin is supple, to facilitate the sutures and early venous return. Severe infection may require a two-stage débridement. Once the recipient site is prepared, the flap is raised with a new set of instruments. Successful harvest of the flap is based on the design of the flap, features of the pedicle, rotation axis, dissection, transfer and fixation on the recipient site, and postoperative care.

DESIGN OF THE FLAP

The design of the flap is based on the knowledge of the course of the arterial pedicle. The size of the flap depends on the turgor of the skin at the donor site. In general, the flap should be slightly larger than the recipient site, but the definitive fixation will be done with some tension to avoid vascular stasis of the capillaries. The design of the flap is relative to the location of the recipient and donor sites. If the donor site is opposite to the recipient site, the pedicle will be reversed. A pivot point like the page of a book, and a sufficient length of pedicle, should be anticipated.

FEATURES OF THE PEDICLE

Only the axial-pattern flap has a fixed pedicle length, which is determined by the distance between the origin of the artery

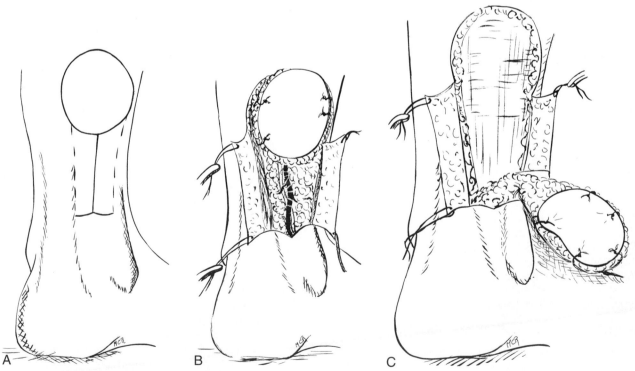

FIG. 104–4. Dissection of a distally based island sural neurocutaneous flap. **A,** design of the flap. The pivot point is located 4 to 5 cm proximal to the tip of the lateral malleolus. **B,** a subcutaneous fascial pedicle is isolated, including the sural vein, the sural nerve, and its arterial network. **C,** this reverse flap is suitable for covering soft-tissue defects of the hind foot.

and its penetration into the flap. On the contrary, an interstitial pattern flap can be raised at different levels of the artery. It is important to understand that, with axial flap, the pedicle is a fixed factor but the size of the flap may vary, whereas, in septal or mesoflap, the main axis is constant but the size of the flap and the length of the pedicle vary in opposite directions. The pedicle of a neurocutaneous flap comprises subcutaneous and fascial tissue (Fig. 104–4).

THE PIVOT POINT (ROTATION OF AXIS) OF THE PEDICLE

Knowledge of the precise location of the pivot point of the pedicle is essential. It generally corresponds to a vascular anastomosis or the emergence of the arterial branch devoted to the flap. The pivot point determines the arc of the coverage of a flap. Arc of coverage is large (i.e., radial forearm flap) for the skin flap, as it depends on the length of the pedicle and the size of the flap. It is only fixed for the true axial flap like the groin flap.

DISSECTION OF THE FLAP

The skin incision is made over the pedicle and half the circumference of the flap. We advocate maintaining a subcutaneous hinge until the blood supply to the flap and the pedicle are well identified as reliable. The flap may be left in place if the pedicle anatomy is not satisfactory. Moreover, the dissection of the pedicle is easier when the physiologic tension of the tissue is maintained. In order to avoid vascular injury to the suprafascial arterial network, the deep fascia is fixed to the dermis with small, adsorbable sutures.

DISSECTION OF THE VASCULAR PEDICLE

The vascular pedicle includes an artery and two venae comitantes, which are sufficient to supply adequate venous drainage. Dissection of the pedicle should maintain a perivascular protective sheath of tissue to avoid spasm and injuries to the vessels. Careful hemostasis by clips and ligatures should be preferred to coagulation.

INSETTING THE FLAP

The donor site and defect are often distant and separated by a skin bridge that can be a retractile scar. In this latter case, the scar should be excised and the pedicle covered immediately with a split-thickness skin graft. If the skin bridge between the recipient and donor site is healthy, there are two possibilities: (a) If the skin is very supple, the pedicle and the flap may be tunnelled and the passage of the flap is made easier by splitting the deep fascia. (b) If the skin is physiologically adherent (e.g., on the medial aspect of the heel), it is preferable to cut the skin and undermine the borders in order to bury the pedicle.

The dorsum of the hands and feet are always difficult to traverse by tunnelling. The skin is supple, but numerous veins make tunnelling risky. Hematoma under an elevated skin bridge may cause thrombosis of the vascular pedicle with necrosis of the flap. Drainage stents, such as a Penrose drain, are put in place between the closure. This allows irrigation under the flap during the postoperative period.

DONOR SITE

The size of the donor-site defect often becomes larger than the area of the flap harvest, owing to retraction of wound edges. This can be reduced by suturing the dermis to the underlying muscles (marsupilization). The time of skin-graft coverage depends on the depth of the defect. It may be preferable to wait a few days to obtain granulation tissue before grafting.

Postoperative Care

The dressing must be comfortable, well-padded, and not too tight, with an opening that allows monitoring of the flap. Elevation is very important; however, the limb must be slightly above the level of the heart because blood pressure decreases quickly with elevation. During the immediate postoperative period, the patient should be quiet and pain free to avoid spasm of small arterioles. The monitoring of the flap is crucial, even for a pedicle island flap. The features to be noted are the color, the capillary filling, and the temperature of the flap. Quite often an island flap is pale or slightly congested. Increasing venous congestion, with progressive appearence of ecchymosis, indicates a venous thrombosis or very significant venous congestion. If neighboring tissues are healthy, this venous congestion of a pedicled flap may be treated by the use of leeches. But the surgeon should keep in mind that use of leeches carries a risk of infection. If the flap is pale and not bleeding, a small incision should be made to determine if there is arterial obstruction resulting from kinking of the pedicle.

When the flap is placed on the lower extremity, the patient must be kept in bed for a few days and not allowed to walk before 2 weeks have elapsed. When the flap is healed, compressive garments are useful to reduce a bulky tissue. Secondary surgery for debulking is usually delayed for at least 6 months.

References

1. McGregor IA, Jackson IT. The groin flap. *Br J Plast Surg* 1972; 25:3.
2. Littler JW. The neurovascular pedicle method of digital transposition for reconstruction of the hand. *Plast Reconstr Surg* 1953; 12:303.
3. Khoo Boo-Chai. John Wood and his contributions to plastic surgery: the first groin flap. *Br J Plast Surg* 1977; 30:9.
4. Shaw DT, Payne RL. One-stage tubed abdominal flap. *Surg Gynecol Obstet* 1946; 83:205.
5. McGregor IA, Morgan G. Axial and random pattern flaps. *Br J Plast Surg* 1973; 26:202.
6. Esser JFS. Island flaps. *Med J New York* 1917; 106:264.
7. Manchot C. *Die hantarterien des menschlichen körpers* (Leipzig, 1889). Translated as: *The cutaneous arteries of the human body.* New York: Springer Verlag, 1983.
8. Salmon M. *Les artères de la peau.* Paris: Masson, 1936.
9. Krizek TJ, Tani T, DesPrez Q, et al. Experimental transplantation of composite grafts by microvascular anastomosis. *Plast Reconstr Surg* 1965; 36:538.
10. Harii K, Ohmori K, Ohmori S. Hair transplantation with free scalp flaps. *Plast Reconstr Surg* 1974; 53:259.
11. Daniel RK, Taylor CI. Distant transfer of an island flap by microvascular anastomoses. *Plast Reconstr Surg* 1973; 52:111.
12. Yang G, Chen B, Gao Y. Forearm free skin flap transplantation. *Med J China* 1981; 61:139.
13. Pontén B. The fasciocutaneous flaps, its use in soft tissue defects of the lower leg. *Br J Plast Surg* 1983; 34:215.
14. Song R, Gao Y, Song Y. The forearm flap. *Clin Plast Surg* 1982; 9:21.
15. Penteado CV, Masquelet AC, Chevrel JP. The anatomic basis of fasciocutaneous flap of the posterior interosseous artery. *Surg Radiol Anat* 1981; 8:209.
16. Katsaros J, Schusterman M, Beppu M. The lateral upper arm flap: anatomy and clinical applications. *Ann Plast Surg* 1984; 12:489.
17. Masquelet AC, Gilbert A. *An atlas of flaps in limbs reconstruction.* London: Martin Dunitz, 1995.

TEN

Practical Concepts
for the Plastic Surgery Practice

105

Basic Medical-Legal Principles in the Practice of Plastic Surgery

Norman M. Cole, M.D., F.A.C.S.

Medicine comprises the art of the prevention, palliation, and healing of illness. As early as 2000 B.C., the Code of Hammurabi documented concern for the quality of medical practice, which was once again emphasized in the Oath of Hippocrates in the 4th century, B.C. According to early English common law, a physician's liability was based on the fact that he was a member of a public calling, much like a shopkeeper.

The exchange of goods and services among individuals has resulted from society's existence. Such exchanges generate rights, obligations, and liabilities between the involved parties. With the rise of commercialism, the physician's role developed from a creation of contract law.

Torts principles and negligence law have supplanted contract law as the dictating doctrines of professional medical liability.

The moral and ethical responsibilities associated with the practice of medicine are well recognized, but the legal obligations between physician and patient are often less well understood. The current medical-legal climate would seem to dictate that the concepts of "duty," "negligence," "proximate cause," and "standard of care" should be included in the education of a surgeon just as are other principles of surgical management. This chapter will provide a brief overview of the legal obligations and risks inherent in the practice of medicine, with particular emphasis on plastic surgery. The information presented is generic and does not address jurisdictional differences. Since it is written by a surgeon and not an attorney, all statements are subject to legal review.

Physician-Patient Relationship

Certain characteristics of the physician-patient relationship make it distinctive. There is a basic difference between the individuals' knowledge bases; the patient carries with him a robe of frailty or vulnerability; the physician's sense of duty governs his actions, and it is hoped that a bond of trust exists.

A physician-patient relationship may be based upon a contract between parties (contractual basis), or on an undertaking to perform (tort basis), or on a combination of the two. For the purpose of personal injury cases, the consensual arrangement reached by the patient and physician "creates a status or relation rather than a contract" (1).

Fault-Based Liability

For the most part, medical malpractice law is founded on a system of loss allocation that is based on the "fault" of the defendant. Liability without fault may be present in cases of res ipsa loquitur, lack of informed consent or breach of contract (e.g. in cases where guaranteed, specific results did not result). Nevertheless, usually some form of unacceptable conduct by the defendant or by someone for whom the defendant is responsible (superior respondeat) occurs.

In the majority of cases, the patient claims that the physician failed to perform according to the required standard of care. Regardless of the contractual or tort basis of the claim, the duty of care is usually the same.

Elements of a Negligence Claim

Legal actions pertaining to injuries coincident with the rendering of medical services are pursued as "personal injury claims." Three conditions (2) must be met if the legal definition of medical negligence is to be proven:

1. A series of events occur during the course of medical treatment.
2. A standard of care appropriate to these circumstances must be established.
3. The events that occurred during the course of medical treatment must then be proven to represent a significant departure from the established standard of care standard established by law for the protection of others against unreasonable risk of harm (3). In order to establish a valid negligence claim, the following elements must exist: (a) a duty of care was owed by the physician to the patient; (b) the physician violated the applicable standard of care; (c) the patient suffered a compensable loss or injury; and (d) such an injury was caused in fact, and proximately caused by the substandard care. The burden of proving the existence of the above mentioned lies with the plaintiff (i.e., the patient or the patient's estate).

Negligence is defined as "conduct which falls below the standard established by law for the protection of others against unreasonable risk of harm" (3). In order to establish a valid negligence claim the following elements must exist: 1) a *duty* of care was owed by the physician to the patient; 2) the physician violated the applicable *standard of care;* 3) the patient suffered a *compensable loss or injury;* and 4) such an injury was *caused in fact* and *proximately caused* by the substandard care. The burden of proving the existence the abovementioned elements lies with the plaintiff (i.e. the patient or the patient's estate).

Duty

CONTRACTUAL CREATION OF DUTY

An expressed contract is created when a physician agrees to treat the patient in exchange for compensation; the courts will infer the presence of an implied contract where circumstances such as the institution of treatment with the patient's consent and with the expectation of compensation from the physician exist. The duty that is created is envisioned as being based on a service contract.

Once a physician-patient relationship is established, the duty of care demanded of a physician is imposed via the enforcement of tort law rather than as a result of any existing contract between the patient and physician. The exception to this premise arises when a special agreement has been created between the two parties, such as the guarantee of a specific result (e.g., the assurance that the surgeon can achieve the result visualized by the patient on a computer image). In the absence of such a special guarantee or agreement, the initial contract is important solely in the establishment of a professional relationship upon which the physician's duty is created.

DUTY CREATED AS A RESULT OF UNDERTAKING TO RENDER MEDICAL CARE

A physician who undertakes to render care to a patient thus creates a professional relationship that carries with it a corresponding duty of care owed to the patient. According to this "undertaking" theory, the existence of the physician-patient relationship and its accompanying duty is not dependent upon payment for the physician's services.

Duty does not prevent the physician from refusing to prescribe treatment or refusing to perform a procedure which the physician does not believe is indicated (4), but the physician cannot refuse to provide care once the professional relationship is established.

Duration of Duty

This duty remains in force until it is terminated in one of the three following ways:

1. *By the patient's request.* The patient may request that records and care be transferred to another physician, and from that point no longer receives care from the physician (5).
2. *By mutual agreement.* If there is no medical need for further services, the patient is informed and the relationship is terminated. Such termination usually requires no written communication to the patient, but an appropriate entry must be placed in the medical record. Referral or transfer of care to another physician with the patient's knowledge and consent can also terminate the relationship (6).
3. *By the physician's request.* A physician may end the relationship, but must meet more exacting requirements to insure continuity of care. The physician is not entitled to terminate the relationship unless reasonable advance notice is first given. The definition of reasonable advance notice depends on the patient's condition and the availability of other suitable care. The patient should be notified far enough in advance for the patient to acquire the effective management of another suitable physician. In

order for the notice to be reasonable, it should apprise the patient of medical status and type of future medical care, including specialized care, needed.

Documentation is required, showing that the patient was duly notified (e.g. "As of 7 days from the receipt of this letter [or some other suitable time interval that conforms to local standards], I will no longer be responsible for your medical care"). The letter should be registered, and a return receipt requested. An attorney acquainted with the requirements for terminating services to patients should be consulted regarding specifics that may apply to the surgeon's own region or jurisdiction (7).

Abandonment

Unless the relationship is terminated by one of the alternatives listed above, the physician remains obligated to provide needed care to the patient. This obligation is without regard for any financial considerations. The inability or failure of the patient to pay for services rendered does not relieve the physician of the "duty" to continue to provide medical care (8). Failure to respond to the medical needs of a patient because of unpaid bills may meet the legal definition of *abandonment,* a departure from the recognized standard of care; if damages occur, abandonment may result in a judgment against the physician (9).

When the professional relationship between physician and patient is terminated unilaterally by the physician without reasonable notice or justification, or is unreasonably interrupted by a failure to treat the patient, the legal definition of abandonment has been met. For various professional or personal reasons, a physician may need to find a substitute physician to act in his absence. If, without justification, a competent substitute physician is selected to care for the patient and harm proximally results as a result of the substitution, the physician may be liable if notice is not given in sufficient time for the patient to engage a physician of the patient's choice (10).

If the physician prematurely terminates the patient's continuing need for care, the patient has been *intentionally abandoned* and the physician may also be liable for breach of contract. In such cases of conscious abandonment, the fact that the relationship was terminated may establish the physician's fault.

A patient's failure to return for follow-up care does not relieve the physician of the obligation to provide follow-up care. If such follow-up care is necessary to achieve a satisfactory result or maintain adequate control of a disease process, the physician has a responsibility to notify the patient of the need for continuing care (11).

Standard of Care: The Nature of the Duty Owed

Individuals must abide by certain standards of behavior in order to prevent avoidable injuries to others. If an injury occurs as a result of a deviation from these standards, the victim may bring action against the responsible party and may also be entitled to compensation.

Conduct is judged based on objective criteria. It is not sufficient that a physician perform to utmost potential and with utter good faith. Rather, the physician must conform to the standard of a reasonable person *under like circumstances* (12). The standard that we as physicians are held to differs from that of the reasonable-person standard based on the following premises: (a) physicians are expected to possess and implement knowledge and skill in their professional practice that surpasses that of ordinary individuals; (b) the possession of such skill and knowledge has normally been evaluated as a result of professional standards set by the profession.

LEGAL DEFINITION (13)

(A physician is) under a duty to use that degree of care and skill which is expected of a reasonably competent practitioner in the same class to which he belongs, acting in the same or similar circumstances.
. . . (L)ocality is merely one factor to be taken into account in applying general professional standards. . . (T)he standard should be established by the medical profession itself and not by lay courts. . .
. . . (T)he evidence may include the elements of locality, availability of facilities, specialization or general practice, proximity of specialists and special facilities, as well as other relevant considerations.

PROFESSIONAL STANDARDS AND EXPERT TESTIMONY REQUIREMENT

The existence of a deviation from the standard of care must be proven as a result of expert testimony. The testimony of an "expert" is generally considered legally mandatory in medical negligence cases. Failure on the part of the plaintiff to provide expert testimony may result in a summary judgment in favor of the defendant physician without regard for any other circumstances in the claim. Only on very rare occasions is expert testimony not required. One example is that of *res ipsa loquitur* claim (it speaks for itself) in which acts of negligence are so obvious that courts have held that jurors can understand them without expert help (14). Another example is the claim in which the physician openly admits liability and blame either at the time of the event or in subsequent testimony (15).

Since specialists are examined by national certifying boards, specialists will generally be held to a national standard that permits testimony by experts from locales well outside the defendant's community (16). Defendant physicians are held only to the standards of care that the *average careful and prudent practitioner of their specialty would be expected to meet under the same circumstances* (17).

Whereas the events, or series of events, that occur in any given claim may be a matter of record, the *standard or care* appropriate to the circumstances can only be established through the testimony of a recognized "medical expert." The medical expert must not only testify as to the standard of care but also be willing to testify that the events of the claim represent a deviation from the established standard of care. It is not enough merely for the medical expert to testify as to what he would have done. The "medical expert" should possess the credentials and qualifications to establish the standard of care and, is usually, but not always, from the defendant's own specialty. Medical experts from other specialties may testify, but defendant physicians are usually held only to the standards that apply to their specialty or to their level of expertise (18).

Time Frame of Reference

For the purposes of establishing negligence, a defendant's conduct will be evaluated in terms of the state of medical science and the professional standards as they existed at the time of the allegedly wrongful conduct (19).

Geographic Frame of Reference

The courts used to define the standard of care of the medical profession based on a reference to a limited geographical setting. This "strict locality rule" is now followed in only a small number of jurisdictions (20). The rule is objectionable, based on the potential effect of maintaining small pockets of substandard practices in certain locales and on limiting the number of available expert witnesses.

"Respectable Minority" and "Error in Judgment"

In order to allow for differing viewpoints and opinions, the courts have developed a "respectable minority" rule. "(A) physician does not incur liability merely by electing to pursue one of several recognized courses of treatment" (21). Additionally, secondary to the fact that medicine is not an exact science, the "error in judgment" concept has been developed. This rule holds that a physician who otherwise follows the applicable professional standards should not be found liable merely because the decision turns out to have been the wrong one. This "error in judgment" rule doesn't determine the outcome of a case. Rather, this rule is given to the jury in their instructions. One court has observed, "(e)rrors in judgment which occur with the best intentions constitute negligence if they result from a failure to use reasonable care" (22).

"Best Judgment" Rule

Some courts have held that it is not enough for a physician to comply with the professional standards of conduct. "If a physician fails to employ his expertise or best judgment. . ., he should not automatically be freed from liability because in fact he adhered to acceptable practice. . . . (A) physician should use his best judgment and whatever superior knowledge, skill and intelligence he has" (23).

CIRCUMSTANTIAL EVIDENCE AND RES IPSA LOQUITUR

Negligence may be proven in two different ways. It may be proven through the use of *direct evidence,* where the series of events that led to the injury and its accompanying negligence are explained. Additionally, negligence may be proven indirectly via *circumstantial evidence.* This indirect method of establishing negligence is referred to as the doctrine of *res ipsa loquitur,* "the thing speaks for itself."

Three elements must be present for the doctrine of *res ipsa loquitur* to apply. The insult must have:

1. resulted from an event that ordinarily doesn't occur in the absence of negligence.
2. (been) caused by an agency or instrumentality under the exclusive control or management of the defendant.
3. occurred under circumstances indicating that the injury was not due to any negligence or voluntary act on the part of the plaintiff (24).

The most common factual pattern in which the doctrine of *res ipsa loquitur* applies involves allegation of surgical sponges or instruments being left inside a patient. Additionally, courts have been more than willing to apply the doctrine to cases involving burns or trauma to parts of the patient's body not in the immediate operative field (25).

Vicarious Liability

Besides being responsible for one's own actions, the physician may be legally responsible and held liable for the actions or omissions of others. For this doctrine of *vicarious liability* to be present, two conditions must be met:

1. A required relationship must exist between parties 1 and 2. This usually comprises that of an employer/employee relationship. Other relationships, such as "borrowed servants" relationships and partnership relationships, are also included.
2. The second requirement is that party 2 must have been acting within the contemplated *scope of the relationship when the tort was committed.* In an employer/employee relationship, the employee must have been acting within the "scope of his employment."

A physician may occasionally be held vicariously liable for the malpractice of another physician. These situations include those in which (a) one physician is the employee of another; (b) two or more physicians are partners or satisfy the requirements to be deemed members of a "joint enterprise"; and (c) when one physician is held to be a "borrowed servant" of another physician (26).

"BORROWED SERVANT" RULE

The "borrowed servant" rule states: "A servant directed or permitted by his master to perform services for another may become the servant of such other in performing the services" (27). This theory applies to support staff such as residents, interns, nurses, and medical technicians, among others. The main question that has to be answered is whether a master/servant relationship existed between the physician and the support staff despite the absence of a traditional employment relationship. Borrowed servant status depends upon a finding that the physician possessed the *required degree of control* over the staff person or resident.

In order to impose the threat of vicarious liability here, it must be shown that:

1. the support staff person was negligent.
2. the physician possessed the required degree of control over the staff support person.
3. the assistant was acting within the scope of his role as an assistant.

Direct negligence on the part of the physician need not be proven.

RESPONSIBILITY FOR OTHER PHYSICIANS

Many physicians may be involved in the performance of an operation besides the primary surgeon: anesthesiologists, residents, and interns, among others. The courts have been reluctant to characterize the participation of other specialists as that of borrowed servants. In the affirmation of the verdict for a surgeon, the court held that the surgeon could not be held vicariously liable for the actions of the anesthesiologist over whose performance she or he had (in the absence of evidence to the contrary) no control or right to control (28).

RESPONDENT SUPERIOR THEORY

If one physician is employed by another, the supervising or employer physician can be held liable for the actions of the employed physician. If the physician is found to be an "independent contractor," the employer/employee relationship vanishes. Whenever there exists a formal relationship and involvement of wages and the *right to control the manner of performance,* as in a master/servant or employer/employee relationship, vicarious liability may be applied (29).

PARTNERSHIPS AND PROFESSIONAL CORPORATIONS

A physician may be held vicariously liable for the torts of another physician who is a partnership member for conduct committed in the scope of partnership activities. Partners may also be held vicariously liable for the wrongdoings of the employees of the partnership (30).

Causation Test

The time-honored test of causation is the "but for" or *sine qua non* test. Causation exists when the injury or loss would not have occurred "but for" the defendant's negligent conduct. An alternate test for causation has been that of the defendant's tortious conduct having been a "substantial factor" in bringing about the injury. Causation must be established by the standard of proof of a preponderance of the evidence. This requires that the plaintiff prove that it was "more likely than not" that the defendant's negligence caused the harm (31).

Proximate Cause

In addition to proof of negligence and proof of damages, the plaintiff is required to prove that the two are *directly related,* which is known as proximate cause (32).

Damages

In addition to proving negligence, a claim for personal injury must establish proof of "damages." The plaintiff must show that damages have occurred that can be translated into monetary relief or retribution. The loss of income and/or the cost of care and treatment that results from a temporary or permanent disability due to negligence comprise economic losses. Claims for noneconomic losses such as "pain and suffering" may also be made. Proof of the existence of damages is essential to a medical liability claim. Even in the face of proven negligence, judgments have not been awarded unless damages occurred (33).

JUDGMENT

When a claim of damages causally related to medical negligence is proven, the plaintiff will be entitled to a judgment that is usually monetary in nature and is satisfied through a transfer of assets from the defendant to the plaintiff. Unless there is some other source of compensation, such as medical liability insurance, the defendant's personal assets will be used to satisfy the judgment.

Medical Liability Insurance

To protect personal assets, physicians generally carry medical liability insurance. Premiums for such insurance vary widely according to risk, which is influenced by geography, specialty, and previous claims. Surgical specialties are rated by underwriters as possessing significantly higher risks than medical specialties. Plastic surgery is rated as a high-risk specialty because of the specialty's high frequency of claims, even though paid claims show relatively low average severity (i.e., size of award) (34).

In addition to providing compensation to the plaintiff, the insurance company also covers legal expenses coincident with the claim. Consequently, the insurance carrier generally reserves the right to choose the defense attorneys. Through its claims adjustors, the insurance company may also provide advice and attempt to influence decisions regarding the defense of a claim and/or settlement. The physician's rights with regard to settlement and defense strategy may vary between carriers. Therefore, each physician must be familiar with the limitations and restrictions of the individual policy.

A physician may wish to employ a private attorney independently to advise and assist in the defense. If the claim is for an amount that exceeds the physician's insurance coverage, a private attorney should be retained to defend that portion of the claim for which the insurance carrier is not liable (35).

In acquiring and maintaining medical liability insurance, one should become knowledgeable regarding the types and amounts of coverage available. The "basic" medical liability policy establishes limits of liability on the part of the carrier: a maximum amount that will be provided for "each event" (i.e., claim) and a maximum amount that will be covered for "all events" for any given year in which the policy is in effect. These limits may be expressed as $100,000/$300,000 limits, or some similar combination. Most companies have maximum limits for the liability covered on the "basic" policy. When, in the physician's judgment, these limits are insufficient to meet exposure, the physician may wish to obtain additional insurance (known as an "umbrella" policy) that will provide coverage in excess of basic coverage. A basic policy must be in effect before an underwriter will provide an umbrella policy.

TYPES OF COVERAGE

Coverage types vary between companies and can be influenced by the medical-legal climate in any given locality. "Occurrence" policies cover the physician for any occurrence (i.e., that occurs during the period of time that the policy was in effect, regardless as to when the claim is made). Occurrence policies are particularly desirable in cases in which the statute of limitations may be extensive, such as in the treatment of children, when claims may be filed even after adulthood for medical events that were allegedly mismanaged during childhood. Since the statute of limitations begins at the time of *discovery* of the alleged medical negligence, which may not be at the time of the actual procedure, occurrence policies are advantageous in that coverage for these events is maintained in perpetuity, even though the claim may be filed many years after the treatment rendered and even though the physician may not be currently insured by the original carrier.

"Claims made" policies provide coverage exclusively for claims that are filed during the period that the policy is in effect, and only if the incident occurred while the physician was continuously insured under the "claims made" policy. If the policy is dropped, the insurance carrier's liability is ter-

minated. A claim filed at a later date on behalf of an event that occurred during the period that the "claims made" policy was in effect will not be covered. Retired physicians and/or physicians who change insurance companies will not be covered for claims that arise from previous events, even though they occurred during the time that the "claims made" policy was in effect. In such an event, the company may offer "prior acts" coverage or a "reporting endorsement" (commonly known as a "tail"), which provides insurance for claims that occur prior to or beyond the "claims made" coverage. The premium for such supplemental coverage is at the insurer's discretion and is based on their actuarial estimate of the potential continuing risk to which the physician may be exposed for events that occurred in the physician's past practice experience.

"Going Bare"

Some physicians believe that medical liability insurance may be an invitation for claims and think that plaintiffs will be less likely to pursue a claim against a physician who does not carry insurance. Individuals who do not carry medical liability insurance are "going bare." Physicians who go bare are encountering increasing difficulties in obtaining hospital staff privileges. The bylaws of many hospitals dictate that its staff personnel must carry a minimum level of medical liability insurance in order to be eligible for staff membership.

Irrevocable Trusts

Should a physician have the right to determine the measures that will be taken to provide compensation to a medically injured patient? Should a physician be forced to carry medical liability insurance if the physician has developed some other suitable compensation alternative? A willing physician may place personal assets at risk as long as the assets available are adequate to meet the potential damages. An alternative to carrying "basic" medical malpractice insurance that appears to meet these requirements is called an "irrevocable trust" (36).

Actions That May Affect Coverage

Medical liability policies must be examined carefully and exclusions from coverage duly noted. A physician may invalidate coverage if he or she fraudulently concealed actions that were related to (or were in any way responsible for) a medical negligence claim. Some carriers use very restrictive language within their policies that may void coverage in cases where physicians have altered medical records to avoid liability. Coverage may be voided if a physician fails to notify an insurance company of a claim or a potential claim. Medical-liability policies generally do not cover fraud, slander, libel, damages arising from unauthorized disclosures, or assault and battery (37).

Insurance companies offer liability coverage on an annual basis and are under no obligation to provide a physician with insurance beyond the end of the termed policy period. Companies are free to set their own premiums, usually subject to review by state insurance commissioners. If these premiums are approved, the physician must be willing to pay the premium or lose coverage. The carrier is also free to determine the nature of coverage to be offered (e.g., "occurrence" vs. "claims made").

The Patient's Right to Information and Self-Determination

REQUIREMENT OF CONSENT

The consent that a patient renders may be implied, and it may also be directly given. The physician must act in good faith in believing that the manifestation of consent accurately reflected the patient's true willingness to undergo the procedure. A consent may be invalidated when it is obtained by duress or misrepresentation concerning the nature or extent of the harm, or when the patient is acting under serious misapprehension of which the defendant is aware concerning such matters (38).

The fact that a patient consents to an operative procedure by one physician does not ordinarily constitute consent to the performance by a substitute physician. The original physician may be found liable (39). Additionally, the substitute physician may be found liable in the absence of a valid consent or emergency situation (40). If a team of physicians are to be involved, this should be explained to the patient and appropriate consents obtained.

Implied Consent

Examination and treatment of patients require the patient's permission and consent. In many instances of medical practice, the consent is "implied" (41) and covers many minor procedures of which the patient is fully aware, such as injections, drawing blood, manual examinations, or any other of the various procedures that make up the daily practice of medicine. The fact that the patient permits these procedures to be done "implies" the patient's consent. Implied consent is present in instances in which immediate treatment is needed to save a life or preserve an individual's well-being. A surgical procedure can be performed without written consent (as in the treatment of a minor, or a patient who is mentally incapacitated) when a parent, spouse, or guardian is unavailable.

Additionally, implied consent is present in the treatment of individuals who are unable to give consent because of unconsciousness or other incapacitating mental or physical conditions. The validity of such implied consents are predicated upon proof that, had treatment been delayed, the patient's health and/or life would have been threatened and a rational, alert, and prudent adult patient would have consented to the procedure (42).

Informed Consent

Patients contemplating elective procedures in which risks are known and alternative treatments are available must be provided information pertaining to these alternatives and risks as well as information describing the consequences, if any, of nontreatment (43). The information must be provided so as to permit the risks to be seen in proper perspective and to accurately transmit *realistic* expectations of the results of treatment (44). The patient must then provide his/her personal consent for the procedure or treatment. Such consent is regarded as "informed" consent and is documented in written form, in which the patient acknowledges that this information was provided and that permission has been granted to perform the procedure. Informed consent is not static but is a continuing process in the patient's treatment, during which updated information must be regularly provided and the original content of the consultation continually reviewed.

Informed consent is never to be construed to be the consent form. No matter how complete or detailed the form, if the information therein has not been clearly transmitted to the patient, the patient is not "informed." Elaborate and lengthy consent forms may be appropriate for some regions and some practices. Short, simple forms written in understandable language with a section in which the patient has written in his/her own hand that they have received the information and have understood it may be equally effective, or more so, in a court of law. The nature of the information provided to the patient must be fully documented in the patient's record.

Informing The Patient

In order for the patient to be properly informed, the following information must be provided:

1. Nature of the disease, injury or deformity
2. Purposes and goals of treatment and consequences of nontreatment
3. Limitations of treatment and consequences of nontreatment
4. Treatment alternatives
5. Risks and complications of treatment

All information modalities should be contemplated as a means to inform and educate patients. While some patients may understand and retain information transmitted verbally, others will be more completely informed by providing additional written material, diagrams, and other appropriate audiovisual presentations. A notation as to the nature of the printed information or visual presentation that was provided should be made in the patient's record. In addition, copies of this supplementary material should be on file to document the information provided, should a question ever arise as to the nature of the information given.

Informed consent or the lack thereof does not possess the pivotal importance to plaintiff attorneys that surgeons often believe. Plaintiff attorneys focus on negligence, causation, and damages. Failure to provide adequate information upon which a patient can make an "informed decision" may reflect an unacceptable standard of care (45), but without the presence of damages, the sole lack of informed consent is not considered by most plaintiff attorneys to be an appropriate basis for a claim. However, in claims in which significant damage has occurred as a result of possible negligence, the lack of adequate "informed consent" can significantly reinforce the plaintiff's claim of negligence.

Some physicians believe that, having informed the patient of the potential for a complication, the patient has no basis for a claim if that complication occurs. No matter how thorough the consultation or how complete the list of complications, the physician does not invoke a claim of immunity for a complication if it occurred as a result of negligence (46). When the patient has been adequately informed, she or he may be more likely to regard and more ready to accept a complication as a known risk regardless of cause; but, if the complication is unexpected, a claim is more likely to occur, even if it can later be proven that the complication was a recognized and accepted risk of the surgical procedure and was not due to negligence.

Despite detailed efforts to inform, patients retain very little of the information provided. Excellent studies have shown that, in a matter of only a few days, the majority of information provided to patients cannot be recalled (47). Even though some patients do not retain the information provided, efforts to inform the patient as completely as possible may be accompanied by a perception on the part of the patient that the physician is concerned, sensitive, and thorough. Transforming the uncertainties and fear of treatment into manageable realities, in which the patient and physician develop an alliance of mutual trust and understanding, may be a major factor in preventing negative reactions to treatment and prove to be a better claim deterrent than a legalistic lists of complications (48).

The basic information upon which informed consent is given must be provided by the physician. The information provided by the physician can then be *supplemented* by associates, residents, nurses, or other qualified individuals, and can be further supplemented by printed material and/or audiovisual presentations.

Validity of Consent

In a landmark decision upholding the right of patients to self-determination, Justice Cardozo (49) wrote, "Every human being of adult years and sound mind has a right to determine what shall be done with his own body. . . ." Strictly interpreted, valid consent for treatment can only be obtained from the patient. Special circumstances or "exceptions" (50) occur when patients are deemed incapable of participating in the consent process. These exceptions include minors, for whom consent must be obtained from a parent; patients who have been adjudicated by a court of law to be incompetent or incapable and for whom a consent must be obtained from the court-appointed guardian; and victims of emergencies, in which delays in treatment could result in a threat to the patient's medical well-being.

The existence of an emergency is determined by a physician and is a matter of medical judgment. Medical judgment, however, is subject to judicial review, and the physician's decision may be overruled. Invoking the emergency exception to obtaining consent should be reserved only for circumstances in which it is impractical to secure consent and when further delay would pose a significant risk to the patient. In situations in which patients cannot participate in decision making, a physician "should, as current law requires, attempt to secure a relative's consent if possible," which is known as a "substitute consent." In the event that no one is available to provide a substitute consent, or when time does not permit locating an appropriate individual, the physician should carefully document the situation that precluded such efforts. Unsuccessful attempts to contact relatives should also be noted. In the absence of consent, it is prudent to obtain and document the opinion of a second physician regarding the necessity of emergency treatment, as long as this second opinion does not result in a delay harmful to the patient (51).

When attempting to obtain a substitute consent, or when advising a family of a patient's condition, the physician must be sensitive to the confidentiality inherent in the doctor-patient relationship. The physician must guard against the disclosure of unnecessary details, facts, or information pertaining to the patient's medical condition to members of the family or "friends" that might later be found to be detrimental to the patient. Disclosures made to anyone without the patient's consent, even in cases of emergency, and even in cases where the information provided was for purposes of obtaining substitute consent, may later be the basis for a claim of "unauthorized disclosure" which, if accompanied by proven damages, could result in a judgment against the physician.

Consents should be written in language that can be understood by the average lay person (52). Studies have shown that, to be effective, consent forms should be worded at no higher that the 7th or 8th grade level (53). Consent forms that list only the technical or medical terminology for a procedure may later be mischaracterized. A plaintiff's attorney may convince a jury that the language used in the form represents the terminology that was used during the consultation (i.e., that it was so technical and so thick with medical terms that no patient could understand what was being said. A thorough consultation provided in language that is easily understood by the average lay person should not be negated by a written consent that contains terms which can only be deciphered by a physician.

Consents must be obtained at a time when the patient is mentally capable of giving consent. Obtaining consent after the patient has received medication that could have altered the patient's mental capacity will invalidate the consent. Where patients appear mentally confused or mentally incompetent but have not been adjudicated incompetent, consent should still be obtained from the patient. Good medical practice would dictate that a responsible family member also be provided with as much information as is necessary to establish "informed consent." A signed statement from the family member to that effect should also be placed in the patient's record. To bypass the "confused patient" and accept consent only from a member of the family may later be complicated by a patient who has regained their senses and brings action not only for a medical misadventure but also for battery resulting from a lack of a valid consent (49,52).

Having obtained consent for treatment, the physician is now obligated to manage the patient within the constraints of the consent provided. A surgeon may extend a procedure beyond that to which the patient agreed, but only if it can be shown that to do otherwise would have jeopardized the patient's medical well-being (54).

The Importance of Medical Records

MEDICAL-LEGAL SIGNIFICANCE

The focus of all medical negligence claims is the medical record. The first documented information that is reviewed by the plaintiff's attorney is the medical record. An attorney's decision to accept or reject the case is usually based on the content and character of the medical record. If a suit is tried, the result for or against the defendant physician will be decided largely on the basis of the medical record. The importance of well-documented, timely, and complete medical records cannot be overemphasized in the defense of medical negligence claims and in its effectiveness in discouraging claims that might otherwise be filed.

A medical record is exactly what the name implies—a record of medical events. The purpose of the medical record is not to provide a defense in a legal action but to facilitate patient care and provide a record of that care. Some defense attorneys have suggested that the record should be written as though it were being read by a jury. Many physicians would disagree. Medical records should be written so as to provide pertinent information to physicians, nurses, technicians, and other health care providers to assist in the coordination of the patient's care. The record should be written so that, if the treating physician were suddenly incapacitated, another physician who previously knew nothing about the patient could immediately take over the patient's care with no interruption in the continuity of that care. A good medical record will, by definition, be a good legal record.

In the course of a medical practice, a physician deals with hundreds of medical problems, many of them having great similarity. When one of the medical problems generates a claim of medical negligence, it is often difficult for the physician to recall from memory specifics relating to the claim. On the other hand, the patient who has filed the suit has probably only dealt with one medical problem that involves the defendant physician. Recollection of the event specifics and details are much more sharply focused in the patient's mind than they could ever be in the mind of the treating physician. It would seem that the patient and the patient's attorney would have a significant advantage. However, that advantage is usually neutralized by the fact that physicians keep contemporaneous written records and patients do not. An accurate, timely, well-documented medical record will always be regarded as carrying greater credibility in the eyes of an attorney and jury than the patient's undocumented recollections of events, most of which occurred months or years previously.

ACCURACY

As medical events occur in the treatment of a patient, words should be carefully chosen that transmit appropriate intent. Words like "inadvertent" to physicians may reflect harmless and unintentional acts, whereas the legal world sees inadvertance as negligence. The physician should be thorough in describing a condition, finding, or situation, but only to the point that it meets the needs of another physician. Long, defensive notes appearing in a record will only alert a perceptive attorney to an unusual occurrence that might otherwise remain insignificant.

Dictated, transcribed, and typewritten reports generate some of the most significant entries in a patient's record. This is a commonly accepted practice throughout hospitals and physicians' offices. Many of these lengthy reports are read very superficially or not at all before being signed by the physician. The signing of a record without an accompanying disclaimer indicates that the physician believes the report is a true and accurate record. In actual practice, transcription errors, typographical errors, inaudible words, unintentional omissions, and the incorrect choice of words to describe a clinical situation occur so frequently that careful line-by-line, word-by-word review of each dictated record should, theoretically, be mandatory before the physician applies a signature. Frequently, physicians fail to do so, and sign incomplete records or records that contain significant inaccuracies with no apparent effort to correct or complete the record. Attorneys may interpret such records as conveying indifference and inattention to detail on the part of the physician, which might further reinforce the attorney's impression that the physician may have also been indifferent and negligent in the medical treatment of their client.

Inaccuracies contained in records must be corrected contemporaneously. A *single* line should be drawn through an inaccurate entry and accompanied by the written correction, date, and physician's initials. It is absolutely essential that, in making a correction, the physician or other health care provider not erase, obliterate, or destroy any portion of the medical record. The words through which the line is drawn must still be legible (55).

Numerous corrections, even though conforming to acceptable standards, that occur following the date that a suit was filed should be avoided. Before undertaking any corrections in a record that is subject to a lawsuit, the defendant physician should consult with the defense attorney as to recommendations regarding inaccurate entries that are present in the medical records.

TIMELINESS

Failure to dictate or write reports immediately may result in significant medical-legal problems for the defendant physician, should the record ever be part of a negligence claim. Records and reports that are dictated days to weeks (or more) after the medical event occurred will be discredited in a court of law. A plaintiff's attorney will convey to the jury that delinquent entries are either:

1. *After the fact* delinquent incident or circumstance descriptions that would satisfactorily explain an injury or complication, and which ordinarily would have no negligence attached, will be characterized as having been made after the surgeon was aware of the injury, and made purposely after the fact so as to diminish liability. Even though all circumstances and all events within a delinquently dictated record may be accurate, and truly reflect the circumstances of the procedure, a question of doubt will be raised as to the validity of these entries because of the timing of the dictation.

2. *Not subject to accurate recall.* A plaintiff's attorney can demonstrate a surgeon's inability accurately to recall events days or weeks later by asking the surgeon to provide details of other events of that particular day (that may have had nothing to do with the medical practice but that may appear to a jury to be events that should be remembered). Once the physician's failure accurately to recall events of the day is established, the jury is then led to believe that the precise events of the surgery could not be accurately remembered either.

Injuries that are largely due to contributory negligence on the part of the patient because of failure to follow instructions following discharge can later be construed by the plaintiff's attorney to be due to inadequate or incomplete discharge instructions on the part of the physician. If these instructions appear only on a discharge summary that is dictated days to weeks after the physician would have been aware that the patient had failed to follow instructions, the discharge instructions appearing in the discharge summary will be discredited, even though it may be a true and accurate reflection of the instructions provided.

LEGIBILITY

For a medical record to perform the function for which it was intended, the entries must be legible and easily interpreted by other health care providers participating in the patient's care. Some physicians take perverse pride in the fact that their handwriting is illegible. Some believe that there is security in illegible handwriting because it can only be interpreted by the writer. However, illegible entries give an opposing attorney an opportunity to raise questions about every illegible entry and imply to the jury that these illegible entries actually say something other than what the physician is claiming or that the defendant physician is interpreting these entries to meet the physician's particular needs under the circumstances of the suit. Such inferences provide an opportunity for the plaintiff's attorney to suggest to a jury that the defendant physician may not be honest. This can be even more detrimental to a physician's defense than a demonstration of negligence.

Never obliterate an entry in the medical record. Any entry that has been rendered illegible provides the opposing attorney an opportunity to suggest to the jury that the obliterated entry contained the exact information that would have proven the defendant physician's negligence beyond a doubt when, in fact, the information obliterated may have been of rather minor significance. Nothing that the defendant physician may thereafter relate to the jury as having been contained in the obliterated entry will change the perception within the jury's mind that the obliterated entry was much more damaging.

VALIDITY

The jury must believe that the record is a true and accurate representation of the circumstances that occurred contemporaneous with the treatment. Accepted methods to correct inaccuracies within a record were described earlier in this chapter. Additions, deletions, or alterations of any kind made to a record without proper notation may, if proven, void a physician's malpractice insurance coverage and will *frequently* result in a verdict against the physician. Technology is currently available that can determine the point in time in which entries have been made as well as decipher entries which have been altered or rendered illegible to the naked eye. Medical records that have been found to have been altered without proper notation may attract a plaintiff's attorney, even though the case has no significant merit. If an altered record is proven to exist *the whole focus of the claim may be shifted from the alleged act of negligence to the question of the honesty and integrity of the physician.* If it can be shown that a physician has altered a record in an effort to avoid liability, juries will consider the physician dishonest. Plaintiff's attorneys are very aware that juries do not accept dishonesty in physicians and in such instances frequently choose to punish the physician with awards to the plaintiff which may actually have very little to do with the alleged act of negligence. An incomplete record or one with numerous inaccuracies can be defended much more easily than a record that has been surreptitiously altered.

Keeping the Patient Out of the Attorney's Office

Greater socioemotional overtones are present in medical-legal claims than in other personal injury claims. Some lawsuits may be triggered by events that have nothing to do with technical errors or negligence. In many cases the patient's first visit to the attorney's office may be prompted by an emotional reaction to what the patient believes to be mis-

treatment, rather than any definite awareness of a medical mistake.

Anger in response to perceived indifference, lack of concern, sympathy, or attention is often the precipitating emotion that causes a patient to first seek legal advice. A plaintiff's attorney welcomes angry clients and wishes to learn what the physician did to make the patient angry. The circumstances can eventually be transmitted to a jury in hopes of making the jury angry as well.

When a patient consults an attorney, the attorney then has the opportunity to search the medical record for a basis for suit. The attorney may find a basis that otherwise may never have been discovered and, ironically, may be completely unrelated to the patient's reason for seeking legal advice. If the patient is sufficiently angry with the physician, the patient may accept any basis for a claim as a means of punishing the physician for the physician's "wrongdoing." **The single most effective way to prevent malpractice claims is to keep the patient out of the attorney's office.**

Factors that Cause Patients to Consult an Attorney

In addition to anger, financial hardship generated by injury, disease, surgery, complications, or financial pressure from a physician or hospital for payment of delinquent bills, especially following an unfavorable result, can result in a lawsuit. The patient may not be aware of any specific acts of medical negligence. Financial pressure may prompt the patient to seek legal advice in hopes of uncovering medical negligence that might serve as a basis for obtaining financial relief.

"Surprise" occurring as a result of an unexpected complication may cause patients to seek legal advice. Even though the complication may later be shown to have occurred without any negligence on the physician's part, the unexpected nature of the complication may cause the patient to believe otherwise. Such events can frequently be prevented through greater emphasis on the informing process, covered earlier in this chapter. Information provided before surgery will be regarded by the patient as "informed consent"; the exact same information provided after surgery will be regarded as "excuses."

Disappointment can also prompt a patient to consult an attorney if expectations from treatment remain unmet. If the expectations were unrealistic, or if the physician provided overly optimistic assurances, the fault may lie with the physician's inability to communicate. Failure to meet expectations may not be a basis for a claim of negligence, but the disappointment resulting from such a failure may cause the patient to consult an attorney, thereby permitting the attorney to review the record and possibly uncover an act of medical negligence that might have otherwise remained unformulated.

IDENTIFYING THE PATIENT POSSIBLY PLANNING TO SEEK LEGAL ADVICE

Expressions of personal dissatisfaction by a patient are the most direct evidence of a patient who may eventually seek legal advice. Other patients may demonstrate more subtle signs of dissatisfaction. Expressions of distress over a complication out of proportion to the event, or persistent focus on unmet expectations and an unwillingness to accept that "nothing more can be done" may be characteristics of patients who are likely to consult an attorney.

A dissatisfied patient who fails to return for follow-up care is frequently a patient who has sought medical attention elsewhere and/or plans to consult an attorney.

A litigious patient may display resentment over the need for additional surgery to correct a complication especially, if additional costs will occur. Such a patient may demonstrate inability to understand how a complication could occur without "something having gone wrong." Hostile statements made to the office or hospital staff, or to other patients, should alert the physician and staff to a patient who may be considering legal action. Patients are inclined to express dissatisfaction to others before expressing it to the physician. The staff should be aware of this and convey any information that will assist the physician in the reduction or modification of legal exposure.

Anger or frustration over a bill, billing techniques, or the handling of insurance claims may precede a visit to an attorney's office. The patient will almost certainly seek legal advice following an unfavorable result if pressure is applied for payment of the bill or if the bill is turned over to a collection agency. Hospitals are particularly prone to push for the collection of delinquent accounts even in cases in which patient dissatisfaction can be shown to be due to hospital-based negligence. Hospital-directed claims will almost always name the treating physician and therein involve the physician in a claim that might possibly have been avoided through a more temperate management of hospital accounts. Physicians must *personally* monitor the handling of accounts of dissatisfied patients or patients with unfavorable results. This may include making inquiries of hospital billing departments as to the status of the patient's hospital account. Hospital administrators must be informed of dissatisfied patients or patients with unfavorable results to permit judgments to be made as to how the account should be managed, depending in part on the medical-legal implications of the event.

Dissatisfied patients who begin to appear for visits accompanied by relatives or friends (when previously the patient came to the office alone) may represent individuals who need the support of others to reinforce their contention that mistreatment has occurred and that consulting an attorney is justified.

Any inferences made to a physician suggesting that the patient may be considering legal action against some other medical provider should alert the physician and staff to the potential for being involved, even though the patient may make assurances to the contrary. All assurances may be negated once an attorney has an opportunity to review the case. Particularly difficult problems occur if one provider has supported the patient's contention that another provider may have been negligent, especially if such support was provided in hopes of deflecting liability.

MANAGING THE PATIENT POSSIBLY PLANNING TO SEEK LEGAL ADVICE

The physician must not wait for the patient to generate enough courage to express dissatisfaction. The physician may already be aware of dissatisfaction through information gleaned from others, or as demonstrated through information gleaned from others, or as demonstrated through behavior patterns outlined above. Early and direct intervention on the part of the physician in exposing the problem, and shared decision-making in its resolution, provide several advantages to the physician:

1. The physician is permitted to take the initiative by having already prepared recommendations and a plan of management to address the problem. This is preferable to having to develop them "on the spur of the moment" in a confrontational situation generated by the patient.
2. Time is minimized for the patient to "dwell" on the problem or exaggerating the problem.
3. The patient is deprived of the initiative, thereby minimizing the patient's opportunity to develop an organized complaint.

Dissatisfied patients sometimes find it easier to express their concerns and disappointments in writing. Such letters deserve immediate attention. Writing letters in response to patient dissatisfaction is sometimes a more effective method of reacting than telephone calls or face-to-face confrontation, which can be intimidating to some patients. A letter gives the patient tangible evidence of the physician's concern. A letter can also be used by the patient to refute the contentions of family members or friends that the physician is indifferent or uncaring. The letter should be structured so as to express concern and sensitivity, but lengthy explanations or excuses should be avoided. The patient should be invited to return to the office and discuss the problem with the physician personally.

Dissatisfied patients should also be urged to obtain a second opinion. If the patient is willing, such arrangements can be made by the treating physician, but the appearance of one physician "covering" for the other should be avoided. Patients may wish to make their own arrangements; in any case, the treating physician should offer to send a medical summary with the patient.

SEEING ANOTHER PHYSICIAN'S DISSATISFIED PATIENT

Second opinions are often sought by patients with unfavorable results. Seeing another physician's dissatisfied patient is one of the most difficult challenges that a physician will encounter in medical practice. Skillful management may diffuse a potential lawsuit. Conversely, lawsuits that might otherwise have been avoided have been filed because of remarks made by a consultant that were later found to be based on incomplete information and unwarranted assumptions.

When a physician sees another physician's dissatisfied patient for the first time, the consultant must exercise caution in accepting the patient's account of the events of treatment until such time that records can be obtained from the treating physician. The patient's authorization must be provided before the consultant can obtain information regarding previous treatment. Contacting the treating physician without patient authorization could be regarded as a violation of confidentiality. Frequently, patients do not wish to identify the treating physician. The consultant would be well-advised to inform the patient that proper evaluation of the patient's condition is not possible without obtaining previous records of treatment and without discussing the matter with the original physician. Consultants must be very cautious in accepting patients who persist in not wanting to identify the treating physician or not wanting the treating physician contacted. Such restraints can be used to justify withdrawing from the case (i.e., "While I respect your request for confidentiality, I cannot properly evaluate your case without obtaining information from your original physician.")

During the course of evaluating the patient's condition, the consultant must avoid conveying by attitude, expression, or word that the condition is due to negligence on the part of the treating physician. To do so will establish this perception permanently in the minds of the patient and family. Nothing that may occur thereafter will change this perception. The patient now has a reason to consult an attorney, who will be advised that the treating physician is at fault because the consultant said so. If subsequent review of the patient's records indicates that the treating physician did not deviate from the standard of care and the consultant thereafter testifies to the same, both physicians will appear collusive in the eyes of the patient—the treating physician for having been negligent and the consultant for "covering up."

Consultants who examine dissatisfied patients must concentrate on an objective evaluation of the patient's *current* medical condition and avoid discussions of liability and fault. The patient must be made to understand that the consultant's function is to provide assistance to both the patient and the treating physician for the purpose of modifying the unfavorable result. Efforts by the consultant to influence the patient to focus on a positive remedial treatment plan rather than liability or fault will be in the best interest of all parties.

If the interests of the patient and treating physician would best be served by the patient's returning to the original physician, the consultant must do everything reasonable to encourage this. If the patient does not wish to return to the original physician, the consultant is not obligated to accept the patient. However, if the consultant does accept the patient, she or he will no longer be considered a consultant but rather a treating physician.

Patients who concentrate on placing blame for an unsatisfactory result and seem uninterested in any corrective treatment may have already consulted with an attorney. A patient may seek a consultation on the advice of his attorney and may not indicate the referral source. Unfortunately, once the patient has been seen, the consultant cannot avoid involvement in the lawsuit if one is filed.

INTENSIVE CARE FILE

Some patients are greater medical-legal risks than others and deserve closer monitoring. Establishing an "intensive care file" may be an effective method to monitor such patients.

To establish such a file, the physician must identify patients with unfavorable results, patients with complications, "dissatisfied" patients, and any other patient who appears to represent a particular medical-legal risk. These patients' charts or names can then be segregated into a special file of which each member of the physician's staff is aware.

A strict policy must then be developed by which these patients are monitored at set intervals by the physician or a specifically designated member of the staff in regard to:

• Current status
• Date last seen
• Adequacy and completeness of records
• Security of records (protection from fire and theft)
• Need for second opinion
• Attitudes/reactions, both of patient and patient's family
• All telephone conversations—written records
• Any special preparation needed for the next office visit
• Need for continued "intensive care" vs return to regular files

POLICY MANUAL

Misunderstandings, communication errors, and inconsistencies in patient management by the office staff can sometimes generate, or further aggravate, patient dissatisfaction following an unfavorable result. Uniform policies governing the management of records, billing, telephone calls, appointments, and general communication guidelines should be developed by the physician and placed in a policy manual, which may then serve as an effective risk management tool in some practices. Such a manual must be "required reading" for the staff, and may be useful in introducing and teaching risk management concepts and techniques to the staff.

MAIL-O-GRAMS

Using Mail-O-Grams rather than registered letters may be preferable when contacting patients regarding problems with significant medical-legal overtones (e.g., the failure to return for follow-up care). A Mail-O-Gram does not carry the medical-legal stigma of a registered letter and yet projects urgency. A copy of the Mail-O-Gram, which can be placed in the patient's records, is provided to the sender.

PATIENT QUESTIONNAIRE

Confidential patient questionnaires serve not only as an effective risk management device but also as an effective practice development tool. What counts is what the patient thinks—not what the physician, colleagues, or staff think. The questionnaire must be made absolutely confidential and anonymous for "physician's eyes only" by mailing all responses to a P.O. box or to the physician's home. The following suggestions (56) can be varied or supplemented to suit one's own practice:

1. *Communication.* Do patients understand the diagnosis and the course of treatment being proposed? Do they understand what they are supposed to do after leaving the office? Do they feel they have not been told enough, talked down to, or not shown enough respect?
2. *Professional services.* Is the physician thorough enough? Does the physician spend enough time with the patient?
3. *Office.* Does the patient like the setting? Is the office up to date? Is it too crowded? Uncomfortable? Not private enough?
4. *Staff.* Are they courteous? Helpful? Knowledgeable? Confidential, and considerate of privacy? Available?
5. *Practice.* Are services readily available? Do patients have to wait too long to be seen? Do patients wait too long in the waiting room? Are billing and insurance procedures handled satisfactorily?
6. *Does the patient have any other questions?*

Limitations on Liability and Defenses

STATUTE OF LIMITATIONS

Instances of alleged medical negligence must be acted upon by the plaintiff within a defined period of time following the act of negligence or the discovery of the act of negligence. In most cases, failure to institute legal action within this statutory period of time precludes a person from filing a lawsuit. In many jurisdictions, discovery rules are applied to prevent the statute of limitations from precluding the filing of a suit in a situation where the patient would not have known the injury had occurred. In such instances, the statute of limitations begins only at the time that the alleged act of negligence was discovered by the patient, rather than being related to the time that the actual incident occurred.

Unfavorable results related to possible medical negligence must be disclosed to the patient, and the exact date and time that the disclosures were made must be documented in the medical record. The statute of limitations does not begin until the disclosure is made. Any intention to conceal such facts will prevent the statute of limitations from applying until such time that the disclosure is made. In addition, efforts to conceal an injury due to medical negligence may be regarded by the courts as "fraudulent concealment," which could affect medical-liability insurance coverage.

Statutes of limitations in most jurisdictions are shorter for personal-injury claims than statutes covering contract law. Physicians must avoid any statement or any written record that would suggest the patient has been given a "guarantee" in regard to the results of a surgical procedure or medical treatment. Such "guarantees" may be regarded by the courts as contractual agreements and, therefore, subject to the much longer statute of limitations for contracts rather than the shorter statutes for personal injury. Any diagrams, drawings, overlays, computer images, or plans of treatment based on cephalometrics, for example, should have the statement *surgical goal but no guarantee* affixed to the diagram or drawing and possibly initialed by the patient.

Claims of medical negligence have been dropped or dismissed because of the patient's failure to file the suit within the period of time defined by the statute of limitations. The documentation of date and time that the patient was advised of the circumstances of the injury have been crucial in preventing these claims from being pursued.

Managing a Claim

NOTIFY CARRIER

Dissatisfied patients, particularly those who have suggested, through action or attitude, that they are considering legal action, must be reported to the physician's medical-liability carrier. The carrier must also be immediately notified if the patient or an attorney requests a copy of medical records regarding the patient or if the patient and/or an attorney asks for a meeting to fully discuss the medical care rendered and the results obtained. A physician should never meet with an attorney regarding the care rendered to a patient in which there may be a potential negligence claim without notifying and receiving approval from the insured's carrier. The carrier must be notified if the physician receives a letter from an attorney that indicates a patient is considering filing a suit, or upon notification that a suit has been filed. If a physician considers that a significant potential for exposure to a medical negligence claim exists, the carrier should be advised.

A physician who assumes care as a treating physician for a patient who is filing suit against another physician may be contacted by a plaintiff's attorney who asks for an appointment to discuss the patient's condition. Even though the second physician may appear to have no claim exposure, his own liability carrier should be contacted and advised of the attorney's request for the following reasons:

1. Exposure could exist of which the second physician is unaware. A conference with a plaintiff's attorney may provide that attorney with information to that effect that might later prove detrimental to the second physician.
2. The second physician may be covered by the same liability carrier as the physician against whom the suit is being filed. In cases where one policy holder may provide information to a plaintiff's attorney that might prove detrimental to another policy holder, the carrier may wish to have a defense attorney present.

SECURE AND ORGANIZE ALL RECORDS ON THE PATIENT

If a claim seems imminent, locate and organize all the patient's records. Immediately, copies should be made of all records, and the original placed in a secure location to prevent accidental loss or unintentional alteration. Do not make any changes in any records or charts. Do not dispose of any records, x-rays, photographs, or any other material that relate to the patient, whether it be medical or nonmedical.

In assisting the defense attorney, the defendant may create additional notes and narratives to make the written record more understandable. In no instance, should these notes or additions be brought to formal hearings such as depositions or the trial itself. Such notes and information are usually considered "privileged" (i.e., protected by the attorney/client privilege) and are not subject to discovery except when they are brought to formal hearings. Each page containing information pertaining to the claim, but which is not in the patient's records, should be headed by the written statement: "personal communication to my attorney" (insert the defense attorney's name if possible). Review only materials approved by the defense attorney, one's own records, and the hospital records, in order to avoid exposing oneself to new areas of inquiry.

DO NOT DISCUSS THE CASE WITH ANYONE

Do not discuss the case with anyone besides the carrier and defense attorney. Plaintiff's attorneys, through interrogatories and depositions, will ask the identity of any individual with whom the defendant physician has discussed the case. The plaintiff's attorney will then ask these individuals about the conversations, in hopes of finding some variation or inconsistency in the physician's sworn testimony as compared to the dialogue that may have occurred with others. Discussion about the case among codefendants can suggest the appearance of "collusion" and should be avoided unless expressly approved by the defense attorney.

PREPARE TO INVEST TIME

Medical liability claims frequently involve months of preparation and, if the claim progresses, the trial may not occur for several years after it has been filed. The defendant physician must be prepared to invest time in a review of the facts of the case and provide assistance to the defense attorney regarding details that might not be contained in the medical records. Interrogatories must be answered and depositions scheduled that will require significant preparation on the part of the defendant physician. In addition, the defendant physician may be asked to attend depositions taken from other parties involved in the suit, most notably those of the plaintiff and the plaintiff's expert. The plaintiff may choose experts from other cities or states. Attending such depositions may result in considerable inconvenience, expense, and time away from one's practice.

On the road to trial, pretrial conferences and reviews will occur that require additional time. If the claim involves several defendants, additional conferences may be scheduled by the respective defense attorneys so as to better understand each defendant's exposure. If the case proceeds to trial, the trial may last days to weeks. Each day of testimony may be followed by additional conferences to assess the testimony and its effect on the physician's defense.

"Maneuvering" is a way of life in the legal profession. Scheduled depositions that necessitate the cancellation of a day of practice can be canceled by the attorney with little or no notice. As the time investment in the legal process becomes greater and greater, and the time available to practice medicine becomes less and less, defendant physicians become increasingly more willing to settle claims, even those that seem to have little or no merit. Initially, the physician may feel that the medical-liability claim is an assault on the physician's competence, professional skill, and integrity. As the suit drags on, the physician may come to the realization that the greatest threat in a medical-liability claim is in terms of lost time—precious time spent away from patients.

ASSIST THE DEFENSE ATTORNEY

The defense attorney handling the defendant physician's case will, most often, be an expert in the management of medical negligence claims. The attorney may not be familiar with procedures, surgical indications, and other details associated with the medical treatment provided in the defendant's case. *It is the obligation of the defendant physician to provide the necessary background material and understanding of medical treatment* so that the defense attorney is enabled to develop an effective defense. The defendant physician must be prepared to dedicate whatever time is required to do this effectively and completely.

It will be the plaintiff's contention that the defendant physician failed to act in accordance with the prevailing standard of care. The attorney will argue that the defendant failed to utilize the degree of knowledge, care, and skill which would have been exercised by another similarly qualified physician under the same or similar circumstances. The defense attorney must be provided with the necessary medical information to determine if, in fact, there exists a deviation from the standard of care. The defendant physician knows much of this information. It is the defendant's responsibility to convey this information to the defense attorney. Honesty and candor are absolutely essential, and failure to convey all pertinent medical facts and information (even though they may appear unfavorable) will significantly diminish the attorney's ability to understand the case and develop an effective defense. The defendant physician will be asked to provide the names of "experts" who are familiar with the medical discipline in question and who would be willing to review the case. The experts must provide an opinion as to the applicable standard of care and an opinion as to whether a deviation from that standard caused the plaintiff's injury.

The defense of medical-liability claims is a specialty within the practice of law, very much as plastic surgery is a specialty within the practice of medicine. The proper management of a medical-liability claim requires a specialized attorney. The defendant must rely upon the expertise of the attorney if any success is to be expected in the defense. Peculiarities of defending medical negligence claims may only be known to attorneys specializing in this area and may not be easily understood by the defendant physician. It is important that the defendant rely upon the attorney's advice in matters relating to legal theory and the defense strategies most appropriate for the circumstances.

With the increase in the numbers of medical negligence claims, defense attorneys are frequently involved in the defense of more than one case. The attorney's enthusiasm for each case may be significantly tempered by the defendant physician's enthusiasm, cooperation, and willingness to assist. Defendant physicians who demonstrate an indifference, lack of concern, and an unwillingness to invest the necessary time and effort for the development of an appropriate defense may be in danger of generating similar attitudes in the defense attorney.

Interrogatories

Interrogatories are a series of written questions developed for the sole purpose of obtaining information from parties to the suit, witnesses, and other persons who may possess information of interest to that particular case. The defendant physician will be asked to answer questions such as whether he or she has been named in previous lawsuits arising from malpractice or professional negligence. The plaintiff, through an attorney, will ask for the case title and number and the jurisdiction where the legal claim was filed. This information permits review of any testimony or factual information that is a matter of public record. The defendant physician will then be asked to provide the names, addresses, and specialties of every physician with whom the care and treatment of the patient was discussed, from the time that treatment of the patient began until the date of the response to interrogatories. If the defendant has been asked to appear before, or attend, any medical committee or official board of any medical society or hospital for the purposes of discussing the case, the plaintiff has the right to inquire as to these meetings or appearances. The defendant may be asked to provide the names, titles, and publication dates of all medical texts, journals, books, or other written information the defendant plans to use as an authority or reference in defending any of the allegations brought by the plaintiff. The plaintiff has the right to ask for information, including lists of surgical procedures performed by the defendant for the purpose of gaining admission to a hospital staff or certification by a professional group. Inquiries may also be made as to whether the defendant has ever testified in court on a medical malpractice case, even though not a named party. The defendant may be asked to provide information about continuing medical education or qualification requirements for certification to the defendant's specialty board. Hospital affiliations and positions the defendant has held on committees or within administrative hospital bodies may be requested. The plaintiff is also permitted to probe into specifics regarding the defendant's medical-liability insurance.

Depositions

A deposition, or examination before trial (EBT), is part of the legal process called *discovery*. The defendant physician is examined in order to establish the defendant's position with regards to the treatment rendered, as well as to allow the plaintiff to learn new factual avenues to investigate (57). Depositions are usually restricted to obtaining testimony from the named parties and from the experts who will testify at trial.

Physicians may consider the trial the focal point of any medical negligence action. Attorneys, rather, consider the depositions to be of greater importance. To a plaintiff's attorney, the single most important deposition is that of the defendant physician. Many medical negligence claims are significantly influenced by the defendant physician's deposition and therefore physicians must not underestimate the importance of the testimony to be given at this examination. Deposition preparation is very much like board preparation. The defendant physician must be informed, knowledgeable, and familiar with the treatment rendered as well as with all pertinent medical records, x-rays, test results, the medical literature, and any additional data that has been gleaned through discovery and investigation during the claim's course.

The answers provided during the deposition will, in essence, freeze such testimony and "etch it in stone." *Every question* asked has a purpose that relates to the matter at hand. Answers must be precise, audible, accurate, appropriately qualified, and clearly understandable, so there can be no misinterpretation of the question or the answer later at trial. Simple gestures without audible responses are unacceptable. The testimony, once established, is used as the basis for both plaintiff and defense attorneys for trial preparation.

Deposition testimony may hold more weight than trial testimony, because depositions are usually taken well in advance of trial and therefore are closer in time to the events in question. Corrections or changes in testimony at the time of trial, when compared to deposition testimony, will be characterized by the attorney as a reflection of the fact that the defendant was coached or is changing the answers to avoid liability.

Depositions are conducted under oath, outside the courtroom, usually in one of the attorneys offices. The defendant physician must remember that testimony is being provided for informational purposes and not for the justification of treatment. No judge or jury is present to decide whether the defendant is guilty of medical negligence.

The purpose of the defendant physician's deposition, from the plaintiff's point of view, is to:

1. Obtain information.
2. Test the defendant as a witness and determine the positive or negative qualities the physician may possess that would make either a favorable or unfavorable jury impression.
3. Develop inconsistencies and illicit damaging statements from the defendant under oath that might later be used to discredit him or her.

Deposition testimony differs from trial testimony. The purpose of the deposition is discovery. While answers should be as complete as necessary to prevent misinterpretation, they should also be concise and confined as closely as possible to the scope of the question. *Information must not be volunteered when it is not essential to answering the question.* To do so may provide information that was not known to the plaintiff's attorney, thereby permitting "breaking of new ground," which will not only lengthen the deposition but also may provide information that may be detrimental.

Do not guess! If the precise details or information cannot be recalled, the defendant physician (deponent) should answer "I do not remember." If, during the course of events, the answer to the question is remembered or if information is later obtained to provide that answer, it may later be possible to explain at trial that the deponent's memory was refreshed and accurate testimony can then be provided. However, if the deponent has already taken a position on the basis of a guess at deposition, the testimony cannot be changed at trial without the risk of being discredited.

In answering questions, the deponent must consider every factor relevant to the answer and then reach a positive and unequivocal response. Physicians possess scientific minds, and in the desire for absolute truth many physicians tend to equivocate when answering. In the jurors' minds, equivocation conjures negative implications and resultant disbelief.

The attorney must not be permitted to summarize the defendant's testimony in the attorney's own words and then ask for confirmation. The defendant should always answer in his own words so as to avoid contradiction with previous testimony. If a question is asked about documented evidence, the document must be reviewed completely before answering. Deponents must watch for leading questions from attorneys that provide a set of facts that are only partly true, which then place the witness in conflict with previous testimony. If a legitimate mistake is made during deposition, it can be corrected before trial.

The defense attorney may play a very passive role during the deposition that is conducted by the plaintiff's attorney. The defense attorney is present to protect the defendant but doesn't wish to disclose facts or opinions of which the plaintiff's attorney is unaware or divulge information that may reveal the defense strategy.

Trial

Most medical negligence claims do not reach trial. As additional facts and data are obtained through discovery and investigation, the evidence will either influence the plaintiff to drop the suit or influence the defendant to settle. However, claims in which the plaintiff believes the evidence supports the contention that the defendant was negligent and when the offers of settlement (if any) by the defendant are not sufficient to compensate for the injury, the claim will go to trial. Conversely, if the defendant believes that there was no negligence and the plaintiff refuses to drop the suit, the claim will go to trial.

The actual trial may not occur for years after its filing, and a considerably longer time will have elapsed from the time that the alleged negligent act occurred. By the time of trial, the defendant physician will be well acquainted with the facts of the case and with the position of the other principals, including the defense attorney, plaintiff, plaintiff's attorney, and the defense and plaintiff experts. The defendant will have had the opportunity to study the deposition given by the various parties to the suit, including his or her own deposition. The defense attorney, in cooperation with the defendant, will have established the theory and defense plan.

For the well prepared defendant, the trial should be a relatively atraumatic experience, but most physician defendants indicate that trial experience is anything but benign. The courtroom is the legal profession's "operating room." This legal setting can generate the same anxieties for the physician defendant that a surgical suite generates for a patient. In addition to being prepared regarding the facts of the case, the defendant must also be prepared to be a courtroom "figure," whose manner and demeanor will be on display throughout trial and can influence the success or failure of the defense.

Attitudes that project indifference, arrogance, or condescension must be avoided. The defendant must appear concerned, sincere, knowledgeable, and sympathetic.

When testifying as a witness, answers should be provided in a straightforward manner. If the answer is yes or no, the defendant should respond accordingly and avoid trying to expand or evade. Such a self-serving stance will negatively impress the jury. At trial, unlike deposition, testimony must stand the test of a cross-examination in order to permit the jury to judge the witness' credibility. Leading, argumentative, and loaded questions are attempted in cross-examination, whereas such questions would not be broached during a deposition.

The defendant's attention must be directed to the proceedings at all times to reinforce and project the impression of the defendant's concern and interest, but also to enable the defendant physician to assist the defense attorney in matters of fact with regard to medical testimony as it is presented.

The defense attorney will manage events occurring during the trial and will guide the physician defendant accordingly. Much of the proceedings are beyond the control or influence of the defendant physician. This can be quite frustrating for a person who is used to "taking charge." The defendant must largely assume a passive role in the proceedings and rely upon the expertise and experience of the defense attorney.

Other Medical-Legal Encounters

TESTIMONY AS A TREATING PHYSICIAN NOT PARTY TO A SUIT

A physician may be asked to give a deposition regarding treatment of a patient in support of a patient's claim against another party (e.g., in an auto accident, regarding another physician defendant, regarding a manufacturer in a products liability case, or in actions to establish disability compensation). If the physician's testimony might raise a question of medical negligence as to his treatment of the patient, the physician's insurance company should be advised. The insurance company may wish to have an attorney present during the deposition to advise and protect the treating physician.

When testifying as a treating physician of a patient who is bringing suit against another doctor, the treating physician is required only to provide factual information pertaining to treatment. An opinion as to whether the previous physician deviated from the standard of care must be obtained from an "expert" (even though the treating physician may qualify as an expert). If asked to give an opinion as to whether the defendant physician deviated from the standard of care, the treating physician may properly respond "I have no opinion." If, however, the treating physician chooses to give an opinion, that opinion will almost certainly have to be repeated at trial.

EXPERTS

The essential question in medical negligence claims is whether the treatment deviated or departed from the accepted standard of practice. Such a determination will depend on what the expert witnesses testify is the accepted standard or practice under the circumstances. Usually, before a plaintiff's attorney accepts a case, the attorney will ask for a case review by an expert physician, often a physician whom the attorney has used in the past as a consultant. Defense attorneys use consultants in the same capacity. Upon review of the case, the consultant will provide an oral report to the attorney about whether evidence exists that the treating physician deviated from the standard of care. Consultants are not obligated to testify as experts unless they agree to do so.

If the plaintiff's attorney accepts the case, expert testimony will have to be provided that supports the plaintiff's contention that the treatment rendered deviated from the accepted standards. Similarly, the defendant must also provide an expert to support the defendant's position that no deviation existed. If the consultants do not wish to serve as experts, the attorneys must obtain other experts who are willing to appear for deposition called by the opposing party and who are willing to be called as trial expert witnesses by the party paying for the experts' services.

Since jurors have no independent knowledge with which to judge the quality of care as compared to the accepted standards, the testimony of the experts is crucial in the decision of the case. The weight that jurors assign to expert testimony will depend on such factors as (a) the witness' demeanor, background, and qualifications, as well as general persuasiveness; (b) the ability of the witness to hold up under cross-examination; (c) the credibility of the opposing expert testimony; (d) the demeanor of the opposing expert; and (e) such intrinsic evidence as the medical records, x-rays, and laboratory tests, not to mention (f) the testimony of the parties and other witnesses.

Because of the pivotal importance of expert testimony in a medical negligence case, expert witnesses are usually subjected to strenuous cross-examination. The expert's qualifications in terms of training, teaching positions, hospital affiliations, contributions to the literature, and the like, add weight to the expert's opinion. Equally or even more important is the manner in which the expert states the opinion. The opinions expressed must be unequivocal and definitive. If an expert opinion is too speculative and the expert appears unsure, the testimony will usually carry no weight with the jurors.

Defendants, as well as expert witnesses, have to deal with expert questions posed in various forms (58). One of the most dramatic is the long hypothetical question in which the interrogator asks the witness to "assume" certain facts to be true. If the witness disagrees with the truth of the assumptions contained in the hypothetical question, the witness may respond that the question cannot be answered because some of the assumptions stated in the question are not true. If the interrogating attorney insists that the witness assume their truth, the witness should respond: "If everything you asked me to assume were true, which I disagree with and find unlikely, my opinion would be. . . ."

When providing an expert opinion, the witness should also note all the relevant reasoning and data that led to the opinion. Doing so not only demonstrates the expert's knowledge of the medicine involved and of the case but also lends credence to the expert's opinion in the eyes of the jury.

Opposing attorneys will often attempt to impeach the opinions of an expert witness on cross-examination by introducing the contrary opinion of a published authority. This tactic requires the use of medical literature. To do so, the witness must recognize the publication as authoritative, or its author as an authority in the field. If the work or the author is not recognized by the witness as authoritative, the cross-examining attorney is not permitted to use the contrary opinion to impeach the expert witness' opinion. An expert is not compelled to recognize any publication or author, no matter how widely used or famous (59). If the witness feels that a certain text must be acknowledged as authoritative, the answer may still be qualified by a statement to the effect that the witness still does not agree with all the opinions expressed in the text. If, in an attempt to embarrass an expert who refuses to accept any text as authoritative, the cross-examining attorney introduces a large number of texts in an effort to make the witness appear unfamiliar with the literature, the witness should indicate awareness of the existence of the work but not accept it as being authoritative and give reasons.

References

1. *Kennedy v. Parrott,* 243 N.C. 355, 360, 90 S.E. 2d 754, 757 (1956).
2. *Coleman v. California Friends Church,* 81 P 2d 469, 470, Cal 1938; *Schneider v. Little Company,* 151 NW, 588, Mich 1915; *Pike v. Honsinger,* 49 NE 760, NY 1898; "The Standard of Care, Parts I, II, and III," 225 *JAMA* No. 6, page 671, August 3, 1973; 225 *JAMA* No. 7, page 791, August 13, 1973, 225 *JAMA* No. 8, page 1027, August 20, 1973; *Adkins v. Ropp,* 14 NE 2d 727, Ind 1938.
3. Restatement (Second) of Torts 282 (1965).
4. *Suburban Hospital Association v. Mewhinney,* 187 A 2d 671, Md 1963.
5. *Miles v. Harris,* 194 SW 839, Tex 1917.
6. *Engle v. Clarke,* 346 SW 2d 13, Ky 1961.
7. *Dashiell v. Griffith,* 35 Atl 1094, Md 1896; *Capps v. Valk,* 369 P2d 238, Kans 1962.
8. *McNevins v. Lowe,* 40 Ill 209, Ill 1866; *Ritchey v. West,* 23 Ill 329, Ill 1860; *Barnes v. Gardner,* 9 NYS 2d 785, NY 1939.
9. *Stohlman v. Davis,* 220 NW 247, Neb 1928; *Mucci v. Houghton,* 57 NW 305, Iowa 1864; *Groce v. Myers,* 29 SE 2d 553, NC 1944; McIntire, Leon L. The Action of Abandonment in Medical Malpractice Litigation. *Tulane Law Rev* 834, 1962.
10. *Miller v. Dore,* 154 Me. 363, 148 A.2d 692 (1959).
11. *Doan v. Griffith,* 402 SW 2d 855, Ky 1966; *Christy v. Saliterman,* 179 NW 2d 288, Minn 1970; *Welch v. Frisbie Memorial Hospital,* 9 A 2d 761, NH 1939.
12. Restatement 283.
13. *Blair v. Eblen,* 461 S.W.2d 370, 373 (Ky. 1970).
14. "Res Ipsa Loquitur, Parts I–VII," 221 *JAMA* No. 5, page 537, July 31, 1972; 221 *JAMA* No. 6, page 633, Aug 7, 1972; 221 *JAMA* No. 10, page 1201, Sept. 4, 1972; 221 *JAMA* No. 11, page 1329, Sept. 11, 1972; 221 *JAMA* No. 12, page 1441, Sept. 18, 1972; 221 *JAMA* No. 13, page 1587, Sept. 25, 1972; 222 *JAMA* No. 1, page 121, Oct. 2, 1972.
15. Holder AR. *Medical malpractice law.* New York: Wiley, 1975; 60.
16. *Hundley v. Martinez,* 158 SE 2d 159, W Va 1967.
17. "Standard of Care for Specialists, Parts I and II," 226 *JAMA* No. 2, page 251, October 8, 1973; 226 *JAMA* No. 3, page 395, October 15, 1973.
18. Alton WG Jr. *Malpractice: a trial lawyer's advice for physicians.* Boston: Little, Brown, 1977; 4.
19. *Tomer v. Amer. Home Products Corp.,* 170 Conn. 681, 368 A.2d 35 (1976); *Johnson v. Yeshiva Univ.,* 42 N.Y.2d 818, 396 N.Y.S.2d 647, 364 N.E. 2d 1340 (1977).
20. Del.Code Ann. 18 6801 (&) Supp. 1984).
21. *Downer v. Veilleux,* 322 A.2d 82, 87 (Me.1974); *Sprowl v. Ward,* 441 So.2d 898, 900 (Ala. 1983).
22.
23. *Toth v. Comm. Hosp. At Glen Cove,* 22 N.Y.2d 255, 263 & n. 2, 292 N.Y.S.2d 440, 447- 448 & n. 2, 239 N.E.2d 368, 373 & n. 2 (1968).
24. *Loizzo v. St. Francis Hosp.,* 121 Ill.App.3d 172, 76 Ill.Dec, 677, 459 N.E.2d 314, 317 (1984).
25. Annot., 37 A.L.R.2d 464 (1971, Supp. 1984).
26. Franklin M, Rabin R. *Tort law and alternatives: cases and materials.* 4th ed. New York: Foundation Press, 1987; 17.
27. The Restatement (Second) of Agency 227 (1958).
28. *Marvulli v. Elshire,* 27 Cal.App.3d 180. 103 Cal.Rptr. 461 (1972). *Accord Thompson v. Presbyterian Hosp., Inc.,* 652 P.2d 260 (Okla. 1982).
29. Franklin M, Rabin R. *Tort law and alternatives: cases and materials.* 4th ed. New York: Foundation Press, 1987; 17.
30. Crane J, Bromberg A. Bromberg, Law of Partnership 64 (1968).
31. *Miles v. Edward O. Tabor, M.D., Inc.,* 387 Mass. 783, 443 N.E.2d 1302 (1982); *Harvey v. Fridley Med. Center,* 315 N.W.2d 225 (Minn. 1982).
32. "Proximate Cause, Parts I, II and III," *JAMA* No. 9, page 1479, Nov. 29, 1971; 218 *JAMA* No. 10, page 1617, ec. 6, 1971; 218 *JAMA* No. 11, page 1761, Dec. 13, 1971.
33. *Morse v. Moretti,* 403 F 2d 564, CA DC 1968.
34. Sowka MP, ed. *Naic: Malpractice Claims; Final Compilation; Medical Malpractice Closed Claims; 1975-1978.* 350 Bishops Way, Brookfield, WI: NAIC, 1980.
35. Alton WG Jr. *Malpractice: a trial lawyer's advice for physicians.* Boston: Little, Brown, 1977; 144.
36. DeMere M. Comments of a doctor-lawyer on Chapter 54. In: Goldwyn RM, ed. *The unfavorable result in plastic surgery.* Boston: Little, Brown, 1984; 1122.
37. Holder AR. *Medical malpractice law.* New York: Wiley, 1975; 260.
38. Restatement § 892A(2)(a), 892B.
39. *Perna v. Pirozzi,* 92 N. J. 446, 457 A.2d 431 (1983).
40. *Guebard v. Jabaay,* 117 Ill.App.3d 1, 72 Ill.Dec. 498, 452 N.E.2d 751 (1983) (dicta).
41. *Lardon v. Kansas City Gas Co.,* 10F 2d 2634, DC Kans 1926; *Caldwell v. Missouri State Life Insurance Co.,* 230 SW 566; Ark 1921; Cameron, to use of *Cameron v. Eynon,* 3 A 2d 423, PA 1939.
42. Prosser WL. *The law of torts.* 4th ed. St. Paul, MN: West, 1971.
43. *Truman v. Thomas,* 661 P 2d 902, Cal 1980.
44. *Mitchell v. Robinson,* 334 SW 2d 11, Mo 1960.
45. *Truman v. Thomas,* 661 P 2d 902, Cal 1980.
46. *Mull v. Emory University,* 150 SE 2d 276, Ga 1966; *Block v. McVay,* 126 NW 2d 808, SD 1964.
47. Gray BH. An assessment of institutional review committees in human experimentation. *Med Care* 1975; 8:318–328; Golden JS, Johnston GD. Problems of distortion in doctor-patient communications. *Psychiatry and Medicine* 1970; 50:127–148; Lee D, Bowers DG, Lynch JB. Observations on the myth of "informed consent." *Plast Reconstr Surg* 1976; 58:280–282.
48. Gutheil TG, Havens LL. The therapeutic alliance: contemporary meanings and confusions. *Int Rev Psychoanal* 1979; 6:467–681.
49. *Scholoendorff v. Society of New York Hospital,* 195 NE 92, NY 1914.
50. Meisel A. The "exceptions" to the informed consent doctrine: striking a balance between competing values in medical decisionmaking. *Wisconsin Law Review* 1979; 2:413–488.
51. Borak J, Veilleux S. Informed consent in emergency settings. *Ann Emerg Med* 1984; 13:731–735.
52. *Pedesky v. Bleiberg,* 59 Cal Rptr 294, Cal 1967.
53. Grunder TM. On the readability of surgical consent forms. *New Eng J Med* 1980; 302:896. Mohammed MB. Patients' understanding of written health information. *Nurs Reg* 1964; 12:100.
54. *Kennedy v. Parrott,* 90 SE 2d 754, NC 1956; *Russell v. Jackson,* 221 P 2d 516, Wash 1950.
55. Alton WG Jr. *Malpractice: a trial lawyer's advice for physicians.* Boston: Little, Brown, 1977; 81.
56. *Malpractice Digest.* St. Paul Fire and Marine Insurance Co. October 1984; 3.
57. Alton WG Jr. *Malpractice: a trial lawyer's advice for physicians.* Boston: Little, Brown, 1977; 148.
58. Alton WG Jr. *Malpractice: a trial lawyer's advice for physicians.* Boston: Little, Brown, 1977; 203.
59. Alton WG Jr. *Malpractice: a trial lawyer's advice for physicians.* Boston: Little, Brown, 1977; 207.

106

Commonly Used Drugs in Ambulatory Plastic Surgery

Ronald Riefkohl, M.D., F.A.C.S., and Robert Rehnke, M.D.

Of all the surgical specialties, plastic surgery presents the greatest opportunities for the application of local and regional anesthetic techniques. The recent trend toward more outpatient surgery and the demonstrated safety of currently used drugs has resulted in the increased use of these methods.

The performance of accurate surgery is facilitated by a relaxed and well-sedated patient. Achievement of this goal may require drug dosages approaching the upper limits of safety. Therefore, it is important for each surgeon to have a thorough knowledge of the agents administered to the patient.

Perioperative Medications

Although many procedures can be performed with the use of local anesthetics alone, more extensive procedures usually require preoperative and intraoperative pharmacologic intervention. Most surgeons employ two or three drugs with which they are intimately familiar and adjust dosages according to the individual patient and procedure to be performed. Experience has demonstrated that a well-informed patient undergoing surgery in a peaceful environment usually requires less sedation.

In general, preoperative medications will include analgesics and sedatives. This combination results in fewer side effects and easier pharmacologic reversal when necessary.

The most widely used preoperative analgesics are morphine and meperidine. These narcotics help to relieve anxiety while providing analgesia during the administration of local anesthetics. Respiratory depression, a well-known side effect of these agents (particularly in smokers and others with compromised pulmonary status) is predictable. Oxygen-saturation monitoring has been helpful in identifying susceptible patients intraoperatively, thus alerting the surgeon of the possible need for reversal (1,2). Reversal with naloxone, usually administered intravenously at a dose of 0.2 mg (1 ampule), is rapid; yet, occasionally, a repeat dose within 5 minutes is necessary.

Intraoperative Medications

Intraoperatively, synthetic narcotics are most commonly given intravenously to augment local anesthesia. In the 1970s, Fentanyl became the most popular synthetic opiate, and by the late 1980s, drugs such as Sufentanil and Alfentanil were added to this armamentarium. These drugs are seldom used for preoperative medication because of their short duration of action and higher incidence of respiratory depression, sometimes requiring ventilatory support. Sufentanil is 5 to 10 times more potent than Fentanyl and has a longer duration of activity. It is less a respiratory depressant, but can cause bradyarrhythmias and hypotension. Alfentanil has one-third the potency of Fentanyl and has less hypotensive side effects. Its rapid onset and short duration of action make it a popular choice for outpatient surgery (3).

Nausea is a common side effect of all narcotics. Some studies indicate that equianalgesic doses of the various agents produce equal potential for this complication (4). Certain patients do appear more sensitive to one drug or another. Maintaining the patient NPO on the morning of surgery along with the concomitant use of either an antihistamine or phenothiazine will reduce the frequency of this problem.

The most common class of drugs used for perioperative sedation are the benzodiazepines, diazepam (Valium), and midazolam (Versed). They act as potent anxiolytics, hypnotics, and mild muscle relaxants. They also have the important effect of producing antegrade amnesia and increase the threshold for convulsions resulting from overdose of local anesthesia (5). Although both work well in combination with other drugs, midazolam has been found to have distinct advantages. It has been shown to be a more effective anxiolytic, sedative, and amnestic agent (6). It has a shorter half-life—2.3 hours, compared to that of diazepam, with a half-life of 27 to 37 hours (7). It is painless when injected intravenously, has a virtual absence of postinjection phlebitis, and consequently has met with a high degree of patient acceptance (6,8). Midazolam is used as a premedication for surgery at doses of 0.1mg/kg intramuscularly, or 10 to 15 mg orally. It is given intravenously at 0.5–1 mg doses to titrate desired levels of sedation, and can even be used to induce and maintain general anesthesia.

When used alone and given in the appropriate doses, midazolam has remarkably few side effects. Hiccoughs, nausea and vomiting, and coughing are examples, but are present 5% or less of the time (7). However, benzodiazepines are not analgesics, and therefore must be combined with narcotics to counteract intraoperative pain from injection of local anesthetics or inadequate local blocks. This combination, or overdosage, can lead to significant respiratory depression and hypotension. Recently, the benzodiazepine antagonist flumazenil (Anexate) has been introduced. It is a competitive antagonist for the benzodiazepine receptor and acts to reverse sedation, respiratory depression, and amnesia. It is given 0.1 to 0.2 mg intravenously every 2 minutes (not to exceed 3 mg) until the desired response is obtained. Like naloxone, its half-life is short, and repeated doses may be required (3).

Ketamine is a short-acting dissociative anesthetic that provides analgesia and amnesia. Because of its possible side effects, including respiratory depression and dose-related unpleasant hallucinatory phenomena, it remains controversial for use in ambulatory settings.

Propofol (Diprivan), an alkylphenol derivative, is a new intravenous anesthetic particularly well suited for outpatient surgery. It is classified as a sedative hypnotic and can be used for induction and maintenance of anesthesia. Its quick onset of action and rapid recovery time gives an ease of control of depth of anesthesia, which has made it very popular as an adjunct to local anesthesia cases. Intermittent boluses can be given to provide short periods of near-general anesthesia, or while local anesthesia is injected, while a continuous infusion provides general anesthesia comparable to inhaled agents. Recent studies have shown propofol to be equivalent to thiopental for induction and it is also safe for use in children and elderly adults at reduced doses (9,10). It has a quicker recovery time than other intravenous agents (approximately 8 to 30 minutes) and a lower incidence of postoperative drowsiness and confusion (9). Finally, postoperative nausea and vomiting is rare following propofol anesthesia. Side effects include pain on injection, hypotension, and apnea on induction. The addition of 1 ml of 1% lidocaine per 20cc of propofol, plus slow administration to well-hydrated patients, can reduce these side effects.

Local Anesthetics (Table 106–1)

Local anesthetics are thought to act on the inner surface of the nerve-cell membrane by blocking the entrance of sodium into the axoplasm, resulting in a nondepolarizing block (11). Factors determining the time to onset, depth, and duration of block depend upon the general structural characteristics of the agent used and its specific physiochemistry. The local anesthetics are weakly basic tertiary amines that penetrate the nerve while in a lipophilic, uncharged, basic form, yet actually function at the nerve-cell membrane in a charged, quaternary amine form. The relative effect of each agent depends on its inherent physical chemistry as well as the temperature and pH of the tissues into which it is injected. Thus, in a patient with systemic or local acidosis, the onset of anesthesia will be significantly delayed.

The depth of anesthesia is determined by the size of the nerve fibers as well as the concentration of the anesthetic used. As an example, 2% lidocaine is required to obtain an adequate motor block in the arm.

Epinephrine is commonly used to prolong the duration of the anesthetic block by its local vasoconstrictive effect, thus delaying uptake and subsequent metabolism. A 1:200,000 concentration of epinephrine has been shown to provide maximal duration of anesthesia without the added systemic toxicity resulting from higher concentrations (12). This toxicity is augmented when epinephrine is used in conjunction with certain general anesthetics (e.g., halothane). It has been recommended that no more than 10 ml of a 1:100,000 solution be given per 10 minutes in a 70-kg patient, up to a total dose of 30 ml per hour when halothane anesthesia is being used (13).

Local toxicity, in the form of ischemia and necrosis of skin flaps, has been thought to result from the use of epinephrine, although the pathophysiological mechanism is not clear (14). This has led some investigators to evaluate other agents for use as local vasoconstrictors, particularly phenylephrine and vasopressin (15,16). The use of these agents, however, has not gained widespread acceptance and cannot be recommended at this time.

TOPICAL AGENTS: COCAINE AND TETRACAINE

Cocaine was first used as a topical anesthetic by Koller in 1884 (17). Halsted (18) performed the first peripheral nerve blocks with cocaine and did much work to examine the use of cocaine as an infiltration agent, but he subsequently became disenchanted with the lower therapeutic index in this setting. Today, cocaine is employed only topically, usually applied as a 3–4% solution. The maximum absorbed dose should be limited to 100 to 200 mg to avoid cardiovascular collapse. Cocaine has inherent vasoconstrictive characteristics secondary to its ability to block reuptake of norepinephrine, and should not be mixed with vasoconstrictors. It is bactericidal for staphylococcus and most gram-positive organisms, as well as for mycobacteria (19).

An alternative to cocaine is 2% tetracaine mixed with phenylephrine (epinephrine does not penetrate mucous membranes). However, 0.5% tetracaine is preferable as a topical ophthalmic anesthetic.

ESTER-LINKED LOCAL ANESTHETICS: PROCAINE AND CHLOROPROCAINE

The elucidation of the chemical structure of cocaine led to the investigation of additional compounds with similar properties. Procaine (Novocaine) is a benzoic acid derivative with an ester linkage to an amino group, and has been found most useful as a 1–2% solution for infiltration and nerve blocks. The maximum safe dose is 10 to 15 mg/kg. The onset of nerve blockage is fast (approximately 5 to 7 minutes) but lasts only 1 hour. As with other agents, the uptake and duration of block may be prolonged with the addition of epinephrine. Chloroprocaine (Nesacaine) was subsequently de-

Table 106–1
Local Anesthetics

Drug	Supplied As	Maximum Dose	Duration
Cocaine	0.25% solution	100–200 mg	1 hr
Procaine	0.5% solution	10–15 mg/kg	30 min–1 hr
Chloroprocaine	0.5% solution	10–20 mg/kg	1 hr
Tetracaine (topical)	1–3% solution	1.5 mg/kg (up to 150 mg)	2 hr
Lidocaine	0.5–2% solution	4 mg/kg (7 mg/kg with epinephrine)	1–2 hr (2–4 hr with epinephrine)
Mepivacaine	1–2% solution	7 mg/kg (up to 1000 mg/24 hr)	2–3 hr
Bupivacaine	0.25–0.5% solution	175 mg in adult (225 mg with epinephrine)	Up to 12 hr in peripheral nerve blocks

veloped, and is both slightly faster acting than procaine and also somewhat safer. When used as a 1–2% solution, the maximum dose may be increased slightly to 10 to 20 mg/kg.

Allergic reactions to ester-linked anesthetics are sometimes encountered, and are much more common than with amide-linked anesthetics. Generally, however, patients are allergic to either a metabolite of these agents (para-aminobenzoic acid) or to a similar chemical (paraben) used as a preservative in multidose vials. Skin tests are not reliable and are difficult to interpret. It is safer to administer a test dose cautiously. There is cross-reactivity between the various agents in the ester class; thus, in patients allergic to an ester-linked anesthetic, one of the amide-linked anesthetics should be used instead (20).

Procaine and chloroprocaine are metabolized by plasma pseudocholinesterase. A family history of a deficiency of this enzyme contraindicates their use (21).

AMIDE-LINKED AGENTS: LIDOCAINE, MEPIVACAINE, AND BUPIVACAINE

Lidocaine (Xylocaine) was the first member of a new class of local anesthetics that contain an amide instead of an ester linkage. The agents with an amide linkage are metabolized via complex hepatic enzyme systems with subsequent renal excretion of byproducts, therefore necessitating the use of lower dosages in patients with significant hepatic or renal disease.

When lidocaine is mixed with epinephrine, a preservative must be added (sodium bisulfite and methylparaben), to which some patients are allergic. If there is a question of allergy, lidocaine for cardiac use may be combined with injectable epinephrine (22).

Lidocaine may be used in 0.5–2% solutions, and its duration of action may be doubled or tripled from 1 hour to 2 to 3 hours with the addition of 1:200,000 epinephrine. The addition of epinephrine delays the peak blood level of lidocaine. The maximum dose may also be increased from 4 to 7 mg/kg if epinephrine is added. Recent studies appear to indicate the relative safety of using higher doses of lidocaine for suction-assisted lipectomy because of the diminished vascularity of fat and because a portion of the injected lidocaine is subsequently aspirated (23,24).

Mepivacaine (Carbocaine) is used in the same dosage as lidocaine, but is believed to have some inherent vasoconstrictive activity. No more than 1 g of mepivacaine should be administered within a 24-hour period.

Bupivacaine (Marcaine, Sensorcaine) is commonly used for nerve block because the duration of anesthesia is greater than that of lidocaine or mepivacaine. A block lasting 8 to 12 hours may be obtained using a 0.5% solution with epinephrine; the epinephrine is added to allow administration of a greater maximum dose of anesthetic.

The onset of anesthesia with bupivacaine may take up to 30 minutes, so it is frequently combined with faster-acting agents because toxicities of similar-class agents may be additive (25). If the peak blood levels of two agents coincide, the dosage of each agent should be lowered accordingly. If a large amount of anesthetic is required, a drug from each class should be combined (e.g., chloroprocaine with bupivacaine).

The depth of anesthesia depends on the concentration of the agent used, but the toxicity depends on the blood level at any given time. Toxicity is determined by the total dose of drug administered, the rate of absorption by the surrounding tissue, and the rate of metabolism of the agent.

TOXICITY

Toxicity of the local anesthetics involves the neurologic and cardiovascular systems. This toxicity is a direct pharmacologic side effect and not an idiosyncratic reaction. Any patient will eventually develop either seizures or cardiac arrest if administered sufficient doses of a local anesthetic. The proper route of administration of a local anesthetic is of utmost importance because toxic levels may be reached inadvertently. Examples include the premature deflation of a tourniquet after a Bier block, direct intravascular injection, or infiltration into a well-vascularized muscle such as an intercostal. It is possible to avoid serious reactions in most patients, but it is also important to know how to treat them when they do occur.

The therapeutic index for neurologic toxicity may be significantly improved by prior administration of benzodiazepines (21). Epileptics are no more likely to experience seizures with the administration of local anesthetics than are any other patients (26); seizures originating with the use of these drugs occur in the limbic system rather than the cerebral cortex, as is usually the case in epilepsy. Seizures most commonly are preceded by drowsiness, tinnitus, nystagmus, twitching, or tremors; however, bupivacaine often does not produce these warning signs. The seizures caused by local anesthetics are precipitated by hypoxemia and acidosis, in contradistinction to other types of seizures (27). The treatment of seizures includes cardiorespiratory support and administration of intravenous diazepam. If the patient is adequately managed, no permanent sequelae will result (28).

Both lidocaine and bupivacaine are vasodilators; however, there is some evidence that at low concentrations lidocaine has an initial vasoconstrictor effect. Thus, bupivacaine is preferred if vasodilation is specifically desired (29).

Toxicity resulting in cardiac symptoms requires a higher serum level of local anesthetic than that resulting in neurologic symptoms. Lidocaine has been extensively studied and is known to have a negative inotropic effect with prolongation of the refractory period. Cardiac arrest by intractable fibrillation is the end result with massive overdose.

Other problems with these agents are uncommon and relatively minor. Direct intraneural injection may cause a lasting paresthesia (up to 3 months). It is unclear whether this is a chemical or mechanical effect. Local anesthetics do not appear to be at all toxic to skin and fat, but have been shown to produce local myonecrosis with direct intramuscular injection (30).

All local anesthetics cross the placenta and may affect the cardiovascular system of the fetus. Teratogenicity has not been a problem. None of the drugs are specifically indicated or contraindicated in early pregnancy, but certainly minimally effective doses should be used.

References

1. Riefkohl R, Cox EB, Kosanin R, et al. Evaluation of transcutaneous oxygen tension monitoring during cosmetic surgery. *Aesthetic Plast Surg* 1987; 11:117.
2. Singer R, Thomas PE. Pulse oximeter in the ambulatory aesthetic surgical facility. *Plast Reconstr Surg* 1988; 82:111.
3. Waugaman WR, Foster DS. New advances in anesthesia. *Nursing Clinics of North America* 1991; 26(2):451.

4. Ordy JM, Kretchmer HE, Gorry TH, et al. Comparison of effects of morphine, meperidine, fentanyl, and fentanyl-droperidol. *Clin Pharmacol Ther* 1970; 11:488.

5. deJong RH, Bonin JD. Benzodiazepines protect mice from local anesthetic convulsions and deaths. *Anesthesia and Analgesia* 1981; 60:385.

6. White PF, Vasconez LO, Mathes SA, et al. Comparison of midazolam and diazepam for sedation during plastic surgery. *Plast Reconstr Surg* 1988; 81:703.

7. Reves JG, Fragen RJ, Vinik JR, et al. Midazolam: pharmacology and uses. *Anesthesiology* 1985; 62:310.

8. Baker TJ, Gordon HL. Midazolam (Versed) in ambulatory surgery. *Plast Reconstr Surg* 1988; 82:244.

9. Heath PJ, Kennedy DJ, Ogg TW, et al. Which intravenous induction agent for day surgery? *Anesthesia* 1988; 43:365.

10. Mirakhur RK. Induction characteristics of propofol in children. *Anaesthesia* 1988; 43:593.

11. Strichartz G. Molecular mechanisms of nerve block by local anesthetics. *Anesthesiology* 1976; 45:421.

12. Scott DB, Jebson PJR, Braid DP, et al. Factors affecting plasma levels of lignocaine and prilocaine. *Br J Anesth* 1972; 44:1040.

13. Katz RL, Epstein RA. The interaction of anesthetic agents and adrenergic drugs to produce cardiac arrhythmias. *Anesthesiology* 1968; 29:763.

14. Burk RW, Serafin D, Klitzman B. Toxic effects of catecholamines on skin. *Plast Reconstr Surg* 1990; 85:92.

15. Canepa CS, Miller SH, Buck DC, et al. Effects of phenylephrine on tissue gas tension, bleeding, infection, lidocaine absorption. *Plast Reconstr Surg* 1988; 81:554.

16. Davis J, Picon MC, Chouela M. Vasoconstrictor for face-lifting. *Aesthetic Plast Surg* 1988; 12:33.

17. Gay GR, Aba DS, Sheppard CW, et al. Cocaine: history, epidemiology, human pharmacology and treatment. Perspective on a new debut for an old girl. *Clin Toxicol* 1975; 8:149.

18. Olch P, William S. Halstead and local anesthesia. *Anesthesiology* 1975; 42:479.

19. Weinstein MP, Maderazo E, Tilton R, et al. Further observations of the antimicrobial effects of local anesthetic agents. *Curr Ther Res* 1975; 17:369.

20. Aldrete JA, Johnson DA. Allergy to local anesthetics. *JAMA* 1969; 207:356.

21. deJong RH. *Local anesthetics.* Springfield, IL: Charles C Thomas, 1977; 112.

22. Aldrete JA, O'Higgins JW. Evaluation of patients with history of allergy to local anesthetic drugs. *South Med J* 1971; 64:118.

23. Lewis DM, Hepper T. The use of high-dose lidocaine in wetting solutions for lipoplasty. *Ann Plast Surg* 1989; 22:307.

24. Gumucio CA, Bennie JB, Fernando B, et al. Plasma lidocaine levels during augmentation mammoplasty and suction assisted lipectomy. *Plast Reconstr Surg* 1989; 84:624.

25. Moore DC, Bridenbaugh LD, Bridenbaugh PO, et al. Does compounding of local anesthetic agents increase their toxicity in humans? *Anesth Analg* 1972; 51:579.

26. Heinonen J, Takke S, Jarho L. Plasma lidocaine levels in patients treated with potential inducers of microsomal enzymes. *Acta Anesth Scand* 1970; 14:89.

27. Englesson S, Grevsten S. The influences of acid-base changes on CNS toxicity of local anesthetic agents II. *Acta Anesth Scand* 1974; 18:88.

28. deJong RH. *Local anesthetics.* Springfield, IL: Charles C Thomas, 1977; 97.

29. Altura BM, Altura BT. Effects of local anesthetics, antihistamines, and glucocorticoids on peripheral blood flow and vascular smooth muscle. *Anesthesiology* 1974; 41:179.

30. Benoit PW, Belt WD. Some effects of local anesthetic agents on skeletal muscle. *Exp Neurol* 1972; 34:264.

107

Radiation Injury

Jack C. Fisher, M.D., F.A.C.S., and Ross Rudolph, M.D., F.A.C.S.

Plastic surgeons have been thinking and writing about radiation injury for many years. Reconstructive surgical practice too often includes patients who suffer the tissue-destructive complications of ionizing radiation. Furthermore, it is not clear that the occurrence of radiation injury is any less frequent, despite introduction of new methods for administration of ionizing energy.

However, newer techniques of radiation therapy, along with more powerful radiation sources, may have reduced the severity of such injury. In particular, higher energy (6 to 24 MEV) places the maximum energy deeper than the skin, and may have some skin-sparing effect.

Radiation oncologists do not often focus upon tissue injury following therapeutic irradiation. All cancer specialists, surgeons included, prefer to focus on their achievement, not their problems. As the survival experience following cancer treatment improves, all members of the cancer treatment team must consider quality-of-life as well as quantity-of-life issues. The permanent and progressive effects of ionizing radiation can destroy a patient's will to live despite successful control of the malignancy.

Solzhenitsyn makes the point well in his novel *Cancer Ward,* recommended reading for all who treat cancer victims: "I would not care to pay too great a price for the hope of being able to live at some time in the distant future."

What Is Ionizing Radiation?

Radiation takes its origin from the electromagnetic spectrum or from atomic particles. Think of the electromagnetic spectrum (Fig. 107–1) as a continuum of energy bundles ranging from low-frequency, long-wavelength radio waves to high-frequency, short-wavelength x-rays. Atomic particles also yield high-frequency radiation energy. Every component of the electromagnetic spectrum travels at the speed of light (186,282 miles/second). Penetration power varies widely, however. Visible light can penetrate glass. Gamma rays can penetrate the skin and carry enough energy to ionize cells deep to the surface. Ionizing radiation is a specific term referring to energy sources powerful enough to inflict cellular damage.

Particulate sources of radiation also produce ionization damage. Particulate radiation is named according to the atomic particle involved. Biologically significant are alpha particles, beta particles, protons, and neutrons. Unlike electromagnetic sources of radiation, particulate radiation can travel at varying speeds.

All sources of ionizing radiation are very powerful when compared to the binding energies of valence electrons within atoms. Molecular binding energies can be 5 to 10 electron volts, whereas gamma rays generate nearly 1 million electron volts (MEV), and some atomic particles yield as many as 10 MEV.

Biologic Effects of Ionizing Radiation

The basis for tissue injury is ionization damage to individual cells. The biologic effects of irradiation may be direct or indirect.

Direct injury means that a cellular unit reacts adversely to a number of "hits," or energy-absorption events. The number of cells injured by ionization is directly proportional to the density of cells exposed. The severity of a cell's injury is directly related to the amount of nuclear material contained within each cell.

Indirect injury follows ionization of cell water with subsequent liberation of free radicals. These fragmented molecules, once activated, are highly destructive. Free radicals can be either oxidizing or reducing agents that react with water to form cell-toxic peroxides.

The sum of direct and indirect effects can totally destroy a cell, or might only partially interrupt its function. The reproductive capacity of a cell is especially vulnerable to ionizing energy; loss or change of the DNA content means interruption of a cell's destiny. Partial cell injury may lead to replication without separation, or the formation of multinucleated cells, or else to uncontrolled replication of cells that assume a cancerlike appearance.

Atrophy is a convenient term to describe what surgeons see when they observe radiation-damaged skin or a radiation-induced wound. Wound repair is a continuous process because collagen content is constantly turning over in any wound. Collagen formation is dependent on fibroblasts. The source of wound fibroblasts is local and not from the systemic circulation. Therefore, depletion of local fibroblasts in part explains the nonregeneration of irradiated tissue. Observable evidence of radiation damage may be delayed for many years. Withers and colleagues (1) have presented evidence supporting parenchymal cell depletion as the basis for chronic radiation-induced atrophy. Rudolph and co-workers (2) have reported deficits in the function of fibroblasts cultured from radiation wounds.

Vascular Injury

Vascular changes become apparent long after radiation exposure. Mature endothelial cells are not especially radiosensitive, explaining why vascular anomalies rarely can be treated

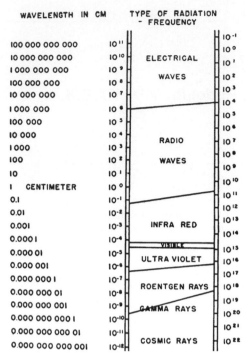

FIG. 107-1. The electromagnetic spectrum.

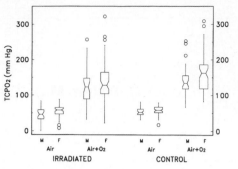

FIG. 107-2. Grouped box-plots of TcPO$_2$ values at irradiated and nonirradiated control skin sites under both ambient air and ambient air + O$_2$ conditions, for 100 patients, separately by sex. (M = males, F = females). The three horizontal lines in each box represent the upper, median, and the lower quartiles, respectively, of the data. The notches in each box approximate a 95% confidence region around the median. The width of each box is proportional to the square root of the sample size of the group it represents. The step value of each box is the height of the box − 1.5. The upper vertical line of each box extends up to the highest value in the data within the step, and the lower vertical line extends down to the lowest value in the data within the step. Data values outside these limits are depicted by small circles. Irradiated and normal control skin have similar TcPO$_2$, whether breathing ambient air or added 100% O$_2$. Inspired O$_2$ produces higher TcPO$_2$, and women have slightly higher TcPO$_2$ than males. (Reprinted from *Cancer* 1994; 74:3063).

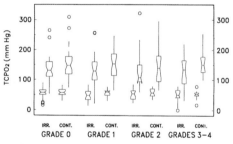

FIG. 107-3. Grouped box-plots of TcPO$_2$ values at irradiated (IRR) and control (CONT) skin sites for all 100 patients, cross-classified by grade of their irradiated skin. For each pair of boxes, starting at the left side of the diagram, the lefthand box is with ambient air breathing and the next higher box to the right is ambient air plus inspired O$_2$ at 6 liters per minute. With increasing grade of skin damage, note that TcPO$_2$ remains level, whether breathing ambient air or with added O$_2$. Skin oxygenation thus remains constant regardless of increasing skin radiation effect. (Reprinted from *Cancer* 1994; 74:3063).

successfully with radiation. Nevertheless, focal necrosis of the vessel wall and hyaline degeneration may lead to eventual occlusion of small vessels.

Plastic surgeons have blamed vascular injury for the complications of surgery involving irradiated tissues. Even the most carefully designed flaps can be lost; granulation tissue does not readily form at the surface of these wounds. However, vascular injury is not a satisfactory explanation, because excellent circulation adjacent to most radiation wounds can be demonstrated by intravenous administration of fluorescein. The delay phenomenon, a sophisticated vascular function, remains intact despite irradiation of skin flaps (3).

Most of the problems experienced after surgery involving irradiated tissue can be better explained by the progressive loss of the fibroblasts so necessary for the proliferative phase of wound healing.

In spite of current dogma, chronically irradiated skin is not hypoxic. In an extensive study of human TcPO$_2$ (transcutaneous oxygen pressure, an excellent indicator of skin oxygenation), Rudolph and others (2) found normal oxygenation even decades after radiation. Neither time since radiation, nor increasing grade of skin radiation damage, were associated with hypoxia (Figs. 107-2, 107-3, 107-4).

Genetic Effect

Ionizing radiation is a potent mutagen. When ionization affects somatic cells, only the patient will experience injury, but when germinal cells are exposed to irradiation, the genetic offspring of those cells might be dysmorphic and dysfunctional.

Radiation can induce either a point mutation or a chromosomal aberration. Point mutations are errors in DNA sequencing not visible by karyotyping, whereas alteration or deletion of one or more chromosomes can be detected by karyotype analysis.

Not all chromosomal injuries are permanent. A fractured chromosome may rejoin without residual expression, or it might join another chromosome with devastating biologic effects.

Carcinogenesis

The carcinogenic potential of ionizing radiation has been recognized for the greater part of this century. Very few years had elapsed following Roentgen's discovery of x-rays before physicians working in the vicinity of x-ray–emitting tubes began to witness changes in the skin of their hands. Unaware of the cumulative effects of radiation, they later experienced skin malignancies as well as a greater frequency of leukemia.

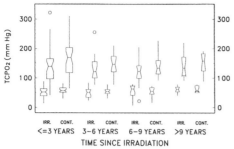

FIG. 107–4. Grouped box-plots of TcPO₂ values at irradiated (IRR) and control (CONT) skin sites for all 100 patients, cross-classified by length of time since they had been irradiated. For each pair of boxes, starting at the left side of the diagram, the lefthand box is with ambient air breathing and the next higher box to the right is ambient air plus inspired O₂ at 6 liters per minute. With increasing time after radiation therapy, TcPO₂ remains level, whether breathing ambient air or with added O₂. Skin oxygenation thus remains constant in spite of increasing time after irradiation. (Reprinted from *Cancer* 1994; 74:306).

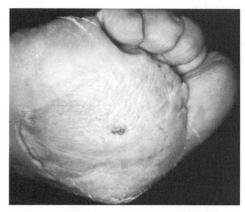

FIG. 107–5. Sacral ulceration appeared on the sole of the foot secondary to chronic irradiation for benign disease (athlete's foot) earlier in life.

Less apparent, and as yet incompletely documented, are the malignancies that develop 20 and 30 years following curative radiotherapy. No good epidemiologic follow-up exists for carcinogenesis following therapeutic radiation, but a review of innumerable individual clinical reports suggest a greater clinical problem than we have been willing to admit.

Most radiation biologists will agree that:

1. Tumors of virtually any variety can be induced by irradiation.
2. All sources of ionizing radiation are carcinogenic.
3. Multiple fractionated doses are more carcinogenic than is a single large dose.

Specific Injuries

SKIN

Prior to 1950, ionizing radiation was even more damaging to skin, because less powerful energy sources penetrated the skin incompletely. Deeper planes were spared, but the germinal cells of the skin absorbed most of the injury.

Since 1950, more potent sources of ionizing energy have been used and are thought to be skin sparing. Deeper tissue layers were more effectively penetrated. Whether this is clinically significant is still hard to determine. Plenty of chronic radiation dermatitis is seen by dermatologists and plastic surgeons, usually 10 to 20 years after radiation therapy.

Early radiation-induced skin changes include erythema, loss of hair, and hyperpigmentation. Radiation skin damage can lead to telangiectasia, greater susceptibility to injury, slower healing, and ulceration.

Whenever multiple skin malignancies develop in patients under 50, possible explanations include excess sun or prior clinical exposure to irradiation for acne or other benign skin dermatoses (Fig. 107–5). Modern safeguards have diminished the frequency of skin cancer among employees who work near sources of ionizing radiation.

Longstanding radiation ulcers may undergo malignant change, just as with any chronic wound. A longstanding wound whose basis is osteomyelitis, or a nonhealed burn, or prior irradiation, can all be likely site for neoplasia. Biopsy

of these wounds is an important first step in their management.

ORAL CAVITY

Following therapy for oral cavity carcinoma, dryness of the mouth is a common and unpleasant after effect. Patients with oral cavity carcinoma often select radiation in preference to surgery. After experiencing the side effects, they may look back with regret and wish they had selected another form of treatment.

The teeth are continually bathed in a bacterial environment made worse by frequent sugar intake. Patients with oral malignancy might therefore suffer an unstable dentition even before irradiation begins. A dentist can play an essential role whenever radiation is selected for oral cancer management.

Surgery for head and neck malignancy may include use of complex skin and muscle flaps for reconstruction. Flap viability depends on a functioning microvasculature as well as adequate parenchymal cells. Whenever flaps or mucosal suture lines break down, patients may be at risk for orocutaneous fistulae or major vessel exposure, leading to risk of serious hemorrhage (Fig. 107–6).

Combined therapy protocols may place patients at risk for surgical complications, particularly when irradiation precedes surgery. Surgeon and radiotherapist alike must take into account a patient's desired quality of life before committing to certain treatment combinations.

BREAST

We are seeing a rewakening of interest in primary irradiation for breast malignancy. It is well documented that survival is comparable to those who elect mastectomy (4). What is less well understood is the frequency of tissue injury long after ionizing radiation. Radiation oncologists, like surgeons, traditionally focus on survival, not on complications. The available outcome data report a low frequency of tissue reactions (5). However, plastic surgeons continue to see patients who suffer disappointing deformities following primary radiation for breast cancer. Women with large breasts seem to be at greater risk for fibrosis, telangiectasia, progressive breast shrinkage, and skin breakdown.

Misuse of radiation as an adjuvant to mastectomy has led to breakdown of chest-wall integrity, mediastinal exposure, chronic pain, and narcotic dependency (Fig. 107–7). The National Surgical Adjuvant Breast Project has demonstrated no advantage to survival or longevity when irradiation is added to mastectomy for treatment of breast cancer (6) (Fig. 107–8).

Reconstructive techniques are available for repair of painful chest-wall defects. Essential for success is the introduction of a new blood supply, using muscle flaps or omentum (7).

PELVIS

Uterine cervical cancer is the most common indication for administration of ionizing radiation to the pelvic region. For

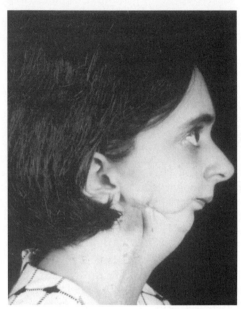

FIG. 107–6. Severe hypoplasia of the lower face is shown after irradiation for benign lymphangioma during infancy.

patients with earlier stages of this disease, there is no therapeutic advantage of surgery over radiation. The spectre of a surgical operation is fearsome, which means that most women choose pelvic irradiation. Greater use of cytologic diagnosis means earlier cancer detection, which also means we are producing a population of women cured of uterine cancer who might suffer a lifetime of radiation sequelae.

The incidence of proctitis, cystitis, sexual dysfunction, and acetabular arthritis are probably higher than commonly believed. Plastic surgeons see the worst of these problems: sacral ulceration (Fig. 107–8). Gynecologists treat the vaginitis, urologists the bladder dysfunction, general surgeons the proctitis, and orthopedic surgeons the hip disability. No single practitioner currently keeps track of all pelvic complications.

Reconstruction for the Radiation-Induced Wound

This brief chapter cannot list every technique used to repair radiation wounds. However, the following principles apply to most challenges:

1. The most common indication for surgery is unrelenting pain, usually requiring heavy narcotic analgesia. After wound excision and flap repair, patients report prompt pain relief, often without signs or symptoms of narcotic withdrawal.
2. For any longstanding wound, always rule out recurrent cancer or a new malignancy. Biopsy first! Remember that patients with radiation wounds may be convinced they suffer recurrent cancer until your biopsy and reassurance informs them they don't.
3. Complications are the rule, not the exception. Warn your patient in advance.
4. Don't excise a radiation wound now and repair it later. The resulting wound will not likely form granulation tis-

FIG. 107–7. **A,** painful ulceration and chondritis secondary to elective postmastectomy adjunctive irradiation. **B,** immediate pain relief and narcotic withdrawal occurred after wide resection of inflamed costal cartilages with repair of defect using omental flaps and skin grafting.

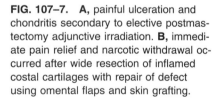

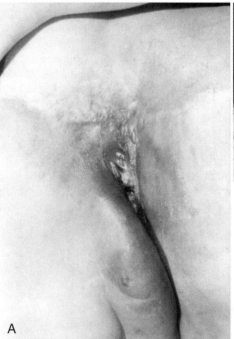

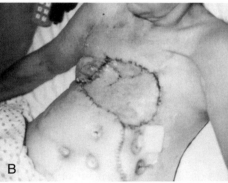

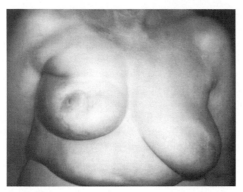

FIG. 107–8. Primary irradiation of left breast for malignancy. The result is categorized as satisfactory by the radiotherapist, yet the left breast is contracted and fibrotic in relation to the normal but ptotic right breast.

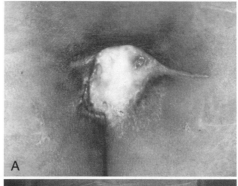

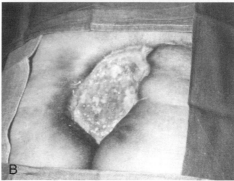

FIG. 107–9. A, sacral ulceration after paralysis following irradiation for prostatic carcinoma. **B,** larger defect after necrosis of rotation flap taken from skin adjacent to wound. Tissue injury in a radiation field is always more widespread than clinical signs would indicate.

sue or contract. Excise these defects only when your flap is ready for transfer into the defect. Wound stability may require potent topical antibacterials (silver sulfadiazine, mafenide acetate) to limit bacterial proliferation. Meanwhile, don't forget to provide lots of emotional support throughout the prolonged course of treatment that most radiation injuries require.

5. The zone of injury will always be more extensive than is clinically apparent.

6. You cannot wait for granulation tissue nor rely on skin grafting to achieve a durable surface. Skin grafts are parasitic and do not bring with them a new blood supply. Grafts applied after wound excision might succeed, but more often fail when the wound is the result of irradiation.

7. Random-pattern flaps taken from adjacent to the defect are least likely to succeed. Radiation scatter effect is more widespread than the dimensions of the original treatment port.

8. Arterial flaps are preferable, but select them with care. The tips of arterial flaps are often dependent on a healthy subdermal plexus.

9. Myocutaneous flaps have an advantage, but their use is not without risk of complication. The abundant blood supply of the muscle is just what the wound needs, but successful adherence of these flaps depends upon adequate excision of radiation-damaged tissue. Failure to excise the wound widely enough can mean nonadherence of your flap.

10. In planning surgery, whether ulcer removal or through intact skin, avoid tension! Remember that radiated skin has normal oxygenation but diminished ability to heal. Putting a healthy flap into an irradiated wound is like putting sod on concrete. Wound complications are often preventable by proper design; avoid wound tension, and protect edematous flaps from gravity's pull by tissue support.

11. Since radiation damages cells, provide "cellular nutrition." To compensate for common borderline nutrition, especially in patients with cancer or painful ulcers, prescribe vitamins C and B and zinc, and encourage a high-protein diet. Postoperatively, use nasal oxygen at 4 min-

utes at normal atmospheric pressure, to enhance collagen synthesis by fibroblasts, as well as leukocyte bacterial killing. Hyperbaric oxygen may also be useful, especially in treating osteoradionecrosis.

12. Whichever flap is selected for coverage, make certain the pedicle is a permanent one. A free microvascular flap can bring with it an instant augmentation of blood supply, as well as a new population of parenchymal cells critical for healing.

13. Don't forget the omentum, a valuable source of highly vascular tissue for filling extensive radiation defects. Omentum can be transferred long distances on the right or left epiploic artery pedicle. Omentum may also be transferred as a free flap. Omental flaps should be covered with split-skin grafts at the time of transfer, or a few days later when flap viability is certain.

14. Considering the magnitude and the risk of most efforts to close a radiation wound, conservative management might be the wisest choice in some cases. When pain is not a dominant feature or when a patient's lifestyle is not significantly altered, then local wound management seems the wiser course.

The Surgeon and the Radiation Oncologist

The choice of optimum treatment for a given malignancy will sometimes be a debate in tumor board discussions. Advocacy is influenced strongly by an individual therapist's perception of the benefits and side effects of his or her own form of treatment. Surgeons prefer surgery because it is what they do best. Radiation oncologists are usually willing to administer radiation because that is the only form of therapy at their disposal. End results data reflect the bias of the interpreter, and patients are often left out of this dialogue. We are not yet in the habit of defining accurately the short-term and long-term sequelae of each form of treatment, allowing for the patient's wishes to be included in the transaction. Take notice that patients now demand more information in advance; therefore, we must seek accurate data regarding late outcomes of therapeutic irradiation.

The Plastic Surgeon's Role in Prevention of Radiation Wounds

We can manage these difficult problems surgically. We can also make an effort to diminish the frequency of radiation injuries. Here are four ways each of us can help:

1. Discourage the use of ionizing irradiation for benign disease, a practice that continues. It is quite simply not in the best interests of a young person to be exposed to ionizing energy for a keloid, for benign skin disorders, or for a congenital hemangioma that will surely undergo spontaneous involution (Fig. 107–9).
2. Anticipate radiation injuries earlier in the course of treatment. Under some circumstances, radiation therapy is very well justified, but the risk of tissue breakdown can be high. Whenever the skin is thin, or if prior surgery has interrupted normal blood supply, or when repeat courses of therapy are given, the plastic surgeon should intercept the problem early and offer his reconstructive skills before a wound develops.

3. Continue to participate on tumor boards, where the reconstructive surgeon enjoys the opportunity to force consideration of the long-term sequelae of all treatment options.
4. Finally, demand from clinical investigators and our journal editors reports of late outcomes following cancer treatment. Publications must provide valid expressions of all late effects—including some definition of a patient's quality of life rather than the time-honored declaration of survival time. If a publication does not, make your opinions known to the editor.

References

1. Withers HR, Peters LJ, Kogelnik HD. The pathobiology of late effects of irradiation. In: Meyn RE, Withers HR, eds. *Radiation biology in cancer research.* New York: Raven Press, 1980; 439.
2. Rudolph R, VandeBerg J, Schneider JA. Slowed growth of cultured fibroblasts from human radiation wounds. *Plast Reconstr Surg* 1988; 82:669.
3. Fisher JC, Hurn I, Rudolph R, et al. The effect of delay on flap survival in an irradiated field. *Plast Reconstr Surg* 1984; 73:99.
4. Hellman S, Harris JR, Levene MB. Radiation therapy of early carcinoma of the breast without mastectomy. *Cancer* 1980; 46:988.
5. Harris JR, Levene MB, Svensso G, et al. Analysis of cosmetic results following primary radiation therapy for stages I and II carcinoma of the breast. *J Radiat Oncol Biol Phys* 1979; 5:57.
6. Fisher B, Redmond C, Fisher E, et al. Ten-year results of a randomized clinical trial comparing radical mastectomy and total mastectomy with or without radiation. *N Eng J Med* 1985; 312:674.
7. O'Brien B. Microvascular free flap and omental transfer. In: *Microvascular reconstructive surgery.* Edinburgh, London, New York: Churchill Livingstone; 1977; 205.
8. Rudolph R, Tripuraneni P, Koziol J, et al. Normal transcutaneous oxygen pressure in skin after radiation therapy for cancer. *Cancer* 1994; 74:3063.
9. Rudolph R. Complications of surgery for radiotherapy skin damage. *Plast Reconstr Surg* 1982; 70:179.

108

Psychologic Understanding and Management of the Plastic Surgery Patient

Thomas Pruzinsky, Ph.D., and Milton T. Edgerton, Jr. M.D., F.A.C.S.

Mastering the art of plastic surgery requires a deep appreciation of the degree to which physical appearance affects self-concept and well-being. Understanding and managing the psychologic concerns of plastic surgery patients is essential for problem prevention (1,2), including reducing the likelihood of patient dissatisfaction and malpractice litigation (3,4). More important, this understanding facilitates achieving the primary mission of plastic surgery—maximizing patient quality of life. If surgeons steadily develop their skills in understanding patients' psychologic concerns, they and their patients will be richly rewarded with the fruits of the "magic" of plastic surgery—the ability to change patients' psyche in a positive way by improving their appearance (2).

This chapter describes the information and skills plastic surgeons need to understand and manage patient psychological concerns by addressing three topics:

1. Defining body image and describing how it is central to understanding the motivations for, and impact of, plastic surgery.
2. Reviewing critical psychologic issues in cosmetic surgery, including assessing patient expectations, screening for psychopathology, insuring informed consent, and evaluating postoperative psychologic responses to surgery.
3. Reviewing critical factors in treating patients undergoing reconstructive surgery, including: describing patterns of psychologic response to reconstructive surgery; suggesting constructive methods of patient referral for psychiatric evaluation and treatment; defining factors influencing patient response to disfigurement; and advocating for the use of all available resources to maximize psychologic rehabilitation.

Body Image and Plastic Surgery

The ultimate goal of plastic surgery is to alter the patient's body image (i.e., to change their subjective perception of their body (5) and to improve the patient's quality of life (6)). To fully understand the power, beauty, and "magic" of plastic surgery, and to be effective in managing the psychologic concerns of patients, the surgeon must understand body image (2).

A critical facet of body image is the degree to which it is directly related to feelings about self (7). Stated simply, if we feel positive about our bodies, we are more likely to feel positively about ourselves and our lives. The most important disease treated by plastic surgeons is the feelings associated with deformity (8), including a sense of personal inadequacy that strikes at the heart of identity—the sense of self.

Robert Goldwyn (9) reminds us that ". . . the word *patient* is derived from *pati,* Latin for 'to suffer'" (p. 10) and that suffering is not confined to physical pain and loss of function. For plastic surgery patients, suffering is largely the result of a negative body image. The plastic surgeon's professional mission is to relieve this suffering by facilitating the patient's creation of a more positive body image (5,10,11).

CHANGING NEGATIVE BODY IMAGE

Psychologic changes brought about by plastic surgery focus on reducing the negative feelings an individual has about physical appearance. Specifically, plastic surgery facilitates changes in body-image cognition, emotion, and behavior (5,10,11).

Body Image Cognition

Body-image cognition refers to the thinking that all individuals engage in regarding their appearance (10,11). These cognitive processes may include self-talk (e.g., "My nose is really ugly"), images (pictures the patient has of self-appearance in own mind), or beliefs about appearance (e.g., "If I am disfigured [have small breasts, etc.], then I cannot be happy") (10,11). If surgery results in positive changes in appearance, individuals can then begin to think differently about themselves (i.e., change the way they talk to, imagine, or believe in themselves). However, the surgical change in appearance must be positive in the eyes of the patient.

Body image is, by definition, subjective (8). You cannot know how someone feels about their body on the basis of evaluating their objective appearance. This point is central to understanding and managing all plastic surgery patients; *perception of appearance is completely subjective, and changes in appearance are "improvements" only if the patient evaluates them as such.*

Body Image Emotions

Negative thinking patterns (or their positive and adaptive counterparts) can dramatically influence emotions (10–12). If I consistently engage in self-talk that is derogatory (e.g., "My nose is disgusting"), have a visual image of myself as "ugly," and believe that I am unlovable, my emotions will be directly affected. Depending upon the situation, I may become depressed, resigned, angry, or anxious as a result of this pattern of thinking. Current psychologic techniques can change negative patterns of thinking regarding one's body, which can lead to change in negative patterns of feeling (10–12).

Body Image Behavior

Patterns of negative thinking and emotion are invariably associated with patterns of maladaptive behavior (10, 11). Patients who think they are ugly, and who feel ashamed of their appearance, are likely to develop negative patterns of social interaction (e.g., social withdrawal). Many levels of social interaction can be affected by negative patterns of body image cognition and emotions, including nonverbal behavior during everyday communication and sexual functioning. For example, women with breast disfigurement may believe that "I am not attractive to my partner," feel ashamed of their appearance, and therefore avoid any kind of sexual contact. Positive changes in patterns of thinking can set the stage for, and be facilitated by, positive changes in behavior (e.g., increased positive social interaction) (10–12).

SUMMARY

The motivation to undergo plastic surgery is a sense of disease and body image discomfort that strikes at the heart of an individual's sense of identity. Fully understanding the motivations for, and the effects of, plastic surgery requires insight into how the individual's subjective perception of his body affects his thinking, emotion, and behavior. By creating changes in physical appearance the patient perceives as positive, surgeons set the stage for patients to change their patterns of thinking, emotion, and behavior. Most important, they have helped individuals to change their identity and overall quality of life.

Cosmetic Surgery Patients: Psychologic Issues

The critical variables essential to understanding and caring for the psychologic needs of cosmetic surgery patients include: (a) understanding patient expectations, (b) screening for the most common forms of psychopathology, (c) assessing patients' evaluation of surgical risk and benefit, and (d) evaluating the postoperative psychologic impact of surgery (13). All four sets of variables are essential to consider. Shortcuts for the sake of clinical efficiency are possible, but only at the cost of compromising clinical effectiveness.

ASSESSING PATIENT EXPECTATIONS

Cosmetic surgery patients have three distinct types of expectations (13). They obviously have expectations regarding the desired changes in appearance. Additionally, they have explicit or implicit expectations regarding how they will respond emotionally to surgery (i.e., psychologic expectations) and how others will respond to them (i.e., social expectations).

Understanding all three sets of expectations serves to structure preoperative patient evaluation. The relevant information can be elicited relatively quickly and with little intrusiveness. Failure to evaluate any of these expectations increases the likelihood of patient dissatisfaction. By evaluating expectations, the surgeon conveys concern for the patient's total well-being, thus laying a solid foundation for the development of a positive professional relationship. There is nothing more fun-

damental to psychologic understanding and managing patients than paying close and constant attention to the patient-physician relationship (9).

Surgical Expectations

It is imperative that patients have clear and realistic expectations regarding the surgical changes they desire. The ability to distinguish between "realistic" and "idealistic" expectations regarding surgical outcome is highly predictive of patient satisfaction with surgical outcome (5). Recent research strongly suggests that ". . . idealistic expectations are pathognomic of potential problems postoperatively" (5, p. 199). Additionally, creating high patient expectations through advertising, or by compiling ". . . a flattering portfolio of excellent results for prospective patients to review. . ." (5, p. 200) risks increasing the probability of some patients being disappointed postoperatively (5).

A fundamental and seemingly obvious principle of psychologic management is that the patient's subjective evaluation of the surgical outcome determines the ultimate impact of cosmetic surgery (i.e., the degree to which the patient's quality of life is improved). This fundamental observation leads to the admonition against surgeons imposing their own aesthetic standards on patients. The surgeon must view the outcome of the operation through the eyes of the patient, not from the perspective of objective aesthetic standards or the surgeon's subjective perception. It is the patient's subjective perception of the surgical outcome that is the gold standard by which the success of surgery is measured (5).

We were reminded of this fundamental principle recently when evaluating a male patient who underwent rhinoplasty for a posttraumatic deformity (to straighten the nose) but who did not expect a reduction in the dorsal hump. At the time of the initial preoperative consultation there was only a brief discussion of the hump reduction (which was undertaken) and an extended discussion of chin augmentation (which the patient did not request, want, or undergo). The patient was partly dissatisfied with the postoperative nasal appearance. In this instance, the surgeon undertook the "reasonable" (but wrong) approach of reducing the prominent hump "while he was there"; however, this was not in keeping with the patient's expectations. The patient was pleased with the postoperative nasal straightening but not with nasal reduction.

Positive changes in appearance are defined as "positive" by the patient. Suggestions for surgical improvements not requested by the patient (e.g., those offered by the surgeon or family members) should be undertaken with only the greatest of care, if at all, and only after multiple preoperative evaluations. Additionally, patients who have vague, nonspecific requests for surgical change, or those willing to defer the definition of change to the surgeon, should be approached with great caution.

Psychologic Expectations

All patients seeking cosmetic surgery are motivated to change their body image (i.e., to change the psychologic experience of their body and achieve a reduction in body-image dysphoria). Having obtained a clear understanding of surgical expectations, and assuming these are reasonable, the surgeon should make a statement similar to the following: "All of my patients have hopes about how they are going to feel after surgery. How do you imagine you will feel after undergoing the operation? We know surgery can change how you look, but how do you think the operation might change your life?"

Many patients will respond with a reply similar to the following: "I will feel better about myself." The surgeon should inquire further about the nature of the motivations and emotions leading up to the request for surgery. For example, the surgeon can ask: "How has your appearance affected the way you feel about yourself?" "How long have you been thinking about having surgery?" "When did you first start to think about it?" "Why do you want surgery now and not a year ago or a year in the future?" "In what way has your appearance affected your behavior?" "How do you expect to feel, think, or act differently after surgery?" "In what specific situations do you believe you will be more comfortable after having the operation?"

Answers to such questions provide the surgeon with some of the information necessary to ascertain if the patient has reasonable expectations. Even more important, such questions provide insight into the patient's overall psychologic functioning and may reveal any current or past psychopathology.

Social Expectations

To understand the patient's social expectations, it is helpful to know how the individuals closest to the patient feel about the operation (14,15). How does the patient expect the important people in his life will respond to the operation? Are they supportive? Are they in any way responsible for the patient wanting the surgery? If a patient is being "pushed" by a family member, or if a patient is going against the advice of a close family member, these factors can significantly influence the patient's ultimate reaction to the operation. Preoperative discussion of these issues can be productive, particularly if the patient is hoping to change the behavior of someone else as a result of undergoing surgery (e.g., to win someone's affection) (14,15).

Summary

Any indication that patient expectations regarding the surgical, psychologic, or social outcome of surgery are problematic warrant a more intensive patient evaluation. In many instances, surgeons may want to insure clear communication regarding expectations by routinely scheduling multiple preoperative patient evaluations. In some instances, the psychologic safety and efficacy of providing surgery may be questioned. In those instances, a more complete psychologic evaluation is required.

SCREENING FOR PSYCHOLOGIC DISORDERS

Most cosmetic surgery patients do not evidence psychopathology. However, a significant minority present with some form of psychologic disorder that requires a more complete psychologic evaluation and that may affect the decision to undertake surgery. Disorders that may be encountered include: Body Dysmorphic Disorder, Personality Disorders, and Eating Disorders (DSM-IV). Other psychologic problems encountered in cosmetic surgery patients include depression, alcohol abuse, and anxiety. These will be reviewed later.

Body Dysmorphic Disorder (BDD)

Patients with Body Dysmorphic Disorder (BDD) are well known to plastic surgeons (16–18). The defining feature of BDD is that the patient has an intensely negative emotional response to some aspect of their appearance, despite the fact that there is little or no evidence for objective deformity (18). These patients often present with the classic contraindications for cosmetic surgery, including minimal deformity (19), multiple consultations with plastic surgeons, an obsessive focus on appearance, and emotional volatility.

Currently, there are no accurate estimates of the incidence of BDD in the population of cosmetic surgery patients (18). Additionally, the intensity of symptom presentation is widely variable. A subgroup of patients appear to have psychotic features, making the differential diagnosis of BDD from somatic delusions critical to consider (18).

BDD patients are invariably challenging to the surgeon and require special management and tremendous amounts of consultation time. Psychiatric input into the evaluation and possible treatment of BDD patients is absolutely necessary. The challenge of differential diagnosis (e.g, psychotic versus nonpsychotic symptom presentation), issues of patient competency to make medical decisions and to provide informed consent, possible alternative or adjunctive approaches to treatment, and predictions regarding the safety and efficacy of undertaking surgery with these patients are all areas in which the psychiatric consultation is mandatory (18).

Many surgeons choose to eliminate these patients from their practices, believing that they cannot be helped with surgery, and lacking experience in treating such patients. However, extensive clinical experience has demonstrated that many individuals with similar symptoms can be helped with a well-structured program of surgical-psychologic evaluation and intervention (20). The resources to conduct such programs are not widely available, and there are some important differences of opinion regarding treatment strategies and efficacy (21). However, plastic surgeons have a professional obligation to address the needs of these long-suffering patients (22).

Personality Disorders

Experienced observers of the psychologic functioning of plastic surgery patients have described specific and unique patterns of maladaptive patient responses to stress (1,4). Napoleon (4) identified the most common personality types observed in plastic surgery, including patients with Narcissistic, Dependent, and Borderline personality features.

Patients with Narcissistic personalities are among the most common in plastic surgery (4). In addition to being arrogant, they have a grandiose sense of self-importance and a belief they are special, and they also feel entitled to special treatment (18). Their hypersensitivity to any social slight, fragile self-esteem, and belief that there should be "automatic compliance" with their expectations, places them at increased risk for negative responses to even minor problems (e.g., small complications, brief delays) (18). They are more likely to seek legal recourse for the "wrongs" that have been done to them (4). When their very strong needs for approval and praise are unfulfilled, patient management problems ensue. These patients must be handled with special care, because they respond negatively to any "perceived" slight. However, if given the full attention they feel they deserve, and if there are no violations of their expectations, they will respond positively to the surgery.

Patients with Dependent Personality are usually passive individuals who look to other people to make their decisions, take responsibility for them, and to provide reassurance (18). They are often very reluctant to express their real feelings or thoughts because of their desperate need to obtain the approval of others (18). "When all is going well such people are amiable, obliging, and a pleasure to be around" (1). However, they are at increased risk for postoperative disappointment if they do not clearly express their expectations for the outcome of surgery. Additionally, under the stress of surgery they can become very "needy," demanding, and childlike (1), sometimes alternating between angry outbursts (often directed at support staff) and tearful apologies (to the surgeon). "They require expressions of warmth and concern" (1).

Plastic surgery patients with borderline personality characteristics are among the most challenging to manage (5). By definition, these individuals are emotionally volatile, unstable, and impulsive (18). This personality type is likely to be the least satisfied with surgery (4). Additionally, for these individuals, even small complications can result in ". . . a catastrophe of immense proportions" (4, p. 202). It also appears that they are more likely to initiate legal action (4). Of greatest clinical relevance to their management is that patients with borderline personality features often enter into the patient-physician relationship with an extremely positive (albeit inflated) evaluation of the surgeon. The scenario of patient idealization is a theme that is evident when analyzing the dynamics of plastic surgery malpractice claims (4).

Characteristically, the initial patient-surgeon contact had been one where the surgeon was idealized in the eyes of the patient. In each case, this idealization transformed into hatred postoperatively. The transformation from "all good" to "all bad" had begun, but was not "caused," by a postoperative medical complication in each malpractice claim. Idealization, therefore, can be an early warning of problems to come. (4, p. 206)

Therefore, surgeons should be even more cautious when encountering patients who place them on a "pedestal." This idealization may indicate inflated and unachievable expectations (regarding all aspects of care) and may indicate the presence of borderline personality disorder.

Evaluating patient personality functioning is very challenging. It is most effectively accomplished by monitoring the patient-surgeon relationship. Clues to predicting patient management problems are often evident on the basis of how the patient makes the surgeon feel. If the surgeon begins to feel irritated, angry, or uncomfortable, or if the surgeon has an atypical emotional response to a patient, this can be an important stimulus to "step back" and scrutinize the patient's psychologic functioning. Additionally, the physician should play close attention to the emotional reactions of trusted staff members to specific patients. Individuals with personality disorders often elicit conflict among staff members who ordinarily interact well together. In general, if a patient is eliciting significant negative attention from those involved in their care, this is an important clue to devote even greater amounts of time and attention to psychologic issues.

Eating Disorders

As many as 8% of the female adolescent and young adult population in the United States have some symptoms of Anorexia Nervosa and/or Bulimia Nervosa (23). These young women are preoccupied with their physical appearance and experience body image distortions (18). They engage in dieting and extreme forms of appetite and weight control. As a general rule, they take great efforts to keep their symptoms hidden.

Some of these individuals seek out plastic surgery and are most likely to request body sculpting procedures, liposuction, and breast related operations (24,25). Some patients may request changes in facial appearance (e.g., reduction of enlarged parotid glands).

The problem with providing these young women with surgery is that the procedures only addresses a symptom of a much larger problem with body dissatisfaction and distortion. Though they are likely to be pleased with the surgical outcome, it is not clear that surgery results in an overall improvement in quality of life or a fundamental change in body image. When surgeons suspect that a young woman requesting surgery may have an eating disorder, they should directly address their concern.

EVALUATING PATIENT PERCEPTION OF SURGICAL RISK AND BENEFIT

The primary reason to undertake the risks inherent in any surgical procedure is the physical and psychologic benefit of the operation. "The weighing of risks and benefits for cosmetic surgery is directly related to the patient's psychologic expectations for cosmetic surgery, and therefore, in effect, it is a requirement of the informed consent process to discuss these expectations" (26, p. 69).

Therefore, in the initial evaluation of cosmetic surgery patients, it is essential to review their evaluation of surgical risk and benefit (26). How well does the patient understand and remember the explanation of the risks described by the surgeon, and how does he weigh these in comparison to the expected benefits of surgery? The surgeon must focus on the risks of surgery (including postoperative discomfort, risk of minor and serious complications, changes in sensory functioning, and the permanent impact of surgical scars) and how these are evaluated in relation to the expected benefits.

SUMMARY

Remember that the only indication for cosmetic surgery is to improve emotional health. Thus, effective management of cosmetic surgery patients requires that attention be given to psychologic factors. In addition to the patient types already described, some others require extra attention, including women desiring removal of breast implants, adolescents, patients requesting multiple surgical procedures (4,27), and some male patients (13). Each of these groups of individuals is likely to be somewhat more psychologically vulnerable than the typical cosmetic surgery patient.

Furthermore, attention given to psychologic factors should extend to evaluating patient response in the postoperative period. Inevitably, there are a minority of patients who are dissatisfied with a less-than-ideal surgical outcome.

In this situation, the wise advice of Robert Goldwyn (9) should be followed, that is, admit the reality, make a very clear plan for addressing the problem, enlist the patient's support, and be sure that you are readily available to the patient.

For those patients who are dissatisfied despite a technically successful surgery, retrospective analysis often reveals that one of the factors already discussed (e.g., violations of implicit or explicit expectations or patient psychopathology) resulted in the patient dissatisfaction (28). These patients should receive a great deal of attention (9) and be given appointments at times when the surgeon will not be rushed and can devote their full attention to the patient. The surgeon must resist the natural tendency to withdraw emotionally from these individuals. In some instances, a surgical and/or psychiatric consultant will be of great help in addressing patient concerns.

Reconstructive Surgery Patients: Critical Psychologic Issues

Plastic surgeons contribute to the psychologic adaptation of reconstructive surgery patients by adapting their professional style of interaction to the patient's particular emotional response, identifying problematic psychologic responses and, when necessary, providing compelling and compassionate referral for psychiatric evaluation and treatment. Patients greatly appreciate surgeons taking a genuine interest in their psychosocial functioning in addition to minimizing disfigurement and maximizing function. Critical psychologic factors to consider when caring for reconstructive surgery patients are presented in Table 108–1.

Table 108–1
Psychological Management of Reconstructive Surgery Patients

General Principles of Psychological Management
1. Clarify expectations regarding the anticipated outcome, challenges and limitations of surgical reconstruction.
2. Seek first to understand patients' unique concerns, and only then give reassurance and information.
3. Identify common patterns of psychological response and evaluate impact on overall functioning.
4. When necessary, provide additional supportive interventions and compassionate, convincing psychiatric referral.

Psychological Responses to Disfigurement and Surgical Reconstruction
Anxiety
Depression
Substance abuse
Regression and dependency
Denial

Factors Influencing Psychological Response
Etiology of disfigurement
Extent and salience of disfigurement
Patient developmental stage

Interventions to Enhance Patient Rehabilitation
Support groups
Image enhancement
Social skills training
Body image therapy

GENERAL PRINCIPLES OF PSYCHOLOGIC MANAGEMENT

Some helpful general principles for managing the psychologic concerns of reconstructive surgery patients include the following:

1. Ideally, surgeons assist patients and families in creating realistic expectations for the process and outcome of surgical reconstruction in the most consistent and compassionate manner possible. The surgeon's challenge is to maintain the delicate balance between hope and surgical reality.

    Describing the process and outcome of surgical reconstruction is beyond the task of obtaining informed consent for any specific procedure. Rather, repeated and accurate description of the final surgical outcome (to the degree this is possible) and the entire process of surgical reconstruction is essential to striking the balance between hope and reality. The difficulties and shortcomings of the reconstruction must be discussed when patients can assimilate the information, and with language the family understands. Repeating information may be necessary, and will cultivate the trust and understanding essential to establishing the patient-physician relationship.

2. The most powerful step in establishing the patient-physician professional relationship is to follow a basic rule for highly effective human relations: "Seek first to understand and only then to be understood" (29). Surgeons are advised to practice the seemingly obvious principle of seeking first to understand clearly each patient's unique concerns before providing information or reassurance. "Facile, nonspecific reassurance can undermine the physician-patient relationship, as the patient is likely to feel the physician is out of touch with and not really interested in what they are actually feeling" (30, p. 585).

3. The plastic surgeon can significantly enhance their ability to care for patients by learning to identify and effectively respond to the most common patterns of psychologic reactions—including anxiety, depression, and substance abuse, as well as denial and regression.

4. Surgeons can develop effective responses to these patient reactions. Depending on the particular situation, the surgeon can provide an increased level of psychologic support, treat the symptoms of emotional distress, or refer the patient for psychiatric evaluation and treatment.

How surgeons refer patients for psychiatric consultation dramatically influences patient compliance with the recommendation. A critical step toward creating a convincing and compassionate referral for psychiatric evaluation (for reconstructive and cosmetic surgery) is for the surgeon to have complete confidence in the psychiatrist's ability to provide services tailored to plastic surgery patients.

To complete this prerequisite, surgeons should establish a long-term relationship with a psychiatric consultant who will evaluate the full spectrum of plastic surgery patients and who is familiar with the professional literature on the psychologic aspects of plastic surgery. Taking these steps will reduce the discomfort shared by many surgeons (2) in recommending psychiatric evaluation to patients.

In general, it is most helpful to establish a relationship with a psychiatrist (as opposed to a clinical psychologist or clinical social worker) because of the need for the consultant to evaluate the patient's medical history, the possible role of medications in causing or exacerbating psychologic symptoms, and, if necessary, to prescribe psychotropic medications.

When surgeons refer patients for psychiatric evaluation, they should do so ". . . with the same attitude and for the same reasons as in the referral to, for example, a cardiologist" (1). The surgeon can explain exactly why the referral is needed and not ". . . fumble around or use euphemisms such as "nerve doctor" or "another specialist" (1). "Call the psychiatrist a psychiatrist" (1). It is also essential to convey to the patient that you are doing what you believe to be in their best interests (1). Remind the patient that all deformities cause some emotional distress and some problems in adaptation.

PSYCHOLOGIC RESPONSE TO DISFIGUREMENT AND SURGICAL RECONSTRUCTION

Plastic surgeons regularly encounter predictable patterns of psychologic response to disfigurement and surgical reconstruction, including (a) anxiety, (b) depression, (c) substance abuse, (d) regression and dependency; and (e) denial.

Anxiety

Anxiety is common in plastic surgery patients. Some patients experience anxiety regarding anesthesia or worry that surgical reconstruction will not be completed (30). For some patients, anxiety is triggered by providing personal information or being physically examined, which are routine for the medical staff but stressful for many patients (30). Some patients fear loss of control and/or pain (30).

There are many forms of anxiety response, ranging in intensity from mild to severe. Surgeons should monitor patient symptoms of physiologic overarousal, worry, and generalized tension, and evaluate the degree to which these impact patient functioning (e.g., sleep patterns).

One anxiety disorder of particular relevance to patients who have sustained traumatic injury is posttraumatic stress disorder (PTSD). The symptoms of PTSD include reexperiencing the trauma (e.g., dreaming about or having flashbacks of the traumatic event) (18). Patients report symptoms of increased arousal (e.g., sleep difficulties, or unusual levels of irritability, anger, or tension). Some patients experience symptoms involving the ". . . avoidance of stimuli associated with the trauma and the numbing of general responsiveness" (18, p. 428). Such patients avoid talking about the trauma, in addition to avoiding any stimuli associated with the trauma (e.g., avoiding automobiles if they were injured in one). They may also report the "inability to recall an important aspect of the trauma" (18, p. 428). Posttraumatic stress disorder symptoms are common in individuals sustaining hand injury (31,32), burn injury (33,34), and facial trauma. For some patients, onset of symptoms occurs long after the trauma (i.e., 6 months or more) (18). For all patients experiencing PTSD symptoms, there is great personal suffering and a negative effect on rehabilitation. The surgeon can begin to relieve this suffering by identifying and labeling the symptoms and providing the appropriate intervention.

Interventions for Anxiety Responses

Much patient anxiety can be relieved through proper use of reassurance and information. "Knowing the patient's specific fears leads the physician to the appropriate therapeutic interventions. . . . If the physician wrongly presumes to know why the patient is anxious without asking, then the patient is likely to feel misunderstood" (30, p. 585).

In some instances, even when reassurance and information directly address the patient's specific concern, it is still not enough to quell patients' anxieties. In these instances, benzodiazepines can be helpful for short-term relief of anxiety symptoms; however, great care should be taken in their use (30). They have potential for physical and psychologic dependence and can exacerbate PTSD symptoms. They also have a synergistic effect with alcohol, which some individuals use to reduce symptoms of tension and sleep difficulties. Any long-term (i.e., greater than 2 weeks) prescription of antianxiety medication should be monitored by a psychiatrist because of the potential for coexisting psychiatric disorder (e.g., depression) requiring different forms of treatment (30).

Deciding to recommend psychiatric consultation is based on the patient's anxiety response. Is it beyond what would be considered "normal" (e.g., some worry/tension regarding anesthesia or the surgical outcome) (30). This determination is often difficult to make.

Anxiety is usually a symptom of psychiatric disorder when it remains unrealistic or out of proportion despite the physician's clarification and reassurance. Other signs that anxiety requires psychiatric intervention are sustained disruption of sleep or gastrointestinal functions, marked autonomic hyperarousal (tachycardia, . . . sweating), and panic attacks. Psychiatric consultation should always be requested when anxiety fails to respond to low doses of benzodiazepines, is accompanied by psychosis, or renders the patient unable to participate in their medical care. . . . (30, p. 585)

Depression

Major depression is experienced by as many as 1 out of 4 women over the course of a lifetime, in addition to being quite common in men and individuals with a medical illness (18). Plastic surgeons regularly encounter individuals with clinical levels of depression.

It is essential to recognize symptoms of depression so the patient can be referred for the effective treatments currently available. Failure to identify and treat symptoms of depression can result in unnecessary patient suffering and negatively affect patient rehabilitation. In the most serious instances, this failure can result in patient suicide.

The defining characteristics of depression include: depressed mood, loss of interest in usual activities, significant weight loss or gain (5% change), changes in sleep patterns, loss of energy, persistent fatigue, feelings of worthlessness, recurrent thoughts of death (including suicidal thoughts and preoccupation with any death-related topic), increased agitation/restlessness, as well as inability to concentrate or make decisions (18). The patient may report these symptoms, or they may be observed by the family, physician, or other member of the health care team.

It is important to specify that there is no one defining symptom of depression. Rather, depression is most accurately described as a syndrome involving changes in mood, thinking, and biologic functions (sleeping, eating, sex) that negatively affects the individuals daily functioning (18).

A challenge in managing depression is distinguishing between "normal" depression (i.e., a reasonable emotional response to trauma or illness) and depression requiring treatment.

Patients experiencing normal degrees of depression retain their abilities to communicate, make decisions, and participate in their own care when encouraged to do so. Depression usually constitutes a psychiatric disorder when depressed mood, hopelessness, worthlessness, withdrawal, and vegetative symptoms (e.g., insomnia, anorexia, fatigue) are present and out of proportion to the coexisting medical illness. Urgent psychiatric referral should always be obtained when the patient is thinking about suicide . . . or has depression with psychotic symptoms. Psychiatric consultation should also be obtained if less serious depression fails to improve with the physician's support and reassurance, if antidepressant medication is needed, or if patients remain too depressed to participate in their own health care and rehabilitation (30, p. 587).

It is recommended that plastic surgeons not conduct the psychopharmacologic treatment of depression; because of the many developments in medication management and the critical issues of differential diagnosis, this is best addressed by a psychiatrist. However, it is essential that surgeons maintain a willingness to monitor the treatment so that the patients do not feel abandoned.

Alcohol Abuse

Plastic surgeons regularly encounter individuals with alcohol-related problems. Some reconstructive surgery patients, particularly those with a family history of substance abuse or depression, may use alcohol to "self-medicate" the negative feelings often associated with disfigurement and the stress of undergoing reconstructive surgery. Alcohol use also plays a role in placing some individuals at risk for sustaining injury, and can negatively impact rehabilitation (35).

The critical features of alcohol dependence include the continued use of alcohol despite knowledge that social, psychologic, or physical problems result from this use (18). Additional signs include the individual spending an inordinate amount of time engaging in alcohol use or neglecting to perform important social roles as a result of alcohol use (18). Individuals with alcohol problems may also manifest tolerance or withdrawal symptoms (18).

Some clues that a patient may be having problems with alcohol include the smell of alcohol on a patient during consultation or a comment from a family member. If the surgeon is concerned that an alcohol problem may exist, it is reasonable to inquire by simply stating "I do not want to intrude on your life, but I am concerned and would like to be of help if I can. I am wondering if you are having any difficulties related to alcohol."

Four screening questions, defined as the CAGE questionnaire (36), are very helpful in identifying individuals with an alcohol-related problem:

1. Cut down. Have you ever felt that you should cut down on your drinking?
2. Annoyed. Have other people annoyed you by criticizing your drinking?
3. Guilt. Have you ever felt guilty about drinking?
4. Eye-opener. Have you ever taken a drink in the morning to steady your nerves or to get rid of hangover? (36)

If the patient answers yes to any one of these questions, a more complete evaluation is warranted. However, the most difficult challenge in evaluating alcohol abuse is that patients, families, and physicians are prone to deny alcohol-related problems and choose to ignore signs and symptoms that are evident. It is not the surgeon's responsibility to ensure that patients obtain evaluation or treatment. However, it is the surgeon's responsibility to recognize and respond to signs that may be evident, to review the above screening questions, and to present the availability of evaluation and treatment options in a compelling and compassionate manner.

Additional Psychiatric Problems

In addition to the psychologic responses already described, there are many others evident in reconstructive surgery patients. For example, some patients become extremely dependent and emotionally regressed when under pre- or postoperative stress (1,30). These patients behave in a childlike manner, often requiring massive amounts of support and reassurance. Other patients will evidence denial of their illness or disfigurement (1,30). Denial can be adaptive in some reconstructive surgery patients (30). If patient denial does not interfere with treatment, there is no reason to intervene. However, when patient denial can lead to harm, then the surgeon needs to address it, most likely by enlisting the help of both the family and a psychiatric consultant.

Other psychiatric problems encountered by plastic surgeons include delirium, dementia, substance withdrawal, and prolonged pain-management problems. Additionally, patients may be suspected of malingering (i.e., lying for the purposes of gaining money, workmen's compensation, or some other external gain) or factitious disorder (i.e., disorders that are self-created in order to take on the sick role) (37). These disorders are all occasionally encountered by most plastic surgeons. Psychiatric referral is essential for each.

Factors Influencing Psychologic Adaptation to Disfigurement

Psychologic adaptation to disfigurement and surgical reconstruction is unique for each individual and is influenced by many factors including the etiology, salience and extent of the disfigurement, as well as the individual's age and gender.

ETIOLOGY OF DISFIGUREMENT

Plastic surgeons generally need to provide more emotional support to patients with an acquired disfigurement than to patients with congenital disfigurement. Many psychologic challenges are inherent in adapting to congenital disfigurement. However, it is more psychologically disruptive to sustain a traumatic disfigurement than to have congenital disfigurement.

With congenital anomalies, there is time to incorporate the malformation into a sense of self. The individual may not like what is reflected in the mirror, but recognizes the image as his/her own, for better or worse. Further, there is a lifetime to prepare for the problems of being identifiably different. The trauma patient has had a lifetime of looking one way, and now must cope with looking both different and worse (38, p. 249).

Changes in appearance, body image, and identity, along with stresses inherent in surgical treatment, make it necessary that the surgeon spend extra time to ensure that patients with acquired disfigurement are understood and their concerns addressed. It is also more likely that they will present with acute symptoms of emotional disturbance (e.g., anxiety, depression, substance abuse) requiring psychiatric intervention.

SALIENCE AND EXTENT OF DISFIGUREMENT

There is no way to predict which patients will require increased psychologic support on the basis of the salience or the extent of their disfigurement. It is well known that there is no necessary correlation between the extent of disfigurement and the degree of emotional response (39).

The consistent negative social response to facial disfigurement (40) and the unique functional and aesthetic impact of hand injuries are massive challenges to psychologic adaptation (41). However, consistent with the subjectivity of body image responses, some individuals with a disfigurement hidden from view can be dramatically affected. For example, the impact of mastectomy and breast reconstruction is well documented (1), as are the problems with breast burns (42). However, the impact of "hidden injuries" is not necessarily limited to those areas of the body that are emotionally loaded (e.g., breasts and genitals) (42,43).

DEVELOPMENTAL STAGE AND GENDER

A few generalizations can be made regarding developmental stage and psychologic adaptation to disfigurement. Disfigurement acquired before 2 years of age, and which does not progress over time, is more likely to result in psychologic adaptation similar to that of individuals with congenital deformities (4). School-age children and adolescents with a congenital or acquired disfigurement are more likely to experience increases in social and psychologic disruption (44).

Predictions regarding psychologic adaptation in relation to gender are very difficult to make. Females are subject to, and have internalized, more stringent standards regarding physical appearance, making it more likely that adapting to disfigurement will be difficult. However, women are able to more readily adapt to body changes than males (45). At present, no clear generalizations can be made, except that it is not safe to assume that adjustment to disfigurement is necessarily more difficult for women.

SUMMARY

Many additional factors can influence patients' psychologic adaptation. Perhaps one of the most important is the degree of social support experienced by the patient. This support can come from family, friends, the community, the physician, and ideally from many available sources. In general, patients with traumatic disfigurement, who have little social support and poor pre-injury social and psychologic functioning, are in greatest need of psychologic intervention.

Rehabilitation Interventions for Reconstructive Surgery Patients

Many reconstructive surgery patients who do not have identifiable psychiatric disturbances or profound negative psychologic reactions still experience the emotional challenges inherent in having any form of disfigurement. Much can be done to facilitate their rehabilitation, including making available the following resources: (a) networking and support groups, (b) techniques of image enhancement, (c) social skills interventions, and (d) body image therapy. Plastic surgeons play a pivotal role in ensuring that patients obtain these rehabilitation services.

NETWORKING AND SUPPORT GROUPS

Many patient support groups and networks are currently available and are valuable in providing patients with information and emotional support. For example, for those individuals with a facial disfigurement, there are numerous resources, which are often designed to serve specific populations (e.g., the Phoenix Society for burn survivors, and SPOHNC, a support group for people with oral and head and neck cancer). A helpful compilation of resources is available (46).

SOCIAL SKILLS TRAINING

Many individuals with facial disfigurement have difficulty in establishing positive patterns of interpersonal communication. These difficulties are largely due to the negative social reaction of those who are not disfigured. However, the patient's maladaptive patterns of coping may also contribute to this social strain (47).

Whatever the source of social strain, the responsibility for improving patterns of interpersonal relations falls to the individual with disfigurement (39). Successful programs for teaching social skills to cope with disfigurement exist (47–49). One well-developed program, "Changing Faces," has been found to reduce social anxiety and improve self-confidence (50), and led to the development of the Disfigurement Recovery Unit at Frenchlay Hospital in Bristol, England. Similar services must be made accessible to all patients who desire to learn disfigurement-related rehabilitation.

IMAGE ENHANCEMENT

Image enhancement techniques, utilizing corrective cosmetics, personal grooming techniques, and development of effective nonverbal behavior, exist for individuals with disfigurement. These techniques have been integrated into a well-developed program by Barbara Kammerer Quayle at the Center for Image Enhancement, in cooperation with Department of Plastic Surgery at Ranchos Los Amigos Medical Center. The Image Enhancement Center provides interventions focussing on the use of corrective cosmetics, color analysis, color coordination, and the development of communication skills. Image Enhancement facilitates the rehabilitation of individuals with facial disfigurement by providing effective techniques the individual can use to reduce the negative social response to their disfigurement and empowering the individual to take control over their own body image.

BODY IMAGE THERAPY

One set of techniques that has great potential for facilitating positive rehabilitation of individuals with any form of disfigurement is based on recently developed body image therapies (10,11). For individuals who habitually engage in negative and critical thinking about their appearance, who believe themselves to be unlovable as a result of their disfigurement, or who experience persistent and debilitating body image behaviors or emotions, these interventions hold promise. Future plastic surgery rehabilitation programs will effectively employ these techniques to enhance the positive changes in appearance brought about by plastic surgery.

Conclusion

Plastic surgeons have the magnificent ability to improve patient appearance, body image, and overall psychologic functioning. By developing their abilities to understand and manage the psychologic dynamics of patients, surgeons can more effectively facilitate patient improvements in quality of life.

References

1. Goin JM, Goin MK. Psychological understanding and management of the plastic surgery patient. In: Georgiade NG, et al., eds. *Essentials of plastic, maxillofacial, and reconstructive surgery.* 2nd ed. Baltimore: Williams & Wilkins, 1987; 1127.
2. Goin JM, Goin MK. *Changing the body: psychological effects of plastic surgery.* Baltimore: Williams & Wilkins, 1981.
3. Macgregor FC. Cosmetic surgery: a sociological analysis of litigation and a surgical specialty. *Aesthe Plas Surg* 1984; 8:219.
4. Napoleon A. The presentation of personalities in plastic surgery. *Ann Plast Surg* 1993; 31:193.
5. Pruzinsky T, Edgerton MT. Body image change and cosmetic plastic surgery. In: Cash TF, Pruzinsky T, eds. *Body images: development, deviance, and change.* New York: Guilford Press, 1990; 217.
6. Pruzinsky T. The psychology of plastic surgery: advances in evaluating body image, quality of life, and psychopathology. *Advances Plast Surg* 1995; 12:11.
7. Pruzinsky T, Cash TF. Integrative themes in body image. In: Cash TF, Pruzinsky T, eds. *Body images: development, deviance, and change.* New York: Guilford Press, 1990; 337.
8. Edgerton MT. Deformity is a disease. *Transactions and Studies of the College of Physicians of Philadelphia* 1973; 41:124.
9. Goldwyn RM. *The patient and the plastic surgeon.* 2nd ed. Boston: Little, Brown, 1991.
10. Cash TF. *What do you see when you look in the mirror?* New York: Bantam Books, 1995.
11. Cash TF. *Body-image therapy: a program for self-directed change.* New York: Guilford, 1991.
12. Freedman R. Cognitive-behavioral perspectives on body image change. In: Cash TF, Pruzinsky T, eds. *Body images: development, deviance, and change.* New York: Guilford Press, 1990; 272.
13. Pruzinsky T. Body image and cosmetic plastic surgery: critical factors in patient assessment. In: Thompson JK, ed. *Body image, eating disorders, and obesity: a practical guide for assessment and treatment.* Washington, DC: American Psychological Association (in press).
14. Wengle HP. The psychology of cosmetic surgery: old problems in patient selection seen in a new way. Part II. *Ann Plast Surg* 1986; 16:487.
15. Edgerton MT, Knorr NJ. Motivational patterns of patients seeking cosmetic (aesthetic) surgery. *Plast Reconstr Surg* 1971; 13:136.
16. Jerome L. Body dysmorphic disorder: a controlled study of patients requesting rhinoplasty (letter to the editor). *Am J Psychiatry* 1992; 149:577.
17. Phillips KA. Body dysmorphic disorder: the distress of imagined ugliness. *Am J Psychiatry* 1991; 148:1138.
18. American Psychiatric Association. Diagnostic and statistical manual of mental disorders. 4th ed. Washington, DC: American Psychiatric Association, 1994.
19. Edgerton MT, Jacobson WE, Meyer E. Surgical-psychiatric study of patients seeking plastic (cosmetic) surgery: ninety-eight patients with minimal deformity. *Br J Plast Surg* 1960; 13:136.
20. Edgerton MT, Langman MW, Pruzinsky T. Plastic surgery and psychotherapy in the treatment of 100 psychologically disturbed patients. *Plast Reconstr Surg* 1991; 88:594.
21. Phillips KA, McElroy SL, Lion JR. Letter to the editor commenting on "Plastic surgery and psychotherapy in treatment of psychologically disturbed patients" (Edgerton, Langman, & Pruzinsky, 1992). *Plast Reconstr Surg* 1992; 90:333.
22. Edgerton MT. The plastic surgeon's obligation to the emotionally disturbed patient. *Plast Reconstr Surg* 1975; 48:551.
23. Yager J. Eating disorders. In: Stoudemire A, ed. *Clinical psychiatry for medical students.* Philadelphia: JB Lippencott, 1993; 355.
24. McIntosh VV, Britt E, Bulik CM. Cosmetic breast augmentation and eating disorders. *N Z Med J* 1994; 107:151.
25. Yates A, Shisslak CM, Allender JR, et al. Plastic surgery and the bulimic patient. *Int J Eat Disorder* 1988; 7:557.
26. Pruzinsky T. Psychological factors in cosmetic plastic surgery: Recent developments in patient care. *Plast Surg Nurs* 1993; 13:64–71, 119.
27. Groenman NH, Sauer HC. Personality characteristics of the cosmetic surgical insatiable patient. *Psychotherapy & Psychosomatics* 1983; 40:241.
28. Macgregor FC. Patient dissatisfaction with results of technically satisfactory surgery. *Aest Plast Surg* 1981; 5:27.
29. Covey SR. *The seven habits of highly effective people.* New York: Simon & Schuster, 1989.
30. Levenson JL. Psychiatric aspects of medical practice. In: Stoudemire A, ed. *Clinical psychiatry for medical students.* Philadelphia: JB Lippencott, 1994; 580.
31. Grunert BK, Devine CA, Matloub HS, et al. Flashbacks after traumatic hand injuries: prognostic indicators. *J Hand Surg* 1988; 13:125.
32. Grunert BK, Matloub HS, Sanger JR, et al. Treatment of posttraumatic stress disorder after work-related trauma. *J Hand Surg* 1990; 15:511.
33. Couremanche DJ, Robinow O. Recognition and treatment of posttraumatic stress disorder in the burn victim. *J Burn Care Rehab* 1989; 10:247.
34. Patterson DR, Carrigan L, Questad KA, et al. Post-traumatic stress disorder in hospitalized burn patients. *J Burn Care Rehabil* 1990; 11:181.
35. Pires M. Substance abuse: the silent saboteur in rehabilitation. *Nurs Clin N Am* 1989; 24:291.
36. Ewing JA. Detecting alcoholism: The CAGE questionnaire. *JAMA* 1984; 252:1905.
37. Mendez-Fernandez MA. The factitious wound: plastic surgeon beware. *Ann Plast Surg* 1995; 34:187.
38. Pertschuk M. Objective change of objective disfigurement. In: Cash TF, Pruzinsky T, eds. *Body images: development, deviance, and change.* New York: Guilford Press, 1990; 237.
39. Macgregor F. *After plastic surgery: adaptation and adjustment.* New York: Praeger, 1979.
40. Macgregor FC. Facial disfigurement: problems and management of social interaction and implications for mental health. *Aesthet Plast Surg* 1990; 14:249.
41. Grunert BK, Maksud DP. Psychological adjustment to hand injuries: nursing management. *Plast Surg Nurs* 1993; 13:72.
42. Willis-Helmrich JJ. Reclaiming body image: the hidden burn. *J Burn Care Rehab* 1992; 13:64.
43. Breslau AJ. The hidden burn. *The Icarus File* 1989; 7:1.
44. Stoddard FJ. Body image development in the burned child. *J Am Acad Child Psychiat* 1982; 21:502.
45. Fisher S. *Development and structure of the body image.* Hillsdale, NJ: Lawrence Erlbaum, 1986.
46. Wilson B. Resources for people with facial difference, 1995. Let's Face It, Box 711, Concord, MA 10742.
47. Bull R, Rumsey N. *The social psychology of facial appearance.* New York: Springer-Verlag, 1988.
48. Fiegenbaum W. A social training program for clients with facial disfigurations: a contribution to the rehabilitation of cancer patients. *Int J Rehab Research* 1981; 4:501.
49. Kapp-Simon KA, Simon DJ. *Meeting the challenge: a social skills training program for adolescents with special needs.* Chicago: University of Illinois at Chicago Press, 1991.
50. Robinson E, Rumsey N, Partridge J. An evaluation of social skills training for facially disfigured people. Unpublished manuscript, 1994.

109

Aesthetic Restorative Prosthetics

Jane Lupton Bahor, A.S.

In a society where physical beauty is glorified and rewarded, where physically attractive people are envied and emulated, it is increasingly important to offer disfigured persons treatments that normalize appearance, address psychological issues and promote occupational and societal rehabilitation (1).

The goals of making patients feel better, function better, and look better are shared by surgeon and prosthetist alike. There is no question that the skillful autogenous reconstruction of malformed or ablated tissues is preferable to prosthetics whenever possible. However, in situations where surgical restoration may be delayed or inadvisable, restorative facial and somato prosthetics can enhance the physical and psychologic healing of patients suffering disfigurement.

Factors Affecting Surgical Reconstruction

There are a multiplicity of factors that affect surgical reconstruction, including:

- Age of patient
- Reluctance of the patient or family for surgery
- General physical condition such as allergies, diabetes mellitus, kidney disease, heart disease, lung disease
- Immunodeficiencies from chemotherapy or disease
- Poor vascular condition of defect site
- Irradiated tissue or ongoing radiation therapy
- Extensive scarring/history of keloiding/lack of viable tissue (large defect area)
- Condition of potential tissue donor sites/risk of donor site morbidity
- Patient prognosis/history of past recurrence of tumor/type of tumor
- Position of critical nerves

A custom prosthetic restoration made from moulage can be fabricated within 6 to 8 weeks after ablative surgery, when edema has subsided and initial healing has taken place. If prosthetic restoration is a possibility from the initiation of treatment planning, a presurgical visit to the prosthetist is helpful. An early prosthetic consultation can assure a patient that a high-quality, lifelike anatomic restoration can be produced that will enhance their appearance and function. A plan of action, an offering of comfort in addressing their loss, and a thorough discussion of their expectations will help patients to accept their treatment, even if reconstructive surgery is delayed, or impossible.

Extraoral Facial Prosthetics

An extraoral facial prosthesis created by a skillful anaplastologist (2) or maxillofacial prosthodontist (3) may be used as a temporary or permanent device to replace all or portions of an ablated or malformed orbit, nose, or auricle. Addition cured silicone rubber elastomer is the preferred material for most prosthetists because it is inert, easily processed and colored, has a lifelike appearance, and is waterproof and durable.

RETENTION

The status of the defect site can adversely affect retention. A poorly conceived closure in a nasal defect, leaving the superior helical rim when deleting the auricle, or closing an orbital exenteration with a muscle flap (4) can greatly affect the aesthetic and retentive outcome of the finished prostheses.

Traditionally, surgical and ostomy adhesives have been used to retain facial prostheses to the skin (Figs. 109–1, 109–2). These adhesives, along with adhesive removers, have a detrimental effect on all prosthetic materials, resulting in discoloration and disintegration of fragile margins. Adhesive application and removal is often challenging for the elderly and the young, or for those with poor eyesight and other physical disabilities.

Dependency on adhesives is alleviated by mechanical retention using anatomic tissue undercuts, cooperative retention with other prosthetic devices, and bone-anchored implant (osseointegrated) retention.

Mechanical retention can be accomplished by creating a silicone insert behind an orbital or nasal prosthesis. The insert may be in the form of a hollow bulb that is squeezed to fill the orbital or nasal cavity, or a silicone lip extending into the defect. The insert must be flexible and smooth or it will cause irritation during its application and removal. Mechanically retained prostheses work well in patients who have had no recent radiation to the defect site, or who have a deep orbital defect or a nasal defect that is well lined with a split-thickness skin graft.

Nasal or orbital defects may also be lined with polymethylmethacrylate (PMMA) keepers (Fig. 109–3). Made from the master moulage of the patient's defect, these plastic inserts follow the configuration of the defect area and contact marginal skin. The keeper insert carries rare-earth magnets on its outer surface. Adhesive is applied to the back of the keeper, which in turn is adhered to the skin. The facial pros-

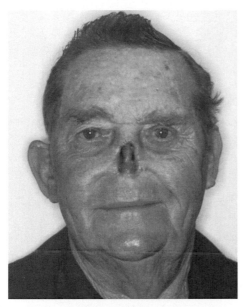

FIG. 109–1. Total nasal defect resulting from squamous cell carcinoma.

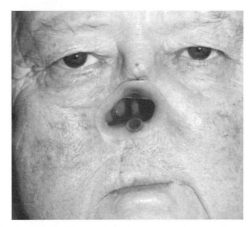

FIG. 109–3. Acrylic "keeper" with rare-earth magnets, adhered to the patient's skin. (Courtesy of Gregory G. Gion, Maxillofacial and Somato Prosthetics, 10501 N. Central Expressway, Suite 311, Dallas, TX 75231.)

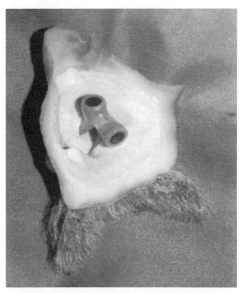

FIG. 109–4. Posterior of prosthesis, showing magnets correlating to keeper magnets. (Courtesy of Gregory G. Gion, Maxillofacial and Somato Prosthetics, 10501 N. Central Expressway, Suite 311, Dallas, TX 75231.)

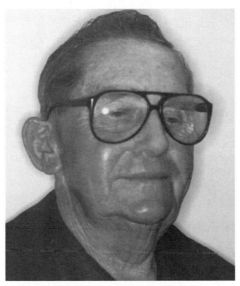

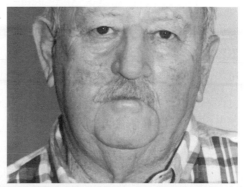

FIG. 109–2. Silicone nasal prosthesis retained by adhesives (prosthesis: Jane Bahor).

thesis, with corresponding magnets, is placed on the keeper (Fig. 109–4). In this manner, a minimum of adhesive is required to retain the device. Strong adhesive is applied to the easily cleaned acrylic keeper and the margins of the silicone prosthesis are preserved (Figure 109–5).

The concept of magnet retention may also be used when a maxillary obturator communicates with a nasal, orbital, or cheek resection. Magnets placed on an acrylic bar imbedded in the facial prosthesis can correspond with magnets on the superior aspect the maxillary obturator bulb. The patient inserts the denture, then applies the extra oral prosthesis. This system works particularly well when used in conjunction

FIG. 109–5. Total nasal prosthesis in position on acrylic keeper. Very light adhesive or petroleum jelly holds thin margins to the skin. (Courtesy of Gregory G. Gion, Maxillofacial and Somato Prosthetics, 10501 N. Central Expressway, Suite 311, Dallas, TX 75231.)

with intraoral implant retention for the denture. The stabilized denture keeps the facial prosthesis from moving during mastication and speech.

OSSEOINTEGRATED RETENTION SYSTEMS

The term *osseointegration* was coined by Per-Ingvar Branemark, a Swedish orthopedist who observed the phenomena in the l950s while doing research in tissue-implant surface relationships. Branemark defines osseointegration as "a direct structural and functional connection between organized living bone and the surface of a load-bearing implant" (5). Although the nature of the biologic association between the implants and living tissue is still being studied, the experiences of the Branemark team over the last 30 years of placing implants in bone has proven that their surgical techniques and product designs offer safe, predictable outcomes in clinical applications.

With this technology it is possible to create prostheses for patients who were virtually untreatable in the past. The fear of dislodgment is alleviated, as the prosthesis is either clipped to a bar or retained by magnets held to an implant-retained abutment. Since application and removal of adhesives isn't necessary, the silicone prosthesis lasts longer and can be designed with thinner, less noticeable margins.

SURGICAL TECHNIQUE/OSSEOINTEGRATED IMPLANTS

In most cases, percutaneous abutments attached to osseointegrated titanium fixtures can be placed in two outpatient surgeries under local anesthesia. The first stage is the placement of the fixtures in the bone; the second stage places titanium abutments through the skin. Within 1 month after the second-stage surgery, the finished prosthesis may be loaded. It is possible for most patients to wear an adhesive-retained prosthesis during the time between the first and second stages.

The craniofacial implant is made of commercially pure titanium, precisely machined, threaded, and cleaned to decrease any unwanted molecules on the implant surface. Meticulous attention to detail in the handling and placement of the fixtures will influence the establishment and maintenance of osseointegration. The implant is placed as gently as possible, with limited drilling at slow speeds with sharp bits and profuse irrigation to minimize damaging heat to the bone. Instrumentation is currently available to keep tissue temperatures under 33° C (6) during drilling, while tapping the bone at the precise depth of the fixture being used (Fig. 109–6).

The craniofacial fixtures are shorter and wider (3.5 mm) than the flangeless dental implant screws intended for the mandible. Jensen, Brownd and Blacker describe the use of the longer 5–7 mm dental implants for the midfacial region for greater load-bearing capacity (7). A careful evaluation of bone thickness using CT scan is useful when considering placement of any implant fixture (8).

The location of the fixtures is established before surgery. A clear acrylic template with openings over the fixture sites is provided by the anaplastologist or prosthodontist. Team planning will insure that the abutment screws and retention framework do not interfere with the anatomic accuracy of the silicone restoration. Two fixtures are necessary in the mastoid to hold a typical aural prosthesis. A minimum of three fixtures are needed for the orbital area (Figs. 109–7, 109–8, 109–9) with two to three fixtures for nasal defects. An extra

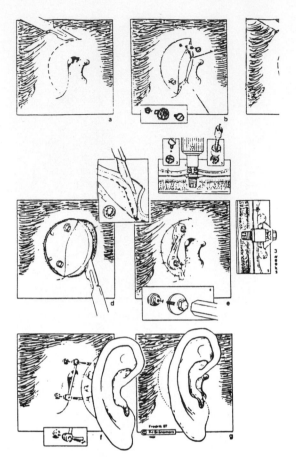

FIG. 109–6. Surgery for the bone-anchored auricular prosthesis. **A,** skin incision. **B,** preparation and threading of holes in the mastoid area and insertion of the fixtures. **C,** incision closed and the implants left unloaded for 3 to 4 months. **D,** exposure of the implants and a reduction in subcutaneous tissue. **E,** suturing of the thinned skin flap in place and punching of holes over the fixtures. Securing of cylinders and attachment of healing caps. **F,** construction of a bar for retention of the prosthesis. **G,** the auricular silicone prosthesis in place. (Courtesy of Anders Tjellstrom, MD, PhD, Department of Otolaryngology, Sahgrens Hospital, University of Göteburg, Göteburg, Sweden.)

fixture is sometimes placed in irradiated bone because the incidence of rejection of the implant increases in patients who have had radiation therapy.

During surgery, the skin is elevated over the planned fixture site. A curvilinear incision is made approximately 1.0 to 1.5 cm from the proposed site and is carried through to the periosteum with the flap reflected and retracted. A second incision through the periosteum is made, and the periosteal flap reflected to the bone. The bone is marked using a burr through the prepared acrylic template. The fixture site is slowly widened with a spiral drill accomplishing 3,000 rpm under constant irrigation. The site is then tapped, with visual bleeding in the drilled bone essential during this stage. The flanged fixture is slowly installed and tightened without irrigation using a hand wrench. A cover screw is inserted into the fixture to prevent bone growth over the top of the implant. The periosteal flap is repositioned and the skin flap thinned, then sutured to close.

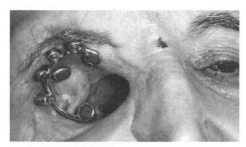

FIG. 109–7. Four Brannemark implants and abutments in the superorbital rim hold a gold bar with magnet retention elements. (Courtesy of Gregory G. Gion, Maxillofacial and Somato Prosthetics, 10501 N. Central Expressway, Suite 311, Dallas, TX 75231.)

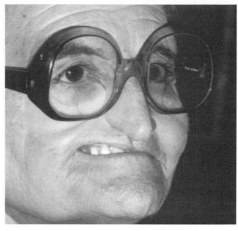

FIG. 109–9. Prosthesis secured by magnets to Brannemark implants. Glasses help to disguise the margins of the orbital defect. (Courtesy of Gregory G. Gion, Maxillofacial and Somato Prosthetics, 10501 N. Central Expressway, Suite 311, Dallas, TX 75231.)

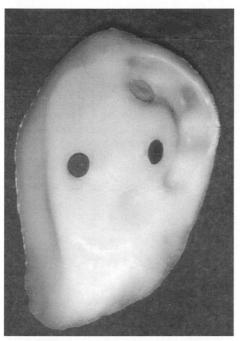

FIG. 109–8. Corresponding magnets on the posterior of the prosthesis allow easy placement by the patient. (Courtesy of Gregory G. Gion, Maxillofacial and Somato Prosthetics, 10501 N. Central Expressway, Suite 311, Dallas, TX 75231.)

Patient selection and education is essential to the success of the procedure because the abutments must be cleaned and maintained by the patient. Without complete cooperation by the wearer and meticulous treatment planning by the surgeon, prosthodontist, and anaplastologist, the success of transcutaneous fixtures cannot be guaranteed.

CUSTOM FABRICATED IMPLANTS

Alloplastic craniofacial implants may be custom made for surgical insertion to obturate bone loss and to restore contour. Custom fabricated implants in the craniofacial region reduce surgery time and eliminate the use of autopolymerizing methylmethacrylate in the operating arena (12). Traditionally, materials used by anaplastologists and prosthodontists have been heat-cured, medical-grade silicone elastomers and heat-cured PMMA. Using palpation, moulage, radiograph, and scans, the prosthetist designs a model of the implant, then processes the form from the appropriate material.

Unpigmented, heat-vulcanized PMMA, cured for a minimum of 6 to 10 hours at 160° F, bench-cooled 24 hours, soaked in hot water, (13) polished, perforated, and sterilized, would seem to be the least problematic of the alloplastic alternatives (14). However, the difficulty with any moulage-generated contour implant is its failure to conform precisely to the underlying surface of the bone. Sized, prefabricated implants or autogenous bone or cartilage grafts may be equally unsatisfactory in this regard (15). Any modifications in the operating room can be costly in terms of surgical time and final outcome.

A recent development in the accuracy of prefabricated custom prosthetic implants has come with the advent of reformatted CT data fed into a CAD/CAM milling machine that replicates the bony structures, usually the skull, in a three-dimensional model. The resultant life-sized anatomic model is then used to create templates that are translated into plastic or rubber implants that very accurately seat over existing bone. The implant is then sterilized and surgically inserted, with a minimum of alteration needed (15).

Implants are allowed to rest for 3 months before the second operative procedure (9). It has been shown that premature loading of an implant may result in fibrous tissue formation instead of bone formation at the implant site (10). The second surgical procedure involves exposing the original fixtures and connecting the titanium abutments. Punch holes over the osseointegrated fixtures allow the abutments to penetrate the skin. Most critical in this stage is the thinning of the overlying skin. It is imperative with transcutaneous abutments that free skin movement around the implants be prevented (11) because this can be a source of inflammation or infection. Healing caps are secured to the abutment tops and a figure-of-eight pressure dressing is applied around the abutments and caps. This dressing can be eliminated in 7 to 10 days with fitting of the prosthesis to commence in 2 weeks to 1 month.

Several commercial companies provide the computer-generated skull and will also provide the custom-made implants in either heat-vulcanized silicone rubber (16) or heat-processed PMMA (17).

Controversy regarding the biocompatability of silicone and PMMA continues (18–25). With any implant materials, extreme care must be taken by surgeon and prosthetist to use approved, and proven, substances in the most conscientious manner possible.

Somato Prosthetics

Conventional prostheses for total amputations of the hands and feet are well known. In an effort to meet patient expectations of physical realism, prosthetists and anaplastologists have attempted to replace missing or mutilated extremities in lifelike custom prostheses.

Upper-extremity patients are particularly sensitive to the final aesthetic outcome of their treatment. People view their hands more than any other part of their bodies. The hands are intimately tied to personal perceptions of competency, craftsmanship, sensuality—even machismo. The emotional impact of hand injuries in both men and women cannot be underestimated. A team approach, utilizing the skills of the surgeon, occupational therapist, psychologist/nurse clinician, and prosthetist/anaplastologist can help meet the complex needs of these patients. What is possible, what is predictable, and what is practical must be thoroughly understood by the treatment team, the patient, and the family in order for treatment to work.

In digital amputations where there is a minimum of 2 cm of proximal phalanx remaining distal to the adjacent web space, a reinforced silicone prosthesis can be made to stretch over the residual finger and hold on by suction. Surgically tapering the amputated digit toward the distal allows for a normal-shaped prosthesis. The prosthetic digits are typically filled from the end of the amputation to the fingertip, allowing some translated sensation to be passed to the end of the residual finger when the artificial finger is tapped (Figs. 109–10, 109–11, 109–12).

Prostheses of this type offer passive function only. They are useful in proportion to the length and usefulness of the residual finger. Although artificial digits can restore the hand aesthetically, the prosthesis wearer must be highly motivated to use them (26). Occupational therapy is recommended for patients receiving more than one restoration per hand. Strengthening exercises and repetition tasks are helpful in training a patient to use prosthetic digits (27,28).

In more mutilating injuries of the hand, creative means must be employed to restore certain types of function while preserving the appearance of the hand. Partial hand prostheses that cover all or part of the hand and arm can be fabricated in latex, polyvinylchloride resin (PVC), or silicone rubber. Either pulled, zipped, or strapped on, these prostheses can help patients perform a variety of passive functional chores. In the case of total thumb amputation, a splint can be devised to hold a realistic silicone thumb that will serve as an oppositional post (Fig. 109–13).

Various somato prostheses including breasts, leg fillers, and prosthetic covers for conventional prostheses; feet and toes are possible using the same techniques and materials.

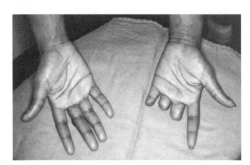

FIG. 109–10. Multiple digit loss from industrial injury. (Photo courtesy of Jane Bahor.)

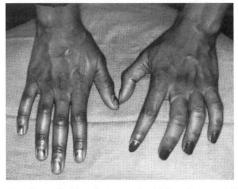

FIG. 109–12. Dorsal side of restored middle, ring, and little fingers of left hand (prostheses: Jane Bahor).

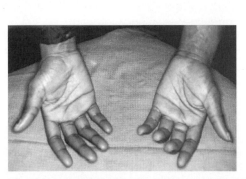

FIG. 109–11. Palmar side of restored middle, ring, and little fingers of left hand (prostheses: Jane Bahor).

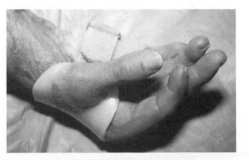

FIG. 109–13. Silicone prosthesis attached to polypropylene splint to provide an oppositional post (prosthesis: Jane Bahor).

Support Groups

Patients suffering disfigurement need special support and understanding. Let's Face It, a support group for the facially disfigured, offers an excellent resource manual for patients and practitioners. Organization names, addresses, and telephone numbers are available through this manual, as well as appropriate tapes and publications (29). Amputee support groups exist in every state and can be tapped through local prosthetic facilities or through the Amputee Coalition of America (30) and the American Amputee foundation (31).

References

1. MacGregor FC. Facial disfigurement: problems and management of social interaction and implications for mental health. *Aesthetic Plast Surg* 1990; 14:249.
2. Anaplastology: def. Artificial anatomical reconstruction as a science or branch of knowledge. American Anaplastology Association, 690 Market St., Suite 920, San Francisco, CA 94104; (415)399-1938.
3. American Academy of Maxillofacial Prosthetics, c/o Jonathan Wiens, DDS, 6177 Orchard Lake Rd., Suite 120, W. Bloomfield, MI 48033; (810)855-6655.
4. Gion G. Orbital prostheses. In: McKinstry RE, ed. *Fundamentals of facial prosthetics*. Arlington, VA: ABI Publications 1995; 121.
5. Holt GR. Osseointegrated Implants in oro-dental and facial prosthetic rehabilitation. *Otolaryngol Clin of North America* 1994; 27:1001.
6. Eriksson E, Branemark PI. Osseointegration from the perspective of the plastic surgeon. *Plast Reconstr Surg* 1994; 93:626.
7. Jensen OT, Brown DC, Blacker J. Nasofacial prostheses supported by osseointegrated implants. *International J Oral Maxillofac Implants* 1992; 7:203.
8. Schaaf N, Kielich M. Implant-retained facial prostheses. In: McKinstry RE, ed. *Fundamentals of facial prosthetics*. Arlington, VA: ABI Professional Publications 1995; 169.
9. Tolman D, Desjardins R. Extraoral application of osseointegrated implants. *J Oral Maxillofac Surg* 1991; 49:33.
10. Tjellstrom A. Osseointegrated systems and their applications in the head and neck. *Ann Otolaryngol Head Neck Surg* 1989; 3:39.
11. Seals R, Cortes AL, Parel S. Fabrication of facial prostheses by applying the osseointegration concept for retention. *J Prosthetic Dentistry* 1989; 61:712.
12. Mizunuma K, Kawai T, Yasugi, et al. Biological monitoring and possible health effects in workers occupationally exposed to methyl methacrylate. *International Arch Occupational Environmental Health* 1993; 65:227.
13. Shintani H, Tsuchiya T, Hata Y, et al. Solid phase extraction and HPLC analysis of toxic components eluted from methylmethacrylate dental materials. *J Analytical Toxicology* 1993; 17:73.
14. Jerolimov V, Krhen J, Besisc J. The role of residual monomer in PMMA powder and methods of polymerization in the finding of residual monomer in poly(methymethacrylate) denture base. *Acta Stomatologica Croatica* 1993; 25:17.
15. Binder W, Kuge A. Reconstruction of posttraumatic and congenital facial deformities with 3-D computer-assisted custom designed implants. *Plast Reconstr Surg* 1994; 94:775.
16. Implantech Associates, Inc. (facial implants) 7100 Hayvenhurst Ave., Suite 207, Van Nuys, CA 91406.
17. Biomet, Inc., PO Box 587, Warsaw, IN 46581-0587, distributed by Lorenz Surgical, PO Box 18009, Jacksonville, FL.
18. White MI, Smart LM, Macgregor DM, et al. Recurrent facial oedema associated with a silicone-rubber implant. *Brit J Dermatol* 1991; 125:183.
19. Leeson MC, Lippitt SB. Thermal aspects of the use of polymethylmethacrylate in large metaphyseal defects in bone. A clinical review and laboratory study. *Clin Orthop* 1993; 295:239.
20. Wanivenhous A, Lintner F, Wurnig C, et al. Long-term reaction of the osseous bed around silicone implants. *Arch Orthop Traum Surg* 1991;110:146.
21. Vasey FB, Espinoza LR, Martinez-Osuna P, et al. Silicone and rheumatic disease: replace implants or not? *Arch Dermatol* 1991; 127:907.
22. Pinto PW. Cardiovascular collapse associated with the use of methylmethacrylate. *AANA J* 1993; 61:613.
23. Chang C, Merritt K. Microbial adherence on polymethylmethacrylate (PMMA) surfaces. *J Biomed Mater Res* 1992; 26:2977.
24. Peters W, Smith D, Lugowski S, et al. Implants have elevated levels of blood silicon compared with control patients? *Ann Plast Surg* 1995; 34:343.
25. Kasper C, Chandler P Jr. Talc deposition in skin and tissues surrounding silicone gel–containing prosthetic devices. *Arch Dermatol* 1994; 130:48.
26. Alison A, Mackinnon S. Evaluation of digital prostheses. *J Hand Surg* 1992; 17A:923.
27. Medelson R, Burech J, Polack EP, et al. The psychological impact of traumatic amputations. *Hand Clin* 1986; 2:577.
28. Roseschein RA, Domholdt E. Factors related to successful upper extremity prosthetic use. *Prosthet Orthot International* 1989; 13:14.
29. Resources for people with facial difference: Let's Face It, Box 711, Concord, MA 01742-0711; (508)371-3186.
30. Amputees Coalition of America: (800)355-8772.
31. National Association of Amputees: (501)666-2523.

Index

Page numbers italicized indicate figures.

Vinorelbine, 420
Violence, mandibular fracture and, 377–378
Virginal breast hypertrophy, 720
Viscosity of blood, skin flap survival and, 25–26
Vitamin A, in wound healing, 7
Vitamin C, in wound healing, 7
Vitamin E
    breast nodules and, 771
    in wound healing, 7–8
Volar advancement flap, fingertip injury and,
    994–995
Volar pad of fingertip, 992
Volar subluxation of metacarpophalangeal joint,
    arthritis and, *1033*, 1034
Volar wrist ganglion, 1047
von Langenbeck cleft palate repair, 243
Von Recklinghausen disease, hand and, 1060
VP-16, 420
V-Y advancement flap
    eyelid reconstruction and, 484, *485*
    fingertip injury and, 994
    hand injury and, 960
    midfoot ulcer and, 1148
V-Y repair for cleft palate, 243
V-Y skin flap, 21, *22*

Wall
    abdominal, 793–794
    chest
        breast asymmetry and, 723
        embryology of, 716–717
        mediastinitis and, 829–835, *830–834*
        TRAM flap and, 786
    pharyngeal, 267–268
Wardill-Kilner cleft palate repair, *243*
Wart, 1048–1049
Warthin tumor, 157, *524*
Washio flap, 467
Wassmund maxillary osteotomy, 326, *326–327*,
    328
Web, thumb hypoplasia and, 987
Webbed penis, 846
Webster intra-areolar incision for gynecomastia,
    824
Webster perialar crescentic advancement flap,
    463
Wedge osteotomy for clinodactyly, 985

Weight, eyelid, 517
Wharton duct stone, 407
Wheal and flare reaction to injectable collagen,
    631–632
Wheelchair, pressure sore and, 1111, 1112
Whistle deformity, *250*
White-head, 118
Whitlow, herpetic, 1083–1084, *1084*
Wire fixation
    hand fracture and, 1091–1092
    replantation of hand and, 974
Wire osteosynthesis, 390, *390*
Witch's chin deformity, 559, *605*
Wolffian duct, 842
Wound
    burn, 202, *202*
    Dupuytren disease and, 1043–1044
    foot ulcer and, 1146–1147
    hand fracture and, 1092
    hand reconstruction and, 958–959
    lower extremity reconstruction and,
        1138–1141
    pressure sore, 1111–1121; *see also* Pressure
        sore
    replantation and, 975–976
    surgical
        closure of, 12
        preparation of, 10–11
        skin graft for, 13–14
    types of, 3
Wound healing, 4–8
    nose reconstruction and, 474
    rheumatoid arthritis and, *1022*
    scar revision and, 111–118, *112–116*
    of skin graft, 17
    tendon injury of hand and, 1001–1002
    trauma and, 106–109
W-plasty, 115–116, *116*
Wrap-around flap for toe-to-thumb transfer,
    1074, *1076*, 1076
Wrightington classification of arthritis of wrist,
    1027, *1027*
Wrinkles
    blepharoplasty and, 587–588
    chemical peel for, 622–629, *625–628*
    dermabrasion for, 618
    facelift for; *see* Facelift
    facial, *554*

Wrist
    arthritis of, 1026–1027, *1027*
        fusion for, 1030–1031
    ganglion of, 1046, 1047
    nerve entrapment and, 1016
    neuroma of, 1018
    radial clubhand and, 980–981
Wuchereria bancrofti, 885–888, *887*, *888*

Xanthogranuloma, juvenile, 145
Xanthoma, 145, *145*
Xanthoma tuberosum, 1055
Xenogeneic bone, 41
Xenograft, bone, 39
Xeroderma pigmentosa, 123
Xylocaine
    Dupuytren disease and, 1043
    lipoplasty and, 694

Y chromosome, 855–856
YAG laser for tattoo, 103
Yellow nail syndrome, 1125

Zephiran, 208
Zone
    of coagulation, 198
    of hand, *1004*, 1004–1005
    of hyperemia, 198
    of stasis, 198
Zovirax, 629
Z-plasty, 12
    cleft lip and, 249, *250*
    for cleft palate, 269
    scar revision and, 115, *116*
Zyderm injectable collagen, 629–632
Zygoma, Le Fort fracture and, 368–369
Zygomatic arch
    facial osteotomy and, 298
    Goldenhar syndrome and, 294
Zygomatic fracture
    clinical assessment of, 343, *344*, 345
    management of, 361, *362*, 363
Zygomatic major muscle, 561

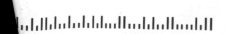